THE
AMERICAN
MEDICAL
ASSOCIATION

ENCYCLOPEDIA
OF MEDICINE

THE
AMERICAN
MEDICAL
ASSOCIATION

ENCYCLOPEDIA
OF MEDICINE

MEDICAL EDITOR
Charles B. Clayman, MD

Random House
New York

The information in this encyclopedia reflects current
medical knowledge. The recommendations and
information are appropriate in most cases; however,
they are not a substitute for medical diagnosis. For
specific information concerning your personal
medical condition, the AMA suggests that you
consult a physician.

The names of organizations, products, or alternative
therapies appearing in this encyclopedia are given for
informational purposes only. Their inclusion does not
imply AMA endorsement, nor does the omission of any
organization, product, or alternative therapy indicate
AMA disapproval.

Library of Congress Cataloging-in-Publication Data
Main entry under title:

The American Medical Association
encyclopedia of medicine.

Includes index.
1. Medicine, Popular—Dictionaries.
I. American Medical Association.

RC81.A2A52   1989   610'.3'21—dc19   88-29693
ISBN 0-394-56528-2

Manufactured in the United States of America

Computerset by M. F. Graphics Limited, England
Reproduction by Mandarin Offset Limited, Hong Kong
98

PREFACE

Medicine has changed a great deal in recent years. First, technological advances such as magnetic resonance imaging, PET scanners, and endoscopes have transformed methods of diagnosis. Second, the development of new treatments—including transplants, implants, laser surgery, lithotripsy, and angioplasty—has widened the range of disorders that can be treated safely and effectively. New drugs have also extended medicine's capabilities, or made possible safer and more effective treatments than their predecessors.

However, probably the most important change has been the recognition by the medical profession that today's patients are not prepared to be merely passive recipients of medical care. Today, people want to be involved in decisions that affect their health; they want to know not only what is wrong with them, but also what the choices of treatment are, and what risks are involved. Recognizing this, most physicians now try to spend more time with patients and their families explaining the problems and options available.

This medical encyclopedia has been produced by the American Medical Association to help you understand the language of medicine. It provides clear, illustrated explanations of how the body works and also gives detailed information on all of the common diseases (and many of the less common ones). Furthermore, in contrast to many popular medical books, this encyclopedia does not expound an individual author's theory or market any "breakthrough" treatment or diet. What this book provides is a clear, systematic account of state-of-the-art, validated, medical knowledge—reviewed and endorsed by expert physicians selected by the American Medical Association.

We hope you will use this volume in the best of health.

James H. Sammons, MD
Executive Vice President
American Medical Association

THE AMERICAN MEDICAL ASSOCIATION

James H. Sammons, MD · *Executive Vice President*
John T. Baker · *Vice President, Publishing*
Heidi Hough · *Director, Office of Consumer Books*
Kathy Kaye · *Managing Editor*
Brenda A. Clark · *Staff Assistant*

EDITORIAL STAFF

Charles B. Clayman, MD · *Medical Editor*
Heidi Hough · *Editor-In-Chief*
Robin Fitzpatrick Husayko · *Editor*
James Ferris · *Assistant Editor*
Julie S. Ferris · *Assistant Editor*
Brenda A. Clark · *Editorial Assistant*
Frank D. Campion · *Consulting Editor*

ACKNOWLEDGMENTS

Mary Banas
Joaquin Chang
Gary Hubler, RPh
Lynne Lamberg
Kenneth F. Lampe, PhD

Jacqueline Martin
Mary Ann McCann
William Smith
Michaela Sullivan-Fowler
Bonnie B. Wilford

Alliance for the Mentally Ill of Greater Chicago
American Dental Association
American Dietetic Association
American Osteopathic Association
American Podiatric Association
American Society of Plastic and Reconstructive Surgeons, Inc.
Mallinckrodt Institute of Radiology
National Organization for Women, Chicago Chapter
Public Health Service, US Department of Health and Human Services
University of Washington School of Medicine

Editorial Director Amy Carroll; **Managing Editor** Ruth Midgley; **Editors** Andrea Bagg, Stephen Carroll,
Robert Dinwiddie, Mary Lindsay, Ricki Ostrov, Martyn Page, Jillian Somerscales, Frances Williams,
Robert M. Youngson; **Editorial Secretary** Pat White; **Managing Art Editors** Chez Picthall, Denise Brown;
Art Editor Caroline Murray; **Designers** Tina Hill, Tracy Timson, Lydia Umney, Peter Cross, Gail Jones,
Melissa Gray, Sarah Ponder, Sandra Archer; **Picture research** Sandra Schneider; **Production** Rupert Wheeler

MEDICAL CONSULTANTS

EMERGENCY FIRST-AID TECHNIQUES

Use this quick-reference list to find illustrated first-aid boxes containing step-by-step instructions for performing emergency techniques.

SYMPTOM CHARTS

Use this quick-reference list to find question-and-answer flow charts that indicate the possible causes and significance of many common symptoms.

CONTENTS

HOW TO USE THE ENCYCLOPEDIA

This highly illustrated encyclopedia is an authoritative guide to all aspects of medicine. For swift and easy reference, encyclopedia entries are arranged alphabetically and longer entries are subdivided into sections, each with a descriptive subheading. Information within entries is presented in clear, concise language. Technical or unfamiliar medical terms are generally explained as they appear.

The main body of the encyclopedia, the **A to Z of Medicine**, contains more than 5,000 entries covering a vast range of medical and medically related topics. It is obviously impossible in a one-volume compendium to provide separate entries for every medical term, but many additional terms and topics are discussed within relevant entries. The **Index** refers you to all such items as well as to the major entries themselves.

The encyclopedia also contains a full-color introductory section, **Medicine Today**, which gives useful information on staying healthy and describes the latest advances in diagnosis and treatment. At the back of the book, additional information on generic and brand-name drugs is contained in the **Drug Glossary.** There is also a list of telephone numbers, many of them toll free, for a wide range of **Self-help Organizations.**

HOW TO FIND THE INFORMATION YOU WANT

All entries in the **A to Z of Medicine** and in the **Index** are arranged alphabetically using the "letter-by-letter" system. In this system, any spaces or punctuation in the entry titles are ignored. *Sick building syndrome* is thus followed by *Sickle cell anemia* and then by *Sick sinus syndrome* – the fifth letter gives the order.

When the name of a topic consists of more than one word, begin by looking up what seems to be the key word. Thus, for information on general anesthesia you will find what you want under the heading *Anesthesia, general.* If the key word is not obvious, you may find it easier to turn first to the **Index,** although many alternative topic names and common abbreviations are included as short cross-reference entries within the main part of the book.

You will also find cross-references within the entries themselves. These are indicated by italics and take several forms, which are explained in the annotated illustration below.

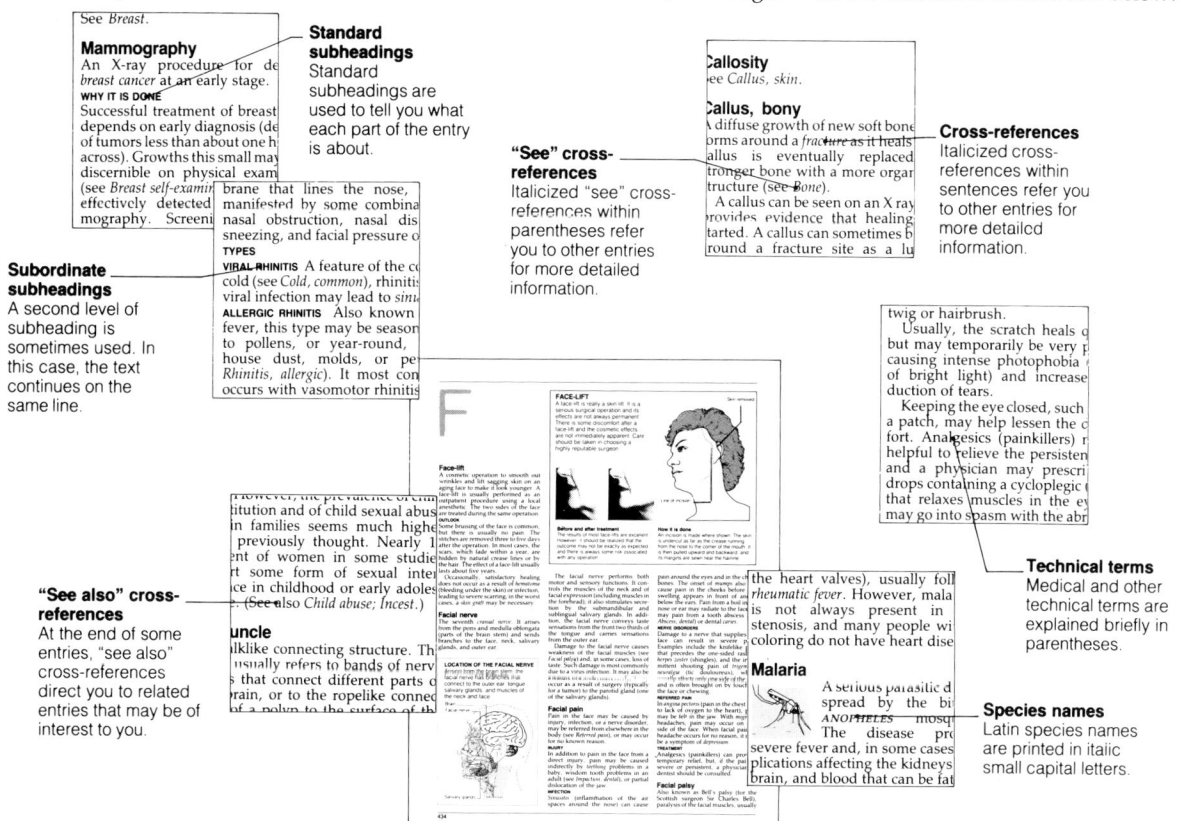

Standard subheadings
Standard subheadings are used to tell you what each part of the entry is about.

Subordinate subheadings
A second level of subheading is sometimes used. In this case, the text continues on the same line.

"See also" cross-references
At the end of some entries, "see also" cross-references direct you to related entries that may be of interest to you.

"See" cross-references
Italicized "see" cross-references within parentheses refer you to other entries for more detailed information.

Cross-references
Italicized cross-references within sentences refer you to other entries for more detailed information.

Technical terms
Medical and other technical terms are explained briefly in parentheses.

Species names
Latin species names are printed in italic small capital letters.

HOW TO FIND INFORMATION ON SYMPTOMS

The A to Z of Medicine contains individual entries on a wide range of physical and psychological symptoms. In general, you will find the main description of a particular symptom under its common name, if it has one. For example, *Vomiting* is the main entry and *Emesis*, the medical term for vomiting, is a short cross-reference entry. Alternative names for symptoms also appear in the **Index**.

Symptom charts

The question-and-answer symptom charts will help you understand the significance of common symptoms that have no obvious cause. Each chart singles out possible causes of the symptom, refers you to relevant entries in the encyclopedia, and suggests appropriate action, if any. Start at the top of the chart and answer "yes" or "no" to the series of carefully selected questions until you reach the box that advises you on your particular problem. For the page numbers of all symptom charts, consult page 8.

Title and description
The title of each symptom chart is followed by a brief description of the symptom in nontechnical language.

The questions
Each question is phrased so that it requires either a "yes" or "no" reply. Follow your "yes" or "no" answer to the appropriate next question and continue until you reach the box with advice on your problem.

Warning
Warning boxes draw your attention to potentially serious symptoms and give practical advice.

Cancer warning
"Cancer watch" boxes alert you to the possibility of cancer if you have certain symptoms.

CANCER WATCH
Recurrent abdominal pain (especially in people over 40) may indicate cancer, especially if the symptoms are newly developed and are accompanied by a change in eating or bowel habits. **Consult your physician without delay!**

Other information
Some symptom charts have additional boxes containing self-help advice or information directed at particular groups of people.

Fever in children
...usually caused by infection ...or bacterium. However, a ...lso become feverish if ...become overheated. Do ...pirin; use an aspirin ...A raised temperature ...hild's forehead to feel hot ...increased sweating and a ...ling of being sick. Normal ...e may vary from 97 to ...37.5°C). Minor ...within this range are no ...oncern if your child seems otherwise well.

• If your baby's temperature rises above 102°F (39°C), whatever the suspected cause, call your physician at once. High temperatures can lead to seizures in some babies.

Emergency! Get medical help now!
This instruction indicates that the problem may be life-threatening and needs immediate medical attention. Call for an ambulance or, if you are certain that the person can be moved safely, take him or her to the nearest hospital emergency room.

Consult/call your physician without delay!
You should telephone your physician at once, either to discuss the problem over the telephone or to arrange for an early appointment at the physician's office.

Consult your physician
This instruction means that you should make an appointment to see your physician about the problem. Haste is not, however, essential.

Cross-references
When appropriate, end boxes cross-refer you to encyclopedia entries for further information.

Irritation of the stomach is the most likely cause of the pain. However, there is also a possibility of an ulcer. Consult your physician.

— See • *Gastritis*
• *Peptic ulcer*

Dull aches or cramps are often associated with menstruation. Discuss with your physician.

Discuss with your physician
You should mention the problem to your physician on your next visit, but there is no need for a special appointment.

11

HOW TO FIND INFORMATION ON DISORDERS

The **A to Z of Medicine** contains individual entries on all major and many minor disorders. There are also general entries covering groups of disorders, such as *Genetic disorders*, or disorders that affect different parts of the body in different ways, such as *Cancer*. These group entries provide an overview and explain the basic disease processes. Specific forms, such as *Hemophilia* or *Breast cancer*, are covered in separate entries. Group entries contain cross-references to more specific entries. If you look up certain group entries in

the **Index**, you will find references to disorders in those groups.

Consult the **Index**, too, if you fail to find an entry on a specific disorder within the **A to Z of Medicine**. You may find that the disorder has another name. For example, if you look up decubitus ulcer in the **Index** you will be directed to the encyclopedia entry on *Bedsores*—decubitus ulcer and bedsore are different names for the same condition. In other cases, the **Index** will show you that a specific disorder is discussed within a more general entry. For

example, conductive deafness is included in the entry on *Deafness*.

Disorder boxes

Entries on the main organs and body parts are accompanied by boxed summaries of the various disorders that may affect them. These disorder boxes help you see at a glance the types of problems most often associated with a particular organ or body part. They also cross-refer you to entries on specific disorders and investigation techniques.

Cross-references
Italicized cross-references direct you to entries on specific disorders for more information.

Subheadings
Different disorders are grouped under standard subheadings, allowing you to see at a glance the problems most likely to affect a particular body part.

DISORDERS OF THE BREAST
Problems involving the breasts are usually minor and respond readily to treatment. The most important . causes of problems are infection, tumors, and hormonal disturbance.

INFECTION
This is uncommon except during breast-feeding. Nursing mothers may suffer from *mastitis* (inflammation of the breast), usually due to a blocked milk duct. An *abscess* may follow if mastitis is not treated.

TUMORS
A *breast lump* may be a *cyst* (a fluid-filled sac), a *fibroadenoma* (a thickening of the milk-producing glandular tissue) or other benign tumor, or, rarely, *breast cancer*.

HORMONAL DISORDERS
It is common for women to notice that before *menstruation* their

breasts become bigger and lumpy. Such lumps are swollen milk glands that shrink when menstruation is over. More common are breast pain and tenderness, which often occur just before menstruation or from taking hormones.

In men, *gynecomastia* (unusual breast development) may result from hormonal disturbance or treatment with certain drugs. Hormones may also cause the rare disorder *galactorrhea* (abnormal milk production).

INVESTIGATION
Disorders of the breast may be discovered during *breast self-examination* or by your physician during a physical examination. Special investigations for the breast are *biopsy* and *mammography*.

Fibroadenoma
• a common benign tumor

Cancer
• a malignant growth

Cyst
• a collection of fluid

Abscess
• a collection of pus

Nipple
• discharge

Galactorrhea
• abnormal production of milk

Mastitis
• inflammation of tissue

Illustrations
Some disorder boxes have an annotated illustration showing areas most likely to be affected by different disorders.

Investigation box
A summary of investigation techniques is given here, including italicized cross-references to entries on diagnostic procedures.

HOW TO FIND INFORMATION ON ANATOMY AND PHYSIOLOGY

All body systems (e.g., *Biliary system*) and major organs and body parts (e.g., *Brain* and *Coccyx*) have individual entries in the **A to Z of Medicine**. There are also entries on the senses (e.g., *Vision*) and on other body processes (e.g., *Breathing* and *Blood clotting*). Anatomy and physiology entries explain how the healthy body works and provide a background for understanding medical disorders.

Most anatomy and physiology entries are accompanied by illustrated boxes. Annotated illustrations show the main structural features of body parts, the location of different body parts in relation to each other, and, for physiology entries, the main stages in important body processes.

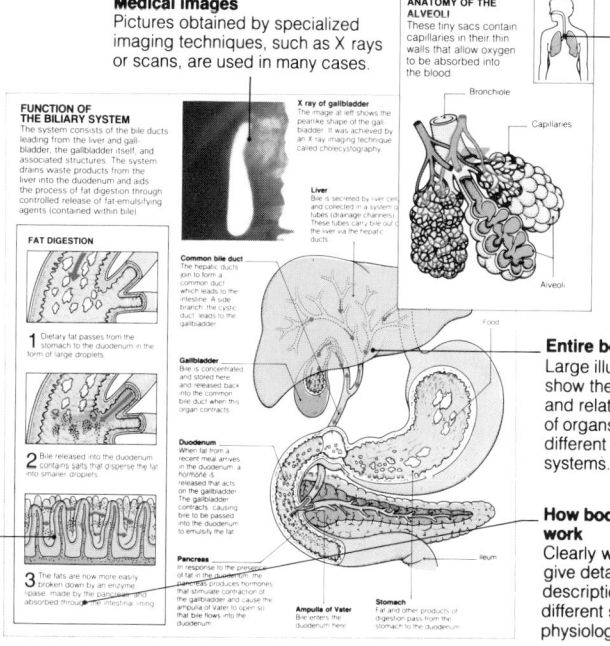

Medical images
Pictures obtained by specialized imaging techniques, such as X rays or scans, are used in many cases.

FUNCTION OF THE BILIARY SYSTEM
The system consists of the bile ducts leading from the liver and gallbladder, the gallbladder itself, and associated structures. The system drains waste products from the liver into the duodenum and aids the process of fat digestion through controlled release of fat-emulsifying agents (contained within bile).

FAT DIGESTION

1 Dietary fat passes from the stomach to the duodenum in the form of large droplets.

2 Bile released into the duodenum contains salts that disperse the fat into smaller droplets.

3 The fats are now more easily broken down by an enzyme, lipase, made by the pancreas and absorbed through the intestinal lining.

X ray of gallbladder
The image at left shows the pearlike shape of the gallbladder. It was achieved by an X ray imaging technique called cholecystography.

Anatomical drawings
Detailed drawings, often with cutaway sections, show the structure of body parts.

ANATOMY OF THE ALVEOLI
These tiny sacs contain capillaries in their thin walls that allow oxygen to be absorbed into the blood

Location diagrams
Most anatomy boxes include a diagram showing the part's position within the body.

Entire body systems
Large illustrations show the structure and relative position of organs within different body systems.

How body systems work
Clearly written captions give detailed descriptions of the different stages in physiological processes.

HOW TO FIND INFORMATION ON MEDICAL TESTS

Many different tests for diagnosing or monitoring medical conditions have individual entries within the **A to Z of Medicine.** Many of these entries are illustrated by step-by-step diagrams.

More general information on tests is given in the entry headed *Tests, medical.* This entry is accompanied by a table that shows the tests used to investigate different parts of the body and directs you to individual entries within the encyclopedia. You can also find out which tests are used to investigate a particular part of the body by consulting the investigation section of the disorder box for that body part.

Entries on specific disorders in the **A to Z of Medicine** cross-refer you to entries that describe the tests used to diagnose and monitor them.

Illustrations showing techniques
Clear illustrations show a test's most important stages, including, for example, where a needle is inserted in the body or how samples are prepared for testing.

Step-by-step text
Concise captions describe the various stages in each test, including what happens to the patient and how test samples are analyzed in the laboratory.

PROCEDURE FOR CHROMOSOME ANALYSIS

1 Fetal cells are obtained by amniocentesis or by chorionic villus sampling; or white blood cells are obtained from the blood of the baby, child, or adult being tested.

2 These cells are suspended in a medium containing substances that encourage the cells to divide. Chemicals are then added that stop the cells from dividing at a stage where their chromosome content is most easily visible.

3 The cells are then spread on a microscope slide, stained, and a selected few (in which the chromosomes are clearly visible and well separated) have their nuclei photographed or are closely examined through a high power microscope.

4 The chromosomes are matched up or cut out from the photographic print and arranged into the 22 pairs of autosomes together with the sex chromosomes. Study of these reveals any abnormalities.

Test results
Diagrams, photographs, and captions explain the results of the test.

HOW TO FIND INFORMATION ON SURGICAL PROCEDURES

Surgical procedures are described either in individual entries or in the treatment section of disorder entries. In many cases, entries are accompanied by illustrated boxes.

Individual entries on surgical procedures are included under their generally accepted medical names. In many cases, these names are self-explanatory—*Heart-lung transplant* or *Hernia repair,* for example.

If you do not know the name of a particular procedure, look up the encyclopedia entry on the disorder for which it is a treatment, where you will find a description of, or a cross-reference to, the appropriate procedure. Alternatively, consult the **Index,** which lists some popular names. For example, if you look up *Stomach, removal of,* you will be referred to the encyclopedia entry on *Gastrectomy.*

Surgery in progress
True-to-life drawings show surgical procedures in progress and provide an accurate representation of current surgical practice.

Incision sites
A red line superimposed on a photograph of the relevant part of the body shows the position and shape of the surgeon's incision.

HEART-LUNG TRANSPLANT
In this procedure, both the heart and lungs of a patient are removed and replaced with organs taken from a brain-dead donor. The removed heart can sometimes be given to another patient.

1 The donor heart and lungs must be healthy and the lungs must match the size of the patient's chest, as measured by chest X rays.

2 In both donor and patient, the heart and lungs are reached via an incision made in the breastbone, and the chest is opened up.

HOW IT IS DONE
Heart and lungs must be removed from both donor and patient; the donor organs then are inserted into the patient.

Site of incision

3 The patient is connected to a heart-lung machine. It takes over the function of heart and lungs, oxygenating blood taken from the venae cavae and pumping it back to the body via the aorta.

Trachea
Aorta
Right atrium/Vena cava

4 In both patient and donor, heart and lungs are removed through cuts in the trachea, aorta, and where the heart connects to the venae cavae. The blood vessels linking donor heart and lungs are left intact.

Tracheal reconnection
Aortic reconnection
Right atrium/Vena cava reconnection

5 Insertion of the donor organs into the patient is, in some respects, easier than in the heart transplant, since fewer reconnections have to be made. The main reconnections are between the patient's and donor's tracheas and aortas and between the right atrium of the donor heart and the patient's venae cavae.

Equipment
Detailed illustrations show the workings of special equipment, such as a heart-lung machine.

Step-by-step text and illustrations
Explanatory captions and anatomically correct illustrations take you through the most important stages of surgical procedures. Large numbers show the sequence of events and help you follow the different stages.

WHY IT IS DONE
Subject to availability of a donor, a heart-lung transplant can offer hope to someone who is dying of an end-stage chronic lung disease, whether or not he or she is also suffering from heart disease. Diseases treated include *emphysema, cystic fibrosis, sarcoidosis,* or *interstitial pulmonary fibrosis.* The heart-lung transplant operation has a better success record than that of lung transplant alone.

These sections were taken from a healthy lung (at left) and an emphysematous lung; transplanting of heart and lungs may give an emphysema patient new hope.

Reasons for surgery
Different medical images – such as photographs, X rays, or scans – of diseased tissue show why operations are necessary.

HOW TO FIND INFORMATION ON DRUGS

The **A to Z of Medicine** contains individual entries on all major drug groups (from *ACE inhibitor drugs* to *Vasodilator drugs*) and on the most important generic drugs (from *Acebutolol* to *Zidovudine*). Other informa-tion on drugs can be found in general entries, such as *Drug, Drug dependence*, and *Drug poisoning*.

The **Drug Glossary** gives concise information on almost 3,000 generic and brand-name drugs, showing the generic equivalents of brand-name drugs, and identifying the drug groups to which individual drugs belong. Each glossary entry cross-refers you for more information to the **A to Z of Medicine**.

Drug charts
Selected entries on individual drugs are accompanied by an illustrated chart that summarizes important information about the drug.

Group to which the drug belongs

Forms in which the drug is available

Availability on prescription or over-the-counter

Availability as a generic or under a brand name only

Generic name
Injection
Intravenous infusion
Suppository
Inhaler
Drops
Applicable symbols are printed in red.
Transdermal patch

Digoxin
DIGITALIS
Tablet Capsule Liquid
Prescription needed
Available as generic

Tablet   Capsule   Liquid   Powder   Cream or ointment

Drug group charts
Most drug group entries are accompanied by a chart showing examples of common drugs within the group.

Group name

Division within the main drug group

Generic examples

Antirheumatic drugs

COMMON DRUGS

Corticosteroid drugs
Dexamethasone Prednisolone

Immunosuppressant drugs
Azathioprine Chlorambucil

Others
Gold Penicillamine

WARNING
Sudden withdrawal of corticosteroid drugs may cause serious illness or death. Always inform a physician you are taking or have recently taken corticosteroids.

Drug warning
Warning boxes draw your attention to the possible dangers associated with taking particular types of drugs.

HOW TO USE THE ENCYCLOPEDIA IN AN EMERGENCY

EMERGENCY FIRST-AID TECHNIQUES

Turn to page 8 for the page numbers of emergency first-aid boxes.

Lifesaving and other, less urgent, first-aid techniques are explained in easy-to-follow first-aid boxes. These boxes accompany relevant entries within the **A to Z of Medicine**. All first-aid boxes have a distinctive red border and a special heading. A list of first-aid boxes describing emergency techniques, with their page numbers, is given on page 8.

WARNING
Warning boxes contain essential advice and indicate when professional help should be sought.

DO NOT
- rub the affected parts
- attempt to burst blisters
- warm the affected area with direct heat
- allow the victim to walk on a frostbitten foot

WARNING
Frostbite is often accompanied by hypothermia, which must be treated first. Proper medical atten-tion should be sought promptly, but first aid should be given immediately.

DO NOT
These boxes tell you what not to do when treating an injured person.

Step-by-step
First-aid techniques are clearly described in numbered sequences of text and illustrations.

Close-ups
More detailed illustrations show you exactly what to do.

Distinctive appearance
Bold red borders and special headings make first-aid boxes easy to find.

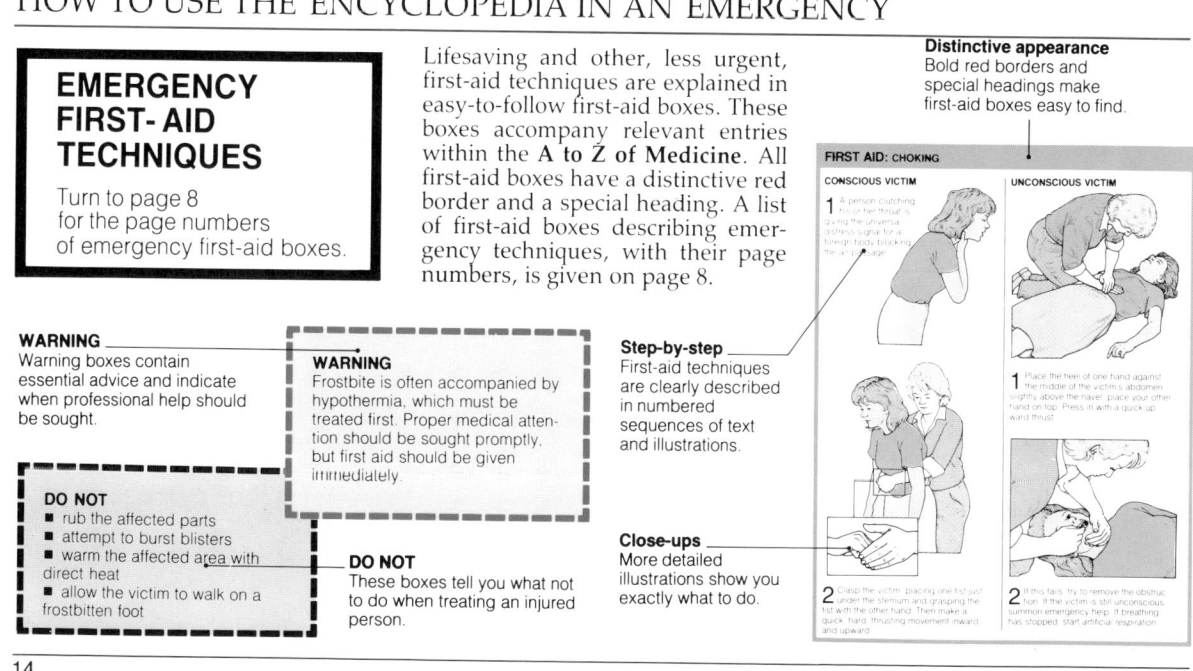

FIRST AID: CHOKING
CONSCIOUS VICTIM   UNCONSCIOUS VICTIM

MEDICINE
TODAY

PROGRESS IN MEDICINE

People living in developed countries today have the opportunity to be healthier than ever before. Our understanding of how the body works has broadened rapidly in the last few years, paralleled by equally dramatic improvements in medical technology. As a result of this progress, a person's chances of staying healthy into old age depend increasingly on following expert advice on a healthy life-style, making full use of preventive techniques such as vaccination and screening tests, and seeking medical advice from your physician at the first sign of illness.

This section of the encyclopedia presents an overview of recent developments in preventive health care, diagnosis, treatment, prenatal technology, and new diseases. It also discusses human potential, including the ways in which we can maximize it.

One important area of advancement in medical science is computer imaging. Computers can now provide images of the interior of the body that are based on various types of scanning techniques, such as X rays, radioactive isotopes, ultrasound, or magnetic resonance. These images—which may be two- or three-dimensional, and even colored to highlight selected features (e.g., specific tissues)—can give

physicians almost as much information as they would be able to obtain through an exploratory operation on the chest or abdomen. In some cases, such as the functional "maps" of tissue metabolism provided by PET scanning, the images provide information that cannot be obtained even by direct examination.

A second major area of advancement has been in medical treatment. As recently as the 1970s, major surgery usually required an incision large enough for the surgeon to get his or her hands into the body. Today, the emphasis in surgery is on less invasive techniques, such as extracorporeal lithotripsy, a noninvasive procedure that uses ultrasound to shatter stones in the body, and endoscopic surgery, in which a viewing tube is passed into the body through a natural orifice or through a tiny incision, directed to the target structure, and then used as a guide through which instruments are passed to enable the physician to perform the surgery. Electrocautery and the use of lasers permit bloodless surgery. As a result of these and other advances in anesthesia, the use of antibiotic drugs, and the monitoring of various body functions, medical treatment today is safer and more effective.

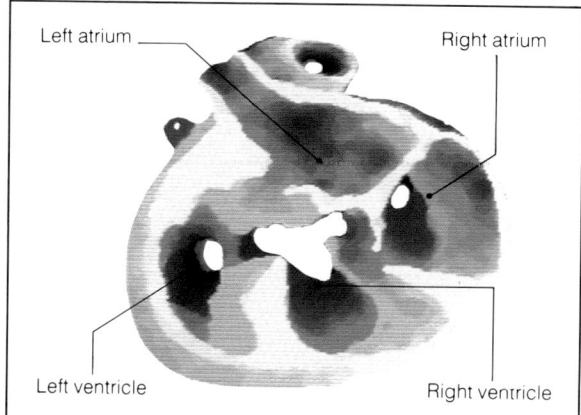

Left atrium — Right atrium

Left ventricle — Right ventricle

Three-dimensional magnetic resonance imaging (3-D MRI)
The image of a section through the heart showing its four chambers (above) was obtained by the recently developed technique of 3-D MRI. This technique, which is noninvasive and without known risk to the patient, gives more accurate and detailed images than could be obtained by other means. As a result, any structural abnormalities are often immediately apparent when the images are examined.

Surgery
Despite trends toward less invasive methods of treatment, conventional surgery (right) is still as important as ever. Significant growth areas include transplants, implants, and repairing damaged or obstructed blood vessels. These operations, along with the removal of cancers, will probably be performed in the future much as they are today, although there will be refinements in anesthesia and postoperative care.

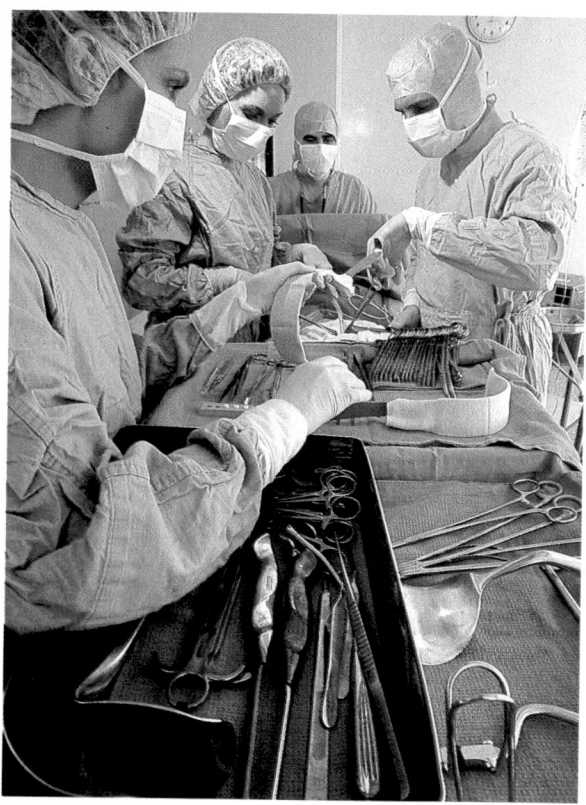

STAYING HEALTHY

Today, most children in developed countries are healthier than ever before; a majority can expect to live well beyond the age of 70. These achievements are partly due to improvements in public health, such as the provision of safe water supplies and sewage disposal systems, adequate housing, and good nutrition, and partly to improvements in medical care.

The health of women today can be carefully monitored before and during pregnancy, and during the birth of the baby. After birth, the newborn infant is closely examined and, if necessary, provided with specialized care.

Throughout infancy and childhood, children are immunized against infections and given vision and hearing tests, as well as tests for physical and mental development. As a result, any problems can be detected and treated promptly.

In the US and Europe, the principal causes of death or disability in youth and middle age are preventable.

World health
Not all countries have high standards of health. In many developing countries, infant mortality is high, principally because many people do not have access to safe water, adequate food, or basic health care (see diagram, right).

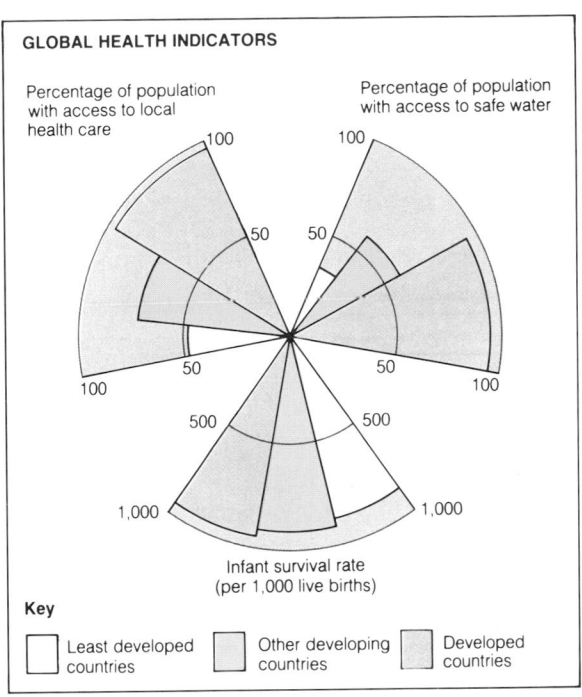

GLOBAL HEALTH INDICATORS

Percentage of population with access to local health care

Percentage of population with access to safe water

Infant survival rate (per 1,000 live births)

Key

Least developed countries

Other developing countries

Developed countries

Childhood infectious diseases
The photomicrograph (above) shows the bacterium *BORDETELLA PERTUSSIS*, the cause of pertussis (whooping cough). In developed countries, this and other potentially serious childhood diseases (such as measles, poliomyelitis, and diphtheria) have been brought under control by immunization. In developing countries, such diseases are still common; the World Health Organization is working to combat this problem by making immunization available to all children.

In early adult life, most deaths are due to accidents or violence; other important causes include suicide, and complications of drug abuse and sexual habits (notably AIDS). In addition, the risk of developing the principal serious disorders of middle age—coronary heart disease and cancer—is reduced by following a healthy life-style and avoiding known health hazards, especially tobacco and alcohol.

Even though following a healthy life-style minimizes an individual's chance of developing life-threatening disease, people living healthy lives may still become ill, either because they have an inborn susceptibility to a disorder or simply by chance. As understanding of the genetic basis of disease improves, screening tests for familial inherited disorders will become wider ranging.

Physicians strongly advise people to become aware of the regular manner in which their bodies function. This includes monitoring bowel habits, appetite, and sleep patterns. When a change in body function is noted, advice should be sought promptly from your physician. Early attention to any illness aids treatment and promotes cure.

Avoiding premature death is not the only benefit to be gained from following a healthy life-style. The quality of life can also improve: the body's natural aging processes are slowed, and physical and mental vigor are retained for much longer.

PERSONAL HEALTH CARE

An individual's health is determined partly by inheritance and partly by external factors. Health and longevity tend to run in families, so a person whose grandparents lived beyond the age of 80 is likely to do the same. However, this is not always the case. Even the intrinsically healthiest body can be damaged by neglect or external factors, especially by unwise use of drugs, including tobacco and alcohol. With the AIDS epidemic still spreading, avoidance of illicit intravenous drugs and sexual promiscuity and adherence to "safe" sex practices are essential for the maintenance of good health.

For many people, however, these "do nots" are less important than three positive keys to a healthy lifestyle: a sound, balanced diet, a positive attitude, and regular, vigorous exercise.

Diet and exercise

For most of history, diseases associated with diet were due to vitamin or mineral deficiencies, or simply to prolonged semi-starvation. In developed countries today, however, the main dietary threat to health is caused by excess: many people overeat, and almost everybody consumes too much saturated fat. Research has shown that variations around the world in the rates of heart disease and some cancers are primarily due to differences in diet. Most Americans consume too much dairy fat, animal fat, and sugar but consume insufficient vegetables and grains. Asian people tend to eat more fish, grains, vegetables, and fruit and so have a healthier diet.

However, over the past few years, a dramatic improvement in our understanding of food and diet has taken place and the dietary habits of many people in the US and Europe have begun to improve. A growing number of people now eat larger amounts of vegetables, fruit, and cereals and have substituted unsaturated fats and oils for dairy fats. In addition, the consumption of fatty meats has declined. According to researchers, these changes have contributed to a significant decrease in the incidence of heart disease in people in many—but not all—developed countries. Nevertheless, many people in the US and other developed countries continue to eat

Health and exercise
Physical exercise, such as running (above), can reduce the risk of coronary heart disease, but only if it is vigorous enough to stimulate the heart and is performed three or more times a week for at least 20 minutes each session.

Types of exercise
The table (right) compares the value of various activities for improving three main aspects of health and fitness—heart and lung efficiency, joint suppleness, and muscle power. The average calorie consumption rate of each activity is also given.

THE FITNESS VALUES OF VARIOUS ACTIVITIES

Activity	Calories	Heart and lung fitness	Joint suppleness	Muscle power
Easy walking	60	Minimal	Minimal	Minimal
Light housework	90	Minimal	Fair	Fair
Light gardening (weeding, etc.)	90	Minimal	Fair	Fair
Golf (flat course)	90	Minimal	Fair	Minimal
Brisk walking	100	Fair	Minimal	Fair
Badminton	115	Fair	Good	Fair
Gymnastics	140	Fair	Excellent	Fair
Heavy gardening (digging, etc.)	140	Fair	Good	Excellent
Dancing	160	Fair	Good	Minimal
Easy jogging	160	Good	Minimal	Fair
Tennis	160	Good	Good	Fair
Skiing (downhill)	160	Good	Good	Fair
Skiing (cross-country)	180	Excellent	Good	Fair
Football	180	Good	Fair	Good
Racquetball or handball	200	Good	Good	Fair
Brisk jogging	210	Excellent	Fair	Fair
Bicycling	220	Excellent	Fair	Good
Swimming	240	Excellent	Excellent	Excellent

Key

- Calories consumed in 20 minutes of activity
- Value in improving heart and lung fitness
- Value in improving joint suppleness
- Value in improving muscle power

- Excellent (4 boxes)
- Good (3 boxes)
- Fair (2 boxes)
- Minimal (1 box)

RECOMMENDED DAILY DIETARY ALLOWANCES (RDAS) OF SELECTED VITAMINS

	Birth to 6 months	6 months to 1 year	1 to 3 years	4 to 6 years	7 to 10 years	11 to 14 years	15 to 18 years	19 to 22 years	23 to 50 years	51+ years	Extra needed pregnancy	Extra needed breast-feeding
Folic acid (mcg)	30	45	100	200	300	400	400	400	400	400	400	100
Niacin (mg)	6.0	8.0	9.0	11	16	M 18 F 15	M 18 F 14	M 19 F 14	M 18 F 13	M 16 F 13	2.0	5.0
Pyridoxine (mg)	0.3	0.6	0.9	1.3	1.6	1.8	2.0	M 2.2 F 2.0	M 2.2 F 2.0	M 2.2 F 2.0	0.6	0.5
Riboflavin (mg)	0.4	0.6	0.8	1.0	1.4	M 1.6 F 1.3	M 1.7 F 1.3	M 1.7 F 1.3	M 1.6 F 1.2	M 1.4 F 1.2	0.3	0.5
Thiamine (mg)	0.3	0.5	0.7	0.9	1.2	M 1.4 F 1.1	M 1.4 F 1.1	M 1.5 F 1.1	M 1.4 F 1.0	M 1.2 F 1.0	0.4	0.5
Vitamin A (mcg) 1	420	400	400	500	700	M 1,000 F 800	M 1,000 F 800	M 1,000 F 800	M 1,000 F 800	M 1,000 F 800	200	400
Vitamin B$_{12}$ (mcg)	0.5	1.5	2.0	2.5	3.0	3.0	3.0	3.0	3.0	3.0	1.0	1.0
Vitamin C (mg)	35	35	45	45	45	M 50 F 60	60	60	60	60	20	40
Vitamin D (mcg) 2	10	10	10	10	10	10	10	7.5	5.0	5.0	5.0	5.0
Vitamin E (mg) 3	3.0	3.0	5.0	6.0	7.0	8.0	M 10 F 8.0	M 10 F 8.0	M 10 F 8.0	M 10 F 8.0	2.0	3.0

1 RDA expressed in mcg of retinol (a form of vitamin A). 1 mcg of retinol (a unit called a retinol equivalent, or RE) equals 6 mcg of beta-carotene (another form of vitamin A).

2 RDA expressed in mcg of cholecalciferol (one of the forms of vitamin D). 10 mcg of cholecalciferol equals 400 international units (IU) of vitamin D.

3 RDA expressed in mg of alpha-tocopherol (one of the forms of vitamin E). 1 mg of alpha-tocopherol equals 1 alpha-tocopherol equivalent (1 alpha-TE).

RECOMMENDED DAILY DIETARY ALLOWANCES (RDAS) OF SELECTED MINERALS

	Birth to 6 months	6 months to 1 year	1 to 3 years	4 to 6 years	7 to 10 years	11 to 14 years	15 to 18 years	19 to 22 years	23 to 50 years	51+ years	Extra needed pregnancy	Extra needed breast-feeding
Calcium (mg)	360	540	800	800	800	1,200	1,200	800	800	800	400	400
Iodine (mcg)	40	50	70	90	120	150	150	150	150	150	25	50
Iron (mg)	10	15	15	10	10	18	18	M 10 F 18	M 10 F 18	10	30-60	**A**
Magnesium (mg)	50	70	150	200	250	M 350 F 300	M 400 F 300	M 350 F 300	M 350 F 300	M 350 F 300	150	150
Phosphorus (mg)	240	360	800	800	800	1,200	1,200	800	800	800	400	400
Zinc (mg)	3.0	5.0	10	10	10	15	15	15	15	15	5.0	10

A Iron requirements while breast-feeding are approximately the same as those for nonpregnant women, but additional iron may be recommended for two to three months after the birth to replenish iron stores depleted by pregnancy.

UNITS
mg = milligrams (thousandths of a gram)
mcg = micrograms (millionths of a gram)

Vitamins and minerals
The tables (above) give recommended daily allowances (RDAs) of vitamins and minerals for which amounts have been established; when different, the RDAs for males and females are denoted by M and F.

an unhealthy diet, so diet-related diseases continue to be a major problem.

While food is the body's energy source, people who engage in little exercise can easily become overweight by eating more than they "burn off" in physical activity. Regular exercise (at least three times a week) keeps the heart, lungs, muscles, and bones in good health and slows down the aging process. A person who is in good physical condition at the age of 60 can achieve up to 80 percent of the level of physical exertion that he or she could achieve in the mid-20s. Regular exercise improves the circulation in the heart and muscles and provides increased stamina. Exercise as simple as regular, brisk walking also maintains the density of bones, thus reducing the risk of developing osteoporosis ("thinning" and weakening of the bones) and fractures. A person who exercises regularly is less likely than a person who does not exercise sufficiently to have a heart attack or to die from a heart attack if one occurs.

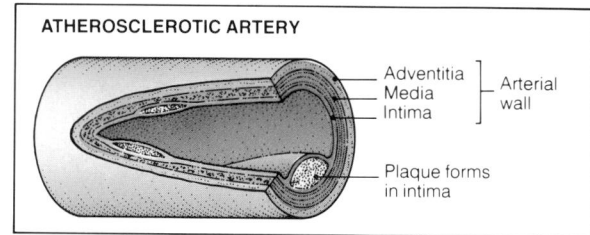

Left main coronary artery

Narrowed section of artery

Diet and atherosclerosis

The colored angiogram of the heart (left) shows narrowing of a coronary artery, a cause of coronary heart disease. Such narrowing can critically reduce the heart's blood supply during exertion; the narrowed section may even become blocked by a blood clot, causing a heart attack. The narrowing of coronary, and other, arteries is usually due to atherosclerosis, the deposition of fatty plaques in the arteries (see diagram below). The risk of atherosclerosis is linked closely to the amount of cholesterol in the blood, which, in turn, is linked to the dietary intake of fats.

ATHEROSCLEROTIC ARTERY

Adventitia
Media
Intima
Arterial wall

Plaque forms in intima

Smoking and drinking

The full extent of the damage to health caused by smoking tobacco and drinking alcohol is gradually being revealed with continuing research. It has become apparent that many people drink regularly and heavily without being recognized as the alcoholics they have become.

Alcohol is a major contributing factor in traffic accidents and drownings. It plays an important role in domestic violence, sexual assaults, and other violent crimes. Furthermore, there is growing evidence that young people who drink heavily are more likely to experiment with other addictive drugs. Alcohol is a significant cause of ill health. Regular heavy drinking can damage the liver (eventually leading to cirrhosis), heart, stomach, and esophagus. It also leads to brain damage, resulting in impairment of motor and

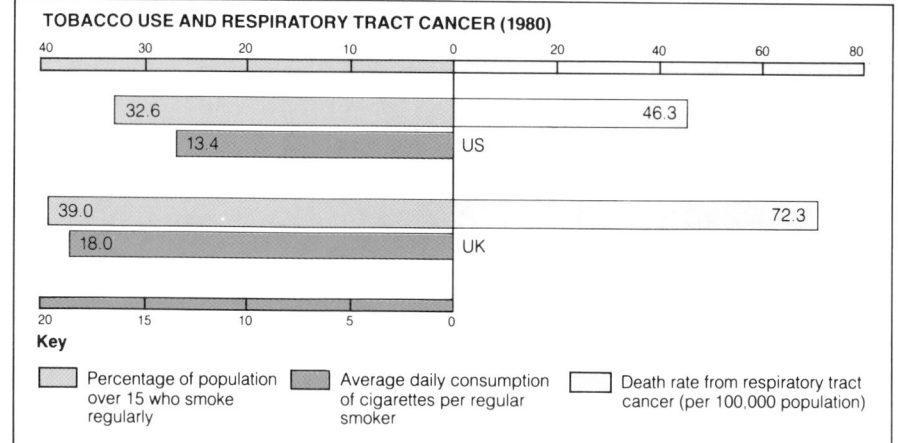

TOBACCO USE AND RESPIRATORY TRACT CANCER (1980)

	US	UK
Percentage of population	32.6	39.0
Death rate	46.3	72.3
Average daily consumption	13.4	18.0

Key

Percentage of population over 15 who smoke regularly

Average daily consumption of cigarettes per regular smoker

Death rate from respiratory tract cancer (per 100,000 population)

Tobacco smoking and mortality

It is now well established that smoking can cause cancer; it is also known that, the more a person smokes, the greater the risk. The relationship between smoking and deaths from respiratory tract cancer is shown in the chart (left). In the US in 1980, 32.6 percent of adults smoked, averaging 13.4 cigarettes per person per day; the death rate from respiratory cancer was 46.3 per 100,000 people. In the UK in 1980, 39 percent of adults smoked, averaging 18 cigarettes per person per day; the death rate from respiratory cancer was 72.3 per 100,000 people.

intellectual capabilities. Drinking during pregnancy can damage the unborn child, causing the mother to give birth to a physically and intellectually maldeveloped baby.

The adverse effects of tobacco are almost as extensive and destructive as those of alcohol. The link between smoking and lung cancer is well known. Moreover, smokers face a substantially greater risk of premature death from coronary heart disease.

It has been demonstrated that people who smoke suffer more angina (chest pain due to inadequate blood supply to the heart muscle) as well as a more recently described phenomenon in which the heart muscle is deprived of oxygen without any angina. This latter, "silent" form of coronary heart disease could be a major factor in the sudden death that can occur with this disease.

Smoking has also become the primary cause of chronic bronchitis and emphysema. It has been linked with ulcers of the stomach and duodenum, and cancers of the cervix and bladder. Smoking during pregnancy, like drinking during pregnancy, damages the developing fetus.

Although smoking is a hazard to the health of smokers themselves, it is also a threat to the health of nonsmokers, particularly children. Recent research has demonstrated that nonsmokers who are exposed to tobacco smoke—as may occur in a household with both smokers and nonsmokers—face an increased risk of respiratory disorders such as bronchitis and lung cancer.

Smoking and emphysema

Although not all smokers get lung cancer, most do develop chronic bronchitis and emphysema. In emphysema, continual irritation by smoke causes progressive damage to the lung tissue. The alveoli (the tiny air sacs across which oxygen and carbon dioxide interchange occurs) first burst and then merge to form fewer, larger sacs with less surface area (see diagrams below). As a result, the working volume of the lungs is progressively reduced, causing breathlessness.

THE EFFECTS OF EMPHYSEMA ON THE LUNGS

Normal lung tissue
- Bronchiole
- Blood capillaries
- Normal alveoli

Emphysematous lung tissue
- Alveolar damage due to emphysema

HEALTHY TISSUE

CIRRHOTIC TISSUE

Effects of alcohol on the liver

The photomicrographs above show healthy liver tissue (left) and liver tissue damaged by alcoholic cirrhosis (right). In the healthy liver, the cells are arranged regularly; in the cirrhotic liver, the regular cell arrangement is disrupted by fibrous scar tissue (the blue areas in the photomicrograph). The scar tissue develops as a result of destruction of liver cells by alcohol. The liver attempts to compensate by growing new cells, but in some areas the damage is so great that nonfunctioning scar tissue develops instead. With continued alcohol use, increasing amounts of scar tissue are formed; eventually it affects so much of the liver that normal liver function cannot be maintained.

Alcohol and mortality

There is a close link between alcohol and death from cirrhosis. In 1980, average intake in the US was about 660 glasses of beer (or equivalent) per person; cirrhosis deaths were 13.6 per 100,000 people. This compares with 1,025 glasses of beer (or equivalent) per person and 28.5 cirrhosis-caused deaths per 100,000 people in France.

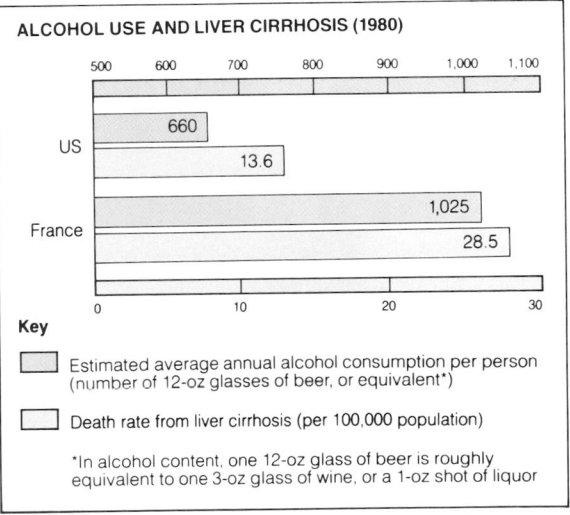

ALCOHOL USE AND LIVER CIRRHOSIS (1980)

| | 500 | 600 | 700 | 800 | 900 | 1,000 | 1,100 |

US — 660 / 13.6
France — 1,025 / 28.5

(scale 0, 10, 20, 30)

Key

☐ Estimated average annual alcohol consumption per person (number of 12-oz glasses of beer, or equivalent*)

☐ Death rate from liver cirrhosis (per 100,000 population)

*In alcohol content, one 12-oz glass of beer is roughly equivalent to one 3-oz glass of wine, or a 1-oz shot of liquor

PREVENTIVE MEDICINE

Many common and serious diseases cause no symptoms in their early stages. This is particularly true of cancer, which often does not produce symptoms until it is beginning to or has already spread to other areas of the body. However, many of these tumors can be detected by simple, reliable tests. Treatment can then arrest or minimize the progress of the disease. Periodic screening tests for cancer become important after age 40, particularly among people in high-risk groups.

Regular check-ups

The most important medical check-ups are for weight and blood pressure. Both tend to increase with age, but a sustained rise above a normal range for a particular age increases the risk of disorders such as heart and kidney disease and stroke, and may warrant treatment. A physical examination should also include checking the eyes, ears, throat, and skin, and an assessment of the condition of all major organ systems of the body (cardiovascular-respiratory, gastrointestinal, genitourinary, musculoskeletal, and neurological). For women who have been sexually active, a cervical smear (Pap test) is included. In addition, middle-aged women should have a mammogram, every two years for those over 40 and annually after the age of 50. A dental examination should also be performed at least once a year.

During a routine check-up, the physician may ask questions designed to screen for a variety of disorders. He or she may also inquire about your life-style, including your diet, sleeping patterns, sexual activity, exercise program, alcohol and tobacco consumption, and whether you use any other addictive drugs.

MEASURING BLOOD PRESSURE

Stethoscope

Blood pressure gauge

Inflatable cuff

Blood pressure
Blood pressure is measured by using an inflatable cuff attached to a pressure gauge, and a stethoscope to listen for sounds of blood flow that indicate maximum (systolic) and minimum (diastolic) pressure. A healthy young adult has a blood pressure of about 110/75, which rises to about 130/90 by age 60.

Screening high-risk groups

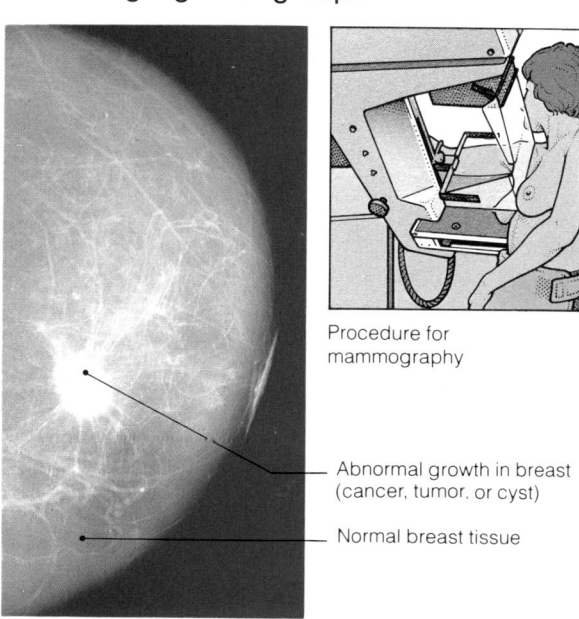

Procedure for mammography

Abnormal growth in breast (cancer, tumor, or cyst)

Normal breast tissue

The medical tests outlined above apply to all adults, irrespective of their medical history. Other specialized tests are recommended for people from families in which a particular disease is prevalent. For example, if a blood relative has had a heart attack before 50, you should tell your physician, who may want to measure the levels of lipids (LDL, HDL, and total cholesterol and triglycerides) in your blood. Coronary heart disease in early middle age almost always indicates an inherited disorder associated with raised lipid levels in the blood, but is a condition that can be treated by a combination of diet and drugs. Similarly, if your mother, father, sister, or brother has had bowel cancer, you should consult your physician about

Mammography
This procedure uses low-dose X rays to image the breasts in screening for cancer (see diagram, left). The mammogram (far left) shows a white area toward the center of the image; such "shadows" may indicate a cancer, but in most cases the cause is a noncancerous tumor or cyst. When a mammogram reveals an abnormality, a sample of the abnormal tissue may be taken for microscopic examination.

when to have regular tests for the presence of blood in your feces and a proctosigmoidoscopic examination. Detection of bowel cancer in its early stages usually enables surgery to be performed with an excellent prospect of a cure.

People who have worked in certain industries have an increased risk of developing some forms of cancer. Workers who have been in regular contact with amine dyes should make sure they have regular tests for bladder cancer.

Other high-risk groups, such as middle-aged men with vague chest discomfort or those about to embark on an exercise program, may be advised to have an exercise stress test to assess the condition of the heart. Liver function tests may be recommended to detect any early evidence of liver damage associated with alcohol consumption. In addition, people who have spent a long period in tropical countries may be advised to undergo special screening tests for tropical diseases.

ECG TREADMILL STRESS TEST

Electrodes

ECG machine

Treadmill

Electrocardiography (ECG)
The ECG treadmill stress test (right) is a widely used test for evaluating chest pain. Electrodes are taped to the chest and connected to the ECG machine, which makes a continuous recording of the heart's electrical activity while the patient walks on a treadmill. The walking speed is then increased to the maximum the patient can tolerate. If the ECG trace remains normal during maximum exertion, it is unlikely that the person has a serious heart disorder.

Immunization and preventive drug treatment

Until as recently as the 1940s, deaths in infancy from infectious diseases, such as diphtheria, measles, and pertussis (whooping cough), were relatively common, even in some developed countries. Today, however, vaccines are available against many potentially fatal diseases, and most children in developed countries are routinely immunized against not only diphtheria, measles, and pertussis, but also against typhoid, poliomyelitis, tetanus, rubella, and mumps. Vaccines are also available against tuberculosis and some types of meningitis.

People planning to travel to a foreign country should ensure that their immunizations are current and should also be immunized against any other diseases (such as cholera, yellow fever, and hepatitis) that may exist in the region to be visited. A vaccine has yet to be developed against malaria, one of the most common tropical diseases. However, prophylactic treatment with an antimalarial drug such as chloroquine can help protect against the disease. Development of drug-resistant forms of malaria in some parts of the world requires the traveler to discuss plans with his or her physician. It is also advisable to take other preventive measures, including using insect repellents, wearing protective clothing, and sleeping under a mosquito net.

Preventing malaria
Malaria is caused by infection with protozoal parasites called plasmodia. The parasites enter the body by passing down through the proboscis (circled in the photograph above) of female ANOPHELES mosquitoes while they suck blood. Travelers to malarial regions can protect themselves against the disease by taking preventive antimalarial drugs (beginning a few days before entering a malarious area), which affect the parasites in the liver before they can cause symptoms. In recent years, control of malaria has become more difficult, partly because the parasites have developed resistance to certain antimalarial drugs, and partly because the mosquitoes have become resistant to many insecticides.

DIAGNOSING DISEASE

Accurate diagnosis of disease is one of the most important aspects of medicine. Without knowing the identity of a disorder, a physician can only relieve symptoms, such as pain or fever. Indeed, medicine consisted largely of a collection of remedies for specific symptoms and injuries until the fifth century BC, when the Greek physician Hippocrates (c.460-c.377 BC) attempted to identify and describe the course of a disease along with its symptoms.

A diagnosis enables the physician to make a prognosis—an estimate of the outcome of a certain disorder. The concepts of diagnosis and prognosis led physicians to identify diseases from the medical history, the patient's account of the illness. The history remains an essential element in diagnosis. It should be followed by a systematic physical examination in which the physician looks for further signs that can help confirm the underlying cause of the disorder.

Despite these developments, diagnosis remained mostly guesswork until the 17th century, when anatomists and pathologists began to study the body's structure and the changes in organs and tissues that were caused by specific diseases. The invention and development of the microscope led to a greater understanding of the body's structure and function, and to understanding how organs and tissues are affected by disease. The 19th century brought another major advance in the history of diagnosis with the discovery that microorganisms (e.g., bacteria and fungi) can cause disease. This discovery led to the development of the germ theory of disease by, among others, the French microbiologist and chemist Louis Pasteur (1822-1895) and the German bacteriologist Robert Koch (1843-1910). The germ theory of disease is generally regarded as one of the greatest achievements of medical and biological science.

Today, physicians still rely heavily on the patient's medical history to arrive at a diagnosis. Success in making a diagnosis is augmented by the physical examination and by myriad biochemical, immunological, and microbiological tests. Physicians also have access to the interior of the patient's body in ways previously unimagined. Modern techniques such as ultrasound, endoscopy, body scanning (such as CT scanning and magnetic resonance imaging), and biopsy provide detailed, accurate information

Computers and diagnosis
Many diagnostic scanning techniques, such as CT scanning and MRI, use computers to image the body (above). Computers can enhance scanning images to highlight specific features.

Diagnosing communicable diseases
Because of rapid air transport, a person with a rare infectious disease may develop the first symptoms anywhere in the world. When physicians suspect such an illness, the patient is treated in strict isolation and samples are cultured in a high-security environment (such as the one shown at left) to determine the causative microorganism.

about internal organs with only minimal risk and discomfort to the patient.

Many advances in diagnosis would not have been possible without developments in other disciplines. For example, most modern scanning techniques depended on the development of the computer to process the information. These and other major landmarks in the history of diagnosis are listed in the chart below.

Medical thermometer
The Italian physician Sanctorius (1561-1636) devised the first medical thermometer in 1612 (right). An adaptation of Galileo's air thermometer, it consisted of a globe-shaped top that was placed in the mouth, a coil graduated with glass beads, and a bulbous bottom immersed in a bowl of water.

LANDMARKS IN DIAGNOSIS

Date	Development
c.400 BC	**Disease concept.** Introduced by Greek physician Hippocrates.
1612	**Medical thermometer.** Devised by Italian physician Sanctorius.
c.1660	**Light microscope.** Single-lens microscope developed by Dutch naturalist Antonj van Leeuwenhoek, who discovered microorganisms with it. A practicable compound microscope was not developed until the 19th century.
1810	**Stethoscope.** Invented by French physician René Laennec.
1850-1900	**Germ theory of disease.** Proposed by French scientist Louis Pasteur and developed by German bacteriologist Robert Koch.
1895	**X rays.** Discovered by German physicist Wilhelm Roentgen. He also produced the first X-ray picture of the body.
1905	**X-ray contrast medium.** First demonstrated (in retrograde pyelography) by Jean Athanese Sicard in Paris.
1906	**Electrocardiograph (ECG).** Invented by Dutch physiologist Willem Einthoven.
c.1932	**Transmission electron microscope (TEM).** Constructed by German scientists Max Knoll and Ernst Ruska.
1938	**Cardiac catheterization.** First performed by George Peter Robb and Israel Steinberg in New York.
1957	**Fiberoptic endoscopy.** Pioneered by South African-born physician Basil Hirschowitz at the University of Michigan.
1973	**CT scanner.** Invented by British engineer Godfrey Hounsfield of EMI Laboratories, England, and South African-born physicist Allan Cormack of Tufts University, Massachusetts.
1975	**Monoclonal antibodies.** Large-scale production method developed by Argentinean-born scientist César Milstein at the Medical Research Council Laboratories, England.
1976	**Chorionic villus sampling.** Developed by Chinese gynecologists as an aid to the early diagnosis of genetic disorders.
1981	**MRI scanner.** Developed by scientists at Thorn-EMI Laboratories, England, and Nottingham University, England.
1985	**PET scanner.** Developed by scientists at the University of California.

X rays
Shortly after his discovery of X rays in 1895, the German physicist Wilhelm Roentgen (1845-1923) made the first X-ray picture of the human body (above). The picture shows his wife's hand, with the ring she was wearing.

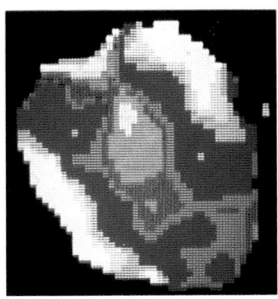

PET scanning
This technique, developed in 1985, enables the functioning of organs to be studied. For example, the image of a normal heart (above) shows the left ventricle pumping blood into the aorta; the image has been computer-colored so that the areas containing the greatest amounts of blood are shown in purple and gray.

MODERN DIAGNOSTIC TECHNIQUES

In the 19th century, physicians usually had to wait until an autopsy had been performed on a patient before they could determine whether or not their diagnosis had been correct. Today, the body's internal organs can be studied during life with minimal risk or no risk to the patient. Physicians use imaging techniques, including X rays, ultrasound, CT scanning, radioisotope scanning, and MRI (magnetic resonance imaging); endoscopy (using a fiberoptic tube to view directly the interior of hollow organs such as the lungs, stomach, bladder, or some joints); and biopsy (examination under a microscope of a small sample of tissue that has been removed from an organ by surgery, by a needle, or via an endoscope).

X rays

A type of electromagnetic radiation with extremely short wavelengths, X rays are invisible and cause no sensation when passed through tissue (although they may damage the skin and internal organs and may cause cancer many years later). When X rays pass through the body, they are absorbed more by dense structures, such as bone, than by softer tissues. Thus, when an X-ray beam is focused onto photographic film behind the patient, shadows of variable intensity are cast on the film, producing the X-ray image.

Chest X rays
Because the lungs are full of air, they offer little resistance to X rays. A radiograph of the chest (left) gives a clear picture of the ribs, heart, and major blood vessels. A "shadow on the lungs" may be caused by an area of infection (such as from tuberculosis), a tumor, or an inhaled foreign body.

Digital subtraction angiography

Because many organs have a relatively uniform consistency, their structure does not show up on conventional X rays. One solution is angiography—injecting a radiopaque dye into blood vessels to make them visible on X rays. In digital subtraction angiography, images before and after injection of the dye are computer-processed to remove confusing detail and produce a clear image.

Digital cardiac imaging
Digital subtraction angiography can be used to visualize the coronary arteries. The digital cardiac imaging unit (left) has four screens to monitor the introduction of radiopaque dye and to display the arteries (seen here on three of the screens).

CT scanning

Conventional X rays and angiograms are essentially shadow photographs, but CT scanning uses X rays in a completely different way. Multiple beams of X rays are passed through the part of the body being examined, and their degree of absorption is recorded by sensors. The scanner moves around the patient, emitting and recording X-ray beams from every point on the circle. The resulting data are then analyzed by a computer, which uses the variations in absorption of the X rays to construct an image.

CT scan through the trunk
The CT scan (right) shows a cross section through the trunk of the body at the level of the kidneys. The image has been colored by computer to make the internal structures (the most important of which are labeled) more clearly visible.

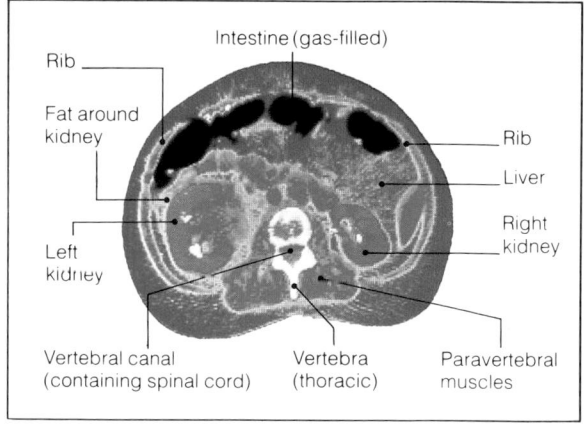

Rib

Intestine (gas-filled)

Fat around kidney

Rib

Liver

Right kidney

Left kidney

Vertebral canal (containing spinal cord)

Vertebra (thoracic)

Paravertebral muscles

Three-dimensional bone imaging

Conventional CT and MRI scanners provide physicians with a computer-generated cross-sectional image that corresponds to a slice through the body (as shown at the bottom of the previous page). However, a surgeon treating a patient with a badly damaged bone or joint sometimes requires more information than can be provided by such an image. In this situation, a powerful computer may be used to generate a three-dimensional image, such as the one shown of a damaged shoulder joint (right), which reveals that the shoulder blade has been broken into several fragments. Such images give surgeons vital information for planning treatment, enabling them to "see" precise details of the damage before undertaking an operation to repair it. Furthermore, because the operation can be planned in advance in great detail, it can be performed more quickly. Three-dimensional imaging is especially valuable for visualizing injuries of the hip, shoulder, rib cage, and skull.

Radionuclide scanning

In conventional radiography and CT scanning, the images produced depend on physical differences (notably in density) among body structures. Imaging by radionuclide scanning utilizes another approach. In this technique, radioactive chemicals are introduced into the body; the radiation emitted by the organs or tissues, which take up the chemicals, is detected and analyzed by an instrument known as a gamma camera. The amount of radiation emitted by a part of the body depends mainly on the level of metabolic activity of its constituent cells. Thus, cells that are dividing rapidly (which occurs within cancerous tissue) show up in some cases as "hot spots" on radionuclide scans.

The substances used in radionuclide scanning are usually either radioactive forms of elements that are normally found in the body, such as iodine, or synthetic radioactive elements, such as technetium. The substance may be swallowed by the patient or injected into the bloodstream; the radiation emitted is then measured by scanning the part of the body being investigated (or, in some cases, the whole body) with a gamma camera. The levels of radiation involved in this technique are very low, usually considerably lower than those to which the body is exposed in a series of conventional X rays.

Radionuclide bone scanning

The radionuclide bone scan (left) shows a front view of the complete skeleton of a healthy person. Bone scanning is an essential step in assessing treatment for some types of cancer, such as breast cancer, because it can reveal whether or not the cancer has spread beyond its primary site and developed secondary growths (metastases) in the bones. If such growths are present—indicated by bright "hot spots" on a bone scan—then removal of all the cancer cells by surgery alone is not usually possible. In this situation, surgery is usually confined to simple removal of the primary tumor; cytotoxic drug therapy is carried out to eradicate the secondary growths. In cancer of the prostate, where spread to the skeleton is common, estrogens (female sex hormones) are given to men for pain relief.

MRI

Unlike X-ray radiography, CT scanning, and radionuclide imaging, MRI (magnetic resonance imaging) does not employ potentially harmful ionizing radiation. Instead, it exploits the natural behavior of the protons (nuclei) of hydrogen atoms when they are subjected to a very strong magnetic field and radio waves. As a result of this stimulation, the protons emit radio signals, which are detected and computer-processed to generate an image. The most abundant sources of protons in the body are the hydrogen atoms in water molecules; an MRI scan therefore reflects differences in the water content of tissues.

Superficially, MRI scans look like CT scans. However, CT scans usually show little differentiation in soft tissues; MRI scans show more of the detailed structure because of differences in water content within these tissues. For example, white and gray matter in the brain are relatively poorly differentiated in CT scans, while they are distinct and well-defined in MRI scans.

NORMAL CHEST SCAN

ABNORMAL CHEST SCAN

Diagnostic MRI scanning
The two MRI scans (right) show cross sections through the chest. The upper scan, which reveals a healthy chest, shows the lungs (the large black areas in the center) and ribs (the crescent-shaped red-yellow areas toward the edge). In comparison, the lower scan shows a tumor in the left lung. The tumor is indicated by the increased amount of blue in the image of that lung and by the lung's small size.

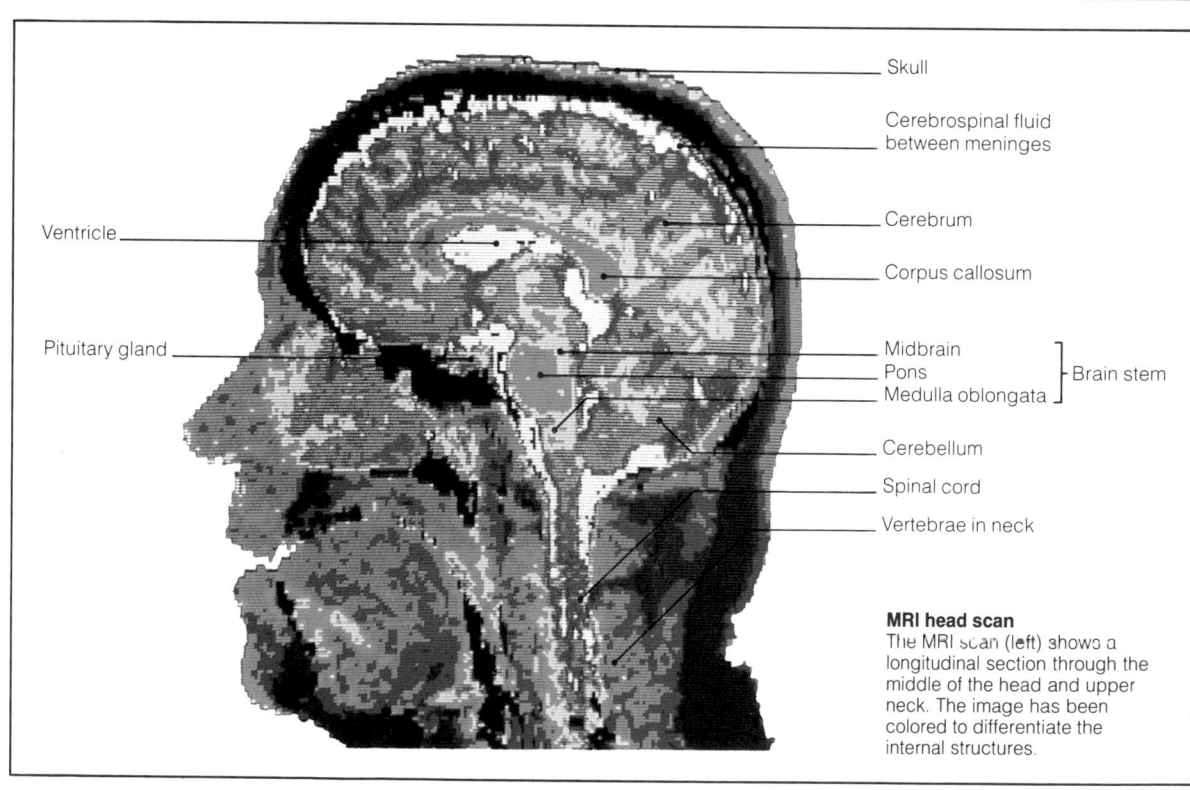

Skull

Cerebrospinal fluid between meninges

Cerebrum

Corpus callosum

Ventricle

Pituitary gland

Midbrain
Pons   } Brain stem
Medulla oblongata

Cerebellum

Spinal cord

Vertebrae in neck

MRI head scan
The MRI scan (left) shows a longitudinal section through the middle of the head and upper neck. The image has been colored to differentiate the internal structures.

HOW MRI WORKS

Radio-wave source

Magnet

Radio-wave detector

The MRI scanner

An MRI scanner consists of a massive electromagnet, a radio-wave emitter, and a radio-wave detector. These instruments are arranged around a central tunnel in which the patient lies, and are connected to a computer and display screen. The electromagnet is extremely powerful. It is able to create a magnetic field up to about 60,000 times that of the Earth's magnetic field.

Scanning plane

Scanning plane

When the patient is inside the machine, it is set up to scan a plane ("slice") of the body.

The scanning process

Scanning begins when a plane of the body has been selected for imaging. First, the electromagnet is turned on. Normally, the protons (nuclei) of the body's hydrogen atoms point randomly in different directions, but under the influence of the scanner's powerful magnetic field they align themselves in the same direction (diagram, top right). Next, the radio-wave source emits a powerful pulse of radio waves, the effect of which is to knock the protons out of alignment (diagram, middle right). However, milliseconds later, the protons realign themselves, emitting faint radio signals as they do so; these signals are picked up by the scanner's radio-wave detector (diagram, bottom right). A computer then processes the radio signals to produce an image of the plane of the body being scanned, such as the "slice" through the chest shown in the photograph (bottom right). Computer software enables three-dimensional images to be derived from MRI.

Magnet   Proton

Radio-wave source   Radio-wave stimulation

Radio-wave detector   Radio-wave emissions

PET scanning

PET (positron emission tomography) scanning is a development of radionuclide scanning and resembles it in many ways. Both techniques use a radioactive substance introduced into the body to produce an image that reflects the level of activity of tissues. However, radionuclide scanning usually produces an image analogous to a conventional X-ray picture; PET scanning gives a cross-sectional image that is analogous to a CT scan.

In PET scanning, a substance that takes part in metabolic biochemical processes is labeled with a radioisotope to make it radioactive; it is then injected into the bloodstream. The substance is taken up by the most metabolically active areas of tissue. In the tissue, the substance emits positrons. The positrons, in turn, release photons, which are then detected by an array of sensors around the patient. The sensors are linked to a computer, which calculates the origins of the photons to construct an image of the distribution of the substance within the tissues.

PET scanning is currently being utilized for investigating brain tumors, locating the origin of epileptic activity, and studying the brain function in various mental illnesses. It is anticipated that PET scanning will be used for other organs.

PET brain scanning

The PET scan (above) of a section through a normal brain has been colored to show levels of protein synthesis (high levels are indicated by pink, red, and orange, intermediate levels by yellow and green, and low levels by blue). In this scan, methionine (an essential amino acid) was used to show protein synthesis. Other brain functions can be imaged by using different substances—such as radioactively labeled glucose to show carbohydrate metabolism.

Biochemical analysis

Body fluids contain thousands of different chemicals. A healthy body maintains the concentration of each substance within clearly defined normal limits. However, in disease, the level of a body chemical may be abnormally high or low; detecting this abnormality by biochemical analysis can help in diagnosis.

A physician may order biochemical tests on samples of blood, urine, and other body fluids, such as spinal fluid, saliva, or sweat, when confirming a diagnosis. These tests may be part of a diagnostic investigation in which the chemical constituents of body fluids are checked primarily to confirm an illness that the physician suspects may exist based on the patient's description of his or her symptoms. The tests may also be used to assess the function of a particular organ, such as the liver or kidneys.

In recent years, the automation of equipment used for analysis has made biochemical testing faster and more accurate. New analytical techniques have been developed that make it possible to measure infinitesimal amounts of substances, such as hormones, in a person's body fluids.

Protein analysis
Fast protein liquid chromatography (above) is one of the many laboratory techniques that provides physicians with rapid, accurate measurement of substances in the blood and other body fluids. This technique is used to separate the individual protein constituents of a complex mixture so that they can be identified and quantified by, for example, measuring differences in their molecular sizes, electrical charges, and motility.

Diagnostic ultrasound

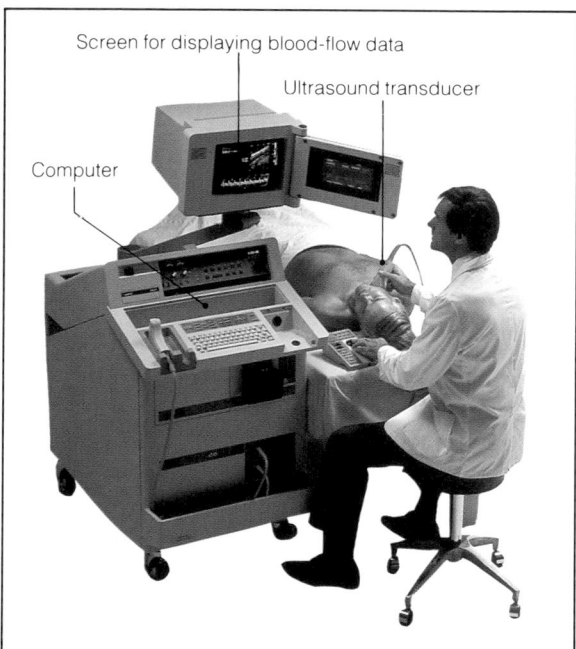

Screen for displaying blood-flow data

Ultrasound transducer

Computer

Angiodynography
This noninvasive ultrasound technique utilizes the Doppler effect to investigate blood flow. The photograph (above) shows the technique being used to examine blood flow through the neck. The physician places a transducer (an ultrasound emitter and detector) against the patient's neck; a computer processes ultrasound echo data to produce an image of the blood flow on a display unit.

The diagnostic use of ultrasound is based on the principle of sonar, in which sound waves are used to locate underwater objects by their echoes. In diagnostic ultrasound, a device called a transducer is placed on the skin and transmits inaudible high-frequency sound waves into the body, where they are reflected by the internal structures. The transducer detects these echoes, which are converted to numerical data and then displayed directly on a screen or analyzed by computer to produce an image of the structures.

In contrast to X rays, which are potentially harmful, ultrasound is thought to be completely safe—a belief based on 30 years' use on hundreds of millions of patients with no evidence of any ill effects. Ultrasound is especially useful in obstetrics because it enables the physician to examine the fetus at no known risk to either the woman or her developing child.

A modification of the basic ultrasound technique makes use of the Doppler effect (the change in pitch that occurs when a sound source is moving relative to the detector) to give information about the rate of blood flow through blood vessels. This procedure, known as angiodynography, enables the physician to detect narrowing of blood vessels or turbulence in the flow of blood.

Another ultrasound procedure, known as echocardiography, provides information about the heart, including the structure and flexibility of heart valves, the condition of the heart muscle, and the flow of blood within the heart.

Biopsy

Biopsy, the examination of a sample of tissue removed from a living patient (in contrast to necropsy, the examination of tissue after death), is a valuable aid in establishing a precise diagnosis. Samples of muscle, liver, kidney, lung, and other tissues may be removed safely and simply by passing a needle through the skin and into the target organ or tissue, sometimes using ultrasound, CT scanning, or fluoroscopy to help guide the needle. Tumors and cysts in organs such as the breast, ovary, testis, or thyroid can be sampled in the same way. Once obtained, the tissue sample may be examined under a microscope and subjected to a variety of biochemical tests, thereby yielding a diagnosis that is accurate.

Normal ovarian tissue

Malignant teratoma

Ovarian biopsy sample
Tissue samples removed by biopsy may be examined under a light microscope or, occasionally, under a scanning electron microscope. The scanning electron micrograph (left) of a sample of ovarian tissue shows a malignant teratoma (a type of ovarian cancer) invading the tissue of the ovary.

Endoscopic investigation

Early endoscopes were simply rigid or partially rigid tubes, sometimes with complex lens systems and interior lighting, and were of limited use. In the late 1950s, the introduction of fiberoptics enabled endoscopes to be completely flexible, thereby greatly increasing their versatility. Today, many specialized endoscopes are available, enabling physicians to view directly virtually any structure in the body, including the digestive tract, nasal sinuses, lungs, bladder, abdominal cavity, and joints. In addition, many endoscopes can be fitted with attachments that enable samples of tissue to be taken for biopsy or surgical procedures to be carried out.

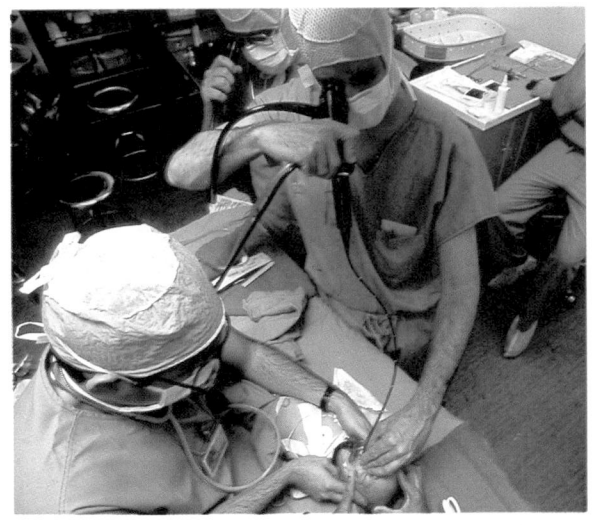

Bronchoscopy
Using a bronchoscope, a type of endoscope designed for looking at the lungs, physicians examine an infant who has breathing difficulty (right). During this procedure, fluid and debris may also be removed from the air passages.

Genetic analysis

Recent advances in genetics have allowed the genetic defects responsible for certain inherited disorders to be identified and detected. When there is a family history of an inherited disorder, such as muscular dystrophy or Down's syndrome, or when a couple has had a child with such a disorder, tests may be performed early in pregnancy to discover whether or not the fetus has the genetic defect. The tests involve removing cells from the membranes or fluid around the fetus, culturing the cells, and then analyzing their gene content by examining the chromosomes under a microscope. As a result of genetic analysis and elective termination of pregnancy, the frequency of some inherited disorders has been reduced. Parents at risk of having a baby with an inherited defect may (with genetic counseling and prenatal testing) be able to reassure themselves about the fetus's health.

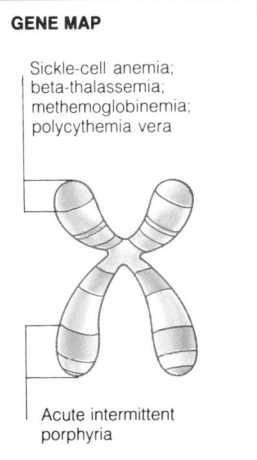

GENE MAP

Sickle-cell anemia; beta-thalassemia; methemoglobinemia; polycythemia vera

Acute intermittent porphyria

Gene mapping
Every normal cell in the body contains 46 chromosomes (except the sex cells—eggs and sperm—which have only 23 each). Each chromosome carries several thousand genes; geneticists are now able to pinpoint the locations of many of the individual genes that, when defective, cause inherited disorders. For example, the gene map (left) of chromosome 11 shows the locations of gene defects responsible for the inherited blood disorders sickle cell anemia, beta-thalassemia, methemoglobinemia, and polycythemia vera, and the metabolic disorder acute intermittent porphyria.

TREATING DISEASE

Until well into this century, most of the advances in medical science focused on understanding the nature of diseases rather than their treatment. The exception was surgery, which had made considerable progress since the introduction of general anesthesia in the 1840s, antiseptic procedures in the 1870s, and blood transfusions in the early 1900s. Physicians, however, had at their disposal few effective drugs with which to work, and they could do little to cure, or even slow the progress of, most diseases.

The situation changed dramatically in the 1930s with the introduction of antibacterial drugs, advances in the production of synthetic drugs, and the development of drugs that act on the body's metabolic processes. Thereafter, progress was (and still is) rapid, as scientists developed an ever wider range of effective drugs and improved methods of drug production. Important landmarks in the development of treatment methods are listed in the accompanying charts on this page and the next.

Drugs from plants
Traditionally, plants were the source of many useful drugs, including the antimalarial drug quinine, from the bark of the CINCHONA tree (called Jesuits' bark, shown above), the painkiller morphine, from poppies, and the heart drug digitalis, from the foxglove plant.

Paul Ehrlich (1854-1915)
A German bacteriologist and pioneer of chemotherapy, Ehrlich introduced (in 1911) salvarsan, the first drug to be prepared for treating the cause of a specific disease—in this case, syphilis.

LANDMARKS IN DRUG DEVELOPMENT

Date	Development
1666	**Quinine.** British physician Thomas Sydenham popularized use of Jesuits' bark (containing quinine) for treating malaria.
1785	**Digitalis.** Use of digitalis to treat heart failure described by British physician William Withering.
1796	**Smallpox vaccination.** The first vaccination to be performed, by British physician Edward Jenner. The first true vaccine (consisting of weakened microorganisms)—against chicken cholera—was developed in 1880 by French scientist Louis Pasteur.
1805	**Morphine.** Extracted from opium and used to relieve pain by German pharmacist Friedrich Sertürner.
1899	**Aspirin.** Developed as a drug by German scientist Felix Hoffmann.
1911	**Salvarsan.** Introduced by Paul Ehrlich to treat syphilis.
1928	**Penicillin.** Antibacterial action first recognized by British bacteriologist Alexander Fleming. It was produced as a drug in 1940, by Australian-born British pathologist Howard Florey, and German-born British biochemist Ernst Chain.
1935	**Sulfonamides.** Antibacterial action discovered by German pharmacologist Gerhard Domagk.
1951	**Oral contraceptive.** Developed by American physicians Gregory Pincus and John Rock, and the Austrian-born American chemist Carl Djerassi.
1959	**Librium (chlordiazepoxide).** The first benzodiazepine minor tranquilizer, introduced by Swiss pharmaceutical company Hoffmann-LaRoche.
1962	**Nethalide (pronethalol).** The first beta-blocking heart drug, developed by scientists at Imperial Chemical Industries, England.
1984	**Genetically engineered human insulin.** Developed by scientists at Genentech, California.
1986	**Zidovudine (originally called AZT).** Introduced for treating AIDS after development by scientists at Burroughs Wellcome Research Laboratories, North Carolina.

LANDMARKS IN SURGERY

Date	Development
1545	**Basic surgical principles.** Established by French surgeon Ambroise Paré.
1842	**General anesthesia.** First operation using general anesthesia performed by American surgeon Crawford Long, who used ether. In 1845, American dentist Horace Wells used nitrous oxide ("laughing gas") as an anesthetic. In 1847, British obstetrician James Simpson introduced chloroform anesthesia.
1870	**Antiseptic surgery.** Pioneered by British surgeon Joseph Lister, who used a carbolic acid (phenol) spray during surgery to help prevent infection.
1901	**Blood groups.** ABO blood groups discovered by Austrian pathologist Karl Landsteiner, so establishing the basis for safe transfusions.
1951	**Coronary artery bypass graft.** First attempted by Canadian surgeon Arthur Vineberg at the Royal Victoria Hospital, Montreal, Canada.
1955	**Kidney transplant.** First successful kidney transplant (between identical twins) performed by team of American surgeons—led by Joseph Murray—of the Harvard Medical School, Massachusetts.
1967	**Heart transplant.** First human heart transplant performed by South African surgeon Christiaan Barnard at the Groote Schuur Hospital, Capetown, South Africa.
1976	**Coronary angioplasty.** Introduced by Swiss surgeon Andreas Grüntzig at the University Hospital, Zurich, Switzerland.
1987	**Fetal tissue transplant.** First transplant of fetal brain tissue into brains of patients with Parkinson's disease performed by research groups in Mexico, the US, and Europe.

LANDMARKS IN OTHER FORMS OF TREATMENT

Date	Development
c.1270	**Eyeglasses.** Thought to have been invented in Italy. Contact lenses were invented in 1887, by Swiss optician Eugen Frick.
1817	**Dental plate.** Introduced by American dentist Anthony Plantson.
1891	**Baby incubator.** Introduced by French physician Alexandre Lion.
1901	**Hearing aid (electric).** Developed by American inventor Miller Reese Hutchinson. The first truly miniature hearing aid introduced in 1952 by the Sonotone Corporation.
1945	**Kidney dialysis machine.** Developed by Dutch surgeon Willem Kolff to treat patients with renal failure.
1978	**"Test-tube baby."** The first (Louise Brown) born in England as a result of in vitro fertilization (IVF) techniques developed by British gynecologist Patrick Steptoe and embryologist Robert Edwards.
1979	**Shock-wave lithotripsy.** Pioneered by researchers at the University Hospital, Munich, West Germany.

Early surgery
Boring a hole in the skull to relieve pressure on the brain (above) dates from prehistoric times. Moreover, archaeological evidence suggests that some patients survived this early form of surgery.

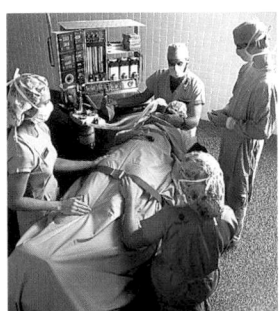

Anesthesia and surgery
A successful surgical operation (above) relies to a great degree on anesthesia. Introduced in the 1840s, anesthetics not only free the patient from pain and restless agitation, but also give the surgeon more time to perform the operation.

Endoscopic surgery
A view through an endoscope of a damaged knee joint is shown in the photograph (above). Endoscopes enable surgeons to directly examine, and perform operations on, internal body structures.

MODERN SURGICAL TREATMENT

Until about the 1940s, most surgery consisted of excision—cutting out abnormal tissue or structures that were diseased or damaged. The primary exception was orthopedics, in which surgeons were attempting to encourage the healing of bones by employing rods, pins, and immobilization. Since then, surgery has been transformed by technological advances such as the operating microscope, the laser scalpel, and the endoscope. Today, many operations emphasize repair or replacement rather than excision.

Transplant surgery

Bone marrow transplants
These transplants replace malignant or defective marrow. A syringe is used to suck out healthy marrow from the donor's hipbone (shown above). This marrow is then injected into the recipient's bloodstream, which carries it to the bones. Drugs that suppress the immune system are given to prevent rejection of the transplanted marrow, but they make the recipient vulnerable to infection. Thus the patient must remain in an isolation unit until the new marrow "takes."

Experience with skin grafting in World War II demonstrated that the body's immune system attacks tissue from another person (causing rejection) in the same way that it attacks microorganisms. Therefore, when transplant surgery began in the 1950s, there were two challenges—the technical task of replacing a diseased organ with a healthy one, and preventing the rejection of the transplanted organ. Because drugs that prevent rejection also suppress the immune system, they lower the body's resistance to infection. Consequently, many early transplant recipients survived the operation but died from infection. Gradually, the technical problems were overcome, first with kidney transplants and later with heart and liver transplants. Improved immunosuppressant drugs were then developed, notably cyclosporine. As a result, the success rate for transplants is generally high. The primary problem today is the lack of available organ donors. Another technical and ethical problem that is currently the subject of much discussion is the use of fetal tissue and organs for transplantation.

Surgical implants

There are four main problems in replacing a part of the body with an artificial implant. First, the implant must be sufficiently inert so as not to provoke the immune system to reject it. Second, it must also be tough enough to last for many years. Third, a means must be found to secure the implant in position. Fourth, scrupulous operative techniques are necessary to prevent infection. Today, these problems have largely been solved, and most implants are successful; hip joint replacements last for 10 years or more in 70 to 80 percent of cases. Furthermore, a wide range of implants is now available—joints, heart valves, lenses for the eye, sections of blood vessels, and replacements for parts of the skull.

Heart valve implants
Damaged heart valves may be replaced by synthetic substitutes (or by valves from a pig or a cadaver). The photograph (left) shows a synthetic heart valve being sewn in place.

Hip joint replacement
The colored X ray (right) shows an artificial hip joint in place. Replacing the hip joint—which is usually done when it has been damaged by arthritis—is one of the most successful types of implant surgery.

Microsurgery

In microsurgery, surgeons use a specially designed microscope, tiny instruments, and delicate sutures (stitches) to perform operations on minute structures, such as small nerves or blood vessels. One of the major advantages of microsurgery is that more of the tiny blood vessels and nerves can be preserved, minimizing damage to the tissues being repaired and thus reducing the amount of scar tissue formed.

Today, microsurgical techniques are used in many operations on the eye or ear. These techniques are also used in operations that involve the joining of blood vessels, such as in reconstructive surgery when the tiny arteries and veins of skin and muscle flaps are sewn together. Microsurgery has also enabled surgeons to reattach severed fingers, toes, complete limbs, and even the two sections of a vas deferens separated in a vasectomy.

Microsurgical operations
In the photograph (right), two surgeons perform a delicate microsurgical operation. Each is looking into a binocular eyepiece of an operating microscope, which is used to magnify the structures being operated on (such as tiny blood vessels). The surgical instruments are also magnified so that the surgeons can achieve the extreme precision necessary for the operation to be successful.

Laser surgery

A laser produces a narrow beam of intense energy that surgeons can use as a "light knife" to cut through tissue (while simultaneously cauterizing blood vessels), usually without causing damage beyond the target area. Lasers are used in many operations on the eye, especially those on the retina, and are also used to seal bleeding arteries in peptic ulcers, to destroy tumors, and to remove some skin blemishes.

LASER TREATMENT

Protective goggles

Fiberoptic cable from laser source

Laser beam

Removing skin blemishes
Lasers are effective at removing certain skin blemishes, such as birthmarks that are due to excessive growth of blood vessels in the skin. In such treatment (shown right), the physician and patient wear goggles to protect their eyes.

Endoscopic surgery

Endoscopes are used not only for diagnosis, but also for performing certain surgical procedures. Special attachments such as scissors or a wire loop snare may be fitted to remove tumors, and sharp-toothed forceps may be used to grasp and remove foreign bodies. Other operations for which endoscopes are used include shattering stones in the urinary tract and repairing torn cartilages in joints.

Endoscopic surgery is generally safer and easier to perform than conventional surgery that requires an incision. It also causes less tissue damage, producing less discomfort and a quicker recovery for the patient.

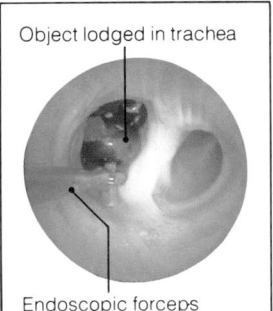

Object lodged in trachea

Endoscopic forceps

Removing foreign objects
The photograph (left), taken through an endoscope (a fiberoptic viewing tube), shows the removal of an inhaled object (the top of a martini stirrer) from the windpipe of a young child. The forceps that are being used to grasp the object have been passed through a special channel in the endoscope. The forceps are operated by remote manipulation.

DRUG TREATMENT

The medicinal herbs and plants that provide physicians with drugs have been identified over thousands of years. More recently, advances in drug production have helped pharmacologists and biochemists develop an immense range of new synthetic drugs.

Before any substance is approved for use as a drug, it is tested for effectiveness and safety. Only after satisfactory evidence has been made available to the Food and Drug Administration can a drug be approved for marketing.

Drugs from natural sources

PLANT SOURCES

Poppy seed pod

Opium poppy
(Papaver somniferum)

Deadly nightshade
(Atropa belladonna)

In medicine, most drugs that were originally derived from plants have now been replaced by pure preparations of the active ingredients. For example, some of the refined derivatives of opium include morphine sulfate, codeine, and papaverine. Plants continue to be a valuable source of new substances that might prove to be effective drugs.

Drugs from plants
Morphine and atropine were once obtained directly from seed pods of the opium poppy and from deadly nightshade, respectively. Today, purified forms are available.

Antibacterials and antibiotics

The first drugs effective against bacterial infections were the chemical-based antibacterials salvarsan (introduced in 1911) and the sulfonamides (developed in the 1930s). Antibiotics (originally derived from molds or fungi, rather than chemicals) were introduced in the 1940s, when penicillin became available as a drug (although its antibacterial activity was recognized in 1928). Since then, numerous other antibacterials and antibiotics have been discovered; physicians today have a wide range of effective drugs from which to choose.

Penicillin
The photograph (right) shows a culture of the mold *PENICILLIUM NOTATUM*. This species was an early source of the antibiotic penicillin; today, synthetic forms of the drug are usually used.

Vaccines

Vaccination dates from 1796, when Edward Jenner inoculated against smallpox, but vaccines against other potentially lethal diseases were not developed until this century. Today, vaccines are available to give protection against measles, mumps, diphtheria, poliomyelitis, tetanus, pertussis, rubella, and other, less common, diseases such as hepatitis, typhoid, typhus, rabies, cholera, and yellow fever.

Vaccination in developing countries
Many infectious diseases (such as measles) that have been brought under control in developed countries remain a major cause of death in developing countries. To reduce such deaths, a variety of international agencies run mass vaccination programs (left).

Synthetic drugs

Many drugs that were originally derived from natural sources are now produced synthetically in the laboratory. Such production ensures that the drugs are of consistent potency (drug extracts from natural sources tend to vary in strength) and that they are available when required.

Furthermore, recent advances in our understanding of the functioning of the body have made it possible to "tailor-make" drugs for specific purposes, rather than relying solely on synthetic analogues of natural substances. For example, propranolol was developed specifically to block the action of the natural hormones epinephrine and norepinephrine on the heart and blood vessels. This blocking effect is useful in treating some cases of high blood pressure, angina, or abnormal heart rhythms. Cimetidine was tailor-made to treat ulcers by reducing the stomach's acid-secreting response to histamine.

Drugs may also be synthesized to supplement hormones or other body chemicals that are produced in insufficient amounts due to disease. One example is the synthetic drug levodopa, which is given to counteract the deficiency of the natural chemical dopamine that occurs in Parkinson's disease. Drugs developed in this purposeful way to meet particular needs may be further modified chemically to increase their potency and duration of action, or to reduce possible adverse effects.

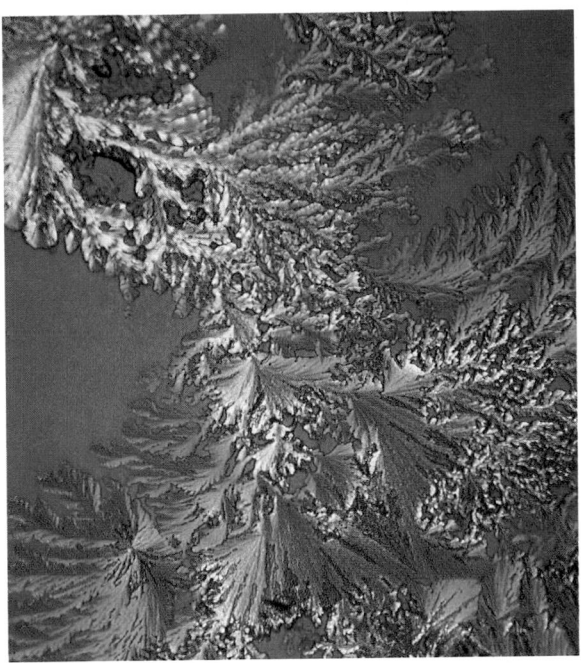

Synthetic hormones
Many hormones that are used therapeutically are produced synthetically. Epinephrine (shown in a polarized light photomicrograph, above) is used to counteract cardiac arrest and control bleeding in surgery.

Genetically engineered drugs

This recently developed technique for modifying the genetic structure of living organisms could revolutionize medicine. However, much more research is needed to explore its full potential. To date, its principal medical use has been to produce human forms of hormones and other natural body chemicals that can be used to treat certain metabolic disorders. One example is the use of genetically engineered human insulin to treat diabetes mellitus (cattle insulin was once used, but it is not well tolerated by some people with diabetes). Other substances produced by genetic engineering include human growth hormone (used to treat pituitary dwarfism), factor VIII (used to treat hemophilia), and erythropoietin (used to treat some forms of anemia).

Although technically difficult to achieve, producing a human hormone (or other body chemical) by genetic engineering is simple in theory. The gene that instructs human cells to produce the hormone is identified, isolated, and inserted into the genetic material of a microorganism such as a bacterium or yeast. The microorganism is then cultured in large vats so that it multiplies and produces large amounts of the hormone for commercial purposes.

Genetically engineered Insulin
Genetic engineering can force bacteria to produce human insulin. The insulin gene is obtained (by removing it from human DNA, then purifying it) and spliced into the DNA of a bacterium, causing it to produce human insulin. The bacterium is then cultured for large-scale insulin extraction.

OTHER METHODS OF TREATMENT

Drug treatment and surgery are still the primary divisions of medical care, but technological advances have become so specialized in recent years that some types of treatment have become separate branches of medicine. Examples include the various forms of intensive care (e.g., medical, coronary, surgical, and neurosurgical). These newer forms of treatment often require specialized medical and nursing staff.

Intensive care

Some patients require continuous monitoring of their body functions—heart rate and rhythm, breathing rate, blood pressure—so that any deterioration in their condition can be detected and treated immediately. Many patients who are seriously ill also must be given fluids, nutrition, and medication intravenously, and some may require a ventilator to help them breathe. Monitoring of a patient's condition is best provided in an intensive-care unit (or, for a patient who has had or is suspected of having a myocardial infarction, a coronary-care unit), which has the necessary equipment and is staffed around the clock by specially trained hospital personnel.

A TYPICAL INTENSIVE-CARE UNIT

Blood pressure monitor · ECG monitor · Intravenous equipment · Defibrillator · Ventilator · Urinary catheter

Intensive-care facilities
An intensive-care unit contains all the equipment needed to continuously monitor vital body functions and to maintain a stable condition in the patient. Such units are also equipped to deal with any medical crises that may arise, such as ventricular fibrillation (rapid, random beating of the lower heart chamber), which may require a defibrillator to restore a normal heart beat.

Radiation therapy

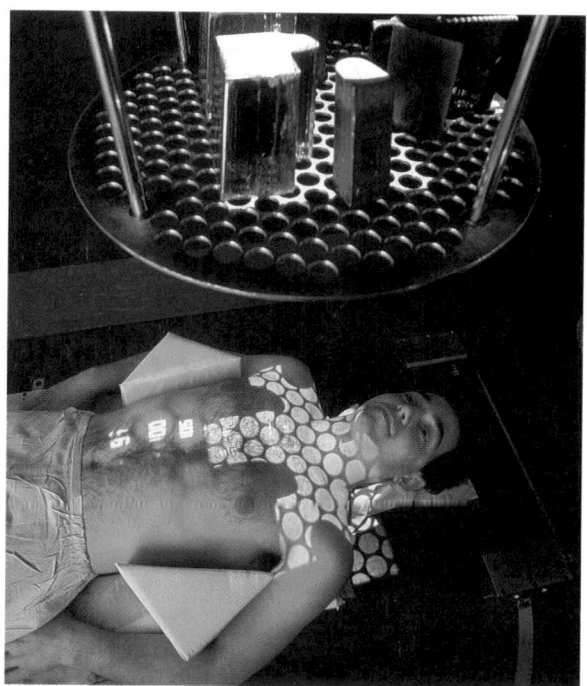

The use of X rays and implants of radium (a naturally radioactive substance) to treat cancers dates from the turn of this century. Today, X rays are still used in radiation therapy (also known as radiation oncology), but the range of treatment has been greatly expanded to include other forms or sources of radiation (e.g., neutron beams or radioactive varieties of substances such as iodine or yttrium). It is now also possible to focus radiation beams more accurately, thereby concentrating them on the tumor and minimizing damage to surrounding healthy tissue.

Radiation may be used alone to treat some tumors—such as basal cell carcinoma and certain tumors of the pituitary gland—but it is more often used in combination with surgery, chemotherapy, or both. The choice between radiation and surgery may depend on the stage of the tumor. In some cases, the results of surgery or radiation are the same.

X-ray therapy
The photograph (left) shows a patient about to receive X-ray therapy to treat cancer. The illuminated disks are the areas that will be irradiated; the pattern is determined by the arrangement of lead blocks on the metal platform (which shields the lungs from excessive radiation) below the source of the X rays.

Dialysis

A person whose kidneys fail will die within a few days unless impurities that accumulate in the blood are removed, either by a kidney dialysis machine or by peritoneal dialysis.

In hemodialysis, a dialysis machine removes impurities by filtering the patient's blood through a semipermeable membrane immersed in a special dialysis solution. The procedure takes a few hours and the patient visits a dialysis unit for each treatment. In peritoneal dialysis, the patient's abdominal cavity lining is used to filter impurities from the blood into the dialysis solution (which is passed in and out of the abdomen through a tube).

Dialysis may be necessary for only a few days if kidney failure is temporary, but it is also effective as a long-term treatment for permanent kidney failure. In most of the latter cases, the best remedy for the patient's condition is a kidney transplant.

Lithotripsy

Lithotripsy is a noninvasive procedure in which ultrasound is used to pulverize stones in the body. This technique seems likely to replace surgery as the treatment for certain kidney stones and is currently under investigation in the treatment of gallstones that cause symptoms. In lithotripsy, repeated pulses of high-energy ultrasound waves are focused on a stone to break it down into tiny particles that can be passed out of the body via the urine (with kidney stones) or via the feces (with gallstones).

EXTRACORPOREAL LITHOTRIPSY
- Arm for positioning shock-wave emitter
- Ultrasound shock-wave emitter
- Location display screen
- Control unit
- Ultrasound location transducer
- Movable couch

Shock-wave treatment of stones
Kidney stones or gallstones may be treated by extracorporeal lithotripsy. This technique involves focusing ultrasound shock waves on a stone until it breaks into tiny fragments that can be passed out of the body. The patient lies on a couch or in a water bath. The physician pinpoints the position of the stone with a fluoroscope or an ultrasound location transducer, and the patient and shock-wave emitter are placed in position for treatment. The stone is then subjected to shock waves until it is pulverized.

Incubator

Babies born prematurely are small and have internal organs that have not fully matured. Additionally, many basic reflexes and physiological functions, such as those that regulate body temperature, are not fully developed. For this reason, a newborn weighing less than 3.5 pounds is usually placed in an incubator, where the temperature, humidity, oxygen, and the baby's vital functions can be monitored.

Caring for premature babies
Improved neonatal care has increased the survival rate of premature babies. Today, babies weighing as little as 1.5 pounds can often be kept alive until they reach a safe size.

Psychiatric treatment

In earlier days, people with mental disorders were incarcerated in remote mental asylums. Today, most individuals are treated in units within general hospitals or in community settings. In addition, new drugs can sometimes transform the outlook for patients with severe mental disorders such as schizophrenia. Drug therapy—often combined with psychotherapy—now enables many people to resume varying degrees of activity within the community. There have also been developments in psychotherapy; the types now available include traditional, Freudian-based psychoanalysis, group therapy, and counseling.

PRENATAL TECHNOLOGY

Since the turn of the century, improvements in medical care have resulted in a dramatic decline in infant and childhood mortality in developed countries. Currently, infant mortality is more of a socioeconomic problem. The greatest difficulties are encountered with teenage pregnancies, which are associated with little or no prenatal care. Infants born today in developed countries have a 98 percent chance of growing up healthily. There has also been much progress in prenatal medicine as the understanding of genetics, fertility, pregnancy, and embryonic development has increased. As a result, prospective parents can now be counseled on such matters as the likelihood of their children having a genetic disorder or, if there is a problem with fertility, how to maximize the chance of conception.

PROCEDURES BEFORE CONCEPTION

To maximize the chance of having a successful pregnancy and a healthy baby, a couple should examine their health habits before pregnancy occurs. Both partners—but especially the woman—should eat a balanced diet and should avoid alcohol, tobacco, and all drugs except those taken in consultation with a physician. Women with metabolic disorders, such as diabetes mellitus, should ensure that their condition is controlled. Advice should be sought if either partner is aware of a disorder that runs in his or her family.

Genetic counseling

About one child in 50 is born with a physical, metabolic, or mental defect. Many of these defects are due to an abnormality in one or more of the genes inherited from the parents. In some cases, the parents are unaware that one (or, rarely, both) of them carries a defective gene. Occasionally, the defect is a new one that is caused by a genetic mutation occurring during the formation of the sperm or ovum. Sometimes, however, a couple planning a family know that one or more of their relatives have had children with a genetic disorder. In such cases, the couple should seek genetic counseling before their first pregnancy. The counselor can often perform tests to determine if there is a risk of a genetic disorder being passed on to the children and, if that is a possibility, may be able to quantify the risk involved. This allows the couple to make an informed decision as to whether they wish to continue with the pregnancy.

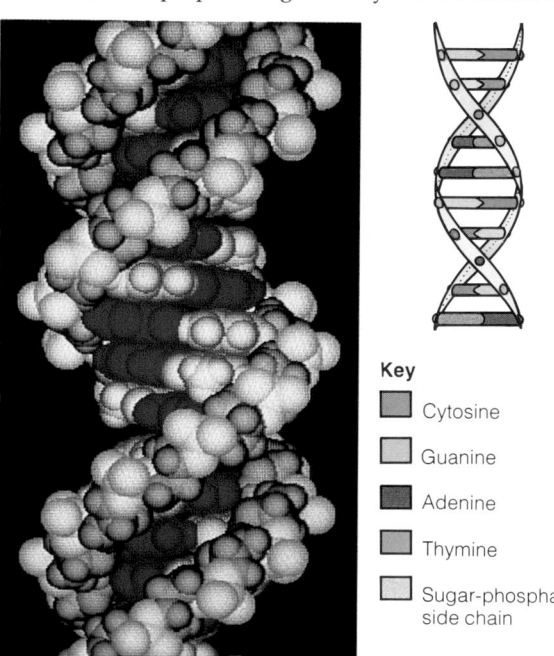

Key
- Cytosine
- Guanine
- Adenine
- Thymine
- Sugar-phosphate side chain

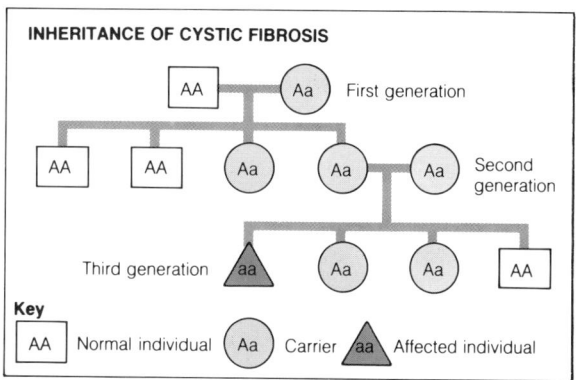

INHERITANCE OF CYSTIC FIBROSIS

AA — Aa First generation

AA   AA   Aa   Aa   Aa Second generation

Third generation aa   Aa   Aa   AA

Key
AA Normal individual   Aa Carrier   aa Affected individual

DNA and genetic disorders
DNA is a large, double-helix molecule (see computer-generated model, far left) consisting of two sugar-phosphate side chains linked by the bases cytosine, guanine, adenine, and thymine (diagram, near left). It carries the 50,000-plus genes that control cellular activities. Thus, a defective gene may disrupt cellular function and lead to a heritable disorder, such as cystic fibrosis (see diagram, above). People with the faulty gene (**a**) in a single dose (**Aa**) are carriers of cystic fibrosis but do not suffer from the disorder; a double dose (**aa**) is necessary for the disease to develop.

Treating infertility

Approximately one in every 10 couples finds it difficult to have children. In about 40 percent of such cases, the man is subfertile or infertile; in another 40 percent, the woman has a fertility disorder. In the remaining 20 percent, both partners have some degree of infertility. Methods employed to improve the likelihood of pregnancy include microsurgery to repair damaged fallopian tubes in women or to reverse vasectomy in men; drugs or hormones to stimulate ovulation in women or improve male fertility; and in vitro fertilization ("test-tube baby") techniques, although the success rate for this procedure remains low.

Viability
The photomicrograph (right) shows a six-day-old fertilized ovum surrounded by remains of sperm (in pink). Even though the ovum has been fertilized, it will not necessarily develop into a fetus; about half of all pregnancies probably terminate naturally within the first month due to a genetic or developmental fault.

PRENATAL DIAGNOSIS

Major developmental or genetic defects occur in more than one in 50 pregnancies. Some result in stillbirths; in others, the baby is born alive. Advances in prenatal diagnosis have made it possible to identify certain major defects early in pregnancy. For some cases in which the fetus has a serious disorder of the brain and/or spinal cord (e.g., anencephaly or spina bifida), treatment is not possible. The same is true for chromosomal defects, such as the one that produces Down's syndrome. In other cases, including certain defects of the fetal heart or kidney, or blood disorders such as hemolytic disease of the newborn, early diagnosis enables treatment to be given even before the baby is born. Early diagnosis also alerts the obstetrician and pediatrician to the need for specialized care of the baby immediately after birth.

Ultrasound scanning

Ultrasound scanning is part of the care given to many pregnant women. The scanning technique, which uses the echoes of high-pitched sound waves to construct an image of the fetus, is considered harmless and causes no discomfort. The ultrasound image enables the obstetrician to identify multiple pregnancies, to measure the size of the fetus (enabling its age to be assessed), and to detect certain physical and developmental defects (such as anencephaly, spina bifida, or some congenital heart abnormalities) early in the pregnancy.

Arm
Head   Leg
Body
Uterine wall

Fetal ultrasonography
A fetus can be imaged by ultrasound as early as the 12th week of pregnancy. The procedure (shown in the photograph above) usually takes about 15 minutes, and the woman is conscious throughout. It involves passing a transducer (a device that emits and receives ultrasound pulses) over the woman's abdomen; a computer then processes the ultrasound data to produce an image, which is displayed on one or more screens. An example of a fetal ultrasound image—of a 12-week-old fetus—is shown (far left), with a diagram to help interpret the image (left).

Fetoscopy

Ultrasound provides relatively clear images of a developing fetus, but in some cases it is necessary to examine the fetus directly or to carry out minor procedures on him or her. These procedures can be performed by fetoscopy, in which a fetoscope (a type of endoscope, or fiberoptic viewing tube) is passed into the woman's uterus through a small incision in her abdomen.

The direct access that fetoscopy gives allows any external fetal abnormalities, such as spinal column defects, facial clefts, or limb defects, to be assessed; it also enables samples of skin or blood to be taken from the fetus for tests. By attaching special instruments to the fetoscope, the physician can perform a variety of procedures, such as transfusing blood into the fetus to treat anemia. The fetoscope also allows some types of disorders (such as obstruction of the urinary tract) to be surgically corrected.

Viewing the fetus
The view of a fetus (right) was obtained using a fetoscope (fiberoptic viewing tube). The procedure carries a small risk of inducing miscarriage, so it is performed only when an obstetrician needs more information or access than is possible with other methods.

Amniocentesis and chorionic villus sampling

Performing amniocentesis
The photograph (above) shows a woman undergoing amniocentesis to remove a sample of amniotic fluid for analysis. Before the fluid is removed, an ultrasound scan is performed to determine the positions of the fetus and placenta. A local anesthetic is then usually applied to a small area of the abdomen, and a hollow needle is inserted through the abdominal wall and into the uterus, taking care to avoid the fetus and placenta. About half an ounce of fluid is sucked out by a syringe attached to the needle.

Amniocentesis and chorionic villus sampling can be used to diagnose certain fetal abnormalities early enough in pregnancy for elective abortion to remain a feasible option. However, because these procedures carry a small risk of inducing miscarriage, they are recommended only when there are good medical reasons for doing so, such as when the woman is older than 35 or when there is a family history of a chromosomal abnormality.

Amniocentesis involves removing and testing a sample of the amniotic fluid that surrounds the fetus. The procedure cannot be done before about the 16th to 18th week of pregnancy because there is not enough amniotic fluid before this time.

The amniotic fluid contains fetal cells, which are cultured to provide chromosomes for a karyotype analysis (a preparation of the chromosomes suitable for identifying chromosomal abnormalities). It may take two to three weeks to culture a chromosome sample, which means that results are not usually available until the 18th to 20th week of pregnancy. The amniotic fluid also contains various chemicals, the levels of which may be measured to test for other, nonchromosomal disorders of the fetus. For example, raised levels of alpha-fetoprotein may indicate a neural tube defect, such as spina bifida.

Chorionic villus sampling is another method of diagnosing fetal abnormalities due to chromosomal defects. Unlike amniocentesis, it is not suitable for detecting nonchromosomal abnormalities. In chorionic villus sampling, a small sample of tissue from the fetal side of the placenta is removed; the cells in the sample (which are genetically identical to those of the fetus) then undergo chromosomal analysis, which can usually be done immediately. Chorionic sampling can be done as early as eight to nine weeks into pregnancy (or later, if necessary). It thus gives results earlier than amniocentesis and permits a safer elective abortion if this course of action is chosen.

Chromosomal analysis
The set of chromosomes (right) from fetal cells has three rather than the normal two chromosomes in number 21. This genetic abnormality causes Down's syndrome.

PRENATAL TREATMENT

While advances in examining the fetus have been used to diagnose extremely severe defects, these same techniques have opened up possibilities for treating certain fetal disorders. The best-known example is treatment of hemolytic disease of the newborn due to Rh incompatibility.

This disorder occurs if the woman's blood is Rh negative and she is carrying a baby whose blood is Rh positive and she has previously been sensitized to Rh-positive blood. The woman can be sensitized through miscarriage, elective abortion, amniocentesis, a previous full-term pregnancy, or a blood transfusion of Rh-positive blood. In each situation except the last, Rh-positive blood has passed from the fetus to the Rh-negative woman. During subsequent pregnancies, the woman produces antibodies directed against the fetus's Rh-positive blood cells because her immune system recognizes the Rh-positive blood cells as "foreign." The fetal blood cells are destroyed by the maternal antibodies, resulting in the development of profound anemia.

If the fetus is found to be severely anemic before he or she is mature enough to be delivered safely (about 30 weeks' gestation), one or more blood transfusions are given via a fetoscope (fiberoptic viewing tube). The blood is transfused into one of the blood vessels in the umbilical cord. Alternatively, blood may be injected directly into the heart of the fetus via a needle passed through the mother's abdominal wall and into the uterus. This technique is called intracardiac transfusion and relies on accurate visualization of the fetus with ultrasound scanning. Although these measures carry some risk of inducing a miscarriage, the risk is usually justified because the ultimate outlook is excellent if the fetus can be kept alive long enough for birth to be feasible.

Sometimes, ultrasound tests show the presence of a defect in the fetus's urinary system, causing obstruction and pressure on the kidneys. In these circumstances, a fetoscope may be used to perform a simple operation to relieve the pressure and thus limit any damage to the kidneys.

Hemolytic disease (anemia) of the newborn
This disease typically occurs when a woman with Rhesus (Rh)-negative blood carries a baby with Rh-positive blood (see diagram, right). The first such pregnancy is usually normal. In subsequent pregnancies in which the fetus is Rh positive, maternal antibodies destroy fetal red blood cells, causing potentially fatal anemia. This anemia may be treated by fetal blood transfusions or prevented by injecting a woman who has Rh-negative blood with anti-D serum after childbirth. The serum prevents the woman's immune system from developing antibodies against Rh-positive blood.

RHESUS INCOMPATIBILITY

First pregnancy

Subsequent pregnancies

Rh-negative mother

Rh-positive baby

At birth, baby's blood enters mother's circulation

Antibodies against Rh-positive blood formed in mother

Antibodies cross placenta and destroy red blood cells of subsequent Rh-positive babies

NEW DISEASES

In general, any disease is most dangerous to a human society upon first exposure; within a few generations, natural selection encourages the survival of individuals who have some natural resistance. When Europeans began colonial expansion in the 15th cen- tury, they brought new diseases (such as smallpox and measles) to the colonized lands; these diseases killed millions of indigenous inhabitants. The col- onizers themselves were killed by diseases that they encountered for the first time.

EMERGENCE OF NEW DISEASES

New diseases in this century have been of three main types: those caused by microorganisms that have only recently infected humans, such as AIDS, Marburg disease, and Lassa fever; diseases that have existed for a long time but which have been identified only recently, including legionnaires' disease and cam- pylobacter food poisoning; and conditions associated with contemporary industrial society, such as asbestosis, liver disease in smelters, drug addiction, and radiation-linked disorders.

AIDS

First recognized in 1982 as a distinct illness in young homosexual men, AIDS is now seen as having some features in common with other viral diseases, such as hepatitis B. Human immunodeficiency virus (HIV), the causative agent of AIDS, may be transmitted by sexual contact (heterosexual or between male homosexuals), blood-to-blood contact, or from a pregnant woman to her unborn child. Infection with HIV follows an unpredictable and, as yet, not completely mapped course. Some of those infected develop full-blown AIDS and die within a short time; others remain in apparent good health (but are infectious) for many years.

Scientists have learned a great deal about AIDS since it was first recognized, but they still have not found a cure or a vaccine, although treatment with

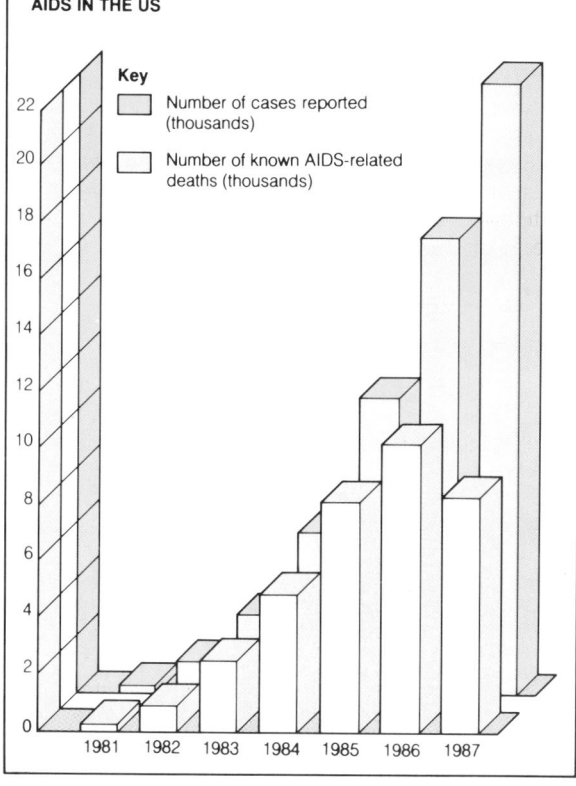

AIDS IN THE US

Key
- Number of cases reported (thousands)
- Number of known AIDS-related deaths (thousands)

(chart, values on y-axis: 0, 2, 4, 6, 8, 10, 12, 14, 16, 18, 20, 22; x-axis years: 1981 1982 1983 1984 1985 1986 1987)

Incidence of AIDS in the US
The photomicrograph at left shows the virus (orange) budding from an infected lymphocyte (blue). Infection with HIV may last for years without causing symptoms, and it is not yet known whether full-blown AIDS develops in all of those infected. Also, recently developed treatment can slow the progress of AIDS, with the result that, although the number of cases increased annually between 1981 and 1987, the number of AIDS-related deaths fell in 1987 (see chart, above).

certain antiviral drugs (such as zidovudine) does slow the progression of HIV infection. Educational programs have advocated following "safe" sex practices and, for intravenous drug users, ensuring that needles and syringes are sterile, in the hope that it may control or reduce the risk of infection. However, any forecast regarding the control of AIDS relies on assumptions about public awareness and changes in behavior, and on how soon medical prevention and treatment of the disease is achieved.

Other new diseases

In developed countries, good nutrition, safe drinking water, proper sanitation, and immunization have conquered most of the previously fatal diseases, such as typhoid and diphtheria. However, many people today live and work in large, air-conditioned buildings, a modern environment that exposes them to disorders that were previously unknown, such as legionnaires' disease. In addition, windowless rooms, certain food additives, and agricultural chemicals can cause disorders that may initially puzzle physicians because their features do not correspond to any of the classic disease patterns.

Genuinely new infectious diseases are rare—AIDS is the best known example, but others include Marburg disease (a potentially fatal viral infection transmitted to humans from certain species of monkey) and Lassa fever (a serious viral infection that is acquired from a type of rat). More commonly, a new disease is identified and subsequently discovered to have existed for some time. For example, once the cause of legionnaires' disease had been identified as a bacterium, research revealed that outbreaks of the disease had occurred over the previous 40 years—

Legionnaires' disease
LEGIONELLA PNEUMOPHILA (right), one of the bacteria that causes legionnaires' disease (a form of pneumonia), was discovered after the 1976 outbreak of the disease among members of an American Legion convention. The bacterium thrives in warm, moist conditions; infection occurs by inhaling contaminated water droplets, usually from poorly maintained air-conditioning systems. Person-to-person transmission has not been demonstrated.

much earlier than the 1976 outbreak at an American Legion convention in Philadelphia that gave the disease its name. Similarly, Lyme disease (an infection that causes skin disorders and arthritis) was first recognized in 1975 in Lyme, Connecticut, but is now thought to have been in existence before that time. As time passes, it is believed that other unreported illnesses will be revealed and proved to have been present unrecognized for years.

Radiation and disease

Chernobyl aftermath
The explosion at Chernobyl in 1986 destroyed a nuclear reactor (to the right in the photograph, above) and released a radioactive cloud that spread across much of Europe. Experts have calculated that, outside the immediate disaster area, a person exposed to radioactive fallout received about as much radiation as that from a chest X ray.

In recent years, events such as the catastrophes at Three Mile Island in 1979 and Chernobyl in 1986 have focused public attention on the hazards of radiation. However, the principal existing sources of radiation for the average person in the Western hemisphere are medical X rays and radioactive chemicals used in medicine, which together account for more than 90 percent of the radiation to which most people are exposed. The remaining 10 percent comes from natural sources of radiation, such as certain rocks and cosmic rays. Exposure to excessive amounts of radiation produces an acute illness that is fatal within a few weeks from the time of exposure. Therapeutic radiation may be accompanied by an acute form of radiation sickness that gets better within weeks.

Advances in medical technology have enabled conventional X rays to be replaced in many circumstances by nonhazardous imaging methods, such as ultrasound, MRI, and endoscopy. Moreover, the use of computers has enabled far lower doses of radiation to be employed in the different medical imaging procedures that do rely on radiation—such as CT scanning and PET scanning.

HUMAN POTENTIAL

Humans are an adaptable species, able to survive under a wide range of environmental conditions and physical and psychological stresses. One of the hallmarks of the human species is the ability not only to adapt to different conditions but also to modify existing conditions to suit human requirements. Much of this survival ability is a result of our species' ability to think, solve problems, and communicate. This allows us to construct a knowledge base that is passed from one generation to the next.

BIOLOGICAL LIMITS

All creatures have a natural lifespan—that is, the age at which death occurs due to natural degeneration of the vital organ system. For humans, the average lifespan seems to be about 87 years, and the maximum lifespan is thought to be about 115 years. Improvements in nutrition and health care have gradually increased the proportion of people that live to an advanced age, but it seems unlikely that further such improvements will increase the maximum lifespan. This is because maximum lifespan, like maximum height or maximum intelligence, is determined genetically. Improving living conditions can therefore be expected to increase only the proportion of people that nears the maximum lifespan, rather than increasing the maximum lifespan itself.

Life expectancy
The increase in life expectancy over recent decades (see chart, right) is mainly due to fewer people dying prematurely from disease, rather than to an increase in maximum lifespan. The gender difference in life expectancy is probably due to more men than women smoking earlier in this century.

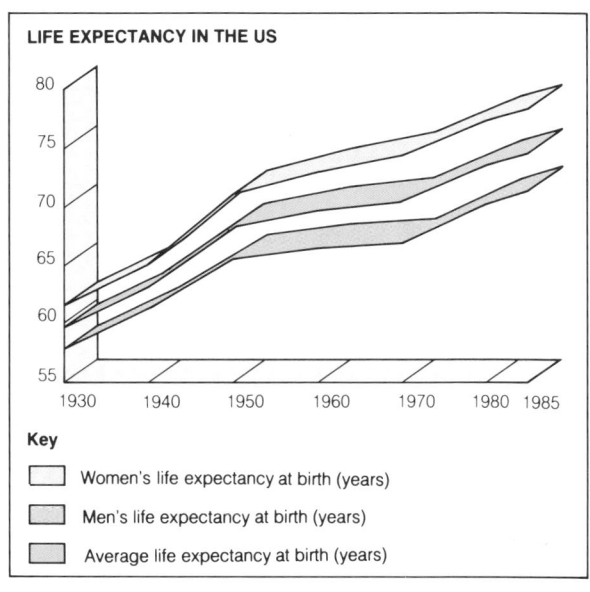

LIFE EXPECTANCY IN THE US

Key
- Women's life expectancy at birth (years)
- Men's life expectancy at birth (years)
- Average life expectancy at birth (years)

Environmental constraints

Although humans now inhabit almost every region of the Earth, the environmental conditions that are compatible with basic human life (that is, without the benefits of modern technology) are quite restricted. In general, vital basic activities such as farming and hunting require average temperatures of between about 15°F and 105°F, and average annual rainfall of some 15 to 20 inches—although some primitive peoples survive in areas with climatic extremes outside these limits. The development of modern technology also means that life in extreme environments is relatively easily sustainable.

Another environmental constraint is altitude. The higher a place is above sea level, the "thinner" the air,

Hazards of space
Modern technology has enabled humans to survive in environments to which they are not biologically adapted, such as deep space. However, technology has not yet overcome all of the problems of space travel. High levels of radiation, the adverse effects of weightlessness on bones, muscles, and the cardiovascular system, and the psychological stress of long journeys are still health hazards for astronauts.

and the faster a person must breathe to get enough oxygen into the blood. People who are born and live at high altitudes—such as those in the Andes and Himalayas—become acclimatized to thin air, but visitors from low altitudes may become acutely or fatally ill if they ascend quickly to altitudes over about 10,000 feet. A person with a respiratory disorder may have difficulty breathing even at 5,000 feet. Sustained human life seems impossible above about 20,000 feet. Mountaineers who have spent long periods above this altitude have found that their health progressively deteriorated—even though they were fully

acclimatized. Such deterioration is due to a progressive increase in the red blood cell count and a rise in the pressure of blood in the lungs.

There has been no evidence that moderate acceleration or speed is harmful to health. With specially designed acceleration couches, the human body is able to withstand the extreme g-forces that occur during a spacecraft launch. The degree to which health may deteriorate during prolonged periods in outer space—as a consequence of high levels of radiation and the adverse effects of weightlessness—is not yet fully known.

Physical constraints

In this century, athletic records have been broken repeatedly, an achievement that is due to several factors. First, the physical size and conditioning of young people increased until about the 1960s in most Western countries; this process has now virtually ceased, although it is continuing in some developing countries. Second, more young people today have access to sporting facilities, so the pool of talent has been enlarged. Finally, training and coaching methods have improved, as has the intensity of training undertaken by many athletes. However, despite these changes and the ever greater efforts made by athletes, breaking records in many sports is becoming increasingly difficult. Competitive efforts to extend physical limits and sports records have resulted in the unfair and physically dangerous practice of body building through the use of anabolic steroid drugs.

 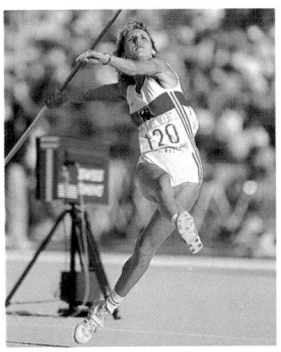

Physical sporting requirements
In javelin throwing (above) size and physical strength are advantageous. Thus, top men and women throwers tend to be tall, heavy, and muscular. However, on average, men are larger and stronger than women, which may explain why they consistently outperform women in the sport (see chart, below left).

Sex differences and sporting achievements
Because of their greater size and muscle bulk, men have a natural physical advantage over women in strength sports. This advantage is shown by world records for javelin throwing (see chart, near right), in which there has been a continual improvement in the performances of men and women, but no reduction in the performance difference between the sexes. Conversely, in stamina sports, size and muscle bulk are generally not advantageous. As a result, the performance difference between men and women has steadily decreased in many such events, such as the marathon (see chart, far right). Whether or not women will ever match—or even better—men in these sports remains open to question. Women do outperform men in many sports that are predominantly skill dependent, such as horse jumping.

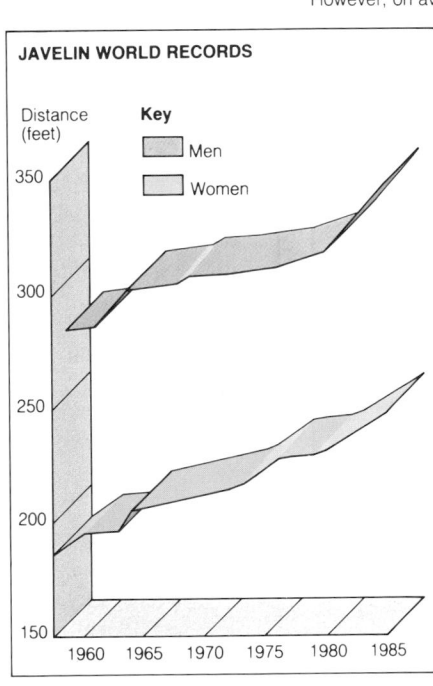

JAVELIN WORLD RECORDS

Distance (feet)

Key
Men
Women

350

300

250

200

150

1960 1965 1970 1975 1980 1985

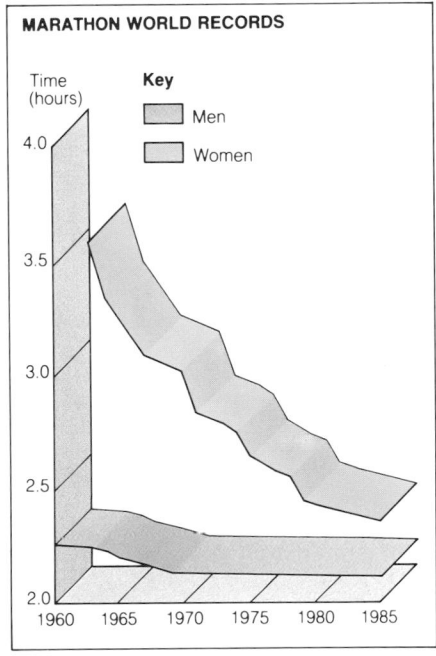

MARATHON WORLD RECORDS

Time (hours)

Key
Men
Women

4.0

3.5

3.0

2.5

2.0

1960 1965 1970 1975 1980 1985

OPTIMIZING HUMAN POTENTIAL

Good nutrition and living conditions, absence of disease, a healthy, progressive mental attitude on the part of the parents, and a stable family relationship all contribute to a child's development. As a result, children who suffer physical and/or emotional deprivation tend not to develop to the full potential allowed by their genes and are thus, in a sense, victims of their environment.

With continuing economic growth, better nutrition, and improved prevention of childhood diseases, each generation, ideally, should include a greater proportion of children who achieve their full genetic potential for physical and mental development. However, measurements of these features in successive generations have revealed a gradual slowing of the rate of improvement in most Western countries, which raises the question of whether the natural limits of development are being reached.

Genetic modifications

Many diseases are due to genetic defects. In some cases, such a "defect" has advantages. For example, it is theorized that the gene responsible for sickle cell disease gives some protection against malaria because the malaria parasite does not invade the distorted sickle cell. Thus the person with sickle cells is not vulnerable to malaria but is at risk of dying from sickle cell disease. However, most genetic defects do not have beneficial effects, so it is desirable to eliminate them. In communities that have a high incidence of a particular genetic disorder, screening of young adults may enable carriers to be identified or affected pregnancies to be terminated; this approach has reduced the incidence of Tay-Sachs disease (a brain disorder) in some Jewish communities.

Modifying the body's defenses
The body's defenses against cancer—T-lymphocyte cells, which are shown attacking a cancer in the electron micrograph (right)—are relatively inefficient. In the future, it may be possible to improve these defenses by using genetic engineering, although much research is still needed.

Environment and development

Maximizing development
Children who have plenty of mental stimulation seem to develop more rapidly than those raised in a boring environment. Some scientists also believe that maximizing mental development in early life leads to an overall increase in mental abilities.

By the age of 5 years, a child's brain is 80 percent of its adult size. The brain's rapid physical growth is paralleled by equally rapid development of mental abilities and physical coordination. By the age of 5, most children can speak fluently; have an understanding of time; can write several letters of the alphabet; and can walk, run, and jump.

Just as optimum physical growth requires good nutrition, so optimum mental development requires an intellectually stimulating environment. Children thrive best in a secure setting with plenty of contact with adults and other children, a wide range of toys and other objects to play with, and encouragement to explore, investigate, and learn as part of play. Children born in the 1970s and 1980s have scored better on intelligence tests than those born earlier, probably in part as a result of improvements in both their physical and mental environments.

THE A TO Z
OF MEDICINE

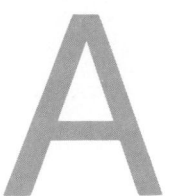

Abdomen

The area of the body between the lower border of the ribs and the upper border of the thighs. The contents of the abdominal cavity, separated from the *thorax* (chest) by the *diaphragm*, include organs of the *digestive system* and *urinary system*. The *pelvis* (the bones surrounding the lower part of the abdomen) contains the organs of the *reproductive system*.

STRUCTURE

The abdominal wall is made up of muscle, and of layers of skin, connective tissue, and fat of varying thickness. The *peritoneum*, a thin, two-layered membrane, lines the abdominal cavity and covers the stomach, intestine, and other organs.

The abdomen is protected from behind by the spinal column and lower ribs. It is vulnerable in the front, where the internal organs are covered only by the abdominal wall.

Abdomen, acute

The medical term for persistent, severe abdominal pain of sudden onset, usually associated with rigidity, guarding (voluntary contracting of the abdominal muscles), vomiting, and fever. Acute abdomen is purely a working diagnosis and usually requires urgent medical investigation. The precise cause of the abdominal pain is diagnosed by careful physician assessment and backed up by specialized tests and X rays. Occasionally, a *laparotomy* (surgical exploration of the abdomen) or a *laparoscopy* (internal examination of the abdomen using a viewing tube) is necessary.

CAUSES AND TREATMENT

The most common cause of acute abdomen is *peritonitis* (inflammation of the membrane that lines the abdomen). Inflammation of any structure in the abdomen may lead to peritonitis—for example, *salpingitis* (inflammation of the fallopian tubes); intestinal disorders, such as an inflamed appendix (see *Appendicitis*), *Crohn's disease*, or *diverticular disease*; or a perforated *peptic ulcer*. Abdominal injury may also be the cause.

Other possible causes of acute abdomen include urinary disorders, such as a stone in the ureter (see *Calculus, urinary tract*), a stone in the duct that drains the gallbladder (see *Gallstones*), and disorders that stretch the outer covering of the liver (such as *hepatitis*) or of the kidneys.

All of these conditions produce similar symptoms. The muscular wall of the abdomen goes into spasm and becomes rigid, and pain is generally first felt near the site of inflammation; later, it tends to become generalized or may temporarily disappear if an abscess ruptures.

Treatment depends on the underlying cause, but, with prompt diagnosis, the prospects for successful treatment are excellent.

Abdominal pain

Discomfort in the abdominal cavity, between the upper border of the thighs and the lower border of the ribs. Accompanying symptoms may include belching, nausea, vomiting, rumbling and gurgling noises, and flatulence (gas).

CAUSES

Minor degrees of abdominal pain are experienced by everybody at some time, and often the cause is easily recognized—for example, overeating, eating too much spicy food, or drinking too much alcohol. Abdominal discomfort may also occur with *diarrhea* or *constipation*.

Many women experience pelvic or lower abdominal pain during part of their menstrual cycles. The pain may occur before or during a period, or around the time of ovulation. Occasionally, this pain is due to a gynecological disorder such as *endometriosis* (fragments of uterine lining that have developed in other regions of the abdomen).

A common cause of pain very low in the abdomen is a urinary infection, especially in women, causing *cystitis* (inflammation of the bladder).

Abdominal pain can have a psychological origin. For example, it may result from anxiety, such as that felt by a child starting a new school or an adult changing jobs.

Spasm, or stretching, of internal organs can result in a wavelike pain known as colic. Intestinal colic, often associated with swelling of the abdomen and flatulence, can occur when the muscles lining the intestine go into spasm (as, for example, in *irritable bowel syndrome*). Colic may also develop as the result of blockage of the gallbladder, bile duct, or urinary tract, usually by a stone. It can also occur in an *ectopic pregnancy*, in which the fetus develops not in the uterus but in one of the fallopian tubes.

LOCATION OF THE ABDOMEN

The abdomen is bounded by the lower ribs at the top and the pelvis below. The illustration shows the position of the abdominal organs in an adult woman.

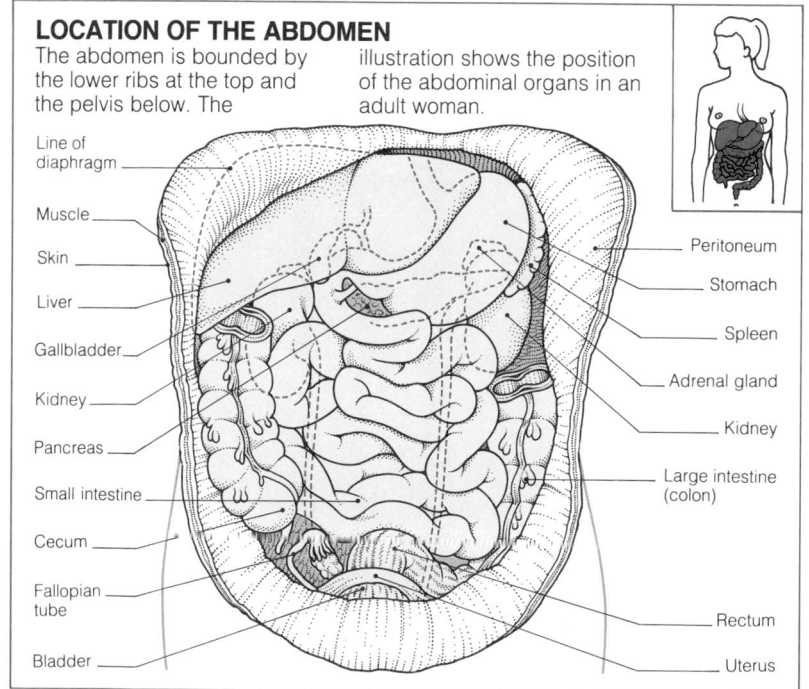

Line of diaphragm
Muscle
Skin
Liver
Gallbladder
Kidney
Pancreas
Small intestine
Cecum
Fallopian tube
Bladder

Peritoneum
Stomach
Spleen
Adrenal gland
Kidney
Large intestine (colon)
Rectum
Uterus

A

ABDOMINAL PAIN

General or localized pain between the bottom of the rib cage and the groin that has occurred within the last 24 hours. See also Recurrent abdominal pain chart.

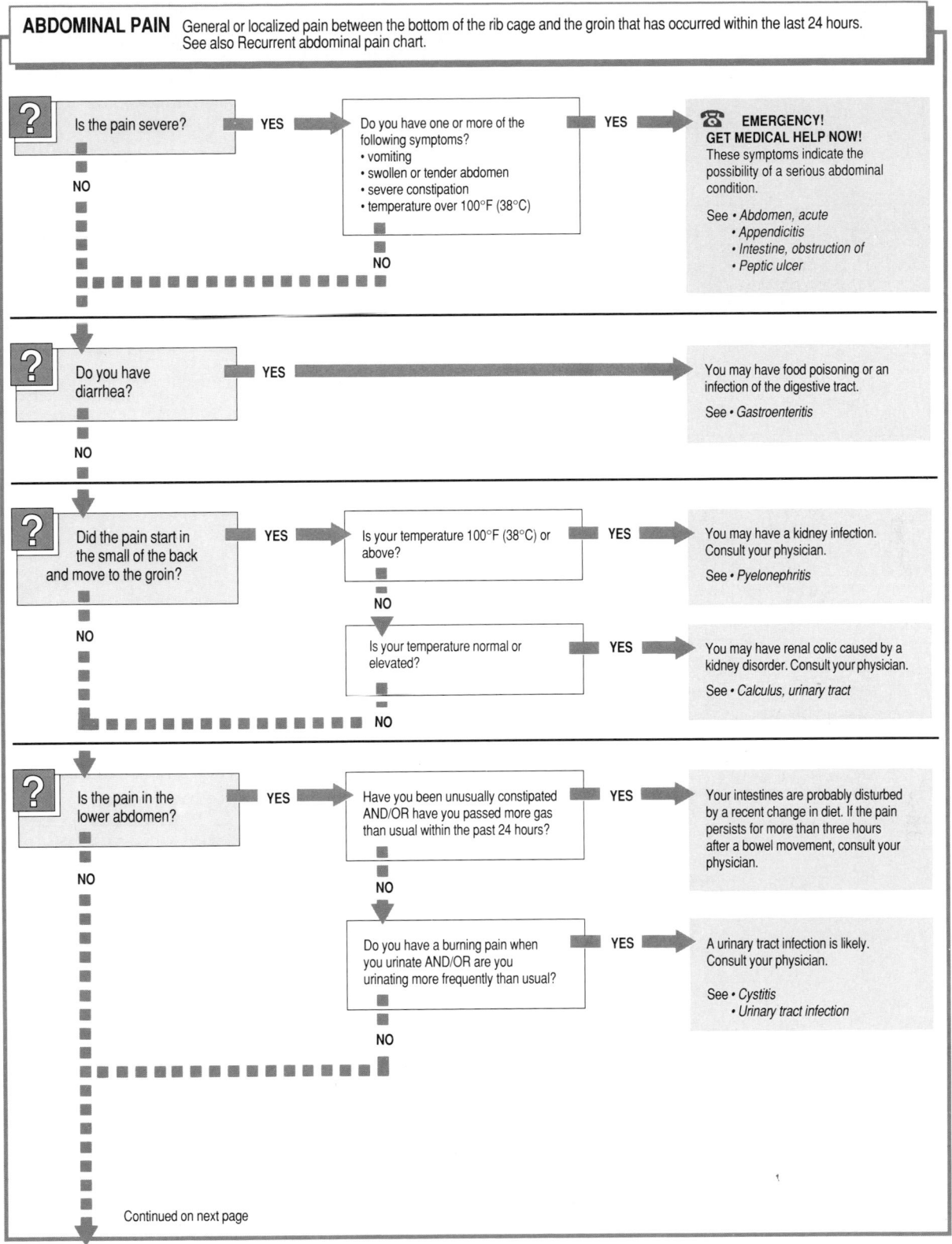

? Is the pain severe?

NO

YES →

Do you have one or more of the following symptoms?
• vomiting
• swollen or tender abdomen
• severe constipation
• temperature over 100°F (38°C)

NO

YES →

☎ **EMERGENCY!**
GET MEDICAL HELP NOW!
These symptoms indicate the possibility of a serious abdominal condition.

See • *Abdomen, acute*
• *Appendicitis*
• *Intestine, obstruction of*
• *Peptic ulcer*

? Do you have diarrhea?

NO

YES →

You may have food poisoning or an infection of the digestive tract.

See • *Gastroenteritis*

? Did the pain start in the small of the back and move to the groin?

NO

YES →

Is your temperature 100°F (38°C) or above?

NO

YES →

You may have a kidney infection. Consult your physician.

See • *Pyelonephritis*

Is your temperature normal or elevated?

NO

YES →

You may have renal colic caused by a kidney disorder. Consult your physician.

See • *Calculus, urinary tract*

? Is the pain in the lower abdomen?

NO

YES →

Have you been unusually constipated AND/OR have you passed more gas than usual within the past 24 hours?

NO

YES →

Your intestines are probably disturbed by a recent change in diet. If the pain persists for more than three hours after a bowel movement, consult your physician.

Do you have a burning pain when you urinate AND/OR are you urinating more frequently than usual?

NO

YES →

A urinary tract infection is likely. Consult your physician.

See • *Cystitis*
• *Urinary tract infection*

Continued on next page

A

Is the pain mainly just below the ribs on the right side and have you been vomiting?

YES → You may have a gallbladder disorder. Consult your physician.

See • *Cholecystitis*
• *Gallstones*

NO

Do you have pain on one side only AND does your skin feel sensitive along the site of the pain?

YES → You may have a nerve infection. Consult your physician.

See • *Herpes zoster*

NO

WARNING

Severe abdominal pain
Severe and continuous abdominal pain requires immediate medical attention in the following cases:
• if it persists for more than four hours
• if it is accompanied by vomiting
• if the abdomen is swollen and tender
• if it is accompanied by faintness, drowsiness, or confusion

Waiting for medical attention
While waiting for medical help to arrive, do not eat or drink anything in case you need to undergo surgery immediately. Do not take aspirin to relieve the pain or drink alcohol; they can further inflame an irritated stomach and, in some circumstances, cause dangerous internal bleeding.

Did the pain follow a bout of heavy drinking or excessive eating?

YES → The lining of your stomach is probably inflamed. Consult your physician.

See • *Gastritis*

NO

Is the pain in the center of the upper abdomen?

YES → Is it a dull cramping pain accompanied by rumbling and gurgling AND/OR nausea?

YES → Overeating or tension is a likely cause of abdominal pain, especially if it occurs soon after a meal.

See • *Indigestion*

NO ■ ■ ■ ■ ■ ■ ■ ■ ■ ■ ■ ■ ■ NO

Are you a woman and do you have intermittent lower abdominal cramping pains?

YES → Are you having a menstrual period?

YES → Dull aches or cramps are often associated with menstruation. Discuss with your physician.

NO

Could you be in the first three months of pregnancy AND/OR have you noticed any vaginal bleeding?

YES → ☎

Consult your physician without delay!
A serious complication, such as a threatened miscarriage or ectopic pregnancy, is a possibility.

See • *Ectopic pregnancy*
• *Miscarriage*

NO

NO

Continued on next page

Continued on next page, column 2

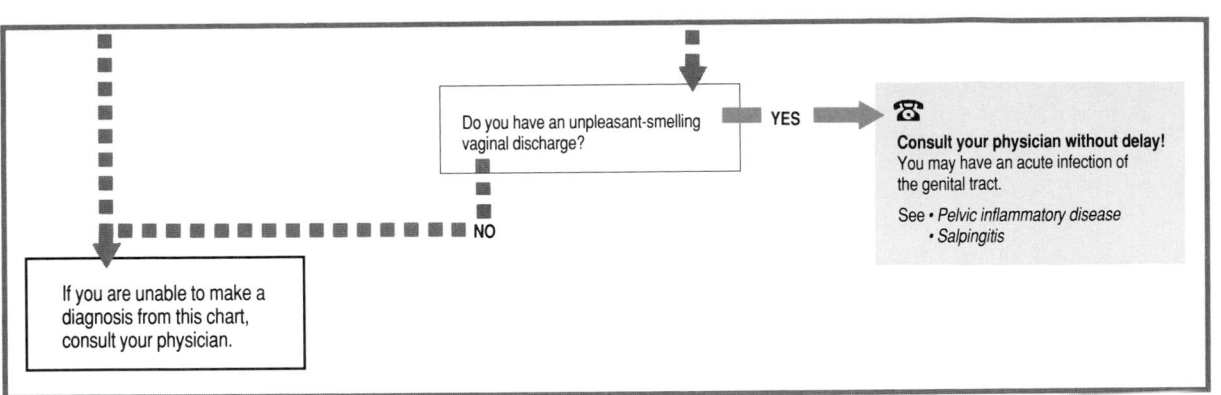

Do you have an unpleasant-smelling vaginal discharge?

YES → ☎

Consult your physician without delay!
You may have an acute infection of the genital tract.

See • *Pelvic inflammatory disease*
• *Salpingitis*

NO

If you are unable to make a diagnosis from this chart, consult your physician.

RECURRENT ABDOMINAL PAIN   Abdominal pain that has recurred over a week or more.

Pain mainly above the waist

? Do you sometimes get a burning pain in the center of your chest, especially when you are bending over or lying down?

YES →

Leakage of acid into the esophagus may be causing the pain. This may occur when there is a relaxation of the muscle at the junction of the esophagus and the stomach.

See • *Heartburn*
• *Hiatal hernia*

NO

? Does the pain come in waves mainly in the upper right side of the abdomen?

YES → Is your temperature 100°F(38°C) or above?

YES →

You may have an inflamed gallbladder. Consult your physician.

See • *Cholecystitis*

NO

NO

Is the pain temporarily relieved by antacid medicine for indigestion?

YES →

Irritation of the stomach is the most likely cause of the pain. However, there is also a possibility of an ulcer. Consult your physician.

See • *Gastritis*
• *Peptic ulcer*

NO

Is the pain mainly just below the ribs on the right side?

YES →

Stones in the duct that connects the gallbladder to the digestive tract may be the cause of this type of pain, especially if you have felt nauseated or have vomited. Consult your physician.

See • *Gallstones*

NO

Continued on next page

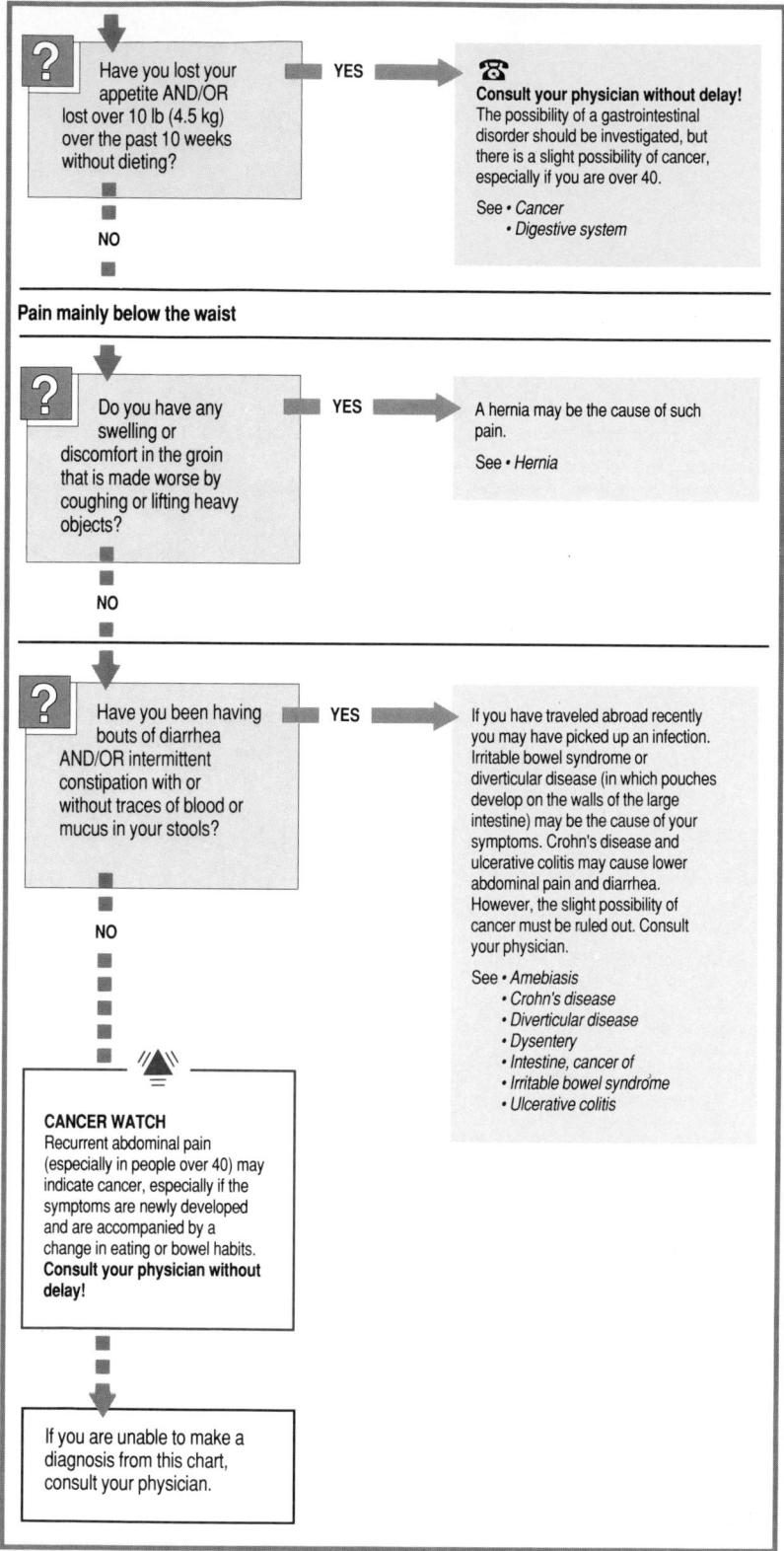

? Have you lost your appetite AND/OR lost over 10 lb (4.5 kg) over the past 10 weeks without dieting?

YES →

☎ **Consult your physician without delay!**
The possibility of a gastrointestinal disorder should be investigated, but there is a slight possibility of cancer, especially if you are over 40.

See • *Cancer*
   • *Digestive system*

NO

Pain mainly below the waist

? Do you have any swelling or discomfort in the groin that is made worse by coughing or lifting heavy objects?

YES →

A hernia may be the cause of such pain.

See • *Hernia*

NO

? Have you been having bouts of diarrhea AND/OR intermittent constipation with or without traces of blood or mucus in your stools?

YES →

If you have traveled abroad recently you may have picked up an infection. Irritable bowel syndrome or diverticular disease (in which pouches develop on the walls of the large intestine) may be the cause of your symptoms. Crohn's disease and ulcerative colitis may cause lower abdominal pain and diarrhea. However, the slight possibility of cancer must be ruled out. Consult your physician.

See • *Amebiasis*
   • *Crohn's disease*
   • *Diverticular disease*
   • *Dysentery*
   • *Intestine, cancer of*
   • *Irritable bowel syndrome*
   • *Ulcerative colitis*

NO

⚠ **CANCER WATCH**
Recurrent abdominal pain (especially in people over 40) may indicate cancer, especially if the symptoms are newly developed and are accompanied by a change in eating or bowel habits. **Consult your physician without delay!**

If you are unable to make a diagnosis from this chart, consult your physician.

An increase in the amount of acid formed in the stomach may be associated with the development of a *peptic ulcer*, which produces a recurrent gnawing pain temporarily relieved by food, milk, or antacids.

Another possible cause of abdominal pain is infection, such as *pyelonephritis* (infection of the kidneys) or *pelvic inflammatory disease* (infection of the uterus and fallopian tubes). Pain may also be due to *ischemia* (lack of blood supply), as occurs, for instance, when a *volvulus* (twisting of the intestine) obstructs blood vessels or when a clot forms in one of the intestinal blood vessels.

Tumors affecting any of the abdominal organs can cause pain by stretching the lining of the organ, by pressing on surrounding structures, or by ulcerating, perforating, or rupturing.

In rare cases, disorders of organs outside the abdomen can cause abdominal pain. For example, right lower lobe pneumonia may produce pain in the upper right abdomen that mimics acute appendicitis.

TREATMENT
Abdominal pain can sometimes be relieved by simple measures, such as drinking milk, applying a heating pad to the affected area, or taking an antacid (to neutralize excess stomach acid), an antispasmodic, or an analgesic (painkiller). If none of these methods alleviates the pain, or if the pain is severe or recurs, a physician should be consulted.

Severe pain with sweating, paleness, or dizziness sometimes indicates a serious disorder that may require immediate surgical attention. Urgent attention is also necessary if the pain is accompanied by persistent vomiting, by vomiting of blood (which may appear brown), by passing of blood-stained or black feces, or by feeling weak or faint.

Similarly, prompt medical attention should be obtained if abdominal pain lasts for more than about six hours or is not relieved by vomiting.

Abdominal pain accompanied by weight loss without dieting or by a change in bowel habits—sudden constipation or attacks of diarrhea—may indicate a serious disorder and should be investigated by a physician.

INVESTIGATION
The physician makes a diagnosis based on the patient's detailed description of the pain and its relationship to eating, urinating, and bowel movements, along with a thorough physical examination of the person.

DIAGNOSING ABDOMINAL PAIN

The physician conducts a physical examination and listens to the patient's description of the pain. More investigations, such as blood tests or X rays, may be carried out. If the diagnosis is still in doubt, gastroscopy, laparoscopy, or colonoscopy may be performed.

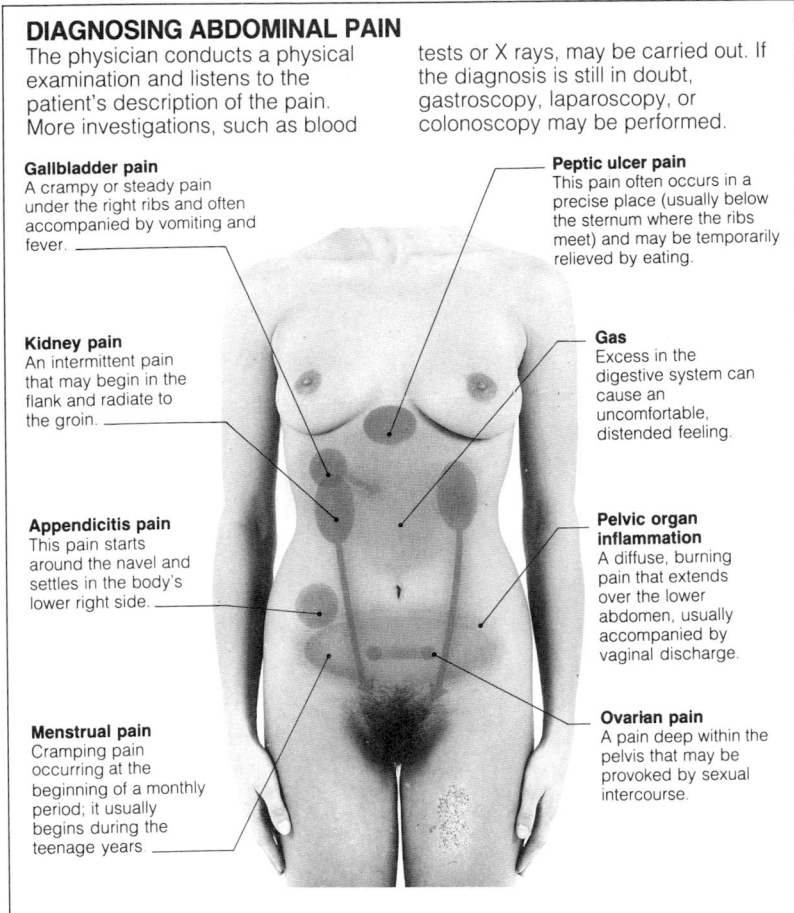

Gallbladder pain
A crampy or steady pain under the right ribs and often accompanied by vomiting and fever.

Kidney pain
An intermittent pain that may begin in the flank and radiate to the groin.

Appendicitis pain
This pain starts around the navel and settles in the body's lower right side.

Menstrual pain
Cramping pain occurring at the beginning of a monthly period; it usually begins during the teenage years.

Peptic ulcer pain
This pain often occurs in a precise place (usually below the sternum where the ribs meet) and may be temporarily relieved by eating.

Gas
Excess in the digestive system can cause an uncomfortable, distended feeling.

Pelvic organ inflammation
A diffuse, burning pain that extends over the lower abdomen, usually accompanied by vaginal discharge.

Ovarian pain
A pain deep within the pelvis that may be provoked by sexual intercourse.

If there is any doubt about the diagnosis, further investigations may be carried out. The investigations may include a urine test, blood tests, X rays, and *ultrasound scanning*.

If the cause still cannot be diagnosed after such tests, endoscopic examination (looking into a body cavity with a viewing tube) may be necessary. This may take the form of *gastroscopy* (inspecting the stomach and duodenum), *colonoscopy* (inspecting the large intestine), or laparoscopy (inspecting the contents of the abdominal cavity). In some cases, the diagnosis can be confirmed only by an exploratory operation on the abdomen, known as a *laparotomy*.

Abdominal swelling

Distention of the abdomen due to a number of causes. Abdominal swelling is the natural result of *obesity* and of enlargement of the uterus during pregnancy, generally noticeable after about 12 weeks.

Some causes of abdominal swelling are harmless. Gas in the stomach or intestine may cause uncomfortable bloating distention of the whole abdomen. Many women experience lower abdominal distention due to temporary water retention just before a menstrual period.

Other causes may be more serious. For instance, *ascites* (accumulation of fluid in the abdomen) may be a symptom of underlying *cancer*, *heart* disease, *kidney* disease, or *liver* disease; the swelling may also be caused by *intestinal obstruction* or an *ovarian cyst*.

INVESTIGATION AND TREATMENT

Diagnosis of the underlying cause may involve abdominal X rays or *ultrasound scanning* to look for abnormalities in the size or shape of the internal organs or for signs of intestinal obstruction. If ascites is present, some of the fluid may be drained for examination. Occasionally, a *laparotomy* (surgical exploration of the

abdomen) or *laparoscopy* (internal examination of the abdomen using a flexible viewing tube) may also be necessary. (See chart, next page.)

Abdominal X ray

An X-ray examination of the abdominal contents. An abdominal X ray is usually one of the first steps in the investigation of suspected abdominal disease (after the physician takes a careful medical history and performs a physical examination).

Because organs are not completely opaque to X rays, only the outlines are visible. The radiologist can see, however, whether any organ is abnormally enlarged and is able to spot swallowed foreign bodies within the digestive tract. Useful information is also gained by studying patterns of fluid and gas. Distended loops of bowel containing collections of fluid often indicate an obstruction (see *Intestine, obstruction of*); gas found outside the intestine indicates intestinal *perforation*.

Calcium, which is opaque to X rays, is present in most kidney stones (see *Calculus, urinary tract*) and also in some *gallstones*; they can sometimes be detected on an abdominal X ray. Some aortic *aneurysms* contain calcium and therefore are visible.

Abdominal X rays often need to be followed by other procedures that give more detail, such as *endoscopy*, *ultrasound scanning*, *CT scanning*, *barium X-ray examinations*, or *intravenous pyelography*.

Abducent nerve

The sixth *cranial nerve*. The abducent nerve supplies just one muscle of each eye, the lateral rectus muscle, which is responsible for moving the eye outward. The abducent nerve originates in the pons (part of the *brain stem*) and emerges from the brain immediately below it. From this point, it extends through the skull, eventually entering the back of the eye socket through a gap between the skull bones.

As a result of its long path inside the skull, the abducent nerve is often damaged in fractures of the base of the skull, or by a disorder such as a tumor that distorts the brain. Such damage may give rise to *double vision* and a convergent *strabismus*.

Abduction

Movement of a limb away from the central line of the body, or of a digit away from the axis of a limb. Muscles that carry out this movement are called abductors. (See also *Adduction*.)

A

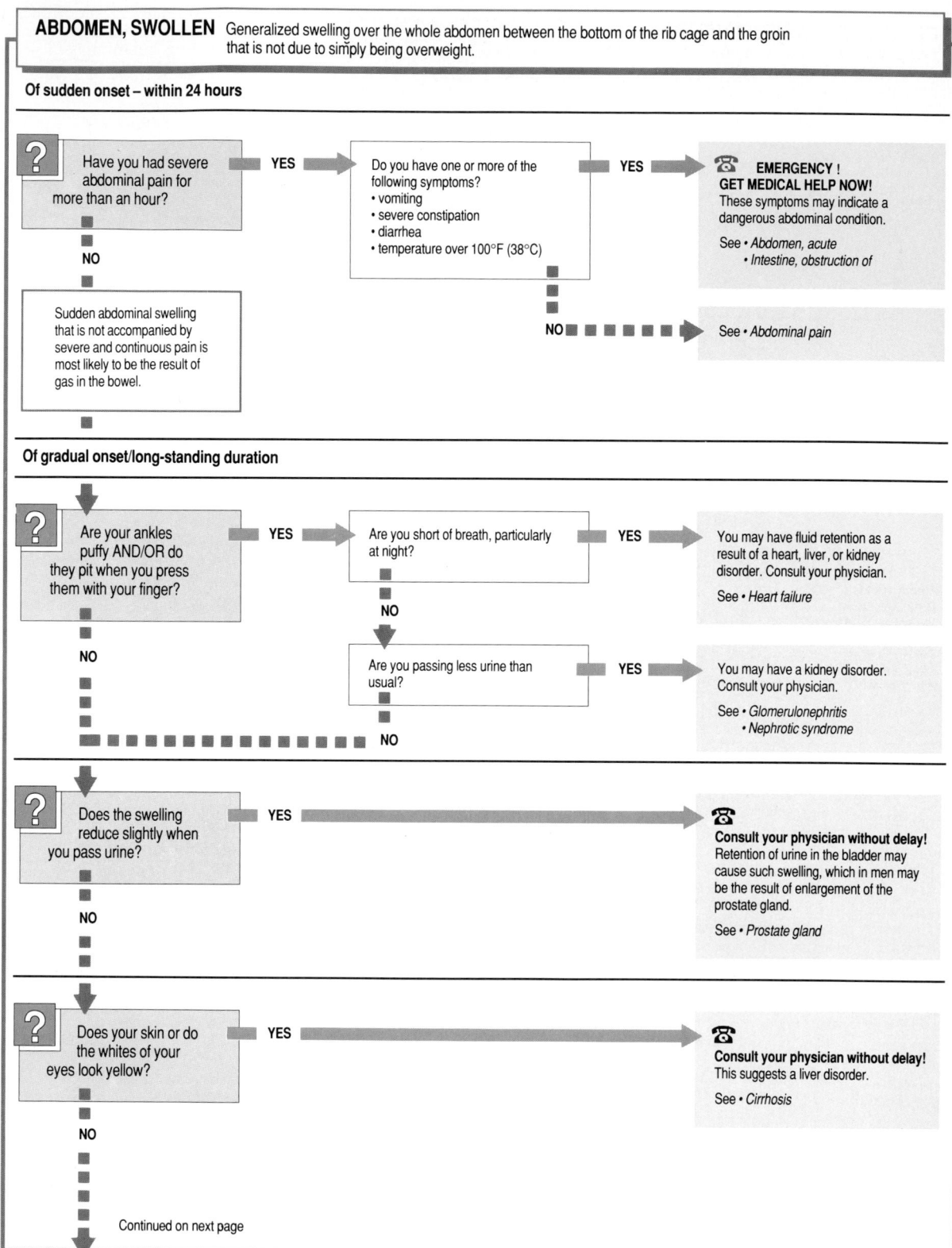

ABDOMEN, SWOLLEN Generalized swelling over the whole abdomen between the bottom of the rib cage and the groin that is not due to simply being overweight.

Of sudden onset – within 24 hours

? Have you had severe abdominal pain for more than an hour?

YES ➡ Do you have one or more of the following symptoms?
• vomiting
• severe constipation
• diarrhea
• temperature over 100°F (38°C)

YES ➡ ☎ **EMERGENCY !**
GET MEDICAL HELP NOW!
These symptoms may indicate a dangerous abdominal condition.

See • *Abdomen, acute*
    • *Intestine, obstruction of*

NO

Sudden abdominal swelling that is not accompanied by severe and continuous pain is most likely to be the result of gas in the bowel.

NO ➡ See • *Abdominal pain*

Of gradual onset/long-standing duration

? Are your ankles puffy AND/OR do they pit when you press them with your finger?

YES ➡ Are you short of breath, particularly at night?

YES ➡ You may have fluid retention as a result of a heart, liver, or kidney disorder. Consult your physician.

See • *Heart failure*

NO

NO ⬇ Are you passing less urine than usual?

YES ➡ You may have a kidney disorder. Consult your physician.

See • *Glomerulonephritis*
    • *Nephrotic syndrome*

NO

? Does the swelling reduce slightly when you pass urine?

YES ➡ ☎
Consult your physician without delay!
Retention of urine in the bladder may cause such swelling, which in men may be the result of enlargement of the prostate gland.

See • *Prostate gland*

NO

? Does your skin or do the whites of your eyes look yellow?

YES ➡ ☎
Consult your physician without delay!
This suggests a liver disorder.

See • *Cirrhosis*

NO

Continued on next page

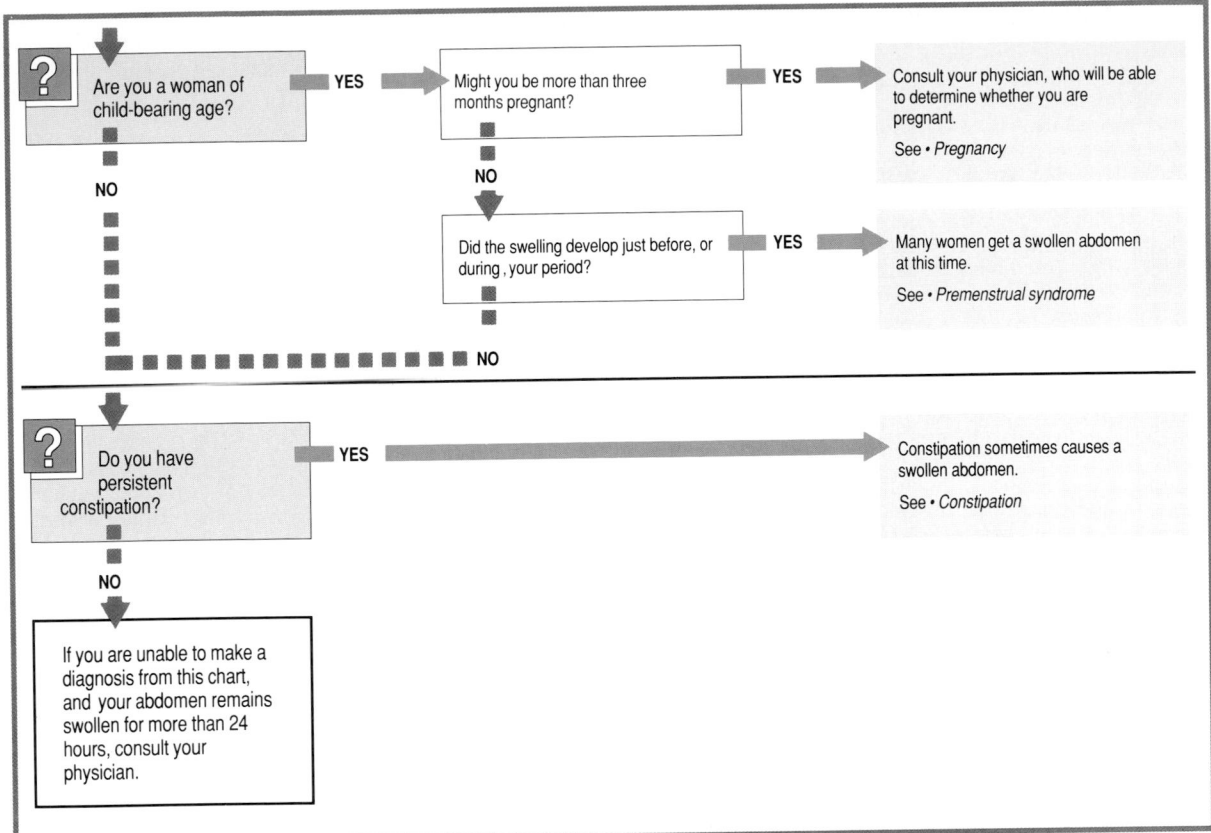

Ablation

The removal of dead or diseased tissue by excision (cutting away with a sharp instrument), freezing (see *Cryosurgery*), *radiation therapy*, burning (see *Diathermy*), or *laser treatment*. Ablation of the thyroid gland is achieved with radioactive iodine isotopes.

Abnormality

A physical deformity or malformation, a behavioral or mental problem, an alteration in function of a tissue or an organ, or a variation from normal in cells or tissues.

Abortifacient

An agent that causes *abortion*. Various substances have been claimed to cause abortion, such as large amounts of castor oil or gin, but none of these is effective. In medical practice, derivatives of local hormones called *prostaglandins* are used to induce abortion; they cause softening and widening of the cervix (neck of the uterus) and muscular contractions of the uterus. They are usually administered in the form of suppositories, placed high in the vagina, or by intravenous infusion.

Abortion

In medical terminology, the word abortion denotes either spontaneous abortion (see *Miscarriage*) or medically induced termination of pregnancy (see *Abortion, elective*).

Abortion, elective

Medically induced termination of pregnancy. Up to the 12th week of pregnancy, an elective abortion in the US is a private matter between a woman and her physician. After the 12th week, state laws may regulate abortion in ways that are related to maternal health. After the 24th week of pregnancy, state laws may regulate and even prohibit abortion except in cases where the life or health of the woman is threatened. An abortion is described as a therapeutic abortion if it is carried out to save the life or health of the mother.

MEDICAL REASONS FOR ABORTION

A physician may recommend an abortion for conditions affecting either the woman or the fetus. In the woman, examples of conditions that may worsen during pregnancy and possibly become life-threatening include severe heart disease, chronic kidney disease, and cancer, especially of the breast or cervix.

Fetal conditions, revealed by *ultrasound scanning*, *amniocentesis*, or *chorionic villus sampling*, include severe developmental defects incompatible with normal life (such as *anencephaly*) and serious *chromosomal abnormalities* (such as *Down's syndrome*). Termination may also be recommended if the woman contracts *rubella* (German measles) during the early stages of pregnancy; this virus can severely damage the baby, especially his or her eyes, ears, and heart. Certain other infections in the woman may also damage the fetus. Termination is recommended if the mother has been infected by the *AIDS* virus because it can be transmitted to the baby.

HOW IT IS DONE

EARLY ABORTION Vacuum suction techniques are the simplest and safest means of terminating an early pregnancy. Within two weeks of a missed period, before pregnancy has been confirmed, *menstrual extraction* (an office-based suction procedure) can be carried out. However, vacuum suction curettage is the most commonly used method. It is performed between the seventh and 12th week of pregnancy at a clinic or in a hospital outpatient department.

The procedure may be performed with either a general or a local anesthetic. If local anesthesia (paracervical block) is used, it may be supplemented by an intravenous narcotic or tranquilizer. The cervix is dilated with curved metal rods, and a narrow plastic tube is then inserted into the uterus. The outer end of the tube is connected to a suction machine, which sucks out the fetal and placental tissue into a vacuum bottle. After this procedure, which usually takes less than 10 minutes, the gynecologist scrapes the lining of the uterus with a curet (a spoonlike instrument) to make sure that no placental tissue has been left behind. The tissue is analyzed in a laboratory to confirm that a pregnancy existed and that the tissue appears complete, since an *ectopic pregnancy* or abdominal pregnancy would require more surgery.

Recovery is fast, although strenuous activity should be avoided for several days. There is usually some bleeding, and sometimes mild cramps, for up to a week. A normal period starts four to six weeks after the termination. Sexual intercourse can be resumed after two or three weeks.

LATE ABORTION Between 12 and 15 weeks, either the suction procedure used in early abortion or the evacuation procedure described below may be recommended, depending on the facilities available. After the 15th week, it is normally considered safer to perform an abortion by causing the uterus to contract so that the fetus is expelled, as in natural labor. Contractions are induced by introducing saline solution or, more commonly, a *prostaglandin* hormone into the uterus. This may be done either by injection directly through the woman's abdomen into the amniotic fluid or by infusion, via the cervix, into the gap between the amniotic sac (the membrane that surrounds the fetus) and the uterine wall. Alternatively, a vaginal suppository containing prostaglandin may be placed high in the vagina.

It usually takes about 12 hours for the fetus to be expelled, during which time the woman is given analgesics (painkillers). She remains in the hospital for 24 to 48 hours after completion of the termination to be monitored for complications.

COMPLICATIONS

If termination is performed in a well-equipped clinic or hospital by a qualified gynecologist, complications are few. Infection, resulting in a condition called septic abortion, or serious bleeding occurs in fewer than 1 percent of cases. Mortality is less than one per 100,000 when abortion is performed before the 13th week, rising to three per 100,000 after the 13th week. (For comparison, maternal mortality for full-term pregnancy is nine per 100,000.) Multiple terminations may increase the risk of miscarriage in subsequent pregnancies, although there is little evidence that a single termination has any effect on future fertility.

Illegal abortions, although rare in the US, are common worldwide; they carry a high risk of complications, including perforation of the uterus, septic abortion, and severe bleeding. Infertility or death often result.

Abrasion, dental

The wearing away of enamel, often accompanied by the wearing away of dentin (the layer beneath the enamel) and cementum (the bonelike tissue that covers the tooth root), usually through overvigorous brushing. The areas most commonly affected are the root surface and the front surfaces of the canine and premolar teeth where they emerge from the gum. The depressions produced by abrasion are often sensitive to very cold or hot food and may require use of a desensitizing dentifrice and/or protection with a *bonding* agent or *filling*.

Abreaction

The process of becoming consciously aware of repressed thoughts and feelings. In Freudian theory, abreaction ideally occurs via *catharsis*, the open expression of emotions associated with the forgotten memories. The term abreaction is sometimes used interchangeably with catharsis but, in its strictest sense, is the result of catharsis. Abreaction is an important part of *psychotherapy* and is more easily achieved when a recent, specific traumatic event is the source of the patient's symptoms.

Abscess

A collection of pus formed as a result of infection by microorganisms, usually bacteria. The pus is formed from destroyed tissue cells, from leukocytes (white blood cells) that have been carried to the area to fight infection, and from dead and live

microorganisms. The abscess may enlarge or subside, depending on whether the microorganisms or leukocytes gain the upper hand. Usually, a protective lining (pyogenic membrane) gradually forms around the abscess.

TYPES

Abscesses may develop in any organ and in the soft tissues beneath the skin in any area. Common sites include the breast (see *Mastitis*) and gums (see *Abscess, dental*). Rarer sites include the liver (see *Liver abscess*) and the brain (see *Brain abscess*).

Common sites for abscesses under the skin include the axilla (armpit) and the groin; these two areas have a large number of lymph glands that are responsible for fighting infection. A collar-button abscess is one in which a small abscess cavity under the skin connects via a sinus (channel) to a much larger one in deeper tissues.

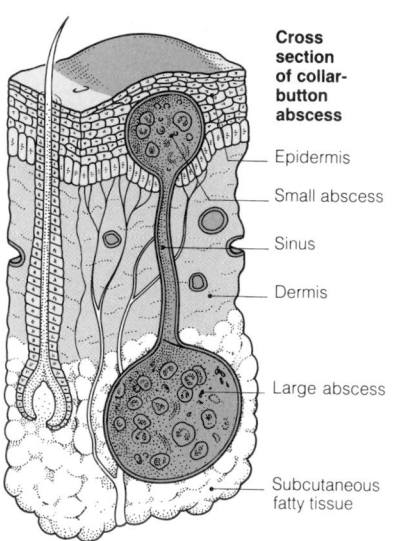

Cross section of collar-button abscess

- Epidermis
- Small abscess
- Sinus
- Dermis
- Large abscess
- Subcutaneous fatty tissue

CAUSES

Common bacteria, such as staphylococci, are the most common cause, although the bacillus responsible for tuberculosis is an important abscess-forming type. Fungal infections sometimes cause abscesses, while amebae (single-celled animal parasites) are an important cause of liver abscesses (see *Amebiasis*). The infection usually reaches an organ via the bloodstream or penetrates tissues under the skin via an infected wound or bite.

SYMPTOMS AND SIGNS

Symptoms of discomfort or pain depend mainly on the site of the abscess, though most larger ones, since they are a source of infection within the body, cause fever (sometimes with chills), sweating, and malaise. Abscesses close to the skin usually cause inflammation with redness, increased skin temperature, and tenderness. Tuberculous abscesses are the exception; hence their description as cold abscesses.

DIAGNOSIS
The presence of an abscess within an organ may be apparent from symptoms and signs. Occasionally the diagnosis is confirmed by imaging techniques, such as *CT scanning*, *MRI*, or *radionuclide scanning* (using radioactively labeled white blood cells or the element gallium, which becomes concentrated in regions where pus has recently formed).

TREATMENT
Antibiotics are usually prescribed to treat a bacterial infection, antifungal drugs to treat fungi, and antiamebic drugs to treat amebiasis. However, the lining of the abscess cavity tends to reduce the amount of drug that can penetrate the source of infection from the bloodstream. The cavity itself therefore requires draining by making a cut in the lining and providing an escape route for the pus, either through a drainage tube (see *Drain, surgical*) or by leaving the cavity open to the skin.

OUTLOOK
Many abscesses subside after drainage alone; others subside after drainage and drug treatment. Occasionally, their presence within a vital organ, such as the liver or brain, damages enough surrounding tissue to cause some permanent loss of normal function.

Abscess, dental
A pus-filled sac in the tissue around the root of a tooth.

CAUSE
An abscess may occur when bacteria invade the pulp (the nerves and blood vessels that fill the central cavity of the tooth), causing the pulp to die. This most commonly happens as a result of dental *caries*, which destroy the tooth's enamel and dentin, allowing bacteria to reach the pulp. Bacteria can also gain access to the pulp when a tooth is injured. Bacteria enter either directly through a fracture or along damaged blood vessels. The infection in the pulp spreads into the surrounding tissue to form an abscess.

Abscesses can also result from *periodontal disease*, in which bacteria accumulate in the deep pockets that form between the teeth and gums.

SYMPTOMS AND SIGNS
The affected tooth aches or throbs and biting or chewing is usually extremely painful. The gum around the tooth is tender and may be red and swollen. An untreated abscess eventually erodes a sinus (small channel) through the jawbone to the gum surface, where it forms a gumboil (swelling). The gumboil may burst, discharging foul-tasting pus into the mouth, which usually lessens the pain. As the abscess spreads through surrounding tissues and bone, the glands in the neck and the side of the face may become swollen. Eventually, symptoms of infection, such as headache and fever, may develop.

TREATMENT
It is always best to try first to save the tooth. To do this, the abscess is drained by drilling through the crown of the tooth and into the pulp cavity to allow the pus to escape. The pulp cavity is then carefully cleaned and disinfected. An antibiotic may be prescribed if the infection has spread beyond the tooth. When the infection has cleared, the cavity is filled with dental cement (see *Root canal treatment*), sealed, and crowned.

When an abscess is caused by diseased pulp and the infection cannot be cleared with endodontic treatment, it is necessary to extract the tooth. However, this is a last resort. Extraction removes the source of infection and drains the abscess. Antibiotics are usually prescribed to clear any residual infection.

An abscess in a periodontal pocket can usually be treated by passing a probe into the pocket and gently scraping away infected material; sometimes it is necessary to make a small incision in the pocket to reach the abscess. If there is loss of bony support and periodontal ligament attachment due to severe periodontal disease, a dental *extraction* may need to be performed.

Absence
In medical terminology, a temporary loss or impairment of consciousness that occurs in some forms of *epilepsy*, typically petit mal seizures.

Acanthosis nigricans
A rare, untreatable condition characterized by thickened dark patches of skin in the groin, armpits, neck, and other skin folds. It may occur in young people as a genetic, inherited disorder, or as the result of an endocrine disorder, such as Cushing's

syndrome. It is also seen in people with carcinomas (malignant tumors) of the lung and other organs. The affected skin, which is thickened, rough, and may itch, is gray to black.

Pseudoacanthosis nigricans is a much more common condition, usually seen in dark-complexioned people who are overweight. In this form, the skin in fold areas, such as the groin, armpits, or neck, is both thicker and darker than the surrounding skin; there is usually excessive sweating in these areas. The condition may improve with dieting.

Access to care
A phrase used to describe a nation's medical system. Access refers both to the geographic accessibility of physicians and facilities, and the financial accessibility of medical services (i.e., the availability of funding provided individually, governmentally, charitably, or by insurance that would enable a person to pay for available needed medical care).

The degree of access in a medical system affects its cost; various attempts have been made to control costs through the regulation of access. Cost-sharing devices (making the patient financially responsible for a share of the fee or service) are regarded as a means of controlling access and, ultimately, overall costs.

Accident-prone
A tendency to have numerous mishaps as a result of some personality trait. Many psychologists doubt that the concept is valid, even though studies have shown that accidents are not distributed evenly among the population according to the laws of chance. A small group of people do seem to have more accidents, but this group changes constantly from study to study and no psychological test can isolate it.

Accidents may be slightly more common in aggressive and nonconforming men. However, emotional stress is probably the most important factor. Cycles of accidents seem to occur in the months after stressful "life events" regardless of the personality of the person involved.

Accidents
In people 1 to 37 years old, accidents are now the leading cause of death in the US. Accidental injuries, burns, drownings, and poisonings account for more than half of all deaths in youths aged 15 to 24 and for a quarter

CAUSES AND INCIDENCE OF ACCIDENTAL DEATH

In young people (up to 37 years), accidents are the leading cause of death. Burns, drownings, poisonings, and motor vehicle accidents are the most common causes. The very young and the very old are at greatest risk in their homes. The age groups in between tend to be victims of accidents elsewhere.

FIVE MOST COMMON CAUSES OF ACCIDENTAL DEATH BY AGE (Rates per 100,000 in each age group)

Age	0–1	1–4	5–14	15–24	25–44	45–64	65–74	75+	All ages
Most common cause	Choking 6.1	Motor vehicle 8.0	Motor vehicle 6.7	Motor vehicle 37.0	Motor vehicle 21.4	Motor vehicle 15.4	Motor vehicle 17.4	Falls 65.7	Motor vehicle 19.7
2nd	Motor vehicle 5.7	Drowning 4.8	Drowning 2.1	Drowning 4.2	Drowning 2.6 and Poison 2.6	Falls 4.0	Falls 10.1	Motor vehicle 25.2	Falls 5.2
3rd	Suffocation 4.5	Fires, burns 4.7	Fires, burns 1.4	Firearms 1.3		Fires, burns 2.3	Fires, burns 4.0	Choking 10.6	Drowning 2.7
4th	Fires, burns 3.8	Choking 0.9	Firearms 0.7	Poison 1.2	Falls 1.4 and Fires, burns 1.4	Drowning 1.9	Medical complications 3.9	Medical complications 9.0	Fires, burns 2.2
5th	Drowning 2.5	Falls 0.6	Falls 0.3	Fires, burns 1.1		Poison 1.5	Choking 3.6	Fires, burns 8.1	Poison 1.5

Accident mortality by age
Certain accidents are more common than others among different age groups. The very young are most likely to die from choking on bits of food or small objects, while the elderly are more likely to die as a result of falling in the home.

Incidence of fatal accidents by age
Among all age groups from infancy through the early 40s, accidents are the single most important cause of death.

ACCIDENTAL DEATHS AS A PROPORTION OF ALL DEATHS (1982)

Age		Non-accidents	Accidents
75+		874,454	14,898
65–74		457,596	8,224
45–64		394,196	15,907
25–44		82,480	25,135
15–24		20,665	21,306
5–14		5,121	4,504
1–4		4,826	3,084
0–1		41,377	1,024
All ages		1,880,715	94,082

of all deaths in those aged 25 to 44. Accidents also cause much long-term physical and mental handicap; for every accident resulting in death, there are almost 10 that cause either major or minor disability.

Motor vehicle accidents are the most common cause of accidental death, accounting for 50 percent of the total. Nevertheless, the number of vehicle-related deaths has decreased in recent years. The introduction of lower speed limits in 1973 contributed to a steady decline in death rates (taking into account miles driven and number of cars owned). In the last few years there has been a decline in the actual number of deaths. This may be due in part to the raising of the drinking age in many states. Alcohol is an important factor in at least half of all fatal motor vehicle accidents. Another factor may be the introduction of mandatory seat belt laws in a growing number of states.

The home appears to be the most dangerous place for both the elderly and the very young. Falls are the second leading cause of death overall; in the elderly, they take first place. Twice as many people 75 years and older die from falls as from motor vehicle accidents. Most of these falls take place in the home while the victim is going about his or her everyday activities. Young people usually suffer only a bruise when they fall, but, in the elderly, bones are much more brittle and more than one third of the falls in those over 74 years old result in fracture of the spine, hipbone (femur), or wrist. Death often follows as a result of complications associated with the fracture.

Up to the age of 1 year, the most important cause of accidental death is choking on a morsel of food or an object placed in the mouth. Death from smothering by bedclothes, plastic bags, or other material is another major home hazard for infants.

THE MECHANISM OF ACCOMMODATION

In a normal, healthy eye, light reflected from a near object is brought into focus on the retina by a process called accommodation. Focusing is achieved by an automatic change in lens shape.

Focusing on a near object
To bring a near object into sharp focus, the ciliary muscles contract and the lens becomes more convex in shape.

Focusing on a distant object
The lens focused on a distant object is thin, flat, and completely relaxed.

The young and the old are also particularly vulnerable to death from burns or asphyxiation as a result of house fires. One third of these victims are under 4 or over 75.

The third leading cause of accidental death is drowning. Eighty percent of the victims are male and most are under 45. Drowning most often occurs when victims are swimming or playing in water. However, it can also result from boating accidents or from falling into water near docks, bridges, or shores. At home, most drownings occur in the family's or a friend's swimming pool. For the very young, the bathtub is also a hazard.

For those 25 to 44, poisoning is almost as common a cause of death as drowning. In many cases, it is due to drug overdose, and suicide may be suspected. If it cannot be proved, the death is classified as accidental.

Accidents at work resulting in death have steadily decreased since the beginning of the century; they now account for less than 2 percent of all accidental deaths.

Accommodation
Adjustment, especially the process by which the eye adjusts itself to focus on near objects. At rest, the eye is focused for distant vision, with the lens relatively thin and flat. To make it possible to focus on a nearer object, the ciliary muscle of the eye contracts, allowing the elastic lens to become thicker and more convex.

With age, the lens loses its elasticity and, as a result, accommodation becomes increasingly difficult. This results in a form of farsightedness called *presbyopia*.

Accreditation
A device traditionally used by medical organizations to maintain and upgrade the standards of medical care through the granting or withholding of approval for teaching institutions, hospitals, and their programs.

Early in this century, the process became more effective as the states began to require graduation from an "accredited" medical school as a condition of licensure. In the very early part of this century, the *American Medical Association* led in the evaluation of medical schools; it was joined later in the accreditation of medical schools by the Association of American Medical Colleges. The American College of Surgeons began the early monitoring of the medical capabilities of hospitals. The accreditation process continues, but the various accrediting bodies now have a broader base, including a wider variety of organizations.

Acebutolol
A *beta-blocker* commonly used in the treatment of *hypertension* (high blood pressure), *angina pectoris* (chest pain due to impaired blood supply to heart muscle), and certain types of *arrhythmia* (irregular heart beat).

ACE inhibitor drugs

Captopril Enalapril

A group of *vasodilator drugs* introduced in 1981. ACE inhibitors (*angiotensin-converting enzyme inhibitors*) are used to treat *hypertension* (high blood pressure) and *heart failure* (reduced pumping efficiency), usually when other drugs have been ineffective. They are sometimes prescribed with other drugs such as *diuretic drugs* or *beta-blocker drugs*.

HOW THEY WORK
ACE inhibitors block the action of the enzyme that converts angiotensin (a protein present in the blood) from an inactive form, angiotensin I, to an active form, angiotensin II, which constricts (narrows) blood vessels. By reducing production of angiotensin II, ACE inhibitors reduce constriction of blood vessels, making it easier for blood to flow through them, and thus reducing blood pressure.

POSSIBLE ADVERSE EFFECTS
These include nausea, loss of taste, headache, dizziness, and a dry cough. The first dose may reduce blood pressure so dramatically that the patient collapses; treatment is therefore often started in the hospital.

Acetaminophen

ANALGESIC

Tablet Capsule Liquid Rectal suppository

Available over-the-counter

Available as generic

A drug widely used since 1955 as an *analgesic* (painkiller). Acetaminophen is used to treat mild pain (for example, headache or toothache) and to reduce fever. Unlike *aspirin*, it does not cause stomach irritation or bleeding and so is particularly useful in the treatment of people who suffer from *peptic ulcer* or who cannot tolerate aspirin. Acetaminophen may also be used with safety to treat children. It was first introduced in the US in liquid form for infants and children. Acetaminophen does not have an anti-inflammatory effect, however, and so is less effective than aspirin as a treatment for joint pain in *arthritis*.

POSSIBLE ADVERSE EFFECTS
Taken in normal doses, nausea or a rash rarely occur. An overdose of acetaminophen may permanently damage the liver and can be fatal.

Acetazolamide

A type of *diuretic drug* known as a carbonic anhydrase inhibitor. Acetazolamide is used in the treatment of *glaucoma* (raised pressure in the eyeball) and, occasionally, to prevent or treat symptoms of *mountain sickness* (headache or weakness occurring at high altitudes).

During treatment with acetazolamide, adverse effects may include lethargy, nausea, diarrhea, weight loss, and impotence.

Acetic acid

The colorless, pungent, organic (carbon-containing) acid that gives vinegar its characteristic sour taste. In medicine, acetic acid is an ingredient of antiseptic jellies that are used to restore the acidity of the vagina in some types of vaginal infections.

Acetohexamide

An oral *hypoglycemic drug* used to treat non-insulin-dependent *diabetes mellitus*. Acetohexamide stimulates the secretion of *insulin*, a hormone that lowers the blood glucose level by increasing glucose absorption by cells.

Acetylcholine

A type of *neurotransmitter* (a chemical that transmits messages between nerve cells or between nerve and muscle cells). Acetylcholine (sometimes abbreviated to ACh) is the neurotransmitter at all nerve-muscle junctions as well as at many other sites in the nervous system. The actions of acetylcholine are called cholinergic actions; these actions are blocked by *anticholinergic drugs*.

Acetylcysteine

A *mucolytic drug* used in the treatment of chronic *bronchitis* and as an antidote for *acetaminophen* overdose.

HOW IT WORKS

Inhaled by *nebulizer*, acetylcysteine makes the mucus in sputum less sticky and therefore easier to cough up. To be effective as an antidote to acetaminophen poisoning, acetylcysteine must be taken by mouth within a few hours of the overdose; it works by reducing the amount of toxic substances produced during the breakdown of acetaminophen, thus reducing the risk of liver damage.

POSSIBLE ADVERSE EFFECTS

In rare cases, vomiting, rash, or increased breathing difficulty may occur when acetylcysteine is taken by nebulizer. Vomiting is common when this drug is taken by mouth.

Achalasia

A condition in which the muscles in the wall of the *esophagus* and the sphincter (valve) between the esophagus and stomach fail to relax after swallowing to permit food to enter the stomach.

Food normally stimulates the muscles in the wall of the esophagus to begin a series of contractions that pushes food toward the stomach. In achalasia, the sphincter does not relax to allow food to pass from the esophagus to the stomach, and the lowest part of the esophagus becomes narrowed and blocked with food.

INCIDENCE AND CAUSE

This rare condition can occur at any age, but is unusual before the age of 15. The underlying cause is unknown.

SYMPTOMS AND SIGNS

Symptoms include difficulty and pain with swallowing and pain in the lower chest and upper abdomen. Regurgitated food that may have been swallowed a day or two earlier may cause a foul taste and bad breath. The ability to swallow gradually deteriorates until there is difficulty swallowing liquids as well as solids.

DIAGNOSIS

A barium swallow (a type of *barium X-ray examination*) will show abnormal, ineffective movement of the esophageal wall and varying degrees of dilatation of the esophagus, as well as narrowing at the lowest end of the esophagus and failure of the sphincter to open after swallowing. *Gastroscopy*, in which a narrow viewing tube is passed down the esophagus, is used to check for *cancer* of the lowest end of the esophagus.

In achalasia, the pressure in the area of the lower esophageal sphincter is markedly elevated; pressure recordings taken while the patient swallows reveal that the esophageal sphincter is incompletely relaxed.

TREATMENT

Drug therapy may rarely help the symptoms of achalasia by relaxing the muscles at the lower end of the esophagus. If drug treatment fails, or if the symptoms worsen, it is possible to widen the esophagus for prolonged periods by passing a slender rubber bag down it and filling the bag with air or water to stretch the muscles (see *Esophageal dilatation*).

There is a surgical procedure that cuts some of the muscles at the stomach entrance to widen the passageway for food. Swallowing may return to normal, but the person may experience *acid reflux*.

Achilles tendon

The tendon that pulls up the back of the heel. It is formed from the calf muscles (the gastrocnemius, soleus, and plantar muscles) and attached to the *calcaneus* (heel bone). The tendon is named for the legendary Greek hero Achilles, who was vulnerable only in the heel.

Minor injuries to the tendon are common. They are usually due to overexercise, faulty running technique, or wearing incorrect footwear (particularly sport shoes with "tendon protectors"). All of these can cause inflammation of the tendon (*tendinitis*) and tearing of the tendon fibers. These conditions usually clear up with rest and physical therapy.

Violent stretching of the Achilles tendon can cause it to rupture. In such cases, surgical repair of the tendon may be necessary.

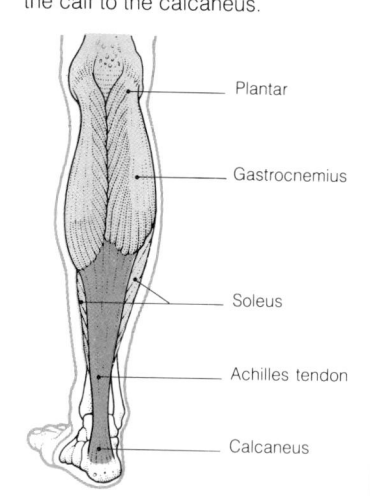

LOCATION OF THE ACHILLES TENDON
The tendon runs from the base of the calf to the calcaneus.

- Plantar
- Gastrocnemius
- Soleus
- Achilles tendon
- Calcaneus

Achlorhydria

Absence of stomach acid secretions. This may be due to chronic atrophic *gastritis* or to an absence or malfunction of parietal, acid-producing cells in the internal lining of the stomach.

About one in every 20 normal people has achlorhydria without symptoms. Achlorhydria in itself is no cause for concern. It is, however, a feature of pernicious anemia, a blood disorder caused by defective absorption of vitamin B_{12} from the stomach (see *Anemia, megaloblastic*) and is present with some stomach cancers.

Achondroplasia

A rare disorder of bone growth, present from birth and leading to *short stature* (once called dwarfism). The affected bones are mainly the long bones of the arms and legs. The cartilage that links each bone to its epiphysis (growing area at its tip) is converted to bone too early, thus preventing further limb growth. Most other bones are able to grow normally.

Affected individuals have short, strong limbs, a well-developed trunk, and a head of normal size except for a somewhat protruding forehead.

INCIDENCE AND CAUSES

In the US and Europe, about two to three persons per 100,000 are achondroplastic. The condition is caused by a gene defect of the dominant variety (see *Genetic disorders*), although exactly how the gene defect leads to the disorder of bone growth is not known.

The children of achondroplastics each have a 50 percent chance of inheriting the defective gene and also of being achondroplastic. However, the parents of most achondroplastics are of normal stature. In these cases, the abnormality has arisen from a new gene defect, or *mutation*.

SYMPTOMS AND OUTLOOK

Achondroplasia is usually obvious at birth or during the first year of life, when there is already a noticeable stunting of the limbs relative to the size of the head. Growth of the limb bones slows and stops during childhood, and no treatment is available to alter the outlook. Intelligence and sexual development are not affected. Life span is close to normal.

Acid

Chemically, an acid is defined as a donor of hydrogen ions (atoms of hydrogen with a positive electrical charge). A wide variety of substances are acids. They include corrosive, mineral acids, such as sulfuric acid (used in automobile batteries) and hydrochloric acid (produced by the stomach lining), and organic acids, such as acetic acid (found in vinegar) and citric acid (found in lemon juice).

When mixed with, or dissolved in, water, acid molecules dissociate (split up) to release their constituent ions; all acids release hydrogen as the positive ion (positively charged ions are called cations, negatively charged ones are called anions). In addition, many acids react with some metals to release hydrogen gas. (See also *Acid-base balance*; *Alkali*; *Burns*.)

Acid-base balance

A combination of mechanisms that ensures that the body's fluids are neither too *acid* nor too alkaline (*alkalis* are also called bases). The body functions healthily only when its fluids are close to chemical neutrality.

Body metabolism involves the conversion of sugars and fats into energy, a process that uses oxygen and produces carbon dioxide (which forms carbonic acid when dissolved in water) and organic acids such as lactic and pyruvic acids. This produces fluctuations in the acidity and alkalinity of the blood and other body fluids.

To maintain normal acid-base balance, the body has three mechanisms: buffers, breathing, and the activities of the kidneys. Buffers are substances in the blood that tend to neutralize acid or alkaline wastes. Rapid breathing increases the rate at which carbon dioxide is eliminated from the blood, thereby making it less acid; conversely, slow breathing allows the blood to become more acid. The kidneys help maintain a constant acidity level in the blood by regulating the amounts of acid or alkaline wastes in the urine.

Disturbances of the acid-base balance result in *acidosis* (excessive blood acidity) or *alkalosis* (excessive blood alkalinity).

Acidosis

A disturbance of the body's *acid-base balance* in which there is an accumulation of acid or loss of alkali (base). There are two types of acidosis: metabolic and respiratory.

CAUSES

In metabolic acidosis, an increased amount of acid may be produced. Ketoacidosis, a form of metabolic acidosis, occurs in uncontrolled *diabetes mellitus* and, to a lesser degree, in starvation. Metabolic acidosis may also be caused by bicarbonate loss through severe diarrhea. In kidney failure there is insufficient excretion of acid in the urine. An overdose of aspirin, which is acidic itself and also causes an increase in acids produced by the process of cell metabolism, is a fairly common cause of metabolic acidosis.

Respiratory acidosis occurs when breathing fails to remove enough carbon dioxide from the lungs, which causes increased blood acidity because the excess carbon dioxide remains in the blood, where it dissolves to form carbonic acid. Impaired breathing leading to respiratory acidosis may be due to conditions such as *bronchitis*, bronchial *asthma*, or *airway obstruction*.

Acid reflux

Regurgitation of acidic fluid from the stomach into the *esophagus* (the tube connecting the throat with the stomach). It is associated with heartburn (a burning pain in the chest), and often leads to *esophagitis* (inflammation of the esophagus).

Mild acid reflux is common and of no serious significance. It may occur in pregnancy and often affects people who are overweight.

Acid reflux is attributed to inefficiency of the muscular valve at the lower end of the esophagus, which permits regurgitation of the acidic fluid. Repeated episodes of discomfort may indicate the presence of a *hiatal hernia*, a weakness in the diaphragm that permits part of the stomach to protrude into the chest.

Acne

A chronic skin disorder caused by inflammation of the hair follicles and the sebaceous glands.

TYPES

The most common type of acne is acne vulgaris, which mainly affects adolescents. Tropical acne affects young whites on unaccustomed exposure to hot, humid environments. Infantile acne, a rare condition affecting male infants, is associated with subsequent severe acne vulgaris in the teen years. Chemical acne is caused by exposure to certain chemicals and oils and results in acne in unusual sites, such as the legs. Chloracne is a form of acne caused by exposure to chlorinated hydrocarbon chemicals; many cases occurred following a severe explosion at a factory in Seveso, Italy, in 1976.

Severe acne
An example of cystic acne, with widespread scarring across the back. Few cases are as extensive as this.

A

INCIDENCE

Acne almost always begins during puberty, although it may develop later in life; most adolescent boys and many girls have some acne.

CAUSE

Acne spots are caused by the obstruction of the follicle by sebum (the oily substance secreted by the sebaceous glands in the skin). When a plug of sebum becomes trapped in the follicle, bacteria multiply and the follicle becomes inflamed. The cause of the change in sebum at puberty is uncertain but it seems to be linked with increased levels of *androgen hormones* (male sex hormones). There may also be a genetic factor, since acne can run in families.

Some drugs may bring on or aggravate existing acne (for example, corticosteroids and androgens, which increase oil production by the skin). Other drugs that can aggravate acne include barbiturates, isoniazid, rifampin, bromides, and iodides.

Oil and grease may also cause acne. The natural oil from the scalp may cause acne around the hairline. Regular contact with mineral or cooking oil, as in restaurant kitchens, can make the condition worse. Cosmetics with oily bases are also associated with an increased tendency to acne.

SYMPTOMS

Acne occurs in areas that have a high concentration of sebaceous glands, mainly the face, center of the chest, upper back, shoulders, and around the neck. The most common acne spots are comedones (blackheads), milia (whiteheads), pustules, nodules (firm swellings below the skin), and cysts (larger firm swellings in the skin). As each spot heals, others tend to appear. The healing spots often fade to a pink mark that usually disappears altogether, although some spots, particularly the cystic ones, may leave scars. Acne scars often appear as small, depressed pits. Occasionally, as with other scars, keloids (overgrowths of scar tissue) may form.

PREVENTION

There are many myths about the prevention of acne, particularly relating to diet. There is no evidence that diet plays any part in causing acne. For example, there is little point in avoiding sweets such as chocolate. Although washing affected areas does not prevent acne, it may keep it from spreading. The skin should be washed twice daily; more frequent washing is unnecessary, since washing simply removes surface oil.

TREATMENT

There is no instant cure for acne, although many treatments are available to relieve it. Topical (applied to the skin) treatments act by unblocking the pores and removing the sebum. They also help to promote healing. Topical applications that are most often used include benzoyl peroxide, retinoic acid, antibiotic lotions, and sulfur-containing creams. Ultraviolet light is often beneficial in treating acne. Exposure to natural sunlight is helpful, and artificial ultraviolet light may be used to treat more severe cases. The spots should not be picked or squeezed; this can worsen the condition and can lead to scarring.

If topical treatment has failed, long-term therapy with oral antibiotics often helps. The antibiotics are prescribed regularly for up to six months at a time. They have an effect not only on the bacteria in the skin but may also have a direct effect on inflammatory cells in acne lesions, as well as on sebum production.

A recent development in the treatment of acne is the use of retinoid drugs. These drugs are prescribed only for severe acne when antibiotics and other measures have not helped. Retinoid drugs reduce oil production and have a drying effect on the skin, but must be taken cautiously because they may cause liver damage and other serious problems.

Acne cysts can often be treated by intralesional therapy (direct injection of a drug into the acne spots), which also helps to reduce scarring. In cases of severe, extensive scarring, *dermabrasion* (removal of the top layer of affected skin) can help improve the cosmetic appearance.

OUTLOOK

Acne improves slowly over a period of time, often clearing up by the end of the teenage years. With modern treatment, no one should have severe, scarring acne.

Acoustic nerve

Also called the auditory nerve, the acoustic nerve is the part of the *vestibulocochlear nerve* (the eighth *cranial nerve*) concerned with hearing.

Acoustic neuroma

A rare, benign tumor arising from supporting cells that surround the eighth cranial (auditory or acoustic) nerve, usually within the internal auditory meatus (the canal in the skull through which the nerve emerges into the inner ear).

INCIDENCE AND CAUSES

Acoustic neuromas constitute about 5 to 7 percent of primary *brain tumors*. They most commonly occur in people between the ages of 40 and 60 and are slightly more common in women than in men. In the US, about four to five cases per million population per year are diagnosed. Usually the cause is unknown. In some cases, however, tumors simultaneously affect the nerves on both sides of the head and may be part of a widespread *neurofibromatosis*, a disease characterized by changes in the nervous system, skin, and bones.

SYMPTOMS AND DIAGNOSIS

Acoustic neuroma can cause *deafness*, *tinnitus* (noises in the ear), loss of balance, and pain in the affected ear. As the tumor enlarges, it may compress the brain stem and cerebellum, causing *ataxia* (loss of coordination). As it expands, it presses on the fifth cranial nerve, causing pain in the face, or on the sixth cranial nerve, causing double vision.

Diagnosis is made by *hearing tests* and tests of balance, such as the *caloric test* or *electronystagmography*, followed by X rays or *CT scanning* to visualize the internal auditory meatus.

TREATMENT

The tumor is treated by surgical removal. Before the operation, a CT scan or MRI is used to show the location of the tumor and its approximate size, so that the surgeon can decide on the best route for removal. The results of surgery depend on the size of the tumor; in many cases, hearing can be preserved with no damage to the acoustic nerve. Occasionally, numbness and weakness of part of the face result from unavoidable damage to other surrounding nerves.

Acrocyanosis

A condition in which the hands and feet turn blue, may become cold, and sweat excessively. Acrocyanosis is caused by spasm in small blood vessels and is usually aggravated by cold weather.

Acrocyanosis is distantly related to a more serious circulatory disorder, *Raynaud's disease*, in which the skin of the fingers and toes may be damaged by chronically reduced blood flow.

Acrodermatitis enteropathica

A rare, inherited disease in which the skin of the fingers and toes, and the anal, mouth, and scalp area of infants, is reddened, ulcerated, and covered with pustules.

Acrodermatitis enteropathica is caused by an inability to absorb enough zinc from food. The addition of zinc supplements to the diet leads to quick improvement.

Acromegaly

A rare disease characterized externally by abnormal enlargement of the skull, jaw, hands, and feet.

CAUSE AND SYMPTOMS

Acromegaly is caused by excessive secretion of *growth hormone* from the anterior pituitary gland at the base of the brain and is the result of a benign tumor (see *Pituitary tumors*).

If such a tumor develops in a person within the first 10 years of life, the result is *gigantism* (in which growth is accelerated) and not acromegaly. More commonly, the tumor develops after growth in the long bones of the limbs has stopped. This leads to acromegaly, although it may take several years before the symptoms and signs appear.

Appearance of acromegaly
The woman in profile at left shows many of the typical features of acromegaly—including lengthening of the face, enlargement of the jaw and nose, and general coarsening of the facial features.

Symptoms and signs of acromegaly include enlargement of the hands and feet, coarsening of the facial features, enlargement of the ears and nose, a jutting jaw, and a long face. Sufferers may notice a gradual increase in ring, shoe, glove, and hat size, and deepening or huskiness of the voice. Other possible symptoms are those common to any tumor in the brain, such as headache and visual disturbances.

DIAGNOSIS AND TREATMENT

If acromegaly appears to be developing in a person, the level of growth hormone in the blood is measured before and after a quantity of glucose has been administered. Glucose usually suppresses growth hormone secretion; if it has no effect on the blood level of the hormone, this confirms uncontrolled secretion of the

hormone by the pituitary gland. *CT scanning* or *MRI* may reveal a tumor or overgrowth of the pituitary gland.

In some cases the drug bromocriptine may cause the pituitary tumor to regress; alternatively, the tumor may be treated by *radiation therapy* or removed surgically.

Acromioclavicular joint

The joint between the outer end of the clavicle (collarbone) and the acromion (the bony prominence at the top of the shoulder blade).

INJURIES TO THE JOINT

Injuries to the joint are rare. They are usually due to a fall on the shoulder and may result in subluxation (partial dislocation with the bones still in contact) or, rarely, dislocation (complete displacement of the bones).

In subluxation, the synovium (joint lining) and the ligaments around it are stretched and bruised, the joint is swollen, and the bones are felt to be slightly out of alignment. In dislocation, the ligaments are torn, the swelling is greater, and the bone deformity is pronounced. In both subluxation and dislocation, the joint is painful and tender, and movement of the shoulder is restricted.

Subluxation is treated by resting the arm and shoulder in a sling. If the pain and tenderness persist, an injection of a corticosteroid and a local anesthetic into the joint often helps.

Dislocation requires a strapping around the clavicle and elbow to pull the outer end of the clavicle back into position. The strapping is usually left on for three weeks.

LOCATION OF THE ACROMIOCLAVICULAR JOINT
The joint lies at the junction of the outer end of the clavicle and the acromion.

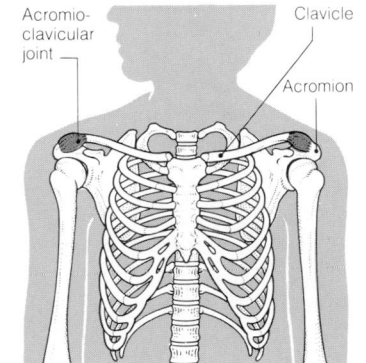

Acromio-clavicular joint

Clavicle

Acromion

Osteoarthritis (degeneration of the joint), which makes shoulder movement painful, can develop if the joint suffers repeated injuries.

Acroparesthesia

A medical term used to describe tingling in the fingers or toes (see *Pins and needles sensation*).

ACTH

The commonly used abbreviation for adrenocorticotropic hormone (also called corticotropin), which is produced by the anterior part of the *pituitary gland* and stimulates the adrenal cortex (outer layer of the *adrenal glands*) to release various *corticosteroid hormones*. ACTH is also necessary for the maintenance and growth of the cells of the adrenal cortex.

ACTIONS

ACTH stimulates the adrenal cortex to increase production of the hormones *hydrocortisone* (cortisol), *aldosterone*, and *androgen hormones*. Most important of these is its stimulation of hydrocortisone production.

ACTH production is partly controlled by the *hypothalamus* (an area in the center of the brain) and partly by the level of hydrocortisone in the blood. When ACTH levels are too high, hydrocortisone production is increased; this, in turn, suppresses the release of ACTH from the pituitary gland. If ACTH levels are too low, the hypothalamus releases its hormones, stimulating the pituitary gland to increase ACTH production. This action stimulates the adrenal cortex to form hydrocortisone.

ACTH levels increase in response to stress, emotion, injury, infection, burns, surgery, and a decrease in blood pressure.

DISORDERS

A tumor of the pituitary gland can cause excessive ACTH production which, in turn, leads to overproduction of hydrocortisone by the adrenal cortex, resulting in *Cushing's syndrome*. Insufficient ACTH production due, for example, to hypopituitarism (underactivity of the pituitary gland), is rare. When it does occur, it causes *adrenal failure*.

MEDICAL USES

ACTH is used to treat inflammatory disorders such as *arthritis*, *ulcerative colitis*, and some types of *hepatitis*. It has also been employed to induce remissions in *multiple sclerosis* but its efficacy is uncertain. ACTH is also used to diagnose disorders of the adrenal glands.

Acting out

Impulsive actions that reflect unconscious wishes. The term is most often used by psychotherapists to describe behavior during analysis when the patient "acts out" rather than reports fantasies, wishes, or beliefs. Acting out can also occur outside of psychoanalysis as a reaction to frustrations encountered in everyday life. In this case it usually takes the form of antisocial, aggressive behavior that may be directed toward oneself or others. Typical behavior includes wrist-cutting, stealing, or impulsively starting new relationships; these activities cannot, however, always be explained in terms of acting out.

Actinic

Pertaining to changes caused by the ultraviolet rays in sunlight, as in actinic *dermatitis* (inflammation of the skin) and actinic *keratosis* (roughness and thickening of the skin), both of which are caused by overexposure, especially in the Southwest.

Actinomycosis

 An infection caused by *ACTINOMYCES ISRAELII* or related actinomycete bacteria. These bacteria resemble fungi and cause diseases of the mouth and jaw, pelvis, and chest.

TYPES

The most common form of the disease affects the mouth and jaw. A painful swelling appears, usually on the jaw. Small openings later develop on the skin of the face and discharge pus and characteristic yellow granules. Poor oral hygiene may contribute to this form of the infection.

Another form of actinomycosis, affecting the pelvis, occurs in women and may cause lower abdominal pain, fever, and bleeding between menstrual periods. This form of the infection has been associated with the use of *IUDs* that do not contain copper. Rare forms of actinomycosis affect the appendix or lung.

DIAGNOSIS AND TREATMENT

A diagnosis of actinomycosis is usually confirmed by the presence of the granules. Treatment with large doses of penicillin is usually successful, although, in severe infections, medication may need to be continued for several months.

Acuity, visual

See *Visual acuity*.

Acupressure

A derivative of *acupuncture* in which pressure instead of a needle is applied to meridians (set points on the body).

Acupuncture

A branch of Chinese medicine in which needles are inserted into a patient's skin as therapy for various disorders or to induce anesthesia.

Traditional Chinese medicine holds that the Chi (life force) flows through the body along meridians (channels); blockage in one or more of these meridians is believed to cause ill health. Acupuncturists aim to restore health by inserting needles at appropriate sites, known as acupuncture points, on the affected meridians.

A cautious view is taken of acupuncture by orthodox medical practitioners, but some use it to complement other treatments.

HOW IT WORKS

Research suggests that acupuncture causes the release within the central nervous system of morphinelike substances, *endorphins*, which act as natural analgesics (painkillers). It has also been suggested that acupuncture may work by inducing a form of hypnosis or because insertion of the needles stimulates peripheral nerves, acting as a distraction from or a counterirritant to the original pain.

WHY IT IS DONE

Acupuncture has been used successfully as an anesthetic for dental procedures and surgical operations, and also during labor and delivery (including cesarean sections). Some practitioners use acupuncture to reduce pain after operations and also to relieve chronically painful conditions, such as arthritis, that are not responding to standard treatments.

It is claimed to be particularly effective for conditions of the muscles, bones, joints, eyes, heart, and the digestive, respiratory, and nervous systems; it is also claimed to help treat addiction, depression, and anxiety.

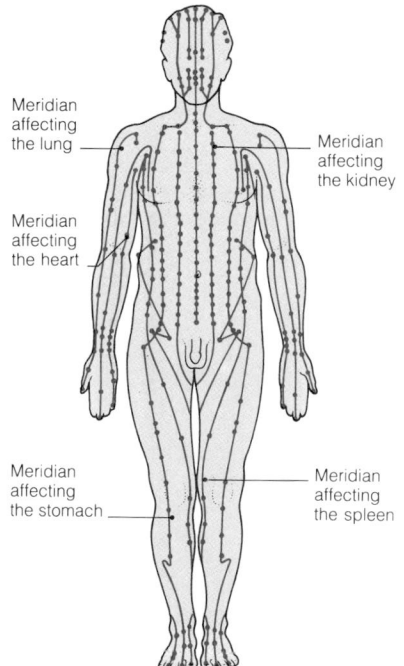

Meridian affecting the lung

Meridian affecting the kidney

Meridian affecting the heart

Meridian affecting the stomach

Meridian affecting the spleen

Acupuncture meridian lines

There are 14 major acupuncture meridians, each considered to affect a particular part of the body. Each meridian contains numerous acupuncture points (sites at which needles may be inserted).

HOW IT IS DONE

The traditional Chinese physician recognizes that accurate diagnosis is essential so that the acupuncturist knows which acupuncture points to use. Diagnosis in traditional Chinese medicine is made by examination of the patient's 12 pulses (six in each wrist). Each pulse is believed to give information about the health of a particular body region.

The precise disorder being treated or the degree of anesthesia required determines the temperature of the needle used, the angle of insertion, whether needles are twisted or vibrated while inserted, the speed of insertion and withdrawal, and the length of time the needles remain in position. Some practitioners pass a mild current through the needle to act as a stimulant in unblocking the meridian; others inject homeopathic remedies into the acupuncture point.

RISKS

Currently there are few legal checks on acupuncturists in the US and no formal qualification is necessary to practice. Infection is a possible risk but good practitioners avoid this with scrupulous sterilization techniques. It is rare that a blood vessel, body cavity, or organ is punctured.

Some people find that they experience a temporary exacerbation of their symptoms immediately following acupuncture treatment. Others experience lightheadedness, drowsiness, or exhilaration, although these feelings disappear soon after the treatment session has ended.

Acute

A term used to describe a disorder or symptom that comes on suddenly. Acute conditions may or may not be severe, and they are usually of short duration. (See also *Chronic*.)

Acyclovir

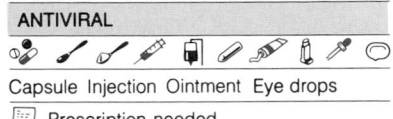

ANTIVIRAL			
Capsule	Injection	Ointment	Eye drops

📋 Prescription needed

🔒 Not available as generic

A drug introduced in 1982 and used in the treatment of the virus that causes *herpes simplex* infections. Acyclovir is also used in the treatment of *herpes zoster* (shingles). Acyclovir also has some effect against *cytomegalovirus* and *Epstein-Barr virus* infections. To be effective, acyclovir must be prescribed soon after infection; it does not prevent attacks from recurring but does reduce their severity.

POSSIBLE ADVERSE EFFECTS

Adverse effects are uncommon. Acyclovir ointment may cause skin irritation or rash. Taken by mouth, acyclovir may cause headache, dizziness, nausea, or vomiting. In rare cases, acyclovir injections can cause kidney damage.

Adam's apple

A projection at the front of the neck, just beneath the skin, that is formed by a prominence on the thyroid cartilage, part of the larynx (voice box). It enlarges in males at puberty.

Addiction

Physiological and psychological dependence on and craving for a chemical substance (see *Alcohol dependence*; *Drug dependence*).

Addison's disease

A rare disorder in which symptoms are caused by a deficiency of the corticosteroid hormones *hydrocortisone* and *aldosterone*, normally produced by the adrenal cortex (part of the adrenal glands). The disease is named for the English physician Thomas Addison (1793-1860). It was invariably fatal before hormone treatment became available in the 1950s.

CAUSES

Addison's disease can be caused by any disease process that destroys the adrenal cortices. The most common cause is an *autoimmune disorder*, in which a person's immune system produces antibodies that attack the adrenal glands. *Tuberculosis* of the adrenal glands, once the main cause, is now very rare.

In addition to the deficient production of aldosterone and hydrocortisone, excessive amounts of ACTH and other hormones are poured out by the pituitary gland. Included among these hormones is one that increases the synthesis of melanin pigment in the skin.

SYMPTOMS AND DIAGNOSIS

Addison's disease generally has a slow onset and chronic course, with symptoms developing gradually over months or years. However, acute episodes, called Addisonian crises, can also occur; they are brought on by infection, injury, or other stresses. During these crises, the adrenal glands cannot increase their production of aldosterone and hydrocortisone, which normally help the body to cope with stress.

The symptoms of Addisonian crises are mainly due to aldosterone deficiency (which leads to excessive loss of sodium and water in the urine), extreme muscle weakness, dehydration, *hypotension* (low blood pressure), confusion, and coma.

Symptoms of the chronic form of Addison's disease include tiredness, weakness, vague abdominal pain, and weight loss. A more specific symptom is darkening of the skin in the creases of the palms and pressure areas of the

body, and most particularly in the mouth. The darkening is caused by excessive production by the pituitary of the hormone that stimulates melanin production.

Diagnosis is generally made if the patient fails to respond to an injection of ACTH, which normally stimulates the secretion of hydrocortisone.

TREATMENT

Treatment of acute Addisonian crises involves monitoring blood pressure and heart rate during the rapid infusion of saline, and supplementary doses of hydrocortisone and fludrocortisone to correct the sodium deficiency and dehydration. Long-term treatment of the disease requires replacement of the deficient hormones with *corticosteroid drugs*.

Because patients with Addison's disease cannot increase their output of corticosteroid hormones in response to stress, they are at risk during stressful situations such as infection, surgery, or injury. Their physicians must instruct them in the use of increased doses of corticosteroid drugs at such times so that the body mechanisms that fight infection and promote healing are not impaired.

Adduction

Movement of a limb toward the central line of the body, or of a digit toward the axis of a limb. Muscles that carry out this movement are often called adductors. The opposite movement is called *abduction*.

Adenitis

Inflammation of a gland, particularly of a lymph gland. Cervical adenitis (swollen, tender lymph glands in the neck) occurs in certain infections (especially *tonsillitis*) caused by streptococcal bacteria, and in infectious *mononucleosis*. In the past, adenitis was often due to scrofula (tuberculosis infection of the cervical lymph nodes).

Mesenteric lymphadenitis is inflammation of the lymph glands in the peritoneum (the membrane that encloses the intestines) caused by a viral infection. The symptoms of mesenteric lymphadenitis—mainly abdominal pain and tenderness—may mimic those of appendicitis and may require an exploratory operation to confirm a diagnosis.

Treatment of adenitis may include the use of analgesics (painkillers), hot compresses, or a heating pad, and, if a bacterial infection is suspected, antibiotic drugs. The inflammation usually subsides within a few days.

LOCATION OF THE ADAM'S APPLE
This projection at the front of the neck, beneath the skin, is formed by a prominence on the thyroid cartilage.

Trachea _____ | _____ Thyroid cartilage

A

Adenocarcinoma

The technical name for a malignant tumor, or cancer, of a gland or glandular tissue, or a tumor of which the gland-derived cells form glandlike structures. An adenocarcinoma arises from epithelium, the layer of cells that lines the inside of an organ.

Cancers of the colon (the main part of the large intestine), breast, pancreas, and kidney are usually adenocarcinomas, as are a proportion of cancers of the cervix, esophagus, salivary glands, and many other organs. (See *Intestine, cancer of; Pancreas, cancer of; Kidney cancer.*)

Adenoidectomy

Surgical removal of the *adenoids*, usually performed on a child with abnormally large adenoids that are causing recurrent infections of the middle ear or air sinuses. The operation is often performed in conjunction with *tonsillectomy*.

Adenoidectomy is generally an operation with minimal aftereffects. The patient usually can begin to eat normally the following day.

Adenoids

Two swellings at the back of the nose, above the tonsils, made up of *lymph nodes* (tissues that contain lymphocytes, which are white cells that help fight infection). These nodes form part of the body's defense against upper respiratory tract infections; they tend to enlarge during early childhood, a time when infections of this type are common.

DISORDERS

In most children, adenoids shrink after the age of about 5 years, disappearing altogether by puberty. In some children, however, they become even larger and obstruct the passage from the nose to the throat, causing snoring, breathing through the mouth, and a characteristically nasal voice. They can also block the eustachian tube (which connects the middle ear to the throat), causing infection and deafness.

Obstruction to the flow of secretions behind the nose can result in rhinitis (infection of the nose), which can spread to the middle ear (see *Otitis media*) and the air sinuses behind the nose (see *Sinusitis*).

DIAGNOSIS AND TREATMENT To discover whether ear, nose, and throat infections are being caused by abnormally enlarged adenoids, the physician usually inspects the back of the throat using a mirror with a light attached. Infections usually respond to antibiotics; if infections recur frequently, *adenoidectomy* (surgical removal of the adenoids) may be advised.

Adenoma

A benign, noncancerous tumor arising from the epithelium (cell layer lining the inner surface) of any gland, forming a benign glandlike tumor or cyst.

Adenomas of endocrine glands (those that secrete hormones directly into the bloodstream), such as the pituitary, thyroid, and adrenal glands and pancreas, can cause disease resulting from excessive hormone production. Pituitary adenomas, for example, can result in *acromegaly* or *Cushing's syndrome*.

Adenomatosis

An abnormal condition of glands in which they are affected either by *hyperplasia* (overgrowth) or by the development of numerous *adenomas* (benign tumors).

Adenomatosis may simultaneously affect two or more different endocrine glands, such as the adrenal, parathyroid, and pituitary glands and pancreas. (See also *Adrenal tumors; Parathyroid tumors.*)

ADH

The abbreviation for antidiuretic hormone (also called vasopressin), which is released from the posterior part of the *pituitary gland* and acts on the kidneys to increase their reabsorption of water into the blood.

ACTIONS

ADH reduces the amount of water lost in the urine and helps control the body's overall water balance. Water is continually being taken into the body in food and drink and is also produced by the chemical reactions in cells. Conversely, water is continually being lost in urine, sweat, feces, and in the breath as water vapor. ADH helps maintain the optimum amount of water in the body.

ADH production is controlled by the *hypothalamus* (an area in the center of the brain), which detects changes in the concentration and volume of the blood. If the blood concentration increases (i.e., contains less water), the hypothalamus stimulates the pituitary gland to release more ADH. If the blood is too dilute, less ADH is produced and, as a result, more water is lost from the body in the urine.

DISORDERS

Various factors can affect ADH production and thus disturb the body's water balance. For example, alcohol reduces ADH production by direct action on the brain, resulting in temporarily increased production of urine. This may also occur in *diabetes insipidus*, a disorder in which there is either insufficient production of ADH in the pituitary gland or, rarely, failure of the kidneys to respond to ADH.

The reverse effect, water retention, may result from temporarily increased ADH production after a major operation or accident. Water retention may also be caused by the secretion of ADH by some tumors, especially of the lung.

DRUG THERAPY

Synthetic ADH is given via the nose or by injection to treat diabetes insipidus. High intravenous doses cause narrowing of blood vessels and may stop bleeding from *esophageal varices*. Adverse effects include abdominal cramps, nausea, headache, drowsiness, and confusion.

Adhesion

Fibrous tissue within the body that joins normally unconnected parts. Although sometimes present from birth, adhesions are usually scar tissue formed after inflammation.

The most common site of adhesions is the abdomen, where they often form after *peritonitis* (inflammation of the abdominal lining), or following surgery as part of the natural healing

---

LOCATION OF THE ADENOIDS

These two glandular swellings are found at the back of the nasal passage above the tonsils. Adenoids are sometimes implicated in *sleep apnea*.

Nasal cavity

Tongue

Adenoids

Tonsil   Trachea

process. Abdominal adhesions infrequently bind together loops of intestine, resulting in intestinal obstruction (see *Intestine, obstruction of*). In such cases, an operation is usually required to cut the fibrous tissue and free the intestinal loops.

Adipose tissue

A layer of fat just beneath the skin and around various internal organs. After puberty, the distribution of superficial adipose tissue differs in males and females. Adipose tissue makes up a larger proportion of total body weight in women than it does in men.

Distribution of adipose tissue
In adult males, adipose tissue accumulates around the shoulders, waist, and abdomen; in women, it accumulates on the breasts, hips, and thighs.

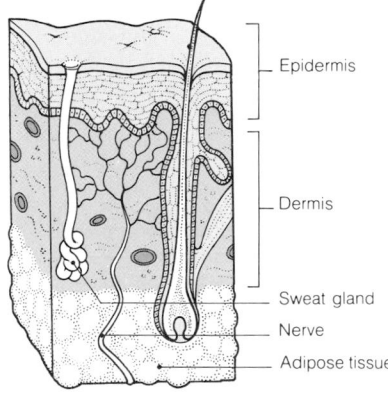

Epidermis

Dermis

Sweat gland

Nerve

Adipose tissue

FUNCTIONS AND DISORDERS

Adipose tissue is built up from fat deposited as a result of excess food intake, thus acting as an energy store; excessive amounts of adipose tissue produce *obesity*. The tissue acts as an insulator against loss of body heat, particularly in babies. Adipose tissue helps absorb shock in areas subject to sudden or frequent pressure, such as the buttocks and feet. It also surrounds and cushions the heart, kidneys, and other internal organs.

Adjuvant

A substance that enhances the action of another substance in the body. The term is usually used to describe an ingredient added to a *vaccine* to increase the production of antibodies by the immune system, therefore enhancing the vaccine's efficiency in conferring immunity. Adjuvant

chemotherapy is the addition of treatment with cytotoxic (anticancer) drugs to the surgical removal of a tumor.

Adlerian theory

A discipline of psychology set forth by the Austrian psychiatrist Alfred Adler (1870-1937).

Adolescence

The period between childhood and adulthood. Broadly speaking, adolescence corresponds to the teen years. A complex stage of personality development and psychological upheaval, adolescence overlaps with, but is not the same as, *puberty*. Puberty is the period of hormonally regulated development when the secondary sex characteristics appear, marking the onset of physical and sexual maturity.

FEATURES

Adolescence is a time of much change for the individual and for the adolescent's family. The adolescent must come to terms with the body's physical changes and with the fact that family and society no longer expect or tolerate childish behavior. During adolescence, the adult's self-identity is formed. This involves achieving independence and emotional separation from parents, understanding adult sexual roles, and learning to use increased aggressive drive. Adolescence is also a time of forming attitudes and opinions.

Adolescents would like to be independent but many must still rely on adults for emotional and financial support. Parental conflicts often arise when adolescents demand increased independence before their parents consider them ready for it.

During the process of achieving an adult identity, the adolescent ceases to define himself or herself only in terms of the adults who are at home and at school, which is what a child does. He or she may seek other figures (such as pop stars) as role models or leaders and may rebel against parental standards and family. Adolescents experiment with views and opinions, with allegiances to peer groups and gangs, and with political movements. They may adopt outrageous fashions of dress, appearance, and behavior.

Sexual experimentation occurs in fantasy and in reality, alone and with others. Gender identity may be questioned; this may be the time that a person first realizes that he or she is homosexual. Often during adolescence, homosexual behavior occurs temporarily. Coming to terms with

sexual drives may be influenced by the adolescent's perception of his or her parents' relationship.

PROBLEMS

Common patterns of adolescent behavior include moodiness, loss of interest in school, fluctuating school performance, and, in extreme cases, truancy. Adolescents worry tremendously about their physical appearance, acne, their changing body shape, and whether they are physically attractive. They may feel nervous, depressed, and withdrawn, and may become painfully shy and lacking in confidence. Often they feel very unsure of their personal identity, suffering a so-called "identity crisis." There may be a strong sense of alienation from parents, who may feel they can no longer talk to their children.

Some adolescents are overassertive and strive prematurely for independence. Rebellion against parents is often exaggerated in adolescents who were overdependent on, or overprotected by, their parents during childhood (such as those with a chronic physical illness). Childhood deprivation that has resulted in weak *bonding* between child and parents can also lead to extreme rebelliousness. On the other hand, a teenager who remains too dependent may remain stuck in adolescence and not grow enough to make his or her own decisions or to form new relationships outside the family.

Aggressive drives that are not controlled and used constructively can lead to outbursts of bad temper or other undesirable behavior. Delinquency is common in adolescents from all backgrounds, but is usually a transient phase if dealt with by a mixture of firmness and understanding.

Adolescents (and children who are younger) may become involved in drug abuse for experimentation, for kicks, or commonly because of peer group pressure. Those youngsters who take drugs to relieve anxiety or depression are more likely to become dependent. Recently, solvent abuse (glue sniffing) has become widespread, particularly among boys.

A high proportion of adolescents with serious or prolonged psychological and behavioral problems, particularly drug abuse and delinquency, are from disturbed or deprived home environments where there is poverty, marital disharmony, alcoholism, or psychiatric disturbance in the parents. Unsocial behavior is also more likely in adolescents who have had behavioral problems (see *Behavioral problems in children*).

Adolescents are often referred for specialized advice because parents or teachers are worried about their behavior. Only a small percentage of those referred need psychiatric medicines and/or hospitalization. Most have temporary problems that resolve on their own. Psychological problems underlie the development of *anorexia nervosa*. Major psychotic illnesses—*schizophrenia* and *manic-depressive illness*—are almost never seen before adolescence, although "identity crisis" may mimic psychosis temporarily. Love problems and family problems can provoke suicidal attempts in disturbed adolescents.

Maintaining communication with their offspring is highly important but not always easy for parents. Parents should give practical help on problems such as acne and diet and never laugh off or underestimate seemingly minor problems; this may undermine the adolescent's confidence. The most valuable support a parent can give the adolescent is encouraging self-confidence. Confidence will provide a firm foundation for coping with the increasing pressures and responsibilities of adult life.

ADP

Abbreviation for adenosine diphosphate, the chemical that takes up energy released during biochemical reactions to form *ATP* (adenosine triphosphate), the main energy-carrying chemical in the body. When ATP releases its energy, ADP is reconstituted. (See also *Metabolism*.)

Adrenal failure

Insufficient production of hormones by the adrenal cortex. It can be acute (of sudden onset) or chronic (of more gradual onset). When chronic adrenal failure is due to a disease or damage to the adrenal gland itself, it is called *Addison's disease*. It can, however, also result from reduced stimulation of the adrenal cortex by *ACTH*, a hormone produced by the pituitary gland (see *Adrenal glands* disorders box).

Adrenal glands

A pair of endocrine glands (glands that secrete hormones directly into the bloodstream). Small and triangular, they sit on top of the kidneys.

Each adrenal gland can be divided, anatomically and functionally, into two distinct organs. The outer region is the adrenal cortex. It secretes *cor-*

ANATOMY OF THE ADRENAL GLANDS

Also sometimes called the suprarenal glands, the adrenal glands are situated on top of the kidneys. Each one is divided into two regions: the adrenal cortex (which secretes hormones that affect the metabolism) and the adrenal medulla (which is part of the sympathetic nervous system).

ticosteroid hormones that have important effects on the body's *metabolism* (the way in which energy stores and food are used), on chemicals in the blood, and on characteristics such as hairiness and body shape.

The smaller, inner region of the gland is the adrenal medulla, which is part of the *sympathetic nervous system*, the body's first line of response and defense against physical and emotional stresses.

FEEDBACK MECHANISM

The rate at which many glands produce hormones is influenced by other hormones, especially those secreted by the pituitary gland and the hypothalamus. If too much hormone is produced, negative feedback mechanisms act on the hypothalamus and pituitary so that they produce less of their stimulating hormones; thus reducing the target gland's activity. If too little hormone is produced, the feedback weakens, leading to increased production of the stimulating hormones.

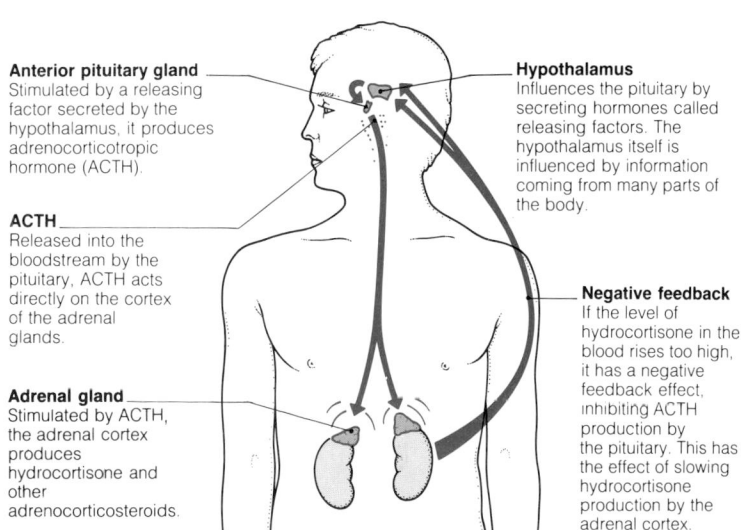

Anterior pituitary gland
Stimulated by a releasing factor secreted by the hypothalamus, it produces adrenocorticotropic hormone (ACTH).

ACTH
Released into the bloodstream by the pituitary. ACTH acts directly on the cortex of the adrenal glands.

Adrenal gland
Stimulated by ACTH, the adrenal cortex produces hydrocortisone and other adrenocorticosteroids.

Hypothalamus
Influences the pituitary by secreting hormones called releasing factors. The hypothalamus itself is influenced by information coming from many parts of the body.

Negative feedback
If the level of hydrocortisone in the blood rises too high, it has a negative feedback effect, inhibiting ACTH production by the pituitary. This has the effect of slowing hydrocortisone production by the adrenal cortex.

DISORDERS OF THE ADRENAL GLANDS

Excessive or deficient production of hormones by the adrenal glands can occur in a variety of ways. These disorders are uncommon, but may be serious. Disturbed hormone production by the adrenal cortex is more common than disturbance of the adrenal medulla.

CONGENITAL DEFECTS

Congenital *adrenal hyperplasia* affects about one newborn baby in 10,000. The adrenal cortex is unable to synthesize sufficient hydrocortisone and (sometimes) aldosterone, and the baby is ill or fails to thrive. As a side effect of the reduced hydrocortisone production, the glands are stimulated to produce androgens (male sex hormones) in excess; this can cause masculinization of female babies.

TUMORS

Growths in the adrenal glands are rare and generally lead to excess hormone production. Excess secretion of aldosterone causes *aldosteronism,* a condition characterized by thirst and high blood pressure. Excess secretion of hydrocortisone causes *Cushing's syndrome,* which is characterized by muscle-wasting and obesity of the trunk. Androgens may also be produced to excess, causing masculinization in females.

Tumors of the adrenal medulla include *pheochromocytoma* and *neuroblastoma.* Excess epinephrine and norepinephrine are secreted, causing a rise in blood pressure.

AUTOIMMUNE DISORDERS

Deficient production of hormones by the adrenal cortex is called *adrenal failure*; if due to disease of the adrenal glands themselves, it is called *Addison's disease.* The most common cause of Addison's disease is an autoimmune process (in which the body's immune system attacks its own tissues). Addison's disease can take a chronic course, characterized by weakness, weight loss, and skin darkening, or an acute form (Addisonian crisis or acute adrenal failure), in which the patient may become confused and comatose.

INFECTION

Destruction of the adrenal glands by *tuberculosis* was once a major cause of Addison's disease; it is now uncommon compared with autoimmune causes. The onset of infection or other acute illness can precipitate acute adrenal failure in someone with Addison's disease.

IMPAIRED BLOOD SUPPLY

Loss or obstruction of the blood supply to the adrenals, sometimes as a result of arterial disease, is another possible cause of Addison's disease or acute adrenal failure.

OTHER DISORDERS

In many cases disturbed activity of the adrenals is caused not by disease of the glands, but by an increase or decrease in the blood level of hormones that influences their activity.

Hydrocortisone production by the adrenal cortex is controlled by the secretion of *ACTH* (adrenocorticotropic hormone) by the pituitary gland. A tumor or other disorder of the pituitary, or tumors elsewhere in the body, can cause excess ACTH secretion, leading to too much hydrocortisone being produced by the adrenals and, hence, leading to Cushing's syndrome. Pituitary disease is, in fact, the most common cause of Cushing's syndrome.

Destruction or removal of the pituitary has the opposite effect, stopping ACTH secretion, preventing stimulation of the adrenal cortex, and leading to adrenal failure.

INVESTIGATION

Suspected disturbance of adrenal function is investigated by measurement of the levels of hormones such as hydrocortisone, aldosterone, epinephrine, and ACTH in the blood plasma and/or urine.

Tests may also be carried out to measure the effects of an injected substance that would normally modify the production of a hormone. Such tests can help localize the underlying cause of the disorder—for example, to distinguish Cushing's syndrome due to an adrenal tumor from that due to pituitary disease.

If disease of the adrenal glands themselves is suspected, the glands may be imaged by such techniques as *CT scanning, arteriography, radionuclide scanning,* or intravenous *pyelography* (which is more likely to show any downward displacement of the kidney by an adrenal gland tumor). If a tumor or overgrowth of a gland is present, it will usually be detectable by one of these techniques.

THE ADRENAL CORTEX

The adrenal cortex is made up of three distinct zones, visible under a microscope. The outermost zone secretes the hormone *aldosterone,* which inhibits the amount of sodium excreted in the urine, maintaining blood volume and blood pressure.

The inner and middle zones together secrete the hormones *hydrocortisone* (also called cortisol) and corticosterone, as well as small amounts of *androgen hormones* (hormones that stimulate the development of male sex characteristics). Hydrocortisone is the most important human corticosteroid, controlling the body's use of fats, proteins, and carbohydrates. Hydrocortisone and corticosterone also have the effect of suppressing inflammatory reactions in the body and also, to some extent, the activities of the *immune system.*

Like the other endocrine glands, the adrenal cortices secrete hormones directly into the blood; the amount is governed by other hormones made in the hypothalamus and pituitary.

The rate of hydrocortisone secretion, controlled by the release of *ACTH* (adrenocorticotropic hormone) by the pituitary gland, varies throughout the 24-hour cycle, being minimal at midnight, rising to a peak at around 6:00 AM, and then falling slowly during the day.

Emotion, stress, and injury are potent stimulators of ACTH and hydrocortisone release; without hydrocortisone, the body is unable to recover properly from stress.

THE ADRENAL MEDULLA

The adrenal medulla is closely related to nervous tissue and secretes the hormones *epinephrine* and *norepinephrine* in response to stimulation by sympathetic nerves. These nerves are most active at times of stress.

A

The release of these hormones into the circulation produces effects similar to sympathetic nerve stimulation. The heart rate and force of contraction increases so that more blood can be pumped around the body, and the airways of the lungs are widened to make breathing easier. The hormones constrict blood vessels in the intestines, kidneys, and liver, and widen blood vessels supplying the skeletal muscles. Consequently, more blood is supplied to the active muscles and less to the internal organs.

Adrenal hyperplasia, congenital

A rare disorder, present at birth, caused by the deficient production of the hormones *hydrocortisone* and *aldosterone* by the adrenal glands and overproduction of *androgen hormones* (male sex hormones).

CAUSES

Most cases result from a gene defect (see *Genetic disorders*), causing lack of an enzyme required by the adrenal cortex to make hydrocortisone. Instead, the materials normally used to make hydrocortisone are channeled into manufacturing androgens, which are produced to excess.

The disorder affects about one in 10,000 babies and is the most common cause of ambiguous genitals at birth.

SYMPTOMS

Symptoms, which vary considerably in severity, are caused by excess androgens and the deficiency of hydrocortisone and aldosterone.

In the most severe forms, a female infant is born with what appears to be a penis and scrotum. Within a few days, vomiting and dehydration occur. Similar symptoms occur in male babies except that the genitals appear normal.

In less severe cases, a considerable delay may occur before the syndrome is recognized. In girls, the clitoris may enlarge to form what appears to be a small penis, and other male characteristics develop, such as deepening of the voice and absence of menstruation at puberty. In boys, puberty may occur early. Untreated, the condition causes infertility in both sexes.

DIAGNOSIS AND TREATMENT

The diagnosis is suggested by the signs and symptoms at birth or later in childhood or adolescence and is confirmed by the measurement of corticosteroid hormones in the blood and urine. *Ultrasound scanning* will show the adrenals to be enlarged but with no tumor present.

Treatment consists of replacing the missing hormones. If the condition is recognized and treatment started early, normal sexual development and fertility usually follow. (See also *Hermaphroditism*; *Sex determination*.)

Adrenaline

See *Epinephrine*.

Adrenal tumors

Rare malignant or benign tumors within the adrenal gland that usually secrete hormones to excess.

Aldosterone-secreting and hydrocortisone-secreting tumors of the adrenal cortex cause, respectively, primary *aldosteronism* (also called Conn's syndrome) and *Cushing's syndrome*.

Excess secretion of epinephrine and norepinephrine from the adrenal medulla may be caused by two types of adrenal tumors—*neuroblastoma* or *pheochromocytoma*. The tumors cause *hypertension* (high blood pressure) and sweating attacks.

Surgical removal of a tumor, or even a whole adrenal gland, often results in cure of the conditions caused by the excess hormone secretion. (See also *Adrenal glands* disorders box.)

Adrenocorticotropic hormone

See *ACTH*.

Adrenogenital syndrome

See *Adrenal hyperplasia, congenital*.

Aerobic

Requiring oxygen to live and grow. Humans and almost all other forms of life are dependent on oxygen for "burning" foods to produce energy (see *Metabolism*). Because of this dependence, they are described as obligate aerobes. In contrast, many bacteria have fundamentally different metabolisms and thrive without oxygen (some of them are even killed by it); such microorganisms are described as *anaerobic*. There are also some bacteria and yeasts (called facultative aerobes) that flourish in oxygen but can also live without it.

Aerobics

Exercise in which the body is able to meet the muscles' increased demand for oxygen continuously during increased activity. Aerobic means "requiring air to live."

Oxygen is necessary to release energy from the body's stores of fat, glycogen (starchy storage material), and sugars. In aerobic exercises, a constant supply reaches the muscles.

Unexercised muscle

Unhealthy muscle   Fat deposits

Exercised muscle

Healthy muscle

Good flow of oxygen

Benefits of aerobic exercise
Regular aerobic exercise improves the condition of the muscles. The supply of blood-carrying oxygen to the muscles is increased and the cells' capacity to use oxygen is consequently enhanced.

During aerobic exercises, such as swimming, jogging, and cycling, the rate at which oxygen reaches the muscles keeps pace with the rate at which it is used up. Because of this continual replenishment, the activity can be sustained for long periods. In contrast, anaerobic exercises rely on a different series of biochemical reactions to obtain energy from the stores of sugar and fat in muscle. The waste products of anaerobic exercise are acidic and, as they accumulate in muscles, the muscles become fatigued. Brief high-intensity exercises are anaerobic and can be performed for only short periods.

BENEFITS OF AEROBIC EXERCISE

To benefit your health, aerobic exercises should involve the large muscles of the trunk, upper body, and legs and need to be performed continuously for 20 minutes at least three times a week.

When performed regularly, aerobic exercises improve stamina and endurance. They encourage the growth of capillaries (small blood vessels), thus improving the supply of blood to the cells. They also increase the size and number of mitochondria (the energy-producing part of muscle cells), thus improving the cells' capacity to use oxygen and increasing the amount of oxygen that the body can use in a given time.

The condition of the heart is also improved as the body becomes more fit. The heart rate becomes slower during both exercise and rest, the heart muscle becomes thicker and stronger, and the stroke volume (the amount of blood pumped with each beat) is increased. As a result of these changes, the heart must do less work to achieve the same level of efficiency.

For all-around fitness, which includes strength and suppleness, other types of exercise should be performed as well as aerobics. (See also *Exercise; Fitness.*)

Aerodontalgia
Sudden pain in a tooth brought on by a change in surrounding air pressure. Flying at a high altitude in a lowered atmospheric pressure can cause a pocket of air within the dental pulp chamber to expand and irritate the nerve in the root. Common sources of aerodontalgia are improperly fitted fillings, inadequately filled root canals, and the presence of pulpitis (inflammation of the pulp).

Aerophagia
Excessive swallowing of air. This can occur during rapid eating or drinking or it can be caused by anxiety. It may also be a deliberate action to relieve indigestion by inducing belching. After *laryngectomy* (surgical removal of the larynx), voluntary aerophagia is used to produce esophageal speech.

Affect
Inner feelings at a particular moment; mood. This Freudian term is sometimes used to describe the mood as perceived by another person. Normal affect varies according to personality and setting. A person whose responses to events seem flat—so that nothing excites, nothing angers—is said to have a shallow, flattened, or reduced affect; this characteristic may be a sign of a mental disorder (see *Affective disorders*).

Affective disorders
Mental illnesses dominated by a disturbance of affect (mood). Affective disorders include various degrees of *mania* (elation and excitement) and *depression*, as well as *manic-depressive illness* (swings of mood between the two). The disorders may be psychotic (involving loss of contact with reality) or neurotic (involving no loss of contact with reality) and are sometimes the result of another physical or psychiatric illness.

Affinity
The attraction between chemicals that causes them to bind together, as, for example, between an *antigen* (a protein that stimulates the body to produce antibodies against it) and an antibody (see *Immune response*). The term is also used in microbiology to describe a physical similarity between organisms (e.g., viruses); it is used in psychology to describe an attraction between two people.

Aflatoxin
 A poisonous substance produced by *ASPERGILLUS FLAVUS* molds, which contaminates stored foods, especially grains, peanuts, and cassava. Aflatoxin has been found to cause liver cancer in laboratory animals and is believed to be one of the factors responsible for the high incidence of this cancer in tropical Africa and Asia.

Afterbirth
Common name for the *placenta*, the structure that provides the link between the circulations of the woman and fetus.

Afterpains
Contractions of the uterus that continue after childbirth. Afterpains are normal and indicate that the uterus is shrinking as it should. They are common during the first few days after delivery and are particularly painful during breast-feeding. Afterpains disappear after a few days but may require analgesics (painkillers).

Agar
 An extract of certain seaweeds with properties similar to those of gelatin. Its full name is agar-agar. It is sold to soften and give bulk to feces in cases of constipation, and to relieve indigestion and heartburn because of its bland, soothing properties. It is also used as a gelling agent in media for growing bacterial *cultures*.

Age
Of medical significance in diagnosis and in determining treatment, age is usually measured chronologically (in terms of the period of time since birth). However, age can also be measured in terms of physical, mental, or developmental maturity.

PHYSICAL AGE
Physical age can be measured even before birth. The age of a fetus is measured in terms of gestational age. Estimation of gestational age is important in neonatal pediatrics for identifying those babies who are too small for their gestational age and who may have problems because of their low birth weight. Gestational age can be assessed from the date of the woman's last menstrual period and by the size of her pregnant uterus. More accurate determination is made by measuring the size of the fetus by *ultrasound scanning*. The gestational age of a newborn baby can be estimated to within about two weeks by physical examination.

Children vary greatly in the rate at which they develop and grow, but their physical age is a measure of maturity that provides a common scale of development that can be used throughout the long period of growth. In adults, physical age is difficult to assess other than through physical appearance. Physical age can be estimated after death by the state of certain organs, particularly by the amount of atheroma (fatty deposits) lining the arteries.

The most useful measure of physical development in children is bone age. Bone age measures how much the bones of a body area have matured, as seen on an X ray. Measures such as height and weight are less useful as age standards because they vary greatly among individuals of the same chronological age. In contrast, all healthy individuals reach the same adult level of skeletal maturity and each bone passes through the same sequence of changes of shape as it grows.

Assessment of bone age is particularly useful in investigating delayed puberty or *short stature* in children. A prediction of the final adult height can be made by the physician if the chronological age, bone age, and current height are known.

Dental age is another, though less useful, measure of physical maturity. It can be assessed by counting the number of teeth that have erupted (see *Eruption of teeth*), and by comparing the amount of dental calcification (as seen on X rays) with standard values in much the same way as bone age is measured.

MENTAL AND DEVELOPMENTAL AGE
Mental age is assessed by comparing scores achieved in intelligence or achievement tests with standard scores for different chronological ages (see *Intelligence tests*).

A young child's age can be expressed in terms of developmental level. Patterns of normal development have been described for children from birth to the age of 5 years in the fields of speech, vision, hearing, and motor skills (principally walking and delicate hand-eye coordination). Specific tasks in these fields are achieved at certain ages (see *Child development*).

Agenesis

The complete or partial absence at birth of an organ or component of the body, caused by failure of development in the embryo.

Agent

Any substance or force capable of bringing about a biological, chemical, or physical change. An agent can also be a person acting on behalf of someone else. (See also *Reagent*.)

Agent Orange

A preparation of the toxic chemical dioxin, used as a defoliant in the Vietnam War (see *Defoliant poisoning*).

Age spots

Blemishes that appear on the skin with increasing age. Most common are seborrheic warts, which are brown or yellow, slightly raised spots that can occur at any site and sometimes get caught on clothing. Also common in the elderly are freckles, keratoses (small, wartlike blemishes caused by overexposure to the sun), and De Morgan's spots (cherry angiomas), which are red, pinpoint blemishes that occur on the trunk.

Treatment is usually unnecessary for any of these age spots apart from keratoses, which may progress to skin cancer. Freezing the keratoses with liquid nitrogen is the usual treatment; they may also be removed surgically using a local anesthetic.

Most spots are harmless but any unexplained blemish, or one that grows rapidly or bleeds, should be seen by your physician because of the possibility of skin cancer.

Ageusia

Lack or impairment of the sense of taste (see *Taste, loss of*).

Aggregation

The clumping of blood cells. Aggregation of platelets (small, sticky blood particles) takes place when a blood vessel is damaged, forming the first stage of *blood clotting* and thus helping to plug the injured vessel. Aggregation, however, can also have adverse effects. It con-

tributes to the formation of atheroma (the fatty substance that accumulates inside arteries and causes *atherosclerosis*) and thrombi (blood clots), which can cause *thrombosis*.

In the treatment of disorders in which thrombosis plays a part—coronary heart disease, for example—drugs such as aspirin, dipyridamole, or sulfinpyrazone may be prescribed to reduce aggregation.

Aggression

A general term for a wide variety of acts of hostility that are outside the range of normal social behavior.

CAUSES

Among animals, aggression serves to protect the species by way of self-defense and in defense of food, territory, and the young. In humans, there seem to be other factors, perhaps based on the needs of prehistoric survival. Some see it as resulting from frustration, lack of affection, and the attitudes of parents; others consider it part of the creative urge.

EEG studies show changes in brain-wave patterns in people who are continuously aggressive. Aggression centers (for example, the amygdaloid area) have been described. Brain disease (such as a tumor) or head injury may sometimes result in aggressive behavior. Even so, such outbursts do seem to be related to events; the person does not start fights for no reason at all, but rather overreacts aggressively to problems.

Androgens, the male sex hormones, seem to promote aggression, whereas estrogen, the female sex hormone, actively suppresses it. Age is another factor, since aggression is more common in adolescence and the early 20s, but becomes increasingly rare the older people get. People truly do seem to mellow with age.

Psychiatric conditions associated with aggressive outbursts are *schizophrenia* (especially the catatonic and paranoid types), *antisocial personality disorder*, *mania*, and abuse of amphetamines or alcohol. *Temporal lobe epilepsy*, *hypoglycemia*, and *confusion* due to physical illness are other, less common, medical causes. *Dementia*, whether associated with *Alzheimer's disease* or *alcohol dependence*, may remove control of aggression.

Aging

The physical and mental changes that occur in a person over time. The aging process is sometimes seen as bringing with it only frailty and increased

vulnerability to disease and injury, but many societies value their old people for their wisdom and experience and recognize other virtues that often come with age (e.g., patience and acceptance).

BIOLOGICAL AGING

All animals have a finite life span, and the maximum for humans seems to have changed little since biblical times. Very few people live beyond 100 years, and the average life span in the absence of disease seems to be about 85 years.

Gerontologists have yet to agree on the biological processes that underlie aging. Among the many theories are the "worn template" concept—that every time cells divide, the copying mechanism is more likely to introduce errors; the accumulated toxins theory, according to which the body is gradually poisoned by the accumulation of chemicals it cannot excrete; and the immune surveillance theory, which postulates that there is a progressive decline in the immune system's ability to detect and destroy microorganisms and developing tumors.

Aging is associated with degenerative changes in various organs and tissues, such as the skin, bones, joints, blood vessels, and nervous tissue (see chart). These changes may be accelerated by factors such as smoking, excessive alcohol consumption, poor diet, insufficient exercise, and excessive exposure of the skin to strong sunlight.

Nevertheless, the provocative evidence of 90 year olds who have smoked and drunk alcohol all their lives shows that an important factor determining life expectancy is genetic. Just as a person's height is determined by the interaction of his or her diet with the genetic potential inherited from the parents, so life span depends to a large extent on heredity.

NORMAL CHANGES

As people age, they discover that their physical performance declines, although not by as much as is often believed. A 60 year old who has always exercised regularly may retain some 80 percent of the physical strength and stamina that he or she had at the age of 25. However, the natural decline in lung function limits exertion past the age of about 60. Wound healing and resistance to infection also decline.

Sexual activity past the age of 60 is variable. Prolonged abstinence tends to lead to loss of libido and potency, whereas those who have remained

THE PRACTICAL EFFECTS OF AGING

In the body, aging is associated with loss of elasticity in the skin, blood vessels, and tendons. There is also progressive decline in the functioning of organs such as the lungs, kidneys, and liver. Mechanical wear and tear causes cumulative damage to certain organ systems. Brain cells, specialized kidney units, and many other body structures are never replaced after they have reached maturity.

EFFECTS OF AGING

Organ or tissue	Natural effects	Accelerated by
Skin	Loss of elastic tissue causes skin to sag and wrinkle. Weakened blood capillaries cause skin to bruise more easily.	Exposure to sun; smoking.
Brain and nervous system	Loss of nerve cells leads to reduction in ability to memorize or to learn new skills. Reaction time of nerves increases, making responses slower.	Excessive consumption of alcohol and other drugs; repeated head trauma (for example, from boxing).
Senses	Some loss of acuity in all senses, mainly due to loss of nerve cells.	Overexposure to loud noise; smoking.
Lungs	Loss of elasticity with age, so that breathing is less efficient.	Air pollution; smoking; lack of exercise.
Heart	Becomes less efficient at pumping, causing reduced tolerance to exercise.	Excessive use of alcohol and cigarettes; a fatty diet.
Circulation	Arteries harden, causing poor blood circulation and higher blood pressure.	Lack of exercise; smoking; poor diet.
Joints	Pressure on intervertebral disks causes height loss; wear on hip and knee joints reduces mobility.	Athletic injuries; being overweight.
Muscles	Loss of muscle bulk and strength.	Lack of exercise; starvation.
Liver	Becomes less efficient in processing toxic substances in the blood.	Damage from alcohol consumption and virus infections.

Hip joint in young person
The X ray shows the rounded head of the thigh bone (femur) separated by cartilage from the surrounding hip socket.

Hip joint in elderly person
This X ray of an osteoarthritic hip shows almost complete degeneration and disappearance of the cartilage in the joint.

Elastic fibers

Young skin
The outer skin layer has an appreciable thickness. The deeper layers contain numerous collagen fibers, which give the skin elasticity.

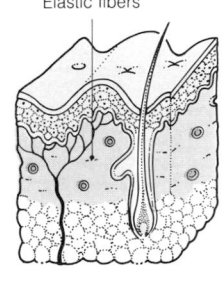

Older skin
The outer layer has become thinned, wrinkled, and prone to injury. There are fewer elastic fibers in the deeper layers.

sexually active often find little, if any, decline in their sex life.

As with physical performance, certain of our mental abilities inevitably deteriorate with age. Most people over 60 experience "benign forgetfulness," finding greater difficulty in such things as recalling names or telephone numbers. Many people find this change frightening, but, in fact, about 80 percent of people older than 80 are not demented.

AGING AND SOCIETY

In the twentieth century there have been dramatic changes in the age structure of Western societies because infant and childhood mortality has declined markedly. Today, few adults under the age of 50 die from natural causes (accidental death is now much more frequent in young adults than death from disease). The result has been a substantial increase in the proportion of people who live beyond the age of 65; the proportion living to beyond 75 continues to increase. However, today about one third of people older than 75 have some disability that restricts their daily lives in some way; improvements in preventive medicine are likely to bring about a decrease in this proportion in the future.

Agitation

Restless inability to keep still, usually due to underlying anxiety or tension. Agitated people may pace up and down, pluck at clothes or sheets, wring their hands, and start tasks without completing them. Because they cannot relax or concentrate, agitated people constantly repeat such aimless activities.

Agitation is usually caused by worry over a particular situation—a father anxiously awaiting the birth of his child, for example. Persistent agitation is also seen in *anxiety disorders*, especially when there is an underlying physical cause such as alcohol withdrawal. Depressive illness (see *Depression*) in older people is usually accompanied by severe agitation. Phenothiazines, antidepressants, and other drugs may also be a cause of the agitation.

A

Agnosia

An inability to recognize objects despite adequate sensory information about them reaching the brain via the eyes or ears or through touch. For an object to be recognized, the sensory information about it must be interpreted, which involves recall of memorized information about similar objects. Agnosia is caused by damage to areas of the brain involved in these interpretative and memory recall functions. The most common causes of such brain damage are *stroke* and *head injury*.

TYPES AND SYMPTOMS

Agnosia is usually associated with just one of the main sensations: vision, hearing, or touch. For example, an object may be recognizable by hearing and sight but not by touch. Some people, after a stroke that damages the right cerebral hemisphere, may seem unaware of any disability in their affected left limbs. This is called anosognosia or sensory inattention.

TACTILE AGNOSIA is an inability to recognize by touch alone objects that are placed in the hands, despite adequate sensation in the fingers.

VISUAL AGNOSIA is an inability to recognize and name objects despite normal vision. Affected people may be able to describe the color, shape, and size of an object but cannot name what they see or indicate its use.

AUDITORY AGNOSIA is an inability to recognize familiar sounds despite normal hearing.

OUTLOOK

There is no specific treatment for agnosia but some of the lost interpretative ability may return over time.

Agoraphobia

Fear of going into open spaces and of entering shops, restaurants, or other public places. The condition often overlaps with *claustrophobia* (fear of enclosed spaces), another *phobia*.

The thought of visiting a public place or mixing with many other people fills sufferers with such dread that they avoid going out as much as possible. Sufferers fabricate any of a number of excuses for their friends and family to remain at home. If they do venture out, they may have a *panic attack*, which leads to further restriction of their activities. Eventually, agoraphobics become completely housebound. People seek psychiatric treatment for agoraphobia more often than for any other phobia and are usually successfully treated by psychotherapy and antidepressants.

Agraphia

Loss of or reduced ability to write, despite normal function of hand and arm muscles, caused by damage to parts of the cerebrum (the main mass of the brain) concerned with writing.

CAUSES

Writing depends on a complex sequence of mental processes, including the selection of words, recall from memory of how these words are spelled, formulation and execution of the hand movements required, and visual checking that written words match their representation in the brain. These processes probably take place in a number of connected brain areas. Agraphia may be caused by damage to various parts of these areas (usually within the left cerebral hemisphere) and can be of different types and severity. The most common reasons for such damage are head injury, *stroke*, and *brain tumors*.

Agraphia rarely occurs on its own. It is often accompanied by *alexia* (loss of the ability to read) or may be part of an expressive *aphasia* (general disturbance in the expression of language).

TREATMENT AND OUTLOOK

There is no specific treatment for agraphia. Over time, following a stroke or other event that has caused brain damage, some of the lost writing skills may return.

Ague

An outdated term for malaria or other diseases causing fever in which the sufferer alternately feels excessively hot and shiveringly cold.

AIDS

A deficiency of the *immune system* due to infection with *HIV* (human immunodeficiency virus). In its present form, AIDS (acquired immune deficiency syndrome) appears to be new to the human population. As yet, there is no curative treatment and no vaccine for AIDS, but the symptoms and complications variably respond to antibiotics, antiviral agents, radiation therapy, and anticancer drugs.

INCIDENCE

AIDS is not present in all individuals who are infected with HIV. The proportion of those infected whose condition progresses to AIDS has varied widely in different countries and in different risk groups. Every year, AIDS will develop in between 1 and 5 percent of people infected with HIV, but there is some evidence that in a few infected people (less than 1 percent) both the virus and the antibodies

eventually disappear from the blood, suggesting that the body has fought off the infection.

Once AIDS has been diagnosed, the condition is considered fatal. By the end of the 1980s, close to 100,000 men, women, and children in the US had been diagnosed as having AIDS and about half of them had died.

The main risk groups are homosexual or bisexual men and people who inject themselves with drugs using unsterile needles and syringes. Many hemophiliacs also became infected in the early 1980s as a result of receiving infected blood products, but this route of infection is now closed by better screening of blood and treatment of blood products. Other risk groups include heterosexual contacts of infected individuals, children of infected women, and people who have received infected transfusions.

HISTORY

In 1981, the Centers for Disease Control (CDC) in Atlanta, Georgia, was alerted to reports of cases of a rare lung infection in previously healthy homosexual men in Los Angeles and then in New York. Infection was found to be with PNEUMOCYSTIS CARINII, a protozoan organism that had previously caused pneumonia only in patients with suppressed immune defenses.

Later, cases of a rare tumor (*Kaposi's sarcoma*) were reported in young homosexual men. Kaposi's sarcoma was recognized as a slow-growing skin tumor previously seen in Africa and also in the US, where it mainly affected elderly men. In the AIDS cases, the tumor behaved much more aggressively and was found in parts of the body besides the skin.

Soon it appeared that there was a rapidly increasing epidemic of conditions associated with depression of the immune system—most being *opportunistic infections* (i.e., infections that do not usually affect people with efficient immune defenses).

These conditions were observed not only in male homosexuals, but also in intravenous drug users and hemophiliacs, suggesting that transmission was related to blood as well as to sexual activity. An infective cause seemed likely and, in 1984, French and American researchers identified the responsible virus. It was named LAV (lymphadenopathy-associated virus) by the French and HTLV III (human T-cell lymphotropic virus, strain III) by the Americans. In 1986, the virus was renamed HIV.

A

CAUSES AND PREVENTION OF AIDS

AIDS is caused by the human immunodeficiency virus (HIV) (right), which consists of some nucleic acid (genetic material) inside two protective shells and an outer envelope. Full-blown AIDS develops in only some people infected with HIV.

Surface proteins
Outer envelope
Outer shell
Inner shell
Nucleic acid

HIV (the AIDS virus)
The electron micrograph at left shows a human immunodeficiency virus (HIV) particle erupting from an infected human lymphocyte (cell of the immune system).

HOW HIV (THE AIDS VIRUS) AFFECTS THE IMMUNE SYSTEM

In a person with a healthy immune system, various types of lymphocytes combat disease organisms.

In a person infected with HIV, the immune system is weakened; in some cases, this may lead to AIDS.

NORMAL IMMUNE SYSTEM

T4-lymphocytes
Disease organisms

1 Disease organisms entering the body alert T4-lymphocytes and other immune system components.

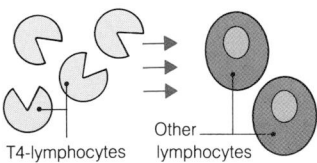

Other lymphocytes
T4-lymphocytes

2 The T4-lymphocytes help regulate the response of other lymphocytes (cells of the immune system).

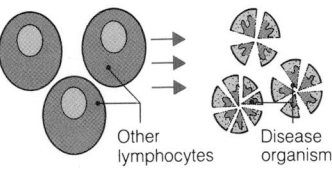

Other lymphocytes
Disease organisms

3 These lymphocytes then counterattack and destroy the disease organisms by various mechanisms.

IMMUNE SYSTEM IN AIDS VICTIM

HIV
T4-lymphocytes

1 HIV (the AIDS virus) multiplies within, and ultimately may destroy, the body's T4-lymphocytes.

Disease organisms
Destroyed T4-lymphocytes

2 When disease organisms invade, immune responses may fail, due to absence of the vital T4-lymphocytes.

Disease organisms

3 The disease organisms may then overwhelm the immune system and lead to the features of AIDS.

RECOMMENDATIONS FOR PREVENTING THE SPREAD OF AIDS

- Do not have sexual intercourse with persons known or suspected of having AIDS, with many people, or with people who have had many partners.

- Do not use intravenous (IV) drugs. If you use IV drugs, do not share needles or syringes.

- Do not have sex with people who use IV drugs.

- People with AIDS or who have had positive HIV antibody test results may pass the disease on to others and should not donate blood, plasma, body organs, other tissues, or sperm. They should not exchange body fluids during sexual activity.

- There is a risk of infecting (or being infected by) others through sexual intercourse, sharing needles, and, possibly, exposure of others to saliva through oral-genital contact or "wet" kissing. The effectiveness of condoms in preventing infection with HIV is not proved, but their consistent use may reduce transmission, since exchange of body fluids is known to increase risk.

- Toothbrushes, razors, or other implements that could become contaminated with blood should not be shared.

A

HOW AIDS HAS BEEN CONTRACTED IN THE US

Cases (%)

60%

Male homosexual activity
This has accounted for the most cases.

16%

Needle-sharing by drug abusers
The number of cases is increasing in this second largest group of AIDS victims.

3%

Received infected blood or blood product transfusions
This is no longer a significant mechanism of transmission in the US.

2%

Male-to-female sexual transmission
In the US, this has accounted for relatively few AIDS cases, but the percentage from this cause is rising.

2%

Female-to-male sexual transmission
Again, this has accounted for relatively few AIDS cases, but the percentage from this cause is rising.

1%

Mother-to-child via placenta
A baby born to a woman who has AIDS or who has tested positively for HIV antibodies has a high risk of being infected.

13%

Multiple risk factors
This group consists of victims with more than one risk factor—mainly homosexual males who have also shared needles.

3%

Other/unknown
This group, many of them hospital workers, contracted AIDS by another means (e.g., needle injury) or by unknown means.

NO-RISK ACTIVITIES

Touching
AIDS virus cannot be transmitted by social contact such as shaking hands.

"Dry" kissing
Kissing without exchange of saliva poses no risk of virus transmission.

Embracing
There is no risk of transmitting the virus by embracing or cuddling.

Sharing utensils
The virus cannot be transmitted by sharing a glass or cutlery.

Giving blood
Only sterile needles are used for taking blood from donors in the US.

Other contact
The virus cannot be caught from toilet seats or other objects.

THE EFFECTS OF THE VIRUS

The virus infects a cell known as the T4 or T-helper lymphocyte, which is crucial for the regulation of the immune mechanisms. The infected cell may die or the virus may remain dormant in the cell, with the possibility of reactivation later. Many infected individuals have no sign of disease; they are "asymptomatic carriers." Or they have vague complaints, such as weight loss, fevers, sweats, or unexplained diarrhea. People in this group have been referred to as having AIDS-related complex (ARC).

In its most severe form, HIV infection interferes with the immune system to make the individual susceptible to a variety of infections and cancers, such as Kaposi's sarcoma and lymphoid tumors (see *Lymphoma*).

METHODS OF TRANSMISSION

HIV has been isolated from blood, semen, saliva, tears, nervous system tissue, breast milk, and female genital tract secretions. However, only semen and blood have been proved to transmit infection.

The major methods of transmission are sexual contact (penis to anus, vagina, or mouth), blood to blood (through transfusions or needle sharing in addicts), and from woman to fetus. Other rare methods are through accidental needle injury, artificial insemination by donated semen, and kidney transplantation.

"Casual" or household spread does not occur. The infection is not spread by touching or hugging, by breathing the same air, or by sharing cutlery or crockery. Heterosexual transmission

does occur. By the late 1980s, this mode of transmission accounted for approximately 4 percent of all known cases in the US. In Africa, AIDS affects men and women equally; heterosexual transmission plays a more important role for unknown reasons.

SYMPTOMS AND SIGNS

Individuals infected with the virus may have no symptoms; others experience a short-lived illness, sometimes resembling infectious *mononucleosis*, when they first become infected. Medical examination of patients without symptoms may reveal abnormalities, most commonly lymph gland enlargement.

Minor features of HIV infection include skin disorders such as seborrheic *dermatitis* (skin inflammation particularly affecting the face). More severe features include marked weight loss, diarrhea, fever, and oral *candidiasis* (thrush).

Other infections that are more common or more severe in HIV-infected patients include *herpes simplex* infections, *shingles*, *tuberculosis*, salmonellosis, and shigellosis. HIV may also affect the brain, causing a variety of neurological disorders including dementia.

The features of full-blown AIDS include cancers, such as Kaposi's sarcoma and lymphoma of the brain, and infections, such as *pneumocystis pneumonia*, severe *cytomegalovirus* infection, *toxoplasmosis*, diarrhea caused by CRYPTOSPORIDIUM or ISOSPORA, candidiasis, disseminated *strongyloidiasis*, *cryptococcosis*, and chronic herpes simplex.

DIAGNOSIS

HIV infection may be suspected in someone with lymph gland enlargement or unexplained weight loss if the person is in a high-risk group.

Confirmation of HIV infection involves testing a blood sample for the presence of antibodies to HIV. Testing for the virus itself is more difficult. A positive HIV antibody test result indicates exposure to the virus; most antibody-positive individuals are virus carriers. Any positive reaction is rechecked by other tests for full confirmation. A negative test result may occur in someone who has very recently come into contact with the virus; a negative result should be followed by repeated testing after six months if the individual is at risk.

Diagnosis of full-blown AIDS is based on positive results for the HIV antibody test and Western blot (a confirmatory test), along with observation of the characteristic infections and tumors.

PREVENTION OF INFECTION

Until a cure or vaccine is found, prevention is the most important measure against AIDS. Risks can be reduced by practicing *"safe" sex*.

Anyone who feels that he or she may have been exposed to the virus can request a blood test, although it is wise to obtain counseling first on the advisability of the test and implications of the result. A person who knows that he or she has been infected should alter his or her sexual life-style to avoid transmitting the virus. An uninfected person should also adopt safe sex procedures to avoid becoming infected.

Safe sex techniques involve reducing the number of sex partners;

ideally sex should be restricted to partners whose sexual histories are known. Unprotected anal and vaginal intercourse should be avoided. Hugging, mutual masturbation, and "dry" kissing are safe. Saliva may contain the virus but is unlikely to be important in transmission; the risk of "wet" kissing with saliva exchange is unknown. If penile penetration occurs, a condom should be worn. Spermicidal jellies seem to inactivate the virus and should be used as lubricants. The risk of oral sex is not fully known, but ejaculation into the mouth should be avoided.

Intravenous drug users should avoid sharing needles to prevent spread of infection; their sexual partners may also be at risk.

In Africa, prostitutes show a high rate of infection. Although rates are much lower in the US, prostitutes are a potential means of spread. They should be encouraged to require use of condoms to protect themselves and their clients.

There is a small risk to hospital and other health workers when handling infected blood products or needles. The risk of transmission by needles in hospitals has, however, been lower than expected; it is minimized if care is taken with all procedures involving sharp instruments, including careful disposal of contaminated materials.

People in risk groups are advised against donating blood and semen. All donated blood, organs, and semen are screened for HIV antibodies.

TREATMENT

There is no cure for AIDS. Supportive treatment is available only for its complications. Pneumocystis pneumonia is treated with antibiotics (such as pentamidine or trimethoprim-sulfamethoxazole), but troublesome side effects often occur and the infection often recurs. Treatment of Kaposi's sarcoma by radiation therapy or anticancer drugs is rarely curative.

Several antiviral drugs, such as zidovudine (AZT) and acyclovir, are being used to treat patients with AIDS and those with HIV infection. Zidovudine has serious side effects, but it does slow the progression of HIV infection. Full assessment will come only after more patients have been treated for long periods.

OUTLOOK

Research is continuing on other methods of attacking the virus or halting its effects. In laboratory tests, several drugs have inhibited an enzyme essential for viral multiplica-

tion, but these drugs have failed in clinical trials or have been drastically limited by severe side effects.

While research into drug treatment for AIDS continues, the failure of medical science to achieve curative treatment for other viral infections makes anything approaching a cure unlikely in the near future.

Medical prevention is possible if a vaccine against HIV can be developed. A successful vaccine has been developed against feline leukemia virus, which bears similarities to HIV, so the technology for vaccine development is available and work is progressing with this intent.

AIDS-related complex

A combination of weight loss, fever, and enlarged lymph nodes in a person who has been infected with *HIV* (the *AIDS* virus), but does not actually have AIDS itself. Many people with AIDS-related complex (ARC) will eventually have the features of AIDS.

Air

The colorless, odorless mixture of gases that forms the Earth's atmosphere. Air consists of 78 percent *nitrogen*, 21 percent *oxygen*, small quantities of *carbon dioxide* and other gases, and some water vapor.

The balance among the various atmospheric gases is maintained largely by the mutual needs of animals and plants. Animals use oxygen and produce carbon dioxide as a waste product; plants use carbon dioxide and release oxygen in a process called photosynthesis. The level of carbon dioxide in the atmosphere is gradually increasing as a result of extensive deforestation and the large-scale burning of fossil fuels. This disturbance of the atmospheric balance is causing concern among scientists because of its potentially disastrous consequences for all life on this planet. (See also *Pollution*.)

Air conditioning

Any system that controls the purity, humidity, and temperature of the air in a building. Air conditioning is essential to the sanitation of hospitals, but is also important in maintaining hygienic conditions in hotels, offices, and other large buildings.

WHY IT IS USED

Air conditioning acts both on the air already in rooms and on air drawn in from outside, filtering out dust, pollen, smoke, bad smells, and excess moisture, and either cooling or heat-

A

ing the air to keep it at a comfortable temperature. In this way, air conditioning helps prevent heat disorders, such as *prickly heat*, headaches, nasal congestion, and chest disorders. By bringing in air from outside, which has been filtered and exposed to the antiseptic effect of ultraviolet light, air conditioning also reduces the risk of airborne infections and of allergies.

Hospital sterile units, used for nursing high-risk patients, have air conditioning units fitted with special bacterial filters that minimize the risk of spreading infection.

DISORDERS

Despite its generally beneficial effects, air conditioning may be responsible for certain disorders. For example, some outbreaks of *legionnaires' disease* (a type of pneumonia) have been linked to contaminated air conditioning systems; and humidifier fever (a lung disease that causes fever, coughing, and breathing difficulty) is thought to be caused by the spread of infectious microorganisms (usually fungi) by air conditioning. Air conditioning has also been blamed for some cases of *sick building syndrome*, which is attributed to the physical working environment; it produces headache, irritability, and loss of energy.

Air embolism

Blockage of a small artery by an air bubble brought to the site of obstruction by the flow of blood.

An air *embolism* is a rare event. The air usually has entered the blood circulation via a vein in the course of an injury or an accident during a surgical procedure. It can also occur as a result of a pressure accident (as can occur when scuba diving or flying), causing rupture of lung tissues and escape of the air bubbles.

Air pollution

See *Pollution*.

Air swallowing

See *Aerophagia*.

Airway

Collective term for the passages from the openings of the mouth and nose to the alveoli (air sacs in the lungs) through which air enters and leaves the lungs. The airway is made up of the nasal passages, oral cavity, upper part of the pharynx (throat), larynx (voice box), trachea (windpipe), bronchi (main airways in the lungs), and bronchioles (airways off the bronchi that end with the alveoli).

The term airway is also applied to an *endotracheal tube*, the artificial airway inserted into the trachea in a person who is under general anesthesia, and to the incision through the neck and into the trachea made in a *tracheostomy* operation. (See *Respiratory system*.)

Airway obstruction

Narrowing or blockage of the respiratory passages. The obstruction may be due to a foreign body, such as a piece of food, that becomes lodged in part of the upper airway and may result in *choking*. Certain diseases or disorders, such as *diphtheria*, affect the airway and can cause obstruction. Additionally, a spasm of the muscular walls of the airway, as occurs in *bronchospasm* (a feature of *asthma* and *bronchitis*), results in *breathing difficulty*. (See also *Artificial respiration*; *Lung* disorders box.)

Akathisia

An inability to sit still, occurring occasionally as a side effect of an *antipsychotic drug* used to treat mental disorders such as schizophrenia and depression. Less commonly, akathisia occurs as a complication of *Parkinson's disease* or as a manifestation of *hysteria*.

Akinesia

Complete or almost complete loss of movement. Akinesia may be due to paralysis (loss of power) in a group of muscles caused by damage to the nerves that supply them (for example, after a *stroke*). It may also occur in the presence of normal power but with rigidity (stiffness) of muscles (for example, in *Parkinson's disease*).

Albinism

A congenital condition (present from birth) characterized by a lack of the pigment melanin that gives color to the skin, hair, and eyes. Although rare, albinism occurs in all races. Affected individuals (albinos) suffer visual problems and a tendency to have skin cancers.

TYPES

In oculocutaneous albinism (the most common type), the hair, skin, and eyes are all affected. There are at least two main forms. In the more severe form, the skin and hair are snowy white throughout life (although the tips of the hairs may turn slightly yellow with age). In the less severe type, the skin and hair are white at birth but darken slightly with age, and numerous freckles develop on sun-exposed skin parts. In both forms, the

Appearance of albinism
The condition is caused by lack of melanin pigment in the skin, hair, and eyes.

Albinism in an African boy
Albinism is found in people of all races, although it occurs only rarely.

eyes are affected by *photophobia* (intolerance to bright light), *nystagmus* (abnormal flickering movements), and, frequently, *strabismus* (squint) and *myopia* (nearsightedness).

Other rare types of albinism affect only the skin and hair or the eyes.

CAUSES AND INCIDENCE

The gene defects responsible for the two main forms of oculocutaneous albinism show an autosomal recessive pattern of inheritance (see *Genetic disorders*). In most cases, the parents have normal skin coloring; they are carriers of the gene defect in a hidden form. If a normally pigmented couple has an albino child, any subsequent children generally have a one in four chance of also being affected.

The overall prevalence of oculocutaneous albinism is low in the US and Europe—less than five people per 100,000 are affected. The prevalence is much higher in certain parts of the world (for example, about 20 persons per 100,000 are affected in southern Nigeria).

COMPLICATIONS AND TREATMENT

SKIN The most serious complication of oculocutaneous albinism derives from the lack of melanin, which normally protects the skin against harmful radiation in sunlight. The skin cannot tan, ages prematurely, and is prone to cancers on sun-exposed areas (see *Skin cancer*).

EYES The visual problems of albinos, such as photophobia and nystagmus, can cause great difficulties, particularly with reading at school. Expert assessment and treatment should be sought at an early age; glasses are usually needed, preferably tinted to help reduce photophobia.

Albumin

The most abundant protein in the body. Albumin is made in the liver from amino acids that have been absorbed from digested protein in the small intestine.

Albumin has several important functions. It helps retain substances (such as calcium, some hormones, and certain drugs) in the circulation by binding to them and thereby preventing their being filtered out by the kidneys and excreted in the urine. Albumin is also important in regulating the movement of water between tissues and the bloodstream by *osmosis* (the attraction of water to an area with a higher concentration of salts or proteins). See also *Albuminuria*.

Albuminuria

The presence of the protein *albumin* in the urine; a type of *proteinuria*. Normally, the glomerulus (filtering part of the kidney) does not allow albumin to pass through it and into the urine, so albuminuria usually indicates a failure of the kidney's filtering mechanism. Such a failure may be due to a kidney disorder, such as *glomerulonephritis* or *nephrotic syndrome*, or it may be a sign that the kidneys have been damaged by *hypertension* (high blood pressure).

Albumin in the urine can be detected by a simple test, providing a valuable preliminary screening for kidney disease.

Albuterol

A *bronchodilator drug* used in the treatment of *asthma*, chronic *bronchitis*, and *emphysema* (a lung disorder). Albuterol relaxes the muscles in the bronchi and in the wall of the uterus. It is currently under investigation for use in the prevention of premature labor.

Alcohol

A colorless liquid produced from the fermentation of carbohydrates by yeast. Also known as ethanol or ethyl alcohol, alcohol is the active constituent of alcoholic drinks such as beer, wine, and spirits. In medicine, alcohol is used as an antiseptic and a solvent. *Methanol*, also known as methyl alcohol or wood alcohol, is a related substance obtained from distilling wood and is highly poisonous.

Alcohol is used by most adults in developed countries, where the number of women and young drinkers has greatly increased in recent years. Recently its use has become common in developing countries as well.

Any society where alcohol is freely used and available is invariably afflicted by the problems of acute alcohol intoxication (drunkenness), *alcohol dependence* (habitual, compulsive, long-term heavy drinking), and *alcohol-related disorders* including liver disorders, heart disease, *hypertension*, *neuropathy*, and *Wernicke-Korsakoff syndrome*. Alcohol is also an important factor in vehicular and industrial accidents, domestic violence, marriage breakdown, child abuse, and other types of crime.

EFFECTS

The effect of alcohol on the *central nervous system* (the brain and spinal cord) is as a depressant, decreasing its activity and thus reducing anxiety, tension, and inhibitions. Taken in moderate amounts, it gives the drinker a feeling of relaxation and confidence that may enable him or her to socialize more easily. However, any feeling of heightened mental and physical efficiency is illusory. Tests have shown that even a low level of alcohol in the blood slows reactions. The more alcohol drunk, the more concentration and judgment are impaired. At the same time, the drinker's confidence is increased—a potentially lethal combination while driving. If excessive amounts are drunk, poisoning or intoxication results, with effects ranging from euphoria to unconsciousness (see *Alcohol intoxication*).

In addition to significantly altering mood and behavior, alcohol has various other effects on the body. As a result of peripheral *vasodilation* (widening of the small blood vessels), the face becomes flushed and the drinker feels warm, although in fact a greater amount of body heat is lost. Small amounts of alcohol increase the flow of gastric juices and therefore stimulate the appetite and aid digestion—although large amounts over a long period can cause erosive *gastritis* (inflammation of the stomach lining with superficial, surface ulcers) and hematemesis (vomiting blood).

The quantity of urine passed increases (over and above that expected from the intake of drink), because the production of *ADH* (antidiuretic hormone) is inhibited. Heavy drinkers thus often become dehydrated; great thirst, a dry tongue, and a hangover may be associated with the effects of alcohol.

Finally, the effects of alcohol on sexual behavior are as summarized by William Shakespeare: "It provokes the desire but it takes away the performance."

TOLERANCE

Habitual drinkers acquire a tolerance to alcohol. This means that, to obtain the same effects, they gradually must increase the amount they drink. The liver breaks down alcohol at a faster rate, necessitating a greater intake to achieve the same level in the blood. At the same time, nerve cells in the brain become less and less responsive to a given amount of alcohol. Paradoxically, however, after years of drinking, many alcoholics experience a reduced tolerance.

Alcohol dependence

An illness characterized by habitual, compulsive, long-term, heavy consumption of alcohol and the development of withdrawal symptoms when drinking has stopped suddenly. The description "alcohol dependence" is generally preferred medically to "alcoholism," but the terms are virtually synonymous.

INCIDENCE

The incidence of alcohol dependence has been rising throughout the world for many years. Statistics on the extent of the problem are difficult to quote with any certainty. Rough estimates indicate there are approximately five million alcohol-dependent persons in the US (one in 50 of the population) and another seven million who have some trouble controlling their consumption of alcohol.

CAUSES

There is no single cause of alcohol dependence. Three causative factors interact in the development of the illness: personality, environment, and the addictive nature of the agent (i.e., the drug alcohol). Thus, if all other factors (such as the availability of alcohol) are equal, then inadequate, insecure, or immature personalities are more at risk than more emotionally mature individuals.

Inherited, genetic factors probably play a part in causing dependence in some cases but it is now widely

A

ALCOHOL AND THE BODY

Alcohol is a drug and, even in small amounts, its effects on the body are noticeable. Problems arise when people fail to take into account the effects of alcohol on tasks requiring coordination (such as driving), when they become intoxicated, or when they become dependent on the drug. Alcohol dependence can cause early death and is a major factor in crime, marital breakdown, child abuse, accidents, and absenteeism. Prolonged heavy drinking that stops short of dependence still may cause a wide variety of diseases, such as *cirrhosis* of the liver and *cardiomyopathy*.

Alcohol in blood
(milligrams per 100 milliliters)

Maximum legal driving limit (most states)

Time 12   2 PM   4 PM   6 PM   8 PM   10 PM

Cumulative effects of alcohol

It takes some time for the body to eliminate even small amounts of alcohol. For instance, if a person has two drinks at lunchtime and then has one or two more drinks early in the evening, his or her cumulative blood alcohol level could be over the legal limit for driving even though several hours have passed.

EFFECTS OF INCREASING BLOOD ALCOHOL LEVELS

Concentration (milligrams per 100 milliliters)	Observable effects
30–50	Flushed face, euphoria, talkativeness, increased social confidence
150–200	
50–150	Disturbed thinking and coordination, irritability, reduced self control, irresponsible talk and behavior
200–350	
150–250	Marked confusion, unsteady gait, slurred speech, unpredictable shows of emotion and aggression
350–500	
250–400	Extreme confusion and disorientation, difficulty remaining upright, drowsiness, delayed or incoherent reaction to questions progressing to coma (a state of deep unconsciousness from which the person cannot be aroused)
500–700	
400–500	Risk of death due to arrest of breathing (although habitual drinkers may survive even such high levels)
700+	

Occasional social drinker

Alcoholic/problem drinker

Alcohol levels in different drinks

Alcoholic drinks come in many forms and contain varying levels of pure alcohol. It can be very difficult to estimate alcohol intake because the strengths of drinks vary. The standard measures shown here contain approximately equal amounts of pure alcohol.

Beer	**Wine**	**Sherry**	**Whiskey**
8 ounces (5 percent)	4 ounces (10 percent)	2 ounces (20 percent)	1 ounce (40 percent)

LONG-TERM EFFECTS ON THE BODY

Persistent heavy drinking eventually damages body tissues; the main effects are shown below.

Liver
The liver is the main organ responsible for metabolizing alcohol from the blood; it manifests many of the long-term effects of heavy drinking. These effects include fatty liver, hepatitis, cirrhosis, and liver cancer.

Cirrhotic liver
In this condition, commonly caused by heavy drinking, bands of scar tissue form in the liver, impairing its function.

Brain and nervous system
Alcohol depresses the central nervous system. Prolonged alcohol abuse permanently impairs brain and nerve function.

Skin
Alcohol causes facial flushing, which becomes constant in heavy drinkers.

Heart and circulation
Prolonged heavy drinking can cause coronary heart disease, hypertension, heart failure, and stroke.

Digestive system
Irritation from large amounts of alcohol can cause gastritis and ulcers.

Urinary system
Alcohol acts as a diuretic, increasing urine output. Prolonged heavy drinking can cause renal failure.

Reproductive system
Alcohol increases sexual confidence, but high levels cause impotence.

A

DEATHS FROM ALCOHOL-RELATED CAUSES IN THE US (1980–1983)

Cause	Deaths	1980	1981	1982	1983
Alcoholic cirrhosis of liver		9,166	8,567	7,893	7,571
Alcohol dependence		4,350	4,207	3,914	4,002
Alcoholic liver damage		1,812	1,782	1,752	1,753
Alcoholic fatty liver		1,166	951	961	1,027
Alcohol abuse		889	771	768	835
Acute alcoholic hepatitis		794	785	687	725
Alcoholic cardiomyopathy		650	647	664	711
Alcohol psychosis		454	453	389	346
Toxic effects of alcohol		385	384	412	341
Total		19,666	18,547	17,440	17,311

This table lists deaths that are known to be wholly attributed to a specific alcohol-related cause. Many other causes are omitted because they are only partly related to alcohol consumption. The most obvious omissions are fatalities suffered as a result of motor vehicle accidents. Alcohol also often contributes to accidents in the home.

believed that any person, irrespective of environment, genetic background, or personality, can become alcoholic if he or she drinks heavily for a prolonged period.

Environmental factors are important, especially the ready availability, affordability, and widespread social acceptance of alcohol in the individual's national culture and among the people he or she associates with at work and during leisure hours. Thus alcoholism is much more common in certain countries, occupations, and social groups than in others.

Stress is another important factor. Many formerly moderate drinkers begin to drink excessively at times of bereavement. Women may turn to drink when their adolescent children leave home. Hormonal factors may also play a role in heavy drinking among women.

Once social and/or psychological factors have induced heavy drinking, the discovery that taking alcohol in the morning relieves the withdrawal symptoms induced by the previous night's drinking tends to accelerate the development of dependence.

ALCOHOL AND PREGNANCY

The damage that alcohol can cause a fetus has been recognized only recently. Drinking more than two drinks per day (for example, two 1-ounce glasses of spirits, two 4-ounce glasses of wine, or two 8-ounce glasses of beer) increases the chance of *fetal alcohol syndrome*. This disorder consists of facial abnormalities such as *cleft lip and palate*, heart defects, abnormal limb development, and lower-than-average intelligence. This level of drinking also increases the risk of miscarriage. Occasional binge drinking may cause the same effects even if the mother drinks little otherwise. Because a proportion of the alcohol from any drink reaches the baby, there is a risk that drinking even small amounts may disrupt normal development (causing, for example, low birth weight).

Fetal alcohol syndrome
An affected baby is abnormally short, has small eyes and a small jaw, and may have heart defects or a cleft lip and palate. He or she may suck poorly, sleep badly, and be irritable.

DEVELOPMENT OF DEPENDENCE

The development of alcohol dependence can be divided into four main stages, which merge imperceptibly. The time scale of these changes may be from five to 25 years, although the average is about 10 years.

In the first phase, tolerance (being able to drink more alcohol before experiencing its ill effects) develops in the heavy social drinker. Entering the second phase, the drinker experiences memory lapses relating to events occurring during the drinking episodes. The third phase is characterized by loss, or lack, of control over alcohol; the drinker can no longer be certain of discontinuing drinking whenever he or she wants to. The final phase starts with prolonged binges of intoxication, with the drinker suffering observable mental or physical complications.

Some people halt their consumption, temporarily or permanently, during one of the first three phases.

SYMPTOMS AND EFFECTS

BEHAVIORAL SYMPTOMS are varied and can include any combination of the following: furtive behavior (such as hiding bottles); aggressive or grandiose behavior; personality changes (such as irritability, jealousy, uncontrolled anger, selfishness); frequent change of jobs; constant promises to self and others to give up drinking; changes in drinking pattern (for example, switching to early-morning drinking, or changing from beer to spirits); neglect of food intake and personal appearance; and lengthy periods of intoxication.

PHYSICAL SYMPTOMS can also be varied. The drinker may exhibit any of the following: nausea, vomiting, or shaking in the morning; abdominal pain; cramps; numbness or tingling; weakness in the legs and hands; irregular pulse; redness and enlarged capillaries in the face; unsteadiness; confusion; poor memory; and incontinence. After sudden withdrawal of alcohol, the dependent person may experience *delirium tremens* (severe shakes, hallucinations, and convulsions).

In addition, alcohol-dependent persons are more susceptible than others to a wide variety of specific physical and mental diseases and disorders (see *Alcohol-related disorders*).

Combinations of physical, mental, personality, and often financial stresses lead to difficulties at work and at home for the alcoholic. Often, the person's marriage suffers. Suicide threats and attempts may occur.

A

PREVENTION

Steps for avoiding the development of alcohol dependence include the following: keep to safe limits of alcohol intake as recommended by medical authorities; drink slowly instead of gulping; and never drink for relief of anxiety, tension, or depression, or on an empty stomach. No person should ever feel embarrassed about refusing an alcoholic drink.

TREATMENT

Many alcoholics require detoxification (medical help in getting over their physical withdrawal symptoms when they stop drinking). Detoxification is followed by long-term treatment. No single form of treatment is best for all alcoholics. Sometimes psychological, social, and physical treatments may be combined.

PSYCHOLOGICAL TREATMENTS involve *psychotherapy* and are now commonly and more reasonably carried out in groups (see *Group therapy*). There are various types of group therapy, using different techniques.

SOCIAL TREATMENTS include help with problems at work and, in particular, the inclusion of family members in the treatment process.

PHYSICAL TREATMENT is needed only by some alcoholics. It generally includes the use of disulfiram, a drug that sensitizes the drinker to alcohol so that he or she is afraid to drink because of unpleasant symptoms.

Alcoholics are strongly advised to use the self-help fellowship of organizations (i.e., *Alcoholics Anonymous*), where the alcoholic greatly benefits from meeting fellow sufferers who share their experiences.

Alcoholics Anonymous

A worldwide fellowship of people who readily admit to being alcoholics and who help each other stay sober. Alcoholics Anonymous (AA) was started in 1935 in the US and now consists of an estimated 67,000 local groups and over 1.5 million members in 92 countries. In the US alone there are more than 1 million members, with at least one group in all but the smallest towns and several groups in large cities. Contact addresses can be found in telephone directories.

Membership is open to anyone who has a drinking problem and has a desire to become and/or to continue to stay sober. There is no membership fee; the organization relies on voluntary contributions from members. Members are of all races, nationalities, and occupations, and range from

people whose health, careers, and relationships were totally destroyed by alcoholism to those who sought help at a much earlier stage of the illness. AA is not affiliated with any sect, political party, institution, or other organization. It has a policy of cooperation with other organizations that fight alcoholism.

Local AA meetings are of two types. At open meetings, which anyone (including members' families) can attend, speakers describe their lives as alcoholics and the effect AA has had in helping them refrain from drinking. At closed meetings, which only members can attend, new members are invited to describe their drinking problems and their difficulties abstaining. Other members who have had the same experiences suggest methods of staying sober and ways in which other problems can be surmounted. A program of recovery is suggested. Many members find that helping other alcoholics is the best way to remain sober themselves.

Members of AA do not reveal the names of other members to people outside AA. The fellowship does not keep membership records, monitor or attempt to control its members, engage or sponsor research on alcoholism, dispense drugs or psychiatric treatment, or provide detoxification, nursing, social services, or vocational counseling.

Alcohol intoxication

The common condition, also known as drunkenness, that results from drinking an excessive amount of alcohol over a relatively short period (usually about 30 minutes to several hours). Alcohol causes acute poisoning if taken in sufficiently large amounts. It depresses the activity of the central nervous system (the brain and spinal cord), leading to loss of normal mental and physical control. In extreme cases, a person who drinks a large amount of alcohol over a short period may lose consciousness and even die.

SYMPTOMS

The effects of a large alcohol intake depend on many factors, including physical and mental state, body size, social situation, and acquired tolerance (see *Alcohol*). Thus, a person may become "jocose, lachrymose, bellicose, or comatose" (cheerful, tearful, argumentative, or unconscious). There are wide individual variations. The important factor, however, is the blood alcohol level (see chart).

TREATMENT

For intoxication that stops short of coma, no treatment is required. Recovery takes place naturally as the alcohol in the person's body is gradually broken down.

If a drinker lapses into a coma, medical attention should be sought, particularly if the person is known or suspected to be diabetic or to have been taking another drug, whether prescribed by a physician (such as a sedative) or illicit (such as cocaine) in addition to alcohol. The person's clothing should be loosened and the mouth and back of the throat checked to make sure there is no obstruction to breathing. No attempt should be made to make the person drink water or make him or her vomit. If breathing stops, *artificial respiration* should be carried out until breathing restarts or medical help arrives.

For the chronic mental, physical, and social effects of long-term heavy drinking, see *Alcohol dependence* and *Alcohol-related disorders*.

Alcoholism

See *Alcohol dependence*.

Alcohol-related disorders

Apart from the many health and social problems that may result from *alcohol dependence*, and the high accident rate associated with *alcohol intoxication*, people who consume large quantities of alcohol are susceptible to numerous physical and mental disorders.

Alcohol consumption can lead to tissue damage and disease by any, or a combination, of three main mechanisms. First, alcohol or its breakdown products from metabolism can have a direct toxic or irritant effect on cells and tissues. Second, many alcoholics eat little or no nutritious food—alcohol satisfies their calorie requirements and at the same time reduces appetite through an irritant effect on the stomach. However, it provides no protein, vitamins, or minerals. Consequently, chronic alcoholics are prone to diseases caused by nutritional deficiency, particularly deficiency of *vitamin B_1* (thiamine).

Third, a continual high level of alcohol in the blood and tissues can cause wide-ranging disturbances in body chemistry. These disturbances can lead to *hypoglycemia* (reduced glucose in the blood) and *hyperlipidemia* (increased fat), which may contribute to malfunction and disease of such organs as the heart, liver, and blood vessels.

ALCOHOL-RELATED DISORDERS

Cancer	High alcohol consumption increases the risk of cancers of the mouth, tongue, pharynx (back of the throat), larynx (voice box), and esophagus, probably due to irritant action. In each of these cancers, alcohol	consumption along with smoking produces a much higher total risk of cancer than the sum of their separate risks. The risk of *liver cancer*, along with most types of liver disease, is also higher among alcoholics.
Liver damage and disease	Liver diseases caused by a high alcohol consumption include *fatty liver*, alcoholic *hepatitis*, *cirrhosis*, and liver cancer. They develop in sequence over a period of years. It is thought that a breakdown product of alcohol (acetaldehyde) has a toxic effect on liver cells and is the main cause of these diseases, although nutritional deficiency may also play some part.	The risk of alcoholic hepatitis and cirrhosis developing increases in proportion to the amount of alcohol consumed and the number of years of high consumption; liver cancer develops in about one in five sufferers of cirrhosis. However, about one third of heavy drinkers never get liver disease and in another third, only a fatty liver develops.
Nervous system disorders	Thiamine (vitamin B₁) deficiency, also known as *beriberi* (which disturbs nerve functioning), may develop in alcoholics. The effect of severe deficiency on the brain produces *Wernicke's encephalopathy*, with symptoms such as confusion, disturbances of speech and gait, and eventual coma. *Korsakoff's*	*psychosis* may also occur. The effect on the peripheral nervous system (nerve pathways outside the brain and spinal cord) produces polyneuropathy, with symptoms such as pain, cramps, numbness, tingling, and weakness in the legs and hands. Injections of thiamine and resumption of a normal diet can produce a dramatic cure.
Heart and circulatory disorders	Severe thiamine deficiency in alcoholics can cause *heart failure* (reduced pumping efficiency of the heart), usually combined with *edema* (fluid collection in the tissues). A high alcohol consumption also	increases the risk of coronary heart disease, of *hypertension* (high blood pressure) and of suffering a *stroke*. Heavy drinkers of certain beers risk *cardiomyopathy*.
Other physical disorders	Other physical diseases and disorders associated with a high alcohol consumption include *gastritis*, *pancreatitis*, and *peptic ulcer*, all probably linked	to an irritant action of alcohol. Heavy drinking during pregnancy carries a risk of the baby being born with *fetal alcohol syndrome*.
Psychiatric illnesses	Alcoholics are more likely than others to suffer from *anxiety* and *depression* (frequently related to financial, work, or family problems) and from paranoia. They are also more likely to	have *dementia* (irreversible mental deterioration) develop. The incidence of *suicide* attempts and actual suicide is also higher among alcoholics.

Alcohol, rubbing

A liquid preparation, consisting mainly of ethyl alcohol, that has a soothing and hardening effect when applied to the skin. It is widely used before injections as an *antiseptic* and may also be used to prevent bedsores and to protect the soles of the feet before a long walk or run.

Aldosterone

A hormone secreted by the adrenal cortex (part of the adrenal gland) that is important in the control of blood pressure and the regulation of sodium and potassium concentration.

Aldosterone acts on the kidney to decrease the amount of sodium lost in the urine; the sodium is reabsorbed from urine before it leaves the kidney and replaced in the urine by potassium. The sodium carries water with it, increasing the blood volume and raising the blood pressure.

The production of aldosterone is stimulated mainly by the action of *angiotensin* II, a chemical produced by the enzyme renin released by the kidneys. Its production is stimulated by the action of *ACTH*, produced by the pituitary gland.

Aldosteronism

A disorder caused by the excessive production of the hormone *aldosterone*. It can be caused by a tumor of the adrenal gland (called Conn's syndrome) or by a disorder that has reduced the flow of blood through the kidney, which leads to overproduction of *renin* and angiotensin, and, in turn, to excessive aldosterone production. *Heart failure* and *cirrhosis* of the liver can cause reduced blood flow through the kidney.

SYMPTOMS
Symptoms are directly related to the actions of aldosterone. Too much sodium is retained in the body, leading to elevated blood pressure; at the same time, excess potassium is lost in the urine. The low potassium level causes tiredness and muscle weakness and impairs kidney function, leading to overproduction of urine and thirst due to fluid loss.

DIAGNOSIS AND TREATMENT
The diagnosis is suggested by a combination of *hypertension*, a raised level of sodium in the blood, and a low level of potassium.

Treatment in all cases includes restriction of salt in the diet and use of the diuretic drug spironolactone. This drug blocks the action of aldosterone on the kidneys, leading to increased loss of sodium from the body, lowered blood pressure, and reduced loss of potassium. With Conn's syndrome, the tumor may be surgically removed.

Alexia

Word blindness; the inability to recognize and name written words, thus severely disrupting the ability to read in a person who was previously literate. The disability is caused by damage (e.g., by a *stroke*) to part of the cerebrum and is a much more severe reading disability than *dyslexia*.

Alienation

Feeling like a stranger, even when among familiar people or places, and being unable to identify with a culture, family, or peer group. Alienated people feel unhappy and uncertain and may turn to unusual religions or alternative life-styles in their search for the meaning of life.

Deprived groups such as immigrants or the poor may feel distanced from the society in which they live as a result of cultural differences, language difficulties, or financial problems. Alienation is also a common feeling among adolescents, made worse by parental neglect or friction, and is sometimes an early symptom of *schizophrenia* or part of a *personality disorder*. Feelings of alienation are thought to be a contributing cause of suicide, attempted suicide, and inner-city violence.

Alignment, dental
The movement of teeth by braces or fixed *orthodontic appliances* to correct *malocclusion* (incorrect bite).

Alimentary tract
The tubelike structure that extends from the mouth to the anus (see *Digestive system*). It is also known as the alimentary canal.

Alkali
Also known as a base, an alkali is chemically defined as a donor of hydroxyl ions (an atom of hydrogen linked to an atom of oxygen and having an overall negative electrical charge). Alkalis include a variety of substances, some of which are corrosive. Examples of alkalis include caustic soda (sodium hydroxide); lime (calcium oxide); various bicarbonates, such as bicarbonate of soda; and *antacids*, such as aluminum hydroxide, used to neutralize stomach acid in the treatment of peptic ulcers. (See also *Acid*; *Acid-base balance*; *Burns*.)

Alkaloids
A group of nitrogen-containing substances isolated from plants for use as a drug (for example, *morphine*, *codeine*, and *nicotine*) or as a poison (for example, strychnine).

Alkalosis
A disturbance of the body's *acid-base balance* in which there is an accumulation of alkali (base) or loss of acid.
CAUSES
There are two types of alkalosis: metabolic and respiratory. In the former, the increase in alkalinity may be caused by taking too much antacid or by losing a large amount of stomach acid as a result of severe vomiting.

Respiratory alkalosis is caused by a reduction in the level of carbon dioxide in the blood (carbon dioxide dissolves in the blood to form carbonic acid). This reduction is caused by *hyperventilation* (deep, fast breathing), which may occur during a panic attack or at high altitudes as a result of lack of oxygen. (See also *Acidosis*.)

Allergist
A physician who diagnoses and treats any form of *allergy*. The allergist conducts tests to determine the agents to which a person is allergic. Once the offending agent or agents have been identified, the allergist can recommend ways to avoid exposure, may attempt to build up the patient's immunity through inoculations of tiny amounts of the allergen, and may put the patient on a regimen of medication to control the reactions.

Allergy
A collection of disease symptoms caused by exposure of the skin to a chemical, of the respiratory system to particles of dust or pollen, or of the stomach and intestines to a particular food, which in the majority of people causes no symptoms.

Allergies are inappropriate or exaggerated reactions of the *immune system* and occur only on second or subsequent exposures to the offending agent, after the first contact has sensitized the body. Many common illnesses, such as *asthma* and allergic *rhinitis* (hay fever), are caused by allergic reactions.
TYPES AND CAUSES
The function of the immune system is to recognize *antigens* (foreign proteins) contained on the surfaces of microorganisms (such as viruses and bacteria) and to form *antibodies* (also called immunoglobulins) and sensitized white blood cells (called *lymphocytes*) that will interact with these antigens when next encountered, leading to destruction of the microorganisms.

In allergies, a similar process occurs, except that the immune system forms antibodies or sensitized lymphocytes against harmless substances—because these allergens (as they are called) are misidentified as potentially harmful antigens.

The inappropriate or exaggerated reactions seen in allergies are termed *hypersensitivity* reactions and can have any of four different mechanisms (termed Types I through IV hypersensitivity reactions). Most well-known

allergies are caused by the Type I variety (also known as anaphylactic or immediate hypersensitivity).
TYPE I HYPERSENSITIVITY REACTIONS Common allergens that can cause Type I reactions include flowers, grasses, and tree pollens, animal dander (tiny particles of skin and hair), house dust, house-dust mites, yeasts, certain drugs and foods, and constituents of bee and wasp venom. Of the food allergens, the most common are milk, eggs, shellfish, dried fruits, nuts, and certain food dyes.

These allergens provoke the immune system to produce specific antibodies, belonging to a type called immunoglobulin E (IgE), which coat cells (called mast cells or basophils) present in the skin and the lining of the stomach, lungs, and upper respiratory airways. When the allergen is encountered for the second time, it binds to the IgE antibodies and causes granules in the mast cells to release several different chemicals, which are responsible for the symptoms of the allergy.

Among the chemicals released is histamine, which causes blood vessels to widen, fluids to leak into tissues, and muscles to go into spasm. Symptoms may be restricted to the skin (itchy swelling or rash), upper airways (inflammation or mucus secretion, sneezing in hay fever, and spasm and narrowing of the airways in asthma), eyes (inflammation), or stomach and intestines (vomiting and diarrhea). Or the symptoms may affect several organs, especially when the allergies are to injected drugs, insect venom, or some foods. Particular illnesses associated with Type I reactions include asthma, hay fever, *urticaria* (hives), *angioedema*, *anaphylactic shock* (a severe, generalized allergic reaction), possibly atopic *eczema*, and many types of food allergy producing immediate symptoms.
TYPES II THROUGH IV HYPERSENSITIVITY REACTIONS These reactions have different mechanisms from Type I reactions (see *Hypersensitivity*) and are less often implicated in allergies. However, Type III reactions are responsible for a type of lung disease called allergic *alveolitis* (which includes *farmers' lung*) and for the skin swellings that occur after booster vaccinations. Type IV reactions are responsible for contact *dermatitis* (a rash caused by contact with substances such as nickel, elastic, detergents, and cosmetics).

It is not known why certain individuals and not others get allergies,

ALLERGY AND THE BODY

An allergy is an inappropriate response (causing troublesome symptoms) to substances that, in most people, cause no response. The response is mainly to harmless substances that come in contact with the skin, respiratory airways, or the eye's surface. In diagnosing an allergy, the individual's medical history is important. The physician needs to know whether the symptoms vary according to the time of day or the season, and whether there are any pets or other likely sources of allergens in the home.

THE MOST COMMON ALLERGENS

Airborne		Foods	
	Grass pollens		Dairy products
	Tree pollens		Eggs
	Spores from molds		Strawberries
	House-dust mites		Fish and shellfish
	Animal dander		Cereals

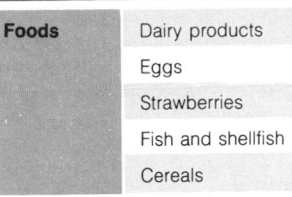

Pollen
Airborne pollen from plants (especially from grasses and trees) may trigger an allergic reaction; symptoms appear during the warmer months. The most common reaction is allergic rhinitis (hay fever), which occurs when pollen is breathed in and irritates the nasal lining.

Animal dander
It is often assumed that allergy results from contact with animal hair. In fact, allergy is caused by flakes of dead skin (dander).

Feathers
Bedding containing feathers may produce an allergic reaction. Instead, use pillows and quilts containing synthetic stuffing.

Mites in house dust
Fragments of mites and their feces in house dust may cause an allergic reaction. Keeping the house dust-free helps.

DIAGNOSING SKIN ALLERGY

Tests are performed to identify specific reactions to allergens. Small amounts of various substances are applied to the skin. A wheal indicates sensitivity to a particular allergen.

Conducting a patch test
Three different allergens are put on a patch (above left) and taped to the skin.

Results are (above right): no reaction; mild inflammation; severe contact dermatitis.

THE ORIGIN OF AN ALLERGY

The immune system is sensitized when it is exposed to an allergen (steps 1 to 3). Symptoms occur when allergens are met again (step 4).

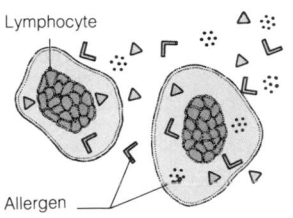

Lymphocyte

Allergen

1 Allergens enter the body and are recognized by lymphocytes (blood cells that form part of the body's immune system).

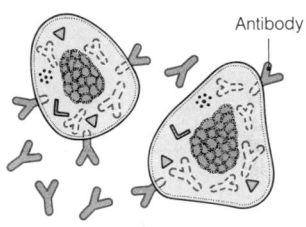

Antibody

2 A few days to weeks later, the lymphocytes produce antibodies specific to the allergens.

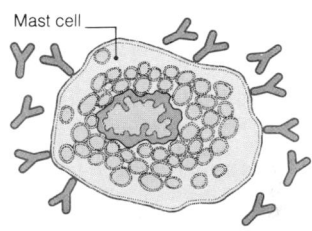

Mast cell

3 The antibodies attach to cells in the tissues called mast cells, which contain granules of histamine.

Allergens

Histamine

4 Binding of allergens to antibodies on the surface of mast cells leads to the release of histamine and to the symptoms of allergy.

although about one person in eight seems to have an inherited predisposition to have allergies (see *Atopy*).

Certain mild deficiencies of the immune system are associated with allergy. Environmental conditions are sometimes involved; a child living in a house with a cat or dog may slowly become sensitized to the pet and an allergic reaction such as hives or asthma may develop. Exposure to some viruses may precipitate or increase allergic responses. Emotional factors are also thought to contribute to allergic diseases such as asthma.

TREATMENT

Immunotherapy can be valuable for people who suffer allergic reactions to insect venom, house-dust mites, and some pollens. Gradually increasing doses of the allergen are given to promote the formation of antibodies that will then block future adverse reactions. The therapy is effective in about two thirds of the cases, but usually requires two to three years of treatment. It can produce mild side effects, such as itching, swelling, or rashes; occasionally, more serious side effects occur, such as bronchospasm or anaphylactic shock. Low-dosage, long-acting methods of desensitization are being researched.

Drug treatment for allergic reactions includes the use of *antihistamine drugs*, which relieve the symptoms (the itching produced by an insect bite, for example). Most available antihistamine drugs are sedative, which is particularly useful in treating the itching due to eczema because they permit the sufferer to sleep more soundly. Several of the newer antihistamines do not cause drowsiness.

Other drugs, such as cromolyn sodium and *corticosteroid drugs*, can be taken regularly to prevent symptoms from developing. Corticosteroid creams are useful for treating eczema, but prolonged use on the same area can damage the skin. In severe allergic diseases, such as asthma, the use of oral corticosteroids may be necessary.

Whenever possible, the most effective treatment for allergy of any kind is avoidance of the relevant allergen. For example, anyone with an allergy to eggs should avoid eating eggs or any dishes containing eggs as an ingredient, and should check the recipes of dishes consumed in restaurants or at parties. If pollen is the allergen, it may be harder to avoid; measures such as keeping car windows closed while driving and closing bedroom windows at night afford some protection.

Allopathy

A term that describes conventional medicine as practiced by a graduate of a medical school or college granting the MD degree. (See also *Homeopathy*.)

Allopurinol

A treatment for *gout* that works by reducing *hyperuricemia* (raised levels of uric acid in the blood). Allopurinol does not relieve pain in acute attacks but does reduce their frequency.

POSSIBLE ADVERSE EFFECTS

These include itching, rash, and nausea. Occasionally, during the first few months of treatment, allopurinol increases the frequency of gout attacks. *Colchicine* may be prescribed to counteract this effect.

Alopecia

Loss or absence of *hair*, which is usually noticeable only on the scalp but which may occur at any hair-bearing site on the body.

TYPES

HEREDITARY ALOPECIA This includes male pattern baldness, the most common form of alopecia. Normal hair is lost initially from the temples and crown, where it is replaced by fine, downy hair. The affected area gradually becomes wider as the line of normal hair recedes. This pattern of hair loss is inherited; it usually affects men, although young women and women who have passed the menopause are occasionally affected.

Stages in male pattern baldness
In this common form of alopecia, the man loses hair first from the temples and from the crown; the bald area then gradually widens.

Other hereditary forms of hair loss are rare. They may be due to an absence of hair roots or to abnormalities of the hair shaft, causing it to snap under the normal effects of sun, wind, shampooing, and combing.

GENERALIZED ALOPECIA In this rare form of alopecia, the hair falls out in large amounts, leaving a nearly invisible covering over the entire scalp. Such hair loss occurs because all the hairs simultaneously enter the resting phase and then fall out about three months later. Regrowth occurs when the cause is corrected.

Causes include various forms of stress, such as an operation, fever, prolonged illness, or *chemotherapy*.

LOCALIZED ALOPECIA This may be due to permanent damage to the skin—for example, by burns or *radiation therapy*. Another common cause of hair loss is trauma to the hair roots. Trauma may be due to excessive pulling of the hair to produce a particular hairstyle or, rarely, to a nervous disorder in which sufferers pull out their hair.

Fungal infection of the scalp (see *Tinea*) may cause a localized hair loss due to breakage of weakened hair shafts. Other skin diseases, such as *lichen planus, lupus erythematosus*, and *skin tumors*, may also be responsible. The bald skin always looks abnormal in conditions such as these and hair stubble can usually be seen in the affected area.

Alopecia areata is a disorder characterized by localized areas of hair loss in which the bald skin looks and feels normal. The cause is unknown.

Alopecia universalis is a rare, permanent form of alopecia areata that causes all the hair on the scalp and the body to be lost, including the eyelashes and eyebrows.

Wigs and toupees are often used to disguise alopecia affecting the scalp. *Hair transplants* are sometimes successful as a permanent method of replacing the lost hair.

Alpha-fetoprotein

A protein produced in the liver and gastrointestinal tract of the fetus and by some abnormal tissues in adults.

ALPHA-FETOPROTEIN IN PREGNANCY

Alpha-fetoprotein (AFP) is excreted in the fetal urine into the *amniotic fluid* (in which the fetus floats in the uterus); the fluid is then swallowed by the fetus, which introduces AFP into the fetal digestive system. Most of the AFP is broken down in the fetal intestine, but some passes from the fetus' circulation. AFP can be measured in the maternal blood from the second quarter of pregnancy onward, peaking between weeks 15 and 20 and then slowly decreasing.

Raised levels of AFP are found in some cases of fetal abnormality and occasionally when the fetus is normal. In *neural tube defects* (such as *spina bifida* or *anencephaly*), excess AFP may leak into the amniotic fluid. AFP levels are also raised in certain kidney abnormalities and can result from impaired breakdown in the intestine if the fetus cannot swallow properly because of malformation of the esophagus.

AFP levels are also raised in multiple *pregnancy* and in threatened or actual *miscarriage*. They may misleadingly appear to be raised when there has been an error in the calculation of gestation dates. AFP levels may be unusually low in pregnancies in which a baby has *Down's syndrome*.

TESTING AFP LEVELS IN PREGNANCY Ideally, pregnant women should be offered prenatal screening by measurement of blood AFP and *ultrasound scanning* at about 16 weeks. Scanning accurately dates the pregnancy, may show multiple pregnancy, and may show certain fetal abnormalities. If the blood AFP level is raised, the test is repeated one week later. If the second result is also raised, the woman may be carrying a baby with a neural tube defect. An ultrasound scan may strengthen or confirm the suspicion. *Amniocentesis* (removal of a small amount of the fluid surrounding the fetus) may be performed, and further measurements of AFP may be made on the sample. If the level is significantly raised, the chances that the woman is carrying an affected baby are high; a termination of pregnancy (see *Abortion, elective*) may then be considered.

About 10 percent of cases of neural tube defect are missed during screening because AFP levels are not significantly raised in every case. Conversely, in about five cases per 1,000 in which both amniotic fluid and blood levels of AFP are raised, the fetus is normal.

AFP IN ADULTS
In adults, AFP is produced in certain abnormal tissues. Levels are commonly raised in patients with hepatoma (see *Liver cancer*) and in those with malignant *teratoma* of the testes or ovaries. Some patients with cancer of the pancreas, stomach, and lung also have raised levels. Because it is present in abnormal quantities in some cancers, AFP is known as a "tumor marker." However, AFP levels are also raised in some benign conditions, including viral and alcoholic *hepatitis* and in *cirrhosis*.

AFP levels can be used to monitor the treatment of hepatomas and teratomas; increasing levels after surgery or chemotherapy are a useful indicator of tumor recurrence.

Alpha-tocopherol

The most potent of the tocopherols, an alcohol that is the main active constituent of *vitamin E*. It is fat-soluble and occurs in many foods. Deficiency of alpha-tocopherol is rare.

Alprazolam

A member of the family of *benzodiazepine drugs* used to treat *anxiety*, *panic attacks*, and *phobias*.

Alprostadil

A *prostaglandin drug* given to newborn infants who have certain types of congenital *heart disease* (such as *tetralogy of Fallot*, in which blood flow to the lungs is impaired). Alprostadil keeps open the ductus arteriosus—which normally closes after birth—and thus provides an alternative route for blood to reach the lungs. The ductus arteriosus links the aorta (the main artery carrying blood to the body) to the pulmonary artery (which takes blood to the lungs). Alprostadil, which is given by *intravenous infusion*, is used as a temporary measure until heart surgery can be performed.

Alprostadil also improves blood flow in general and is currently under investigation as a treatment for *Raynaud's disease* (a circulatory disorder affecting the hands and feet).

ALS

Amyotrophic lateral sclerosis (see *Motor neuron disease*).

Alternative medicine

Any medical system based on a theory of disease or its treatment that is incompatible with the orthodox science of medicine as it is taught in medical schools. Complementary medicine, by contrast, is the use by orthodox physicians of treatment techniques, such as *acupuncture* or manipulation, that are not generally included among orthodox therapies. In complementary medicine these alternative techniques are used empirically, that is, they are used in circumstances in which experience has suggested they may be effective, although the mechanism of their action may be unknown or uncertain.

Every society has its *folk medicine* and traditional healers who use methods and beliefs handed down through the generations. In some cultures, such as in China (see *Chinese medicine*), textbooks of traditional medicine date back several thousands of years. Some systems, such as acupuncture and *acupressure*, are based on theories of disease that emphasize internal balances.

Many cultures contain traditions of *herbal medicine*, plant-based remedies for common complaints. Some plants have properties recognized by orthodox medicine.

European folk medicine, based on the four humors described by the ancient Greeks and on ordinary herbal medicine, was transformed by the scientific discoveries of the eighteenth and nineteenth centuries.

The early nineteenth century brought the development and flourishing of many new alternative systems, including *chiropractic*, *homeopathy*, and *naturopathy*. The popularity of these alternative practices declined from the 1930s to 1950s with the successes of orthodox medicine—notably vaccines, antibiotics, diuretics, antidepressants, and advances in anesthesia and surgery. In the last decade, however, a small but increasing number of people have questioned the ability of orthodox medicine to provide all the answers. Numerous new and rediscovered disciplines, such as *aroma therapy* and naturopathy, have won a following without conclusive scientific confirmation.

Many alternative practitioners are sympathetic listeners who give sensible advice backed by treatments that have, at the very least, a powerful placebo effect. The opposition by orthodox physicians to alternative therapies is based on the principle that the first step in the treatment of any disorder is accurate diagnosis, which itself requires extensive medical knowledge. Treatment of symptoms without knowing their cause may be disastrous if an underlying remediable but progressive condition has not been recognized. Some herbal remedies, although based on natural ingredients, may cause adverse reactions in some people and might also be dangerous if taken at the same time as conventional medicines.

Altitude sickness

See *Mountain sickness*.

Aluminum

A light metallic element that is abundant in various minerals, such as bauxite. Aluminum is also found in relatively low concentrations in the body, though it is not known to have any useful function and is almost certainly harmful.

Sources of ingested aluminum include antacids, cooking utensils and foil, antiperspirants, some baking powders, and food additives such as potassium alum (used to whiten flour) and aluminum calcium silicate (used to keep table salt running freely). Most of the aluminum that is taken into the body is excreted. The remainder is stored in the lungs, brain, liver, and thyroid gland.

ADVERSE EFFECTS

Industrial processes in which aluminum aerosols are used (i.e., aluminum processing, pottery making, and explosives manufacturing) are associated with various lung diseases, including *fibrosis* of the lungs and *emphysema*.

Aluminum hydroxide is widely used in *antacids* for the treatment of peptic ulcers and acid indigestion; prolonged use can cause weakness, tiredness, and loss of appetite. Some people get an allergic reaction to the aluminum chloride contained in *antiperspirants*, resulting in *dermatitis* (itchy, inflamed skin).

Aluminum-induced *dementia* (a form of mental disorder) has developed in some patients undergoing *dialysis* (artificial purification of the blood, used to treat kidney failure) due to the aluminum content of the water used. However, the condition can be prevented by adequate monitoring procedures. There is no convincing evidence linking aluminum with *Alzheimer's disease*.

Alveolectomy

See *Alveoloplasty*.

Alveolitis

Inflammation of the alveoli (tiny air sacs) in the lungs, with thickening of their walls. Alveolitis reduces the elasticity of the lungs during breathing and reduces the efficiency of transfer of gases between the lungs and the surrounding blood vessels.

CAUSES

There are a number of causes of alveolitis. The most common is an allergic reaction to an inhaled dust of animal or plant origin, often containing fungal spores. This allergic alveolitis may be related to occupation. Examples include *farmers' lung* (caused by spores from moldy hay), *bagassosis* (spores from moldy bagasse, a material used in cardboard manufacture), and bird breeders' lung (caused by particles from bird droppings).

Fibrosing alveolitis may be an *autoimmune disorder*, in which the body's defenses produce antibodies against its own tissues, in this case the lung tissues. The exact cause of this disorder is unknown, although in some cases it occurs with other autoimmune disorders such as systemic *lupus erythematosus* or *rheumatoid arthritis*.

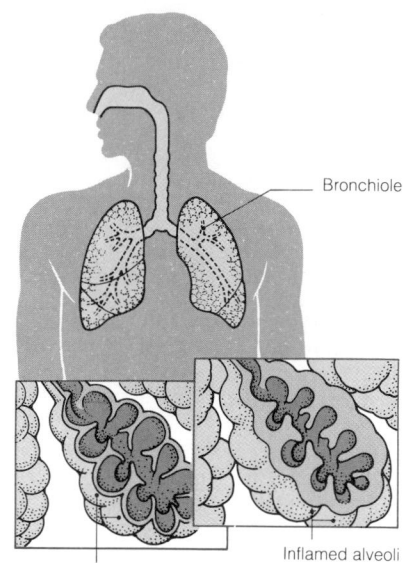

Normal alveoli

Inflamed alveoli

Signs of alveolitis

The alveoli become inflamed and their walls thicken, causing the lungs to become less elastic and less efficient.

Radiation alveolitis is inflammation caused by exposure to radiation, usually as a rare complication of *radiation therapy* treatment for lung or breast cancer.

SYMPTOMS AND DIAGNOSIS

Alveolitis usually causes a dry cough and breathing difficulty on exertion.

A chest X ray usually shows mottled shadowing across the lungs. Blood tests may be performed to show specific antibodies to an allergen or as evidence of an autoimmune disorder. *Pulmonary function tests* will demonstrate reduced lung capacity without obstruction to airflow through the bronchi. A lung *biopsy* may be performed to examine an area of damaged lung tissue under the microscope and may be the only way to make a conclusive diagnosis.

TREATMENT AND OUTLOOK

The conditions of some people with alveolitis show improvement on a course of *corticosteroid drugs*. In fibrosing alveolitis, a low dose of corticosteroids may be continued indefinitely as a maintenance treatment; in other types, the benefit of corticosteroids will apply only to a short course.

If the cause of allergic alveolitis is recognized and avoided before any damage occurs, there is often no permanent disability. In fibrosing alveolitis, however, the lung damage progresses despite treatment, causing increasing breathing difficulty and, sometimes, respiratory failure. (See also *Hypersensitivity*; *Pneumonitis*.)

Alveoloplasty

Dental surgery to remove protuberances and to smooth out other uneven areas from tooth-bearing bone in the jaw prior to fitting dentures. Alveoloplasty is carried out on people whose alveolar ridge underlying the gums would not otherwise be even enough for dentures to be fitted easily or worn comfortably.

HOW IT IS DONE

Minor alveoloplasty may require only local anesthesia but in most cases the patient is given a general anesthetic. An incision is made in the gum, which is peeled back to expose the uneven bone. The bone is either reshaped with large bone forceps or filed down to the required shape. The gum is then replaced and stitched together.

Some bruising and swelling of the mouth may occur, just as it sometimes does after a tooth is extracted. The gum usually heals within two weeks.

Alveolus, dental

The bony cavity or socket that supports each tooth in the jaw.

Alveolus, pulmonary

One of a group of minute, balloonlike sacs at the end of a bronchiole (one of the many small air passages in the

ANATOMY OF THE ALVEOLI

These tiny sacs contain capillaries in their thin walls that allow oxygen to be absorbed into the blood.

Bronchiole

Capillaries

Alveoli

lungs). Inhaled oxygen is absorbed into the bloodstream by capillaries in the thin wall of each alveolus, and carbon dioxide passes the other way (from the blood into the lungs) to be breathed out. There are about 300 million alveoli in each lung.

Alzheimer's disease

A progressive condition in which nerve cells degenerate in the brain and the brain substance shrinks. Alzheimer's disease is the single most common cause of *dementia*. Although originally classified as a "presenile" dementia, Alzheimer's disease is now known to be responsible for 75 percent of dementia cases in those over 65 years old. Because of the increasing numbers of elderly citizens, interest and research into the causes and treatment of Alzheimer's disease have greatly expanded in recent years. The progress of the disease (which, in most cases, represents several years of intellectual and personal decline until death) cannot be arrested.

Brain scan in Alzheimer's disease
The volume of the brain substance (gray area) has shrunk markedly. Its normal outline is shown by the dotted line.

CAUSES

The cause of Alzheimer's disease is unknown, although a number of theories have been proposed, ranging from the effects of a chronic infection to those of toxic poisoning by a metal such as aluminum. There is known to be a reduced level of *acetylcholine* and other brain chemicals in people with Alzheimer's disease. A genetic factor is also a possibility; the disease is more common in those with *Down's syndrome*, and 15 percent of the victims of Alzheimer's disease have a family history of the disease, occasionally with a dominant pattern of inheritance (in which children with one affected parent have a 50 percent chance of inheriting the disease).

INCIDENCE

Onset is rare before the age of 60, but thereafter increases steadily with age. Up to 30 percent of people over the age of 85 are affected.

SYMPTOMS AND SIGNS

The features of the disease vary among individuals, but there are three broad stages. At first the patient notices his or her increasing forgetfulness and may try to compensate by writing lists or by soliciting the help of others. Problems with memory often cause the patient to feel anxious and depressed, but these symptoms frequently go unnoticed.

Forgetfulness gradually shades into a second phase of severe memory loss, particularly for recent events. Victims may remember long-ago events, such as their schooldays and young adulthood, but they are unable to recall yesterday's visitors or what they saw on television. They also become disoriented as to time or place, losing their way even on familiar streets; their concentration and ability to calculate numbers declines and *dysphasia* (inability to find the right word) is noticeable. Anxiety increases, mood changes are sudden and unpredictable, and personality changes soon become apparent.

In the third stage, patients become severely disoriented and confused. They may also suffer from symptoms of *psychosis*, such as *hallucinations* and paranoid *delusions*. Symptoms are worsened by the patient's disorientation and memory losses and are usually most severe at night. Signs of nervous system disease begin to emerge, such as primitive *reflexes* (involuntary actions that occur normally in newborn babies) and incontinence of urine and feces. Some patients become demanding, unpleasant, and sometimes violent, and lose all awareness of social norms. Some become docile and somewhat helpless. They neglect personal hygiene and may wander purposelessly. Eventually the burden for caring relatives becomes impossible, and full-time hospital care and nursing are often inevitable. Once the patient is bedridden the complications of bedsores, feeding problems, and pneumonia make life expectancy very short.

DIAGNOSIS

Alzheimer's disease can be definitely diagnosed only by examination of the brain, either by brain *biopsy* or after death. Not only is the brain shrunken in size, but under the microscope it is possible to observe a loss of nerve cells, specks of brain debris, and tangles of nerves resembling pieces of unwound string.

In the absence of any absolute diagnostic test for the disease during life, the diagnosis is a clinical one. An *EEG* (recording of brain-wave patterns) will show increasingly slow waves, but will add nothing by itself to that which is clinically apparent. *CT scanning* and *MRI* of the brain show evidence of reduced cerebral size. Mental status tests indicate a decrease in the person's intellectual ability.

Some 10 percent of people with symptoms of dementia have a reversible disease (such as *hypothyroidism*, pernicious anemia or vitamin B_{12} deficiency, a tumor, or subdural *hematoma*). Routine investigations should be carried out to ensure that any treatable diseases are noted. It is also not uncommon for the elderly to have a depressive pseudodementia, in which the patient appears to be demented but is actually suffering from the effects of *depression*.

TREATMENT

There is no specific treatment for the disease itself apart from the provision of suitable nursing and social care for both victim and relatives. Keeping the victim well nourished, exercised, and occupied helps alleviate anxiety and personal distress, especially in the earlier stages when the person is still sufficiently aware of his or her condition. Tranquilizing medication can often improve difficult behavior and help the patient sleep.

Counseling of victims' families can help to prevent problems, such as physical abuse of the afflicted person, and can minimize disruption of family life. Provision of suitable day-care facilities (where patients stay temporarily to give families a break), personal care facilities (where patients live in a structured environment until inpatient care is necessary), and inpatient care for advanced cases all can help ease the burden on families.

OUTLOOK

With the increasing numbers of elderly people, the pressure on public health care services is becoming intense. Ideally, care is best provided at home, but this may be impossible. Although efforts are being made to expand facilities, a shortage of suitable places exists for elderly people with dementia. Research into drug therapy is continuing.

AMA

See *American Medical Association*.

A

Amalgam, dental

A material used to fill teeth, consisting of an alloy of mercury with one or more other metals. Amalgam is soft enough to be easily workable by the dentist but sets rapidly (within 24 hours) into a hard, strong solid; it is thus ideal for use as a filling, especially for back teeth (see *Filling, dental*).

Amantadine

An *antiviral drug* used in the prevention and treatment of *influenza* A. Amantadine more recently has been used to help relieve symptoms of *Parkinson's disease*.

Amaurosis fugax

Brief loss of vision, lasting for periods of seconds to minutes, usually caused by the temporary blockage of small blood vessels in the eye by tiny *emboli* (particles of solid matter such as cholesterol crystals and particles of clotted blood). These emboli are carried in the bloodstream from diseased carotid arteries in the neck or, rarely, from the heart. Sufferers typically experience a loss or dimming of vision, in one eye only, that is like a shade being pulled down or up.

Attacks may be infrequent or may occur many times a day. This symptom should never be ignored since it is a clear warning that the person is at increased risk of *stroke* or *coronary heart disease*. Medical investigation, with special attention to the state of the arteries, is urgently needed.

Amaurotic familial idiocy

A term covering a range of rare inherited disorders, of which the best known is *Tay-Sachs disease*. In these conditions, the nervous system suffers progressive degeneration and atrophy, with early involvement of the optic nerves and retinas, leading to blindness. Brain involvement causes mental deterioration. The conditions are incurable but are exceedingly uncommon. They may be diagnosed early in pregnancy and termination of the pregnancy may be considered.

Ambidexterity

The ability to perform manual skills, such as writing or using cutlery, equally well with either hand because there is no definite *handedness* (preference for using one hand). Ambidexterity is an uncommon and often familial trait.

Amblyopia

A permanent visual acuity defect in which there is usually no structural abnormality in the eye. In many cases there is now known to be a failure in the linkup of nerve connections in the visual pathway between the retina and the brain. The term is also sometimes applied to toxic or nutritional causes of decreased visual acuity, as in tobacco-alcohol amblyopia.

If normal vision is to develop during infancy and childhood, it is essential that clear, corresponding visual images are formed on both retinas so that compatible nerve impulses pass from the eyes to the brain. If no images are received, normal vision cannot develop. If images from the two eyes are very different, one will be suppressed to avoid double vision, and normal vision may not develop in one of the eyes.

CAUSES

The most common cause of amblyopia is *strabismus* (squint) in very young children, in which only one eye points at a selected object while the different image from the other eye is suppressed. Failure to form normal retinal images may also result from congenital *cataract* (opacity of the internal lens of the eye at birth), and severe, unequal, focusing errors in a young child, such as when one eye is normal and the other eye has an uncorrected large *astigmatism*, causing a blurred retinal image. Toxic and nutritional amblyopia may result from damage to the retina and/or optic nerve.

TREATMENT AND OUTLOOK

It is important to treat amblyopia at an early age; after the age of 8, amblyopia usually cannot be remedied. For amblyopia due to strabismus, patching (covering up the good eye to force the deviating eye to function properly) is the usual treatment. Glasses and/or surgery to place the deviating eyes in the correct position may be necessary. Glasses may also be necessary to correct severe focusing errors. Congenital cataracts may be removed.

Ambulance

A vehicle for conveying sick, injured, or disabled people. There are two types of ambulance: nonemergency ambulances (medi-cars or vans) and emergency ambulances.

A medi-car or van is designed for people traveling to outpatient departments at hospitals and to day-care clinics. The van usually has eight to 10 seats and an elevator for moving wheelchairs.

The emergency ambulance responds to 911 calls, taking accident victims and severely ill people to the hospital. In addition to stretchers, it contains many items useful in emergency situations, including oxygen, intravenous fluids, ECG equipment, a cardioversion unit with paddles (to treat heart attack victims), analgesics, splints, and dressings.

Ambulatory care

Medical care given without the patient being admitted to a hospital.

Ambulatory surgery

Surgery done without the patient being admitted to a hospital. Ambulatory surgery may, however, be performed in the outpatient section of a hospital. It is also performed in physicians' offices, or in outpatient surgical centers specially designed for cases in which an overnight stay in a hospital is not necessary.

Amebiasis

An infection caused by a tiny animal parasite, *ENTAMOEBA HISTOLYTICA*, which lives in the human large intestine. The infection is characterized by persistent moderate to severe diarrhea and, occasionally, the development of abscesses in the liver or, more rarely, in the brain.

INCIDENCE

Amebiasis is prevalent in poor countries where standards of public hygiene and sanitation are low. Although it can be acquired anywhere, most cases in the US and other developed countries occur among travelers who have recently returned from developing countries in the tropics or subtropics.

About 5,000 to 10,000 cases are diagnosed per year in the US, leading to about 20 deaths annually.

CAUSES

ENTAMOEBA HISTOLYTICA is an ameba, a type of single-celled animal that multiplies by simple division and moves around in the intestine, scavenging for small morsels of food and bacteria. The life cycle of this organism, and method by which it is spread from one person to another, is shown in the diagram.

Many people (few in the US) carry *ENTAMOEBA HISTOLYTICA* in their intestines and excrete amebic cysts but have no symptoms, probably because the strain of amebae they carry is harmless. Other strains, for unknown reasons, invade the intestinal wall,

THE CYCLE OF AMEBIASIS

The parasite *ENTAMOEBA HISTOLYTICA* lives in the large intestine, where it multiplies; sometimes protective cysts develop. Passed out in feces, the cysts can survive long periods before the next host acquires them.

The infection is spread by drinking water or eating food contaminated with cysts

Once swallowed the cyst wall breaks down and amebae parasitize the large intestine

The amebae develop protective capsules forming cysts which are passed out in feces

In the large intestine the amebae thrive and multiply by simple division

causing bleeding and mucus secretion into the intestines and diarrhea—an illness called amebic dysentery. Ulcers are formed in the intestinal wall and sometimes the amebae gain access to the bloodstream, by which they travel to the liver to form abscesses. Brain infection is rare.

PREVENTION
Travelers to countries where sanitary standards are low can reduce their chances of acquiring amebiasis by drinking only water that has been bottled or boiled (water-purifying tablets are ineffective against amebic cysts) and by not eating uncooked vegetables (especially lettuce) or unpeeled fruit.

SYMPTOMS
The diarrhea caused by amebiasis may vary from two or more rather loose stools per day, accompanied by rumbling pains in the stomach, to full-blown dysentery, with high fever and the frequent passage of watery, bloody diarrhea.

The symptoms of amebic liver abscess are shaking chills, fever, weight loss, and painful enlargement of the liver. Abscesses may develop in people who have never had digestive tract symptoms.

TREATMENT
Treatment of all forms of amebiasis is with drugs such as metronidazole or iodoquinol, which effectively kill the parasite within a few weeks, leading to full recovery. Occasionally, it is necessary to drain a liver abscess.

Amebic dysentery

See *Amebiasis*.

Amebicides

A group of drugs used to treat *amebiasis* (an infection caused by amebae). Some amebicides (for example, iodoquinol) act only on amebae in the intestine. Others, such as *chloroquine* and *metronidazole*, also destroy amebae in other tissues, such as the liver.

Amelogenesis imperfecta

An inherited condition of the teeth in which the enamel is either abnormally thin or deficient in calcium. Affected teeth may be pitted and discolored (see *Discolored teeth*), and, depending on the type of imperfection, may be more susceptible to dental *caries*.

Amenorrhea

Absence of menstrual periods. Primary amenorrhea is defined as failure to start menstruating by the age of 16. Secondary amenorrhea is the temporary or permanent cessation of periods in a woman who has menstruated regularly in the past.

PRIMARY AMENORRHEA The main cause of primary amenorrhea is a delay in the onset of puberty. A delay of this type may be natural, or, in rare cases, it may result from a disorder of the *endocrine system*. This may be the direct result of a *pituitary tumor*; the indirect result of other hormonal disorders, such as *hypothyroidism* (underactivity

of the thyroid gland), an *adrenal tumor*, or *adrenal hyperplasia*; or it may occur for no known reason. A rare cause of delayed puberty is *Turner's syndrome*, in which one female sex chromosome is missing.

In some cases, menstruation fails to take place because the vagina or uterus has been absent from birth, or because there is no perforation in the hymen (the membrane across the opening of the vagina) to allow the menstrual blood to escape.

SECONDARY AMENORRHEA The most common cause of secondary amenorrhea is pregnancy.

Periods may temporarily cease after a woman has stopped taking the birth-control pill. This temporary cessation of menstrual flow usually lasts for only six to eight weeks, but it may persist for a year or longer. Secondary amenorrhea can also be the result of interference with the release of hormones due to emotional stress, depression, *anorexia nervosa*, or drugs.

Rarely, periods may stop as a result of the same disorders of the endocrine system that can cause primary amenorrhea. Another possible cause of secondary amenorrhea is a disorder of the *ovary*, such as *polycystic ovary* or a tumor of the ovary (see *Ovary, cancer of*).

Amenorrhea occurs permanently after the *menopause* or after a *hysterectomy* (surgical removal of the uterus).

INVESTIGATION
Investigation of amenorrhea usually includes a physical examination, blood tests to measure hormone levels, *laparoscopy* to inspect the ovaries, *CT scanning* of the skull to exclude the possibility of a pituitary tumor, and *ultrasound scanning* of the abdomen and pelvis to exclude an adrenal gland or ovarian tumor.

TREATMENT
Some women with either primary or secondary amenorrhea may choose not to have treatment, but in every case the cause should be identified. If an *ovarian cyst* or tumor is the cause, it requires removal. Anorexia nervosa, too, needs treatment because of its long-term threat to health. If a woman with amenorrhea wants treatment and the cause is related to the endocrine system, ovulation can usually be induced by treatment with *clomiphene* or *gonadotropin hormones*.

American Medical Association

The largest physician organization in American medicine, with approximately 279,000 members (1986) and an annual budget of approximately $133 million. Its members, nearly all of whom pay annual dues of $375, tend to be physicians engaged in patient care. Although the AMA is a federation of state and county medical societies, it provides representation in its policy-making body for many other medical groups, such as medical specialty societies, hospital and staff physicians, the deans of medical schools, residents, medical students, and physicians in the armed services, the Veterans Administration, and the US Public Health Service.

The house of delegates meets twice a year to debate issues, make policy, take positions, and elect officers. Officers include a president, who serves a one-year term, and a board of trustees, which makes policy decisions between the meetings of the house. An executive vice-president serves as a chief executive, overseeing a staff of more than 1,000 employees, most of them based at AMA headquarters in Chicago.

Ametropia

Optical defect of the eye that alters *refraction*. (See *Hyperopia*; *Myopia*; *Astigmatism*; *Presbyopia*.)

Amiloride

A potassium-sparing *diuretic drug*. Combined with loop or thiazide diuretic drugs, amiloride is used in the treatment of *hypertension* and *edema* due to *heart failure* or to *cirrhosis* of the liver.

Amino acids

 A group of chemical compounds that forms the basic structural units of all *proteins*. Each amino acid molecule consists of nitrogenous amino and acidic carboxyl groups of atoms linked to a variable chain or ring of carbon atoms.

Individual amino acid molecules are linked together—by chemical bonds, called *peptide* bonds, between the amino and carboxyl groups—to form short chains of molecules called *polypeptides*. Hundreds of polypeptides are, in turn, linked together—also by peptide bonds—to form a protein molecule. What differentiates one protein from another is the arrangement of the amino acids.

There are 20 different amino acids that make up all the proteins in humans. Of these, 12 can be made by the body; they are known as nonessential amino acids, because they do not need to be obtained from the diet. The other eight, the essential amino acids, cannot be made by the body and must be obtained from the diet.

The 20 amino acids that make up proteins also occur free within cells and in body fluids. In addition, there are more than 200 other amino acids that are not found in proteins but which play an important part in chemical reactions within cells.

Aminoglutethimide

An *anticancer drug* that, in 1987, was under investigation as a treatment for certain types of breast cancer and for endocrine gland tumors.

Aminophylline

BRONCHODILATOR VASODILATOR		
Tablet Liquid Injection Rectal suppository		
📋 Prescription needed		
💊 Available as generic		

A drug used in the treatment of *asthma*, chronic *bronchitis*, and other respiratory disorders.

HOW IT WORKS
Aminophylline relieves breathing difficulty by widening the bronchi in the lungs. It also increases the production of urine and dilates (widens) blood vessels, which improves blood flow from the heart.

POSSIBLE ADVERSE EFFECTS
Unless the dose is carefully controlled, adverse effects, such as nausea, vomiting, headache, dizziness, and palpitations, may occur. During long-term treatment, blood tests may be carried out to monitor the level of aminophylline in the body.

Aminosalicylic acid

A drug existing in three distinct chemical forms. Para-aminosalicylic acid is an *antibacterial drug* used with other drugs to treat *tuberculosis*. Two forms (4-aminosalicylic acid and 5-aminosalicylic acid) are under investigation for use in the treatment of inflammatory bowel diseases such as *ulcerative colitis*.

Amitriptyline

An *antidepressant drug,* amitriptyline also has a sedative effect; it is useful in the treatment of *depression* accompanied by *anxiety* or *insomnia*.

Possible adverse effects include dry mouth, blurred vision, dizziness, drowsiness, and hot flashes, all of which may disappear if the dosage is reduced. Amitriptyline usually takes between two and six weeks to become fully effective.

Ammonia

A colorless, pungent gas that dissolves in water to form an alkaline solution (see *Alkali*). Ammonia consists of one nitrogen atom linked to three hydrogen atoms. Although it is poisonous, ammonia is produced by the body; it plays a valuable role in maintaining the *acid-base balance*.

In severe liver damage, the capacity of the liver to convert ammonia to *urea* is diminished. This leads to a high level of ammonia in the blood, which is thought to be a cause of the impairment of consciousness that occurs with liver failure.

Amnesia

Loss of the ability to memorize information and/or to recall information stored in memory. Memory can be divided into short-term and long-term: in the former, material is retained for seconds or minutes only, in the latter, it is retained indefinitely. In most amnesic conditions, the storage of information in long-term memory and/or the recall of such information is impaired.

CAUSES
Amnesia is caused by damage or disease of brain regions concerned with memory functions. Possible causes of such damage include head injuries (including concussion), degenerative disorders such as *Alzheimer's disease* and other forms of *dementia*, infections such as *encephalitis*, thiamine deficiency in alcoholics leading to *Wernicke-Korsakoff syndrome*, and also *brain tumors*, *strokes*, and *subarachnoid hemorrhage*. Amnesia can also occur in some forms of psychiatric illness (in which there is no apparent physical damage).

With many types of amnesia, the patient has a gap in memory extending back for some time from the moment of onset of the brain damage. This is called retrograde amnesia and is principally a deficit of recall. Usually the memory gap gradually shrinks over time. A patient may additionally (or alternatively) be unable to store new information in the period following damage to the brain. The resultant gap in memory, called an anterograde amnesia, extends from the moment of onset of the amnesia to the time when long-term memory resumes (if it ever does). This gap in the memory is usually permanent.

Amniocentesis

A diagnostic procedure in which a small amount of *amniotic fluid* is withdrawn from the amniotic sac, the membrane that surrounds the fetus in the uterus.

WHY IT IS DONE

The amniotic fluid contains cells and chemicals from the fetus that can be analyzed to detect fetal abnormalities, such as *Down's syndrome*, which is a chromosomal abnormality. Amniocentesis can also help detect other chromosomal abnormalities, sex-linked disorders (such as *hemophilia*), metabolic diseases (such as *Tay-Sachs disease*), or developmental disorders (such as *spina bifida*). It is also used to assess fetal disorders such as *hemolytic disease of the newborn* and *respiratory distress syndrome*.

Amniotic sac

Placenta

Amniotic fluid

Fetus   Uterus

Procedure for amniocentesis
A needle is introduced through the abdomen and uterine wall into the amniotic sac; a sample of amniotic fluid is then drawn.

HOW IT IS DONE

Genetic amniocentesis is usually performed between the sixteenth and eighteenth week of gestation. *Ultrasound scanning* is used to estimate the age and position of the fetus, the placental site, and the amount of amniotic fluid. A needle is then inserted through the abdomen and uterine wall into the amniotic sac, avoiding the fetus and placenta. A syringe is attached to the needle and about 20 to 30 ml of fluid is removed.

A local anesthetic is occasionally used. The woman can usually go home soon after the procedure but is advised to rest for 24 hours.

RESULTS

The amniotic fluid may be analyzed biochemically and a chromosome *culture* performed to test for fetal abnormalities such as Down's syndrome and spina bifida.

Chromosome cultures take up to four weeks, so any results may not be available until about 20 weeks' gestation. The sex of the fetus is also determined by the chromosome analysis and the woman should indicate whether or not she wishes to receive this information.

COMPLICATIONS

There is a slight increased incidence of threatened miscarriage and early rupture of the membranes after amniocentesis (older studies show a risk of 1 to 2 percent; more recent studies show a risk of about 0.5 percent). For these reasons, amniocentesis is usually recommended only for women over the age of 35 (who are more likely to have a child with Down's syndrome) or when there are other compelling medical reasons, such as a family history of a chromosomal abnormality. (See also *Chorionic villus sampling*.)

Amnion

The membranous sac that surrounds the *embryo* and fills with watery *amniotic fluid* as pregnancy advances. The outside of the amnion is covered by another membrane called the chorion.

Amnioscopy

Another name for *fetoscopy*, direct observation of the fetus and amniotic fluid by means of an *endoscope* (viewing tube) passed through the pregnant woman's abdomen into the uterus.

Amniotic fluid

The clear fluid or "waters" that surround the fetus in the uterus throughout pregnancy. The fluid is contained within the amniotic sac (a thin membrane).

The fetus floats in the amniotic fluid and, in the early months of pregnancy, can move about freely while still remaining attached by the umbilical cord to the placenta (the organ that nourishes the fetus during pregnancy). The amniotic fluid cushions the fetus against pressure from internal organs and protects it from any injury from the mother's movements.

The fluid is produced by the cells that line the amniotic sac and is constantly circulated. It is swallowed by the fetus, absorbed into its bloodstream, then excreted by the fetal kidneys as urine. Amniotic fluid

is 99 percent water. The remainder consists of dilute concentrations of the substances found in blood plasma, along with cells and *lipids* (fats) that have flaked off from the fetus.

Amniotic fluid appears during the first week after conception and gradually increases in volume until the tenth week, when the increase becomes very rapid. By 35 weeks' gestation the volume of fluid is about 2 pints. Thereafter it slowly declines until it is just over 1 pint at term.

In a small number of women, excessive fluid is formed; this is known as *hydramnios* or polyhydramnios. Less frequently, insufficient amniotic fluid is formed (a condition called *oligohydramnios*).

Amniotomy

Artificial rupture of the amniotic membranes (breaking of the waters) performed for *induction of labor*.

Amoxapine

A tricyclic *antidepressant drug*. Amoxapine has a weaker sedative effect than many antidepressant drugs and is used when they have caused daytime drowsiness. Amoxapine may cause dry mouth and constipation before the dosage is adjusted.

Amoxicillin

A *penicillin*-type *antibiotic drug* used to treat a wide variety of infections, including *bronchitis*, *cystitis*, *gonorrhea*, and ear and skin infections.

An allergic reaction to amoxicillin may cause a blotchy rash and, rarely, fever, swelling of the mouth, itching, and breathing difficulty.

Amphetamine drugs

COMMON DRUGS

Dextroamphetamine Methamphetamine

A group of *stimulant* drugs that has an *appetite suppressant* effect.

In the past, amphetamine drugs were commonly prescribed to treat *obesity*; this use has been largely abandoned today because of dependence problems and abuse.

Amphetamines are now used mainly in the treatment of *narcolepsy* (abnormal daytime sleepiness).

HOW THEY WORK

Amphetamine drugs stimulate the secretion of *neurotransmitters* (chemicals released by nerve endings), such as *norepinephrine*, which increase nerve activity in the brain and make a person wakeful and alert.

A

POSSIBLE ADVERSE EFFECTS

Taken in high doses, amphetamines can cause tremor, sweating, palpitations, anxiety, and sleeping difficulties. Delusions, hallucinations, high blood pressure, and, rarely, seizures may also occur. Prolonged use may cause *tolerance* and physical dependence (see *Drug dependence*).

ABUSE

Amphetamines are abused for their stimulant effects; their manufacture and distribution are governed by the Controlled Substance Act.

Amphotericin B

A drug used to treat fungal infections. Minor infections of the eyes, ears, or skin are treated with drops, lotions, or creams. Life-threatening infections, such as *cryptococcosis* and *histoplasmosis* are treated with injections.

Adverse effects are likely only when amphotericin B is given by injection; these include vomiting, fever, headache, and, rarely, seizures.

Ampicillin

A *penicillin*-type *antibiotic drug* used to treat infections including *cystitis*, *bronchitis*, and ear infections. Ampicillin is also useful in the treatment of *gonorrhea*, *typhoid fever*, and *biliary system* infections.

Some people have an allergic reaction to ampicillin. This may cause rash, diarrhea, and, rarely, fever, swelling of the mouth and tongue, itching, and breathing difficulty.

Amputation

Surgical removal of part or all of a limb, usually to prevent *gangrene* (death and decay of tissues) or infection. Until the introduction of antibiotics in the early 1940s, amputation was a common operation, especially in wartime; it was the only means of preventing gangrene when an open fracture (one in which the broken bone is exposed) became infected.

WHY IT IS DONE

Today, the use of antibiotics to treat infected wounds means that amputation is restricted mainly to severe cases of arterial disease. Eighty-five percent of the 25,000 amputations performed in the US each year are carried out on patients with *peripheral vascular disease*, in which a combination of *atherosclerosis* and *thrombosis* may completely block the blood supply to a limb, causing gangrene.

Amputation may be performed to prevent the spread of bone cancer or malignant *melanoma* (a skin cancer).

HOW IT IS DONE

Before the operation, the surgeon decides where on the limb to operate; the tissue at the amputation site must be healthy if the wound is to heal rapidly. Investigative techniques used at this stage include *angiography* (injection into an artery of a solution visible on X ray) and *thermography* (recordings of surface temperatures of the body with a heat-sensitive camera).

During the operation, skin and muscle are cut below the level at which the bone is to be severed to create flaps that will later provide a fleshy stump. Blood vessels are tied off, the bone is sawed through, the area is washed with saline, and the flaps of skin and muscle are stitched over the sawed end of bone to form a smooth and rounded stump.

While amputating, the surgeon tries to ensure that nerves are severed well above the stump, reducing the risk of pressure pain when a prosthesis (see *Limb, artificial*) is fitted. But, despite every precaution, a painful *neuroma* (a benign tumor of nerve tissue) sometimes develops in the stump.

In an amputation at the ankle (Syme's amputation), the tough skin of the heel pad is retained to cover the stump. The patient can then place weight on the stump without necessarily having to use a prosthesis.

Amputations below the knee are now more satisfactory than before. Newer techniques for shaping the stump make it easier to fit a prosthesis, and new prostheses, attached by suction rather than straps, are easier to put on and take off.

RECOVERY PERIOD

As the wound heals, bandaging and plaster casts are used to mold the stump to a shape suitable for accepting a prosthesis. The stump is usually swollen for about six weeks after the operation and a permanent prosthesis can be fitted only after it has settled down to a stable size. The patient is usually helped to move around using a temporary prosthesis during this period to avoid becoming unaccustomed to walking.

For some time after an amputation, some patients have the unpleasant sensation that the amputated limb is still present—a phenomenon known as "phantom limb."

OUTLOOK

The prospect of a person who has had a leg amputation remaining mobile afterward depends on several factors: age, attitude, general health, the amount of limb lost, and whether the pressure of a prosthesis on the stump causes pain. Some healthy people lead almost as active lives as they did before, but many older people become confined to *wheelchairs*.

Amputation, congenital

Absence of the lower part of a limb from birth (see *Limb defects*).

Amputation, traumatic

Loss of a finger, toe, or limb through injury. (See also *Microsurgery*.)

Amyl nitrite

A *nitrate drug* once prescribed to relieve *angina pectoris* (chest pain due to impaired blood supply to the heart muscle). Because amyl nitrite frequently causes adverse effects (including headache, hot flashes, palpitations, and restlessness) it has been largely superseded by other drugs.

Amyl nitrite is sometimes abused for its effect of intensifying pleasure during orgasm.

Amyloidosis

An uncommon disease in which a substance called amyloid, which contains protein and starch, accumulates in tissues and organs.

CAUSES

Amyloidosis may occur for no known reason, when it is called primary; more commonly, it is a complication of some other disease, when it is called secondary. Conditions that may lead to amyloidosis include *rheumatoid arthritis*, *multiple myeloma* (a cancer of bone marrow), and *tuberculosis* or a pyogenic (pus-generating) process such as chronic osteomyelitis. Exactly why amyloid is deposited in any of these circumstances is not known.

SYMPTOMS AND SIGNS

Amyloid may accumulate in any organ. The symptoms and signs of amyloidosis vary, depending on which part of the body is involved. The liver, kidney, tongue, spleen, and heart are often affected. The organs become enlarged and may have a rubbery consistency and a waxy, pink or gray appearance if examined.

Accumulation of amyloid in the heart may result in *arrhythmias* (disturbances of the heart beat) and *heart failure* (reduced pumping efficiency). If the stomach and intestines are affected, symptoms such as diarrhea may develop and the lining of these organs may become ulcerated. The joints may be affected.

Primary amyloidosis is often characterized by deposits of amyloid in the skin. Slightly raised, waxy spots appear, usually clustered around the armpits, groin, face, and neck.

Some forms of amyloidosis are inherited. These forms of the disease tend to involve the nervous system. Symptoms include peripheral *neuropathy*, postural *hypotension*, urinary or fecal *incontinence*, and reduced *sweating*. Death may result from *renal failure* caused by deposits of amyloid in the kidneys.

DIAGNOSIS AND TREATMENT
Diagnosis depends on microscopic examination of a *biopsy* sample of tissue from the affected organ.

There is no treatment, but secondary amyloidosis may be arrested or even reversed when the underlying disorder is treated.

Amyotrophic lateral sclerosis

See *Motor neuron disease.*

Amyotrophy

Shrinkage or wasting away of a muscle, caused by a reduction in the size of its constituent contractile fibers and leading to weakness. It is usually due to poor nutrition, reduced use of the muscle (as when a limb is immobilized for a long period), or disturbance to the muscle's blood or nerve supply, as can occur in *diabetes mellitus* or *poliomyelitis*.

Anabolic steroids

See *Steroids, anabolic.*

Anaerobic

Capable of living and growing without oxygen. Many important bacteria are anaerobes and thrive in the intestinal canal or in tissue with a poor supply of oxygenated blood. These species can cause various diseases, including *food poisoning*, *tetanus*, *gangrene*, and a form of diarrhea (pseudomembranous enterocolitis).

Some human body cells are capable of limited anaerobic activity. For example, when muscular exertion is so strenuous that oxygen is used faster than the blood circulation can supply it, the muscle cells can temporarily work anaerobically. When this happens, lactic acid is produced as waste (instead of the carbon dioxide from *aerobic* activity). Compensation for this anaerobic activity (converting the lactic acid to glucose) requires oxygen, which explains why we need to continue to breathe rapidly after vigorous exertion. The deficit of oxygen that builds up in the muscles during exercise is known as the oxygen debt.

Anal dilatation

A procedure for enlarging the anus. Anal dilatation is used to treat conditions in which the anus becomes too tight, such as *anal stenosis* and *anal fissure*. It is also used as a treatment for *hemorrhoids*. Anal dilatation can be performed using general anesthetic by a surgeon, using fingers or an anal dilator, or by the patient, using a dilator and lubricating jelly.

Anal discharge

The loss of mucus, blood, or pus from the anus. *Hemorrhoids*, *anal fissures* (tears in the anal margin), and *proctitis* (inflammation of the rectum) all can cause anal discharge. The production of mucus from the anus tends to irritate the surrounding skin and may cause pruritus ani (*itching* of the anus). Anal discharge can be temporarily relieved by warm, shallow baths.

Analeptic drugs

Drugs that stimulate breathing, used in the treatment of *apnea* (absent breathing) in a newborn infant. Analeptics, which include doxapram and nikethamide, are occasionally used to treat *respiratory failure* caused by a drug overdose and to hasten recovery from a general anesthetic. Analeptics work by stimulating the respiratory center, a group of nerve endings in the brain stem that control the rate and volume of breathing.

Anal fissure

A fairly common anal disorder caused by an elongated ulcer that extends upward into the anal canal from the anal sphincter. The fissure probably originates from a tear in the lining of the anus caused by the passage of hard, dry feces.

SYMPTOMS
There is usually pain during defecation and the muscles of the anus may go into spasm. There may be a small amount of bright red blood on the feces or the toilet paper.

TREATMENT
The tear often heals naturally in the course of a few days, although spasm of the anal muscles may delay healing. Treatment of recurrent or persistent fissures usually includes *anal dilatation* (a procedure to enlarge the anus) and a high-fiber diet, including whole-grain products, fruits, vegetables, and plenty of fluids, to soften the feces. Fissures usually heal within a few days after such treatment, but, if this treatment is unsuccessful, surgery to remove the fissure may be necessary.

Anal fistula

An abnormal channel connecting the inside of the anal canal with the skin surrounding the anus.

CAUSES
A fistula is occasionally an indication of *Crohn's disease*, *colitis*, or *cancer* of the large intestine. However, in most cases it results from an abscess (which develops for unknown reasons in the anal wall) that discharges pus both into the anus and out onto the surrounding skin.

A fistula is treated surgically by opening the channel, removing the fistulous lining, and draining the abscess of thin pus. The operation is performed using a general anesthetic.

Analgesia

Loss of pain sensation. Analgesia differs from *anesthesia* (loss of all sensation) in that the person's sensitivity to touch is still preserved. (See also *Analgesic drugs*.)

Analgesic drugs

COMMON DRUGS
Nonnarcotic
Acetaminophen Aspirin Sodium salicylate
Narcotic
Codeine Meperidine Morphine Pentazocine Propoxyphene

> **WARNING**
> Over-the-counter (nonnarcotic) analgesics should be used only for 48 hours before seeking medical advice. If pain persists, becomes more severe, recurs, or differs from pain previously experienced, consult your physician.

Drugs that relieve pain. The two main types of analgesics are nonnarcotic (most of which contain *aspirin*, aspirinlike substances, or *acetaminophen*) and narcotic (which are related to *morphine*).

WHY THEY ARE USED
Nonnarcotic analgesics are useful in the treatment of mild or moderate pain (for example, headache or toothache). For more severe pain, a preparation combining one of the weaker narcotic analgesics (such as *codeine*) with a nonnarcotic analgesic (such as aspirin) is usually prescribed. The most potent narcotic analgesic drugs are used only when other preparations would be ineffective.

HOW THEY WORK
When body tissues are damaged (for example, by injury, infection, or

HOW ANALGESICS WORK

When tissue is damaged (for example, by injury, inflammation, or infection) the body produces prostaglandins. These substances combine with opiate receptors (specific sites on the surface of cells in the brain and spinal cord). As a result, a signal is passed along a series of nerve cells to the brain, where the signal is interpreted as pain by brain cells. Analgesics (except for acetaminophen) work either by preventing the production of prostaglandins or by blocking pain impulses in the brain and spinal cord. Acetaminophen works by blocking the pain impulses in the brain itself. This action prevents the perception of pain.

Action of narcotics
When tissue damage occurs, the body produces prostaglandins, chemicals that trigger the transmission of pain signals (above). Normally, the pain signal is transmitted between brain cells, but narcotic drugs (below) combine with opiate receptors to prevent the signals from actually reaching the brain.

Action of nonnarcotics
Nonnarcotic drugs block the production of prostaglandins (the chemical released in response to tissue damage). This action prevents stimulation of the nerve endings so that no pain signal passes on to the brain. As a result, these drugs provide pain relief.

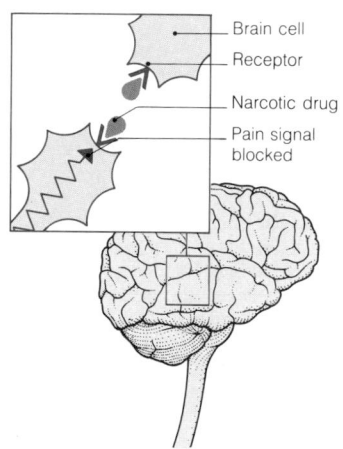

inflammation), they produce *prostaglandins*, chemicals that trigger the transmission of pain signals to the brain. Nonnarcotic analgesics (except acetaminophen) work by preventing prostaglandin production. Acetaminophen blocks the pain impulses in the brain itself, thereby preventing the perception of pain.

Narcotic analgesics act in a similar way to *endorphins* (substances formed within the body that relieve pain). They block pain impulses at specific sites (called opiate receptors) in the brain and spinal cord.

POSSIBLE ADVERSE EFFECTS
Adverse effects are uncommon with acetaminophen. Aspirin may irritate the stomach lining and cause nausea, pain, and, occasionally, a peptic ulcer. Nausea, vomiting, drowsiness, constipation, and breathing difficulties may occur with narcotic analgesic drugs. The stronger types may also produce euphoria.

ABUSE
The euphoric effects produced by some narcotic analgesics have led to their abuse. In most cases, long-term abuse causes *tolerance* and physical dependence (see *Drug dependence*). Both the manufacture and the distribution of strong narcotic analgesics are governed by the Controlled Substance Act.

Anal stenosis
A tightness of the anus, sometimes referred to as anal stricture, which makes it too small to allow the normal passage of feces. This often leads to constipation and pain during defecation. Anal stenosis can be a congenital abnormality. It may also be caused by a number of conditions in which scarring has occurred, such as *anal fissure, colitis,* or cancer of the anus. It sometimes occurs after surgery on the anus—for example, to treat *hemorrhoids*. It is treated by *anal dilatation* (a

procedure to enlarge the anus), which in some cases may be performed by the patient.

Anal stricture
See *Anal stenosis.*

Analysis, psychological
See *Psychoanalysis.*

Analysis, scientific
Determination of the identity of a substance or of the individual chemical constituents of a mixture. Analysis may be qualitative, as in determining whether or not a particular substance is present, or it may be quantitative, that is, measuring the amount or concentration of one or more constituents. (See also *Assay.*)

Anaphylactic shock
A rare, severe, frightening, and life-threatening allergic reaction. It is a Type I hypersensitivity reaction (see *Allergy*) that occurs only rarely in people in whom an extreme sensitivity to a particular substance (or allergen) has developed. The reaction occurs most commonly after an *insect sting* or as a reaction to an injected drug—for example, penicillin, anti-tetanus serum, a local anesthetic, or during *immunotherapy* for an allergy. Less commonly, the reaction occurs after a particular food or drug has been taken by mouth.

Entry of the allergen into the bloodstream provokes the release of massive amounts of histamine and other chemicals with effects on body tissues. The blood vessels widen, with a sudden severe lowering of blood pressure. Other symptoms include an itchy, raised rash (hives), bronchospasm (constriction of the airways in the lungs), pain in the abdomen, swelling of the tongue or throat, and diarrhea.

FIRST AID AND TREATMENT
If a person becomes severely ill or collapses soon after an insect sting or an injection, medical help should be summoned immediately.

The victim should be laid down and the legs raised to improve blood flow to the heart and brain. An injection of *epinephrine* is often lifesaving and must be given as soon as possible.

People who have suffered previous severe reactions to insect stings, drugs, or foods should carry a preloaded syringe of epinephrine, so that they can inject themselves (if still conscious) or can have the dose administered promptly by someone familiar with the method of injection. Otherwise, medical help should be awaited. If the person's breathing or heart beat stops, measures should be employed to restart them (see *Cardiopulmonary resuscitation*).

Apart from epinephrine, medical treatment administered by a physician may include *antihistamine drugs* and *corticosteroid drugs*.

Individuals who have suffered anaphylactic reactions to insect venom may respond to a course of immunotherapy, although this procedure itself carries a risk of repetition of the anaphylaxis and should be carried out only by a physician with a supply of epinephrine and other emergency medications at hand.

Anastomosis

A natural or artificial connection in the body; a communication between two tubular cavities or blood vessels that may or may not normally be joined.

A natural anastomosis usually takes the form of two blood vessels joining (see *Arteriovenous fistula*). Surgical anastomosis is used to treat various disorders. For example, if an artery is blocked by *thrombosis* (clot) or *atheroma* (fat deposits), an operation may be performed to remove the blockage and directly hook up the two ends of the vessel. Alternatively, an operation to bypass the blockage may be performed by joining a synthetic substitute or a section of a vein from the patient to the artery above and below the obstruction. Or, the internal mammary artery in the chest wall may be joined beyond the narrowing directly to a coronary artery.

Another common use of surgical anastomosis is to treat intestinal obstruction; a section of intestine is cut out and the healthy ends joined. To bypass this same area, two openings are made in a loop of the intestine (one either side of the defective area) and the openings joined.

Anatomy

The structure of the body of any living thing, and the scientific study of it. The science of human anatomy dates back to ancient Egyptian times and, together with *physiology* (the functioning of the body), forms the foundation of all medicine. The primary source of information for anatomists is dissection of human corpses.

The ancient Greek physician Galen produced many medical treatises containing some anatomical descriptions that are still in use today, but his work is also full of gross errors. It was not until 1543 that the first accurate, comprehensive anatomical text, "De Humani Corporis Fabrica" ("On the structure of the human body"), was produced by the Flemish scientist Andreas Vesalius.

BRANCHES OF ANATOMY

Anatomy as a scientific study today is subdivided into many branches. They include comparative anatomy (the study of the differences between human and animal bodies), surgical anatomy (the practical knowledge required by surgeons, especially recognition of the surface markings of internal organs and the pattern of blood vessels within them), *embryology* (the study of structural changes that occur during the development of the embryo and fetus), systematic anatomy (the study of the structure of particular body systems, such as the urinary system), and *cytology* and *histology* (the microscopic study of, respectively, cells and tissues).

DESCRIPTIVE TERMS

In textbook descriptions of human anatomy, the body is assumed to be standing upright, with the arms hanging down and the palms facing forward. The body is divided by the median (or sagittal) plane into right and left halves, and by the coronal plane into front (anterior or ventral) and rear (posterior or dorsal) halves.

Every anatomical structure is scientifically named in Latin, but today many anatomists prefer to use simpler terms when they exist. For example, the main blood vessel in the thigh is usually called the femoral artery rather than the arteria femoralis.

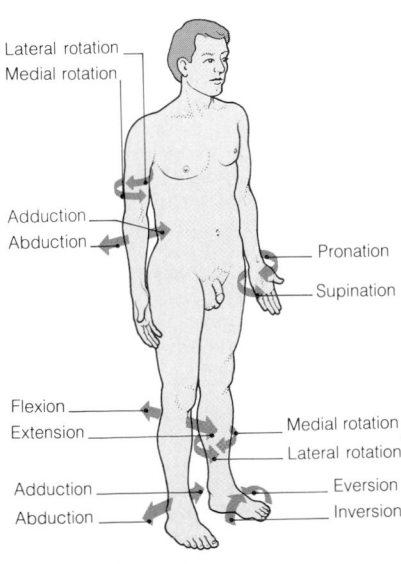

Joint movements
Flexion bends and extension straightens a joint; abduction moves a body part away from, adduction toward, the median plane. Rotations are movements around a long axis.

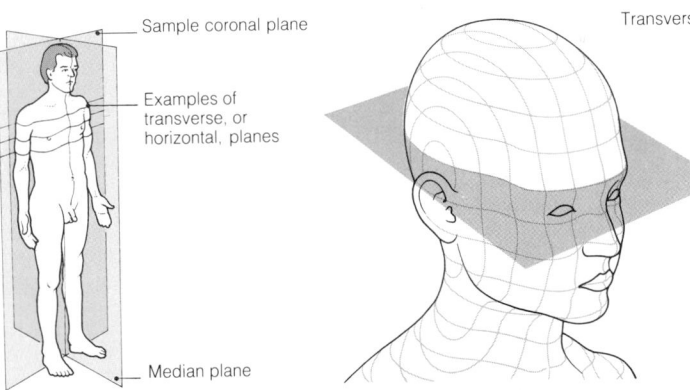

Planes through the body
Different body movements and sections through the body may be described by reference to various planes. The median plane divides the body evenly into right and left halves. Coronal planes are vertical planes at right angles to the median plane; the coronal plane most often referred to divides the body into front and back halves. Transverse planes are horizontal slices through the body.

Transverse plane through head
Computerized tomographic (CT), MRI, and other scans of the head are often taken in one or a series of transverse planes. One such scan is shown at left.

A

Ancylostomiasis

See *Hookworm infestation*.

Androgen drugs

A group of drugs that has effects similar to the *androgen hormones*; one of the most important of these hormones developed as a drug is *testosterone*.

Androgen drugs are used in the treatment of male *hypogonadism* (underactivity of the testes) to stimulate the development of sexual characteristics, such as growth of facial and pubic hair, enlargement of the genitals, and deepening of the voice. This treatment improves libido and potency but does not increase the production of sperm.

Androgen drugs are also used to stimulate production of new blood cells by the bone marrow in aplastic *anemia*. They also may occasionally be used in the treatment of certain types of *breast cancer*.

Androgen drugs are commonly used by athletes and bodybuilders wishing to increase muscle bulk and strength, but this practice is condemned by physicians due to doubts concerning the drugs' benefits and the risk of adverse effects.

POSSIBLE ADVERSE EFFECTS

Adverse effects include fluid retention, weight gain, increased levels of cholesterol in the blood, and, rarely, liver damage. When taken by women the drugs can cause deepening of the voice and other male characteristics. Because androgen drugs affect sexual development of babies, they are not prescribed during pregnancy or breast-feeding. They are prescribed with caution during adolescence because they may prematurely halt the growth of the long bones.

Androgen hormones

A group of hormones that causes *virilization* (the development of male secondary sexual characteristics), such as the growth of facial hair, deepening of the voice, and increase in muscle bulk.

FORMATION

Androgens are produced by specialized cells in the testes in males and in the adrenal glands in both sexes. The ovaries secrete very small quantities of androgens until the menopause. The most active androgen is *testosterone*, which is produced in the testes. Androgens produced by the adrenal glands are less active than testicular androgens, and have no significant masculinizing effects unless produced to excess.

The production of androgens by the testes is controlled by certain pituitary hormones, called *gonadotropins*. Adrenal androgens are controlled by *ACTH*, another pituitary hormone.

EFFECTS

Androgens stimulate the appearance of male secondary sexual characteristics at puberty, including enlargement of the penis and growth of facial and body hair. Androgens have what is called an anabolic effect, that is, they raise the rate of protein synthesis and lower the rate at which it is broken down. This increases muscle bulk, especially in the chest and shoulders, and accelerates growth, especially during early puberty. At the end of puberty, androgens cause the long bones to stop growing.

Androgens also promote aggression, a characteristically male trait. They stimulate sebum secretion, which, if excessive, causes *acne*. In early adult life, androgens promote male-pattern baldness. Absence of androgens protects against male-pattern baldness.

ANDROGEN DEFICIENCY

Adult males may be deficient in androgens if their *testes* are diseased or if the pituitary gland fails to secrete gonadotropins. Such men are termed "hypogonadal." Results of androgen deficiency include decreased body hair and beard growth, smooth skin, a high-pitched voice, reduced sexual drive and performance, underdeveloped genitalia, and lack of muscle development.

ANDROGEN EXCESS

Overproduction of androgens may be the result of adrenal disorders (see *Adrenal tumors*; *Adrenal hyperplasia, congenital*), of testicular tumors (see *Testis, cancer of*), or, rarely, of androgen-secreting ovarian tumors (see *Ovary, cancer of*).

In adult males, excess androgens accentuate male physical characteristics. In boys, they cause premature sexual development. Initially they increase bone growth but adult height is reduced because they cause the long bones to stop growing.

In females, excess androgens cause virilization, that is, the development of masculine features such as increase in body hair, deepening of the voice, enlargement of the clitoris, and *amenorrhea* (absence of menstruation).

Anemia

A condition in which the concentration of the oxygen-carrying pigment *hemoglobin* in the blood is below normal. Hemoglobin molecules are carried inside red *blood cells* and function to transport oxygen from the lungs to the tissues. Under normal circumstances, stable hemoglobin concentrations in the blood are maintained by a strict balance between red cell production in the bone marrow and red cell destruction in the spleen. Anemia may result if this balance is lost.

By far the most common form of anemia worldwide is due to a deficiency of iron, an essential component of hemoglobin. However, there are numerous other causes of anemia, which is not a disease itself but a feature of many different diseases and disorders.

TYPES AND CAUSES

Red blood cells are formed in the bone marrow over a period of about five days from less specialized cells called stem cells. During this time, the cells change their appearance and accumulate hemoglobin. The red cells released from the bone marrow into the blood are called reticulocytes. Over a few days reticulocytes mature into adult red blood cells. The adult cells circulate in the bloodstream for about 120 days; they age and are eventually trapped in small blood vessels (mainly in the spleen) and destroyed. Some cell components, including iron, are recycled for use in new cells.

The various forms of anemia can be classified into those caused by decreased or defective production of red cells by the bone marrow and those caused by decreased survival of the red cells in the blood (see illustrated box on types and causes).

SYMPTOMS

The symptoms common to all forms of anemia result from the reduced oxygen-carrying capacity of the blood. Their severity depends on how low the hemoglobin concentration in the blood is. Normal blood hemoglobin concentrations are between 14 to 16 g/100 ml for men and 12 to 14 g/100 ml for women. Concentrations below 10 g/100 ml can cause headaches, tiredness, and lethargy. Concentrations below 8 g/100 ml can cause breathing difficulty on exercise, dizziness due to reduced oxygen reaching the brain, *angina pectoris* due to reduced oxygen supply to the heart muscle, and palpitations as the heart works harder to compensate. General signs include pallor, although this is not a reliable indicator of the severity of the anemia. Symptoms also depend upon the speed of development of an anemia. The slowly developing form is toler-

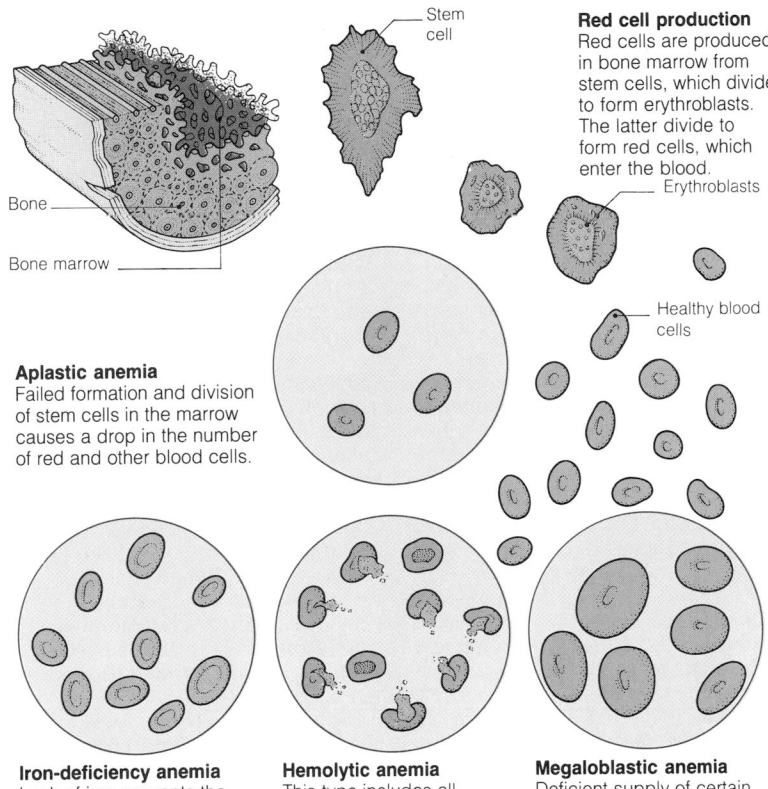

TYPES AND CAUSES OF ANEMIA

Anemia results either from reduced or defective production or from an excessively high rate of destruction of oxygen-carrying red blood cells.

Four of the main types are shown below, but anemia can have many other causes (such as various forms of leukemia).

Stem cell

Red cell production
Red cells are produced in bone marrow from stem cells, which divide to form erythroblasts. The latter divide to form red cells, which enter the blood.

Erythroblasts

Bone

Bone marrow

Healthy blood cells

Aplastic anemia
Failed formation and division of stem cells in the marrow causes a drop in the number of red and other blood cells.

Iron-deficiency anemia
Lack of iron prevents the bone marrow from making sufficient hemoglobin for the red cells. The cells produced are small and pale-centered and have a reduced oxygen-carrying capacity.

Hemolytic anemia
This type includes all anemias in which the rate of red cell production is normal or high but in which the cells are destroyed much faster than normal.

Megaloblastic anemia
Deficient supply of certain vitamins causes the bone marrow to produce red cells that are larger than normal and have a reduced oxygen-carrying capacity.

ated well until it becomes advanced; the sudden development of anemia causes immediate symptoms depending on the degree of blood loss.

Other symptoms may occur with particular forms of anemia. For example, some degree of *jaundice* occurs in most types of hemolytic anemia, because the high rate of destruction of red cells leads to increased bilirubin in the blood.

DIAGNOSIS
Anemia is diagnosed from the patient's symptoms and by the measurement of a low level of hemoglobin in the blood. To establish the type and cause of the anemia, a sample of blood is first examined

under the microscope, the numbers of different types of blood cells are counted, and their appearance is noted (see *Blood count*; *Blood smear*). A low proportion of reticulocytes suggests that the cause is decreased production of red cells; a high proportion of reticulocytes suggests that cells are being destroyed at a high rate. The size of the red cells—whether small, normal, or large—provides further clues. With some specific forms—for example, *sickle-cell anemia* (a type of hemolytic anemia)—some of the red cells have an abnormal shape.

Other investigations that may help the diagnosis include examination of cells in the bone marrow by means of a

bone marrow biopsy and measurement of the levels of substances such as folic acid, bilirubin, and vitamin B_{12} in the blood. Sometimes, more investigations must be carried out to establish the exact cause.

Treatment is aimed at correcting, modifying, or diminishing the mechanism or process that is leading to defective red cell production or reduced red cell survival. Treatment tends to be more straightforward for anemias caused by deficiencies (iron deficiency and megaloblastic anemias) than for those caused by inherited disorders or other disease processes (thalassemia and many types of hemolytic anemia).

Anemia, aplastic

A rare but important type of *anemia* in which the red cells, white blood cells, and platelet cells in the blood are reduced in number. Aplastic anemia is caused by failure to produce stem cells, the earliest form of all blood cells, in the *bone marrow*.

CAUSES AND INCIDENCE
Treatment of cancer with *radiation therapy* or *anticancer drugs* can interfere with the marrow's cell-producing capacity, as can certain viral infections and other drugs. In these cases, the bone marrow usually recovers and resumes normal production of cells once the cause is removed.

Long-term exposure to the fumes of benzene (a constituent of gasoline) or insecticides has been implicated as a cause of more persistent aplastic anemia, while a moderate to high dose of nuclear radiation (from radioactive fallout or nuclear explosions) is another recognized cause. In some people, aplastic anemia develops for no known reason—a condition that is known as primary or idiopathic aplastic anemia.

Aplastic anemia is most common around the age of 30.

SYMPTOMS
A low level of red blood cells may result in symptoms common to all types of anemia. Deficiency of white cells increases susceptibility to infections, while deficiency of platelets may lead to bruising easily, bleeding gums, or nosebleeds.

DIAGNOSIS
The disorder is usually suspected from the results of a blood test, particularly a *blood count*, and is confirmed by a *bone marrow biopsy*, in which a small sample of marrow is removed and examined for the presence or absence of blood-forming cells.

A

When aplastic anemia is due to infection or treatment for cancer, transfusions of red cells and platelets are given until the marrow returns to its normal state.

In persistent aplastic anemia, *bone marrow transplantation* may be carried out if a suitable donor is available. The donor must be someone whose tissue type closely matches that of the patient genetically (usually a brother or a sister).

OUTLOOK

Recovery usually occurs in mild forms of the disease. However, without bone marrow transplantation, severe aplastic anemia frequently is fatal.

Anemia, hemolytic

A form of *anemia* (reduced level of the oxygen-carrying pigment *hemoglobin* in blood) caused by the premature destruction of red cells in the bloodstream—a process known as hemolysis. Bone marrow has the capacity to increase red cell production approximately sixfold over normal rates. Anemia results only if the shortening of the red cell life span is sufficiently severe to overcome the marrow's reserve capacity.

TYPES AND CAUSES

Hemolytic anemias can be classified according to whether the cause of the problem is inside the red cell, in which case it is usually an inherited condition, or outside the cell, in which case it is usually acquired later in life.

RED CELL DEFECTS Hemolysis due to disorders within the red cell results from an abnormal rigidity of the cell membrane (the envelope that surrounds the cell). This causes the cell to become trapped at an early stage of its life span in the smaller blood vessels (usually of the spleen) and eventually be destroyed by macrophages (types of white blood cell).

The abnormal rigidity may result from an inherited defect of the cell membrane (as in hereditary *spherocytosis*), from a defect of the hemoglobin within the cell (as in *sickle-cell anemia*), or from a defect of one of the cell's enzymes. There are only two chemical processes occurring in red cells that are essential to their survival—one that provides energy and one that helps protect the cell from chemical damage. The last process is of great importance; a deficiency of one of the enzymes that catalyzes the process, called glucose-6-phosphate dehydrogenase, is a common cause of hemolytic anemia. A variety of it is

very common among blacks in the US and results from exposure to many types of drugs, including antibiotics and antimalarials (see *G6PD deficiency*). Another variety, in which hemolysis occurs after eating a certain type of bean, is most common in Greece (see *Favism*).

DEFECTS OUTSIDE THE RED CELL Hemolytic anemias resulting from defects outside the red cell fall into three main groups. First are disorders in which red cells are destroyed by mechanical buffeting (for example, when the lining of the blood vessels is abnormal, when the blood flows past artificial surfaces such as replacement heart valves, or in conditions in which a blood clot has formed inside the blood vessel). In all these conditions the otherwise normal red cell is physically disrupted by mechanical forces.

A second group of conditions is one in which red cells are destroyed by antibodies produced by the *immune system* and directed against the red cells. These immune hemolytic anemias may occur if foreign blood cells enter the bloodstream, as during an incompatible blood transfusion, or if the immune system becomes defective and fails to recognize the body's own red cells. This is a type of *autoimmune disorder*. Commonly, the reaction is triggered by a drug such as methyldopa. In *hemolytic disease of the newborn*, the baby's red cells are destroyed by antibodies produced by the mother.

In a third group of conditions, the red cells are destroyed by microorganisms in the blood. By far the most important cause is *malaria*.

SYMPTOMS AND DIAGNOSIS

People with hemolytic anemia may have symptoms common to all types of anemia (such as pallor, headaches, fatigue, and shortness of breath on exertion) or symptoms specifically due to the hemolysis (such as *jaundice*, caused by an excessive concentration in the blood of bile pigments formed from red cell destruction).

The diagnosis of hemolytic anemia depends on microscopic examination of the blood (see *Blood smear*), which often shows abnormally large numbers of immature red cells and, with some specific types, red cells that are abnormally shaped. The patient's racial background and medical history may also help establish the diagnosis.

TREATMENT

Some inherited causes of hemolytic anemia can be controlled by removing the main site of destruction of the red

cells—the spleen (see *Splenectomy*). Others, such as G6PD deficiency and favism, are largely preventable through avoidance of the drugs or foods that precipitate hemolysis.

Treatment of hemolysis caused by mechanical buffeting of red cells relies on reducing the disruptive forces. Those caused by immune or autoimmune processes can often be controlled through the use of *immunosuppressant drugs*.

More specific treatments may be required in particular cases—for example, the use of antimalarial drugs in hemolysis caused by malaria. Transfusions of red blood cells, or exchange transfusions of whole blood, are sometimes required for emergency treatment of severe life-threatening anemia.

Anemia, iron-deficiency

The most common form of *anemia* (a reduced level of the oxygen-carrying pigment *hemoglobin* in the blood); it is caused by a deficiency of iron, an essential constituent of hemoglobin.

Iron-deficiency anemia develops if insufficient iron is available to the bone marrow, where hemoglobin is manufactured and packaged into red blood cells. Anemia occurs when iron loss, along with any extra demand for iron required for growth, exceeds iron gained from the diet.

Small losses of hemoglobin and iron occur normally from the body through occasional minor bleeding; in women of childbearing age, these losses are much greater due to menstrual blood loss. Small amounts of iron are also shed in skin cells as they peel off from the body surface and tiny amounts are lost when red blood cells are destroyed at the end of their life span (most of the iron is efficiently repackaged into new red cells).

Because of their menstrual blood losses, women of childbearing age tend to have low, or no, built-up stores of iron and thus tend to become anemic more quickly in the event that iron losses exceed iron intake. The advent of pregnancy stops the menstrual losses but is replaced by an even greater drain on iron stores (from the baby); hence, pregnant women are at particular risk.

CAUSES

INCREASED LOSSES The main cause of iron-deficiency anemia is loss of iron at a greater rate than normal as a result of bleeding that is abnormally heavy or persistent. It may be caused by disease or by particularly heavy periods (see *Menorrhagia*). The diseases most commonly responsible for persistent bleeding are those of the digestive tract, such as erosive *gastritis*, *peptic ulcer*, *stomach cancer*, *inflammatory bowel disease*, and sometimes *hemorrhoids*. Prolonged treatment with aspirin and aspirinlike *nonsteroidal anti-inflammatory drugs* (NSAID) can cause gastrointestinal bleeding. In some countries, *hookworm infestation* of the digestive tract is an important cause.

Blood lost from the lower part of the intestine and from the rectum is bright red and usually noticed when feces are passed. If the bleeding is in the stomach or upper intestine, it is invisible; when it is excessive, it usually makes the feces black.

Bleeding may also take place in urinary tract disorders (such as *kidney tumors* or *bladder tumors*, *cystitis*, and *prostatitis*), when it colors the urine.

INSUFFICIENT INTAKE The second most common cause of iron deficiency is poor absorption of iron from the diet, usually as the result of surgical removal of part or all of the stomach (see *Gastrectomy*) but also sometimes due to *celiac sprue*, a digestive disorder of the small intestine.

The third possible, and the least common, cause is a diet that does not provide enough iron. Those most affected are old people who live alone and who eat a generally poor diet, and children and pregnant women, because of their extra needs. Women should be sure to have an iron-rich diet and may be prescribed iron tablets during pregnancy.

Foods containing iron
Foods such as fruit, whole-grain bread, beans, lean meat, and green vegetables are good sources of iron that help prevent iron-deficiency anemia.

SYMPTOMS
The symptoms are those of the underlying cause (for example, symptoms accompanying a peptic ulcer that bled), along with those common to all forms of anemia—fatigue and headaches, sometimes a sore mouth or tongue, brittle nails, and, in severe cases, breathlessness and pain in the center of the chest.

DIAGNOSIS AND TREATMENT
The diagnosis is made from the measurement of a low level of hemoglobin in the blood and from a *blood smear* test that usually shows the red blood cells to be smaller than normal. When the cause is not clear, investigations such as fecal analysis (for evidence of blood) and *barium X-ray examination* (to find digestive tract disorders) are carried out.

Treatment is for the underlying cause, along with a course of iron tablets or injections (or syrup for children) to build up the depleted iron stores and correct the anemia.

Anemia, megaloblastic
An important type of *anemia* (reduced level of the oxygen-carrying pigment *hemoglobin* in blood), caused by a deficiency of vitamin B_{12} or another vitamin, folic acid. Either of these deficiencies seriously interferes with the production of red blood cells in the bone marrow; the red blood cells that are formed are enlarged and deformed and are known as macrocytes.

CAUSES
VITAMIN B_{12} DEFICIENCY Vitamin B_{12} is found only in food of animal origin, such as meat, fish, and dairy products. It is absorbed from the small intestine after first combining with a chemical called intrinsic factor, produced by the stomach lining. In most diets, there is much more vitamin B_{12} than the body requires; the excess is stored in the liver, where it can last for a few years. If a person on a normal diet acquires a vitamin B_{12} deficiency, it is due not to lack of the vitamin but to an inability to absorb it.

The most common cause of such a deficiency is called pernicious anemia; it is caused by failure of the stomach lining to produce intrinsic factor, usually because of an *autoimmune disorder*, in which antibodies are produced that block the production of intrinsic factor. Pernicious anemia has a tendency to run in families, to start in middle age, and to affect women more than men. It is sometimes associated with other disorders, such as *diabetes mellitus* or *myxedema*. Total gastrectomy (removal of the stomach) prevents intrinsic factor production by removing its source.

Other causes of malabsorption of the vitamin include removal of part of the small intestine (where vitamin B_{12} is absorbed) and *Crohn's disease*.

Bone marrow in megaloblastic anemia
In this microscopic view, some of the large cells are abnormal red cell precursors (megaloblasts)

In a minority of cases, vitamin B_{12} deficiency is the result of a vegan diet, which excludes eggs and dairy products as well as meat and fish.

FOLIC ACID DEFICIENCY Present to some extent in many foods, folic acid is found mainly in green vegetables and liver. However, unlike vitamin B_{12}, it is not stored in the body in large amounts; therefore, a constant supply is needed (and pregnant women require supplements). For this reason, the usual cause of deficiency is a poor diet. The disorder is most common in the poor and in old people living by themselves. It may also occur in people with alcohol dependence.

Deficiency can also be caused by anything that interferes with the absorption of folic acid from the small intestine (e.g., disorders such as *Crohn's disease* and *celiac sprue* or removal of part of the small intestine).

SYMPTOMS
Many people with mild megaloblastic anemia have no symptoms. In others, symptoms may include any or all of the following: tiredness, headaches, a sore mouth and tongue, weight loss, and, in pernicious anemia, *jaundice*, shown by a slight yellow tint to the skin. In severe cases there may also be breathlessness, chest pain, and sometimes loss of balance and tingling in the feet due to damage to the nervous system from lack of the vitamins.

DIAGNOSIS
The anemia is usually first suspected following *blood tests* that show a low level of hemoglobin, a preponderance of large red blood cells, and low levels of either vitamin B_{12} or folic acid or both. The disease is confirmed if a *bone marrow biopsy* (removal of a small sample of marrow for analysis) reveals the presence of large numbers of megaloblasts. Tests may also be carried out to discover an underlying cause in cases where it is not clear.

Pernicious anemia is sometimes diagnosed by a special test, the Schilling test, in which the absorption of vitamin B_{12} into the bloodstream is measured with the vitamin first unbound and then bound to intrinsic factor. If the vitamin is found to be absorbed only when bound to intrinsic factor, it confirms the cause as pernicious anemia.

TREATMENT

When megaloblastic anemia is due to poor diet, it can be remedied by adopting a normal diet and taking a short course of vitamin B_{12} injections or folic acid tablets.

In cases when the deficiency is due to inability to absorb the vitamin, it can sometimes be remedied by treating the underlying cause, but often the power of absorption is lost permanently. A lifelong course of replacement injections or tablets of vitamin B_{12} or folic acid is then required.

Anemia, pernicious

One of the main types of anemia caused by vitamin B_{12} deficiency. See *Anemia, megaloblastic*.

Anencephaly

Absence at birth of the brain, cranial vault (top of the skull), and spinal cord. Most affected infants are stillborn or survive only a few hours. Anencephaly is detectable early in pregnancy by measurement of *alphafetoprotein*, by *ultrasound scanning*, and by *amniocentesis*; if anencephaly is detected, termination of the pregnancy may be considered.

Anencephaly is due to a failure in development of the neural tube, the nerve tissue in the embryo that eventually develops into the spinal cord and brain. Maldevelopment of the neural tube may also result in *spina bifida* and *hydrocephalus*. These abnormalities are collectively known as *neural tube defects* and seem likely to have similar causes. Anencephaly occurs in about five in every 1,000 pregnancies, but only in about one third of these does the pregnancy continue to term.

Anesthesia

Literally, the absence of all sensation. It may occur in an area of the body after nerve tissues are damaged by injury or disease. Rarely, anesthesia may be a result of extreme arousal, as in the case of boxers or soldiers who do not notice painful blows or wounds. Psychological factors may be responsible for numbness, particularly in the hand or foot (see *Conversion disorder*). Anesthesia is also induced artificially to abolish pain during surgical procedures and childbirth.

Two types of anesthesia are used for medical purposes. Under local anesthesia (see *Anesthesia, local*), the patient remains conscious and sensation is abolished in only part of the body. This is usually accomplished by injection of drugs that temporarily interrupt the nerve supply from the region to be anesthetized. Local anesthetics can also be given in the form of eye drops, sprays, skin creams, and suppositories. It may be possible to produce local pain relief by using *acupuncture*; this technique is widely used in China, but is rarely used by Western practitioners, who have less success with it.

Using general anesthesia (see *Anesthesia, general*), the patient is rendered unconscious and maintained in this state by being given a combination of drugs that are either injected intravenously or inhaled. These drugs affect all parts of the body but have their main sites of action in the brain and spinal cord.

Anesthesia, dental

Loss of sensation induced in a patient to prevent pain during dental treatment or dental surgery. Most dental procedures are carried out using local anesthesia; general anesthesia is usually reserved for surgical procedures and special cases.

LOCAL ANESTHESIA

For minor restorative work, such as fillings, some patients and dentists choose no anesthesia; otherwise, a local anesthetic (for example, lidocaine or procaine) is injected into the gum at the site that is being treated. Sometimes it is not possible to inject directly into the area to be treated because the gum is painfully inflamed or because there is a risk of spreading an infection in the gum. In these cases, the anesthetic is injected into or around the nerve a short distance away from the site of operation, a procedure known as a peripheral *nerve block*. Topical anesthetics on the gums are often used in conjunction with injected anesthetics.

SEDATION

In addition to receiving a local anesthetic, a patient who is abnormally anxious, agitated, or uncooperative may need to be calmed by sedation. To sedate the patient, an antianxiety agent is given orally or intravenously, or through inhalation.

These antianxiety agents include tranquilizers, nitrous oxide (laughing gas), and barbiturates.

GENERAL ANESTHESIA

The most common use for general anesthesia is in surgical procedures such as periodontal (gum) surgery and multiple tooth extractions. General anesthesia is also used for young children, for people who are allergic to local anesthetics or who have extremely sensitive teeth, and for those who are unable to cooperate due to, for example, a mental disorder or physical handicap.

For relatively short dental surgery, general anesthesia is given by an injection of a barbiturate, such as methohexital or thiopental, into a vein, with a mixture of nitrous oxide and oxygen being given during surgery to maintain anesthesia.

For longer or more complicated procedures, general anesthesia is carried out as it is for other surgery (see *Anesthesia, general*).

Anesthesia, general

Loss of sensation and consciousness induced in a patient, most often to prevent pain and discomfort during surgery. The state of general anesthesia is produced and maintained by an *anesthesiologist*, who gives combinations of drugs by injection, inhalation, or both. The anesthesiologist is also responsible for the preanesthetic assessment of patients, their safety during surgery, and their recovery during the postanesthetic period.

HISTORY

Until the middle of the nineteenth century, pain relief during surgery relied on natural substances such as alcohol, opium, and cannabis. However, the relief obtained was often inadequate and short-lived. It was not until the 1840s that solutions began to be found to the problem of inducing unconsciousness in a manner that was safe, easily maintained for long periods, and reversible. *Ether* was first demonstrated successfully in Boston in 1846, where a tooth was extracted without pain while the patient was breathing ether. Soon after, the anesthetic properties of chloroform and nitrous oxide were discovered, heralding a new era in surgery.

WHY IT IS DONE

The primary objectives of general anesthesia are to abolish pain, awareness, muscle tone, and cardiovascular reflexes in the patient to make conditions suitable for surgery or diagnostic procedures and easier for the patient.

TECHNIQUES FOR GENERAL ANESTHESIA

The main phases in the administration of a general anesthetic are induction (bringing on unconsciousness), maintenance, and emergence (returning the patient to consciousness). Some of the main stages are shown below. Often, to allow surgical manipulation, a muscle relaxant must be given in addition to anesthetic gases or injections. Because the relaxant temporarily paralyzes the breathing muscles, the patient's lungs must be ventilated artificially.

DRUGS USED IN GENERAL ANESTHESIA

Type	Action	Examples
Drugs given as premedication	Relax patient, abolish pain, reduce saliva and mucus formation	Diazepam, morphine, atropine
Induction agents	Induce unconsciousness	Thiopental sodium
Anesthetic gases and volatile agents	Induce and/or maintain unconsciousness	Nitrous oxide, halothane, enflurane, isoflurane
Analgesics	Abolish pain	Morphine, fentanyl
Muscle relaxants	Relax muscles	Pancuronium, vecuronium
Reversal agents	Reverse muscle relaxation	Neostigmine

1 Before the operation, the anesthesiologist talks to and examines the patient and assesses his or her fitness for anesthesia and surgery. He or she also answers the patient's questions.

2 Before the operation, premedication may be given. It may include a drug that relieves pain or anxiety and one that prevents excessive salivation.

Anesthesiologist

Assistant

Gas mask

Gas cylinder pressure meters

Hoses carrying anesthetic gas supply

6 While surgery is in progress, the patient is kept at a level of anesthesia deep enough to be unaware of the operation. The composition of the gas mixture, and the patient's heart rate, breathing, blood pressure, temperature, blood oxygenation, and exhaled carbon dioxide are continuously monitored.

3 The induction agent is usually given via a cannula inserted into a vein. The cannula is left in position so that other drugs can be given rapidly if needed.

4 Sometimes, anesthesia is induced or maintained with gases delivered by mask. If no muscle relaxant is used, the patient may be able to continue breathing naturally.

5 In other cases, a breathing tube is inserted for delivery of the anesthetic gases. If a muscle relaxant is used, artificial ventilation is necessary.

A

COMPLICATIONS

The likelihood of any complications occurring depends on the preoperative condition of the patient, the anesthetic technique used, and the nature of the operation performed.

General anesthesia is associated with many possible complications necessitating the administration of several powerful drugs. Complications include *hypotension* (low blood pressure), cardiac *arrhythmia* (irregular heart beat), *myocardial infarction* (heart attack), inhibited respiration, *airway obstruction*, life-threatening febrile (feverish) reactions, allergic reactions, nausea, vomiting and *aspiration* (inhaling vomit into the lungs), *hypoxia*, physical injury (such as chipped teeth, muscle cramps, and brain damage), and death.

AWARENESS DURING ANESTHESIA It is possible, though rare with modern anesthetic techniques, for patients to remain aware of events during surgery but, because of muscle relaxants, to be unable to signal this distressed state to the anesthesiologist. The concentrations of anesthetic agents required to produce adequate anesthesia in the majority of patients are well documented. In addition, the anesthesiologist can detect an inadequate level of anesthesia by noting physical signs, such as increased sweating, tearing, and salivation, and irregular breathing, changes in muscle tone, spontaneous eye movements, and increases in the patient's heart rate and blood pressure.

Anesthesia, local

Loss of sensation induced in a limited region of a person's body to prevent pain during examinations, diagnostic procedures, treatments, and surgical operations. Local anesthesia is produced by the administration of drugs that temporarily interrupt the action of pain-carrying nerve fibers.

HOW IT IS DONE

For minor surgical procedures, such as stitching of small wounds, local anesthesia is usually produced by direct injection into the area to be treated. When it is necessary to anesthetize a large area, or when local injection would not penetrate deeply enough into body tissues, a *nerve block* may be used. For a nerve block, nerves at a point remote from the area to be treated are injected (i.e., the palm of the hand may be anesthetized by injecting points near the elbow, which blocks the ulnar and median nerves). This is known as regional anesthesia.

LOCAL ANESTHETICS

Drug	Common uses	How taken	Action
Benzocaine	To treat skin irritation, toothache, teething pains, hemorrhoids	Cream, ointment, spray, gel, liquid	Rapid action, short duration
Bupivacaine	As a nerve block (e.g., epidural anesthesia)	Injection	Medium action, long duration
Cocaine	Formerly used for minor surgical procedures on eye, ear, nose, and throat	Liquid, spray	Rapid action, short duration
Lidocaine	To treat skin irritation, relief of pain during dental treatment, nerve blocks (e.g., epidural anesthesia)	Cream, ointment, spray, injection	Rapid action, medium duration
Procaine	For relief of pain before surgical and dental treatment	Injection	Slow action, short duration
Tetracaine	For anal irritation, relief of pain during dental treatment and throat examinations, minor surgical procedures on the eye	Cream, ointment, spray, liquid, eye drops	Rapid action, medium to long duration

Nerves can also be blocked as they branch off from the spinal cord, as in *epidural anesthesia*, which is widely used during childbirth, and spinal anesthesia (see *Spinal block*), which is used mainly for surgery of the lower limbs and lower abdomen.

Some parts of the body that are permeable to local anesthetic drugs can be anesthetized by applying an anesthetic drug directly to the area. The throat, larynx, and respiratory passages can be sprayed before *bronchoscopy*, and the urethra can be numbed with a gel for performing *catheterization* or *cystoscopy*. A cream has been developed that is rubbed onto the skin so that injections will be painless. Other applications include lozenges for sore throats, and ointments or rectal suppositories for relieving hemorrhoids.

For some procedures, particularly if the patient is anxious, a sedative is given with the local anesthetic.

COMPLICATIONS

Patients can have adverse reactions to the anesthetic drug if the dose is too high or has been absorbed too rapidly. Such reactions include dizziness, loss of consciousness, seizures, and cardiac arrest. In rare cases, people have an allergic reaction to the drug itself. During major (epidural and spinal) blocks, reduced activity of the blocked sympathetic nervous system may result in hypotension and reduced blood flow to the brain and heart. Infections at the site of injection range from inconsequential to life-threatening (e.g., meningitis). Certain local anesthetics may cause long-term nerve damage.

Anesthesiologist

A specialist who administers the drugs that "put you to sleep" during an operation. Anesthesiologists also assess the condition of a patient's heart, lungs, and circulation before he or she is sent into the operating room. They decide what type and how much anesthesia is needed, determine the patient's position on the operating table, watch for signs of trouble, and decide what actions should be taken if an emergency develops. An anesthesiologist is also responsible for monitoring the progress of the waking patient and watching for any developing complications in the recovery room after surgery. In many institutions the anesthesiologist is responsible for respiration therapy.

Aneurysm

Ballooning of an artery due to the pressure of blood flowing through a weakened area. The weakening may be due to disease, injury, or a congenital defect in the artery wall.

TYPES

Some of the common types, sites, and shapes of aneurysm are shown in the illustrated box.

A dissecting aneurysm, usually associated with atherosclerosis, is a condition in which a longitudinal, blood-filled split forms within the lining of the wall of an artery—usually the aorta—and spreads so that extensive areas of the vessel are weakened. There is usually severe pain and the vessel may rupture. When the aneurysm is located in the arch or ascending aorta and dissects into the pericardium (membrane surrounding the heart), the pressure of the blood around the heart may be fatal because it prevents the heart from beating. If an abdominal aorta ruptures, it hemorrhages behind the peritoneum (outside the abdominal cavity).

The heart wall may also develop an aneurysmal swelling after weakening of the muscle from *myocardial infarction* (heart attack). Such aneurysms seldom rupture but they often interfere with the efficient pumping action of the heart.

A traumatic aneurysm is one caused by mechanical injury that weakens the blood vessel wall.

CAUSES

There are several reasons why aneurysms form. One is congenital weakness of the muscular middle layer of an artery; normal blood pressure causes dilation (ballooning) of the blood vessel wall at the weak point. *Marfan's syndrome*, a condition in which the middle layer of the wall of the aorta is defective, often leads to aneurysm just above the heart. The arterial wall can also be weakened by inflammation, as in *periarteritis nodosa*.

The great majority of aneurysms of the aorta—usually in the lower part of the vessel—are caused by atherosclerotic (see *Atherosclerosis*) weakening of a segment of the wall. Aneurysm of the ascending aorta once commonly resulted from untreated *syphilis* but this is now rare. Aneurysms of smaller vessels (mycotic aneurysms) may occur in septicemia as a result of local infection of the wall of the artery.

SYMPTOMS AND SIGNS

Symptoms vary according to the type, size, and location of the swelling.

TYPES OF ANEURYSM

An aneurysm forms when pressure from the blood flow causes a weakened artery wall to distend or forces blood through a fissure.

Aneurysms can form anywhere in the body, although the most common sites are the aorta and the arteries supplying the brain.

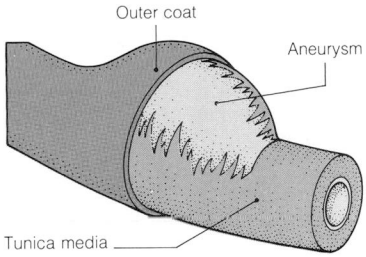

Common aneurysm
This type forms when the tunica media, the artery's middle wall, is weakened; the strong force of the blood flow distends the wall of the artery.

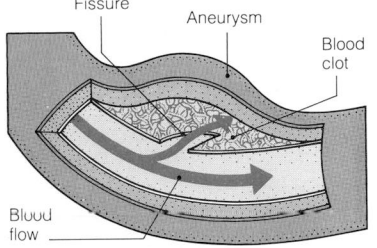

Dissecting aneurysm
This type occurs when there is a fissure in the internal wall of the artery; blood forced through the fissure forms a swelling.

Cerebral (or berry) aneurysm
A swelling where the arteries branch at the brain's base, often caused by congenital weakness.

Saccular aneurysm
A balloon-shaped distention of part of an artery's wall, often seen in aortic aneurysms just above the heart.

Fusiform aneurysm
A distention around an artery's circumference, tapered at both ends, often seen in lower aortic aneurysms.

Cerebral aneurysms may persist for many years without causing symptoms, but the close proximity of so many important neurological structures makes them very dangerous. Sudden enlargement and bursting of a berry aneurysm produces obvious symptoms and signs, such as paralysis of eye movement, drooping of the lid, dilation of the pupil, neck rigidity, severe headache, and unconsciousness (symptoms similar to those of a stroke).

Pressure from an aneurysm on surrounding structures may cause damage, especially within the confined space of the skull.

Aneurysms may rupture, sometimes causing fatal blood loss, or, in the case of cerebral aneurysms, severe damage to the brain structure (see *Subarachnoid hemorrhage*).

Aneurysms of the thoracic (chest) part of the aorta are usually accompanied by hoarseness (due to pressure on the esophagus or a nerve controlling a vocal chord), difficult swallowing, and chest pain that may be mistaken for myocardial infarction (heart attack). Abdominal aortic aneurysm is sometimes visible as a throbbing swelling and may also cause backache.

DIAGNOSIS

X rays will sometimes reveal an aneurysm in a larger blood vessel, but *angiography* provides more detailed information. In the case of cerebral aneurysms, valuable information may be obtained from *CT scanning* or *MRI*.

A

TREATMENT AND OUTLOOK

This varies with the site of the aneurysm and the age and health of the patient. Nonurgent surgery for aortic aneurysms of the chest offers an 80 to 90 percent chance of survival; emergency surgery carries a high risk. A ruptured aneurysm in the chest always requires surgery, but the outlook is poor. Ruptured or enlarged aneurysms require urgent surgery (see *Arterial reconstructive surgery*). If cerebral aneurysm causes symptoms, surgery is recommended if possible.

Angel dust

One of the common names for phencyclidine, an illicit drug taken for its hallucinogenic properties. Adverse effects of the drug include respiratory depression, agitation, muscle rigidity, vomiting, and convulsions; several deaths have also been reported.

Angiitis

See *Vasculitis*.

Angina

A term that describes a strangling or oppressive heaviness or pain. Angina has become synonymous with the heart disorder *angina pectoris* (chest pain caused by lack of oxygen to the heart muscle, usually a result of poor blood supply). Other types of angina include abdominal angina (abdominal pain after eating caused by poor blood supply to the intestines) and Vincent's angina, pain caused by inflammation of the mouth (see *Vincent's disease*).

Angina pectoris

Pain in the chest and arms or jaw due to a lack of oxygen to the heart muscle, usually when the demand for oxygen is increased during exercise and at times of stress.

CAUSES

Inadequate blood supply to the heart is usually due to *coronary heart disease*, in which the coronary arteries are narrowed by *atherosclerosis* (fat deposits on the walls of the arteries). Other causes include coronary artery spasm, in which the blood vessels narrow suddenly for a short time but return to normal with no permanent obstruction, *aortic stenosis* (narrowing of the aortic valve), and *arrhythmias* (abnormal heart rhythm).

Rare causes of angina pectoris include severe *anemia*, which reduces the oxygen-carrying efficiency of the blood, and *polycythemia* (increased numbers of red blood cells), which thickens the blood, causing it to slow its flow through the heart muscle. *Thyrotoxicosis* (excessive production of thyroid hormones) can precipitate angina pectoris by making the heart work much harder and faster than its blood supply will permit.

INCIDENCE

This very common condition may occur at any time in men. It is common in men in their fifties, but has been known to occur after the age of 30; in women it usually starts later in life.

SYMPTOMS

The chest pain varies from mild to severe and is often described as a sensation of pressure on the chest. It usually starts in the center of the chest but can spread to the throat, upper jaw, back, and arms (usually the left one) or between the shoulder blades.

The pain usually comes on when the heart is working harder and requires more oxygen—for example, during exercise, when under stress, in extremes of temperature, or during milder exercise soon after a meal. Typically the pain develops at the same point in daily activities—for example, the third flight of stairs on the climb to the office, or halfway up the hill to the stores—and is relieved by a short rest.

Other symptoms may include nausea, sweating, dizziness, and breathing difficulty. These symptoms are usually characteristic of angina pectoris, but somewhat similar symptoms can be caused by *esophagitis* (inflammation of the esophagus), spasm of the esophagus, arthritis in the upper spine or rib cage, or a pulled muscle in the chest wall.

A prolonged and usually more severe attack of angina pectoris may be due to *myocardial infarction* (heart attack), in which the heart muscle is permanently damaged.

DIAGNOSIS

Angina pectoris cannot be diagnosed with certainty by a physical examination; more tests are necessary. Tests usually include an ECG (measurement of the electrical activity in the heart) while the patient is at rest and a *cardiac stress test* (an ECG performed while the patient is exercising enough to cause chest pain—for example, while walking on a treadmill). The resting ECG will show no signs of the angina (unless it is occurring), but may show former heart damage.

Blood tests may be performed to look for an underlying cause, such as *anemia* or *hyperlipidemia* (abnormally high levels of fat in the blood, which can cause *atherosclerosis*).

TREATMENT

Initial treatment attempts to control the symptoms. It is important to stop smoking; nicotine and carbon monoxide contribute to the progressive development of coronary heart disease and make the symptoms worse. Overweight people should lose weight to reduce stress on the heart during exercise.

Attacks of angina pectoris may be prevented and treated by *nitrates* (nitroglycerin), which increase the flow of blood through the heart muscle and improve blood flow around the body. If nitrates are not effective, or are causing severe headaches due to an increased blood flow through the brain, other drugs may be used, including *beta-blockers* and *calcium channel blockers*.

If *hypertension* (high blood pressure) is found during examination, it is treated with antihypertensive drugs to reduce the work of the heart in pumping out blood. Other specific causes can also be treated—for example, arrhythmias with antiarrhythmic drugs and hyperlipidemia with a low-fat diet and/or drugs.

Drug treatment can control the symptoms of angina pectoris for many years but it cannot cure the disorder. If attacks become more severe, more frequent, or more prolonged, despite drug treatment, and if there is angiographic evidence of advanced narrowing of vessels, then *coronary artery bypass* surgery or *angioplasty* may be performed to reestablish blood flow to the heart muscle.

OUTLOOK

The effect of angina pectoris on lifestyle depends on the severity of the underlying disease and the effectiveness of drug treatment or surgery. Some people are able to lead a normal life apart from some restriction on strenuous exercise. Others are severely disabled and can do very little for themselves.

Angioedema

An allergic reaction, also known as angioneurotic edema. It is similar to *urticaria* (hives) and characterized by large, well-defined swellings, of sudden onset, in the skin, larynx (voice box), and other areas. These swellings may last several hours or days if they are left untreated.

INCIDENCE AND CAUSES

Angioedema primarily affects young people (especially those in their twenties) and those with a general tendency toward allergies (see *Atopy*).

The most common cause is a sudden allergic reaction to a food, such as eggs, strawberries, or seafood. Less commonly, it results from allergy to a drug (such as penicillin), a reaction to an insect sting or bite, or from infection, emotional stress, or exposure to animals, molds, pollens, or cold conditions. There is also a hereditary form of the disease.

SYMPTOMS
Angioedema may cause very sudden difficulty breathing, speaking, and swallowing accompanied by obvious swelling of the lips, face, and neck.

Angioedema of the throat and the larynx may be life-threatening because it can block the airway, causing *asphyxia* (suffocation). If the gastrointestinal tract is involved, colic, nausea, and vomiting may occur.

TREATMENT
Severe cases are treated with injections of *epinephrine* and may require intubation (passage of a breathing tube via the mouth into the windpipe) or *tracheostomy* (surgical creation of a breathing hole in the windpipe) to prevent suffocation. *Corticosteroid drugs* may also be prescribed to be taken intravenously or by mouth. In less severe cases, *antihistamine drugs* often relieve symptoms.

Angiography
A procedure that enables blood vessels to be seen on film after the vessels have been filled with a contrast medium (a substance that is opaque to X rays).

WHY IT IS DONE
Angiography is used to detect diseases that alter the appearance of the blood vessel channel. These diseases include *aneurysms* (weakening of the blood vessel wall and ballooning of the vessel itself), and narrowing or blockage from *atheroma* (fatty deposits) or from a thrombus or embolus (clot). Angiography is also used to detect changes in the pattern of blood vessels that lead to tumors and to organs that have been injured. By noting the abnormal arrangement of blood vessels, the physician can evaluate the extent of disease and plan treatment accordingly.

TYPES
Carotid angiography is sometimes performed on patients suffering from *transient ischemic attacks* (symptoms of *stroke* lasting less than 24 hours) to see whether there is a blockage or substantial narrowing in one of the carotid arteries (in the neck), which supply blood to the brain. Cerebral

Angiogram of a normal kidney
Contrast medium is passed through the catheter into the kidney's arterial system and a series of X-ray pictures is taken.

Digital subtraction angiography
Here, the normal kidneys are revealed more clearly because the computer eliminates unwanted information.

angiography is used to demonstrate the presence of an aneurysm within the brain or to help visualize a brain tumor prior to surgery. Angiography of the coronary arteries, often combined with cardiac *catheterization*, is carried out to identify the sites of narrowing or blockage in arteries, which may be treated by *coronary artery bypass* or balloon *angioplasty*.

HOW IT IS DONE
Contrast medium is usually injected into the vessel to be examined through a fine catheter (flexible plastic tube) inserted into the femoral artery at the groin, the brachial artery just over the elbow, or the carotid arteries that run up the neck.

To insert the catheter, the skin and tissues around the artery are numbed with local anesthetic and then a needle is inserted through the skin into the artery. A long, thin wire with a soft tip is inserted through the needle, the needle is removed, and the catheter is then threaded over the wire into the blood vessel. Under X-ray control, the tip of the catheter is further guided into the vessel to be examined and contrast medium is injected. A rapid sequence (or movie) of X-ray pictures is taken so that the flow along the vessels can be studied.

Angiography can take from as little as a few minutes to as long as two or three hours.

DIGITAL SUBTRACTION ANGIOGRAPHY
This type of angiography uses computer techniques to process images and subtract, or remove, unwanted background information, leaving only an image of the blood vessels being studied. This technique makes it possible to use a much smaller amount of contrast medium (sometimes injected intravenously), which makes the procedure somewhat safer; in

some cases, it removes the need for direct injection of contrast medium into vessels not accessible by catheter. However, the detail provided is not always as good as in conventional angiography.

RISKS
The contrast medium usually produces a sensation of warmth lasting a few seconds; it may be felt to a greater degree in the part of the body that has been injected. Allergy to the contrast medium is a more serious side effect, but with new contrast agents the risk of a severe reaction is less than one in 80,000 examinations.

Damage to blood vessels can occur at the site of puncture, anywhere along the vessel during passage of the catheter, or at the site of injection.

With digital subtraction angiography, the risks are considerably reduced because the catheter does not need to be passed as far into the blood vessels, thus lessening the possibility of damage or blockage.

OUTLOOK
Angiographic techniques have, in the last few years, been adapted to allow not only diagnosis, but certain types of treatment that, in some cases, eliminate the need for surgery. For example, small balloons can be inflated at the tip of a catheter to expand a narrowed or blocked segment of artery (balloon angioplasty), foreign material can be injected to reduce or shut off blood supply to a tumor (see *Embolism, therapeutic*), and medication to control bleeding or treat tumors can be infused directly into the blood supply to individual organs.

Angioma
A benign tumor made up of blood vessels (see *Hemangioma*) or lymph vessels (lymphangioma).

Angioplasty, balloon

A technique for treating stenosis (narrowing) or occlusion (blockage) of a blood vessel or heart valve by introducing a balloon into the constricted area to widen it.

WHY IT IS DONE

Balloon angioplasty is used in the treatment of *peripheral vascular disease* to increase or restore the flow of blood through a significantly narrowed artery in a limb; it is also used in the treatment of stenosis of the coronary arteries (see *Coronary heart disease*).

COMPLICATIONS

There is a slight risk of damaging the artery or valve during this procedure and immediate surgery may be required. Prolonged interruption of blood supply to an area of the heart, when the balloon is inflated, can lead to *myocardial infarction* (heart attack). The mortality for balloon angioplasty is about the same as for a coronary artery bypass graft.

RESULTS

In the US, coronary balloon angioplasty is successful in improving the condition of about two thirds of the patients treated with it. In three quarters of these cases the improvement continues after a year; in the remainder, stenosis recurs in the affected vessel, but angioplasty may be repeated successfully.

Angioplasty of peripheral vessels is most successful in treating the iliac and femoral arteries, particularly when the area of stenosis or occlusion is small. After five years, 85 to 90 percent of iliac arteries treated by angioplasty remain free of stenosis. For femoral arteries, the success rate is 50 to 70 percent after two years.

Angiotensin

The name of two related proteins involved in regulating blood pressure. The first of these, angiotensin I, is itself inactive and is converted to the second, active form, angiotensin II, by the action of a converting enzyme. Angiotensin II causes narrowing of the small blood vessels in tissues, resulting in an increase in blood pressure. It also stimulates the release from the adrenal cortex (the outer part of the *adrenal glands*) of the hormone *aldosterone*, which also causes an increase in blood pressure.

Certain kidney disorders can increase the production of angiotensin II, causing *hypertension* (high blood pressure). Whatever the cause of the hypertension, it may be treated with drugs that are known as *ACE inhibitors* (angiotensin-converting enzyme inhibitors), which reduce angiotensin II formation.

Animal experimentation

The use of living animals in research and safety testing to provide information about biological science and to increase knowledge about human physiology or behavior. Animal experimentation is most prolific in developed countries, where medical standards are high and there is intense concern for public health and safety.

The species most extensively used in animal experimentation are rats and mice, which are bred for laboratory research. Less than 1 percent of experiments involve cats, dogs, farm animals, nonhuman primates, frogs, fish, and birds.

LEGISLATIVE CONTROLS

Animal experimentation is controlled by law in most countries but the controls vary in their stringency. Governments must balance pressures for very tight controls against the weight of medical and scientific opinion, which maintains that animal experiments are indispensable to health and safety.

TYPES OF EXPERIMENTS

The experiments for which animals are used fall into several groups. One group consists of experiments to test the safety of nonmedical substances, such as pesticides, cleaning chemicals, and cosmetics, before they are released for public use.

Another group includes the many medical experiments in which a condition in an animal corresponds to a human disease. This provides the

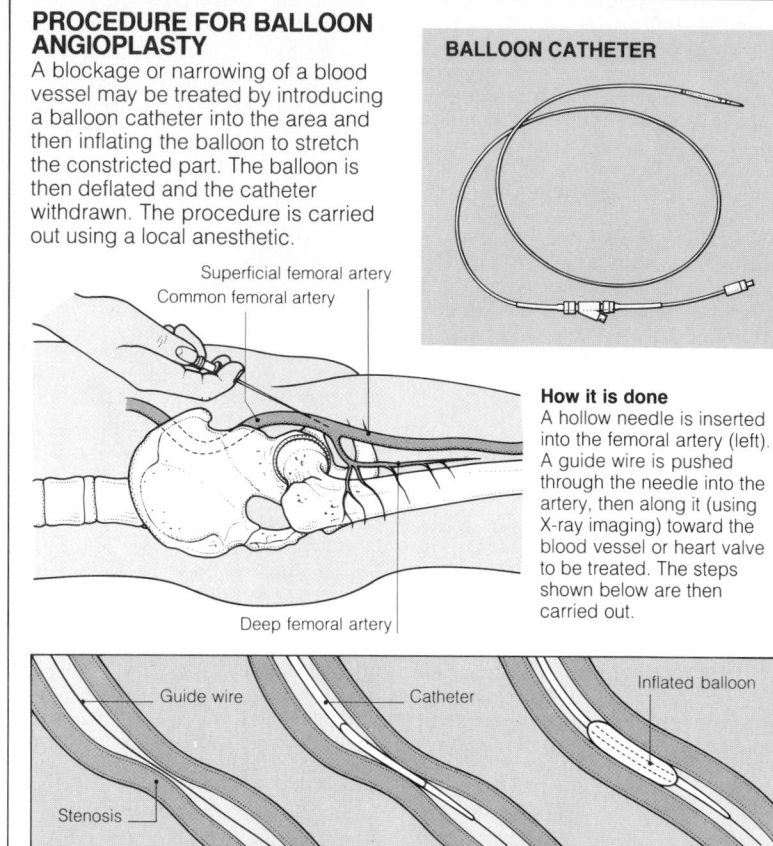

PROCEDURE FOR BALLOON ANGIOPLASTY

A blockage or narrowing of a blood vessel may be treated by introducing a balloon catheter into the area and then inflating the balloon to stretch the constricted part. The balloon is then deflated and the catheter withdrawn. The procedure is carried out using a local anesthetic.

BALLOON CATHETER

Superficial femoral artery
Common femoral artery
Deep femoral artery

How it is done
A hollow needle is inserted into the femoral artery (left). A guide wire is pushed through the needle into the artery, then along it (using X-ray imaging) toward the blood vessel or heart valve to be treated. The steps shown below are then carried out.

Guide wire — Catheter — Inflated balloon
Stenosis

1 The thin guide wire is maneuvered through the arteries (using X-ray control) until it is just past the stenosis (narrowing) to be treated.

2 A balloon-tipped catheter (top right) is then threaded over the guide wire and pushed along it until it reaches the narrowed area.

3 A sausage-shaped balloon at the end of the catheter is inflated and deflated a few times to widen the narrowed part, then withdrawn.

potential for testing new treatments to discover cures for the disease in the animal and therefore in humans.

Other experiments are performed to discover new drugs and medical procedures or to develop new substances for use in the environment.

ETHICAL OBJECTIONS

Campaigners for animal rights point out that animals suffer in many of these experiments. Sometimes the suffering is an implicit part of the research, as in research to study the mechanism of pain or to create models of painful conditions on which to test analgesics (painkillers). Some of the conditions or effects being studied necessarily cause illness, stress, or pain, such as infecting animals with disease or studying the irritant or poisonous effects of chemicals.

Two safety tests, often required by law, have received considerable criticism from protest groups and scientists alike. One test is the LD50 test, which measures acute toxicity (short-term poisonous effects) by estimating the dose that would kill 50 percent of the animals in a test group. The other test is the Draize test, which measures irritant damage of chemicals and substances to eyes and skin.

BENEFITS

Experiments on animals have contributed greatly to the advancement of science and have specifically produced benefits to humanity by virtue of new medical and surgical treatments. In the past 30 years, smallpox has been eradicated and the incidence of polio and other infections has been reduced enormously as a result of vaccines produced after such testing.

Antibiotics developed using animal experiments have also prolonged and saved many lives. It has been estimated that the reduction in infant mortality as a result of antibiotics has alone saved half a million lives. Drugs for the treatment of noninfectious disorders, such as arthritis, diabetes, and hypertension (high blood pressure), are also the result of animal-based research. Surgical treatments may also be developed in animals; the success of transplant operations and microsurgery techniques are notable recent advances.

ALTERNATIVES

Alternatives to animal experiments have been developed and are used whenever possible. Laboratory tests using cultured cells or tissues have replaced many experiments that once involved animals. Other alternatives involve the use of simple organisms, such as bacteria or yeasts, or the computerized or mathematical modeling of an experiment.

New techniques have also led in some cases to the replacement of animals as a source of vaccines and hormones. Cell culture techniques have now almost replaced the use of animals in vaccine production, while genetically engineered bacteria and yeasts are increasingly used to produce substances, such as insulin, that were once derived only from animals.

However, even with these newer methods, it is dangerous—and illegal—not to undertake confirmatory studies on animals before releasing the drug or vaccine in question.

Animals, diseases from

See *Zoonoses*.

Anisometropia

Unequal focusing power in the two eyes, usually due to a difference in size and/or shape in the eyes. For example, one eye may be normal and the other myopic (nearsighted) or hyperopic (farsighted), or there may be astigmatism in one eye.

Significant anisometropia may cause visual discomfort. Although glasses may give clear vision in each eye, if significant anisometropia exists, the images on the retinas will be of different sizes, which can be disturbing. There is no entirely satisfactory remedy, but contact lenses minimize the effect. Full correction may not be prescribed in severe cases because the resulting perception of differences in image size could cause discomfort.

Ankle joint

The hinge joint between the talus (uppermost bone in the foot) and tibia (shin). The talus fits between the two bony protuberances on either side of the ankle. Strong ligaments on each side of the joint provide support and prevent overmovement. The ankle allows upward and downward movements of the foot. Other movements, such as tilting and rotation, take place around joints in the foot itself.

DISORDERS

An ankle *sprain* is one of the most common of all injuries. It usually results from the foot twisting over onto its outside edge, which produces overstretching and bruising of the ligaments on the outside of the ankle. Very severe sprains may cause extensive tearing of the ligaments, which requires surgical repair.

LOCATION OF THE ANKLE JOINT
This hinge joint is formed where the top of the talus fits in between the lower ends of the tibia and fibula.

Tibia
Fibula
Talus
Ligament
Calcaneus

Excessive or violent twisting of the ankle can cause a combined fracture and dislocation (called *Pott's fracture*), in which the fibula (outer of the two bones of the lower leg) breaks above the ankle, and either the tibia breaks or the ligaments tear, resulting in dislocation of the ankle.

Ankylosing spondylitis

An inflammatory disease affecting joints between the vertebrae of the spine and the sacroiliac joints (joints between the spine and the pelvis).

CAUSES

In most cases the cause of this condition remains unknown. A related disorder is preceded either by *colitis* (inflammation of the intestine) or *psoriasis* (a skin disease).

INCIDENCE

Ankylosing spondylitis affects less than 1 percent of the population, is more common in men than women, and has its onset between the ages of 20 and 40 years. It also seems to run in families. A genetic marker or tissue type (HLA-B27) is found much more often in people with this condition than in the rest of the population.

SYMPTOMS

Ankylosing spondylitis usually starts with discomfort in the lower back and hips, with pain and stiffness worse after resting. Typically, exercise helps reduce the stiffness.

Other symptoms include pain in the chest (from the joints between the spine and the ribs), loss of appetite, tiredness, and, occasionally, redness and pain in the eyes due to *iritis*

A

(inflammation of the iris). In about one fifth of patients, other joints may be inflamed—for example, the hips, knees, and ankles. Inflammation of tissues around the heel can cause pain and tenderness.

In time, the inflammation in the spine can lead to *ankylosis* (permanent stiffness and limitation of motion) and *kyphosis* (curvature of the spine). Movement is restricted and expansion of the chest is often limited.

DIAGNOSIS
Back pain and stiffness that is worse in the morning and relieved by exercise is suggestive of this condition. Other causes of back pain are usually mechanical and improve with resting.

Blood tests can be performed to measure inflammation and to indicate the presence of the HLA-B27 antigen on white blood cells. At the onset, X rays of the back may be normal, but later in the disease ankylosis is shown by loss of space between joints and bony outgrowths.

TREATMENT
There is no curative treatment but symptoms may be reduced by a program of heat, massage, and supervised exercise. Regular daily exercise (such as swimming) is essential to keep the back muscles strong. To prevent curvature of the spine, patients are taught breathing exercises and exercises to improve posture; they are also advised to lie facedown during the night. Anti-inflammatory drugs may be prescribed to reduce the pain and stiffness.

OUTLOOK
The inflammatory process tends to become less active with age. With treatment, most people suffer only minor deformity of the spine and are able to lead a normal life.

Ankylosis
Complete loss of movement in a joint caused by degeneration and fusion of the bony surfaces. This may be due to injury, infection, or inflammation. Ankylosis may also occur as a result of a surgical fusion of a diseased joint to correct deformity or to alleviate persistent pain.

Anodontia
Failure of some or all of the teeth to develop. Anodontia may be due to congenital absence of tooth buds or may be the result of damage to developing tooth buds caused by infection or systemic disease. Both primary and permanent teeth, or permanent teeth only, may be affected.

If only a few teeth are missing, a *bridge* can fill the gap; if all the teeth are missing, a *denture* is needed.

Anomaly
A deviation from what is accepted as normal, especially as a result of a birth defect such as a limb malformation.

Anorexia
The medical term for loss of appetite (see *Appetite, loss of*).

Anorexia nervosa
An eating disorder characterized by intense fear of being fat, by severe weight loss, and, in time, by *amenorrhea* (absence of monthly periods). Sufferers have a distorted body image and "see" themselves as fat even when they are of normal weight or even emaciated. Anorexia nervosa primarily affects teenage and young adult women and occasionally young men. Popularly known as the "slimming disease," it is difficult to treat and sometimes fatal.

CAUSES
There is much debate as to the causes of anorexia nervosa. Many anorectics seem to be part of very close, constricted families, having a special relationship with one of the parents. Anorectics are often highly conforming people and anxious to please, even obsessional in their habits. As their bodies change with puberty, anorectics try to take control over their lives by dieting stubbornly. It seems as if they do not wish to grow up and are trying to keep their childhood shapes. The exercise of control also helps anorectics compensate for a general sense of ineffectiveness.

Others have suggested that anorexia is a true *phobia* about putting on weight, which leads to a special fear of eating foods containing fats or carbohydrates. Hormonal changes related to weight loss and amenorrhea have led some physicians to regard anorexia as a physical illness caused by a disorder of the *hypothalamus* (part of the midbrain concerned with hunger, thirst, and sexual development). It is likely that these changes are secondary to the starvation.

Changes in fashion may also be a contributing factor; the disorder seems to have increased in the last 30 years, during which slimness has become closely identified with beauty. In the US and Europe, most women diet at some time, especially models, athletes, and dancers, all of whom are more prone to the disorder. About one

in 100 young, middle-class women have anorexic symptoms, although the figure is five times greater in the "at-risk" groups.

Some physicians see anorexia merely as a symptom rather than a separate disease, citing *depression, personality disorder*, or even *schizophrenia* as the real cause. However, despite the numerous cases of anorexia, it is frequently difficult to identify any such underlying cause.

SYMPTOMS AND SIGNS
The most obvious sign is emaciation (extreme thinness), with one third or more of the body's weight being lost. Starvation causes certain biochemical disorders and the balance of sex hormones is disrupted; amenorrhea develops as a result of these changes. A number of other physical changes and characteristic behavior patterns occur. They may indicate a person is suffering from anorexia.

FEATURES OF ANOREXIA NERVOSA

Weight loss
Overactivity and obsessive exercising
Tiredness and weakness
Lanugo (babylike) hair on body, thinning of hair on head
Extreme choosiness over food
Binge eating
Induced vomiting
Use of laxatives to promote weight loss

The anorectic often feels intensely hungry, although hunger pains are denied. Food and weight dominate the anorectic's thinking to an extreme degree; drug and alcohol abuse occasionally occur.

TREATMENT
The characteristic stubbornness and ability of anorectics to cause discord between health care professionals and family members has shown that anorectics are usually best treated in the hospital by a team experienced in managing the disorder.

Treatment is usually based on a closely controlled refeeding program, combined with individual *psychotherapy* or with *family therapy*. Unless a strict watch is kept on feeding, patients tend to hide or secretly throw away food. Often, a system of rewards

A

is organized, so that for every pound of weight gained the anorectic is allowed more privileges, such as having visitors or watching a favorite TV show.

Drugs may be needed if there is a clear depressive or other illness. Chlorpromazine is often helpful in the early stages to calm patients and promote weight gain. Once they have achieved a more normal weight, patients may need to continue psychotherapy for months or years.

OUTLOOK

Relapses are common whenever there is the slightest stress and about half of hospital patients still have symptoms for many years. Five to 10 percent of patients treated for anorexia nervosa in a hospital later die from starvation or suicide.

Anorgasmia

Inability to achieve orgasm (see *Psychosexual dysfunction*).

Anosmia

Loss of *smell*.

Anoxia

A medical term that means literally a complete absence of oxygen within a body tissue—for example, the brain or a muscle. Anoxia causes a disruption of cell *metabolism* (chemical activity) and cell death unless corrected within a few minutes.

Anoxia is a very rare occurrence, whereas *hypoxia* (the reduction of oxygen supply to a tissue) is a more common disorder.

Antacid drugs

COMMON DRUGS

Aluminum hydroxide Magnesium hydroxide Sodium bicarbonate

WARNING
Antacid drugs should not be taken regularly except under medical supervision as they may suppress the symptoms of a more serious disorder or provoke serious complications.

A group of drugs taken to relieve the symptoms of *indigestion, heartburn, esophagitis* (inflammation of the esophagus), *acid reflux* (regurgitation of stomach acids into the esophagus), and *peptic ulcer*.

TYPES

Antacid drugs usually contain compounds of *magnesium* or *aluminum*, which have a long-lasting effect, or

sodium bicarbonate, which produces a rapid, short-lived effect. Some antacid drugs also contain dimethicone (to relieve flatulence), alginate (to help prevent heartburn), or a local anesthetic (used in esophagitis to numb pain).

HOW THEY WORK

Antacid drugs neutralize stomach acids, an action that helps prevent or relieve inflammation and pain in the digestive system. Antacid drugs also give the stomach lining time to heal when it has been damaged by a peptic ulcer and is sensitive to normal amounts of stomach acid.

POSSIBLE ADVERSE EFFECTS

Since aluminum may cause constipation, and diarrhea may occur with magnesium, these ingredients are often given together to avoid these effects. A person taking sodium bicarbonate may experience fluid retention and, because this substance combines with acid to produce gas, bloating and belching. Antacid drugs should not be taken with other medication without the advice of a physician because they interfere with the absorption of other drugs.

Antepartum hemorrhage

Vaginal bleeding after the beginning of the third trimester of pregnancy.

CAUSES AND INCIDENCE

Antepartum hemorrhage is most commonly due to a defective placenta, the organ in the uterus that sustains the developing fetus. The placental problem may be *placenta previa* (a low-lying placenta), in which the placenta is close to the birth canal, a placental abruption (detachment of part of the placenta from the wall of the uterus), or bleeding from the edge of a normally sited placenta. Bleeding can also be caused by *cervical erosion* or lesions of the cervix or vagina.

Antepartum hemorrhage occurs in about 3 percent of all pregnancies.

SYMPTOMS

The bleeding is often painless but, when the placenta has become partly separated from the uterus, there may be abdominal pain.

INVESTIGATION AND TREATMENT

The physician may be able to ascertain whether the fetus is alive by listening for a heart beat and the woman will be admitted to the hospital. There, the fetus' heart beat will be monitored and the position of the placenta will be located by *ultrasound scanning* (not by a physical examination, which could damage a low-lying placenta).

If bleeding is not heavy, it is necessary only to keep a careful watch on

the condition of the woman and baby. In cases of severe bleeding, the woman is given an *intravenous infusion* and sometimes blood transfusions. When bleeding is severe the baby may be starved of oxygen, in which case immediate delivery is essential, sometimes by *cesarean section*.

When delivery is not necessary, the woman usually stays in the hospital for at least 48 hours. If the woman is felt to be at risk of more bleeding, which could endanger her or the baby, she sometimes stays in the hospital until delivery. Otherwise, if the bleeding has stopped and the conditions of woman and baby are considered satisfactory, the woman is allowed to go home—though her condition is carefully monitored for the remaining weeks of the pregnancy.

COMPLICATIONS

Because of good obstetric care, mortality of women and babies today is low. Death of the baby is more likely than maternal death; it is caused by lack of oxygen or by prematurity if bleeding triggers labor.

Anterior

Relating to the front of the body. In human *anatomy*, the term is synonymous with *ventral*.

Anthracosis

A medical term for coal workers' *pneumoconiosis*, a lung disease of workers in the coal industry caused by inhalation over many years of small amounts of coal dust. It is likely that all people living in large industrial cities have a mild form of anthracosis.

Anthralin

WARNING
Anthralin should not be applied to raw or blistered areas of skin.

A drug used to treat *psoriasis* (a skin disorder caused by excessive skin cell production). Anthralin, which is prescribed as an ointment or a cream, works by slowing the rate at which skin cells multiply. This effect is sometimes boosted by ultraviolet light treatment (see *Phototherapy*).

POSSIBLE ADVERSE EFFECTS

Skin inflammation causing redness and irritation is a common reaction; it may be relieved by the application of a *corticosteroid drug*. The skin around patches of psoriasis can be protected from inflammation by applying petroleum jelly.

Anthralin may stain clothing and, temporarily, the skin and hair. It is therefore advisable to wear gloves and old clothes when applying the drug.

Anthrax

A serious bacterial infection of livestock, occasionally spread to people. The most common type of human infection—in the skin—is readily treatable. Anthrax is rare today, mainly due to widespread vaccination of livestock, but some serious epidemics have occurred in animals and humans in some developing countries, usually due to lapse of control programs.

CAUSES AND INCIDENCE
Anthrax is caused by a bacterium, *BACILLUS ANTHRACIS*. It produces spores that can survive dormant for many years in soil and animal products but are capable of reactivation. Animals become infected by grazing on contaminated land.

People may become infected by handling materials from animals that have died of anthrax, by inhaling spores contained in these materials, or by eating infected meat.

In the US, human cases of anthrax are extremely rare. There was one case in 1980 and six cases in 1978.

SYMPTOMS AND TREATMENT
The most common site of human anthrax infection is the skin; the bacterium enters via a scratch or sore when contaminated animal material is handled. A raised, itchy, area develops at the site of entry, progressing to a large blister and finally to a black scab, with swelling of the surrounding tissues.

If infected meat is eaten, the symptoms are those of severe *gastroenteritis*, with fever, diarrhea, and vomiting. If anthrax spores are inhaled, the result may be a severe form of *pneumonia*. Anthrax is curable in its early stages with penicillin.

Antianxiety drugs

A group of drugs used to relieve symptoms of *anxiety*. *Benzodiazepines* and *beta-blockers* are the two main types of antianxiety drugs. Other drugs used to treat anxiety include *antidepressant drugs* and, rarely, *barbiturate drugs*.

WHY THEY ARE USED
Antianxiety drugs are used to provide temporary relief from anxiety when it limits a person's ability to cope with everyday life. In most cases, the underlying disorder is best treated by *counseling* or *psychotherapy*.

Antianxiety drugs are sometimes used to calm a person before surgical treatment (see *Premedication*) or before a public performance.

HOW THEY WORK
Benzodiazepines promote mental and physical relaxation by reducing nerve activity in the brain. Beta-blockers work by reducing the physical symptoms of anxiety, such as shaking and palpitations.

POSSIBLE ADVERSE EFFECTS
Long-term drug treatment with benzodiazepines should be ended gradually due to a risk of physical dependence (see *Drug dependence*).

Antiarrhythmic drugs

A group of drugs used to treat different types of *arrhythmia* (irregular heart beat). Antiarrhythmic drugs include *beta-blockers, calcium channel blocker drugs, digitalis drugs,* and *disopyramide*. The choice of drug depends on the type of arrhythmia.

WHY THEY ARE USED
An arrhythmia can reduce the pumping efficiency of the heart, causing breathlessness, dizziness, and chest pain. Antiarrhythmic drugs relieve these symptoms and, in some cases, restore normal heart beat.

HOW THEY WORK
The heart's pumping action is governed by electrical impulses. Some antiarrhythmic drugs work by altering these impulses within or on their way to the heart. Others affect the response of the heart muscle to the impulses received.

Antibacterial drugs

A group of drugs used to treat infections caused by *bacteria*. Antibacterial drugs share the actions of *antibiotic drugs* but, unlike antibiotics, have always been produced synthetically.

The largest group of antibacterial drugs are the *sulfonamide drugs*, used mainly for the treatment of *urinary tract infection*.

Antibiotic drugs

COMMON DRUGS
Aminoglycosides *Gentamicin Streptomycin*
Cephalosporins *Cefaclor Cephalexin*
Penicillins *Amoxicillin Penicillin V*
Tetracyclines *Doxycycline Oxytetracycline*
Others *Erythromycin Neomycin*

> **WARNING**
> You must inform your physician of any previous allergic reaction to an antibiotic drug. Always complete a course of antibiotics or the infection may return.

A group of drugs used to treat infection caused by *bacteria*. Originally derived from molds and fungi, antibiotic drugs are now made synthetically.

HOW ANTIBIOTICS WORK
Antibiotic drugs are either bactericidal (killing bacteria) or bacteriostatic (halting bacterial growth, allowing the immune system to cope with the infection). Penicillin drugs and cephalosporin drugs are bactericidal; these drugs work by disrupting bacterial cell walls.

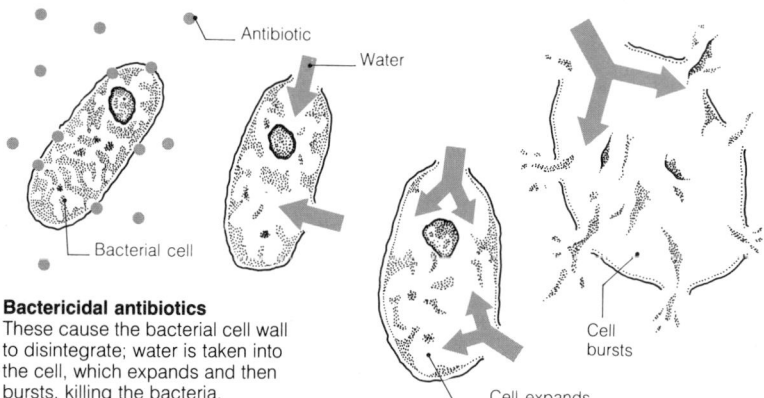

Bactericidal antibiotics
These cause the bacterial cell wall to disintegrate; water is taken into the cell, which expands and then bursts, killing the bacteria.

TYPES

Some antibiotic drugs are effective against only certain types of bacteria. Others, known as broad-spectrum antibiotics, are effective against a wide range of bacteria. The choice of antibiotic drug depends on both the type of bacteria and the site of the infection. This choice is most effectively made by growing a culture of the bacteria and checking its sensitivity to various types of antibiotic.

More than one antibiotic drug may be prescribed to increase the efficiency of treatment and to reduce the risk of antibiotic resistance.

WHY THEY ARE USED

Antibiotic drugs help fight infection either when the body has been invaded by harmful bacteria or when bacteria present within the body multiply uncontrollably. They also prevent infection in cases when the *immune system* is impaired or when there is a risk of *endocarditis* (inflammation of the lining of the heart).

ANTIBIOTIC RESISTANCE

Some bacteria develop resistance to a previously effective antibiotic drug. Resistance may occur if a type of bacteria develops a method of growth that is not disrupted by the effects of the drug or if it begins to produce an enzyme that breaks down or inactivates the drug.

Resistance is most likely to develop if a person fails to take an antibiotic drug as directed or during long-term treatment. Some powerful antibiotic drugs are available to treat severe infections resistant to the commonly prescribed antibiotic drugs.

POSSIBLE ADVERSE EFFECTS

Apart from side effects typical of each specific group, most antibiotic drugs can cause nausea, diarrhea, or a rash. Antibiotic drugs may kill bacteria naturally present in the body and fungi may grow in their place, causing oral, intestinal, or vaginal *candidiasis* (thrush). Some people occasionally experience a severe allergic reaction, causing facial swelling, itching, or breathing difficulty.

Antibody

A protein that is manufactured by lymphocytes (a type of white blood cell) to neutralize an *antigen* (foreign protein) in the body. Bacteria, viruses, and other microorganisms commonly contain many antigens; antibodies formed against these antigens help the body neutralize or destroy the invading microorganisms. Antibodies may also be formed in response to *vac-*cines, thereby giving immunity against some infections. Antibodies are also known as *immunoglobulins*.

In some cases, inappropriate or excessive formation of antibodies leads to illness. The body's response to certain substances may lead to *allergy*, as in *asthma* or *eczema*. Antibodies against antigens in skin grafts or organ transplants may result in rejection. In some disorders, antibodies are formed against the body's own tissues, resulting in an *autoimmune disorder*, such as some forms of *arthritis* and the *collagen diseases*. (See also *Immune response*.)

Antibody, monoclonal

An artificially produced *antibody* that neutralizes only one specific *antigen* (foreign protein).

Monoclonal antibodies are produced in the laboratory by stimulating the growth of large numbers of antibody-producing clones. (A clone is a group of cells that is genetically identical, or an individual member of such a group.) In effect, this cloning process enables antibodies to be tailor-made so that they will react with a particular antigen.

Monoclonal antibodies are used in the diagnosis and treatment of some forms of cancer.

Anticancer drugs

COMMON DRUGS

Cytotoxic
Azathioprine Chlorambucil Cyclophosphamide Doxorubicin Fluorouracil Melphalan Mercaptopurine Methotrexate

Sex hormone-related
Aminoglutethimide Diethylstilbestrol Ethinyl estradiol Medroxyprogesterone Megestrol Nandrolone Tamoxifen

Drugs used to treat *cancer*. They are particularly useful in the treatment of *lymphomas*, *leukemias*, and cancer affecting the ovary and testis. These drugs are sometimes used after surgery or *radiation therapy*.

TYPES

Most anticancer drugs are cytotoxic drugs (drugs that kill or damage cells). Others are synthetic forms of sex hormones and substances related to these hormones (e.g., *androgen drugs*, *estrogen drugs*, and *progesterone drugs*).

Anticancer drugs are often prescribed in combination to maximize their effects. The choice of drugs depends on the type of cancer, its stage of development, and the general health of the patient.

HOW THEY WORK

All anticancer drugs kill cancer cells by preventing them from growing and dividing. Some cytotoxic drugs work by damaging the cells' *DNA*. Others block the chemical processes in the cell necessary for growth.

Sex hormones stimulate the growth of certain cancers (for example, estrogen stimulates some types of breast cancer). Substances related to these hormones may inhibit growth by blocking their stimulatory effect. The growth of other cancers is sometimes disrupted by a synthetic sex hormone given in high doses. Cancer of the prostate gland, for example, may be treated with *diethylstilbestrol* (DES), an estrogen drug.

POSSIBLE ADVERSE EFFECTS

In the early stages of treatment, nausea, vomiting, and diarrhea may occur and be sufficiently serious to make hospitalization necessary.

Anticancer drugs may alter the rate at which noncancerous cells grow and divide. This effect may cause alopecia (hair loss) and reduce the number of blood cells produced by the bone marrow, causing *anemia*, increased susceptibility to infection, and/or abnormal bleeding. Regular blood tests are usually carried out to monitor blood cell production.

To minimize adverse effects, anticancer drugs are usually given in short courses with time between each course to enable noncancerous cells to recover from the drugs' effects.

Anticholinergic drugs

COMMON DRUGS

Atropine Benztropine Diphenhydramine Orphenadrine Procyclidine Propantheline Scopolamine

A group of drugs that blocks the effects of *acetylcholine*, a chemical released from nerve endings in the parasympathetic division of the *autonomic nervous system*. Acetylcholine triggers activity in a number of reactive cells. For example, it stimulates muscle contraction, increases secretions in the mouth and lungs, and slows the heart beat.

WHY THEY ARE USED

Anticholinergic drugs are used in the treatment of *irritable bowel syndrome* and certain types of urinary *incontinence* (see also *Antispasmodic drugs*). They are given in the treatment of *Parkinson's disease*, *asthma*, and bradycardia (abnormally slow heart beat) and are also used before an examina-

HOW ANTICHOLINERGICS WORK

Acetylcholine combines with a receptor on the cell's surface. This interaction stimulates activity in that cell (e.g., contraction of a muscle fiber or secretion of a fluid). Anticholinergic drugs block the stimulatory action of acetylcholine by combining with the acetylcholine receptors. This action produces, for example, muscle relaxation (e.g., in the bladder, intestine, and bronchi) and dries up secretions in the mouth and lungs. Anticholinergic drugs are used to treat asthma.

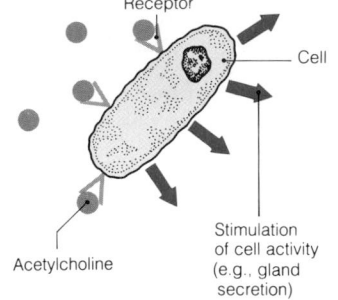

Receptor

Cell

Acetylcholine

Stimulation of cell activity (e.g., gland secretion)

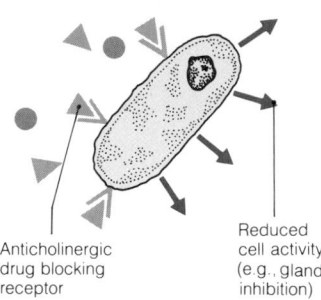

Anticholinergic drug blocking receptor

Reduced cell activity (e.g., gland inhibition)

tion of or surgical procedure on the eye. Anticholinergic drugs are also helpful as a *premedication* before general *anesthesia* and in the treatment of *motion sickness*.

POSSIBLE ADVERSE EFFECTS
Anticholinergic drugs may cause dry mouth, blurred vision, abnormal retention of urine, and confusion.

Anticoagulant drugs

COMMON DRUGS

Dicumarol Heparin Warfarin

> **WARNING**
> Many drugs, such as aspirin and alcohol, may increase the risk of an anticoagulant drug causing abnormal bleeding. Always consult your physician before taking any other drug during anticoagulant treatment.

A group of drugs used to treat and prevent abnormal *blood clotting*. They are used to treat *thrombosis*, and may be used to prevent and treat *stroke* or *transient ischemic attack*. Anticoagulant drugs are also prescribed to prevent the development of abnormal blood clotting after major surgery (especially heart valve replacement) or during hemodialysis (see *Dialysis*).

HOW THEY WORK
Heparin increases the effect of antithrombin III, an enzyme that blocks the activity of other enzymes—known as coagulation factors—that are needed for blood to clot. This drug is given by injection and begins to work within a few hours.

Other anticoagulant drugs are taken by mouth and begin to act within a day. They work by reducing the production of some coagulation factors.

By disrupting the blood clotting mechanism, anticoagulant drugs prevent an abnormal blood clot from forming. When a blood clot already exists, anticoagulant drugs stop it from enlarging and reduce the risk of an *embolus* breaking off and blocking another blood vessel. Unlike *thrombolytic drugs*, they do not dissolve blood clots that have already formed.

POSSIBLE ADVERSE EFFECTS
Anticoagulant drugs in high doses may cause abnormal bleeding in different parts of the body. As a result, regular *blood clotting tests* are carried out to monitor treatment.

Anticonvulsant drugs

COMMON DRUGS

Carbamazepine Clonazepam Diazepam Ethosuximide Phenobarbital Phenytoin Primidone Valproic acid

> **WARNING**
> Never suddenly stop taking an anticonvulsant drug after long-term treatment; the dose should be reduced gradually or symptoms may return.

A group of drugs used in the treatment of *seizures* (see also *Epilepsy*). Anticonvulsant drugs are taken on a regular basis to reduce the frequency and severity of seizures and as an emergency treatment to stop a prolonged seizure. Anticonvulsant drugs are also given to prevent seizures following a serious head injury or some types of brain surgery; they may be given to a child with a high fever who has a history of febrile seizures (see *Seizure, febrile*).

The choice of drug is largely determined by the type of seizure. In long-term treatment of certain types of seizure, more than one anticonvulsant drug may be needed. Even in people taking regular anticonvulsant medication, an occasional seizure may occur. The frequency with which these seizures occur determines, in part, whether the dose of a medication is increased, another drug added, or the entire drug program is changed.

HOW THEY WORK
Seizures are caused by an abnormally high level of electrical activity in the brain. Anticonvulsant drugs have an inhibitory effect that neutralizes this excessive electrical activity and the spread of this activity throughout areas of the brain.

POSSIBLE ADVERSE EFFECTS
These include reduced concentration, impaired memory, poor coordination, and fatigue. Such effects are usually monitored by regular blood tests.

Antidepressant drugs

COMMON DRUGS

Tricyclics
Amitriptyline Amoxapine Doxepin Imipramine

Monoamine oxidase inhibitors (MAOIs)
Isocarboxazid Phenelzine

Others
Lithium Maprotiline Trazodone

> **WARNING**
> Food and drink containing tyramine (e.g., cheese and red wine) and certain drugs may produce a potentially fatal rise in blood pressure if taken during treatment with an MAOI. Always tell your physician if you are taking an MAOI.

Drugs used in the treatment of *depression*. Antidepressant drugs are prescribed when depression lasts longer than a few days, causing symptoms such as lethargy, loss of appetite or sex drive, or a feeling of despair. The two main types are tricyclic antidepressant drugs and monoamine oxidase inhibitors.

HOW THEY WORK
Some antidepressant drugs trigger the release of chemicals in the brain that

stimulate nerve activity. Others, notably tricyclic antidepressants and monoamine oxidase inhibitors, prolong the active life of these chemicals after their release. Antidepressant drugs usually take at least ten days to have any beneficial effect and up to eight weeks to become fully effective.

POSSIBLE ADVERSE EFFECTS
Most antidepressant drugs can cause dryness of the mouth, blurred vision, dizziness, drowsiness, constipation, and difficulty with urination; these symptoms often improve as treatment continues. An antidepressant drug overdose may cause abnormal heart rhythm, seizures, coma, and, occasionally, death.

Antidiarrheal drugs

COMMON DRUGS

Narcotics
Codeine Diphenoxylate with atropine Loperamide

Bulking agents
Kaolin Methylcellulose Psyllium

> **WARNING**
> Do not take antidiarrheal drugs regularly except under medical supervision because they may mask a serious underlying disorder.

A group of drugs used to treat *diarrhea*; they are either *narcotic* substances or bulking agents.

WHY THEY ARE USED
Antidiarrheal drugs may be recommended if diarrhea persists for more than 24 to 48 hours. They are often prescribed while the cause of persistent diarrhea is being investigated, especially if the diarrhea is severe and debilitating. Antidiarrheal drugs are given to help regulate bowel action in people with a *colostomy* or *ileostomy*.

HOW THEY WORK
Narcotic antidiarrheal drugs affect the muscles in the wall of the intestine. This action slows the passage of the feces and allows more time for water to be absorbed into the bloodstream. As a result, both the fluidity and frequency of bowel movements are reduced. Bulking agents (such as fiber in the diet) absorb water from the feces, making them more solid.

POSSIBLE ADVERSE EFFECTS
Antidiarrheal drugs may cause constipation. If diarrhea is caused by an infection, these drugs may delay recovery by slowing the elimination of the microorganisms. Prolonged use of a narcotic antidiarrheal may cause

physical dependence (see *Drug dependence*), producing nausea, abdominal pain, and diarrhea if the drug is suddenly stopped. Bowel obstruction may result if bulking agents are used without sufficient water. Obstruction of the bowel may also occur if a narrowing exists in the bowel.

Antidiuretic hormone
See *ADH*.

Antidote

A substance that neutralizes or counteracts the effects of a poison. The antidote for acid is alkali, and vice versa. A chemical antidote works by combining with a poison to form an innocuous substance, or in some way blocking or diverting the action of the poison. A mechanical antidote prevents the absorption of poison.

Antiemetic drugs

COMMON DRUGS

Anticholinergics
Scopolamine

Antihistamines
Dimenhydrinate Meclizine Promethazine

Phenothiazine antipsychotics
Fluphenazine Perphenazine Prochlorperazine Promazine

Others
Dronabinol Metoclopramide

> **WARNING**
> An antiemetic drug should not be taken regularly except under medical supervision as it may mask a serious underlying disorder.

A group of drugs used to treat *nausea* and *vomiting* caused by *motion sickness*, *vertigo*, *Meniere's disease*, *radiation therapy*, or certain drugs (especially *anticancer drugs*). Some antiemetic drugs are also used to treat severe vomiting during pregnancy.

Drugs from this group are seldom prescribed to treat food poisoning because it is believed that vomiting enables the body to rid itself of harmful substances.

HOW THEY WORK
Some antiemetic drugs reduce nerve activity at the base of the brain and thereby suppress the vomiting reflex. Antihistamine drugs and also anticholinergic drugs reduce the vomiting associated with vertigo by suppressing nerve activity in the balance center in the inner ear. Other antiemetic drugs prevent vomiting by

relaxing the muscles in the lower part of the stomach. This action enables the stomach contents to pass into the small intestine.

POSSIBLE ADVERSE EFFECTS
Many antiemetic drugs cause drowsiness. Some must not be taken during pregnancy because they may damage the developing fetus.

Antifreeze poisoning

Most antifreeze contains ethylene glycol or methanol (methyl alcohol), both of which are poisonous when drunk. Antifreeze poisoning is rare. Most of the 50 or so deaths each year in the US occur in alcoholics (who use antifreeze as a substitute for alcoholic drinks); some people commit suicide by this method.

SYMPTOMS AND TREATMENT
Drinking small amounts of antifreeze initially produces the same effects as alcohol intoxication. When a large amount has been ingested, vomiting, stupor, seizures, and coma occur successively within a few hours; within 24 to 36 hours, acute *renal failure* occurs. If the antifreeze contains methanol, blindness may also result.

Any person believed to have drunk antifreeze needs immediate medical help. Until help arrives, the person, if conscious, should be given a small amount of alcohol (approximately two shots of liquor), which reduces the rate at which antifreeze is metabolized and becomes toxic in the body.

Hospital treatment may include gastric *lavage* (pumping out the stomach) and giving *diuretic drugs*, alcohol, and bicarbonate (by drip into a vein) to correct excess acidity in the body fluids.

Antifungal drugs

COMMON DRUGS

Amphotericin B Ciclopirox Clotrimazole Econazole Griseofulvin Ketoconazole Miconazole Nystatin Tolnaftate

A group of drugs prescribed to treat infections caused by *fungi*. Antifungal drugs are commonly used to treat different types of *tinea*, including tinea pedis (athlete's foot), tinea cruris (jock itch), and tinea capitis (scalp ringworm). They are also used to treat *candidiasis* (thrush) and rare fungal infections (such as *cryptococcosis*) that affect internal organs.

Antifungal preparations are available as tablets, lozenges, suspensions, creams, injections, and vaginal suppositories.

HOW THEY WORK

Antifungal drugs damage the cell walls of fungi, causing chemicals essential for normal function and growth to escape. The fungal cells are unable to survive without these chemicals and die.

POSSIBLE ADVERSE EFFECTS

Preparations applied to the skin, scalp, mouth, or vagina may occasionally increase irritation. Antifungal drugs given by mouth or injection may cause more serious side effects, including damage to the kidney or to the liver.

Antigen

A substance that can trigger an *immune response*, resulting in production of an *antibody* as part of the body's defense against infection and disease. Many antigens are foreign proteins (those not found naturally in the body); they include microorganisms, toxins, and tissues from another person used in organ transplantation.

Antihelmintic drugs

COMMON DRUGS

Niclosamide Niridazole Piperazine Praziquantel Pyrantel Thiabendazole

A group of drugs used in the treatment of *worm infestations*. The body's *immune system* does not deal with worms effectively and, as a result, persistent infestations are common. Antihelmintic drugs eliminate worms from the body and prevent the complications (such as *anemia*, vitamin deficiency, or intestinal obstruction) that occur when worm infestation persists. Different types of antihelmintic drugs are used to treat infestation by different types of worms.

HOW THEY WORK

Antihelmintic drugs either kill or paralyze worms. These drugs cause intestinal worms to pass out of the body in the feces by preventing them from gripping onto the intestinal walls. To hasten this process, laxatives are occasionally prescribed with antihelmintic drugs.

Antihelmintic drugs kill worms in other tissues by making them more vulnerable to attack by the immune system. Once these worms have been killed, they may require surgical removal along with any cysts that the worms have caused.

POSSIBLE ADVERSE EFFECTS

Adverse effects include nausea, vomiting, abdominal pain, headache, dizziness, and rash.

Antihistamine drugs

COMMON DRUGS

Chlorpheniramine Diphenhydramine Promethazine Terfenadine Trimeprazine Triprolidine

> **WARNING**
> Do not drive or operate potentially dangerous machinery while taking an antihistamine drug until you are certain that the treatment is not causing dizziness or drowsiness or impairing your coordination.

A group of drugs that blocks the effects of *histamine*, a chemical released during an allergic reaction (see *Allergy*).

WHY THEY ARE USED

Antihistamine drugs are used in the treatment of *urticaria* (hives) and other rashes to relieve itching, swelling, and redness. Drugs of this type are also used in the treatment of allergic *rhinitis* (hay fever) to relieve sneezing and a runny nose.

Antihistamine drugs are sometimes included in *cough remedies* and *cold remedies* because they dry up nasal secretions and suppress the nerve centers in the brain that trigger the cough reflex.

Antihistamine drugs are also used as *antiemetic drugs* because they suppress the vomiting reflex.

Because most antihistamine drugs have a sedative effect, they are sometimes used to induce sleep, especially when itching keeps the sufferer awake at night.

Antihistamine drugs may be given by injection in an emergency to aid in treating *anaphylactic shock* (a severe allergic reaction).

HOW THEY WORK

Antihistamine drugs block the effect of histamine on tissues such as the skin, eyes, and nose. Without drug treatment, histamine would dilate (widen) small blood vessels, resulting in redness and swelling of the surrounding tissue due to leakage of fluid from the circulation. Antihistamines also prevent histamine from irritating nerve fibers, which would otherwise cause itching, and prevent it from stimulating nerve activity in parts of the brain.

POSSIBLE ADVERSE EFFECTS

Most antihistamines cause drowsiness and dizziness. Other possible side effects include loss of appetite, nausea, dry mouth, blurred vision, and difficulty passing urine.

Antihypertensive drugs

COMMON DRUGS

ACE inhibitors
Captopril Enalapril

Beta-blockers
Atenolol Metoprolol

Calcium channel blockers
Nifedipine Verapamil

Diuretic drugs
Chlorthalidone Hydrochlorothiazide

Vasodilator drugs
Hydralazine Minoxidil Prazosin

Others
Clonidine Methyldopa

> **WARNING**
> Never stop taking antihypertensive drugs suddenly as this may cause a dramatic rise in blood pressure with serious results.

A group of drugs used in the treatment of *hypertension* (high blood pressure) to prevent complications such as *stroke*, *myocardial infarction* (heart attack), *heart failure* (reduced pumping efficiency), and kidney damage. Antihypertensive drugs are also used to relieve symptoms, such as tiredness and dizziness, caused by hypertension.

HOW THEY WORK

Beta-blockers reduce the force of the heart beat, thereby lowering the pressure of blood flow into the circulation. *Diuretic drugs* increase the amount of salts and water excreted in the urine, but the way in which they lower the blood pressure is not entirely clear. Other types of antihypertensive drugs cause the blood vessels to dilate (widen), which allows the blood to circulate more easily throughout the body.

POSSIBLE ADVERSE EFFECTS

Apart from side effects typical of specific groups, all antihypertensive drugs may cause dizziness and fainting by lowering the blood pressure too much.

Anti-inflammatory drugs

Drugs that reduce the symptoms and signs of *inflammation*. (See *Nonsteroidal anti-inflammatory drugs*; *Corticosteroid drugs*; *Analgesics*.)

Antiperspirant

COMMON DRUGS

Aluminum chloride Aluminum chlorohydrate

A drug applied to the skin in the form of a lotion, cream, or spray to reduce excessive sweating.

WHY IT IS USED

An antiperspirant is used to prevent the accumulation of sweat, which usually occurs under the arms. When sweat remains on the skin, it creates a moist environment in which bacteria can thrive. The bacteria break down the chemicals in the sweat, causing body odor.

High concentrations of antiperspirants are sometimes prescribed to treat *hyperhidrosis* (abnormally profuse sweating). Results of this treatment are variable.

HOW IT WORKS

An antiperspirant reduces the production of sweat by the sweat glands and blocks the ducts that drain sweat onto the surface of the skin.

POSSIBLE ADVERSE EFFECTS

Antiperspirants may cause skin irritation and a burning or stinging sensation. Such effects are more common when high concentrations are used. If the irritation persists when a lower dose is used, treatment should be stopped to prevent *dermatitis*. (See also *Deodorants*.)

Antipsychotic drugs

COMMON DRUGS

Phenothiazines
Chlorpromazine Fluphenazine
Perphenazine Thioridazine Trifluoperazine

Others
Haloperidol Lithium Thiothixene

A group of drugs used to treat *psychoses* (mental disorders involving loss of contact with reality), particularly *schizophrenia* and *manic-depressive illness*. Antipsychotic drugs enable many people suffering from mental illness to live relatively normal lives outside mental institutions.

Antipsychotic drugs are also used to calm or sedate people with other mental disorders (such as *dementia*) who have become highly agitated or aggressive.

Antipsychotic drugs include *phenothiazine drugs* and various other drugs, including *lithium*, which is used specifically to treat the symptoms of *mania* (abnormal elation and overactivity).

HOW THEY WORK

Most antipsychotic drugs block the action of dopamine, a *neurotransmitter* acting on the brain. Lithium is thought to reduce the release of *norepinephrine*, another neurotransmitter.

POSSIBLE ADVERSE EFFECTS

Most antipsychotic drugs can cause drowsiness, lethargy, *dyskinesia* (jerky movements of the mouth, face, and tongue), and *parkinsonism* (a disorder with symptoms similar to those of *Parkinson's disease*). Other possible side effects include dry mouth, blurred vision, and difficulty passing urine. Lithium may cause nausea, diarrhea, tremor, rash, weight gain, and muscle weakness.

Antipyretic drugs

Drugs that reduce fever, such as *aspirin* and *acetaminophen*.

Antirheumatic drugs

COMMON DRUGS

Corticosteroid drugs
Dexamethasone Prednisolone

Immunosuppressant drugs
Azathioprine Chlorambucil

Others
Gold Penicillamine

A group of drugs used in the treatment of *rheumatoid arthritis* and types of arthritis caused by other *autoimmune disorders* (disorders in which the body's immune system attacks its own tissues)—for example, systemic *lupus erythematosus*. Antirheumatic drugs are prescribed when *nonsteroidal anti-inflammatory drugs* (NSAIDs) fail to relieve joint pain and stiffness or when the disease is causing progressive deformity and disability.

HOW THEY WORK

Antirheumatic drugs limit the damage caused by the immune system by suppressing either the production or activity of white blood cells. Each type of drug works in a different way, but all antirheumatics damp down the inflammation caused by the autoimmune reaction and prevent or slow down the degeneration of the cartilage that lines joints.

The effectiveness of each type of antirheumatic drug varies according to the individual. Beneficial effects may not appear for several weeks.

POSSIBLE ADVERSE EFFECTS

All antirheumatic drugs may cause serious adverse effects. For example, gold and penicillamine may cause kidney damage, chloroquine may damage the eyes, and *immunosuppressant drugs* may cause blood disorders. Regular medical examinations, including blood and urine tests, are carried out during treatment to monitor toxic effects.

Antiseptics

Chemicals applied to the skin to destroy bacteria and other microorganisms and thus prevent *sepsis* (infection). Antisepsis (the use of antiseptics to prevent infection) is not the same as asepsis, which is the creation of a germ-free environment (see *Aseptic technique*). Antiseptics are milder than *disinfectants*, which decontaminate inanimate objects but are too strong to be used on the body.

Antiseptic fluids are generally used for bathing wounds, whereas creams are applied to wounds before they are dressed. Among the more commonly used antiseptics are iodine, hydrogen peroxide, and thimerosal.

Antiserum

A preparation containing antibodies that combine with specific *antigens* (foreign proteins), usually components of microorganisms (such as viruses or bacteria). Such antibody-antigen interaction leads to the inactivation or destruction of the microorganisms. Antiserum samples are prepared from the blood of animals or humans who have been injected with killed, or live but harmless, strains of particular viruses or bacteria—in other words, people who have already been immunized against these organisms.

Antiserum is usually used, along with *immunization*, as an emergency treatment when someone has been exposed to a dangerous infection such as *lassa fever* and has not previously been immunized against the infection. The antiserum helps to provide some immediate protection against the infective microorganisms while full immunity is developing.

Such measures are not as effective in preventing disease as earlier (pre-exposure) immunization.

Antisocial personality disorder

Failure to conform to social norms of behavior. The category of antisocial personality is relatively new and was devised to provide clear guidelines for diagnosing psychiatric illness. In the past, people displaying antisocial behavior were classified in a number of ways, such as "sociopaths" or "psychopaths," but it was argued that these labels described character traits rather than specific illnesses causing a change in personality or behavior.

DIAGNOSIS

For a person to be diagnosed as suffering from this type of disorder, the antisocial behavior must have started

A

DIAGNOSIS OF ANTISOCIAL PERSONALITY DISORDER

Four areas of behavior are considered: performance at work and school, childhood behavior, personal life, and personal relationships. There must be a positive rating in all four areas.

1

Performance at work and school
Constant changing of job, persistent unemployment for no good reason, regular absences from work, and poor school performance would give someone a positive rating in this category.

2

Childhood behavior
A positive rating would be assigned when three or more of the following have occurred: truancy, rule-breaking, or expulsion; lying, stealing, or running away, excessive drinking, vandalism, juvenile court appearances, or precocious sexual activity.

3

Personal life
A positive rating in this category would be assigned if two or more of the following apply: arrests, separations, or divorces; getting into fights; regular drunkenness; money troubles; periods of homelessness.

4

Personal relationships
Inability to form or maintain close relationships with family, friends, or sexual partners is evidence of a lack of personal warmth. If insufficient concern for others seems to be the cause, a person would get a positive rating.

---

before the age of 15 and must not be a result of mental handicap or obvious illness. Since there must be evidence of persistent disturbance over a period of time, the term cannot be used to describe anyone under 18 years old.

TREATMENT

Given such categories, it is clear that behavior is being judged. The aim of treatment is to alter behavior; this may include residence in *therapeutic communities*, *behavior therapy*, various forms of *psychotherapy*, and participation in community help programs. There is a clear overlap with legal punishment, since criminal activity is common, but the debate as to whether people with this disorder are "bad" or "mad" remains unsolved.

Antispasmodic drugs

COMMON DRUGS

Belladonna Dicyclomine

A group of drugs that relaxes spasm in smooth (involuntary) muscle in the wall of the intestine or bladder. Antispasmodic drugs are used in the treatment of *irritable bowel syndrome* and *irritable bladder*.

Antispasmodic drugs may have an anticholinergic action (that is, they work by blocking the action of *acetylcholine*, a chemical that is released from nerve endings that stimulates muscle contraction).

Adverse effects of antispasmodic drugs include dry mouth, blurred vision, and difficulty passing urine. (See also *Anticholinergic drugs*.)

Antitoxin

Any of a variety of commercially prepared substances, each of which contains *antibodies* that can combine and neutralize the effect of a specific toxin released into the bloodstream by bacteria (such as those that cause *tetanus* and *diphtheria*).

Antitoxins are prepared by inoculating animals, usually horses, with specific toxins that provoke the animal's immune system to produce antibodies that will neutralize the toxins. Extracts of the animal's blood are used as the antitoxin.

Antitoxins are usually administered by injection into a muscle, under the supervision of a physician. Occasionally, an antitoxin may cause an allergic reaction; rarely, it causes an *anaphylactic shock* (severe allergic reaction) requiring emergency treatment.

Antitussive drugs

Drugs that prevent or relieve *cough*. (See *Cough remedies*.)

Antivenin

A specific treatment for snake, scorpion, spider, or other venomous animal bites. Antivenin is pre-

pared by inoculating animals, usually horses, with small but increasing amounts of venom from a particular poisonous animal. This provokes the production of *antibodies* that will neutralize the poisons in the venom. A preparation containing these antibodies or antivenins can then be produced from samples of the horse's blood.

In the US, commercial antivenins are available against all types of pit viper (rattlesnakes, cottonmouth, and copperhead) and for coral snake bites. Antivenins for treating the bites of snakes originating outside the US and various scorpions, spiders, fish, and jellyfish can be obtained from zoos and veterinarians.

Antiviral drugs

COMMON DRUGS

Acyclovir Amantadine Idoxuridine Trifluridine Zidovudine

A group of drugs used in the treatment of infection by a *virus*. Drugs that kill viruses have proved difficult to develop because viruses live only within body cells and there is a danger that antiviral drugs will damage the host cell as well as the virus. To date, no drugs have been developed that can effectively eradicate viruses and cure the illnesses that they cause.

Immunization is at present more important than drug treatment in fighting serious viral infections. However, some drugs have already proved successful in treating a few viral infections, particularly those caused by *herpes* viruses. Antiviral drugs reduce the severity of these infections but may not eliminate them completely, so attacks may recur. Other antiviral drugs are currently being developed and used (e.g., to treat AIDS).

HOW THEY WORK

Most antiviral drugs destroy viruses by disrupting chemical processes necessary for viruses to grow and multiply within cells. Some antiviral drugs prevent viruses from actually penetrating cells.

POSSIBLE ADVERSE EFFECTS

Antiviral drugs against AIDS carry a high risk of causing anemia due to bone marrow damage. Most other antiviral drugs rarely cause side effects. Antiviral creams and ointments may irritate the skin, causing redness. Antiviral drugs given by mouth or injection can cause nausea and dizziness, and, rarely, in long-term treatment, kidney damage.

Antral irrigation

Irrigation of the antrum (also called the maxillary sinus), one of the nasal sinuses, to diagnose and treat persistent *sinusitis*.

WHY IT IS USED

Antral irrigation is used when sinusitus persists after an adequate course of medical therapy, consisting mostly of antibiotics and decongestants, and sometimes dental consultation. Antral irrigation allows a firm diagnosis of infection to be made and sometimes cures the infection.

The normal drainage channel from the antrum into the nose is usually at least partially blocked in chronic sinusitis, so that infected material builds up within the cavity. Antral irrigation creates a temporary opening that allows the contents to be flushed out through the natural opening.

HOW IT IS DONE

A cannula (hollow, flexible tube) is inserted into the antrum, guided by a trocar (sharp, pointed rod). The trocar enters through the nose or under the upper lip. The trocar is withdrawn, leaving the cannula in place. A syringe is then attached to the cannula and the contents of the sinus are sucked out and sent to the laboratory for bacteriological culture to identify the organism responsible for the infection and to test sensitivity to antibiotics.

A large syringe filled with warm saline is attached to the cannula and the antrum is thoroughly washed out by injecting the solution into the cavity and having it flow out through the natural sinus opening. This is repeated until the fluid is clear.

RESULTS

Unless the sinusitis has been present for so long that permanent damage to the mucosa (lining of the sinus) has occurred, antral irrigation may be curative. If the infection fails to resolve after several weeks, and an irrigation confirms that the antrum is still infected, more surgery to enlarge the drainage channel may be required.

Anuria

Complete cessation of urine production by the kidneys; the extreme of oliguria (reduced urine production).

Failure to pass urine is an indication of a serious problem in the urinary tract because, even when a person is severely dehydrated, some urine is produced. Much more common than anuria as a cause of failure to urinate is a complete blockage to the flow of urine—due, for example, to an enlarged *prostate gland*, *bladder tumor*, or urinary tract calculus (stone). True anuria may be due to oxygen depletion as a result of reduced blood flow through the kidneys, as occurs in *shock*, or to severe kidney damage, resulting in acute *renal failure* or tubular necrosis.

Anuria requires urgent investigation to establish the cause and may require dialysis. Untreated, it leads to *uremia* (excess waste products in the blood) and death.

Anus

The canal at the end of the alimentary tract through which feces are expelled from the body. About 1.5 inches (4 cm) long, the anus is an extension of the

STRUCTURE OF THE ANUS

A canal at the end of the alimentary tract, with internal and external sphincters to open and close the orifice.

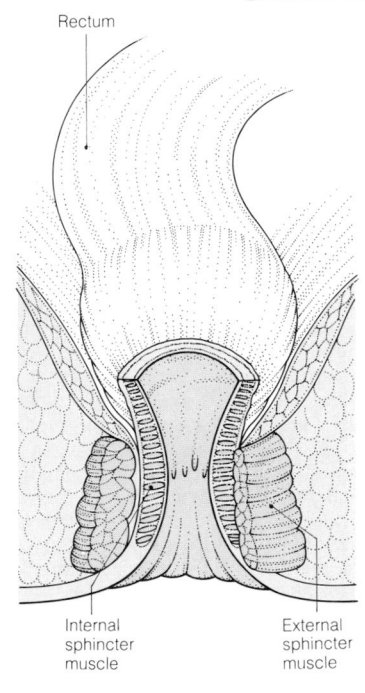

Rectum

Internal sphincter muscle

External sphincter muscle

rectum as it passes backward and downward through the pelvic floor. The orifice at the end of the anal canal is only open during defecation—at other times it is kept closed by the muscles of the anal sphincter. These muscles are arranged in two layers, the internal sphincter, which cannot be controlled voluntarily, and the external sphincter, which can be relaxed at will for defecation. (See also *Digestive system*.)

Anus, cancer of

A rare cancer of the skin of the anus that is not usually related to the cells occurring in cancer of the intestine.

In the early stages of anal cancer there may be a swelling at the outside of the anus as well as some bleeding and discomfort. Surgical removal of the cancer is the usual treatment.

Anus, imperforate

A rare congenital abnormality, detected and treated at birth, in which the anal opening appears to be covered over.

TYPES

The two main types of imperforate anus, high and low, depend on whether or not the bowel ends above or below the pelvic floor. In the high type, the anal canal fails to develop and there is no connection between the rectum and the anus. Many of the normal anal structures, such as the muscles, are missing and the disorder is associated with other abnormalities, especially of the urinary organs. The low type may have only a skin covering at the anal opening.

TREATMENT

Treatment for high imperforate anus involves major surgery to open up the end of the rectum and join it to the anus. This operation is usually successful and the long-term outlook is good. In some cases, a *colostomy* may be needed.

Treatment for low imperforate anus usually involves surgical removal of the skin over the anus. *Anal dilatation* (enlargement of the anus) may be needed for several months afterward.

Anxiety

An unpleasant emotional state ranging from mild unease to intense fear. The anxious person usually feels a sense of impending doom, although there is no obvious threat, and has certain physical and psychological symptoms. A certain amount of anxiety is normal and serves to improve our performance. However, anxiety becomes a symptom when it starts to inhibit thought and disrupt normal activities of daily life.

SYMPTOMS AND SIGNS

The most common symptoms relate to the chest. They include palpitations (awareness of a more forceful or faster heart beat), throbbing or stabbing pains, a feeling of tightness and inability to take in enough air, and a tendency to sigh or overbreathe (see *Hyperventilation*).

Tension of the muscles leads to headaches, spasms in the neck, back pains, grasping too tightly, and an inability to relax. Restlessness, tremor of the hands, and a sense of tiredness are also common.

Gastrointestinal symptoms include dryness of the mouth, a feeling of distention, diarrhea, nausea, changes in appetite, constant belching, and difficulty swallowing. Some sufferers may actually vomit or have severe pain mimicking serious illness.

There are also certain, socially obvious symptoms, such as sweating, blushing, and pallor, or the constant need to urinate or defecate. Dizziness, hyperventilation (deep and fast breathing), sighing, yawning, belching, and the light-headedness that results occur especially in public and are related to fears. Paresthesia (a pins and needles sensation) and a fixed spasm of the arms can result from hyperventilation, which prevents the muscles from functioning by depriving them of carbon dioxide.

People with anxiety usually have a constant feeling that something bad is going to happen. They may fear that they have a chronic or dangerous illness—which is reinforced by the physical symptoms outlined above—or that the health or safety of family and friends is in danger. Fear of losing control is also common. This fear leads to increasing dependence on others, irritability, a sense of fatigue, and a state of being easily frustrated. Inability to relax may lead to difficulty getting to sleep and constant waking during the night. Frightening dreams often occur.

A particularly strange yet common symptom is that of *depersonalization* (the sense of being cut off from oneself) or the related *derealization* (the sense of being cut off from the world). These symptoms can begin suddenly and last for a long time, leading people to fear they are going mad.

CAUSES

Three different areas of research have contributed theories for the cause of anxiety. Physiological measures show that anxious individuals have a raised level of *arousal* in the central nervous system, so that they react more excitedly and adapt more slowly to events. This feeling also leads to physical symptoms, such as palpitations, which themselves are unpleasant and reinforce the anxiety.

Psychoanalytical ideas derive from Freud, who coined the term "anxiety neurosis" and believed that anxiety stems from repressed unresolved childhood experiences. Originally, anxiety was thought to be due to unsatisfied sexual needs, but the importance of *bonding* and child-parent separations has now led to theories based on the fear of losing loved objects. Unconscious conflict can also lead to anxiety.

Behavioral psychologists describe anxiety as a learned response to, for example, pain or mental discomfort. The anxiety initially serves to drive people to improved learning and performance, but eventually becomes a habit that is brought on by the slightest difficulty. It thus impairs performance and thought, though people become so deeply conditioned that they cannot control it.

ANXIETY AND ILLNESS

Symptoms of anxiety usually result from an *anxiety disorder*, or are part of another psychological disorder, such as *hypochondriasis*, *depression*, or a type of *psychosexual disorder*. However, because the symptoms of anxiety mimic the symptoms of so many other diseases, the physician tries to avoid reinforcing the patient's anxiety, which can lead to numerous unnecessary consultations and treatments—including surgery. People with anxiety disorders ideally are referred for psychotherapy to determine the real causes of their fears.

Anxiety disorders

A group of mental illnesses in which symptoms of anxiety are the main feature. Anxiety disorders include a number of specific syndromes, though there is considerable overlap among them and boundaries are not always clear.

Anxiety disorders are common, affecting roughly 4 percent of the population, mainly younger adults; the disorders occur equally in men and women and heredity is a contributing factor. Symptoms tend to vary during the course of the illness.

TYPES

Generalized anxiety disorder (the traditional "anxiety neurosis") is diagnosed if the patient has had at least one definite period of anxiety, accompanied by at least one physical or psychological symptom that impairs normal activity. *Panic disorders* are characterized by sudden, intense attacks of panic (extreme, unreasonable fear and anxiety), while *phobias* are dominated by irrational fears that lead to avoidance of certain situations or objects, such as open spaces or spiders. *Posttraumatic stress disorder* is associated with a serious specific event, such as rape, and symptoms include reliving the event in dreams and a general feeling of numbness and lack of involvement. The main features of *obsessive-compulsive behavior* are recurrent and persistent thoughts and ritualized, repetitive behavior.

TREATMENT

Treatment of anxiety disorders is most effective when there is an identifiable and justified reason for stress. Treatment is more successful in people who have stable, underlying personalities. Reassurance, *counseling*, and *psychotherapy* are used, as are *antianxiety drugs* (especially *benzodiazepine drugs*).

Aorta

The main *artery* of the body. The aorta arises directly from the left ventricle (lower chamber of the heart) and supplies oxygenated blood to all other arteries except the pulmonary artery (which carries deoxygenated blood from the heart to the lungs).

DISORDERS

Like other arteries, the aorta can become narrowed as a result of *atherosclerosis* (fat deposits on the walls), which often causes *hypertension* (high blood pressure). There are also specific aortic disorders, notably *coarctation of the aorta* (in which the aorta is abnormally narrow at birth) and *aortitis* (inflammation of the wall of the aorta), a rare condition associated with untreated *syphilis* and *ankylosing spondylitis* (inflammation of the joints of the spine).

Both aortitis and atherosclerosis can cause an aortic *aneurysm* (a balloonlike swelling of the vessel wall), which may require surgery to correct impaired blood flow and to remove the risk of rupture and fatal blood loss. (See also *Arteries, disorders of*; *Circulatory system*.)

Aortic insufficiency

Leakage of blood through the aortic valve, resulting in a backflow of blood into the left ventricle (lower chamber of the heart).

CAUSES

Failure of the aortic valve to close correctly may be due to a congenital abnormality. Another cause of aortic insufficiency is *aortitis* (inflammation of the aorta), which occurs in some people who have bacterial *endocarditis* of the aortic valve (in which the bacteria destroy the valve leaflets). This condition can occur in intravenous drug users. Aortic insufficiency is also found in untreated *syphilis*, *ankylosing spondylitis* (inflammation of joints in the spine), and *Marfan's syndrome* (a congenital disorder of connective tissues). *Rheumatic fever* was once a common cause of aortic incompetence but this infection has become very rare. Atherosclerosis is associated with both aortic insufficiency and *aortic stenosis*.

SYMPTOMS AND SIGNS

Aortic insufficiency may not cause any symptoms. It is sometimes found during a routine medical examination; the physician hears a murmur (abnormal heart sound) over the front of the chest wall to the left of the breastbone.

The heart compensates for the backflow of blood into the left ventricle by working harder, until the combination of hypertrophy (muscle thickening) and dilation (ballooning) of the left ventricle wall leads to *heart failure* (reduced pumping efficiency); this results in breathing difficulty and *edema* (fluid retention).

DIAGNOSIS

A *chest X ray* may show white patches of calcium in the area of the aortic valve, an enlarged heart, and dilation of the aorta.

An *ECG* (measurement of the electrical activity of the heart) may show evidence of thickening of and strain on the left ventricle.

Echocardiography (imaging heart structures by measuring the pattern of deflection of sound waves from them) will show the diameter of the valve opening and the diameter of the aortic ring, a thickening of the wall of the left ventricle, and reduced movement of the aortic valve. Doppler echocardiography shows the blood flow across the valve.

A cardiac catheter (flexible tube inserted into the heart through blood vessels) can be used to demonstrate the degree of insufficiency; a radiopaque dye is injected into the heart through the catheter and X-ray pictures taken (see *Catheterization, cardiac*). The information provided by preoperative catheterization studies is not substantially different from that provided by the aforementioned noninvasive studies (those not requiring penetration within the body).

TREATMENT

Heart failure resulting from aortic insufficiency can be treated with diuretics to remove retained fluid from the lungs. Heart valve surgery to

---

LOCATION AND STRUCTURE OF THE AORTA

From its origin at the left ventricle, the aorta passes upward, curves behind the heart, and runs downward, passing through the thorax (chest) and into the abdomen, where it terminates by dividing into two common iliac arteries. The aorta is thick-walled and large in diameter (about 1 inch, or 2.5 cm, at its origin) to cope with the high pressure and large volume of blood that passes through it. The thick walls of the aorta have an elastic quality that helps even out the peaks and troughs of pressure that occur with each heart beat.

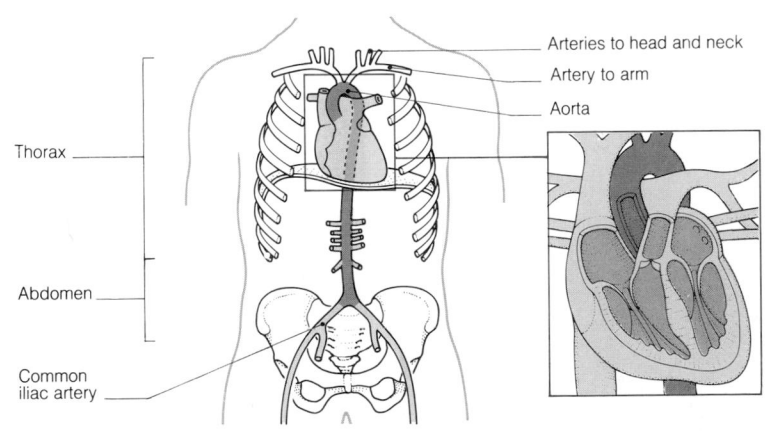

Thorax

Abdomen

Common iliac artery

Arteries to head and neck

Artery to arm

Aorta

replace the damaged valve may not be required for many years from the time of diagnosis; it is considered when symptoms develop or substantial changes in the valve occur.

Aortic stenosis

Narrowing of the aortic valve opening, causing obstruction of blood flow into the circulation. This makes the heart work harder and causes the muscle in the wall of the left ventricle (lower chamber) to thicken.

CAUSES

The most common cause is deposition of calcium on the aortic valve, usually associated with *atherosclerosis*. Aortic stenosis may also be due to a rare congenital abnormality. Another cause is *cardiomyopathy* (heart muscle disease in which thickening of the heart muscle may lead to narrowing of the aortic valve). In the past, *rheumatic fever* was a common cause of heart valve damage; today it is rare.

SYMPTOMS AND SIGNS

Aortic stenosis may not cause any symptoms. It is sometimes found during a routine medical examination; the physician hears a murmur (abnormal heart sound) over the front of the chest wall to the right of the breastbone and sometimes up into the neck. Symptoms, when they do occur, include fainting attacks, lack of energy, chest pain on exertion (*angina pectoris*), and breathing difficulty. Other signs include a weak pulse felt at the wrist and *cardiomegaly* (heart enlargement) at a late stage.

DIAGNOSIS

A *chest X ray* may show white patches of calcium in the area of the aortic valve. The heart may also appear enlarged on an X ray.

An *ECG* (measurement of the electrical activity of the heart) may show evidence of thickening of and strain on the left ventricle.

Echocardiography (imaging heart structures by measuring the pattern of deflection of sound waves from them) usually reveals the diameter of the valve opening and thickness of the valve leaflets, abnormal movement within the aortic valve, and thickening of the left ventricle walls. *Doppler* studies can confirm and quantitate the reduced flow across the valve.

A cardiac catheter (a flexible tube inserted into the heart through blood vessels) can be fitted with a pressure-measuring device to measure the degree of aortic stenosis; the difference in pressure on either side of the valve reflects the severity of the stenosis. The information provided by preoperative catheterization studies is not substantially different from that provided by the aforementioned *noninvasive* studies (those not requiring penetration within the body).

TREATMENT

Before developments in *heart valve surgery*, the outlook for people with aortic stenosis was gloomy; once symptoms developed, the predicted life span was only a year or so. Now, provided that valve replacement is done before irremediable damage to the left ventricle, the outlook is good.

Aortitis

Inflammation of the aorta, the large artery that carries blood from the heart to supply all parts of the body except the lungs. It is a rare condition occurring in people with *arteritis* (inflammation of arteries) or untreated *syphilis* and in some people with *ankylosing spondylitis* (inflammation of joints of the spine).

Aortitis may cause part of the aorta to widen and its walls to become thinner. This may then lead to the formation of an *aneurysm* (a swelling of the artery), which may burst and cause severe, sometimes fatal, blood loss. Aortitis may also damage the ring surrounding the aortic valve, leading to *aortic insufficiency*. This allows regurgitation of blood back to the heart, which can cause *heart failure*.

Aortography

A procedure that allows the aorta and its branches to be seen on X-ray film after injection with contrast medium (a substance opaque to X rays).

WHY IT IS DONE

Aortography is used to detect aortic *aneurysm* (weakening of the wall and ballooning of the vessel) and to investigate *peripheral vascular disease* before surgery.

HOW IT IS DONE

Contrast medium is usually injected into the aorta through a fine catheter (flexible plastic tube) inserted into the femoral artery at the groin or the brachial artery just inside of the elbow (see *Angiography*). In people with severe arterial disease, the major arteries may be blocked and the contrast medium may have to be injected directly into the lumbar aorta through a hollow needle.

COMPLICATIONS

There is a small risk of allergic reaction to the contrast medium. Damage to a vessel during puncture or catheterization can also occur.

Aperient

A mild laxative. (See *Laxative drugs*.)

Apgar score

A system devised by Virginia Apgar, an American anesthesiologist, to assess the condition of a newborn baby. Five features are scored at one minute and at five minutes after birth. The features are respiratory effort, heart rate, color, muscle tone, and motor reactions. The most important features are the infant's attempts to breathe and the infant's heart rate. In general, if these two are satisfactory, the other features are as well. Each feature is scored from 0 to 2, making a total of 10 possible points. A low total score of 0 to 3, which will occur if the baby does not breathe or if the heart rate is too slow, means the child needs urgent resuscitation. A score of 7 to 10 indicates a well baby.

APGAR CHART

Sign	0	1	2
Color	Blue, pale	Body pink; extremities blue	Completely pink
Respiratory effort	Absent	Weak cry; irregular breathing	Good strong cry; regular breathing
Muscle tone	Limp	Bending of some limbs	Active motion; limbs well-flexed
Reflex irritability	No response	Grimace (response to stimulation)	Cry
Heart rate	Absent	Slow (below 100 beats per minute)	Over 100 beats per minute

All too often anxious parents attach undue importance to the Apgar score. The score was originally intended to try to quantitate the enormous changes a newborn goes through in the first few minutes of life and help direct appropriate care. Certainly a very low score (0 to 4) means emergency care is needed. However, middle scores (5 to 7) do not indicate a damaged baby or some lack in the prenatal care.

Aphakia

The absence of the crystalline lens from the eye. Aphakia occurs if the lens has been surgically removed, as in *cataract surgery*, or if it has been destroyed by a penetrating injury and subsequently absorbed into the aqueous humor (the fluid within the eyeball). Removal of cataracts produces aphakia in both eyes.

Aphakia causes severe loss of focusing in the affected eye or eyes and requires correction by lens implants, contact lenses, or glasses.

Aphasia

A disturbance of previously acquired language skills caused by cerebral dysfunction; aphasia affects the ability to speak and write, and/or the ability to comprehend and read. Strictly, aphasia is a complete absence (and dysphasia a disturbance) of these communication and comprehension skills, but the distinction between the two terms is not useful.

The difficulty with speech expression in aphasia is different from that caused by disease or damage to the parts of the body involved in the mechanics of speech (see *Dysarthria*; *Dysphonia*). The comprehension difficulties are not due to defective hearing or sight.

Related disabilities that may occur as a feature of aphasia or, more rarely, by themselves, are *alexia* (word blindness) and *agraphia* (writing difficulty).

CAUSES

A *stroke* or a *head injury* is the most common cause of brain damage leading to aphasia.

Language function within the brain lies in the dominant cerebral hemisphere (see *Cerebrum*). Two particular areas in the dominant hemisphere, called Broca's and Wernicke's areas (named after their discoverers) and the pathways connecting the two, are known to be important in language skills. Damage to these areas is the most common cause of aphasia.

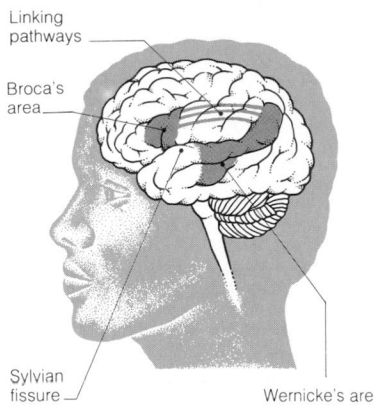

Linking pathways
Broca's area
Sylvian fissure
Wernicke's area

Language function and the brain
Damage to two particular areas (and the pathways between them) in the dominant cerebral hemisphere results in aphasia.

TYPES AND SYMPTOMS

BROCA'S (EXPRESSIVE) APHASIA Damage to Broca's area causes difficulty in the expression of language. Speech is nonfluent, slow, labored, with loss of normal rhythm. The few words uttered do tend to be meaningful.

WERNICKE'S (RECEPTIVE) APHASIA Damage to Wernicke's area causes difficulty in comprehension. Speech is fluent but, because of the impaired comprehension, its content is disturbed, with many errors in word selection and grammar, indicating that "internal speech" is impaired. Writing is also impaired and spoken or written commands are not understood.

GLOBAL APHASIA In global aphasia there is a total or near total inability to speak, write, or understand spoken or written words. This is usually caused by widespread damage to the dominant cerebral hemisphere.

NOMINAL APHASIA This is restricted to a difficulty in naming objects or in finding words, although the person may be able to choose the correct name from several offered. Nominal aphasia may be caused by generalized cerebral dysfunction or damage to specific language areas.

TREATMENT AND OUTLOOK

Some recovery from aphasia is usual after a stroke or head injury, although the more severe the aphasia, the less the chances of recovery. *Speech therapy* is the main treatment. (See also *Speech*; *Speech disorders*.)

Apheresis

Also called pheresis, a procedure in which blood is withdrawn from a donor and then reinfused after selected components, such as platelets, white blood cells, or plasma, have been separated and removed. (See also *Blood donation*.)

Aphonia

Total loss of the voice, usually sudden in onset and caused by emotional stress. A physician examining the larynx (voice box) would see that the vocal cords fail to meet as normal when the patient tries to speak, though they come together when the person coughs. Otherwise, there is no detectable abnormality in the larynx.

There is no treatment other than reassurance and *psychotherapy*. The sufferer's voice usually returns as suddenly as it disappeared.

Disease or damage to the larynx, as, for example, in *laryngitis* (inflammation of the larynx) or following surgery to remove a laryngeal cancer, normally causes only partial loss of voice production, known as *dysphonia*.

Aphrodisiacs

Substances thought to stimulate erotic desire and enhance sexual performance. Aphrodisiacs are named for Aphrodite, the ancient Greek goddess of love.

Various substances have been used as "love potions" over the centuries—honey, ginseng, ginger, strychnine, rhinoceros horn, and oysters, among many others. In fact, no substance has a proven aphrodisiac effect, although virtually anything may produce the desired results if the person taking it believes strongly enough that it will work. Alcohol can encourage sexual desire; it is a mental depressant and usually removes inhibitions. However, a high level of alcohol in the blood can impair sexual performance.

Probably the best known "aphrodisiac" is Spanish fly, which consists of powdered, dried beetles of the species LYTTA VESICATORIA. The substance's active ingredient, cantharidin, irritates the lining of the bladder and urethra (the tube between the bladder and outside) and may, in some cases, cause *priapism* (persistent erection). Spanish fly is potentially dangerous; some men have died as a result of using it.

Other substances used for their purported aphrodisiac effects include marijuana, yohimbine (a chemical obtained from the bark of the West African yohimbe tree), and amyl nitrite (a drug once used to treat angina). There is no scientific evidence that any of these is effective, and amyl nitrite may reduce blood pressure to dangerously low levels.

The male sex hormone *testosterone* is sometimes regarded as a sexual stimulant but, in normal men, it actually reduces sperm production. However, in men who have a testosterone deficiency, the hormone may restore both libido and potency.

Aplasia

Incomplete or reduced growth and development of any organ or tissue. For example, in bone marrow aplasia, the rate of cell division in the bone marrow is considerably reduced, leading to reduced formation of blood cells of one or all types (see *Anemia, aplastic*). A number of birth defects—for example, the presence of one or more stunted limbs (see *Phocomelia*)—are due to incomplete organ formation during prenatal development.

Aplastic anemia

See *Anemia, aplastic*.

Apnea

Cessation of breathing either temporarily (for a few seconds to a minute or two) or for a prolonged period, which is life-threatening.

CAUSES

Breathing is an automatic process controlled by the respiratory center in the brain stem. The respiratory center sends nerve impulses to the muscles in the chest that regulate lung expansion and contraction.

Prolonged apnea can occur if the brain stem is damaged by a *stroke*, by a *transient ischemic attack* (symptoms of stroke lasting less than 24 hours), or by a head injury. Prolonged apnea can also occur as an effect of certain drugs or as the result of *airway obstruction*, usually by food, drink, vomit, or a small inhaled object.

Deliberate temporary apnea occurs in *breath-holding attacks* and in underwater swimmers. Nondeliberate temporary apnea can also occur, usually during sleep (see *Sleep apnea*).

Another type of apnea occurs in *Cheyne-Stokes respiration*, which is characterized by cycles of deep, rapid breathing alternating with episodes of breath stoppage.

Apnea requires investigation and treatment of the underlying cause. Treatment may be aimed at relieving any airway obstruction. It may also include the use of respiratory stimulants if the respiratory center in the brain stem is affected.

Apocrine gland

A gland that discharges cellular material in addition to the fluid it secretes. The term is usually applied to the type of *sweat glands* that occur only in hairy areas of the body and appear after puberty.

Aponeurosis

A wide sheet of tough, fibrous tissue that acts as a tendon (i.e., attaches a muscle to a bone or a joint).

Apoplexy

An outdated term for a *stroke* (interruption of blood flow within the brain), resulting in sudden loss of consciousness, paralysis, or loss of sensation. The usual cause of apoplexy is rupture of a brain artery or blockage by a clot.

Apothecary

An obsolete term for a *pharmacist*.

Appendectomy

Surgical removal of the appendix to treat acute *appendicitis*.

WHY IT IS DONE

Appendectomy is carried out to prevent the inflamed appendix from bursting and causing *peritonitis* (inflammation of the abdominal lining) or an abdominal abscess.

Acute appendicitis is often difficult to diagnose and, sometimes, because of the dangerous complications that can develop from the condition, a *laparotomy* (an exploratory operation on the abdomen) is performed even when appendicitis is only suspected. In this case, the appendix, which has no apparent useful function in humans, is removed even if it is normal to prevent the possibility of appendicitis in the future.

HOW IT IS DONE

If there is time before the operation, the patient is started on a course of antibiotics to prevent the operative wound from becoming infected, an ever-present risk in appendectomy. Next, the physician makes a small incision in the abdomen (see box).

If the appendix has burst, the abdominal cavity in the area is washed out with saline (salt solution) and a plastic drainage tube is inserted into the infected area through another small incision to drain off pus.

Appendectomy may take from 10 minutes to more than an hour to perform, depending on the problems and complications involved.

COMPLICATIONS

Infection is the most common postoperative complication of appendectomy. The infection frequently involves the wound in the abdominal wall; it may also involve localized peritonitis or abscess at the site of appendix removal.

PERFORMING AN APPENDECTOMY

The patient is given a general anesthetic. A small incision is made in the lower right abdomen, above the groin, revealing the cecum (the chamber that links the small and large intestine), to which the appendix is attached.

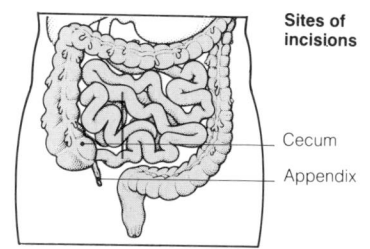

Sites of incisions

Cecum

Appendix

1 The appendix is carefully and gently brought to the surface of the draped abdomen, clamped, tied off at the base (where it joins the cecum), and cut off.

2 The stump is tied with a suture, sometimes touched with phenol, inverted, and tucked into the cecum with a suture to prevent fluid from leaking into the abdomen.

RECOVERY PERIOD

Following an uncomplicated appendectomy, the patient is usually able to drink and eat light food within 24 hours of the operation. If a drainage tube has been inserted, it is removed after about 48 hours; the wound seals itself. Normally, the patient can go home after two or three days. Stitches are removed seven to 10 days after the operation (an outpatient procedure). Normal physical activities can usually be resumed after two or three weeks. If there are complications, recovery may take much longer.

Appendicitis

Acute inflammation of the appendix, which is a common cause of abdominal pain and *peritonitis* (inflammation of the lining of the abdominal cavity) in children and young adults.

CAUSES

The cause is not always known, but appendicitis is sometimes due to obstruction of the appendix by a lump of feces or, occasionally, by worms in *pinworm infestation*. The closed end of the appendix beyond the obstruction becomes inflamed, swollen, and infected. This may lead to *gangrene* (tissue death) of the appendix wall, which may perforate (burst).

INCIDENCE

Appendicitis affects about 200 per 100,000 people per year in the US. Although anyone can get appendicitis, it is rare in the very young and the very old. It is the most common abdominal surgical emergency in the Western world but is comparatively rare in developing countries.

SYMPTOMS

The first symptom is usually vague discomfort just above and around the navel. Within a few hours this gradually develops into a sharper, more localized pain. This pain is usually most intense in the lower right-hand side of the abdomen. If the appendix descends behind the cecum over the brim of the pelvis, appendicitis may cause little abdominal pain, but severe pain on rectal examination. If it impinges on the ureter, there may be bloody urine passed.

The pain and abdominal tenderness characteristic of appendicitis are usually accompanied by a slight fever, loss of appetite, nausea, vomiting, a coated tongue, and foul breath, sometimes preceded by constipation. Anyone who has sudden abdominal pain and other symptoms of appendicitis should consult a physician without delay.

DIAGNOSIS

Diagnosis can sometimes be difficult because the symptoms of appendicitis are similar to those of many other abdominal disorders. Nonspecific abdominal pain (also called mesenteric adenitis), which is common in childhood and often follows a viral respiratory tract infection, has symptoms and signs that resemble those of appendicitis. Disorders of the right fallopian tube and ovary, *Crohn's disease*, and right-sided *pyelonephritis* (inflammation of the kidney) can also mimic appendicitis. Sometimes a *laparotomy* (surgical investigation of the abdomen) is necessary to confirm or exclude the diagnosis.

COMPLICATIONS

If treatment is delayed, the inflamed appendix may perforate, releasing its contents into the abdomen. This causes peritonitis. In some cases, the omentum (fold of peritoneum covering the intestines) envelops the inflamed appendix; this prevents the spread of infection and results in a localized abscess around the appendix. Peritonitis or an abscess causes a high swinging fever (sometimes with chills) as well as increasing pain that recurs hours or a day or so following the abrupt cessation of pain (which occurs when the appendix ruptures) and tenderness in the abdomen.

TREATMENT

The usual treatment is *appendectomy* (surgical removal of the appendix). If an abscess of the appendix is suspected, drainage of the abscess and an appendectomy may be delayed until the infection has been reduced by large doses of antibiotics.

Appendix

A narrow, small, finger-shaped tube branching off the large intestine that has no known function. In adults it is usually about 3.5 inches (9 cm) long, with a thick wall, narrow cavity, and a lining similar to that of the intestine. It contains a large amount of lymphoid tissue, which provides a defense against local infection.

The appendix projects out of the first part of the colon at the lower right-hand side of the abdomen. It may lie behind the cecum (the first part of the large intestine), but in some people descends over the brim of the pelvis, lies below the cecum, or lies in front of or behind the ileum (part of the small intestine). Its varying position partly determines the set of symptoms produced by acute *appendicitis* (inflammation of the appendix).

Appetite

A desire for food; a pleasant sensation felt in anticipation of eating, as opposed to *hunger*, a disagreeable feeling caused by the need for food.

Appetite, which is regulated by two parts of the brain (the hypothalamus and the cerebral cortex), is learned by enjoying a variety of foods that smell, taste, and look good. Ideally, it combines with hunger to ensure that the correct amount of a wide range of foods is eaten to promote health, to produce growth in children, and to maintain a proper weight in adults.

Appetite may be lost as a result of various disorders, both physical and psychological (see *Appetite, loss of*).

Appetite, loss of

Known medically as anorexia, loss of appetite is usually temporary and due to an emotional upset or minor feverish illness. Persistent loss of appetite may be a symptom of a more serious underlying physical or psychological disorder and requires investigation by a physician.

CAUSES

In adolescents and young adults, loss of appetite may be due to *anorexia nervosa* (rejection of food due to psychological causes), or to abuse of drugs, particularly the abuse of

LOCATION OF THE APPENDIX

In the lower right-hand side of the abdomen, the appendix may lie behind the cecum, or in front of or behind the ileum.

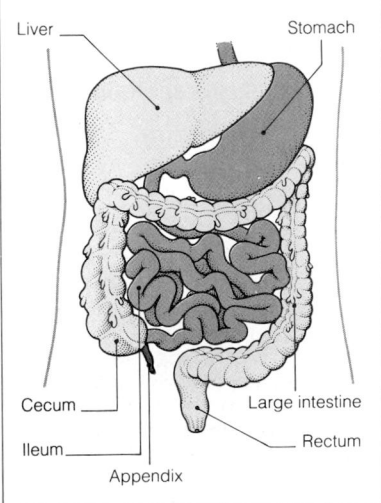

Liver — Stomach — Cecum — Large intestine — Ileum — Rectum — Appendix

amphetamine drugs. Depression or anxiety can cause loss of appetite at any age.

Among possible physical causes are a *stroke, brain tumor*, or a brain injury that has damaged the hypothalamus or cerebral cortex, the parts of the brain that control appetite. Other physical causes include intestinal disorders, such as *gastritis* (inflammation of the stomach lining, common in alcoholics), a stomach tumor (see *Stomach cancer*) or a *gastric ulcer*, and liver disorders, such as *hepatitis*. Many infectious diseases, notably *influenza*, also cause loss of appetite.

Between the ages of about 2 and 4, some children go through a phase of refusing food. If there are no other symptoms, this period of food refusal should be regarded as a normal part of child development.

For a person who is otherwise healthy, a period of two or three days without food is not harmful, provided that plenty of nonalcoholic fluids are taken. However, if there are other health problems, particularly *diabetes mellitus*, or if regular medication is being taken, a physician should always be consulted.

All cases of loss of appetite that last for more than a few days should be investigated by a physician. Appetite generally returns to normal once any underlying illness has been treated. (See also *Appetite stimulants*.)

Appetite stimulants

There are no known drugs that safely and effectively stimulate the appetite. Lost appetite usually returns when an underlying illness subsides. A variety of drugs (including alcohol and elixirs containing small quantities of iron, quinine, and strychnine) have been prescribed, without benefit.

Appetite suppressants

COMMON DRUGS
Diethylpropion Fenfluramine Mazindol Phenmetrazine Phentermine Phenylpropanolamine

A group of drugs that reduces the desire to eat food. Appetite suppressants may be used in the treatment of *obesity*, along with advice on diet and exercise. These drugs are thought to suppress appetite by affecting the *hypothalamus* (part of the brain).

POSSIBLE ADVERSE EFFECTS
Adverse effects include dry mouth, dizziness, palpitations, nervousness, restlessness, and difficulty getting to sleep. Symptoms usually disappear after a few days of treatment.

Taking an appetite suppressant regularly for more than six weeks may lead to dependence (see *Drug dependence*). Newer appetite suppressants are less addictive than the *amphetamine drugs* that used to be prescribed.

Apraxia

An inability to carry out purposeful movements despite normal muscle power and coordination. Apraxia is caused by damage to nerve tracts within the cerebrum (the main mass of the brain) that translate the idea for a movement into an actual movement. People with apraxia usually know what they want to do but appear to have lost the ability to recall from memory the sequence of actions necessary to achieve the movement. The damage to the cerebrum may be caused by a direct *head injury*, infection, *stroke*, or *brain tumor*.

TYPES AND SYMPTOMS
Various forms of apraxia are known, each related to damage within different parts of the brain. A person with ideomotor apraxia is unable to carry out a spoken command to make a particular movement—for example, to lick his or her lips—but at another time can be observed making precisely the same movement unconsciously.

Agraphia (difficulty writing) and expressive *aphasia* (severe difficulty speaking) are special forms of apraxia.

TREATMENT AND OUTLOOK
Recovery from events such as a stroke or head injury, and from accompanying syndromes such as apraxia, is highly variable. Usually some deficit remains and it may require considerable effort and patience for the person to relearn lost skills.

APUD cell tumor

A growth, sometimes called an apudoma, composed of cells that produce various hormones. These cells—amine precursor uptake and decarboxylation (APUD) cells—are similar, even though they occur in different parts of the body.

Some tumors of the thyroid glands, pancreas, and lungs are APUD cell tumors, as are a *carcinoid* tumor and *pheochromocytoma* (an adrenal tumor).

Arachnodactyly

Long, thin, spiderlike fingers and toes that sometimes occur spontaneously but are characteristic of *Marfan's syndrome*, an inherited connective tissue disease.

Arachnoiditis

An uncommon condition characterized by chronic inflammation and thickening of the arachnoid mater, the middle of the three meninges (membranes that cover and protect the brain and spinal cord).

Arachnoiditis may develop up to several years after an episode of *meningitis* (infection of the meninges) or *subarachnoid hemorrhage* (bleeding beneath the arachnoid). It may be a feature of diseases and disorders such as *syphilis* or *ankylosing spondylitis*, or may result from trauma or procedures such as *myelography* (injection of radiopaque dye into the spinal canal followed by X rays). Usually, however, no cause is found.

The signs and symptoms vary with the extent of the disorder. It may cause headache, epileptic seizures, blindness, or slowly progressive spastic paralysis (difficulties with movements due to increased muscle tension) affecting both legs or all four limbs. There is no effective treatment.

ARC

Abbreviation for *AIDS-related complex*. (See also *AIDS*.)

Arcus senilis

A gray-white ring in the cornea, at the front of the eye, that occurs almost invariably during old age. The ring overlies the outer rim of the iris and is encircled by a narrow zone of unaffected cornea. Arcus senilis is caused by degeneration of fatty material within the cornea.

Arcus senilis
The arcus senilis is the lighter ring that overlies the edge of the iris (the colored part of the eye).

Arcus senilis develops gradually during adult life, usually starting in the lower part of the cornea, then appearing in the upper part, before affecting the sides to form a complete ring. It never spreads to the center, does not affect eyesight, and is not believed to be related to health.

A similar phenomenon in the young is called arcus juvenilis; this condition may be associated with the metabolic disorder *hyperlipidemia*.

Aroma therapy

A range of treatments using aromatic oils extracted from plants. Many ancient civilizations, particularly the Chinese, documented the use of essential oils in treating different disorders. Recently, interest in aroma therapy has been rekindled along with other alternative therapies (see *Alternative medicine*). Practitioners claim that the treatment can be used for a range of disorders, but that it is particularly effective in *psychosomatic* and stress-related disorders.

The patient describes his or her symptoms to the therapist, who chooses the most appropriate oil or oils from a prepared range. The oil is applied in small quantities through massage or is inhaled or incorporated into creams or lotions. Very occasionally the oil is taken internally.

There is no conclusive scientific evidence that the benefits achieved are greater than those achieved by the power of suggestion.

Arousal

The awakening of a person from unconsciousness or semiconsciousness. Physicians test the depth of unconsciousness in a patient who may be suffering, for example, from concussion, a drug overdose, or alcohol intoxication with reference to the amount of stimulus required for arousal. Stimuli used include speech, a pinprick, and pressure on the Achilles tendon, which lies at the back of the ankle.

The term arousal is also used to describe any state of heightened awareness, such as that caused by sexual stimulation or fear.

Arousal is regulated by the reticular formation within the *brain stem*.

Arrhenoblastoma

A rare tumor of the ovary, also called andreoblastoma, that occurs in young women. Although the tumor is benign, it secretes androgens (male sex hormones) that cause *virilization* (the development of male sex characteristics). Treatment is by surgical removal of the affected ovary.

Arrhythmia, cardiac

An abnormality of the rhythm or rate of the *heart beat*. Arrhythmia is caused by a disturbance in the electrical impulses to the heart (see box).

TYPES

Arrhythmias can be divided into two main groups: the tachycardias, in which the rate is faster than normal (greater than 100 beats per minute), and the bradycardias, in which the rate is slower than normal (fewer than 60 beats per minute). The rhythm may be regular, as in the normal heart beat, with each beat of the atria being followed by one beat of the ventricles, or it may be irregular. The beat may originate at the sinus node or some other area of the heart.

TACHYCARDIAS

In *sinus tachycardia*, the rate is raised (100 to 160 beats per minute), the rhythm is regular, and the beat originates in the sinoatrial node. *Supraventricular tachycardia* is faster (with a rate of 120 to 200 beats per minute), the rhythm is regular, and the beat may arise anywhere in the conducting tissue above the ventricles. When rapid, irregular heart beats (120 to 200 per minute) originate in the ventricles, it is called *ventricular tachycardia*.

In *atrial flutter*, the atria beat regularly and very rapidly (200 to 400 beats per minute), but not every impulse reaches the ventricles, which beat at a rate of about 100 to 200 beats per minute. Totally uncoordinated beating of the atria at about 300 to 500 beats per minute is called *atrial fibrillation* and produces completely irregular ventricular beats. Any isolated irregular beat is called an *ectopic beat* (which does not necessarily indicate the presence of an abnormality).

BRADYCARDIAS

A slow, regular beat is called *sinus bradycardia*. In *heart block*, the conduction of electrical impulses through the heart muscle is partially or completely blocked, leading to slow, irregular beating. Periods of bradycardia alternate with periods of tachycardia due to a fault in impulse generation (see *Sick sinus syndrome*).

CAUSES

A common cause of arrhythmia is *coronary heart disease*. In this condition, vessels supplying blood to the heart

---

CARDIAC ARRHYTHMIA

Any disorder that interferes with the generation or transmission of impulses through the heart's electrical conducting system (below) can lead to a disturbance of cardiac rate or rhythm. These ECG recordings show two kinds of arrhythmia: sinus bradycardia and atrial fibrillation.

Sinoatrial node
This is the heart's natural pacemaker from which electrical impulses originate. The impulses spread over the atria, causing them to contract.

Left ventricle

Right ventricle

Right atrium

Left atrium

Atrioventricular node
Impulses from the sinoatrial node travel to this second node, from which they spread to the ventricles, causing contractions that follow the atrial beats.

1 second

1 second

Sinus bradycardia
The heart rate is slow but the rhythm normal, with each atrial beat (small rise) followed by a ventricular beat (spike). Sinus bradycardia is common in athletes, but can also be caused by hypothyroidism.

Atrial fibrillation
The atria beat rapidly and irregularly. Ventricular beats (spikes) do not follow each atrial beat and are irregularly spaced. This arrhythmia is common in the elderly and people with hyperthyroidism.

A

are narrowed by *atheroma* (fatty deposits) and are unable to supply sufficient blood to the conducting tissue, which becomes damaged. Arrhythmias due to coronary heart disease come on more frequently after a *myocardial infarction* (heart attack).

Sinus tachycardia may be a normal response to exercise or stress; likewise, sinus bradycardia often occurs in healthy athletes.

Caffeine and other drugs can cause tachycardia in some individuals. Amitriptyline and other antidepressants can cause serious cardiac arrhythmias if taken in high doses.

SYMPTOMS
Sudden onset of tachycardia can cause palpitations, with the individual becoming aware of an abnormally fast heart beat. Any sudden arrhythmia can cause faintness or dizziness due to reduction of blood flow to the brain. If a bradycardia reduces the flow of blood to the lungs, breathing difficulty may occur. If there is underlying heart disease, arrhythmia may lead to *angina pectoris* (chest pain due to reduced blood supply) or *heart failure* (reduced pumping efficiency).

DIAGNOSIS
The physician makes a preliminary assessment by feeling the patient's pulse and listening to the heart.

The type of arrhythmia is confirmed by an *ECG*, which shows the pattern of electrical activity within heart muscle. In some cases, if the arrhythmia is intermittent, it may be necessary to make continuous ECG recordings for 24 hours using a portable monitor.

TREATMENT
There are many different drugs that can be used to treat arrhythmias (see *Antiarrhythmic drugs*). When an arrhythmia occurs suddenly after a myocardial infarction, *defibrillation* (administration of an electric shock to the heart) may be required.

Artificial *pacemakers* can be used to stimulate heart beat in cases of heart block. Pacemakers usually consist of a small generating unit implanted under the skin of the chest wall that passes electrical impulses to the heart by means of electrodes.

Arsenic
A metallic element that occurs naturally in its pure form and as various chemical compounds. The term arsenic is popularly used to refer to the poisonous trioxide. Arsenic is present in trace amounts in water and many foods and, as a result, most

people have minute quantities in their bodies, particularly in their hair and in their skin.

POISONING
Arsenic has been used intentionally to murder, but most poisoning occurs industrially or through accidental ingestion, particularly in rural areas, where arsenic is an important constituent of some pesticides.

Arsenic poisoning may be acute or chronic. Acute poisoning primarily affects the lining of the intestine, producing painful symptoms of sudden onset. The victim experiences nausea, vomiting (sometimes with blood stains), diarrhea, excessive sweating, and burning of the throat, followed by collapse and death if untreated.

Chronic poisoning is usually first noticeable as weakness, tiredness, scaly skin, *keratosis* (changes in skin pigmentation), and swelling of the lining of the mouth. *Neuropathy* (degeneration of nerves) then sets in, which produces tingling, then numbness in the hands and feet.

INVESTIGATION AND TREATMENT
Arsenic poisoning, once suspected, may be confirmed by urine analysis. Treatment of acute poisoning includes gastric *lavage* (pumping out the stomach), replacement of lost fluids, treatment of shock and pain, and administration of dimercaprol, a drug that helps to remove the poison from the body. Chronic poisoning is also treated with dimercaprol.

Arterial reconstructive surgery
Operation to repair arteries that are narrowed, blocked, or weakened.

WHY IT IS DONE
Arterial reconstructive surgery is most often performed to repair arteries narrowed or blocked by *atheroma* (fatty deposits) in arterial disease. It is also used to repair *aneurysms* (balloonlike swellings at areas of weakness) that may be congenital or may be due to *atherosclerosis*. Arteries that have been damaged by injury can also be repaired surgically.

HOW IT IS DONE
A narrowed or blocked section of artery can be bypassed by sewing in a length of vein—usually taken from the patient's leg—above and below the constricted area. This technique is most often used for coronary arteries (see *Coronary artery bypass*).

For damaged arteries elsewhere in the body, it is more common to cut out the affected section and replace it with an artificial tube or a section of vein taken from another part of the body.

OUTLOOK
Arterial reconstructive surgery is generally successful, depending on the age and health of the patient. Aortic reconstruction carries an operative death rate of up to 5 percent; untreated, larger aortic aneurysms may eventually rupture, however, and the risks of emergency surgery are much higher. (See also *Angiography; Angioplasty, balloon; Endarterectomy*.)

Arteries, disorders of
Disorders of the arteries may take the form of abnormal narrowing (which reduces blood flow and may cause tissue damage), complete obstruction (which may cause tissue death), or abnormal widening and thinning of an artery wall (which may cause rupture of the blood vessel).

TYPES
ATHEROSCLEROSIS Affecting most adults to some extent, atherosclerosis (fat deposits on the artery walls) is the most common arterial disease. It can involve arteries throughout the body, including the brain (see *Cerebrovascular disease*), the heart (see *Coronary heart disease*), and the legs (see *Peripheral vascular disease*). It is the main type of *arteriosclerosis*, a group of disorders that causes thickening and loss of elasticity of artery walls.

HYPERTENSION High blood pressure is another common cause of thickening and narrowing of arteries. It predisposes people to coronary heart disease and increases the risk of having a *stroke* as well as *renal failure*.

ARTERITIS This is a group of disorders in which inflammation of artery walls causes narrowing and sometimes blockage (see *Arteritis*).

THROMBOSIS A thrombus (blood clot) may form within an artery, causing partial or complete obstruction of the blood flow. Thrombosis usually occurs in areas already damaged by atherosclerosis or aneurysm.

EMBOLISM Obstruction of an artery by an embolus (usually a fragment of thrombus that has broken off from a larger vessel or the wall of the heart, although it may consist of fat particles from a bone fracture or an air bubble from decompression sickness).

ANEURYSM Thinning and swelling of an artery wall, this may occur in arteries damaged by atherosclerosis or as a congenital defect. In the aorta, an aneurysm may be due to *aortitis* (inflammation of the aorta wall), which may be part of a generalized arteritis or, rarely today, due to untreated syphilis.

RAYNAUD'S DISEASE This is a disorder involving intermittent spasm of small arteries in the hands and feet, usually due to cold. This obstruction of blood flow causes a change in skin color, numbness, and a pins and needles sensation. Occasionally, if the obstruction lasts, skin damage with the formation of an ischemic ulcer (see *Ischemia*) may result.

TREATMENT
Embolism and thrombosis of arteries may be treated with thrombolytic drugs (tissue plasminogen activator or streptokinase) that will dissolve the clot, and then may be prevented with *anticoagulant drugs* or by surgery to remove the obstruction (see *Embolectomy*). The various forms of arteritis (except those caused by syphilis) often respond to treatment with corticosteroid drugs. Aneurysms and arterial damage may sometimes be repaired surgically (see *Arterial reconstructive surgery*).

Arteriography
Another name for *angiography*.

Arteriole
A blood vessel that branches off an *artery* to link it to a *capillary*. Arterioles are intermediate in size and structure between arteries and capillaries. However, arterioles have proportionately more smooth muscle in their walls; their nerve supply allows the arterioles to be constricted or dilated to meet variations in the blood-flow needs of the tissues they supply.

Arteriopathy
Any abnormal condition or disorder of an artery. (See *Arteries, disorders of.*)

Arterioplasty
Surgical repair of an artery (see *Arterial reconstructive surgery*).

Arteriosclerosis
A group of disorders that causes thickening and loss of elasticity of artery walls. *Atherosclerosis* is the most common type of arteriosclerosis. Different types include medial arteriosclerosis (in which muscle and elastic fibers from the lining of large and medium-sized arteries are replaced by fibrous tissue) and Monckeberg's arteriosclerosis (in which there are deposits of calcium within the lining of the arteries).

Arteriovenous fistula
An abnormal communication or malformation between an artery and a vein that may occur congenitally or as a result of injury or infection. It can also be created surgically to provide an easy route of access into the bloodstream. The technique is useful in performing *dialysis*.

If the fistula is close to the skin surface, it may cause a small pulsating swelling. If several fistulas are present in the lungs, they can impair the uptake of oxygen into the blood, cause *cyanosis* (blue skin color), cause breathing difficulty on exertion, and sometimes cause *hemoptysis* (coughing up blood).

If an isolated fistula is causing symptoms, it is usually cut away, the channel restored, and the ends of the blood vessels sutured (stitched). If there are large numbers of fistulas, surgery is not practicable. Some arteriovenous malformations in inaccessible areas of the brain are treated with proton-beam radiation (see *Radiation therapy*).

Arteritis
Inflammation of the artery wall, causing narrowing or complete obstruction of the affected arteries, reduced blood flow, and, in some cases, thrombosis (blood clot formation) and damage to tissues.

Buerger's disease includes an arteritis that affects the limbs, causing pain, numbness, and, in severe cases, *gangrene* (death of tissue).

Periarteritis nodosa, an *autoimmune disorder* (in which the body's defense mechanism against disease attacks its own tissues), can affect arteries in any part of the body, causing symptoms such as abdominal and testicular pain, chest pain, breathing difficulty, and tender lumps under the skin.

Temporal arteritis affects arteries in the scalp over the temples, causing headache and scalp tenderness; if the retinal artery is affected, there is a risk of permanent blindness.

A very rare type of arteritis is Takayasu's arteritis. The cause is unknown but thought to be autoimmune (the body's defense mechanisms attacking its own tissues—in this case, the artery walls). Takayasu's arteritis usually affects young women and involves the arteries that branch from the first part of the aorta into the neck and arms.

Artery
A blood vessel that carries blood away from the heart. Systemic arteries carry blood from the left ventricle (lower chamber) of the heart, through the aorta (the largest artery in the body), to all parts of the body except the lungs. The pulmonary arteries carry blood from the right ventricle of the heart to the lungs. Pulmonary arteries are shorter, thinner-walled, and contain blood under a lower pressure than systemic arteries.

STRUCTURE AND FUNCTION
Arteries are pliable tubes with thick walls that enable them to withstand the high blood pressure to which they are subjected every time that the heart muscle beats.

STRUCTURE OF AN ARTERY
An artery's walls consist of three layers: a smooth, inner lining, a thick, muscular, elastic, middle layer, and a tough, fibrous, outer covering. Veins have thinner walls and most contain valves.

Artery

Thin, elastic layers

Tough, outer layer

Muscular, middle layer

Inner coat

Vein

Inner coat

The structure of arteries helps even out the peaks and troughs of blood pressure caused by the heart beat, so that the blood is flowing at a relatively constant pressure by the time it reaches the smaller blood vessels. These smaller vessels include the *arterioles*, which branch directly off the artery. The arterioles connect to the even smaller *capillaries*. (See also *Arteries, disorders of.*)

Arthralgia
A term meaning pain in the joints. (See *Joint*; *Arthritis.*)

A

Arthritis

Inflammation of a joint, characterized by pain, swelling, stiffness, and redness. Arthritis is not a single disorder but the name of joint disease from a number of causes. The arthritis may involve one joint or many, and can vary in severity from a mild ache and stiffness to severe pain and, later, joint deformity.

TYPES AND CAUSES

OSTEOARTHRITIS Also known as degenerative arthritis, this is the most common type of arthritis. It results from wear and tear on the joints, evolves in middle age, and most commonly troubles older people.

RHEUMATOID ARTHRITIS The most severe type of inflammatory joint disease, this is an *autoimmune disorder* in which the body's *immune system* acts against and damages joints and surrounding soft tissues. Many joints—most commonly those in the hands, feet, and arms—become extremely painful, stiff, and deformed.

STILL'S DISEASE Juvenile rheumatoid arthritis; it is most common in children under the age of 4. It usually clears up after a few years but even then may stunt growth and leave the child with permanent deformities.

SERONEGATIVE ARTHRITIS This is a group of disorders that causes symptoms and signs of arthritis in a number of joints, although blood test results for rheumatoid arthritis are negative. It can be associated with skin disorders (such as *psoriasis*), inflammatory intestinal disorders (such as *Crohn's disease*), or autoimmune disorders.

INFECTIVE ARTHRITIS Also known as septic or pyogenic arthritis, this is joint disease caused by the invasion of bacteria into the joint from a nearby

Arthritis in the hands
Severely deformed joints in the hands of an elderly woman who is suffering from rheumatoid arthritis.

infected wound or from *bacteremia* (infection in the bloodstream). The infected joint usually becomes hot as well as painful and swollen.

Arthritis may also occur as a complication of an infection elsewhere in the body, such as *chickenpox*, *rubella* (German measles), *mumps*, *rheumatic fever*, or *gonorrhea*; it may also be a complication of *nonspecific urethritis*, in which case the joint inflammation forms part of *Reiter's syndrome*.

ANKYLOSING SPONDYLITIS In this arthritis of the spine, the joints linking the vertebrae become inflamed and the vertebrae fuse. The arthritis may spread to other joints, often the hips.

GOUT This disorder is associated with a form of arthritis in which uric acid (one of the body's waste products) accumulates in joints in the form of crystals, causing inflammation. It usually affects one joint at a time.

DIAGNOSIS

The diagnosis is made from the patient's symptoms and signs. To discover the cause, fluid may be withdrawn through a needle from an affected joint. This fluid may then be examined microscopically for the presence of microorganisms, or uric acid or other crystals. Sometimes a *culture* is made from the fluid so that it can be analyzed for any infection.

X rays may be carried out to reveal the type and extent of damage to joints. *Blood tests* can reveal the presence of proteins typical of rheumatoid arthritis, a high level of uric acid indicative of gout, or sometimes a high *ESR* (erythrocyte sedimentation rate), indicating inflammation.

TREATMENT

There are specific treatments for the different types of arthritis—for example, *antibiotic drugs* for septic arthritis, *anti-inflammatory drugs* for treating rheumatoid arthritis and osteoarthritis, and allopurinol for gout. Many other drugs are used to treat different forms of arthritis, but none seems able to effect a cure.

In a severe attack of arthritis affecting several joints, a few days' bed rest will help settle the inflammation; individual joints can be splinted to reduce the pain, and heat and supervised exercises help keep the deformity in the joints to a minimum. Obese people with arthritis in weight-bearing joints should lose weight.

Diseased joints that have become extremely painful, unstable, or deformed may require *arthroplasty* (replacement of the joint with an artificial substitute) or *arthrodesis* (fusion of the bones in the joint).

OUTLOOK

Arthritis has many forms and varies widely in its effects. Only a few sufferers become severely disabled. Most are able to lead productive lives, although activity may need to be altered to preserve joint function.

Arthrodesis

A surgical procedure in which the two bones in a diseased joint are fused to prevent the joint from moving.

WHY IT IS DONE

If pain and deformity in a diseased joint are so severe that they cannot be relieved by drugs, splinting, and physical therapy (as can occur in *rheumatoid arthritis*), or if a joint has become unstable, usually as the result of an injury, some form of surgery is required. In most cases, the operation of first choice is *arthroplasty* (reconstruction of a diseased joint using artificial replacements), since this procedure retains movement in the joint. When arthroplasty is not feasible or fails, arthrodesis is used.

HOW IT IS DONE

A local anesthetic may be all that is required for a small joint, such as a finger. Otherwise, general anesthetic is used. The technique of the operation varies according to the joint being treated, but in most cases cartilage (smooth, shock-absorbing tissue) is removed from the ends of the two bones, along with a surface layer of bone from each. The two ends are then joined so that, when fresh bone cells grow, the ends will fuse. The bones may need to be kept in position with plates, rods, or screws; a *bone graft* may also be carried out.

In arthrodesis of the knee or ankle, additional immobilization of the joint—by transfixing it with pins inserted through the skin—may be necessary to keep the area stable until healing is complete.

RECOVERY PERIOD

Complete union of the bones can take up to six months but is usually much quicker. In some cases the bones fail to fuse, but often this is irrelevant because fibrous tissue fills the gap between them and is strong enough to provide the same effect and strength as bone fusion.

OUTLOOK

One advantage of arthrodesis over arthroplasty is that, once performed, it needs no regular surveillance or further care; the patient can be reasonably certain that the problem with the joint has been solved permanently.

Arthrography

A diagnostic technique for examining the interior of a damaged joint by injecting into it a radiopaque solution (one visible on X ray). The procedure is gradually being replaced by *ultrasound scanning* and *arthroscopy*.

Arthrogryposis

See *Contracture*.

Arthropathy

A medical term for *joint* disease.

Arthroplasty

Replacement of a joint or part of a joint by metal or plastic components. *Hip replacements* were the first operations of this type to be introduced and are still the most successful and often performed. Replacement of other joints, including the knee (see *Knee joint replacement*), finger (see *Finger joint replacement*), shoulder, and elbow, is also routine.

The first attempts to replace part of a damaged hip joint with a man-made substitute were made in the 1930s. In the 1960s, hip replacement operations were revolutionized by developments on three fronts. First, metal and plastic materials were developed that were strong enough to allow a good level of activity while being to some extent self-lubricating; second, cement was used to help fix the artificial joint to the bones; and third, the risk of infection in the joint—a very serious complication—was virtually eliminated by performing the surgery in an operating room in which the air is filtered and all members of the surgical team wear all-enveloping clothing.

These principles have now been applied to the full range of replacement joints. Engineers and orthopedic surgeons are still developing and improving replacements for the knee and shoulder, which are more complex than the hip.

Arthroscopy

Inspection through an *endoscope* (a flexible viewing tube) of the interior of a joint, usually for the purpose of diagnosing a condition affecting that joint. Arthroscopy has rapidly become one of the most frequently performed procedures in orthopedic surgery, thanks to the development of modern lens systems and brighter lighting by means of fiberoptics.

WHY IT IS DONE

Arthroscopy is most frequently used to inspect the inside of the knee joint. Many conditions affecting the knee do

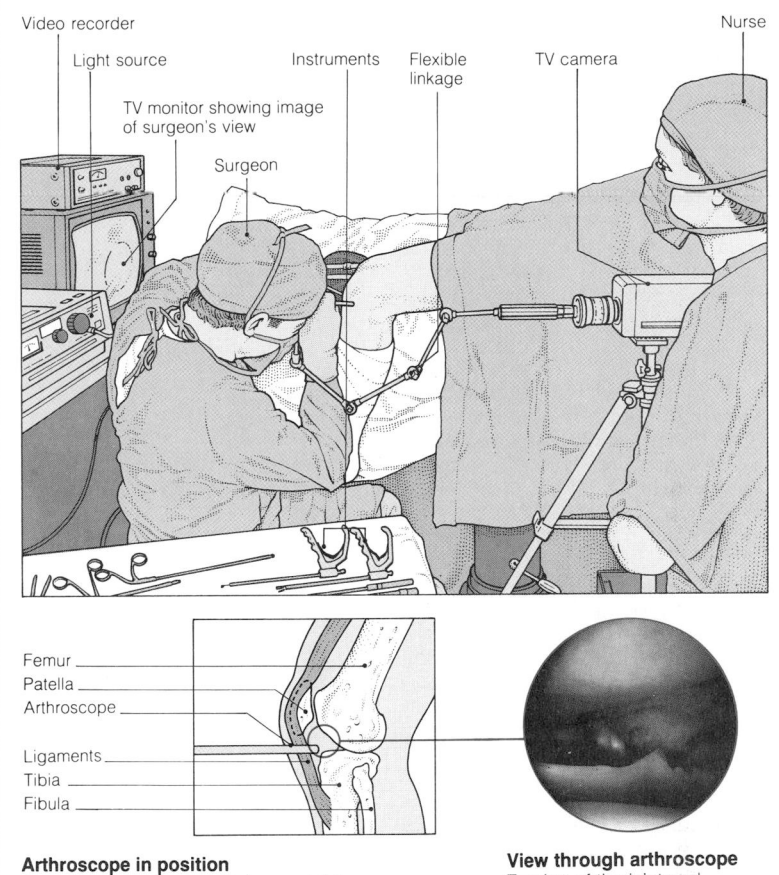

HOW ARTHROSCOPY IS DONE

The procedure is usually performed using a general anesthetic, but sometimes a *nerve block* is used. The joint is distended by injecting air or a saline solution; the instrument is inserted into the joint through a small skin incision. While watching through the endoscope, the surgeon can probe or lift structures to check for damage.

Video recorder
Light source
TV monitor showing image of surgeon's view
Surgeon
Instruments
Flexible linkage
TV camera
Nurse

Femur
Patella
Arthroscope
Ligaments
Tibia
Fibula

Arthroscope in position
An arthroscope is a steel tube containing optical fibers, a lens, and a light source.

View through arthroscope
Tearing of the joint and cartilage lining is shown.

not show up on X rays and are difficult to diagnose on the basis of symptoms alone. Arthroscopy allows the surgeon to see the surfaces of the bones that come into contact in the joint, the ligaments and cartilages within the joint, and the synovial membrane that lines the internal surface of the joint capsule. Specimens of these structures can be removed for examination and analysis.

A new and exciting development is the application of arthroscopic surgery techniques. Instruments that fold down as they are passed through a channel in the arthroscope enable surgeons to carry out some procedures that formerly necessitated opening up the knee. Procedures include removal of damaged cartilage, repair of torn cartilage and ligaments, and shaving or drilling the surface of the patella (kneecap). Arthroscopic surgery substantially reduces the time a patient needs to stay in the hospital, and the time an athlete is unable to participate in his or her sport.

Artificial insemination

The introduction of semen into the cervix (opening of the uterus) by means of an instrument instead of through sexual intercourse, with the aim of inducing conception and pregnancy. Artificial insemination was first carried out in the US in 1866. About 10,000 babies are born here annually as a result of the procedure.

TYPES

There are two principal types of artificial insemination. AIH (artificial insemination using the husband's semen) is the use of semen from the woman's permanent sexual partner. It is usually employed for couples who are unable to have intercourse, either because of psychosexual difficulties, such as impotence, or because of physical injury or deformity. Occasionally, it may be used when the husband has a low sperm count or a low volume of ejaculate or if the acid in the woman's vagina creates a hostile environment for the sperm. It is also used when semen has been stored from a man who is to undergo medical treatment (such as chemotherapy or radiation therapy) that may make him sterile. AID (artificial insemination using a donor's semen) is the use of semen from an anonymous male donor. It is available to couples if the man is infertile, has a genetic disease, or may be a carrier of such a disease. It may also be used by a woman who wants children but has no male partner.

HOW IT IS DONE

Both AID and AIH are carried out at centers that are specially staffed and equipped to obtain and store semen from donors, to carry out the insemination, and to give counseling before and after the procedure.

Donors must be in good health and are usually screened for as many physical and mental disorders as possible. However, there is no safeguard against the use of sperm from a carrier of a genetic disease.

Fresh semen is usually used for AIH. For AID, the semen is frozen in liquid nitrogen and then stored; before it is used it is tested to exclude the presence of any infection-causing microorganisms. The viruses causing *hepatitis B* and *AIDS* have been transmitted through AID. As a result, all stored semen is placed in quarantine until the donor has been tested for antibodies to these viruses and until test results have been negative on two occasions three months apart.

Insemination is carried out by injecting semen into the cervix with a small syringe. Two or three inseminations are carried out during the two to four optimum days for conception in the woman's menstrual cycle and, unless pregnancy occurs, they are repeated for up to five more cycles.

RESULTS

When fresh semen is used, the success rate of artificial insemination in bringing about pregnancy over a six-month period is 60 to 70 percent. With frozen semen, the success rate is 55 percent.

Artificial kidney

Common name for the machine used in renal *dialysis*.

Artificial respiration

Forced introduction of air into the lungs of someone who has stopped breathing (see *Respiratory arrest*) or of someone whose breathing is inadequate. Artificial respiration may be administered by the mouth-to-mouth or mouth-to-nose method. It may also be given by the use of ventilating equipment administered by skilled technicians (see *Ventilation*).

WHY IT IS DONE

Artificial respiration should be started as soon as possible after someone has stopped breathing; delay in breathing for more than six minutes can cause death. When someone has stopped breathing there is no rise-and-fall movement of the chest or abdomen, the face becomes blue-gray, and no exhaled breath can be felt. When there is no breathing, it is likely that the

---

FIRST AID: ARTIFICIAL RESPIRATION

1 If possible, send for medical help, but start resuscitation immediately—do not waste time loosening clothing around the neck unless there is obvious strangulation. Lay the victim on his or her back on a firm, rigid surface. Quickly clear the mouth and airway of any foreign material with your fingers.

2 If there does not appear to be any neck injury, gently tilt the victim's head backward and maintain it in the midline by placing one hand under the back of the neck and lifting upward. Place the heel of the other hand on the victim's forehead and press downward so that the chin is elevated.

3 Using the hand that is placed on the victim's forehead, pinch the victim's nostrils, using your thumb and index finger. Take a deep breath. Place your open mouth tightly around the victim's open mouth and blow air from your lungs into the victim's lungs. Stop blowing when the victim's chest is expanded.

4 Remove your mouth and turn your head toward the victim's chest. Listen for air leaving his or her lungs and watch the chest fall. Give four quick breaths, taking a deep breath between each one. Continue at the rate of 12 breaths per minute, until you see the victim beginning to breathe on his or her own.

heart has stopped beating. If no pulse can be felt in the wrist or neck, cardiac compressions should be carried out in conjunction with artificial respiration (see *Cardiopulmonary resuscitation*).

When breathing is weak or shallow, movements of the chest are minimal and hardly any breath can be felt. If breathing is not restored, the brain is deprived of oxygen; permanent brain damage or death can result.

HOW IT IS DONE

MOUTH-TO-MOUTH RESUSCITATION This is the simplest and most effective method of introducing air into the victim's lungs (see illustrated box). The method is safe to use on a person whose breathing is weak, shallow, or labored. Time your exhalations with the victim's inhalations.

MOUTH-TO-NOSE RESUSCITATION If the victim has a facial injury, it may be difficult for you to breathe into his or her mouth. In such cases, follow steps 1 and 2 shown in the box, left. Remove your hand from the back of the victim's neck and close his or her mouth by lifting the chin. Take a deep breath and seal your mouth around the victim's nose. Blow strongly into the nose. Remove your mouth and hold the victim's mouth open with your hand, so that air can escape. Repeat as for mouth-to-mouth resuscitation every five seconds.

RESUSCITATION OF BABIES AND CHILDREN The method of resuscitating a baby or young child is basically the same as the method of resuscitating an adult, except that you will find it easier to seal your mouth over both the mouth and nose of the child. Do not tip the child's head back very far, because a child's neck and airway are more fragile than an adult's. Blow gentle breaths of air into the lungs, one breath every two to three seconds (20 to 30 breaths per minute) until the child's chest starts to rise.

Artificial sweeteners

Synthetic substitutes for sugar used by people on reducing diets, by diabetics, and by the food industry.

Saccharin is 500 to 600 times sweeter than cane sugar (though it has a sour aftertaste) and has no calories. Saccharin has been associated with bladder cancer in animal experiments but the risk of it causing cancer in humans is negligible. (Cyclamate, another artificial sweetener, was banned in the late 1960s after it had been proved to cause cancer in animals.)

Aspartame is about 200 times sweeter than sugar—although its sweetness

is destroyed by prolonged heating— and is virtually calorie free. It has no known adverse effects when taken in normal quantities but in excess may cause neurological disorders.

Although saccharin and aspartame are often recommended for use in reducing diets, they are of questionable value because they do nothing to reduce the craving for sweet foods.

Sorbitol, which occurs naturally in certain fruits, is another sugar substitute. It is used by diabetics but its high caloric value (about 140 Calories per ounce) makes it unsuitable for use in reducing diets. One problem with using sorbitol is that its poor absorption from the intestine into the bloodstream may cause diarrhea by pulling fluid into the bowel channel.

Asbestosis

 A chronic lung disease caused by inhaling fibers of asbestos, a heat-resistant and insulating material. Those affected are mainly workers employed in the mining of asbestos, the manufacture of asbestos products, or in the building industry. Asbestosis is probably the single most important work-related lung disease.

CAUSES AND INCIDENCE

Asbestos fibers penetrate and irritate the outer parts of the lung, causing inflammation and, over the years, *pulmonary fibrosis* (thickening and scarring of the lung tissue). An extended period (20 years or more) may elapse between exposure to the dust and onset of the disease.

In the US, it is estimated that more than one million people have been exposed to significant levels of asbestos fibers. Fewer than 10 new cases of asbestosis are diagnosed per 100,000 population each year; the incidence is higher in areas where there has been a heavy concentration of asbestos-related industry.

PREVENTION

Recently there has been a far greater awareness of the dangers of working with asbestos and workers are regularly screened by *chest X rays*. If the X-ray films show any shadows on the lungs, the person is advised to stop working with asbestos, even if there are no symptoms.

SYMPTOMS AND COMPLICATIONS

Breathlessness is the main symptom; it becomes increasingly severe as the disease develops. There may also be a dry cough and a feeling of tightness in the chest. Eventually, *respiratory failure* develops.

Asbestos fiber in lung
The term asbestos refers to any of a group of fibrous minerals that can cause lung disease.

Asbestosis sufferers have a higher-than-average risk of acquiring *tuberculosis* and *lung cancer*, particularly if they smoke cigarettes. Exposure to asbestos may also be a predisposing factor in the development of lung cancer (without asbestosis) and of *mesothelioma* (a tumor of the lung covering), especially in smokers.

DIAGNOSIS AND TREATMENT

Along with chest X rays, *pulmonary function tests* are used in diagnosis to measure breathing efficiency. Once asbestosis has developed, there is no effective treatment; the disease usually causes disability and death.

OUTLOOK

Since the middle 1970s, asbestos has been replaced, wherever possible, by other materials, such as glass fiber. Along with rigorous screening, this should produce a reduction in the incidence of the disease.

Ascariasis

A worm infestation, common worldwide and especially in the tropics. The parasite responsible, *ASCARIS LUMBRICOIDES*, is a pale, cylindrical, tapered roundworm, between six and 15 inches in length in adult form, which lives in the small intestine of its human host. One or several worms may be present, but symptoms usually occur only in people with heavy worm infestations.

INCIDENCE AND CAUSES

Ascariasis affects up to 80 to 90 percent of the population in poorer countries, where children living in rural areas are prone to heavy infestations. In developed countries, such as the US, about 1 percent of the population may have a light infestation at any one time, although few people are aware of the presence of worms.

A

LIFE CYCLE OF THE ASCARIASIS WORM

The person becomes infested by swallowing the eggs. They hatch into larvae in the intestine, then travel via the wall of the intestine and the blood to the lungs, up the windpipe, and are swallowed back to the small intestine. There they become adult worms.

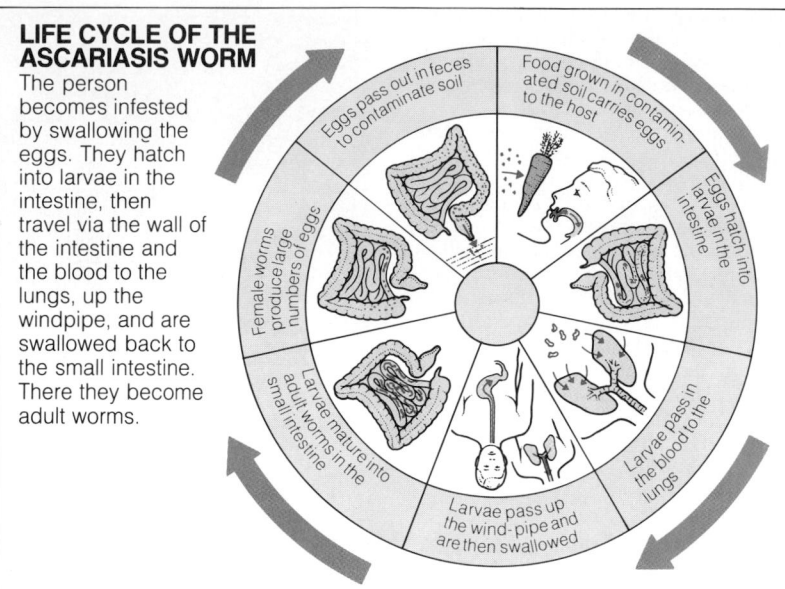

The life cycle of the worm and the mechanism by which the infestation is acquired are shown above.

In some dry, windy climates, airborne eggs may be swallowed after being blown into the mouth.

SYMPTOMS

Light infestations may cause either no symptoms or occasional nausea, abdominal pain, and irregular bowel movements. A worm may be passed via the rectum or vomited.

A heavy load of worms may compete with the host for food, leading to malnutrition and anemia, which in children can retard growth.

DIAGNOSIS AND TREATMENT

Ascariasis is diagnosed by finding the worm's eggs in a person's feces during microscopic examination.

The infection is treated with *antihelmintic drugs*, such as piperazine, which is highly effective in a single dose. The worms are passed via the rectum some days after the drug is taken. The patient usually makes a complete recovery.

Ascites

An excess of fluid in the peritoneal cavity—the space between the two layers of membrane, or peritoneum, that line the inside of the abdominal wall and the outside of the abdominal organs. A few gallons of fluid may be present, which causes distention.

CAUSES

Ascites may occur in any condition that causes generalized *edema* (excessive accumulation of fluid in the body

tissues). The most important of these conditions are congestive *heart failure*, *nephrotic syndrome*, and liver *cirrhosis*.

Ascites may occur in *cancer* if metastases (secondary growths) from lung, breast, or intestinal tumors are deposited on the surface of the peritoneum. Ascites also occurs in cases of *tuberculosis* infecting the abdomen, a rare disease today.

SYMPTOMS AND TREATMENT

In addition to abdominal swelling and discomfort, ascites may cause difficulty breathing due to pressure on and immobilization of the diaphragm, the sheet of muscle that separates the thorax (chest) and the abdomen.

Ascites is detected during physical examination. Diagnosis of the cause involves the physician performing a careful history and physical examination and removing and analyzing a sample of ascitic fluid via a sterile needle inserted through the abdominal wall. The fluid is examined under the microscope for malignant cells. Its color, turbidity (opacity), and chemical composition also help identify whether the cause is due to inflammation or a condition such as cirrhosis.

Treatment depends on the precise cause of the ascites, but in many cases includes bed rest, and fluid and salt (sodium) restriction. Alcohol is eliminated when liver disease is implicated. *Diuretic drugs*, particularly spironolactone, may be prescribed.

If the ascites causes discomfort or breathing difficulty, fluid can be drained from the peritoneal cavity.

Ascorbic acid

The chemical name for *vitamin C*.

Aseptic technique

The creation of a germ-free environment, mainly by the use of *sterilization*, to protect a patient from infection. Aseptic sterilization is distinct from antisepsis, which is the destruction of germs by chemicals (*antiseptics*).

WHY IT IS DONE

Aseptic technique is needed for any procedure in which there is a danger of introducing infection into the body. The patient can be contaminated from four main sources: other people, instruments, the patient himself or herself, and the air. To prevent such contamination, aseptic technique is used for surgery in an operating room as well as for minor office procedures, such as inserting a urinary catheter or stitching a wound. Aseptic technique is also needed when caring for patients with suppressed immune systems (such as those being treated for leukemia) and for those who have reduced natural defenses against infection (see *Isolation*).

HOW IT IS DONE

All people who come in contact with the patient must scrub their hands and wear presterilized gowns and disposable gloves and masks. Instruments are sterilized beforehand in an *autoclave* and placed on a cart covered with sterile material.

The area of the patient that is to be operated on is cleaned with antiseptic solutions of iodine or hexachlorophene, and the surrounding skin is covered with sterile drapes. In addition, before operations on the intestine, the bowel is cleared by giving laxatives and sometimes enemas to prevent any contamination of the abdominal area by feces.

Throughout the procedure, care is taken to place used, possibly contaminated, instruments well away from sterile instruments and dressings.

In an operating room it is important to keep the air and the room scrupulously clean. The windows remain closed and the only air that enters the room is through a special ventilation system that purifies the air and maintains it at a certain humidity.

Aspergillosis

 Infection caused by aspergillus, a fungus found in old buildings or decaying plant matter. It is an occasionally fatal, *opportunistic infection* (one caused by organisms that are usually harmless to healthy people but that produce illness in those whose resistance is reduced.

Aspermia

Failure to produce or ejaculate sperm. (See *Ejaculation, disorders of*.)

Asphyxia

The medical term for suffocation. Asphyxia may be due to obstruction of a large airway, usually by a foreign body (see *Choking*), to a lack or falling levels of oxygen in the surrounding air (as occurs when a closed plastic bag is put over the head), or to poisoning with a gas such as carbon monoxide that interferes with the uptake of oxygen into the bloodstream.

The person initially breathes more rapidly and strongly to try to overcome the lack of oxygen in the blood. There is also an increase in heart rate and blood pressure.

TREATMENT

First-aid treatment consists of *artificial respiration* after first moving the person into the open air and clearing the airway of any obstruction. Untreated asphyxia causes death.

Aspiration

The withdrawal of fluid or tissue from the body by suction. The term also refers to the act of breathing in a foreign body, usually food or drink.

Aspiration *biopsy* is the removal of tissue or fluid for examination by suction through a needle attached to a syringe. The procedure is used mainly to obtain cells from a fluid-filled cavity (such as a breast cyst); from the bone marrow (see *Bone marrow biopsy*); or from internal organs, when a narrow needle is guided to the site of the biopsy by *CT scanning* or *ultrasound scanning*. The cells obtained are examined under a microscope, particularly for any evidence of cancer.

Aspiration pneumonia is inflammation of the lungs that results from inhalation of foreign material; this material could be vomit inhaled during induction of anesthesia or during a coma, or infected secretions from the nose or throat.

Aspirin

ANALGESIC (NONNARCOTIC)
Tablet Capsule
Available over-the-counter
Available as generic

An *analgesic drug* (painkiller) that has been used for more than 80 years to treat disorders such as headache, menstrual pain, and muscle ache. Because aspirin has an anti-inflammatory action, it is particularly useful in treating joint pain and stiffness caused by *osteoarthritis* and other types of arthritis. Aspirin also reduces fever and is therefore included in a number of *cold remedies*.

In small doses it reduces the stickiness of platelets (blood particles involved in clotting). This has led to its use in preventing *thrombosis* (abnormal blood clots) in some individuals at risk of having a *stroke* or *myocardial infarction* (heart attack).

HOW IT WORKS

Aspirin reduces the production of certain *prostaglandins* (hormonelike chemicals) that can be responsible for inflammation, pain, fever, or clumping of platelets.

POSSIBLE ADVERSE EFFECTS

In children there is a slight risk of *Reye's syndrome* (a rare brain and liver disorder). Aspirin should not be given to children except under close medical supervision; acetaminophen should be used instead.

Aspirin may cause irritation of the stomach lining, resulting in indigestion or nausea. These side effects may be reduced by taking the drug with food or by taking a coated tablet that does not release the drug until it reaches the intestine. Prolonged use of aspirin may cause bleeding from the stomach due to *gastric erosion* (disruption of the surface lining of the stomach) or *peptic ulcer* (a deeper penetration of the wall of the stomach or duodenum).

Assay

Analysis of a substance to determine its presence or effects. A qualitative assay determines only whether or not a substance is present, whereas a quantitative assay determines the actual amount present.

Biological assays (called bioassays) are concerned mainly with measuring the response of an animal or specific organ to a drug or hormone. They are used, for example, to assess the side effects of a particular drug. (See also *Immunoassay*.)

Assignment

One way in which a physician is reimbursed for services to patients enrolled in Medicare. If a physician wishes to receive direct payment from Medicare and is willing to allow that organization to determine the amount of payment, he or she may elect assignment. The patient agrees to have Medicare benefits assigned to the physician. By assignment, the patient and physician effectively agree to accept Medicare's determination of a "reasonable charge" for the services rendered. Medicare reimburses the physician directly for the services, but pays only 80 percent of the "reasonable charge" as determined by a formula. The physician may bill the patient for the remaining 20 percent.

As an alternative, the physician may refuse assignment and bill a Medicare patient for a fee the physician determines himself or herself. The patient may submit the bill to Medicare (through the insurance company that handles Medicare's billing locally) and expect as reimbursement 80 percent of Medicare's predetermined "reasonable charge."

Astereognosis

An inability to recognize objects by touch when they are placed in one hand—even though there is no defect of sensation in the fingers or any difficulty holding the object. Testing for astereognosis is part of any detailed examination of the central nervous system. Astereognosis is either left-sided or right-sided; tactile recognition is normal on the other side. If both sides are affected, the condition is called tactile *agnosia*.

Both astereognosis and tactile agnosia are caused by disease or damage to parts of the cerebrum (the main mass of the brain) concerned with recognition by touch.

Asthenia

A term meaning loss of strength and energy (see *Weakness*).

Asthenia, neurocirculatory

See *Cardiac neurosis*.

Asthma

Recurrent attacks of breathlessness, characteristically accompanied by wheezing when breathing out and varying in severity from day to day and from hour to hour. The illness frequently starts in childhood and tends to clear up or become less severe in early adulthood.

LIVING WITH ASTHMA

Breathlessness and wheezing in asthma is caused by narrowing of the bronchioles (small airways in the lungs). Breathing is most difficult and wheezing most pronounced when the sufferer is breathing out because the lungs collapse to expel air. This causes further narrowing of the bronchioles. Inflammation of the linings of these bronchioles causes an increased production of sputum (phlegm), which makes the obstruction worse. A dry cough often develops as the sufferer attempts to clear the airways.

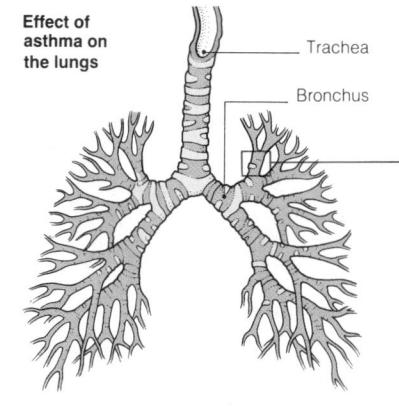

Effect of asthma on the lungs

Trachea

Bronchus

TREATMENT OF AN ASTHMA ATTACK
Attacks are treated by inhalation of a bronchodilator drug from an inhaler or from a nebulizer.

Using an inhaler
To use the inhaler correctly, exhale first; then take in a slow, deep breath while you release the drug by depressing the canister. Two puffs should increase air flow within 15 minutes.

INHALER

Pressurized canister

Mouthpiece

Obstructed bronchiole
Before treatment, airflow is obstructed by a narrowing of the bronchiole.

Healthy bronchiole
Inhalation of the bronchodilator widens the bronchiole and improves airflow.

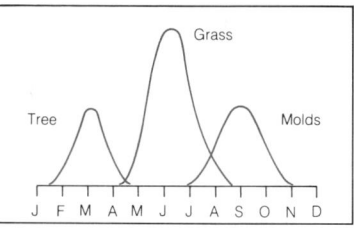

Tree

Grass

Molds

J F M A M J J A S O N D

Seasonal asthma
When symptoms occur only during a few months, the cause is likely to be allergy to pollen or spores.

The familiar form of asthma is more correctly called bronchial asthma; this use of the full name distinguishes it from a condition associated with wheezing caused by heart failure (see *Asthma, cardiac*).

Although asthma frequently begins early in life (most people have their first attack before the age of 5), it can develop at any age.

CAUSES
Asthma is of two main types: extrinsic, in which an allergy (usually to something inhaled) triggers an attack, and intrinsic, in which there is no apparent external cause.

The most common allergens responsible for asthma are pollens, which often also cause allergic *rhinitis* (hay fever). Other common allergens include house dust, house-dust mites, animal fur, dander, or feathers. Extrinsic asthma may also be triggered by a respiratory infection (such as a cough, cold, or bronchitis), by exercise (especially in cold air), by tobacco smoke or other air pollutants, and by allergy to a particular food or drug (most commonly aspirin).

Intrinsic asthma tends to develop later in life than extrinsic asthma, with the first attack often following a respiratory tract infection. Emotional factors, such as stress or anxiety, may precipitate attacks.

PREVALENCE
About one in 20 of the overall population is asthmatic but the prevalence among children is much greater—about one in 10.

Heredity is a major factor in the development of extrinsic asthma. Asthma seems to be becoming more common in the US and other developed countries.

SYMPTOMS
Asthmatic attacks vary greatly in their severity, ranging from a slight breathlessness to respiratory failure. Attacks may be most frequent in the early morning.

The main symptoms are breathlessness, wheezing, a dry cough sometimes brought on by exercise, and a feeling of tightness in the chest.

During a severe attack, breathing becomes increasingly difficult, causing sweating, rapid heart beat, and great distress and anxiety. The sufferer cannot lie down or sleep, may be unable to speak, breathes rapidly, and wheezes loudly.

In a very severe attack, the low amount of oxygen in the blood may cause *cyanosis* (blue-purple discoloration) of the face, particularly the lips, and the skin may become pale and clammy. Such attacks may be fatal. In 1979, more than 1,800 people died as a direct result of an asthma attack; an additional 4,400 people died of asthmatic complications.

PREVENTION
Although there is no cure for asthma, attacks can be prevented to a large extent. For sufferers of extrinsic asthma, tests are available to discover whether any of the common allergens is responsible for triggering attacks; if a specific cause is discovered, steps can be taken to avoid it. For example, if pollen is the cause, the person will need to avoid gardens, parks, and the countryside during the pollen season. If the house-dust mite is responsible, mattresses (in which the mites flourish) should be enclosed in airtight

plastic covers and the home should be kept as free of dust as possible.

Immunotherapy (a course of injections of the allergen) can be performed but has a limited success rate. Much more successful in preventing attacks are prophylactic (preventive) drugs, such as cromolyn sodium and inhaled *corticosteroid drugs*. To be effective, they must be taken several times daily, usually through an inhaler.

TREATMENT

Once an attack has started, a prophylactic drug has limited effects and a *bronchodilator* (a drug that relaxes and widens the airways), such as albuterol, must be used. Most asthmatic people learn to administer the drug themselves with a hand-held plastic inhaler (see illustration).

An inhaler loses its effectiveness after a certain period (the date is marked on the container), so it is essential for the asthmatic person to renew his or her supply regularly. Oral theophylline preparations are also used preventively for their bronchodilating properties.

EMERGENCY PROCEDURE

Most attacks of asthma either pass naturally or can be controlled by use of a bronchodilator. In some cases, however, an attack may be so severe that it fails to respond to the recommended dose of the drug. In this case, the dose should be repeated. If it has no effect, a physician should be seen or the person taken to the hospital.

Emergency treatment at home or in the hospital may include the administration of oxygen, a corticosteroid, and a bronchodilator through a nebulizer or an intravenous injection of aminophylline. If these measures are ineffective (which is rare), the patient requires a *ventilator*, which forces air or oxygen under pressure into the lungs.

OUTLOOK

More than half of affected children grow out of asthma completely by the age of 21. In a large proportion of the remainder, attacks become decreasingly severe as they grow older. With modern drug treatment, even people who suffer repeated attacks as adults can expect to live a normal life. In most cases, quality of life need not be impaired (demonstrated by the success of world-class athletes who have had asthma).

Asthma, cardiac

Difficulty breathing caused by fluid collection in the lungs that causes bronchospasm and wheezing. This response is usually due to reduced pumping efficiency of the left side of the heart (see *Heart failure*), causing congestion and increased pressure within the blood circulation through the lungs and fluid collection.

Although cardiac asthma has a different cause from the more familiar bronchial asthma, the two conditions have similar symptoms, including wheezing and breathing difficulty. A chest X ray may show fluid in the lungs. Treatment is primarily for heart failure but may include use of bronchodilator drugs.

Astigmatism

A condition in which the front surface of the cornea of the eye is not truly spherical. Although the eye is perfectly healthy, the corneal surface has discrepancies in the curvature, so that magnification in one direction is greater than in others.

A minor degree of astigmatism is normal and glasses are not necessary to correct it. More severe astigmatism causes blurring of lines set at a particular angle. A person with astigmatism might see horizontal lines clearly but vertical lines blurred, or the blurring may occur in an oblique meridian.

TREATMENT

Ordinary "spherical" eyeglass lenses cannot correct astigmatism. Lenses are needed that have no optical power in the normal meridian but appropriate curvature in the others. These cylindrical lenses must be framed at a precise angle.

Hard contact lenses bridge over the anomalous corneal curve and present a perfect spherical surface for focusing; they give excellent vision in astigmatism. Ordinary soft lenses tend to mold to the astigmatic curve, but special "toric" soft lenses are available to treat this condition.

Astringent

COMMON DRUGS

Aluminum acetate Potassium permanganate Silver nitrate Zinc sulfate

A substance that causes tissue to dry and shrink by reducing its ability to absorb water. Astringents are widely used in *antiperspirants* and skin tonics. They are also used to promote healing of broken or inflamed skin. Astringent drugs are used to treat *otitis externa* (inflammation of the ear canal) and watering of the eye due to minor irritation. Astringents may cause burning or stinging when applied.

Astrocytoma

A type of malignant *brain tumor*. Astrocytomas are the most common type of *glioma*, a tumor arising from the glial (supporting) cells within the nervous system, and are composed of cells called astrocytes.

Astrocytomas most commonly develop within the cerebrum (the main mass of the brain). Although all types are very serious, they are classified in four grades (I through IV) according to their rate of growth and malignancy. A grade I astrocytoma is a slow-growing tumor that may spread widely throughout the brain but may be present for many years before causing symptoms. A grade IV astrocytoma is a very fast-growing tumor that causes rapid development of disabling symptoms.

Symptoms are similar to those seen with other types of brain tumor. Diagnosis is made after the physician performs a history, physical examination, *CT scanning* or *MRI* and, often, *angiography*. Few astrocytomas can be completely surgically removed.

Asylum

An outdated term for an institution that provides care for those who are mentally ill.

Asymptomatic

A medical term that means without *symptoms*—those indications of illness noticed by the patient (as distinct from *signs*, which are observed by the physician). Examples of conditions that may be asymptomatic include *hypertension* (high blood pressure), which is usually discovered during a routine blood pressure test, and *diabetes mellitus*, which is often diagnosed from a blood or urine test. Most disorders are asymptomatic in their early stages. In the case of cancer, much effort has been made to devise screening tests to detect tumors at the asymptomatic stage.

Asystole

A term meaning absence of the heart beat (see *Cardiac arrest*).

Ataxia

Incoordination and clumsiness, affecting balance and gait, limb or eye movements, and/or speech.

CAUSES

Ataxia may be caused by damage to the *cerebellum* (part of the brain concerned with coordination) or to the nerve pathways that carry information to and from the cerebellum.

Possible causes include injury to the brain or to the spinal cord. In adults, ataxia may be caused by drug or alcohol intoxication (the most common cause), by a *stroke* or *brain tumor* affecting the cerebellum or brain stem, by a disease of the balance organ in the ear, or by *multiple sclerosis* or other types of nervous system degeneration. In rare cases, it is a result of untreated *syphilis*. In children, causes of ataxia include acute infection, brain tumors, and the inherited condition *Friedreich's ataxia*.

SYMPTOMS

Symptoms depend on the site of damage within the nervous system, although an awkward gait is common to most forms. The typical ataxic gait is lurching and unsteady, like a drunk, with the feet widely placed. If the damage is to nerves that carry sensory information from joints and muscles to the cerebellum, sensory ataxia results. In such cases, the person's unsteadiness is much worse when the eyes are closed. Damage to parts of the brain stem concerned with the control of eye movements often cause *nystagmus* (jerky eye movements).

Damage to the cerebellum itself usually causes *dysarthria* (slurred speech) as well as an unsteady gait. Sometimes, if damage is confined to one side of the cerebellum, incoordination is confined to the limbs on the same side and is often accompanied by a tremor in the limbs during purposeful movements. When walking, the person often has a tendency to veer or fall toward the affected side. Other features may include decomposition of complex actions into their component parts, producing jerky, puppetlike movements, and "overshoot" when attempts are made to touch or pick up objects.

DIAGNOSIS AND TREATMENT

Discovery of the cause of ataxia may be helped by *CT scanning* or *MRI*. Treatment depends on the cause.

Atelectasis

Collapse of part or all of a lung caused by obstruction of the bronchus (the main air passage through the lung) or the bronchioles (smaller air passages). When this happens, air already in the lung cannot be breathed out and, instead, is absorbed into the blood, leading to the collapse of all or part of the lung. After collapsing, the lung loses its elasticity and cannot take in air; consequently, the blood passing through it can no longer absorb oxygen or dispose of carbon dioxide.

In an adult, atelectasis is usually not life-threatening, since unaffected parts of the lung (or, if the whole lung has collapsed, the other lung) expand to compensate for the loss of function in the collapsed area. However, when a lung collapses in a newborn baby—as the result of mucus blocking the bronchus—the baby's life is at risk. (For lung collapse caused by a perforation in the pleura, the outer covering of the lung, see *Pneumothorax*.)

CAUSES AND INCIDENCE

The bronchus is usually obstructed by one of four mechanisms. First, secretions of mucus in the bronchus or bronchioles may accumulate and cause blockage. This can happen after an abdominal or chest operation that has made the dispersal of mucus by coughing difficult due to pain; as a possible complication of general anesthesia; in a baby at birth; in *asthma*; or in certain infections, such as *pertussis* (whooping cough) in children or chronic *bronchitis* in adults.

Second, an accidentally inhaled *foreign body*, such as a peanut, may stick in the bronchus; this is more common in children than in adults. Third, a benign or malignant *tumor* in the lung may press on the bronchus. Fourth, enlarged lymph glands (which occur in *tuberculosis*, other lung infections, or some forms of *cancer*) may exert pressure on the airway.

SYMPTOMS, DIAGNOSIS, AND TREATMENT

The main symptom is breathing difficulty. There may also be a cough and chest pain, depending on the underlying cause.

The condition is diagnosed when the physician carefully examines the chest and takes *chest X rays*. Treatment is directed to deal with the cause of the blockage. If the cause is an accumulation of mucus, chest clapping, deep breathing, coughing, and *postural drainage* will be used.

Once the obstruction has been removed, the collapsed lung usually reinflates gradually, although some areas of it may be permanently damaged or scarred.

Atenolol

A *beta-blocker* commonly used in the treatment of *hypertension* (high blood pressure), *angina pectoris* (chest pain due to impaired blood supply to heart muscle), and certain types of *arrhythmia* (irregular heart beat).

Atheroma

Fatty deposits on the inner lining of an artery that can cause *atherosclerosis*.

Atherosclerosis

A disease of the arterial wall in which the inner layer thickens, causing narrowing of the channel and thus impairing blood flow.

The narrowing is due to the formation of *plaques* (raised patches) in the inner lining of the arteries. These plaques consist of low-density lipoproteins (see *Fats and oils*), decaying muscle cells, fibrous tissue, clumps of blood platelets, *cholesterol*, and sometimes calcium; they tend to form in regions of turbulent blood flow and are found most often in people with high concentrations of cholesterol in the bloodstream. The number and thickness of plaques increase with age, causing loss of the smooth lining of the blood vessels and encouraging the formation of thrombi (blood clots). Sometimes fragments of thrombi break off and form *emboli*, which travel through the bloodstream and block smaller vessels.

INCIDENCE

Atherosclerosis is responsible for more deaths in the US than any other single condition. Atherosclerotic heart disease involving the coronary arteries is the most common single cause of death, accounting for one third of all deaths (see *Coronary heart disease*); atherosclerotic interference with blood supply to the brain (causing stroke) is the third most common cause of death after cancer. Atherosclerosis also causes a great deal of serious illness by reducing the blood flow in other major arteries, such as those to the kidneys, the legs, and the intestines.

CAUSES

Certain risk factors increase the probability that atherosclerosis will develop. These risk factors are cigarette smoking, *hypertension* (high blood pressure), male gender, obesity, physical inactivity, a high serum cholesterol level, family history of arterial disease, and, possibly, an anxious or aggressive personality.

The risk of atherosclerosis increases with age, probably in part because of the length of time it takes for the plaques to develop. The influence of gender can be illustrated if men are compared with premenopausal women. In the group aged 35 to 44, coronary heart disease kills six times as many men as women.

PREVENTION

Modifications of the risk factors, especially early in adult life, can markedly reduce the probability that atherosclerosis will develop or will at

ARTERIAL DEGENERATION IN ATHEROSCLEROSIS

Atherosclerosis is narrowing of the arteries caused by plaques on their inner linings. These plaques are composed mainly of fats deposited from the bloodstream. They disrupt the normal flow of blood through the affected artery. Men are affected earlier than women because premenopausal women are protected by natural estrogen hormones.

RISK FACTORS

Cigarette smoking

Hypertension

Male gender

Obesity

Physical inactivity

Diabetes mellitus

Heredity

Aggressive personality

X ray showing atherosclerosis
The leg arteries shown here appear as bright channels. One is narrowed at a point corresponding to the dark gap.

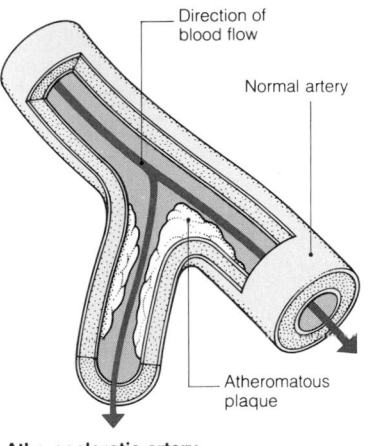

Direction of blood flow

Normal artery

Atheromatous plaque

Atherosclerotic artery
A deposit of atheromatous plaque disrupts normal blood flow through the artery at the point where it branches. This occurs because of the greater level of turbulence in this area.

---

least delay its manifestations. Smoking should be stopped, blood pressure checked regularly, and hypertension treated. Diet should be low in saturated fat and obesity avoided. If cholesterol levels remain high despite diet therapy, drug therapy for this condition may be warranted. Meticulous control of diabetes is important. Regular exercise is of great value in maintaining the health and efficiency of the heart and circulation.

SYMPTOMS
Unfortunately, atherosclerosis produces no symptoms until the damage to the arteries is severe enough to restrict blood flow. Restriction of blood flow to heart muscle due to atherosclerosis can cause *angina pectoris*. Restriction of blood flow to the muscles of the legs causes intermittent *claudication* (pains in the legs brought on by walking and relieved by rest). Narrowing of the arteries supplying blood to the brain may cause *transient ischemic attacks* (symptoms and signs of a *stroke* lasting less than 24 hours) and episodes of dizziness.

DIAGNOSIS
A general medical history and examination will reveal a great deal about the health of the circulation, but special investigation may be necessary. The flow of blood within an artery can be demonstrated by *angiography* (X rays after injection of a radiopaque dye), or, less invasively, by *Doppler* ultrasound velocity detection, or by *plethysmography* (a technique that produces a tracing of the pulse pattern).

TREATMENT
Medication is unsatisfactory in treating atherosclerosis since the damage has already been done. *Anticoagulant drugs* have been used to try to minimize secondary clotting and embolus formation, but have little or no effect on the progress of the disease. *Vasodilator drugs* are helpful in providing symptom relief but are of no curative value.

Surgical treatment is available for those unresponsive to medical treatment or in certain high-risk situations. Balloon *angioplasty* can open up narrowed vessels and promote an improved blood supply. The blood supply to the heart muscle can be restored by a vein graft bypass (see *Coronary artery bypass*). Large atheromatous and calcified arterial obstruction can be removed by *endarterectomy*, and entire segments of diseased peripheral vessels can be replaced by woven plastic tube grafts (see *Arterial reconstructive surgery*).

Athetosis

A nervous system disorder, characterized by slow, writhing involuntary movements, most often seen in the head, face, neck, and limbs. The movements commonly include facial grimacing, with contortions of the mouth and lips. Often, the person also has difficulty balancing and walking. In some cases the muscles are abnormally flaccid (floppy), while in others they are spastic (tight).

Very commonly athetosis is combined with *chorea* (involuntary fidgety movements)—a combination called choreoathetosis. Both conditions arise from damage to the *basal ganglia*, clusters of nerve cells deep within the brain that are concerned with the control of movements. Causes include damage to the brain prior to or around the time of birth (see *Cerebral palsy*), *encephalitis* (brain infection), degenerative disorders such as *Huntington's chorea*, or certain drugs such as phenothiazines or levodopa derivatives. If drug treatment is the cause, the abnormal movements may stop when the drug is withdrawn.

Athlete's foot

A common skin condition in which the skin between the toes becomes itchy and sore, may crack and peel away, and occasionally blisters. The fourth and fifth toe webs are most often involved. Athlete's foot is rare in young children and is associated with wearing shoes and sweating; it is rare where most people go barefoot.

CAUSES
Athlete's foot is usually caused by a dermatophyte (fungal) infection called tinea pedis. Secondary infection occurring through skin cracks is bacterial.

TREATMENT

Athlete's foot sometimes clears up without medication. Careful drying of the affected area is necessary; wearing dry cotton socks or sandals may help. Disinfecting the floors of showers and locker rooms helps control the spread of infection.

Most fungal infections respond to treatment with antifungal creams, such as tolnaftate, miconazole, or compound undecylenic acid.

Athlete's foot
The typical appearance shows fissuring in the cleft between the fourth and fifth toes. There is usually an annoying itch.

Atony

Complete loss of tension in a muscle, so that the muscle is completely flaccid (floppy). Atony can occur in some nervous system disorders or after injury to nerves. The arm muscles may become atonic after injury to the *brachial plexus* (nerve roots in the neck passing into the arm).

Atopy

A predisposition to various allergic reactions. Atopic individuals have a tendency to suffer from one or more allergic-based disorders, such as *asthma*, *eczema*, *urticaria* (hives), and allergic *rhinitis* (hay fever).

The mechanism that causes the predisposition is not fully understood, although various theories have been proposed. There is some evidence that atopy may be caused in the first few weeks of life by the absorption into the body of abnormally high levels of *antigens* (substances foreign to the body, capable of becoming allergens). This could be due to a breakdown in the normal mechanisms by which potential allergens are prevented from penetrating surfaces, such as the lining of the intestines or the airways in the lungs; or it could be due to excessively high exposure to potential allergens—babies born during the grass pollen and house-dust mite seasons are more likely than the average person to become atopic.

There is also a distinct genetic, or inherited (familial), basis to atopy—the relatives of atopic individuals are much more likely than the average person to be atopic (even after allowance is made for bias caused by similarities of environment).

ATP

The abbreviation for adenosine triphosphate, the chief energy-carrying chemical in the body. (See also *ADP*; *Metabolism*.)

Atresia

The absence or closure of a body opening or canal, present at birth and caused by a failure of development while in the uterus. Examples are *biliary atresia*, in which the bile ducts between the liver and duodenum are absent; *esophageal atresia*, in which the esophagus comes to a dead end; pulmonary atresia, in which the pulmonary artery between the right side of the heart and the lungs is closed off; and anal atresia, in which the anal canal is narrowed and shut off. Most forms of atresia require surgical correction early in life.

Atrial fibrillation

A type of irregular heart beat (see *Arrhythmia, cardiac*) in which the atria (upper chambers of the heart) beat irregularly and very rapidly (300 to 500 beats per minute). Not all these beats pass through the atrioventricular node (the impulse carrier between the atria and the ventricles, the lower chambers of the heart). As a result, the ventricles beat irregularly at a rate of 80 to 160 beats per minute.

CAUSES

Atrial fibrillation can occur in almost any form of long-standing heart disease in which there is enlargement of the atria. It is common in rheumatic heart disease (see *Rheumatic fever*), *thyrotoxicosis*, and atherosclerotic heart disease.

SYMPTOMS AND SIGNS

Sudden onset of atrial fibrillation can cause *palpitations* (awareness of fast heart beat) or *angina pectoris* (chest pain due to reduced blood supply). The inefficient pumping action of the heart in *heart failure* can reduce the output of blood into the circulation by as much as 30 percent. *Embolism*, in which blood clots in the atria enter the bloodstream and become lodged in an artery, can occur. This is most serious when it affects the main artery to the lungs (*pulmonary embolism*) or an artery in the brain (*stroke*).

DIAGNOSIS

The pulse is irregular in rate and strength and does not correspond with the heart rate; many heart beats that can be heard when the chest is listened to fail to reach the wrist because the heart has contracted prematurely when only partly filled. The diagnosis of atrial fibrillation is confirmed by an *ECG*, which shows the electrical activity within the heart.

TREATMENT

The first step usually is to control the heart rate by giving *digoxin* or, in certain instances, intravenous verapamil. If the fibrillation is of recent onset, treatment is directed at remedying the cause—for example, removal of the thyroid or drug treatment for thyrotoxicosis, or replacement of heart valves damaged by rheumatic heart disease. When recent onset atrial fibrillation persists, it can often be reversed by *defibrillation* (a short electrical shock applied to the heart).

If atrial fibrillation is long-standing, or is combined with severe heart disease, the likelihood of reversing it is small. In this case, control of the heart rate with digoxin is continued and *beta-blockers* are sometimes also used. *Anticoagulant drugs* may also be given to reduce the risk of embolism.

Atrial flutter

A type of irregular heart beat (see *Arrhythmia, cardiac*) in which the atria (upper chambers of the heart) beat very rapidly at 200 to 400 beats per minute. At these rates the atrioventricular node, the conducting mechanism between the atria and the ventricles (lower chambers of the heart), is unable to respond to every beat. As a result, the ventricles beat only once to every two, three, or four beats of the atria. The condition generally occurs in people over 40 who have severe heart disease.

Some people with atrial flutter have no symptoms; others may complain of palpitations (an awareness of a fast heart beat). The condition can lead to *heart failure* (reduced pumping action of the heart) or *angina pectoris* (chest pain due to reduced blood supply).

When treatment is urgent, *defibrillation* (electric shocks delivered to the heart) is effective. For nonurgent treatment, digoxin may be prescribed by the physician.

Atrial natriuretic peptide

A substance produced in the muscular wall of the atria (upper chambers of the heart). It is released into the bloodstream in response to an increase in atrial muscle tension caused, for example, by *heart failure* (reduced pumping action of the heart) or by some types of *hypertension* (high blood pressure).

The chemical increases the amount of sodium excreted in the urine; sodium draws water out with it, decreasing the volume of water in the circulation and helping to lower the blood pressure. Atrial natriuretic protein also lowers the blood pressure by causing blood vessels to dilate (widen) so that blood can flow more easily.

Children with congenital heart disorders causing heart failure (see *Heart disease, congenital*) have high levels of atrial natriuretic peptide. These levels fall after successful surgery to correct the abnormality.

Atrium

Either of the two (right and left) upper chambers of the *heart*.

ANATOMY OF THE ATRIUM
The left atrium receives oxygenated blood from the pulmonary veins; the right atrium receives deoxygenated blood from the venae cavae.

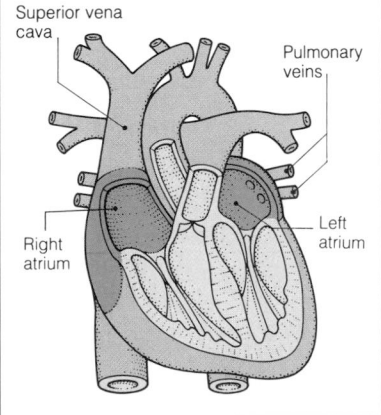

Atrophy

Shrinkage or wasting away of a tissue or organ due to a reduction in the size or number of its cells. Atrophy is commonly caused by disuse (such as when a limb has been immobilized in a plaster cast) or by inadequate cell nutrition due to poor blood circulation. Atrophy may also occur during prolonged serious illness, when the body needs to use up the protein reserves in the muscles. Other, less common, causes include nerve damage that partly or completely immobilizes part of the

body, and lack of a specific *enzyme* or *hormone* that stimulates growth of a cell or an organ.

Atropine

ANTICHOLINERGIC				
Tablet	Liquid	Injection	Ointment	Eye drops

Prescription needed

Available as generic

A drug used to treat *uveitis* (inflammation of the iris) and *corneal ulcer*. Atropine is also used in young children to dilate (widen) the pupil of the eye for examination.

It is given as a *premedication* before general *anesthesia* to reduce secretion from the lungs and is also used as an emergency treatment for bradycardia (abnormally slow heart beat).

Combined with an *antibacterial drug* and an *analgesic* (painkiller), atropine is occasionally prescribed for antispasmodic effects to relieve the symptoms of *urinary tract infection*.

POSSIBLE ADVERSE EFFECTS
Adverse effects include dry mouth, blurred vision, abnormal retention of urine, and, in the elderly, confusion. Atropine eye drops are rarely given to adults because they cause disturbance of vision lasting two to three weeks and may precipitate acute glaucoma in a susceptible person.

Attachment

An affectionate bond between individuals, especially between parent and child (see *Bonding*), or between a person and an object, as in the case of young children and security objects such as a blanket or a doll. The attachment gives emotional satisfaction.

The term attachment is also used to note the joining of a muscle or tendon to a bone.

Attending physician

A hospital term that refers to the physician who has the principal responsibility and authority for the care of a patient who has been admitted. Residents, who may perform a number of procedures necessary for the patient's care, do so under the direction and supervision of the attending physician.

Audiogram

A graph produced as a result of certain *hearing tests* that shows at what level of intensity (loudness) an individual can hear sounds of different frequencies.

Audiologist

A specialist in defining and treating hearing and speech-related problems. Audiologists are not physicians and thus cannot treat infections or other diseases. They conduct *hearing tests* to determine the degree of damage done to the hearing ability by injury or disease. Audiologists also can recommend *hearing aids* and train people to overcome problems related to hearing loss or speech impediments. Audiologists often test and work with children in schools.

Audiology

The study of hearing, especially of impaired hearing that cannot be corrected by drugs or surgery.

Audiometry

Measurement of the sense of hearing. The term often refers to specific *hearing tests* in which a machine is used to electronically produce sounds of a defined intensity (loudness) and frequency (pitch) and in which the hearing in each ear is measured over the full range of normally audible sounds.

Auditory nerve

Also called the acoustic nerve, the part of the *vestibulocochlear nerve* (the eighth *cranial nerve*) concerned with the sense of hearing.

Aura

A peculiar "warning" sensation that precedes or marks the onset of a *migraine* attack or a seizure in a person suffering from *epilepsy*.

An epileptic aura may be a distorted perception, such as a hallucinatory sound or smell, or a sensation of movement in part of the body. One type of attack (in people with temporal lobe epilepsy) is often preceded by a vague feeling of discomfort in the upper abdomen, sometimes accompanied by borborygmi (rumbling, gurgling bowel sounds) and followed by a sensation of fullness in the head.

A migraine attack may be preceded by a feeling of elation, unusual well-being, excessive energy, or drowsiness. The sufferer recognizes these as warning signs of an attack. Thirst or a craving for sweet foods may develop. An attack of migraine may also be heralded by flashing lights seen before the eyes, blurred or tunnel vision, or difficulty speaking. Weakness, numbness, or tingling of one half of the body may occur. As these symptoms subside, the migraine headache pain begins.

Auranofin

A *gold* preparation used as an *antirheumatic drug* in the treatment of people with *rheumatoid arthritis*. Auranofin, unlike other gold preparations, is effective when it is taken by mouth.

Auricle

Another name for the *pinna*, the external flap of the ear. The term was also once used as a synonym for *atrium* (one of the two upper chambers of the heart). Small, earlike appendages of the atria are still called auricles.

Auscultation

The procedure of listening to sounds within the body to assess the functioning of an organ or to detect the presence of disease. The sounds are heard through a stethoscope.

To listen to the heart, the physician places the stethoscope at four points on the chest, corresponding to the location of the heart valves. With the patient sitting up, in a semireclining position, or lying on his or her left side, the physician listens for any abnormality in the rate and rhythm of the heart beat and for heart *murmurs* or other abnormal *heart sounds* that may indicate a possible heart defect or *heart valve* disorder.

When listening to the lungs, the physician places the stethoscope on many different areas of the front and back of the chest. The patient breathes normally and then takes deep breaths while the physician compares the sounds of the air movement on the left and right sides. Abnormal sounds, or rales, can indicate *pneumonia*, *bronchitis*, or *pneumothorax*. Additional sounds (called crepitations) which resemble crackling or bubbling, are caused by fluid in the lungs. Wheezing sounds result from spasm of the airways, usually as a result of *asthma*. In *pleurisy*, a scratching sound can be heard, produced by inflamed areas of the lung rubbing together.

The physician also tests for vocal resonance by asking the patient to whisper something. The sound produced is louder if there is pus in the lung (e.g., as a result of pneumonia) because sound is transmitted better through this medium than through normal air-containing lung tissue.

Blood vessels near the skin surface (usually the carotid artery in the neck, abdominal aorta, and renal artery) can be listened to for bruits (sounds made by turbulent or abnormally fast blood circulation). They occur when blood vessels are narrowed by *atheroma* (fatty deposits) or widened (such as by an *aneurysm*), or when heart valves are narrowed or damaged (such as in *endocarditis*).

The abdomen is auscultated for borborygmi (very loud sounds made by the movement of air and fluid in the intestines) and abnormal bowel sounds. The former may have no significance; the latter may indicate *intestinal obstruction*.

PROCEDURE FOR AUSCULTATION

A physician's examination often includes auscultation—listening to sounds within the body using a stethoscope. Some organs make sounds during normal functioning.

Examples are the movement of fluid through the stomach and intestine, the opening and closing of heart valves, and the flow of air through the lungs and airways. However, the presence of abnormal sounds usually indicates disease of that tissue. The obstetrician listens to the baby's heart beat as part of routine examination during pregnancy.

STETHOSCOPE

The heart
The stethoscope is usually placed at four places on the chest overlying the sites of the heart valves. The physician listens for the presence of murmurs, clicks, and extra heart sounds that indicate disease of a heart valve.

Using a stethoscope
The end is held against the skin. The diaphragm picks up most noises, while the bell detects quiet, deep noises.

Carotid artery and abdominal aorta
The physician may listen to the flow of blood through a blood vessel that passes just beneath the skin. The presence of a bruit usually indicates abnormal narrowing or widening of an artery.

The abdomen
The physician may listen to the abdomen for the sounds made by movement of fluid through the intestine. A disorder of the intestine may cause these sounds to be absent, abnormal, or very loud.

The lungs
The physician places the stethoscope over several different areas of the chest and back to listen to sounds made during breathing. In addition to comparing the sounds made by each lung, the presence of crackles and dry or moist wheezes indicates various types of lung disease.

Autism

A condition in which children fail to form relationships with others. The term was originally used to describe active withdrawal from relationships, such as occurs in *schizophrenia*, but is not generally used in this sense today.

INCIDENCE

Autism is rare, occurring in about two to four out of every 10,000 children. Nearly three times more boys than girls are affected, and it seems more common among the higher social classes. Autism is by definition evident before the age of 30 months and is usually apparent within the first year of life.

CAUSES

The precise causes of autism are unknown, but evidence points to a physical basis. Because about one quarter of autistic children have signs of a neurological disorder and epileptic seizures develop in nearly one third in adolescence, it is likely that there is a subtle form of brain damage. The earlier theory that a lack of warmth from parents was a cause is now rejected. At the most, parents may react to the stress of coping with a disturbed child.

SYMPTOMS AND SIGNS

Often, autistic children are normal for the first few months of life before becoming increasingly unresponsive to parents or other stimuli. The first sign may be resistance to being cuddled, with the child screaming to be put down when picked up, even if hurt or tired.

The child remains aloof from parents and others and fails to form relationships. He or she avoids eye-to-eye contact, prefers to play alone, and is often indifferent to the feelings of others and to social conventions.

Extreme resistance to change of any kind is an important feature. The child reacts with severe tantrums to alteration in routine or interference with activities. Rituals develop in play and often the child becomes attached to unusual objects or collections, or obsessed with one particular topic or idea. This wish for sterile "sameness" makes it very difficult to teach the autistic child new skills.

Delay in speaking is very common. The autistic child lacks the ability to understand or copy speech or gestures and responds to sounds inappropriately. Even when speech is acquired, it is immature, unimaginative in content, and has a robotlike sound. The child often makes up words and echoes what has been said.

There may be other behavioral abnormalities, such as walking on tiptoe, flicking or twiddling fingers for hours on end, rocking, self-injury, sudden screaming fits, and *hyperactivity*. Unusual fears and difficulty learning manual tasks are also common in autistic children.

Despite all these bizarre symptoms, appearance and muscular coordination are normal. Sometimes autistic children have an isolated special skill, such as an outstanding rote memory or musical ability.

TREATMENT

There is no known effective treatment. Special schooling, support and *counseling* for parents and families, and sometimes *behavior therapy* (for example, to reduce violent self-injury) can be helpful. Medication is useful only for specific problems, such as *epilepsy* or *hyperactivity*.

OUTLOOK

Outlook depends on IQ and language ability. Only about one sixth of autistic children can lead any form of independent life; the majority need special care, sometimes in an institution.

Autoclave

Apparatus that produces steam at high pressure within a sealed chamber; the resulting high temperature of the water vapor destroys microorganisms. Autoclaving is used in hospitals as a means of sterilizing surgical equipment (see *Sterilization*).

Autoimmune disorders

Any of numerous disorders, including *rheumatoid arthritis*, insulin-dependent *diabetes mellitus*, and systemic *lupus erythematosus*, caused by a reaction of the individual's *immune system* against the organs or tissues of his or her own body.

The function of the immune system is to respond to invading microorganisms (e.g., bacteria or viruses) by producing antibodies or sensitized lymphocytes (types of white blood cell) that will recognize and destroy the invaders. Autoimmune disorders occur when these reactions unexplainably take place against the body's own cells and tissues, producing a variety of disorders.

The disease-producing processes in autoimmunity are termed *hypersensitivity* reactions; there are a variety of types. Hypersensitivity reactions also occur in *allergy*, which is a related phenomenon. Both are inappropriate responses of the immune system, except that, with allergy, the response is to substances from outside the body. People who have allergies are thought by some to be susceptible to autoimmune disorders.

CAUSES

The immune system normally distinguishes "self" from "nonself." Some lymphocytes are capable of reacting against self, but these lymphocytes are generally suppressed. Autoimmune disorders occur when there is some interruption of the normal control process, allowing lymphocytes to escape from suppression, or when there is an alteration in some body tissue so that it is no longer recognized as "self" and is consequently attacked. The exact mechanisms causing these changes are not fully understood, but bacteria, viruses, and drugs may play a role in triggering an autoimmune process in someone who already has a genetic (inherited) predisposition.

It is speculated that the inflammation (infectious or toxic) initiated by these agents somehow provokes in the body, along with the usual inflammatory response, a "sensitization" to the involved tissues.

TYPES

Autoimmune processes can have various results—for example, slow destruction of a particular type of cell or tissue, stimulation of an organ into excessive growth, or interference in its function. Organs and tissues frequently affected include the endocrine glands (such as the thyroid, pancreas, and adrenal glands), components of the blood (such as the red blood cells), and the connective tissues, skin, muscles, and joints.

Specific autoimmune disorders are frequently classified into organ-specific and non-organ-specific types. In organ-specific disorders, the autoimmune process is directed mainly against one organ. Examples (with the organ affected) include *Hashimoto's thyroiditis* (thyroid gland), pernicious *anemia* (stomach), *Addison's disease* (adrenal glands), and insulin-dependent *diabetes mellitus* (pancreas).

In non-organ-specific disorders, autoimmune activity is widely spread throughout the body. Examples include systemic *lupus erythematosus* (SLE), *rheumatoid arthritis*, and *dermatomyositis*. Some autoimmune diseases fall between the two types. Patients may experience several organ-specific or non-organ-specific diseases simultaneously. However, there is little overlap between the two ends of the spectrum.

FUNCTIONS OF THE AUTONOMIC NERVOUS SYSTEM

The autonomic nervous system is responsible for controlling the involuntary body functions, such as sweating, digestion, and heart rate. The system affects smooth muscles, such as those of the airways and the intestines, rather than the striated muscles, which are under the body's voluntary control.

SYMPATHETIC SYSTEM

Dilates pupils

Inhibits salivation

Dilates bronchi

Accelerates heart rate

Inhibits gastric juice production

Inhibits digestive process

Relaxes bladder muscles

Stimulates secretion of epinephrine and norepinephrine

Contracts rectum

Medulla oblongata

Cranial nerves

Ganglia chain

Cervical nerves

Thoracic nerves

Lumbar nerves

Sacral nerves

Spinal cord

PARASYMPATHETIC SYSTEM

Contracts pupils

Stimulates salivation

Constricts bronchi

Slows heart rate

Stimulates gastric juice production

Speeds up digestive process

Contracts bladder muscles

Relaxes rectum

The autonomic nervous system

The autonomic nervous system is divided into two subsidiary systems: the sympathetic nervous system and the parasympathetic nervous system. The sympathetic system is the one that is primarily concerned with preparing the body for action; it dominates at times of stress or excitement. The sympathetic system stimulates functions such as heart rate and sweating, and dilates the blood vessels to the muscles so that more blood is diverted to them. Simultaneously, it subdues the activity of the digestive system. In contrast, the parasympathetic nervous system is concerned mainly with the body's everyday function of excreting waste products; this system dominates during sleep. The parasympathetic system slows the heart rate and stimulates the organs of the digestive tract. Most of the time, activity is balanced between the two systems, with neither dominating. Both of the systems play an important part in sexual arousal and orgasm in both men and women.

TREATMENT

The first principle in treating any autoimmune disorder is to correct any major deficiencies. This may involve replacing hormones, such as thyroxin or insulin, that are not being produced by a gland. Alternatively, it may involve replacing components of the blood by transfusion.

The second principle is to diminish the activity of the immune system; this necessitates a delicate balance, controlling the disorder while maintaining the body's ability to fight disease in general. The drugs most commonly used are *corticosteroid drugs*. More severe cases can be treated with other more powerful *immunosuppressant drugs* such as cyclophosphamide, methotrexate, and azathioprine, but all of these drugs can damage rapidly dividing tissues, such as the bone marrow, and so are used with caution. Drugs that act more specifically on the immune system (for example, by blocking a particular hypersensitivity reaction) are being devised.

Automatism

A state in which behavior is not controlled by the conscious mind. The individual carries out movements and activities without being aware of doing so, and later has no clear memory of what happened. The episodes, which are uncommon, start abruptly and usually last a few seconds or minutes at the most.

Automatisms are the primary symptom of psychomotor *epilepsy*; this diagnosis can be confirmed by *EEG*. Other causes include *dissociative disorders, hysteria, alcohol intoxication* or *drug abuse, brain disorders*, and *hypoglycemia*.

Autonomic nervous system

The part of the *nervous system* that controls the involuntary, seemingly automatic, activities of organs, blood vessels, glands, and a variety of other tissues in the body. The autonomic nervous system consists of a network of nerves divided into two parts: the *sympathetic nervous system* and the *parasympathetic nervous system*.

In general, the sympathetic nervous system heightens activity in the body—quickening the heart beat and breathing rate as if it were preparing the body for a *fight or flight response*. The parasympathetic system has the opposite effect.

The two systems act in conjunction and normally balance each other. However, during exercise or at times of stress or fear, the activity of the sympathetic system predominates, while during sleep the parasympathetic system exerts more control.

SYMPATHETIC NERVOUS SYSTEM

The sympathetic nervous system consists of two chains of nerves that pass from the spinal cord throughout the body to the organs and other structures they control. Into these tissues the nerve endings release the *neurotransmitter* chemicals *epinephrine* and *norepinephrine*. The system also stimulates the release of epinephrine from the adrenal glands into the bloodstream.

Among the most important effects produced by the neurotransmitters of the autonomic system are accelerating and strengthening the heart beat, widening the airways, dilating the blood vessels in muscles and constricting those in the skin and abdominal organs (to increase blood flow through the muscles), decreasing the activity of the digestive system, dilating the pupil of the eye, and producing the contractions in the male urethra by which sperm are ejaculated at orgasm.

PARASYMPATHETIC NERVOUS SYSTEM

The parasympathetic nervous system is composed of one chain of nerves that passes from the brain and another that leaves the lower spinal cord. The nerves are distributed to the same organs and structures that are supplied by the nerves of the sympathetic system. The parasympathetic nerves release the neurotransmitter *acetylcholine*, which has the opposite effects of those produced by epinephrine and norepinephrine. The parasympathetic nervous system also helps to produce and maintain erection of the penis in sexually aroused men.

EFFECT OF DRUGS

Certain disorders can be treated by giving drugs that affect the autonomic nervous system. *Anticholinergic drugs*, for example, block the effect of acetylcholine, which can reduce painful muscle spasms in the intestine. *Beta-blocker drugs* block the action of epinephrine and norepinephrine on the heart and thus slow the rate and force of its beat.

Autopsy

A postmortem examination of the body, sometimes required by statute, sometimes not. In instances of unnatural death or death under suspicious circumstances, states require an autopsy to be performed by the county coroner (not necessarily a physician) or the medical examiner, who is a physician with qualifications in pathology. Some states require a report to the medical examiner in the case of any death occurring outside a hospital. When the cause of death is not suspicious, but when examination of the organs after death will be useful for research or teaching, hospitals and physicians must seek the next-of-kin's permission for an autopsy.

Autosuggestion

Putting oneself into a receptive hypnotic-type state as a means of stimulating the body's ability to help itself. The idea that symptoms could be relieved merely through attitude was put forth by a Frenchman at the end of the nineteenth century. He observed that, if people accepted a physician's suggestion that a treatment would be effective, it was often enough to make it so. It was thought that people could try to make suggestions to themselves with equally effective results.

As an aid to achieving the necessary relaxed state for successful autosuggestion, the repetition of the key phrase "Every day in every way, I am getting better and better" was advocated. Although autosuggestion enjoyed only brief popularity, some techniques used today are based on its premise. For example, in one method used to control anxiety symptoms, people are taught muscular relaxation (biofeedback) techniques and then learn to summon up calming imagery or thoughts.

Aversion therapy

An outdated form of *behavior therapy* in which unpleasant stimuli, such as electric shocks, are applied to suppress unwanted behavior (e.g., alcoholism or drug addiction).

Aviation medicine

The medical specialty concerned with the physiological effects of flight and the causes and treatment of medical problems during air travel. Aviation medicine covers assessment of the fitness of passengers and crew to fly, the management of medical emergencies in the air, the consequences of special types of flight (for example, in helicopters and spacecraft), and the investigation of aircraft accidents.

EFFECTS OF REDUCED OXYGEN

Increasing altitude causes a fall in air pressure and with it a fall in the pressure of oxygen. *Hypoxia* (a seriously reduced oxygen concentration in the blood and tissues) is the single most serious threat to anyone who flies.

In healthy air travelers, the oxygen saturation of the blood falls from nearly 100 percent to about 60 percent at 10,000 feet. To avoid the development of hypoxia, airliners are kept at a pressure equivalent to an altitude of about 6,000 feet during flight, although the cruising altitude may be as high as 39,000 feet (even higher in a Concorde). This means that the cabin pressure is about 30 percent less than at ground level but much higher than the outside pressure. Any sudden failure of the aircraft's pressure hull leads to a rapid fall in cabin pressure, with a risk of hypoxia and *decompression sickness*. Rapid decompression in civil aircraft is extremely rare, but passengers and crew are provided with oxygen masks for use in emergencies while the aircraft descends to a safe altitude.

ANXIETY AND HYPERVENTILATION
Hypoxia or, more commonly, anxiety during flight can lead to *hyperventilation* ("overbreathing"). In this condition, increased breathing efforts lead to excess loss of carbon dioxide, which alters the acidity of the body and gives rise to symptoms such as tingling around the mouth, muscle spasms, and light-headedness. The symptoms of hyperventilation are themselves likely to increase anxiety.

Although flying can be an exhilarating experience, many people are anxious at some stage of a flight; others suffer an acute fear of flying and may need mild preflight sedation. If the symptoms of hyperventilation develop, the treatment is to rebreathe air from a paper bag held over the nose and mouth, which reduces the loss of carbon dioxide.

DECOMPRESSION SICKNESS
Aviators' decompression sickness has the same causes as the condition that affects scuba divers and deep tunnel workers (see *Decompression sickness*). It is not a risk for passengers on normal flights, except when there is a marked, rapid depressurization in the cabin or when a passenger has recently been exposed to pressure changes—in most cases due to scuba diving (which should be avoided in the 24 hours prior to a flight).

PRESSURE EFFECTS ON BODY CAVITIES
The changes in cabin pressure during a flight affect the body's gas-containing cavities, principally the middle ears, facial sinuses, lungs, and intestines. When pressure drops dur-

CONDITIONS AFFECTING PASSENGER SUITABILITY FOR AIR TRAVEL

Conditions	Comments
Have a lung disease (such as chronic bronchitis or emphysema) Have a severe anemia Have a heart condition (such as angina pectoris, heart failure, or recent heart attack)	The lowered cabin pressure (and thus the oxygen level) at higher altitudes aggravates an already impaired ability to oxygenate the blood or tissues and may cause severe respiratory distress or collapse. Seek your physician's advice. Flying may be possible, if you are able to walk 50 yards without breathlessness or chest pain.
Have had a recent stroke	Seek your physician's advice. You may need to wait some weeks before flying.
Have had recent surgery to inner or middle ear, abdomen, chest, or brain, a recently collapsed lung, or a fractured skull	Seek your physician's advice. You may need to wait before flying to avoid damage to your hearing mechanism or from expansion of gas trapped in the chest, abdomen, or skull.
Are pregnant	No flying after 34 to 36 weeks on most airlines.
Are newborn	An infant should not fly until at least 48 hours old.
Have psychiatric disorders	May need trained escort.
Have an infectious disease, or terminal illness, or are vomiting	May be refused entry to aircraft. Check with airline.

ing ascent, the volume of gas in these cavities expands; on descent, the gas volume decreases as pressure rises.

On ascent, unless there is a catastrophic fall in pressure, air from the lungs is harmlessly released via the windpipe, air in the large intestine and stomach can also escape freely (although trapped gas in the small intestine can give rise to a feeling of fullness), and air in the middle ears and sinuses can leave via ducts linking them to the back of the nose.

It is during descent that pressure changes in the ears and sinuses may fail to keep up with cabin repressurization. Unless preventive measures are taken, this may lead to pain and, rarely, damage (see *Barotrauma*).

ACCELERATION AND DECELERATION
The accelerational forces experienced by civil aircraft passengers are mild, even during takeoff and descent, and no precautions are necessary other than the wearing of a seat belt. Military aircraft pilots, on the other hand, may experience severe accelerations, frequently in an upward direction, and must wear special suits and use a reclined seat to prevent pooling of blood in the feet, which causes immediate loss of consciousness.

OTHER EFFECTS
The problem of *motion sickness* is usually less for air than for road or sea

travelers. Affected passengers may benefit from one of the antimotion sickness preparations available.

Air travel has made possible the rapid crossing of several time zones within a short period. This can affect sleep-waking cycles, causing tiredness and reduced mental performance, often at inconvenient times of the day (see *Jet lag*).

FITNESS TO FLY
Most aircraft passengers are well able to tolerate travel in the comfort of a pressurized cabin. Those with preexisting disorders, however, are advised to seek medical advice before undertaking a journey by air, especially if the condition is likely to be made worse by even the mild hypoxia induced at normal cabin pressures.

AVIATION MEDICINE SPECIALISTS
Most large airlines have a medical department staffed by physicians, trained in aviation medicine, who are responsible for the health care of the airline staff. The physicians also give advice on the transportation of sick passengers, the provision of training and equipment to deal with illness during a flight, and the maintenance of airline hygiene.

Avoidant personality disorder
A term that describes the characteristic behavior of people whose

sensitivity to criticism affects their entire lives. Such people see the most innocent behavior as "getting at" them, do not make friends easily, and have a limited social life. They have a very low opinion of themselves, constantly downgrade their personal accomplishments, and easily become anxious and depressed over their supposed shortcomings.

Unlike those with a *schizoid personality disorder*, those with avoidant personality disorder want to have a social life and are often desperate to be loved and accepted. They may also have a form of social *phobia*, avoiding situations in which they might be drawn into relationships with other people and thus risk possible humiliation or rejection.

This disorder usually extends from childhood and is said to be quite common. Long-term *psychotherapy* or *counseling* may help, as does the maturity that comes with age.

Avulsed tooth

A tooth that has become completely dislodged from its socket as the result of an accident. The tooth should be carried to the dentist immediately in a glass of milk or cool water, or in a loosely wrapped, damp cloth. The dentist will reimplant the tooth into the socket as rapidly as possible, and immobilize it with a splint (see *Reimplantation, dental*). If the tooth is reimplanted within 30 minutes of the accident, it will reattach itself to the socket in 90 percent of the cases. After 90 minutes, the success rate falls to about 70 percent.

Avulsion

The tearing away of a body structure from its point of attachment. Avulsion may be due to an injury, such as a severe ankle sprain in which the ligaments on the outside of the ankle are stretched so much that a small fragment of bone is torn from its attachment point to the two bones in the lower leg.

Alternatively, avulsion may be performed deliberately as part of a surgical procedure. In the treatment of *varicose veins*, for example, the stripping of veins from the leg is described as an avulsion.

Axilla

The medical name for the armpit.

Ayurvedism

Asiatic Indian herbal medicine (see *Indian medicine*).

Azatadine

An *antihistamine drug* used in the treatment of *urticaria* (hives) and insect bites to relieve itching, swelling, and redness of the skin. Azatadine is also given to help relieve nasal congestion in allergic *rhinitis* (hay fever).

Possible adverse effects include dry mouth and blurred vision. Azatadine has a strong sedative effect, which may cause drowsiness during the day; it is useful if persistent itching is disturbing sleep at night.

Azathioprine

IMMUNOSUPPRESSANT
🥄 ✏️ ⬗ 🖊️ 🗐 ✎ 🧴 🧴 🔬 ⬭
Tablet Injection
📄 Prescription needed
🔒 Not available as generic

A drug used in the treatment of severe *rheumatoid arthritis* and other *autoimmune disorders* (disorders in which the *immune system* attacks the body's own tissues). Azathioprine is prescribed when other treatments (for example, *corticosteroid drugs* and other *antirheumatic drugs*) fail to slow the progress of the disease or to improve symptoms. Azathioprine is also among the drugs used to prevent the rejection of a transplanted organ (see *Transplant surgery*).

HOW IT WORKS

Azathioprine reduces the efficiency of the body's immune system by preventing lymphocytes (a type of white blood cell) from multiplying. Lymphocytes destroy proteins not normally found in the body and, in autoimmune disorders, attack proteins that the immune system considers to be foreign.

POSSIBLE ADVERSE EFFECTS

Abnormal bleeding and increased susceptibility to infection may occur as a result of reduced blood cell production.

Azoospermia

The absence of sperm from semen; an important cause of *infertility* in males. Azoospermia may be congenital or may develop later in life. The condition is thought to affect about one male in 100.

CAUSES

Congenital azoospermia may be the result of a chromosomal abnormality, such as *Klinefelter's syndrome* (the presence of an extra sex chromosome); failure of the testes to descend into the scrotum; absence of the vas deferens (the ducts that carry sperm from the testes to the seminal vesicles, the sacs where sperm is stored before ejaculation); or *cystic fibrosis*, a genetic disorder that affects the lungs and pancreas that may also cause defects of the vas deferens. *Orchitis* caused by mumps may result in azoospermia, although, more often, some abnormal sperm persist.

In some males, puberty fails to take place, usually because the pituitary gland produces an insufficient amount of *follicle-stimulating hormone* (FSH), which is necessary for sperm production. In other males, puberty occurs but the testes fail to function properly. This disorder may also cause azoospermia.

The most common cause of azoospermia in later life is *vasectomy*, the sterilization operation in which the vas deferens are cut and tied off. Another cause is blockage of the ducts, which may follow a sexually transmitted disease, tuberculosis, or surgery on the groin (usually performed to repair a hernia or to lower undescended testes in a boy).

Azoospermia can also develop because of a temporary or permanent failure of the testes to produce sperm. This can follow radiation therapy, accidental radiation, treatment with particular drugs (especially anticancer drugs and the antidiarrheal drug sulfasalazine), and prolonged exposure to heat, insecticides, or industrial chemicals. In some cases, production of sperm ceases permanently for no known reason.

DIAGNOSIS

The diagnosis is made by analyzing at least two samples of semen, given a month apart, for the presence of sperm. Other tests are carried out to discover or confirm the cause. Blood samples are analyzed for evidence of chromosomal abnormalities or measured for levels of FSH. A *biopsy* of cells from the testes that gives a normal result indicates that the cause is a blockage; X rays can reveal the site.

TREATMENT AND OUTLOOK

Injections of FSH may cause puberty to develop and surgery can sometimes unblock ducts closed by infection; most other causes of azoospermia are untreatable. Most men with azoospermia who wish to become parents must do so through *artificial insemination* by using donor sperm (AID) or adoption.

AZT

The abbreviation for azidothymidine, the former name for *zidovudine*.

Babesiosis

An infectious disease caused by a parasitic protozoan (a type of single-celled microorganism). The disease is transmitted to humans by the bites of ticks that have picked up the protozoa from infected animals, such as rodents or horses.

Human infection is rare but cases have been reported in Europe and in the offshore islands of New England during the summer months. Avoidance of tick-infested areas and prompt removal of any attached ticks further reduces the already slim chances of infection.

Symptoms include fever and chills and closely resemble those of *malaria* (which is caused by a similar parasite). No specific treatment is available. Most patients recover without treatment, although intensive hospital care may be required in cases where infection is severe.

Babinski's sign

A reflex movement in which the big toe bends upward when the outer edge of the sole of the foot is scratched. Babinski's sign indicates damage or disease of the brain or the spinal cord.

Baby blues

A common name for a mild form of depression that is likely to occur after childbirth. It almost always disappears without treatment, but can develop into a more serious illness. (See *Postpartum depression*.)

Baby Doe case

A celebrated legal case involving the medical care of infants born with severe physical handicaps. In 1983 the Department of Health and Human Services began requiring that the maximum of resources be used to preserve life in such cases.

Traditionally, the decision to preserve the life of the severely handicapped was determined after consultation among the physician, the child's family, and, often, the family

minister. Acting as one of the plaintiffs, the AMA prevailed in the Supreme Court in a challenge of the federal government's intervention in such decisions, involving as they do many difficult ethical, moral, and economic considerations.

Bacampicillin

A common penicillin-type antibiotic. (See *Penicillin drugs*.)

Bacilli

Rod-shaped *bacteria*. They are responsible for many diseases, including diphtheria, dysentery, tetanus, and tuberculosis.

Bacitracin

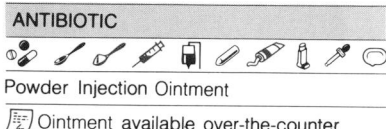

ANTIBIOTIC

Powder Injection Ointment

Ointment available over-the-counter

Available as generic

An *antibacterial drug* active against many of the bacteria that cause skin and eye infections. It is often used in combination with other antibiotics, such as neomycin and polymyxin B, that complement its antibacterial activity.

Bacitracin is usually applied to the skin as a powder or ointment and to the eye in the form of an ointment. It is not absorbed into the bloodstream when taken by mouth and is therefore given by injection when used to treat a severe infection.

Kidney damage is a possible adverse effect and bacitracin is therefore used only for severe infections that have not responded to other more common antibiotics.

Back

The area from the shoulders to the buttocks. The back is supported by the spinal column (see *Spine*), which is bound together by ligaments and supported by muscles that also control posture and movement.

Back disorders

Problems involving the back are numerous. They arise from a number of causes affecting the *spine*, and can involve disorders of bones, muscles, ligaments, tendons, nerves, and joints in the spine. These disorders can cause *back pain* with or without *sciatica*—pain in the buttock and down the back of the leg. (See also *Spine* disorders box.)

Back pain

Most people suffer from back pain at some time in their lives. In many cases it is labeled "nonspecific back pain" and no exact diagnosis is made because the pain resolves with rest and because analgesics (painkillers) are used before any tests such as X rays are performed.

CAUSES

Nonspecific back pain is one of the largest single causes of lost working days through illness in the US. People most likely to suffer from back pain are those whose jobs involve much heavy lifting and carrying, or those who spend long periods sitting in one position or bending awkwardly. Overweight people are also more prone to back pain—their backs carry a heavier load and they tend to have weaker abdominal muscles, which help provide back support.

Nonspecific back pain is thought to be due to a mechanical disorder affecting one or more structures. The disorder may be a ligament strain, a muscle tear, damage to a spinal facet joint, or a *disk prolapse*.

In addition to pain from a damaged structure, spasm of surrounding muscles will cause additional pain and tenderness over a wider area and can cause temporary *scoliosis*.

Abnormalities of a facet joint and disk prolapse can both cause *sciatica* (pain in the buttock and down the back of the leg into the foot), resulting from pressure on a sciatic nerve root as it leaves the spinal cord. Coughing, sneezing, or straining will increase the pain. Pressure on the sciatic nerve can cause "pins and needles" in that leg and weakness in muscles activated by the nerve. Rarely, pain can radiate down the femoral nerve on the front of the thigh.

Osteoarthritis in the joints of the spine can cause persistent back pain. *Ankylosing spondylitis* causes back pain and stiffness with loss of back mobility. *Coccygodynia* (pain and tenderness at the base of the spine) can occur after a fall in which the coccyx has struck the ground, during pregnancy, or for unknown reasons.

Fibrositis is a controversial term used to describe pain and tenderness in muscles usually in the back. It is often worse in cold and damp weather and is occasionally associated with feeling sick. Unlike other causes of back pain, fibrositis is not accompanied by muscle spasm or restriction of back movement. It often responds to nonsteroidal anti-inflammatory drugs.

BACKACHE Pain and/or stiffness in the back that may be continuous or intermittent.

Of recent origin

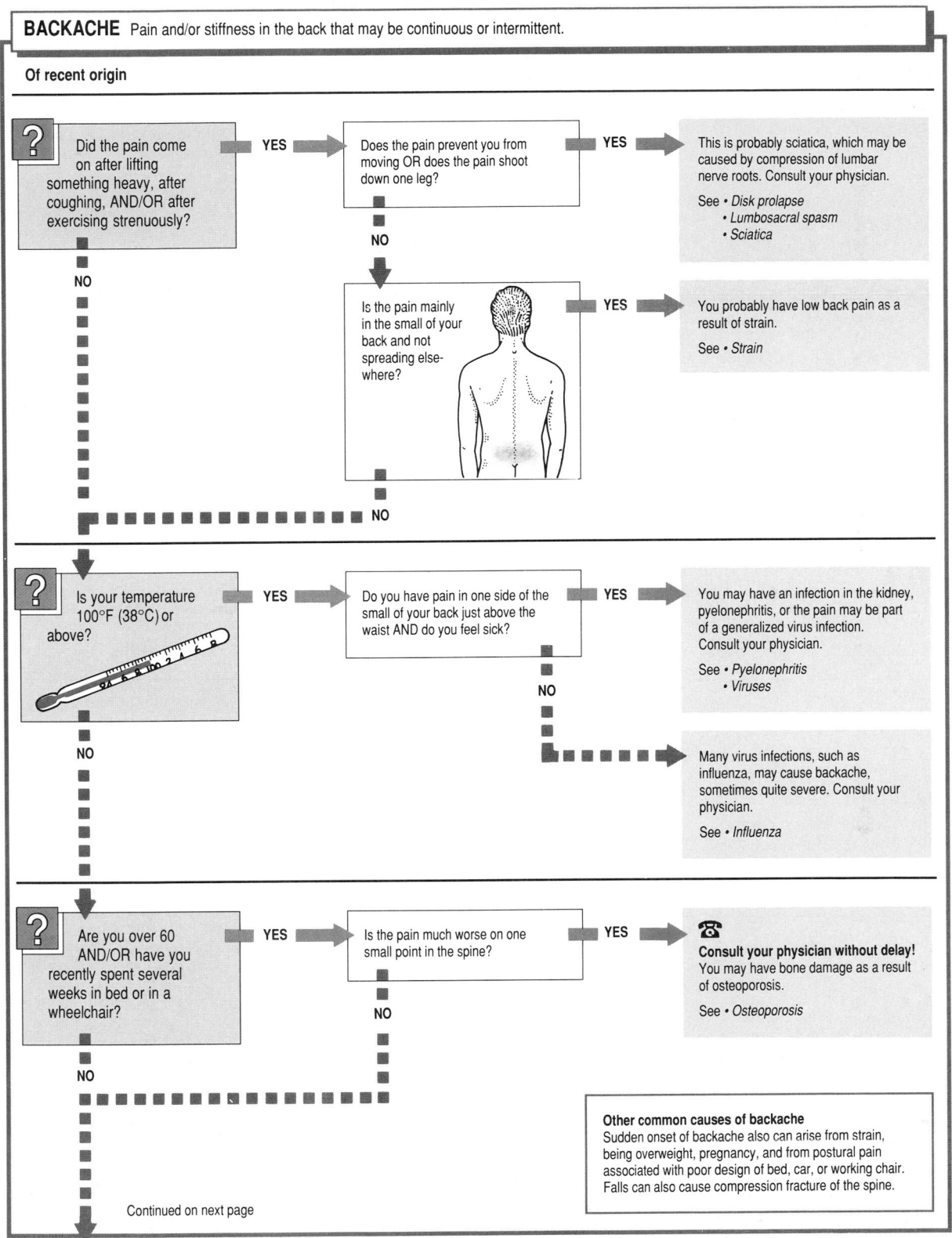

Did the pain come on after lifting something heavy, after coughing, AND/OR after exercising strenuously? — **YES** → Does the pain prevent you from moving OR does the pain shoot down one leg? — **YES** → This is probably sciatica, which may be caused by compression of lumbar nerve roots. Consult your physician.

See • *Disk prolapse*
• *Lumbosacral spasm*
• *Sciatica*

NO → Is the pain mainly in the small of your back and not spreading elsewhere? — **YES** → You probably have low back pain as a result of strain.

See • *Strain*

NO

Is your temperature 100°F (38°C) or above? — **YES** → Do you have pain in one side of the small of your back just above the waist AND do you feel sick? — **YES** → You may have an infection in the kidney, pyelonephritis, or the pain may be part of a generalized virus infection. Consult your physician.

See • *Pyelonephritis*
• *Viruses*

NO → Many virus infections, such as influenza, may cause backache, sometimes quite severe. Consult your physician.

See • *Influenza*

NO

Are you over 60 AND/OR have you recently spent several weeks in bed or in a wheelchair? — **YES** → Is the pain much worse on one small point in the spine? — **YES** → ☎ **Consult your physician without delay!** You may have bone damage as a result of osteoporosis.

See • *Osteoporosis*

NO

Other common causes of backache
Sudden onset of backache also can arise from strain, being overweight, pregnancy, and from postural pain associated with poor design of bed, car, or working chair. Falls can also cause compression fracture of the spine.

Continued on next page

151

B

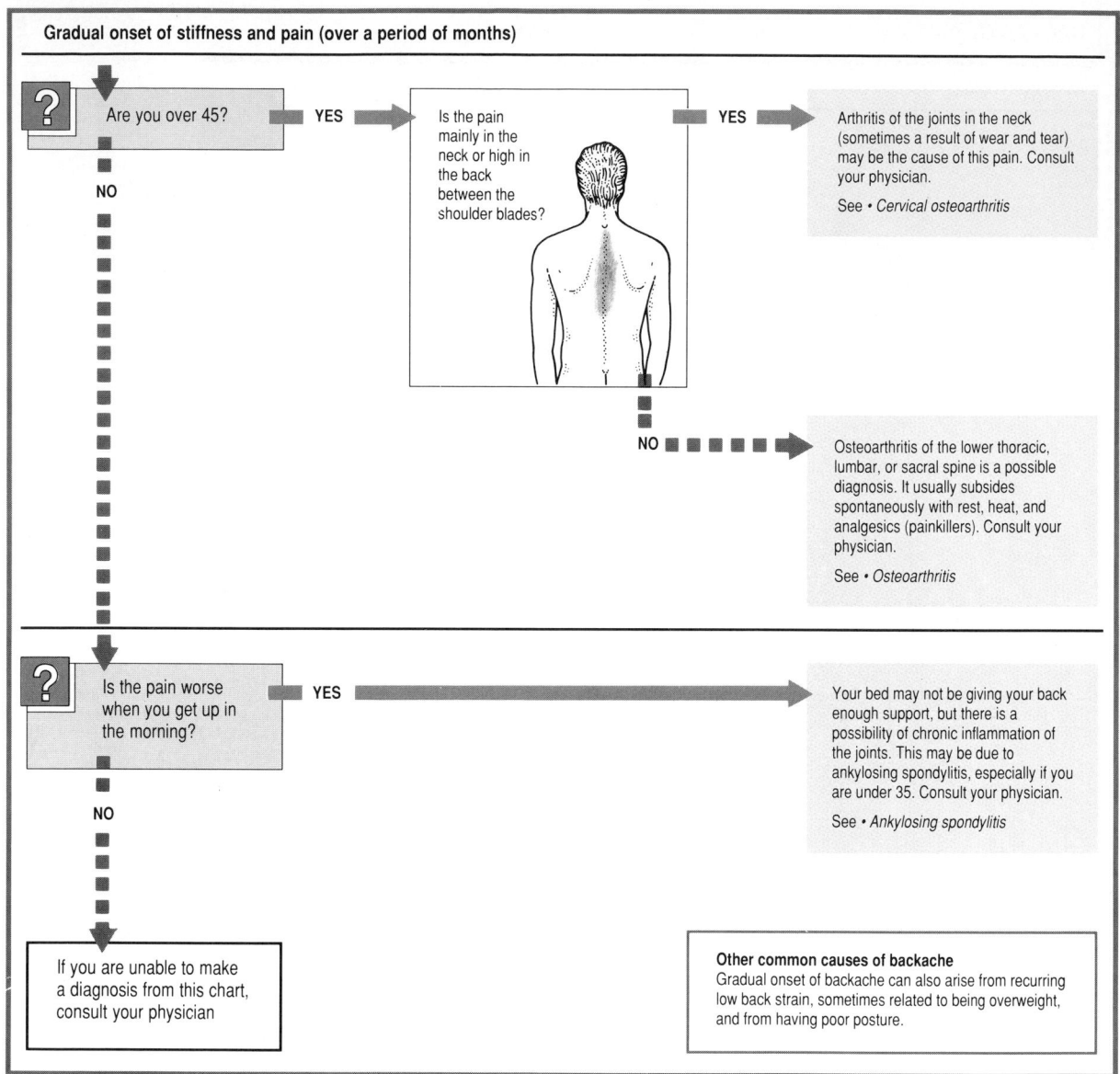

Gradual onset of stiffness and pain (over a period of months)

? Are you over 45? — **YES** →

Is the pain mainly in the neck or high in the back between the shoulder blades? — **YES** →

Arthritis of the joints in the neck (sometimes a result of wear and tear) may be the cause of this pain. Consult your physician.

See • *Cervical osteoarthritis*

NO

NO →

Osteoarthritis of the lower thoracic, lumbar, or sacral spine is a possible diagnosis. It usually subsides spontaneously with rest, heat, and analgesics (painkillers). Consult your physician.

See • *Osteoarthritis*

? Is the pain worse when you get up in the morning? — **YES** →

Your bed may not be giving your back enough support, but there is a possibility of chronic inflammation of the joints. This may be due to ankylosing spondylitis, especially if you are under 35. Consult your physician.

See • *Ankylosing spondylitis*

NO

If you are unable to make a diagnosis from this chart, consult your physician

Other common causes of backache
Gradual onset of backache can also arise from recurring low back strain, sometimes related to being overweight, and from having poor posture.

Pyelonephritis can cause back pain with pain and tenderness in the loin, fever, chills, and pain when passing urine. Cancer in the spine can cause persistent back pain that disturbs sleep and is unrelieved by rest.

SELF-HELP
Back pain and sciatica may improve by resting in bed on a firm mattress or a board. Analgesics (painkillers) and the application of heat to the back can help the pain. If the pain persists, is very severe, or is associated with weakness in a leg or problems with bladder control, a physician should be consulted without delay.

INVESTIGATION
Examination of the back may show tenderness in specific areas and loss of motion of the back. Weakness or loss of sensation in the legs implies pressure on a nerve root; this requires prompt investigation.

X rays of the spine may show narrowing between the spinal disks, osteoarthritis, osteoporosis, ankylosing spondylitis, compression fracture, stress fracture, bone *metastasis*, or *spondylolisthesis* (displacement of vertebrae). X rays will not reveal ligament, muscle, facet joint, or disk damage. To reveal pressure on a nerve

root (for example, due to prolapse of a disk), *myelography*, *CT scanning*, or *MRI* is performed.

TREATMENT
If a specific cause is found for back pain, treatment will be for that cause. Acute, nonspecific back pain is treated with periods of rest and use of analgesic drugs (painkillers). Chronic nonspecific back pain is more difficult to treat. Treatment may include taking aspirinlike medication, *anti-inflammatory drugs*, or *muscle-relaxant drugs*; *acupuncture* or spinal injection; or exercise, spinal *manipulation*, wearing an elastic *brace*, or spinal surgery.

B

BACK PAIN

Most people experience back pain some time in their lives, but in most cases it is not serious and the problem corrects itself before investigation takes place. However, some kinds of back pain can be related to a specific disorder. In the diagram below, you will find the most common sites affected by back pain.

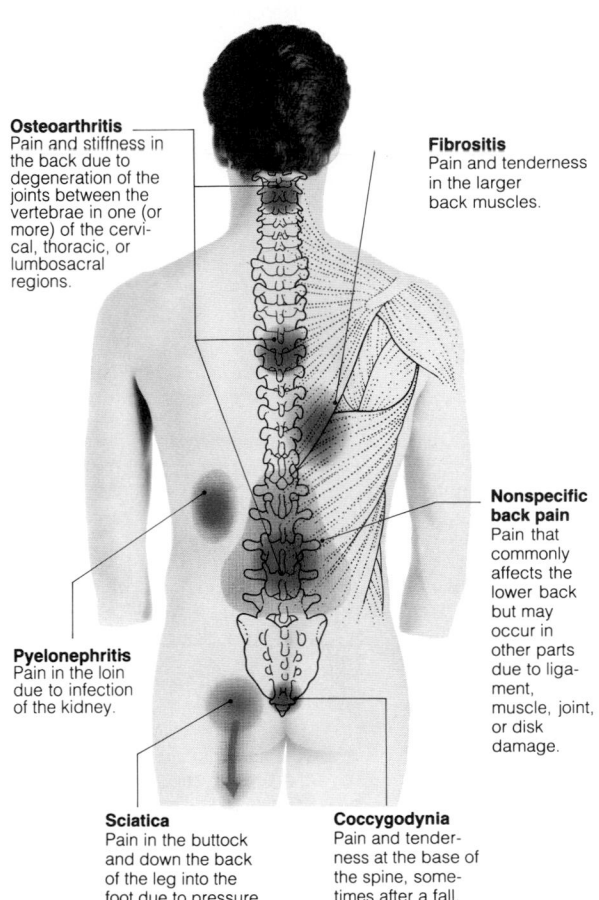

Osteoarthritis
Pain and stiffness in the back due to degeneration of the joints between the vertebrae in one (or more) of the cervical, thoracic, or lumbosacral regions.

Fibrositis
Pain and tenderness in the larger back muscles.

Pyelonephritis
Pain in the loin due to infection of the kidney.

Nonspecific back pain
Pain that commonly affects the lower back but may occur in other parts due to ligament, muscle, joint, or disk damage.

Sciatica
Pain in the buttock and down the back of the leg into the foot due to pressure on a nerve.

Coccygodynia
Pain and tenderness at the base of the spine, sometimes after a fall.

REDUCING STRAIN ON THE BACK

Don't push a heavy object in front with straight arms; this puts strain on the back.

Do push backward; the strain is taken by the legs instead.

Don't slouch; the lower back is pushed out at an angle, resulting in strain.

Do sit up straight, with the spine resting against the chair back.

Don't lift with straight legs and curved back; this puts strain on the lower back.

Do lift with the back straight and knees bent, which transfers strain to the legs.

Baclofen

MUSCLE RELAXANT
Tablet
Prescription needed
Not available as generic

A *muscle relaxant* that blocks nerve activity in the spinal cord. It relieves muscle spasm and stiffness that have been caused by brain or spinal cord injury, *stroke*, or neurological disorders such as *multiple sclerosis*. Baclofen does not cure the underlying disorder but it allows other treatment to be carried out. Often, it makes walking and performing tasks with the hands easier.

To reduce the risk of side effects such as drowsiness and muscle weakness, the dose is usually increased slowly under medical supervision until the desired effect is achieved.

Bacteremia

The presence of bacteria in the bloodstream. Bacteremia occurs for a few hours after many minor surgical operations and may also occur with infections such as tonsillitis.

In people with abnormal heart valves due to a congenital defect or previous rheumatic fever that has scarred the valves, the bacteria may cause *endocarditis*. Also, if a person's immune system has been weakened by illness or a major operation, bacteremia may lead to *septicemia* and shock.

Bacteria

A group of single-cell *microorganisms*, some of which cause disease. Commonly known as "germs," bacteria have been recognized as a cause of disease for a century now but we still do not fully understand why some

B

people become ill while others remain well when exposed to the same sources of infection. Abundant in the air, soil, and water, most bacteria are harmless to humans. Some, indeed, are beneficial, such as those that live in the intestine and help to break down food. Types of bacteria that cause disease are known as pathogens.

Bacteria were discovered in the seventeenth century, with the introduction of the microscope, but it was not until the mid-nineteenth century that the French chemist Louis Pasteur established beyond doubt that they were the cause of many diseases.

Bacteria are only one of various types of microorganisms that produce disease in man. The others are classified into eight main groups: *viruses, chlamydiae, mycoplasmas, rickettsiae, fungi, protozoa, parasites* (eggs and larvae), and *ectoparasites*.

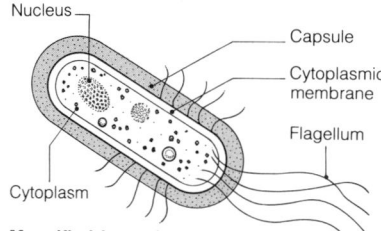

Magnified bacterium
A typical bacterial cell enlarged to approximately 20,000 times its normal size.

Staphylococcus
(causes boils)

Streptococcus
(causes sore throat)

Salmonella typhosa
(causes typhoid fever)

Spirochaeta
(causes syphilis)

Common types of bacteria

TYPES
Pathogenic (disease-producing) bacteria are classified, on the basis of shape, into three main groups: cocci (spherical), bacilli (rod-shaped), and spirilla (spiral-shaped).

Among the wide range of diseases that are caused by cocci are pneumonia, tonsillitis, bacterial endocarditis, meningitis, toxic shock syndrome, and various conditions affecting the skin.

Bacilli produce diseases that include leprosy, tuberculosis, dysentery (i.e., typhoid, shigellosis, campylobacter,

or salmonellosis), whooping cough, tetanus, diphtheria, legionnaires' disease, and botulism.

The third, and smallest group of bacteria, spirilla, is responsible for syphilis, yaws, leptospirosis, and Lyme disease.

GROWTH, MOVEMENT, REPRODUCTION
The bacteria that colonize the human body thrive in warm, moist conditions. Some are aerobic—that is, they require oxygen to grow and multiply—and so they are most commonly found near the surface, on the skin or in the respiratory system. Anaerobic bacteria thrive where there is no oxygen—deep within tissue, the colon, or deep wounds.

Many bacteria are naturally static and, if they move around the body, do so only on currents of air or fluid. Some, however, such as salmonella (responsible for food poisoning and typhoid) are highly motile, moving through fluid by lashing with their flagella (whiplike, filamentous tails).

Bacteria reproduce by dividing into two cells, which in turn divide, and so on. Under ideal conditions (exactly the right temperature and sufficient nourishment for all cells), this division can take place every 20 minutes, an extremely rapid rate of reproduction. After only six hours one bacterium can have multiplied to more than one quarter of a million. This very rarely happens, however, because ideal conditions rarely occur and in a healthy individual the body's *immune system* destroys the invading bacteria.

As well as dividing, some types of bacteria—such as, for example, clostridia (responsible for botulism, tetanus, pseudomembranous colitis, and anthrax)—also multiply, in a more restricted way, by each producing a spore, a single new bacterium that is protected by a tough membrane and can survive high temperatures, dryness, and lack of nourishment.

HOW BACTERIA ENTER THE BODY
Bacteria can enter through the lungs if droplets breathed, coughed, or sneezed out by an infected person are inhaled. Diseases contracted in this way include tuberculosis, diphtheria, and whooping cough.

The digestive tract can become infected if contaminated food is eaten. Bacteria may be brought to food by flies or by contaminated hands.

Microorganisms that enter the genitourinary system include those causing sexually transmitted diseases (e.g., syphilis, pelvic inflammatory disease, and gonorrhea).

Bacteria penetrate the skin in various ways: through hair follicles, as in boils; through surface cuts or abrasions, as in erysipelas; or through deep wounds, as with tetanus.

HOW BACTERIA CAUSE DISEASE
Bacteria produce poisons that are harmful to human cells. If they are present in sufficient quantity and the affected person is not immune to them, disease results. Some bacteria release poisons known as endotoxins, which can cause fever, hemorrhage, and shock. Others produce exotoxins, which account for the major damage in diseases such as diphtheria, tetanus, and toxic shock syndrome.

RESISTANCE BY THE BODY
The body's first means of preventing invasion by harmful bacteria are the substances hostile to bacteria in the skin, lining of the respiratory tract, digestive tract, and genitourinary system. The eyes are protected by an enzyme in the tears, and the stomach secretes hydrochloric acid, which kills many bacteria in food and water.

If the bacteria break through this defense, two types of white blood cell attack them: neutrophils engulf and destroy many of the bacteria, and lymphocytes produce antibodies against them. The antibodies attack the bacteria directly. After an infection, antibodies remain in the blood for a considerable time—many years in the case of smallpox, rubella (German measles), typhoid, and scarlet fever—so that any further attacks of the disease are usually prevented or are mild.

TREATMENT OF BACTERIAL DISEASE
The response of the immune system to bacterial illness is sometimes enough by itself to bring about recovery, but in many cases medical treatment is necessary. The main form of treatment is *antibiotic drugs*, either by mouth or by injection. Some, such as penicillin, destroy the invading bacteria; others, such as tetracycline, prevent them from multiplying further, permitting the immune system to overcome the invaders.

Some diseases—among them diphtheria, tetanus, botulism, and gas gangrene—are treated by the injection of an antiserum. This is a fluid taken from the blood of a horse (or, less commonly, a person) that has been given a series of immunizing injections and whose blood therefore contains antitoxin against the disease.

Superficial inflammation and infected wounds may be treated with antiseptic solutions.

PREVENTION

Immunity to certain bacterial diseases (for example, diphtheria, typhoid, whooping cough, and tetanus) can be acquired by active *immunization* (injection with weakened or killed forms of the bacteria or their poisons).

People with infections should take steps to prevent their spread; those with respiratory infections should keep away from crowded places to prevent the possibility of droplet infection, and should always use a handkerchief when coughing or sneezing. Food handlers should be meticulous about their health and personal hygiene.

Any wound should be washed with an antiseptic solution to destroy bacteria, and then covered with a clean, dry dressing.

Bactericidal

A substance that kills bacteria. (See *Antibacterial drugs*.)

Bacteriology

In medicine, this is the study of *bacteria* that cause disease. The pioneer of this science was the French chemist Louis Pasteur (1822-1895), who was the first to prove that bacteria are the cause and not the result of illness. He was followed by the German physician Robert Koch (1843-1910), who not only discovered a large number of the bacteria responsible for particular diseases but also laid down the principles for isolating and identifying disease-producing bacteria on which modern bacteriology is based.

METHODS OF IDENTIFYING BACTERIA

To discover which bacterium is causing a disease, it must be isolated. A throat swab or a specimen of urine, feces, blood, spinal fluid, sputum, or pus is first taken from an infected person. This material is then examined by one of three main methods.

STAINING The application of special stains makes it possible to look at and differentiate different bacteria under the microscope. In a sample treated with Gram's stain, for example, staphylococci, the cause of many abscesses as well as toxic shock syndrome, or streptococci would be seen to turn purple, whereas many bacteria, such as salmonella, which causes diarrhea, would turn red.

CULTURE For this method of examination, the sample material is introduced into a nutrient, where the bacteria multiply. Different antibiotics are introduced and their effects studied (see panel).

CULTURING AND TESTING BACTERIA

1 The bacteria are introduced onto a nutrient plate (i.e., agar or blood agar) and incubated at body temperature.

2 Any bacteria present multiply rapidly to form visible colonies that can be studied under the microscope and identified by different patterns of growth.

3 To test sensitivity to specific antibiotics, disks of different antibiotics are placed within the colonies of bacteria.

4 Any clear areas around each disk indicate that the bacteria are being killed by a particular antibiotic.

ANTIBODY TESTING This is done by extracting serum from the blood of an infected person and adding it to a sample of the type of bacteria suspected of causing the infection. If the suspicion is correct, antibodies against the bacteria already present in the serum will visibly clump together with the bacteria in the sample.

Bacteriostatic

A term used to describe a substance that stops the growth or multiplication of bacteria. (See *Antibacterial drugs*.)

Bacteriuria

The presence of bacteria in the urine. A small, harmless number of bacteria may be found in the urine of many healthy people, so bacteriuria is worrisome and of significance only if more than 100,000 colonies are present in each milliliter (1/30 of an ounce) of urine, or 100 bacterial colonies per milliliter if white blood cells (pus cells) are also present. This level of bacteriuria accompanies infection of the bladder, urethra, or kidneys.

Bad breath

See *Halitosis*.

Bagassosis

An occupational disease affecting the lungs of workers who handle paper and other products made from sugarcane bagasse (the fibrous residue of sugarcane after the juice has been extracted). Bagassosis is one cause of an allergic *alveolitis*, a reaction of the lungs to inhaled dust containing fungal spores.

Acute attacks usually develop four to five hours after inhalation of dust. The symptoms may include shortness of breath associated with wheezing, fever, headache, and cough; typically they last no more than 24 hours. Repeated exposure to dust may lead to permanent lung damage, chronic sickness, and weight loss. Bagassosis is a recognized industrial hazard; protective measures taken by industry have now made the disease rare.

Baker's cyst

A collection of fluid that forms a firm, walnut-sized lump behind the knee. The fluid-filled *bursa* (sac) is created by a backward "ballooning out" of the membrane covering the knee joint. Baker's cysts are caused by increased pressure within the knee due to a persistent *effusion* (secretion of fluid)—for example, in a joint affected by *rheumatoid arthritis*.

B

The cyst is usually painless and may remain for months or disappear spontaneously. Occasionally a Baker's cyst may rupture. Fluid then seeps down between the layers of the calf muscles and may cause pain and swelling.

Diagnosis may be assisted by *arthrography* (imaging of the joint with X rays after injection of radiopaque material). Treatment may consist simply of a supportive bandage, although occasionally the cyst requires surgical removal.

Balance

The ability to remain upright and move without falling over. Keeping one's balance is a complex process that relies on a constant flow of information about body position to the brain. Integration of this information and a continual flow of instructions from the brain allow various parts of the body to perform the changes needed to maintain balance.

Information about body position comes from three sources: the eyes (which give visual information about the body's position relative to its surroundings), sensory nerves in the skin, muscles, and joints (called proprioceptors, which provide information about the position and movement of the different parts of the body), and the three semicircular canals of the labyrinth in the inner ear (which detect movements and the speed of head movements). The portion of the brain called the cerebellum collates this information and instructs muscles to contract or relax.

DISORDERS

Various disorders can affect balance, particularly disorders of the inner ear, such as *labyrinthitis* (inflammation of the labyrinth) and *Meniere's disease* (abnormally high pressure of fluid in the labyrinth). In some cases, *otitis media* (inflammation of the middle ear) may also affect the inner ear and disturb balance. These disorders also cause *dizziness* or *vertigo*.

Damage to nerve tracts in the spinal cord, which carry information from proprioceptors, may occur as a result of tabes dorsalis (a complication of *syphilis*), spinal tumors, vascular disorders, or nerve degeneration due to deficiency of vitamin B_{12}. These disorders produce a distinctive, wide-based, clumsy gait.

A tumor or stroke that affects the cerebellum may cause not only clumsiness of the arms and legs, but also speech disorders and other features of impaired muscular coordination.

Balance billing

See *Assignment.*

Balanitis

Inflammation of the glans (head) of the penis and sometimes the foreskin as well. The main symptom is a painful or itchy glans, and the entire area may be red and moist. Causes include infection with bacteria or fungi, injury from a tight foreskin, or irritation by chemicals in clothing or contraceptive cream. Infection may be the result of poor hygiene, but fungal infections such as *candidiasis* (thrush) are usually contracted from a sexual partner. Uncircumcised men are more susceptible than those who are circumcised.

Washing the penis, applying a soothing cream (your physician will recommend one), and taking a course of antibiotics will relieve the symptoms. (See also *Phimosis.*)

Baldness

See *Alopecia.*

Balloon catheter

A type of *catheter* with one or more balloons, which, when inflated, keep the catheter in place or apply pressure on an organ or vessel.

USES

The oldest and simplest type, the Foley catheter, is used to drain the bladder. This catheter is passed into the bladder and water is injected into one channel to inflate the balloon, which prevents the catheter from dropping out of or being pulled out of the urethra. Urine flows out of the bladder through a second channel.

Balloon catheters are infrequently used when a blood vessel has been blocked by an *embolus* (blood clot). The end of the catheter is passed through the clot, the balloon is inflated, and, when the catheter is withdrawn, the balloon pulls the clot out with it. This is called a balloon *embolectomy.*

A type of balloon catheter with a sausage-shaped balloon is used to expand narrow arteries. In many cases this technique, known as balloon *angioplasty,* avoids the need for surgery, although narrowing of the vessel may recur.

Another use of the balloon catheter is to treat bleeding *varices* (enlarged veins in the esophagus or stomach), a life-threatening complication of some kinds of liver disease. The tube is passed down the esophagus and into the stomach, where a balloon at the tip keeps the tube in position. Another balloon higher up the tube is inflated

TYPES OF BALLOON CATHETER

Irrigation tube for fluid to wash out bladder

Sterile water tube

Tube to drain urine from bladder

Embolectomy catheter

Inflatable balloon

Urinary catheter

to compress the veins; this usually stops or controls the bleeding until the patient can be prepared for surgery.

Recently, balloons have been developed that can be placed by the catheter into a blood vessel, inflated with a quick-setting durable material, detached, and left in permanent position, thereby completely shutting off blood flow in that vessel. These catheters are used to control bleeding or to starve a tumor of its blood supply.

Balm

A soothing or healing medicine applied to the skin.

Bandage

A strip of fabric used to keep *dressings* in position, to apply pressure, to control bleeding, or to support a *sprain* or strain. Roller bandages are the traditional type of bandage and still the most widely used. Tubular gauze bandages are a newer type that are in many ways quicker and easier to apply than roller bandages. They are, however, more expensive and require a special applicator. Tubular gauze bandages are mainly used for small cuts, grazes, and burns on parts of the body that are awkward to bandage, such as a finger. Triangular bandages are used to make *slings* that support limbs. (See also *Wounds.*)

FIRST AID: APPLYING BANDAGES

TUBULAR BANDAGE

1 Cut a length of tube gauze about two and a half times the length of the finger and put it all onto the applicator. Push the applicator over the finger and hold onto the end of the gauze.

2 Still holding the gauze end on the finger, gently pull back the applicator, leaving the tube of gauze in position. Then twist it once or twice, but not more, or you may impair circulation.

3 Push the applicator back onto the finger; again, hold onto the two gauze ends, then pull it off again leaving two layers in position. Secure the ends of the gauze with tape.

ROLLER BANDAGE

1 Place the end of the bandage on the arm and hold it firmly while you make a straight turn with the rolled end to secure it.

2 Work up the limb, making a series of spiral turns so that each successive turn covers two thirds of the previous one.

3 Complete the bandaging with a straight turn, cut off the spare bandage roll, and secure the end with a safety pin, adhesive tape, or bandage clip.

Bandaging equipment
Shown, from top left, are two crepe and two gauze roller bandages, a bandage clip, safety pins, a roll of tubular bandage and applicator, and a triangular bandage.

Barbiturates

COMMON DRUGS

Amobarbital Pentobarbital Phenobarbital Secobarbital Thiopental

> **WARNING**
> Barbiturates may be habit-forming or fatal if taken with large amounts of alcohol.

A group of *sedative drugs* that works by depressing activity within the brain. Barbiturates were formerly in wide use as antianxiety drugs, sleeping drugs, and anticonvulsants. Today, their use is strictly controlled because they are habit-forming and widely abused. Overdosage can be fatal, particularly with alcohol.

WHY THEY ARE USED
Phenobarbital is still often used in the treatment of *epilepsy* (see *Anticonvulsant drugs*), and thiopental remains a drug of choice for inducing anesthesia (see *Anesthetics, general*). However, *benzodiazepines* and other nonbarbiturate drugs have now largely replaced barbiturates in the treatment of sleeplessness and anxiety (see *Sleeping drugs; Antianxiety drugs*). Barbiturates that are used today to treat sleeplessness include amobarbital, pentobarbital, and secobarbital.

HOW THEY WORK
The sedative action of barbiturates is produced by molecules of the drug passing through the membrane walls of the nerve cells within the brain. The drug blocks the conduction of stimulatory chemical signals and reduces the ability of the cells to respond.

Barbiturates, especially phenobarbital, also reduce the sensitivity of brain cells to abnormal electrical activity. This action is beneficial in the treatment of epilepsy because it reduces the likelihood of seizures.

POSSIBLE ADVERSE EFFECTS
Adverse effects include excessive drowsiness, staggering gait, and, in some cases, excitability. The depressant effect on the brain (including suppression of the respiratory center) is dangerously increased by alcohol.

Barbiturates are likely to produce dependence if used for longer than four weeks; withdrawal effects (which may include sleeplessness, twitching, nightmares, and convulsions) may occur when regular treatment is suddenly stopped. Tolerance, in which increasingly large doses are needed to produce the same effect, often develops. (See also *Drug dependence*.)

B

Barium X-ray examinations

A group of procedures used to detect and follow the progress of some diseases of the gastrointestinal tract. Powdered barium sulfate mixed with water is passed into the part of the tract that needs to be examined and *X-ray* pictures of the area are taken. Because barium, a metallic chemical, is impervious to X rays, it provides an image of the tract on the X-ray film.

WHY THEY ARE DONE

Barium X rays are among the studies used to diagnose the cause of pain or difficulty in swallowing, abdominal pain, blood-stained vomit, bleeding from the rectum, a change in bowel habits, persistent diarrhea or con-stipation, and unexplained weight loss. In many instances they have been replaced or supplemented by *endoscopy*. Disorders that can be detected include narrowing or inflam-mation of the esophagus, disorders of the swallowing mechanism, hiatal hernia, stomach and duodenal ulcers and tumors, inflammatory bowel

---

BARIUM X-RAY PROCEDURES

BARIUM SWALLOW, MEAL, AND INTESTINAL FOLLOW-THROUGH

1 No food or drink is permitted for six to nine hours beforehand.

2 At the examina-tion, the patient swallows a glass of barium mixed with a flavored liquid, or is given a piece of bread or a cookie soaked in barium if a disorder of the swallowing mecha-nism is being investigated.

3 The X-ray technician then takes X-ray pictures. For a barium swallow, the patient stands; for a barium meal, the patient lies on the table in different posi-tions; for a barium follow-through, the patient lies on the right side and X rays are taken at intervals until the barium has progressed through the small intestine.

BARIUM SMALL-BOWEL ENEMA

1 No food or drink is permitted for nine hours beforehand.

2 At the examination, the patient lies down and the X-ray technician passes a fine tube through the mouth or nose, down through the stomach and duodenum, and into the small intestine.

3 Barium is then passed down the tube directly into the small intestine.

BARIUM ENEMA

1 For successful examination, the large intestine needs to be as empty and clean as possible, since feces can obscure or simulate a polyp or tumor. For this reason the patient's intake of food and fluids is sometimes restricted for a few days before the examination, and laxatives are given.

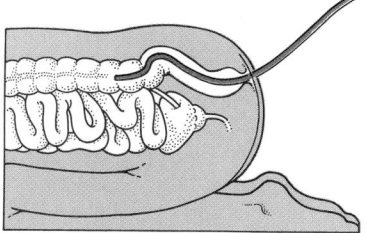

2 The patient is positioned on the X-ray table.

3 The X-ray technician introduces barium into the intestine through a tube inserted in the rectum.

X-RAY TECHNIQUES

There are two different techniques.

Double-contrast technique

Air, as well as barium liquid, is introduced into the tract. As a result, the barium does not fill the tract but forms only a film on its inner surface. This provides an image of small, surface abnormalities that would not be visible using the single-contrast technique.

Single-contrast technique

The section of intestine is filled with barium liquid, which provides an outline image that shows up prominent abnor-malities.

disease, diverticular disease, Crohn's disease, celiac disease, and colonic tumors and polyps.

HOW THEY ARE DONE

Barium X-ray examinations are generally carried out on an outpatient basis, and no anesthetic is required. A fluorescent screen connected to the X-ray machine enables the radiologist to follow the progress of the barium through the gastrointestinal tract, and to see the abnormalities outlined by the barium. Permanent records of the examination are provided by X-ray photographs or video recordings.

Because barium sulfate liquid dries out as water is absorbed in the colon, it often causes constipation. Patients may therefore need a fiber-rich diet, plenty to drink, and in some cases laxatives to get rid of the chemical.

TYPES OF EXAMINATION

Different types of barium X-ray examination are used to investigate the gastrointestinal tract.

BARIUM SWALLOW, BARIUM MEAL, BARIUM FOLLOW-THROUGH These types are used to investigate disorders of the upper gastrointestinal tract: barium swallow for the esophagus, barium meal for the lower esophagus, stomach, and duodenum, and barium follow-through for the small intestine.

In a barium swallow examination, the patient usually takes in enough air with the barium to facilitate double-contrast imaging. If a double-contrast barium meal examination is required, it is necessary to give carbonated barium, usually with gas-producing tablets or granules. Double-contrast is usually not possible for follow-through as it is too difficult to introduce air into this part of the tract.

Barium swallow and meal take about 10 minutes to perform; follow-through may last up to five hours.

BARIUM SMALL-BOWEL ENEMA Also known as enteroclysis, this single-contrast X-ray technique provides a more detailed examination of the small intestine than the barium follow-through because more barium reaches the area. Sedation may be necessary because the procedure, which takes 20 to 25 minutes, can cause some discomfort.

BARIUM ENEMA This barium technique is used to investigate disorders of the lower gastrointestinal tract: the large intestine and rectum. For a single-contrast image, the large intestine is filled with diluted barium liquid. For a double-contrast examination, a smaller quantity of thicker barium liquid is introduced, followed by air. The whole procedure lasts about 20 minutes, and in most cases causes only mild discomfort.

After the examination, a small amount of barium is expelled from the body immediately, and the rest is excreted later in the feces. (Procedures for all barium X rays are given in the panel, opposite.)

Barotrauma

Damage or pain mainly affecting the middle ear and facial sinuses caused by the effects of a change in atmospheric pressure. Air travelers are the largest group at risk, but scuba divers face similar problems, with an additional risk of damage to the lungs (see *Scuba-diving medicine*).

CAUSE

When an aircraft ascends to cruising height, cabin pressure is usually reduced by about one third. A "popping" sensation may be felt as air, trapped at ground level pressure in the middle ears and sinuses, escapes via the eustachian tubes and sinus ducts (which, respectively, link the middle ears and sinuses to air passages at the back of the throat).

When the aircraft descends, cabin pressure is increased again and becomes greater than the pressure within the ears and sinuses. Some pain may be felt as the eardrum is pushed inward. To ease this, air needs to be reintroduced into the middle ears and sinuses to equalize the internal and external pressures. This can be achieved by vigorous swallowing or an action similar to bearing down with the mouth closed and nose pinched—the Valsalva maneuver.

If the sinus ducts or eustachian tubes are blocked with mucus, as during a head cold, equalizing pressure in this way can be difficult or impossible. Minor damage can occur if equalization is prevented or delayed, or if the Valsalva maneuver is carried out overenthusiastically. The damage usually involves rupture of tiny blood vessels in the walls of the middle ears, or in the membranes lining the inside of the sinuses.

Changes in pressure sufficient to rupture the eardrum are unlikely during ordinary airline flights but may be suffered by scuba divers or high altitude pilots (see *Eardrum, perforated*).

Increased air pressure

Eardrum bulging inward

Reduced air pressure

Blocked eustachian tube

Mechanism of barotrauma
The diagram above shows the location of the middle ear and pressure changes when the eustachian tube is blocked and there is an increase in surrounding air pressure.

PREVENTION

Anyone with a severe head cold should avoid flying if possible. If flying is unavoidable, a decongestant nasal spray should be used shortly before descent. Air travelers should also know how to perform the Valsalva maneuver. Infants should be breast- or bottle-fed during descent; the baby's sucking and swallowing produces the same effect as the Valsalva maneuver.

SYMPTOMS

Pain in the ears, or over the cheekbones and forehead, during aircraft descent is a warning of pressure differences. Minor pressure damage in the middle ear, called barotitis, may cause continued pain, some hearing loss, and *tinnitus* (ringing in the ears) for a few days; pressure damage within the facial sinuses, called barosinusitis, may also cause pain, and possibly a discharge of mucus or blood for a couple of days.

TREATMENT

In most cases, no treatment is necessary and symptoms wear off within hours or days. However, if an infection is present, these symptoms may become aggravated and persist for several days. If sinus pain persists or a discharge from the nose is noticed, suggesting infection, medical advice should be sought. Treatment with antibiotic drugs, decongestant drops or nasal sprays, or sometimes *antral irrigation* may be required. (See also *Ear; Sinus; Aviation medicine*.)

Barrier cream

A cream used to protect the skin against the effects of irritant substances and of excessive exposure to water, which may occur when the hands are washed frequently. (See also *Spermicides*.)

Barrier method

Method of preventing pregnancy by blocking the passage of sperm to the woman's uterus. (See *Contraception, barrier methods*.)

Bartholin's glands

A pair of oval, pea-sized glands whose ducts open into the vulva (the folds of flesh that surround the opening of the vagina). During sexual arousal these glands secrete a fluid that lubricates the vulval region.

DISORDERS

Infection of Bartholin's glands causes bartholinitis, in which an intensely painful red swelling forms at the opening of the ducts. Treatment is with antibiotics, analgesics (painkillers), and warm baths.

If the infection develops into an *abscess*, the gland is cut open and drained—an outpatient procedure that requires only a local anesthetic. Should abscesses recur, an operation may be performed either to convert the duct into an open pouch or to remove the gland altogether.

If an infection narrows the duct by scarring, the gland may not be able to empty, and a Bartholin's cyst, a painless swelling of the duct, may form. The cyst may become repeatedly infected, in which case the same treatment as for a recurrent abscess is needed. Even if both are removed or destroyed by infection, the other glands in the vagina are capable of secreting adequate lubricants.

BARTHOLIN'S GLANDS
These glands are located on either side of the entrance to the vagina.

Vagina

Vulva

Anus

Bartholin's glands

Bartonellosis

A disease transmitted by the bite of a sand fly carrying the bacterium *BARTONELLA BACILLIFORMIS*. It is found only on the western slopes of the Andes.

The illness has two distinct forms. The first, Oroya fever, starts about three weeks after the bite and is characterized by fever, anemia, and joint pain. The second, milder form consists of crops of spots on the face and limbs. Treatment with antibiotics rapidly brings about a full recovery.

Avoidance, for travelers to the Andes, is through the use of insect repellents, insecticides, and protective clothing. (See *Insect bites*.)

Basal cell carcinoma

A type of skin cancer that occurs most commonly on the face or neck. The cells of the tumor closely resemble, and are possibly derived from, cells in the basal (innermost) skin layer.

INCIDENCE

Basal cell carcinoma is the most common skin cancer in the US with an overall incidence of about 150 cases per 100,000 population per year.

Fair-skinned persons over 50 are the most commonly affected (dark and black-skinned people are affected only rarely). The incidence also increases significantly in those with outdoor occupations and living in sunny climates—such as Arizona and Texas, or Queensland, Australia, where over half the white population has had a basal cell carcinoma by age 75.

CAUSE

Direct skin damage from ultraviolet radiation contained in sunlight is thought to be the cause in most cases. Dark-skinned people are protected by the higher amounts of the ultraviolet radiation-absorbing pigment, melanin, in their skin.

SYMPTOMS

Over 90 percent of basal cell carcinomas occur on the face, often at the side of an eye or on the nose, but the tumor can appear virtually anywhere on the body. It starts as a small, flat nodule and grows slowly, eventually breaking down at the center to form a shallow ulcer with raised edges.

Unless treated, the growth gradually invades and bites deeper into surrounding tissues.

Fortunately, basal cell carcinomas virtually never metastasize (spread to other parts of the body).

Diagnosis is made by microscopic examination of cells from the tumor.

PREVENTION

Individuals at risk, particularly fair-skinned people, should avoid overexposure to strong sunlight through the use of protective clothing and headgear, and sunscreen containing para-aminobenzoic acid (PABA).

TREATMENT AND OUTLOOK

The tumor can be destroyed by *radiation therapy* or removed by surgical excision, and this usually gives a complete cure. New tumors may, however, develop in people who do not take adequate preventive measures. (See also *Sunlight, adverse effects of; Squamous cell carcinoma; Melanoma, malignant*.)

Basal ganglia

Paired nerve cell clusters in the brain, deep within the *cerebrum* and upper part of the *brain stem*. They play a vital part in producing smooth, continuous muscular actions and in stopping and starting movement.

Disease or degeneration of the basal ganglia and their connections may lead to the appearance of involuntary movements, trembling, and weakness; the best known examples are *Parkinson's disease* and *chorea*.

LOCATION OF BASAL GANGLIA
These groups of nerve cells sit above the brain stem and under the cerebrum.

Cerebrum

Basal ganglia

Brain stem

Cerebellum

Baseball elbow

Either of two types of injury to the elbow that can occur as a result of playing baseball.

The first and more common injury is caused by repeated overstraightening of the elbow, either when pitching or batting the ball. This results in damage to the cartilage that lines the joint. Loose flakes of cartilage may then interrupt the free movement of the elbow, friction between exposed areas of bone can cause pain on elbow movement, and the eroded bony surfaces may form into osteophytes (bony spikes) that further disrupt joint movement.

Surgery to remove flakes of cartilage and trim osteophytes can help restore joint movement, but, if the individual continues to play baseball without altering his or her pitching or batting technique, the problems will return.

The second type of injury (an avulsion fracture) results from sudden straightening of the elbow at high speed when pitching. This action can cause a piece of cartilage or bone to be torn off at the point where the tendon of the biceps muscle is attached to the joint. The injury leaves the person with weakness when bending or rotating the elbow. It is treated by stitching the end of the tendon back onto its attachment to the joint. Healing normally takes about four to eight weeks. (See also *Tennis elbow; Golfers' elbow*.)

Baseball finger
Injury to the fingertip caused by a heavy blow to the end of the finger that forces the tip from a straight into a bent position. The injury, also called mallet finger, can occur in any sport where a ball (e.g., a baseball, softball, football, or basketball) strikes the finger in this way.

The sudden bending of the extended finger may tear the tendon on the back of the finger, or, if the tendon doesn't "give," pull off a fragment of bone. In either case, the fingertip is left bent. Treatment is with an external splint or the insertion of a temporary wire through the bones to hold the finger straight. The injury heals over a period of two to three months.

Battered baby syndrome
Injuries to a child that suggest repeated physical assault. They often include bruises, burns, and fractures. Usually the full extent of past injuries is apparent only when the child is examined and the complete skeleton is X rayed. (See *Child abuse*.)

B cells
See *Lymphocyte*.

BCG vaccination
A vaccine that provides immunity against *tuberculosis*. BCG is prepared from an artificially weakened strain of bovine (cattle) tubercle bacilli, the microorganisms responsible for the disease. The initials BCG stand for "bacille Calmette-Guérin," after the two Frenchmen who developed the vaccine in 1906.

WHY IT IS DONE
In the US, vaccination is usually given only to people who are likely to be exposed repeatedly to tuberculosis infection and who respond negatively to a tuberculin skin test, showing they have not naturally become immune. BCG vaccination is sometimes recommended shortly after birth—for example, if someone in the family has tuberculosis.

HOW IT IS DONE
The vaccine is usually injected into the upper arm. Six to twelve weeks later a small pustule appears. This normally heals completely, leaving a small scar. The tuberculin skin test is repeated two to three months after vaccination. If it proves negative, the vaccination should be repeated.

An occasional complication is development of a chronic ulcer because the pustule fails to heal.

Beclomethasone

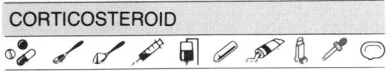

CORTICOSTEROID
Inhaler Nasal spray
Prescription needed
Not available as generic

A *corticosteroid drug* prescribed as a nasal spray to relieve the symptoms of allergic *rhinitis* and as an inhaler to treat *asthma*. Beclomethasone controls nasal symptoms by reducing inflammation and mucus production in the nose. In asthma, it helps to reduce wheezing and coughing by reducing inflammation in the bronchi. It also reduces the severity and frequency of asthma attacks. However, once an attack has started, this drug will not help relieve symptoms because it takes several hours to have any effect.

Beclomethasone is given primarily to people whose asthma does not respond to *bronchodilators* alone. Side effects may include hoarseness, throat irritation, and, rarely, fungal infections in the mouth. Irritation may be prevented by thoroughly rinsing the mouth and gargling with water after each inhalation.

Becquerel
See *Radiation* units box.

Bed bath
Method of washing a person who is confined to bed. To give a bed bath, wash and dry a small area at a time.

Bedbug

Flat, wingless, brown insect 0.20 inch (5 mm) long and 0.12 inch (3 mm) wide. Bedbugs live in furniture, especially beds, and floors during the day and emerge at night. They rarely transmit disease but their bites may become infected.

Bedpan
A metal, plastic, or fiber container into which a patient confined in bed can defecate and, if female, urinate. A *urinal* is used for male patients. In the past, bedpans and urinals were used routinely, but today, unless the patient is immobile, the use of the toilet or a bedside *commode* is considered to be less stressful.

Bed rest
A term used to describe periods spent in bed. It may be an essential part of treatment in certain illnesses, such as rheumatic fever, and for some types of injuries, such as a fractured vertebra.

Bed rest may involve various risks for the patient, among them muscle wasting, *bedsores*, weakness, depression, and calcium loss leading to bone demineralization and urinary tract *calculi* (stones). Those recovering from an operation are at special risk of developing deep vein thrombosis and, for the elderly in particular, hypostatic pneumonia is also a threat. To prevent these problems, patients today are encouraged to be physically active while in bed and are made to get out of bed sooner than in the past.

Bedridden
A term describing a person who is unable to leave bed due to illness or injury. Most likely to be confined to bed in this way are the very elderly, the terminally ill, or those paralyzed as the result of an accident.

Beds
Special beds for nursing sick or injured patients, used in hospitals and sometimes in the home.

TYPES
STANDARD HOSPITAL BED This bed is made of metal to allow it to be disinfected, mounted on wheels for

B

ease of movement, jointed to allow tilting in any direction, and adjustable in height. The higher position is used for nursing procedures; the lower position allows the patient to get in and out of bed easily. A firm mattress provides support for the patient during procedures and is generally more comfortable.

TURNING FRAMES These beds, including the Stryker frame and the Foster frame, enable patients with extensive burns, multiple injuries, pelvic and spinal fractures, or spinal cord injuries to be turned with a minimum of handling and without disturbing body alignment. The patient lies prone or supine on a canvas-covered frame. When turning is required, a second canvas is placed on top of the patient, both canvases (with the patient sandwiched between) are rotated through 180 degrees, and the top canvas is then removed.

REVOLVING CIRCULAR BED This bed is used for the same purposes as manual turning frames, but allows the patient to be placed in a variety of sitting or standing positions at any angle between vertical and horizontal. It is particularly useful in patients with spinal cord injury who may develop hypotension (fall in blood pressure) when sitting or placed upright after being immobilized in a horizontal position for a long period. Gradual rehabilitation of patients is also facilitated because they can adjust gradually from lying flat to standing upright, while remaining supported.

AIRBEDS AND WATERBEDS Beds with air- or water-filled mattresses can help prevent bedsores by providing uniform support for the patient's whole body. Airbeds are more commonly used than waterbeds because they are lighter and more comfortable for patients. A modern type of airbed, the ripplebed, has a small motor that alternately fills and empties coils inside the mattress with air, creating a rippling effect. Continuous motion stimulates the patient's circulation, which, it is claimed, helps keep the skin healthy and less prone to sores.

BALKAN FRAME This type of bed is used for the attachment of traction apparatus. It incorporates a hanging bar so that the patient can pull himself or herself up.

Bedsores

Also known as decubitus ulcers or pressure sores, these are ulcers that develop on the skin of patients who are bedridden, unconscious, or

---

PREVENTING BEDSORES

Once a bedsore has developed it will heal only if pressure on it is minimized, so good nursing care of a bedridden, immobile patient is crucial. The patient's position should be changed at least every two hours and it is important to wash and dry pressure areas carefully, especially if there is incontinence. Barrier creams can be used for additional protection.

Air flow

Ripple bed mattress
A rippling effect is created by pumping air in and out of the mattress, so stimulating the circulation.

Cushions and pillows
These can be used to relieve pressure by placing them between the knees and under the shoulder.

Sheepskins
A sheepskin under the buttocks and booties under the heels relieve pressure.

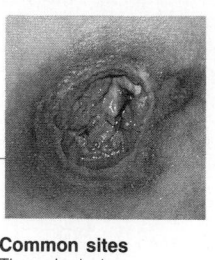

Common sites
These include the shoulders, elbows, lower back, hips and buttocks, knees, ankles, and heels.

---

immobile. They commonly affect victims of stroke or spinal cord injuries that result in a loss of sensation. Constantly wet skin, caused by incontinence, may also be a factor.

Bedsores start as red, painful areas that become purple before the skin breaks down, developing into open sores. Once the skin is broken, they often become infected, enlarge, deepen, and are very slow to heal.

TREATMENT
Deep, chronic ulcers may require treatment with antibiotics, packing with plastic foam, and possibly *plastic surgery*. New medications for topical application to the skin are constantly being evaluated.

Bed-wetting

The common name for lack of bladder control at night. (See *Enuresis*.)

Bee stings

See *Insect stings*.

Behavioral problems in children

Behavioral problems are seen occasionally in all children; specialist management is called for when they become frequent and disrupt school and/or family life. Enuresis (bed-wetting), sleep difficulties, tantrums, feeding difficulties, truancy, disobedience, stealing, jealousy, aggressive attitudes toward siblings, and alcohol and drug abuse are all common problems. When a particular form of disturbed behavior continues for a long time or forms part of a larger pattern, it has become a cause for concern. Almost inevitably, however, stressful external events, such as moving, changing schools, peer pressure, birth of a sibling, divorce, remarriage, hospitalization, chronic disease in family or child, unemployment, or death in the family may produce periods of problem behavior.

TYPES OF PROBLEM, BY AGE

Babies up to 18 months	Sleeping and feeding difficulties, colic, crying
Toddlers and small children 1-4 years	Head-banging, tantrums, biting, breath-holding attacks, separation anxiety, poor social interaction, difficulty changing from one activity to another, toilet-training problems
Early childhood 4-8 years	Nail-biting, thumb-sucking, aggression, clinginess, anxiety about illness and death, nightmares, enuresis
Middle childhood/ adolescence 9-18 years	Lying, stealing, smoking, truancy, disobedience, aggression, low achievement in school, drug or alcohol use, running away, sexual promiscuity

MANAGEMENT

BABIES Most problems resolve themselves over a matter of months; your physician will discuss any concerns you may have. (See *Crying in infants; Colic, infantile; Feeding, infant.*)

TODDLERS Parents need to be realistic and consistent in their expectations, and should provide some room for decision sharing. Toilet-training should be delayed until a child is physically and emotionally ready; separations should be carefully planned. Parents who exercise adequate self-control provide the best model for a toddler. (See *Breath-holding attacks; Toilet-training.*)

EARLY CHILDHOOD Parents should reward good behavior rather than punish bad behavior, which tends to exaggerate difficulties or create new ones. Close cooperation is needed between home and playgroup/school because children often exhibit bad behavior in only one place. (See *Enuresis; Nightmares; Thumb-sucking.*)

MIDDLE CHILDHOOD/ADOLESCENCE Firm, but not punitive, parental treatment can help the child at this stage. If the child's difficulties persist and there are stressful events happening in the

family, this may be a useful time to seek professional advice. Drug or alcohol use (or suspicions of) necessitates immediate medical attention.

OUTLOOK

Parents who find a baby difficult to care for may be better able to cope with an older child. When an older child's behavior is linked to a deterioration in the family situation, improvements can be expected when circumstances improve. Whether family problems persist or are resolved, professional advice should be sought if the child's behavior continues to be difficult. Even when the family situation is satisfactory, worried parents can benefit from the reassurance that professional advice can bring.

Behaviorism

American school of psychology founded by John Broadus Watson, PhD, early this century. He argued that, because behavior, rather than experience, was all that could be observed in others, it should constitute the sole basis of psychology.

Behavior therapy

A collection of techniques for treating mental disorders based on changing abnormal behavior rather than attempting to analyze underlying causes. Behavior therapy can be effective in the treatment of phobic and obsessional disorders and certain kinds of sexual and marital problems. Behavior therapy deals with eliminating the symptom without affecting the underlying psychological cause. Often, it is not the procedure but the unspoken relationship with the therapist performing the behavior modification that is really important.

The concept of behavior modification originated with animal psychologists, but the techniques have been expanded and refined by psychiatrists in the last decade. Treatment relies on two basic ideas: that repetition of a feared experience under safe conditions will render it less threatening, and that desirable behavior can be encouraged by using a system of rewards. Aversion therapy—using punishment to discourage undesirable behavior—was used in the past, particularly in the treatment of alcoholics and drug addicts.

TYPES

EXPOSURE THERAPY Also called desensitization, this consists of exposing the patient in stages to the cause of his or her anxiety. At the same time, the patient is taught to cope

with anxiety symptoms by using relaxation techniques. The intensity of the anxiety-provoking stimulus is gradually increased until the patient is able to deal with the situation.

FLOODING Instead of being introduced to the cause of the phobia in stages, the patient is confronted with the anxiety-provoking stimuli at once, but with the support of the therapist. The patient remains in this situation until the feelings of anxiety eventually disappear.

RESPONSE PREVENTION The patient is prevented from carrying out an obsessional task. This technique is used in combination with other methods.

MODELING The therapist acts as a model for the patient, performing the anxiety-provoking activity first, so that the patient may copy.

HOW IT IS USED

TREATMENT OF PHOBIC DISORDERS This is dependent on exposure therapy. In *agoraphobia* (fear of open spaces), the patient is reassured that he or she can cope outside the house, and then the therapist accompanies him or her on a short journey, providing emotional support. The patient uses relaxation techniques to help cope with anxiety. Gradually, the distance traveled from home is increased, and the therapist withdraws from the treatment as the patient gains confidence.

Flooding techniques are especially useful in treating fears of objects. A patient who is frightened of dogs might be placed in a room with a number of dogs until the fear disappears.

TREATMENT OF OBSESSIONAL RITUALS This consists of three different aspects: prevention, exposure, and modeling. For example, a patient with a hand washing compulsion would be prevented from carrying out the washing rituals. At the same time, exposure to materials that the patient might consider contaminated is encouraged, the therapist acting as a model by touching the "contaminated" objects first.

TREATMENT OF MARITAL AND SEXUAL PROBLEMS This is based on partners rewarding each other for pleasing behavior. (See *Marital counseling; Sex therapy.*)

Behçet's syndrome

A rare disorder of which the most frequent symptom is recurrent mouth ulcers, which are more severe than the common (aphthous) ulcers in the mouth. Other major symptoms are ulcers on the genitals, eye inflammation, rashes, arthritis, and venous thrombosis. Less common manifestations include intestinal ulcers, arterial *aneurysms, epididymo-orchitis,* and neuropsychiatric symptoms. Behçet's syndrome was first described by the Turkish dermatologist Hulusi Behçet (1889-1948).

The cause of the disorder is unknown. It is uncommon in the US, but more common in some Middle Eastern countries.

The diagnosis relies on three or more of the major characteristic symptoms being present. Treatment is difficult and may require use of *anticancer drugs* or *corticosteroid drugs*. The condition becomes chronic in many patients.

Belching

The noisy return of air from the stomach through the mouth. Swallowing air is usually a nervous habit of which the person is unaware. It also may be due to eating or drinking too much too quickly.

Each time a person belches, he or she swallows air, which makes further belching more likely. Sometimes, belching helps alleviate discomfort caused by indigestion or acid *dyspepsia*. During pregnancy, belching very briefly helps relieve nausea and heartburn, which disappear following delivery of the baby.

Belladonna

An extract of the deadly nightshade plant, containing *alkaloids* including atropine, which has been used in medicine since ancient times. Women used to apply belladonna to their eyes to dilate the pupils (the name in Italian means beautiful lady). In modern medicine belladonna alkaloids are used as *antispasmodics* in the treatment of gastrointestinal disturbances. (See *Anticholinergic drugs*.)

Bell's palsy

Another name for *facial palsy*.

Bendroflumethiazide

One of the thiazide group of *diuretics* used to treat *hypertension* (high blood pressure) and *heart failure* (reduced pumping efficiency).

Bends

A term popularly applied to all forms of *decompression sickness* suffered by divers who surface too rapidly, or sometimes more specifically to the severe bone and joint pains that are a common symptom.

The origin of the term "bends" is uncertain, but it may have referred to

the diver being literally bent double in pain, or to the slight easing of pain achieved by flexing an affected joint.

Benign

The term used to describe a relatively mild form of a disease. More specifically, a benign tumor will not spread throughout the body, whereas a *malignant* tumor may.

Benoxaprofen

A *nonsteroidal anti-inflammatory drug* (NSAID) introduced in the early 1980s. It proved very effective in the treatment of arthritis. Unfortunately, in some users, it caused photosensitization (rash when exposed to sunlight). More seriously, its use was associated with a number of deaths, mainly in the elderly, from liver damage. It was therefore withdrawn from the market.

Benzodiazepine drugs

Among the best-known and most widely prescribed drugs in the world, benzodiazepines are used mainly as *tranquilizers* for the control of symptoms due to *anxiety* or *stress* and as sleeping tablets for *insomnia*.

WHY THEY ARE USED

For the regular treatment of anxiety, benzodiazepines are given for short periods to promote mental and physical relaxation. They reduce feelings of agitation and restlessness, slow mental activity, and relax the muscles.

Most benzodiazepines also have a strong sedative effect and help to relieve *insomnia*. They cause drowsiness and sleep when given in a higher dose than that used to treat anxiety.

Benzodiazepines are used in the management of alcohol withdrawal and in the control of *epilepsy*.

HOW THEY WORK

Benzodiazepines promote sleep and relieve anxiety by depressing brain function. By interfering with chemical activity in the brain and nervous system, they reduce the communication between nerve cells. This leads to a reduction in brain activity, which varies in proportion to the amount of drug taken.

POSSIBLE ADVERSE EFFECTS

Minor adverse effects include daytime drowsiness, dizziness, and forgetfulness. Benzodiazepines may also cause unsteadiness and may slow reactions thus impairing the ability to drive or operate machinery.

The main risk of benzodiazepines is that regular users may become psychologically and physically depen-

dent on them. For this reason, they are usually given for courses of two to three weeks or less. When benzodiazepines are stopped suddenly, withdrawal symptoms, such as excessive anxiety, nightmares, and restlessness, may occur. When they are taken for longer than two weeks, they are therefore withdrawn gradually under medical supervision.

Benzodiazepines have been abused for their sedative effect and so they are prescribed with caution.

Benzoyl peroxide

An *antiseptic* agent used in the treatment of *acne*.

Bereavement

The death of a loved relative or friend and the emotional reaction following such a loss. A bereaved person's feelings will vary in intensity according to his or her level of maturity and the nature of emotional problems or conflict in the bereaved person prior to the loss. Also involved is the nature and quality of the bereaved person's relationship with the deceased and the kind of relationship they shared before the death. The expression of grief is individual to each person, but there are recognized stages of bereavement, each one characterized by a particular attitude.

STAGES OF BEREAVEMENT

Numbness, hallucinations, and an unwillingness to recognize the death are defense mechanisms against admitting and therefore accepting the loss and associated pain. Numbness is the pervading feeling that enables the bereaved person to get through the funeral arrangements, family gatherings, and applications for pensions and insurances. It can last anywhere from three days to three months. Often, the reality of the death does not penetrate completely at this time, and many people continue to behave as if the dead person were still alive. Hallucinations, too, are a common experience among the recently bereaved. They may consist of a sense of having seen or heard the dead person, or of having been aware of his or her presence. This comforts some people but others find it disturbing.

Depression is a reaction to loss. Once the numbness wears off and the bereaved person can know and feel that a loss has occurred, he or she may be overwhelmed by feelings of anxiety, anger, and despair that can develop into a depressive illness (see *Depression*). Gastrointestinal disturbances and mental disorders are not uncommon, nor is attempted suicide, which is an abnormal expression of grief. An increase in the intake of alcohol, tranquilizers, and other drugs is common, but may cause problems. Insomnia, malaise, agitation, and tearfulness are normal.

ACCEPTANCE Gradually, but usually within two years, the bereaved person adjusts to the loss and begins to make positive plans for the future. This process can involve periods of pain and despair (sometimes mourning occurs in "waves"), alternating with ones of enthusiasm and interest; eventually, positiveness usually triumphs over despair. Research suggests, however, that the death of a spouse may increase the mortality for people in every age group, although there is little consistent information on the length of survival after widowhood. Survival may depend on whether the bereaved can develop or tries to develop other relationships.

SUPPORT AND COUNSELING
Family and friends can often provide the support a bereaved person needs, but sometimes other factors can impede the recovery process. Outside help may be required and may be given by a social worker, health visitor, clergy, or self-help group (the number of self-help groups is increasing in the US). For some people, however, the care of a psychiatrist is necessary when depression, apathy, and lethargy obstruct any chance of recovery. In these cases, specialized *counseling* and *psychotherapy* should be encouraged by family and friends. (See also *Stillbirth*.)

Beriberi

A metabolic disorder resulting from a lack of thiamine (vitamin B_1) in the diet. The illness is seen only in people who are starving or on an extremely restricted diet (such as alcoholics). Breast-fed babies can develop beriberi if their mother's milk is seriously deficient in thiamine as a result of severe dietary restriction.

CAUSES
Thiamine, found in whole-grain cereals, meat, green vegetables, potatoes, and nuts, is essential for the metabolism of carbohydrates. Without it, the brain, nerves, and muscles (including the heart muscle) cannot function properly.

INCIDENCE
Beriberi occurs among underfed populations in developing countries. The illness was once a major problem in the Far East among people subsisting on rice from which the thiamine-rich outer layer had been removed, but improved milling has led to a dramatic decline in the disorder.

In developed countries, the illness is restricted to chronic alcoholics, those living in extreme poverty, and elderly people on a very poor diet.

SYMPTOMS AND SIGNS
Two forms of the illness—"dry" and "wet" beriberi—are recognized. In dry beriberi, the thiamine deficiency mainly affects the nerves and skeletal muscles. Symptoms include numbness, a burning sensation in the legs, and wasting of the muscles. In severe cases, the patient becomes emaciated, virtually paralyzed, and bedridden.

In wet beriberi, the main problem is *heart failure* (inability of the heart to keep up with its task of pumping blood). This in turn leads to congestion of blood in the veins, and *edema* (swelling caused by fluid collection) in the legs and sometimes the trunk and face. Other symptoms include poor appetite, rapid pulse, and breathlessness. As the heart failure worsens, breathing becomes difficult and, without medical treatment, the patient will die.

DIAGNOSIS AND TREATMENT
The diagnosis is usually obvious from the symptoms and environmental factors; it can be confirmed by a test of the thiamine level in the blood.

Treatment consists of thiamine, given orally or by injection, which brings a rapid and complete cure.

Berylliosis

An occupational disease caused by the inhalation of dust or fumes containing beryllium, a metallic element that, with its compounds, is used in high-technology industries, such as nuclear energy, electronics, and aerospace.

Short exposure to high concentrations of beryllium may lead to an episode of severe *pneumonitis* (lung inflammation) characterized by coughing and breathlessness. Exposure over many years to smaller concentrations may lead to more permanent lung and liver damage. The lung changes may lead eventually to severe breathlessness after the slightest exertion.

Treatment with *corticosteroid drugs* can help alleviate the symptoms of berylliosis, but does not alter the course of the illness. The main emphasis is on preventing the disease through adequate protection against beryllium fumes.

Beta-blocker drugs

COMMON DRUGS

Cardioselective
Acebutolol Atenolol Metoprolol

Noncardioselective
Nadolol Oxprenolol Propranolol

WARNING
Do not suddenly stop taking a beta-blocker; a severe recurrence of your previous symptoms and a significant rise in blood pressure may result.

A group of drugs, also known as beta-adrenergic blocking agents, prescribed principally to treat heart disorders. They have been used since the 1960s and, although other, newer drugs have been found to treat many of the conditions for which they are effective, beta-blockers are still prescribed widely today.

WHY THEY ARE USED
Beta-blockers are used in the treatment of *angina pectoris* (chest pain due to a lack of oxygen in the heart muscle), *hypertension* (high blood pressure), and cardiac *arrhythmia* (irregular heart beat). They are sometimes given after a *myocardial infarction* (heart attack) to reduce the likelihood of further damage to the heart muscle.

Beta-blockers may also be given to prevent *migraine* attacks and to reduce the physical symptoms of *anxiety* (such as palpitations, tremor, and excessive sweating). They may be given to control symptoms of *thyrotoxicosis* (overactive thyroid gland). A beta-blocker is sometimes given in the form of eye drops in the treatment of *glaucoma* (raised fluid pressure in the eyeball) to lower the fluid pressure.

HOW THEY WORK
See explanatory box, overleaf.

POSSIBLE ADVERSE EFFECTS
By reducing heart rate and air flow to the lungs, beta-blockers may reduce an individual's capacity for strenuous exercise, although this may not be noticed if physical activity is already limited by heart problems.

Beta-blockers may worsen the symptoms of asthma, bronchitis, or other lung disease. They may also reduce blood flow to the limbs and thus aggravate peripheral vascular disease.

If long-term treatment with beta-blockers is abruptly withdrawn, there may be a sudden severe recurrence of the patient's symptoms and a significant rise in blood pressure. These problems can be avoided by gradually decreasing the dosage.

HOW BETA-BLOCKERS WORK

Beta-blockers block beta-receptors—specific sites on body tissues where *neurotransmitters* (chemicals released from nerve endings) bind. There are two types of beta-receptor: beta$_1$-receptors found in heart tissue and beta$_2$-receptors found in the lungs, blood vessels, and other tissues. The neurotransmitter chemicals epinephrine and norepinephrine are released from nerve endings in the *sympathetic nervous system*, the part of the involuntary nervous system that enables the body to deal with stress, anxiety, and exercise. These neurotransmitters bind to beta-receptors to increase the force and speed of the heart beat, to dilate the airways to increase air flow to the lungs, and to dilate blood vessels.

Cardioselective beta-blockers combine predominantly with beta$_1$-receptors; noncardioselective beta-blockers combine with both types.

Beta-blockers slow heart rate and reduce the force of contraction of the heart muscle. These effects can be used to slow a fast heart rate and regulate abnormal rhythms.

Beta-blockers prevent angina pectoris attacks by reducing the work performed by the heart muscle and so the heart's oxygen requirement. High blood pressure is reduced because the rate and force at which the heart pumps blood into the circulation is lowered.

The effect of blocking beta-receptors on tissues elsewhere in the body is to reduce the muscle tremor of anxiety and an overactive thyroid gland. Beta-blockers can help to reduce the frequency of migraine attacks by preventing the dilation of blood vessels surrounding the brain, which is responsible for the headache. In glaucoma they lower pressure in the eye by reducing fluid production in the eyeball.

Cardioselective beta-blockers
These beta-blockers occupy beta$_1$-receptors on heart tissue and have only a mild effect on beta$_2$-receptors in the bronchi of the lungs. These drugs are used in the treatment of heart disorders to reduce the work load of the heart,

thus slowing the rate and reducing the force of contractions. They are less likely than other beta-blockers to cause breathing difficulty.

Types of beta-receptors
Beta$_1$-receptors occur mainly in the heart muscle; beta$_2$-receptors are found in the lungs, blood vessels, and certain tissues. Beta-blocker drugs bind to beta-receptors, thereby blocking neurotransmitters.

Betamethasone

CORTICOSTEROID

Tablet Syrup Injection Cream Spray

Prescription needed

Available as generic

Betamethasone is used in the treatment of inflammation. It is used to treat *eczema* and *psoriasis* and to reduce the severity and frequency of *asthma*. To be effective as a treatment for asthma, it must be inhaled regularly. Betamethasone is also prescribed to treat allergic *rhinitis*.

As a tablet, betamethasone is used to treat severe cases of asthma and *arthritis*. It is also occasionally used to reduce cerebral edema (swelling in the brain) and, in women about to deliver prematurely, to lessen the risk to the baby of developing *respiratory distress syndrome*.

POSSIBLE ADVERSE EFFECTS
Adverse effects are unlikely to occur when betamethasone is inhaled or used as ear drops. This is because the dose that reaches the bloodstream is low. A higher dose may be absorbed when the drug is applied to the skin and for this reason it is only prescribed as a short-term treatment for skin disorders and the user is advised to apply it sparingly. Even when used with caution, betamethasone can cause thinning of the skin. It may also aggravate a skin infection and is therefore sometimes prescribed with an antibiotic if skin infection is present. Taking betamethasone tablets for a prolonged period or in high doses can cause adverse effects typical of other *corticosteroid drugs*.

Bezoar

A ball of food and mucus, vegetable fiber, hair, or other indigestible material, in the stomach. Bezoars are rare in adults except after partial *gastrectomy* (removal of part of the stomach). Trichobezoars (composed of hair) occur in children who nibble at, or pull out and swallow, their hair, or in adult patients who have severe emotional disturbances.

Bezoars can cause loss of appetite, constipation, nausea and vomiting, and abdominal pain. If they pass into the intestines they may cause an obstruction. Bezoars are diagnosed by means of a *barium X-ray examination* or *gastroscopy* (passage of a viewing tube down the digestive tract), and are removed by washing out the stomach (see *Lavage, gastric*), by use of a pincer attachment to the gastroscope, by surgery, or by use of drugs to digest the protein portion of the bezoar.

A low-fiber diet may help prevent recurrent bezoars in affected adults.

Bi-
The prefix meaning two or twice, as in bilateral (two-sided).

Bicarbonate of soda
See *Sodium bicarbonate.*

Biceps muscle
The name, meaning "two heads," given to a muscle originating at one end as two separate parts, which then fuse. The biceps in the upper arm bends the arm and rotates the forearm; the biceps muscle at the back of the thigh bends the leg and extends the thigh.

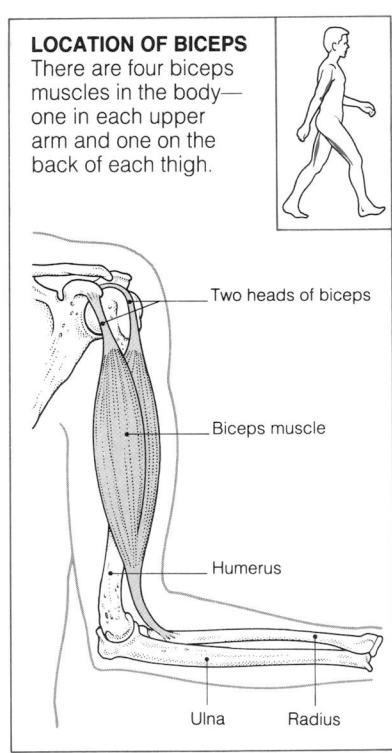

LOCATION OF BICEPS
There are four biceps muscles in the body—one in each upper arm and one on the back of each thigh.

Two heads of biceps

Biceps muscle

Humerus

Ulna   Radius

Bicuspid
The term meaning to have two cusps (curved, pointed structures) used to describe certain *heart valves* and *teeth*.

Bifocal
A term used to describe a lens with two different focal lengths. Glasses with bifocal lenses correct the eyes for both close and distant vision.

Bilateral
Affecting both sides of the body, or affecting both organs if they are paired (e.g., both ears in bilateral deafness).

Bile
A liquid secreted by the liver. It carries away waste products formed in the liver and helps break down fats in the small intestine during digestion.

The main constituents of bile, apart from waste products (such as the pigments *bilirubin* and biliverdin, which give the liquid its greenish-brown color) are *cholesterol* and bile salts. It is the bile salts that aid in the breakdown and absorption of fats.

Bile passes out of the liver via the bile ducts and is then concentrated and stored in the gallbladder until, after a meal, it is expelled and enters the small intestine by way of the common bile duct. Bile is normally excreted from the body in the feces, which it colors dark brown. (See also *Biliary system.*)

Bile duct
Any of the ducts by which bile is carried from the liver, first to the gallbladder and then to the duodenum (the first section of the small intestine).

STRUCTURE
The bile duct system starts as tiny tubular canals called canaliculi that surround the liver cells and collect the bile. Canaliculi join together to form a network of cholangioles of ever-increasing size, which emerge from the liver, on the underside, as the two hepatic ducts.

These ducts join within or just outside the liver to form the common hepatic duct and, shortly after the junction, another duct known as the cystic duct branches off to the gallbladder. This lies in a hollow on the undersurface of the liver. The continuation of the common hepatic duct past the junction with the cystic duct is known as the common bile duct. This leads directly into the duodenum. (See also *Biliary system.*)

Bile duct cancer
See *Cholangiocarcinoma.*

Bile duct obstruction
A blockage or constriction of any of the ducts that carry bile from the liver to the gallbladder and then to the duodenum (see *Biliary system*).

This results in *cholestasis* (accumulation of bile in the liver), and the development of *jaundice* due to

accumulation of *bilirubin* in the blood. Prolonged obstruction over many years can lead to secondary *biliary cirrhosis*, a serious type of advanced liver disease.

CAUSES
The bile ducts can become blocked or narrowed for a variety of reasons. *Gallstones* are perhaps the most common cause. They have usually formed in the gallbladder and escaped into the common bile duct.

A tumor of the pancreas can compress the lower end of the common bile duct, and occasionally cancers of other organs may spread to the biliary system and cause obstruction. Cancer of the bile ducts, *cholangiocarcinoma*, is a very rare cause of blockage.

Other causes include trauma, including injury during gallbladder operations, *cholangitis* (inflammation of the bile ducts), and, in the Far East, the entry of various flukes or worms into the ducts.

SYMPTOMS
All patients develop "obstructive" jaundice, characterized by pale-colored feces (due to lack of the normal bilirubin content) and dark urine (excess bilirubin content) as well as the yellow skin coloration. Some patients complain of itching caused by the presence of bile salts in the skin.

Other symptoms depend on the cause of the biliary obstruction—for example, abdominal pain with gallstones or weight loss with many types of cancer.

DIAGNOSIS AND TREATMENT
Liver function tests show any blockage, which can be confirmed by *ultrasound scanning* and *cholangiography* or *ERCP*.

Treatment consists of removing the cause of the obstruction if possible—by surgery or by means of an attachment to an *endoscope* (viewing instrument) passed down the digestive tract and up the common bile duct. When the obstruction is due to cancer too advanced for surgical removal, the obstruction is usually bypassed to relieve the jaundice. A loop of intestine may then be joined to the gallbladder or biliary system above the blockage. Another possibility is to push a tube through the blockage, either from the intestinal side using an endoscope or with catheters from the liver side of the duct under X-ray viewing. The tube is left in place for bile to flow through.

Bilharziasis
An alternative name for the tropical parasitic disease *schistosomiasis*.

B

Biliary atresia

A rare disorder, present from birth, in which the bile ducts, either outside or inside the liver, fail to develop or have developed abnormally. As a result, bile cannot flow through the ducts to the duodenum (the first part of the small intestine) and becomes trapped in the liver (see *Cholestasis*). Unless treated, secondary *biliary cirrhosis* will develop and may prove fatal.

The main signs of biliary atresia are deepening *jaundice*, which usually appears a few days after birth and persists more than two weeks, together with the passing of dark-colored urine and pale feces.

DIAGNOSIS AND TREATMENT

If biliary atresia is suspected, blood tests and *liver biopsy* (removal and examination of a small sample of the organ) are performed. These tests rule out *hepatitis* or other causes of jaundice in the newborn infant. An operation is then performed to examine the liver and bile ducts directly. If this confirms the diagnosis of biliary atresia, surgery is done to bypass the ducts by joining a loop of small intestine directly to the liver. If the bypass operation fails, or if the jaundice recurs, a *liver transplant* is the only possible treatment.

FUNCTION OF THE BILIARY SYSTEM

The system consists of the bile ducts leading from the liver and gallbladder, the gallbladder itself, and associated structures. The system drains waste products from the liver into the duodenum and aids the process of fat digestion through controlled release of fat-emulsifying agents (contained within bile).

FAT DIGESTION

1 Dietary fat passes from the stomach to the duodenum in the form of large droplets.

2 Bile released into the duodenum contains salts that disperse the fat into smaller droplets.

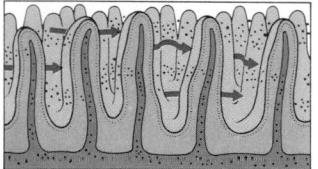

3 The fats are now more easily broken down by an enzyme, lipase, made by the pancreas, and absorbed through the intestinal lining.

X ray of gallbladder
The image at left shows the pearlike shape of the gallbladder. It was achieved by an X-ray imaging technique called cholecystography.

Liver
Bile is secreted by liver cells and collected in a system of tubes (drainage channels) These tubes carry bile out of the liver via the hepatic ducts.

Common bile duct
The hepatic ducts join to form a common duct, which leads to the intestine. A side branch, the cystic duct, leads to the gallbladder.

Gallbladder
Bile is concentrated and stored here and released back into the common bile duct when this organ contracts.

Duodenum
When fat from a recent meal arrives in the duodenum, a hormone is released that acts on the gallbladder. The gallbladder contracts, causing bile to be passed into the duodenum to emulsify the fat.

Pancreas
In response to the presence of fat in the duodenum, the pancreas produces hormones that stimulate contraction of the gallbladder and cause the ampulla of Vater to open so that bile flows into the duodenum.

Ampulla of Vater
Bile enters the duodenum here.

Stomach
Fat and other products of digestion pass from the stomach to the duodenum.

Food

Ileum

Biliary cirrhosis

An uncommon variety of liver *cirrhosis* that results from disease or defects of the bile ducts.

There are two types: primary and secondary biliary cirrhosis. Both types are characterized by *cholestasis* (accumulation of bile in the liver), which impairs liver function.

PRIMARY BILIARY CIRRHOSIS

Here, the bile ducts within the liver become inflamed and destroyed. The cause is unknown, but the disease seems to be associated with a malfunction of the *immune system*. Middle-aged women are the group most commonly affected.

The first symptom is itching, followed later by *jaundice*, an enlarged liver, and sometimes abdominal pain, fatty diarrhea, and *xanthomatosis* (the appearance of fatty deposits under the skin). *Osteoporosis* may develop. Over a number of years the patient may develop other symptoms of liver cirrhosis and *liver failure*.

The disease is diagnosed by *liver function tests*, by *liver biopsy*, and by *cholangiography* or *ERCP*. Drug treatment has been aimed mainly at relieving symptoms, such as itching, and minimizing complications. A *liver transplant*, if available, provides the only long-term cure.

SECONDARY BILIARY CIRRHOSIS

This results from prolonged *bile duct obstruction* or *biliary atresia* (absence or abnormality of the bile ducts from birth). The symptoms and signs include abdominal pain and tenderness, liver enlargement, fevers and chills, and sometimes blood abnormalities. Treatment is as for bile duct obstruction or biliary atresia.

Biliary colic

A severe pain in the upper right quadrant of the abdomen usually caused by the gallbladder's attempts to expel *gallstones* or the movement of a stone in the bile ducts. The pain, which is extremely severe and can mimic that of a heart attack, often lasts up to an hour; it may radiate to the right shoulder or penetrate through to the center of the back from the tip of the breastbone. Injections of an analgesic (painkiller) and an *antispasmodic drug* may be given to relieve the colic. Tests such as *cholecystography* or *ultrasound scanning* are usually carried out to determine whether gallstones are definitely present; if they are, *cholecystectomy* (removal of the gallbladder) may be considered.

Biliary system

The organs and ducts by which bile is formed, concentrated, and carried from the liver to the duodenum (the first part of the small intestine). It removes waste products from the liver and carries bile salts, necessary for the breakdown and absorption of fat, to the intestine.

Bile is secreted by the liver cells and collected by a system of tubes that mirror the blood supply to the organ. This network of bile-drainage channels carries the bile out of the liver by way of the hepatic ducts, which join together to form a common duct, running into the duodenum by way of a controlled opening called the ampulla of Vater. Bile does not run directly into the duodenum but is first concentrated and then stored until needed in the gallbladder, a pear-shaped reservoir lying in a hollow under the liver, to which it gains access by way of the cystic duct.

When food is eaten, the presence of fat in the duodenum causes the secretion of a hormone, which opens the ampulla of Vater and causes the gallbladder to contract, squeezing stored bile via the cystic and common bile ducts into the duodenum. Bile salts act to emulsify fat, breaking it down to a kind of milk of microscopic globules, which are easily absorbed in the small intestine.

DISORDERS

The main disorder of the gallbladder is the formation of *gallstones*, which can have multiple complications affecting the entire biliary system (see *Gallbladder* disorders box). The main disorders of the bile ducts are congenital *biliary atresia* (absence or abnormality of the bile ducts from birth) and *bile duct obstruction*, which may itself be caused by gallstones or by other causes, such as cancer. Bile duct obstruction can have important complications affecting the liver.

Biliousness

A term commonly and erroneously used to describe nausea or vomiting. More accurately, biliousness describes a condition in which bitter bile is brought up to the mouth from the stomach.

Bilirubin

The main pigment found in *bile*. It is produced by the breakdown of *hemoglobin*, the red pigment in blood cells. Bilirubin is responsible for the brown color of feces and is the pigment associated with jaundice.

Billings' method

A technique (also called mucus inspection method) in which a woman notes changes in her normal vaginal discharge to predict the time of ovulation for *contraception* or *family planning*.

Billroth's operation

A type of partial *gastrectomy* (surgical removal of the lower part of the stomach) devised by the Viennese surgeon Theodor Billroth. It was the first successful operation on the stomach and is still one of the standard operations today for the treatment of peptic ulcer and certain types of gastric tumor.

Binet's test

The first *intelligence test* that attempted to measure higher mental functions rather than more primitive abilities, such as reaction times. It was devised by Alfred Binet and Theodor Simon for French schoolchildren in 1905.

Binge-purge syndrome

A feature of the psychiatric illness *bulimia*, characterized by the ingestion of large quantities of food and their elimination by induced vomiting or through abuse of laxatives. (See also *Anorexia nervosa*.)

Bio-

A prefix that describes a relationship to life, as in biology, the science of life.

Bioavailability

The amount of a drug that enters the bloodstream and thus reaches the tissues and organs around the body, usually expressed as a percentage of the dose given. In this way, the effectiveness of various means of administration or types of preparation can be compared. For instance, intravenous administration produces 100 percent bioavailability since the drug is injected directly into the bloodstream. Drugs given by mouth have a much lower bioavailability, because only a proportion of the drug can be absorbed through the digestive system; some drugs may be broken down in the liver before reaching the general circulation.

Preparations that have the same bioavailability are said to be "bioequivalent." (See also *Drugs*.)

Biochemistry

A science that studies the chemistry of living organisms, including human beings. The human body is made up of millions of cells that require nutrients and energy, and which grow, multiply, and die. The chemical processes that provide their energy, eliminate their wastes, repair damage, and lead to growth and normal and abnormal cell division are all studied by biochemists.

Life is maintained by a huge number of chemical reactions, which are carried out inside cells and are linked in a complex way. These reactions make up the body's *metabolism*, which has two main aspects. The reactions that produce energy by breaking down food, energy stores, and body structures are known as catabolism. The reactions that build up body structures and energy stores are known as anabolism. These processes are controlled largely by *hormones*—simple chemicals secreted into the bloodstream by the *endocrine glands*—and are actually carried out by *enzymes* (biological catalysts).

Some vital chemical processes occur in every cell in the body; others are confined to specialist organs. (When cells of the same type mass together they form a particular type of *tissue*, which makes up organs such as the heart.) For instance, after digestion, the chemical constituents of food are carried in the portal vein to the liver for storage and chemical manipulation. In addition to regulating the amount of fluid in the body, the kidneys control the amounts of minerals and other basic materials in the blood.

There is a constant interchange between fluids, which move in and out of the cells, and blood and urine. As a consequence, biochemists can learn about the chemical changes going on inside cells from measurements of the various minerals, gases, enzymes, hormones, and proteins contained in blood and urine. Such tests are used to make diagnoses, to screen people for disease, and to monitor the progress of a disease and its treatment. The most important biochemical tests are *blood tests*, such as *liver function tests*, *kidney function tests*, and parts of *urinalysis*.

Biofeedback training

A technique in which a person uses information about a normally unconscious body function, such as blood pressure, to gain conscious control over that function.

WHY IT IS USED

Biofeedback training may help in the treatment of stress-related conditions, including certain types of hypertension, anxiety, and migraine.

HOW IT IS DONE

The physician connects the patient to a recording instrument that can measure one of the unconscious body activities: blood pressure, pulse rate, body temperature, muscle tension, the amount of sweat on the skin, brain waves, or stomach acidity. The patient receives information (feedback) on the changing levels of these activities from alterations in the instrument's signals—a flashing light, a fluctuating needle, or a sound changing its tone.

After some experience, the person starts to become aware of how he or she is feeling whenever there is a change in the recording instrument's signal. Relaxation techniques may also be used to bring about a change in the signal; the instrument's response may indicate which methods of relaxation are most effective.

With time, the patient learns to change the signals by consciously controlling the body function being tested. Once acquired, control can be exercised without the instrument.

Example of biofeedback training
Here, a patient learns to relax using a device that monitors sweatiness of the palm.

Biomechanical engineering

A discipline that applies engineering principles and methods to the human body to explain how it functions and to treat disorders. Joint movements, the reaction of bone to stress, and the flow of blood are among the body activities that can be looked at in terms of these principles. Practical applications are varied and include the design of artificial joints, renal dialysis machines, and artificial heart valves.

Biopsy

A diagnostic test in which tissue or cells are removed from the body for examination under the microscope.

Most of these procedures are minor and require no sedation, but some require anesthesia. Biopsy is an accurate method of diagnosing many illnesses, including cancer.

The term "biopsy" is also commonly used by the public for the cell or tissue sample itself (although the term "biopsy specimen" is more correct).

WHY IT IS DONE

Microscopic examination of tissue (*histology*) or cells (*cytology*) usually gives a correct diagnosis. Biopsy is valuable for discovering whether a tumor is benign or malignant, since the malignant tumor usually has many features that clearly distinguish it from a benign tumor. In the case of a malignant tumor, biopsies of the surrounding tissue and the lymph nodes can be done to determine whether the cancer has spread. Another important use of biopsies is to determine the cause of unexplained infections and inflammations.

HOW IT IS DONE

SKIN OR MUSCLE BIOPSY This consists of cutting away a small piece of skin or muscle for analysis. The skin or muscle biopsy is a straightforward procedure that requires only a local anesthetic.

NEEDLE BIOPSY A needle is inserted through the skin and into the organ or tumor to be investigated. The needle may be fitted with a cutting tip to help remove a piece of tissue for microscopic examination. Aspiration biopsy is another type of needle biopsy in which the cells that are sucked from a tumor are examined cytologically. In most cases only a local anesthetic is required.

Until recently, if the target area could not be felt through the skin, or the organ was not accessible by endoscopic biopsy (see below), the physician would have to work "blindly," relying only on experience and a knowledge of anatomy, so that deep-needle biopsy was almost never done. Today, "guided" biopsy, using *ultrasound scanning* or *CT scanning* to precisely locate the tissue to be biopsied and follow the progress of the needle, makes the procedure far more accurate, safe, and productive. In addition, the recent use of very fine needles for biopsies allows for safe sampling of tumors in organs such as the salivary glands and pancreas, in which sampling with larger needles was considered dangerous.

ENDOSCOPIC BIOPSY An *endoscope* (instrument with a viewing lens) is passed into the organ to be investigated and an attachment (forceps to remove tissue and brushes to remove cells) is used to take a sample.

The procedure, which usually requires sedation, is used to take samples from the lining of accessible hollow organs, such as the colon, esophagus, stomach, and bladder.

OPEN BIOPSY This is part of an operation, usually requiring a general anesthetic, in which the surgeon opens a body cavity, such as the chest or abdomen, to reveal a diseased organ or tumor, and removes a sample. Open biopsy is carried out when neither guided nor endoscopic biopsy is possible, or when it is likely that the organ or tumor will require removal. After a tissue sample has been taken, prompt analysis of it can enable the surgeon to remove the diseased area immediately.

EXCISIONAL BIOPSY If a lump is found in the skin or an organ, such as the breast, the surgeon may remove it completely and send the whole specimen for laboratory examination. For lesions (abnormalities) discovered only through *mammography*, the abnormal area may first be identified for the surgeon with the use of injected dye or fine wire probes.

OBTAINING A RESULT

When an immediate diagnosis is essential (for example, to enable breast cancer to be operated on without delay), the tissue can be prepared for staining in a few minutes by freezing or by smearing cells onto slides to study their cytologic features. The more time-consuming, wax-embedded techniques are also carried out for later examination.

In the investigation of infections and inflammations, tissue is sometimes tested with specific antibodies, or tissue *culture* may be required.

The electron *microscope* is used with some kidney biopsies and to distinguish the cell origin of certain tumors. Special enzyme and antibody *staining* techniques are also used in certain cases as well as other histochemical stains performed directly on the fixed and wax-embedded tissues. All of these procedures prolong the time required to make an exact diagnosis but allow for greater accuracy and more precise information about prognosis of certain diseases and tumors.

Biorhythms

A term used to describe all of the physiological functions that vary in a rhythmic way (e.g., the menstrual

BIOPSY PROCEDURES

ASPIRATION BIOPSY

1 The area is usually first numbed with local anesthetic, although occasionally a general anesthetic is required. A needle attached to a syringe is then inserted into the cyst or tumor to be investigated and cells are sucked out to be examined cytologically.

2 Before examination, the fluid is sometimes spun at high speed in a centrifuge and a small amount is placed on a slide.

3 The cells are then fixed (preserved) and finally stained for viewing. The cytologist examines individual cells for abnormalities, paying particular attention to the size, shape, and structure of the nucleus.

Cells as seen through microscope

TISSUE BIOPSY

1 The area is first numbed with a local anesthetic and a section of tissue is cut away. The wound is then stitched.

2 The tissue is then embedded in wax so that it is given a firm consistency suitable for slicing. This process usually takes 24 hours.

3 The tissue is then cut into ultrathin slices and transferred to a slide. The pathologist conducts an examination, looking for distortion or alteration of tissue structure.

Tissue sample as seen through microscope

ENDOSCOPIC BIOPSY

If an area of abnormal tissue is to be removed for further examination, the forceps attachment, shown here, is passed through an endoscope to remove the piece of tissue.

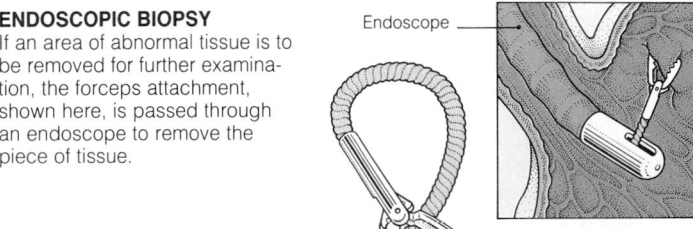

Endoscope

Forceps attachment

The forceps attachment removing a tissue sample from a stomach.

B

cycle, which repeats itself about every 28 days in fertile women).

Most biorhythms are based on a twice-daily or circadian (24-hour) cycle. Our bodies are governed by an internal clock, itself regulated by *hormones*—chemicals secreted into the bloodstream by the *endocrine glands*. Periods of sleepiness and wakefulness are influenced by the level of melatonin, secreted by the pineal gland in the brain. Release of melatonin is stimulated by darkness and suppressed by light. When the normal regular division between night and day is distorted by air travel to a distant time zone, the body's internal clock is disrupted and the result is *jet lag* (the symptoms of which, research suggests, may be relieved by the administration of melatonin).

Cortisol, secreted by the adrenal glands, also reflects the sleeping and waking states, being low at bedtime and high during the very early morning waking hours.

The applications of biorhythms are still being explored. For example, many asthmatics feel worse in the morning due to the cyclic release of hormones. This finding has implications for the management of their condition, and research groups are studying the optimum time of day for the administration of *bronchodilators* and other drugs that interact with functions subject to body rhythms.

Bipolar disorder
An illness that varies between opposite extremes. The principal example is *manic-depressive illness*.

Birth
See *Childbirth*.

Birth canal
The passage, extending from the dilated, effaced cervix (neck of the uterus, which becomes the uterus "mouth" during labor) to the introitus (vaginal opening), through which the baby passes during *childbirth*.

Birth control
Control of the number of children born by preventing or lessening the frequency of conception. Birth control can refer to the narrow area of using natural or artificial means to prevent pregnancy. In a broader sense it refers to control of family or population size by limiting births.

Most people in the US and other developed nations regulate childbirth, so that the population growth rate has

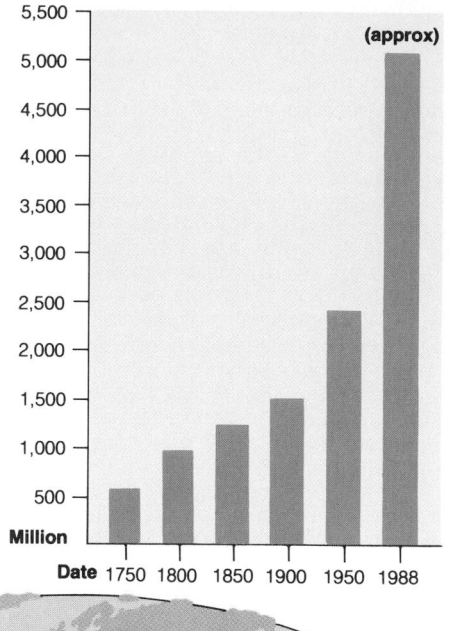

WORLD POPULATION
The rapid rate of population growth is a major problem. Reduction in infant and child mortality, due to better sanitation and disease control, has increased the number of people reaching their reproductive years. Because the world's population is doubling every 35 years, the task of adequately feeding, educating, and employing people is becoming increasingly difficult.

World population growth
The chart at right shows growth from 1750 to 1988.

Distribution by continent
The diagram below shows the 1984 population of each continent, given also as percentages of total world population.

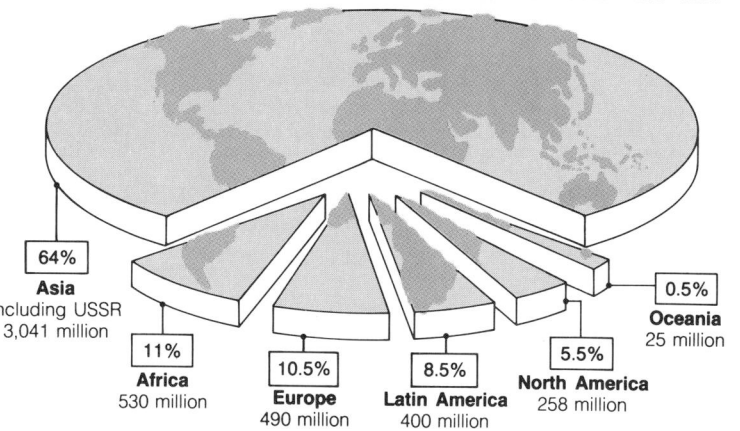

64%
Asia
including USSR
3,041 million

11%
Africa
530 million

10.5%
Europe
490 million

8.5%
Latin America
400 million

5.5%
North America
258 million

0.5%
Oceania
25 million

now slowed in Western countries and in many nations in the Far East. *Family planning* means that men and women can choose if and when to have children; *contraception* provides a means of preventing unwanted pregnancies. Other medical methods of preventing births include abortion (See *Abortion, elective*) and *sterilization*. Political and social pressures are applied to couples in some countries by governments eager to reduce population growth.

Birth defects
Abnormalities obvious at birth or detectable early in infancy. Also called congenital defects, they encompass both minor abnormalities, such as *birthmarks*, and serious disorders such as *spina bifida* (a failure of the spinal column to close completely). About 2

percent of babies born in the US have a defect but only about half of them require treatment.

CAUSES
Birth defects may be due to one or more known causes, but unknown factors also play a part. Among the recognized causes are the following.
CHROMOSOME DEFECTS Some children are born with more or fewer than the normal 23 pairs of *chromosomes* (threadlike structures in cell nuclei that carry the information necessary for normal development)—or there are extra or missing bits of chromosomes, as in *Down's syndrome* (see *Chromosomal abnormalities*).
GENETIC OR HEREDITARY DEFECTS These types of defects may be inherited from one or both parents (see *Genes; Genetic disorders*).

Examples of genetic defects obvious at birth are *achondroplasia* and *albinism*.

DRUGS AND OTHER HARMFUL AGENTS Some drugs can damage the fetus if taken by the mother in early pregnancy, the most notorious being *thalidomide*, a sedative widely prescribed in the late 1950s and early 1960s.

Smoking by the mother can harm the fetus; the ingredients in tobacco smoke stunt the baby's growth. Alcohol can have the same effect and may also affect the development of the face and brain (see *Fetal alcohol syndrome*). Drugs and chemicals that can harm the fetus in this way are collectively called *teratogens*.

IRRADIATION Accidental irradiation of the embryo in early pregnancy—for example, if the mother is X-rayed or receives *radiation therapy* for cancer—can cause abnormalities. However, care is taken to avoid these procedures or to prevent radiation from reaching the embryo if the woman is known to be (or might be) pregnant.

Radiation damage to the unborn child from atomic radiation or radioactive fallout (following a nuclear explosion or leak from a nuclear reactor) is more than just a theoretical risk of modern living. Heavy doses of radiation (as occurred at Hiroshima in 1945, for example) can cause serious mental and physical handicaps at birth, such as *microcephaly*. Even very small doses of radiation increase the child's risk of developing leukemia later in life (see *Radiation hazards*).

MATERNAL INFECTIONS Certain illnesses during pregnancy can cause birth defects. If a woman who has not been immunized against *rubella* (German measles) contracts the disease during the first three months of pregnancy, there is a 50 percent chance that her child will suffer brain, eye, ear, or heart abnormalities. Other types of infection, such as *toxoplasmosis*, may cause inflammation of the eyes, spleen, liver, and other important organs in the fetus.

PHYSICAL FACTORS IN THE UTERUS If the developing baby has too little fluid around it, its limbs may become distorted. *Talipes* (clubfoot) is thought to occur in this way.

Apart from defects of known cause, many others occur, the causes of which are unknown. Among the more common are abnormalities of the brain and spinal cord. In the embryo these structures develop from a simple, fluid-filled tube of nerve tissue. Interference in development can lead to *spina bifida* and *hydrocephalus*.

BIRTH DEFECTS (for every 100,000 babies born live)

Defect	Number	Cause
Congenital heart disease	700	Multifactorial
Mental deficiency (without structural defect)	300	Multifactorial
Pyloric stenosis (structural stomach defect)	300	Multifactorial
Anencephaly (no brain)	200	Multifactorial
Spina bifida	150	Multifactorial
Down's syndrome	150	Chromosome abnormality
Cleft lip and palate	150	Multifactorial
Hypospadias	150	Multifactorial
Clubfoot	100	Multifactorial
Congenital hip dislocation	100	Multifactorial
Congenital deafness	70	Multifactorial
Cystic fibrosis	50	Recessive gene
Turner's syndrome	20	Chromosome abnormality
Hereditary spherocytosis	10	Dominant gene
Albinism	5	Recessive gene

The heart and blood vessels in a fetus develop from what in the embryo is a central muscular tube. If the development of this cardiovascular system is impaired, a congenital heart disorder may result—for example, patent ductus arteriosus, septal defect, transposition of the great vessels, or tetralogy of Fallot (see *Heart disease, congenital*).

Other common defects include *cleft lip and palate*, both of which result from a failure of the two halves of the fetal face and palate to join completely.

PREVENTION

Steps can be taken to minimize the risk of an abnormal child being born. For example, before starting a family, *genetic counseling* should be obtained if either parent has relatives who have genetic or hereditary abnormalities. All women should make sure they are immune to rubella.

A woman should not smoke during pregnancy and should drink alcohol in moderation only. Unless prescribed by a physician, drugs of any kind should be avoided during the first three months of pregnancy.

Various tests may be carried out when there is a possibility that a fetus may have some defect.

Tests include *amniocentesis* (taking a sample of amniotic fluid from the uterus), blood tests to detect the level of *alpha-fetoprotein* (AFP) in the mother, *chorionic villus sampling* (removing a sample of tissue from the placenta), and *ultrasound scanning*.

Birth injury

Damage sustained during birth. All babies suffer at least minor trauma, leading to bruising or swelling of the scalp, during a vaginal delivery. The swelling is sometimes marked (see *Cephalhematoma*) if delivery is by *vacuum extraction* or *forceps*.

More serious injury can occur during a complicated delivery, particularly if the baby is premature, is born by *breech delivery* (born bottom-first), or is too big to pass easily through the mother's pelvis. Birth injuries are less common today, partly because more babies are now being delivered by *cesarean section*.

In breech deliveries, nerves in the shoulder region are sometimes injured, causing temporary paralysis in the arm. The face, likewise, may be paralyzed temporarily if the facial nerve is traumatized by forceps. Broken bones such as the clavicle (collarbone), humerus (upper arm bone), and particularly the ribs, are another hazard of difficult deliveries. The bones usually heal easily.

Many cases of *cerebral palsy*, *mental retardation*, and *epilepsy* were attributed to birth injury, but it is now considered that these problems are more often due to prenatal factors. Poor nutrition, smoking, maternal alcohol intake, bleeding during pregnancy, and prematurity are among the various factors that can lead to brain damage in a baby. (See *Birth defects; Brain damage*.)

B

Birthmark

An area of discolored skin present from birth. The most common birthmarks are freckles and moles, also called melanocytic *nevi* (brown to blue-gray skin patches of various types), which are malformations of pigment cells. Strawberry marks (bright red, usually protuberant areas) and port-wine stains (purple-red, flat, often large areas) are *hemangiomas* (malformations of blood vessels). Strawberry marks often gradually disappear after the age of 6 months, but port-wine stains seldom fade. In rare cases (the *Sturge-Weber syndrome*), port-wine stains are associated with abnormalities in the blood vessels of the brain.

Unsightly moles can be removed from late childhood onward by *plastic surgery*. Port-wine stains can now be caused to fade by *laser treatment*; the most successful results have been in young people.

Very rarely, a mole may develop into a type of skin cancer called a malignant *melanoma*. A mole that is large or irregular or suddenly starts to change in appearance or bleed is a cause for suspicion.

Birthmark
Strawberry marks—a common type of birthmark caused by malformation of blood vessels—are usually bright red, protuberant, and spongy.

Birth weight

The average full-term infant weighs 7.5 pounds at birth. Very few babies weigh less than 5.5 pounds (2,500 g) or more than 9.5 pounds (4,500 g).

A baby's birth weight depends on a number of factors, including the size and racial origin of the parents. Small parents tend to have small babies, and Asian infants tend to be smaller than white ones. Baby boys weigh, on the average, 8 ounces more than baby girls.

Babies who weigh less than 5.5 pounds at birth are classified as "low birth weight." About one half of these babies are small due to *prematurity*—

that is, they were born before the 37th week of pregnancy. Others are small because they have been undernourished in the uterus, where the placenta was insufficient because the mother had *preeclampsia* or smoked heavily during pregnancy.

Oversized babies are often born to mothers who have *diabetes mellitus*.

During the first few weeks of life, babies lose up to 10 percent of their birth weight, but thereafter should steadily gain weight.

Bisexuality

Sexual interest in members of both sexes that may or may not involve sexual activity. Between what are regarded as being the two ends of the human sexuality spectrum—exclusive heterosexuality and exclusive homosexuality—there exists a continuous spectrum of bisexuality. Sexuality is determined by a person's sexual desires as well as his or her actual sexual behavior. Thus, the term bisexual includes those who suppress homosexual desires and behave exclusively as heterosexuals.

Sexual preference may vary during a person's lifetime. Alfred Kinsey, who conducted a broad study of human sexual habits in the US during the 1940s, developed a scale that allowed him to rate the relative amounts of heterosexual and homosexual activity and/or responses during different periods in an individual's life. He concluded that, at some stage in their adult life, half the population engaged in both heterosexual and homosexual activity, or reacted sexually to persons of both sexes.

Bismuth

A metal, the salts of which are used in various drug preparations including tablets and suppositories to treat *peptic ulcer*, *hemorrhoids* (piles), and inflammatory diseases of the intestine. Bismuth salts adhere to ulcers of the stomach and duodenum and form a protective coating, thus promoting healing. Preparations containing bismuth salts taken by mouth may color the feces black, simulating the presence of blood in the feces. Darkening of the tongue and nausea and vomiting may also occur. Certain bismuth salts enter the bloodstream and may be associated with abnormal behavior patterns.

Bite

See *Occlusion*.

Bites, animal

Any injury inflicted by the mouthparts of an animal—from the tiny puncture wounds of blood-sucking insects to the massive injuries caused by shark or crocodile attacks.

The bites of venomous snakes, other venomous animals, and insects cause special problems (see *Snake bites*; *Venomous bites*; *Insect bites*).

INCIDENCE
The greatest number of animal attacks worldwide come from dogs, mainly strays. In the US, more than 1 million people annually are bitten badly enough by a dog to seek hospital treatment. A small number of deaths each year result from dog bites, and also from the bites of other domestic animals, such as cattle, horses, pigs, and sheep.

Wild animals that have killed or caused serious injuries to humans include bears, buffalo, wolves, hyenas, wild pigs, lions, tigers, elephants, rhinoceroses, and hippopotamuses. Small mammals such as rodents cause less extensive injury, but they often have razor-sharp teeth and there is a high risk of infection.

About 100 shark attacks occur worldwide each year, of which half are fatal. In Africa, more than 1,000 people annually die from crocodile attacks. Other aquatic creatures capable of a serious bite include barracuda, groupers, and moray and conger eels.

THE MAIN HAZARDS
TISSUE DAMAGE The mouth's function is to obtain food and prepare it for digestion. Teeth, especially those of carnivores, are well adapted to tearing, crushing, and macerating tissues and bones, and can inflict severe and extensive mechanical injury.

BLOOD LOSS Severe injuries and lacerations to major blood vessels can sometimes lead to serious blood loss and physiological *shock*.

INFECTION An animal's mouth is heavily populated with bacteria and other microorganisms that thrive on food residue and debris. These organisms can produce serious secondary infection, especially in wounds where there is already extensive tissue damage. *Tetanus* is a particular hazard of animal bites.

RABIES In countries in which rabies occurs, any mammal may potentially harbor the virus and transmit it by its bite (see *Rabies*). Worldwide, dog bites are by far the most common source of human infection. In the US, however, there is relatively little rabies in dogs.

In 1983, for example, there were 132 cases in dogs compared with 168 cases in cats, from a total of 5,880 cases of animal rabies in the entire country. Skunks, raccoons, and bats accounted for most of the remainder (5,101).

TREATMENT
For anything more serious than a minor bite or scratch—or if there is any possibility of rabies—treatment should be sought. It usually includes wound cleaning and exploration (under anesthesia, if necessary). The wound will usually be left open and dressed, rather than stitched, as a closed wound tends to encourage the multiplication of bacteria transmitted by bites. Preventive antibiotic treatment, and an antitetanus injection, may also be given.

If possible, the animal that inflicted the bite should be held and checked for rabies. Sometimes, an antirabies vaccine or serum may have to be given. (See also *Bites, human*.)

Bites, human
Wounds caused by one person biting another. In general, wounds from human bites are more serious than those from animal bites due to higher complication and infection rates.

CAUSES
People bite each other more often than might be supposed—commonly in the course of fights or domestic arguments, or as part of a general pattern of *child abuse*. In New York in 1982, 10 percent of all bites were human. Occasionally, bite wounds occur unintentionally, such as in fistfights where a person is punched in the teeth, or as a result of sexual play.

HAZARDS
Human bites rarely cause serious tissue damage or blood loss. However, infection from any of the range of microorganisms (viruses and bacteria) in the mouth is as likely, or even more likely, than with animal bites, particularly if the bite is deep. There is a risk of *tetanus* infection.

The viruses responsible for *hepatitis B*, *herpes simplex*, *AIDS*, and *rabies* are present in the saliva of those affected by these illnesses. Transmission of hepatitis B and AIDS by a bite has never been documented but is a theoretical hazard. Human cases of rabies are extremely rare, and the risk of being bitten by a human victim would be generally confined to physicians and nurses.

TREATMENT
Treatment for any bite that penetrates the skin is as for an animal bite.

Black death
The medieval name for bubonic *plague*. One feature of the disease is bleeding beneath the skin with the formation of dark blue or black bruises. This, along with the fact that in medieval times the disease was fatal in over 50 percent of the cases, accounts for the name.

Black eye
The bruised appearance of the skin around the eye following an injury. Any direct blow damages the numerous small blood vessels beneath the skin, causing blood to leak and collect there.

Because the skin around the eyes is loose and transparent, bruising is darker in this area than on other parts of the body. A cold compress held over the eye will reduce inflammation and help relieve the discomfort.

Blackhead
A semisolid, black-capped plug of greasy material blocking the outlet of a sebaceous (oil-forming) gland in the skin. Blackheads occur most commonly on the face, chest, shoulders, and back, alone or in groups, and are associated with increased sebaceous gland activity, which is normal in adolescents. They are a characteristic feature of certain types of *acne*.

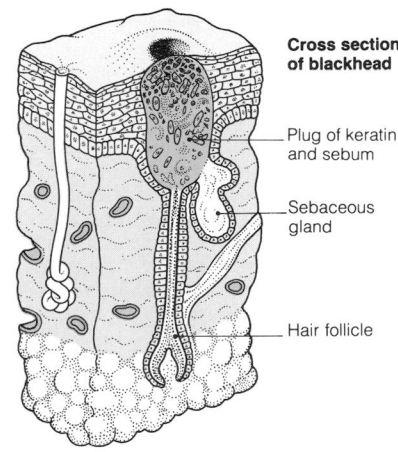

Cross section of blackhead

Plug of keratin and sebum

Sebaceous gland

Hair follicle

Blackout
A common term for loss of consciousness or syncope. (See *Fainting*.)

Black teeth
See *Discolored teeth*.

Blackwater fever
An occasional and life-threatening complication of falciparum *malaria* (the most dangerous form of the disease). The condition is brought on by a sudden increased rate of destruction of red blood cells. The breakdown products of the cells find their way via the kidneys into the urine and cause it to darken, hence "blackwater." Other symptoms include loss of consciousness (cerebral malaria), fever, chills, and vomiting.

Bladder
The hollow, muscular organ that acts as a reservoir for urine. The adult bladder can hold a pint or more of urine. It lies behind the pubic bone, hidden within and protected by the pelvis.

The bladder walls consist of muscle and an inner lining called urinary epithelium. At the back are the two ureters, which carry urine to the bladder from the kidneys. At the lowest point within the bladder—the neck—is the opening into the urethra; this is normally kept tightly closed by a sphincter (circular muscle).

FUNCTION
The bladder's function is to collect and store urine until it can be expelled from the body at a suitable time.

Full control over bladder function takes some years to develop. In infants, bladder emptying is an entirely automatic or *reflex* reaction. When the bladder fills and stretches beyond a certain point, signals are sent to the spinal cord. Nerve centers in the spinal cord then cause the urethral sphincter to relax and the main bladder muscle to contract, thus expelling urine via the urethra.

As the child grows, he or she gradually develops the ability to delay emptying. Stretching of the bladder is registered consciously (as discomfort) in brain centers, which, if desired, can then send signals suppressing the emptying reflex. Eventually, the bladder becomes so stretched that the urge to pass urine is overwhelming.

Children vary in the age at which they achieve perfect bladder control and, in particular, night-time control. Most children are dry at night by the age of 5 years, but some take longer (see *Enuresis*).

Defective bladder function, leading to problems such as *incontinence* and *urine retention*, has various causes. (See *Bladder* disorders box.)

Bladder cancer
See *Bladder tumors*.

Bladder tumors
Growths originating in the urinary epithelium (inner lining) of the blad-

B

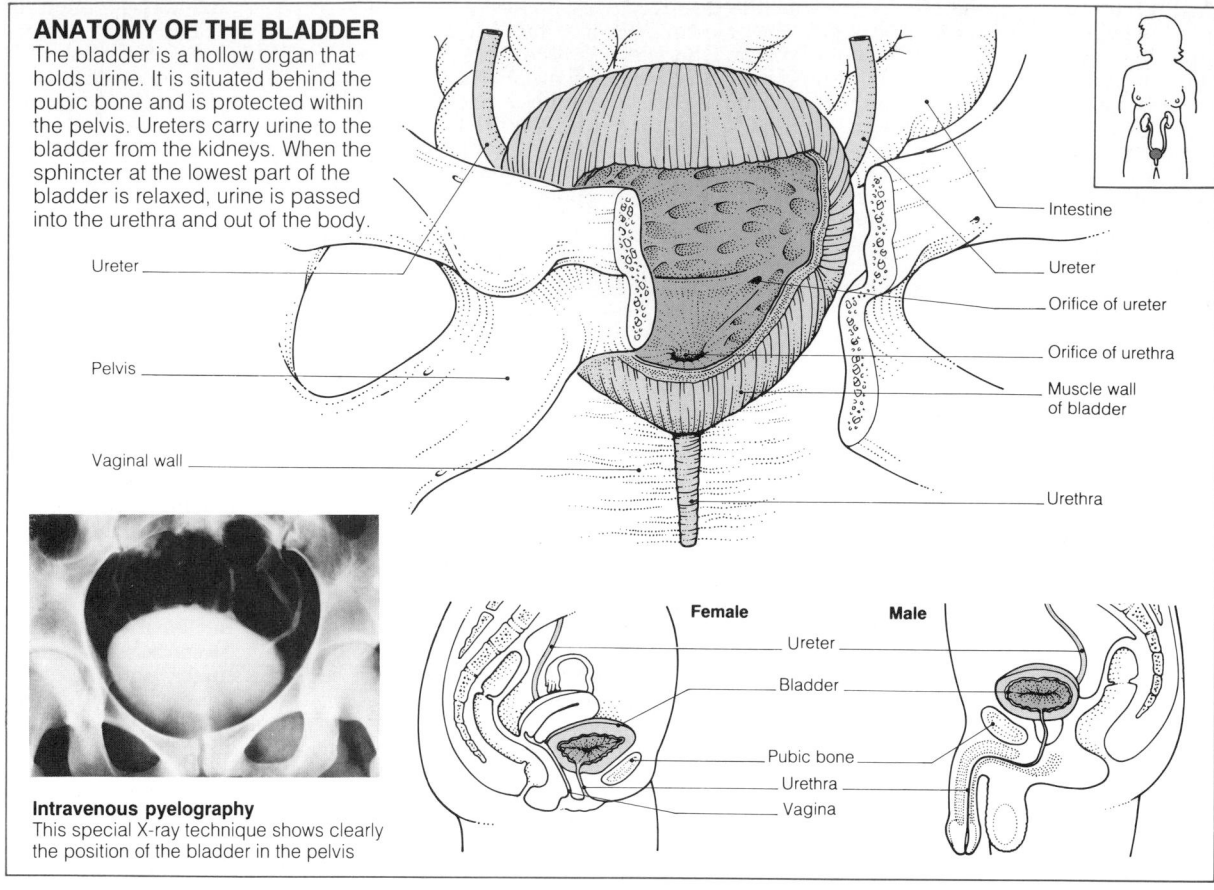

ANATOMY OF THE BLADDER

The bladder is a hollow organ that holds urine. It is situated behind the pubic bone and is protected within the pelvis. Ureters carry urine to the bladder from the kidneys. When the sphincter at the lowest part of the bladder is relaxed, urine is passed into the urethra and out of the body.

Ureter

Pelvis

Vaginal wall

Intestine

Ureter

Orifice of ureter

Orifice of urethra

Muscle wall of bladder

Urethra

Female   Male

Ureter

Bladder

Pubic bone

Urethra

Vagina

Intravenous pyelography
This special X-ray technique shows clearly the position of the bladder in the pelvis

der. Many bladder tumors are benign *papillomas* (small wartlike growths), but these tend to recur, and eventually one or more may become cancerous. Malignant growths tend to spread inward, into the bladder cavity, but may also spread through the bladder wall to nearby organs, such as the rectum, sigmoid colon, prostate gland, or uterus, and to the lymph glands and the bones of the pelvis.

INCIDENCE AND CAUSES

Bladder cancers account for about 4 percent of all cancers diagnosed in the US, with about 15 new cases (leading to about four deaths) per 100,000 population per year. If papillomas are included, the incidence is higher. Almost three times as many men as women are affected, and the average age at diagnosis is 65 years.

Certain groups are at increased risk, notably smokers and workers in the dye and rubber industries. Exposure to carcinogenic (cancer-inducing) substances used in these industries or in tobacco smoke is the presumed cause in these groups. The disease is

also common in areas of the tropics where the parasitic infection *schistosomiasis* is prevalent.

Avoiding smoking is the principal means of reducing the personal risk of bladder tumors. The incidence of occupational bladder cancer has been reduced by protective measures in the industries concerned and by regular screening of those who have been exposed in the past.

SYMPTOMS

Hematuria (blood in the urine) is the main symptom. Passing urine is usually painless, but a bladder infection may develop, and it then becomes painful and frequent. Sometimes, a tumor may obstruct the entry of a ureter into the bladder, causing back pressure and pain in the kidney region or may obstruct the urethral exit, causing difficulty in passing urine.

DIAGNOSIS AND TREATMENT

Bladder tumors are diagnosed primarily by *cystoscopy* (passage of a slim viewing tube up the urethra into the bladder) and by *biopsy*. If the tumor is still in its early stages, it is usually cut

out or treated by *diathermy* (heat destruction), via the cystoscope. Tumors recur in 80 percent of cases, so regular cystoscopy checkups are needed. Recurrences may be treated with surgery or *anticancer drugs*.

In the case of a more widely spread cancer, treatment is usually a combination of *radiation therapy* and more drastic surgery to remove the bladder (see *Cystectomy*).

OUTLOOK

This varies according to what stage the growth has reached when first diagnosed. If a tumor is diagnosed and treated early, the patient's long-term prospects are excellent (with regular follow-up checkups). If, however, it has spread beyond the bladder wall, the chances of survival for more than five years are not good.

Blastomycosis

A rare infection caused by breathing in a fungus, BLASTOMYCES DERMATITIDIS, found in wood and soil. The infection occurs mainly in the eastern part of the US and Canada.

DISORDERS OF THE BLADDER

The most important causes of bladder problems are infection, tumors, urinary tract *calculi* (stones), or impairment of the bladder's nerve supply.

INFECTION

Infection of the bladder, better known as *cystitis*, is particularly common in women, mainly because of the much shorter female urethra, which provides less of a barrier to bacteria. In men, infection is usually associated with obstruction to the flow of urine from the bladder by, for example, tumors of the bladder or prostate (the gland situated around the bladder neck in males). In some parts of the tropics, the parasitic worm infection *schistosomiasis* (bilharziasis) is a common cause.

TUMORS

Bladder tumors may be benign or malignant and are more common in men than in women. They are usually painless in the early stages and may cause *hematuria* (blood in the urine) or obstruction to the outflow of urine from the bladder. The latter may also be caused by a tumor of the prostate and result in partial or complete *urine retention* and stagnation in the bladder.

Tumors of the spinal cord may affect the nerves controlling the bladder, leading either to retention or *incontinence* (involuntary bladder emptying or leakage).

CALCULI

Calculi (stones) in the bladder, caused by the precipitation from solution of substances present in the urine, are an uncommon problem in the US. They mainly affect men and usually result from urinary retention and/or a long-standing urinary tract infection. In some other parts of the world, such as Southeast Asia, they are more common and are often associated with a low-protein diet.

Cancer
• a growth that can arise from any part of the bladder wall

Urethral stricture
• narrowing that can be due to infection or trauma

Infection
• causing inflammation of bladder wall

Stone
• can block urethral opening

Enlarged prostate
• causing slow urination

INJURY

Injury to the bladder is uncommon. It may occur, however, if the pelvis is fractured when the bladder is full. Such injury typically occurs in traffic accidents. The bladder ruptures and urine leaks into the abdominal and pelvic cavities.

Damage to the nerves involved in bladder control may severely disrupt bladder filling and emptying, causing either incontinence or urinary retention, depending on the site of the injury. In the US, the most common cause of such damage is spinal cord injury due to motorcycle and automobile accidents or to bullet wounds. Nerves controlling the bladder may also be damaged by a prolapsed intervertebral disk.

OTHER DISORDERS

Disturbance of bladder control can also result from nerve degeneration found in conditions such as *diabetes mellitus* or *multiple sclerosis*.

An unstable or *irritable bladder* is a common condition in which the urge to empty the bladder occurs frequently. It is not fully understood but is sometimes associated with a *urinary tract infection* or prolapse of the uterus. Many other underlying conditions, most com- monly tension or anxiety, can cause frequent urination.

Failure to achieve bladder control by the age of 4 or 5 is termed *enuresis* (bed-wetting); this may be due to a treatable physical cause, such as urinary tract infection, or to emotional problems but more often results from delayed maturation of the nervous system.

INVESTIGATION

Many different methods are used to investigate bladder disorders. Urinary tract infection is diagnosed by culturing a urine sample. The bladder can be viewed directly by means of *cystoscopy*. X-ray studies include a voiding *cystourethrogram*, which shows only the bladder, and intravenous *pyelography*, which provides a picture of the whole urinary tract. *Cystometry* is a technique for measuring bladder capacity in relation to changing pressure.

The infection may cause acute pneumonia or a more chronic illness affecting the lungs, skin, and bones. It cannot be passed from one person to another. Treatment is with *antifungal drugs*, such as amphotericin B or ketoconazole.

Bleaching, dental

A cosmetic procedure for lightening endodontically treated or nonvital "dead" teeth that have become discolored (see *Discolored teeth*). The surface of the affected tooth is painted with oxidizing agents and may be exposed to special heat or light.

Bleb

A tiny *blister*. A common cause is the injection of a small amount of fluid under the outer layer of skin—for example, in the tuberculin skin test.

Bleeder

A term used to describe anyone who suffers from a *bleeding disorder*, which may be congenital or acquired.

Bleeding

Loss of blood from the *circulatory system* caused by damage to the blood vessels or by a *bleeding disorder*, which may be visible (external) or concealed (internal). Rapid loss of more than 10

B

percent of the blood volume can cause symptoms of shock with faintness, pallor, and sweating.

CAUSES
The most common cause of bleeding is an injury. The speed with which blood flows from a cut depends on the type of blood vessel damaged—it usually oozes from a capillary, flows from a vein, and spurts from an artery. If an injury does not break open the skin, blood collects around the damaged blood vessels close under the skin to form a *bruise*.

Damage to internal blood vessels may be the result of inflammation, infection, an ulcer, or a tumor. Any lost blood that mixes with other bodily fluids such as sputum or urine will be noticed quite readily; bleeding in the digestive tract may make vomit or feces appear darker than usual because the blood is partially digested. Internal bleeding, however, may not become visible but may gradually progress to where severe anemia is present.

Bleeding without injury usually requires investigation. The exceptions are an occasional *nosebleed* (epistaxis) and bleeding during *menstruation*. The amount of blood lost during menstruation varies and is only a problem if bleeding becomes very heavy or frequent, when it might lead to iron-deficiency *anemia*.

Bleeding disorders

Conditions that are associated with bleeding without injury or abnormally prolonged and excessive bleeding after injury.

Bleeding disorders are the result of one or more defects in the three mechanisms by which bleeding is normally stopped (see *Hemostasis* and *Blood clotting*). These mechanisms are blood coagulation, the plugging of damaged blood vessels by platelets, and the constriction of blood vessels.

Coagulation defects tend to cause deep bleeding into the gastrointestinal tract, the muscles, and the joint cavities, while defects of the platelets or blood vessels produce superficial bleeding into the skin, gums, or lining of the intestine or urinary tract. However, bleeding may occur anywhere with these defects.

COAGULATION DEFECTS
These defects usually result from too little of one or more of the enzymes (called coagulation factors) that take part in blood clotting, or from the enzymes being abnormal. The defect causes the blood to clot very slowly and produces clots that are weak and do not seal blood vessels securely. Coagulation defects may be congenital (present from birth) or acquired later in life.

CONGENITAL The main congenital coagulation defects are *hemophilia*, *Christmas disease*, and *von Willebrand's disease*. In each of these, one of the coagulation factors is either absent from the blood or is present in only small amounts.

Hemophilia and Christmas disease are similar disorders, resulting from deficiencies of two different coagulation factors, called factor VIII and factor IX, respectively. They are inherited as sex-linked disorders (see *Genetic disorders*), which means that normally only males are affected. In the US, about 10 people per 100,000 have hemophilia and about two people per 100,000 have Christmas disease.

Von Willebrand's disease is also a factor VIII defect but affects both sexes roughly equally. About five persons per 100,000 are affected.

Individuals with any of these disorders may bleed internally without warning and often have recurrent bleeding into joints such as the knee or elbow. The severity of the bleeding is variable.

ACQUIRED Deficiency of one or more coagulation factors may develop at any age as a result of severe liver disease, digestive system disorders that prevent the absorption from the diet of *vitamin K* (required to make some coagulation factors), or the use of *anticoagulant drugs*, such as warfarin, that prevent normal production of these enzymes. As with congenital bleeding disorders, a severe bleeding tendency may result.

One particularly complex coagulation disorder is disseminated intravascular coagulation (DIC); it may be triggered by a variety of circumstances. First there is aggregation of platelets and clotting within small blood vessels. Subsequently, coagulation factors are used and broken up in the blood faster than they can be replaced by the liver, and severe bleeding may result. Paradoxically, sometimes anticoagulants are given to interfere with the clotting activity, but this very serious condition generally does not improve until the underlying problem (for example, an infection or cancer) is brought under control.

Coagulation defects are investigated by *blood-clotting tests* such as the prothrombin time. Treatment of these disorders is based on giving the patient infusions of the missing coagulation factor or factors in fresh blood or fresh frozen plasma. Since these factors come from human blood, transmission of some viral infections (for example, hepatitis B or AIDS) is possible. Attempts are made to reduce the risk of contaminating viruses, such as the hepatitis B or AIDS virus, by checking for the presence of antibodies against the virus and, if they are present, discarding the blood or blood products.

PLATELET DEFECTS
Bleeding caused by a defect in the platelet system is usually due to too few of these cells in the blood—a condition called *thrombocytopenia*. The main features are surface bleeding into the skin and gums, which usually appears in the skin as multiple small bruises called *purpura*.

Occasionally, platelets are normal in number but function abnormally with resultant bleeding. Such defects may be inherited, may be associated with the use of many drugs (including aspirin), or may be a complication of certain bone marrow disorders such as myeloid *leukemia*.

Platelet defects are investigated by blood clotting tests such as bleeding and clotting times and various other tests of platelet aggregation (clumping). Whatever the cause, the main treatment of platelet disorders consists of transfusions of platelets from single donors or from "pools" (obtained from several normal blood transfusions). The transfusions need to be given daily until the underlying defect has been corrected and the body is producing its own healthy platelets again.

BLOOD VESSEL DEFECTS
Abnormal bleeding caused by blood vessel defects is rare today. In the past, *scurvy* (vitamin C deficiency) was a frequent and often fatal disorder of this type, affecting sailors, polar explorers, and anyone with a diet lacking fresh fruit and vegetables. Today, mild scurvy is occasionally seen in elderly people on a poor diet. Elderly people and patients on long-term *corticosteroid drugs* may also suffer mild abnormal bruising due to loss of skin support to the smallest blood vessels. These conditions are mild and treatment is rarely required.

Bleeding gums
See *Gingivitis*.

Bleeding, treatment of
The body's response to internal or external loss of blood is to contract the damaged blood vessels and to cause blood to clot at the site of injury. At the same time, blood flow may be reduced in the skin and muscles to make sure that the brain, kidneys, and other vital organs are adequately supplied. Loss of a large volume of blood quickly causes a dramatic fall in blood pressure accompanied by weakness, confusion, pallor, and sweating as the body tries to compensate; this state is known as *shock*.

First-aid measures have two objectives: to minimize blood loss and to help the body cope with the loss.

PROFESSIONAL TREATMENT
When bleeding is severe, infusions of saline solution and plasma preparations may be given to help replace fluids lost from the circulation. If a large amount of blood is lost, *blood transfusion* may also be required. Large wounds may need closing with *sutures* (stitches), which are effective in stopping bleeding from scalp injuries and also reduce the risk of scarring. If bleeding within the abdomen is suspected following an accident, *CT scanning* and/or exploratory surgery may be needed. If bleeding within the skull is compressing the brain, a hole will be drilled in the skull in order to relieve the pressure.

Severe bleeding may require treatment in the operating room. During operations, bleeding from small blood vessels is controlled by clamping them with forceps and then either tying them or sealing them with *diathermy*, the application of a high frequency electric current.

Blepharitis
Inflammation of the eyelids, with redness, irritation, and scaly skin at the lid margins. Older patients sometimes call marginal blepharitis "granulated eyelids." The patient may note burning and discomfort in the eyes and flakes or crusts on lashes. Occasionally, the surface of the eye may also be inflamed and red. In some cases the roots of the eyelashes become infected, and small ulcers form. Blepharitis is common, tends to recur, and is sometimes associated with dandruff or eczema of the scalp.

The problem can often be cleared up by removing the scales with cotton moistened with warm water. Mar-

FIRST AID: TREATING BLEEDING

SIMPLE CUT

1 Wash your hands before dealing with the cut. Then, if the cut has dirt in it, rinse it lightly under lukewarm running water until it is clean, being careful not to touch the spout.

2 Dab the cut gently (to dry it) with sterile gauze. Then dress it with an adhesive dressing.

DEEP CUT

1 Raise the injured part and support it. Put a sterile dressing on the wound and apply firm pressure to control bleeding.

2 If blood seeps through, do not remove the dressing as this may disturb clots and restart bleeding. Put other dressings on top of the first one and bandage all dressings snugly.

ginal blepharitis frequently recurs, requiring more treatment. Ulcerated eyelids need the attention of your physician. Severe cases of blepharitis can lead to corneal problems.

Blepharoplasty
A cosmetic operation to remove wrinkled, drooping skin from the upper and/or lower eyelids. The operation is usually done using local anesthesia and takes about one and a half hours. Normally, the patient can go home the same day.

WHY IT IS DONE
As a person grows older, the skin loses some of its fat, and much of its elasticity, becoming droopy and creased. This process may be accelerated by grief, worry, or sudden loss of weight. As a result, the eyelids become baggy. Removing the excess skin can result in a greatly improved appearance.

HOW IT IS DONE
On the upper lids a horizontal fold of skin is removed from the center of each lid so that the resultant scar runs in a natural crease line. On the lower lids the incision is made just below the

Appearance before (inset) and after blepharoplasty
The operation involves removal of a crescent-shaped section of skin and underlying fat from each eyelid.

B

eyelashes, so that the scar will be in the shadow of the lashes and extend into a smile wrinkle.

RECOVERY PERIOD

After the operation, ice packs and pads soaked with witch hazel solution are applied to both eyes, to reduce swelling and bruising. The patient is advised to repeat these applications at home. Swelling usually subsides within three days but bruising may last for two weeks.

Some of the stitches are removed three to five days after the operation, the rest seven to 10 days after. The scars usually fade to fine, unnoticeable marks within six to 12 months of the operation.

Blepharospasm

Involuntary prolonged contraction of one of the muscles that controls the eyelids, causing almost complete closure. It may be due to *photophobia* (sensitivity of the eyes to light), *blepharitis, anxiety,* or *hysteria.* Treatment is aimed at remedying the cause.

Blind loop syndrome

A condition leading to diarrhea with pale yellow, foul-smelling, bulky feces (called steatorrhea) that are difficult to flush away, along with general sickness, tiredness, and weight loss. The syndrome is caused by a redundant area or dead end in the small intestine, called a blind loop, which is usually the result of surgery but may be congenital (existing at birth).

Because there is not a constant flow of the bowel contents through the loop, its contents stagnate. Bacteria that are not the ordinary dominant inhabitants of the bowel multiply. They spread into other areas of the intestine where they interfere with absorption of nutrients, including fat and vitamin B_{12}.

Treatment with an antibiotic, usually a tetracycline, may be successful. If not, surgery to remove the blind loop usually cures the condition.

Blindness

Total or partial inability to see. Generally, blindness refers to a severe loss of vision that cannot be corrected with ordinary *glasses.* More commonly, vision is impaired to the extent that it markedly hinders everyday activities. Such partial loss—which may develop slowly or suddenly, according to the cause—can affect central vision, peripheral (side) vision, or both. The definition of blindness may vary by agency, but in the US it is usually defined as corrected *visual acuity* of 20/200 or less in the better eye, or a *visual field* of no more than 20 degrees in the better eye.

A person suffering from loss of central vision is usually aware of the fact, since it prevents reading and discernment of fine detail. However, loss of peripheral vision may pass unnoticed by the sufferer until it is well advanced, when it causes clumsiness of movement.

INCIDENCE

It is estimated that over 40 million people in the world are partially or totally blind. Vitamin A deficiency alone accounts for blindness in millions of children living in the poor countries of Africa, Asia, and South America.

In the US, about 214 persons per 100,000 are registered as legally blind, though the definition varies.

CAUSES

Blindness may result from injury, disease, or degeneration of the eyeball, of the optic nerve or nerve pathways connecting the eye to the brain, or of the brain itself.

EYEBALL Normal vision depends on the uninterrupted passage of light from the front of the eye to the light-sensitive retina at the back. Anything that obstructs the passage of light rays from the retina can cause blindness (see *Eye; Vision*).

Various disorders may impair the transparency of the cornea at the front of the eye. In *Sjögren's syndrome,* an inability to produce tears leads to *keratoconjunctivitis sicca,* which, if severe, causes the cornea to cloud over. Other causes of a cloudy cornea include *vitamin A* deficiency, accidental chemical damage, and injury. Ulcers on the cornea can also cause blindness since, when healed, they leave scars (see *Cornea* disorders box).

The common causes of such ulcers are severe attacks of certain infections, among them *ophthalmia* neonatorum

---

AIDS FOR THE BLIND

There are many ways in which life can be made easier for the blind person, and there are now a number of specially designed and adapted devices available. These include braille writers, mathematical apparatus, and home appliances, as well as aids for helping the blind person get around outside the home.

Liquid level indicator
This device measures liquid being poured into a cup or glass. Two sets of prongs are connected to a bleeper. A short set of prongs measures almost to the top, while the long set measures small amounts in the bottom. A bleep sounds when the liquid contacts the prongs.

Pocket watch
Strengthened hands and raised dots make it easier for a blind person to "read" numerals: three dots are at 12, two are at 3, 6, and 9, and one is at each of the other hour positions.

Pocket braille maker
This frame produces braille on one side of the paper. A special pointed stylus is used to make the braille indentations; a stencil keeps the stylus in the right place. The braille can be read without removing the paper from the frame.

(inflammation of the conjunctiva in newborn babies), *trachoma* (most common in hot, overcrowded regions), *herpes simplex*, and bacterial ulcers.

Inflammation of the iris, ciliary body, or choroid—a condition known as *uveitis*—can be caused by infections such as *tuberculosis*, *sarcoidosis*, *syphilis*, *toxocariasis*, or *toxoplasmosis*, but such inflammation frequently occurs for no known reason.

Cataract (cloudiness of the lens) is a common cause of blindness. It is usually the result of the lens deteriorating in old age, but is occasionally present from birth or develops during childhood.

Diabetes mellitus, *hypertension*, or injury can cause bleeding into the fluid that makes up the bulk of the eyeball. In *hyphema* blood enters the aqueous humor (watery substance) in front of the lens. *Vitreous hemorrhage* is bleeding into the jellylike vitreous humor behind the lens.

Disorders of the retina are a common cause of blindness. They include the age-related *macular degeneration* (degeneration of the central area of the retina, which occurs in old age), *retinopathy* due to diabetes or hypertension, *retinal artery occlusion* (blockage of the blood supply to the retina), *retinal vein occlusion*, *retinal detachment*, tumors such as *retinoblastoma* and malignant *melanoma* of the eye, and *retinal hemorrhage* (bleeding into the retina), caused by diabetes, hypertension, vascular disease, or injury.

In *glaucoma*, a common cause of blindness, pressure in the eyeball causes degeneration of the nerve fibers of the optic nerve disk. Many types of glaucoma exist; the more common types can cause loss of peripheral vision (side vision), which may be unnoticed until the disease is well advanced. *Amblyopia* ex anopsia (lazy eye from disuse in childhood) is subnormal vision that is associated with *strabismus* (misalignment of the eyes) or *anisometropia* (unequal focus between the eyes).

OPTIC NERVE AND NERVE PATHWAYS The light energy received by the retina is transformed into nerve impulses that travel along the optic nerve and nerve pathways into the brain. Conduction of these impulses may be impaired by pressure from a tumor in the orbit (the bony cavity that contains the eyeball) or in the brain; by interference with the blood supply to the optic nerve, which can be caused by diabetes mellitus, hypertension, tumors, injuries, or *temporal arteritis*; by *optic neuritis* (inflammation of the optic nerve that may occur in *multiple sclerosis*); or by toxic and nutritional deficiency amblyopia (optic neuropathy) caused by the poisonous effects of certain chemicals or by the lack of certain nutrients.

BRAIN Nerve impulses from the retina eventually arrive in a region of the *cerebrum* called the visual cortex. The nerve impulses are analyzed and interpreted to provide conscious images. Blindness can be caused if there is pressure on the visual cortex from a *brain tumor* or *brain hemorrhage* or if a *stroke* reduces blood supply to the visual cortex.

Finally, apparent blindness can be related to *hysteria*, a reaction to severe stress in which physical symptoms develop without there being any physical cause.

DIAGNOSIS AND TREATMENT

Anyone who suffers loss of vision, whether partial or complete, should consult a physician immediately. Various types of *vision tests* can be carried out.

Often, the cause can be ascertained by direct examination of the eye, including ophthalmoscopy, slit-lamp examination, tonometry, and perimetry. Electrical activity produced in the brain following visual stimulation can be measured by visual potentiometry (see *Evoked responses*). The age and medical history of the patient, the patient's account of the development of the sight loss, and other signs and symptoms, may provide important clues to the diagnosis. In a few cases, *ultrasound scanning*, *CT scanning*, or *MRI* may be performed to look for any abnormalities in the eyes, orbits, structures around the optic nerves, or brain. *Fluorescein angiography* (a technique for photographing the inside of the eye) may be used to study the retina and choroid.

Treatment depends on the underlying cause once discovered. If not correctable, and the loss of vision meets an agency's definition of blindness, certain services may be available. (See also *Color vision deficiency*; *Night blindness*; *Onchocerciasis*, also known as river blindness.)

Blind spot

The small, oval-shaped area on the retina of the eye where the optic nerve joins the eyeball. The area is not sensitive to light because there are no light receptors (nerve endings responsive to light) present there.

LOCATION OF BLIND SPOT
The blind spot is a minute area on the retina that lacks light receptors and so is not light-sensitive.

Blind spot · Retina · Optic nerve · Light rays

To demonstrate the presence of the blind spot, mark an X on a piece of paper and a dot 6 inches to the right. While holding the paper at arm's length, shut your left eye and look at the X with your right eye. Slowly move the paper toward you until the dot disappears. This is the point at which the dot has entered your right eye's blind spot.

Blister

A collection of fluid beneath the outer layer of the skin that forms a raised area, usually oval or circular in shape. Large blisters (more than a half inch in diameter) are sometimes called bullae; small blisters are called vesicles.

The fluid in a blister is serum that has leaked from blood vessels in underlying skin layers after minor damage. The fluid is usually sterile, and the blister provides valuable protection to the damaged tissue.

CAUSES

Common causes of blisters are *burns* (including *sunburn*) and friction—for example, from an ill-fitting shoe.

A number of skin diseases also can cause blisters. These include *eczema*, *impetigo*, and *erythema multiforme* (in which blistering is usually seen only in severe forms), and *pemphigoid*, *pemphigus*, and *dermatitis herpetiformis* (collectively called "bullous" disorders), in which blistering is the most important feature of the disease. Blisters also occur in the congenital disease *epidermolysis bullosa* and in some types of *porphyria*.

B

Small blisters develop at an early stage in the rashes of the viral infections *chickenpox, herpes zoster* (shingles), and *herpes simplex*; these blisters contain infectious virus particles that may spread the infection elsewhere or to another person.

TREATMENT

A blister is best left to heal on its own. It should not be burst, because the underlying damaged tissue could become infected. In the case of large, troublesome, or unexplained blisters, consult your physician. Bullous disorders are potentially serious and expert advice is needed.

Blocked nose

See *Nasal congestion*.

Blocking

Inability to express true feelings or thoughts, usually as a result of emotional or mental conflict. In Freudianbased psychotherapies, blocking is regarded as originating from the repression of painful emotions in early life. Successful treatment is thought to depend on putting patients in touch with these unconscious feelings.

A very specific form of thought blocking occurs in *schizophrenia*. In this disorder, trains of thought are persistently interrupted involuntarily, to be replaced by totally unconnected new ones. (See also *Psychotherapy*.)

Blood

The sticky red fluid that circulates in our veins and arteries. Its main function is to act as the body's transport system, but it also has a major role in the defense against infection.

Blood also contains ingenious mechanisms to halt its own loss from the body; it seals damaged blood vessels, protects the injury with a clot, and helps to repair the damage (see *Hemostasis; Blood clotting; Wounds*).

The average-sized adult has about 10 pints of blood. At rest, 10 pints a minute are pumped by the heart via the arteries to the lungs and all other tissues, then returned to the heart in veins, in a continuous circuit (see *Circulatory system*). During exercise the heart may pump blood at a rate of 40 pints or more a minute.

Almost half the volume of blood consists of cells, which include red blood cells (or erythrocytes), white blood cells (or leukocytes), and platelets or thrombocytes (see *Blood cells*). The remainder is a fluid called plasma, which contains dissolved proteins, sugars, fats, and minerals.

BLOOD CELLS

The main function of red blood cells is to act as containers for the pigment and protein *hemoglobin*. Hemoglobin carries oxygen from the lungs to the tissues, where it is exchanged for the waste product carbon dioxide (see *Respiration*). White blood cells play an important part in the defense against infection by viruses, bacteria, fungi, and parasites, and in inflammation of any cause (see *Immune system*). Platelets are essential to arrest bleeding and repair damaged blood vessels. They clump together to block small holes, and these clumps release chemicals that begin the process of blood clotting.

PLASMA

Blood plasma is a straw-colored fluid, consisting mainly of water (95 percent) with a salt content very similar to seawater. Levels of its many other dissolved constituents vary from time to time. Measurements of these constituents are useful to physicians in the diagnosis of disease states (see *Blood tests; Liver function tests*). Important constituents of plasma include the following.

NUTRIENTS These substances are transported to the tissues after absorption from the intestinal tract or following release from storage depots such as the liver. Nutrients include sugars (principally glucose), fats, amino acids required by cells to make proteins, and various vitamins and minerals. Immediately after a meal that is rich in fats, the plasma has a milky appearance as a consequence of its high fat content.

WASTE PRODUCTS The main product of tissue metabolism is urea, which is transported in the plasma to the kidneys; abnormally high blood urea levels occur in *renal failure*. The waste product from the destruction of hemoglobin is a yellow pigment called bilirubin. This is normally removed from the plasma by the liver and turned into bile. Bilirubin levels become abnormally high in liver disease, or in hemolytic *anemia*, where there is excessive destruction of red blood cells. Bilirubin causes the yellow color of the skin and eyes and the dark urine in patients with *jaundice*.

PROTEINS These include substances such as fibrinogen, that are involved in the processes of coagulation and clotting, and others that act to inhibit coagulation (see *Blood clotting*). Plasma proteins, such as *immunoglobulins* (see also *Antibodies*), and complement (bacteria fighters) are part of the immune system. Another type of plasma protein is *albumin*. The large size of the protein molecules prevents them from escaping from the blood into the tissues; this helps to "hold in" the water content of blood (by osmotic pressure) and thus maintain blood volume.

HORMONES The hormones are chemical messengers transported in the blood from various glands to their target organs. (See *Endocrine system*.)

Blood cells

Cells present in blood for most or part of their life span. These include red blood cells, which make up about 40 percent by volume of normal blood, and white blood cells and platelets, which make up less than 5 percent of the total volume.

All types of blood cells are formed within the bone marrow by a series of divisions from a single type of cell called a stem cell.

RED BLOOD CELLS

 These are also called RBCs, red blood corpuscles, or erythrocytes. They carry oxygen from the lungs to the tissues, where oxygen is exchanged for carbon dioxide (see *Respiration*).

FORMATION RBC formation from stem cells in the bone marrow takes about five days. It requires an adequate supply of nutrients, including iron, amino acids, and the vitamins B_{12} and folic acid. The rate of RBC formation is influenced by a hormone called erythropoietin, which is produced by the kidneys.

Cells just released into the bloodstream from the marrow are called reticulocytes; over two to four days, these develop into mature RBCs. Reticulocytes are easily recognized in blood by means of special staining techniques, and a count of their numbers provides physicians with a helpful estimate of the rate at which RBCs are being formed (see *Blood count; Blood smear*).

STRUCTURE AND FUNCTION One cubic millimeter of blood contains about 5 million RBCs, each of which is doughnut-shaped, about 7.5 thousandths of a millimeter in diameter, and much thicker around the edge than at the center. This shape gives the cell a relatively large surface area, which assists it in absorbing and releasing oxygen molecules. The shape also allows the cell to distort and so helps it squeeze through narrow blood vessels.

CONSTITUENTS OF BLOOD

Blood is pumped around the body in veins and arteries, transporting oxygen from the lungs to the tissues, and carbon dioxide from the tissues to the lungs. Blood also carries nutrients such as sugars, fats, and proteins that have been absorbed from the intestine, and hormones produced by a variety of glands. Waste products that are released from cells are carried in the blood to be broken down in the liver or excreted from the kidneys.

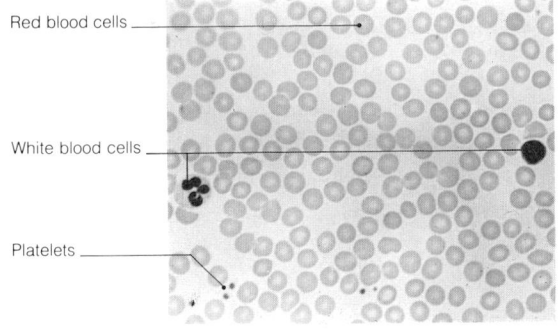

Normal blood smear
This is the appearance of normal blood under a microscope. The dominant feature is the abundance of red blood cells, which make up almost half the blood volume. Two stained white blood cells (a granulocyte at left and a lymphocyte) can be seen; the platelets are the tiny dark particles.

Red blood cells

White blood cells

Platelets

White blood cells
These cells protect the body against infection and fight it when it occurs. They are bigger than red blood cells but fewer in number. Each of the three main types (granulocytes, monocytes, and lymphocytes) plays a different role in dealing with infection.

Monocyte

Granulocyte　Lymphocyte

Platelets
The smallest type of blood cell produced in the bone marrow; they play an important part in blood clotting.

Plasma
The fluid part of the blood that consists mostly of water. It carries substances such as proteins, fats, glucose, and salts.

Red blood cells
These doughnut-shaped cells are formed in the bone marrow and carry oxygen from the lungs to the rest of the body. They have a large surface area and a flexible shape.

Each cell is packed with large quantities of *hemoglobin*, a protein that contains iron. Hemoglobin is found in all animals—from insects and worms to birds, fish, and mammals—and is highly efficient at "binding" (combining chemically) with oxygen when the oxygen concentration is high (in the lungs), and releasing the oxygen again when the oxygen concentration is low (in the tissues). Oxyhemoglobin, formed when oxygen combines with hemoglobin, is responsible for the bright red coloration of oxygenated blood; the unbound (oxygen-free) hemoglobin in venous blood accounts for its darker color.

Each RBC also contains *enzymes*, minerals, and sugars, which give energy to maintain shape, structure, and elasticity (see *Cell*; *Metabolism*).

The surface structure of RBCs varies slightly among individuals, and this provides the basis for classifying blood into groups (see *Blood groups*).

AGING AND DESTRUCTION RBCs normally circulate in the blood for about 120 days, which is also their life span when removed for blood transfusion (within three to four weeks blood in blood banks contains a significant proportion of dead cells and must be discarded). As cells age, their internal chemical machinery wears out, they lose elasticity, and they become trapped in small blood vessels in the spleen and other organs; they are then destroyed by a type of white blood cell called a macrophage (see *Phagocyte*). Most components of the hemoglobin molecules are reutilized but some are broken down to a waste product called *bilirubin*.

DISORDERS Abnormalities can occur in the rate at which RBCs are formed or destroyed, in the number of RBCs in the blood, and in their shape, size, and hemoglobin content, causing various forms of *anemia* and *polycythemia* (see *Blood* disorders box).

WHITE BLOOD CELLS

 These are also called WBCs, white blood corpuscles, or leukocytes; their principal role is to protect the body against infection and to fight infection when it occurs. The WBCs are bigger than RBCs (up to 15 thousandths of a millimeter in diameter) but much less numerous (about 7,500 per cubic millimeter of blood). They generally spend a much shorter part of their life span than RBCs in the blood itself. There are three main types of WBC, known as granulocytes, monocytes, and *lymphocytes*.

GRANULOCYTES WBCs of this type are also called polymorphonuclear leukocytes. Under the microscope, they are seen to contain granules and have an oddly shaped nucleus. Granulocytes are themselves of three types, called neutrophils, basophils, and eosinophils. Of these, the most important, making up 60 percent of all WBCs, are neutrophils, which are responsible for isolating and killing invading bacteria (pus consists largely of neutrophils). The action of neutrophils in swallowing bacteria has led to their being called phagocytes (literally "engulfing cells"). Neutrophils remain in the blood for only about six to nine hours before moving through blood vessel walls into the tissues, where they survive for a few more days. Eosinophils play a part in allergic reactions and increase in numbers in certain parasitic infections.

MONOCYTES Also a type of phagocyte, these circulate in the bloodstream for about six to nine days and play an important part in the *immune system*.

LYMPHOCYTES Many of these are formed in the lymph glands rather than the bone marrow. They play a central role in the immune system, roving around the body between the bloodstream, lymph glands, and channels between the lymph glands.

T-type lymphocytes are responsible for the delayed hypersensitivity phenomena (see *Allergy*) and produce substances called lymphokines, which affect the function of many cells. T-type lymphocytes also moderate the activity of other lymphocytes called B-type cells. These lymphocytes form the antibodies that protect us against second attacks of diseases (e.g., measles). Individual lymphocytes survive for anywhere between three months and 10 years.

DISORDERS The *leukemias* are disorders in the numbers and maturity of WBCs. WBCs may also be too few in number (see *Blood disorders*). In *AIDS*, the T-lymphocytes are infected by a virus,

which results in dysfunction and increased risk of certain types of infection and cancers.

PLATELETS

 These are the smallest type of blood cell (two to three thousandths of a millimeter in diameter), more numerous than WBCs but less numerous than RBCs (about 250,000 per cubic millimeter of blood). Like other blood cells, they originate from stem cells in the bone marrow; they survive in blood for about nine days.

FUNCTION Platelets circulate in the blood in an inactive state, but under certain circumstances they begin to stick to blood vessel walls and adhere to each other. These activities are important in *hemostasis* (the arrest of bleeding) and in *blood clotting*. The same processes can also lead to the unwanted formation of thrombi (clots) in intact blood vessels (see *Thrombosis*), and to fatty deposits on blood vessel walls (see *Atheroma*). Because of their role in the formation of clots, platelets are sometimes also known as thrombocytes.

DISORDERS Abnormal platelets, or a lack of platelets, can lead to some types of *bleeding disorder*.

BLOOD CELLS IN DIAGNOSIS
Microscopic examination of blood preparations may reveal not only blood cell abnormalities characteristic of various diseases, but also healthy variations in the numbers of WBCs produced in response to infections. For example, the number of neutrophilic WBCs is raised in response to bacterial infections. The same is true of lymphocytes in some viral infections. The blood cell "picture" (numbers, shapes, and appearance of the various types) is thus of value to physicians in disease diagnosis (see *Blood count; Blood smear*).

Blood clotting
Solidification of blood. Blood begins to clot within seconds of the skin being cut. The clot helps seal the damaged blood vessels, which also contract to keep loss of blood to a minimum. Blood clotting is not always helpful, however. Thrombi (clots) formed inside major blood vessels are the cause of many heart attacks, strokes, and other disorders (see *Thrombosis*).

The blood clotting process has two parts (see illustration, below).

To prevent the formation of clots inside healthy blood vessels, the

---

HOW BLOOD CLOTS
Clotting describes the solidification of blood anywhere in the body. Clotting occurs almost immediately at the site of a cut and helps limit blood loss by sealing damaged blood vessels. However, if abnormal clotting occurs in major blood vessels, heart attacks, strokes, and other disorders may occur. The clotting process has two main parts—platelet activation and the formation of fibrin filaments.

Red blood cells enmeshed in fibrin filaments
Fibrin is formed by a chemical change from a soluble protein, fibrinogen, which is present in the blood. The fibrin molecules aggregate to form long filaments, which enmesh blood cells (see left) to form a solid clot. The conversion of fibrinogen to fibrin is the last step of the "coagulation cascade," a series of reactions in the blood triggered by tissue injury and platelet activation.

Platelet | Fibrin | Clot | Epidermis | Dermis | White blood cell | Red blood cell

1 Platelets are activated by coming into contact with damaged blood vessel walls, where they become sticky and then clump at the site of injury and adhere to the damaged blood vessel wall.

2 Chemicals released by platelets and damaged tissues stimulate coagulation factors within the blood to form filaments of fibrin at the site of injury.

3 The fibrin filaments enmesh the platelets along with red and white blood cells.

4 Once the cut blood vessel is plugged by the mass of fibrin, platelets, and red and white blood cells, the fibrin filaments contract to form a solid clot.

blood also contains mechanisms that act to discourage clotting and dissolve clots. These balance the pro-clotting mechanisms; normally, the balance is tipped in favor of clot formation only when a blood vessel is damaged.

PLATELET AGGREGATION

Platelets have to be "activated" before they will clump together. This occurs when they come into contact with damaged blood vessel walls or artificial surfaces (such as glass), when blood flow is turbulent, or when platelets are acted on by certain chemicals secreted into the blood.

Once activated, platelets first become sticky, adhering to surfaces. They then change shape from disks into spiny spheres, enmeshing with each other. Finally, they release chemicals that activate other platelets, start the process of coagulation, and cause blood vessels to contract.

COAGULATION

Blood coagulation is triggered by chemicals released either by activated platelets or by tissues (following injury). Fibrin formation—the end product of coagulation—is the result of a complex series of reactions in the blood plasma called the "coagulation cascade." With each step in the cascade, a coagulation factor in the plasma is converted from an inactive to an active form.

The active form of the factor then activates several molecules of the next factor in the series—and so on until, in the final step, a factor called fibrinogen is converted into fibrin.

Provided all the participating factors are present, the activation of just one molecule of the first factor in the series can lead to the explosive production of up to 30,000 molecules of fibrin at the site of injury.

The factors involved in the coagulation cascade are numbered I, II, and V to XIII. Factor I is fibrinogen and factor II, its immediate precursor in the cascade, is called prothrombin. Most of the coagulation factors are made in the liver, which needs an adequate supply in the diet of *vitamin K*, found in green vegetables, for the manufacture of certain ones.

ANTICLOTTING MECHANISMS

Separate mechanisms act to prevent unwanted platelet activation and coagulation. Activation is inhibited mainly by a chemical known as prostacyclin (a type of *prostaglandin*), which is secreted by healthy blood vessel walls.

Coagulation is discouraged by various mechanisms. First, a number of inhibitory enzymes (types of protein) circulating in the blood neutralize activated coagulation factors. The most important of these is called antithrombin. Second, another series of enzymes is activated at the same time as the coagulation cascade. These enzymes form a substance called plasmin that breaks down fibrin (see *Fibrinolysis*). In addition, blood flow tends to discourage coagulation by washing away active coagulation factors from areas where they are being formed, and the liver deactivates any excess coagulation factors.

DEFECTS AND DISORDERS

Defects can occur for a wide variety of reasons in the clotting (or anticlotting) mechanisms, tipping the balance either in favor of a tendency to bleed or to form clots.

Some people carry a genetic defect that prevents them from producing sufficient amounts of one of the coagulation factors. In other cases, abnormally few platelets are made, insufficient vitamin K (required to make certain coagulation factors) is absorbed from the diet, or excessive amounts of the enzymes that inhibit coagulation of blood are produced. Abnormal bleeding may then result (see *Bleeding disorders*).

On the other hand, sometimes the balance is tipped abnormally in favor of coagulation and clotting. Possible causes include an increase in the levels of coagulation factors (as can occur in late pregnancy or when using some oral birth-control pills), a decrease in the level of enzymes that inhibit coagulation (as can occur in some forms of liver disease), or a sluggish blood flow through a particular area. The result may be abnormal clot formation (see *Thrombosis*).

Conditions in which there is a tendency for clot formation are often treated with *anticoagulants* such as heparin or warfarin. Heparin exerts its anticoagulant effect by increasing the level of antithrombin, which neutralizes activated coagulation factors; warfarin works by disrupting the production of coagulation factors. Because of the delicate balance between clotting and anticlotting mechanisms in blood, the use of these drugs has to be monitored frequently. Otherwise severe or persistent bleeding may develop.

Blood-clotting tests

Tests performed to screen for and diagnose *bleeding disorders*. These disorders usually result from deficiencies or abnormalities of the blood platelets or of blood coagulation factors (see *Blood clotting*).

Bleeding disorders caused by low numbers of platelets are detected by a *blood count* in conjunction with a test of the bleeding time.

Bleeding time may be measured by nicking the earlobe or puncturing the fingertip and timing the interval before bleeding stops. The normal range is three to eight minutes. Reduced platelet activity results in a prolonged bleeding time.

Various tests are used to assess the activity of blood coagulation factors—the most frequently performed being prothrombin time and partial thromboplastin time (named after two coagulation factors). The time taken for the patient's blood to clot is measured after addition of calcium and other factors that promote the coagulation process; the results are compared with the time taken for normal blood to clot under the same conditions. Abnormal results may indicate deficiency of a specific coagulation factor, as occurs in *hemophilia*, or of many coagulation factors, as in liver disease.

Anticoagulant therapy is designed to prolong the prothrombin time (clotting time) in order to reduce the risk of thrombosis (clotting) in susceptible subjects. People taking anticoagulants should have regular clotting tests to ensure that their therapy is adequate but not excessive, which could cause life-threatening bleeding.

Blood count

Also called complete blood count, this test measures hemoglobin concentration, and the numbers of red blood cells, white blood cells, and platelets in one cubic millimeter of blood. The proportion of various white blood cells is measured and the appearance of red and white cells is noted.

This is the most commonly performed blood test, important for diagnosing *anemia* and other conditions in which the number of blood cells is abnormally high (such as white blood cells in *leukemia* or red blood cells in *polycythemia*) or abnormally low (such as platelets in *thrombocytopenia*).

About 1 to 2 ml of blood are required for a blood count, which is usually performed in a laboratory by an automatic computerized analyzer, such as a Coulter counter.

Blood culture

See *Culture*.

DISORDERS OF THE BLOOD

Abnormalities can occur in any of the components of blood—the red blood cells (RBCs), white blood cells (WBCs), platelets, and numerous constituents of plasma.

Anemia (a deficiency of the red cell pigment *hemoglobin* and a consequent reduction in the blood's oxygen-carrying capacity) is by far the most common blood disorder. It has many different possible causes. In *polycythemia* there are too many red blood cells. In *leukemia* excessive numbers of immature white blood cells crowd out the normal cells from the bone marrow.

Defects in the platelets and in the clotting mechanisms may lead to any of various *bleeding disorders*. Unwanted clot formation (*thrombosis*) may result from circumstances that overactivate the clotting mechanisms.

Deficiencies of the proteins in blood plasma include hypoalbuminemia (*albumin* deficiency) and agammaglobulinemia (gamma globulin deficiency). Known causes of blood disorders include the following.

GENETIC DISORDERS

In these disorders there is an inherited abnormality in the production of some component of blood. People with *sickle cell anemia* and *thalassemia* produce an abnormal type of hemoglobin that makes their red blood cells more fragile; those with *hemophilia* fail to produce enough of one of the proteins involved in blood clotting. Disorders of this kind are present from birth and continue throughout life.

Sickle cell anemia
In this genetic (inherited) disorder, the red blood cells are abnormally fragile and have a characteristic sickle shape.

NUTRITIONAL DISORDERS

Loss of regular amounts of blood over an extended period may mean that iron (required to make hemoglobin) is lost faster than it can be replaced in the diet (see *Anemia, iron-deficiency*).

If insufficient amounts of the vitamins B_{12} or folic acid reach the bone marrow, it produces fewer red blood cells, which are abnormally large (see *Anemia, megaloblastic*). The vitamin deficiency may be due to a poor diet or, more often in developed countries, to a failure to absorb vitamin B_{12} correctly from the intestinal tract.

INFECTION

Multiplication of bacteria in the blood with the production of toxins is termed *bacteremia* and *septicemia*.

Many other microorganisms (i.e., viruses, fungi, protozoa, and other parasites) may infect the blood at some stage in their life cycle. Some organisms (notably those responsible for *malaria*) may actually attack and destroy red blood cells and so cause anemia (see *Anemia, hemolytic*).

TUMORS

All types of leukemia are the result of a type of cancer of the bone marrow, causing overgrowth of abnormal white blood cells and destruction of the healthy marrow. In *polycythemia* vera, a similar process occurs, except that mainly red cells are produced to excess. Another type of bone marrow cancer called *multiple myeloma* can cause an excess of certain proteins in the blood plasma.

POISONS

Carbon monoxide directly impairs the functioning of red blood cells by displacing oxygen bound to hemoglobin within the cells. Lead poisoning causes defective red blood cell production. Some snake and spider venoms destroy red cells and/or provoke clotting. *Septicemia* describes the presence of poisons produced in the blood by bacteria; toxemia describes the presence of metabolic poisons in the blood.

DRUGS

Certain drugs can cause blood abnormalities as a side effect. For example, co-trimoxazole, thiazide diuretics, and carbimazole may depress the production of white blood cells and/or platelets; chloramphenicol and sulfonamides may

Cold agglutinin disorder
This is a rare blood disorder in which the body develops antibodies to its own red blood cells, causing them to clump together. This effect is especially marked in cold conditions when the clumps of cells reduce blood flow to the limbs.

depress all blood cell production; methotrexate and phenytoin may interfere with red cell production.

Too high a dose of *anticoagulant drugs* can cause a bleeding tendency through excessive disruption of clotting mechanisms.

RADIATION

High doses of radiation (received at the time of therapy or from nuclear explosions or radioactive leaks from nuclear reactors) can severely damage the bone marrow, causing depression of all blood cell production (see *Anemia, aplastic*).

OTHER DISORDERS

Albumin—an important protein in the blood plasma—may become deficient either as a result of liver disease (reduced production) or kidney disease (loss of albumin in the urine).

Liver disease may also cause *hyperbilirubinemia* (excess bilirubin in the blood), anemia, and deficiencies of some of the clotting factors. Kidney disease causes *uremia* (excess urea in the blood), sometimes anemia (possibly due to decreased production of the hormone erythropoietin), and also complex changes in blood chemistry.

INVESTIGATION
Blood disorders are investigated principally by various *blood tests*, such as the *blood count*, *blood smear*, and *blood clotting tests*.

Blood donation

The process of giving blood so that it can be used in *blood transfusion*. Usually whole blood is taken from the donor and broken down later into components for storage. Recently, a new method called apheresis has been introduced, which involves extracting only a specific blood component from the donor. Whole blood donation takes about 45 minutes, including the medical check, while apheresis takes about two and a half hours.

Any healthy adult can potentially be a blood donor. Volunteer donors are first interviewed about their medical history. Anyone who has had anemia, cancer, heart disease, malaria, or hepatitis, or who has been exposed to the AIDS virus may be disqualified. Pregnant women are also disqualified. A blood sample taken from a finger or earlobe is then tested for anemia; body temperature, pulse, and blood pressure are also checked.

Most regular donors of whole blood give blood three or four times a year, but those with rare blood groups may be asked to give once every two months. Donors may safely give blood by apheresis as often as twice a week, provided a whole blood donation is not made between procedures.

HOW IT IS DONE

WHOLE BLOOD DONATION While the donor lies down and relaxes, a needle attached to a tube is inserted into the forearm. Up to a pint of blood (about one tenth of the total volume in the circulation) is slowly withdrawn into a plastic bag containing anticoagulant to prevent the blood from clotting. Most people feel fine after giving blood. A few may feel faint or sick and should rest or lie down for a few minutes. All donors should avoid strenuous exercise for about five hours after giving blood and should drink plenty of water and fruit juices.

The blood is taken to a local transfusion center, where it is tested for hepatitis B virus, syphilis, and antibody to HIV (the AIDS virus). The blood will not be used for transfusion if any of these is present. After being classified into blood groups, the blood is stored in a blood bank, either whole or separated into different components (see *Blood products*).

APHERESIS This technique allows only a blood component, such as plasma, platelets, or white cells, to be withdrawn from the circulation. About a pint of the donor's blood is taken from one arm, circulated through a closed, sterile separator system, and then returned to the other arm minus the component being collected. This withdrawal and return is repeated six to eight times, and collects the same amount of component normally requiring six to eight donors. Because only a single donor may be required to provide a patient with a sufficient quantity of a particular component, the risk of reaction or hepatitis transmission is reduced.

Blood gases

A test for determining the acidity-alkalinity (pH) and the concentrations of oxygen, carbon dioxide, and bicarbonate in the blood.

Blood oxygen and carbon dioxide values are useful in the diagnosing and monitoring of *respiratory failure*. Bicarbonate and acidity reflect the *acid-base balance* of the body. This may be disturbed in conditions such as diabetic ketoacidosis, aspirin poisoning, or repeated vomiting.

Modern apparatus can measure blood gases quickly using a few drops of blood, but full information requires samples to be taken from an artery as well as a vein and possibly from the interior of the heart.

Blood groups

Systems of classifying blood according to differences in the antigenic (able to provoke an immune reaction) make-up of red blood cells. Blood group typing is essential for a safe blood transfusion.

TYPES

ABO GROUPS Attempts in the nineteenth century and earlier at transfusing blood from one living person to another were sometimes successful but sometimes caused serious illness and even death. In 1900 the German pathologist Karl Landsteiner began mixing blood taken from different people and found that some mixtures were "compatible" while others were not. He discovered two types of marker proteins, or antigens, on the surface of the red blood cells—these he called A and B. According to whether a person's blood contains one or other antigen, both, or neither, it is classified as type A, B, AB, or O. Landsteiner found that the fluid part of the blood contained antibodies—anti-A and anti-B—that reacted with the protein markers.

The most common of the ABO blood groups is O, followed by A, then B, and finally AB. The precise frequency of each group differs among races.

BLOOD GROUP COMPATIBILITY

		Donor blood group			
		A	B	AB	O
Recipient blood group	A	▲	●	●	▲
	B	●	▲	●	▲
	AB	▲	▲	▲	▲
	O	●	●	●	▲

Key	▲ Compatible	● Incompatible

RHESUS FACTORS Another blood-group system, the Rhesus factors (Rh factors), was discovered in 1940 by Landsteiner during experiments on Rhesus monkeys. This system involves several antigens, the most important of which is factor D. This factor is found in the blood of 85 percent of people, who are called Rh positive, while 15 percent lack the factor and are Rh negative. Individuals are therefore classed as, for example, "O positive" or "AB negative" on the basis of their ABO and Rh blood groups. The main importance of this group is in pregnancy in Rh-negative women since, if the baby is Rh positive, the mother may form antibodies against the baby's blood (see *Hemolytic disease of the newborn*). Rh-negative women are given antibodies directed against factor D after delivery to prevent the development of anti-D antibodies in the mother, which would cause hemolytic disease of the newborn in Rh-positive infants. Transfusion of Rh-positive blood into an Rh-negative patient can also cause a serious reaction if the patient has had previous blood transfusions that contained the RH antigen.

OTHER GROUPS

Since the discovery of the ABO and Rh factors, about 400 other antigens have been identified, but, since these various antigens are widely scattered throughout the population, these rarely cause transfusion problems.

USES

TRANSFUSION AND CROSS MATCHING The ABO and Rh groups are used to categorize blood stored in blood banks so that if a patient who is, for example, A positive, needs a transfusion he or she can be given A-positive blood from the bank. In practice, however, each unit (about a pint) of blood to be given is first tested against a small sample of the patient's blood to exclude the small possibility that the two might be incompatible because of a reaction due to one of the other blood groups. This test is known as cross matching and takes a short time to perform. In an emergency, unmatched blood of the appropriate group may need to be given. (See *Blood transfusion*.)

ANTHROPOLOGY The ABO blood groups are found in all people, but the frequency of each group varies with race and geographical distribution. Study of blood groups can therefore aid anthropologists who are involved in investigating, for example, early population migrations.

PATERNITY CASES The blood group of an individual is determined by the genes inherited from his or her parents. Identification of blood group can be used in a paternity case to establish that a man could not have been the father of a particular child. It cannot

be shown positively that a man is the father by blood grouping, but, with modern techniques of gene analysis, paternity can now be proved with virtual certainty.

CRIMINAL INVESTIGATION Blood found at the scene of a crime can be grouped according to the various red blood cell antigens present. Although techniques are not yet sophisticated enough to allow positive identification of a specific individual, it is possible to exclude suspects if one of the red blood cell antigens does not match. Because ABO antigens are inherited, they occur in other tissue fluids, such as semen and saliva. Analysis of blood groups can also be useful in *forensic medicine* (the interrelation of medicine and the law).

INHERITED DISORDERS Some blood groups are associated with particular disorders. For example, blood group

A has been found to be more common in people suffering from cancer of the stomach. People who have blood group O are apparently more susceptible to peptic ulcer.

Blood loss
See *Bleeding, treatment of*.

Blood poisoning
A common name for *septicemia* or toxemia, a serious, often life-threatening illness caused by multiplication of bacteria and their formation of poisons or toxins in the bloodstream. Septicemia may be a complication of an infection (i.e., an infected wound or burn). It was formerly a feared and fatal complication of childbirth (see *Puerperal sepsis*). In some infective conditions, profound shock—called *septic shock*—may be caused by toxins released by bacteria. (See also *Bacteremia*.)

Blood pressure
The pressure of the blood in the main arteries, which rises and falls as the heart and muscles of the body cope with varying demands—exercise, stress, and sleep. Two types of pressure are measured. Systolic, the highest, is the pressure created by the contraction of the heart muscle and the elastic recoil of the aorta (great artery) as blood surges through it. Diastolic is when the ventricles relax between beats; it reflects the resistance of all the small arteries throughout the body and the load against which the heart must work. The pressure wave transmitted along the arteries with each heartbeat is easily felt as the *pulse*.

MEASURING BLOOD PRESSURE
A soft rubber cuff is inflated around the upper arm until it is tight enough to stop the flow of blood. The cuff is then gradually deflated until, by listening to the main artery through a stethoscope, the blood can first be heard as a beat forcing its way along the main artery in the arm. This is recorded as the systolic pressure. The cuff is then deflated further until the beat disappears and the blood flows steadily through the now open artery—giving the diastolic pressure.

Blood pressure may also be measured by miniature devices attached to an artery or by a continuous recording while an individual leads his or her daily life.

Blood pressure is recorded by giving the systolic pressure and diastolic pressure, expressed as millimeters of

mercury (mm Hg). This is because the earliest equipment used a glass column filled with mercury to measure the pressure directly. Today, some sphygmomanometers use a

spring gauge with a round dial. A healthy young adult has a blood pressure reading of about 110/75, which often normally rises with age to about 130/90 at age 60.

CHANGES IN BLOOD PRESSURE
Raised or lowered blood pressure can be caused by various factors. During pregnancy it tends to rise but then returns gradually to its previous level after birth. Certain drugs also affect blood pressure as a side effect. During the day (below) a normal person's blood pressure fluctuates according to activity. Hypertension (abnormally high blood pressure) is treated with weight loss, sodium restriction, drugs, and modification of life-style.

Waking and getting up cause blood pressure to rise.

Vigorous exercise raises blood pressure.

Getting tense or smoking makes blood pressure rise.

Systolic

Diastolic

S

D

180
160
140
120
100
80
60

Time 7 AM   8   9   10   11   12   1 PM   2

Blood products

After *blood donation*, blood is stored either whole or separated into its various components. Each product has a particular use in *blood transfusion*.

WHOLE BLOOD

Used to restore blood volume following sudden severe bleeding—for instance, after a traffic accident or during major surgery. Whole blood keeps three to four weeks after donation.

PACKED RED CELLS

Prepared by removing part of the liquid plasma. Concentrated red cells are used to treat patients with some forms of chronic anemia that have not responded to drug treatment. They provide the necessary hemoglobin without overloading the recipient with fluid, which can result in or aggravate heart failure. The cells can also be used to treat babies with *hemolytic disease of the newborn* ("Rhesus" babies).

WASHED RED CELLS

Blood that has had the white blood cells and/or plasma protein removed, thus reducing the chances of allergic reaction in patients, such as those with chronic anemia, who require transfusions over a long period.

FROZEN RED CELLS

Red cells can be preserved for long periods if stored at very low temperatures. This technique is used to preserve red cells belonging to rare blood groups.

PLATELETS

Extracted from whole blood and concentrated, they play an important part in normal blood clotting. Their low level in some blood disorders causes the patient to bruise easily and suffer internal bleeding. If necessary, platelets from several donors can be given during one transfusion.

WHITE BLOOD CELLS

Granulocytes, a type of white blood cell, can be separated from normal blood, or from the blood of patients with chronic granulocytic leukemia (who have an excess of these cells). Patients with life-threatening infections accompanied by abnormally low levels of granulocytes may be treated with granulocytes if they are not responding to antibiotics.

FROZEN FRESH PLASMA

Prepared by separating and freezing plasma as soon as possible after blood collection. Rich in clotting factors, fresh plasma is used to correct many types of bleeding disorders.

PLASMA PROTEIN SOLUTIONS

The liquid part of any whole blood not used within three weeks of collection that is converted into a concentrated solution of albumin (the main protein in plasma). The solution can be stored for long periods. Its chief use is in treating shock, resulting from severe blood loss, until whole blood compatible with the patient's blood group becomes available.

Purified albumin preparations are used to treat the nephrotic syndrome (a kidney disorder causing albumin loss in the urine) and chronic liver disease (in which production of albumin is deficient).

CLOTTING FACTORS

Concentrates of clotting factors VIII and IX can be prepared for the treatment of hemophilia and Christmas disease. Because blood from many donors is required to produce one small batch of clotting factor, it must be heat-treated to reduce the risk of hepatitis or AIDS transmission.

IMMUNOGLOBULINS

Antibodies (immunoglobulins) occur in the blood of patients recovering from certain viral diseases, such as rubella or hepatitis B, and in those who have recently been immunized—for example, against tetanus. These antibodies can be concentrated from plasma taken from such patients and used to protect people who are unable to produce their own antibodies or who have recently been exposed to a viral disease. This technique of inferring immunity is known as passive *immunization*.

A similar blood product, anti-D immunoglobulin, is obtained from the blood of patients sensitized to the Rh blood group factor. If given to an Rh-negative mother within 60 hours of her giving birth to an Rh-positive baby, it will prevent *hemolytic disease of the newborn* in her future babies.

Blood smear

A test that involves smearing a drop of blood onto a glass slide so that it can be examined under a microscope. The blood smear is stained with special dyes to make the blood cells show up more clearly.

The shape and appearance of blood cells are inspected for any abnormality, such as sickle-shaped red blood cells in sickle cell disease or abnormal lymphocytes in infectious mononucleosis. The relative proportions of the different types of white blood cells can also be counted. This examination, called a differential white cell count, may be helpful in diagnosing infection or leukemia. Blood smears are also used in diagnosing infections, such as malaria, in which the parasites can be seen inside the red blood cells.

Blood smears are usually done with a complete *blood count*.

Blood tests

Analysis of a sample of blood that gives information on its cells and proteins and any of the chemicals, antigens, antibodies, and gases that it carries. Since blood is the main transport system of the body, such tests can be used to check on the health of major organs, as well as on respiratory function, hormonal balance, the immune system, and metabolism.

TYPES

There are three types of blood test.

HEMATOLOGICAL TESTS These tests involve looking at the components of the blood itself, examining the numbers, shape, size, and appearance of cells, and testing the function of clotting factors. The most important hematological tests are *blood count*, *blood smear*, and *blood clotting tests*.

BIOCHEMICAL TESTS These look at chemicals in the blood, such as sodium, potassium, uric acid, and urea, and at vitamins, gases, digested foods, and drugs. (See *Acid-base balance*; *Kidney function tests*; *Liver function tests*.)

MICROBIOLOGICAL TESTS In these tests, the blood is examined for microorganisms, such as bacteria, viruses and viral particles, fungi, and parasites, and for antibodies that form against them. (See *Culture*.)

HOW THEY ARE DONE

The most convenient site for taking a blood sample is a vein at the bend in the elbow. A tourniquet is applied to the upper arm, and the blood is withdrawn through a needle into a syringe. The procedure causes only mild discomfort. Up to 20 ml of blood may be required, but, as the circulation contains 4 to 5 liters, loss of this small proportion has no harmful effect. If only a few drops are needed, they may be obtained by pricking a finger. Some tests require arterial blood, which is taken from the wrist or the groin. Obtaining such blood is a more difficult procedure that may cause some discomfort.

The sample may be allowed to clot, leaving its clear serum for examination, or an anticoagulant may be added to allow study of the cells and clotting factors. The sample is then sent to the laboratory, where one or more of the hundreds of available tests are performed. In some laboratories, modern computerized analyzers are used to perform many different tests simultaneously on one small sample of blood. The printed results compare each value with the accepted normal range for that test. Each laboratory produces its own normal ranges that depend on the method and the ingredients of the test, and sometimes on the age and sex of the patient.

Blood transfusion

The infusion of large volumes of blood or blood components directly into the bloodstream, done mainly to remedy severe blood loss or to correct anemia.

Before the discovery of the major *blood groups* earlier this century, blood transfusion was a hazardous procedure, often causing severe reactions and even death. Growing knowledge of the complex properties of blood and its components has now made transfusion a safe procedure, although still not without possible complications.

WHY IT IS DONE

Blood transfusion may be needed by a patient who has bled severely after an accident or has lost a lot of blood during an operation. It may also be required after internal bleeding—for example, from a bleeding peptic ulcer. Chronic anemia that does not respond to medication may require treatment by blood transfusion (for example, in conditions such as thalassemia and leukemia).

In an exchange transfusion, nearly all of the recipient's blood is replaced by donor blood. It is most often needed in *hemolytic disease of the newborn* ("Rhesus babies") when abnormally high levels of bilirubin in the blood might cause brain damage.

HOW IT IS DONE

Before transfusion, blood must be cross matched to ensure compatibility. This procedure involves taking a sample of the recipient's blood, identifying the blood group, and matching it with suitable donor blood. This is done by mixing some of each blood sample on a microscope slide and examining it to make sure there are no antibodies in the recipient's plasma that would damage the donor blood cells. Blood can usually be cross matched in one hour or less. If the patient is losing blood very rapidly, it may not be possible to wait. In this case, O Rh-negative blood that has not been cross matched ("universal donor"), plasma protein solution, or an artificial plasma substitute may be given to the patient until tested blood becomes available.

Blood is transfused into an arm vein. Usually, each unit (about 1 pint) of blood is given over one to four hours; in an emergency 1 pint may be given in a couple of minutes. The amount of blood required depends on how much has been lost or on the severity of anemia. Usually, if transfusion is needed, more than one unit is given to justify the risks entailed in giving blood. During transfusion, the patient's pulse, blood pressure, and temperature are measured regularly, and, if there is any sign of a reaction, the transfusion is stopped.

COMPLICATIONS

If blood has not been cross matched reliably, antibodies in the recipient's blood may cause incompatible donor cells to hemolyze (burst). The most severe reactions can result in *shock* or kidney failure. Less severe reactions can produce fever, chills, a rash, or delayed anemia. Transfusion reactions can also occur as a result of allergy to transfused white cells, plasma proteins, or platelets.

Infections, such as hepatitis B, AIDS, syphilis, and malaria, can occur if donor blood has not been adequately screened. All blood for transfusion is now carefully tested and the risk of infection is very low.

In elderly or severely anemic patients transfusion can overload the circulation, leading to heart failure. *Diuretics*, which cause fluid loss, may need to be given simultaneously to avoid this. In patients with chronic anemia who require regular transfusion over many years, excess iron may accumulate (a condition called hemosiderosis) and cause damage to various organs, such as the heart, liver, and pancreas. Dangerous buildup of iron can be relieved by giving the drug deferoxamine.

Blood vessels

A general term for arteries, veins, and capillaries. (See *Circulatory system*.)

Blue baby

An infant with a cyanotic (blue-purple) complexion caused by a relative lack of oxygen in the blood. This is usually due to a structural defect of the heart or of the major arteries leaving the heart. The defect allows some of the deoxygenated blood returning to the right side of the heart to be pumped straight back into the general circulation instead of first going to the lungs to receive oxygen. Such defects can usually be corrected surgically. (See *Heart disease, congenital*.)

Blue bloater

A term physicians use to describe the appearance of some patients with the lung disease *emphysema*, with or without chronic *bronchitis*.

The person appears cyanotic (blue-purple) because of a deficiency in oxygen reaching the bloodstream from the lungs and appears bloated because of *edema* (swelling caused by fluid collection) in body tissues, mainly due to *heart failure* resulting from the lung damage.

Other patients with emphysema may have an alternative appearance known as *pink puffer*.

Blue Cross/Blue Shield

A private, not-for-profit health insurance association. The first local Blue Cross plan, covering hospital charges, began in 1929. Blue Shield's plans, to cover physicians' charges, were started a few years later by groups of physicians, in many cases by medical societies. The Blue Cross and Blue Shield associations merged in 1983. Blue Cross/Blue Shield plans in the US provide health insurance for more than 77 million people.

Blurred vision

A common term used to indicate a decrease or distortion of vision, or indistinct, fuzzy, or misty visual images. Blurred vision should not be confused with *double vision* (diplopia). Blurred vision can occur in one or both eyes, for episodes of varying lengths of time, and develop gradually or suddenly. Sometimes only part of the field of vision is affected. The need for proper glasses is probably the most common cause of blurred vision. Any change in vision should be brought to the attention of your physician.

CAUSES

Vision may be impaired, or blindness caused, by damage, disease, or abnormalities affecting the tear film, cornea, iris, lens, aqueous or vitreous humor, retina, or the nerve pathways behind the eye. These nerve pathways may be damaged by tumor, head injury, or *stroke*.

Many people notice gradual changes in near vision from the age of 40 onward—their vision for close work and for reading close-up becomes less sharp. They may also have problems with small print. Generally, distance vision does not worsen after age 40. After age 40 or 45, people generally need reading glasses or bifocals for close-up reading to correct the blur. This is due to *presbyopia* (decreased ability to focus close-up). If a person has been myopic (near-sighted), he or she may be able to take off the glasses to see close-up objects after age 40.

Blurred vision is most commonly due to refractive errors. They include *myopia* (nearsightedness), *hyper-metropia* (farsightedness), and *astigma-tism* (unequal curvature of the front of the eye). These defects can easily be rectified by glasses or contact lenses.

Blushing

Brief reddening of the face and sometimes the neck caused by the dilation of the blood vessels close to the surface of the skin. Blushing is usually an involuntary reaction to embarrassment. Some women blush during *menopause* due to changes in hormonal activity (see *Hot flashes*). Flushing of the face occurs in association with the *carcinoid syndrome*.

Board certification

Formal recognition of a physician's qualifications in a medical specialty by one of the 23 organizations belonging to the American Board of Medical Specialties. To become board-certified in a medical specialty (i.e., dermatology, pediatrics, or surgery), a physician must usually complete an extended residency, demonstrate experience, complete special studies, and pass an exhaustive examination.

The 23 specialty boards, in addition to giving general certification, grant certification in 46 subspecialties (i.e., gastroenterology, hematology, or child psychiatry) after further study, experience, and examination.

The specialty boards consist of 15 to 25 physicians, representing the specialties and subspecialties in a given field, physicians in related fields and, often, physicians representing general medical organizations.

Body contour surgery

Operations performed to remove excess fat, skin, or both, from various parts of the body, especially the abdomen, thighs, and buttocks. Diet and exercise are the proper means of reducing the fat content of the body, and surgery is not a substitute. Operations may improve appearance where accumulations of fat or excess skin persist in certain areas after successful weight control.

ABDOMINAL WALL REDUCTION

In this contouring operation, often called abdominoplasty, excess skin and fat are removed from the abdomen. After the abdomen decreases in size, such as following weight loss or pregnancy, there remains an excess of skin in some people. These people may benefit from surgery.

The operation is carried out using general anesthesia and requires a hospital stay of from two to three days. The surgeon makes a horizontal "bikini" incision in the skin as low down on the abdomen as possible, then cuts upward between the fat and muscle layers. The flap of skin and fat is pulled down and the excess is removed. Sometimes, when the amount to be removed is particularly large, a vertical incision is required in addition to the horizontal one.

At the end of the operation the skin is stitched together. Drains are inserted into the wound and left in place for several days to prevent the risk of blood or serum collecting, which can lead to infection. The patient may sit on a chair soon after the operation, but should walk with the trunk slightly flexed for several weeks. Avoidance of tension on the wound will help minimize the size of the scar.

Despite care taken with movement after the operation, the final scar is often not as narrow as the patient and surgeon would like. In addition, the umbilicus (navel) usually must be moved to a higher position (with a resulting scar around it) because it has been pulled down with the flap during the operation.

REDUCTION OF THIGHS AND BUTTOCKS

In these operations, fat and skin are removed from the area of the crease separating these regions. The scar is planned to be in the "stocking-seam line," but the scars are often wide and unattractive and often end up in an undesired location. The wounds occasionally fail to heal properly, and the final appearance may not be symmetrical. Patients with generalized excess fat do not see improvement. Some people who ask for this operation may have a tilted pelvis because of prominent buttock muscles. Buttock and thigh reduction surgery yields a less satisfactory result than most other types of cosmetic plastic surgery operations.

SUCTION LIPECTOMY

To overcome the problem of noticeable scars, instruments have been developed to remove fat through "key-hole" incisions. A suction instrument is inserted through a small skin incision and moved back and forth under the skin to break up large areas of fat, which can then be suctioned through the instrument. However, because of the plentiful blood supply within the fat, there may be significant blood and fluid loss, which must be treated by the physician to prevent shock or anemia. In addition, the total amount of fat that can be removed at one time is limited. Suction lipectomy is useful in improving the appearance of people who have localized areas of excess fat, such as occurs on the hips, but cannot be used as a substitute for weight control. Minor irregularities and dimpling of the skin commonly occur after surgery.

Body odor

The smell caused by sweat on the skin surface. Sweat itself has no odor, but, if it remains on the skin for a few hours, bacterial decomposition may lead to body odor. The sweat may also smell strongly after garlic, curry, or other spicy foods are eaten. Bacterial decomposition of sweat occurs most noticeably in the armpits and around the genital area, because the *apocrine glands* in these areas contain proteins and fatty materials favorable to the growth of bacteria. Sweat from other areas of the body is mainly salt water, which does not encourage bacteria to form. Feet are an exception because they are subject to warm, airless conditions for hours on end—so making them a perfect environment for bacteria and fungi.

PREVENTING BODY ODOR

If body odor is a problem, the most effective treatment is to wash all over at least once daily. After washing, the use of a deodorant containing an antiperspirant will prevent sweat from reaching the surface of the skin.

Boil

An inflamed, pus-filled area of skin, usually an infected hair follicle (the tiny pit from which a hair grows). Common sites include the back of the neck, and moist areas such as the armpits and groin. A more severe and extensive form of a boil is a *carbuncle*.

The usual cause of boils is infection with the bacterium STAPHYLOCOCCUS AUREUS. Some people carry this organism in their nose or other sites; in many cases the source of an infection cannot be traced.

SYMPTOMS

A boil starts as a red, painful lump. As it swells it fills with pus and becomes rounded, with a yellowish tip (head). Recurrent boils may occur in people

B

with known or unrecognized *diabetes mellitus* or other conditions in which general body resistance to bacterial infection is impaired.

TREATMENT

Do not burst a boil, as this may spread the infection. A hot compress applied every two hours will relieve discomfort and hasten possible drainage and healing. Taking showers, instead of bathing, reduces the chances of spreading the infection.

If the boil is large and painful, consult your physician. He or she may prescribe an antibiotic, or may open the boil with a sterile needle to allow the pus to drain.

Occasionally, large boils have to be lanced using a surgical knife. This is usually done with a local anesthetic.

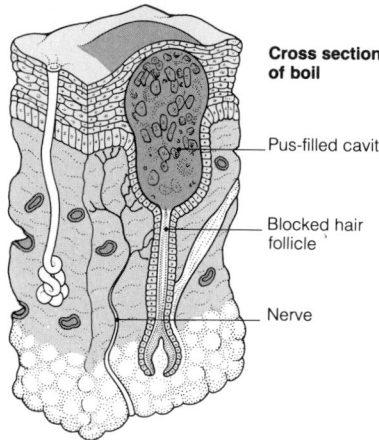

Cross section of boil

Pus-filled cavity

Blocked hair follicle

Nerve

Bolus

A soft mass of chewed food, ready to be swallowed, produced by the action of the tongue, teeth, and saliva. In this form, food is easily swallowed and passed through the esophagus.

A bolus also describes the rapid injection into a vein of a relatively large dose of a drug.

Bonding

The process by which a strong psychological tie is established between a parent and newborn child. Bonding is essential for a baby's healthy emotional development.

Ideas about bonding were first developed from studies of geese, monkeys, and other animals. Goslings were observed attaching themselves to and following the first moving object they saw after birth. Monkeys deprived of their mothers failed to develop normal maternal instincts. But most monkeys in the experiment developed normally when

The bonding process
By maintaining eye-to-eye and frequent physical contact, bonding gradually becomes established.

given an inanimate mother substitute, especially a furry one that could be held and cuddled.

Bonding is a reciprocal process in which baby and parent respond to each other's gestures and expressions. A failure to bond may occur if a baby is sick or premature and has to be taken from his or her parent (by being placed in an incubator directly after birth), but most babies bond normally with special attention at a later stage. Bonding problems may occur if a new parent's own early family experiences failed to provide a good model of parent-infant interaction. However, such people can be taught successful ways to interact with their newborns.

Lack of bonding may increase the risk of neglect or child abuse and may lead to delayed mental development, depression, and inability to develop satisfactory relationships in adulthood. Most studies indicate that employed mothers can bond as successfully as nonemployed mothers and that children can fare well with more than one primary caregiver (of either sex) as long as all caregivers are loving and consistent.

Bonding, dental

The correction of tooth defects by using plastic materials, porcelain, or acrylic. The effects of bonding can be preventive (as with the use of sealants) or restorative.

WHY IT IS DONE

Bonding is used to treat teeth that are fractured, chipped, too widely spaced, malformed, or badly stained. Bonding is also used to close small gaps between front teeth, restore decayed back teeth, and, in some cases, substitute for a crown. Bonding has been used to protect exposed roots and is increasingly used to attach *orthodontic appliances*. Its use may also

make the teeth less sensitive to variations in temperature. One type of bonding, which incorporates sealants, is preventive in nature. Sealants, which are made of plastic, help prevent decay in the deep grooves of molars by keeping out bacteria.

HOW IT IS DONE

In many cases, bonding procedures require no anesthesia or drilling. Bonding techniques involve securing a plastic or porcelain material to the surface of the tooth. First, the dentist applies a weak acid solution to the tooth, creating a roughened surface to which the bonding material can adhere. This technique is sometimes called acid-etching. The liquid bonding material (resin) is then applied to the rough surface.

If a portion of a tooth needs to be rebuilt or a missing part replaced, a composite resin is shaped on the tooth and then hardened.

If work is being done on the front teeth or on badly stained teeth, a porcelain or acrylic laminate veneer may be bonded to the tooth's surface. For this procedure the enamel is acid-etched and an adhesive resin is attached. Finally, the preshaped laminate veneer is positioned on top of the resin.

EFFECTIVENESS

With bonding, the structure and appearance of teeth can be improved. Results of the bonding procedure last for about five years, so the procedure requires renewing. In addition, bonding is weaker than natural tooth enamel, so it chips more easily. Bonded areas may also become stained by certain foods and beverages. Because crowns are more durable than bonding materials, crowns may be more suitable for repairing badly damaged back teeth. Poorly aligned teeth may require orthodontic treatment.

Bone

The structural material of the body's framework, or *skeleton*. Bone contains calcium and phosphorus, which make it hard and rigid; the arrangement of bone's fibers makes it resilient.

STRUCTURE

The surface of bone is covered with periosteum, a thin membrane that contains a network of blood vessels and nerves. Beneath the periosteum is a hard, dense shell of compact, or ivory bone. Inside this shell the bone is cancellous or spongy. The central cavity of hollow bones and the meshes of spongy bone contain a fatty tissue,

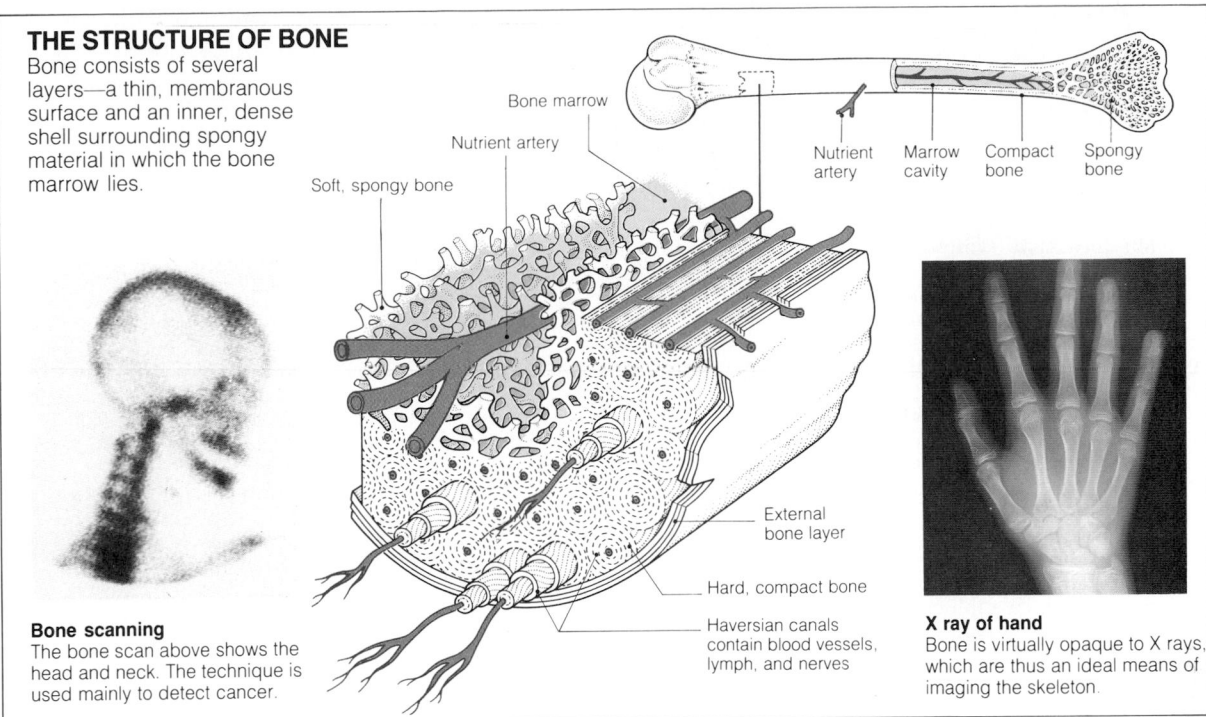

THE STRUCTURE OF BONE

Bone consists of several layers—a thin, membranous surface and an inner, dense shell surrounding spongy material in which the bone marrow lies.

Bone marrow

Nutrient artery

Soft, spongy bone

Nutrient artery

Marrow cavity

Compact bone

Spongy bone

External bone layer

Hard, compact bone

Haversian canals contain blood vessels, lymph, and nerves

Bone scanning
The bone scan above shows the head and neck. The technique is used mainly to detect cancer.

X ray of hand
Bone is virtually opaque to X rays, which are thus an ideal means of imaging the skeleton.

bone marrow, in which the red and most white blood cells and platelets are formed.

The hard structural part of bone underneath the periosteum is formed of columns of bone cells known as haversian canals. These are important for the nutrition, growth, and repair of the bone. The direction of the canals corresponds with the mechanical forces acting on the bone. Bone is insensitive; any sensation comes from the nerves in the periosteum.

FUNCTIONS

The long, short, flat, and irregular bones of the skeleton provide a rigid framework for the muscles; the muscles form surface coverings of the cavities that protect the body's organs (the heart and lungs in the bony thoracic cavity and the brain in the skull). Bones, with the joints and muscles, form the locomotor system.

GROWTH

The growth of bone is a balance between the activity of its two constituent cells, osteoblasts and osteoclasts. Osteoblasts encourage the deposit of the mineral calcium phosphate on the protein framework of the bone. Osteoclasts remove mineral from the bone. The actions of these cells are controlled by hormones: growth hormone secreted by the pituitary gland, the sex hormones estrogen and

testosterone, the adrenal hormones, parathyroid hormone, and the thyroid hormone thyrocalcitonin. These hormones also maintain the calcium level in the blood within close limits; any fall below the normal range affects the nerves and muscles.

Most bones begin to develop in the embryo during the fifth or sixth week of pregnancy, taking the form of cartilage. This cartilage begins to be replaced by hard bone, in a process known as *ossification*, at around the seventh or eighth week of pregnancy; the process is not complete until early adult life. At birth many bones consist mainly of cartilage, which will ossify later. The ends of the long bones are separate from the shaft, allowing the bones to grow. Some small bones of the hands and feet consist entirely of cartilage. Many of the bones of the skull do not begin life as bone. They are known as membranous bones.

Bone abscess

A localized collection of pus in a bone (see *Osteomyelitis*).

Bone cancer

Malignant growth in bone. Bone cancer may originate in the bone itself (primary bone cancer) or, more commonly, be a result of cancer that has spread from elsewhere in the body

(secondary bone cancer). The growth replaces bone, causing pain and sometimes swelling. It also makes the bone more likely to fracture without preceding injury. Bone cancer that affects the spine may cause collapse or crushing of vertebrae, damaging the spinal cord, and thus causing weakness or paralysis of the affected limbs.

PRIMARY BONE CANCER

The most common type of this rare form of cancer is *osteosarcoma*, which most frequently affects the leg bones of children and young adults. Symptoms of osteosarcoma are pain, tenderness, and swelling, typically just above or just below the knee. X rays, bone scans (see *Bone imaging*), and *biopsy* will confirm the diagnosis.

Other, even rarer, types of primary bone cancer include *chondrosarcoma* (originating from cartilage) and *fibrosarcoma* (from fibrous tissue). Cancer can also start in bone marrow (see *Ewing's tumor; Multiple myeloma*).

The treatment of osteosarcoma, chondrosarcoma, and fibrosarcoma depends on the extent to which the disease has spread. If it is confined to bone, amputation may be recommended. Alternatively, *radiation therapy* or *chemotherapy* may be used to control the tumor. With modern drugs, the outlook has improved and many patients have benefited.

SECONDARY BONE CANCER

Secondary, or metastatic, bone cancer, is more common than primary bone cancer; it usually occurs later in life. The cancers that spread readily to bone are those of the breast, lung, prostate, thyroid, and kidney. Bone metastases occur commonly in the vertebrae, pelvis, ribs, and skull.

In secondary bone cancer, pain is usually the main symptom and is often worse at night. Affected bones are abnormally fragile and may fracture, even without preceding injury. Such a fracture (a pathological fracture) may be the first indication that a person has cancer.

Imaging studies will confirm the presence of secondary bone cancer. If the original site of the cancer is not obvious, further tests may be needed to identify it.

Secondary bone cancers from the breast and prostate often respond to hormone therapy. Growth of prostate tumors may be inhibited with estrogen or hypothalamic hormones and in some breast tumors by *hormone antagonists*. Sometimes the most effective treatment is removal of the endocrine glands (ovaries, testes, or adrenals). Pathological fractures may require orthopedic surgery, with pins and plates inserted in the bone.

Bone cyst

A cavity in a bone, usually filled with fluid. It typically develops at one end of a long bone. The presence of a cyst is often discovered by chance after there has been a bone fracture at the site of the cyst. A minor operation that involves scraping the cyst and filling the cavity with bone chips usually cures the condition.

Bone graft

An operation in which a small piece of bone is taken from one part of the body to repair bone damage in another part. The bone graft is attached to the defective bone, and provides a bone growth stimulating protein. Although the bone graft eventually dies, it acts as a scaffold upon which new bone can grow.

WHY IT IS DONE

A bone graft has four main uses: to encourage a fracture to heal, to restore bone lost through injury, to replace bone removed surgically because of disease, and to provide a peg to join the bones of a diseased or unstable joint. A bone graft may also be used in cosmetic surgery to improve the shape of the face and skull.

DISORDERS OF THE BONE

Bone is affected by the same types of disorders as other body tissues, but its hard, rigid structure makes for extra complications. If a bone receives a direct blow or suffers from repeated stress it may *fracture*. If it becomes infected (for instance, due to *osteomyelitis* or a *bone abscess*), the resulting inflammation may interfere with the blood supply, leading to death of part of the bone.

GENETIC DISORDERS

Several genetic (inherited) conditions may affect bone growth; these include *achondroplasia* and *osteogenesis imperfecta*. People with these are usually of *short stature*.

NUTRITIONAL DISORDERS

Lack of calcium and vitamin D in the diet may result in *rickets* in children and *osteomalacia* in adults; in both conditions the bones become soft and lose their shape.

HORMONAL DISORDERS

If the pituitary gland produces excess growth hormone before puberty, there is an overgrowth of bones and other organs leading to *gigantism*. Excess parathyroid hormone causes *bone cysts*. *Osteoporosis* is also frequently due to other hormonal disturbances.

TUMORS

Several different types of benign and malignant growth can affect bones (see *Bone tumor*; *Bone cancer*).

DEGENERATION

Degenerative disorders of bone become more common in old age. In *osteoarthritis* there is wearing of the bone surface in a number of joints.

AUTOIMMUNE DISORDERS

Here the body's *immune system* attacks its own tissues. The main autoimmune disorder that may affect bones is *rheumatoid arthritis*.

OTHER DISORDERS

Paget's disease involves thickening of the outer layer of the bones while the inside becomes spongy.

INVESTIGATION

Bone disorders are investigated by techniques such as *X rays*, *CT scanning*, and *radionuclide scanning*, by *biopsy*, and by biochemical *blood tests* to look for any abnormalities in the levels of hormones or nutrients such as calcium and vitamin D.

HOW IT IS DONE

The bone from which the graft is to be taken is exposed and a portion removed. The most common sources are the iliac crests (upper part of the hip bones). These bones contain a large amount of cancellous bone, the inner, spongy part, which is especially useful for getting grafts to "take." Other sources are the ribs, which provide curved bone, and the ulna (in the forearm), which provides excellent bone pegs.

The bone that needs treatment is exposed and the graft fixed to it with screws or wires. After the area has been stitched, it is put into a plaster cast to keep the graft in place.

RECOVERY PERIOD

Bruising and pain at the site from which the graft was taken clear up within a week or two, and the only large scars left are those where bone has been taken from the iliac crests. X rays are taken to check the progress of healing, which usually is well under way after about six weeks.

Most bone graft operations succeed in permitting formation of new bone as strong and efficient as the old.

Bone imaging

Technique for providing pictures that show bone structure or function, used for the detection of disease or injury of the bone.

TYPES

Because *X rays* are more fully absorbed by bone than by other tissues, X-ray images show bone structure clearly. This makes them ideal for diagnosing fractures and injuries and also for revealing tumors and infections that cause changes in bone structure. A more detailed examination of small changes or abnormalities hidden by surrounding structures is provided by *tomography* (taking X-ray pictures at different depths of the structure being examined) or *CT scanning*. Magnetic resonance imaging (*MRI*), which is tomographic imaging using extremely high voltage magnets, shows tumors and infections and the effect of diseased bone on surrounding muscles, ligaments, and fat. Either CT scanning or MRI is useful in looking for *disk prolapse* in people with low back pain.

Radionuclide scanning is used to reveal bone function—the rate of blood flow to the bone and of cell activity within it. The technique is used mainly to determine whether cancer has spread to bone. It also can give useful information on bone injuries, infections, tumors, arthritis, and on metabolic bone diseases, such as rickets.

Bone marrow

The soft fatty tissue found in bone cavities; it may be red or yellow. Red bone marrow is a blood-producing tissue present in all bones at birth. During the teens, it is gradually replaced in some bones by less active yellow marrow. In the adult, red marrow is confined chiefly to the spine, sternum, ribs, clavicle (collarbone), scapulae (shoulder blades), hipbones, and skull bones.

Red bone marrow is the factory for most of the *blood cells*—all of the red cells and platelets and most of the white cells. Stem cells within the red marrow are stimulated to form blood cells by erythropoietin, a hormone originating in the kidney. The blood cells go through various stages of maturation in the red marrow before they are ready to be released into the circulation. Yellow marrow produces some white cells, but is composed mainly of connective tissue and fat.

Sometimes marrow fails to produce the normal amount of blood cells, as in aplastic *anemia* or when it has been displaced by tumor cells. It may overproduce only certain blood cells, as in *polycythemia* and *leukemia*.

Bone marrow biopsy

A procedure to obtain a sample of cells from the bone marrow (aspiration biopsy) or a small core of bone with marrow inside (trephine biopsy). Microscopic examination of the bone marrow gives information on the development of the various components of blood and on the presence of cells foreign to the marrow. It is useful in the diagnosis of many blood disorders, including anemia, leukemia, bone marrow failure, and certain infections. It can also show whether bone marrow has been invaded by lymphoma or cells from other tumors. Trephine biopsy requires a long, thick needle for removal of the bone core,

usually from the iliac crest. Trephine is used when tumor growth makes aspiration impossible, or when bone marrow structure needs to be examined. Bone marrow biopsy may be performed repeatedly to monitor the response of a disease to treatment.

Bone marrow transplant

The technique of using normal bone marrow to replace malignant or defective marrow in a patient. In allogeneic bone marrow transplantation (BMT), healthy bone marrow is taken from a donor who has a very similar tissue type to the recipient's—usually a brother or sister. In autologous BMT the patient's own bone marrow is used. Either type of BMT should be done only in centers specializing in this procedure.

WHY IT IS DONE
Because the procedure itself carries certain risks, BMT is used only in the treatment of potentially fatal blood and immune disorders, including severe aplastic anemia, leukemia, severe combined immunodeficiency and inborn errors of metabolism.

HOW IT IS DONE
ALLOGENEIC BMT (See box, overleaf.)
AUTOLOGOUS BMT Bone marrow is taken from the patient (usually someone with a malignant disease) while his or her disease is in remission (not active) and stored by *cryopreservation* (a tissue-freezing technique). Before freezing, the marrow may be treated in an attempt to eliminate any remaining malignant cells. This method remains investigational for most conditions. If the disease recurs, the stored bone marrow can be thawed and reinfused into the patient, after destroying all his or her bone marrow as in allogeneic BMT.

COMPLICATIONS
Infection can be a major problem during the recovery period, and isolation nursing procedures must continue for about four to six weeks until the new marrow is producing adequate numbers of white blood cells.

In allogeneic BMT, the other dangerous complication is the rejection process known as *graft-versus-host disease* (GVHD). GVHD occurs when lymphocytes in the donor bone marrow recognize their new host (recipient) environment as foreign. Symptoms include rash, jaundice, and diarrhea. *Immunosuppressant drugs*, such as *cyclosporine*, prevent and treat rejection.

Complications may continue to arise for long periods after BMT.

Bone tumor

A swelling of bone. Bone tumors may be *benign* or *malignant* (see *Bone cancer*). There are different types of benign bone tumors. The most common is *osteochondroma*, a mixed swelling of bone and cartilage that often begins in childhood. Other types are *osteoma*, a smooth, rounded bone swelling, and chondroma (see *Chondromatosis*), which is made up of cartilage cells and occurs mainly in the hands or feet. Osteoma and chondroma are painless and may affect any bone in the body. No treatment is necessary unless the tumor becomes very large or unsightly, or if pressure on other structures (such as arteries or nerves) causes symptoms. In such cases, the tumor can be removed surgically.

Another type of benign tumor of bone is the giant cell tumor, or osteoclastoma. This tumor occurs in young adults, usually in the arm or leg. The giant cell tumor is painful and tender and should be removed.

Booster

A follow-up dose of *vaccine* given to reinforce the effect of the first.

Borborygmi

Name for the audible bowel sounds that are a normal part of the digestive process. They are caused by movement of air and fluid through the intestine. In some people they may be accentuated during times of anxiety.

Borborygmi may be affected by some disorders of the *intestine*, and physicians listen to the bowel sounds as an aid to diagnosis.

Borderline personality disorder

A form of personality organization falling between neurotic and more primitive psychotic levels. Someone with a borderline personality disorder is usually incapable of maintaining stable relationships; mood changes are often rapid and inappropriate. Frequent, angry outbursts are common, as are impulsive, self-damaging acts such as gambling, shoplifting, or suicide attempts.

Boric acid

A weak *antiseptic* that may still be used in some antifungal skin lotions and ophthalmic ointments.

Bornholm disease

One of many names for epidemic *pleurodynia*, an infectious disease characterized by severe chest pains and fever.

PERFORMING A BONE MARROW TRANSPLANT

Normal bone marrow is used to replace malignant or defective marrow. In the allogeneic procedure, healthy marrow is taken from a donor. In the autologous procedure, the patient's own healthy marrow is used.

With one sibling there is a 25% chance of finding a compatible donor.

With three siblings there are three opportunities for a 25% chance of finding a donor.

Finding a donor

The more siblings one has, the greater the chance of finding a donor. With three or more siblings, the chances are good.

HOW IT IS DONE

1 Before transplantation, all the recipient's marrow is destroyed by treatment with drugs or radiation. Destroying the marrow kills any cancer cells there.

3 After aspiration, the bone marrow is transfused intravenously into the patient. The bone marrow cells find their way through the circulation into the patient's marrow cavities, where they start to grow.

SITES OF BONE MARROW

Red or yellow in color, bone marrow is a soft, fatty tissue found in the cavities of bones. In newborn babies, red bone marrow is present in all bones; during the teen years, most is replaced by yellow marrow. The marrow used for transplants is red.

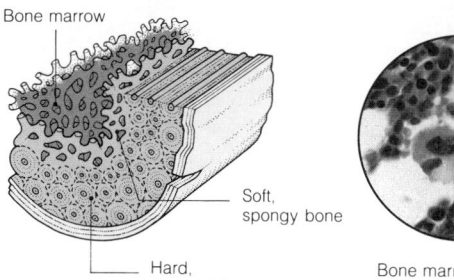

Bone marrow

Soft, spongy bone

Hard, compact bone

Bone marrow seen under the microscope

Surgeon

Assistant

Anesthesiologist

2 Using general anesthesia, bone marrow is aspirated from the donor's iliac crests and/or sternum. Only 20 to 50 ml is removed, since the transplanted marrow grows quickly to occupy the bone spaces.

ASPIRATION BIOPSY

A hollow aspiration needle is introduced into the bone (iliac crests or sternum). A stylet (a thin, sharp lance) is passed through the needle and advanced (using small, twisting movements) through the bone cortex. The stylet is removed. Bone marrow is sucked out from the cortex into a syringe connected to the needle.

Stylet

Aspiration needle

Syringe

Sternum

Iliac crest

B

Bottle-feeding

A method of infant feeding using a formula usually based on modified cow's milk. Although *breast-feeding* is recommended where possible, many parents choose bottle-feeding for the convenience, certainty, and flexibility it offers. With bottle-feeding, there is no fluctuation in the quality or quantity of the milk, the baby's intake can be measured and regulated, and the mother's presence is not necessary.

PREPARING THE FEEDING

The formula must be measured accurately and made to the correct strength with water as instructed on the container. Some formulas may be purchased "ready-to-feed." No extra formula, sugar, or cereal should be added. Overconcentrated milk may injure a baby's kidneys and the extra calories may make him or her fat.

It is essential that strict hygienic rules be observed when preparing infant feedings because bacteria-causing infections thrive in warm milk. All equipment should be cleaned thoroughly and sterilized using one of two methods.

ASEPTIC STERILIZATION

This technique involves sterilizing all bottles, nipples, and caps before use by immersing them in boiling water. The feeding is then prepared using boiled water and can be used immediately after it cools to a lukewarm temperature.

TERMINAL STERILIZATION

This method involves sterilizing the prepared milk along with the bottles in a special steam sterilizing unit or saucepan. Up to six feedings—enough for one day—may be prepared at once and

---

BOTTLE-FEEDING

The parent's back should be supported firmly with feet flat on the floor. The baby should be cradled snugly with the head supported well above the level of the stomach. Eye contact should be maintained.

Types of bottle
Bottles, and their nipples, come in various shapes and sizes. Some come ready-filled with prepared formula.

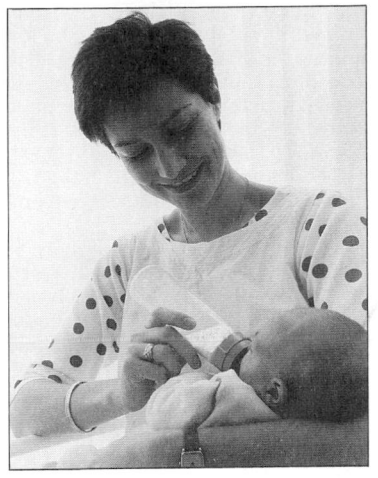

Technique
The bottle must be kept tilted and the flow of milk maintained at a good rate but not so fast as to cause choking.

---

stored in the refrigerator. The feeding may be warmed for use by standing the bottle in a pan of hot water, or by placing it in an electric warmer. Do not use a microwave oven; this method of warming may alter the nutritional value of the formula. Any unused milk must be discarded immediately.

PROBLEMS

If feedings are carefully prepared, equipment sterilized, and bottles given with warmth and cuddling, problems should be rare. However, parents should guard against overfeeding; the correct amount for an infant is based on his or her birth weight and ideal growth rate.

A more serious long-term problem for some bottle-fed infants concerns the amino acids found in cow's milk. Early exposure to these amino acids (which are not present in breast milk) may sensitize the infant to cow's milk protein and result in allergic reactions in later life. If there is a history of allergy in the family, feeding an infant with a nonmilk formula may be recommended to prevent future allergic reaction. Consult your physician. (See also *Feeding, infant*.)

Botulism

A rare but serious form of poisoning caused by eating improperly canned or preserved food contaminated with a toxin, the most potent poison known to man, produced by the bacterium *CLOSTRIDIUM BOTULINUM*, which causes progressive muscular paralysis and other disturbances of the central and peripheral nervous system.

CAUSES

CLOSTRIDIUM BOTULINUM is found in soil and untreated water in most parts of the world and is harmlessly present in the intestinal tracts of many animals, including fish. It produces spores that resist boiling, salting, smoking, and some forms of pickling. These spores, which multiply only in the absence of air, cannot normally infect humans, but thrive in improperly preserved or canned food

where they produce the toxin. If such food is eaten, absorption of even minute amounts of toxin can lead to severe poisoning.

The foods most commonly responsible are home-preserved canned vegetables, cured pork and ham, and smoked or raw fish. Factory-canned foods are implicated occasionally, but are usually safe.

In infants, botulism can be contracted by another mechanism. The bacterium, which enters the intestinal tract in water or food (such as honey), colonizes the intestine, produces its toxin there, and causes a type of *hypotonia* (reduced muscle tone) known as the floppy infant syndrome. Botulism can also occur if the *CLOSTRIDIUM BOTULINUM* bacteria in the soil enter skin broken during an injury.

INCIDENCE

Botulism is more common in the US than anywhere else in the world (due to the popularity of preserving food at home). However, in an average year there are approximately 20 reported cases of food-borne botulism (causing fewer than 10 deaths), as many as 250 cases of infant botulism, and fewer than five cases of wound botulism in the entire country.

PREVENTION

Anyone who preserves food at home should make sure they sterilize it by pressure cooking at 250°F (120°C) for 30 minutes. Bulging cans or off-smelling preserved foods should not be taste-tested but should be discarded or investigated by health authorities.

SYMPTOMS AND TREATMENT

Symptoms of food-borne botulism usually first appear between eight and

B

36 hours after eating contaminated food. Symptoms include difficulty swallowing and speaking, nausea, vomiting, and double vision. Death occurs in about 70 percent of untreated cases and is usually due to suffocation caused by paralysis of the respiratory muscles. Prompt treatment with an antitoxin brings the risk of death down to less than 25 percent. (See also *Food poisoning*.)

Bougie
A soft flexible rod used to stretch narrowed passages in the body, particularly in the urethra and esophagus. The name is derived from the French word for candle, because bougies were often made from wax.

Bowel
A common name for the *intestine*.

Bowel movements, abnormal
See *Feces, abnormal*.

Bowel sounds
See *Borborygmi*.

Bowen's disease
A very rare skin disorder that sometimes becomes cancerous. The disorder consists of a flat, regular-shaped, patch of red, scaly skin, usually on the face or hands. Treatment consists of removing the diseased patch of skin surgically or destroying it by freezing or by *cauterization*. It is unlikely to recur. A person who has had Bowen's disease is much more likely than the average person to develop cancer of the lung, kidney, or large intestine later in life, therefore he or she should have periodic medical checkups to look for these.

Bow leg
An outward curving of bones in the legs. Bow legs are common in very young children and are a normal part of development. The curve usually straightens as the child grows, but, if the bowing is severe or persists beyond age 6, a physician should be consulted. A corrective operation may be needed.

Rarely, leg deformity is a result of bone disease, particularly *rickets* (a vitamin D deficiency) in children.

Brace, orthopedic
An appliance worn to support part of the body or hold it in a fixed position. One application is to correct or halt the development of a deformity. For example, a deformed spine is prevented from curving further by a rigid brace that fits closely to the back, chest, and pelvis.

A brace may also help the movement of a limb when movement would otherwise be impossible. For example, a person who has lost the ability to flex the foot upward, and, as a result, drags the toes on the ground with each step, can be fitted with a device (called a foot-drop splint) that keeps the foot permanently at right angles to the leg and thus allows walking. Some braces are used to relieve pain. The use of braces should be monitored because misuse can lead to weakness and joint stiffness.

Braces, dental
See *Orthodontic appliances*.

Brachialgia
Pain or stiffness in the arm. It is often accompanied by pain, tingling, or numbness of the hands or fingers, and weakness of hand grip. It may indicate an underlying disorder such as *frozen shoulder* or nerve compression from *cervical osteoarthritis*.

Brachial plexus
A collection of large nerve trunks that pass from the lower part of the cervical spine and upper part of the thoracic spine down the arm. These nerve trunks divide into the musculocutaneous and axillary, median, ulnar, and radial nerves that control muscles in and receive sensations from the arm and hand.

INJURIES
Injuries to the brachial plexus are an important and fairly common cause of partial or complete loss of movement and sensation in the arm. Damage to the brachial plexus sometimes occurs during birth, with an increased risk in breech delivery. In adults, a common cause of brachial plexus injury is a fall from a motorcycle.

Injury is usually a forcible separation of the neck and shoulder, due to a fall pushing the shoulder downward or to a blow to the side of the neck that stretches or tears upper nerve roots in the plexus. Damage to these roots causes paralysis in muscles of the shoulder and elbow.

Injury to lower nerve roots in the plexus, causing paralysis of muscles in the forearm and hand, can result from a forcible blow that lifts the arm and shoulder upward. In severe injuries, both upper and lower roots are damaged, producing complete paralysis of the arm.

TYPES OF BRACES
Braces are worn to support a part of the body or a limb or to keep a limb in a certain position. Braces also can help limb movement that would otherwise be difficult. A brace allows a person recovering from an injury or operation to exercise.

Wrist brace
Used to support a painful or weak wrist and as an alternative to surgery in the treatment of carpal tunnel syndrome. A wrist brace is usually made of plastic with foam padding.

Knee brace
Provides control of ligament instability while allowing the natural action of the knee. Knee braces are often used by athletes.

Spinal brace
Helps sufferers of chronic low back pain. The brace encircles the abdomen like a corset, preventing painful movement and decreasing the load on the lower spine. Braces are usually made of elastic material reinforced with metal or plastic.

Paralysis may be temporary if the stretching was not severe enough to actually tear nerve fibers.

TREATMENT The treatment of a brachial plexus injury depends on the extent of nerve damage, which is reflected in the amount of movement possible in the arm and shoulder. Electrical activity in the muscles, shown by *EMG* (electromyography) demonstrates those nerves that are still intact. *Myelography* (X-ray examination of the spinal cord after injection of a contrast medium) is used to assess nerve root damage. Sometimes, the exact situation will not be known until the neuroanatomy is inspected during the course of a repair operation.

Nerve roots that have been torn can be repaired by nerve grafting, a procedure done under a microscope, often with good results. If a nerve root has become separated from the spinal cord, attempts at repair will not restore function.

In the event of permanent paralysis of a particular group of muscles in the arm, function can be improved by doing a muscle or tendon transfer operation to provide an alternative structure to perform a particular movement. Physiotherapy, with exercises continued at home, will help restore function after a successful nerve graft operation and can reduce *contractures* in paralyzed muscles.

DISORDERS
Apart from injuries, the brachial plexus can be affected by the presence of a *cervical rib* (extra rib), infections, tumors, or *aneurysms*.

Bradycardia

An adult heart rate of below 60 beats per minute. Most people have a beat rate of between 60 and 100 beats, the average being 72 to 78. Many athletes and healthy people who exercise regularly and vigorously have bradycardia that is perfectly normal. In others, however, it may indicate an underlying disorder such as *myxedema* (an underactive thyroid gland) or *heart block*. Bradycardia may also be an effect of *beta-blockers*. Profound or sudden bradycardia may cause symptoms such as loss of energy, weakness, and fainting attacks.

Braille

A system of embossed dots that enables blind people to read and write. It was developed by the Frenchman Louis Braille and is now accepted for all written languages, music, mathematics, and science.

Example of Grade I braille
In this system, each letter is represented by its own pattern of dots.

The braille system is based on six raised dots, which can be arranged in different combinations to form 63 symbols. There are two types. In Grade I, each symbol represents an individual letter or punctuation mark. In Grade II, symbols represent common letter combinations or words. This second form is more widely used.

Brain

The major organ of the *nervous system*, located in the *skull*. The brain is the organ of thought, speech, and emotion, but its primary role is as the body's control center.

The brain and spinal cord constitute the *central nervous system* (CNS). The CNS controls basic functions such as rate of heartbeat, breathing, and body temperature. The brain receives, sorts, and interprets sensations from the nerves that extend from the CNS to every other part of the body; it initiates and coordinates the motor output involved in activities such as movement and speech.

The nerve pathways that control internal body functions, such as heart rate, temperature, sweating, and digestion, are called the *autonomic nervous system*.

The nerve pathways that carry sensations to the brain from the sense organs and messages from the brain to the muscles initiating movement are called the somatic nervous system.

Three main structures are easily recognized: the *brain stem, cerebellum,* and, above the brain stem, the large forebrain, much of which consists of the *cerebrum* (see illustration overleaf). Extending from the brain are 12 pairs of *cranial nerves*; some of these have a sensory function, some a motor function, and some have both.

BRAIN STEM AND CEREBELLUM
These parts of the brain are the oldest in evolutionary terms, and their structure and function differ little between humans and other mammals. The brain stem is concerned mainly with control of vital functions, such as breathing and blood pressure, and the cerebellum with muscular coordination, balance, and posture.

Both brain regions operate below the level of consciousness by *reflex* action, in which any particular stimulus or pattern of stimuli evokes a preprogrammed or automatic response. The brain stem and cerebellum receive sensory information (about temperature, pressure, position, or pain) from sensory receptors scattered throughout the body. The brain stem and cerebellum then transmit the appropriate response— for example, to muscles in the blood vessels to change blood pressure.

FOREBRAIN
The forebrain consists of a central group of structures and nerve nuclei (nerve cell groups) on the top of the brain stem and, enclosing these, the relatively huge cerebrum.

CENTRAL STRUCTURES These act mainly as links between parts of the cerebrum above and brain stem below. They include the two egg-shaped *thalami* which serve as relay stations for sensory information to the cerebrum. Beneath them, the *hypothalamus* is a tiny region involved in the regulation of body temperature, thirst, and appetite; it also influences sexual behavior, aggression, and sleep. The hypothalamus has close connections with the *pituitary gland*, which produces hormones that affect other glands and in this way controls growth, sexual development, metabolism, fluid balance, and many other physiological variables. Encircling the thalami, a further complex of nerve centers, the *limbic system*, is thought to be involved in the handling of emotions, some memory functions, and olfactory (smell) sensations.

CEREBRUM The two hemispheres that make up the cerebrum project upward and outward from the center of the forebrain to form an almost continuous egg-shaped mass. It constitutes nearly 70 percent of the weight of the entire nervous system.

The surfaces of the hemispheres are folded into deep clefts so that only one third of the total surface is visible. Certain of the sulci (fissures) separating gyri (folds) are particularly noticeable and divide the surface into distinct lobes—occipital, parietal, temporal, and frontal—named after the main bones of the skull that overlie them. The two halves of the cerebrum are connected by the corpus callosum.

The cerebral cortex (the outer surface of the cerebrum) consists of gray matter, with nerve cells arranged in six layers. This is the region of conscious thought, movement, and sen-

B

STRUCTURE OF THE BRAIN

The brain has three main parts—the brain stem (an extension of the spinal cord), the cerebellum, and the forebrain, much of which consists of the two large cerebral hemispheres. Each hemisphere consists of an outer layer, or cortex, which is rich in nerve cells and called gray matter, and inner areas rich in nerve fibers, called white matter. The surface of each hemisphere is thrown into folds called gyri separated by fissures called sulci. The two hemispheres are linked by a thick band of nerve fibers, the corpus callosum. Deep within the forebrain are various central structures, which include the thalamus, hypothalamus, basal ganglia, and pituitary gland.

The brain has a consistency like jelly and, in adults, weighs about 3 pounds. It is protected by membranous coverings, the meninges, within the skull.

Lobes

These are broad surface regions of each hemisphere that are named after the overlying bones of the skull. The four main regions are the frontal, parietal, temporal, and occipital lobes.

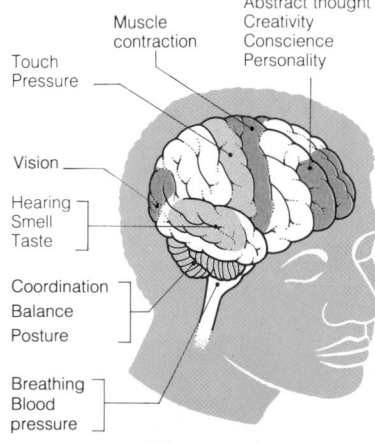

Special areas

Some brain areas are associated with specific functions—for example, the occipital lobe with vision, and the cerebellum with balance and coordination. Touch and pressure sensation is perceived within the postcentral gyrus. Muscle movements are controlled from the precentral gyrus; speech is controlled from an area in the frontal lobe of the dominant hemisphere.

Angiography

This technique makes blood vessels clearly visible. The angiogram above shows the main blood supply to the brain—the carotid artery and its branches.

Magnetic resonance imaging

This technique is used mainly to reveal abnormalities that are otherwise undetectable. In the MRI scan above, the white mass to the upper right is a tumor.

CT scanning

The CT scan above shows a "slice" through the head. The nose and eyeballs are visible at right; the small circular area in the center is the brain stem.

sation. It operates much like more primitive parts of the brain, except that incoming sensory information undergoes a much more detailed analysis. Various conscious factors, including perception, memory, thought, and decision-making, are interposed between the reception of sensory information and the output of a motor response. Actions initiated by output from the cortex—speech, movement, writing—can be highly complex in form.

Beneath the cortex, much of the cerebrum consists of tracts of nerve fibers forming "white matter"; these tracts connect various areas of the cortex to each other and to nerve centers in the center of the forebrain and brain stem. Deeper within the hemispheres are groups of cells named the *basal ganglia*; they are connected to the brain stem and cerebellum and are involved in relaying and modifying motor output from the cerebral cortex, signaling and coordinating movements to skeletal muscles.

Though the cerebrum is symmetrical in appearance, some higher activities such as speech and writing are controlled from one cerebral hemisphere, the dominant one. In right-handed people this is the left hemisphere; even in left-handed people the left side is usually dominant. The nondominant side is important in visual/spatial orientation and may be involved in artistic appreciation and creative thought.

PROTECTION AND NOURISHMENT
The whole of the brain and spinal cord is encased in three layers of membranes, called the *meninges*. The *cerebrospinal fluid* circulates between two of these layers and also within the four main brain cavities called *ventricles* (one in each cerebral hemisphere, a third in the center of the forebrain, and a fourth in the brain stem). This cerebrospinal fluid helps nourish the brain and also helps cushion it from trauma when the head is moved quickly or receives a blow.

The brain as a whole also has an extensive blood supply. Blood comes from a circle of arteries fed by the internal *carotid arteries* (which run up each side of the front of the neck to enter the base of the skull) and from two vertebral arteries that run parallel to the spinal cord. The brain receives about 20 percent of the cardiac output. (See *Brain* disorders box, overleaf; *Vision; Hearing; Smell; Pain; Consciousness; Thought; Memory; Speech; Intelligence; Perception; Psychology.*)

Brain abscess
A collection of pus, surrounded by inflamed tissues, in the brain or on its surface. Along with *brain tumors* and other space-occupying brain abnormalities, abscesses cause symptoms due to raised pressure and local damage to nerve tracts. The most common sites are the frontal and temporal lobes of the *cerebrum* in the forebrain.

CAUSES AND INCIDENCE
Brain abscesses, except with head injury, almost always result from the spread of infection from elsewhere in the body. About 40 percent of abscesses result from middle ear or sinus infections. Other causes include infection following a penetrating brain injury and blood-borne infection, most commonly in patients with acute bacterial *endocarditis* and certain *immunodeficiency disorders*. Abscesses that are due to blood-borne infection are often multiple.

SYMPTOMS
The most common symptoms are headache, drowsiness, and vomiting. There may also be visual disturbances, fever, epileptic seizures, and symptoms caused by local brain damage—for example, partial paralysis or speech disturbances.

DIAGNOSIS AND TREATMENT
The diagnosis is suggested by *CT scanning* or *MRI* (magnetic resonance imaging) of the brain. Treatment consists of a high dosage of antibiotics and usually surgery. A hole may need to be made in the skull (see *Craniotomy*) and the abscess is then either drained or removed; antibiotic drugs are also given.

OUTLOOK
Brain abscesses prove fatal in about 10 percent of cases, and the remaining patients often suffer some residual impairment of brain function. *Epilepsy* is common, so *anticonvulsant drugs* are often prescribed following removal or drainage of the abscess. (See also *Brain tumors; Brain hemorrhage; Brain syndrome, organic.*)

Brain damage
Degeneration or death of nerve cells and tracts within the brain. Damage may be localized to particular areas of the brain—causing specific defects of brain function, such as loss of coordination or difficulty with speech—or may be more diffuse, causing mental or severe physical handicap.

DIFFUSE DAMAGE
The most important cause of diffuse brain damage is prolonged cerebral *hypoxia* (not enough oxygen reaching the brain). This may occur during birth; a baby's brain cannot tolerate a lack of oxygen for more than about five minutes. At any age, hypoxia may occur as a result of *cardiac arrest* (stoppage of the heart) or *respiratory arrest* (cessation of breathing), and from causes such as poisoning, drowning, electric shock, or *status epilepticus* (prolonged convulsions).

Diffuse damage may also occur through the accumulation in the brain of substances poisonous to nerve cells—as in *phenylketonuria* (unless treated early) or *galactosemia*. Diffuse damage may also be a result of inhaling or ingesting environmental pollutants such as lead or mercury compounds (see *Minamata disease*).

Other possible causes include infections of the brain, such as *encephalitis* or, very rarely, vaccine damage following immunization.

LOCALIZED DAMAGE
Localized brain damage can occur as a result of *head injury*, especially penetrating injuries, at any age. It occurs later in life as a result of *stroke, brain tumor,* or *brain abscess*.

At birth, local damage to the *basal ganglia* (deep within the brain) caused by a raised blood level of *bilirubin* (formed from the destruction of blood cells in *hemolytic disease of the newborn*) leads to a condition called *kernicterus*, which is characterized by disorders of movement and sometimes mental deficiency. The basal ganglia may also be damaged by carbon monoxide.

SYMPTOMS AND TREATMENT
Brain damage that occurs before, during, or after birth may result in *cerebral palsy*, a condition characterized by paralysis and abnormal movements and often associated with mental retardation and sometimes deafness.

Victims of head injury, stroke, or other causes of localized or diffuse brain damage may also be left with any of a range of handicaps, including disturbances of movement, speech, or sensation, mental handicap, or epileptic seizures.

Nerve cells and tracts in the brain and spinal cord do not recover their function if they have been destroyed (nerves in the limbs or trunk regenerate slowly after being cut or crushed). Nevertheless, some improvement may be expected after brain damage as the victim learns to use other parts of the brain and other muscle groups in the body. Treatment often involves teamwork on the part of physicians and specialists in *physical therapy, speech therapy,* and *occupational therapy*.

DISORDERS OF THE BRAIN

Defects and disorders of the brain have much the same causes as disease in other body organs. One special feature of the brain, however, is that it is packed inside a rigid casing, the skull, so any space-occupying *brain abscess*, *brain tumor*, or *hematoma* (large blood clot) following a *head injury* or *brain hemorrhage* creates raised pressure that impairs the function of the whole brain. Another special feature is that brain cells destroyed through injury or disease cannot be replaced, so the loss in function can be more difficult to reverse.

Some diseases and defects in the brain are localized in a small region and may thus have a specific effect—for example, *aphasia* (speech loss). More often, damage is more diffuse and, because the brain has so many related functions, the symptoms can be varied and numerous.

CONGENITAL DEFECTS

Babies may be born with brain defects due to genetic or chromosomal disorders, as in *Down's syndrome*, *Tay-Sachs disease*, or *cri du chat syndrome* (all of which are associated with mental deficiency). Structural defects that arise during fetal development may be fundamental and untreatable, as in *microcephaly* (small head), or fatal, as in *anencephaly* (congenital absence of the brain). Others are potentially correctable, even while the fetus is still in the uterus, as in *hydrocephalus* (water on the brain).

IMPAIRED BLOOD AND OXYGEN SUPPLY

These are two of the most important causes of brain dysfunction because brain cells can survive only a few minutes without oxygen. *Hypoxia* (lack of oxygen) affecting the brain as a result of asphyxiation during the process of birth is one of the causes of *cerebral palsy*. Later in life, cerebral hypoxia can result from accidents such as choking or from arrest of breathing and heart beat following electrocution or drowning.

From middle age onward, the most important affliction of the brain is *cerebrovascular disease* impairing blood supply to one or several brain regions. If an artery within the brain becomes blocked or ruptures leading to hemorrhage, the result is a *stroke*.

Meningioma
● a tumor of the meninges

Brain tumor
● a growth

Abscess
● a collection of pus

Thrombosis
● causes infarction

Hematoma
● a blood clot

Infection
● encephalitis or meningitis

Hypoxia
● a lack of oxygen

INJURY

Although protected by the skull, the brain may be damaged by heavy blows to the head or following skull fracture as a result of falls, high speed impacts, bullet wounds, or other physical violence (see *Head injury*).

INFECTION

Infection within the brain, called *encephalitis*, or of the membranes surrounding the brain, called *meningitis*, is uncommon today. Meningitis is usually caused by a bacterial infection. Encephalitis can be caused by any one of numerous viruses, of which the best known and most dangerous are the *rabies* and *herpes simplex* viruses.

An abscess (localized pocket of infection) in the brain may result from spread of infection from the ear, sinuses, or elsewhere in the body (see *Brain abscess*).

TUMORS

Tumors that affect the brain may be primary (arising from tissues inside the skull) as in *gliomas*, *meningiomas*, *acoustic neuromas*, and *pituitary tumors*, or secondary (arising from cancer cells that have spread through the bloodstream from tumors in the lungs, breasts, or elsewhere). See *Brain tumors*.

DEGENERATION

Multiple sclerosis, a progressive disease of unknown cause in which the nerve sheaths (composed of myelin) are destroyed, starts most commonly in early adulthood.

Degenerative brain diseases, such as *Alzheimer's disease* (a type of dementia) and *Parkinson's disease*, are particularly important causes of disability among the elderly.

OTHER DISORDERS

Disorders characterized by their symptoms rather than any obvious cause include *migraine*, *narcolepsy* (excessive episodic sleepiness), and idiopathic *epilepsy* (epilepsy of unknown cause), though epileptic seizures can also have specific causes, such as a tumor or infection.

Disorders of thought, emotion, or behavior are generally described as psychiatric or *mental illnesses*. Often, there is no obvious physical brain defect or disorder, although, with many important mental illnesses, such as *depression* and *schizophrenia*, there seems to be an underlying disturbance of brain chemistry. Some psychiatric illnesses, collectively called organic *brain syndromes*, by definition have a physical cause.

INVESTIGATION

Many different procedures may be used to investigate disorders of the brain. A full physical *examination* will include assessment of brain function by means of tests of mental abilities and state, sensation, movement, muscle tone, and reflexes. Electrical activity within the brain may be measured by means of an *EEG*. Physical abnormalities may be looked for using *brain imaging* techniques, such as *angiography*, *CT scanning*, or *MRI*. A *lumbar puncture* may be performed to look for evidence of bleeding or infection.

Brain death
The irreversible cessation of all functions of the entire brain, including the *brain stem*. The recognition of brain death, as defined above, has allowed physicians to certify death in situations where the lungs and heart continue to function (with machine assistance) but where death has occurred based on the absence of brain function. (See also *Death*.)

Brain failure
See *Brain syndrome, organic*.

Brain hemorrhage
Bleeding within or around the brain, caused either by trauma or spontaneous rupture of a blood vessel. There are four possible types: *subdural hemorrhage, extradural hemorrhage, subarachnoid hemorrhage*, and *intracerebral hemorrhage*.

Extradural and subdural hemorrhages usually result from a blow to the head (see *Head injury*); symptoms may include headache, drowsiness, confusion, and paralysis on one side of the body. These symptoms may develop within hours in extradural hemorrhage but possibly over months in subdural hemorrhage. Hospital treatment is urgently required.

Subarachnoid and intracerebral hemorrhage usually occur spontaneously (i.e., without any head injury) and are the result of rupture of *aneurysms* or small blood vessels in the brain. Middle-aged and elderly persons with untreated *hypertension* (high blood pressure) are at highest risk. Subarachnoid hemorrhage is characterized by a sudden violent headache and/or sudden loss of consciousness. Intracerebral hemorrhage is one of the three main types of *stroke*; symptoms may include sudden collapse, speech loss, and paralysis of the facial muscles or of an arm or leg. Both subarachnoid and intracerebral hemorrhages are emergencies.

Brain imaging
Obtaining pictures of the brain to detect injury or disease. The introduction of computerized scanning has revolutionized this field.

TYPES
CONVENTIONAL X-RAY TECHNIQUES The simplest and longest established method of obtaining images of the brain is to take *X-ray* films. X rays reveal distortion or erosion of the bony skull caused by a fracture, tumor, *aneurysm*, or abscess. Unless the brain substance itself is calcified in

SITES OF BRAIN HEMORRHAGE
Hemorrhages within the skull fall into four main categories—extradural, subdural, subarachnoid, and intracerebral hemorrhages—according to the site of the bleeding in relation to the brain and its protective coverings, the meninges. The causes and effects of the bleeding and the outlook of the patient vary among the categories.

Skin
Subcutaneous layer
Skull
Dura mater
Arachnoid
Pia mater
Brain
Subarachnoid

Extradural   Subdural   Intracerebral

Intracerebral hemorrhage
This brain section shows a mass of blood in the left hemisphere.

a localized area due to disease, the plain X ray cannot detect disease of the brain matter.

Angiography involves injecting a dye into one of the arteries supplying the brain, and then taking X-ray pictures. This technique shows up the blood vessels in the brain, and is used to investigate subarachnoid hemorrhage, aneurysms, abnormalities of the blood vessels, and other disorders of the circulation.

SCANNING TECHNIQUES *CT scanning* was first conceived in 1971 specifically to study the brain. Unlike the conventional X-ray procedure, this method gives images of the brain substance itself. It gives especially clear pictures of the ventricles (the fluid-filled cavities of the brain) and can reveal tumors, blood clots, strokes, aneurysms, and abscesses. Contrast dye is often administered to help differentiate normal from abnormal brain tissue.

MRI produces better images of the brain than CT scanning. It is especially helpful in showing tumors of the posterior fossa (back of the skull). MRI does not involve radiation.

Radionuclide scanning uses radioactive isotopes to detect tumors, abnormalities of the blood vessels, and other lesions. It has been largely replaced by CT scanning and MRI.

Ultrasound scanning is used only in premature or very young babies because ultrasound waves cannot penetrate the bones of a mature skull.

Ultrasound scanning is particularly useful in detecting hydrocephalus and ventricular hemorrhage in premature babies and, because no radiation is involved, repeated scans can be performed safely.

PET scanning combines the use of radionuclides with CT scanning and gives information on activities in different parts of the brain.

Brain stem
The lowest section of the brain, which acts partly as a highway for messages traveling between other parts of the brain and the spinal cord, but also connects with ten of the 12 pairs of *cranial nerves* and controls basic functions such as breathing, vomiting, and eye reflexes. The activities of the brain stem are below the level of consciousness and operate largely on an automatic basis.

STRUCTURE
From the spinal cord upward, the brain stem consists of three main parts, called medulla, pons, and midbrain. Attached to the back of the brain stem is a separate brain organ, the *cerebellum*, concerned principally with balance and with coordinated movement. Running longitudinally through the middle of the brain stem is a canal, widening in the pons and medulla into a cavity, the fourth *ventricle* of the brain, which contains the circulating *cerebrospinal fluid*.

MEDULLA The medulla resembles a thick extension of the spinal cord. It

B

LOCATION OF THE BRAIN STEM
A 3-inch-long stalk of nerve cells and fibers joins the upper part of the spinal cord with the rest of the brain.

Midbrain

Cerebrum

Pons

Medulla

Cerebellum

Spinal cord

contains the *nuclei* of the ninth to twelfth cranial nerves and thus receives and relays taste sensations from the tongue and relays signals to muscles involved in speech and in tongue and neck movements. It also contains the vital centers—groups of nerve cells involved in the automatic regulation of heart beat, breathing, blood pressure, and digestion—and sends and receives information regarding these functions via the tenth cranial or *vagus nerve*.

Many of the tracts running through the medulla cross over in its lower portion so that the right side of the body links up with the left side of the brain and vice versa.

PONS This is considerably wider than the medulla and contains thick bundles of nerve fibers that connect with the cerebellum, which lies directly behind. The pons also contains the nuclei for the fifth to eighth cranial nerves and thus relays sensory information from the ear, face, and teeth, as well as the signals that move the jaw, adjust facial expressions, and produce some eye movements.

MIDBRAIN This is the smallest section of the brain stem, above the pons. It contains the nuclei of the third and fourth cranial nerves, which control eye movements and the size and reactions of the pupil. It also contains cell

groups such as the substantia nigra and red nuclei, which are involved in coordinating limb movements.

RETICULAR FORMATION Scattered throughout the brain stem are numerous nerve cell groups collectively known as the reticular formation. The reticular formation is believed to act as a watchdog on sensory information entering the brain, alerting the higher brain centers to new or important sensory stimuli that may require a conscious response. Our sleep/wake cycle is controlled by the reticular formation. Many *hypnotic drugs* (sleeping pills) and stimulants are believed to exert their actions by affecting this part of the brain.

DISORDERS
The brain stem is susceptible to the same disorders that afflict the rest of the central nervous system. Damage to the medulla's vital centers is rapidly fatal, while damage to the reticular formation may cause coma. Damage to specific cranial nerve nuclei can have specific effects—*facial palsy* in the case of the seventh cranial (facial) nerve and tongue-wasting with the twelfth cranial (hypoglossal) nerve. Degeneration of the substantia nigra in the midbrain is thought to be a cause of *Parkinson's disease*.

Brain syndrome, organic
Disturbance of consciousness, intellect, or mental functioning of organic (physical) as opposed to psychiatric origin. Possible causes include degenerative diseases (such as *Alzheimer's disease*), metabolic imbalances, infections, medication, toxins, vitamin deficiencies, or the effects of trauma, stroke, or tumor.

SYMPTOMS
In acute organic brain syndrome, symptoms range from slight confusion to stupor or coma, and may also include restlessness, disorientation, memory impairment, hallucinations, and delusions (see *Delirium*). The chronic form results in a progressive decline in intellect, memory, and behavior (see *Dementia*).

TREATMENT
Treatment relies on identifying and, if possible, dealing with the underlying cause. Treatment is more likely to be successful with the acute form. In chronic cases, irreversible *brain damage* may already have occurred.

Brain tumor
Abnormal growth in or on the brain. Although not always malignant, all brain tumors are serious because of

the buildup of pressure in the brain and compression of adjoining brain areas as the tumor expands.

TYPES
Brain tumors may be primary growths arising directly from tissues within the skull or metastases (secondary growths) spread via the bloodstream from tumors elsewhere in the body, most commonly the lungs or breasts.

The cause of primary brain tumors is not known. About 60 percent are *gliomas* (frequently malignant), which arise from the brain substance. Other primary tumors include *meningiomas*, arising from the meningeal membranes that cover the brain, *acoustic neuromas* arising from the acoustic nerve, and *pituitary tumors* arising from the pituitary gland, all of which are benign. Certain brain tumors mainly affect children and are often situated in the back of the brain. Included among these are two types of glioma called *medulloblastoma* and cerebellar *astrocytoma*.

Secondary growths, or metastases, are always malignant and may be found in more than one organ.

INCIDENCE
In the US, about six new cases of primary brain tumor, leading to about four deaths, are diagnosed per 100,000 population per year. They occur most commonly around the age of 50 years, although a significant number of children are also affected; about one child in 3,000 dies from a primary brain tumor before the age of 10 years.

In addition, about 30 persons per 100,000 annually die of cancer that includes metastases in the brain.

SYMPTOMS
Brain tumors cause symptoms by several mechanisms. Compression of brain tissue or nerve tracts within the vicinity of the tumor may cause muscle weakness, loss of vision, or other sensory disturbances, speech difficulties, and, in about one fifth of cases, epileptic seizures.

The presence of an expanding tumor can increase pressure within the skull, causing headache, vomiting, visual disturbances, and impaired mental functioning. If the circulation of cerebrospinal fluid is obstructed by the tumor, *hydrocephalus* (water on the brain) may result.

DIAGNOSIS
Many different techniques are used to locate the site of a brain tumor and to establish the extent of its spread. The most important are *CT scanning*, magnetic resonance imaging (*MRI*), special *X-ray* studies, and *angiography*.

TREATMENT

When possible, tumors are removed by surgery after opening the skull (see *Craniotomy*), but many malignant growths are inaccessible or too extensive for removal. The outlook in these cases is poor; fewer than 20 percent of patients survive for a year. In cases where a tumor cannot be completely removed, as much of it as possible will be cut away to relieve pressure in the brain. *Radiation therapy* or *anticancer drugs* may also be given. *Corticosteroid drugs* are often prescribed to reduce tissue swelling around a tumor, thus relieving symptoms.

Bran

 The fibrous outer covering of grain. Eating bran regularly, either in breakfast cereals or added to food, raises *fiber* intake. This helps prevent constipation and thus lessen the risk of intestinal disease.

Branchial disorders

Branchial disorders include branchial cyst and branchial fistula.

A branchial cyst is a soft swelling that appears on the side of the neck in early adult life. The swelling contains a puslike or clear fluid that is rich in cholesterol. Diagnosis is made by identifying cholesterol crystals in a few drops of the fluid drawn from the cyst by means of a needle and syringe. Treatment is by surgical removal.

A branchial fistula is an abnormal passage between the back of the throat and the external surface of the neck, where it appears as a small hole usually noted at birth. Like a branchial cyst, the fistula results from an abnormality of fetal development. If the hole in the neck does not extend to the back of the throat, it is termed a branchial cleft sinus; it may be present at birth or may form if a branchial cyst becomes infected and ruptures. A branchial fistula or a branchial cleft sinus may discharge mucus or pus. If this is troublesome, the fistula or sinus can be excised (cut away).

Brash, water

Sudden filling of the mouth with tasteless saliva. It is not to be confused with *acid reflux* (the regurgitation of gastric juices), which has an unpleasant, sour taste. Water brash is usually accompanied by other symptoms such as abdominal pain before a meal. It usually indicates a disorder of the upper gastrointestinal tract, such as a *duodenal ulcer*.

Braxton Hicks' contractions

Short, relatively painless contractions of the uterus during pregnancy. These contractions allow the uterus to grow and also help circulate blood through the uterine vessels. In early pregnancy, they may be felt by a physician performing an internal examination. In late pregnancy, they may be felt by the woman and seen by looking at the abdomen. Sometimes they are mistaken for labor pains, although they occur as isolated contractions, have no effect on the cervix, and are not as uncomfortable as true labor.

Breakbone fever

 A tropical, mosquito-spread, viral illness also known as *dengue*. One symptom is severe joint and muscle pain, hence the name "breakbone fever."

Breakthrough bleeding

Vaginal bleeding or staining ("spotting") between periods when taking an oral birth-control pill, especially the minipill. Breakthrough bleeding is most common during the first few months of taking the pill, when the body is adjusting to alterations in hormone levels. Loss of blood during pregnancy, or when an oral birth-control pill is not being taken, may be a symptom of an important underlying disorder (see *Vaginal bleeding*).

Breast

In addition to its primary function of nourishing a baby with milk, the female breast is a secondary sexual characteristic. It has always been regarded by society as a symbol of femininity, beauty, and eroticism. The size, shape, and appearance of breasts vary more than almost any other part of the body. Men's breasts are immature versions of women's breasts.

STRUCTURE

The female breast consists mainly of 15 to 20 lobes of milk-secreting glands embedded in fatty tissue. The ducts of these glands have their outlet in the

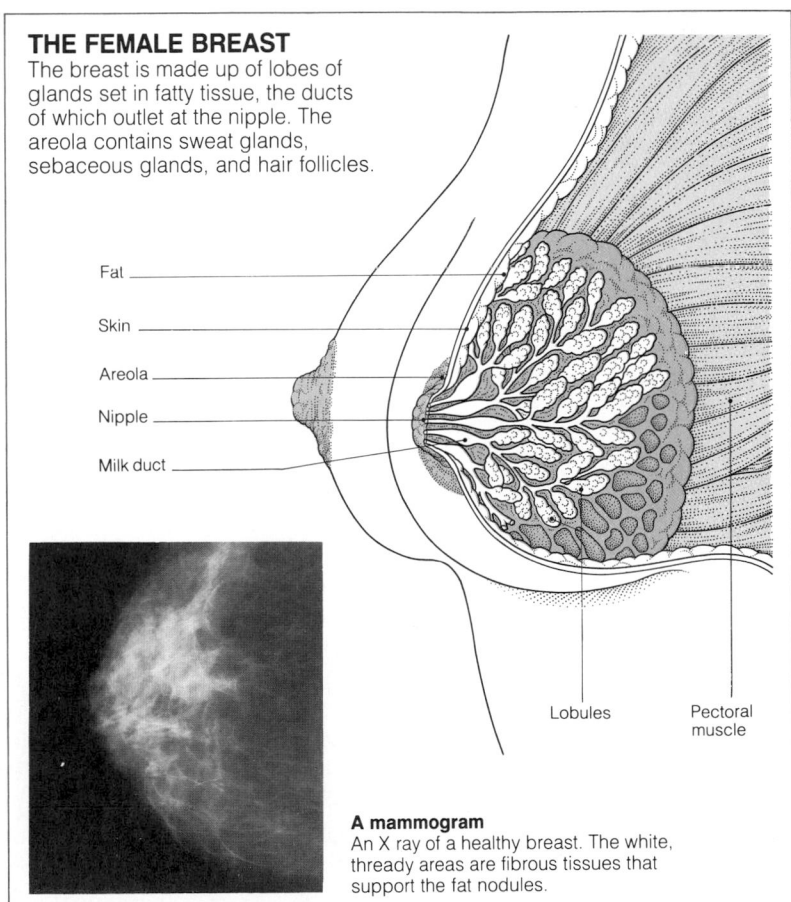

THE FEMALE BREAST
The breast is made up of lobes of glands set in fatty tissue, the ducts of which outlet at the nipple. The areola contains sweat glands, sebaceous glands, and hair follicles.

Fat

Skin

Areola

Nipple

Milk duct

Lobules

Pectoral muscle

A mammogram
An X ray of a healthy breast. The white, thready areas are fibrous tissues that support the fat nodules.

nipple, which is surrounded by the areola, the circular area of pigmented skin. The breast contains no muscle, but bands of fine ligaments that weave between the fat and lobules are attached to the skin and determine the breast's height and shape.

The skin over the breast is somewhat smoother, thinner, and more translucent than over much of the rest of the body. The areola skin is particularly thin, and contains sweat glands, sebaceous glands, and hair follicles. The nipple is very sensitive to the touch; contraction of its muscle fibers results in erection, a sign of sexual arousal or cold.

The size and shape of the breasts of mature women vary not only between individuals, but also vary at different times of a woman's life—during the menstrual cycle, during pregnancy and lactation, and after the menopause, for instance.

FUNCTION

During pregnancy estrogen and progesterone, secreted in the ovary and placenta, cause the milk-producing glands to develop and become active and the nipple to enlarge. Just before or after childbirth the glands in the breast produce a watery fluid called colostrum, which contains proteins and antibodies to protect the sucking baby against infection. Within about three days the colostrum is replaced with milk, whose production is stimulated by the hormone prolactin, released from the anterior pituitary gland (see also *Breast-feeding*).

BREAST DEVELOPMENT

The breasts, which are modified sweat glands, start to grow from mammary buds when the fetus is about 5 months old. At birth there is a nipple with rudimentary milk ducts. At *puberty*, a girl's breasts begin to develop—the areola swells and the nipple enlarges. This is followed by an increase in the production of glands and fat, which enlarges the breast. Ultimately the breast becomes rounded in shape and the areola gradually flattens.

Breastbone

A common name for the *sternum*.

Breast cancer

The most common cancer in women: one woman in every 14 develops breast cancer and one in every 20 dies from it. Fewer than one in every 100 breast cancers are in men.

Mortality from breast cancer (taking account of age) has hardly changed this century, but, in the early 1980s, research studies in Sweden and the Netherlands suggested that deaths could be cut by about one third by mammographic screening of whole populations of women. Other studies indicate the great importance of breast examination by the physician and patient in diagnosing breast cancer in its early stages.

CAUSES AND INCIDENCE

Current theories of the cause of breast cancer are focused on hormonal influences. The incidence of breast cancer is known to be raised in women whose menstrual periods began when they were young and those whose menopause was late; in those who had no children or had their first child in their late 20s or 30s; and in those with mothers or sisters who had breast cancer. Diet also plays a part. The disease is rare in Japan, which has a low fat diet, but Japanese women living in the US and eating an American diet have the same rate of breast cancer as Americans. Tall, heavy women have more breast cancer than short, thin ones. Breast cancer may also be more common among women who have previously had nonmalignant cysts and tumors removed from their breasts.

There is no agreement on the part played by the oral birth-control pill in the cause of breast cancer. Some groups believe that women who take the pill in their teens have a slightly increased risk; others claim that it is protective. At present the evidence suggests that any increase in breast cancer from the pill, if at all, is small—and that it is outweighed by the effect of the pill in lowering the incidence of cancers of the ovary and uterus.

SYMPTOMS

The most common site of a malignant breast tumor is the upper, outer part of the breast. The lump is usually felt rather than seen, and in most cases is not painful. Other symptoms include a dark discharge from the nipple, retraction (indentation) of the nipple, and an area of dimpled, creased skin over the lump. In 90 percent of cases only one breast is affected.

DIAGNOSIS

Monthly examination of the breasts (see *Breast self-examination*) should enable a woman to detect at an early stage any new or changed breast lump or any change in her nipples. The breast examination is important and should routinely be done by internists and gynecologists. In addition, X rays of the breasts, called mammograms, are recommended for high-risk women (i.e., women with a family history of breast cancer) at age 40 and should be repeated every three to five years thereafter, or sooner, when advised. This procedure, called *mammography* is also of value for all women over 50 years old.

A woman who discovers a lump in her breast should report it to her physician immediately. A mammogram may be appropriate at this time. If the physician suspects that the lump is merely a *cyst* (a fluid-filled tissue sac), it can be aspirated (i.e., the fluid can be withdrawn) and may disappear completely. Where there is a possibility that the lump may be a malignant tumor, a *biopsy* will be carried out. This may be an outpatient procedure in which breast tissue is withdrawn with a hollow needle, causing little discomfort, or an operation to remove all or part of the lump; in either case the suspect tissue will be examined under the microscope.

If cancer is discovered, blood tests, X rays, and scanning will determine whether the disease has spread to other parts of the body.

TREATMENT

The high mortality from breast cancer is because the disease has spread beyond the breast when first detected. Surgical removal of the tumor achieves a cure in one third of women with early breast cancer. Studies have shown survival is not improved by extensive operations (such as radical *mastectomy*); many surgeons recommend *lumpectomy*, the simple removal of the tumor, combined with *radiation therapy* or *anticancer drug* therapy, or both. The extent of the primary treatment is influenced by the woman's age, the size of the tumor, whether or not there are signs of spread to the lymph nodes under the arm, and the sensitivity of the tumor cells to hormones as determined in the laboratory by a technique called estrogen receptor testing.

Tests carried out at the time of the initial diagnosis may show that the cancer is in the bones, liver, or other organs. Evidence of *metastasis* may develop years after apparently successful treatment. In either case, treatment with *anticancer drugs* and hormones usually relieves symptoms and prolongs life.

OUTLOOK

If cancer is treated at an early stage the outlook is optimistic; either a complete cure or many years of good health can be expected. Regular checkups are needed to detect any recurrence or

DISORDERS OF THE BREAST

Problems involving the breasts are usually minor and respond readily to treatment. The most important causes of problems are infection, tumors, and hormonal disturbance.

INFECTION

This is uncommon except during breast-feeding. Nursing mothers may suffer from *mastitis* (inflammation of the breast), usually due to a blocked milk duct. An *abscess* may follow if mastitis is not treated.

TUMORS

A *breast lump* may be a *cyst* (a fluid-filled sac), a *fibroadenoma* (a thickening of the milk-producing glandular tissue) or other benign tumor, or, rarely, *breast cancer*.

HORMONAL DISORDERS

It is common for women to notice that before *menstruation* their breasts become bigger and lumpy. Such lumps are swollen milk glands that shrink when menstruation is over. More common are breast pain and tenderness, which often occur just before menstruation or from taking hormones.

In men, *gynecomastia* (unusual breast development) may result from hormonal disturbance or treatment with certain drugs. Hormones may also cause the rare disorder *galactorrhea* (abnormal milk production).

INVESTIGATION

Disorders of the breast may be discovered during *breast self-examination* or by your physician during a physical examination. Special investigations for the breast are *biopsy* and *mammography*.

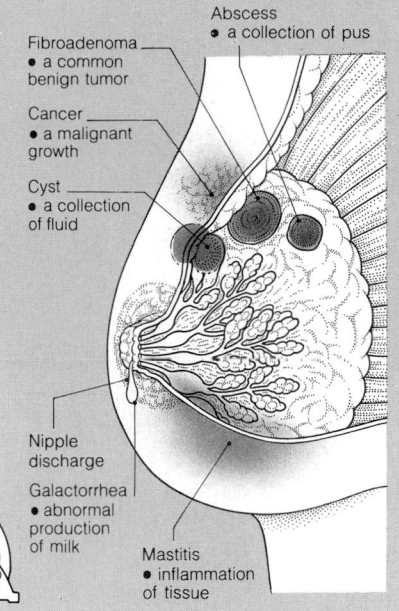

cancer in the other breast. Breast self-examination should be carried out monthly and mammograms should be performed periodically. If the cancer recurs, it can be controlled for many years by drugs, radiation therapy, and, in some cases, further surgery.

Breast enlargement

See *Mammoplasty*.

Breast-feeding

The natural method of infant feeding from birth to weaning. Human milk contains the ideal balance of nutrients for the human baby and provides valuable antibodies to protect the child against infections, such as *gastroenteritis*. Breast-feeding also provides the mother and child with a physical closeness that strengthens the bond between them.

HOW TO BREAST-FEED

Ideally, the baby should be put to the breast as soon after delivery as possible. Once sucking has begun, the mother should ensure that the whole of the areola (the dark area around the nipple) is in the baby's mouth. This helps to stimulate flow and can prevent soreness caused by the baby chewing on the nipple. In the first few days after birth, the baby should be encouraged to suck frequently, but for only a few minutes at a time. This provides him or her with valuable colostrum, and also stimulates the breasts so that a consistent and plentiful milk

supply is established. During the first few weeks a baby should be fed on demand to make sure that the milk supply is maintained. Babies may want to nurse from once every hour or two to once every three or four hours.

PROBLEMS

Engorged (overfull) breasts are common in early lactation; they are uncomfortable and can prevent the baby from sucking properly. Expression of milk, either manually or with a *breast pump*, usually helps.

Sore or cracked nipples, often a problem in the early weeks, may be relieved by using a nipple shield. Alternatively, the milk may be expressed and given by bottle.

MANAGING BREAST-FEEDING

The mother should wear comfortable, loose, front-opening clothes and a nursing bra that provides good support. She should rest her back, firmly cradling the baby in the crook of her arm, with the baby's head well above the stomach level.

Front-opening bra

Prolactin, released and carried in the bloodstream, maintains milk secretion

Nerve impulse stimulated by sucking baby

B

A complication of breast-feeding is infection leading to an abscess, indicated by soreness and inflammation on the surface of the breast. Early antibiotic treatment may mean that breast-feeding can continue.

Sometimes breast-feeding problems have an emotional basis. A few women regard their breasts as having a primarily sexual function and find the whole feeding process distasteful. Others fear feeding may spoil the shape of their breasts and may resent the intensive commitment to the child that breast-feeding requires.

A woman whose baby always seems unsatisfied after feedings may doubt the quality or quantity of her milk. If she is in good health, eating a nutritious diet, and getting enough rest, then her milk supply should be adequate, and she may simply need reassurance and encouragement. Sometimes, despite continuing efforts by the mother, the baby remains hungry or the process of feeding is painful. A change to *bottle-feeding* is the likely answer, and should not be seen as failure or a reason for guilt. (See also *Feeding, infant.*)

Breast lump

Any mass, cyst, or swelling that can be felt in the breast tissue. At least 80 percent of lumps are benign; the remainder may be malignant. All breast lumps need assessment.

POSSIBLE CAUSES

The most common cause of a breast lump is fibrocystic disease, also known as chronic *mastitis* or fibroadenosis, in which one or more cysts (fluid-filled tissue sacs) and thickening of milk glands develop. Occurring mainly in women between the ages of 30 and 50, fibrocystic disease usually causes one or both breasts to become lumpy and tender in the week or so before a menstrual period starts.

Another common type is found most often in young women and usually results in a single lump called a *fibroadenoma*. This benign growth is usually round, firm, and rubbery, causes no pain, and can be moved around beneath the skin using the fingertips.

There are also several less common forms of breast lump: *breast cancer*, lipoma, intraductal papilloma, and cystosarcoma phylloides.

A lipoma is a benign, painless tumor, made up of fatty tissue, that sometimes changes the size and shape of the breast.

An intraductal papilloma is a wart-like growth within a duct of the milk-producing glands. The most common symptom is a discharge from the nipple, either clear or dark or bloody; there may be a pea-sized lump beneath the nipple. Intraductal papillomas are harmless but may become malignant.

A cystosarcoma phylloides is a tumor of connective tissue that can grow to an enormous size very quickly. Again, it is usually benign and only rarely becomes malignant.

SEEKING MEDICAL ADVICE

All women should examine their breasts each month (see *Breast self-examination*) to detect any significant changes. If a new lump or a change in a known lump is detected, or there is any discharge from a nipple, a physician should be seen.

DIAGNOSIS AND TREATMENT

Since a physical examination cannot reveal whether or not a growth is benign, tests (including *mammography*, needle aspiration *biopsy*, or tissue biopsy) will be arranged.

If fibrocystic lumps cause discomfort, they can be drained in a simple outpatient procedure if they are fluid-filled or be removed surgically if they are fibrous. Fibroadenomas, intraductal papillomas, and cystosarcoma phylloides are usually removed because it cannot be ascertained whether or not a lesion is benign and they continue to grow if they are left. All except very small lipomas are also usually removed. For the treatment of malignant tumors, see *Breast cancer*.

Breast pump

A simple device, consisting of a rubber bulb and a glass or plastic tube and reservoir, that is used to draw milk

Using a breast pump
Both parts of the pump must first be sterilized. The opening is placed firmly over the nipple to form a tight seal. The bulb is squeezed rhythmically until milk comes out.

Bulb

Milk

from the breasts. The pump is used to relieve overfull breasts during early lactation and to express milk for future use. Most pumps are hand-operated but electric ones are available.

Breast reconstruction
See *Mammoplasty*.

Breast reduction
See *Mammoplasty*.

Breast self-examination

A visual and manual examination of the breasts carried out by a woman to detect lumps and other changes that might indicate the presence of early breast cancer. Although *mammography* (breast screening) has been shown to be more effective, it is not universally available. Self-examination is still important and should be carried out at about the same time monthly.

WHY IT IS DONE

Breast cancer is the leading cause of death among women aged 35 to 54 years. It is curable, however, if diagnosed at an early stage. Self-examination allows early changes and small lumps to be detected.

Breast tenderness

Soreness or tenderness of the breasts, often accompanied by a feeling of fullness in one or both breasts. Breast tenderness is relatively common just before menstruation (see *Premenstrual syndrome*), in early pregnancy, or during *breast-feeding*. Otherwise, it is comparatively rare and, in the absence of other symptoms, such as a *breast lump*, *nipple* discharge, or hot, inflamed skin over the breast, it is unlikely to be due to a serious underlying *breast disorder*. Malignant breast tumors are usually painless. Most cases of breast tenderness are thought to be due to hormonal changes (especially increased levels of *estrogen*) affecting the cells of the breast, causing them to retain excess fluid. This explains why the birth-control pill causes, or makes worse, breast tenderness in some women. Conversely, very low dose oral contraceptives may reduce breast tenderness in some women. Tenderness during breast-feeding may be due to engorgement with milk or to *mastitis* (inflammation of breast tissue as a result of infection).

Treatment of premenstrual breast tenderness may include dietary restriction of sodium and, when benefits justify the risk, *diuretics* (to reduce fluid retention) before each

B

EXAMINING YOUR BREASTS

1 Once a month, after your period, examine your breasts. With arms by your side, look in a mirror and get to know their general appearance, shape, and size. Be alert to changes.

2 Raise each arm in turn above your head, looking for changes in appearance. Turn from side to side, looking at the outline of the breasts for any changes.

3 Gently squeeze the nipples to see whether there is any discharge.

4 Examine the skin surface for peculiarities. Orange-peel texture could indicate the presence of a lump.

5 Lie on your back with a pillow under your shoulders and head, your arm by your side. Using the flat of your hand, work around the outer parts of the breast in a clockwise direction.

6 Raise your arm above your head and examine the inner parts of the breast. Stretching the tissue makes detection of lumps easier. Feel also along the top of the collarbone and into the armpit.

---

period or the regular use of danazol (a drug that reduces changes in hormone levels) for a few months.

Breath-holding attacks

Periods during which a toddler holds his or her breath, usually as an expression of frustration or anger. Psychologists believe that children may unconsciously bring on these attacks to exert control over their parents. In some children, the attacks occur as a response to pain.

The child usually begins to cry, then holds his or her breath, becoming red or even blue in the face after a few seconds. The child may faint temporarily, but breathing quickly resumes as a natural reflex, ending the attack. Breath-holding sometimes results in twitching that resembles an epileptic seizure. However, a true epileptic seizure occurs with no obvious warning and is not preceded by breath-holding. Although breath-holding attacks may be alarming to parents, they are harmless.

CAUSES AND INCIDENCE
Breath-holding attacks occur in 1 to 2 percent of toddlers. They are most common between the ages of 1 and 2 years, particularly in children with determined personalities. Children at this age are just beginning to see themselves as individuals and are trying to determine the extent of their

power over the environment. They may quickly learn that breath-holding attacks annoy or frighten parents, and use them as a means of manipulation.
MANAGEMENT
Breath-holding attacks should, as far as possible, be ignored. If the child is rewarded by gaining increased attention from parents, then he or she will continue to have attacks. As soon as the child realizes there is nothing to be gained, the attacks will stop. Firm, patient, and consistent handling will also help in avoiding attacks. The attacks will usually stop in any case by the age of 5 years, but, if they are causing parental anxiety, the physician should be consulted.

Breathing
The process by which air passes into and out of the lungs to allow the blood to take up oxygen and dispose of carbon dioxide (see *Respiration*). Breathing is controlled by the respiratory center in the brain stem; no conscious effort is needed to inhale and exhale air, but the depth and rate of breathing can be altered voluntarily. During exercise, when the heart and muscles need more oxygen, reflexes lead to a rapid increase in the breathing rate. This can vary in an adult from 13 to 17 breaths per minute at rest up to 80 breaths per minute during vigorous exercise. A newborn baby breathes at a rate of approximately 40 breaths per minute.
HOW AIR ENTERS THE LUNGS
When air is inhaled (inspiration), the diaphragm, which is dome shaped when relaxed, contracts and flattens. The muscles between the ribs contract and pull the rib cage upward and outward. This movement increases chest volume, causing the lungs to expand

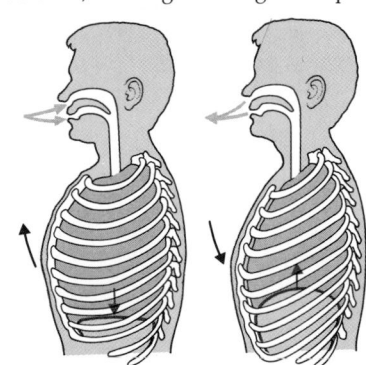

Inhaling and exhaling
When inhaling, the diaphragm flattens; the rib cage is pulled up and out. When exhaling, the diaphragm relaxes; the rib cage sinks.

and suck in air. When air is exhaled (expiration), the chest muscles and diaphragm relax, causing the rib cage to sink and the lungs to contract, squeezing out air.

The lungs do not fill completely during inhalation or empty completely during exhalation. In normal, quiet breathing only about one tenth of the air in the lungs passes out to be replaced by the same amount of fresh air. This new air (tidal volume), mixes with the stale air (residual volume) already held in the lungs.

A man's lungs hold about 1.5 gallons (6 liters) of air at one time, and a woman's lungs about 1 gallon (4.25 liters). At rest, about 0.1 gallon (0.4 liter) of air is taken into the lungs during normal inspiration; a deep breath can take in up to 0.8 gallon (3 to 4 liters) of air.

Breathing difficulty

Breathing difficulty is a change in the rate and depth of breathing. This happens when the effort required to breathe is increased, or when breathing movement is causing pain. Accompanying symptoms may include a feeling of tightness in the chest, coughing, wheezing, or chest pain.

Breathing difficulty may be due to any condition that affects the airflow into and out of the lungs, the transfer of oxygen from lungs to the blood, the circulation of blood through the lungs, or control of breathing by the brain stem. Breathing difficulty can occur at rest or when the body needs more oxygen during exercise or illness.

LACK OF FITNESS
The heart and lungs of an unfit person cannot respond adequately to the increased need for oxygen, so the increased effort needed to breathe causes discomfort. This problem can be overcome by fitness training.

OVERWEIGHT
Overweight people often experience difficulty breathing during exertion, partly because they are unfit and partly because of the increased effort needed to carry extra weight. In the very obese the brain-stem breathing center may not function efficiently and this may cause irregular breathing patterns (pickwickian syndrome).

ANXIETY
Severe anxiety during times of stress or tension can bring on attacks of *hyperventilation*. These attacks are associated with a feeling that one cannot get a good breath, itself leading to further overbreathing.

BRAIN-STEM DAMAGE
Damage to the breathing center in the brain stem due to a *transient ischemic attack* or a head injury can reduce or increase breathing activity. This may also happen as a side effect of certain drugs. In certain instances, a *ventilator* may be required.

ALTITUDE SICKNESS
This can cause breathlessness because there is less oxygen present in the surrounding air, so the lungs have to work harder to give the body sufficient oxygen. Swelling of the brain and fluid filling the lungs are serious stages of altitude sickness.

ANEMIA
When there is a shortage of red *blood cells* there is insufficient *hemoglobin* to carry oxygen around the body. If anemia is severe, the lungs need to work harder to supply the body with oxygen, resulting in breathlessness.

CIRCULATION DISORDERS
Breathing difficulty intensified upon exertion may be caused by a reduced circulation of blood through the lungs. This may be due to *heart failure*, where the heart pumps blood less efficiently, to blockage of blood vessels in the lungs by a blood clot (see *Pulmonary embolism*), or to increased pressure in the arteries within the lungs (see *Pulmonary hypertension*).

AIRWAYS BLOCKAGE
Breathing difficulty due to airflow obstruction may be caused by chronic *bronchitis* (in which mucus and thickened walls block the airways), by *asthma* or allergic reaction (where there is constriction of the lungs), or by *lung cancer* (in which a *tumor* blocks a large airway).

LUNG DAMAGE
Breathing difficulty may also be due to inefficient transfer of oxygen from the lungs into the bloodstream. This can be a result of damage to lung tissue, which may be temporary as in *pneumonia*, or a result of a *pneumothorax* (collapsed lung), pulmonary *edema* (fluid in the lung), or *pleural effusion* (fluid around the lung). Lung damage may also be permanent as in *emphysema*, where the walls of the *alveoli* are destroyed.

PAIN
Any pain in the chest that is made worse by chest or lung movement can make normal breathing difficult and painful. A fractured rib, for example, results in pain at the fracture site during breathing or movement of the torso. Pleurisy is associated with pain in the lower chest and often in the shoulder tip of the affected side.

Breathing exercises

Techniques for learning to control the rate and depth of breathing, used in therapy and to aid relaxation.

WHY THEY ARE DONE
PHYSICAL THERAPY Breathing exercises are often recommended for people with chronic chest diseases, such as bronchitis. They can also help people with anxiety disorders who breathe too deeply and rapidly and as a result disturb the chemical composition of their blood.

Breathing exercises are important after operations, when patients often breathe shallowly and are afraid to cough because of pain. In these circumstances, poor ventilation and the buildup of secretions can lead to collapse of segments of the lung or to collapse of a lobe of the lung, particularly in patients who are overweight or smokers. Deep breathing promotes coughing and keeps the lungs clear.

Many patients undergoing chest or upper abdominal surgery are given a device that, upon deep inhalation, causes three plastic balls to rise. This breathing exercise is called incentive spirometry and it promotes deep breathing and chest clearing.

RELAXATION In yoga, deep rhythmic breathing is used to achieve a state of relaxation. During labor and childbirth, breathing exercises relax the mother, help control contractions, and reduce pain.

HOW THEY ARE DONE
The person is taught to inhale through the nose, expanding the chest. He or she then exhales fully through the mouth, while contracting the abdominal muscles.

Hand lying on chest should hardly move

Hand lying on stomach should rise first

Practicing breathing
This exercise can be done unsupervised. A second person may apply gentle pressure to the chest or abdomen to help you become aware of the muscle groups used.

BREATHING DIFFICULTY Rapid breathing, or pain or tightness in the chest that makes you aware of your breathing.

B

? Has the breathlessness come on suddenly? → **YES** → Do you have pain in the chest AND/OR is breathing painful? → **YES** → See • *Chest pain*

NO ↓

WARNING
If someone is having severe difficulty breathing AND/OR if there is a bluish coloring around the lips, this is an EMERGENCY requiring immediate medical attention.

Is your temperature 100°F (38°C) or above AND/OR do you have a cough? → **YES** → ☎
Call your physician without delay!
A chest infection, such as pneumonia or acute bronchitis, is the likely cause of your symptoms. This can be dangerous, especially for the elderly, the very young, and those in poor health.

See • *Bronchitis*
• *Pneumonia*

NO ↓

Have you been awakened at night by an attack of breathlessness AND/OR have you been coughing up frothy white or pink sputum (phlegm)? → **YES** → ☎
Call your physician without delay!
A dangerous buildup of fluid in the lungs, perhaps as a result of heart disease, is a possibility. Sit upright in a chair and try to stay calm; this will make breathing easier for you until help arrives.

See • *Edema*

NO ↓

Have you recently been confined to bed through illness or injury? → **YES** → ☎ **EMERGENCY!**
GET MEDICAL HELP NOW!
A blood clot in the lung is a possibility, especially if you have also coughed up bloody sputum (phlegm).

See • *Pulmonary embolism*

NO ↓

Has the attack of breathlessness come on at a time when you are feeling tense or under great stress? → **YES** → ☎
Call your physician without delay!
Panic attacks caused by severe anxiety often result in hyperventilation. If this is the first time you have experienced such symptoms, or if you are in any doubt as to their cause, call your physician now.

See • *Hyperventilation*
• *Panic attack*

NO ↓

Continued on next page

211

B

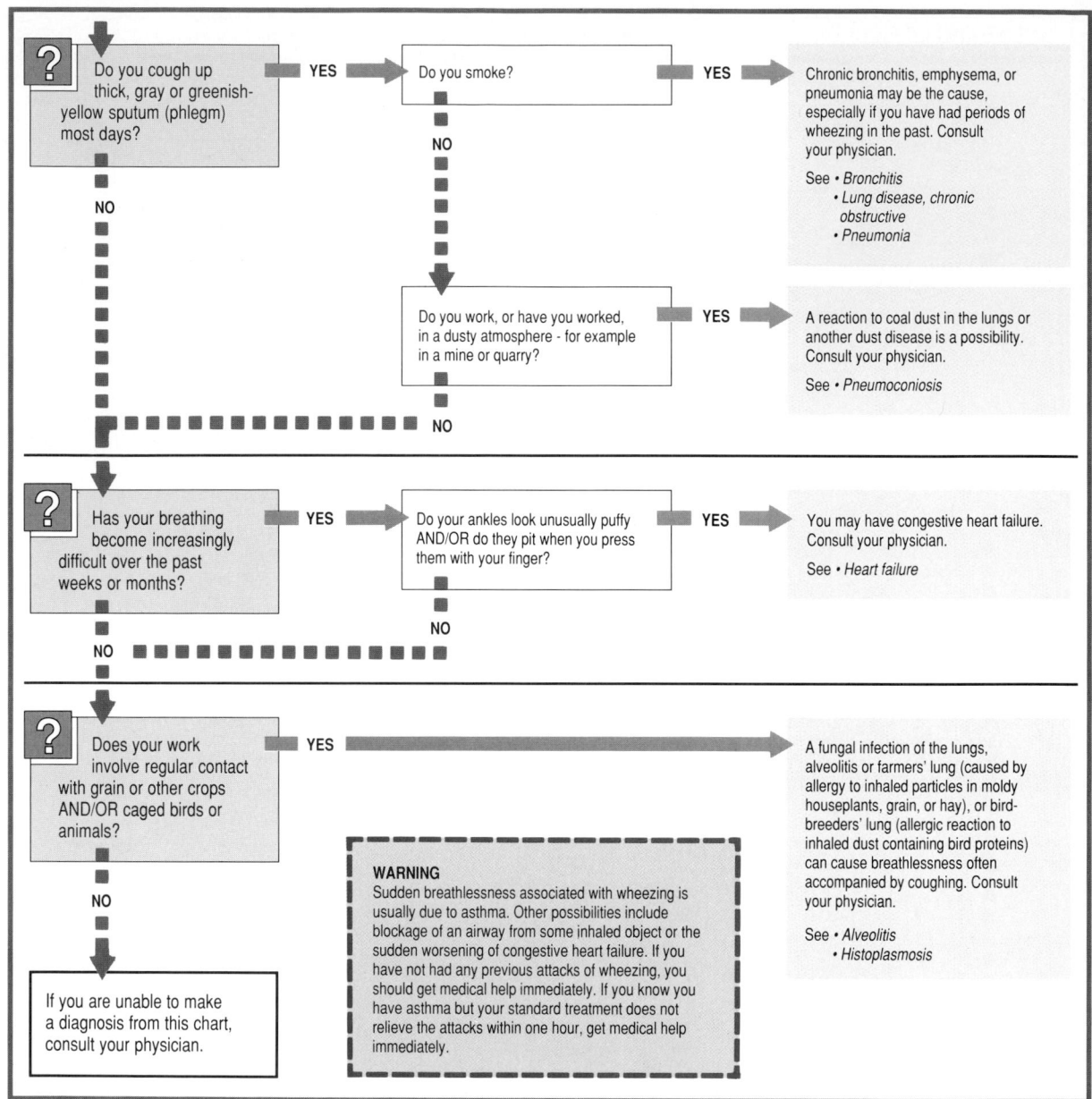

Do you cough up thick, gray or greenish-yellow sputum (phlegm) most days?

YES → Do you smoke? → **YES** → Chronic bronchitis, emphysema, or pneumonia may be the cause, especially if you have had periods of wheezing in the past. Consult your physician.

See • Bronchitis
• Lung disease, chronic obstructive
• Pneumonia

NO

NO

Do you work, or have you worked, in a dusty atmosphere - for example in a mine or quarry? → **YES** → A reaction to coal dust in the lungs or another dust disease is a possibility. Consult your physician.

See • Pneumoconiosis

NO

Has your breathing become increasingly difficult over the past weeks or months? → **YES** → Do your ankles look unusually puffy AND/OR do they pit when you press them with your finger? → **YES** → You may have congestive heart failure. Consult your physician.

See • Heart failure

NO

NO

Does your work involve regular contact with grain or other crops AND/OR caged birds or animals? → **YES** → A fungal infection of the lungs, alveolitis or farmers' lung (caused by allergy to inhaled particles in moldy houseplants, grain, or hay), or bird-breeders' lung (allergic reaction to inhaled dust containing bird proteins) can cause breathlessness often accompanied by coughing. Consult your physician.

See • Alveolitis
• Histoplasmosis

NO

WARNING
Sudden breathlessness associated with wheezing is usually due to asthma. Other possibilities include blockage of an airway from some inhaled object or the sudden worsening of congestive heart failure. If you have not had any previous attacks of wheezing, you should get medical help immediately. If you know you have asthma but your standard treatment does not relieve the attacks within one hour, get medical help immediately.

If you are unable to make a diagnosis from this chart, consult your physician.

Breathlessness
The need to breathe air in and out of the lungs very quickly. This is part of exercise or exertion in healthy people and not a cause for concern. The body requires more oxygen, so the lungs work harder. However, if breathlessness develops for any other reason it is a *breathing difficulty* that indicates some underlying disorder.

Breech delivery
Birth of a baby bottom-first instead of the usual head-first delivery.

By around the 32nd week of pregnancy, most babies have assumed a head-down position in the uterus, but about 3 to 4 percent take up breech presentation with the head at the top of the uterus. Often, one of two twins may present as a breech. At 34 weeks, some obstetricians try to turn a baby with a breech presentation into the head-down position.

If this attempt fails, the baby is left in the breech presentation until delivery. A breech delivery adds to the problems of mother and baby because the baby's bottom does not mold a passage through the birth canal as efficiently as the head. Usually, an *episiotomy* will be performed to ease the baby's passage, and *forceps* are commonly used to ensure smooth emergence of the head.

If a baby with a breech presentation has a large head or the mother's pelvic girdle is small, delivery by *cesarean section* may be decided upon before she goes into labor. Some physicians recommend cesarean section for most breech babies, particularly if the baby is feet-first (footling presentation) or if a woman has not had a previous vaginal delivery, as there is an increased risk to the baby. In other instances, the decision is based on the results of *fetal heart monitoring*.

Delivering a breech baby
The buttocks are delivered first and then the legs. An episiotomy may be performed before the head is delivered.

Bridge, dental
False teeth (usually no more than four) attached to natural teeth on either side of a gap left by a missing tooth or teeth. Some bridges are removable. Unlike a *denture*, a bridge has no baseplate (artificial gum). Bridges are usually made of platinum or gold alloy faced with porcelain, but those at the back of the mouth may consist of only gold or gold-platinum alloy.

As with a denture, a bridge is fitted to fill any gap in the mouth to enable the person to bite properly, speak clearly, and avoid problems resulting from shifting or drifting of the remaining natural teeth. People who wear bridges usually do not have the option of wearing a denture.

Bright's disease
Another name for the kidney disease, *glomerulonephritis*, first described by the English physician Richard Bright (1789-1858).

Brittle bones
A term used to describe bones with an increased tendency to fracture. Brittle bones are a feature of the disorder *osteoporosis* (thinning of the bones), which is common in postmenopausal women and may occur in people confined to bed, on corticosteroid drugs, or with hormonal disorders. In *osteomalacia* (a vitamin D deficiency disease), the bones become soft, with an increased tendency both to deform and fracture.

A rare cause of brittle bones is the inherited connective tissue abnormality *osteogenesis imperfecta* (sometimes called brittle-bone disease). The disease is associated with blue sclerae (whites of the eyes) and with an increased susceptibility to many fractures throughout life.

Broken blood vessels
Any small, widened blood vessel visible beneath the skin surface, most commonly on the cheeks. Sometimes called a broken vein, it is the natural result of heavy alcohol consumption over many years, or of loss of supporting tissues in the skin due to overexposure to the sun. More rarely, a connective tissue disease, such as systemic *lupus erythematosus*, is the cause. Broken blood vessels may also be a feature of the facial redness seen in *rosacea*. Often, however, there is no obvious cause.

Broken blood vessels need not be any cause for concern. The only means of removal is *electrodesiccation*—electrical destruction of the upper layers of the skin—administered by a dermatologist. The procedure is successful only in some cases.

Broken tooth
See *Fracture, dental*.

Bromides
Substances formerly prescribed as sedatives in the treatment of *anxiety* or as anticonvulsants in the treatment of *epilepsy*. They are no longer prescribed due to their unpleasant side effects, which include loss of libido (sex drive), acne, tremor, and confusion.

Bromocriptine
By inhibiting the secretion of the hormone, prolactin, from the pituitary gland, bromocriptine is helpful in treating conditions associated with excessive prolactin production. Such conditions include *galactorrhea* (abnormal milk production by the breast), some types of female and male infertility, severe premenstrual breast discomfort, and benign pituitary tumors that cause *acromegaly* (abnormal tissue and bone growth). Bromocriptine is also used to suppress lactation in women who do not wish to breast-feed.

A few years after its development in the 1960s, bromocriptine was found to be effective for relieving the symptoms of *Parkinson's disease*. The reason is that it has almost the identical characteristics of dopamine, the chemical that is lacking in the brain of someone with Parkinson's disease. Bromocriptine is now widely used to treat those in the advanced stages of the disease when other drugs have failed or are unsuitable.

Serious adverse effects are uncommon when the drug is given in low doses. Nausea and vomiting, the most

---

FITTING A BRIDGE
The most common type of bridge consists of one or more false teeth attached to a crown on each side of a gap. The natural teeth are shaped to receive the crowns, which are then cemented into place.

1 Two complete teeth are missing. A bridge of two false teeth and three crowns can be attached.

2 The three healthy teeth are shaped so that they can receive the crowns on either side of the gap.

3 A cast-metal subframe made from an impression is tried out in the mouth and any necessary alterations are made.

4 The finished bridge is in position, showing the new porcelain teeth cemented to the metal base.

common problems, can be minimized by taking bromocriptine with meals. In rare cases, it may cause ulceration of the stomach. When taken in high doses, bromocriptine may cause drowsiness and confusion.

Bronchiectasis

A lung disorder in which one or more bronchi (the branching air passages that connect the windpipe to the lungs) are distorted and stretched, with a damaged lining. The abnormality usually occurs in childhood and results in chronic lung infections that may extend into later life.

CAUSES AND INCIDENCE

Bronchiectasis was formerly common and usually caused by childhood chest infections such as measles, whooping cough, tuberculosis, and severe bacterial pneumonias. As these infections have been controlled by immunization and antibiotics, so the incidence of bronchiectasis has plummeted. Bronchiectasis is now virtually extinct among children in the US and other developed countries.

When bronchiectasis occurs today, the cause is more often a congenital bronchial defect or blockage of a bronchus by a foreign body.

SYMPTOMS

The main symptom of chronic lung infection in bronchiectasis is a daily cough that produces large amounts of dark green sputum (phlegm) containing pus and occasionally flecked with blood. The sputum causes bad breath. If the disease is extensive it causes shortness of breath.

DIAGNOSIS AND TREATMENT

The diagnosis is usually made from the symptoms present. Occasionally a chest X ray or *bronchography* (X rays of the bronchi after they have been injected with a special dye) may be used to determine exactly how the bronchi have been affected.

Symptoms can usually be controlled by antibiotics and postural drainage; the patient is taught to lie in a position so that the pus and fluid drain from the affected segment or segments of lung and can then be coughed up.

If severe symptoms persist despite these measures, surgery may be recommended to remove the damaged lung areas.

Bronchiolitis

An acute viral infection of the lungs, mainly affecting babies and young children, in which the bronchioles (the smaller airways that branch off the bronchi) become inflamed.

CAUSES AND INCIDENCE

The most common cause of bronchiolitis is the respiratory syncytial virus (RSV), but various other viruses may also be responsible. Adult bronchiolitis may follow *bronchitis*, brought on by an influenza virus.

Winter epidemics of bronchiolitis tend to occur every two or three years, affecting thousands of children in the US. The viruses responsible can be transmitted from one person to another in airborne droplets, and a virus that may cause only a moderate head or chest infection in an adult can cause severe bronchiolitis in an infant. Hence, when suffering from a severe head or chest infection, contact with a baby is best kept to a minimum.

SYMPTOMS

The symptoms are a cough, shortness of breath, and, in severe cases, a cyanotic (blue-purple) complexion due to shortage of oxygen. The physician will also often hear crepitations (bubbling noises) in the lungs through a stethoscope.

TREATMENT

If a baby or young child has a cold and a cough that suddenly worsens, leading to rapid and labored breathing, a physician should be consulted. Sometimes no treatment is necessary, but, in more severe cases, the child may be admitted to the hospital, where oxygen and respiratory therapy (to clear the mucus from the bronchioles) is given.

Antibiotics and *corticosteroid drugs* (commonly used to treat bronchiolitis in adults) are ineffective against the viral infection, but antibiotics may nevertheless be prescribed to prevent any secondary bacterial infection. Occasionally, the child needs to be put on an artificial *ventilator* until normal breathing is restored.

With prompt treatment, even the most severely affected children usually recover completely within a few days.

Bronchitis

Inflammation of the bronchi, the airways that connect the trachea (windpipe) to the lungs, resulting in a persistent cough that produces considerable quantities of sputum (phlegm). Two forms of the disease are recognized acute bronchitis (of sudden onset and short duration) and chronic bronchitis (persistent over a long period and recurring over several years). Both are more common in smokers and in areas with high atmospheric pollution.

ACUTE BRONCHITIS

This form comes on suddenly and usually clears up within a few days, except in those with a low resistance to infection, such as frail, elderly people and people with lung disease.

CAUSES AND INCIDENCE

Acute bronchitis is usually a complication of a viral infection such as a cold or influenza, but may also be caused by the effect of air pollutants. Bacterial infection may cause acute bronchitis or occur as a further complication of acute bronchitis with other causes.

Attacks occur most often in winter. In addition to smokers, those most susceptible are babies, the elderly, and people with lung disease.

SYMPTOMS

The inflammation of the mucosal lining of the bronchi causes swelling and congestion, and pus is formed. The main symptoms are wheezing, breathlessness, and a persistent cough that produces yellow or green sputum. There may also be discomfort behind the sternum (breastbone) and a raised temperature.

TREATMENT

Symptoms may be relieved by humidifying the lungs, either using a humidifier in the home, or by inhaling steam directly (be careful—inhaling steam that is too hot can cause serious burns). Drinking plenty of fluids is the best expectorant.

Most acute bronchitis clears up without further treatment and causes no further trouble. Complications such as *pneumonia* and *pleurisy* are exceptional. However, a physician should be consulted in any of the following cases: if there is severe breathlessness, if there is no improvement after three days, if blood is coughed up, if the temperature is above 101°F (38.3°C), or if the patient has underlying lung disease.

If your physician suspects there is a bacterial infection, antibiotics will be prescribed, but these are of no use if the infection is caused by a virus.

CHRONIC BRONCHITIS

Bronchitis is regarded as chronic when sputum is coughed up on most days during at least three consecutive months in at least two consecutive years. The disease commonly results in widespread narrowing and obstruction of the airways in the lungs. It often coexists with (and may contribute to the development of) another lung disease, *emphysema*, in which the alveoli (air sacs) in the lungs become distended. Chronic bronchitis and emphysema together are sometimes called chronic obstructive lung disease (COLD) or chronic obstructive pulmonary disease (COPD).

CAUSES AND INCIDENCE

Cigarette smoking is the main cause. It stimulates the production of mucus in the lining of the bronchi and thickens the bronchi's muscular walls and those of the bronchioles (smaller airways in the lungs), resulting in narrowing of these air passages. The passages then become more susceptible to infections, which cause further damage. Atmospheric pollution can have the same effect.

Approximately 3,000 persons per 100,000 in the US suffer from chronic bronchitis. Most are over 40 and male sufferers outnumber female sufferers two to one. The disease is most prevalent in industrial cities and in smokers, and is more common in manual and unskilled workers than among white collar workers (even after adjusting for differences in smoking habits). Chronic obstructive lung disease accounts for about 30 deaths per 100,000 in the US per year.

SYMPTOMS AND COMPLICATIONS

The symptoms are the same as in acute bronchitis—cough, breathlessness, and, rarely, chest pain—except that they are persistent instead of clearing up, and there is usually no fever. This persistence of symptoms also distinguishes the disease from chronic *asthma*, in which wheezing and breathlessness vary in severity from hour to hour and day to day.

As the disease progresses, often with the development of emphysema, the lungs become more resistant to the flow of blood, resulting in *pulmonary hypertension* (increased pressure in the arteries that supply blood to the lungs), and in strain on the right side of the heart due to its increased work in pumping blood through the lungs. The patient may become a *pink puffer*, with severe breathlessness. Sometimes, heart failure develops, further reducing the oxygen in the blood and causing a cyanotic (blue-purple) complexion. *Edema* (swelling caused by fluid collection) then develops in the legs and ankles due to the back pressure in blood vessels as a result of the heart failure. Patients with this condition are called *blue bloaters*.

Those with chronic bronchitis usually have two or more episodes of acute viral or bacterial infection of the lungs every winter. Occasionally, blood may be coughed up, requiring urgent medical investigation to exclude the possibility of *lung cancer*.

PREVENTION

A reduction in atmospheric pollution in some cities over the last few decades has helped reduce the incidence of chronic bronchitis, but the crucial advice is that smoking is by far the most common cause of chronic bronchitis. Most cases of chronic bronchitis could be prevented if people stopped smoking. Waiting until symptoms develop may be too late to halt the course of the disease.

DIAGNOSIS AND TREATMENT

Before starting treatment, the physician may decide the patient's condition requires investigation by chest *X rays*, *blood tests*, *sputum* analysis, and *pulmonary function tests*.

To relieve breathlessness, the physician may prescribe an inhaler containing a *bronchodilator* (a drug that relaxes and widens the bronchi). In certain specific cases, the patient may benefit from inhaling oxygen from oxygen cylinders or an oxygen concentrator kept at home. Efforts may be made to help the patient cough up sputum; to treat or prevent any bacterial lung infection, antibiotics may be given.

The disease often shows an inexorable progression with increasing shortness of breath leading to early retirement; eventually the sufferer may become housebound.

Bronchoconstrictor

A substance that causes narrowing of the airways in the lungs. Bronchoconstrictors such as *histamine* or dinoprost (a *prostaglandin*) are sometimes given by inhalation to provoke an attack of *asthma* in order to confirm the diagnosis or to test the effectiveness of a *bronchodilator drug*.

Bronchodilator drugs

COMMON DRUGS

Sympathomimetics
Albuterol Ephedrine Epinephrine Isoproterenol Metaproterenol Terbutaline

Anticholinergics
Ipratropium

Xanthines
Aminophylline Theophylline

> **WARNING**
> If your inhaler is not helping your symptoms, call your physician.

A group of drugs that widen the airways in the lungs.

Under certain conditions the bronchioles (narrow airways) become narrowed, either as a result of contraction of the muscle in their walls and/or as a result of mucus congestion within them. Narrowing of the bronchioles obstructs the flow of air into and out of the lung and causes breathing difficulty. Bronchodilator drugs are prescribed to widen the bronchioles, which increases the flow of air and improves breathing.

TYPES

There are three principal types: sympathomimetic drugs, anticholinergic drugs, and xanthine drugs. Sympathomimetics are primarily used for the rapid relief of breathing difficulty. Anticholinergics and xanthine drugs are more often used for the long-term prevention of attacks of breathing difficulty.

WHY THEY ARE USED

Bronchodilators may be prescribed for any condition in which there is a reduced flow of air into the lungs, as in chronic *bronchitis*, although they are of little benefit when damage to the bronchioles from repeated infections is severe. Most commonly, however, they are used in the treatment of asthma, both to relieve attacks that are in progress and to try to prevent such attacks from occurring. Some people find it helpful to take an extra dose of their bronchodilator immediately before an activity likely to provoke an attack of breathlessness. Drugs can be given by *inhaler* or in tablet form and one or a combination of drugs may be prescribed. In a severe attack of asthma that has not responded to an inhaler, bronchodilators can be given by *nebulizer* (a type of inhaler that uses air and/or oxygen under pressure to propel a watery suspension of the drug into the lungs) or by injection.

POSSIBLE ADVERSE EFFECTS

Bronchodilators can have a variety of minor side effects especially if taken in large doses or very frequently. Because sympathomimetic drugs stimulate the sympathetic branch of the autonomic nervous system which controls heart rate, they may sometimes cause palpitations and trembling. Anticholinergic drugs have the side effects typical of all drugs of this type, including dry mouth, blurred vision, and difficulty passing urine. Xanthine drugs may cause headaches and, like adrenergics, may cause palpitations. When bronchodilators are inhaled they are not absorbed by the body in large amounts and therefore do not commonly cause serious side effects. However, because of their possible effect on

HOW BRONCHODILATORS WORK

Bronchodilator drugs relax muscles surrounding bronchioles. Sympathomimetic and anticholinergic drugs interfere with nerve signals passed to the muscles through the autonomic nervous system. Xanthine drugs relax muscle in the bronchioles by a direct effect on the muscle fibers but their precise action is not known.

When bronchioles become narrow following contraction of the muscle layer and swelling of the mucous lining, the passage of air is impeded. Bronchodilators act on the nerve signals that govern muscle activity. Sympathomimetics enhance the action of neurotransmitters that encourage muscle relaxation. Anticholinergics block the neurotransmitters that trigger muscle contraction.

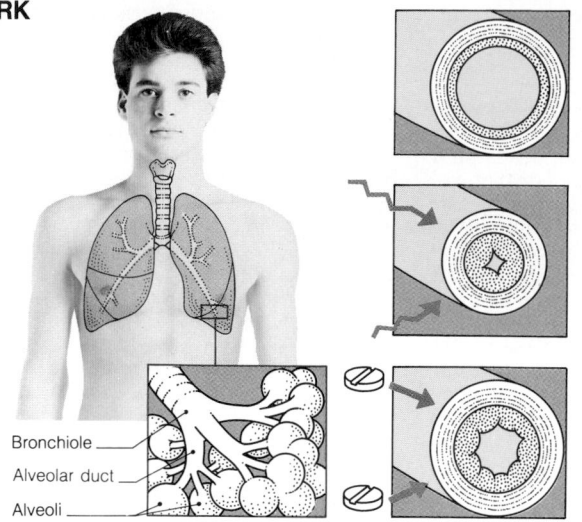

Bronchiole
Alveolar duct
Alveoli

Normal bronchioles
The muscle surrounding the bronchioles is relaxed, leaving the airway open.

Asthmatic spasm
The muscle contracts and the lining swells, narrowing the airway.

After drug treatment
The muscles relax, opening the airway, but the mucous lining remains swollen.

heart rate, sympathomimetic and xanthine drugs are prescribed cautiously for those with heart problems, high blood pressure, or an overactive thyroid gland. Anticholinergic drugs may not be suitable for men with enlarged prostate glands or for people who have a tendency to glaucoma.

Bronchography

An X-ray procedure for examining the bronchi, the main air passages of the lungs. Bronchography was formerly used to diagnose the disease *bronchiectasis*, but has now largely been replaced by other imaging techniques, such as *CT scanning* or lung *tomography*, and by using *bronchoscopy*.

HOW IT IS DONE
After the patient has been given mild sedation and/or a local anesthetic, contrast medium (an iodinated substance opaque to X rays) is introduced into the lung through a hollow flexible tube (either a cannula or a bronchoscope). X-ray pictures are then taken of the bronchi to detect any deformities in them. When the procedure is finished the contrast medium is partly coughed up and partly absorbed into the bloodstream.

Bronchopneumonia

The most common form of *pneumonia*, differing from pneumococcal or lobar pneumonia in that inflammation is spread throughout the lungs in small patches rather than confined to one lobe. It is often the cause of death in chronically ill patients.

Bronchoscopy

Examination or treatment of the bronchi, the main airways of the lungs, by means of a hollow tube or fiberoptic viewing tube with a light and lens attached.

WHY IT IS DONE
The two main uses of bronchoscopy are to aid in diagnosing and treating certain lung disorders. Apart from inspecting the bronchi for abnormalities, diagnostic procedures include collecting samples of mucus, obtaining cells from the outermost distant airways of the lungs, and taking biopsy specimens (small samples of tissue), all for analysis or microscopic examination. The bronchoscope is also sometimes used in a type of X-ray investigation called *bronchography*.

PERFORMING BRONCHOSCOPY

There are two kinds of bronchoscope. The rigid type is passed into the bronchi via the mouth and requires anesthesia. The flexible, fiberoptic bronchoscope (a narrower tube formed from light-transmitting fibers) can be inserted through either the mouth or nose. It is used after giving only a light sedative and/or local anesthetic and it reaches farther into the lungs. Both types of bronchoscope can be fitted with forceps, and the instrument also has attachments for performing laser therapy and cryosurgery. (See also *Endoscopy*.)

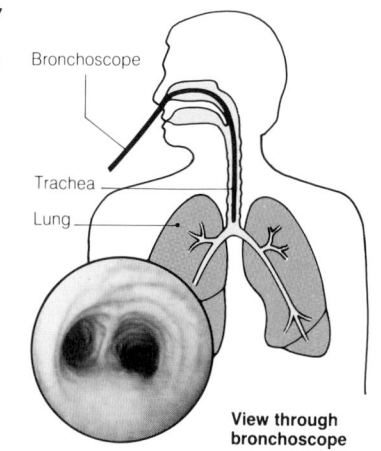

Bronchoscope
Trachea
Lung

View through bronchoscope

THE BRONCHOSCOPE

Control lever

Insertion tube

Forceps — various forceps can be attached; this one has a basket for removing small, hard objects

Eyepiece

Among the various forms of treatment possible are the removal of thick secretions of mucus or inhaled foreign bodies, destruction of growths, and the sealing off of damaged blood vessels. The last two are carried out by *laser treatment*, *diathermy*, or *cryosurgery* by means of attachments to the bronchoscope.

Bronchospasm

Temporary narrowing of the bronchi (airways into the lungs) caused by contraction of the muscles in the lung walls, by inflammation of the lung lining, or by a combination of both.

Contraction and relaxation of the airways is controlled by the autonomic nervous system. Contraction may also be caused by the release of substances during an allergic reaction.

When the airways are narrowed, flow of air out of the lungs causes wheezing or coughing. The most common cause of bronchospasm is *asthma*, though other causes include respiratory infection, chronic lung disease (including *emphysema* and chronic *bronchitis*), *anaphylactic shock*, or an allergic reaction to chemicals.

Bronchus

The air passage into the lungs. Each lung has one main bronchus, originating at the end of the trachea (windpipe), that is divided into smaller branches known as segmental bronchi. These then further divide into bronchioles.

Bronchus, cancer of

See *Lung cancer*.

Brown fat

A special type of fat, found in infants and some animals, but not in healthy adults. It is located between and around the scapulae on the back. Brown fat is a source of calories and so is useful in helping infants maintain a constant body temperature.

Brucellosis

A rare, bacterial infection caught from farm animals that causes fever.

CAUSES AND INCIDENCE

Three types of bacteria can cause the disease: BRUCELLA ABORTUS, B. MELITENSIS, and B. SUIS. These bacteria affect cattle, goats, and pigs, respectively. People who work with animals are at highest risk of infection. The bacteria enter the bloodstream through a cut or are breathed in. Up to 200 cases of brucellosis occur in the US each year.

In areas where milk pasteurization is not the rule—for example, Latin America and the Mediterranean—the disease can also be caught from drinking or eating unpasteurized dairy products from infected animals.

SYMPTOMS

The acute form of brucellosis consists of a single bout of high fever, shivering, widespread aching, and drenching sweats, which last for a few days. Other symptoms include headache, poor appetite, backache, weakness, and depression.

Sweating occurs by night as well as by day and can cause severe dehydration unless plenty of fluids are taken. The mental depression is sometimes severe; the patient may feel suicidal. In rare, untreated cases an acute attack is severe enough to cause sometimes fatal complications, such as *pneumonia* or *meningitis*.

In chronic brucellosis, bouts of the illness recur over months or years.

PREVENTION

The disease in livestock—and thus also human infection—is controlled by immunizing herds that have first been checked to guarantee that they are not infected. Infected animals are usually destroyed.

DIAGNOSIS AND TREATMENT

A definite diagnosis is made from blood tests. Treatment consists of tetracyclines, co-trimoxazole, or other *antibiotic drugs*, and the patient is advised to rest. After apparent recovery, the illness sometimes recurs a few months later, necessitating another course of treatment.

Bruise

A discolored area under the skin, caused by leakage of blood after injury. At first, the blood appears blue or black; then the breakdown of *hemoglobin* turns the bruise yellow.

To reduce the pain and swelling of a large bruise, place a cloth soaked in ice-cold water over it for 10 minutes. If a bruise does not fade after about one week, or if bruises appear for no apparent reason or are severe after only minor injury, a physician should be consulted as these may be signs of a *bleeding disorder*. (See also *Purpura*; *Black eye*.)

Bruits

The sounds made in the heart, arteries, or veins when blood circulation becomes turbulent or flows at an abnormal speed. This happens when blood vessels become narrowed by disease (as in *arteriosclerosis*), when

heart valves are narrowed or damaged (as in *endocarditis*), or if blood vessels dilate (as in an *aneurysm*). Bruits are usually heard through a *stethoscope*.

Bruxism

Rhythmic grinding or clenching of the teeth. This habit, which may develop at any age, usually occurs during sleep, but is sometimes done unconsciously when a person is awake. There are two underlying causes: unresolved stress and emotional tension, and some minor discomfort or unevenness when the teeth are brought together.

Continued bruxism may cause considerable wearing away and loosening of the teeth, and stiffness in the jaw. If the underlying problems cannot be resolved, a biteplate worn at night will minimize the damage.

Bubonic plague

The most common form of *plague*, characterized by the appearance of a bubo (swollen lymph node) in the groin or armpit early in the illness.

Buccal

An anatomical term, from the Latin word for cheek, relating to the cheek or mouth.

Buck teeth

Prominent upper incisors (front teeth), which protrude from the mouth and are often splayed out at an angle to each other. Buck teeth are easily damaged and may be susceptible to decay because they are not moistened by saliva.

CAUSES

The malpositioning of the teeth is probably an inherited trait rather than

Buck teeth
Apart from the usually undesirable appearance protruding upper teeth produce, the upper and lower incisors do not meet satisfactorily. This produces stress on the jaw joint that can cause problems. A plaster cast of buck teeth is shown.

B

acquired—for example, by faulty eating habits. Often, the person's upper jaw is relatively large compared with the lower jaw, and the lips do not close over and exert a controlling influence on the position of the teeth. Rarely, the malpositioning may be the result of an abnormally large tongue gradually displacing the teeth forward. In many cases, there is an overall crowding of teeth within the upper jaw.

TREATMENT
Orthodontic treatment involves gradually coaxing the teeth back into position with a removable brace, or, in more extreme cases, with a fixed appliance (see *Orthodontic appliances*). To create room for the incisors, other crowded teeth may sometimes need to be extracted.

Budd-Chiari syndrome
A rare disorder in which the veins draining blood from the liver become blocked or narrowed. Blood then accumulates in the liver, which swells. The blockage leads to serious *liver failure*, and to *portal hypertension* (back pressure in the blood vessels due to slowed blood flow through the liver).

Treatment is aimed at removing the cause of the vein obstruction—which may be a blood clot, pressure on the veins from a liver tumor, or a congenital abnormality of the veins. In most cases, however, treatment has only a limited effect, and, unless a *liver transplant* can be performed, most patients die within two years.

Buerger's disease
A rare disorder, also called thromboangiitis obliterans, in which the arteries, nerves, and veins in the legs, and sometimes those in the arms, become severely inflamed. Narrowing of the arteries blocks off blood supply to the toes and fingers, eventually causing *gangrene*.

The disease occurs mainly in men under the age of 45 who smoke heavily. Most have a history of *phlebitis* (a type of vein inflammation). The main symptom is pain in the hands and feet; victims suffer cold sensitivity, with the hands turning white, then blue, then red (see *Raynaud's disease*) in cold conditions.

Sufferers must stop smoking to halt progress of the disease. *Vasodilators* (drugs that widen the blood vessels) may be prescribed, but are rarely, if ever, effective. If *gangrene* (tissue death) develops, the affected limb, toes, or fingers almost always have to be amputated.

Bulimia
An illness characterized by bouts of gross overeating usually followed by self-induced vomiting. These activities are often kept secret, so the exact prevalence of the illness is not known, but most sufferers are girls or women between the ages of 15 and 30.

CAUSES
Bulimia is often, though not always, a variant of another psychiatric disorder, *anorexia nervosa*, in which dieting is carried out to excess. In both illnesses there is a morbid fear of fatness. After months or years of eating sparsely, an anorectic may develop a constant craving for food and begin to binge—but the fear of becoming overweight remains and prompts the vomiting. Sometimes, large doses of *laxatives* are used as well as, or instead of, vomiting in an effort to expel food as quickly as possible.

Occasionally, a woman develops bulimia without a previous history of anorexia.

SYMPTOMS
Bulimics may be of normal weight or only slightly underweight, although some remain extremely thin. Bingeing and vomiting may occur once or several times a day. In severe cases, this can lead to dehydration and loss of potassium from the body, causing symptoms such as weakness and cramps. Gastric acid contained in vomit may damage the teeth. The sufferer is often highly distressed about her compulsive behavior and as a result may be depressed and sometimes suicidal.

TREATMENT AND OUTLOOK
Once the bulimic has been persuaded to accept it, treatment is similar to that given for anorexia nervosa. It consists of supervision and regulation of eating habits, *psychotherapy* aimed at improving emotional maturity, and, sometimes, the use of *antidepressant drugs*. To be successful, treatment usually must be given in a hospital over several weeks. In many patients there is a risk of relapse weeks or even months after their treatment has ended. (See also *Appetite*; *Obsessive-compulsive behavior*.)

Bulla
A large air- or fluid-filled bubble, usually in the lungs or skin.

In young adults lung bullae are usually congenital defects (abnormalities present from birth). In later life they develop in patients with the lung disease *emphysema* as the result of overdistention and coalescence of the alveoli (tiny air sacs) in the lungs.

A bulla in the skin is simply a large, fluid-filled *blister*.

Bundle-branch block
See *Heart block*.

Bunion
A firm, fluid-filled pad, or *bursa*, overlying the inside of the joint at the base of the big toe (which can become inflamed and very painful).

The underlying cause of the bunion is hallux valgus, an abnormal outward projection of the joint and inward turning of the toe.

HOW BUNIONS FORM
A bunion results from rubbing of a shoe against an abnormal outward projection of the joint at the base of the big toe (a hallux valgus), leading to irritation and inflammation. The joint abnormality is often itself due to the wearing of narrow, pointed shoes with high heels, although it can also result from an inherited weakness in the joint.

Valgus deformity of the joint between the first metatarsal bone and the adjoining phalanx.

TREATMENT

To remedy a small bunion, wear well-fitting shoes and a special toe pad or corrective sock that straightens the big toe and keeps it in position. Large bunions may require surgery to remove the swollen tissue; in some cases the big toe may have to be completely remodeled.

Unless treated, a bunion will get worse. People with recurring bunions should see a foot specialist.

Buphthalmos

Larger than normal eyeball due to *glaucoma*. In infants, increased pressure inside the eyeball due to glaucoma can result in abnormal eye development. Treatment usually involves surgery to reduce pressure.

Burkitt's lymphoma

A cancer of lymph tissues that is characterized by an enlarging tumor or tumors within the jaw and/or the abdomen.

INCIDENCE

Burkitt's lymphoma is confined almost exclusively to children living in low-lying, moist, tropical regions of Africa and New Guinea. A few cases have occurred among a wider age group in North America and Europe.

CAUSE

The growths are believed to be an abnormal response to a common virus, the Epstein-Barr virus. The distribution of the disease in Africa closely follows that of *malaria*; it is theorized that malaria in childhood alters the body's immune response to the Epstein-Barr virus, which triggers growth of the lymphoma.

TREATMENT

Injections of *anticancer drugs*, such as cyclophosphamide, or treatment by *radiation therapy* gives complete or partial cure in about 80 percent of cases. (See also *Lymphoma*.)

Burns

Each year in the US 2 million people are burned or scalded badly enough to need medical treatment, and about 70,000 require admission to a hospital. Burns are most common in children and older people; many are due to accidents in the home, which are usually preventable.

TYPES

The skin is a living tissue; even brief heating above 120°F damages its cells.

FIRST-DEGREE BURNS These burns cause reddening of the skin and affect only the epidermis, the top layer of the skin. Such burns heal quickly, but the

CARE OF BURN PATIENTS

Burn patients need specialized nursing care. Sterile linen should be used with sterile starch powder sprinkled on it. Drafts should be avoided and room humidity should be controlled. The revolving circular bed is useful in the treatment of burn patients since it can be moved into many different positions and stopped at any angle.

The revolving circular bed

Degrees of burns
Burns are divided into three categories, depending on the depth of damage to the skin. First-degree burns affect the epidermis and skin may peel; second-degree

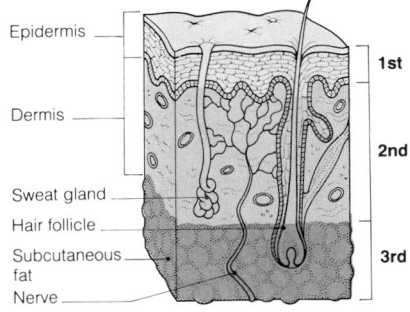

Skin surface area
This is a rough guide to what percentage each area represents of the total skin area (percentages do not total 100 due to rounding).

burns cause the formation of blisters (above left); third-degree burns destroy the whole of the skin's thickness and require special treatment.

PRIMARY CAUSES OF FIRE AND BURN DEATHS, 1980

Cause	Number	% of total
House fire	4,509	75
Fire, other buildings	292	5
Ignition of clothing	364	6
Ignition of highly flammable material	105	2
Hot substances	194	4
Other causes	552	9
Total (percentages do not total 100 due to rounding)	6,016	101

B

FIRST AID: TREATING BURNS

MINOR BURNS

1 Immerse the burned area immediately in cold, running water.

2 Or apply a cold-water compress (a clean towel or handkerchief) until the pain diminishes.

3 Remove any watches, bracelets, rings, belts, or constricting clothing from the area before it begins to swell.

4 Dress the area with a clean (if possible, sterile), nonfluffy material.

MAJOR BURNS

1 If a person's clothing is on fire, douse the victim with water or wrap him or her in a blanket and place on the ground.

2 Do not remove clothing that is stuck to the wound, but cover any exposed burned areas with a dry, clean, nonfluffy cloth to stop infection; secure with a bandage.

DO NOT
- use adhesive dressings on burns
- apply butter, oil, or grease
- apply lotions or creams
- prick blisters with a pin or otherwise interfere with the injured area
- use fluffy materials on wounds

damaged skin may peel away after a day or two. A *sunburn* is an example.

SECOND-DEGREE BURNS These damage the skin more deeply, causing blisters. However, some of the dermis (deep layer of the skin) is left to recover, and these burns usually heal without scarring, unless they are very extensive.

THIRD-DEGREE BURNS These burns destroy the full skin thickness. The affected area will look white or charred, and, if the burn is very deep, muscles and bones may be exposed. Even if very localized, these burns will need specialist treatment and skin grafts to prevent scarring.

ELECTRICAL BURNS These can cause extensive damage with minimal external skin damage. Since they can also cause heart damage, electrical burns require evaluation by a physician.

EFFECTS AND COMPLICATIONS

Extensive first-degree burns (such as sunburn) cause pain, restlessness, headache, and fever, but they are not life-threatening.

In second- or third-degree burns affecting more than 10 percent of the body surface, the victim will be in *shock* with a low blood pressure and rapid pulse. This is caused by the loss of large quantities of fluid (and its constituent proteins) from the burned area. It may be fatal if not treated by intravenous fluid replacement.

When skin is burned, it can no longer protect the body from contamination by airborne bacteria. The infection of extensive burns may cause fatal complications if effective antibiotic treatment is not given.

Victims who have inhaled smoke may develop swelling and inflammation of the lungs and may need specialist care for burns of the eyes. People who die in burning buildings usually suffocate long before their bodies are burned.

PROFESSIONAL TREATMENT

The burn will be either lightly dressed with an antibacterial dressing or left exposed to promote healing, with every effort made to keep the skin area scrupulously clean by reverse *isolation* nursing. If necessary, analgesic drugs (painkillers) will be given; antibiotics will be given if there is any sign of the wound being infected. Shock is treated by giving intravenous fluids through a drip inserted into a vein, usually in the arm.

For extensive second-degree burns, skin-grafting will be used early in the treatment to minimize scarring. Third-degree burns always require skin grafting if scarring is to be avoided.

Extensive burns may require repeated operations by a plastic surgeon.

Length of hospital stay can vary from a few days in some cases to many weeks in the case of severe and extensive burns. Extensive burns are usually treated at a burn center.

Burping

Another term for *belching*.

Burr hole

A hole made in the skull by a special drill with a rounded tip (burr). The hole permits access to the brain and the tissues surrounding it. The hole is made to relieve pressure on the brain, often resulting from the accumulation of blood between the inside of the skull and the brain after a head injury. The burr hole relieves the pressure, which can be fatal, by allowing the blood to drain. Burr holes also permit biopsy of the brain, injection of gas or drugs, drainage of abscesses or cysts, and placement of electrodes.

Bursa

A small, fluid-filled sac that acts as a cushion at a pressure point in the body—often near joints, where a tendon or muscle crosses either bone or other muscles. The most important bursae are around the knee, elbow, and shoulder.

A *bunion* is a bursa near the toe.

Bursitis

Inflammation of a *bursa*, causing it to swell and be painful.

Bursitis is usually the result of pressure, friction, or slight injury to the membrane surrounding the joint. Prepatellar bursitis ("housemaid's knee") is caused by prolonged kneeling on a hard surface, tibial tubercle bursitis ("clergyman's knee") from kneeling on a more upright surface, and olecranon bursitis ("student's elbow") from prolonged pressure of the elbow point against a desk or table. Another common form is subdeltoid (of the shoulder) bursitis, which, if left untreated, may result in "frozen shoulder."

The treatment is usually rest; often the bursitis will subside after a few days, with the fluid being reabsorbed into the bloodstream. Applying an ice-pack may help relieve pain.

Infection may be treated with antibiotics and drainage. The physician may apply a pressure bandage to stop the fluid from reforming. An injection of a *corticosteroid drug* may also be given.

In rare, recurrent cases, bursectomy (a minor operation to remove the bursa) may be performed. Using general anesthesia, a small incision is made in the skin over the bursa, and the lining of the bursal sac is completely removed to prevent it from regrowing.

Bursitis of the elbow
This condition produces a fluid-filled swelling around the point of the elbow.

Bypass operations

Procedures to bypass the blockage or narrowing of an artery or vein or any part of the digestive system.

TYPES
Arteries can become blocked or narrowed by *atheroma*. Those most often affected are the carotid arteries (in the neck), the coronary arteries (in the heart), and the iliofemoral vessels (leading to the legs). These blocks can be bypassed using sections of artery or vein (taken from the patient) or using synthetic tubing.

Surgeons have attempted to bypass blocked arteries in the brain by joining points above the blockage to an artery in the neck. Known as extracranial-intracranial bypass, it has had little success, and is now rarely used.

Veins are bypassed most often in patients with diseases of the liver that cause portal hypertension (increased pressure in the veins draining the intestinal tract) and bleeding esophageal varices (enlarged veins in the lower esophagus). These bypasses are called *shunts*.

Intestinal bypasses are most commonly employed in patients with cancer. If tumor growth is too extensive for surgical removal, symptoms may be relieved by joining the sections of gut at either side of the blockage. Bypass for other conditions has been largely abandoned. An obstructed bile duct may be diverted into the intestine lower down the digestive tract. Intestinal bypass operations for treatment of obesity have largely been replaced by operations to reduce the capacity of the stomach. (See also *Coronary artery bypass*.)

Byssinosis

An industrial disease of the lungs caused by allergy to an unknown agent in the dust produced during the processing of flax, cotton, hemp, or sisal. It produces a feeling of tightness in the chest and shortness of breath that may become chronic. In the US, preventive measures in the textile industry have lowered the incidence of the disease, but it is common in India and other developing countries.

At first, symptoms are most pronounced at the start of the working week, but gradually they become troublesome on every working day. In chronic byssinosis (the risk of which is increased by smoking), the sufferer is short of breath even when away from work. *Respiratory failure* may eventually develop when lung damage has become extensive.

Drugs used to treat asthma, such as *bronchodilators*, can relieve symptoms, but the answer to the problem is prevention. This is achieved by treatment of raw textiles before processing, reduction of dust levels, and the wearing of face masks.

In the US, people who suffer from byssinosis have a statutory right to government compensation.

Common bypass locations
The carotid and coronary arteries and the iliofemoral vessels are the usual locations for bypasses.

Carotid artery

Coronary artery

Iliofemoral artery

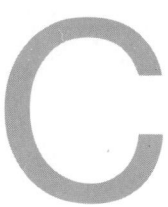

and kola nuts. Several popular drinks contain caffeine, notably coffee. In medicine, caffeine is sometimes combined with certain analgesics.

Cachexia
An appearance of profound illness and massive weight loss, usually due to either extreme starvation or a serious underlying disease such as cancer or tuberculosis.

Cadaver
A dead human body used as a source of transplant organs or preserved for anatomical study and dissection.

Cadmium poisoning
Poisoning by the fumes or dust of this tinlike metal, which is an industrial hazard. Cadmium varies in its effects according to the duration and severity of exposure. Exposure can lead to urinary tract *calculi* (stones), *renal failure* in severe cases, or inflammation in the lungs progressing to severe *emphysema*. In Japan, many cases of severe cadmium poisoning have occurred when people have eaten rice contaminated with industrial effluent. Cadmium poisoning can also be caused by eating vegetables grown in cadmium-rich soil, and by foods stored in cadmium-lined containers.

It is known that cadmium accumulates in the body (especially in the kidneys) throughout life. Cadmium has been implicated in causing high blood pressure, but this has not been proved in man. Minute amounts of cadmium may be essential for health.

Café au lait spots
Pale, coffee-colored patches, usually oval, and up to 3 inches across, that may develop anywhere on the skin. They usually have no significance, but the presence of several café au lait spots is sometimes a sign of *neurofibromatosis*, a hereditary disorder of the sheaths that surround nerve fibers. In such cases there are commonly (in addition to the café au lait spots) multiple small nodules in and on the skin.

Caffeine
A stimulant that occurs naturally in coffee beans, tea leaves, cocoa beans,

CAFFEINE LEVELS (mg per cup)	
Tea, weak	50
Tea, strong	80
Coffee, weak	80
Coffee, strong	200
Cocoa	10-17
Cola	43-75

The strength and method of preparation determine exact amounts of caffeine present (in mg per cup).

USES AND ABUSES
Few people consume so much caffeine that they experience unpleasant side effects, but some people are particularly sensitive and feel side effects from relatively small amounts.

People who regularly consume large amounts of caffeine (more than five cups of coffee a day) often find their system has adapted to this amount of caffeine so that their *tolerance* to the substance increases; the result is that they must increase their intake to continue any stimulant effect. Furthermore, if such people go without caffeine for some time—as little as a few hours in some cases—they may suffer withdrawal symptoms, such as tiredness, headaches, and

EFFECTS OF CAFFEINE ON THE BODY
Within a few minutes of consuming caffeine-containing drinks or tablets, there is a stimulant effect on all organs and tissues. Caffeine acts directly on individual cells by affecting the chemical reactions within them; it acts indirectly by increasing the release, from the adrenal glands into the circulation, of *epinephrine* (adrenaline) and norepinephrine (noradrenaline), hormones that stimulate cell activity.

Brain
Small amounts of caffeine stimulate the brain cells, helping to reduce drowsiness and fatigue. Concentration is improved and reactions are speeded up. Large amounts cause overstimulation, anxiety, irritability, and restlessness. This is why consuming caffeine before going to bed can cause insomnia and a hangover in the morning, with excessive fatigue and drowsiness on waking.

Skeletal muscles
Stimulation by caffeine may improve their performance during exercise, but excessive stimulation of the skeletal muscles can cause twitching.

Heart
With small amounts of caffeine, the heart muscle is stimulated, augmenting its pumping action. This causes the blood to circulate faster and blood pressure to increase for a short time. Too much caffeine results in overstimulation of the heart muscle and can result in palpitations.

Stomach
While small amounts of caffeine can actually help digestion by increasing production of stomach acid, too much can cause abdominal pain and nausea.

Kidneys
Caffeine action on the kidneys increases the production of urine.

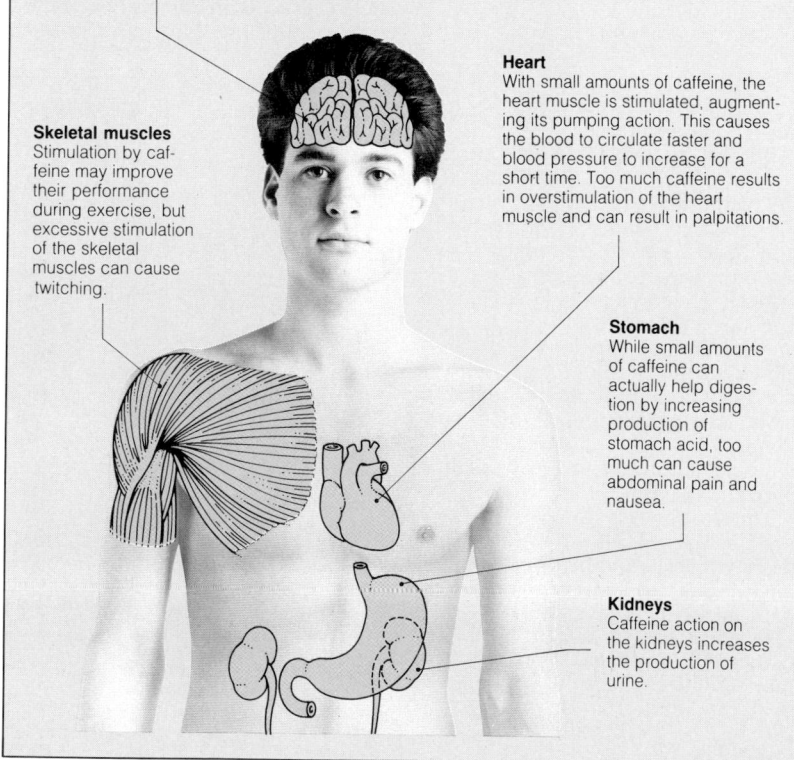

irritability due to their physical and psychological dependence on the drug (see *Drug dependence*).

Because of increasing concern about the undesirable effects of caffeine, there has been a general decrease in its consumption in recent years. Moreover, because it can improve short-term athletic performance, caffeine has been included in the list of drugs banned in sports competitions (see *Sports, drugs and*).

The medical use of caffeine has also recently been reevaluated, in particular its inclusion in some combination analgesics. Caffeine was originally included in such preparations because it was thought to enhance their painkilling action, but studies indicate that it may not have this effect. Caffeine is combined with *ergotamine* in several drugs for the early preventive treatment of migraine.

Calamine

A pink substance consisting of zinc oxide and ferric oxide that is applied to the skin in the form of ointments, lotions, or dusting powders. It has a protective, cooling, and drying effect, and is used to relieve skin irritation and itching arising from *dermatitis, eczema, poison ivy, insect bites,* and *sunburn*. It is sometimes combined with topical local anesthetics, such as benzocaine (see *Anesthesia, local*), and with *corticosteroid drugs* or *antihistamine drugs*, which reduce any accompanying inflammation. Bandages impregnated with calamine are sometimes used to protect leg ulcers.

Calcaneus

The heel bone, which can be fractured as a result of falling from a height onto the heels. Minor fractures of this bone usually do not cause problems and are treated by putting the foot and leg in a cast. A more serious fracture, with compression of the bone, may cause permanent damage to the joints in the foot that are involved in turning the foot in and out. This usually leads to pain and stiffness in the foot that is aggravated by walking.

The *Achilles tendon* is fixed to the back of the heel bone and controls the up and down movement of the foot. The point at which the tendon joins the bone may be strained by excessive or prolonged stress from the pull of the tendon—for example, in some *running injuries*. In children this area of bone is still growing and occasionally becomes inflamed and painful (see *Osteochondrosis*).

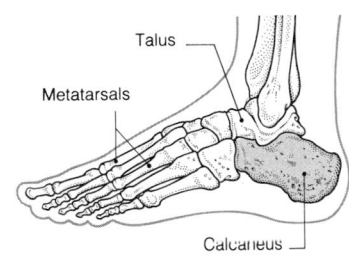

LOCATION OF THE CALCANEUS
This is the largest tarsal bone, projecting backward beyond the leg bones.

Talus

Metatarsals

Calcaneus

Tendons in the sole of the foot (see *Aponeurosis*) are fixed under the heel bone; the associated muscles are important in supporting the arches of the foot. Inflammation around these tendons (as in plantar *fasciitis*) causes pain and tenderness under the heel when standing or walking. A calcaneal spur (a bony protrusion from this part of the calcaneus) is sometimes seen on X rays of the foot in plantar fasciitis, but the spurs are also found on X rays of healthy feet.

Calciferol

An alternative name for vitamin D_2 (see *Vitamin D*); it is also known by the name ergocalciferol.

Calcification

The deposition of calcium salts in body tissues. Calcification is normal in bone and teeth formation and is necessary for the healing of fractures. Calcification can occur in an injured muscle and is common in arteries affected by *atherosclerosis*. It may also occur if the blood calcium level is raised as a result of a disorder of the parathyroid gland.

Calcification, dental

The deposition of calcium crystals in developing teeth. Calcium and phosphorous salts are brought to the teeth, where the crystals make up 96 percent of tooth enamel and 70 percent of dentin. Calcification of primary teeth begins in the fetus between three and six months; calcification of permanent teeth (other than wisdom teeth) begins between birth and 4 years.

Abnormal calcification occurs in amelogenesis imperfecta, an inherited disorder of the enamel (see *Hypoplasia, enamel*). The affected teeth have a thin, grooved covering due to incomplete

calcification. Another cause of abnormal calcification is the ingestion of high levels of fluoride (see *Fluorosis*).

Calcinosis

A condition in which there is abnormal deposition of calcium salts in various tissues (such as the skin) of the body, and in connective tissues including cartilage and tendons. Calcinosis tends to be associated with an underlying disorder of the connective tissue, such as *scleroderma* or *dermatomyositis*. The term "calcinosis" is usually combined with another word to signify which part of the body is affected—for example, calcinosis cutis affects the skin (and is apparent as nodules in the skin). (See also *Calcification; Calcium*.)

Calcitonin

A hormone produced by the thyroid gland. It controls the level of calcium in the blood by slowing the rate at which calcium is lost from bones.

WHY IT IS USED

A synthetic form of calcitonin is used to treat *Paget's disease*, in which the bones grow abnormally and become deformed, causing pain and an increased risk of fracture. Given by injection, calcitonin halts abnormal bone formation in about a week and can relieve pain within a few months.

Calcitonin is also used to treat *hypercalcemia* (abnormally high levels of calcium in the blood) caused by overactivity of the parathyroid glands or by cancer of the bone. Calcitonin helps relieve the nausea and vomiting that results from hypercalcemia by quickly reducing the level of calcium in the blood. It may be prescribed with a *corticosteroid drug* that decreases the calcium level in the blood.

POSSIBLE ADVERSE EFFECTS

Calcitonin does not generally cause any troublesome adverse effects. Gastrointestinal reactions, such as nausea, vomiting, and diarrhea, usually diminish with continued use.

Calcium

 The most abundant mineral in the body— about 2 to 2.5 pounds (0.9 to 1.1 kg) in an average-

C

sized person—with several important functions. Calcium is essential for the functioning of cells, for muscle contraction, for the transmission of nerve impulses from nerve endings to muscle fibers, and for blood clotting. In the form of calcium phosphate it makes up the hard basic constituent of teeth and bones.

The main dietary sources of calcium are milk and dairy products, eggs, fish, green vegetables, and fruit.

CONTROL OF CALCIUM LEVELS

Vitamin D and certain hormones help control the overall amount of calcium in the body by regulating the amount of calcium absorbed from food, and the amount removed from the body by the kidneys (which filter excess calcium from the blood and excrete it in the urine).

Control of calcium levels is achieved by the actions of two hormones: parathyroid hormone (produced by the parathyroid glands) and calcitonin (produced by the thyroid gland). When the level of calcium in the blood is too low, the parathyroid glands release more parathyroid hormone, which raises the blood calcium level by helping to release calcium from the enormous reservoir of the mineral in the bones. When the blood calcium level is too high, the thyroid gland releases more calcitonin, which counteracts the effects of parathyroid hormone and lowers the calcium level.

DISORDERS OF CALCIUM METABOLISM

Some people have too little calcium in the blood, a condition known as hypocalcemia. The most common cause is vitamin D deficiency, due to a poor diet or, occasionally, lack of sunshine. Rarer causes include chronic kidney failure (which leads to a poor absorption of calcium from the diet), *hypoparathyroidism* (in which insufficient parathyroid hormone is produced), and unintentional removal of the parathyroid glands during thyroid surgery.

In mild cases hypocalcemia is symptomless. In severe cases it causes *tetany* (cramplike spasms in the hands, feet, and face) due to the effect of low blood calcium on muscle activity. Hypocalcemia may also lead to softening of the bones. In children this softening takes the form of *rickets*; in adults it takes the form of *osteomalacia*.

Too much calcium in the blood (hypercalcemia) is rarer. It is most commonly due to cancer (or the treatment of certain cancers) that has spread to the bones and caused excessive release of calcium into the blood.

Other causes include *hyperparathyroidism* (in which too much parathyroid hormone is produced), excessive vitamin D in the diet (as may occur by taking huge doses of vitamins), and certain inflammatory disorders (such as *sarcoidosis*). Hypercalcemia can result in depression and kidney stones. (See also *Calcium channel blockers; Mineral supplements*.)

Calcium channel blockers

COMMON DRUGS

Diltiazem Nifedipine Verapamil

A relatively new class of drug used in the treatment of *angina pectoris* (chest pain due to an inadequate blood supply to heart muscle), *hypertension* (high blood pressure), and certain types of cardiac *arrhythmia* (irregular heart beat).

HOW THEY WORK

In the treatment of angina pectoris and high blood pressure, calcium channel blockers work by interfering with muscle contraction. They prevent the movement of calcium across the membrane that lines muscle cells, which is an essential part of the mechanism of muscle contraction. As a result of this interference, the walls of the muscles relax and dilate. This action decreases the work of the heart's blood pumping, reduces the pressure of blood flow through the body, and improves the circulation of blood through heart muscle.

Calcium channel blockers also slow the passage of nerve impulses through heart muscle, which helps correct certain types of arrhythmia.

POSSIBLE ADVERSE EFFECTS

Adverse effects of calcium channel blockers are mainly related to their action of increasing blood flow through tissues. These effects include headaches, facial flushing, and dizziness (usually on standing). Such effects, however, generally disappear with continued treatment.

Calculus

A deposit on the teeth (see *Calculus, dental*) or a small, hard, crystalline mass formed from substances that have precipitated gradually from a fluid, such as bile or urine. The usual sites for such calculi are the gallbladder and bile ducts (see *Gallstones*), and the kidneys, ureters, or urinary bladder (see *Calculus, urinary tract*). Stones may be symptomless or may cause severe pain and require removal, dissolving, or shattering.

Calculus, dental

A hard, crustlike deposit found on the crowns and roots of teeth. Also known as tartar, calculus is formed when mineral salts from saliva are deposited in existing *plaque*. These minerals, mainly calcium and phosphorus, make up about 70 percent of the calculus; the rest is organic material and bacteria. Calculus commonly occurs on the inside surfaces of the lower incisors and on the outer surfaces of the upper molars—areas close to the duct openings of the salivary glands.

TYPES

Supragingival calculus, which forms above the gum margin on the crowns of teeth, is white or yellowish unless stained. Subgingival calculus, which forms below the gum margin, is more evenly distributed around all the teeth. Brown or black, possibly because of breakdown products of blood from the inflamed gums, it is visible if the gum is gently parted from the tooth and may show through the gum as a dark area. Both types of calculus are hard, and therefore difficult to remove; the subgingival variety may be more difficult to remove because of its location and degree of calcification.

EFFECTS AND TREATMENT

Being porous, calculus is impossible to keep clean and continually becomes covered by plaque. The irritant effect of toxins in plaque and calculus causes progressive inflammation and destruction of the gums and supporting structures of the teeth (see *Periodontitis*). Any calculus should be completely removed on a regular basis by professional *scaling*. Careful *oral hygiene*, professional cleaning, and elimination of stagnation areas, such as poorly finished fillings, should diminish or slow its recurrence.

Calculus, urinary tract

A stone that has formed or is present in the kidneys, ureters, or bladder, caused by precipitation from a solution of substances in urine.

INCIDENCE

Calculi differ in their incidence according to their site of origin. Kidney and ureteral stones are more common than bladder stones in developed countries and are three times more common in men than in women. In the US each year, about 100 persons per 100,000 are hospitalized with a ureteral calculus. Stones occur with different frequency in different sections of the country and the world.

Stones tend to be a recurrent problem; about 60 percent of patients treated for a stone develop another within seven years. The incidence is highest in the summer months, perhaps because we sweat more and pass a more concentrated urine.

COMPOSITION AND CAUSES

KIDNEY AND URETERAL STONES There are various types of kidney and ureteral stones; their composition is sometimes related to a specific cause. In the majority of cases, there is no identifiable underlying cause, although mild chronic dehydration (for example, due to inadequate water consumption in a hot climate) may play a part.

About 70 percent of kidney and ureteral stones consist mainly of calcium oxalate and/or phosphate. Oxalate is an end product of body *metabolism* and is present naturally in the urine. The salt it forms with calcium has a low solubility (dissolves poorly). An abnormally high level of oxalate in the urine encourages stone formation and may be related to a diet containing food or drinks with a high content of oxalic acid—for example, rhubarb, spinach, leafy vegetables, and coffee. Stones containing calcium are sometimes the first evidence of a disturbance of metabolism associated with *hyperparathyroidism*.

About 20 percent of calculi are termed infective stones and are linked with chronic infections of the urinary tract. These calculi consist of a combination of calcium, magnesium, and ammonium phosphate and are associated with a high ammonium content and alkalinity of the urine produced by the action of bacteria on urea (a substance in urine). In the kidney, an infective stone may fill the entire network of urine-collecting ducts and the top part of the ureter, forming a large, oddly shaped calculus.

Stones consisting mainly of uric acid comprise about 5 percent of the total and may occur in people with *gout*, people with some cancers, and people with chronic *dehydration*.

Other, uncommon types of stone occasionally occur. Those formed from the amino acid cysteine are most notable and affect people with a particular inherited metabolic disorder.

BLADDER STONES In poorer countries, bladder stones usually develop as a result of a diet low in phosphate and protein. In developed countries, such as the US, they result from obstruction to the flow of urine from the bladder and/or a long-standing urinary tract infection; they almost exclusively

URINARY TRACT CALCULI

Symptoms vary according to the site of the stone. Small stones in the kidney often cause no symptoms until they start to pass down the ureter, resulting in *renal colic*, a sudden pain in the flank that moves toward the groin. The pain is acute, sharp, and intermittent and may cause nausea and vomiting. There may also be hematuria (blood in the urine). Bladder stones, which affect men far more often than women, can cause difficulty in passing urine, a poor flow rate, and dribbling. Some stones may be associated with recurrent episodes of *urinary tract infection*. Any obstruction to urine flow may result in rapid kidney damage and acute severe infection termed *pyelonephritis*.

Ureter Kidney

Bladder

Bladder stones
The stones at top all came from a patient with an enlarged prostate gland obstructing urine flow. At bottom is a cross section through a much larger stone.

Staghorn calculus
Stones of this type form within and fill the pelvis of the kidney (at the top of the ureter). They are linked with urinary tract infection.

affect men. The composition of bladder stones varies according to the acidity or alkalinity of the urine, but in the US the most common type consists of calcium oxalate.

DIAGNOSIS

Investigation of a suspected calculus usually starts with examination of the urine, which may reveal red blood cells and the presence of crystals. The degree of acidity or alkalinity of the urine may reflect the type of stone involved. About 90 percent of urinary tract calculi are visible on X rays, which will show the site of the stone; this can be confirmed by intravenous or retrograde *pyelography*. These techniques also indicate any obstruction of the urinary tract above the stone, which can be monitored by *ultrasound scanning*. If a metabolic disorder is a suspected cause of the stone, chemical analysis of the blood and urine may be performed to look for high levels of calcium, phosphate, or urate.

TREATMENT

Renal colic is treated with bed rest, pain relief using a narcotic analgesic (painkiller), and adequate fluid intake to encourage the passage of the stone through the ureter, bladder, and urethra. The majority of stones less than 0.2 inch (5 mm) in diameter are passed in the urine at home with relatively few problems.

With larger stones, or if an infection or obstruction to urinary flow is present, surgical treatment may be needed to prevent damage to the kidney. The traditional method of removing stones from the ureter and from the junction between the ureter and kidney is by surgery using general anesthesia. Stones in the bladder and lower ureter can be crushed and removed by *cystoscopy* (passage of a viewing tube and crushing device up the urethra into the bladder) or by ureterorenoscopy (passage of the same type of tube into the ureter).

In recent years new methods for removing kidney and ureteral stones have evolved and dramatically changed the way in which they are treated. Ultrasonic *lithotripsy* involves the use of an ultrasonic probe through a telescopic tube to help break up stones that are too large to be removed whole. More advanced is the extracorporeal shock-wave lithotriptor, which is used to disintegrate kidney stones by focusing a shock wave on the stone from outside the body.

If a stone is thought to have developed because of some metabolic disorder, the patient may be prescribed a diet, and possibly drugs, to lower the content in the urine of the substance from which the stone is formed; it may also be necessary for the patient to maintain a high fluid intake. These methods may act to dissolve an existing stone and may help prevent recurrences.

Stones associated with hyperparathyroidism are treated by methods appropriate to their location; the parathyroid gland tumor that is usually responsible for the condition is removed.

Calendar method

A method of *contraception*, also called the rhythm method, that entails abstaining from sexual intercourse around the time of ovulation, which is predicted on the basis of the length of previous menstrual cycles.

The calendar method is unreliable because a woman's cycle may vary, and thus the time of ovulation can be estimated only approximately. There are now more scientific and effective contraceptive methods of this type. (See *Contraception, periodic abstinence*.)

LOCATION OF CALF MUSCLES
The gastrocnemius and soleus join to form the Achilles tendon.

Gastrocnemius muscle

Soleus muscle

Achilles tendon

Calcaneus

Calf muscles

Muscles extending from the back of the knee to the heel. The gastrocnemius muscle starts behind the knee and forms the bulky part of the calf. Under it is the soleus muscle, which starts lower down from the back of the *tibia* (shin). These muscles join to form the *Achilles tendon*, which connects them to the heel.

Contraction of the calf muscles pulls the heel up to produce a springing movement through the toes. This movement is important in walking, running, jumping, and hopping.

Pain can occur because of *cramp*, *sciatica* (inflammation of one of the long nerves in the leg), or, more rarely, *claudication* (cramplike leg pain) or deep vein *thrombosis*.

Caliper splint

An orthopedic device used to exert control on a deformed leg or to support a leg weakened by a muscular disorder, making it possible for the person to stand and walk. A caliper splint consists of one or two vertical metal rods attached to leather or metal rings worn around the limb. A caliper splint extending only below the knee is sufficient to control the position of the ankle. Longer splints may be jointed to allow knee movement.

Callosity

See *Callus, skin*.

Callus, bony

A diffuse growth of new soft bone that forms around a *fracture* as it heals. The callus is eventually replaced by stronger bone with a more organized structure (see *Bone*).

A callus can be seen on an X ray and provides evidence that healing has started. A callus can sometimes be felt around a fracture site as a lumpy deformity. As healing continues, the original shape of the bone is restored.

Callus, skin

An area of thickened skin, caused by regular or prolonged pressure or friction. Manual laborers develop calluses on the palms of their hands, joggers on the soles of their feet, and guitarists on the tips of their fingers.

Calluses may also develop if body weight is borne unevenly—for example, if there is a *contracture* (persistent deformity) affecting one foot. A *corn* is a callus on a toe.

TREATMENT
If a callus on the foot becomes troublesome or painful, a podiatrist should be consulted. He or she can pare away the thickened skin in layers with a scalpel. Calluses caused by foot deformities almost always recur unless the underlying problem is corrected—either surgically or by using a molded insole in the shoe.

Caloric test

A method of discovering whether a person with *vertigo* (dizziness) and hearing loss has a diseased labyrinth (part of the inner ear). If so, *nystagmus* (reflex flickering of the eyes) stops sooner than normal or is absent.

Checking for nystagmus
The outer-ear canal is flooded with water at varying temperatures, which induces convection currents within the lateral or horizontal semicircular canals. This stimulates them with resulting nystagmus, which is noted and its duration measured.

Calorie

A measure of energy. Strictly, it is the amount of energy needed to raise the temperature of 1 g of water by 1°C. In medicine and dietetics, the energy content of foods and the energy used to perform various activities is measured in units called kilocalories, which are equal to 1,000 calories. These two units are often confused because both are referred to as calories. However, the medical unit is abbreviated as Cal (with a capital "C") or kc, whereas the ordinary, "small" calorie is abbreviated as cal (with a small "c").

When the daily calorie intake is the same as the amount of energy expended, a person's weight remains constant. If intake exceeds expenditure, weight is gained; if expenditure exceeds intake, weight is lost. In general, fatty foods contain the most calories per unit weight while carbohydrate and protein have equal calories per unit weight, 56 percent less than fat. (See also *Calorimetry; Diet and disease*.)

Calorie requirements

See *Energy requirements*.

Calorimetry

A method of discovering the *calorie* (energy) value of foodstuffs by burning them in a container.

Direct calorimetry is the usual method of calculating the calorie value of small amounts of a particular foodstuff. This calorie value may then be converted to the number of calories in a typical serving. After being weighed and placed in a special sealed container, called a bomb calorimeter, the food is ignited; the calorimeter is then immersed in a known volume of water. The rise in the temperature of the water when the foodstuff is completely burned up gives the calorie value.

Cancer

Any of a group of diseases in which symptoms are due to the unrestrained growth of cells in one of the body organs or tissues. Most commonly, malignant tumors develop in major organs, such as the lungs, breasts, intestines, skin, stomach, or pancreas, but they may also develop in the nasal sinuses, the testes or ovaries, or the lips or tongue. Cancers may also develop in the blood cell-forming tissues of the bone marrow (the *leukemias*) and in the lymphatic system, muscles, or bones. Cancer is the second most common cause of death in the US, accounting for about one fifth of the total (the most common is heart disease).

Cancers are not the only type of abnormal growth, or *neoplasm*, that occur in the body. However, a cancer differs from a *benign* tumor, such as a *wart* or a *lipoma*, in two important ways. As it grows, it spreads and infiltrates the tissues around it and may block passageways, destroy nerves, and erode bone. Cells from the cancer may spread via the blood vessels and lymphatic channels to other parts of the body, where these *metastases* form new, satellite tumors that grow independently.

INCIDENCE

Cancer is a process that has affected humans since prehistoric times and is also common in domestic and farm animals, birds, and fish. Apart from childhood cancers, which may be associated with events during pregnancy, such as exposure to radiation, most cancers are a feature of aging.

CAUSES

The growth of a cancer begins when the *oncogenes* (genes controlling cell growth and multiplication) in a cell or cells are transformed by agents known as *carcinogens*.

Once a cell is transformed into a tumor-forming type (malignant transformation), the change in its oncogenes is passed on to all offspring cells. A small group of abnormal cells is thus established, and they divide more rapidly than the normal surrounding cells. Usually the abnormal cells show a lack of *differentiation*—that

Chemical and environmental factors

Smoking

Familial factor

Normal cells

Viral factor

Alcohol and dietary factors

Cancer cells

Susceptibility to cancer
A person's susceptibility to cancer is determined by his or her genetic makeup, which is inherited. The triggers that may provoke cancerous changes in susceptible individuals range from sunlight and viruses to alcohol, chemi-cals in environmental pollutants, tar in tobacco smoke, and dietary factors such as fat. Two, three, or more such triggers may interact to cause cancers in the skin or internal organs.

is, they no longer perform the specialized task of the cells of their host tissue—and may escape the normal control of hormones and nerves. Thus, they are in effect parasites, contributing nothing to their host tissue but continuing to consume nutrients.

Years may pass before the growth of cells becomes large enough to cause symptoms, although the rate of growth varies according to the tissue of origin. Current estimates suggest that some cancers of the lung and breast have been present for more than five years before they cause symptoms. During this "occult" phase, metastases may be seeded in the liver, lungs, bones, or brain, and, in these circumstances, surgical cure is impossible because the cancer has already spread far beyond the primary site of origin.

CANCER-CAUSING AGENTS
The table gives a rough estimate of the contribution of various agents or behaviors to the causation of cancers. Smoking is particularly implicated in lung and bladder cancers, alcohol in cancers of the tongue, pharynx, and esophagus. Sexual and reproductive behavior affects the risk of cervical cancer (the more sexual partners a women has, the higher the risk) and of breast cancer (having children while relatively young protects against this cancer). Note the importance of dietary factors.

CANCER-CAUSING AGENTS

Agents	% of all cancers
Natural constituents of food (estimate)	35
Tobacco	30
Sexual and reproductive history	7
Occupational hazards	4
Alcohol	3
Food additives	1
Unknown	20

C

INCIDENCE OF CANCER

The likelihood of cancer developing varies with age. A 20 year old has a very low likelihood of it developing by the age of 30, but the risk roughly doubles between 30 and 40, and doubles again for each decade thereafter. Whatever the cause of death in someone aged 90, careful examination of the internal organs will often reveal a small cancer that may not have caused any symptoms. Localized cancer of the prostate is an almost universal finding in elderly men. Thus, while cancer seems to be much more common than in the past, this is mostly due to the increasing numbers of old people in the population.

CANCER WARNING SIGNS

Cancer may cause a variety of minor symptoms. Any that persist for several days should be checked by a physician. The earlier a cancer is diagnosed, the better the chance of there being a cure.

Rapid weight loss without apparent cause

A scab, sore, or ulcer that fails to heal within three weeks

A blemish or mole that enlarges, bleeds, or itches

Severe recurrent headaches

Difficulty swallowing

Persistent hoarseness

Coughing up bloody sputum (phlegm)

Persistent abdominal pain

Change in shape or size of testes

Blood in urine, with no pain on urination

Change in bowel habits

Lump or change in breast shape

Bleeding or discharge from nipple

Vaginal bleeding or spotting between periods or after menopause

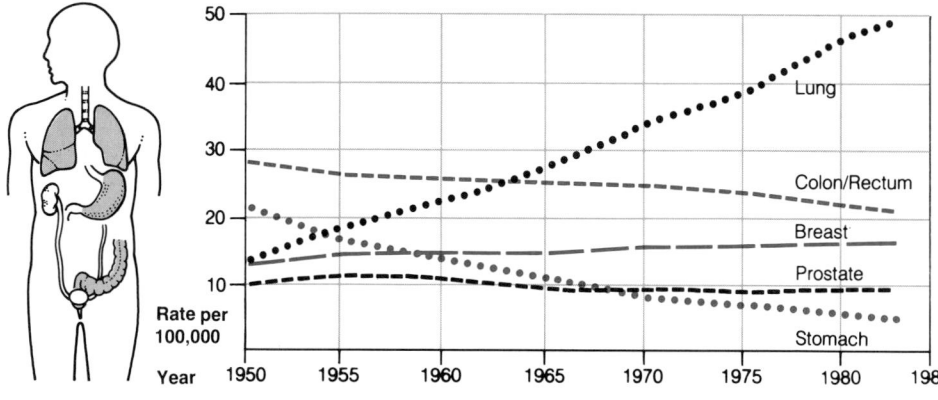

Trends in incidence of different types
In the past 30 years there has been little change in the incidence of cancers of the intestines, breast, and prostate. But stomach cancer has become less frequent because of improved diet, and lung cancer has become more common because of the dramatic increase in smoking.

WORLD INCIDENCE RATES FOR COMMON CANCERS

Site of origin of cancer	% affected in high-incidence area by age 75	Low incidence area
Skin	20 Queensland, Australia	Bombay, India
Esophagus	20 Northeast section of Iran	Nigeria
Lung and bronchus	11 England	Nigeria
Stomach	11 Japan	Uganda
Cervix	10 Colombia	Jewish Israel
Prostate	9 US (blacks only)	Japan
Liver	8 Mozambique	England
Breast	7 British Columbia, Canada	Non-Jewish Israel
Colon	3 Connecticut	Nigeria
Uterus	3 California	Japan
Mouth	2 Bombay, India	Denmark
Rectum	2 Denmark	Nigeria
Bladder	2 Connecticut	Japan
Ovary	2 Denmark	Japan
Nasopharynx	2 Chinese Singapore	England
Pancreas	2 Maori New Zealand	Bombay, India
Larynx	2 São Paulo, Brazil	Japan
Pharynx	2 Bombay, India	Denmark
Penis	1 Parts of Uganda	Jewish Israel

Incidence of breast cancer
Breast cancer most commonly affects women over the age of 30 and the incidence rises rapidly with age. At age 30, the rate is 20 per 100,000; at age 80, the rate is 260 per 100,000.

C

SYMPTOMS

The range of symptoms that may be produced by cancers is vast, depending on the site of the growth, the tissue of origin, and the extent of the growth. Symptoms may be a direct feature of the growth (e.g., lumps or skin changes) or derived from obstruction or bleeding into passageways, such as the lung airways, gastrointestinal tract, or urinary tract, or from disruption of the function of a vital organ. Tumors pressing on or disturbing nerve tracts can cause nervous system disorders and pain. Some tumors lead to the overproduction of hormones, with complications and effects far distant from the site of the growth. Unexplained weight loss is a feature of many types of cancer.

Some important warning signals that always warrant investigation by a physician are shown in the accompanying table.

DIAGNOSIS

Both the means of diagnosing cancer at an early stage (when the chances of cure are highest) and the range of treatments available have improved dramatically in the past decade.

Screening tests (for early breast cancer, cancer of the cervix, and intestinal cancer) have cut mortality from these tumors. For most tumors, however, diagnosis generally occurs after the appearance of symptoms, is based on the physician's examination of the patient, and is confirmed by microscopic examination of tissue cells obtained by *biopsy*; cancer cells look different from the normal cells of the host tissue. New scanning and imaging techniques give more information while causing less discomfort to the patient.

There are four main types of tests: cytology tests, imaging techniques, chemical tests, and direct inspection.

OUTLOOK

Almost half of all cancers are today cured completely, and cure and survival rates for various years after diagnosis continue to improve. For disease of certain organ systems, the diagnosis of a cancer may actually provide a better outlook than some of the alternative diagnoses. Cure and survival rates and the chances of recurrence do, however, vary markedly according to the organ or tissue affected.

For more information on cancers of individual organs—their incidence, causes, symptoms, treatment, and outlook—refer to the organ in question (e.g., *Breast cancer; Lung cancer; Stomach cancer*).

TREATMENT OF CANCER

The treatment of many cancers is still primarily surgical; excision of an early tumor will often give a complete cure. Because there may be small, undetectable metastases at the time of operation, surgery is commonly combined with *radiation therapy* and *anticancer drugs*. The aim of these treatments is to suppress, or arrest, the rate of cell division in any tumor cells left after surgery. Anticancer drugs often have unpleasant side effects because it is sometimes difficult to target specific drugs effectively, and normal cells and tissues may be disrupted along with the tumor cells.

Before radiation therapy
The photograph shows a skin cancer in front of the ear before treatment.

After radiation therapy
This was the appearance a few weeks later, after a course of radiation therapy.

TYPES OF CANCER TEST

Cytology tests	These tests reveal the shedding of abnormal cells. One example is the *cervical smear test* (Pap smear), an investigation in which cells are scraped from the cervix and examined microscopically to	detect potential or early cancer of the cervix. Another example is the urine cytology test, periodically carried out on those working in manufacturing industries where bladder cancer is a known risk.
Imaging techniques	These can sometimes reveal early cancerous changes in tissue. A notable example is the special low-dose X-ray technique used in *mammography* to detect early cancer of the breast. Research	with *ultrasound scanning*, which produces images of internal organs, suggests that it may provide a means of screening for cancer of the ovary.
Chemical tests	These tests can reveal the presence of substances indicative of cancer—for example, microscopic amounts of blood in	the feces and high levels of the enzyme acid phosphatase in the blood.
Direct inspection	Inspection of the interior of organs subject to cancer is usually carried out with an *endoscope* (a tube with a viewing lens), which is passed into the organ to be examined. Examples of this technique are	*colonoscopy, gastroscopy, cystoscopy,* and *laparoscopy.* These procedures are usually carried out only when clinical suspicion has been aroused.

Cancerphobia

An intense fear of developing cancer, out of proportion to the actual risk, so that the sufferer's behavior and lifestyle are significantly altered. Instead of paying sensible attention to diet and prevention (such as giving up smoking), the cancerphobe adopts extreme behavior (prolonged washing rituals, avoidance of social contact, bizarre eating habits) typical of *obsessive-compulsive behavior*. If the person experiences any symptoms (e.g., skin problems, constipation, or difficulty swallowing), he or she is convinced that they are signs of cancer. *Psychotherapy* may be of benefit. (See also *Phobia*.)

Cancer screening

Tests carried out on groups of people to detect cancer at an early stage. To warrant their use, screening tests must have a high rate of accuracy, must be safe, and must cause minimal discomfort. There must also be an effective treatment available. Screening tests are most effectively carried out among persons particularly susceptible to cancer.

In theory, regular annual checkups, including radiological and laboratory tests, might be expected to detect cancers at an early, treatable stage. In practice, several of the more common cancers—notably lung and stomach cancers—are rarely detected by screening tests before they cause symptoms. Nevertheless, in the past decade, screening tests have been developed for cancers of the cervix, breast, ovary, gastrointestinal tract, bladder, and prostate, and they are saving lives (see previous page).

Cancrum oris

A condition, also called *noma*, in which ulcers and tissue destruction occur within and around the mouth. It commonly affects malnourished children in poor tropical countries.

Candidiasis

Infection by the fungus CANDIDA ALBICANS, often within the vagina or, less commonly, on other areas of mucous membrane, such as inside the mouth or on moist skin. The infection is also known as thrush or moniliasis.

CAUSES AND INCIDENCE

The fungus that causes candidiasis grows in ecologic equilibrium in the vagina and mouth. Its growth is kept under control by the bacteria usually present in these organs. If a course of antibiotics destroys too many of the bacteria, or if the body's resistance to infection is lowered, as it is in *AIDS* and in patients being treated with *immunosuppressant drugs*, the fungus may multiply and overgrow. Certain disorders, notably *diabetes mellitus* and the hormonal changes that occur in pregnancy or when taking birth-control pills, may also encourage growth of the fungus.

Candidal infection of the penis is more common among uncircumcised than circumcised men, and may result from sexual intercourse with an infected partner. The condition can spread from the genitals or mouth to other moist areas of the body, such as the skin folds in the groin or under the breasts in women. In infants, candidiasis sometimes occurs in conjunction with *diaper rash*.

SYMPTOMS

Vaginal candidiasis may cause a thick, white, "cottage cheese" discharge from the vagina and/or itching and irritation in the area, which may cause discomfort when passing urine. Some women have no symptoms.

Infection of the penis usually results in *balanitis* (inflammation of the head of the penis). If the fungus spreads within the mouth, it produces sore, creamy-yellow, raised patches. Candidiasis in skin folds and as part of diaper rash takes the form of an itchy red rash with flaky white patches.

DIAGNOSIS AND TREATMENT

Candidiasis is diagnosed by examination of a sample of the white discharge or patches. If the cause proves to be CANDIDA ALBICANS, the physician will prescribe an *antifungal drug*, such as nystatin, clotrimazole, miconazole, or econazole nitrate. The drugs are usually prescribed in the form of a vaginal suppository or a cream for skin application.

OUTLOOK AND PREVENTION

Antifungal drugs usually clear up the trouble, but the infection may recur—sometimes as a result of reinfection by a sexual partner. Hence, treatment of both partners is preferable. People with a tendency to skin candidiasis should keep the skin as dry as possible, and women who take birth-control pills and suffer from candidiasis should consider changing to another method of birth control.

Canine tooth

See *Teeth*.

Canker sore

A small, painful ulcer that heals without help, occurring alone or in a group on the inside of the cheek or lip or underneath the tongue.

INCIDENCE

Minor canker sores affect about 20 percent of the population at any given time. They are most common between the ages of 10 and 40 and affect women more than men. The most severely affected people have continuously recurring ulcers; others have just one or two ulcers per year.

SYMPTOMS

Each ulcer is usually small and oval with a gray center and a surrounding red, inflamed halo. The ulcer usually lasts for one to two weeks.

CAUSES

The ulcer may be a hypersensitive reaction to hemolytic streptococcus bacteria. These organisms have been isolated repeatedly from canker sores. Other factors often associated with the occurrence of canker sores are trauma (such as an injection or a toothbrush abrasion), acute stress, and allergies (such as allergic *rhinitis*). In women, ulcers are most common during the premenstrual period. Ulcers may also be more likely to occur if other members of the family suffer from recurrent ulceration.

TREATMENT

The ulcers will heal by themselves if left alone. Topical painkillers may ease the pain and healing may be hastened by a corticosteroid ointment or a tetracycline mouthwash. The ulcer may also be covered with a waterproof ointment to protect it.

Cannabis

Any of the numerous psychoactive preparations derived from the hemp plant CANNABIS SATIVA (such as hashish and *marijuana*).

Cannula

A plastic or metal tube with a smooth, unsharpened tip for inserting into a blood vessel, lymphatic vessel, or body cavity to introduce or withdraw fluids. The physician first punctures the site with a long, thin needle, slides the cannula over it, and then withdraws the needle. Alternatively, he or she may insert a trocar (sharp-pointed rod) inside the cannula and remove it once the vessel has been entered. Cannulas are frequently used for *blood transfusions* and *intravenous infusions* and for draining *pleural effusions*. In certain circumstances, such as when blood is required for testing over a period of time, the cannula may be left in place for several days.

Cap, contraceptive

A barrier method of contraception in the form of a latex rubber device placed directly over the cervix to prevent sperm from entering. (See *Contraception, barrier methods*.)

Capgras' syndrome

The *delusion* (false belief) that a relative or close friend has been replaced by an impostor. Also known as the "illusion of doubles," Capgras' syndrome is seen most frequently in paranoid *schizophrenia*, but also occurs in organic disorders (see *Brain syndrome, organic*) and *affective disorders*.

Capillary

Any of the vessels that carry blood between the smallest arteries, or arterioles, and the smallest veins, or venules (see *Circulatory system*). Capillaries form a fine network throughout the body's organs and tissues. It is through the thin capillary walls that blood and cells exchange their constituents (see *Respiration*).

Capillaries have a diameter of approximately ten thousandths of a millimeter—not much wider than the red blood cells that flow through them. Their walls are permeable to substances such as oxygen, glucose, and water, which can thus move freely between the blood and the tissue fluid that surrounds all cells.

STRUCTURE OF CAPILLARIES
These minute blood vessels have permeable walls to allow transfer of oxygen, glucose, and water from blood to tissues.

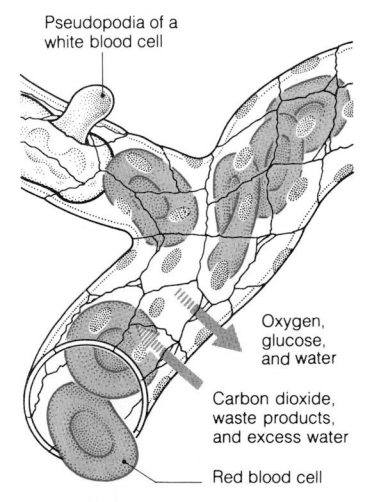

Pseudopodia of a white blood cell

Oxygen, glucose, and water

Carbon dioxide, waste products, and excess water

Red blood cell

The capillaries are not open to blood flow all the time; they open and close according to different organs' requirements for oxygen and nutrients. Thus, when running, most of the capillaries in the leg muscles are open, but at rest many are closed. The opening and closing of skin capillaries plays an important role in *temperature* regulation. Blood flow through each capillary is controlled by a tiny circle of muscle at its entrance.

DISORDERS
Because of their thin walls, capillaries are fragile. A direct blow to an area of the body can often rupture capillaries under the surface of the skin. Bleeding from them will cause swelling and bruising (around the eye this can cause a black eye).

Capillaries become more fragile in the elderly, in people taking high doses of steroids, and in victims of *scurvy* (vitamin C deficiency). These groups all have a tendency to *purpura* (small black and blue-purple areas of bleeding under the skin).

Capillary angiomas are benign tumors of the capillary wall that may be present at birth or may develop later in life. They may cause a red patch of variable size and shape on the skin and mucous membranes.

Capitation

A method of reimbursement based on constant dollar amounts per person rather than on variable fees reflecting services performed. For example, a group of physicians, contracting to provide medical services for the employees of a company, may charge the company so much per month per employee, collecting a capitation fee (so much "per head") rather than fees for the actual services rendered.

Capping, dental

See *Crown, dental*.

Capsule

A hard or soft shell, usually made of gelatin, that contains a dose of medication. Capsules are taken by mouth and have two main advantages over solid tablets. First, their elongated shape makes them easy to swallow. Second, they make it easier for patients to take solid or liquid medications that would have an unpleasant taste or smell if not administered in capsule form.

Some capsules have a special coating to prevent the release into the stomach of drugs that may have an irritant effect. Others are designed to release their contents into the small intestine at a slow steady rate so that a drug need be taken only once or twice a day.

Capsulitis

See *Bursitis*.

Captopril

The first member of a new class of drugs, the *ACE inhibitors*, used in the treatment of *hypertension* (high blood pressure) and *heart failure*.

Caput

Latin for head. The word caput is also used to refer to the face, skull, and all associated organs, to the origin of a muscle, or to any enlarged extremity, such as the caput femoris, the head of the femur (thighbone). However, the term most commonly refers to the caput succedaneum, a soft swelling in the scalp of newborn babies. It occurs as a result of pressure on the baby's head during labor and usually disappears after a few days.

Carbachol

A drug that mimics some of the actions of the *neurotransmitter* (chemical released from nerve endings) *acetylcholine*. It is used mainly as eye drops to treat *glaucoma* (raised pressure within the eyeball).

Carbamazepine

ANTICONVULSANT									

Tablet

Prescription needed

Not available as generic

An *anticonvulsant drug*, introduced in 1960, chemically related to tricyclic *antidepressant drugs*.

WHY IT IS USED
Carbamazepine reduces the likelihood of seizures caused by abnormal nerve signals in the brain and is mainly used in the long-term treatment of *epilepsy*. It has less sedative effect than other anticonvulsants.

Carbamazepine is also prescribed to relieve *neuralgia* (the intermittent severe pain caused by damage to or irritation of a nerve). Carbamazepine is also occasionally prescribed to treat certain psychological or behavioral disorders, such as *mania*.

POSSIBLE ADVERSE EFFECTS
There may be some sedative effect, especially if alcohol is drunk while taking carbamazepine.

C

Carbohydrates

A group of substances that provides the body with one of its two main sources of energy (the other is *fat*) and is an essential ingredient of a healthy diet. Sugar and starch are probably the most familiar carbohydrates.

TYPES AND SOURCES

There are three main types of carbohydrate, differentiated by their chemical structure.

Monosaccharides	glucose, galactose, fructose
Disaccharides	sucrose, lactose, maltose
Polysaccharides	starch cellulose

Types of carbohydrates
Monosaccharides are the simplest, consisting of a single saccharide molecule. Disaccharides consist of two saccharide molecules linked together. Polysaccharides consist of a long chain of many saccharide molecules. The most important carbohydrate is starch.

Cereals and vegetables contain sugars, starch, and cellulose and are known as unrefined (complex) carbohydrate foods; they usually also contain vitamins and a little protein. Refined carbohydrate foods, such as white table sugar, are virtually pure energy sources; they usually contain neither cellulose nor other nutrients. Complex carbohydrates should constitute 50 to 60 percent of the diet.

CARBOHYDRATE METABOLISM

Before they can be used by the body, complex carbohydrates must be broken down to simple monosaccharide sugars—glucose, galactose, and fructose. This is accomplished by *enzymes* in saliva and other digestive juices. The enzymes break down polysaccharides into the monosaccharides glucose, galactose, and fructose. Cellulose is unaffected by digestive enzymes and passes out of the body largely unchanged.

The monosaccharides are then absorbed through the intestinal wall and into the bloodstream for distribution throughout the body. Certain cells, such as brain cells and red blood cells, must have glucose to survive. Some of the glucose is used immediately by these cells, which "burn" it in a series of biochemical reactions to generate energy and heat (see *Metabolism*). The rest of the glucose is conveyed to the liver, muscles, and fat cells where it is converted into *glycogen* (animal starch) and fat for storage. When more energy is needed, this glycogen is converted back to glucose, which reenters the bloodstream for distribution around the body. Fat cannot be converted to glucose but can be burned as fuel to save glucose. Unlike glucose, galactose and fructose cannot be used directly by cells and so must first be converted by the liver to glucose; thereafter, the fate of this glucose is the same as that of glucose absorbed directly into the bloodstream from the intestine.

When the blood sugar level is high, such as after a meal, carbohydrate metabolism is primarily controlled by *insulin* secreted by the *pancreas*. Insulin restores the glucose level to normal by stimulating the uptake of unneeded carbohydrate calories by the liver, muscles, and fat for storage as glycogen and fat. In the disorder *diabetes mellitus*, carbohydrate metabolism is disturbed by a deficiency of insulin, and carbohydrates cannot enter most cells for storage.

The action of insulin is balanced by that of glucagon, another pancreatic hormone. When the blood sugar level is low—after fasting overnight or after exercise—insulin secretion slows down and glucagon stimulates the conversion of glycogen to glucose for release into the bloodstream. Epinephrine and corticosteroids, adrenal hormones secreted at times of stress, have the same basic effect as glucagon (i.e., to increase the blood sugar level).

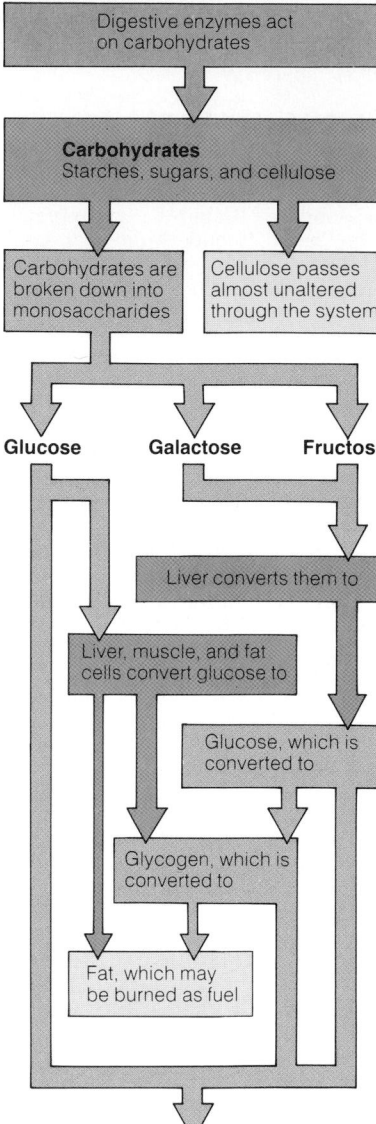

CARBOHYDRATE METABOLISM

Digestive enzymes act on carbohydrates

Carbohydrates
Starches, sugars, and cellulose

Carbohydrates are broken down into monosaccharides

Cellulose passes almost unaltered through the system

Glucose   Galactose   Fructose

Liver converts them to

Liver, muscle, and fat cells convert glucose to

Glucose, which is converted to

Glycogen, which is converted to

Fat, which may be burned as fuel

Glucose is absorbed into the bloodstream for distribution throughout the body or is used directly by body cells

Carbon

A nonmetallic element that is present in all organic molecules, the fundamental molecules of all living organisms. Pure carbon exists in nature as the major constituent of diamonds, coal, and graphite (pencil lead).

Carbon dioxide

A colorless, odorless gas (at normal temperatures) that is present in small amounts in the air and is also important as a by-product of normal metabolism in the body. Cooled and compressed carbon dioxide forms a white solid, *dry ice*, which is used in *cryosurgery*. Carbon dioxide consists of one carbon atom (symbol C) linked to two oxygen atoms (symbol O) and has the chemical formula CO_2.

Carbon dioxide is a waste product of the metabolic reactions that break down various substances, especially carbohydrates and fats, to generate energy. The carbon dioxide is carried by the blood to the lungs, where it is released and breathed out. One of the factors that controls the rate of breathing is the level of carbon dioxide in the bloodstream. When a person exercises strenuously, the amount of carbon dioxide produced increases rapidly, and the resultant high level in the bloodstream causes the person to breathe more rapidly to eliminate the carbon dioxide and take more oxygen into the body.

Carbon monoxide

A colorless, odorless, poisonous gas that is present in the exhaust fumes of oil- or gasoline-powered engines and is also produced by inefficient burning of coal, gas, oil, or propane in domestic heating appliances. It consists of one carbon atom (chemical symbol C) linked to one oxygen atom (symbol O) and has the chemical formula CO.

POISONING

Carbon monoxide is poisonous because it binds with *hemoglobin* (the oxygen-carrying molecule in red blood cells) and prevents it from carrying oxygen. As a result, the tissues are deprived of oxygen and asphyxiation occurs. If inhalation of the gas continues, it may lead to permanent brain damage or even death.

The initial symptoms of carbon monoxide poisoning—which may sometimes be mistaken for those of food poisoning—are dizziness, headache, nausea, and faintness. The most important step in first-aid treatment is to take the victim out into fresh air; continued exposure to the gas will lead to unconsciousness. If the victim has stopped breathing, get emergency medical aid, and give *artificial respiration*. Even if the victim seems to recover completely when taken into fresh air, it is advisable for him or her to consult a physician to make certain that there are no long-term effects.

Carbon tetrachloride

A colorless, poisonous, volatile liquid with a characteristic odor present in some home dry-cleaning fluids and also used as an industrial solvent. It consists of one carbon atom (symbol C) linked to four chlorine atoms (symbol Cl). Carbon tetrachloride has the chemical formula CCl_4.

Carbon tetrachloride is a dangerous chemical; it can cause liver and kidney damage if it is inhaled or drunk. Symptoms of poisoning include headache, nausea, pain in the abdomen, and convulsions.

Carbuncle

A cluster of interconnected *boils* (painful, pus-filled, inflamed hair roots). Carbuncles are usually caused by the bacterium *STAPHYLOCOCCUS AUREUS*; they generally begin as single boils, then spread. Common sites are the back of the neck and the buttocks.

Carbuncles are less common than single boils. They mainly affect people who have a lowered resistance to infection, in particular, diabetics.

TREATMENT

Anyone with a carbuncle should see a physician, who will usually prescribe an antibiotic and recommend the application of hot compresses (cotton soaked in hot salty water) or plasters. These may cause the pus-filled heads to burst, relieving pain. Subsequently, the carbuncle should be covered with a dressing until it has healed completely. Occasionally, incision and drainage (with removal of the core of the carbuncle) are necessary if drainage and healing do not occur on their own.

Carcinogen

Any agent capable of causing *cancer*, such as tobacco smoke, high-energy radiation, or asbestos fibers.

CHEMICAL CARCINOGENS

These form the largest group of carcinogens. Chief among them are the chemicals known as PAH (polycyclic aromatic hydrocarbons). They are found in, among other things, tobacco smoke, pitch, and tar fumes, all of which may cause lung cancer if inhaled over a long period; in solid pitch and tar, which may cause skin cancer in workers who handle them; and in soot, which was responsible for cancer of the scrotum among chimney sweeps in the eighteenth century.

Aromatic amines, which are used in the chemical and rubber industries, are other major chemical carcinogens, and prolonged exposure to them may cause urinary bladder cancer.

PHYSICAL CARCINOGENS

The best known physical carcinogen is high-energy radiation, such as nuclear radiation or X rays. In high doses, radiation usually first causes malignant change in cells, which divide quickly—for example, in the precursors of white blood cells in the bone marrow, causing leukemia. Everyone is exposed to some high-energy radiation from cosmic rays, radioactivity in rocks, and the like, but for many people the main source is X rays used in medical diagnosis.

Exposure over many years to ultraviolet radiation from sunlight can cause skin cancer, particularly in fair-skinned people.

Asbestos fibers are another known physical cause of cancer. White asbestos may cause lung cancer, particularly in workers who experience prolonged exposure to the fibers, who

already have the lung disease *asbestosis*, and who smoke. Blue asbestos and, to a lesser extent, brown asbestos can cause a tumor (mesothelioma) of the cells constituting the membranes that surround certain body cavities and organs. In the case of blue asbestos, this cancer can develop after very little exposure.

BIOLOGICAL CARCINOGENS

Very few biological agents cause cancer in humans. *SCHISTOSOMA HAEMATOBIUM*, one of the blood flukes that causes the tropical disease schistosomiasis, can cause cancer of the bladder, where it lays its eggs. *ASPERGILLUS FLAVUS*, a fungus that contaminates stored grain and peanuts, produces the poison aflatoxin, which is believed to cause liver cancer.

Certain viruses have been associated with cancer. The papilloma virus is believed to be responsible for cancer of the cervix, the hepatitis B virus has been implicated in liver cancer, and the Epstein-Barr virus is considered to be the cause of *Burkitt's lymphoma*, a malignant tumor of the jaw and abdomen that occurs mainly among children in Africa. *Kaposi's sarcoma* is probably caused by *HIV* (human immunodeficiency virus) or by one of the viruses associated with it.

SCREENING

Any substance that could possibly be carcinogenic, such as a food additive, cosmetic, or chemical for use in drugs, must be screened before it is allowed to be manufactured. One major preliminary test is to expose a certain strain of bacteria to the substance, and, if mutation (genetic change) occurs in the bacteria, the substance is regarded as a suspect carcinogen. It is then tested on laboratory animals, such as rats. If an increased incidence of tumors occurs, no license is usually granted to manufacture the substance for public sale.

AVOIDING CARCINOGENS

In industry, known carcinogens are either banned or allowed only if their use is considered essential, if exposure to them is strictly limited, and if regular medical screening is provided for workers using them, as, for example, in the nuclear fuel industry.

Outside of industry, the individual is exposed to very few known, unavoidable, high-risk carcinogens.

Carcinogenesis

The development of a *cancer* (a malignant tumor or blood disease) caused by the action of certain chemicals,

C

viruses, constituents of the diet, radiation, and unknown factors on primarily normal cells.

Cancer-causing factors are called carcinogens. Carcinogens are believed to alter the *DNA* (genetic material) within cells, particularly the structure of certain genes called *oncogenes* that normally control the growth and division of cells. An altered cell divides abnormally rapidly and passes on the changes in its genetic material to all its offspring cells. Thus, a group of cells becomes established that is not affected by the body's normal restraints on growth.

Carcinoid syndrome

A rare condition characterized by bouts of facial flushing, diarrhea, and wheezing. It is caused by an intestinal or lung tumor, called a carcinoid, that secretes excess quantities of the hormone serotonin. Symptoms (profuse diarrhea and intermittent flushing of the skin) usually occur only if the tumor has spread to the liver or affects the lung.

DIAGNOSIS AND TREATMENT

Carcinoid syndrome is diagnosed by measuring the level of a breakdown product of serotonin in the urine. The condition is sometimes treated by removal of the tumor from the lung, intestine, and from the liver as well, if possible. In most cases, surgical treatment is thought unlikely to be helpful, and in these circumstances treatment with drugs that block the action of serotonin may be successful in relieving the symptoms.

Carcinoma

Any malignant tumor (*cancer*) arising from cells in the covering surface layer or lining membrane of a body organ. A carcinoma is thus distinguished from a *sarcoma*, which is a cancer arising in connective tissue, bone, or muscle. Carcinomas include all the most common cancers of the lungs, breast, stomach, skin, cervix, and the like. The terms cancer and carcinoma tend to be used interchangeably but are not strictly synonymous.

Carcinomatosis

The presence of one or more enlarging carcinomas in different sites of the body due to metastasis (spread of malignant cells) from an original malignant tumor. The sufferer experiences weight loss, lack of energy, and other symptoms depending on the site of the metastases (secondary or offspring tumors).

Metastases in the lungs may cause coughing or breathlessness; in the liver they may cause jaundice.

The clinical diagnosis of carcinomatosis may be confirmed by X rays or *radioisotope scanning* of the bones and lungs, by *liver function tests*, or during an operation or autopsy. An operation to remove the primary (original) tumor will not help someone with carcinomatosis unless the primary tumor is producing a hormone that is directly stimulating growth of the metastases. *Chemotherapy* or *radiation therapy* may be given to deal with the metastases, sometimes following removal of a primary carcinoma.

Metastases associated with some cancers (of the testis, prostate, and thyroid glands) may be treated with drugs or hormones, and a prolonged abatement of symptoms is now common. Metastases from lung and intestinal cancers are less amenable to treatment and, in such cases, the outlook is not good.

Cardiac arrest

A halt in the pumping action of the heart due to cessation of its rhythmic, muscular activity.

CAUSES

The most common cause is a *myocardial infarction* (heart attack), but other causes include *respiratory arrest*, *electrical injury*, *hypothermia*, loss of blood, drug overdose, and *anaphylactic shock*.

DIAGNOSIS AND TREATMENT

A person with cardiac arrest collapses suddenly, with loss of consciousness, absence of pulse, and no respiratory movements. A person who is breathing cannot have suffered a cardiac arrest. An absolutely certain diagnosis can be made only by measuring the electrical activity of the heart with an *ECG* machine, but emergency *cardiopulmonary resuscitation* should be started immediately to minimize the risk of irreversible brain damage.

As soon as adequate help arrives—in most hospitals there is a cardiac arrest team on standby to manage such emergencies—the diagnosis can be confirmed by ECG. This test distinguishes between two types of disturbance that can occur in the heart muscle. *Ventricular fibrillation* is the random contraction of individual heart muscle fibers. This abnormal activity may be corrected by *defibrillation* (application of electric shock to the heart).

Asystole is the complete absence of heart muscle activity and is more difficult to reverse. It may respond to

intravenous infusion of *epinephrine* and calcium or in extreme cases to direct injection of epinephrine into the heart. An electrical *pacemaker* may also stimulate the heart in asystole.

In all cases of cardiac arrest the balance of the chemical constituents of the blood is disturbed, making the blood more acidic; an intravenous infusion of sodium bicarbonate is usually given to correct it. Other drugs, such as lidocaine, also can be administered intravenously to stabilize the heart muscle.

OUTLOOK

Between one fifth and one third of patients whose heart beat is restored after cardiac arrest recover sufficiently to leave the hospital (however, a substantial number of these die within the following year). In the remainder, the damage to the heart or brain is too extensive for recovery to be possible.

Cardiac neurosis

Excessive anxiety or fear about the condition of the heart. Cardiac neurosis usually occurs after a *myocardial infarction* (heart attack) or heart surgery. However, it may occur in people who have had no previous heart trouble.

The sufferer experiences symptoms that mimic those typical of heart disease—chest pain, tightness in the chest, lethargy, palpitations, and breathlessness—and may be reluctant to exercise or return to work for fear of bringing on these symptoms. Examination and investigation of the heart by a physician will reveal no physical cause for the symptoms.

Psychotherapy may help the patient overcome fears and anxieties. If it does not, the patient may not be able to return to a normal, active life.

Cardiac output

The volume of blood pumped by the heart in a given time (usually per minute). It can be used as a measure of how efficiently the heart is working. At rest, a healthy adult heart pumps between 2.5 and 5 quarts (2.35 and 4.7 liters) of blood per minute; during exercise this figure may rise to 32 quarts (30 liters) per minute. A low figure during exercise is a sign that the heart muscle is damaged or that major blood loss has occurred.

Cardiac stress test

A type of *fitness* test carried out in people who have chest pain, breathlessness, or palpitations during exercise. The test is used to determine

C

How the test is done
The patient is attached to an ECG machine, which records the pattern of the heart's electrical activity. He or she then performs an exercise, such as walking on a treadmill. A diagnosis of coronary artery disease is confirmed if there are specific changes in the wave pattern shown on the ECG recording as the intensity of the exercise is increased.

whether the cause of these symptoms is *angina pectoris* or another form of *coronary heart disease*.

The test is performed under close medical supervision, with resuscitation facilities immediately available. If at any time the patient has chest pains, becomes breathless, or feels sick, the test is stopped immediately. A cardiac stress test may also be performed with injection of a radioactive isotope, which outlines any damaged area of the heart.

Cardiologist

A specialist in diagnosing and treating problems related to the heart. Guided by symptoms such as shortness of breath, chest pain, or irregular heart rhythm, a cardiologist examines X rays, echocardiograms (see *Echocardiography*), and electrocardiograms (*ECGs*), or runs *cardiac stress tests* to determine the specific cause of a problem. Depending on the results of the tests, the cardiologist may recommend changes in diet or physical activity, prescribe medication, or refer the patient to a *cardiovascular surgeon*.

Cardiology

The study of the function of the *heart*; the investigation, diagnosis, and medical treatment of disorders of the

heart and blood vessels, especially *atherosclerosis* and *hypertension*.

Anatomically and physiologically, the heart occupies a central position in the body. It has a single function—to pump blood first to the lungs and then to the rest of the body—but the sequence of events in each heart contraction is complex. Similarly, many heart disorders are variations of a single disorder. Reduced pumping efficiency can have various underlying causes, including *arrhythmias, coronary heart disease* (in which the blood supply to the heart muscle is impaired), *cardiomyopathy* (in which the muscle itself is abnormal), and *heart valve* disorders. Disease of the lungs and blood vessels can also have adverse effects on heart function. In addition, some babies are born with structural defects of the heart and/or major blood vessels that emerge from it (see *Heart disease, congenital*).

Heart disorders are now the leading cause of death in the US. The study of the heart in health and disease is thus a large part of the training of every physician; family physicians are familiar with the treatment of patients with common disorders, such as coronary heart disease and hypertension. For more expert investigation and treatment, a person with a heart problem may be referred to a cardiologist.

The past 10 years have seen rapid advances in the understanding of heart disease, its investigation, and its treatment.

Cardiomegaly

Enlargement of the heart. In some cases, it takes the form of hypertrophy (thickening) of the heart muscle; in others, one or more of the heart chambers increases in volume (dilatation).

CAUSES

Hypertrophy of the heart muscle occurs in any condition where the heart has to work harder than normal to pump blood around the body. Such conditions include *hypertension* (increased blood pressure associated with increased resistance against which the heart must pump), which causes the wall of the left ventricle to thicken; *pulmonary hypertension* (increased blood pressure in the lungs), in which the wall of the right ventricle thickens; and one type of *cardiomyopathy* (disease of the heart muscle), in which either or both ventricles may thicken.

Dilatation of a heart chamber may be due to heart valve incompetence (failure of a valve to close properly

after a contraction). For example, in *aortic insufficiency*, failure of the aortic valve to close completely allows blood to flood back from the aorta into the left ventricle, eventually enlarging the chamber. Certain types of cardiomyopathy can also lead to swelling of a chamber.

SYMPTOMS

There are no symptoms of the enlargement until a critical point is reached in which added stress (e.g., hypertension, exercise, or infection) may reduce the efficiency of the heart as a pump. *Heart failure* will result, causing breathlessness and swelling of the legs and hands.

DIAGNOSIS AND TREATMENT

Cardiomegaly is diagnosed by a physician from a physical examination, chest X ray, and *ECG* (measurement of electrical impulses in the heart). Treatment is directed at the underlying disorder.

Cardiomyopathy

Any disease of the heart muscle that causes a reduction in the force of heart contractions and a resultant decrease in the efficiency of circulation of blood through the lungs and to the rest of the body. The disease may be infectious (viral), metabolic or nutritional, toxic, *autoimmune*, degenerative, or of unknown cause.

TYPES

Cardiomyopathies fall into the following three main groups: hypertrophic, dilated, and restrictive.

The hypertrophic type is usually a familial (inherited) disorder of unknown cause that leads to an abnormality of heart muscle fibers.

In dilated cardiomyopathy, muscle cell metabolism (chemical activity) is abnormal, and the walls of the heart tend to dilate (balloon out) under pressure. The cause of the abnormal cell metabolism is unknown.

Restrictive cardiomyopathy is caused by scarring of the endocardium (the inner lining of the heart) or by *amyloidosis* (infiltration of the muscle with a starchlike substance).

Heart muscle disorders may also be due to poisoning (e.g., by excessive consumption of alcohol) or to a vitamin or mineral deficiency (for example, lack of vitamin B_1).

INCIDENCE

Cardiomyopathies are less common than other types of heart disease. The specific incidence of the different types is unknown because in many cases there are few or no symptoms. Sometimes the damage to the heart

C

muscle is discovered only at an autopsy following death from an unrelated cause.

SYMPTOMS AND SIGNS

Symptoms usually include fatigue, chest pain, and palpitations due to an increased awareness of heart beat or to an abnormal heart rhythm such as *atrial fibrillation* (fast, irregular contractions of the upper heart chambers).

Heart failure (reduced efficiency of the heart's pumping action) can cause breathing difficulty and edema (swelling of the legs and hands).

DIAGNOSIS

A chest X ray usually shows enlargement of the heart outline. An *ECG* (measurement of electrical activity in the heart) often shows enlarged electrical impulses on the tracing due to heart muscle hypertrophy.

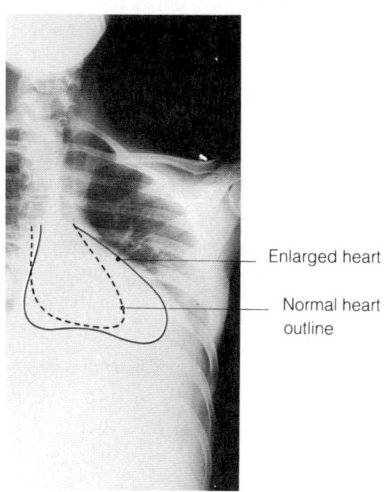

Enlarged heart

Normal heart outline

Chest X ray showing cardiomyopathy
The heart has become much enlarged, due to the heart muscle abnormality.

The diagnosis can be confirmed by examining a *biopsy* sample of heart muscle under the microscope to show muscle cell abnormalities.

TREATMENT

Since the causes remain unknown, there is no specific treatment. Treatment of symptoms may include the use of *diuretic drugs* to control heart failure and *antiarrhythmic drugs* to correct abnormal heart rhythm. For those with alcoholic cardiomyopathy, stopping all intake of alcohol is essential. Immunosuppresive drugs are occasionally helpful.

In many cases, heart muscle function steadily deteriorates, and the only option left, if available, is a *heart transplant*, which has successfully extended life in some individuals.

Cardiopulmonary resuscitation

The administration of the lifesaving measures of external cardiac compression massage and *mouth-to-mouth resuscitation* to someone collapsing with a *cardiac arrest* (cessation of effective heart beat).

It is vital to restore the circulation of oxygen-carrying blood to the brain as quickly as possible because permanent brain damage is likely if the brain is starved of oxygen for more than three to four minutes.

WHEN TO GIVE CARDIOPULMONARY RESUSCITATION

Before starting cardiopulmonary resuscitation it is important to establish that the victim has indeed suffered a cardiac arrest and has not simply fainted. The person will be unresponsive and have little or no breathing motion. Skin color will be pale, or blue-gray, especially around the lips. The person's heart will not seem to be beating. No pulse will be felt in the wrist or neck, and no heart beat will be heard when the chest is listened to. (If the person is breathing, no matter how slowly, then the heart will probably still be beating, even if no pulse can be felt.)

Cardiovascular

Of the heart and blood vessels.

Cardiovascular disorders

Disorders of the heart, blood vessels, and blood circulation. (See *Heart* disorders box; *Arteries, disorders of*; *Veins, disorders of*.)

Cardiovascular surgeon

A surgeon specializing in operations on the heart and the blood vessels to prevent or repair damage caused by, for example, birth defects, clogged arteries, or heart attacks. Procedures performed include *heart valve surgery*, *coronary artery bypass*, and *heart transplant*. Cardiovascular surgeons are generally seen by patients only on referral from other physicians.

Cardioversion

Another name for *defibrillation*.

Carditis

A general term for inflammation of any part of the heart or its linings. Carditis may be a *myocarditis*, inflammation of the heart muscle, usually caused by a viral infection; an *endocarditis*, inflammation of the internal lining of the heart chambers and heart valves, usually due to a bacterial infection; or a *pericarditis* (inflammation of

the outer lining of the heart), possibly with *effusion*. The latter is usually due to a viral or bacterial infection, but may be associated with a *myocardial infarction* (heart attack) or occasionally may be caused by an *autoimmune disorder*, such as systemic *lupus erythematosus* (SLE).

Caries, dental

Tooth decay. The gradual erosion of enamel (the protective covering of the tooth) and dentin (the substance beneath the enamel).

CAUSES

Plaque is the main cause of tooth decay (see illustrated box).

The most common sites of initial decay are the grinding surfaces of the back teeth (which have minute grooves in them), the lateral surfaces of adjacent teeth, and near the gum line. Plaque easily becomes trapped in all these areas.

INCIDENCE

An encouraging sign in industrialized countries over the past 10 to 15 years has been the significant decline (of 35 to 50 percent) in dental caries among children. The evidence suggests that, of the various factors probably responsible, the most important is water fluoridation, which strengthens enamel. The addition of fluoride to toothpaste has also played a part in the reduction of dental caries.

SYMPTOMS AND TREATMENT

Early decay, the most easily treated, usually does not cause any symptoms. The chief symptom of advanced decay is toothache (brought on by eating sweet, hot, or cold food) that increases in severity as the decay progresses. Decay may also cause bad breath.

Treatment consists of drilling away the area of decay and filling the cavity with a dental restoration, usually made of amalgam (a metal alloy) or a cement (composite resin) that matches the color of the tooth (see *Filling, dental*). In cases of advanced decay it may be necessary to remove the infected pulp and replace it with a filling (see *Root canal treatment*) or to extract the tooth (see *Extraction, dental*).

PREVENTION

Our modern diet makes it unlikely that, even by taking the most scrupulous preventive measures at all times, we could avoid dental caries altogether. However, it is possible to reduce the risk of caries considerably by cutting down on the amount (and frequency) of sugar and other refined carbohydrates that is eaten and by practicing good *oral hygiene*.

FIRST AID: CARDIOPULMONARY RESUSCITATION

1 First make sure the airway is clear. Then look and listen for signs of breathing. Listen for air escaping and feel for air flow. Feel for the pulse.

2 If the victim is breathing, place in the *recovery position*. If the victim is not breathing, place on a hard surface and start mouth-to-mouth resuscitation.

3 Pinch the victim's nose shut, take a breath, seal your lips around the mouth, and blow. Your breath contains enough oxygen for the victim's needs.

4 If breathing does not restart and you cannot detect a pulse or heart beat, start cardiac compression. Press with the heel of one hand placed on top of the other.

5 It is vital to apply pressure at the correct point—the lower part of the breastbone. Keep the pressure well clear of the victim's chest area.

6 If you are on your own, the rate of compression should be 80 per minute, with two breaths given after every 15 compressions.

WARNING

Cardiopulmonary resuscitation is a life-support technique that is used in a medical emergency when the victim is not breathing and when it is possible that his or her heart has stopped beating.

Although opening the victim's airway and restoring breathing can be performed effectively at the time of the crisis by following the instructions here, restoring the victim's circulation if the heart has stopped beating (cardiac compression) cannot be learned effectively in a crisis situation.

Cardiac compression, and all phases of cardiopulmonary resuscitation, should be learned through formal instruction. Practicing the technique regularly and taking refresher courses are also recommended.

WITH TWO RESCUERS

If two rescuers are available, one should give mouth-to-mouth resuscitation (one breath every five compressions).

Sixty compressions should be given per minute, with a pause of 1 to 1.5 seconds allowed after every five compressions.

C

CAUSES OF TOOTH DECAY

The primary cause of tooth decay is dental *plaque*, a sticky substance that forms on the teeth. Plaque consists of food remains, mucus-saliva by-products, and the bacteria that live in the mouth. The bacteria feed mainly on the fermentable carbohydrates (simple sugars and starches) in food, and, in breaking them down, create an acid that gradually destroys enamel, forming a cavity. If the process is not checked, the dentin is eroded next, enlarging the cavity and enabling the bacteria to invade the exposed pulp at the center of the tooth.

Severe dental caries
Example of caries affecting the necks of several upper and lower teeth.

 1 Acid produced in the breakdown of food gradually destroys enamel, forming a cavity.

 2 Unchecked, decay spreads to the dentin.

 3 The cavity continues to enlarge, enabling the bacteria to invade exposed pulp at the tooth's center.

 4 If untreated, the infected pulp will die and the tooth will be destroyed.

LOCATION OF CAROTID ARTERY

The common carotid on each side divides to form internal and external branches.

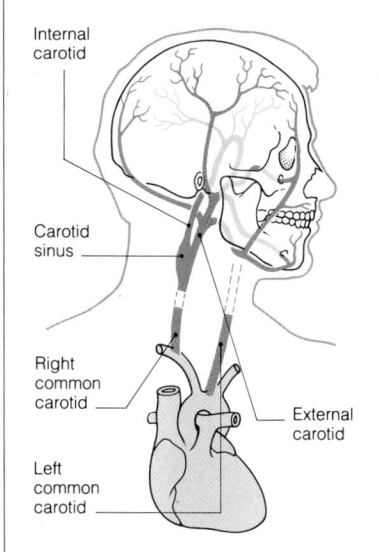

Internal carotid

Carotid sinus

Right common carotid

Left common carotid

External carotid

Sweet food should be eaten only at mealtimes; snacks between meals should be limited. The harmful effects of simple carbohydrates (especially sugars) should be monitored from the beginning of a child's life. Babies should not be given a bottle of milk, fruit juice, or other sugar-containing liquid to comfort them or get them to sleep; this habit can cause extensive early tooth decay.

Teeth need brushing thoroughly each day with fluoride toothpaste. Dental floss should be used to clean between them. A dentist should be visited regularly for checkups. (See also *Oral hygiene*.)

Carisoprodol

A *muscle-relaxant drug* used mainly to treat muscle spasm caused by injury.

Carotene

 An orange pigment found in carrots, tomatoes, and other colored plants, including leafy green vege-tables. Carotene is converted in the liver to vitamin A, which is essential for normal vision and the health of the skin and other organs. Excessive intake of carotene-containing foods, especially carrots, results in carotenemia (high blood levels of carotene). This condition is harmless, but does cause yellowing of the skin, especially of the palms and soles. It can be differentiated from jaundice because the eyes remain white. The abnormal pigment rapidly disappears if carrots or other such plants are omitted from the diet.

Carotid artery

Any of the four principal arteries of the neck and head. There are two common carotid arteries (left and right), each of which divides into two main branches (internal and external).

The left common carotid artery arises from the *aorta*, just above the heart, and runs up the neck on the left side of the *trachea* (windpipe). Just above the level of the *larynx* (voice box) it divides in two, forming the left internal carotid and the left external carotid arteries. The right common carotid artery follows a similar path, but on the right side of the neck. However, it arises from the subclavian artery, which branches off the aorta.

The external carotid arteries have multiple branches, which supply most of the tissues in the face, scalp, mouth, and jaws. The internal carotid arteries enter the skull to supply the brain (via cerebral branches) and eyes (via ophthalmic branches). At the base of the brain, branches of the two internal carotids and the basilar artery join to form a ring of blood vessels called the circle of Willis. Narrowing of these vessels may be associated with *transient ischemic attack* (TIA), while obstruction causes a stroke.

The carotid arteries have two specialized sensory regions in the neck, called the carotid sinus and the carotid body. The former monitors blood pressure; the latter monitors the oxygen content of the blood and helps regulate breathing.

Carpal tunnel syndrome

Numbness, tingling, and pain in the thumb, index, and middle fingers that often worsens at night. The condition may affect one or both hands and is sometimes accompanied by weakness in the thumb(s).

CAUSES AND INCIDENCE

The condition results from pressure on the median nerve where it passes into the hand via a gap (the "carpal tunnel") under a ligament at the front of the wrist. The median nerve carries sensory messages from the thumb and some fingers and also motor stimuli to the muscles in the hand; damage to the nerve causes sensory disturbances, particularly numbness or tingling, and weakness.

Carpal tunnel syndrome occurs most commonly among middle-aged women, usually for no obvious reason. It also occurs more commonly than average in women who are pregnant or have just started using birth-control pills, who suffer from *premenstrual syndrome*, and in people of either sex who suffer from *rheumatoid arthritis*, *myxedema*, or *acromegaly*.

TREATMENT

The condition often resolves itself without treatment. Resting the affected hand at night in a splint may alleviate symptoms. If symptoms persist, a small quantity of a *corticosteroid drug* may be injected under the ligament in the wrist. If this fails to help, surgical cutting of the ligament may be performed to relieve the pressure on the nerve.

Carrier

A person who is able to pass on a disease to others without actually suffering from it. Carriers may transmit infectious diseases to others, or may pass on inherited diseases to their offspring.

A carrier who harbors potentially harmful bacteria or viruses may unknowingly transmit an infectious disease such as typhoid or hepatitis B. The carrier may never have had symptoms of the disease, or may have had an infection in the past with apparently complete recovery.

Inherited disease may be transmitted if a parent who shows no signs of having a particular disease carries a gene for it. For example, a woman who carries the gene for hemophilia does not have the disease herself but may pass it on to her sons.

Cartilage

A type of connective tissue that, although not as hard as bone, forms an important structural component of many parts of the skeletal system, such as the joints. Much of the fetal skeleton is formed entirely of cartilage, which is then gradually converted to bone.

TYPES OF CARTILAGE
The three main types contain different proportions of collagen and vary in their toughness and elasticity.

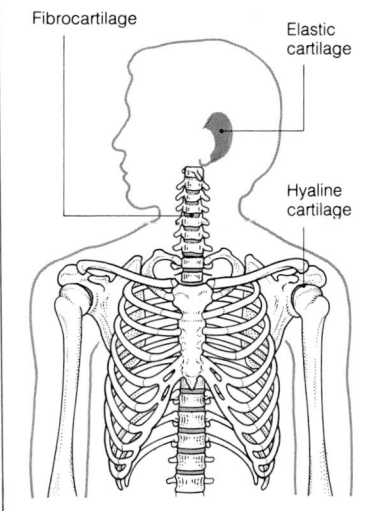

Fibrocartilage

Elastic cartilage

Hyaline cartilage

Cartilage consists of specialized cells called chondrocytes embedded in a matrix, or ground substance, that comprises varying amounts of *collagen*, a gellike substance. There are three main types of cartilage: hyaline, fibrocartilage, and elastic, each with a different proportion of collagen and each with different functions.

TYPES

Hyaline cartilage is a tough, smooth tissue that lines the surfaces of joints, such as the knee, providing an almost frictionless layer over the bony parts of the joint. If the lining becomes worn (as occurs in *osteoarthritis*) or damaged, joint movement may be painful or severely restricted.

Fibrocartilage contains a large amount of collagen and is solid and very strong. It makes up the intervertebral disks between the bones of the spine and the shock-absorbing pads of tissue that are found in joints.

Elastic cartilage is soft and rubbery. It is found in various structures, notably the outer ear and the *epiglottis*.

Cast

A rigid casing applied to a limb or other part of the body to hold a broken bone or dislocated joint so that it will heal in the correct position. Most casts consist of bandages to which wet plaster of Paris has been applied; the plaster is positioned before it sets.

In some cases a half-plaster, known as a back slab, is applied. Held in place with straps, it covers only half the affected limb. It is used if swelling at the site of injury is likely, or as a temporary measure pending the insertion of a pin to secure a broken bone.

Modern fiberglass casts are stronger and lighter than plaster, but are more expensive and difficult to apply.

Castor oil

A colorless or yellow-tinged oil obtained from the leaves of the castor oil plant.

When given by mouth, castor oil irritates the lining of the small intestine and within two to six hours causes a powerful *laxative* action that completely empties the bowel. This effect helps in preparing patients for X rays of the intestine. Castor oil should not be used as a regular treatment of constipation because of its strong, rapid effect.

Zinc and castor oil ointment is an *emollient* used to soothe the skin and keep it moist in conditions such as diaper rash.

Castration

The removal of the testes (see *Orchiectomy*) or ovaries (see *Oophorectomy*). Castration is performed to remove a diseased organ or to reduce the amount of *testosterone* (male hormone produced in the testes) or *estrogen* (female hormone produced in the ovaries) in the body. Castration may be used in the treatment of breast and prostatic cancers since estrogen stimulates the growth of some breast cancers and testosterone stimulates the growth of prostatic cancer. In adults, the procedure has no immediate effect on libido (sexual desire), though in some cases libido may be affected in the long run.

Historically, castration was performed on some male singers during boyhood to preserve a high-pitched voice and on male slaves who guarded Muslim harems.

Catalepsy

A peculiar physical state in which the muscles of the face, body, and limbs are maintained in a semirigid position. Catalepsy may last for many hours, during which time neither the expression nor bodily position will alter no matter how uncomfortable (for example, an upraised arm or bowed trunk). Attempts to change the person's position will meet with resistance or the unyielding adoption of a

C

new position. This state occurs mainly in those with schizophrenia, epilepsy, or hysteria, but may also be caused by some drugs or by various types of brain disease, such as a tumor.

Cataplexy

A sudden loss of muscle tone, causing the victim to collapse, without any loss of consciousness. Cataplexy usually lasts for a few seconds and is triggered by emotions, particularly laughter. A rare cause of sudden involuntary falls, it occurs almost exclusively in those suffering from *narcolepsy* and other *sleep* disorders.

Cataract

Loss of transparency of the lens of the eye. The name arose many centuries ago from the fanciful idea that the whiteness behind the pupil was a kind of waterfall descending from the brain. In fact, the white appearance is due to changes in the delicate protein fibers within the lens, in a manner similar to that occurring in eggs when they are boiled.

Cataract never causes complete blindness, because even a densely opalescent lens will still transmit light. However, with increasing loss of transparency, the clarity and detail of the image is progressively lost. Even at a fairly advanced stage, a cataract may not be apparent to an external observer, and it is only when the front part of the crystalline lens becomes densely opaque that whiteness is visible in the pupil.

Cataract usually occurs in both eyes, but in most cases one eye is more severely affected than the other.

INCIDENCE
Almost everyone over the age of 65 has some degree of cataract, but usually the opacification is minor and often confined to the edge of the lens, where it does not interfere with vision. Opacification tends to progress with age, so that the majority of people over 75 have minor visual deterioration from cataract. Cataract in the elderly is so common that it is considered almost normal.

CAUSE
The majority of cataracts occur in old age; the cause in these cases is unknown. Progressive hardening of the center of the lens and increased permeability to water of the lens capsule (shell) occur in the natural aging process. Both lead to protein changes.

Congenital cataract (present at birth) may be due to maternal infection early in pregnancy, especially with the *rubella* virus, or to toxic effects from drugs taken by the mother. It may be due to *Down's syndrome* or to one of a variety of rare genetic conditions. *Galactosemia*, in which the sugar galactose accumulates in the body, almost always causes cataract unless a galactose-free diet is given.

Cataract may be caused by direct injury to the eye, either penetrating or concussive (caused by a hard blow to the head), and is almost inevitable if a foreign particle enters the crystalline lens. It may be associated with prolonged intake of corticosteroid drugs or caused by poisoning with substances such as naphthalene (found in mothballs) or ergot (formed in stored grain contaminated by a fungus). Severe *diabetes mellitus*, with high blood sugar levels, can be associated with cataract in young people. Finally, almost any form of radiation (other than light), including infrared, microwave, and X rays, can cause cataract to develop.

Cataracts with a known cause are rare compared to the large number of cases that occur in elderly people for no obvious reason.

SYMPTOMS
Cataract is entirely painless and causes only visual symptoms. The onset of these symptoms is almost imperceptible, and progress is nearly always very slow. The increased density in the lens often produces an increase in its light-refracting power so that the person concerned becomes nearsighted. This may temporarily permit a person who was previously hypermetropic (farsighted) to read without using his or her reading glasses. Color values are often disturbed, with dulling of blues and accentuation of reds, yellows, and oranges. The full perception of color is strikingly restored after surgery.

The main symptom, however, is progressive loss of visual acuity with increased blurring of vision. Often the opacities in the lenses cause scattering of light rays and, even at a fairly early stage, this may seriously affect night driving. Many patients, however, are barely aware of these effects and notice only that they cannot see as well as before.

TREATMENT
Once a lens has developed a cataract, there is no possible way of reversing the change and restoring transparency and vision by means of medications. If normal clear images are to be perceived, the lens must be removed and the refracting power of the eye restored either by means of a substitute (implant) lens or with a special type of contact lens. Cataract extraction is one of the less complex and most successful operations in all surgery and the expectation of an excellent result, provided the eye is otherwise healthy, is well over 90 percent. (See also *Cataract surgery*.)

Cataract surgery

Removal of an opacified lens, or *cataract*, from the eye, to restore sight.

WHY IT IS DONE
Cataract extraction is most often performed as soon as the lens opacification has developed to the point where the person feels it seriously affects his or her vision. It is no longer necessary to wait for a cataract to "ripen" (i.e., until its nucleus becomes hard). Ophthalmologists are usually relieved to find that a cataract, and not some other problem, is the cause of visual loss because the results of surgical treatment are now so good.

Together with the cornea at the front of the eye, the lens provides the eye with the light-refracting power needed to see the world in focus (see *Eye*; *Vision*). Once an opacified lens has been extracted, some method must be used to restore the lost focusing power. In the past, patients were forced to wear very strong, highly magnifying glasses, which were heavy and uncomfortable and caused much distortion at the edges of the narrowed field of vision. Such glasses are now seldom necessary; it has become usual during surgery to replace the removed lens with a tiny plastic implant, fixed permanently within the eye.

By taking preoperative measurements of the curvature of the cornea and (using an ultrasonic method) of the length of the eye, it is often possible to calculate the power of the implant lens needed to restore the patient to normal vision. Some patients, however, will need to wear glasses after the operation.

There are still, however, some cataract patients for whom intraocular lens implants are unsuitable. This group consists mainly of people with a history of other eye disease. Some surgeons also advise against intraocular lenses in young people because the life span of the implant has not been established. Contact lenses can offer these people excellent vision postoperatively, and many people now wear such lenses.

PROCEDURE FOR CATARACT SURGERY

In a normal, healthy lens there is no interference to the passage of light rays. Even with peripheral opacities, vision is not limited until the central zone is affected. Dense nuclear opacities, as that shown at right, result in deteriorating vision and cannot be restored to transparency, hence the need for surgical replacement.

1 In preparation for surgery, measurements are taken of the cornea and of the length of the eye, in order to calculate the power of the lens implant needed to restore vision fully. The operation may be performed using general or local anesthesia; there is no pain in either case. Instruments of remarkable delicacy and precision are used to carry out the procedure, usually with the help of microscope magnification.

2 Before the operation, drops are used to widen the pupil so that most of the front surface of the lens is exposed. An incision is made around the upper edge of the cornea using an instrument with a diamond tip.

3 A small quantity of a clear gel (sodium hyaluronate) is injected to maintain a space between the back of the cornea and the lens.

4 A large part of the center of the front capsule of the lens is then removed and the hard nucleus of the lens carefully squeezed out of the eye. The soft remaining parts of the lens are then cleared away, leaving the back of the capsule.

5 The artificial lens implant is slipped into the natural lens capsule; plastic loops hold it in place. The corneal incision is sewn up with fine nylon thread about half the diameter of a human hair.

Surgeons use slightly different techniques, but a typical operation is described in the box at left.

Some surgeons remove the whole lens, in its capsule, by means of a probe that can be made to freeze to the lens. The lens may first be loosened by means of a digestive enzyme injected into the front chamber of the eye. In this case, the implant must be of a type that clips into the pupil or that is fitted in front of the iris. This method can also give excellent results.

Patients are no longer kept in bed after cataract surgery and, indeed, are encouraged to move about freely as soon as possible after the operation. The operation is commonly done today in an operating suite in the ophthalmologist's office. The corneal incision takes about a month to heal, but it is usually about ten weeks before the corneal curvature has ceased to alter. Glasses are not fitted until then.

OUTLOOK

The prospect of developing cataract need no longer cause concern. The results of treatment are usually excellent as long as no other cause of visual deterioration is present.

Catastrophic insurance

Insurance against a financially catastrophic illness. Though the term has not been specifically defined, it generally refers to the sort of health insurance that does not cover routine, moderately expensive procedures, but does protect a patient from the high costs of something such as a coronary artery bypass.

Catatonia

A state characterized by abnormalities of movement and posture. The sufferer's muscles usually become extremely rigid, but at other times he or she may be excessively active. Catatonia is a feature of a rare form of *schizophrenia*; it also occurs in people with certain brain diseases.

Catharsis

The process of expressing or acting out feelings and memories that were previously repressed. The term was originally used by Sigmund Freud, who believed that the revival of "forgotten" memories and the expression of the emotions associated with them could bring relief from anxiety, tension, and other symptoms.

The patient may be hypnotized or given drugs to bring on a suggestive state that allows the traumatic memory to be recalled and the emotions associated with the memory to be openly expressed. *Psychodrama*, which involves dramatic recreation of events, is another method used to help patients achieve emotional release. This cathartic method is claimed to be particularly successful in the treatment of battle fatigue and other forms of combat neurosis. (See also *Psychoanalytic theory*.)

Cathartic

A drug given by mouth or suppository that stimulates movement of the bowels, with production of liquid feces (see *Laxative drugs*).

Catheter

A flexible tube used either for draining fluid from or injecting fluid into the body. The most common type is the Foley catheter, which is used to drain urine from the bladder (see *Catheterization, urinary*). Other types of *balloon catheter* are used for unblocking or stretching open blood vessels, or for controlling bleeding.

A different variety of catheter is used to sample blood from the heart and to inject dye into the blood vessels during X-ray screening (see *Catheterization, cardiac*).

Catheterization, cardiac

A diagnostic test in which a fine tube called a *catheter* is introduced into the heart, via a blood vessel, to investigate its condition. The technique is used to diagnose and assess the extent of congenital heart disease (see *Heart disease, congenital*), *coronary heart disease*, and valvular defects (see *Heart valves*).

HOW IT IS DONE

The procedure, which causes little discomfort, is performed using local anesthesia. A small incision is made in a vein or artery and the catheter introduced through it. The tube is passed along the blood vessel and into the heart. Catheterization of the left side of the heart is carried out via an artery in the thigh or elbow. To investigate the right side of the heart, a vein in the groin or elbow is used.

Once in position, the catheter can measure blood pressure within the heart, withdraw blood to measure its oxygen content, or inject a dye that is opaque to X rays into the cavities of the heart so that X-ray photographs of them can be taken.

If an artery has been used, it is repaired with stitches after the catheter has been withdrawn; if a vein has been used, it is simply tied off.

COMPLICATIONS

Catheterization may disturb the heart rhythm, but, in a person in good physical condition, the rhythm is usually quickly restored to normal. For weaker patients the procedure does carry a slight risk of death from disturbed heart rhythm. However, since the disorders that it is used to investigate are life-threatening, the risk is regarded as acceptable.

Catheterization, urinary

Insertion of a sterile catheter into the bladder to drain urine.

WHY IT IS DONE

Catheterization is most often needed in a person who is unable to empty the bladder normally or who suffers from urinary *incontinence*. It may also be necessary during certain operations in which a bladder distended with urine might obstruct the surgeon's view of surrounding organs. Catheterization is performed in critically ill patients so that urine production can be carefully monitored; it is also used in tests of bladder function, such as *cystometry* and voiding *cystourethrogram*.

HOW IT IS DONE

The outlet of the urethra is cleaned before the catheter is inserted.

If it is not possible to pass a catheter up the urethra (because it is abnormally narrow, for example), a suprapubic catheter is inserted into the bladder through the abdominal wall. The skin of the lower part of the abdomen is cleaned with antiseptic solution, local anesthetic is injected under an area of skin overlying the bladder, and a small incision is made with a scalpel blade. The catheter surrounds a long needle that guides its insertion through this incision into the bladder. When urine flows back through the catheter, the guiding needle is withdrawn, leaving the catheter in place.

RISKS

Despite the use of sterile equipment, surgical gowns, gloves, and face masks, there is a risk of introducing infection into the bladder during catheterization.

Patients with incontinence associated with neurological disorders may have permanent catheters or may be

---

CATHETERIZATION OF THE BLADDER

The catheter is usually passed into the bladder through the urethra. Before this is done, the physician or nurse cleans the surrounding area with antiseptic solution to avoid introducing infection into the urinary tract. The procedure usually takes about ten minutes.

Catheter

Bag

Balloon catheter inflated in position in bladder

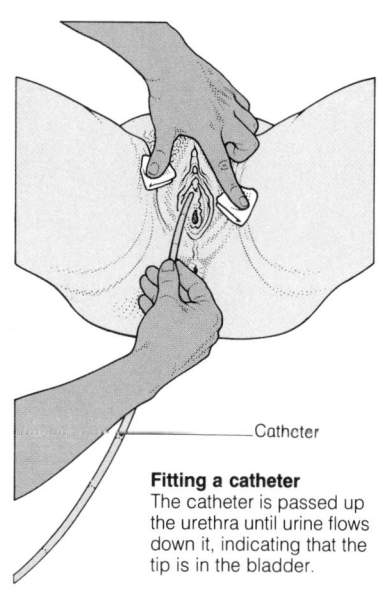

Catheter

Fitting a catheter
The catheter is passed up the urethra until urine flows down it, indicating that the tip is in the bladder.

Self-retaining type
If the catheter is to remain in the bladder, a self-retaining type is used. This catheter has a balloon at its tip that can be inflated and filled with sterile water.

taught to carry out self-catheterization several times a day. Again, there is a substantial risk of infection, which can lead to urinary tract disorders, such as *cystitis* or *pyelonephritis*.

CAT scanning

Computerized axial tomographic scanning, more commonly known as *CT scanning*.

Cat-scratch fever

An uncommon disease that usually develops after a scratch or bite by a cat and is thought to be due to infection with a small bacterium transmitted by the cat. The cat itself is not ill. Three quarters of cases occur in children, and the disorder is more common in autumn and winter.

SYMPTOMS

Symptoms usually appear three to 10 days after a bite or scratch. In some cases there is no apparent break in the skin, although contact with a cat is sometimes reported. The main sign of illness is a swollen lymph node near the scratch. The node may become painful and tender and, in rare cases, it may discharge. A small, infected blister sometimes develops at the original site of skin injury. A fever, rash, and headache may also occur.

DIAGNOSIS AND TREATMENT

The diagnosis is made from a *biopsy* of a small sample of the swollen lymph node and from a skin test using a cat-scratch fever *antigen*. Analgesics (painkillers) may be needed to relieve fever and headache, and if a lymph node or blister is severely infected it may have to be drained. The prognosis is excellent. In most cases, the illness clears up within two months. The cat need not be destroyed.

Cats, diseases from

Cats carry various parasites and infectious organisms that can be spread to humans. Some are specific to cats, others affect dogs as well. A well-cared for cat poses no serious threat to human health, but cat owners should be aware of possible problems.

SPECIFIC DISEASES

Of the rare but serious problems, *rabies* can be contracted by the bite of an infected cat. Sudden unexplained aggression in a cat in any area where the disease is present, or in cats recently imported from such areas, should be treated with suspicion. Have a veterinarian see the animal as soon as possible and call your state health department to determine whether there have been any reported cases of rabies in your area.

Cat-scratch fever is an uncommon illness that usually follows the scratch or bite of a cat. The suspected cause of the illness is a small bacterium that has not yet been identified.

Cats commonly carry the protozoan (single-celled parasite) TOXOPLASMA GONDII, which is the cause of *toxoplasmosis*. A form of the parasite is present in the cat's feces. In most cases, the infection causes few or no symptoms, but, if a woman is infected during pregnancy, the parasites may gain access, via the placenta, to the fetus. Infections in early pregnancy can lead to spontaneous abortion or severe malformation; infections that occur later in pregnancy can cause nervous system disorders and sometimes blindness in early childhood. Pregnant women should not change cat litter boxes.

Cat feces may also carry eggs of the cat roundworm, a possible cause of *toxocariasis*. In very rare cases, a larva from an ingested egg may lodge in an eye, causing deterioration of vision or even blindness. This most commonly occurs in children who have been playing in soil or sand contaminated by infected dog or cat feces.

Of the more common problems, a substantial number of *tinea* (ringworm) fungal infections of the skin—particularly scalp ringworm—probably come from cats. Unlike dogs, cats are little affected by the fungus, but its presence can be demonstrated by examining the fur under ultraviolet light, which causes fluorescence of infected skin and hairs.

Bites from cat *fleas* are more common than is realized; many bites blamed on midges and mosquitoes are actually caused by fleas. The fleas may jump onto humans to feed, particularly in warm weather and if the cat is absent. Bites are most common around the ankles and can be very irritating. Look for these fleas in places, such as beds or chairs, where the cat habitually rests.

Finally, some people develop allergic reactions to dander (tiny scales derived from animal skin and fur and present in the air) and consequently may suffer from *asthma* or *urticaria* when a cat is in the house.

PREVENTION

Serious diseases from cats are easily avoided by good hygiene—in particular, thorough washing of the hands if there is any chance they have been contaminated by cat feces. Young children should be discouraged from playing with cats and other animals, except under supervision, until they have become aware of the risks of poor hygiene. Animals that are obviously ill should be seen by a veterinarian, and routine health care should include regular worming and flea treatment.

HOW CATS TRANSMIT INFECTION

There are three main routes by which an infection or parasitic disease may be spread.

Direct contact
Mites or fungi from the animal's fur may be transferred.

In feces
Worm eggs or parasites contained in feces may contaminate fingers or food.

Bites or scratches
Microorganisms contained in the cat's mouth or on its claws may be transmitted by a bite or scratch.

C

Cauda equina

A collection of nerve roots that descends from the lower part of the spinal cord and occupies the lower third of the spinal canal (the space in the backbone that contains the spinal cord). This "spray" of nerves resembles a horse's tail.

Caudal

Denoting a position toward the lower end of the spine. Caudal literally means "of the tail."

Caudal block

A type of *nerve block* in which local anesthetic is injected into the lower part of the spinal canal. Obstetric and gynecological procedures utilize this form of anesthesia.

Cauliflower ear

A painful, swollen, distorted ear resulting from blows or friction that have caused bleeding within the soft cartilage framework of the pinna (outer ear). The condition occurs most commonly among boxers. In other sports it is prevented by means of a protective helmet (as in football).

Example of cauliflower ear
Deformity of the shape of the ear, with loss of normal folds of skin.

TREATMENT

If the ear swells after injury in a game or fight, an ice pack should be used to reduce the swelling. In severe cases, a physician should be consulted. Blood can be drained from the ear using a needle and syringe, and a pressure bandage applied. Despite these measures, repeated injury will lead to a severely distorted ear, and plastic surgery is sometimes needed to improve the appearance.

Causalgia

A persistent, burning pain, usually in an arm or leg. The skin overlying the painful area may be red and tender or may be cold, blue, and clammy.

Causalgia is usually the result of injury to a nerve by a gunshot wound, a deep cut, or a limb fracture. The pain may be aggravated by emotional factors or by normal sensations, such as touch or a cold breeze.

Treatment is unsatisfactory, but, occasionally, a patient benefits from *sympathectomy*, an operation in which certain nerves are severed.

Caustic

Any substance with a burning or corrosive action on body tissues or that has a burning taste. An example is caustic soda, the common name for sodium hydroxide.

Caustic substances can destroy body tissues and so should not be used without adequate protection, such as rubber gloves. If a caustic chemical is spilled onto the skin or splashed into the eye, wash it off immediately with a gentle stream of running water, taking care not to wash the chemical onto other areas of skin or into the other eye.

Cauterization

The application of a heated instrument or a caustic chemical to tissues to destroy them, to stop them from bleeding, or to promote healing within them. In the past, heat was widely used to destroy hemorrhoids, to stop bleeding during operations, and to treat cervical erosion. It has now been largely replaced by *electrocoagulation* (the use of high-frequency electric current), which is more efficient and easier to use. Chemicals such as silver nitrate are still used to destroy warts.

Cavernous sinus thrombosis

Blockage by a thrombus (blood clot) of a venous sinus (collection of a group of veins) deep within the skull behind an eye socket. Usually it is a complication of a bacterial infection in an area drained by the veins entering the sinus. At first, only the veins behind one eye are affected but, within two or three days, the thrombosis may spread to the sinus behind the other eye. The condition has become rare since the advent of antibiotics to treat bacterial infections.

CAUSES

Among the infections that can lead to the thrombosis are *cellulitis* (a severe skin infection) occurring on the face; an infection of the mouth, eye, or middle ear; *sinusitis* (infection of the air spaces around the nose); and *septicemia* (infection in the bloodstream).

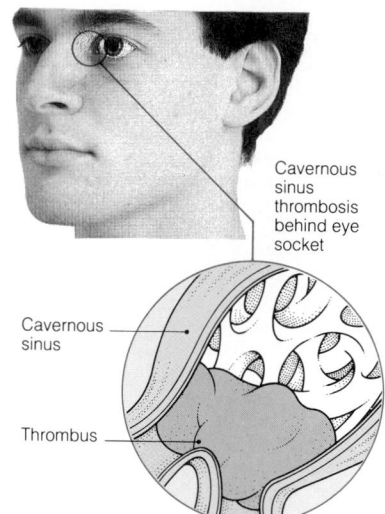

Cavernous sinus thrombosis behind eye socket

Cavernous sinus

Thrombus

Thrombus in cavernous sinus
The cavernous sinus is found behind the eye socket, deep within the skull.

Picking at a small, infected pimple at the angle of the nose may also spread infection to the sinus.

Rarely, the thrombosis is caused by a tumor pressing on the veins or by *polycythemia* (an excessive concentration of red cells in the blood).

SYMPTOMS AND TREATMENT

The symptoms are severe headache, high fever, pain in and above the affected eye, loss of sensation in the cornea and on the forehead due to pressure on the fifth cranial nerve, and *exophthalmos* (protrusion of the eye) due to swelling around and behind the eye. Vision may become blurred and eye movements may be paralyzed due to pressure on the optic nerve and on other cranial nerves controlling the muscles that move the eyes.

The patient is usually critically ill. Treatment is with antibiotics to treat the infection and anticoagulants to help disperse the blood clot. Given promptly, treatment can save vision in the affected eye or eyes; if untreated, blindness will result, and the infection may prove fatal.

Cavity, dental

See *Caries, dental*.

CDC

See *Centers for Disease Control*.

Cecum

The chamber at the beginning of the large intestine and the large intestine's widest part. It takes its name from the

LOCATION OF CECUM
The cecum is situated in the lower right-hand side of the abdomen, linking the *ileum* with the colon via the ileocecal valve.

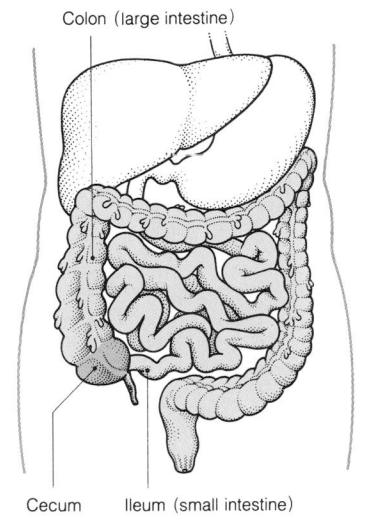

Colon (large intestine)

Cecum   Ileum (small intestine)

Latin word for blind, "caecum," because the large intestine terminates at this point. The *appendix* usually opens into the base of the cecum. (See also *Digestive system*.)

Cefaclor
A common cephalosporin-type antibiotic. (See *Cephalosporins*.)

Celiac sprue

An uncommon condition, known also as gluten enteropathy, in which the lining of the small intestine is damaged by gluten, a protein found in wheat, rye, and certain other cereals. The damage causes *malabsorption* (failure to absorb many important nutrients from the intestine), and the patient loses weight and also suffers from deficiencies of some vitamins and minerals. This can lead to anemia and skin problems. In addition, a large amount of fat and other nutrients remains in the stools, which are bulky and foul smelling.

CAUSE
Exactly how gluten damages the intestinal lining is not fully understood. However, it seems to be due to an abnormal immunological response. The *immune system* becomes sensitized to gluten and reacts in the same way as it would to an infection or foreign body. The abnormal reaction is limited to the intestinal lining, and the practical result is that the villi (frondlike projections) from the lining become flattened. Flattening of the villi seriously impairs their ability to absorb nutrients.

INCIDENCE
The proportion of people affected by the disease varies widely among different countries and populations. The severity of the disease varies, and many people who suffer some damage to the intestinal lining never develop symptoms.

INCIDENCE (per 100,000)

Western Ireland	300
Scandinavia	15
US	60
Africa	0
Asia	0

Celiac sprue tends to run in families—relatives of patients are much more likely than other people to have the disease themselves—which suggests that genetic factors may be involved (see *Genetic disorders*).

SYMPTOMS AND SIGNS
In babies, symptoms usually occur within six months of the introduction of gluten into the diet. The feces become bulky, greasy, pale, and offensive smelling, and the baby loses weight, becomes listless and irritable, and has a lot of gas, which makes the abdomen swell. Defective absorption of iron may lead to iron-deficiency *anemia* and defective absorption of folic acid (a vitamin) may lead to megaloblastic anemia. Vomiting may occur, and sometimes the baby develops acute diarrhea, becoming dehydrated and seriously ill.

In adults, symptoms, which usually develop gradually over months or even years, range from vague tiredness and breathlessness (due to anemia) to weight loss, diarrhea, vomiting, and abdominal pain and swelling of the legs.

In some patients, the damage to the intestinal lining is minimal, but a chronic, distinctive rash called *dermatitis herpetiformis* develops.

DIAGNOSIS
A firm diagnosis is made by means of jejunal *biopsy*, in which a small sample of tissue is taken from the lining of the upper small intestine. Three biopsies may be performed—one when the patient is eating foods containing gluten, another when he or she is on a gluten-free diet, and a third when gluten is again introduced into the diet. A change in the intestinal lining during the second and third stages indicates that gluten is causing the illness. Blood, urine, and feces tests show the level of malabsorption.

TREATMENT AND OUTLOOK
The only treatment required is a lifelong gluten-free diet; all foods containing wheat, rye, or barley must be avoided (many sufferers are also advised to avoid oats).

Specially manufactured substitute foods, including gluten-free bread, flour, and pasta, are available. There is no restriction on meat, fish, eggs and dairy products, vegetables, fruit, rice, and corn.

Within a few weeks of the start of a gluten-free diet, symptoms clear up and the sufferer starts to regain lost weight and to enjoy normal health.

Cell
The basic structural unit of the body. Each person consists of billions of cells, structurally and functionally integrated to perform the nearly infinite number of complex tasks necessary for life.

There is enormous variation among cells in the body. For example, mature red blood cells are only about 7 microns (about 0.0003 inch) across and are so highly specialized for their function of transporting oxygen that they lack some of the internal structures normally found within other cells, such as a nucleus. In contrast, nerve cells may be 3 ft (1 m) or more in length and are specialized to perform their function of transmitting electrochemical messages (nerve impulses).

Despite detailed differences, most human cells are basically similar in structure. Each cell is an invisibly small bag containing a fluid material called cytoplasm, surrounded by an outer skin called the cell membrane. Within the cytoplasm are the nucleus (except in red blood cells) and various other specialized structures, known collectively as organelles.

CELL MEMBRANE
Formed from a double layer of fatty material and proteins, the cell membrane holds the cell together. Its other main function is to regulate the passage of materials into and out of the cell, thereby enabling useful substances (such as nutrients and oxygen) to enter the cell, and waste materials

C

CELL TYPES

Despite their fundamental similarities, the cells of the body are differentiated to perform specific tasks, such as carrying oxygen (red blood cells), destroying invading microorganisms (white blood cells), manufacturing hormones (secretory cells in glands), and so on. Some cells (nerve cells, for instance) cannot be replaced once destroyed, while other cells (those that form fingernails, for instance) continue to function even after death. Cells can be grouped into four main types according to their underlying similarities.

Epithelial cells
Make up the tissues that cover the outside of the body and line the digestive, respiratory, and urinary tracts. The epithelium includes glandular tissue, which is specialized for secretion.

Connective tissue
Includes fat cells, the cells that make cartilage, and the fibrous and elastic tissues that hold the body together.

Muscular tissue
Made up of different types of muscle cells that are specialized to contract.

Cells in the nervous tissue
Conduct electrochemical messages throughout the body.

Microfilament

Villi

Nucleolus

Mitochondrion

Nucleus

Ribosomes

Microtubule

Peroxisome

Nuclear membrane

Cell membrane

Endoplasmic reticulum

Lysosome

Golgi apparatus

(such as carbon dioxide) and substances for use elsewhere in the body (hormones, for example) to leave it. Small molecules pass freely through the membrane, but larger molecules require special molecular transport systems to cross the membrane.

NUCLEUS

The control center of the cell, the nucleus governs all major activities and functions. The nucleus exerts its influence by regulating the amount and types of *proteins* made in the cell. Proteins have two main functions. Large, structural proteins make up the tough building material of the body (such as muscle fibers). Smaller proteins called *enzymes* regulate all functions and activities of the cell.

The *chromosomes* (genetic material of the cell) in the form of DNA (see *Nucleic acids*) are situated in the nucleus. This DNA contains the instructions for *protein synthesis*, which are transmitted by a type of *RNA* to ribosomes (protein producers) in the cytoplasm. It is on the ribosomes that protein synthesis—the linking of various amino acids to form proteins—occurs.

OTHER ORGANELLES

In addition to the nucleus there are various other organelles within the cell, each with a specific role.

The endoplasmic reticulum is a single sheet of membrane twisted into complex folds. The sheet has rough and smooth areas. Rough endoplasmic reticulum is covered with small round "beads"; these are the ribosomes that produce proteins.

Once completed, the proteins are transferred to another membrane system, the Golgi apparatus, which resembles a series of stacked plates. Here protein structures are modified and packaged into vesicles budded from its surface.

Energy is generated (from the breakdown of sugars and fatty acids) by organelles called mitochondria. These are shaped like coffee beans and have a complex, folded inner surface. Cells that have high energy requirements, such as muscle or liver cells, have a large number of mitochondria. Many cell processes involve substances that would damage the cell if they came into contact with the cytoplasm, so they are contained within special vesicles called lysosomes and peroxisomes. Lysosomes are the cell's major digestive structures in which enzymes break down large particles, such as bacteria. Peroxisomes neutralize toxic substances.

CYTOPLASM

Modern cytological techniques have shown that the cytoplasm contains a network of fine tubes (microtubules) and filaments (microfilaments) known as the cytoskeleton. This network gives the cell a definite shape and allows it to move. In addition, microfilaments support microvilli (small projections from the surface of the cell), which help increase the surface area of the cell. Microfilaments also form micromuscles, which can produce contractions and movements of the cell.

Cell division

The processes by which cells multiply. There are two main types of cell division, *mitosis* and *meiosis*. The former gives rise to daughter cells that are identical to the parent cell. The latter gives rise to egg and sperm cells, which differ from their parent cells in that they have only half the normal number of *chromosomes*.

Cellulitis

A bacterial infection of the skin and the tissues beneath it. The most common form is caused by streptococci, which enter the skin via a wound.

SYMPTOMS

The face, neck, or legs are the usual sites. The affected area is hot, tender, and red, and the patient is often feverish and may have chills.

Untreated cellulitis complicating a wound may progress to *bacteremia* and *septicemia* or, occasionally, to *gangrene*. Before the advent of antibiotics the infection was an occasional cause of death. Facial infections may spread to the eye socket. Very rarely, cellulitis occurs after childbirth and may spread to the pelvic organs.

Any form of cellulitis is likely to be more severe in people with reduced resistance to infections, such as diabetics and those with any type of *immunodeficiency disorder*.

TREATMENT

The usual treatment is a penicillin antibiotic (or erythromycin in case of allergy). Drugs may need to be taken for up to two weeks to clear an infection. (See also *Erysipelas*.)

Celsius scale

A temperature scale in which the melting point of ice is zero degrees (0°C) and the boiling point of water is 100 degrees (100°C). On this scale, normal body temperature is 37°C (equivalent to 98.6°F). The scale is named for the Swedish astronomer Anders Celsius (1701-1744). Centigrade is an obsolete name for the same scale.

To convert Celsius to Fahrenheit, multiply by 1.8 (or nine fifths), then add 32. To convert Fahrenheit to Celsius, subtract 32 then multiply by 0.56 (or five ninths). (See also *Fahrenheit scale*.)

0°C	37°C	100°C
32°F	98.6°F	212°F

Cementum

The bonelike tissue that surrounds the root of a tooth (see *Teeth*).

Centers for Disease Control

A part of the US Department of Health and Human Services that is responsible for the analysis and timely reporting of significant variations in the normal patterns of morbidity (the occurrence of diseases) and mortality. In effect, the CDC is the nation's medical watchdog. The centers are located in Atlanta, Georgia.

Centigrade scale

The obsolete name for the *Celsius scale*.

Central nervous system

The anatomical term for the brain and spinal cord, often abbreviated as CNS. The central nervous system works in tandem with the *peripheral nervous system* (PNS), which consists of all the nerves that carry signals between the CNS and the rest of the body.

The overall role of the CNS is to receive sensory information from organs, such as the eyes, ears, and receptors within the body, analyze this information, and initiate an appropriate motor response (for example, moving a muscle).

The analytical stage may be very short and simple for information that goes no further than the spinal cord or lower areas of the brain (see *Reflex*), but may be complex and prolonged for information reaching higher, conscious brain centers.

In anatomical terms the CNS consists of nerve cells or neurons and supporting tissue; the PNS is made up of nerve fibers extending from cells in the CNS. In functional terms, injury or disease to the CNS usually causes permanent disability; recovery is sometimes possible after damage to the PNS has been repaired surgically. (See also *Nervous system*.)

Centrifuge

A machine that separates the different components of a body fluid, such as blood or urine, so that they can be analyzed as an aid to diagnosis. The liquid is placed in a container that is spun at high speed around a central axis, and the centrifugal force (force moving away from the center) separates groups of particles of varying density. Blood, for example, can be separated into red cells, white cells, and its remaining constituents.

Cephalexin

A common cephalosporin-type antibiotic. (See *Cephalosporins*.)

Cephalhematoma

An extensive, soft swelling on the scalp of a newborn infant, caused by bleeding into the space between the cranium (skull) and its overlying fibrous covering, the periosteum. The swelling is due to pressure on the baby's head during delivery, causing rupture of some small blood vessels within the periosteum.

Although slightly alarming, a cephalhematoma is not serious and no treatment is necessary. The swelling should not be handled unnecessarily. It gradually subsides as the blood clot is reabsorbed, although this may take many weeks.

Bilateral cephalhematoma
This baby was born with a cephalhematoma on both sides of the scalp at the back of the head.

Cephalic

Relating to the head, as in cephalic presentation, the head-first appearance of a baby in the birth canal.

Cephalosporins

COMMON DRUGS

Cefaclor Cefadroxil Cefazolin Cefoperazone Cefoxitin Ceftriaxone Cephalexin Cephalothin Cephapirin Cephradine

A group of *antibiotic drugs* derived from the fungus *CEPHALOSPORIUM ACREMONIUM*. Cephalosporins were discovered in Sardinia in 1948. A large number of synthetic cephalosporins have since been produced, the most recent of which are effective against a wide range of infections.

WHY THEY ARE USED
Cephalosporins are widely used to treat ear, throat, and respiratory infections. They are also particularly useful in the treatment of urinary tract infections (which are often caused by bacteria resistant to penicillin-type antibiotics) and are used to treat *gonorrhea* that is resistant to other antibiotics. Cephalosporins are also sometimes used after surgery to reduce the incidence of wound infections.

The drugs in this group may be used in patients allergic to penicillin-type antibiotics. However, approximately 10 percent of those people allergic to penicillins are also found to be allergic to cephalosporins.

HOW THEY WORK
Cephalosporins interfere with the development of bacterial cell walls and inhibit the production of protein within the cells. As a result, the organisms die. However, some bacteria produce an enzyme (a protein that stimulates chemical reactions) called beta-lactamase that can inactivate some of the older cephalosporins. The newer drugs in the group are not affected by this enzyme.

POSSIBLE ADVERSE EFFECTS
Some people who take cephalosporins develop an allergic reaction. Reactions may include rash, itching, fever, and very rarely, *anaphylactic shock* (a severe allergic reaction causing collapse).

Cerebellum

A region of the brain concerned primarily with the maintenance of posture and balance and the coordination of movement.

STRUCTURE
The cerebellum is a rounded structure located behind the *brain stem*, to which it is linked by thick nerve tracts. The cerebellum accounts for about 11 percent of the whole brain weight and, with its convoluted surface, appears similar to the *cerebrum* (the main mass of the brain).

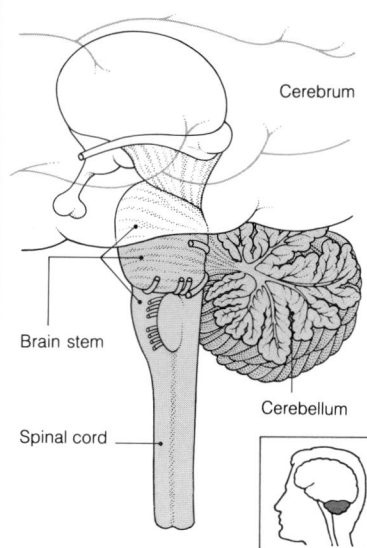

LOCATION OF CEREBELLUM
The cerebellum is found behind the brain stem and is connected to it by nerve tracts.

Cerebrum

Brain stem

Cerebellum

Spinal cord

Outwardly, the cerebellum consists of two hemispheres flanking a small protrusion from the brain stem, the vermis. The cortex (surface) of the hemispheres consists of numerous parallel ridges separated by deep fissures, so that only one sixth of the surface is visible. From the inner side of each hemisphere, three nerve fiber stalks, or peduncles, arise; these link up with different parts of the brain stem. All the signals between the cerebellum and the rest of the brain travel along these nerve tracts.

Microscopically, a cross section of the cerebellum shows the nerve fibers from these tracts fanning out toward the convoluted cortical surface. The cortex itself consists of gray matter (interconnected nerve cells) arranged in three main layers. Prominent among them are large cells in the middle layer, called Purkinje's cells, each of which may interconnect with up to 100,000 other cells.

FUNCTION
Via its connections to the brain stem, the cerebellum receives information from organs such as muscle tendons and the balance organ in the inner ear. Much of this information concerns the body's posture and the state of contraction or relaxation of its muscles. After receiving this information, the cerebellum, working in concert with the *basal ganglia*, "fine-tunes" the orders sent to muscles from the motor cortex in the cerebrum, resulting in smoothly coordinated movements and balance.

DISORDERS
Disease or damage to the cerebellum can result in abnormalities of posture or movement. These include *ataxia* (jerky, staggering gait and other uncoordinated body movements); *dysarthria* (slurred speech); hand tremor and "overshoot" when an attempt is made to grasp or touch something; and *nystagmus* (jerky eye movements, with an inability to fix the gaze in one direction).

Alcohol intoxication impairs cerebellar function and thus may produce symptoms similar to those of cerebellar disease. *Stroke* may cause cerebellar damage, often associated with impairment of the function of one or more *cranial nerves*.

Cerebral hemorrhage

Bleeding within the brain caused by rupture of a blood vessel. (See *Intracerebral hemorrhage*.)

Cerebral palsy

A general term for nonprogressive disorders of movement and posture resulting from damage to the brain in the later months of pregnancy, during birth, in the newborn period, or in early childhood.

A child with cerebral palsy may suffer from *spastic paralysis* (abnormal stiffness and contraction of groups of muscles), *athetosis* (involuntary writhing movements), or *ataxia* (loss of coordination and balance). The degree of disability is highly variable, ranging from slight clumsiness of hand movement and gait to complete immobility. Other nervous system disorders, such as hearing defects or epileptic seizures, may be present. Many affected children are also mentally retarded, although a proportion are of normal or high intelligence.

In the US about two to six babies per 1,000 develop cerebral palsy. There has been only a slight reduction in cases in the past 20 years.

CAUSES
In over 90 percent of cases the damage occurs before or at birth. Probably the most common cause is cerebral *hypoxia* (poor oxygen supply to the brain).

A maternal infection spreading to the baby within the uterus is an occasional cause. A rare cause is *kernicterus*, which results from an excess of bilirubin (bile pigment) in babies with *hemolytic disease of the newborn*. The baby is severely jaundiced, and the bile pigment damages the *basal ganglia* (nerve cell clusters in the brain concerned with control of movement).

Following birth, possible causes include *encephalitis* or *meningitis* (infection of the brain or its protective coverings), or a head injury.

SYMPTOMS

Often cerebral palsy is not recognized until well into the baby's first year. Sometimes, but not always, some of the infant's muscles are initially hypotonic (floppy), and the parents may notice that the baby in some way does not "feel right" when held. There may also be feeding difficulties.

Once the disability is apparent, most affected children fall into one of two groups—a spastic group, in which the muscles of one or more limbs are permanently contracted and stiff, thus making normal movements very difficult, and a smaller, athetoid group, characterized by involuntary writhing movements.

The diplegic child (see below) has delayed development in many movement skills and has difficulty learning to walk. In hemiplegia the limbs on

---

TYPES OF CEREBRAL PALSY

There are three different categories of disability in the spastic group: diplegia, hemiplegia, and quadriplegia.

Diplegia
All four limbs are affected, the legs more severely than the arms.

Hemiplegia
The limbs on only one side of the body are affected, and the arm is usually worse than the leg.

Quadriplegia
All four limbs are severely affected, not necessarily symmetrically.

---

the affected side grow slowly; there may be some sensory loss from the affected side of the body.

In quadriplegia, it may be difficult to know whether the child's arms or legs are the worst affected; mental retardation is usually severe. Often, the child never learns to walk.

The athetoid type of cerebral palsy results from damage to the basal ganglia, due either to birth asphyxia caused by hypoxia or to kernicterus.

Mental retardation, with an IQ below 70, occurs in about three quarters of all people with cerebral palsy, but the exceptions are important and occur particularly among athetoids; many athetoids and some diplegics are highly intelligent.

None of the various types of cerebral palsy is progressive (i.e., they do not worsen), but the features of the condition change as the child gets older, often for the better with patience and skilled treatment.

DIAGNOSIS

Parents of babies who are "at risk" from cerebral palsy—for example, babies born prematurely or during particularly difficult births—are generally encouraged to take the child more frequently for routine checkups by a physician, who will test with particular care for any abnormalities in the baby's muscle tone and reflexes, and for any delay in reaching various developmental milestones (see *Child development*). The diagnosis may rely on a combination of abnormalities.

TREATMENT

Although cerebral palsy is incurable, much can be done to help children affected by it. Abilities need to be recognized and developed to the full, as much stimulation as possible should be offered, and loving patience must always be shown.

Physical therapy is required to teach the child how to develop muscular control and maintain balance. This therapy is often given initially at a special school or clinic and then continued at home, possibly with the use of special equipment.

Inadequate speech can be helped greatly by *speech therapy*. For children who cannot speak at all, sophisticated techniques and devices have been developed to teach them how to communicate nonverbally.

Every attempt is made to place children with mild cerebral palsy in normal schools, but those who are severely affected need the special help available at schools for the physically and/or mentally handicapped.

OUTLOOK

Children with only moderate disability have a near-normal life expectancy and, with the help of social services, most of those who can move around and communicate effectively grow up to lead a relatively independent and normal life.

Cerebral thrombosis

The formation of a clot, or thrombus, in an artery in the brain. The clot may completely block the artery, cutting off the supply of blood and oxygen to a brain area, causing a *stroke*.

Cerebrospinal fluid

A clear, watery fluid that circulates between the ventricles (cavities) within the brain, the central canal in the spinal cord, and the space between the brain and spinal cord and their protective coverings, the meninges. Cerebrospinal fluid contains dissolved glucose, proteins, and salts, and some lymphocytes (roving cells—part of the immune system—that are also found in blood).

Examination of cerebrospinal fluid, usually obtained by *lumbar puncture*, is important in the diagnosis of many conditions affecting the brain and spinal cord, including *meningitis* and *subarachnoid hemorrhage*.

Accumulation of cerebrospinal fluid within the skull during fetal development or in infancy may cause the skull to become enlarged—a condition known as *hydrocephalus*.

Cerebrovascular accident

Sudden rupture or blockage of a blood vessel within the brain, causing serious bleeding and/or local obstruction to blood circulation.

Blockage may be due to *thrombosis* (clot formation) or *embolism* (obstruction by a plug of insoluble material formed and transported from elsewhere in the circulation). Rupture of different blood vessels may cause different patterns of bleeding, e.g., *intracerebral hemorrhage* (within the brain) or *subarachnoid hemorrhage* (around the brain).

Intracerebral hemorrhage, thrombosis, or embolism lead to neurologic features commonly called *stroke*.

Cerebrovascular disease

Any disease affecting an artery within and supplying blood to the brain—for example, *atherosclerosis* (narrowing of the arteries) or constitutional defects or weaknesses in arterial walls causing *aneurysm* (permanent swelling in an

C

artery). The disease may eventually lead to a *cerebrovascular accident* (sudden blockage or rupture of a blood vessel), most commonly leading to the features of *stroke*. Extensive narrowing of blood vessels throughout the brain can be a cause of *dementia*.

Cerebrum

The largest and most developed part of the brain, and the site of most conscious and intelligent activities. The cerebrum consists of two large outgrowths from the upper part of the brain stem (an extension of the spinal cord) called the cerebral hemispheres. Together these growths form an almost continuous mass that envelops much of the rest of the brain.

For size relative to body weight, and also for sophistication, the human cerebrum is unmatched in the animal kingdom, except arguably by that of some marine mammals, such as dolphins. Its complexity dwarfs that of the most advanced man-made machines and, although its structure and function are understood in broad terms, much of its workings remain a complete mystery.

STRUCTURE

Like the rest of the brain, the cerebrum consists of billions of interconnected nerve cells, arranged in layers or in clusters called nuclei, together with nerve fibers, the long filamentous outgrowths from nerve cells along which electrical messages pass to other cells. These fibers are organized into bundles, or nerve tracts, like electrical cables. Both the nerve cells and their fibers lie in a matrix of supporting cells, called glia cells, which provide both physical support and some metabolic requirements (e.g., energy, nutrients, or structural components) for the nerve cells.

Each cerebral hemisphere contains a central cavity, called a ventricle, that is filled with cerebrospinal fluid. Much of the rest of each hemisphere falls into three main layers: an inner layer surrounding the ventricle and consisting of clusters of nerve cells called the basal ganglia, a middle layer of "white matter" consisting mainly of tracts of nerve fibers, and an outer surface layer, the cerebral cortex or "gray matter," which is about 0.3 inches (1 cm) deep and consists of several layers of interconnected nerve cells.

The surface of each hemisphere is thrown into a series of folds, called gyri, separated by fissures called sulci; much of the cortex is hidden within the folds. Broad surface regions, or

lobes, of each hemisphere are named for overlying bones; the four main regions are the frontal, parietal, temporal, and occipital lobes.

The pattern of cortical folding is not precisely the same for everyone, but some of the gyri and sulci are constant and easily recognized on the surface of any brain. They have been given names by anatomists. The parietal and frontal lobes, for example, are separated by the central sulcus, and the temporal lobe from the frontal by the sylvian fissure. The longitudinal fissure is a deep cleft running front to back over the entire surface of the cerebrum, thus separating the two hemispheres. By reference to such landmarks, the location of any point on the surface of the cortex can be specified with some precision.

The nerve fibers forming much of the central white matter in each hemisphere are of three main types: association fibers link areas of cortex within a single hemisphere, projection fibers link areas of the cortex to central brain structures and to the

brain stem below, and commissural fibers, collected into a thick band called the corpus callosum, link the two hemispheres. A continuous stream of information, in the form of electrical impulses, flows along these fibers between groups of nerve cells.

FUNCTION

Much of the sensory information from organs such as the eyes and ears and from sensory receptors in the skin has its final destination in the cerebral cortex, where it is sorted, analyzed, and generally integrated until finally it is perceived as images, sound, touch sensations, and the like. Different levels of analysis are thought to correspond to the distinct layers of neurons in the cortex, with full conscious sensation probably occurring only in the top few layers.

Certain sensory modalities are specifically located within particular cortical regions—for example, visual perception is located within a part of the occipital lobe called the visual cortex. If this part of the brain is seriously damaged, vision is lost completely.

STRUCTURE OF THE CEREBRUM

The cerebrum dwarfs the rest of the brain; much of its surface is hidden in the folds, as shown by the vertical cross section.

Central sulcus

Right hemisphere

Left hemisphere

Gyrus

Longitudinal fissure

Gray matter

Longitudinal fissure

Corpus callosum

Brain stem

Sylvian fissure

Cerebellum

Ventricle

Basal ganglia

Spinal cord

White matter

Touch and pressure sensations are consciously perceived along the postcentral gyrus, immediately behind the central sulcus that divides the frontal and parietal lobes. Other cortical regions, mainly in the temporal lobe, are associated with auditory (hearing), olfactory (smell), and gustatory (taste) sensations, although less specifically so. If these areas are destroyed, sensation is dulled considerably, but not lost altogether. It seems that some primitive sensations (e.g., smell and pain) may be perceived below the level of the cortex.

In addition to sensory areas, there are also specific "motor" areas concerned with the initiation of the signal for movement by the skeletal muscles. The main motor area of the cortex is in the frontal lobe, along the precentral gyrus, immediately in front of the central sulcus. Again, however, it seems that not all movements are initiated from the cortex. Some learned, semiautomatic programs of movement, such as those required for walking, are delegated to lower brain regions, leaving the cortex free to deal with newly formulated, skilled movements.

Linked to the more clearly defined sensory and motor areas are association areas of the cortex, which integrate information from various senses. The association areas also perform functions such as comprehension and recognition, memory storage and recall, arithmetic calculation, thought and decision-making, or are involved in the conscious experience of emotions. Whereas many of the sensory and motor areas are on both sides of the cerebrum (serving the opposite side of the body), some of these other cortical functions are localized to one hemisphere. The "dominant" hemisphere (the left in almost all right-handed and many left-handed people) tends to control logical functions such as word comprehension, language, speech, and numeration, whereas the nondominant hemisphere is concerned with spatial relationships and emotional responses such as color appreciation.

In general, the more complex the function, the less well localized it is. However, the areas responsible for the comprehension of words (heard and read) and for the formulation of speech are located within clearly defined areas of the dominant hemisphere. The comprehension region (Wernicke's area) is close to the part of the cortex concerned with sound perception; the speech region (Broca's area) is close to the motor region that controls the muscles used in speech.

Of all the regions of the cerebrum, the functions of the frontal lobe are the least understood, and for this reason it is sometimes termed a "silent area." Information on the activity of this and some other areas derives mainly from study of the symptoms of local damage or disease.

DISORDERS

Damage to the cerebrum may be the result of direct physical trauma, *intracerebral hemorrhage* or other forms of *stroke*, *brain tumors*, *encephalitis* (brain infection), some types of poisoning, nutritional deficiency, or degenerative processes.

Damage to particular regions may cause specific syndromes. Examples are mental apathy and self-neglect (or other personality change) resulting from frontal lobe damage, or the loss of sensory discrimination, tactile *agnosia* (loss of the ability to recognize objects by touch), and geographic disorientation (losing one's way even in a familiar neighborhood), which may occur with parietal lobe injury. Disease of the temporal lobe may cause *amnesia* (loss of memory), strange hallucinations of smell, sight, and sound, and *aphasia* (loss of verbal comprehension and/or speech) if in the dominant hemisphere. Specific visual defects result from damage to the occipital lobe.

Often, however, cerebral disease causes nonspecific symptoms such as epileptic convulsions or headaches.

Certificate-of-need

A measure aimed at holding down medical costs. In some areas of the US, a certificate-of-need satisfying governmental criteria is required before a health facility, such as a hospital, may be built, expanded, or acquire expensive medical equipment.

Certification

The process of completing the necessary legal documents during the procedure of *commitment* to a mental institution for compulsory detention and treatment. The term is also used to refer to death certification—the formal signing of a statement of cause of death issued by a medical practitioner. In addition, the term is used when a specialty board approves a physician candidate as a specialist. The candidate is then said to be "board certified" (see *Board certification*).

Certification, board

See *Board certification*.

Cerumen

The waxlike yellowish substance commonly found in the external ear canal (see *Earwax*).

Cervical

Relating to the neck or to the cervix (neck of the uterus).

Cervical cancer

See *Cervix, cancer of*.

Cervical erosion

A condition (also called cervical eversion) affecting the cervix (neck of the uterus) in which a layer of cells with a composition similar to that of its inner lining appears on its outside surface—as though the cervix had been turned slightly inside out. The layer of cells contains many that are column-shaped and of a glandular (mucus-forming) type. The term "erosion" is something of a misnomer as there is no loss of tissue or ulceration of the cervix. The cervix may, however, be more fragile and have a tendency to bleed and secrete more mucus.

CAUSES

Some women are born with cervical erosion and have no symptoms. Other causes include injury to the cervix during labor (which may cause glandular tissue to appear on the outer surface of the cervix during healing) and long-term use of oral contraceptives.

SYMPTOMS

Most women with an erosion have no or few symptoms. Those who do have symptoms usually complain of a vaginal discharge, especially in the week prior to a period, or bleeding between periods or after intercourse. Inspection of the cervix shows a reddened area on the surface that may bleed easily when touched. This appearance needs to be distinguished from cervical cancer by means of a *cervical smear test* (Pap smear) and *colposcopy*.

TREATMENT

Only women with symptoms need to be treated (after a cervical smear has been taken and inspected). Treatment by local destruction of glandular tissue includes *cauterization*, *cryosurgery* (freezing), *diathermy* (heat destruction), or *laser treatment*. The areas of destroyed glandular tissue are replaced in time by a layer of normal squamous (flat) cells.

Cervical eversion

See *Cervical erosion*.

Cervical incompetence

Abnormal weakness of the cervix (the neck of the uterus) that can result in recurrent *miscarriages* (spontaneous abortions). Normally, the cervix remains closed throughout pregnancy until labor begins. However, if the cervix is incompetent, it gradually widens from about the 12th week of pregnancy onward because of the weight of the fetus within the uterus.

CAUSES AND SYMPTOMS

Cervical incompetence may be suspected if a woman has had two or more miscarriages after the 14th week of pregnancy. About one fifth of women who have recurrent miscarriages have cervical incompetence.

The physician can detect the widening of the cervical opening by performing an internal pelvic examination. The condition can also be diagnosed by *ultrasound scanning*.

TREATMENT

When a woman with cervical incompetence becomes pregnant, a suture (stitch) is tied, like a purse string, around the cervix. This is performed during the fourth month of pregnancy with an epidural or spinal anesthetic. After the operation, the patient stays in the hospital for a few days, and should rest frequently in bed throughout the remainder of the pregnancy. The suture is left in position until the pregnancy is at or near full term. It is then cut so that the mother can deliver the baby normally.

Cervical mucus method

A form of contraception based on periodic abstinence from intercourse according to changes in the mucus secreted by a woman's cervix. (See *Contraception, periodic abstinence*.)

Cervical osteoarthritis

A degenerative disorder that affects the joints between the bones in the neck and causes neck pain, stiffness, and other symptoms. The affected joints are those between the cervical vertebrae (the neck segments of the spinal column).

Because the degenerative changes are associated with aging, middle-aged and elderly people are mainly affected. Occasionally, the degeneration may be started by an injury—for example, the repeated injury sustained by football players. Almost everyone over the age of 50 has some evidence of cervical osteoarthritis on X-ray imaging. However, in most cases it causes no symptoms or only minor ones.

LOCATION OF CERVICAL RIB
The overdeveloped seventh cervical vertebra forms a rib parallel to a normal one.

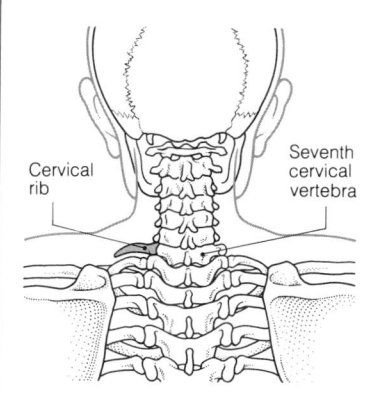

Cervical rib

Seventh cervical vertebra

SYMPTOMS

In addition to pain and stiffness in the neck, there may be pain in the arms and shoulders, numbness and tingling in the hands, and a weak grip. These symptoms are caused by pressure on the nerves that run from the spinal cord into the arms as they pass between the affected vertebrae. The symptoms tend to flare up from time to time, with intervening periods of only mild discomfort.

Other symptoms can include dizziness, unsteadiness, double vision, and headache brought on by turning the head. These are caused by pressure on blood vessels running through the vertebrae up to the brain. Rarely, pressure on the spinal cord itself can cause weakness or even paralysis in the legs, and loss of bladder control.

DIAGNOSIS AND TREATMENT

People with persistent minor symptoms or symptoms that are becoming worse should consult their physicians. X rays will reveal the degenerative changes. If pressure on the spinal cord is suspected, other studies will be performed to decide whether decompression can be accomplished surgically.

Treatment of severe neck pain and stiffness may include resting at home with cervical traction, wet heat, supporting the neck in a collar, and the use of analgesics (painkillers). *Physical therapy* is useful when the pain has eased; it includes *diathermy*, ultrasound, massage, and exercises to improve neck posture and movement.

Cervical rib

A congenital disorder in which the lowest of the seven cervical vertebrae (neck section of the spine) has overdeveloped to form a rib. This rib lies parallel to the normal rib attached to the first thoracic vertebra (see *Spine*). The abnormality varies from a small bony swelling to a fully developed rib and may occur on one or both sides. The cause is unknown.

SYMPTOMS

Often, there are no symptoms and the rib is discovered only when an X ray of the chest or neck is taken for some unrelated reason. Symptoms may develop in early adult life, when the rib begins to press on the lower part of the brachial plexus (the group of nerves passing from the spinal cord into the arm), causing pain, numbness, and a *pins and needles sensation* in the forearm and hand. These symptoms can often be relieved by changing the position of the arm.

DIAGNOSIS AND TREATMENT

Pain and tingling in the hand and forearm have a variety of possible causes, and the presence of a cervical rib, which is easily detected on an X ray, does not necessarily mean that it is the cause. Other possible causes of the pain and tingling include *carpal tunnel syndrome* or a *disk prolapse* (herniated disk) in the neck.

If the cervical rib seems the most likely cause, the symptoms can sometimes be helped by exercises to strengthen the shoulder muscles and improve the posture. Severe or persistent symptoms may require surgery.

Cervical smear test

A test to detect abnormal changes in the cells of the cervix (the neck of the uterus) and thus prevent the development of cervical cancer. The procedure is also known as a Pap smear, for George Papanicolaou, the physician who devised it.

WHY IT IS DONE

The test offers a 95 percent chance of detecting dysplasia (abnormal cell changes) which, if not discovered and treated, could become cancerous.

Cervical smears are also used to detect viral infections of the cervix, such as *herpes simplex* and wart virus infection, and to assess the level of hormones in the body, particularly estrogen and progesterone.

WHEN IT IS DONE

A woman should have a cervical smear within six months of first having sexual intercourse. A second smear should be done six to 12 months

PROCEDURE FOR A CERVICAL (PAP) SMEAR

The procedure is risk-free and the smear test itself takes only a few seconds. It should be done as a matter of routine within six months of first having sexual intercourse, and then six to 12 months after. Thereafter, it should be performed at one- to three-year intervals.

EQUIPMENT USED

Speculum

Plastic gloves

Spatula

Glass slides

Fixative

1 The women lies, preferably on her back, with her arms relaxed. Her legs should be bent up and relaxed so that the knees fall open.

Normal cells as seen under the microscope

Abnormal cells as seen under the microscope

2 The vagina is held open with a speculum; a spatula is used to scrape away some cells, which are examined under the microscope.

later (because of the small chance of missing an abnormality on one smear) and, if no abnormality is found, subsequently at one- to three-year intervals for the rest of her life. More frequent tests may be needed in women who change sex partners often or whose partner changes sex partners frequently.

Most family planning clinics perform cervical smears; women may also be tested by their physicians.

RESULTS

If the cells appear normal, no further treatment is required. If the cells appear abnormal, the smear is graded according to the cervical intraepithelial neoplasia (CIN) classi-fication system: CIN1 (mild dysplasia), CIN2 (moderate dysplasia), or CIN3 (severe dysplasia/early cancer). All abnormal smears are followed by *colposcopy* (examination of the cervix through a system of lenses) and biopsy (removal of small samples of tissue for analysis) of any suspicious areas. There are two types of cervical biopsy: punch and cone. A punch biopsy is the less invasive and is used for diagnostic purposes only (see illustration, next page). Areas confirmed as abnormal by biopsy are treated by *electrocoagulation* or *laser* (both use heat to destroy tissue) or *cryosurgery* (which uses cold to destroy tissue). This treatment is sometimes carried out at the same time as colposcopy if the abnormal area is small and well defined. In pregnancy, treatment is usually delayed until after delivery.

If colposcopy is not available, or if the extent of the severe dysplasia cannot be identified, treatment is by *cone biopsy*, an operation to remove a core of cervical tissue.

Cervicitis

Inflammation of the cervix (the neck and outlet of the uterus). Cervicitis is usually due to a vaginal infection or a sexually transmitted disease, such as *gonorrhea*, a *chlamydial infection*, or genital *herpes*, but infection may also follow injury to the cervix during childbirth or an operation on the uterus. Both acute and chronic forms of the condition may occur.

SYMPTOMS

Acute cervicitis is often symptomless and may not be discovered until the cervix is examined for some other reason. The cervix is inflamed and there may be a discharge from it.

Chronic cervicitis may produce a vaginal discharge, bleeding from the vagina after sexual intercourse or between periods, and pain low in the abdomen, sometimes felt only during sexual intercourse.

COMPLICATIONS

Untreated cervicitis can spread to cause *endometritis* (infection of the lining of the uterus) or *salpingitis* (infection of the fallopian tubes). If a pregnant woman has cervicitis, her baby may be infected during delivery, resulting in neonatal *ophthalmia* (an eye infection leading to blindness), or, less commonly, pneumonia caused by chlamydial infection.

DIAGNOSIS AND TREATMENT

A woman with the symptoms described should see her physician, who will probably examine the cervix

BIOPSY OF THE CERVIX

If a woman has recurrent abnormal smears, colposcopy and biopsy of suspicious areas will be performed. If the abnormal area cannot be seen completely by colposcopy, a larger sample of tissue is removed by cone biopsy. This procedure is used for treatment as well as diagnosis.

View of cervix
The photograph shows the end-on appearance of the cervix after a biopsy specimen has been taken from its tip.

Punch biopsy
If regions of the cervix look abnormal, but not serious enough for full biopsy, minute fragments of the cervix are removed for examination.

Cone biopsy
Using general anesthesia, a cone-shaped piece of the cervix (containing an area with abnormal cells) is removed with a scalpel. The resulting crater is repaired by stitching flaps of tissue over the wound. Alternatively, the wound may be left open and diathermy or freezing used to stop any bleeding. Recently, lasers (left) have been used to destroy abnormal tissue.

---

and take swabs of any discharge so that the microorganism responsible for the discharge can be identified.

Treatment is with antibiotics, such as tetracyclines or penicillin, or antiviral agents, such as acyclovir, depending on the cause of the infection. If symptoms persist, the inflamed area of the cervix may be cauterized by *electrocoagulation*, *cryotherapy*, or *laser treatment* to destroy the infected tissue.

Cervix

A small, cylindrical organ, an inch or so in length and less than an inch in diameter, comprising the lower part and neck of the uterus. The cervix separates the body and cavity of the uterus from the vagina.

The bulk of the cervix consists of fibrous tissue with some smooth muscle. This tissue makes the cervix into a form of sphincter (circular muscle), allowing for the great adaptability in its size and shape required during pregnancy and childbirth.

FUNCTION

After puberty, mucus secreted from the glandular cells in the cervix aids the entry of sperm into the upper cervix, which acts as a sperm reservoir. In the middle of the menstrual month, this mucus becomes less viscous and more favorable for sperm transport. Within the cervix, the sperm are protected and provided with their energy requirements by the mucus.

During pregnancy, the internal muscular fibers increase in size, thus

ANATOMY OF THE CERVIX

The cervix contains a central canal for passage of sperm and menstrual blood, and for childbirth. Both the canal and outer surface of the cervix are lined with two types of cells: mucus-secreting glandular cells and protective squamous cells.

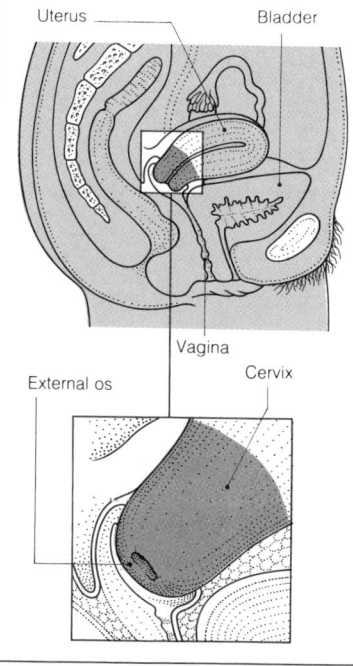

lengthening the cervix, which acts as a barrier for retention of the fetus. Toward the end of pregnancy there is a general shortening of the cervix in readiness for labor and delivery. During labor the central canal widens up to 4 inches in diameter to allow the baby to pass from the uterus. Soon after childbirth the muscles in the cervix contract and the canal returns to its original size.

Cervix, cancer of

Cancer of the cervix (neck of the uterus) is one of the most common cancers affecting women worldwide, and in many areas is becoming more common. Untreated, it may spread directly and through the lymph nodes to most of the organs in the pelvis. The chances of cure depend very much on what stage the cancer has reached when first detected.

TYPES

Cervical cancer is one of the few cancers that has well-defined precancerous stages. Before any cancer appears, abnormal changes occur in cells on the surface of the cervix, referred to as various degrees of dysplasia, which are readily detected by a *cervical smear test* (Pap smear).

Mild dysplasia may later revert back to normal, but any woman who has an abnormal cervical smear should undergo further investigation and possible follow-up smears.

If more severe dysplasia or early cancer is detected, it can be treated and cured completely.

DISORDERS OF THE CERVIX

The cervix (neck of the uterus), with its central position in the female reproductive tract, is susceptible to injury, infections, and tumors.

INJURY

Minor injury to the cervix is common during childbirth, especially if labor has been prolonged or if forceps have been used to deliver the baby's head. These injuries usually take the form of a laceration (tear) in the side wall. Usually they can be repaired immediately after delivery, but rarely they may extend into the tissues surrounding the uterus and lead to internal bleeding, requiring major surgery.

Injury may also occur if the cervical canal is inexpertly dilated (widened) in the process of an abortion, especially if the woman has not had children. However, the risk of such injury is extremely small if the abortion is carried out in a well-equipped hospital or clinic by a qualified gynecologist.

When an injury does occur, there is a danger that the muscle fibers within the cervix will be damaged or weakened, leading to a condition called *cervical incompetence*. The ability of the cervix to retain a fetus in the uterus is impaired, with a risk of miscarriage unless the weakness is repaired.

INFECTION

Cervical infections are common and usually sexually transmitted, but may cause no or few symptoms. *Gonorrhea* and *chlamydial infections* are the two most frequent and are sexually transmitted. These infections may spread to the lining of the uterus or to the fallopian tubes with a risk of causing infertility (see *Cervicitis; Endometritis; Salpingitis*).

Trichomoniasis is another common infection affecting the vagina and cervix; it is also sexually transmitted and caused by a protozoan parasite.

Viral infections of the cervix are becoming more common, especially those due to the human papilloma or wart virus and the herpes simplex virus. These infections are sexually transmitted and are associated with warts or herpetic ulcers in other parts of the reproductive tract (see *Warts, genital; Herpes, genital*). Both have been incriminated in cancerous and precancerous conditions of the cervix.

TUMORS

Growths may be benign or malignant (cancerous). The former are usually present in the form of a polyp.

Malignant growths are always preceded by changes in the surface layer of cells, called cervical dysplasias. These changes can be detected by a *cervical smear test* (Pap smear) and alert the gynecologist to the need for possible further investigation and treatment to prevent a cancer from developing (see *Cervix, cancer of*).

OTHER DISORDERS

Mucus-forming cells typical of those usually found in the cervical canal may appear as a layer on the outer surface of the cervix, causing a tendency to bleed. This relatively harmless condition is readily treated (see *Cervical erosion*).

Wart
● a benign growth caused by a virus

Tear
● a rare occurrence caused by childbirth or abortion

Infection
● causing inflammation of the cervix

Polyp
● a form of benign growth on the cervix

Erosion
● cells normally in the cervical canal appearing on the cervix

Cancer
● a malignant growth arising from abnormal cells in the cervix

INVESTIGATION

Investigation is by means of an internal examination (see *Pelvic examination*), a *cervical smear test*, and, in cases of suspected cancer or a precancerous condition, a *colposcopy*.

CAUSES AND INCIDENCE

Two main types of invasive (malignant) cervical cancer occur before or after the menopause.

SQUAMOUS TYPE This is by far the most common type of cervical cancer and is almost certainly the result of some process that occurs during sexual intercourse, probably transmission of an infectious organism to the cervix from the male partner. Recent evidence suggests that the culprit organism is a strain of the human papilloma, or wart, virus, which can infect the penis (see *Warts, genital*). A woman in a sexual relationship with a man with genital warts has a high risk (about one in three) of developing a precancerous condition of the cervix. For this and other reasons, men with penile warts should seek treatment from their physicians.

There are 45 different strains of the human wart virus, but traces of one in particular, called HPV16, have been found in 90 percent of squamous-type cervical cancers and in 50 to 70 percent of precancerous conditions.

Other factors may predispose to the cancer. Female smokers are at higher risk than nonsmokers, possibly because smoking impairs the *immune system* (defenses against infection) in the vagina, allowing entry and proliferation of a causative virus.

The sexual behavior of a woman and her male partner(s) strongly influences the chances of her developing the disease. The earlier a woman and/or her partner(s) first started having sex, and the greater the number of sexual partners they have had, the higher the risk that she will develop a precancerous condition.

ADENOCARCINOMA The causes of this much rarer type of cervical cancer are unclear. Both sexually active women and those who have never had intercourse are susceptible.

The overall incidence of cervical cancer per 100,000 population in the US is about 17 new cases of cancer, leading to four to five deaths per year. Although the incidence of diagnosed cervical cancer and precancerous conditions has been increasing in the US for several years, the death rate has been decreasing for over 30 years, and should continue to do so due to more widespread, regular, and efficient cervical smear (Pap smear) testing.

SYMPTOMS

The precancerous stages cause no symptoms whatsoever. Symptoms of the malignant stage are also initially few. Eventually, a woman will notice vaginal bleeding or a bloodstained discharge at unexpected times—between periods, after intercourse, or after the menopause.

If left untreated, the cancer spreads from the cervical surface into the deeper parts of the cervix and then out into the pelvic tissues, causing pain. Eventually it enters the bladder, rectum, or surrounding pelvic tissue.

DIAGNOSIS

The precancerous stages are not visible to the naked eye and can be detected only by a cervical smear test or by *colposcopy* (inspection of the cervix under magnified illumination). All sexually active women are advised to have this test soon after their first experience of sexual intercourse, again six to 12 months later, and at regular intervals thereafter.

Diagnosis of more advanced stages may be made from a cervical smear, colposcopy, *cone biopsy*, or from a physician seeing areas of ulceration or cauliflowerlike growths on the cervix after symptoms are experienced.

TREATMENT

If a persistent area of abnormality or localized early cancer is diagnosed by colposcopy and biopsy and can be seen in its entirety, destruction is by *electrocoagulation*, *diathermy*, or *laser treatment* (all of which use heat to destroy tissue), or by *cryosurgery* (which uses cold). All methods except diathermy can usually be carried out painlessly using local anesthesia. Success rates for complete removal after one application of laser or diathermy are about 95 percent. In pregnancy, treatment of precancerous conditions

or early cancer is usually delayed until after delivery.

If an area of abnormality or cancer has spread into the canal, close inspection of a cone biopsy may show that this procedure has removed all the diseased tissue. In all other cases of spreading cancer, treatment will depend on the extent of the spread, the age of the patient, and the physician's recommendation for surgery or radiation therapy.

In more advanced cases, when the tumor has spread to the organs of the pelvis, radiation therapy is given. In specialized centers, radical surgical techniques may be employed for selected patients, in which bladder, vagina, cervix, uterus, and rectum may all be removed.

Survival rates (five or more years after treatment) are about 50 to 80 percent for early spreading cancer, whether treated by surgery or radiation therapy, dropping to 10 to 30 percent for later-stage disease. Among patients selected for radical surgery, the survival rate improves to about 30 to 50 percent.

Cesarean section

An operation to deliver a baby from the uterus through a vertical or horizontal incision in the abdomen. Cesarean section is performed when it is impossible or dangerous to deliver the baby vaginally. In the past 15 years the number of cesarean sections performed in the US has increased dramatically to around 25 percent of all births. This is partly because of the increased safety of the operation, but also because obstetricians fear litigation if a difficult birth leads to complications for the mother or baby.

The procedure is done under anesthetic (see illustrated box, opposite). For the first 24 hours, the bladder catheter remains in place and the patient is given analgesics (painkillers). Usually, the mother can drink 12 hours and eat 24 hours after the operation. The recovery period tends to be much quicker when an epidural rather than a general anesthetic has been used. Barring problems, hospital stay following the operation is a few days.

HISTORY

Cesarean section, which takes its name from the Latin "to cut," was first performed in ancient Rome when it was required by law in the event of maternal death. According to legend, Julius Caesar was born in this way. In the eighteenth century, desperate

women tried to perform the procedure on themselves, but most died in the attempt. Not until the present century has the procedure been considered safe for both mother and child.

Cestodes

The scientific name for *tapeworms*—a group of long, flat, multisegmented parasites. Cestodes live in the intestine, where they may grow to more than 20 ft (6 m) long. Their larvae may infest other parts of the body, such as the brain (causing *cysticercosis*) or muscles. Tapeworms are acquired by eating raw or undercooked meat or fish. They may cause anemia.

Chagas' disease

An infectious parasitic disease found only in parts of South and Central America and spread by certain insects commonly called "conenosed" or "assassin" bugs. The disease is named after the Brazilian physician Carlos Chagas (1879-1934).

CAUSES AND INCIDENCE

The parasites responsible for Chagas' disease are single-celled organisms called trypanosomes, very similar to those that cause *sleeping sickness* in Africa. They live in the bloodstream and can also affect the heart, intestines, and nervous system.

Chalazion

A round, painless swelling on the upper or lower eyelid, sometimes known as a meibomian cyst. It results from obstruction (by its own secretion) of one of the meibomian glands that lubricate the edge of the eyelids. If the swelling is large, the pressure on the cornea at the front of the eye can cause blurring of vision.

A chalazion on the lower lid
Many small chalazions disappear spontaneously. Larger ones may require surgery.

PROCEDURE FOR A CESAREAN SECTION

A cesarean section allows delivery of a baby through a horizontal or vertical cut in the abdominal and uterine walls. The mother is usually given epidural anesthesia, so that she remains conscious during the procedure, but general anesthesia is sometimes used.

HOW IT IS DONE

Vertebra
Spinal cord
Epidural space
Hollow needle

1 Epidural anesthesia involves injection of a local anesthetic into the epidural space surrounding the spinal cord. This numbs the abdomen by deadening the nerves leading to it.

WHY IT IS DONE

The operation is necessary if the baby is unable to fit through the mother's pelvis or shows signs of *fetal distress* (lack of oxygen) before the cervix is fully dilated. Other reasons for performing a cesarean section include a placenta (afterbirth) that is lying close to the cervix (placenta previa), scarring on the uterus from previous surgery for urinary incontinence, unsuccessful induction of labor, *breech* presentation, and *postmaturity*.

Breech presentation

Placenta previa

2 A *catheter* is inserted into the bladder to empty it. The abdomen is then opened, usually through a horizontal incision made just above the pubic bone. This type of cut heals most effectively.

3 The amniotic fluid is drained off by suction. The baby is delivered through an incision in the lower part of the uterus, the umbilical cord is cut, and the afterbirth removed.

4 The incisions in the uterus and abdomen are then sewn up. The mother is given an injection of ergonovine to make the uterus contract and stop any bleeding.

5 The resulting scar is hardly noticeable and comes below the "bikini line."

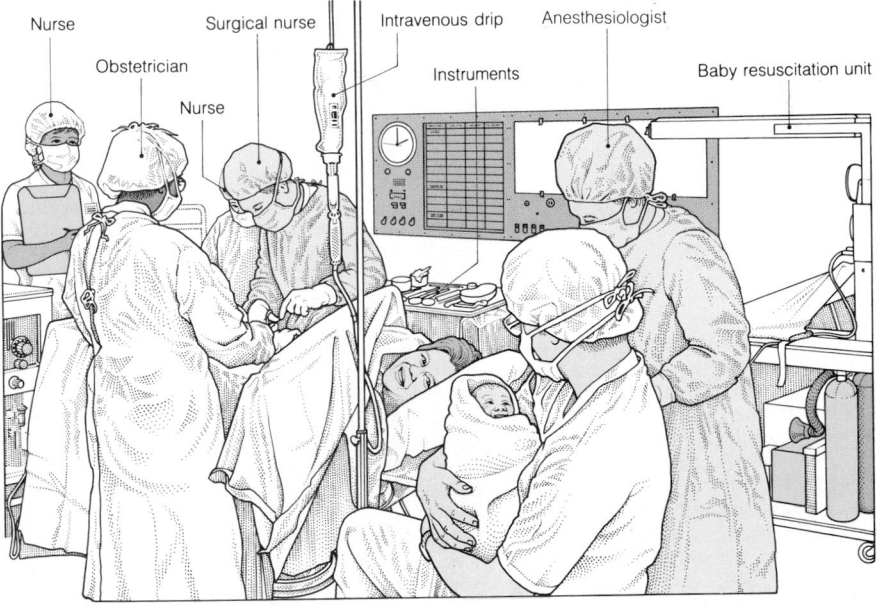

Nurse
Obstetrician
Nurse
Surgical nurse
Intravenous drip
Instruments
Anesthesiologist
Baby resuscitation unit

Chalazions can occur at any age and are particularly common in people suffering from the skin conditions *acne*, *rosacea*, or seborrheic *dermatitis*. If the cyst becomes infected the lid becomes more swollen, red, and painful. About one third disappear without any treatment, but large cysts usually need to be removed surgically using a local anesthetic.

Chancre, hard

An ulcer, usually on the genitals, that develops during the first stage of the sexually transmitted disease *syphilis*.

The chancre usually first appears as a dull red spot some 14 to 30 days after infection. It may occur on the penis, the anus, the vulva (the folds at the entrance of the vagina), or the inside of the vagina. The chancre can also occur on the lips or in the throat if oral sex has taken place. The spot gradually develops into a virtually painless ulcer, about one third of an inch in diameter, with a clearly defined edge and a thick rubbery base.

Diagnosis is made by microscopic examination of a smear of the chancre; blood test results may begin to be positive at this time.

TREATMENT
Any skin or mouth abnormality that might be a hard chancre should be reported to a physician immediately. A course of penicillin injections almost always prevents primary syphilis from developing into the later, more serious stages of the disease.

Chancroid

A sexually transmitted disease common in the tropics; it is characterized by painful ulcers on the genitals and enlarged lymph nodes in the groin. Also known as soft chancre and soft sore, the disorder is caused by the bacterium HEMOPHILUS DUCREYI.

The infection is relatively rare in the US and Europe; most cases that do occur involve sailors or travelers who have had contact with prostitutes in tropical countries.

TREATMENT
Prompt treatment with antibiotics usually clears up the problem. If the disease is left untreated, abscesses can form in the groin area and leave deep scars.

Chapped skin

Sore, cracked, rough skin on areas that have been repeatedly wet, inadequately dried, or exposed to the cold. The hands, face, and lips are most commonly affected.

Chapping occurs when the skin becomes excessively dry due to lack, or removal, of the natural oils that help keep it supple. This tends to happen in cold weather because the oil-secreting glands produce less oil. Repeated washing removes the oils.

Chapped skin can often be prevented by using protective gloves or barrier creams and by drying the skin carefully. Skin that has already become chapped usually responds well to applications of a rich, lanolin-based hand cream or face cream.

Character disorders

See *Personality disorders*.

Charcoal

A form of carbon. Charcoal's main medical use is as an emergency treatment for some types of poisoning and drug overdose.

Charcot-Marie-Tooth disease

An inherited muscle-wasting disease that mainly affects the legs. (See *Peroneal muscular atrophy*.)

Charcot's joint

A joint damaged by injuries that go unnoticed because of a neuropathy (loss of sensation) affecting the joint. Thus, the person cannot tell that certain activities are causing damage. (See *Neuropathic joint*.)

Checkup

See *Examination, physical*.

Cheilitis

Inflammation, cracking, and dryness of the lips. It can be caused by ill-fitting dentures, a local infection, allergy to cosmetics, too much sunbathing, or riboflavin (vitamin B_2) deficiency. In riboflavin deficiency, the corners of the mouth are chiefly affected. Until the underlying problem is remedied, a soothing skin cream will relieve the soreness.

Chelating agents

Chemicals used in the treatment of poisoning by metals such as lead, arsenic, and mercury. They act by combining with these metals to form less poisonous substances, which are usually excreted in the urine at a faster rate. Penicillamine is a commonly used chelating agent.

Chemonucleolysis

The injection of the enzyme chymopapin into a prolapsed intervertebral disk (see *Disk prolapse*) that is pressing on the spinal nerve root, causing *sciatica*. The enzyme dissolves the soft center of the disk, causing it to shrink, thus relieving the pressure on the nerve. Following initial enthusiasm, the frequency with which this procedure is performed seems to be declining. Chemonucleolysis is an alternative to surgical removal of the disk by *laminectomy* or to decompression of the spinal nerve root (see *Decompression, spinal canal*) in patients who have not been helped by conservative measures, such as bed rest or traction.

Chemotherapy

The treatment of infections or malignant diseases by drugs that act selectively on the cause of the disorder, but which may have substantial effects on normal tissue.

Infections are treated by *antibiotics*, which may be bactericidal (killing harmful bacteria) or bacteriostatic (stopping further bacterial growth and allowing the body's immune system to take over and destroy the bacteria). In the same way, *anticancer drugs* act either by destroying tumor cells or by stopping them from multiplying.

One problem with chemotherapy is that natural selection leads to the emergence of resistant bacteria or cells. This effect is minimized by the discriminatory use of antibiotics, and, in cancer chemotherapy, by giving several different types of drugs simultaneously. A further problem with cancer chemotherapy is that the drugs act on all rapidly dividing cells, not just tumor cells. Thus, they affect the bone marrow, the intestinal lining, the hair follicles (sometimes causing baldness), and the mouth, sometimes causing severe side effects. Antibiotics act more selectively because bacteria have a different structure from human cells, making side effects less of a problem for the patient.

Chenodiol

A chemical in *bile* that reduces the amount of cholesterol released by the liver into the bile.

Chenodiol is sometimes prescribed as a treatment for small *gallstones* if they contain mainly cholesterol and no calcium. Treatment takes several months, during which time progress is monitored by *X rays* or *ultrasound scanning* of the gallbladder. Chenodiol may cause diarrhea and, rarely, liver damage. It should not be taken during pregnancy because of possible adverse effects on the fetus.

Chest

The upper part of the body. Known technically as the *thorax*, the chest extends from the base of the neck to the *diaphragm*.

Chest pain

Chest pain usually does not have a serious cause, though occasionally it may be a symptom of a disorder that requires medical attention. The pain may occur in the chest wall (in the skin, underlying muscles, or ribs) or in an organ within the chest.

CAUSES

The most common causes of pain in the chest wall are a strained muscle (which is usually due to exercise) or an injury, such as bruising or a broken rib (due to a blow, fall, or other accident).

Pressure on a nerve root attached to the spinal cord may result in a sharp pain that travels to the front of the chest. This pain may be caused by *osteoarthritis* of, or injury to, the vertebrae, or, more rarely, a *disk prolapse*. Pain in the side of the chest may be due to *pleurodynia* (inflammation of the muscles between the ribs and the diaphragm associated with a viral infection). In rare cases, the viral infection *shingles* can cause pain in the chest wall. The pain, which is severe, runs along the course of a nerve and is followed by a rash of blisters in the *dermatome* (area of skin supplied by the same nerve). Inflammation of the junctions of the bony ribs and their cartilage or the junctions of the cartilage and the breastbone may cause chest pain that increases as the chest cage moves (*Tietze's syndrome*).

Within the chest, pain may be caused by *pleurisy* (inflammation of the pleurae, the membranes surrounding the lungs and covering the inner surface of the chest wall), which may be brought on by *bronchitis, pneumonia*, or, rarely, by *pulmonary embolism* (a blood clot lodged in an artery in the lungs). The pain of pleurisy is worse when the sufferer breathes in.

Malignant tumors of the lung (see *Lung cancer; Mesothelioma*) may cause pain as they grow and press on the pleura and ribs.

Acid reflux, a cause of heartburn, is a burning pain behind the breastbone produced by acid fluid from the stomach being regurgitated into the esophagus. It may occur as a symptom of *hiatal hernia*.

Various heart disorders can cause chest pain. The most common is *angina pectoris*, which is due to the

DIAGNOSING CHEST PAIN

To make an accurate diagnosis of the underlying cause, it is important for the patient to describe the location, quality (i.e., burning, pressing, or sharp), severity, and duration of the pain, any factors that relieve it or make it worse, and any other symptoms, such as breathing difficulty. In addition, the physician will perform a physical examination, including listening to chest sounds with a stethoscope and feeling for areas of tenderness in the chest wall. He or she may also arrange for other diagnostic procedures to be carried out.

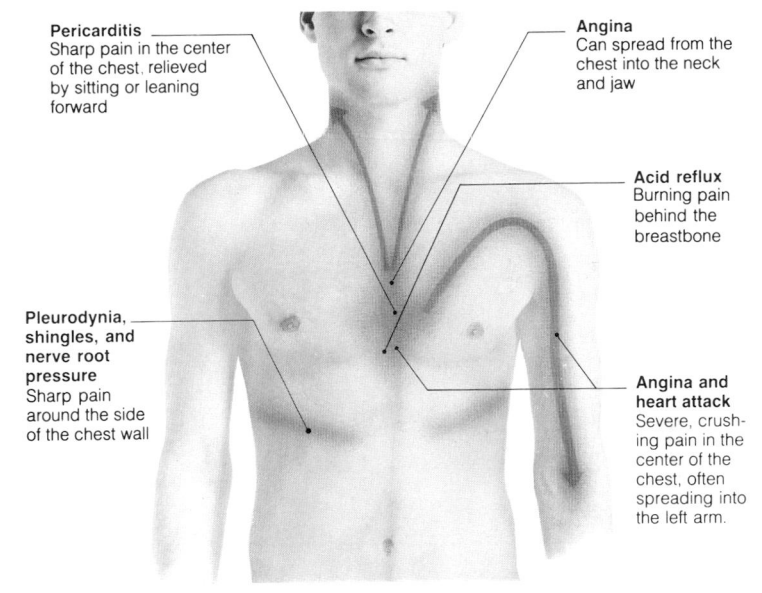

Pericarditis
Sharp pain in the center of the chest, relieved by sitting or leaning forward

Angina
Can spread from the chest into the neck and jaw

Acid reflux
Burning pain behind the breastbone

Pleurodynia, shingles, and nerve root pressure
Sharp pain around the side of the chest wall

Angina and heart attack
Severe, crushing pain in the center of the chest, often spreading into the left arm.

heart muscle receiving too little blood (and therefore oxygen), commonly as a result of *coronary heart disease*. The pain, which resembles that of severe indigestion or of a heavy weight pressing on the chest, is felt in the center of the chest and may spread outward to the throat, jaw, or arms (usually the left one). It usually is associated with effort or some acute stress that places an added work load upon the heart muscle. Stable angina pectoris may be present for many years. *Myocardial infarction* (damage to the heart muscle due to an inadequate blood supply) produces pain in the same areas as angina does but the pain is more severe. This is the crushing pain of a heart attack.

The pain of acute *pericarditis* (inflammation of the pericardium, the membrane that surrounds the heart) is also felt in the center of the chest. In some cases it is severe enough to resemble the pain of a heart attack. It can often be relieved by leaning forward. Acute pericarditis is rare and tends to occur in young adults after or with a viral infection.

Mitral valve prolapse has been associated with many symptoms, including chest pain. The chest pain may be sharp and left-sided. Chest pain may also be a result of anxiety and emotional stress. (See *Hyperventilation; Panic attack*.)

INVESTIGATION AND TREATMENT

Chest pain not associated with a trivial cause (such as bruising from a minor injury) should receive medical attention. Whether or not emergency treatment is necessary depends on the type and location of the pain and on the accompanying symptoms.

The treatment of chest pain depends on the underlying cause. For example, antibiotics may be prescribed for chest pain caused by pneumonia, and surgery may be necessary for the treatment of a malignant lung tumor or for some cases of coronary heart disease.

Chest X ray

One of the most frequently performed medical tests, usually carried out to examine the heart or lungs. The procedure is simple, quick, and painless,

C

CHEST PAIN Pain anywhere between the neck and the bottom of the rib cage that may be dull and persistent, stabbing, burning, or crushing.

? Is the pain crushing AND/OR does it radiate from the center of the chest to the jaw, neck, or arms?

YES → Has pain persisted despite 15 minutes of rest?

YES → ☎ **EMERGENCY!**
GET MEDICAL HELP NOW!
A heart attack is possible.

See • *Myocardial infarction*

NO ↓

Does the pain come on during exertion and have you had previous attacks?

YES → ☎

Consult your physician without delay!
Angina pectoris is the most likely explanation for your pain.

See • *Angina pectoris*
    • *Coronary heart disease*

NO

NO ↓

? Are you short of breath?

YES → Have you recently had an operation, injury, or illness that has kept you in bed?

YES → ☎ **EMERGENCY!**
GET MEDICAL HELP NOW!
This suggests that you may have a blood clot in the lung.

See • *Pulmonary embolism*

NO ↓

Do you have a cough OR is your temperature 100°F (38°C) or above?

YES → ☎

Call your physician without delay!
These symptoms suggest the possibility of pneumonia or bronchitis.

See • *Bronchitis*
    • *Pneumonia*

NO → ☎

Call your physician without delay!
You may have a collapsed lung.

See • *Pneumothorax*

NO ↓

WARNING
Anyone in whom severe chest pain develops for the first time, whether or not he or she feels sick otherwise, should call an ambulance or go to the hospital immediately. This could be a heart attack and is a medical emergency.

Continued on next page

C

? Does the pain worsen when you swallow, bend, or lie down?

YES → You may have heartburn due to reflux esophagitis or hiatal hernia, spasm of the esophagus, or some other esophageal disorder. Consult your physician.

See • *Esophageal spasm*
• *Esophagitis*
• *Hiatal hernia*

NO

? Do you have a burning pain in the lower chest AND/OR the upper abdomen?

YES → Does the pain come on soon after eating or after eating too much or too quickly, or after eating rich, spicy, or fatty foods?

YES → A stomach disorder or some other kind of dyspepsia is the most common explanation for such pain. If it happens regularly, consult your physician.

See • *Indigestion*

NO

NO

? Is the pain on one side only?

YES → Have you recently had a chest injury or a severe cough?

YES → A pulled muscle or injury to the ligaments and cartilages of the rib cage is the most likely cause of your pain.

See • *Sports injuries*
• *Sprain*
• *Strain*

NO

Is the pain region tender to the touch?

YES ↑

NO

Do you have a burning pain in the skin that is unaffected by breathing?

YES → Shingles, a virus infection of the nerves, is a possibility. The appearance of a blistery rash along the site of the pain a few days after the onset of pain will confirm the diagnosis. Consult your physician.

See • *Herpes zoster*

NO

NO

If you are unable to make a diagnosis from this chart, consult your physician without delay.

C

and is normally performed on an outpatient basis. Mobile equipment means that it can also be used (although somewhat less accurately) at the bedside of patients in the hospital, in the homes of immobilized people, and elsewhere.

WHY IT IS DONE

Chest X rays are usually used to confirm a diagnosis in patients suspected of having heart or lung disease, such as lung cancer, tuberculosis, or enlargement of a heart chamber.

HOW IT IS DONE

The X-ray machine contains a film in a large, flat cassette positioned at chest level. The patient stands facing the film cassette with the chest touching it and the chin projecting over the top. The hands are placed on the hips and the elbows swung forward, to move the shoulder blades to the side so that they do not obscure the lungs. A lead apron or screen protects the lower half of the body from radiation.

The patient takes (and holds) a deep breath and the radiographer then passes X rays through the upper trunk for a fraction of a second, from equipment behind the patient. The resultant X-ray picture provides an image not only of the heart and lungs but of major blood vessels, bones and joints, the esophagus, stomach, liver, and other organs and structures.

Cheyne-Stokes respiration

An abnormal pattern of breathing in which the rate and depth of respiration varies rhythmically. Deep, rapid breathing gradually becomes slower and shallower until breathing actually stops for some 10 to 20 seconds. Respiration then resumes, with deep, rapid breathing, and the cycle repeats itself. Each cycle lasts a few minutes.

Cheyne-Stokes respiration may be caused by disease or malfunctioning of the part of the brain that controls breathing (as occurs in some cases of *stroke*, head injury, metabolic dysfunction, or drug overdose). It may also occur as a result of *heart failure* and in some healthy people at high altitudes, especially during sleep.

Chickenpox

A common and mild infectious disease of childhood, characterized by a rash and slight fever. It is sometimes called varicella. Chickenpox is rare in adults; when it does occur it usually takes a more severe form.

INCIDENCE AND CAUSE

Throughout the world, most people have had chickenpox by the age of 10.

The disease is caused by the varicella-zoster virus. Although an attack confers lifelong immunity, the virus remains dormant within nerve tissues after the attack and may cause *herpes zoster* later in life.

The virus is spread from person to person in airborne droplets. Patients are highly infectious from about two days before the rash appears until about a week after.

All healthy children should be exposed to chickenpox so that they can catch the illness at an age when it is no more than an inconvenience. However, adults who have never had the disease should avoid it by staying away from children with chickenpox and also from anyone with shingles. Women in the final stage of pregnancy should be particularly careful since, if they catch the disease, the newborn child may develop a severe attack.

SYMPTOMS

One to three weeks after infection, a rash appears on the trunk, face, under the armpits, on the upper arms and legs, inside the mouth, and sometimes in the windpipe and bronchial tubes, causing a dry cough. The rash consists of a mass of small, red, itchy spots that become fluid-filled blisters within a few hours. After several days the blisters dry out and form scabs. Children usually have only a slightly raised temperature, but an adult may have severe pneumonia with breathing difficulties and fever. Those taking *immunosuppressant drugs* may also have a severe form of the disease.

Rarely, *encephalitis* (inflammation of the brain) occurs as a complication.

DIAGNOSIS AND TREATMENT

Diagnosis is usually obvious from a simple examination of the patient. In most cases rest is all that is needed for complete recovery, which usually takes place within 10 days in children, but over a longer period in adults. Acetaminophen can be taken to reduce fever, and calamine lotion relieves the itchiness of the rash. In severe cases the antiviral drug acyclovir may be prescribed. Children should be discouraged from scratching the blisters, which could lead to secondary bacterial infection (keeping the child's nails short is a good idea).

No vaccine against chickenpox is available or envisaged.

Chigger bite

An intensely irritating, itchy swelling, about half an inch in diameter, caused by the minute larva

of the harvest or red mite. Found on grass and weeds in summer, the mites attach themselves to the legs, particularly the ankles, of humans and feed on the blood. The swelling may become a blister, and sometimes the itching persists for weeks.

Chigoe

A painful, itchy, pea-sized swelling caused by a sand flea (also called the jigger or burrowing flea). When stepped on, the flea penetrates into the skin of the feet, under the toenails, or between the toes.

The chigoe flea lives in sandy soil only in Africa and tropical America. The burrowing fleas are pregnant females, which lay their eggs under the skin.

Avoidance involves wearing shoes or sandals outdoors in tropical countries (this also protects against *hookworms*). In the event of a suspected chigoe infestation, consult a physician. Chigoe fleas should be removed with a sterile needle and the wounds treated with an antiseptic.

Chilblain

See *Pernio*.

Child abuse

Any form of serious mistreatment of a child, whether physical or mental, including the use of a child for sexual gratification. Cases of child abuse today are coming to light with increasing frequency, probably not because such abuse is more widespread, but because there is a greater awareness of the problem.

Child abuse appears to be more common in lower socioeconomic groups, partly because of the greater stress on poor families with low living standards. However, the problem occurs at all levels of society, although it may be less easily recognized in higher socioeconomic classes.

The person injuring the child is usually a parent, but may be a stepparent, a parental friend or lover interest, or someone to whom care of the child has been delegated.

CAUSES

Being ill-treated when young seems to predispose people to abuse their own children by repeating the pattern of their own experience. This is particularly likely if the abused people have become parents at an early age, when they are too immature and inexperienced to cope with the demands made on them by a young child.

Children under age 3 are at greatest risk of abuse (other than sexual) because at this time a child is most demanding and is not yet old enough to be reasoned with.

Alcoholism, drug addiction, or emotional disturbances are other causative factors, since they may lessen a parent's self-control.

PHYSICAL ABUSE

Physical injury is the most readily recognized and diagnosed type of abuse. The National Center for the Prevention of Child Abuse and Neglect estimates that approximately 1 to 2 million children in the US are maltreated each year. Of this number 200,000 are sexually exploited and 200,000 to 300,000 are psychologically abused. An estimated 4,000 children die annually from child abuse.

Inflicting injury on a child is in most cases an impulsive act, the result of a sudden loss of temper. Infants and toddlers may be picked up and shaken vigorously, which can damage the eyes and rupture blood vessels in the brain and eventually cause severe brain damage. Slapping or punching is usually delivered to the head, resulting in black eyes and other facial bruises, cuts on the inner lip, and, less commonly, bone fractures. Injuries of abuse present different characteristics than those that occur accidentally and may reveal to a physician or other examiner that, whatever the reason given for them by the parents, deliberate infliction is the real cause.

Premeditated, repeated physical assault is rare. When it does occur it is a sign that a parent is severely disturbed and that the risks to the child are grave. These types of assaults can lead to multiple fractures, damage to internal organs, and even to death. Such abuse is sometimes accompanied by deliberate neglect, with no attempt made to adequately feed or clothe the child.

A child with nonaccidental injuries is usually admitted to the hospital for full examination and tests. He or she may then be removed from the home while members of the health, social, and probation services, and often a police representative, assess the case and decide on the best course of action. The child's interests remain paramount, but the parents, who may be under considerable stress, should be treated sympathetically.

EMOTIONAL ABUSE OR NEGLECT

Neglect of physical and emotional needs, such as love, stimulation, and guidance, is another form of abuse

recognized only more recently by courts. Such abuse is usually unintentional, arising from the parents' lack of understanding of their child's needs. Intentional abuse indicates that the parents are emotionally disturbed and require psychiatric help.

Indications that a child is being emotionally abused include failure to thrive, slow development, and lack of normal emotional responses. The diagnosis usually is confirmed when the child begins to put on weight and become more responsive after he or she is taken into the hospital for observation. Management of the situation is the same as for physical abuse.

SEXUAL ABUSE

This form of abuse has been increasingly recognized in recent years. Most frequently sexual abuse occurs within the family; usually the victim is a girl, although there is some evidence that indicates adolescent boys may also be at risk. Sexual exploitation of both sexes occurs in pornography and prostitution.

Most cases of sexual abuse consist of a father, close relative, or family friend taking advantage of a girl's affection to obtain sexual gratification from her. This form of abuse is secretive, because of the man's awareness of the gravity of the offense, and morally coercive, because of the power he holds over the girl.

Sexual abuse may come to light because of an obvious complaint from the child, a relative, or friend, or the child may display disturbed behavior or have other symptoms, such as venereal infection. Police, psychiatrists, and social workers usually cooperate in management of the problem, the main aim being to prevent further sexual abuse and to rehabilitate the child through therapy. Although the offender may be convicted, every effort is made to keep the family unit together.

Childbed fever

See *Puerperal sepsis.*

Childbirth

The process by which an infant is moved from the uterus to the outside world. Childbirth normally occurs at between 38 and 42 weeks' gestation (pregnancy), timed from the mother's last normal menstrual period.

In previous centuries women of all social classes commonly died in childbirth; maternal mortality still remains high in developing countries. In Western countries, however,

MATERNAL MORTALITY

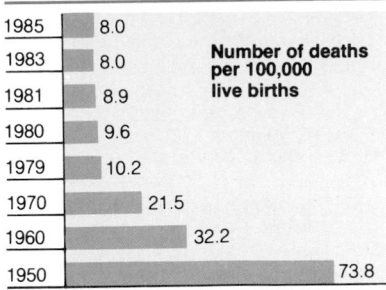

Year	Number of deaths per 100,000 live births
1985	8.0
1983	8.0
1981	8.9
1980	9.6
1979	10.2
1970	21.5
1960	32.2
1950	73.8

Mortality for complications of pregnancy and childbirth in selected years from 1950 to 1983 shows a dramatic decrease.

deaths and complications of childbirth have declined dramatically since the start of this century. Much of this decline is due to improvements in women's general health; the remainder has resulted from advances in the medical treatment of the complications of pregnancy and labor— most notably the availability of blood transfusion and antibacterial drugs.

Although the role of specialized equipment and drugs in improving safety during childbirth cannot be denied, women have become concerned about the increased mechanization of childbirth. Hence, the popularity of "natural childbirth," which advocates the avoidance of unnecessary medical intervention. Hospitals have begun to recognize the right of women to choose the type of birth they prefer (as long as it is compatible with safety). This choice may include the option of having people present during the birth and the type of pain relief, if any, the woman would like to have administered.

More flexibility is also being shown in allowing women to choose the position they prefer for giving birth. For many years, the supine position has been traditional in the US and many European countries. Historically, however, this position is a fairly recent innovation, not introduced until the eighteenth century.

Most hospitals still transfer the mother from the labor ward to a separate delivery room when she is ready to have the baby. Some hospitals now have alternative birthing rooms, where the mother can deliver in a homelike atmosphere with medical facilities at hand.

ONSET OF LABOR

It is often difficult to know when labor has started. During the last three months of pregnancy the uterus starts

C

STAGES OF BIRTH

The time it takes for a baby to be born depends on several factors, but primarily on whether it is a first or later baby. The first stage of labor can take 12 or more hours for a first baby, but only a few hours for a subsequent one. The mother is usually examined vaginally (or, on occasion, rectally) every two to four hours to assess the extent of dilation.

Fetal heart monitoring is performed throughout all stages of labor, and the frequency, strength, and duration of the mother's contractions are recorded.

Once delivered, the baby is usually placed on the mother's abdomen or warmed, dried, and quickly checked by a nurse or pediatrician.

ELECTRONIC FETAL MONITORING

This may be carried out if the fetus is at risk, or as a routine procedure. The detecting device is linked to a monitoring machine.

Printout — Fetal heart rate — Uterine contractions

Detecting devices

Here, the baby's heart beat is picked up by a metal plate strapped to the mother's abdomen (lower belt). A plate beneath the upper belt detects the mother's contractions.

An alternative method is to attach to the baby's head an electrode linked to the monitor by a wire led through the mother's vagina.

THE FIRST STAGE

With the first contractions, the normally thick, tough cervix becomes thinned and softened and is gradually pulled up until it becomes effaced (merged with the walls of the uterus). The cervix then begins to dilate (open) with each contraction. It is fully dilated when the opening is approximately 4 inches (10 cm) in diameter. This stage can take anywhere from a few hours to 12 hours or more for first babies.

Uterus

Cervix

The head emerges
At this point, an episiotomy is sometimes performed to prevent tissues from tearing.

THE SECOND STAGE

As the baby's head descends, it reaches the pelvic floor muscles, which cause the head to rotate until eventually the baby's chin is pointing down to the woman's rectum. As the baby is pushed farther down, the anus and perineum (the area between the genitalia and anus) begin to bulge out, and soon the baby's head can be seen at the opening of the vagina. As the head emerges, the perineal tissues are stretched very thin; sometimes it is necessary to perform an *episiotomy* to prevent the tissues from tearing. As soon as the baby's head emerges, it turns so that it is once more in line with the rest of the baby's body; the physician usually helps this rotation.

With the next few contractions, first one shoulder and then the other is delivered; then the rest of the baby slides out. After delivery, the umbilical cord is clamped and cut.

Final stage of delivery
Once both shoulders are out, the rest of the baby emerges easily.

THE THIRD STAGE

Within three to 10 minutes after the baby's birth, the placenta (afterbirth) is usually expelled. Drugs such as ergonovine or oxytocin may be used to aid in its expulsion, or the placenta may be manually removed by the physician. Any tears or incisions are cleaned and stitched. This may be done while the mother holds her baby.

Placenta — Umbilical cord

Placenta being delivered
The placenta is usually expelled within a few minutes of the baby's birth.

to contract in preparation for the birth, and these *Braxton Hicks' contractions* may be mistaken for the start of labor. However, when contractions become progressively more painful, regular, and at shorter intervals, then labor has probably started. Two other events may also happen. The mucous plug that has blocked the cervical canal during pregnancy may be expelled as a bloody discharge. This is called a "show" and means that the cervix is beginning to stretch. Rupture of the membranes surrounding the amniotic fluid in which the baby floats may occur at any time up to delivery. The leakage of amniotic fluid, called "breaking of the waters," varies from woman to woman. It may be a slow trickle of fluid from the vagina, or it may be a sudden gush.

STAGES OF LABOR

Labor is divided into several stages that are defined as though they are distinct, but which, in reality, can blend into one another. The latent phase (or prelabor) is a time of irregular contractions, when the cervix thins out and may dilate very gradually. This stage can last many hours. The first stage begins with rapid dilatation of the cervix and ends with full dilatation of the cervix.

After the cervix is fully dilated, the second stage begins; contractions become stronger and the women feels the urge to push (by contracting the voluntary muscles of the diaphragm and abdominal wall). She is advised to push only during a contraction.

The third stage of labor—expulsion of the placenta (afterbirth)—usually occurs within three to 10 minutes after delivery of the baby. Sometimes, medication such as ergonovine or oxytocin may be used to aid in the expulsion of the placenta, or the placenta may be removed manually by the physician reaching into the uterus. Any tears or incisions in the vagina are then cleaned and stitched.

Childbirth, complications of

Difficulties and complications occurring after the onset of labor. These complications may be associated with the mother or the baby, or both. Some are potentially life-threatening, especially to the baby, because they may impair its oxygen supply and cause brain damage (see *Fetal distress*).

MATERNAL PROBLEMS

If contractions begin, or if the membranes rupture, before 37 weeks' gestation, premature labor may occur, with the risk of delivery of a small, immature baby who may not be developed adequately to survive (see *Prematurity*). Drugs such as albuterol and ritodrine can sometimes stop premature labor. However, if the gestation period is more than 34 weeks and hospital conditions are suitable, the labor may be allowed to progress. Premature rupture of the membranes can also lead to infection in the uterus, which must be treated with delivery and antibiotics.

Slow progress early in a normal labor is most often the result of failure of the cervix to dilate, usually due to inadequate contractions of the uterine muscles. This is often treated by giving intravenous infusions of synthetic oxytocin to augment the naturally occurring oxytocin that causes the muscles of the uterus to contract during labor.

The mother may tire during a long labor so that she is unable to push strongly enough, or the muscular contractions of the uterus may be ineffective; in these cases *forceps delivery*, *vacuum extraction*, or even *cesarean section* may be required.

A major hazard in childbirth is blood loss. This may occur before the delivery (see *Antepartum hemorrhage*), either because the placenta separates from the wall of the uterus too early or, less commonly, because the placenta lies over the opening of the cervix instead of being attached to the wall of the uterus, a condition called *placenta previa*. Blood loss after the delivery (*postpartum hemorrhage*) is usually due either to failure of the uterus to contract normally after the child has been expelled or to retention of part of the placenta. With blood transfusions, complications from hemorrhage have decreased dramatically in the last 40 years.

In rare instances, women suffer from *eclampsia* (convulsions associated with raised blood pressure) during or just prior to the onset of labor. This is treated by giving anticonvulsant drugs and oxygen and inducing labor or performing a cesarean section.

FETAL PROBLEMS

If the baby is in a malposition (not lying in the normal headdown position in the uterus), vaginal delivery may be difficult or impossible. A baby in the breech position (bottom downward) can be delivered vaginally, although delivery by cesarean section may be preferable (see *Breech delivery*). A baby lying horizontally is always delivered by cesarean section because the arm and shoulder usually become jammed in the pelvis.

Multiple pregnancies (see *Pregnancy, multiple*) may be a problem during delivery because it is often difficult to predict the position of subsequent babies. It is also more likely that such babies will be born prematurely.

FETAL-MATERNAL PROBLEMS

Sometimes the mother's pelvis is too small in proportion to the baby's head (known as cephalopelvic disproportion), making vaginal delivery impossible or hazardous. In these cases, cesarean section is usually necessary.

PAIN RELIEF IN LABOR AND DELIVERY

Method	Why given	Possible effects on baby
Narcotic analgesics	Routine pain relief during labor	Less responsive at birth; respiratory problems, particularly in premature babies
Epidural	Routine pain relief during labor and childbirth, forceps delivery, and cesarean section	Brief drop in fetal heart rate; fetal monitoring is recommended during and after the procedure
Paracervical block	Pain relief during active labor (after the fetal head is engaged)	Drop in fetal heart rate; respiratory problems
Pudendal block	Forceps delivery	None
Local anesthetic into perineum	Forceps delivery, episiotomy, repair perineal tear	None
General anesthesia	Cesarean section	Reduced responsiveness at birth; respiratory problems, particularly in premature babies

C

FIRST AID: EMERGENCY CHILDBIRTH

PREPARING FOR THE BIRTH

1 Summon medical help and reassure the mother. Stay calm—most births are normal and natural.

2 Wash hands and scrub nails under running water. Do not dry them. Wash hands frequently during the birth. Make sure everything you use is clean: bedding, sheets, towels, and cloths.

3 Prepare a flat surface, using a clean sheet or towel, a plastic sheet, or fresh newspaper.

4 Prop the mother up with pillows. Her legs should be bent and apart, and the feet flat.

WARNING
DO NOT attempt to delay the birth by crossing the mother's legs or pushing in the baby's head. This is very harmful.

YOU WILL NEED
- Sterilized scissors (boil for 10 minutes and wrap in clean cloth).
- Clean pieces of string, boot laces, or strips of cloth about 9 inches (22 cm) long for tying the cord.
- Container in case the mother vomits.
- Container or plastic bag for the afterbirth (which must be taken to a physician for examination).
- Sanitary napkins or clean cloth to place over the mother's vagina after the birth.
- Cradle (or a box or drawer) and soft blanket for the baby.

1 As the baby's head emerges, support it with cupped hands. If a membrane covers the face, tear it with your hands and remove quickly. If the cord is looped around the neck, ease it gently over the head. DO NOT touch the baby's head until it is out.

2 Support the shoulders as they emerge. One appears first, the second follows easily if you carefully raise the head. DO NOT pull on the baby's head.

3 Support the body as it comes out. Using a clean cloth, wipe away any mucus or blood from the baby's mouth.

4 If the baby fails to breathe immediately, hold the head lower than the body to drain mucus away. DO NOT slap the baby on the back. Blow hard on the chest or tap the soles of the feet. If these methods fail, start *artificial respiration*.

5 When the cord has stopped pulsating, tie it firmly once 6 to 8 inches (15 to 20 cm) away from the baby and again 2 to 4 inches (5 to 10 cm) away. Cut between the ties with sterilized scissors. Wrap the baby and place on the mother's abdomen.

6 The afterbirth is delivered within 10 minutes. To help control blood flow, place a hand on the mother's abdomen and gently massage the uterus every few minutes until it feels firm. DO NOT pull on the cord to deliver the afterbirth.

Child development

Children acquire physical, mental, and social skills in well-recognized stages called developmental milestones. Although there is wide variation in the rate at which each child progresses, most children develop certain skills by a predictable age.

FACTORS AFFECTING DEVELOPMENT

A child becomes capable of developing certain skills only as his or her nervous system matures. The rate at which maturity occurs is determined genetically for each individual and modified by environmental factors in the uterus and after birth. For instance, girls often begin to walk and/or talk at an earlier age than boys. Premature children miss out on some growing time in the uterus; the time they take to progress should be calculated from the full-term pregnancy date, not the actual date of birth.

Sight and hearing are both crucial to a child's general developmental progress; any defect will affect the child's ability to watch, listen, learn, and imitate. Intelligence also affects a child's development, especially in the acquisition of speech and the ability to coordinate muscles for precise movements, such as holding a pencil.

The home environment plays an important part in developing the child's potential for certain skills. Speaking to and playing with children is essential for language development and for practicing new physical skills. Introducing children to other children at the age of 2 or 3 years provides them with plenty of stimulation.

HOW A CHILD DEVELOPS SKILLS

Reflex actions present at birth gradually disappear as the child learns to perform voluntary actions and develops sufficient muscle strength and control to perform them. Often, the child's actions progress from seemingly unconnected movements to the ability to control part of his or her body. In most children, development begins with control of the head and progresses down the body until control of the arms, trunk, and legs is attained. Walking is achieved in numerous stages, from lying with head raised, to sitting unsupported, to crawling, to toddling, to standing, and, finally, to walking unaided.

A baby begins to develop hand-eye coordination from birth. He or she watches objects, learns to focus and to judge distances, and develops the connection of seeing and doing by watching his or her hands. Both hand-eye and body-limb coordination can

be encouraged in an older child (by practicing ball games, for example).

At birth, a child communicates his or her needs by crying. After vision and hearing are sufficiently well developed, a child watches the parent's mouth intently to learn how to smile and listens to the parent speaking before attempting to imitate sounds. A child is able to concentrate on learning only one skill at a time, often forgetting a recently mastered skill that will appear again some time in the future.

DEVELOPMENTAL MILESTONES

When assessing the development of a child, specialists in child development look at abilities in four main areas: locomotion, hearing and speech, vision and fine movement, and social behavior and play. All children acquire skills in much the same order—for example, a child will not stand before learning to sit. The rate at which these skills are acquired varies enormously; a more detailed professional investigation is necessary (see *Developmental delay*) only if a child's progress is significantly out of line or if the parent is concerned for some other reason. (See next page.)

Child guidance

Multidisciplinary diagnosis and advice for a child who is suffering from emotional or *behavioral problems*. The problems may include poor school performance, disruptive behavior at school or at home, other behavioral problems, breaking the law, or using drugs.

SOURCES OF HELP

Trained professionals and lay workers from a number of fields offer help to such children and their families. A physician will arrange referral to the most appropriate team for assessment and, possibly, therapy.

Psychiatrists are medical doctors with a special interest and training in the field of mental problems. Their techniques may range from *psychotherapy* to treatment with drugs.

Clinical and educational *psychologists* are nonmedical specialists whose main role is diagnosis and assessment by means of intelligence and personality tests. They may also assess a child's progress during treatment. Many clinical psychologists also provide psychotherapy.

Psychiatric social workers are also nonmedical specialists. They are trained to deal with family problems and relationships within the family. In some instances they may be given

legal responsibility for children with severe personality or family problems.

These specialists often work closely together, either in hospital pediatric departments, schools, or special child-guidance clinics, using *counseling, group therapy,* or *family therapy.*

Chill

A shivering attack accompanied by chattering teeth, pale skin, goose bumps, and a cold feeling. It frequently precedes a fever, usually one caused by an infection. Treatment includes drinking plenty of fluids. A physician should be consulted if the condition persists.

Chinese medicine

Most of the various techniques of traditional Chinese medicine are based on the theory that there is a universal life force, called "chi," that manifests itself in the body as two complementary qualities known as "yin" and "yang." According to traditional beliefs, the vigorous yang and restraining yin must be balanced, and the chi must flow evenly for good health. An imbalance in the yin and yang and disruption of the flow of chi produce illness. Traditional Chinese treatments therefore aim to restore the yin-yang balance and normalize the flow of chi. To achieve this aim various techniques have evolved, notably *acupressure, acupuncture,* Chinese *herbal medicine,* and *t'ai chi.*

In general, these treatments are incompatible with orthodox Western medicine and most physicians do not recommend them. However, some techniques may help when standard treatment has not been effective.

Chinese restaurant syndrome

A short-lived illness that some people develop after eating food containing *monosodium glutamate* (MSG). Only about 5 percent of the population is susceptible to it.

SYMPTOMS AND PREVENTION

The most common symptoms, which usually occur within three hours of a meal, are pain in the neck and chest, a hot feeling, heart palpitations, and headache. Nausea, dizziness, and other symptoms have also been reported, and some people compare Chinese restaurant syndrome to the effects of migraine.

The symptoms pass and have no long-term effects. Affected people should avoid food containing MSG as an additive. Many "fast foods" may also contain the additive.

CHILD DEVELOPMENT

LOCOMOTION

By 6 months, babies lift up their heads and chests and roll from front to back and from back to front. They can sit up with support, bounce up and down, and bear weight on their legs if supported.

9-month-old children try to crawl, sit without support, pull themselves up to standing or sitting positions, and step purposefully on alternate feet if supported.

1-year-old children crawl on hands and knees, walk around furniture (holding on), and may walk alone or with one hand held.

At 18 months, children can walk well with feet closer together, can stoop to pick up objects, run with care, walk upstairs with one hand held, and crawl backward downstairs.

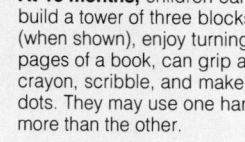

VISION AND FINE MOVEMENT

By 6 months, babies look intently at everything and everybody. They follow moving objects with their eyes and reach out for objects with one or both hands. Objects are transferred from hand to hand and brought to the mouth.

9 month olds are visually very alert. Grasp involves mostly the index and middle fingers. They can manipulate objects with both hands, but have difficulty voluntarily releasing grasped objects.

1-year-old children can grasp small objects well and release grasped objects easily. Both hands are used equally. They can hold a block in each hand and bang the blocks together.

At 18 months, children can build a tower of three blocks (when shown), enjoy turning pages of a book, can grip a crayon, scribble, and make dots. They may use one hand more than the other.

HEARING, UNDERSTANDING, AND SPEECH

By 6 months, babies turn their heads to locate sources of sound and have begun to understand the tone of their mothers' voices. They enjoy making vowel sounds and tuneful noises. They laugh, chuckle, and squeal.

9 month olds listen to sounds and understand "no" and other words. They babble in long strings (making sounds such as ba-ba, da-da, ma-ma) and start using sound to attract attention. (Deaf babies' utterances are monotonous and do not develop in complexity.)

1-year-old children turn when they hear their own names. They have some understanding of how other people feel, know what most household objects are used for, may babble meaningfully to themselves, and may say two or three words.

At 18 months, children comprehend short communications spoken directly to them, but do not understand the difference between statements, commands, and questions. Vocabulary may contain six to 20 words.

SOCIAL BEHAVIOR AND PLAY

6 month olds enjoy looking at their images in mirrors and playing peekaboo games. They can grasp objects and also shake, bang, and otherwise manipulate them. However, they will not look for objects that are shown and then hidden. They are shy with strangers.

9 month olds look for objects that are shown and then hidden, thus showing the beginnings of memory. They imitate hand clapping, wave bye-bye, and show great determination in getting objects. They continue to be shy with strangers.

1-year-old children spend less time putting objects in their mouths and more time releasing objects—throwing them, dropping them, putting them in boxes. They play pat-a-cake and like to be around a familiar adult to whom they demonstrate affection.

At 18 months, children actively explore their homes. They enjoy putting things in and taking things out of boxes and looking at picture books. They use spoons and cups and can take off their shoes and socks. They are also determined, impetuous, selfish, and cannot be reasoned with. They alternate between clinging to a familiar adult and struggling to break free.

C

LOCOMOTION

2 year olds climb furniture and walk up and down stairs (with two feet to each step).

3 year olds can climb with agility, throw and kick balls, ride tricycles, and run around corners.

4 year olds walk up and down stairs with one foot on each step, and can stand, walk, and run on tiptoe.

5 year olds can stand and hop on one foot, and are skillful in rolling, sliding, and swinging.

VISION AND FINE MOVEMENT

2 year olds can build towers of six or seven blocks, can unscrew a lid, and show a definite right- or left-handedness.

3 year olds hold crayons with an adult grasp and can undo buttons, but may need help buttoning them up. Their handedness is clearly established.

4 year olds hold a pencil with a mature grasp, can copy simple letters (i.e., O,T,H, or V), and can build a tower of more than 10 blocks.

5 year olds can match 10 or 12 colors, can copy many more letters, and can draw the full body of a person with a recognizable head and facial features.

HEARING, UNDERSTANDING, AND SPEECH

2 year olds begin to listen to general conversation. They obey simple instructions and can use 50 or more words meaningfully. They constantly talk to themselves and can put two or more words together to communicate.

3 year olds listen to general conversation and enjoy nursery stories. They understand the difference between statements, commands, and questions. They have large vocabularies and speak clearly in sentences, but there may be some errors.

4 year olds can repeat softly spoken words at a distance of three feet. They speak fluently and with correct grammar and can provide their full names, ages, and addresses. They tell long stories, confusing fact and fantasy.

5 year olds enjoy reciting rhymes, telling stories, and having books read to them.

SOCIAL BEHAVIOR AND PLAY

2 year olds ask the names of everything and enjoy participating in nursery rhymes and songs. They ask for food and drink and indicate toilet needs. They begin to play with toys more imaginatively, though they may not like to share them. They are constantly demanding and will throw tantrums if their desires are thwarted.

3 year olds constantly ask questions. They can dress and undress and eat with a fork and spoon. They are dry and clean during the day and sometimes at night. Three year olds can play with toys imaginatively and will share with others. They can be reasoned with and have fewer tantrums. They are also more affectionate to younger siblings.

4 year olds continue to ask questions constantly. They are more independent and skillful in dressing, undressing, eating, and washing. They need to play with other children and can share with others. They can understand past, present, and future.

5 year olds ask the meaning of abstract words. They like to build complex structures out of bricks or other objects. They continue in imaginative and dramatic play. They enjoy companionship and understand the need for rules and fair play. They have an understanding of time and are generally sensible, restrained, and independent.

Chiropody
See *Podiatry*.

Chiropractic
A theory of healing based on the belief that disease results from a lack of normal nerve function. Chiropractic relies on physical manipulation and adjustment of the spine for therapy, rather than on drugs or surgery. Physicians believe that no scientific basis for chiropractic theory has ever been established and that it is ineffective in the treatment of such common ailments as hypertension, heart disease, stroke, cancer, diabetes, and infectious diseases.

Chlamydial infections
Chlamydiae are a group of microorganisms, intermediate in size between bacteria and viruses, that cause various infectious diseases in humans and animals (particularly birds). Like viruses, they can multiply only by first invading the cells of another life-form; otherwise, they behave more like bacteria than viruses and are susceptible to treatment with antibiotic drugs.

Two main species of chlamydiae cause disease in humans. Different strains of CHLAMYDIA TRACHOMATIS are responsible for various genital, eye, and lymph node infections. CHLAMYDIA PSITTACI mainly affects birds, but is occasionally spread to humans as a lung infection.

CHLAMYDIA TRACHOMATIS INFECTIONS

GENITAL INFECTIONS In the tropics, strains of CHLAMYDIA TRACHOMATIS cause the sexually transmitted disease *lymphogranuloma venereum*.

In developed countries, by far the most important impact of CHLAMYDIA TRACHOMATIS is its role as a cause of *nonspecific urethritis* (NSU), or nongonococcal genital infection. This is the most common sexually transmitted disease in the US, and in almost 50 percent of cases it is due to a chlamydial infection.

In men, nonspecific urethritis may cause a discharge from the penis and complications such as swelling of the testes, which, if untreated may lead to infertility. In women, NSU is usually symptomless, but may cause a vaginal discharge or pain on passing urine, and may lead to *cervicitis* (inflammation of the cervix) or cause complications such as *salpingitis* (inflammation of the fallopian tubes). In the US, an estimated 5 to 13 percent of all women have a chlamydial infection of the cervix (which is often symptomless).

Treatment is with antibiotics such as tetracycline or erythromycin and is usually rapidly successful. Treatment of sexual partners is advisable to prevent reinfection.

EYE INFECTIONS A child born to a woman with a chlamydial infection of the cervix may acquire an acute eye infection called neonatal *ophthalmia*.

In parts of Africa and Asia, usually where hygiene is lacking, certain strains of CHLAMYDIA TRACHOMATIS cause the serious eye disease *trachoma*. It is spread from eye to eye by flies and is the most important cause of blindness worldwide.

RESPIRATORY INFECTIONS CHLAMYDIA TRACHOMATIS is a major cause of pneumonia among infants in the US; up to three or four newborn babies per 1,000 are affected, and 50 percent of the children usually also have an eye infection. The main symptoms are breathing difficulty and a staccato cough, but no fever. Treatment is with antibiotic drugs.

CHLAMYDIA PSITTACI

The only disease that can be caused by CHLAMYDIA PSITTACI in humans is a type of pneumonia called *psittacosis*. It is a rare infection, usually contracted from parrots, parakeets, pigeons, or poultry. The disease can be treated with antibiotics, but it may be fatal in elderly and debilitated patients.

Chloasma
A condition, also called melasma, in which blotches of pale, green-brown skin pigmentation appear on the face. Chloasma may occur during pregnancy, around the time of the menopause, or in women who have been taking birth-control pills.

The blotches occur on the forehead, cheeks, and nose, and sometimes merge, forming the "mask of pregnancy." The pigmentation is aggravated by sunlight. It usually fades gradually, but may be permanent or recur in successive pregnancies.

There is no treatment, although avoiding direct sunlight and changing the brand of birth-control pill (if appropriate) may help.

Chloral hydrate
One of the oldest *sleeping drugs* in use today. It is mainly used as a short-term treatment for insomnia, especially in the elderly.

Chlorambucil
An *anticancer drug* used to treat some types of cancer, including Hodgkin's lymphoma and cancer of the ovary.

Chloramphenicol
An *antibiotic drug* widely prescribed as eye drops or an ointment to treat *conjunctivitis* caused by a bacterial infection. In tablet or injection form, chloramphenicol is used only in the hospital for the treatment of serious infections that are resistant to safer antibiotics. Chloramphenicol given in these ways carries a risk of causing aplastic *anemia* (a complete shutdown of the bone marrow's production of red cells, white cells, and platelets).

Chlorate poisoning
Chemicals present in some defoliant weed killers that, if swallowed, cause kidney and liver damage, corrosion of the intestine, and methemoglobinemia (a chemical change in the blood pigment hemoglobin). Even small doses can prove fatal, especially in children. Symptoms of poisoning include ulceration in the mouth, abdominal pain, and diarrhea.

If chlorate poisoning is known or suspected, medical help should be obtained immediately. If these substances have been spilled onto the skin or into the eyes, they should be washed off with plenty of water.

Chlordiazepoxide
A *benzodiazepine drug* used mainly to treat anxiety, but also in the management of alcohol withdrawal.

Chloroform
A colorless liquid producing a vapor that, if inhaled, acts as a general anesthetic (see *Anesthesia, general*). Formerly, it was used widely for operative procedures but it caused a high incidence of liver damage and heart problems and has now been replaced by safer drugs.

Chloroform is still occasionally used as an emergency anesthetic for major first aid or field surgery. Its main use today is as a flavoring and preservative for other medicines.

Chloroquine
A drug used in the prevention and treatment of *malaria* and occasionally as an *antirheumatic drug*.

When taken to prevent malaria, chloroquine is usually prescribed with other drugs to avoid problems of drug-resistant strains. Chloroquine remains the main treatment of acute attacks of malaria.

Chloroquine is used to treat *rheumatoid arthritis* and *lupus erythematosus* that have not responded to other drugs.

Possible side effects are nausea, headache, diarrhea, and abdominal cramps. Long-term treatment (as for rheumatoid arthritis) can damage the retina, causing blindness.

Chlorosis

A severe form of iron-deficiency *anemia* characterized by a yellow-green tinge to the skin. During the nineteenth century and before World War I, chlorosis was a common condition among underfed adolescent girls. This form of anemia has now virtually disappeared.

Chlorothiazide

One of the thiazide group of *diuretic drugs* often used as a treatment for *hypertension* (high blood pressure) and edema (fluid retention). It also reduces the amount of calcium excreted in the urine and is therefore sometimes used to prevent the recurrence of certain types of kidney stone.

Chlorpheniramine

An *antihistamine drug* used in the treatment of allergies such as allergic *rhinitis* (hay fever), allergic *conjunctivitis*, *urticaria* (hives), and *angioedema* (allergic facial swelling). It is also a common ingredient of over-the-counter *cold remedies*.

Chlorpromazine

ANTIPSYCHOTIC		
Tablet Liquid Injection Rectal suppository		
℞ Prescription needed		
Available as generic		

The first *antipsychotic drug* to be marketed. Introduced in the early 1950s, it remains one of the most widely used of this group of drugs. It suppresses abnormal behavior, reduces aggression, and has a tranquilizing effect.

WHY IT IS USED

Chlorpromazine is used in the treatment of schizophrenia, mania, dementia, and other disorders in which confused or abnormal behavior may occur. It does not cure the underlying disorder, but does relieve distressing symptoms.

Another use of chlorpromazine is in the treatment of nausea and vomiting, especially if caused by drug treatment, radiation therapy, or anesthetics.

POSSIBLE ADVERSE EFFECTS

Chlorpromazine sometimes produces serious side effects. These include uncontrollable movements of the face and limbs similar to those in *Parkinson's disease*, slowed reactions, and blurred vision; driving and operating machinery should be avoided. Alcohol should not be drunk when taking chlorpromazine because it increases the sedative effect.

Chlorpropamide

A drug used to treat *diabetes mellitus*. (See *Hypoglycemics, oral*.)

Chlorthalidone

One of the thiazide group of *diuretic drugs*, chlorthalidone is used to treat *hypertension* (high blood pressure) and *heart failure*. It reduces the amount of calcium in the urine and is sometimes used to prevent the recurrence of certain types of kidney stone.

Chlorzoxazone

A *muscle-relaxant drug* used mainly to treat painful muscle spasm caused by injury, strain, or misuse.

Choking

Partial or complete inability to breathe due to an obstruction of the airway, usually by food, drink, or an inhaled or swallowed foreign body. If the blockage is only partial, the choking person can usually inhale enough air to cough out the obstruction. If the airway is completely blocked, the person will be unable to breathe and, unless the blockage is cleared, he or she will die of suffocation.

CAUSES

Choking is caused by blockage of any part of the airway—the pharynx (throat), larynx (voice box), trachea

---

FIRST AID: CHOKING

CONSCIOUS VICTIM

1 A person clutching his or her throat is giving the universal distress signal for a foreign body blocking the air passage.

2 Clasp the victim, placing one fist just under the sternum and grasping the fist with the other hand. Then make a quick, hard, thrusting movement inward and upward.

UNCONSCIOUS VICTIM

1 Place the heel of one hand against the middle of the victim's abdomen, slightly above the navel; place your other hand on top. Press in with a quick upward thrust.

2 If this fails, try to remove the obstruction. If the victim is still unconscious, summon emergency help. If breathing has stopped, start *artificial respiration*.

C

FIRST AID: CHOKING

INFANT

Straddle the baby over your arm with the head lower than the trunk, supporting the head by holding the baby's jaw. Deliver four back blows between the shoulder blades.

CHILD

Place the heel of one hand slightly above the navel and well below the rib cage. Place the other hand on top and press down with a quick, upward thrust.

(windpipe), or bronchi (air passages from the trachea into the lungs). Most cases of choking occur when food or drink "goes down the wrong way," that is, when it enters the trachea (airway) and bronchi instead of passing from the pharynx into the esophagus. Although this can be an alarming experience, it is normally corrected by a bout of coughing.

Obstruction by something that partially blocks the airway is more serious. In adults the cause is usually a fishbone or a piece of meat. In children, who are more vulnerable to this type of choking because their airways are narrower, the obstruction is often a peanut or small plaything, such as a bead. Less commonly, choking may be due to aspiration (inhaling vomit) during a bout of coughing.

TREATMENT
Emergency medical help should be summoned if the obstruction cannot be cleared. The physician will probably try to clear the blockage manually; if this fails, an emergency *tracheostomy* (making an incision into the trachea and inserting a tube through it into the lungs), will be performed. With the airway restored, the physician can then use a laryngoscope, bronchoscope, or esophagoscope (viewing tubes through which instruments can be passed) to locate and clear the obstruction (see *Laryngoscopy*; *Bronchoscopy*; *Esophagoscopy*).

Cholangiocarcinoma
A malignant growth in one of the ducts that carries bile from the liver and gallbladder to the small intestine. The disease is rare, with less than one new case per 100,000 of the population each year in the US. The cause of the cancer is unknown. The main symptoms of cholangiocarcinoma are jaundice and weight loss.

Cholangiography
A procedure that enables the bile ducts to be seen on X-ray film after they have first been filled with a contrast medium (a substance that is opaque to X rays).
WHY IT IS DONE
Cholangiography is used when people who have had their gallbladders removed are suspected of having biliary stones. Biliary stones are similar to gallstones, but they form in the bile ducts instead of the gallbladder. Cholangiography is usually employed as a follow-up to *ultrasound scanning* if it has failed to establish the presence of stones. Cholangiography is also performed during an operation to remove the gallbladder to ensure that no stones have been left behind in the bile ducts. Cholangiography is also useful for diagnosing narrowing or tumors of the bile ducts.
HOW IT IS DONE
The contrast medium may be injected slowly into a vein, in which case the liver will excrete it several hours later in bile into the ducts (in this case, images are somewhat less satisfactory than those obtained by the following methods). Or the contrast medium may be injected directly into the ducts. This is done either through an endoscope (a flexible viewing instrument) passed into the ducts via the mouth, stomach, and duodenum (see *ERCP*), or by means of a long, fine needle inserted through the abdomen into

the liver. Once the ducts have filled, X-ray pictures are taken and any stones are apparent.

Cholangitis
Inflammation of the common bile duct (see *Biliary system*). There are two types: acute ascending cholangitis and sclerosing cholangitis.
ACUTE ASCENDING CHOLANGITIS
This type is usually due to bacterial infection of the duct and its content of bile. It generally occurs with a blockage of the duct—by a gallstone, tumor, following surgery, or, in some parts of the world, infestation of the duct by a worm or fluke (see *Bile duct obstruction*). The infection moves up the duct and may affect the liver.

The main symptoms are recurrent bouts of jaundice, abdominal pain, and chills and fever. Attacks may vary from mild episodes to a severe, life-threatening illness with *septicemia* (spread and multiplication of bacteria in the bloodstream) and *kidney failure* from toxins circulating in the blood.

The infection is usually diagnosed from the patient's symptoms, although investigations such as *liver function tests* and *ultrasound scanning* may also be carried out.

Mild cases are treated with antibiotics and a high intake of fluids. In severe cases, if there is no improvement within 24 hours, the infected material is drained from the bile duct by surgery or endoscopy.

Once the patient has recovered, the cause of the blockage must be determined and appropriate treatment of the cause of the obstruction provided (see *Bile duct obstruction*).
SCLEROSING CHOLANGITIS
In this rare condition, all the bile ducts, within and outside the liver, become narrowed; the liver is progressively damaged. No treatment is available other than the possibility of a *liver transplant*. The drug cholestyramine may relieve itching.

Chole-
A prefix relating to the bile or biliary system, as in cholelithiasis (the formation of stones in the biliary system).

Cholecalciferol
An alternative name for vitamin D_3 (see *Vitamin D*).

Cholecystectomy
Surgery to remove the gallbladder.
WHY IT IS DONE
Cholecystectomy is usually performed to deal with the presence in

PROCEDURE FOR CHOLECYSTECTOMY

If simple removal of the gallbladder is performed, it will take approximately an hour. However, more extensive exploration of the ducts may prolong the procedure.

With the patient under general anesthesia, an incision is made under the rib cage on the right-hand side; the cut may be vertical, horizontal, or oblique, according to the patient's build.

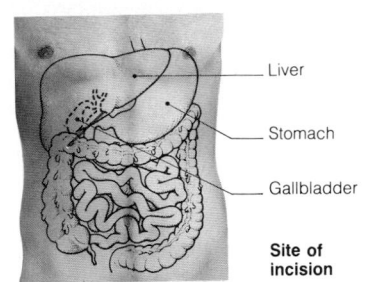

Liver

Stomach

Gallbladder

Site of incision

1 Gallstones, as shown by an ultrasound scan or by a cholecystogram (X-ray image of the gallbladder) such as the one above, increase in prevalence with age.

2 After an incision has been made, the liver is pulled up to expose the gallbladder. The thin membrane covering it is incised so that the cystic duct and artery can be identified.

3 The artery to the gallbladder and the cystic duct leading from it are tied and cut, and the gallbladder is removed. If the person has jaundice, X rays are taken to ensure that there are no stones in the common bile duct. If the X ray reveals the presence of stones, they are removed.

4 Drains are placed under the liver (and in the bile duct if it was opened) and the abdominal incision is closed. The two drains are removed, respectively, 48 hours and eight to 10 days later, after another X ray shows there are no more stones.

the gallbladder of troublesome *gallstones*, often because they are causing recurrent attacks of *biliary colic* (pain). Many surgeons advocate cholecystectomy at an early stage to treat acute *cholecystitis* (infection of the gallbladder). Emergency cholecystectomy is occasionally required for perforation (bursting) or *empyema* (pus formation) within the gallbladder.

Many gastroenterologists believe that gallbladders should not be removed if they contain stones that are not causing any symptoms.

HOW IT IS DONE

Simple cholecystectomy takes almost one hour, but duct exploration may add considerably to this time. Most patients are out of the hospital within five to seven days. (See box.)

RISKS AND OUTLOOK

The chief risk is inadvertent damage to the common bile duct. Severe inflammation sometimes obscures the anatomy and the surgeon may decide it is safer to perform a cholecystostomy (removal of gallstones by opening but not removing the gallbladder).

The outcome of cholecystectomy operations is generally good—symptoms are relieved completely in 90 percent of patients. About three weeks should be allowed for recovery from the operation.

Cholecystitis

Inflammation of the gallbladder, causing severe abdominal pain. There are two types: acute and chronic.

CAUSES

Acute cholecystitis is almost always caused by a *gallstone* obstructing the outlet (cystic duct) from the gallbladder. The trapped bile becomes concentrated by absorption of its water content and causes chemical irritation of the gallbladder walls; this is followed by bacterial infection of the stagnating bile.

Repeated mild attacks of acute cholecystitis can lead to chronic cholecystitis, in which the gallbladder walls thicken and the gallbladder shrinks and ceases to store bile. Whether chronic cholecystitis produces recognizable symptoms that justify surgery is controversial.

SYMPTOMS AND COMPLICATIONS

The main symptom of acute cholecystitis is severe constant pain in the right side of the abdomen, just under the ribs, which worsens on movement. The pain is accompanied by fever and, occasionally, jaundice.

In some people, complications develop. Complications may include *empyema* (in which the gallbladder fills with pus) and *peritonitis* (inflammation of the lining of the abdominal cavity) if the gallbladder bursts. In either event the patient is extremely sick and surgery is urgently needed.

The ill-defined gastrointestinal symptoms attributed to chronic cholecystitis are indigestion, vague pains in the upper abdomen, nausea, and belching. These symptoms may be aggravated by eating fatty food and are not invariably relieved by *cholecystectomy*.

DIAGNOSIS AND TREATMENT

A provisional diagnosis of acute cholecystitis is made by listening to a description of the symptoms and by performing a physical examination. The patient is usually admitted to the

C

C

hospital at once and given analgesics (painkillers), antibiotics, and an *intravenous infusion* to provide nutrients and fluid. *Ultrasound scanning* or *radionuclide scanning* may be used to make a firm diagnosis and exclude other possible causes of the pain, such as a perforated duodenal ulcer (see *Abdominal pain*).

Most cases subside without the need for urgent surgery, but, to prevent recurrences, the patient is usually advised to have a cholecystectomy (surgical removal of the gallbladder), which can be performed either during the initial attack or after an interval of several weeks. The same treatment is usually advised for chronic cholecystitis although the results are less certain. Loss of the gallbladder has little adverse effect on the digestive system.

Cholecystography

An X-ray procedure for examining the gallbladder and common bile duct after they have been filled with a contrast medium (a substance opaque to X rays). The main use of the technique is to detect gallstones, usually as a follow-up procedure to *ultrasound* if this test has failed to enable a definite diagnosis to be made. Cholecystography is not the procedure chosen first to study the gallbladder and is performed much less frequently than it once was.

HOW IT IS DONE

The patient swallows or is injected with contrast medium, which, after about 12 hours, is excreted by the liver into the bile. The opaque bile is stored by the gallbladder, which then shows up when X-ray pictures are taken. Gallstones, which do not absorb the contrast medium, appear on the film as "holes."

Cholera

An infection of the small intestine caused by the bacterium *VIBRIO CHOLERAE* (a vibrio is a comma-shaped bacterium). Cholera results in profuse watery diarrhea that in severe untreated cases can lead to rapid dehydration and death. Infection is always acquired by swallowing food or water that has been contaminated with the vibrio.

HISTORY, CAUSE, AND INCIDENCE

Cholera has been known for centuries in northeast India, where outbreaks of the disease occur regularly. In the nineteenth century, with the opening up of world trade routes and the increase in Muslim and Hindu

pilgrimages, cholera spread throughout the world, causing millions of deaths in a series of epidemics.

For the first half of the twentieth century the disease was confined to Asia, but since 1961 a new pandemic (worldwide epidemic) has spread from Indonesia to much of the rest of Asia, Africa, the Mediterranean, and the Gulf Coast of North America.

A handful of cases occurs in the US in most years, mainly among travelers who have returned from a visit to Asia or Africa. Occasionally, cases crop up in areas bordering the Gulf of Mexico and around the Mediterranean. Usually the victim has eaten shellfish, which appear capable of harboring the vibrio bacterium.

SYMPTOMS

Cholera starts suddenly, between one and five days after infection, with diarrhea, often accompanied by vomiting. Over a pint of fluid may be lost each hour in the diarrhea and, if not replaced, this loss of fluid causes death within a few hours. The fluid loss is brought about by the action of a toxin produced by a bacterium that greatly increases the passage of fluid from the bloodstream into the large and small intestines.

TREATMENT

Cholera is treated by replacing the lost fluid with drinks of water containing the correct proportions of various salts and sugar (see *Rehydration therapy*). If dehydration develops despite fluid replacement by mouth, the patient may be given extra fluid by means of intravenous infusion. Antibiotics, such as tetracycline hydrochloride, can shorten the period of diarrhea and infectiousness to others.

Given adequate rehydration, patients usually make a full recovery. In major epidemics following natural disasters, sufficient supplies of clean water may not be available—or so many people become ill simultaneously that there are few left to nurse the sick.

PREVENTION

Worldwide, cholera is controlled by improving sanitation—in particular by ensuring that sewage is not allowed to contaminate water supplies that will later be used for drinking. Travelers to cholera-infected areas should either restrict themselves to bottled drinks or boil all water before drinking.

A vaccine that provides some protection against the disease is advisable when traveling to Africa and to the Middle and Far East. The protection it

gives is short-lived (six months) and precautions still must be taken with drinking water. Usually, no country insists that travelers arriving directly from the US or Europe have a cholera vaccination certificate, but regulations change from time to time, and a certificate is sometimes required if travel has been via a cholera-infected area. International travelers should check vaccination requirements before departure. (See also *Dysentery*; *Gastroenteritis*; *Typhoid fever*.)

Cholestasis

Stagnation of bile in the small bile ducts within the liver, which leads to a characteristic type of jaundice and to liver disease. The obstruction to the flow of bile may be intrahepatic (within the liver) or extrahepatic (in the bile ducts outside the liver).

CAUSES

Intrahepatic cholestasis may be caused by viral *hepatitis* (inflammation of the liver) or may be a side effect of a number of drugs.

The bile ducts outside the liver can become blocked or constricted for a variety of reasons, including gallstones or tumors (see *Bile duct obstruction*); rarely, the ducts are absent from birth (see *Biliary atresia*).

TREATMENT

Extrahepatic bile duct obstruction and biliary atresia can often be treated surgically to guarantee a free passage of bile from the liver to the duodenum.

Drug-induced cholestasis usually disappears if the causative drug is stopped. In the case of viral hepatitis, there is no specific treatment; the flow of bile improves gradually as the liver inflammation resolves.

Cholesteatoma

A rare but serious condition in which skin cells proliferate and debris collects within the middle ear.

Cholesteatoma usually occurs as a result of a long-standing *otitis media* (middle-ear infection) that has caused the eardrum to burst (see *Eardrum, perforated*). In such cases, skin may grow inward from the ear canal into the middle ear. If the cholesteatoma continues untreated, it may grow and damage the small bones in the middle ear and surrounding bony structures.

Cholesteatoma requires surgical removal either through the eardrum or by mastoidectomy (excision of the mastoid bone behind the ear together with the cholesteatoma). If there is residual deafness, a hearing aid may be required.

Cholesterol

Chemically a *lipid*, cholesterol is an important constituent of body cells. It is also involved in the formation of *hormones* and bile salts and in the transport of fats in the bloodstream to tissues throughout the body. Most cholesterol in the blood is made by the liver from a wide variety of foods, but especially from saturated *fats*. However, some cholesterol is absorbed directly from cholesterol-rich foods, such as eggs and dairy products.

Both cholesterol and fats (triglycerides) are transported around the body in the form of lipoproteins. These are particles with a core, made up of cholesterol and triglycerides in varying proportions, and an outer wrapping of phospholipids and apoproteins ("carrier" proteins).

CHOLESTEROL-RELATED DISEASES

The level of cholesterol in the blood—which can be measured by analysis of a blood sample—is influenced by diet, heredity, and metabolic diseases such as *diabetes mellitus*. There is overwhelming evidence that a high blood cholesterol level increases the risk of developing *atherosclerosis* (accumulation of fatty tissue on the inner lining of arteries), and with it the risk of *coronary heart disease* or *stroke*. Recent research has shown that the risk of developing atherosclerosis can be assessed more accurately by measuring the proportions of different types of lipoproteins in the blood. In general, if most cholesterol in the blood is in the form of high density lipoproteins (abbreviated to HDLs), it seems to protect against arterial disease; conversely, if most cholesterol is in the form of low density lipoproteins (LDLs) or very low density lipoproteins (VLDLs), the risk of disease developing is increased.

A group of genetic metabolic disorders, the *hyperlipidemias*, cause abnormally high levels of LDLs in the blood; people with these disorders are susceptible to heart disease and stroke from an early age. Such people may need treatment with low fat diets and drugs to lower the level of LDLs in their blood. People with relatives who have had a heart attack or stroke before age 50 are at risk and should have their blood checked.

Cholestyramine

A *lipid-lowering drug* used to treat some types of *hyperlipidemia* (high levels of fat in the blood). Cholestyramine reduces the amount of bile and cholesterol absorbed into the blood from the small intestine. By reducing the level of bile in the circulation it increases the amount of cholesterol that can be converted into bile in the liver, thereby reducing high levels of cholesterol in the blood.

Cholestyramine is also used to treat diarrhea caused by abnormal digestion and absorption of fats in disorders such as *Crohn's disease*.

Chondritis

Inflammation of a cartilage, usually caused by mechanical pressure, stress, or injury. For example, in costal chondritis the cartilage between the ribs and the sternum (breastbone) becomes inflamed, usually after being stretched forcibly during a bout of coughing or heavy lifting. This causes tenderness over the sternum and pain if pressure is exerted on the ribs at the front of the chest.

The cartilage lining the hip and knee joints may also be affected, eventually leading to *osteoarthritis*.

Chondro-

A prefix that denotes a relationship to *cartilage*, as in chondroblast (or, alternatively, chondroplast), a cell that forms cartilage. The prefixes chondr-, chondri-, and chondrio- are also used to denote cartilage.

Chondromalacia patellae

A painful disorder of the knee, most commonly affecting adolescents, in which the cartilage directly behind the kneecap is damaged. When (rarely) it occurs in adults it is known as retropatellar arthritis.

CAUSE

The cause is uncertain. One theory is that actions such as bicycling or horseback riding, in which the knee is bent more than it is straight, or certain injuries to the knee, weaken the inner part of the main thigh muscle, the quadriceps. The result is that, when the knee is straightened, the kneecap is tilted; instead of sliding smoothly across the lower end of the thigh bone it rubs against it, roughening the smooth cartilage that covers both of the bones.

SYMPTOMS AND DIAGNOSIS

Pain is felt when the knee is straightened and is particularly bad when using stairs. After examination, the physician may use X rays to confirm the diagnosis.

TREATMENT AND OUTLOOK

Analgesics (painkillers) may be given to relieve tenderness in the knee. Treatment consists of strengthening the inner part of the quadriceps by exercises or electrical stimulation, which usually clears up the problem and the pain. If pain persists, it may indicate considerable damage to the cartilage; surgery may be necessary to alter the angle of the kneecap permanently, thus preventing further friction on the cartilage.

In rare, severe cases the kneecap must be removed—an operation that hinders mobility surprisingly little.

Chondromatosis

A condition in which multiple benign tumors, called chondromas, arise within bones. The tumors consist of cartilage cells and most commonly develop in bones of the hand. They occasionally develop in the pelvis.

Usually the tumors cause no symptoms, but occasionally they lead to thinning of the lining of the bone and a resultant fracture, which may occur on its own without injury.

Chondrosarcoma

A cancerous growth of cartilage that can develop within a bone or on its surface, occurring most commonly within large bones, such as the femur (thigh bone), tibia (shin), and humerus (long bone of the upper arm). Chondrosarcoma is one of the more common types of cancer arising in bone, but bone cancers in the overall population are rare.

Chondrosarcoma usually occurs in middle age and may develop from a benign tumor (see *Chondromatosis; Dyschondroplasia*) or from a previously normal area of bone. It causes pain, swelling, and, occasionally, tenderness. X rays will show an abnormal area of bone. The tumor grows slowly and does not spread elsewhere early in this stage, so that amputation of the bone above the tumor usually results in a permanent cure.

Chondrosarcoma is different from an *osteosarcoma* (cancer of bone cells), which has usually spread to other parts of the body (for example, the lungs) before it causes any symptoms.

Chordee

Abnormal bending or curvature of the penis. Chordee most often occurs in males with *hypospadias*, a congenital defect in which the urethral opening lies on the underside of the penis instead of at the tip. An operation to correct the condition is usually performed when the child is about 3 years old. Untreated chordee may make sexual intercourse very difficult.

C

Chorea

A condition characterized by irregular, rapid, jerky movements, or fidgets, usually affecting the face, limbs, and trunk. These movements are involuntary and, unlike *tics*, they are not predictable, but occur at random. Sometimes they resemble fragments of coordinated movements. They disappear in sleep.

TYPES AND CAUSES

Chorea arises from disease or disturbance of structures deep within the brain, in particular the paired nerve cell groups called the *basal ganglia*. Chorea is a feature of two specific diseases called *Huntington's chorea* and *Sydenham's chorea*. It may also occur in pregnancy, when it is called chorea gravidarum. Chorea may be a side effect of certain drugs, including birth-control pills, neuroleptics (for psychiatric disorders), and those used to treat Parkinson's disease; the choreic movements usually disappear when the drug is withdrawn.

In children with *cerebral palsy*, chorea may be combined with *athetosis*, a continuous writhing movement with the inability to maintain a posture. This combination is called choreoathetosis, and it may also occur as a drug side effect.

TREATMENT

If chorea has occurred as a drug side effect, a physician may withdraw the drug or prescribe a substitute. If there is an underlying disease, the physician may prescribe a drug that inhibits nervous system pathways concerned with movement.

Choreoathetosis

A condition that is characterized by uncontrollable movements of the limbs, face, and trunk, which combine the jerky, rapid fidgets characteristic of *chorea* and the slower writhing movements of *athetosis*.

Choriocarcinoma

A rare malignant tumor that develops from the placenta in the uterus. It is a type of *trophoblastic tumor* (a disorder of the tissues derived from the original placental attachment of the fertilized ovum to the wall of the uterus).

INCIDENCE AND CAUSES

Choriocarcinoma occurs in about one in 20,000 pregnancies, usually as a complication of a *hydatidiform mole* (a benign tumor of the trophoblast). Much less frequently, choriocarcinoma follows an abortion; very rarely, it develops after a normal pregnancy. Sometimes the tumor may

develop months or even years after the pregnancy.

If untreated, the tumor invades and destroys the walls of the uterus and may spread to the vagina and vulva. Distant spread may occur to the liver, lungs, brain, and bones.

SYMPTOMS

The tumor may become apparent because of persistent bleeding from the vagina after an abortion or for more than eight weeks after childbirth. There may be no early symptoms, the disease being suspected and diagnosed only after the cancer has spread to the lungs and caused breathlessness and coughing up of blood, or to the brain, producing mental changes.

Any woman who has had a hydatidiform mole (an abnormal pregnancy resulting from an abnormal ovum) must have regular examinations for at least 12 months after it has been removed to check that she shows no signs of choriocarcinoma.

TREATMENT

Successful treatment depends upon diagnosing the disease at an early stage. Diagnostic tests include *ultrasound scanning* and measurement of blood and urine levels of human chorionic gonadotropin (HCG), a hormone normally produced by the placenta. Abnormally high levels of HCG may occur with choriocarcinoma.

Treatment is with *anticancer drugs*, especially methotrexate or dactinomycin. *Hysterectomy* (surgical removal of the uterus) may be necessary if persistent bleeding occurs despite drug treatment. The use of anticancer drugs has reduced the mortality from this formerly highly lethal cancer from 90 percent to 30 percent.

Chorionic villus sampling

A method of diagnosing abnormalities in the fetus during the first three months of pregnancy. A small sample of tissue is taken from the placenta and analyzed in the laboratory. The outpatient procedure provides earlier results than *amniocentesis*.

WHY IT IS DONE

The procedure is usually performed to determine whether a pregnant woman with a family history or an increased risk of a genetic disease, such as *Down's syndrome* or *thalassemia*, is carrying a child affected by the condition. Because the test can also identify the sex of the fetus, it can be used by a woman who is a known carrier of a sex-linked disease (such as *hemophilia*, which affects half the male

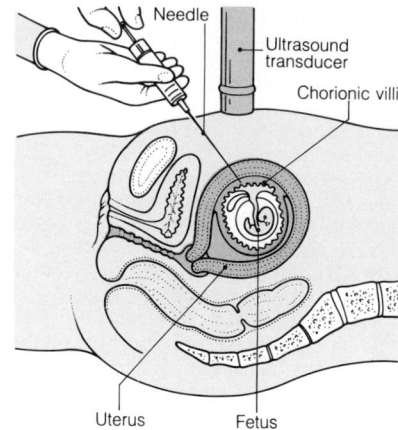

Sampling via the abdomen
A few chorionic villi are sucked through a hollow needle from the placenta.

but few female offspring) to predict the child's odds of having the disease.

HOW IT IS DONE

In some cases the woman is sedated before the sample is taken. The most common method of performing the test is to introduce a tube called a cannula, with a syringe attached, through the vagina and into the uterus. This procedure is controlled by the use of ultrasound or by an endoscope (a viewing tube with a light and lens attached). The syringe is used to suck a few chorionic villi (minute fingerlike projections) from the fetal side of the placenta. The chorionic villi are genetically identical to the fetus.

An alternative method is to insert a hollow needle through the abdominal wall and into the uterus, under ultrasound control, and withdraw some villi through the needle. Both procedures take about half an hour.

Chromosome analysis is done on the cultured villi; cell cultures may be set up if more cells are needed.

RESULTS

If the test reveals genetic abnormalities in the fetus, the parents may choose to terminate the pregnancy (see *Abortion, elective*).

RISKS

The procedure occasionally causes complications, such as perforation of the amniotic sac (the membrane that encloses the fetus), bleeding, and infection. The test itself seems to carry a 1 to 2 percent risk of pregnancy loss. (There is a 3 to 4 percent miscarriage rate in all pregnancies at this stage.) As the procedure becomes more routine, risks should decline.

The advantage lies in the woman's ability to secure an abortion in the first three months of pregnancy if this course is chosen rather than add to the risk to her life by having the abortion later (as is the case when amniocentesis is employed).

Choroid

A layer of blood vessels that lies at the back of the eye behind the retina. Pigment between the blood vessels gives color to the back of the eye that is visible through an *ophthalmoscope* (see *Eye, examination of*). The choroid supplies nutrients and oxygen to the light-sensitive cells in the retina and to surrounding tissues in the eye.

STRUCTURE OF CHOROID

The choroid thickens above and below the lens to form the ciliary body. Ciliary muscles found between it and the lens contract to control the lens' shape.

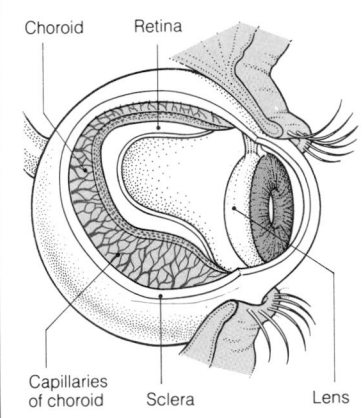

Choroid   Retina

Capillaries of choroid   Sclera   Lens

Choroiditis

Inflammation of the choroid (network of blood vessels that line the back of the eye). It may occur on its own or as part of a generalized inflammation affecting the whole eye. It is commonly caused by infections such as *toxocariasis* or *toxoplasmosis*, more rarely by sarcoidosis, syphilis, and histoplasmosis, or may have no obvious cause.

Treatment may include *corticosteroid drugs* for the inflammation, and *antibiotic drugs* for the eradication of any causative infection.

Christian Science

A religious movement founded by Mary Baker Eddy. Following a near-fatal accident in 1862, she supposedly was healed after reading one of the New Testament healing miracles. Eddy devoted the rest of her life to spreading the ideas of Christian Science. Strict Christian Scientists reject orthodox medicine and will, for example, refuse to allow themselves or members of their families to receive blood transfusions, opting to die rather than break the faith.

Christmas disease

A rare type of *bleeding disorder* caused by a defect in the mechanism of blood coagulation. Christmas disease has very similar features to another bleeding disorder, *hemophilia*, and is sometimes called hemophilia B. It is named for a man named Christmas, the first patient in whom the disease was shown to be distinct from hemophilia, and was first described in 1952.

Both Christmas disease and hemophilia are *genetic disorders* in which there is deficient production of one of the proteins in blood (see *Blood clotting*). In Christmas disease the deficiency is of a protein called factor IX, while in hemophilia the deficiency is of factor VIII.

Chromium

A metallic element that is essential for life because of its vital role in the activities of several *enzymes* (substances that promote biochemical reactions in the body). Chromium is required only in minute amounts (see *Trace elements*); chromium deficiency is unknown. In excess, chromium is toxic, although poisoning is rare. Chromium produces inflammation of the skin and, if inhaled, damages the nose. People exposed to chromium fumes also have a greater risk of developing lung cancer.

Chromosomal abnormalities

Variations from normal in the number or structure of chromosomes contained within a person's cells. In most cases, the chromosomal abnormality is present in all the cells; it may have anything from a lethal to virtually no effect, depending on the particular type of abnormality.

INCIDENCE AND CAUSES

About one in every 200 babies born alive has a chromosomal abnormality. Among spontaneously aborted fetuses, about one in three has such an abnormality; this suggests that most chromosome abnormalities are incompatible with life and that those seen in babies born alive are actually the less serious ones.

The cause in most cases is some fault in the process of chromosome division (see *Chromosomes*), either during the formation of the egg or sperm from which a person is derived, or during the first few divisions of the fertilized egg. Occasionally, one of the parents has an abnormal arrangement of his or her chromosomes.

TYPES

A complete extra set of chromosomes per cell is called polyploidy and is lethal. Other abnormalities can be classified according to whether they involve the 44 autosomes or the two sex chromosomes (see *Chromosomes*). Those affecting the autosomes are slightly less common than sex chromosome abnormalities, but tend to produce more serious and widespread effects.

AUTOSOMAL ABNORMALITIES

An extra autosome means that one of the 22 pairs of autosomes occurs in triplicate instead of as a pair—a phenomenon called *trisomy*. The most common trisomy, occurring in about one in 650 live births, is called *Down's syndrome*; it is due to the presence of three chromosomes labeled number 21. Other trisomies are rare and usually cause multiple physical defects and death soon after birth. All trisomies are more common with advancing maternal age.

Sometimes, a part of a chromosome is missing (for instance, in *cri du chat syndrome*) or an extra bit is present and joined to another chromosome.

All these autosomal abnormalities, as well as others causing physical defects of varying severity, tend to cause mental retardation as well.

Occasionally, a person has a normal chromosomal complement, but part of one autosome is not in its proper position; rather, it is joined to another chromosome—a phenomenon called *translocation*. The person is normal, but some of his or her children may suffer from an abnormality.

SEX CHROMOSOME ABNORMALITIES

About one girl in 2,500 is born with only one X chromosome in her cells instead of two—a condition known as *Turner's syndrome*. The annotation for this is 45 XO, meaning 45 instead of 46 chromosomes, with just a single X chromosome. The condition causes characteristic physical abnormalities, defective female sexual development, and infertility.

All other sex chromosome abnormalities involve extra chromosomes. A boy born with one or more extra X chromosomes has *Klinefelter's*

C

syndrome. The annotation for this is usually 47 XXY or 48 XXXY. Klinefelter's syndrome occurs in about one in 500 male births, although it is often not diagnosed until puberty. The condition causes defective male sexual development, infertility, and, in some cases, mental retardation.

Some women are born with an extra X chromosome (47 XXX) and men with an extra Y chromosome (47 XYY). These people are usually normal physically, but may have an increased risk of mental retardation and perhaps psychological problems. The presence of the extra chromosome is recognized only if a special attempt is made to discover it.

DIAGNOSIS AND TREATMENT

Abnormalities are diagnosed by *chromosome analysis*, which is now possible early in pregnancy using *chorionic villus sampling*. Because of the fundamental nature of these defects—affecting every one of a person's cells—no "cure" is possible. Most babies with autosomal chromosomal defects, apart from those with Down's syndrome, do not survive long. Children and adults with Down's syndrome, although handicapped, can usually integrate well into the community, living at home and even working at a modest job. Hormonal and/or surgical treatment can help correct some of the developmental defects characteristic of Klinefelter's and Turner's syndromes.

Anyone with a child or other member of the family with a chromosomal abnormality should obtain *genetic counseling* to establish the risk of his or her prospective children being affected and also to discuss other considerations of family planning.

Chromosome analysis

Study of the chromosomal material in an adult's, child's, or unborn baby's cells to learn whether a *chromosomal abnormality* is present or to establish its nature.

WHY IT IS DONE

Certain fetuses have a higher-than-average chance of being born with a chromosomal abnormality, in particular if the mother is over 35 years old, if she has previously given birth to a child with a chromosomal defect, or if either the mother or father is known to carry a defect or rearrangement of his or her chromosomes. In such cases, the parents are usually offered, at around the fifteenth week of pregnancy, chromosome analysis of cells that can be obtained from the fetus by a technique called *amniocentesis*. Some centers offer an alternative, *chorionic villus sampling*, which may have greater risks (regarding loss of the fetus), but which can be carried out as early as six to eight weeks into pregnancy.

If no abnormality is found, the test spares the parents any anxiety. If a serious abnormality is discovered, such as one that would lead to the infant having *Down's syndrome*, termination of the pregnancy may be considered, along with *genetic* counseling to assess the chances of a subsequent pregnancy being affected.

Chromosome analysis is also carried out when a baby is stillborn, or is born with physical abnormalities that suggest a chromosome defect. The analysis clarifies the nature and type of defect, which in turn affects the counseling given to the parents.

Finally, analysis of a person's sex chromosomes may be carried out to establish the chromosomal sex of a child with ambiguous genitals (see *Intersex*); to diagnose sex chromosome abnormalities such as *Turner's syndrome* and *Klinefelter's syndrome*; or to investigate *infertility*.

PROCEDURE FOR CHROMOSOME ANALYSIS

1 Fetal cells are obtained by amniocentesis or by chorionic villus sampling, or white blood cells are obtained from the blood of the baby, child, or adult being tested.

2 These cells are suspended in a medium containing substances that encourage the cells to divide. Chemicals are then added that stop the cells from dividing at a stage where their chromosome content is most easily visible.

3 The cells are then spread on a microscope slide, stained, and a selected few (in which the chromosomes are clearly visible and well separated) have their nuclei photographed or are closely examined through a high-power microscope.

4 The chromosomes are matched up or cut out from the photographic print and arranged into the 22 pairs of autosomes together with the sex chromosomes. Study of these reveals any abnormalities.

1 2 3 4 5
6 7 8 9 10 11 12
13 14 15 16 17 18
19 20 21 22 X Y
Male   Female

Chromosomes

Threadlike structures present within the nuclei of cells. Chromosomes carry the inherited, genetic information that directs the activities of cells and, thus, the growth and functioning of the entire body.

All the cells of any one person (with the exception of egg or sperm cells) carry precisely the same chromosomal material. This is because everyone is derived, by a process of cell division, from a single, fertilized egg cell and, with each cell division, the chromosomal material originally present in the fertilized egg is faithfully copied. A rare exception to this rule is seen in people with *mosaicism*, in which some cells contain one set of chromosomal material and other cells contain a slightly different set.

Although most chromosomal material is the same for everyone, certain parts differ from one person to another; these differences make each person (with the exception of identical twins) unique. Chromosomes determine physical characteristics, such as sex, hair texture and color, skin and eye color, nose shape, height, and (probably to a lesser extent) mental abilities and personality.

Each chromosome contains up to several thousand *genes* (hereditary units) arranged in single file along its length. A single gene is responsible for just one small aspect of body chemistry (e.g., enzyme synthesis).

STRUCTURE AND NUMBERS

Chemically, a chromosome consists of an extremely long chain of the hereditary substance deoxyribonucleic acid, or DNA, along with a coating of protein. This combination of DNA and protein is called chromatin. The sequence of chemical units, or bases, in the DNA provides the coded instructions for cellular activities. Each cell contains the chemical machinery for decoding these instructions (see *Genetic code; Nucleic acids*).

Although DNA chains are relatively enormous (compared, for example, with a molecule of water), their long, filamentous shape means that chromosomes cannot normally be seen in cell nuclei, even with the aid of a powerful microscope. But, shortly before any cell divides, its DNA molecules contract (probably by forming into tight coils) and, if cell division is chemically halted and the cell stained with a dye, the chromosomes can be seen with a microscope as dark rods in the nucleus, a few thousandths of a millimeter long.

EGG AND SPERM CELLS

These differ from other body cells in that they contain only 23 chromosomes—one from each of the 22 autosome pairs plus an X chromosome (in the case of an egg) and either an X or a Y (in the case of a sperm). Because they have only half the normal complement, they are said to be haploid, while other cells are called diploid.

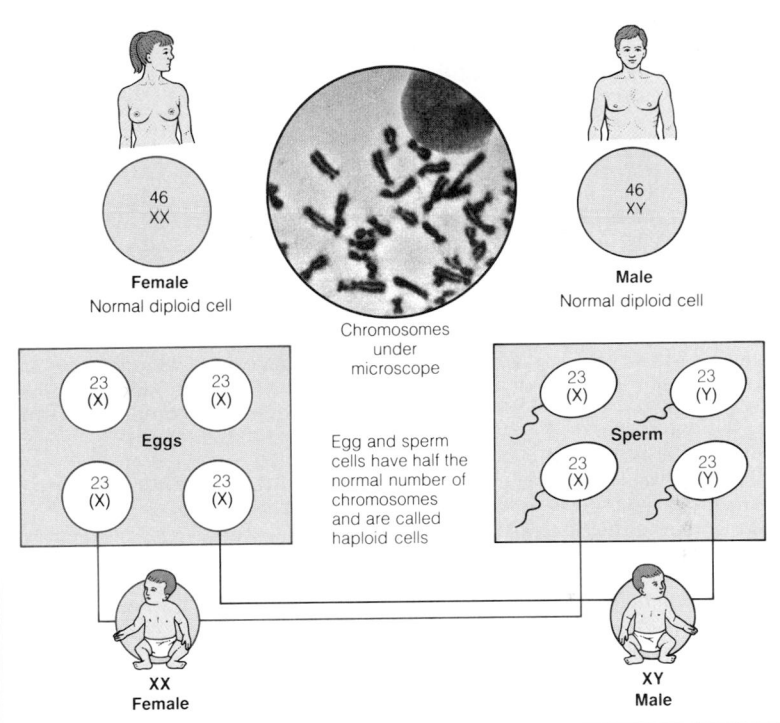

Female
Normal diploid cell

Chromosomes under microscope

Male
Normal diploid cell

Eggs

Egg and sperm cells have half the normal number of chromosomes and are called haploid cells

Sperm

XX
Female

XY
Male

This technique has shown that human cells (with the exception of egg and sperm cells) normally contain 46 chromosomes consisting of 23 pairs.

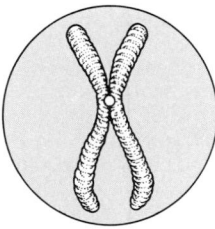

Most chromosomes have a constriction called a centromere that divides them into long and short "arms"

Appearance of chromosomes
This is the appearance just after a chromosome has copied itself. The two copies are joined at the centromere.

AUTOSOMAL AND SEX CHROMOSOMES

Of the 23 pairs of chromosomes, 22 are the same in both sexes and are called autosomal chromosomes. The two members of a pair cannot be told apart under the microscope—being alike in their length, the position of their centromeres, and in other aspects—but at the molecular level they differ slightly, in particular in the sequence of chemical bases in their DNA. One member of each pair is derived originally from a person's mother and the other from the father.

The other two chromosomes are called sex chromosomes. In women they form a pair and are called X chromosomes. Again, they look alike but differ slightly at the molecular level. In men, however, the two sex chromosomes are completely different. One is an X chromosome, but the other is a much shorter chromosome called the Y chromosome. The Y chromosome is believed to provide all the information for the development of male sexual characteristics. In its absence, the female pattern of development occurs.

As with the autosomal chromosomes, one of a person's sex chromosomes (an X) has come originally from the ovum of the mother and the other (an X in girls and a Y in boys) has come from the sperm of the father.

C

CHROMOSOME DIVISION

When a cell divides, its components are duplicated in the two offspring cells (see *Mitosis*); this applies also to the chromosomes. Shortly before division, the DNA in each chromosome is copied (see *Nucleic acids*). This means that, when the chromosomes are viewed just before division, they appear not as single but as double rods, conjoined in the region of their centromeres. This gives all 46 chromosomes (not just the sex chromosomes) an X-shaped appearance in the nuclei. As the normal cell division proceeds—a process known as mitosis—these duplicated chromosomes are pulled apart, dividing at the centromere, so that each daughter cell receives a single copy of each of the usual 46 chromosomes.

When egg or sperm cells are formed (a process known as meiosis) there are two important departures from the norm in the process of chromosome division. First, after the DNA has been copied, but before division takes place, some sections of chromosomal material are exchanged between the two members of all the paired chromosomes. This helps ensure that each of a person's eggs or sperm has a different combination of chromosomal material—and helps explain why all brothers and sisters (except identical twins) have a unique appearance.

The second difference is that, because eggs and sperm get only 23 chromosomes, their formation requires two consecutive divisions—a first one in which the 46 chromosomes in the parent cell are split into two groups of 23 (one group going to each daughter cell), followed by a second division in which the 23 chromosomes in each daughter cell (which at this point are still in duplicate form) are pulled apart. Thus, the original cell gives rise to four separate egg or sperm cells.

DISORDERS

Defective chromosome division during the formation of eggs and sperm—or more rarely during the first few divisions of a fertilized egg—can lead to various *chromosomal abnormalities*. The precise nature of the abnormality can be investigated by detailed *chromosome analysis*.

Chronic

Describing a disorder or set of symptoms that has persisted for a long time. In some disorders, such as chronic active *hepatitis*, the time is specified as six months or longer.

Chronic disorders are usually contrasted with acute ones. In addition to the duration difference between the two, the term acute suggests the presence of symptoms such as high fever, severe pain, or breathlessness, with a rapid change in the patient's condition from one day to the next. By contrast, a person with a chronic infection, such as some forms of hepatitis or a chronic form of *arthritis*, shows little change in symptoms from day to day and may be able, albeit with some difficulty, to carry out his or her regular daily activities.

A person with a chronic disease may experience an acute exacerbation (flare-up) of symptoms. Also, people who have had an acute illness such as a *stroke*, or who have been injured in an accident, may be left with permanent disabilities, but their condition is not chronic. A chronic disorder implies a continuing disease process with progressive deterioration (sometimes despite treatment).

Chronic obstructive lung disease

See *Lung disease, chronic obstructive*.

Cimetidine

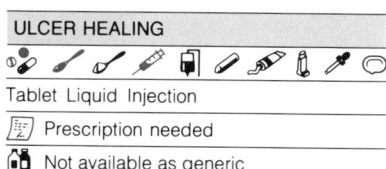

ULCER HEALING
Tablet   Liquid   Injection
📋 Prescription needed
🔋 Not available as generic

An *ulcer-healing drug* related to the *antihistamines*. Introduced in 1976, cimetidine reduces the secretion of hydrochloric acid in the stomach and, by doing so, promotes healing of gastric and duodenal ulcers and reduces esophagitis (inflammation of the esophagus).

Cimetidine generally relieves symptoms within one to two weeks and heals an ulcer in over 75 percent of cases after one to two months. Once the ulcer has healed, a maintenance dose of cimetidine is often prescribed; without such treatment the chance of an ulcer recurring is high.

There is a slight risk that cimetidine may temporarily mask the symptoms of stomach cancer by relieving symptoms in the early stages, thus delaying the diagnosis. It is therefore usually not prescribed for periods longer than two months unless investigations, such as *gastroscopy* and *barium X-ray examinations*, have ruled out the possibility of cancer.

Cimetidine interferes with the breaking down by the liver of certain drugs, such as *anticoagulants* and *anticonvulsants*.

Some people taking cimetidine suffer from confusion, headaches, and dizziness, which usually disappear when the drug is stopped.

Circadian rhythm

Any biological pattern based on a cycle approximately 24 hours long. (See also *Biorhythms*.)

Circulation, disorders of

Conditions affecting the flow of blood around the body. (See *Arteries, disorders of*; *Veins, disorders of*; *Capillary*.)

Circulatory system

The *heart* and blood vessels, which together are responsible for the continuous flow of blood throughout the body. Also called the cardiovascular system, the circulatory system provides all body tissues with a regular supply of oxygen and nutrients and carries away carbon dioxide and other waste products.

STRUCTURE AND FUNCTION

The circulatory system consists of two main parts: the systemic circulation (which comprises the blood supply to the entire body except the lungs) and the pulmonary circulation to the lungs (which is responsible for reoxygenating the blood).

The systemic circulation begins at the left side of the heart, where the left atrium receives oxygen-rich blood from the pulmonary circulation. The blood is ejected from the left atrium to the left ventricle, a powerful pump that sends the blood out through the *aorta*, the body's main artery. Other arteries branching off the aorta carry the blood all over the body, into the arterioles (small arteries) that supply the various organs. The arterioles branch further into a network of capillaries. These extremely fine blood vessels have thin walls to allow oxygen and other nutrients to pass easily from the blood into the tissues, and carbon dioxide and other wastes to pass in the opposite direction.

The capillaries deliver the deoxygenated blood into venules (small veins), which join to form veins. These carry the blood into the *venae cavae*, the body's two main veins, which then return the blood to the right atrium of the heart.

From the right atrium, the blood enters the pulmonary circulation. It passes to the right ventricle, which

CIRCULATORY SYSTEM

The heart and blood vessels create a continuous flow of blood around the body to provide tissues with oxygen and nutrients. The system also removes waste products. The systemic circulation deals with the supply of blood to all parts except the lungs; the pulmonary system reoxygenates the blood.

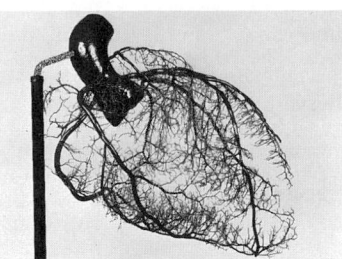

C

Resin cast of coronary arteries

Shown at left is a cast of the arrangement of blood vessels that supply the heart muscle. The larger vessels are the coronary arteries; they branch off the root of the aorta, the massive artery that receives oxygenated blood from the heart. The coronary arteries and their branches supply blood and oxygen to all parts of the heart muscle.

SYSTEMATIC CIRCULATION

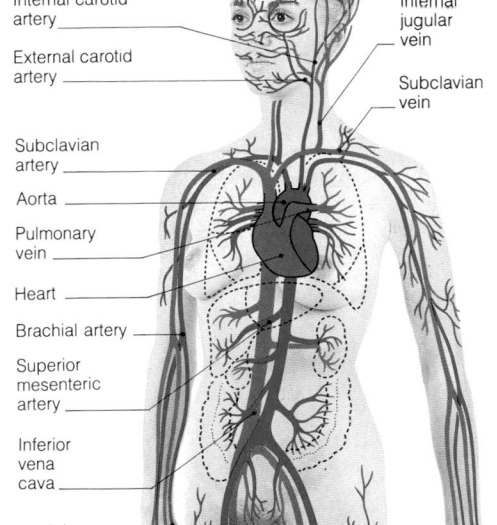

Internal carotid artery

External carotid artery

Subclavian artery

Aorta

Pulmonary vein

Heart

Brachial artery

Superior mesenteric artery

Inferior vena cava

Radial artery

Iliac vein

Femoral artery

Peroneal artery

Internal jugular vein

Subclavian vein

Femoral vein

Great saphenous vein

Small saphenous vein

Key

Oxygenated blood

Deoxygenated blood

PULMONARY CIRCULATION

Trachea

Superior vena cava

Right atrium

Right ventricle

Inferior vena cava

Aorta

Left ventricle

Lung

Aorta

Left atrium

Alveoli

Blood is pumped by the left side of the heart, via arteries, to the body, where it gives up oxygen. It then drains, via the venae cavae, to the right side, is pumped to the lungs, receives oxygen from the alveoli, and returns to the left side.

CAPILLARY NETWORK

All tissues contain a network of tiny blood capillaries. Blood enters these from the arterioles and is drained by venules.

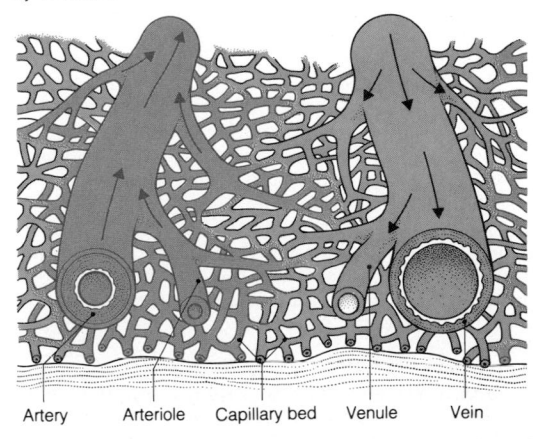

Artery   Arteriole   Capillary bed   Venule   Vein

C

pumps the blood through the pulmonary artery to the lungs. Here, carbon dioxide passes out of the blood, and oxygen enters. The reoxygenated blood then returns through the pulmonary veins to the left atrium of the heart, where it reenters the systemic circulation.

Within the systemic circulation there is a bypass to the liver called the portal circulation. Capillaries carrying nutrient-rich blood from the stomach, intestine, and other digestive organs join to form venules which, in turn, meet to form veins. These then merge to form the portal vein, which conveys the blood to veins, venules, and capillaries in the liver. Nutrients pass from the capillaries into the liver cells for processing and storage or reentry into the general circulation. Blood from the liver continues to rejoin the main systemic circulation via the inferior vena cava.

On its journey from the heart to the tissues, blood is forced along the arteries at high pressure. However, on the return journey through the veins and back to the heart, the blood is at low pressure. It is kept moving by the muscles in the arms and legs compressing the walls of the veins, and by valves in the veins preventing the blood from flowing backward. (See also *Lymphatic system*; *Respiration*.)

Circumcision
Removal of the foreskin of the penis. Circumcision is most often performed on newborn male babies, usually for religious reasons. It may also be carried out on adults.

WHY IT IS DONE
Circumcision is a religious ritual practiced for thousands of years by both Jews and Muslims. In some countries it is also routinely carried out for reasons of hygiene (because circumcision prevents the accumulation of secretions under the foreskin).

Medical reasons for performing circumcision include a tight foreskin that balloons on urination, or recurrent attacks of *balanitis* (infection under the foreskin due to retained secretions). In adults, the foreskin may be removed because it is tight and painful during intercourse, or because of attacks of paraphimosis (painful compression of the shaft of the penis by a retracted foreskin).

HOW IT IS DONE
In newborn babies, the operation takes only a few minutes. The foreskin is pulled forward over the tip of the penis and cut. The outer layer of the remaining foreskin retracts, leaving the glans covered by the thinner, inner layer. This is cut and pulled back. The two layers of the foreskin are then stitched and a waterproof dressing is applied.

In adolescents and adults, circumcision is usually performed using a general anesthetic. The foreskin is pulled back as far as it will go. It is slit along its upper surface and then all around so that it can be removed. The raw edges of the inner and outer layers are stitched, and a dressing is applied. The patient usually goes home the same day.

Circumcision, female
Removal of all or parts of the clitoris, labia majora, and labia minora, sometimes combined with narrowing of the entrance to the vagina. The operation is common in parts of Africa. In the early 1980s it was estimated that more than 84 million women in 30 countries had been circumcised.

There is absolutely no valid medical purpose for the procedure. Circumcision may cause retention of urine, injuries during coitus, and may also lead to frigidity and other psychological problems. Childbirth is likely to be made more hazardous.

There has been a strong move to end the practice, with little success. Legislation prohibiting circumcision in the Sudan was introduced in the 1940s, but has been ineffective.

Cirrhosis
A disease of the liver caused by chronic damage to its cells. Bands of *fibrosis* (internal scarring) break up the normal structure of the liver. The surviving cells multiply to form regeneration nodules (islands of living cells separated by scar tissue). Because these nodules are inadequately supplied with blood, liver function is gradually impaired—for example, the liver no longer effectively removes toxic substances from the blood (see *Liver failure*). The distortion and fibrosis of the liver leads to *portal hypertension* (high blood pressure in the veins from the intestines and spleen to the liver), which can cause serious complications.

INCIDENCE AND CAUSES
In the US, about one in 70 people dies as a direct result of chronic liver disease and cirrhosis—accounting for about 30,000 deaths each year.

Heavy alcohol consumption is the most common cause of cirrhosis both in Europe and the US; it is an increasing problem in most developed countries. The risk relates to the amount of alcohol consumed rather than the type, and women are more susceptible than men (see *Alcohol*).

Hepatitis (inflammation of the liver) can lead to cirrhosis. Chronic viral hepatitis (particularly that due to hepatitis B virus) is the most common cause of cirrhosis in the Middle and Far East and Africa (see *Hepatitis, viral*). A special pattern of liver inflammation called chronic active hepatitis is usually present before the cirrhosis develops (see *Hepatitis, chronic active*). Autoimmune chronic active hepatitis, with similar liver changes but with no obvious viral infection, is found in Europe and the US.

Rarer causes of cirrhosis include diseases and defects of the bile ducts, which can cause primary or secondary *biliary cirrhosis*; *hemochromatosis*, in which increased iron absorption occurs; *Wilson's disease*, in which there is an increase in copper absorption; *cystic fibrosis*, in which the bile ducts become obstructed by sticky mucus; and "cardiac cirrhosis," in which *heart failure* has led to long-standing congestion of blood in the liver.

SYMPTOMS AND SIGNS
There may be no symptoms of cirrhosis; the disease may be discovered initially during a routine medical examination or blood test because of some abnormality. The most common symptoms are mild *jaundice*, *edema* (fluid collection in the tissues), mental confusion, and *hematemesis* (vomiting of blood).

In men, enlargement of the breasts and loss of body hair are thought to be due to an abnormality in the sex hormone balance caused by liver failure associated with cirrhosis.

COMPLICATIONS
There are four main complications associated with cirrhosis and any may be the first sign of the condition. *Ascites* (collection of fluid in the abdominal cavity) can occur because of low protein levels in the blood (see *Albumin*) and high blood pressure in the veins leading to the liver. The high pressure in these veins also leads to *esophageal varices* (enlarged veins in the wall of the esophagus), which can rupture, causing vomiting of blood. *Confusion* and *coma* can result from the accumulation of toxic materials poisonous to the brain that would normally be processed and detoxified by a healthy liver. *Hepatoma* is a primary cancer of liver cells that complicates chronic hepatitis with cirrhosis.

DIAGNOSIS AND TREATMENT

Although the symptoms and signs of cirrhosis, or *liver function tests*, may suggest the diagnosis, the diagnosis is usually confirmed by *liver biopsy*, which may also show features that point to the underlying cause. Special blood tests and *cholangiography* (X rays of the bile ducts) may be performed to exclude the rarer causes.

The cirrhotic process itself can be treated by slowing the process causing liver cell damage. Abstinence from alcohol can lead to substantial improvement, and in some cases specific treatment for the underlying cause may be available. Ascites may be controlled by giving diuretics (drugs that increase the production of urine) and sometimes by reducing salt intake. Bleeding esophageal varices can be obliterated by injecting them with a sclerosant solution (a liquid that blocks off the affected veins) via a gastroscope (see *Gastroscopy*). The pressure in the veins can be reduced by using a *shunt* operation to divert the blood supply away from the engorged, dilated veins.

Confusion can be improved by measures that reduce the level of toxic waste products and other poisonous substances circulating in the blood. Such measures may include reducing the protein intake in the diet and giving special antibiotic treatment to reduce the number of bacteria in the intestines. In some cases a *liver transplant*, if available, may offer the only chance of a long-term cure.

Cisplatin

An *anticancer drug* used especially to treat cancers of the testis and ovary. It is used on its own or in combination with other anticancer drugs.

Cisplatin is being investigated to treat esophageal cancer.

Clap

A slang term used since the 16th century for the sexually transmitted infection *gonorrhea*.

Claudication

Lameness or limping. The term is associated with the Roman Emperor Claudius, who was notably lame. As a medical term it refers to a cramplike pain in one or both legs, which develops on walking and may eventually cause a limp.

The usual cause of claudication is blockage or narrowing of arteries in the legs due to *atherosclerosis* (see *Peripheral vascular disease*). Patients typically find that they have to stop walking after a set distance because of pain in the calves. After a short rest, they may be able to walk on. This is called intermittent claudication.

A rarer cause is spinal *stenosis* (narrowing of the canal carrying the spinal cord), causing pressure on nerve roots that pass into either leg.

Claustrophobia

Intense fear of being in enclosed spaces, such as elevators or small rooms, or of being in crowded areas. Claustrophobia may originate from a previous bad experience involving enclosed spaces (such as being locked inside a closet as punishment). *Psychotherapy* and/or *behavior therapy* is the usual treatment.

Clavicle

The collarbone. There are two of these bones, each slightly curved like an "f," that join the top of the sternum (breastbone) to the scapula (shoulder blade). The clavicles support the arms and transmit forces from the arms to the central skeleton.

The ligaments that link the clavicle to the sternum and scapula are very strong, which explains why the clavicle is rarely dislocated but frequently broken. Most fractures occur as a result of a fall onto the shoulder or an outstretched arm. When the clavicle is broken, the arm tends to sag and must be supported by a *sling* and a figure-of-eight bandage to keep the broken ends together until the fracture has healed, which may require six to 12 weeks of immobilization.

LOCATION OF CLAVICLE
The two f-shaped bones join the top of the sternum (breastbone) to the shoulders and help support the arms.

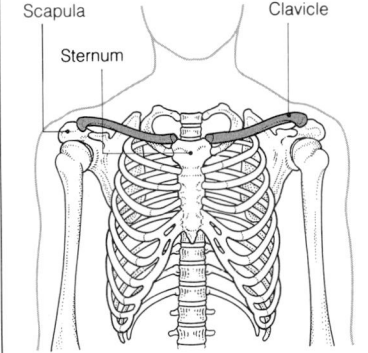

Scapula — Clavicle

Sternum

Clawfoot

A deformity of the foot that includes an exaggerated arch and turning under of the tips of the toes. The disorder may be present from birth or may result from disturbance or damage to the nerve or blood supply to the muscles of the foot.

Clawhand

A deformity of the hand in which the fingers are permanently curled. Clawhand is caused by an injury to the ulnar nerve, which controls some of the muscles involved in hand and finger movements.

Cleft lip and palate

Cleft lip is a vertical, usually off-center split in the upper lip that may be a small notch or may extend up to the nose. In some cases the upper gum is also cleft or notched, and the nose is crooked. Although cleft lip is also sometimes known as hare lip, this term properly refers only to a midline cleft lip, which is extremely rare. In some cases the lip or palate is cleft on both sides of the mouth.

Cleft palate is a gap in the roof of the mouth that runs along its midline, from behind the teeth to the nasal cavity. Many people with cleft palate are partially deaf and may have another *birth defect*.

Cleft lip and palate are present from birth, occurring either singly or together. About one in 600 babies is born with one or both deformities. Of every nine affected babies, two have only a cleft lip, three have only a cleft palate, and four have both. Inheritance is complicated but one third of those affected have relatives with one or both deformities.

DIAGNOSIS AND TREATMENT

All babies are routinely examined for both deformities immediately after birth. Babies with a cleft lip can breast-feed, but those with a cleft palate must be bottle-fed.

Surgery, usually at about 3 months, can restore a cleft lip so that it looks almost normal, and there are rarely any speech defects. A cleft palate is usually repaired at about 1 year; further operations and speech therapy are sometimes necessary.

Clergyman's knee

Inflammation of the bursa (fluid-filled sac) that acts as a cushion at the pressure point over the tibial tubercle (the bony prominence below the knee). The inflammation is caused by prolonged kneeling. (See *Bursitis*.)

C

Climacteric

The *menopause*, which indicates the end of menstruation (and thus fertility) in the female.

Clindamycin

An *antibiotic drug* used to treat serious infections that have not responded to other antibiotics. It is also used in the treatment of infections caused by bacteria (usually staphylococci or pneumococci) that are resistant to more commonly used antibiotics.

Clitoridectomy

An operation to remove the clitoris (see *Circumcision, female*).

Clitoris

Part of the female genitalia. The clitoris is richly supplied with nerves and blood vessels; during sexual stimulation, it swells and becomes even more sensitive.

LOCATION OF CLITORIS

The clitoris is a small, sensitive, erectile organ located just below the pubic bone, partly enclosed within the labia.

Opening of urethra — Clitoris
Labia — Vagina
— Anus

Clofibrate

A drug that reduces high levels of triglyceride (a type of fat) in the blood; it is sometimes used in the treatment of certain types of *hyperlipidemia*. (See *Lipid-lowering drugs*.)

Clomiphene

INFERTILITY

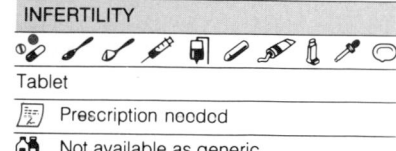

Tablet

Prescription needed

Not available as generic

A drug used to treat *infertility* caused by failure to ovulate in a woman and inadequate sperm production in a man. Multiple births may occur.

USE IN FEMALE INFERTILITY Normal ovulation (the release of a ripened egg from one of the ovaries) is stimulated by the action of two *gonadotropins* (follicle-stimulating hormone and luteinizing hormone) released from the pituitary gland. This secretion is stimulated by chemicals released by the hypothalamus (a part of the brain).

Failure to ovulate, one of the most common causes of infertility, is usually due to an abnormally low production of these gonadotropins. Clomiphene works by blocking the action of estrogens in the hypothalamus. Estrogens normally reduce the output of gonadotropins from the pituitary gland. As a result, the production of gonadotropins is increased and sometimes ovulation is stimulated. Occasionally, clomiphene must be given with gonadotropins before ovulation will occur.

USE IN MALE INFERTILITY Clomiphene is used to stimulate sperm production in some infertile men. Sperm counts are carried out regularly to check for increased sperm production and treatment is usually continued for six to twelve months or until his partner becomes pregnant.

POSSIBLE ADVERSE EFFECTS Minor side effects, some of which may occur in both men and women, include hot flashes, nausea, headache, breast tenderness, and, occasionally, blurred vision. All usually improve when the dose is reduced or if a gonadotropin is also taken. Between 5 and 15 percent of the women who take clomiphene develop ovarian cysts. These cysts shrink when the dose is reduced. Very rarely, alopecia (loss of hair) occurs in people taking the drug.

Clone

An exact copy. In medicine the term usually refers to one of three main types: clones of cells, clones of genes, and clones of organisms.

Clones of cells are all descended from one original cell. Many types of cancer are thought to be cellular clones derived from one abnormal cell. *Monoclonal antibodies* have been used to identify certain types of cancers and infections.

Clones of genes are duplicates of a single gene. Gene cloning is a valuable research tool because it enables numerous copies of a gene to be made so that they can be studied in detail.

Finally, clones of organisms can be produced by removing the nucleus from a cell of one individual and transplanting it into the egg cell of another individual. When this egg matures into a living plant or animal, it contains only the genes of the donor nucleus. To date, this process has been successful only in experiments with simple organisms.

Clonidine

An *antihypertensive drug* (used to treat high blood pressure). Clonidine is sometimes used with a diuretic, especially when the blood pressure is not being controlled by the diuretic alone. Clonidine works by reducing nerve impulses from the brain to the heart and circulatory system. Rarely, an unexpected rise in blood pressure develops when clonidine is given with a beta-blocker.

POSSIBLE ADVERSE EFFECTS

When given in high doses, sudden stopping of the drug may lead to a dangerous rise in blood pressure.

Other possible adverse effects, also usually occurring only in patients on high dosages, include drowsiness, dizziness, dry mouth, and constipation. Such effects often decrease with continued treatment or may require a reduction in dose.

Clonus

An abnormal response of a muscle to stretching. Normally when a muscle is stretched, it responds by contracting once and then relaxing (see *Reflex*). In clonus, stretching sets off a series of contractions of the muscle or muscles in quick succession.

Clonus is a sign of damage to nerve fibers that carry impulses from the motor cortex within the *cerebrum* of the brain to a particular muscle.

One typical example of clonus is called ankle clonus. A physician may demonstrate this type in the course of an examination by forcibly jerking the front of the foot upward, thus stretching the muscles of the calf, which are then triggered into a series of rhythmical contractions.

Clonuslike, or clonic, muscle contractions are also one feature of seizures in grand mal *epilepsy*.

Clorazepate

A drug used mainly in the treatment of anxiety. (See *Benzodiazepine drugs*.)

Closed panel

See *Health maintenance organization*.

Clotrimazole

A drug used to treat yeast and fungal infections, especially *candidiasis*. (See *Antifungal drugs*.)

Clove oil

 A colorless or pale-yellow oil distilled from the dried flower buds of *EUGENIA CARYOPHYLLUS*. Clove oil is sometimes used to relieve flatulent colic, but its main use today is in flavoring pharmaceuticals. Applied externally, it is germicidal and mildly analgesic, and has been used as a domestic remedy for toothache. Repeated application, however, may damage the gums.

Cloxacillin

A penicillin-type antibiotic used to treat infections with staphylococcal bacteria. (See *Penicillin drugs*.)

Clubbing

Thickening and broadening of the tips of the fingers and toes, with increased curving of the fingernails and toenails.

Clubbing is associated with certain chronic lung diseases, including *bronchiectasis*, *lung cancer*, fibrosing *alveolitis*, and lung *abscess*; heart abnormalities that result in *cyanosis* (bluish complexion due to lack of oxygen in the blood); and occasionally with inflammatory bowel diseases such as *Crohn's disease* and *ulcerative colitis*. Rarely, clubbing may be inherited, in which case it is not a sign of any disease. (See also *Spatulate*.)

Clubfoot

A deformity of the foot, present from birth. (See *Talipes*.)

CNS

An abbreviation for *central nervous system* (the brain and spinal cord).

CNS stimulants

Drugs that increase mental alertness. (See *Stimulants*.)

Coagulation, blood

One of the main mechanisms by which blood clots (solidifies). Coagulation involves a complex series of reactions in the blood plasma (the fluid part of blood as distinct from the blood cells). The end result of this process is the formation of an insoluble substance called fibrin, which provides much of the framework for a clot. (See also *Blood clotting*.)

Coal tar

A thick, black, sticky substance, coal tar is a common ingredient of ointments and some medicinal shampoos. These preparations, which often also contain *antiseptics* and *corticosteroids*, are prescribed for skin and scalp conditions such as psoriasis, eczema, and certain forms of dermatitis.

Coarctation of the aorta

An abnormality, present from birth, in which there is a localized narrowing of the aorta (the large artery that supplies blood from the left side of the heart to the rest of the body).

The narrowing usually occurs just past the point where the left subclavian artery (which supplies blood to the neck, head, and the left arm) branches off the aorta. Thus, there is a reduced supply of blood to the lower part of the body, including the legs. In an attempt to compensate, the heart works harder, causing raised blood pressure in the upper part of the body, while the blood pressure in the legs is normal or low.

The cause is unknown. Coarctation of the aorta occurs in about 10 percent of babies born with heart defects (see *Heart disease, congenital*), affecting about one in 2,000 babies overall.

SYMPTOMS AND DIAGNOSIS

The symptoms often first appear in early childhood and depend on the severity of the hypertension. Symptoms may include headache, weakness after exercise, cold legs, and, rarely, breathing difficulty and leg swelling due to *heart failure*.

A physical examination of the child usually reveals the following abnormalities associated with the defect: a murmur (abnormal heart sound), weak or absent pulses in the groin, lack of synchronization between groin and wrist pulses, and higher blood pressure in the arms than in the legs. The diagnosis is confirmed by X rays of the chest that show bulging of the aorta on either side of the narrowed segment, among other abnormalities.

TREATMENT AND OUTLOOK

Surgery is necessary to prevent progressive hypertension, even when there are no symptoms. The narrowed segment of the aorta is removed and the two ends rejoined. The operation is usually performed between the ages of 4 and 8. Despite successful repair, high blood pressure may persist, requiring drug treatment.

Cobalamin

A cobalt-containing complex molecule that forms part of *vitamin B_{12}*.

Cobalt

A metallic element and a constituent of *vitamin B_{12}*. Radioactive cobalt is used in cancer treatment.

Cocaine

A drug obtained from the leaves of a South American plant.

WHY IT IS USED

Cocaine was once used as a local anesthetic (see *Anesthesia, local*), mainly for minor surgical procedures on the eye, ear, nose, or throat. It is sometimes sprayed onto the back of the throat before examination of the lungs or stomach with an *endoscope*. Because of its potential for abuse, cocaine has largely been replaced by other local anesthetics.

The onset of anesthesia is rapid and the effects last for about one hour. Cocaine also constricts blood vessels, helping to localize its effect. However, some cocaine is usually absorbed into the bloodstream; this may interfere with the action of chemical *neurotransmitters* in the brain, possibly producing feelings of euphoria and increased energy.

ABUSE

The effects of cocaine on the brain have led to its abuse. Regular inhaling of the drug can damage the lining of the nose. Continued use can lead to psychological dependence (see *Drug dependence*), and *psychosis* may develop if high doses are taken. Overdose can cause seizures and *cardiac arrest*. "Crack," a purified form of cocaine, produces a more rapid and intense reaction that also wears off very quickly; it has caused deaths due to adverse effects on the heart. (See also *Drug abuse*.)

Coccygodynia

A pain in the region of the coccyx. It usually starts after a fall in which the base of the spine strikes a hard surface, or through prolonged pressure on the coccyx (as can occur when slouching in a chair), or in women who have been in the *lithotomy* position (lying on the back with legs in the air) during childbirth. Occasionally there is no apparent cause.

Treatment may include the application of heat, injections of a local anesthetic, and manipulation, but these measures are not always successful. The pain usually eases in time with or without treatment. In very rare cases of persistent, incapacitating pain, surgical removal of the coccyx may be considered.

Coccyx

A small triangular bone at the base of the spine, positioned in front of the top of the cleft between the buttocks. The coccyx consists of four tiny bones

C

ANATOMY OF COCCYX
This bone at the spine's base consists of four fused bones. It forms, with the sacrum, the back of the pelvis.

Four bones of coccyx fused together

fused together; it is all that remains of the tailbone structure of our evolutionary ancestors.

Along with a much larger bone called the sacrum, which lies above it, the coccyx forms the back section of the pelvis—a bowl-shaped, bony structure that provides protection to organs (such as the uterus and bladder) and supports the upper body.

The coccyx and sacrum can barely move relative to each other, although they do somewhat during childbirth. After middle age they fuse together.

Cochlear implant

A device for treating severe deafness that consists of one or more electrodes implanted by surgery inside or outside the cochlea (an organ in the inner ear that transforms sound vibrations into nerve impulses for transmission to the brain). Unlike a *hearing aid*, which amplifies sounds, the implant receives and passes on electrical signals. It cannot restore normal hearing, but, along with lipreading, allows a greater understanding of speech than is possible by lipreading alone.

WHY IT IS DONE
In rare cases, damage to structures in the cochlea (through disease, injury, or drug poisoning) is so great and the resultant deafness so profound that a hearing aid serves no useful purpose. If some nerve fibers have survived, it is sometimes possible to stimulate them electrically by an implant.

HOW IT IS DONE
An operation is carried out to implant one or more tiny electrodes either inside or outside the cochlea. At the

same time, a miniature receiver is implanted under the skin, either behind the ear or in the lower part of the chest. A wire connecting the electrodes to the receiver is implanted at the same time.

Directly over the implanted receiver, the patient wears an external transmitter, which is connected to a sound processor and a microphone.

OUTLOOK
In general, an implant enables the user to hear the rhythms of speech, and sometimes also the intonation of the voice. Understanding obtained through lipreading is increased, and the deaf person is able to converse more effectively.

However, the usefulness of an implant for any particular person cannot be reliably predicted, and, in this respect, the technique is considered to be investigational. One quarter of patients make extremely good use of the implant and are able to repeat two thirds of simple words in unrehearsed sentences without lipreading. One

Electrodes implanted in cochlea

Subcutaneous fat

Receiver coil

Signals

Transmitter coil — Skin

Microphone (sometimes set into an ear mold)

Speech processor

How a cochlear implant works
Sounds picked up by the microphone are converted into electronic signals by the processor and relayed to the external transmitter, which sends them through the skin to the receiver. The waves then travel along the wire to the electrodes in the cochlea.

quarter can repeat some words without lipreading and one quarter can repeat words only with lipreading. In the remainder, the signal is poor, an electrical fault occurs, or the patient develops an infection.

Codeine

ANALGESIC COUGH REMEDIES ANTIDIARRHEAL		
Tablet	Liquid	Injection
Prescription needed		
Available as generic		

A narcotic *analgesic drug* (painkiller), derived from a poppy plant, in use since the early 1900s. It is not as strong as some other narcotic analgesics and is often combined with other drugs in tablets and mixtures.

WHY IT IS USED
Codeine is most useful in the relief of mild to moderate pain. It is also used as a *cough remedy*, because it suppresses the part of the brain that triggers coughing, and as an *antidiarrheal drug*, because it slows down muscle contractions in the intestinal wall.

POSSIBLE ADVERSE EFFECTS
Codeine may cause dizziness and drowsiness, especially if taken with alcohol. When taken over a long period, codeine may cause constipation and be habit-forming.

Cod-liver oil

A pale yellow oil obtained from the liver of fresh cod. It is a valuable source of *vitamin A* and *vitamin D* and is given to infants as a dietary supplement to ensure the healthy development of bones and skin. Cod-liver oil is available in capsule form and in a malt extract.

Cognitive-behavioral therapy

A method of treating mental disorders based on the idea that the way we think about the world and ourselves (our cognitions) affects our emotions and behavior.

A person suffering from depression may always think that undesirable events are due to his or her behavior and that desirable events are due to chance. The therapist shows the patient that these interpretations are false, suggests more positive ways of thinking, and encourages the patient to try out these new ideas during his or her everyday activities. Because cognitive-behavioral therapy is based on the manner in which each person

C

relates to the environment, it allows treatment to be more specifically tailored to the individual's needs than do the more traditional forms of *behavior therapy*.

Coil

Any of the different types of intrauterine contraceptive devices (see *IUD*).

Coinsurance

A provision in a health insurance policy that requires the patient to pay a predetermined percentage of the various insured medical charges incurred during the life of the policy. (See also *Deductible*.)

Coitus

Sexual intercourse (from the Latin word for a coming together).

Coitus interruptus

The contraceptive technique in which the male partner withdraws his penis from the vagina before ejaculation occurs. This technique is not very reliable as a contraceptive method, because sperm may sometimes be released before orgasm occurs. In addition, coitus interruptus has been blamed for *psychosexual dysfunction* in both men and women. (See also *Contraception*.)

Colchicine

A drug extracted from the autumn crocus, colchicine has been in use since the nineteenth century as a treatment for *gout*. Although it has now been partly superseded by newer drugs, it continues to be used to treat acute and chronic gout and familial Mediterranean fever.

Cold, common

A viral infection that causes inflammation of the mucous membranes lining the nose and throat, resulting in a stuffy, runny nose and sometimes a sore throat and headache.

CAUSES

Almost 200 viruses, all broadly similar in their effects, are known to cause colds. The most common belong to one of two groups—the rhinoviruses and coronaviruses.

Most colds are contracted by breathing in virus-containing droplets that have been sneezed or coughed into the atmosphere or by rubbing the eyes or nose with fingers that have picked up a virus by hand-to-hand contact or by handling contaminated objects, such as playing cards.

INCIDENCE

Almost everyone occasionally gets a cold. The incidence is highest among schoolchildren (who may have as many as 10 colds a year) and declines with increasing age. On average, a young adult has two or three colds per year, an elderly person one or none at all. The reason for this is that children at school are exposed to a host of different viruses to which they have not yet had time to become immune and which they pass to one another. Adults gradually build up immunity against a wide variety of viruses responsible for colds.

Colds are most frequent in winter, probably because people tend to spend more time during these months crowded together indoors in places such as the movies and at parties, where there is a higher chance of viruses being spread.

SYMPTOMS

Most colds are what are popularly known as head colds—that is, infections confined to the nose and throat. The first symptoms are often a tickle in the throat, a watery discharge from the nose, and sneezing. Then the discharge may thicken and become yellow or green and other symptoms may develop—watering eyes, a low-grade fever, a sore throat, a cough, aching muscles and bones, a mild headache, listlessness, and chills.

In some cases, infection spreads to the larynx, windpipe, lungs, sinuses, or middle ear, leading to, respectively, *laryngitis*, *tracheitis*, acute *bronchitis*, *sinusitis*, or *otitis media*. At these sites a more serious secondary bacterial infection may then follow.

Colds can also aggravate existing respiratory disorders, such as asthma and chronic bronchitis, and chronic ear infections. They may also reactivate dormant *herpes simplex* virus, causing *cold sores*.

TREATMENT

Most colds clear up within a week or so. A physician should be consulted only if this fails to happen, if the infection has spread beyond the nose or throat, or if the cold has aggravated a chronic chest infection or ear disorder. If a secondary bacterial infection is suspected, antibiotics will be given.

PREVENTION

Many people believe there are ways of preventing colds—by avoiding exposure to cold drafts and dampness, for instance, or by taking large quantities of vitamin C—but there is no scientific evidence that any such measures work.

OUTLOOK

The search to find a cure for the common cold continues. The two most hopeful possibilities are the drug interferon and synthetic *antigens* (substances that stimulate the immune system to produce antibodies). In volunteer experiments, interferon has proved effective in preventing and reducing the severity of colds, but has caused local inflammation. Research is now centered on finding preparations of interferon that are less toxic.

Cold injury

Localized tissue damage caused by chilling—as distinct from *hypothermia*, which refers to generalized chilling; the two may occur together.

The most serious form of cold injury is *frostbite*, a hazard of very cold, dry conditions. The frostbitten area of skin and flesh is frozen, hard, and white; it is caused either by direct exposure to the air or restriction of the blood supply to the affected area.

Immersion foot is another type of cold injury, occurring when the legs and feet have been cold and damp for many hours or days, and blood supply to the feet has been restricted by tight-fitting footwear.

In established frostbite and immersion foot, the main risk is that blood flow will be slowed so much that the tissues will die, leading to gangrene. Treatment may take several months.

Less serious forms of cold injury include *pernios* (chilblains), caused by rapid skin rewarming after being out in cold weather, and *chapped skin* of the lips, nose, and hands from exposure to cold, windy conditions.

Cold remedies

Many preparations are available over-the-counter to treat different symptoms of the common cold. The main ingredient is usually a mild *analgesic drug* (painkiller), such as *acetaminophen* or *aspirin*, which helps to relieve aches and pains. Other ingredients include *antihistamines* and *decongestants*, which help to reduce nasal congestion, and *caffeine*, which acts as a mild stimulant and is thought to enhance the analgesic effects. *Vitamin C* is frequently included in cold relief products, but there is no evidence that it speeds recovery.

Cold sore

A small skin blister anywhere around the mouth caused by the *herpes simplex* virus. Usually, several such blisters occur together in a cluster.

C

CAUSE AND INCIDENCE

The strain of the virus usually responsible for cold sores is called HSV1 (herpes simplex virus 1). Most people—perhaps as many as 90 percent worldwide—are infected by HSV1 at some time in their lives. The first attack may pass unnoticed or may cause an illness resembling influenza and painful ulcers in the mouth and on the lips—a condition called gingivostomatitis.

Subsequently, the virus lies dormant in nerve cells, but in some people it is occasionally reactivated, causing cold sores. They tend to recur when the person is exposed to hot sunshine or a cold wind, has a cold or other infection, or is feeling run down; women seem more likely to develop cold sores around the time of their menstrual periods. Some people are afflicted regularly throughout the year. Prolonged attacks can occur in patients with an underlying disease that affects their immunity to infection, or in those taking immunosuppressive drugs (transplant or cancer patients, for example).

SYMPTOMS AND TREATMENT

An outbreak is often preceded by a telltale tingling in the lips. The blisters are small at first but soon enlarge, sometimes causing itching, irritation, and soreness. Within a few days they burst and become encrusted, but they usually disappear within a week.

If cold sores are particularly troublesome, a physician may prescribe idoxuridine paint or the antiviral drug acyclovir (by mouth or injection) to soothe them. No effective preventive treatment is available, although some people find that applying a lip salve before sun exposure does help prevent outbreaks.

Colectomy

The surgical removal of part or all of the colon (large intestine).

WHY IT IS DONE

A partial colectomy may be performed to relieve severe cases of *diverticular disease* or to remove either a malignant tumor in the colon or a narrowed part of the intestine that is obstructing the passage of feces. A total colectomy is carried out in cases of *ulcerative colitis* that cannot be controlled with drugs, in long-standing ulcerative colitis in which colonoscopic examination raises the question of a hidden malignancy, and in cases of familial *polyposis*, a rare condition in which potentially malignant growths stud the lining of the colon.

HOW IT IS DONE

In a partial colectomy, the damaged section of the colon is removed and the two ends of the severed colon are joined together; they fuse in a matter of weeks. A temporary *colostomy* (which allows the discharge of feces from the large intestine through an artificial opening in the abdominal wall) may also be required. The temporary colostomy is closed when the rejoined colon has healed.

In a total colectomy the whole of the large intestine is removed; the rectum may be removed or left in place. If the rectum is removed, an *ileostomy* (similar to a colostomy, but involving the small instead of the large intestine) is performed. If the rectum is left in place, the ileum (the lower part of the small intestine) may be joined directly to it—an ileorectal *anastomosis*.

RECOVERY PERIOD

The patient is in the hospital for eight to 12 days. After discharge, it may take up to two months or so at home to recover from the operation. A patient with an ileostomy or colostomy should receive training—before leaving the hospital and preferably from a specialist nurse—on caring for the opening in the abdomen.

OUTLOOK

The bowel usually functions normally after most partial colectomies. If a large section of the colon has been removed, or if the ileum has been joined directly to the rectum, the greatly reduced ability of the intestines to absorb water from the feces can cause diarrhea. Drugs such as codeine phosphate, loperamide, or diphenoxylate may be used to reduce the diarrhea.

Colic

Severe, spasmodic pain that occurs in waves of increasing intensity, reaches a peak, then abates for a short time before returning. The intermittent increase in the pain occurs when the affected part of the body contracts—for example, the bile duct (the tube between the gallbladder and small intestine) or the ureter (the tube from the kidney to the bladder).

Colic in the bile ducts or urinary tract is often the result of obstruction by a stone, but intestinal colic is usually due to an infection or to an obstruction. (See also *Colic, infantile*.)

Colic, infantile

Episodes during which an infant is irritable, cries or screams excessively, and draws up the legs. The baby may be red in the face and may pass gas. Episodes of colic tend to be worse in the evenings and do not respond to the usual means of comforting the infant, such as feeding, cuddling, or diaper changing.

CAUSES

Infantile colic is common, occurring in approximately one in ten babies. It often first appears around the third or fourth week of life. Usually it clears up on its own by the age of 12 weeks, hence its name, "three-month colic." Colic is thought to be due to spasm in the intestines, although there is no proof of this, and the cause of the presumed spasm is unknown.

Babies who have colic are otherwise well. The condition is harmless, although it can be highly distressing to a tired parent. If the baby seems sick between the bouts of colic or has diarrhea, constipation, or a fever, a pediatrician should be consulted as the baby may have a more serious underlying problem.

TREATMENT

Treatment essentially involves waiting for the baby to grow out of the condition. Attempts may be made to distract the baby by diaper changing, cuddling, or bathing. Treatment with *antispasmodic drugs* has been used in the past, but these drugs are now not usually recommended for babies under 6 months of age.

Don't overstimulate your child. Rapid changes coupled with parental anxiety will make the child even more irritable. A common mistake is to feed

TREATING COLIC

Take the baby for a ride in the car

Use white noise in the baby's room (e.g., radio static or an air conditioner)

Place a heating pad (set on a safe, comfortable setting) or a warmed washcloth under the baby's stomach

Place the baby facedown on your knees while stroking his or her back

Put the baby securely in a seat on top of a running washer or dryer (under diligent supervision)

Rock the baby in a rocking chair

Carry the baby in a front sling or pouch (this leaves your hands free)

Give the baby a pacifier

the child every time he or she cries. This causes a bloated stomach and more crying. Overall, rhythmic, soothing activities work best. It is most important that the parent avoid fatigue and exhaustion. A relative, spouse, friend, or sitter should provide some relief.

Colistin

One of the polymyxin group of *antibiotics*. It is used only to treat severe infections that are resistant to other antibiotics, due to a risk of damage to the kidneys and nerve tissue.

Colitis

Inflammation of the colon (the large intestine) causing diarrhea, usually with blood and mucus. Other symptoms may include abdominal pain and fever.

CAUSES

Colitis may be due to infection by a virus, an ameba, or a bacterium such as campylobacter that produces toxins that irritate the lining of the intestine. Other bacteria may directly infect the colon lining, causing colitis.

Antibiotics, especially if taken for a period of more than two weeks, may provoke a form of colitis. Antibiotics kill the bacteria that normally live in the intestine and may allow another type of bacterium, CLOSTRIDIUM DIFFICILE, to proliferate and produce an irritating toxin. Very commonly, prolonged use of antibiotics is associated with diarrhea that may be a direct irritative effect of the drug itself (antibiotic-associated diarrhea).

Ischemia, or impairment of the blood supply to the intestinal wall, which is usually due to *atherosclerosis* (narrowing of blood vessels), is a very rare cause in the elderly.

Ulcerative colitis and *Crohn's disease* are two serious intestinal disorders of unknown origin that usually start in young adulthood.

Other disorders that can cause symptoms similar to those of colitis include *proctitis* (inflammation of the rectum), which may be due to a form of ulcerative colitis or to *gonorrhea* or another sexually transmitted disease; inflammation of an area of colon affected by *diverticular disease*; or an intestinal cancer.

DIAGNOSIS

A physician will usually advise a patient with severe diarrhea to stop eating and to drink only clear fluids (e.g., water, tea, clear soups, and so on). If the diarrhea, with or without blood and mucus, persists for more

than five days despite these measures, the physician will usually send a sample of feces for investigation for parasites, and culture and smear staining for bacteria.

If digital examination of the rectum is normal and no infection is found, the rectum and colon will usually be examined with a sigmoidoscope (viewing tube for examining the rectum and colon, see *Sigmoidoscopy*) to see if there is any inflammation or ulceration of the lining. *Biopsy* samples of inflamed areas or ulcers may be taken and examined under a microscope to look for the changes of ulcerative colitis or Crohn's disease.

A barium enema of the colon may be performed (see *Barium X-ray examinations*) to look for any areas of narrowing or severe inflammation.

TREATMENT

Most infections that can cause a colitis resolve without treatment. Campylobacter infections are sometimes treated with the antibiotic drug erythromycin, amebic infections are treated with metronidazole, and clostridium infections are treated with metronidazole or vancomycin.

Colitis caused by ischemia is treated by surgical excision of the damaged section of colon. Crohn's disease and ulcerative colitis are treated with *corticosteroid drugs* (taken either by mouth or in an *enema* to settle an acute colitis), with different drugs (including sulfasalazine or newer forms of this drug that do not contain sulfa), or by a special diet and vitamin supplements. Surgery does not cure these diseases and is usually reserved for the treatment of complications.

Collagen

A tough, fibrous protein that is the single most common protein in the body. It is the body's major structural protein, forming an important part of tendons, bones, and connective tissues. Because of its tough, insoluble nature, collagen helps hold together the cells and tissues of the body.

Collagen diseases

Two groups of diseases are referred to as collagen diseases—true collagen diseases and connective tissue diseases. True collagen diseases are uncommon, usually inherited, and due to faulty formation of *collagen* fibers. Features of true collagen diseases include thin, slack skin and poor wound healing.

Connective tissue diseases are due to malfunctioning of the immune

system (see *Autoimmune disorders*). This malfunctioning often affects blood vessels and, as a result, produces secondary damage in connective tissues. For this reason, these diseases are sometimes called collagen vascular diseases. They are relatively common, and include *rheumatoid arthritis*, systemic *lupus erythematosus*, *periarteritis nodosa*, *scleroderma*, *dermatomyositis*, and other less clearly defined disorders.

Collarbone

The common name for the *clavicle*.

Collar, orthopedic

A device worn to treat neck pain or instability. A soft collar, usually made of foam, can relieve pain by limiting the movement of the neck, by transferring some of the weight of the head from the neck to the chest, and by providing local warmth.

Stiff collars, commonly made of foam reinforced with plastic, are used when a fractured neck has almost healed but still needs support or when the vertebrae in the neck have otherwise become unstable.

Colles' fracture

A break just above the wrist in the radius (one of the two bones in the lower arm), usually resulting from a fall with the hand outstretched to break the fall. The fracture causes the wrist and hand to be displaced backward. Colles' fracture is the most common fracture in people over 40.

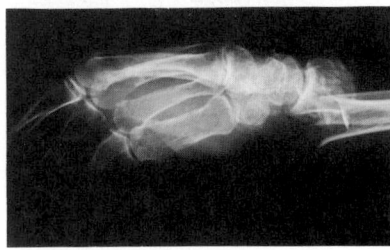

X ray of Colles' fracture
The wrist has been pushed back over the broken bone. This gives a classic "dinner fork" appearance when viewed from the side.

CAUSES AND INCIDENCE

The fracture usually occurs when someone stumbles when walking or slips on an icy sidewalk and puts out a hand to lessen the impact of the fall. Such a fall rarely produces a fracture in a young person, but it may be enough to break a bone weakened by *osteoporosis*, an invariable feature of aging. When a young person suffers a

C

Colles' fracture, it is usually the result of a more violent injury and often extends to the wrist joint itself.

SYMPTOMS

The wrist and hand are displaced and cannot be moved and there is severe pain and swelling in the area.

TREATMENT AND OUTLOOK

In most cases the two ends of the broken bone are manipulated back into position while the patient is under a local or general anesthetic, and a plaster cast is applied. Healing usually takes up to six weeks. When the cast is removed, the wrist may be stiff and exercise may be needed to restore its flexibility.

Minor deformity of the wrist may result from Colles' fracture, but movement of the hand and wrist is not usually impaired. In a young person, however, the more extensive damage may eventually lead to arthritis.

Colloid

A type of liquid similar to a suspension. A suspension—milk, for example—consists of insoluble particles of a substance suspended in a liquid. These particles are large and heavy enough to be separable from the liquid by centrifugation (spinning at high speed). A colloid is basically the same, except that its particles are significantly smaller and lighter than those of a suspension; they can be separated from the liquid part of the colloid only by ultracentrifugation (spinning at extremely high speed).

In medicine, colloid preparations containing *plasma proteins* (proteins in the fluid portion of blood) or certain complex carbohydrate molecules may be given to replace blood lost in cases of *shock* due to severe bleeding or burns. Such colloid preparations are called plasma expanders. Colloids containing gold or the metallic element technetium are used in some *radioisotope scanning* techniques.

The term colloid is also used to refer to the protein-containing material that fills the follicles of the *thyroid gland*.

Colon

The major part of the large intestine. A segmented tube about 2.5 inches (6.4 cm) wide and 4.5 feet (1.4 m) long, the colon forms a large loop, shaped somewhat like a distorted "M," in the abdomen. Its segments, or haustrations, give it an irregular outline.

The colon consists of four sections: the ascending, transverse, descending, and sigmoid colon. The first part, the ascending colon, starts at the

LOCATION OF COLON
A segmented tube within the abdomen, the colon takes the form of a large, roughly M-shaped, loop about 4.5 feet (1.4 m) long and 2.5 inches (6 cm) wide.

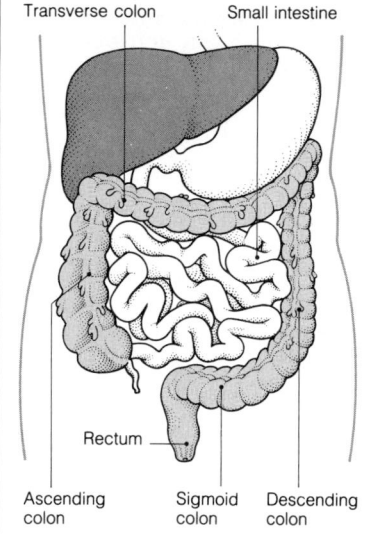

Transverse colon   Small intestine

Rectum

Ascending colon   Sigmoid colon   Descending colon

cecum, in the lower right-hand side of the abdomen, and extends up to a sharp bend just below the liver. This point, called the hepatic flexure, marks the beginning of the transverse colon, which loops across the abdomen, passing below the stomach to the spleen on the left-hand side of the abdomen. Here, there is a sharp downward bend (called the splenic flexure) that marks the start of the descending colon. From this point, the descending colon passes down the left side to approximately the brim of the pelvis, where it adopts an S-shaped course of variable length (the sigmoid colon) to connect with the *rectum* at the lower left-hand side of the abdomen.

STRUCTURE

The colon is a muscular tube with a lubricated inner lining. Its outermost layer, called the serous coat, is a tough, fibrous membrane with a smooth outer surface. This membrane protects the colon from damage when intestinal movements cause it to rub against the abdominal wall.

The muscular coat consists of three bands of longitudinal muscles and an inner layer of circular muscles. Rhythmic contractions and relaxations of these muscles (*peristalsis*)

squeeze the intestinal contents through the colon.

Inside the muscular coat is the third layer, the submucous coat. It consists of *connective tissue*, blood vessels, and lymphatic vessels.

The innermost layer is the mucous coat, which contains numerous tubular glands. These glands produce large amounts of mucus to lubricate the passage of digested material through the colon. Unlike the small intestine, the mucous coat of the colon (and the rest of the large intestine) is not folded into *villi* (tiny, fingerlike projections).

FUNCTION

The functions of the colon are, principally, to absorb water (and also a small amount of mineral salts) from the digested material passing through the colon and to concentrate indigestible waste for expulsion as feces.

When the intestinal contents enter the colon, digestion has been completed and the material is in the form of a liquid. As this liquid passes through the colon, the water and salts it contains are absorbed into the blood vessels in the submucous coat. By the time the intestinal contents pass out of the colon into the rectum, almost all the water has been absorbed and the contents are in the form of feces. (See also *Digestive system*; *Intestine* disorders box.)

Colon and rectal surgeon

A surgeon specializing in operations to correct disorders in or remove diseased tissue from the colon (large intestine) or the rectal area. Operations can range from the removal of *hemorrhoids* to the removal of part of the intestine. Patients are usually referred by another physician.

Colon, cancer of

See *Intestine, cancer of*.

Colon, disorders of

See *Intestine* disorders box.

Colon, irritable

See *Irritable bowel syndrome*.

Colonoscopy

Examination of the inside of the colon (the major part of the large intestine) by means of a long, flexible, fiberoptic viewing instrument called a colonoscope (see *Endoscopy*).

WHY IT IS DONE

Colonoscopy is used to investigate symptoms (such as bleeding from the bowel) and to look for disorders of the colon, such as colitis, polyps (small, benign, grapelike growths), and cancer. Attachments at the end of the instrument enable the physician to take biopsy specimens (remove small samples of tissue for analysis) or brushings for cytologic examination and to remove polyps.

HOW IT IS DONE
The patient takes laxatives for one or two days before the examination to empty the colon of feces. Because the procedure causes a little discomfort, the patient is lightly sedated beforehand. The colonoscope is passed into the colon through the anus and guided along the length of the colon, which the operator examines through a viewing lens. A complete examination of the entire colon can take from 10 minutes to a couple of hours to perform.

Colon, spastic
See *Irritable bowel syndrome*.

Color blindness
See *Color vision deficiency*.

Color vision
The ability to discriminate among different parts of the color spectrum. It is an ability found in some, but not all, animals, and probably developed as an aid to finding or catching food.

THE COLOR SPECTRUM
Light perceived by the human eye consists of electromagnetic radiation

C

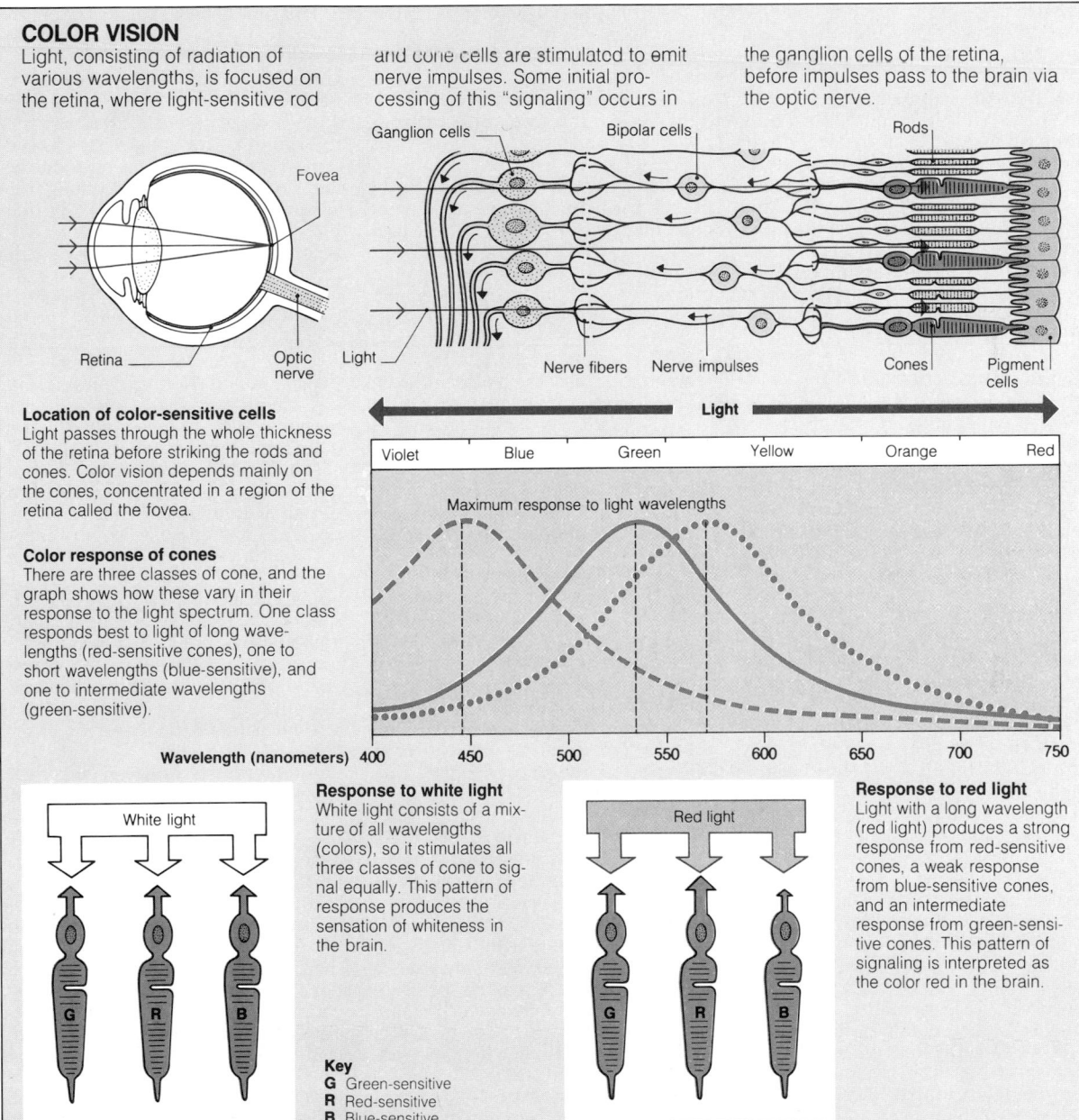

COLOR VISION
Light, consisting of radiation of various wavelengths, is focused on the retina, where light-sensitive rod and cone cells are stimulated to emit nerve impulses. Some initial processing of this "signaling" occurs in the ganglion cells of the retina, before impulses pass to the brain via the optic nerve.

Location of color-sensitive cells
Light passes through the whole thickness of the retina before striking the rods and cones. Color vision depends mainly on the cones, concentrated in a region of the retina called the fovea.

Color response of cones
There are three classes of cone, and the graph shows how these vary in their response to the light spectrum. One class responds best to light of long wavelengths (red-sensitive cones), one to short wavelengths (blue-sensitive), and one to intermediate wavelengths (green-sensitive).

Response to white light
White light consists of a mixture of all wavelengths (colors), so it stimulates all three classes of cone to signal equally. This pattern of response produces the sensation of whiteness in the brain.

Response to red light
Light with a long wavelength (red light) produces a strong response from red-sensitive cones, a weak response from blue-sensitive cones, and an intermediate response from green-sensitive cones. This pattern of signaling is interpreted as the color red in the brain.

Key
G Green-sensitive
R Red-sensitive
B Blue-sensitive

C

(energy waves) with wavelengths between about 400 and 700 nanometers (a nanometer is 40 billionths of an inch). Going from the short to the long end of this spectrum, different wavelengths produce the sensations of violet, blue, green, yellow, orange, and red (colors of the spectrum, or rainbow) when they impinge upon the retina and stimulate nerve signals, which are processed in the rear portion of the brain (occipital lobe).

Light consisting of a single wavelength—pure spectral color—is rare in nature. The light reflected or emitted by most objects consists of a complex mixture of many different wavelengths, known as a spectral mixture. White light consists of a fairly uniform mixture of all wavelengths of the visible spectrum. The number of possible spectral mixtures is infinite, and a major task of the retina and brain is to sort and interpret the information available in order to produce a usefully large but finite number of perceivable colors (which is estimated at several million).

CONE FUNCTION

The light-sensitive cells in the retina are of two main types, rods and cones. Of these types, the rods vary little in their response to different light wavelengths, and thus play little, if any, part in color vision. The cone cells, of which there are roughly four million to seven million per eye, are more concentrated within a central area of the retina called the macula lutea; about 25,000 of the cones are in the central fovea in the center of this area. Consequently, color vision is most accurate for objects viewed directly and is poor at the periphery of vision. Color perception also requires a minimum level of total available light—below this level, only the rods respond, and everything is seen as shades of gray.

When light impinges upon a cone, it causes a structural change in pigment contained within the cone, which in turn causes the cone to emit an electrical impulse. Light of any wavelength and of sufficient intensity, in general, causes all cones to respond to some

extent, but any single cone responds better (i.e., produces impulses more frequently) to certain wavelengths than others. Overall, it has been found that there are probably three classes of cone, responding maximally to light wavelengths of 445, 535, and 570 nanometers. Any particular light wavelength produces a unique overall pattern of response from all the cones together, and consequently any two wavelengths thus produce different patterns of response.

This offers some explanation of how the retina distinguishes light of different wavelengths, but gives few clues as to how information about complex mixtures of wavelengths is sorted, transmitted to the brain, and interpreted. The retina seems to contain other cells that receive, analyze, and compare the signals coming from several classes of cones. Further integration of the signals is accomplished as they are carried to the brain, where additional processing occurs, allowing for the perception of color. (See also *Eye*; *Perception*; *Vision*.)

Color vision deficiency

Any abnormality of the color vision system that causes a person to see colors differently from other people or causes difficulty distinguishing among certain colors. Such deficiencies are of various types and differ markedly in degree. Mild forms of deficiency are by far the most common; people with such mild defects generally have vision that is completely adequate for most purposes. True "color blindness" (monochromatism), in which the world is seen only in shades of black, white, and gray, is extremely rare.

CAUSES AND TYPES

Most cases of color vision deficiency are caused by an inherited defect of light-sensitive pigment in one or more classes of cone cell in the retina of the eye (see *Color vision*) and/or an abnormality or reduced number of the cone cells themselves. Acquired color vision deficiency may occur with certain retinal and optic nerve diseases and degenerations or trauma (injury).

The two common types of hereditary color vision deficiency are reduced discrimination of light wavelengths within the middle (green) and long (red) parts of the visible spectrum. The inherited defects are usually sex-linked (see *Genetic disorders*), which means that the majority of sufferers are male, although

women may carry the defect and pass it on to some of their children.

A further very small group of people have a blue deficiency, called tritanopia, which may be inherited or due to the toxic effects of poisons or drugs on, or degenerative processes of, the retina or optic nerve.

INCIDENCE

Among whites of European origin, about 8 percent of males and less than 1 percent of females have either green or red deficiency. The prevalence is generally lower in people of Asian or American Indian origin and even lower among blacks. The prevalence of both blue deficiency and monochromatism may be as low as one affected person per 100,000.

SYMPTOMS

Most people with defective color vision have no reason to suspect there is anything abnormal about the way they see, because they have no ready access to how other people see the world and because most cases are mild and do not interfere with daily living. Most cases come to light only when a person is noticed making mistakes with color discrimination, such as confusing close shades of colors. Other cases are discovered when the person's color vision is tested.

DIAGNOSIS AND MEASUREMENT

Color vision is commonly tested, usually by means of special color

plates under daylight conditions, during childhood or on entry to professions for which good color discrimination is needed.

More complicated testing, such as arranging sequences of colored chips or use of an anomaloscope, may also be used. The anomaloscope shines a variable mixture of green and red lights, and the person is asked to adjust the mixture until it appears the same as a fixed yellow light. If the adjusted mixture looks far too red or too green to the person with normal vision, the subject of the test is color defective. The severity of the defect is also measurable in this way.

OUTLOOK

People with the common, inherited, types of color deficiency retain the defect for life. It could be important for them to know about the abnormality, especially if considering an occupation that depends on color. The following occupations or careers may be unsuitable: train driver, airplane or marine pilot, electrician, jeweler, commercial artist, color photographer. In particular, the person who is severely color deficient can potentially be dangerous in some jobs (an electrician, for example, if color-coded wires cannot be properly identified). However, the more common mild color vision deficiencies do not interfere with most activities.

C

Colostomy

An operation in which part of the colon (large intestine) is brought through an incision in the abdominal wall and formed into an artificial opening to allow the discharge of feces into a lightweight bag attached to the skin. The colostomy may be temporary or permanent.

WHY IT IS DONE

In a severely ill patient, a temporary colostomy may be carried out as an emergency measure to deal with an obstruction or perforation in the large intestine that is preventing the patient from passing feces. The colostomy is made above the obstruction and, by allowing the feces to discharge, enables the patient to become well enough for a partial *colectomy* (an operation to remove part of the large intestine) to remove the obstruction. A temporary colostomy may also be performed at the same time as a colectomy to allow the repair to the colon to heal without feces passing through it. Temporary colostomies are closed when the rejoined colon has healed.

A permanent colostomy is needed when all or part of the rectum or anus, as well as part of the large intestine (for example, in cases of cancer of the rectum), require removal and normal defecation is no longer possible.

RECOVERY PERIOD

For two or three days after the operation the patient is fed intravenously. After that, the patient is given a light diet and begins to pass feces through the stoma (artificial opening) into a lightweight bag that is attached by adhesive seals to the skin around the stoma. After a bowel movement, the bag is exchanged for a new one.

During this period the patient should receive advice and training—preferably from a specialist nurse—on the care and management of the stoma and on how to apply and change the colostomy bag.

After leaving the hospital, the patient usually needs to convalesce for up to several weeks before returning to normal activities.

OUTLOOK

A person with a colostomy may eventually establish an almost normal bowel routine. The bowel usually discharges feces into the bag once or twice a day; the bag is then changed. The person with a temporary colostomy wears a bag over the stoma until the operation to close it is performed.

A person with a colostomy can expect to lead a normal life once fully recovered from the operation. The co-

---

PROCEDURE FOR COLOSTOMY

An incision is made in the abdominal wall and either a small loop of the colon or (if the rectum and anus have been removed) the severed end of the colon is pulled through. If a loop of the colon is used, an opening is made in it large enough for the feces to pass through. The edges of this opening or the edges of the severed end of the colon are stitched to the skin at the edge of the abdominal incision to create a stoma (artificial opening)

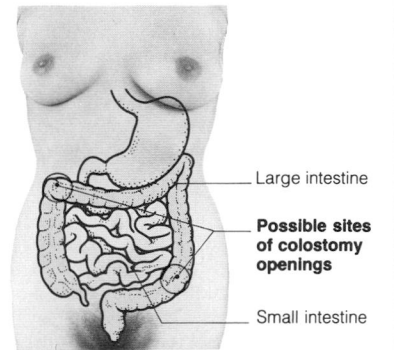

Large intestine

Possible sites of colostomy openings

Small intestine

Diseased part of rectum removed

Open end of bowel brought through to skin surface

Position of colostomy bag
The bag is attached to the skin around the stoma by adhesive seals. After a bowel movement, a new bag is attached.

---

lostomy usually causes no trouble, but occasionally a problem can occur. For example, the colostomy can prolapse (protrude too far from the abdomen) or become narrowed, blocking the passage of feces. In most cases these problems are overcome by surgery.

Colostrum

The thick, yellowish fluid produced by the breasts during late pregnancy and the first few days after childbirth. Colostrum is replaced by mature breast milk the week following birth. Compared with mature breast milk, colostrum contains less fat and sugar, and more minerals and protein. It has a high content of *lymphocytes* (a type of white blood cell) and *immunoglobulins* (antibodies), which help protect the baby from infection.

Colposcopy

Visual inspection of a woman's cervix (neck of the uterus) and vagina under illuminated magnification. A series of lenses is employed that can provide magnification of between five and 25 times.

WHY IT IS DONE

Colposcopy is performed to recognize or exclude the presence of any areas of precancerous conditions or early cancer in the tissues covering the cervix (see *Cervix, cancer of*). Usually, the gynecologist has been alerted by an abnormal *cervical smear test* (Pap smear), by smears that repeatedly show inflammation or infection, or by an abnormal appearance of the cervix during visual inspection at the time of a physical examination.

HOW IT IS DONE

Colposcopy is a painless procedure requiring no anesthetic. With the woman in the lithotomy position (lying on her back with legs apart and supported), the vagina and cervix are exposed using a speculum (an instrument that widens the opening and separates the collapsed walls of the vagina). The exposed tissues are first wiped with a dry sponge; the area is then washed with a solution of either dilute acetic acid or saline. The tissues are visually inspected under magnification to identify any suspicious-looking areas.

C

The applied solution causes any precancerous areas to show up either white (instead of their natural pink state) or with a characteristic surface pattern due to abnormal blood vessels. Once any such areas are seen, a *biopsy* sample of the tissue can be obtained. If, on examination by a pathologist, the tissue sample shows cells typical of severe dysplasia (abnormal growth) or an early cancer, and if the whole of the abnormal area can be seen, local destruction treatment (by *diathermy*, *cryosurgery*, or *laser treatment*) can be employed.

If any of the abnormal area is within the cervical canal, a *cone biopsy* (removal of a conical section of the cervix for inspection) is needed.

Coma

A state of unconsciousness and unresponsiveness distinguishable from *sleep* in that the person does not respond to external stimulation (e.g., shouting or pinching) or to his or her inner needs (e.g., a full bladder).

CAUSES
Coma results from disturbance or damage to areas of the brain involved in conscious activity or the maintenance of consciousness—in particular, parts of the *cerebrum* (the main mass of the brain), upper parts of the brain stem, and central regions of the brain, especially the *limbic system*.

The damage may be the result of a head injury, or of an abnormality such as a *brain tumor*, *brain abscess*, or *intracerebral hemorrhage*; all are shown by brain imaging techniques.

More often, there has been a buildup of poisonous substances that intoxicates brain tissues (due to a drug overdose, advanced liver or kidney disease, acute alcoholic intoxication, or in uncontrolled *diabetes mellitus*) or there has been impairment of blood flow to some brain areas, leading to cerebral *hypoxia* (lack of oxygen). *Encephalitis* and *meningitis* (respectively, inflammation of the brain and inflammation of the brain's protective coverings) can also cause coma.

SYMPTOMS
Varying depths of coma are recognized. In less severe forms, the person may respond to stimulation by uttering a few words or perhaps moving an arm. In severe cases, the person fails to respond in this way to repeated vigorous stimuli. However, even deeply comatose patients may show some automatic responses—they continue to breathe unaided, may cough, yawn, blink, and show roving eye movements, indicating that the lower brain stem, which controls these responses, is still functioning.

Measurement of variations in the depth of coma is important in assessment and treatment. Variations can be recorded by systems that classify the coma according to the person's verbal behavior, the movements he or she makes, and the state of the eyes (whether open, shut, or roving).

A person may remain in a state of deep coma for years, with little or no apparent activity in the cerebrum, but may be still alive because the brain stem is still functioning. By contrast, spread of the damage or disturbance to the lower brain stem may impair the vital functions of coughing, swallowing, and breathing. Artificial ventilation and maintenance of circulation may be needed. Complete irreversible loss of brain-stem function leads to death (see *Brain death*).

Combination drug

One that contains more than a single, active, therapeutic substance. A common example is the antibiotic drug co-trimoxazole, which contains sulfamethoxazole and trimethoprim.

Comedo

Another name for a *blackhead*.

Commensal

A usually harmless bacterium or other organism that normally lives in or on the body. Occasionally, commensals may cause disease, especially in people with impaired immunity.

Commitment

The process by which an individual suffering from a severe mental disorder is legally deprived of his or her freedom. A person is committed if he or she is likely to harm him- or herself or other people. Physicians who have examined the person explain to the court, usually in writing, why they believe he or she should be placed in a mental institution.

Commode

A portable chair that contains a removable toilet bowl in its seat. Commodes are useful for patients who are not confined to bed but who are not mobile enough to use the bathroom.

Communicable disease

Any disease caused by a microorganism or parasite that can be transmitted from one person or animal to another. (See *Infectious disease*.)

Compartment syndrome

A painful cramp caused by compression of a group of muscles during exercise. Usually, the affected muscles are situated in a confined space, so that when they expand slightly during exercise they are thus compressed and the blood flow through them is obstructed. The muscles may have become slightly enlarged before exercise, through intensive training, or possibly through injury.

An example is tibial compartment syndrome, in which muscles on the outer side of the shin expand within their lining and cause a cramp in this area. Usually the pain subsides rapidly when exercise is stopped.

Compensation neurosis

Psychological reaction to injury affected by the prospect of financial compensation. Also called accident or "traumatic" neurosis, the symptoms vary with personality, but headache, dizzy spells, loss of concentration, anxiety, and mild depression are common, as are neurological symptoms, such as pain and tingling in the legs or numbness in the affected part.

Some specialists consider the neurosis to be a genuine and persistent psychiatric reaction; others insist it is an attempt, conscious or unconscious, to manipulate the situation for profit. Repeated medical assessments, legal wrangling, and contradictory experts make this one of the most difficult areas of psychiatric diagnosis. Backing the idea of a genuine organic disorder, recent studies have shown that some people's symptoms persisted over the period of observation even after a satisfactory settlement of their insurance claims.

Complex

A group of related ideas, beliefs, and memories that have great importance emotionally, but which are always unconscious. The term was first used by the early psychoanalysts Sigmund Freud and Carl Jung to sum up psychological states deriving from experiences and relationships in childhood. The *Oedipus complex* is an important example, affecting all levels of adult behavior and attitudes.

Compliance

The degree to which patients follow medical advice. One reason for poor compliance is that patients sometimes do not remember or understand the physician's advice. Good compliance is more likely if the patient knows what to expect from taking the prescribed medicine. It is also important to know whether side effects are possible or likely, under what circumstances any medication should be stopped, and whether a prescribed drug has the potential to interact with other medicines the patient may be taking.

Complication

A disease or condition that results from, and is often more serious than, another condition. For example, in a case of *appendicitis*, the inflamed appendix may burst, spreading infection throughout the abdominal cavity and causing a serious complication called *peritonitis*. The childhood condition *mumps* occasionally has complications that may be serious, particularly *encephalitis* (inflammation of the brain) or *orchitis* (inflammation of the testes).

Sometimes a complication may be the result of treatment. Recovery from a surgical operation, for example, may be complicated by infection of the wound (caused by germs in the skin or in the operating room) or by cross infection from other patients.

Compos mentis

Latin for "of sound mind."

Compress

A pad of sheet lint or linen applied, under pressure, to an area of skin, and held in place by a bandage. The pad may be soaked in ice-cold water or wrapped around ice to provide a cold compress for reducing pain, swelling, and bleeding under the skin immediately after an injury (see *Ice pack*).

Compresses that have been soaked in hot water increase the circulation and are useful for bringing boils to a head. A dry compress may be used to stop bleeding from a wound (see *Bleeding* first-aid treatment box) or may be smeared with medication such as magnesium sulfate to draw pus from an infected area of skin.

Compression syndrome

A collection of symptoms caused by pressure on a nerve or nerves that supply the muscles and carry sensations from a particular area of the body. The symptoms may include numbness, tingling, discomfort, and muscle weakness. The best known is *carpal tunnel syndrome* (which affects the hand), caused by pressure on the median nerve as it passes under a ligament in the wrist.

Compulsive behavior

See *Obsessive-compulsive behavior*.

Computer-aided diagnosis

The physician makes a diagnosis by considering the patient's symptoms and medical history, examining the patient, and, when necessary, making use of imaging procedures, blood tests, and other diagnostic aids. Today, the computer has been added to the list of such aids.

PROBABILITY-BASED SYSTEMS

With probability-based systems the computer is used to store vast quantities of information involving cases of many different disorders. For example, it may be programmed with the details of thousands of cases of stomach pain—giving, for each patient, the exact type, location, and duration of the pain, accompanying symptoms, and relevant medical history, together with the eventual diagnosis. A physician confronted with a new case of stomach pain can enter the details into the computer, which, in a matter of seconds, will compare them with those already stored in its memory. It will then print out a list of the most likely diagnoses.

Although such computers are currently used in comparatively few hospitals, they are proving valuable in the treatment of people isolated from medical services, such as oil-rig crews or deep-sea divers. If someone becomes sick, the computer may be used to diagnose whether the case is an emergency requiring the sick person to be transported to a hospital.

PATTERN-RECOGNITION SYSTEMS

Computers can also be programmed to recognize and interpret visual data. One example is the examination of cells under a microscope. The computer has the ability to recognize abnormal cells. This could be of great future significance in certain types of *blood count* (for example, a differential white blood cell count) and also in *cervical smear tests* (Pap smears), in which cells taken from the cervix are microscopically examined for early signs of cancer. At present, each of the millions of smears taken annually needs examination by a laboratory technician, who can check only a comparatively small number at a time.

Computerized tomography

Another name for *CT scanning*.

Conception

Fertilization of a woman's *ovum* (egg) by a man's *sperm*, followed by implan-

tation of the resultant blastocyst in the lining of the *uterus*. (See also *Contraception*; *Pregnancy*.)

Concussion

Brief unconsciousness, usually lasting only a few seconds, that follows a violent blow to the head or neck. The loss of consciousness is due to disturbance of the electrical activity in the brain, and in most cases is not associated with any damage. Even so, concussion should always be treated seriously and reported to a physician.

Among the more common causes of concussion are traffic accidents, sports injuries, falls, industrial accidents, and blows received in fights.

SYMPTOMS AND TREATMENT

Common symptoms immediately following concussion include: confusion, inability to remember events immediately before the injury, dizziness, blurred vision, and vomiting. The more prolonged the period of unconsciousness, the more severe and persistent symptoms tend to be.

Repeated concussion—as happens, for example, to some boxers—can damage the brain and cause the "punchdrunk" syndrome: impaired concentration, slow thinking, and slurred speech.

Anyone who has been knocked out should see a physician, who will usually advise 24 hours of bed rest, either in a hospital or at home, under observation. The person should not drive a car or play any sport during this time. If new symptoms develop, such as drowsiness, difficulty breathing, repeated vomiting, or visual disturbances, they should be reported to the physician immediately since they could signify damage to a brain area or an *extradural hemorrhage* (bleeding between the skull and the outside of the brain).

The initial symptoms usually start to clear within a few days. If they fail to do so, medical opinion should be sought again, at which time the physician may wish to have the condition further investigated. (See also *Head injury*; *Drop attack*; *Syncope*.)

Conditioning

The formation of a specific type of response or behavior to a specific stimulus in the environment.

TYPES

Theories of conditioning are based largely on the work of the animal psychologists Pavlov and Skinner, whose names are identified with classical and operant conditioning.

C

C

In classical conditioning, if a stimulus that is known to consistently produce a response is paired consistently with a second "neutral" stimulus, eventually the second stimulus alone will produce the response. Pavlov demonstrated this occurrence in dogs. Each time food was presented to the dog, making it salivate, a bell was rung. Eventually the dog would salivate in response to the bell alone. Pavlov noted that the response would generalize to similar stimuli. Thus a dog conditioned to salivate when shown a round object would also salivate, although not as much, when shown an elliptical one. He also found that the conditioned response would eventually fade if not reinforced occasionally with the original neutral stimulus.

In operant conditioning, behavior is determined by rewards and punishments. Skinner placed a hungry rat in a box. It moved randomly about the cage, but occasionally accidentally pawed a lever, which released a pellet of food. Eventually the rat learned to press the lever whenever it wanted food; that is, it became conditioned.

EFFECTS
Behavioral psychologists believe that all behavior is learned in this way, and they regard psychiatric problems as learned behavior patterns. Many neurotic disorders are thought to arise because a previously neutral stimulus becomes associated with an anxiety-provoking stimulus. For example, someone who was punished as a child by being shut in a closet may develop claustrophobia (fear of enclosed spaces) because the enclosed space becomes associated with the fear of punishment. The anxiety may spread to fear of crowds or heights, for example, and does not diminish because it is continually reinforced by behavior; the claustrophobic person avoids using elevators or entering crowded shops.

Treatment for these disorders is based on the same principles of conditioning. A response that has been learned can also be unlearned, or a more appropriate form of behavior can be relearned (see *Behavior therapy*).

Condom
A barrier method of male contraception in the form of a thin latex rubber or plastic sheath placed over the penis before intercourse. Condoms provide both partners with some protection against sexual transmission of disease. (See *Contraception, barrier methods*.)

Conduct disorders
A group of behavioral disturbances, occurring in childhood or adolescence, in which the individual persistently and repetitively violates the rights and privileges of others. These violations may include vandalism, arson, assault, and robbery, as well as less aggressive forms of behavior such as truancy, substance abuse, and persistent lying (see *Behavioral problems in children; Adolescence*).

Condyloma acuminatum
See *Warts, genital*.

Condyloma latum
A small, moist, wartlike growth in the skin. In the second stage of the sexually transmitted disease *syphilis*, several develop at the side of the mouth, around the anus, and around the entrance to the vagina.

Cone biopsy
A surgical technique in which a section of the lower part of the cervix (neck of the uterus) is removed, either in the shape of a cone or a cylinder.

WHY IT IS DONE
A cone biopsy is performed if a woman has had an abnormal *cervical smear test* (Pap smear) or a series of abnormal smears, and if visual inspection of the cervix by *colposcopy* has failed to delineate the exact area of cancer or precancerous conditions (see *Cervix, cancer of*). Sometimes a cone biopsy is performed if a smear test suggests the presence of cancer, but colposcopy has failed to detect any abnormality on the outer surface of the cervix or at the entrance to the canal. In the latter cases there may be a precancerous area or cancer confined to the cervical canal.

Cone biopsy is now being accomplished using *laser* techniques or *cryosurgery*. (See also box on biopsy of the *cervix*.)

Confabulation
The use of a fictional story to make up for gaps in memory. Confabulation differs from lying in that it is motivated by the need to make sense of one's past rather than by a desire to deliberately deceive a listener. The phenomenon occurs most commonly in chronic alcoholics, when it is known as *Wernicke-Korsakoff syndrome*, and in people with head injuries.

Confidentiality
The ethical principle that a physician does not disclose to others information given in confidence by a patient. This concept was introduced by the ancient Greek physician Hippocrates and has been adopted by medical associations in all countries.

The physician's responsibility for maintaining confidential records has become more difficult with modern trends in medical practice. Clinics and health centers may have scores of medical and ancillary staff with access to records. In hospitals with computerized records, thousands of staff members may have such access. In theory everyone working in a medical setting is expected to understand and respect the code of confidentiality. In practice the code seems to be breached only rarely. More sophisticated computer systems make it possible to render the sensitive sections of medical records secure.

The patient's consent to disclosure is required before a physician may give confidential information to an employer, insurance company, or lawyer. When required by law to disclose confidential information, a physician does not have (as lawyers have) any "privilege" that allows refusal. A physician who persists in refusal is in contempt of court.

Physicians who treat children are expected to discuss their findings with the parents. As children mature, a point is reached at which their confidences merit the same respect as those of adult patients. In general, physicians believe that they should respect a child's request for confidentiality.

Most legal systems require physicians to override confidentiality in certain cases. For example, they are required to notify certain health authorities about specified infectious diseases; if patients with certain of these diseases refuse treatment, the health authorities may be informed so that treatment or isolation may be imposed by law. Physicians are generally required to notify the police if they treat gunshot wounds or know of other serious crimes.

Physicians who breach confidentiality without legal justification may be sued in the civil courts; damages may be awarded against them.

Confusion
A disorganized mental state in which the abilities to remember, think clearly, and reason are impaired.

TYPES AND CAUSES
Confusion can be acute or chronic. The acute condition can arise as a symptom of *delirium*, in which the ac-

tivity of the brain is affected by fever, drugs, poisons, or injury. Elderly people are particularly prone to acute confusional states from these causes, especially from certain drugs (e.g., *barbiturates, tranquilizers,* or *alcohol*).

Chronic confusion is often associated with *alcohol dependence,* long-term use of tranquilizers, and certain organic mental disorders such as *schizophrenia.* Chronic confusion is a feature of *dementia,* a brain disorder commonly caused by the progressive degeneration and death of brain cells.

SYMPTOMS AND SIGNS
People who are acutely confused often suffer from terrifying hallucinations and may behave in a violent and abusive manner. However, acute confusion is usually only temporary, and few people remember the events after the attack has passed.

Chronic confusion is generally noticeable from features such as absentmindedness, poor short-term memory, and a tendency for the sufferer to repeat himself or herself. Chronically confused people may also become depressed and frustrated, but they are less likely to become aggressive or violent. Many of the conditions responsible for chronic confusion tend to be slowly progressive.

DIAGNOSIS AND TREATMENT
An accurate diagnosis is essential before confusion can be treated. A detailed description of the symptoms (often from a relative) and a general physical examination will suggest which studies should be performed.

If a treatable cause is found, the appropriate treatment can often produce a marked improvement. Undiagnosable acute confusion may be treated with sedatives. Medicine has little to offer the elderly, chronically confused patient apart from skilled, supervised care.

Congenital
A term that means "present at birth." Thus, a congenital abnormality is a defect that has been present since birth. It may have been inherited genetically from the parents, may have occurred as the result of damage or infection in the uterus, or may have occurred at the time of birth. Congenital abnormalities are often also called *birth defects.*

Note that "congenital" does not mean the same as "hereditary." Not all congenital abnormalities are inherited, and many hereditary diseases (such as *Huntington's chorea*) are not apparent at birth.

Diseases and disorders that are not congenital—for example, most infectious diseases, cancers, and degenerative disorders—are called "acquired."

Congestion
Usually a reference to the accumulation of an excessive amount of blood, *tissue fluid,* or *lymph* in part of the body. A major cause of congestion is an increased flow of blood in the area, as occurs in inflammation. Another possible cause is reduced drainage of blood from the area, as can occur in *heart failure,* venous disorders such as *varicose veins,* and *lymphatic* disorders. (See also *Congestion, nasal.*)

Congestion, nasal
Obstruction of the flow of air through the passages of the nose due to swelling of its lining. Congestion may be accompanied by the accumulation of thick nasal mucus, which further impedes breathing. These two factors produce the familiar feelings of a stuffy, "full" nose, and the frequent desire to blow the nose (which usually has little effect on the congestion).

Nasal congestion is a symptom of the common cold (see *Cold, common*) or hay fever (see *Rhinitis, allergic*). In these conditions, the swelling is due to inflammation of the nasal lining. This inflammation may become persistent in certain disorders such as *sinusitis* or nasal *polyps.*

Congestive heart failure
See *Heart failure.*

Conjunctiva
The transparent membrane covering the sclera (white of the eye) and lining the inside of the eyelids. Cells in the conjunctiva produce a fluid (similar to tears) that lubricates the lids and cornea. Blood vessels within the conjunctiva are normally invisible to the naked eye, but become engorged in *conjunctivitis* (pinkeye) and other inflammatory conditions.

Conjunctivitis
Inflammation of the conjunctiva, causing redness, discomfort, and a discharge from the affected eye.

Conjunctivitis is very common. Each year, at least one person in 50 visits a physician because of this complaint. The common causes are infections (especially in children) and allergy (more common in adults).

INFECTIVE CONJUNCTIVITIS
Most conjunctival infections are caused by bacteria—for example,

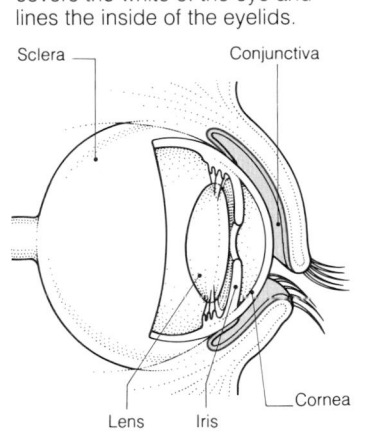

LOCATION OF CONJUNCTIVA
This transparent membrane covers the white of the eye and lines the inside of the eyelids.

Sclera

Conjunctiva

Cornea

Lens   Iris

staphylococci—that are spread by hand-to-eye contact, or by viruses, associated with a cold, sore throat, or illness such as measles. Viral conjunctivitis can occur in epidemics, spreading rapidly (through schools and other group settings).

Newborn babies occasionally acquire a type of conjunctival infection called neonatal *ophthalmia,* caused by spread of infection from the mother's cervix during birth. This type of infection may be with common bacteria, with the microorganisms responsible for *gonorrhea* or genital *herpes,* or may be a *chlamydial infection* (any of which may be present on the mother's cervix without symptoms). The infection may spread to the whole of the baby's eye and can cause blindness.

Keratoconjunctivitis is an inflammation of both the conjunctiva and the cornea; it is often due to a viral infection. In some tropical countries, *trachoma* is a serious form of conjunctivitis caused by a type of chlamydial infection.

ALLERGIC CONJUNCTIVITIS
The following substances can provoke an allergic response of the conjunctiva: cosmetics (such as mascara), contact lens cleaning solutions, and pollen among allergic *rhinitis* (hay fever) sufferers. Prevention is by avoiding the causative substance.

SYMPTOMS AND DIAGNOSIS
All types of conjunctivitis cause redness, discomfort of an itchy, scratchy nature, a discharge, and occasionally photophobia (dislike of bright lights). In infective conjunctivitis the discharge is purulent (containing pus)

and may occasionally stick the eyelids together in the morning. In allergic conjunctivitis the discharge is clear, and the eyelids are often swollen.

Diagnosis is made from the appearance of the eye. If an infection is suspected, swabs may be taken to find out the causative organism, especially in a newborn baby when an exact diagnosis may be needed.

TREATMENT
Warm water is used to wash away the discharge and remove any crusts on the eyelids. In babies the eye may be washed with sterile saline solution.

If an infection is suspected, antibiotic eye drops or ointment (with chloramphenicol, for instance) are instilled into the eye. These will not cure a viral conjunctivitis, which tends to resolve of its own accord.

Allergic conjunctivitis can be helped by the use of antihistamine drops. Occasionally, corticosteroid drops are used, but only when there is definitely no infection present (which could be made worse by corticosteroids).

Connective tissue
The material that holds together the various structures of the body. Some structures are made up of connective tissue, notably *tendons* and *cartilage*. Connective tissue also forms the matrix (ground substance) of *bone* and the nonmuscular structures of *arteries* and *veins*.

Connective tissue diseases
See *Collagen diseases*.

Conn's syndrome
A disorder caused by the secretion of excessive amounts of the hormone aldosterone by a benign tumor of one of the adrenal glands. This upsets the body's salt and water balance, causing *hypertension* (high blood pressure) and symptoms such as thirst, muscle weakness, and excessive passage of urine. (See also *Aldosteronism*.)

Consciousness
An awareness of self and surroundings, so that a person knows what he or she is doing and intends to do. The awareness is dependent on sensations (especially visual and auditory), memories, and experiences.

Such awareness requires intact brain function, particularly within the *cerebrum* (the main mass of the brain) and the reticular system in the *brain stem*. The content of consciousness relies heavily on the functions of the cerebrum—for example, on memory

and the interpretation of sensations—while wakefulness is linked with the reticular system.

Although a person may be conscious, much that goes on within the brain is still below the level of consciousness. In psychological terms this activity is referred to as subconscious activity.

Disturbance of consciousness leads to impaired attention, concentration, and understanding. The thinking becomes slowed and memory fails. There appears to be a lack of direction in thoughts and actions. Although patients can be stimulated to respond, their responses are faulty. As the level of arousal deteriorates, the person may eventually pass into a state of *stupor* and then *coma*.

Consent
The legal term describing a patient's agreement with a physician performing an operation, arranging drug treatment, or carrying out diagnostic tests. Consent is valid only if the patient has been fully informed about the purpose of the procedure, the likely outcome, and both common and rare complications and side effects that may arise.

AVAILABILITY OF INFORMATION
Even as recently as the 1960s many physicians in the US believed it necessary to conceal much of the information about an illness and its treatment from the patient and his or her family. At that time few physicians told patients they had cancer, even when the illness was at an advanced stage, and few told such patients that they would die. Similarly, few physicians discussed the risk of death or serious complications—small but unavoidable—in any surgical procedure requiring an anesthetic, or explained the full range of side effects possible from treatment with a particular drug.

This concealment was justified by the medical profession in the paternalistic belief that the physician knew best, and that patients were unable to understand technical terms or concepts. The consumer rights movements of the 1960s and 1970s swept away such ideas, and physicians now recognize that patients expect full and frank information about illness and its treatment. In the US, a physician has no defense if the patient suffers harm from a foreseeable hazard of treatment that was not disclosed at the time consent was given. In other countries (such as Britain), physicians are still allowed to conceal rare hazards if they

believe that such a policy is in the patient's best interests.

Nevertheless, even in the US the amount of detailed information offered to patients varies from physician to physician. Some distribute printed information sheets before asking patients to sign consent forms, while others discuss the issues at length. Many physicians tell patients that they will answer their questions honestly, but will not force unwanted information on them.

When the investigation or treatment is carried out solely for the patient's benefit the explanations may be fairly brief, but more detail is usually offered when patients are asked to take part in research studies that may be of no direct benefit to them as individuals. Under these circumstances the purpose of the study must be explained along with all its hazards. Consent to a research procedure is invalid if any pressure was placed on the patient (for example, by suggestions that participation in the study would ensure preferential treatment by a surgeon).

WITHHOLDING CONSENT
Consent cannot be given by children or by people with serious mental disorders. Consent may be given (or withheld) on their behalf by parents or relatives. On several occasions in recent years, however, the courts have intervened and overruled the consent of relatives to withhold treatment from newborn children with severe handicaps and from adults with permanent brain damage. This action by the courts is based on the doctrine that the law forbids euthanasia or assisted suicide, whether or not the patient consents or consent is given on his or her behalf. Consent may not be given on behalf of children or the mentally ill for research procedures that would be of no benefit to them as individuals.

Constipation
The infrequent or difficult passing of hard, dry feces. In most cases constipation is harmless, but occasionally it may be a symptom of an underlying disorder, especially if it is of recent onset in an adult over 40. Many people worry that they do not move their bowels often enough, but, in fact, regularity and comfort of bowel action are more important than frequency. However, any persistent change in the pattern of bowel movements should be investigated by a physician to rule out a serious disorder.

C

CONSTIPATION Infrequent or difficult passing of hard bowel movements.

? Have you always tended to suffer from constipation? — **YES** → Do you often resist the urge to move your bowels because you are too busy? — **YES** → This can lead to an eventual loss of normal bowel reflexes. You should try to reestablish a regular habit by always going to the toilet when you feel the urge.

NO

NO ↓ Have you used laxatives regularly for a long time? — **YES** → Overuse of laxatives can eventually make your bowel inactive. Stop taking the laxatives and try adding bran and extra fruit to your diet instead.

See • *Laxative drugs*

NO

Your constipation is probably due to a lack of fluid, fruits, vegetables and whole-grain cereals in your diet. Increase your intake. If no improvement results, consult your physician.

See • *Fiber, dietary*

Dietary fiber
This should be an essential part of everyone's diet because it provides bulk to help the large intestine carry away body wastes. Not only does it help prevent constipation and certain diseases of the large intestine but it may also help lower the level of fats in the body.

? Has defecation become painful? — **YES** → A tear in the lining of the anus or hemorrhoids may cause such pain. Consult your physician.

See • *Anal fissure*
    • *Hemorrhoids*

NO

? Do you have lower abdominal pain? — **YES** → Have you had similar episodes of pain and constipation for many years? — **YES** → You probably have an irritable bowel. Consult your physician.

See • *Irritable bowel syndrome*

NO

☎
Consult your physician without delay!
An irritable bowel or swellings in the walls of the large intestine may cause such symptoms. However, the slight possibility of intestinal cancer also must be ruled out.

See • *Diverticular disease*
    • *Intestine, cancer of*
    • *Irritable bowel syndrome*

NO

Continued on next page

Fiber-rich foods
Fruit, leafy vegetables, potato skins, whole-grain bread and cereals, dried peas and beans, and bran are all examples of high-fiber foods.

C

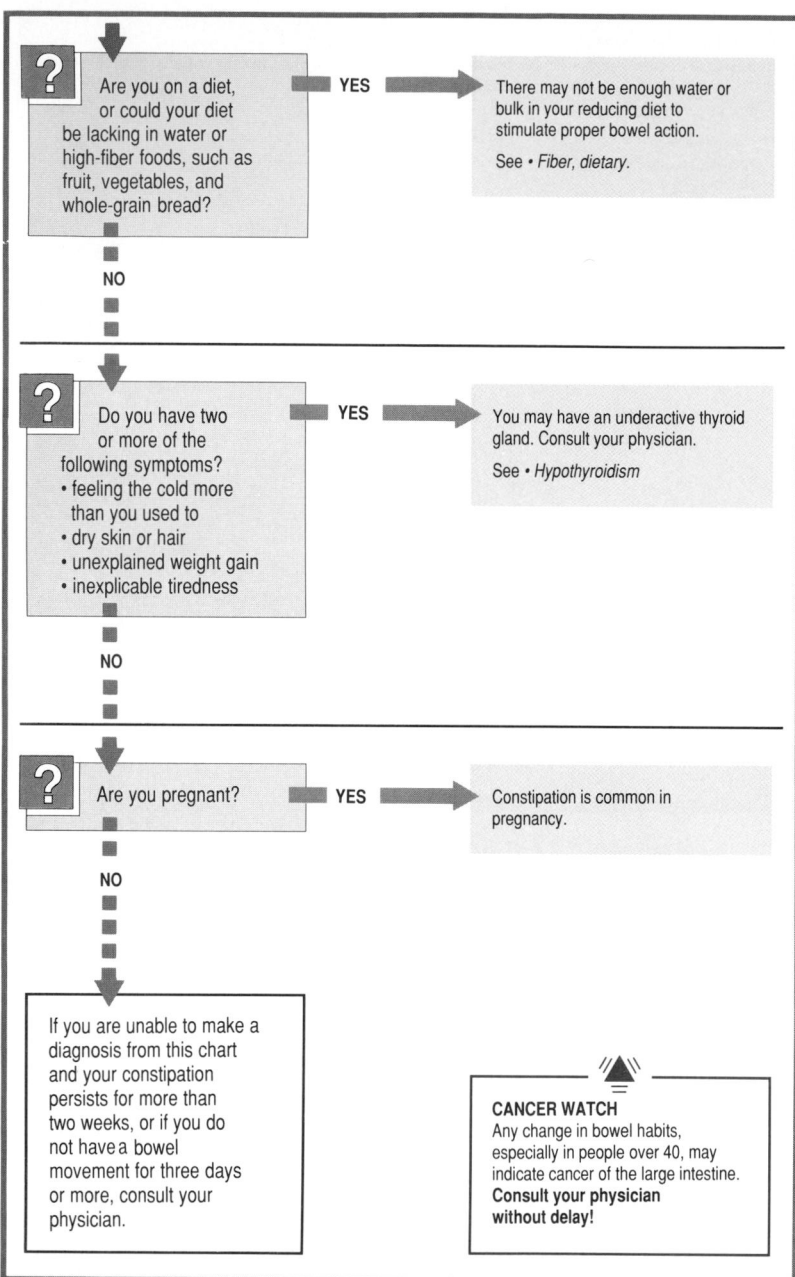

? Are you on a diet, or could your diet be lacking in water or high-fiber foods, such as fruit, vegetables, and whole-grain bread?

YES → There may not be enough water or bulk in your reducing diet to stimulate proper bowel action.

See • *Fiber, dietary.*

NO

? Do you have two or more of the following symptoms?
• feeling the cold more than you used to
• dry skin or hair
• unexplained weight gain
• inexplicable tiredness

YES → You may have an underactive thyroid gland. Consult your physician.

See • *Hypothyroidism*

NO

? Are you pregnant?

YES → Constipation is common in pregnancy.

NO

If you are unable to make a diagnosis from this chart and your constipation persists for more than two weeks, or if you do not have a bowel movement for three days or more, consult your physician.

CANCER WATCH
Any change in bowel habits, especially in people over 40, may indicate cancer of the large intestine. **Consult your physician without delay!**

CAUSES

The most common cause of constipation in Western countries is insufficient *fiber* in the diet. Fiber, which is found in foods such as whole-grain bread, fresh fruit, and vegetables, provides the bulk that the muscles of the colon (large intestine) need to stimulate propulsion of the fecal matter.

Lack of regular bowel-moving habits is another cause. This may be the result of inadequate toilet training in childhood or of repeatedly ignoring the urge to move the bowels. In the elderly the latter is sometimes due to immobility. Another cause of constipation in some elderly people is weakness of the muscles of the abdomen and pelvic floor, which prevents adequate pressure in the attempt to move the bowels.

In people suffering from *hemorrhoids* or an *anal fissure* (a crack, laceration, or tear in the skin around the anus), the pain that results from passing feces can seriously inhibit efforts to initiate bowel movements.

In *irritable bowel syndrome*, the person may experience intermittent constipation, sometimes alternating with diarrhea. In *hypothyroidism*, colonic contractions are reduced, resulting in chronic constipation.

Finally, constipation may be caused by narrowing of part of the colon, due to *diverticular disease* or cancer (see *Intestine, cancer of*).

TREATMENT

In many cases constipation can be cured by following a few simple measures—establishing a regular routine for using the toilet (sometimes facilitated by the use of a glycerin suppository), acting on any urge to move the bowels, avoiding the use of laxatives and purgatives, increasing the amount of fiber in the diet, and drinking more fluids. If constipation continues despite these measures, medical advice should be obtained.

A physician should also be consulted if constipation occurs after years of normal bowel habits, or if it is accompanied by blood in the feces, pain on moving the bowels, loss of a sense of well-being, or weight loss.

A physician usually investigates the condition by obtaining a detailed case history, carrying out a physical examination, and sometimes arranging for tests.

Contact lenses

Very thin, shell-like disks fitted on the cornea (the transparent front part of the eye) to correct defective vision. Contact lenses alter the power of the cornea by replacing the existing outer surface with a plastic surface.

Leonardo da Vinci in 1508 was the first to describe the possibility of using contact lenses. The first lens was made by a German in 1887; it was made of glass and covered the entire front surface of the eye. The conventional small hard lens made of transparent plastic was first introduced in the 1940s and many millions have been used since.

WHY THEY ARE USED

Contact lenses can correct most of the defects in vision for which glasses are prescribed and can correct some conditions that glasses cannot.

Vanity and convenience account for most contact-lens wear. The lenses are almost undetectable when worn. Unlike glasses, these lenses generally do not fall off, do not get covered with rain, and normally do not mist up.

C

Some contact-lens wearers have a particular optical problem or medical condition. For people who are extremely nearsighted or those who have had cataracts removed, glasses can produce considerable distortion of vision, making contact lenses preferable. Contact lenses can also be useful for hiding scars on the surface of the cornea. Patients with irregular corneas (such as may follow corneal disease, corneal trauma, corneal ulceration, and corneal grafting) may be helped by contact lenses.

TYPES

HARD PLASTIC LENSES These give good optical vision, are long-lasting and durable (possibly five years or more of use), inexpensive, and easy to maintain. However, they sometimes are difficult to tolerate and occasionally fall out; severe pain can result if grit gets into the eye and under the lens. When the lenses are removed after prolonged wear, vision with glasses may be temporarily blurred.

HARD, GAS-PERMEABLE LENSES Introduced in the early 1980s, these have the same visual qualities as hard plastic lenses, but are more comfortable and easier to get used to because they allow oxygen to pass through the lens to the eye. However, they are less durable (possibly giving up to five years of wear) and more expensive.

SOFT LENSES Also called hydrophilic lenses (having a strong affinity for water), these are the most comfortable because of their high water content, which can range from 38 to 70 percent. They are usually easy to wear from the beginning, can be worn for long periods, and are ideal for occasional use since the eye generally tolerates them for short periods of time despite infrequent wearing. Classic soft lenses can correct nearsightedness and farsightedness, but not much astigmatism. Being flexible, they mold themselves to the shape of the eye, and thus cannot correct the irregularly shaped cornea that is the cause of astigmatism. However, special types of soft lenses are designed to correct some astigmatism. Other drawbacks include fragility, a shorter life (12 to 18 months), and more complicated maintenance than for hard lenses.

Extremely thin, specially designed soft lenses with a high water content can be worn for periods of up to one month. These extended-wear contact lenses may increase the risks and dangers of infection.

SPECIAL LENSES Rigid, scleral lenses, which cover the whole of the front of

CARE AND INSERTION OF CONTACT LENSES

Hard lenses may require several solutions, one for cleaning, one for wetting, and possibly one for storage. If used, the storage solution is washed off before lens insertion. The wetting solution is used before inserting a lens in the eye.

Care of soft lenses is more complicated. Because the lenses are permeable and absorb any chemi- cals they come in contact with, the solutions must be weaker. Disinfection with a chemical or heating system is required to prevent contamination and infection. Two or three solutions may be necessary, but intermittent cleaning with a third system, such as an enzyme tablet or an oxidizing agent, is also required to remove mucus and protein.

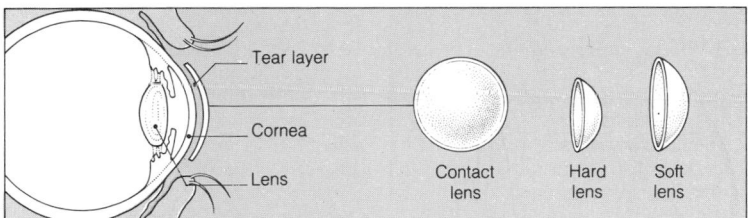

Tear layer · Cornea · Lens · Contact lens · Hard lens · Soft lens

1 Wash your hands thoroughly under running water and carefully rinse off all traces of soap.

2 If you like, use a rubber sucker to remove a hard lens from its container. Rinse the lens thoroughly.

Inverted lens

3 Place the lens on your index finger. If it is a soft lens, make sure that it has not turned inside out. If it has, you will see an out-turned rim.

4 Keep both eyes open, hold the upper lid open, and look straight ahead or at the lens as you bring it up to your eye.

5 Place the lens on your eye. Look downward and then release the lid. If necessary, the lens may be centered by gently massaging the eyelid (the photograph on the right shows a hard lens correctly positioned).

C

the eye, are used to hide disfigured eyes. Hard or soft bifocal contact lenses can be produced, but can be difficult to fit and vision may not be satisfactory. Toric contact lenses (thicker around the outside than in the middle) are used to correct high degrees of astigmatism and can be made in all materials.

PROBLEMS

Contact lens wearers can encounter problems with their lenses. A small group may be unable to wear contact lenses at all, because of hypersensitivity (for example, some hay-fever sufferers and very fair-skinned people), difficult optical requirements, or personal hygiene habits.

Lenses can irritate the eye because of dryness due to problems with tear production, which may be inadequate, especially in older people.

With hard plastic contact lenses, abrasion of the cornea can occur because of too rapid buildup of wearing time during the adaptation period, particularly with a tight-fitting lens. Wearing the contact lens too many hours per day can cause the same problem. Symptoms are pain and tearing. With patching and/or antibiotics applied to the eye, symptoms usually clear up within 24 hours.

A common problem that sometimes occurs with soft lenses is that people develop sensitivity of the eyes and lids, either to the maintenance solutions or to mucus forming on the lens surface itself. Symptoms include decreased lens tolerance, stinging, increased lens movement, increased mucus, and redness of the conjunctiva. The person generally must stop wearing contact lenses for several months and then start again with new lenses and a different type of maintenance solution.

Contact lens wear should be stopped if the eyes become red or infected, if vision is blurred, or if the lenses become uncomfortable.

Contact tracing

A service, provided by boards of health, that aims to control the spread of some infectious diseases.

WHY IT IS DONE

If a person is diagnosed as having a serious infectious disease, it may be possible to identify from whom it was caught and to whom it may have been passed on. If these contacts can be encouraged to have an examination and possible treatment, it can help reduce the spread of the disease. Many contacts do not, in fact, have the

infection; others are infected although they may have no obvious symptoms.

Contact tracing is undertaken for many types of sexually transmitted diseases (STDs), including *syphilis* and *gonorrhea*, and also for infections such as tuberculosis, meningitis, and sometimes some imported tropical diseases such as *Lassa fever*. Contact tracing is not carried out for less serious diseases or those for which the transmission mechanism is indirect or not clearly understood.

HOW IT IS DONE

At clinics involved in the treatment of sexually transmitted or other infections, trained nurses and health workers interview patients after their diagnosis to explain the nature of the disease, mode of transmission, and possible complications if left untreated. In strictest confidence, patients are asked for the names and, when relevant, addresses of contacts. These people may either be primary contacts (from whom they may have caught the disease) or secondary contacts (to whom they may have transmitted the disease).

Patients are not compelled to reveal the names of their contacts, nor are contacts compelled to consult a physician (although they are strongly encouraged to do so). If a patient is deemed to be a real danger to the community, the commissioner of health may legally quarantine the patient. This is rarely necessary.

It is important to remember that the principle of *confidentiality* is maintained throughout, and no patient or employer can be given the name or diagnosis of anyone else involved.

Contagious

A term describing a disease that can be transferred from one person to another by social contact, such as sharing the home or workplace.

Contraception

The control of fertility to prevent *pregnancy*. There are various contraceptive methods that work in differing ways, but their basic action is either to stop the sperm and the ovum from meeting in the fallopian tube (thus preventing conception or fertilization) or to prevent a fertilized ovum from implanting in the lining of the uterus.

METHODS

Contraception may be achieved in the following ways: by avoidance of intercourse; *coitus interruptus*; forms of periodic abstinence; various barrier methods; hormonal methods; postco-

ital methods; *IUDs*; and *sterilization*. Regarded today as highly unreliable, *breast-feeding* was once used as a method of contraception. If it is carried out frequently during both the day and the night, it causes changes in the hormone levels in the body that sometimes prevent ovulation until the baby is weaned.

MEASURING CONTRACEPTIVE EFFECTIVENESS

Contraceptives are measured not so much for their effectiveness as for their failure rate. The failure rate is the rate of pregnancies per 100 woman-years of use (i.e., the number of pregnancies among 100 women using the method for one year, or 50 using it for two years). The lower the failure rate, the more effective and useful the contraceptive. No account is taken of the fact that most failures occur in the first year of use, while the woman is getting used to the method.

There are two ways of defining contraceptive effectiveness: the theoretical, or method, effectiveness; and use effectiveness (i.e., the effectiveness in actual use).

THEORETICAL (METHOD) EFFECTIVENESS This is the effectiveness of a particular contraceptive method when used exactly as prescribed by the manufacturers, the physician, or the clinic. Theoretical failure rates are usually much lower than the failure rates of contraceptives in actual use.

USE EFFECTIVENESS Measures the effectiveness of the method under all circumstances. It takes into account pregnancies resulting from incorrect use (for example, forgetting to take the pill or not putting on a condom correctly). Use effectiveness is almost always markedly lower than theoretical effectiveness in "user-dependent" methods, such as barriers. With "nonuser-dependent" methods, such as IUDs and sterilization, there is less of a difference.

RISKS INVOLVED IN CONTRACEPTIVE METHODS

Risks vary a great deal depending on the method. Perhaps the greatest risk in all cases is failure of the method, which can lead to unwanted pregnancy and all that this entails (such as an elective *abortion*). Other risks include danger to the health or life of the mother or danger to the health of any other children.

Risks inherent in contraceptives themselves must also be weighed against the benefits. Hormonal contraceptives are linked with *cardiovascular* disease, particularly in women over 35 who smoke; IUDs may be associated with an increase in *pelvic*

METHODS OF CONTRACEPTION

There are various methods of contraception: the natural methods, barrier methods, hormonal methods, and postcoital methods. Sterilization interferes with part of the male or female reproductive system to render the individual infertile.

Hormonal method

Pill

Mini-pill

Pill

The pill
Prevents ovulation, changes the cervical mucus to prevent sperm penetration, or alters the uterine lining to prevent implantation.

Hormonal implant
Capsules containing a progestogen are inserted into the arm, where they release progestogen into the blood.

Barrier method

Spermicidal foam and gel

Condom

The condom
A tube-shaped piece of latex rubber that usually has a teat to hold ejaculate. It should be used with spermicide, examined for holes before use, and have all air squeezed out of the tip to prevent bursting. The rim should be held during withdrawal to stop the condom from slipping off.

Barrier method

Sponge

Diaphragm plus spermicide

Caps

Diaphragm in position
Held in place over the cervix by means of a coiled metal spring in its rim, the diaphragm prevents sperm from reaching the cervix.

IUD in position
A small piece of molded plastic with string attached, sometimes with copper or a female hormone added, the IUD is worn in the uterus.

IUDs

STERILIZATION

Offers an almost completely safe and reliable form of birth control, although it is usually irreversible. It has no effect on the production of sex hormones, so a man produces sperm-free semen and a woman produces normal eggs.

Male sterilization (vasectomy)
A surgical operation in which the vas deferens are cut so that sperm cannot pass from testes to penis.

Female sterilization
Two cuts are made below the navel, and a laparoscope is inserted. An attachment to this is used to seal off the tube ends.

Mucosal and temperature methods
The temperature method involves charting the woman's temperature to ascertain whether ovulation has taken place. The mucosal method involves studying the cervical mucus throughout the woman's menstrual cycle.

C

FAILURE RATES OF CONTRACEPTIVES

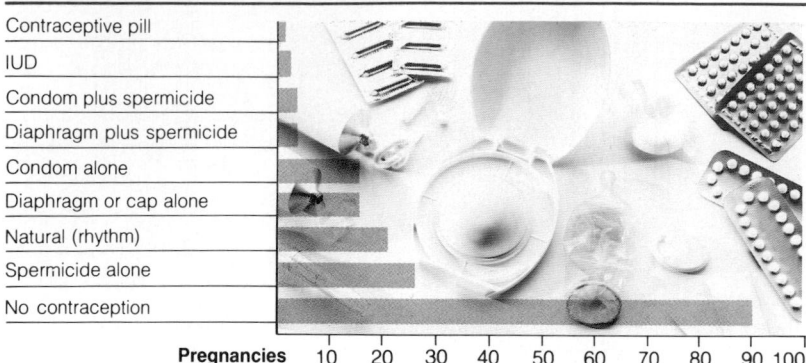

	Pregnancies	10	20	30	40	50	60	70	80	90	100
Contraceptive pill											
IUD											
Condom plus spermicide											
Diaphragm plus spermicide											
Condom alone											
Diaphragm or cap alone											
Natural (rhythm)											
Spermicide alone											
No contraception											

The chart shows the number of pregnancies that can be expected, on average, if 100 healthy young couples use a given contraceptive method (or none at all) for one year. Note that use of the pill or IUD, or barrier methods (condom or diaphragm) combined with spermicide, are all moderately to highly effective contraceptives. Using a barrier method without spermicide, or spermicide alone, is much less effective.

inflammatory disease, particularly in women who have had more than one sex partner; and sterilization carries the risks of any surgical operation.

CONTRACEPTIVE RESEARCH
New forms continue to be investigated although the constraints of licensing authorities, the great cost, and the paucity of funds have slowed the pace. However, a few of the promising lines of research are as follows.

HORMONAL CONTRACEPTION New forms of hormonal contraception include the use of *LH-RH* (a hormone that regulates the release of other hormones that control the ovulatory cycle), which may be given as a nasal spray.

RU-486 The development of this antiprogesterone is quite far advanced and is undergoing clinical trials, sometimes in conjunction with prostaglandins (hormonelike substances that play multiple roles in the body). It seems to act by stopping production of progesterone in the second half of the menstrual cycle, thus preventing implantation of a fertilized ovum in the uterus. It can also be used as a "morning-after" contraceptive.

STEROIDAL VAGINAL RINGS Made of silicone-rubber containing a progestogen, these are at a late stage of development. They are inserted into the vagina and release the progestogen locally, which acts directly on the reproductive organs.

PINPOINTING OVULATION Various methods to determine the exact time of ovulation continue to be researched; this would be of great help in the use of periodic abstinence for contraception.

VACCINES These are being studied, but still present problems. Vaccines are being developed against sperm, against the outer coat of the ovum, and against the hormone that helps maintain a pregnancy.

THE MALE PILL This continues to be researched, but so far without much practical progress. The main problem is that the testes are continually producing millions of sperm, while the ovaries have a definite number of ova present at birth and release only one each month—making suppression of ovulation simpler than suppression of sperm production.

Contraception, barrier methods

The use of a device and/or chemical to block or otherwise prevent sperm from reaching the ovum, thus preventing fertilization and pregnancy. Barrier contraceptives include the condom (placed over the erect penis), and the diaphragm, the contraceptive cap, and the contraceptive sponge, which are all positioned within the vagina. Spermicides are recommended in combination with barrier devices for maximum protection.

Barrier methods, especially condoms, are advisable for people with more than one sex partner because they help prevent the sexual transmission of diseases such as *gonorrhea*, *AIDS*, and *hepatitis B*.

TYPES
CONDOM A sheath of fine, latex rubber or plastic, about 7 inches long, that is usually lubricated for ease of application. A condom normally has a teat at its end to hold ejaculated sperm. Condoms are available over-the-counter in various sizes, colors, and textures and may be precoated with a spermicide.

A condom should be inspected before use to make certain there are no holes or tears, and then carefully rolled onto the erect penis before intercourse. The tip of the condom should be squeezed as it is rolled on, so that no air is trapped in the end (preventing it from bursting when ejaculation occurs). The condom rim should be held close to the penis when it is withdrawn from the vagina, which should occur after orgasm but before the erection subsides.

DIAPHRAGM A hemispherical dome of thin rubber with a coiled metal spring in the rim. It fits diagonally across the front wall of the vagina, with the top part of the rim up behind the cervix (neck of the uterus) and the opposite edge of the rim resting on the ledge above the pubic bone. Diaphragms are available in a range of sizes and must be properly fitted, the size and type being determined by an individual's anatomy. It must be used with a spermicidal agent and be left in place for six hours after intercourse. Without disturbing the diaphragm, additional spermicide should be used if intercourse is repeated within six hours.

CONTRACEPTIVE CAP Smaller and more rigid than the diaphragm, this latex rubber device fits tightly over the cervix (rather than covering the vaginal vault), where it is held in place by suction. There are three types: the cervical cap is thimble-shaped, the vault cap is bowl-shaped, and the vimule cap combines features of both the cervical and vault caps. Caps are often used by women who cannot use diaphragms because of anatomical changes, such as *prolapse* of the uterus or a *cystocele*. As with the diaphragm, a cap must be properly fitted and used with a spermicide. Caps became available in the US in 1988.

SPERMICIDE A range of spermicides is available, including aerosol foams, creams, jellies, pessaries, soluble plastic film, or foaming tablets that are placed in the vagina as near to the cervix as possible. Some preparations are recommended for use with a condom, diaphragm, or cap. Others are intended to be used alone; they are inserted into the vagina using a syringelike applicator. Some should not be used with rubber barrier devices. Spermicides should be applied shortly before intercourse; a fresh application is needed when intercourse is repeated or prolonged.

Pessaries are slightly waxy and bullet-shaped. One pessary is inserted 15 minutes before intercourse. Spermicides must be used in accordance with the manufacturer's instructions since the length of time for which they remain effective varies. They should not be washed away for six to eight hours after intercourse.

CONTRACEPTIVE SPONGE A disposable circular polyurethane foam sponge about 2 inches in diameter and 2 inches thick that is impregnated with spermicide. The sponge incorporates a loop for easy removal. Before being inserted high into the vagina, the sponge should be moistened with water to activate the spermicide. It should be left in position for at least six hours after intercourse.

EFFECTIVENESS

If used consistently and correctly, employing both mechanical and chemical barriers, these methods are highly effective in preventing conception. Failure rates in actual use vary between four and seven pregnancies per 100 woman-years of use for the condom, diaphragm, or contraceptive cap; nine to 16 pregnancies per 100 woman-years of use for the contraceptive sponge; and 30 to 40 pregnancies per 100 woman-years of use for spermicides used alone. (See *Contraception* for definition of woman-years.)

Contraception, hormonal methods

The use by women of synthetic progestogens, sometimes combined with synthetic estrogens, to prevent pregnancy. The best-known hormonal contraceptives are the various types of birth-control pill (see *Oral contraceptives*), but injectable contraceptives and implants are also available.

HOW THEY WORK

Most injectable contraceptives contain progestogens only. These contraceptives are administered every two or three months.

Contraceptive implants consist of six small silicone-rubber capsules containing a progestogen. These are inserted subcutaneously (under the skin) in the upper arm in a fanlike manner and are active for five years, releasing the progestogen steadily into the bloodstream.

Both methods suppress ovulation in most (although not all) menstrual cycles. All hormonal contraceptives act on the cervical mucus to make it thick and impenetrable to sperm. They also cause thinning of the endometrium (lining of the uterus).

Properly used, injectables and implants are extremely effective—the failure rate is about two pregnancies per 100 woman-years (see *Contraception* for definition of woman-years). The return of ovulation is sometimes delayed after stopping injectables, but a woman is fertile soon after implants are removed.

FOR WHOM ARE THEY RECOMMENDED?

Both methods are suitable for most women who want long-term protection against pregnancy and who cannot use estrogens or other hormonal contraceptives or IUDs. Injectable contraceptives are licensed and used in more than 80 countries; the Food and Drug Administration has not yet approved their use in the US.

Their main advantage is their excellent effectiveness and the relative lack of motivation necessary on the part of the user. Side effects include heavy bleeding in the first few months, irregular menstruation, or amenorrhea (cessation of periods). There is sometimes weight gain. Injections have the disadvantage of running their full two or three months of activity in the body after being administered. There is no way of neutralizing their action.

Contraception, periodic abstinence

Avoidance of sexual intercourse during part of the menstrual cycle in an attempt to avoid conception. Abstinence has been practiced with varying degrees of success in many parts of the world for many years. Often referred to as "natural" family planning, the term periodic abstinence describes more accurately what happens when couples abstain from sexual intercourse during those times when fertilization can take place.

TYPES

All forms of periodic abstinence attempt to pinpoint the time of ovulation. The oldest method (the calendar, or rhythm, method) attempted to predict ovulation on the basis of the lengths of previous menstrual cycles; it fell into disrepute because of its high failure rate. More up-to-date are the temperature and the cervical mucus (or Billings) methods. When these two are used together for greater accuracy, they are given the name symptothermal method.

TEMPERATURE METHOD Also known as the basal body temperature method, this involves the woman charting her daily temperature. This should be done at the same time each day—normally first thing in the morning while the body is in an inactive state—and using a special ovulation thermometer marked in fractions of degrees. Provided the woman is well (with no other cause for a rise in temperature), a sustained temperature rise for at least three days means that ovulation has taken place and that it is now considered safe to have sexual intercourse. However, to use this method properly, no intercourse should take place until after the sustained temperature rise has occurred; this can mean abstinence for more than half the cycle.

CERVICAL MUCUS METHOD This involves the observation and charting of the amount and appearance of the mucus secreted by the cervix (neck of uterus) throughout the menstrual cycle. Immediately after menstruation come the dry days when the mucus forms a thick plug that blocks the cervix. The mucus then becomes thick and viscid and appears at the vulva. About the time of ovulation it turns thin, watery, elastic, and slippery and flows more easily. A few days after ovulation it begins to become thick and viscid again, and this state lasts until the start of the next menstrual period. In this method, it is considered contraceptively safe to have sexual intercourse on alternate days during the dry days (alternate so that any semen remaining does not obscure the start of the thin mucus). As soon as any mucus appears, abstinence must begin. This should last until the fourth day after the peak day of the mucus (that is, the fourth day after the last appearance of fertile-type mucus). Intercourse can then continue until the next menstrual period.

SYMPTOTHERMAL METHOD This method combines the temperature and the cervical mucus methods and requires a closely supervised learning period of about six months. Intercourse can still take place during the dry days after the period, but must stop as soon as mucus is felt. It can be resumed only when both the sustained rise in temperature and the four days after peak mucus have been registered—thus giving a double sense of security.

EFFECTIVENESS

All these methods need great motivation on the part of the couple, with a strong commitment to abstain from intercourse when there could be a possibility of pregnancy. None of these methods is suitable for women who normally have irregular cycles, and they should not be used after a pregnancy until the cycle has regularized. Studies have shown the greatest use effectiveness with the

305

symptothermal method—6.24 pregnancies per 100 woman-years.

SIDE EFFECTS

Once the techniques have been mastered and a woman can observe and chart the necessary changes, there are no provable side effects, although there is a supposition that a higher incidence of miscarriages or congenital defects could occur because of fertilization by so-called "aged" sperm of "aged" ova. This supposition has neither been completely proved nor disproved.

Contraception, postcoital

The prevention of pregnancy after sexual intercourse has occurred, normally reserved for emergency situations. Rape of a woman who is not using contraception is a preeminent example; the bursting of a condom during intercourse is another.

Postcoital contraception must be provided very soon after intercourse, especially if the woman is ovulating. There are two main types, but neither of them is 100 percent effective; a woman should have a pregnancy test a month after treatment to ensure that she is not pregnant.

TYPES

HORMONAL CONTRACEPTIVE PROTECTION
This must be started not later than 72 hours after unprotected intercourse. There are two methods: a five-day course of *estrogens* or a short, high-dose course of combined *oral contraceptives*. With the combined medication, often called the "morning-after" pill, two pills containing 250 micrograms of levonorgestrel (a progestogen) and 50 micrograms of ethinyl estradiol (an estrogen) are given at once and the dose is repeated 12 hours later. This sometimes causes nausea and vomiting, and an antiemetic treatment may be needed at the same time.

COPPER-BEARING IUD Insertion of a copper-bearing IUD within five days of unprotected sexual intercourse has been shown to be effective. However, it is not always advisable in women who have never been pregnant; its presence can also be one of the factors associated with an increase in *pelvic inflammatory disease*. Copper-bearing IUDs are not available in the US.

Contraceptive

Any agent that diminishes the likelihood of conception. Contraceptives can be hormonal (as in the oral birth-control pill), chemical (as in spermicides), or mechanical (as in condoms). (See *Contraception*.)

Contractions

The spasms of rhythmic, squeezing muscular activity that affect the walls of the *uterus* during *labor*. These true labor contractions should be distinguished from the *Braxton Hicks' contractions* that are often noticeable during the last few weeks of pregnancy. True contractions are characterized by their regularity and the discomfort they cause. Furthermore, they increase in strength and frequency from the start of the first stage of labor.

Contract practice

See *Corporate practice*.

Contracture

A deformity caused by shrinkage of scar tissue in the skin or connective tissues, or by irreversible shortening of muscles and tendons.

Skin contractures are common after extensive burns and may restrict movement. Other types of contracture may be caused by inflammation of the tendons and fascia (a sheet of fibrous tissue) that support muscle fibers, as in *Dupuytren's contracture*, which affects the hand. Sometimes there is damage to muscle fibers, usually due to ischemia (reduced blood supply). In *Volkmann's contracture*, this damage may be caused by a plaster cast being placed too tightly around a fractured bone in the arm, thus interfering with the circulation.

Contraindication

Any factor in a patient's condition that makes it unwise to pursue a certain line of treatment—such as drug therapy or surgery.

Controlled trial

A method of testing the value of a treatment—such as a new drug—or comparing the effectiveness of different treatments.

WHY IT IS DONE

The effectiveness of a treatment cannot accurately be assessed simply by administering it to a group of sick people and seeing if their conditions improve. With many illnesses, a large proportion of patients tend to get better even if the treatment they are given is useless and harmless. Reasons for this phenomenon include the healing properties of time, the psychological reassurance of a physician, and the fact that both patient and physician believe the treatment will work (the so-called *placebo* effect). A controlled trial is a scientific attempt to unravel the true curative activity of a treatment from the psychological side benefits of "being treated."

HOW IT IS DONE

In a typical controlled drug trial, a randomly selected sample of patients with the illness that the drug is thought to cure is split into two carefully matched groups. One group is given a normal course of the drug—for example, a pill to be taken every day. The other patients—called the control group—are given an identical course of treatment, except that their pills are "dummy," or placebo, tablets, containing none of the drug being tested, but only an inert substance such as starch. Alternatively, the control group may be given a well-established drug treatment but with the drug disguised to appear identical to the test drug.

After a predetermined period, the two groups are medically assessed. If the improvement in the illness has been significantly greater in the patients given the drug over those given the dummy tablets, this suggests that the drug does have a real curative effect. Any benefits of treatment separate from the pharmacological effects of the drug have been accounted for (or "controlled") by comparing the two groups.

To be of any use, controlled trials must be conducted "blind"—that is, the patients do not know whether they are receiving the real or dummy treatment. In a further refinement—the *double-blind* controlled trial—neither the patients nor the physicians who assess them know who is receiving which treatment. The results of trials require detailed and careful statistical analysis before any conclusions can be drawn.

Contusion

Damage to the skin and underlying tissues from a blunt injury such as a fall; the skin may be grazed and the tissues bruised.

Convalescence

The recovery period following an illness or a surgical operation during which the patient regains strength before returning to normal activities. The convalescent period can vary from one or two days (following an infection such as influenza or tonsillitis) to several weeks (following a heart attack or a major operation). At one time special convalescent homes were popular, but today such places are generally reserved for the elderly.

Conversion disorder

A psychological illness in which painful emotions are repressed and unconsciously converted into physical symptoms. The repressed idea is expressed symbolically by the particular bodily symptom. For instance, a paralyzed right arm may represent guilt over an injury that the patient, using that arm, inflicted on another person; mutism (inability to speak) may represent sexual guilt, the mouth symbolizing the vagina.

This disorder serves mainly to relieve anxiety, but the sufferer may also "benefit" by gaining sympathy and avoiding responsibility.

Treatment requires *psychotherapy* involving exploration of the person's history and childhood experiences.

Convulsion

See *Seizure*.

Convulsion, febrile

See *Seizure, febrile*.

Cooley's anemia

One of the principal and most serious forms of *thalassemia*, an inherited blood disorder characterized by production of a defective *hemoglobin* (the protein that carries oxygen in red blood cells).

Copper

A metallic element that forms an essential part of several *enzymes* (substances that promote biochemical reactions in the body). Copper is needed in minute amounts (see *Trace elements*); deficiency is rare.

Copper poisoning is rare, occurring mainly in people who drink homemade alcohol distilled using copper tubing. Symptoms of poisoning include nausea, vomiting, and diarrhea. Copper excess may also result from *Wilson's disease*, an extremely rare inherited disorder of copper metabolism.

Cordotomy

An operation to divide bundles of nerve fibers within the spinal cord.

Cordotomy is performed to relieve persistent pain that has not responded to treatment with strong analgesics (painkillers) or *TENS* (transcutaneous electrical nerve stimulation). In theory, cordotomy can treat pain anywhere in the body, depending on the part of the cord operated on. In practice, however, it is often difficult to locate precisely the nerves responsible for pain in the upper part of the body, and the operation is most frequently performed for pain in the lower trunk and legs, usually on patients with cancer.

Corn

A small area of thickened skin on a toe, caused by the pressure of a tight-fitting shoe. People with high foot arches are affected most, because the arch increases the pressure on the tips of the toes when walking.

If a corn is painful, the obvious solution is to change to shoes that fit more comfortably; the corn should then gradually disappear. Until then, a spongy ring or corn pad—available at drug stores in various sizes—can be placed over the corn to ease pressure. If neither measure is successful, a podiatrist can remedy the problem by paring away the corn with a scalpel. (See also *Bunion*; *Callus, skin*.)

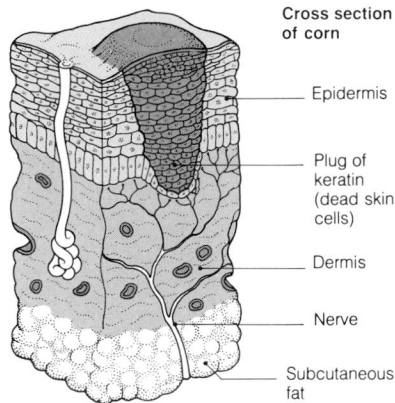

Cross section of corn

Epidermis

Plug of keratin (dead skin cells)

Dermis

Nerve

Subcutaneous fat

Cornea

Front part of the tough outer shell of the eyeball. The cornea is transparent and is shaped like a thin-walled cap or dome. It is about 0.5 inches (12 mm) in diameter, less than 0.04 inches (1 mm) thick, and has a convex front surface like the front of a camera lens. At its circumference it joins the sclera (white of the eye), which is easily seen. The cornea itself, being transparent, is less obvious. The black pupil and the colored iris are visible beneath it.

The cornea performs two main functions; it helps focus light rays onto the retina at the back of the eye and it is a protective cover of the front of the eye. To warn of possible damage, the cornea's surface is extremely sensitive, and small scratches and foreign bodies are thus very painful.

The cornea must be kept moist (by tears), like the inside of the mouth, to remain healthy. This function is performed by the lacrimal gland and the mucus and fluid-secreting cells in the lids and conjunctiva (the thin lining of the rest of the surface of the eye and the inside of the eyelids). The endothelial cells (inner cell layer) in adults cannot reproduce themselves. If they are severely damaged there may be permanent corneal clouding, since they function to pump excess water out of the cornea to keep it clear and transparent.

Corneal abrasion

A scratch or defect in the epithelium (outer layer) of the cornea. The abrasion may be caused by a small, sharp particle in the eye (see *Eye, foreign body in*) or by an injury—for example, by a twig or hairbrush.

Usually, the scratch heals quickly, but may temporarily be very painful, causing intense photophobia (dislike of bright light) and increased production of tears.

Keeping the eye closed, such as with a patch, may help lessen the discomfort. Analgesics (painkillers) may be helpful to relieve the persistent pain, and a physician may prescribe eye drops containing a cycloplegic (a drug that relaxes muscles in the eye that may go into spasm with the abrasion), which makes the eye more comfortable. Antibiotic eye drops are usually also given to prevent any risk of bacterial infection, which could lead to a serious corneal ulceration, abscess, and blindness.

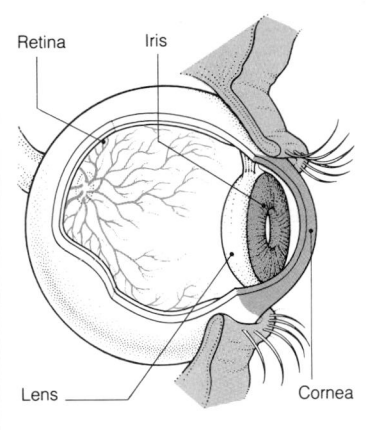

LOCATION OF CORNEA
The cornea is a transparent thin-walled dome forming the front of the eyeball. It consists of five layers of differing thickness.

Retina

Iris

Lens

Cornea

C

DISORDERS OF THE CORNEA

The cornea is a living structure, much like very specialized skin, and is prone to many disorders.

CONGENITAL DEFECTS

These are rare. Microcornea (smaller than normal) or megalocornea (bigger than normal) may occur in one or both eyes. In *buphthalmos,* or "ox-eye," the entire eyeball is enlarged and there is a strong tendency to *glaucoma.* This often leads to haziness of the cornea.

INJURY

Trauma to the cornea is common and is usually minor, a frequent occurrence being a *corneal abrasion* (scratch) caused by a particle in the eye or by overuse of contact lenses. An abrasion may become infected and progress to a *corneal ulcer.* Penetrating corneal injuries can cause scarring with loss of transparency, which may lead to a severe defect of vision.

Chemical injuries to the cornea can result from acid or alkali splashes, the latter being more serious. All contact with corrosive substances is dangerous, and immediate vigorous flushing with large volumes of water is essential if sight is to be saved. The term *keratopathy* can be applied to any corneal disorder, but is also used more specifically for certain types or causes of corneal damage.

Actinic keratopathy is damage to the outer layer of the cornea by ultraviolet light radiation. Exposure keratopathy is the damage done to a cornea deprived of the normal protection afforded by the tear film and the blink reflex.

INFLAMMATION

Keratitis means inflammation of the cornea. However, because the cornea contains no blood vessels, true inflammatory reactions are uncommon.

INFECTION

The cornea can be infected by viruses, bacteria, and fungi. Some of these cause ulceration, which may lead to penetration. *Herpes simplex* is especially dangerous.

NUTRITIONAL DISORDERS

Keratomalacia is the result of vitamin A deficiency and is common in severely undernourished children. The cornea becomes soft and often perforates. Keratomalacia is a major cause of blindness in some tropical countries.

DEGENERATION

Degenerative conditions of the cornea occur mainly in the elderly or may affect generally diseased eyes. The corneal changes include the deposition of calcium, thinning, and spontaneous ulceration.

OTHER DISORDERS

Keratoconjunctivitis sicca (dry eye) occurs when the tear film is inadequate. This is a feature of *Sjögren's syndrome,* the *Stevens-Johnson syndrome,* and various rheumatic disorders. Corneal dystrophies are inborn errors of corneal structure or function that may appear at various ages and may lead to opacification. One form of dystrophy is *keratoconus,* in which the cornea thins and bulges forward into a conical shape. Edema (fluid collection) in the cornea occurs when the endothelium (the inner layer) fails to prevent the internal fluid of the eye from entering the cornea. This may severely affect vision.

INVESTIGATION

Corneal disorders are examined under high magnification, using a slit-lamp microscope. In the majority of cases, the appearance of the various conditions is characteristic and diagnosis is straightforward. Corneal ulcers may require gentle scraping so that samples can be obtained for viral, bacterial, or fungal *culture* in the pathology laboratory.

Corneal abrasions usually heal completely within a few days, but (rarely) they may recur, probably because the new epithelium fails to stick properly to the underlying tissue. Patching the eye, application of bland ointments, and even prescription of a soft "bandage" contact lens may be tried.

Corneal graft

The surgical transplantation of corneal tissue. Most corneal transplants are homografts, meaning the tissue is taken from a human donor and put into the eye of a recipient with a corneal disorder. A much smaller number are autografts, in which a person's cornea is simply repositioned—for example, it may be rotated to a position in which the effect of a scar on the corneal surface is lessened. Donor corneal tissues can now be stored for days for future use. The term "eye bank" is used for the organization that handles the donor corneas.

WHY IT IS DONE

A corneal graft is carried out when a patient has an eye with possible good visual potential (most of the eye is healthy) but with substantially impaired vision caused by a cornea scarred or clouded by fluid collection in the tissues or for other reasons (see *Cornea* disorders box).

HOW IT IS DONE

With the patient under general or local anesthetic, the diseased area of the cornea is excised and replaced with a similarly shaped piece of donor tissue, which is fastened in place with stitches. Most corneal grafts are full-thickness, but, if the back part of the cornea is healthy, the cornea is sometimes split, with only the front, diseased part removed and replaced.

OUTLOOK

The success rate for corneal grafts is high, but depends on the type of corneal disorder (certain corneal problems have lower transplant success

rates than others). Generally, corneal grafts have a much better chance for success than other types of transplant. This is because the healthy cornea is free of blood vessels and there is therefore less access for the white blood cells, which bring about rejection of donor tissue. Matching certain features of the donor's and recipient's immune systems (see *Histocompatibility antigens*) has also improved the success rate of corneal grafts. Unlike other transplants, there is usually no need for the patient to receive immunosuppressant drugs to lessen the chances of rejection.

Corneal ulcer

A break, erosion, or open sore in the outer layer of the cornea, sometimes extending into the underlying stroma (middle layer).

CAUSES

The most common cause is a *corneal abrasion* or scratch, but an ulcer may also be produced by chemical damage, by infection (particularly with the *herpes simplex* or *herpes zoster* viruses), or by various bacteria and fungi.

Certain eye conditions may make an ulcer more likely—for example, *keratoconjunctivitis sicca* (dry eye), eyelid deformities such as *entropion* or *ectropion*, or diminished sensation in the cornea, which more easily permits injury to occur.

SYMPTOMS, DIAGNOSIS, AND TREATMENT

Corneal ulcers are very painful, though chronic ones may become less so. They are easily recognized by a physician instilling some fluorescein dye into the eye and shining a blue light on it; the fluorescein fills the ulcer and reflects back green light.

Superficial, noninfectious ulcers caused by mechanical injury usually heal quickly. If an infection is suspected, swabs will be taken to identify the causative microorganism and the physician will then prescribe a suitable antimicrobial drug. Sometimes, a predisposing eye condition may need to be treated. Noninfectious ulcers that fail to heal quickly sometimes respond to a "bandage" contact lens or a tarsorrhaphy (a temporary joining of the eyelids).

Coronary

Strictly, a term used to describe any structure that encircles like a crown (from "corona," the Latin word for crown). In practice, the term usually refers to the coronary arteries that encircle and supply the heart. In popular usage, coronary often means a *coronary thrombosis* or a *myocardial infarction* (heart attack).

Coronary artery bypass

An operation to circumvent narrowed or blocked coronary arteries by grafting on additional blood vessels to receive blood flow.

Usually, symptoms of coronary heart disease can be controlled by drugs, weight loss (if appropriate), not smoking, and adopting a sensible diet and life-style. If this fails to relieve the symptoms, however, other treatment will be considered. When the disease is localized to one or two segments of artery it may be possible to relieve the blockage or blockages by using a technique called balloon *angioplasty*. In balloon angioplasty a small balloon is passed via catheter through the circulation into the coronary artery. The artery is then distended to stretch the narrowed segment. However, in most cases not re-

sponding to treatment with drugs, bypass surgery may be recommended rather than angioplasty.

HOW IT IS DONE

A decision to operate is based on identification of the sites of blockage using *angiography* (an X-ray technique). The operation itself is performed using general anesthesia. It usually requires two surgeons and lasts up to five hours. The heart is temporarily stopped and the circulation is maintained with a *heart-lung machine* that adds oxygen to the blood outside of the body. The procedure is illustrated on the following page.

RECOVERY PERIOD

After a coronary artery bypass, the patient spends two to four days in an intensive care unit, where his or her heart and other body functions are carefully monitored. Hospital stay is generally about ten to 12 days, and return to work is usually possible after about six weeks.

OUTLOOK

When candidates are appropriately selected, coronary artery bypass offers the patient another chance to feel well again and return to a normal life.

Coronary artery disease

Disease of the arteries that supply blood to the heart muscle, causing damage to or malfunction of the heart. (See *Coronary heart disease*.)

Coronary care unit

A small ward, specially staffed and equipped for the care of acutely ill patients who are suspected of being in the process of or who have suffered a *myocardial infarction* (heart attack involving damage to the heart muscle

from a blockage of one of the coronary arteries). In the unit, patients are kept under close surveillance and given immediate treatment if a complication such as *cardiac arrest* (cessation of heart beat), *arrhythmia* (irregular or very rapid or slow heart beat), or *heart failure* occurs.

A coronary care unit usually holds only five to 10 people, and the ratio of specially trained nurses to patients is high—one-to-one or one-to-two. The ward is equipped with monitoring equipment that provides a continuous record of each patient's heart rhythm, respiratory rate, blood pressure, and so on, and contains specialized equipment for providing treatment, such as *defibrillation* (to restore normal heart rhythm), and *ventilation*.

Coronary heart disease

Damage to or malfunction of the heart caused by narrowing or blockage of the coronary arteries, which supply blood to the heart muscle. Two of the manifestations of coronary heart disease (CHD) are *angina pectoris* (chest pain usually associated with effort or anxiety) and acute *myocardial infarction* (AMI, or heart attack).

INCIDENCE

CHD is an extremely common disorder in developed countries and is the cause of more deaths in the US than any other disorder. Many such deaths occur without warning in middle-aged men and women who are otherwise in good health, although most deaths from CHD are in people over 65.

In the past 20 years deaths and disability from CHD have declined. The mortality from CHD in men aged

DEATH RATES FROM HEART DISEASE (per 100,000 in age group 35 to 74)

The downward sloping graphs for the US probably result from a combination of healthier living and better treatment of heart disease. In the UK, death rates have remained more constant, while Japan has always had a low rate. Note the higher death rates in men.

Key
- – – – – – US male
- • • • • • US female
- – – – – – UK male
- • • • • • UK female
- – – – – – Japan male
- • • • • • Japan female

C

CORONARY ARTERY BYPASS

This is now the most common and successful major heart operation in the Western world. Each year some 500,000 Americans undergo the operation, which can relieve them from dependence on drug treatment for heart disease and restore them to active life.

HOW IT IS DONE

Coronary artery bypass is a major procedure, requiring two surgeons and lasting up to five hours.

1 The first surgeon makes an incision down the center of the patient's chest. The heart is then exposed by opening the pericardium.

2 Simultaneously, several incisions are made in the leg, and a length of vein removed.

Site of incision

3 Before any incisions are made in the coronary arteries, the patient is connected to a heart-lung machine. This takes over the function of the heart and lungs while the surgeon repairs the heart.

Heart-lung machine

4 A section of the vein taken from the leg is then sewn to the aorta and to a point below the blockage. If several arteries are blocked, they can be bypassed by using other sections from the same leg vein.

5 The heart-lung machine is disconnected, allowing blood to flow back into the coronary arteries.

WHY IT IS DONE

Narrowed coronary arteries are unable to supply the heart muscle with a sufficient amount of blood; as a result, it becomes starved of oxygen. This may cause angina (chest pain) or, if the narrowed artery becomes blocked, heart tissue damage. By attaching lengths of a vein taken from the leg to the aorta and to a point below the blockages, the narrowed or blocked sections can be bypassed.

Before the operation

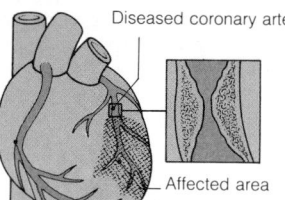

Diseased coronary artery

Affected area

Coronary arteries

After the operation

Bypass

First surgeon prepares heart for bypass

Second surgeon removes vein from leg

Anesthesiologist

Oxygenated blood from heart-lung machine

Superior vena cava (tied off)

Deoxygenated blood to heart-lung machine

Inferior vena cava (tied off)

Pericardium

Aorta

Bypass

Coronary arteries

6 Finally, the breastbone is wired together, and pericardium and chest are sewn up.

35 to 64 declined by 35 percent between 1968 and 1982. Part of this decline is thought to be due to better medical treatment of elevated blood pressure, one of the causes of CHD, and part is due to improved surgical treatment of narrowed coronary arteries. Also, emergency treatment of heart attacks has improved.

CAUSES

CHD is caused by reduction in the blood flow to the heart muscle and to its electrical conducting system, which initiates and coordinates the contractions (beats) of the muscle (see *Heart*). The coronary arteries are first narrowed and may eventually be blocked by plaques (patches) of the cholesterol-rich fatty deposit called *atheroma*. Further narrowing or blockage may be caused by thrombi (blood clots) formed on the roughened surface of the plaques.

The causes of atheroma are numerous and interrelated (see *Atherosclerosis*). In addition to some genetic predisposition and diseases such as *diabetes mellitus* and *hypertension* (elevated blood pressure), the main causes are smoking, lack of exercise, being overweight, and elevated blood cholesterol (which itself is linked in part with a diet rich in dairy and animal fats).

The importance of personality traits, behavior, and stress as causes is still disputed. Some physicians believe that heart attacks are more frequent in people with "type A" personalities. Such individuals are always in a hurry, checking the time, impatient with delays, and interrupting colleagues in mid-sentence—but they are also doers and achievers. There is some evidence that heart attacks occur more frequently in people who are depressed after the death of a relative, loss of a job, or some other adverse life event. The medical consensus is that these psychological and behavioral factors are less important than physical factors—smoking, unhealthy diet, high blood pressure, and lack of exercise.

SYMPTOMS

In its early stages, atheroma of the coronary arteries causes no symptoms. The first symptom is usually either angina pectoris or heart attack.

Angina pectoris is discomfort or pain in the chest, typically brought on by exertion and relieved by rest. The pain is a dull ache in the middle of the chest or a feeling of pressure that may spread up to the neck or down the arms (on the left more often than the right). In some cases the pain occurs only in an arm or in the neck. The characteristic pain comes on predictably after a certain amount of exertion—after walking halfway up the stairs, for instance—and disappears after resting a minute or so.

Angina occurs when the heart muscle is working hard and getting too little blood for the amount of effort being expended. If the blood supply to part of the muscle is cut off completely by a blood clot or spasm in one of the coronary arteries, the result is an acute myocardial infarction (a coronary thrombosis or heart attack)—death of a portion of the heart muscle. The main symptom is intense chest pain of the same type as angina, but not relieved by rest and not necessarily brought on by effort; in addition the victim may become cold, sweat profusely, feel weak and nauseated, or even lose consciousness as the pumping action of the heart is weakened and shock ensues.

Angina and AMI may lead to disturbances in the electrical conduction system of the heart with resulting *arrhythmias* (abnormalities in heart beat) ranging from *ectopic beats* (occasional double beats) to *tachycardia* (rapid beats) and *ventricular fibrillation* (ineffective fluttering of the heart muscle). The latter causes rapid loss of consciousness and is fatal if not treated within a few minutes.

DIAGNOSIS AND INVESTIGATION

An AMI may produce such clear-cut symptoms that the diagnosis is in no doubt. Confirmatory tests may include electrocardiography and measurement of the level of serum creatine kinase enzymes released into the blood by damaged muscle. The conditions of patients who have intermittent attacks of angina are usually assessed by electrocardiography both at rest and during controlled exercise.

When the angina is persistent, severe, changing in quality, or of recent onset, the patient's condition is assessed by various *heart imaging* techniques. These imaging procedures, such as coronary *angiography* (injection of a radiopaque dye into the arteries followed by X ray), give the physician detailed, precise data on the extent of the narrowing of the coronary arteries and any damage to the heart muscle. The data aid in determining whether medical or surgical treatment is best.

TREATMENT

Angina may be relieved by a range of drugs that improves the blood flow through the coronary arteries and/or that reduces the work load on the heart during exercise. These drugs include glyceryl trinitrate and other *nitrates*, *beta-blockers*, *calcium channel blockers*, and peripheral *vasodilator drugs*. Arrhythmias are commonly treated with beta-blockers, calcium channel blockers, and specific *antiarrhythmic drugs*. If the heart's pumping action is weak, it may sometimes be improved by vasodilators or *digoxin*.

If drug treatment fails to relieve the symptoms, or if investigation shows extensive narrowing of the coronary arteries, blood flow may be improved by *coronary artery bypass* surgery (in which a vein graft is used to skip over the narrowed segment) or by transluminal *angioplasty* (in which the narrowed part of the artery is stretched apart when a balloon, passed to the site, is inflated).

An AMI is usually treated initially in a hospital coronary care unit. Treatment may be given with *thrombolytic drugs* in an attempt to dissolve the clot, the affected coronary artery may be widened by angioplasty or may be immediately bypassed by surgery, or treatment may simply be aimed at allowing the heart to recover by a natural process of healing.

OUTLOOK AND PREVENTION

CHD is a disease of middle to old age, but its foundations are laid in the teens and early adult life. The chances of developing the disease can be considerably reduced by an "anticoronary" life-style. The person who has never smoked, exercises regularly, has a normal weight and blood pressure, and eats a prudent diet is unlikely to develop symptoms of CHD until late in life.

Even when symptoms develop, treatment can do a great deal to halt their progression. Studies of patients treated by coronary bypass surgery for disease affecting all the major coronary arteries reveal that 80 to 90 percent are still alive five years after the operation. Survival is even better among those with less extensive disease; they can usually be treated with drugs. Survival is substantially improved in patients who quit cigarette smoking.

Coronary thrombosis

Narrowing or blockage of one of the coronary arteries (which supply blood to the heart muscle) by a thrombus (clot). This causes a section of the heart muscle to die because it has been deprived of oxygen.

C

Coronary thrombosis is one of the main processes involved in *coronary heart disease*, the major cause of death in the US. Sudden blockage of a coronary artery causes an acute *myocardial infarction* (death of a portion of heart muscle). The terms coronary thrombosis and myocardial infarction thus tend to be used interchangeably, but the latter is the more precise medical term for heart attack.

Coroner
A public officer appointed to look into any death in which the cause is unknown, or when it is suspected or known to result from unnatural causes. A coroner is most often called when the deceased was not attended by a physician during the final illness. Other circumstances vary from state to state. If there are any uncertainties about the cause of death, the coroner will order a postmortem examination before issuing a death certificate. If the death is thought to be due to unnatural causes, the coroner will hold an inquest.

Corporate practice
The employment of a physician by a lay-controlled corporation that sells the services of the physician for profit. Because the physician, as an employee, is presumed to owe greater loyalty to the corporation than to the patients, corporate practice has been opposed on ethical grounds. Physician employment by hospitals, health maintenance organizations, and similar providers is regarded as an independent contractor arrangement, the physician being free to make medical decisions independently of the corporation. Under these circumstances, no objections are raised.

Cor pulmonale
Enlargement and strain of the right side of the heart due to chronic lung disease. Damage to the lungs increases resistance to blood flow from the heart through the branches of the pulmonary artery and causes pulmonary hypertension (increased pressure in the pulmonary artery). The resultant "back pressure" strain on the heart may eventually cause right-sided heart failure with *edema* (fluid collection in the tissues). (See *Pulmonary hypertension*.)

Corpuscle
Any minute body or cell, particularly red and white *blood cells* or certain types of nerve endings.

Corset
A device worn on the trunk to treat back pain and spinal injuries or deformities. Soft corsets, usually made of cotton fabric stiffened with plastic or metal, have straps enabling them to be tightened. Most commonly prescribed for back pain, corsets work in the same way as weight-lifters' belts—by exerting increased pressure on the abdomen they take the weight of the trunk off the lower spine. They also restrict painful movements and help keep the back warm.

Rigid corsets are made of plaster or lightweight plastic and must be molded to the body. They immobilize and support the spinal column when it has become unstable as the result of injury or help to correct its faulty alignment, as in scoliosis (curvature of the spine).

Corticosteroid drugs

COMMON DRUGS

Beclomethasone Betamethasone Cortisone Dexamethasone Hydrocortisone Prednisolone Prednisone

> **WARNING**
> Sudden withdrawal of corticosteroid drugs may cause serious illness or death. Always inform a physician you are taking or have recently taken corticosteroids.

A group of drugs similar to the natural corticosteroid hormones produced by the cortex of the *adrenal glands*.

WHY THEY ARE USED
Corticosteroid drugs have a wide variety of uses. They are prescribed as hormone replacement therapy to patients with an inadequate level of natural corticosteroids caused by *Addison's disease* or following surgical removal of the adrenal glands.

Corticosteroid drugs are used in the treatment of inflammatory intestinal disorders, such as *Crohn's disease* and *ulcerative colitis*. *Temporal arteritis* needs urgent treatment with corticosteroids to reduce inflammation in the artery leading to the retina and so prevent blindness.

Other disorders that often improve with corticosteroid treatment include *asthma*, *rheumatoid arthritis*, *eczema*, *iritis* (inflammation of the iris), and allergic *rhinitis* (hay fever). The injection of corticosteroids around an inflamed tendon may relieve pain in disorders such as *tennis elbow*.

Corticosteroid drugs are also used to suppress the immune system to prevent rejection of a transplanted organ (see *Transplant surgery*) and in the treatment of some types of cancer, such as a *lymphoma* or *leukemia*.

POSSIBLE ADVERSE EFFECTS
The incidence and severity of any adverse effects depends on the dosage, the form in which the drug is given, and the length of treatment.

HOW CORTICOSTEROIDS WORK
When given as hormone replacement therapy, corticosteroids supplement or replace natural hormones. Large doses have an anti-inflammatory effect as they reduce the production of prostaglandins. They also suppress the immune system by reducing the release and activity of white blood cells.

Inflamed joint

Inflamed skin

Dilated blood vessels

Increase in white blood cells

Corticosteroids

Reduced inflammation

Blood vessels return to normal

Fewer white blood cells

Adverse effects are uncommon when corticosteroids are given in the form of a cream or by inhaler because only small amounts are absorbed into the bloodstream.

Corticosteroid tablets taken in high doses for long periods may cause *edema* (tissue swelling), *hypertension* (high blood pressure), *diabetes mellitus*, *peptic ulcer, Cushing's syndrome, hirsutism* (excessive hairiness), inhibited growth in children, and, rarely, *cataract* or *psychosis*.

High doses of corticosteroid drugs also increase susceptibility to infection by impairing the body's *immune system* (natural defenses).

Long-term treatment with corticosteroid drugs suppresses the natural production of corticosteroid hormones by the *adrenal glands*. Sudden withdrawal of the drugs may lead to collapse, coma, and death (see *Adrenal failure*).

Corticosteroid hormones

A group of hormones produced by the *adrenal glands* that control the body's use of nutrients and the excretion of salts and water in the urine.

Corticotropin

An alternative name for *ACTH* (adrenocorticotropic hormone).

Cortisol

Another name for *hydrocortisone*, an important corticosteroid hormone produced by the *adrenal glands*.

Cortisone

A synthetic *corticosteroid drug* used to reduce inflammation in severe allergic, rheumatic, and connective tissue diseases. It is also used as a replacement hormone in *Addison's disease*, in which there is a corticosteroid hormone deficiency, and after adrenal gland removal.

Coryza

See *Cold, common*.

Cosmetic dentistry

Procedures to improve the appearance of the teeth. In many cases, these treatments are also necessary to restore or prevent further damage to the teeth and/or gums.

Teeth that are out of alignment can become decayed because the bite is incorrect and because the teeth are hard to keep clean. Such teeth can be moved into proper position by fitting a fixed *orthodontic appliance* (braces) that stays in place over a period of months. Correction is usually best carried out during childhood, when the teeth and jaws are still growing and developing, but can be done in adults as well.

The main use of a *crown* is to restore normal tooth structure and prevent further damage when a tooth is severely decayed or broken. However, crowns can also be important for appearance, particularly when a front tooth is damaged; in this case a porcelain crown is fitted because of its similarity in color to the natural teeth that surround it.

Bonding is a relatively new technique with a wide range of cosmetic uses. It can be used to treat chipped or malformed teeth, to close small gaps between front teeth, or to cover stained or discolored teeth. In some cases it can be used instead of a crown for front teeth.

Teeth that have become discolored because the pulp is dead or has been removed can be treated by *bleaching*.

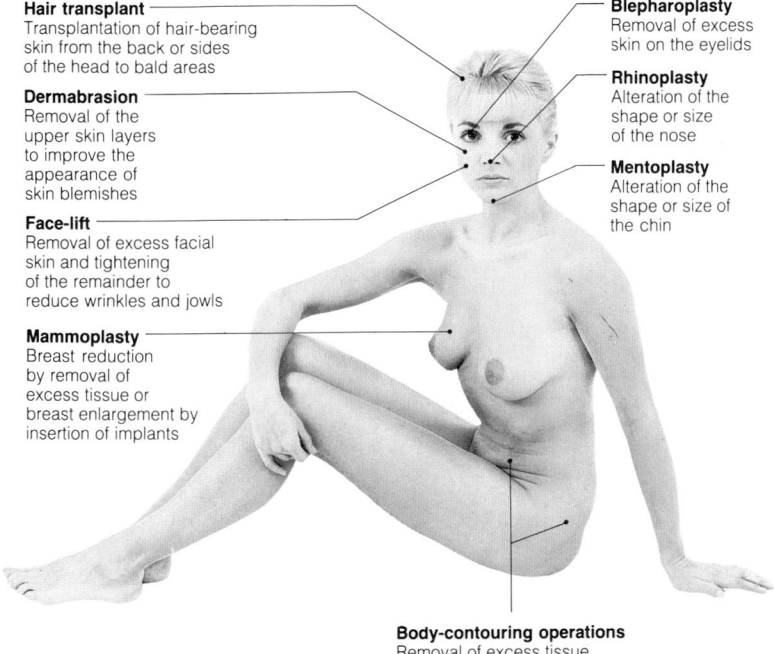

Hair transplant
Transplantation of hair-bearing skin from the back or sides of the head to bald areas

Dermabrasion
Removal of the upper skin layers to improve the appearance of skin blemishes

Face-lift
Removal of excess facial skin and tightening of the remainder to reduce wrinkles and jowls

Mammoplasty
Breast reduction by removal of excess tissue or breast enlargement by insertion of implants

Blepharoplasty
Removal of excess skin on the eyelids

Rhinoplasty
Alteration of the shape or size of the nose

Mentoplasty
Alteration of the shape or size of the chin

Body-contouring operations
Removal of excess tissue and fat to alter body shape

Types of treatment
The different procedures vary as to permanency and satisfactory results.

Cosmetic surgery

An operation performed primarily to improve the appearance of an individual rather than to improve function or cure disease.

WHY IT IS DONE

Cosmetic surgery can improve appearance in a number of ways. Skin blemishes can be removed, and the appearance of an unsightly scar improved. The shape and size of the nose, chin, jaw, or breasts can be altered. Excess skin and fat, and any unsightly creases or marks that come with age or loss of weight, can be removed from the eyelids, face, breasts, or stomach.

An individual's expectations of the benefits of cosmetic surgery are often too great, however. Cosmetic surgery will not produce a dramatic change in personality or cure depression that a person attributes to his or her appearance. Nor can it reproduce an exact replica of someone else's features. Some procedures (such as face-lifts and hair transplants) may need to be repeated over the years; other procedures (such as *body contour surgery*) may result in uneven residual fat and unattractive scarring. Anyone contemplating cosmetic surgery should discuss the operation in detail with his or her physician.

Costalgia

Pain around the chest due to damage to a rib or to one of the intercostal nerves (which run beneath the ribs). A broken rib produces pain and tenderness over the affected part of the rib cage. The pain is made worse by deep breathing and often persists for several weeks after the original injury.

Damage to one of the intercostal nerves is most commonly a result of an attack of the virus infection *herpes zoster* (shingles). The pain is difficult to treat successfully and tends to persist for several months or longer.

Cough

A reflex action to try to clear the airways of mucus, phlegm, a foreign body, or other irritants or blockages. Most coughs are due to irritation of the airways by dust, smoke, or mucus dripping from the back of the nose. However, in some cases a cough may be a symptom of an underlying disorder, most commonly a cold (see *Cold, common*), but sometimes a serious illness such as *lung cancer*.

A cough is said to be productive when it brings up mucus or phlegm, and unproductive, or dry, when it does not.

CAUSES

Among the more common causes of a cough are irritation of the upper respiratory tract—the pharynx (throat), larynx (voice box), and trachea (windpipe)—by inhaled particles, smoke, dust, or gases, or inflammation of these airways (see *Pharyngitis*; *Laryngitis*; *Tracheitis*), usually as a result of a viral infection.

In a child, inflammation of the upper respiratory tract can narrow the airways considerably (a condition called *croup*), causing a barking cough and breathing difficulty. Infection with the bacterium BORDETELLA PERTUSSIS produces a characteristic type of cough (see *Pertussis*).

Bronchitis (inflammation of the bronchi, the air passages into the lungs) produces thick mucus and phlegm and causes severe coughing. The disorder may be brought on by an infection, but is often the result of smoking (see *Cough, smokers'*). In *bronchiectasis* (distortion or dilatation of the bronchi), a large amount of infected phlegm collects in the bronchi, making the sufferer cough persistently in an attempt to bring up the phlegm, which may be associated with bleeding.

Bronchospasm (temporary narrowing of the bronchi) causes a dry cough that is usually worse at night. It is a feature of *asthma*, but also may be due to infection or allergic reaction.

The damage to lung tissues caused by *pneumonia* (inflammation of the lungs due to infection) results in painful coughing that brings up blood-flecked phlegm. Damage to the lungs brought about by pulmonary *edema* (accumulation of fluid in the lungs) produces a cough that is dry at first, but which later may bring up frothy, blood-stained phlegm. The cough associated with viral bronchitis and viral pneumonia is often dry and persistent, and may interrupt sleep.

Various chronic lung infections, notably *tuberculosis* and fungal infections (such as *histoplasmosis*), may cause a cough. Many *pneumoconioses* (dust diseases of the lungs) also cause a cough, which is usually accompanied by shortness of breath.

An inhaled foreign object, such as a peanut, that lodges in the larynx causes violent coughing to relieve *choking*. If the object travels further down and blocks a bronchus, inflammation and mucus will be produced at the site of obstruction, leading to a persistent cough.

Lung cancer and, less commonly, other tumors of the air passages usually first cause a mild cough, then a more severe one that may produce blood-stained phlegm.

Sometimes, especially in children, coughing develops as a nervous reaction to stress.

SELF-HELP

In some cases, a dry cough may be relieved by sucking on throat lozenges or by drinking warm, soothing drinks, such as honey and water. If ineffective, narcotic *cough remedies* afford symptomatic relief, particularly at bedtime to permit sleep.

Productive coughing is the body's way of unblocking airways obstructed by mucus or phlegm and, in such cases, cough suppressants should be avoided since they can do more harm than good. An expectorant cough medication or drinking lots of fluids can help loosen mucus or phlegm if there is difficulty coughing it up.

A physician should be consulted if any cough persists for more than two or three days, is severe, or is accompanied by symptoms such as chest pain, green phlegm, coughed-up blood, or breathing difficulty.

TREATMENT

Treatment depends on the underlying disorder. For example, antibiotics may be given for a bacterial infection, a *bronchodilator* and/or *corticosteroid drugs* for asthma, *breathing exercises* and *postural drainage* (lying in a position that allows mucus to drain from the bronchi) for bronchiectasis and chronic bronchitis, and surgery or *radiation therapy* for cancer.

Coughing up blood

Known medically as hemoptysis, coughing up blood is due to rupturing of a blood vessel in the airways, lungs, nose, or throat. The underlying cause can range from persistent coughing to a serious disorder, such as cancer. Coughed-up blood may be in the form of bright-red or rusty-brown streaks or clots in or on the phlegm, a pinkish froth, or, more rarely, pure blood. The form it takes depends as much on the size of the ruptured blood vessel as on the underlying cause. Because of the possibility of a serious underlying disorder, all cases of coughing up blood require medical assessment.

Coughing up blood should not be confused with blood in the mouth, which is usually due to a nosebleed or to bleeding gums.

CAUSES

The most common cause of coughing up blood is an infection—such as *pneumonia*, *bronchitis*, or *tuberculosis*—in which inflammation of the bronchi (airways into the lungs) and alveoli (air sacs) damages the wall of a blood vessel. Similarly, in *bronchiectasis* the bronchi become enlarged and distorted, which can lead to rupture of a blood vessel and coughing up blood.

Any disorder that causes persistent coughing, such as *tracheitis* (inflammation of the windpipe), can produce hemoptysis as a result of the coughing putting strain on the blood vessels in the airways.

Another cause of coughing up blood is congestion in, and subsequent rupture of, blood vessels within the lungs. Congestion can be due to *heart failure*, *mitral stenosis* (narrowing of the mitral valve in the heart), or *pulmonary embolism* (blood clot lodged in an artery in the lungs).

A malignant tumor can lead to coughing up blood by eroding the wall of a blood vessel in the larynx (voice box), bronchi, or alveoli.

Any *bleeding disorder* (such as *hemophilia*) can also cause hemoptysis.

INVESTIGATION AND TREATMENT

A *chest X ray* may be carried out. Anyone who smokes, who is older than 40, whose chest X rays are abnormal, or who has coughed up blood more than once may need *bronchos-*

COUGH A noisy expulsion of air from the lungs that may produce sputum (phlegm) or be "dry."

C

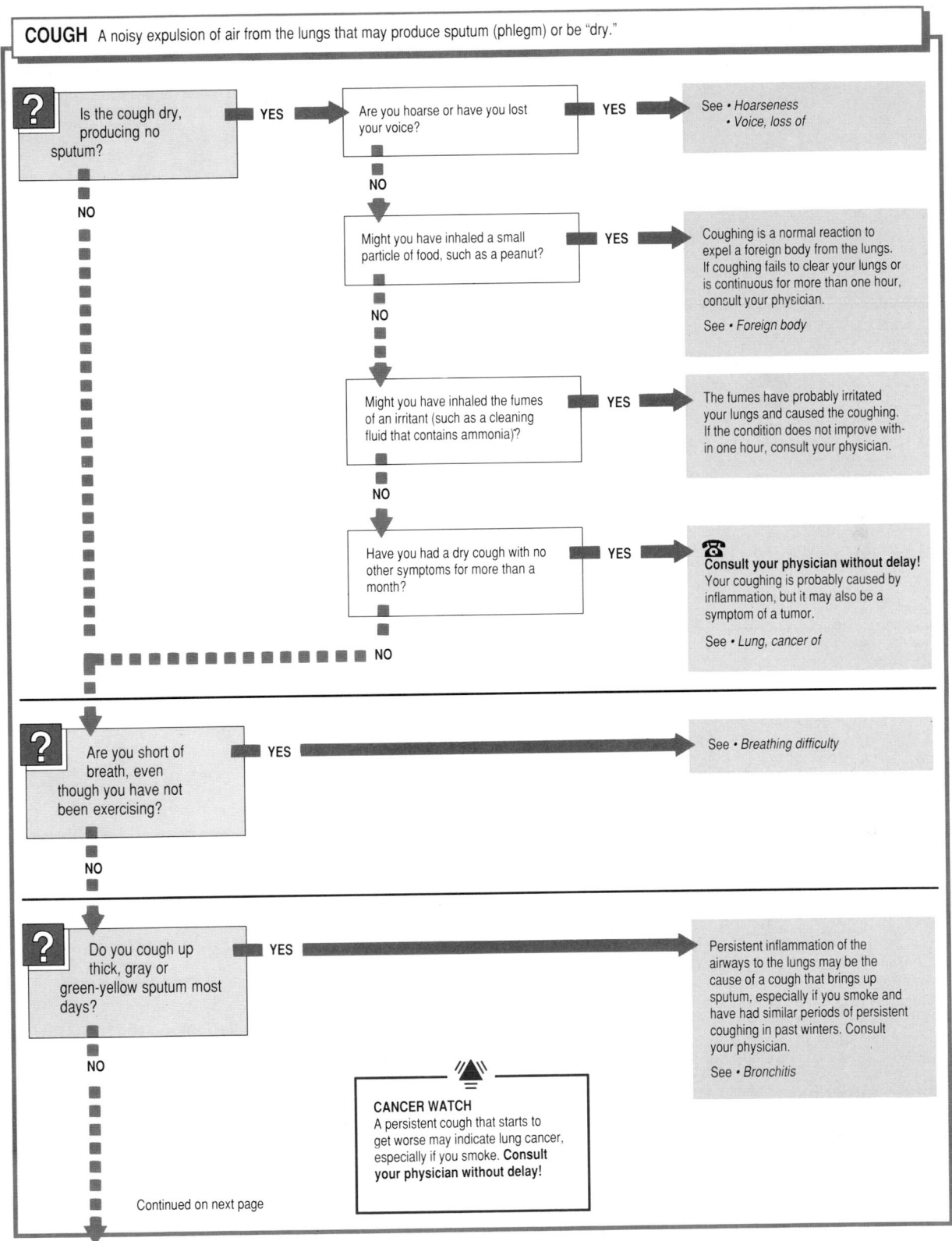

Is the cough dry, producing no sputum?

YES → **Are you hoarse or have you lost your voice?** YES → See • *Hoarseness* • *Voice, loss of*

NO → **Might you have inhaled a small particle of food, such as a peanut?** YES → Coughing is a normal reaction to expel a foreign body from the lungs. If coughing fails to clear your lungs or is continuous for more than one hour, consult your physician. See • *Foreign body*

NO → **Might you have inhaled the fumes of an irritant (such as a cleaning fluid that contains ammonia)?** YES → The fumes have probably irritated your lungs and caused the coughing. If the condition does not improve within one hour, consult your physician.

NO → **Have you had a dry cough with no other symptoms for more than a month?** YES → ☎ **Consult your physician without delay!** Your coughing is probably caused by inflammation, but it may also be a symptom of a tumor. See • *Lung, cancer of*

NO →

Are you short of breath, even though you have not been exercising? YES → See • *Breathing difficulty*

NO →

Do you cough up thick, gray or green-yellow sputum most days? YES → Persistent inflammation of the airways to the lungs may be the cause of a cough that brings up sputum, especially if you smoke and have had similar periods of persistent coughing in past winters. Consult your physician. See • *Bronchitis*

NO →

CANCER WATCH
A persistent cough that starts to get worse may indicate lung cancer, especially if you smoke. **Consult your physician without delay!**

Continued on next page

315

C

Have you had your cough for several weeks or months AND has it been getting more severe?

YES →

☎ **Consult your physician without delay!**
Asthma or chronic bronchitis may be the cause of your symptoms, but the possibility of tuberculosis or lung cancer also exists.

See • *Asthma*
    • *Bronchitis*
    • *Lung, cancer of*
    • *Tuberculosis*

NO

Of recent origin – within the past week.

Is your temperature 100°F (38°C) or above?

YES → **Are you breathless?** YES →

☎ **Call your physician without delay!**
These symptoms suggest that you may have pneumonia.

See • *Pneumonia*

NO

You may have acute bronchitis or a viral infection. Treat the fever. If there is no improvement in 24 to 48 hours, consult your physician.

See • *Fever*

NO

Do you have a runny nose AND/OR a sore throat?

YES →

You probably have a cold. Take analgesics and gargle with salt water.

See • *Cold, common*

NO

If you are unable to make a diagnosis from this chart, consult your physician.

---

copy, a diagnostic procedure in which a flexible viewing tube is passed into the lungs. In about one third of cases, no underlying cause is found.

Treatment depends on the cause, but may include *antibiotic drugs*, *anticoagulant drugs*, and *diuretic drugs*.

Cough remedies

COMMON DRUGS

Expectorants
Ammonium chloride

Cough suppressants
Antihistamines Codeine Dextromethorphan

A bewildering variety of over-the-counter medications is available for treating a *cough*. Most cough remedies consist of a syrupy base to which various active ingredients and flavorings are added.

Two main groups of drugs are used: expectorants, intended for coughs that are producing sputum (phlegm), and cough suppressants, intended for dry coughs. It is important to select the correct type of medication—a cough suppressant taken for a sputum-producing cough may interfere with the coughing up of sputum and may delay recovery.

HOW THEY WORK
Expectorants "loosen" a cough by stimulating the production of watery secretions in the lungs. Some expectorants also have a mucolytic action (a direct effect on the sputum that makes it less sticky).

Cough suppressants act on the part of the brain that controls the coughing reflex. Drugs with this effect include some *antihistamine drugs* and the narcotic analgesic drug *codeine*.
POSSIBLE ADVERSE EFFECTS
All cough suppressants have a sedating effect and may cause drowsiness. Using cough remedies to alleviate the

symptoms of a persistent cough may delay diagnosis of a serious disorder.

Cough, smokers'

A recurrent cough that is very common among smokers, particularly heavy smokers and those who have smoked for a long time. In many instances, the sufferer becomes accustomed to his or her cough and regards it as normal.

Usually, coughing is triggered by the accumulation of large amounts of abnormally thick sputum (phlegm) in the airways (a feature of *bronchitis*), which is caused by inflammation of the airways due to smoking.

TREATMENT

Stopping smoking usually stops the persistent cough, though it does not happen immediately. The longer the person has been smoking, the longer the cough will persist after quitting.

Because of the health hazards of smoking, it is essential for the smoker to consult his or her physician about a cough, particularly if there is any change in its frequency or character. (See also *Tobacco smoking*.)

Counseling

Advice and psychological support given by a health professional and usually aimed at helping a person cope with a particular problem (for example, bereavement or cancer treatment). A more general exploration of a person's feelings and attitudes, not aimed at one particular problem, is sometimes included in the definition.

WHY IT IS DONE

Counseling can help people with problems at school, work, or within the family; provide advice on family planning, abortion, and sexual and marital problems; help people deal with drinking and drug problems; and provide support during life crises.

Counseling methods may be used by caseworkers as a means of history-taking and information gathering. Physicians, too, may use a counseling style when interviewing a patient whose medical problem is complicated by personal circumstances, or when the objectives of the consultation are not clear.

HOW IT IS DONE

Some counseling, especially for genetic disorders (see *Genetic counseling*) or the treatment of cancer, consists mainly of providing personalized information in a setting in which the patient, or client, is encouraged to ask questions and to express any doubts and uncertainties.

The techniques that are used in psychotherapeutic counseling are essentially similar. The counselor encourages the individual to make statements about his or her feelings, experiences, and problems. These statements can then be discussed and explored for inconsistencies as a means of helping the individual develop a greater and more realistic understanding of his or her problems.

Usually, counseling is a one-to-one activity. However, in some situations, such as *sex therapy*, representatives of a particular point of view or gender model may be incorporated (for example, one male and one female counselor). This is termed co-counseling. Counseling may also occur in small groups. (See also *Child guidance*; *Family therapy*; *Marital counseling*.)

Cowpox

An infection caused by the vaccinia virus, which usually affects cows.

An attack of cowpox used to confer immunity against *smallpox* (now presumed to be extinct) because the viruses responsible for the two diseases were very similar. This fact was the basis of smallpox vaccination. Vaccinia virus, which gave its name to "vaccination," continued to be used as smallpox vaccine until smallpox was considered to have been eradicated in the 1970s.

Coxa vara

A deformity of the hip in which the angle between the neck and head (ball) of the femur and the shaft of the femur (thigh bone) is reduced, causing shortening of the leg and a limp.

CAUSES AND INCIDENCE

The most common cause is injury—either a fracture of the neck of the thigh bone or, in adolescence, injury to the developing part of the head of the bone. The deformity can also occur if the bone tissue in the neck of the bone is soft instead of firm, so that it bends under the weight of the body. This softening may be congenital or the result of a bone disorder such as *rickets* or *Paget's disease*.

SYMPTOMS AND DIAGNOSIS

The symptoms are pain and stiffness in the hip and increased difficulty in walking. The disorder is diagnosed by X rays, which reveal the deformity.

TREATMENT AND OUTLOOK

When coxa vara is due to an underlying bone disorder, it can be treated to bring about hardening of the bone tissue; however, little can be done about bone that is soft from birth. To

relieve pain, stiffness, and limping, *osteotomy* is required. The neck of the bone is cut and the two ends are repositioned and secured at the correct angle. This usually eases the condition so that the patient can walk with only minor discomfort.

Crab lice

See *Pubic lice*.

Cradle cap

A condition common in babies in which thick, yellow scales occur in patches over the scalp. Cradle cap is harmless, although it tends to recur.

Cradle cap is a form of seborrheic *dermatitis*, which may also occur on the face, neck, behind the ears, and in the diaper area. The skin in these areas may look red and inflamed.

Appearance of cradle cap
Most prevalent between 3 and 9 months of age, it is not clear why cradle cap occurs, but it is not a result of poor hygiene.

TREATMENT

Rub warm olive or mineral oil into the baby's scalp and leave on overnight. This loosens and softens the scales, which can be gently washed off the next day with a mild, antidandruff shampoo. This procedure may need repeating for a few days until all scales have been loosened. The baby's hair should be brushed daily using a soft-bristled brush. This will also help loosen the scales so they can be removed with a fine-tooth comb. If the condition seems to be worsening or if the skin looks inflamed, a physician should be consulted. A mild corticosteroid cream may be prescribed until the condition improves.

Cramp

Painful spasm in a muscle caused by excessive and prolonged contraction of the muscle fibers. Cramps are a common occurrence and usually last only a few moments.

C

CAUSES

Cramps often occur during or immediately after exercise because of a buildup of lactic acid and other chemicals in the muscles (caused by increased muscular activity) and small areas of muscle fiber damage.

Cramps can also occur during any repetitive movement such as writing (see *Cramp, writers'*), or through sitting or lying in an awkward position. Any condition that causes profuse sweating, such as a fever, heat wave, or prolonged exercise, can lead to cramps in resting muscles; the loss of sodium salts in the sweat disrupts muscle cell activity.

Cramps at night may be due to poor circulation of blood into the legs (see *Peripheral vascular disease*), but often there is no known cause.

TREATMENT

The pain can be helped by massaging or stretching the muscles involved. If cramps occur regularly at night your physician may prescribe a drug containing calcium or quinine, which can help prevent painful recurrences. If cramps persist for longer than an hour they are likely to be due to a more serious medical condition and the attention of a physician should be sought immediately.

Cramp, writers'

Painful spasm in the muscles of the hand, making it impossible to write. In most cases the muscles in the hand are still able to perform other tasks, indicating that the problem may be psychological in origin. Contrary to this theory, however, writers' cramp fails to respond to psychotherapy. The use of muscle relaxants and other drugs has also met with little success in tackling the problem.

The condition sometimes improves if the hand is rested for months, but often it is permanent. Occasionally the other hand becomes affected.

Cranial nerves

Twelve pairs of nerves that emerge directly from the brain—as opposed to the *spinal nerves*, which connect with the spinal cord. All but two of the cranial nerve pairs connect with nuclei in the *brain stem* (the lowest section of the brain). The other two (the olfactory and optic nerves) link directly with parts of the *cerebrum* (the main mass of the brain). All the nerves emerge through various openings in the cranium (skull); many then soon divide into several major branches.

Craniopharyngioma

A tumor of the pituitary gland. The condition is very rare. There are about one or two cases per million population in the US each year.

Symptoms include headaches, vomiting, defective vision, stunted growth, and failure of sexual development. If untreated, the tumor may result in permanent brain damage.

FUNCTIONS OF CRANIAL NERVES

Some cranial nerves are principally concerned with delivering sensory information from organs, such as the ears, nose, and eyes, to the brain. Others carry messages that move the tongue, eyes, and facial (and other) muscles, or stimulate glands such as the salivary glands. A few have both sensory and motor functions. One of the nerves—the tenth cranial, or *vagus nerve*—is one of the most important components of the *parasympathetic nervous system*, concerned with maintaining the rhythmic automatic function of the internal body machinery. It has branches to all the main digestive organs, the heart, and the lungs.

1
Olfactory nerve
Smell

2
Optic nerve
Vision

3, 4, 6
Oculomotor, trochlear, and abducent nerves
Eye movements

5
Trigeminal nerve
Facial sensation and jaw movements

7
Facial nerve
Facial expressions and taste

8
Acoustic (vestibulocochlear) nerve
Hearing and balance

9
Glossopharyngeal nerve
Taste and throat sensations

10
Vagus nerve
Breathing, circulation, and digestion

11
Spinal accessory nerve
Movements of neck and back muscles

12
Hypoglossal nerve
Tongue movements

Craniopharyngiomas are identified by imaging techniques for the brain (see *Brain imaging*) and are usually removed surgically.

Craniosynostosis

The early closure of one or more of the joints between the bones of the cranium (see *Skull*).

Craniosynostosis may occur in a baby affected by a bone disease, such as rickets, in a baby with multiple birth defects, or in an otherwise healthy baby. It may also occur if the baby's brain is abnormally small.

DIAGNOSIS AND TREATMENT

The physician's diagnosis is made from the outward appearance of the skull and by skull X ray. Treatment must be undertaken during the first few months of life to prevent brain damage. An operation is performed to separate the skull bones by cutting away the fused edges and separating the bony plates.

Craniotomy

Removal of part of the skull to carry out an operation on the brain, such as performance of a biopsy, removal of a tumor, or aspiration and drainage of an abscess or blood clot.

After the operation the bone is replaced and the membranes, muscle, and skin are sewn back into position.

Following successful surgery, the patient can usually leave the hospital within a week. He or she will generally experience mild headaches for a time, but little real pain.

Cranium

The part of the *skull* around the brain.

Cream

A thick, semisolid preparation used to apply medications to the skin for therapeutic or prophylactic (preventive) purposes. Creams are useful in the treatment of dry skin conditions because their high water content gives them a moisturizing effect.

Creatinine clearance

See *Kidney function tests*.

Cremation

Burning dead bodies to ash. Typically, the process takes between one and two hours and results in 5 to 7 pounds (2.3 to 3.2 kg) of ash. In some cases certain precautions must be taken before cremation can be performed. For example, if the deceased person was fitted with a pacemaker, it must be removed from the body because of

the risk of an explosion. Also, cremation involves additional formalities, principally to prevent destruction of a body before the possibility of a crime has been ruled out.

Crepitus

The grating sound heard, and the sensation felt, when two rough surfaces rub together. It may be experienced when the ends of a broken bone rub against each other or in *osteoarthritis*, when the cartilage that covers the bony surfaces of a joint has worn away and the roughened areas of the joint grind against each other. The sound is usually loud enough to be heard by the naked ear. Fainter sounds, audible through a stethoscope, are produced when lung *alveoli* rub together—as a result of inflammation due to pneumonia, for example.

Crepitus is also used to describe the sounds made when an area of subcutaneous *emphysema* (air under the skin) or gas *gangrene* (gas within infected tissues) is pressed.

Cretinism

A condition characterized by mental retardation, stunted growth, and coarse facial features. It results from decreased production of the hormone *thyroxine* by the thyroid gland. (See also *Hypothyroidism*.)

Creutzfeldt-Jakob syndrome

A very rare degenerative condition of the brain presumably caused by a slow virus (one that causes no signs of disease until many months or years after the original infection).

In most instances, no source of infection is discovered. However, rarely, infection has been linked with brain surgery when instruments contaminated by the virus have been used, transplantation of an infected cornea, and treatment with growth hormone extracted from pituitary glands after death (current growth hormone preparations are products of genetic engineering and carry no risk).

The condition causes progressive *dementia* and *myoclonus* (sudden

PROCEDURE FOR CRANIOTOMY

Before the operation, all or part of the patient's scalp is shaved. After a general anesthetic has been given, layers of skin, muscle, and membrane are cut away from the skull at the planned operation site and the bone between them is cut with a saw. The lid of bone is then either lifted back on a hinge of muscle or removed completely. The dura (the outer membrane lining the brain) is then opened to reveal the inner membranes and the brain.

Burr holes
A series of burr holes is made. They must be very close together if the bone is thick.

Burr
Skull
Dura
Brain

Brain

Skin hinged back
Flap of skull hinged back

Burr hole   Gigli's saw

Gigli's saw
The cuts between the burr holes are made using Gigli's saw, which is passed between the burr holes using a malleable saw guide.

C

muscular contractions). Muscular coordination diminishes, the intellect and personality deteriorate, and blindness may develop. As the disease progresses, the power of speech is lost and the body becomes rigid. There is no treatment and death usually occurs within three to 12 months of onset.

Crib death
See *Sudden infant death syndrome*.

Cri du chat syndrome
A congenital (present at birth) condition characterized by a catlike cry due to a small larynx. Mental handicap, unusual facial characteristics (such as a wide spacing between the eyes), a small head, and shortness of stature are other typical features.

Cri du chat syndrome is rare and the result of a *chromosomal abnormality*; a portion of one chromosome is missing in each of the affected individual's cells. No treatment is possible. The child needs special care and schooling if he or she survives infancy. (See also *Genetic counseling*.)

Crisis
A term that describes a turning point in the course of a disease (marking the onset of either recovery or deterioration), an emergency, or a distressing time of emotional difficulty (such as divorce or a death in the family). The term was in common use before the advent of antibiotics when patients with lobar *pneumonia* would be watched for the crisis.

Crisis intervention
The provision of immediate advice or help to people with acute personal or sociomedical problems.

Many voluntary organizations have been established to help people in crisis. Help may also be available at walk-in centers or social services departments. In addition to other crisis services, these centers may offer *counseling*, usually with the aim of helping clients cope with crises rather than of providing longer-term help.

Critical
A term used to mean seriously ill, or to describe a crucial state of illness from which it is uncertain whether or not the patient will recover.

Crohn's disease
A chronic inflammatory disease that can affect any part of the gastrointestinal tract from the mouth to the anus.

Crohn's disease may cause pain, fever, diarrhea, and loss of weight.

The most common site of inflammation is the terminal ileum (the end of the small intestine where it joins the large intestine). The intestinal wall becomes extremely thick due to continued chronic inflammation, and deep, penetrating ulcers may form. The disease tends to be patchy; areas of the intestine that lie between diseased areas may appear to be normal, but are usually mildly affected.

CAUSES AND INCIDENCE
The cause is unknown. It may represent an abnormal allergic reaction or may be an exaggerated response to an infectious agent, such as a bacterium or a virus. There is a slight genetic predisposition (inherited tendency to develop the disease).

The incidence of Crohn's disease varies between three and six new cases per year per 100,000 population in most developed countries, including the US; the incidence seems to have increased over the last 30 years. A person may be affected at any age, but the peak ages are in adolescence and early adulthood and after 60.

SYMPTOMS
In young people the ileum (small intestine) is usually involved, and the disease causes spasms of pain in the abdomen, diarrhea, and chronic sickness due to loss of appetite, anemia, and weight loss. The ability of the small intestine to absorb food is reduced. In the elderly, it is more common for the disease to affect the rectum and cause rectal bleeding. In both groups the disease may also affect the anus, causing chronic abscesses, deep fissures (cracks), and fistulas (passageways that create an abnormal link between organs of the body).

Crohn's disease can also affect the colon (large intestine), causing bloody diarrhea. It is rare in the mouth, esophagus, stomach, and duodenum (upper part of the small intestine).

Complications may affect the intestines or may develop elsewhere in the body. The thickening of the intestinal wall may narrow the inside diameter so much that an intestinal obstruction occurs.

About 30 percent of patients with Crohn's disease develop a fistula. Internal fistulas may form between loops of intestine. External fistulas to the skin of the abdomen or the skin surrounding the anus may follow a surgical operation (or rupture of an abscess) and may cause leakage of feces onto the skin.

Abscesses (pus-filled pockets of infection) form in about 20 percent of patients. Many of these abscesses occur around the anus, but some occur within the abdomen.

Complications in other parts of the body may include inflammation of various parts of the eye, severe arthritis affecting various joints of the body, *ankylosing spondylitis* (an inflammation of the spine), and skin disorders (including *eczema*).

DIAGNOSIS
If the symptoms suggest Crohn's disease, a physical examination may reveal tender abdominal swellings that indicate thickening of the intestinal walls. *Sigmoidoscopy* (examination of the rectum with a viewing tube) may confirm the disease's presence in the rectum. X rays using barium meals or barium enemas (see *Barium X-ray examinations*) will show thickened loops of bowel with deep fissures. It may be difficult to differentiate between Crohn's disease that affects the colon and *ulcerative colitis*, a form of inflammatory disease that is limited to the large intestine, but *colonoscopy* (examination of the colon using a flexible viewing tube) and *biopsy* (removal of a piece of tissue for microscopic examination) may help in doubtful cases. Blood tests may show evidence of protein deficiency or *anemia*.

TREATMENT
Sulfasalazine may be given by mouth to try to control the inflammatory process and *corticosteroid drugs* may be given by mouth or as enemas. Severe acute attacks may require admission to the hospital for blood transfusion, intravenous feeding, and treatment with corticosteroid drugs given intravenously. The severity of the disease fluctuates widely, and the patient is usually under long-term medical supervision.

Some patients find that particular foods exacerbate their symptoms. Others may benefit from a high-vitamin, low-fiber diet.

A surgical operation to remove damaged portions of the intestine may be needed to treat chronic obstruction or blood loss. If the small intestine is involved, the surgeon will remove as little of the intestine as possible, seeking only to remove the most affected parts since the surgery is not curative.

If the large intestine is involved, surgery may involve removal of narrowed obstructing segments.

Emergency surgery may be required to deal with an abscess. Simple drainage of an abscess will produce an external fistula, but occasionally the patient is too ill for any further treatment. Surgery may also occasionally be required for obstruction, perforation, or severe bleeding.

OUTLOOK
The disease is chronic and the symptoms fluctuate over many years, "burning out" in time for some patients. Many patients eventually require surgical treatment to deal with the complications of the disease. The recurrence rate after surgery is high, although recurrences may be delayed for many years. Some patients with localized disease remain in normal health indefinitely after surgery and seem to be cured. There is no predisposition to intestinal cancer.

Cromolyn sodium

ALLERGY
⚗️ 🥄 ✏️ 🖊️ 🖊️ 🗃️ 🖊️ 🖋️ 🖌️ 🧪 ⬭
Capsule Inhaler Eye drops Nose drops
📋 Prescription needed
🔒 Not available as generic

A drug used in the treatment of some types of *asthma* and allergic conditions such as allergic *rhinitis* (hay fever), allergic *conjunctivitis*, and *food allergy*. Cromolyn sodium was introduced in the 1970s.

WHY IT IS USED
Cromolyn sodium is commonly given by inhaler to prevent attacks of mild to moderate asthma in children. It is also prescribed for allergic asthma in adults and for asthma induced by exercise or cold air. Cromolyn sodium has a slow onset of action, taking up to four to six weeks of regular dosing to produce its antiasthmatic effect. Its use sometimes permits a reduction in the dosage of other drugs taken to relieve attacks. It is not effective for the relief of an acute asthmatic attack in progress.

Taken as a nasal spray, cromolyn sodium is useful in treating allergic rhinitis. In the form of eye drops, it treats allergic conjunctivitis, and as capsules it can help in some types of food allergy.

HOW IT WORKS
Cromolyn sodium works by blocking the release of *histamine* (a chemical released into the body when an allergic reaction occurs).

POSSIBLE ADVERSE EFFECTS
Side effects are generally mild and rarely require the drug to be stopped. Coughing and wheezing on inhalation may be prevented by using a sym-

pathomimetic *bronchodilator drug* first. Hoarseness and throat irritation can be avoided by rinsing the mouth with water after inhalation.

Crossbite

A type of *malocclusion* in which the lower teeth overlap the upper teeth. In a normal bite, just the reverse is true.

Cross-eye

A type of *strabismus* (squint) in which one eye turns inward relative to the other eye.

Appearance of cross-eye
Most types of cross-eye can, and should, be corrected to improve appearance and vision.

Cross matching

A procedure used to determine compatibility between the blood of someone requiring a *blood transfusion* and that of a blood donor.

Red blood cells from the donor are mixed with serum from the recipient, and red blood cells from the recipient are mixed with serum from the donor. After a short time, the mixtures are examined on a glass slide under a microscope. Clumping together of the red cells to form a small clot indicates the presence of antibodies in the serum, showing that the blood is not compatible. If no clotting occurs, the donor's blood may be safely transfused to the recipient.

Croup

Inflammation and narrowing of the air passages in young children, causing a barking cough, hoarseness, and stridor (a wheezing or grunting noise on breathing in). The condition is very common in children up to the age of about 4 years. In older children and adults, the air passages are too wide and the cartilage in the wall too stiff for any swelling or inflammation to cause the walls to collapse.

CAUSES
Croup is brought on by a viral infection, often a cold, affecting the larynx (voice box), trachea (windpipe), and bronchi (airways into the lung).

Several different types of virus can infect this part of the respiratory system, so one bout of croup does not confer immunity from subsequent attacks; some children are prone to recurrent bouts. Croup tends to occur in outbreaks in late fall and winter.

TREATMENT
Most cases are mild and pass quickly. A parent should remain calm and comfort the child; once soothed, the child will be able to breathe more easily. Providing cool mist for the child to inhale may also help (by utilizing a room humidifier or sitting in the bathroom with the shower running, for example). Cool night air has a beneficial effect as well.

If a child is struggling to breathe or turns blue, medical help should be obtained immediately. The child should be taken to the hospital and there given humidified oxygen in a tent. When breathing is seriously obstructed, treatment involves either passing a tube down the throat or an operation called a *tracheostomy* in which a tube is passed into the throat through the neck to bypass the obstruction. In either case, the tube can usually be removed within 24 hours. Complete recovery takes place within a few days.

Crowding, dental

A type of *malocclusion* that occurs when there is insufficient space along the jawbones to accommodate all the teeth in correct alignment.

Crown, dental

An artificial replacement for the crown of a tooth (the part above the gum) that has become decayed, discolored, or broken. A porcelain crown is usually used on front teeth because of its similarity in color to natural teeth, but back teeth require the greater strength of a crown made from gold or from porcelain fused to metal. (See illustration, next page.)

Cruciate ligaments

Two ligaments in the knee that pass over each other to form a cross (hence their name, from the Latin word "crux," meaning cross). The ligaments form connections between the femur (thigh bone) and tibia (shin) inside the knee joint.

The role of the cruciate ligaments is to prevent overbending and overstraightening at the knee joint. Consequently, if these ligaments are torn, the knee joint becomes unstable and may cause pain.

C

HOW CROWNS ARE FITTED

The tooth is filed to form a peg over which the replacement is fitted. An impression of the peg and natural tooth is taken and a replica made. Using this as a model, the crown is constructed.

Cast full crown

Porcelain fused to metal crown

Porcelain jacket crown

Three-quarter crown

POST CROWNS

If the natural tooth is heavily decayed or has been weakened, a post crown is fitted.

Tooth root
Damaged tooth

1 This tooth is so decayed that a retaining peg cannot be fashioned.

2 The natural crown of the tooth is completely removed.

Tooth trimmed

Gold post in root canal

Crown

3 A post is cemented into the root canal and the crown is cemented over the post.

1 A cracked, heavily filled, or broken tooth can be replaced by a crown.

2 The remaining part of the tooth is shaped to receive the crown.

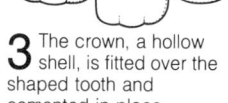

3 The crown, a hollow shell, is fitted over the shaped tooth and cemented in place.

Crush syndrome

Damage to a large amount of body muscle—most commonly as a result of a serious auto accident—causing *renal failure*. Protein pigments released into the bloodstream from the damaged muscles temporarily impair the functioning of the kidney. As a result, some substances normally excreted in the urine build up to toxic levels in the blood. Without treatment the kidney failure may be fatal. Today, treatment by *dialysis* gives the kidneys a chance to recover their function.

Crutch palsy

Weakness or paralysis of muscles in the wrist, fingers, and thumb from a crutch pressed tightly under the arm, caused by pressure on the nerves that supply these muscles. The disorder occurs only after prolonged walking with a crutch that is too tall for the individual. A crutch should fit comfortably under the arm when standing upright, with the hand taking much of the weight.

Crutch palsy can also occur after falling asleep with one arm over the back of a chair with the top of the chair pressed into the armpit. Usually, the person has fallen asleep after a bout of drinking, giving the disorder its common name, Saturday night palsy.

Symptoms usually improve without treatment since the damage to the nerves is temporary. In rare cases, exercises are needed to strengthen the wrist and fingers.

Crying in infants

Occasional crying in a baby is normal behavior—it is the baby's only means of communicating a need. Only when crying is inconsolable or unusual in any way should it be regarded as signifying a problem.

CAUSES

Crying in infants is usually a response to needs or discomforts, such as hunger, thirst, a wet or soiled diaper, tiredness, interrupted sleep, a desire to be comforted, feeling hot or cold, boredom, or separation from parents. Most healthy babies stop crying when their needs are attended to.

Persistent crying, when it is not due to a continually ignored or unrecognized need, may be a baby's reaction to the overwrought state of a parent who is angry, resentful, or overtired. In a minority of cases, crying may be due to illness, commonly ear or throat infections, or to viral fevers. Persistent crying may indicate maltreatment (see *Child abuse*).

TREATMENT

A crying baby should always be attended to. The idea that attending to a crying infant is "giving in" is wrong. Persistent lack of attention is believed to have an adverse effect on emotional development in later life.

If a baby continues to cry after a feeding and a change of diaper, parents should make sure that their child is not too hot or cold, and should try to comfort the baby. A baby sling can be used to provide continuous physical contact. The baby may also prefer being propped up in a chair rather than lying flat, so that he or she can look around.

Parents should try to get as much sleep as possible, and mothers especially should put aside at least one period during the day for relaxation. If the baby cries at night, parents should take turns attending to him or her.

Medical advice is usually necessary only if a baby cries persistently despite all attempts to soothe him or her, if a normally quiet baby starts to cry a lot, if a baby also has diarrhea, vomiting, fever, or seems sick, or if a baby cries only weakly or not at all. Parents should not attribute persistent crying to teething or colic without consulting a physician.

Cryo-

A prefix meaning cold. It is often used to indicate that a procedure uses freezing or low temperatures.

Cryopreservation

The preservation of living cells by freezing. The technique is used chiefly to store human eggs, sperm, and blood for later use.

WHY IT IS DONE

In a woman who is infertile because of blocked fallopian tubes, eggs can be removed from her ovaries, frozen, and stored until they can be used for *in vitro fertilization.*

Treatment of cancer by radiation therapy or chemotherapy carries the slight risk of damaging sperm. If the man wants to retain the option of future fatherhood, a sample of his sperm is collected before treatment and frozen for possible later use in *artificial insemination*. Sperm from donors can also be frozen and used in this way to enable a woman whose husband is infertile to bear a child.

Plasma and blood from rare blood groups can be preserved by freezing and stored in a blood bank for long periods until needed.

HOW IT IS DONE

The cells to be preserved are first immersed in a fluid, usually glycerol. Glycerol enters and surrounds the cells so that they are protected from the normally destructive effect of freezing (see *Cryosurgery*). The temperature is lowered as the concentration of protecting fluid is increased until the final storage temperature of about -290°F (-180°C) is reached.

OUTLOOK

Apart from widespread cryopreservation of cells, there has also been some success with freezing and reusing small areas of tissue, such as the cornea and portions of skin. This has led to much experimental work on the possibility (as yet unfulfilled) of cryopreservation of major organs, such as the heart, liver, and kidneys, taken from people who have recently died, for the purposes of transplantation. This would enable transplants to be carried out on a normal surgical time scale rather than as a race against time, as at present.

Cryosurgery

The use of temperatures below freezing to destroy tissue. The term is also applied to the use of cold during surgery to produce adhesion between an instrument and body tissue. Cryosurgery has been in common use only for the past decade; in many cases it is proving to be a useful alternative to more traditional surgery or radiation therapy.

WHY IT IS DONE

Because cryosurgery causes only minimal scarring, it is particularly valuable for dealing with malignant tumors in the cervix and in major organs, such as the liver or bowel, in which heavy scarring can block vital openings or channels. For cosmetic reasons, it is also the best technique for removing skin cancers, such as basal cell carcinoma, and skin disfigurements, such as birthmarks. Hemorrhoids and other anal lesions can be treated rapidly and effectively.

Cryosurgery is also a good method for handling tiny structures in the eye; it has proved particularly useful in performing *cataract surgery* and for treating *retinal detachment*.

HOW IT IS DONE

Treatment of an internal tumor with cryosurgery is a major operation requiring a general anesthetic. The growth is destroyed in one of two ways—by applying a metal probe cooled to the temperature of liquid nitrogen, about -256°F (-160°C), or by spraying it with liquid nitrogen.

Skin cancers, disfigurements, and hemorrhoids are usually treated in the outpatient department, using a metal probe cooled to the same temperature as above. The procedure is virtually painless, since the extreme cold paralyzes the nerves in the skin as a local anesthetic does. After treatment, a blister develops, which may weep for a few days before healing. Although there is little scarring, the treated area may show up as a patch of paler skin.

Cryptococcosis

A rare infection caused by inhaling the fungus CRYPTOCOCCUS NEOFORMANS. It is found throughout the world, especially in soil contaminated with pigeon droppings. Infection with the fungus may cause *meningitis* (inflammation of the coverings of the brain) or granular growths in the lungs, skin, or elsewhere. Most but not all cases occur in people whose resistance to infection has been drastically lowered by diseases such as *AIDS* and *Hodgkin's disease* or by *immunosuppressant drugs*.

SYMPTOMS

Meningitis is the most usual, and serious, form that the illness takes. Symptoms include headache, stiffness in the neck, fever, drowsiness, blurred vision, and a staggering gait. If the infection is not treated, it may end in coma and death. When the disease attacks the lungs it causes chest pain and a cough, sometimes with sputum (phlegm); there may also be a skin rash of ulcerating spots.

DIAGNOSIS AND TREATMENT

Cryptococcal meningitis is diagnosed from a sample of fluid drawn from the spine. An X ray may be needed to detect any damage to the lungs, and laboratory examination of the sputum, lung *biopsy*, and *bronchoscopy* may be needed.

Most cases in which only the lungs have been infected need no treatment, clearing up of their own accord. When

the meninges have been affected, a combination of the antifungal drugs amphotericin B and flucytosine is usually given for about six weeks. Although these drugs are usually effective, relapses can occur.

Cryptorchidism

A developmental disorder of male infants in which the testes fail to descend normally into the scrotum. (See *Testis, undescended*.)

CT scanning

A diagnostic technique in which the combined use of a computer and *X rays* passed through the body at different angles produces clear cross-sectional images ("slices") of the tissue being examined. CT (computerized tomography) scanning—also known as CAT (computerized axial tomography) scanning or whole body scanning—provides clearer and more detailed information than X rays used by themselves. In addition, CT scanning tends to minimize the amount of radiation exposure.

WHY IT IS DONE

The first CT scanner, which came into operation in 1972, was developed to study the brain. Since then, CT brain scanning has marked a major advance in the diagnosis and treatment of tumors, abscesses, and hemorrhages in the brain, as well as strokes and head injuries. These once required tests, such as *angiography* and ventriculography (an outmoded technique for imaging the ventricles of the brain), that not only were difficult to perform, lengthy, and not always clear-cut in their findings, but also entailed some risk for the patient. CT scanning, on the other hand, is simple, quick, accurate, and carries a modest exposure to radiation.

As well as being essential for the study of the brain, CT scanning is invaluable in investigating disease of any part of the trunk. It is particularly useful for locating and imaging tumors, and for guiding the operator who is performing a needle *biopsy*.

RESULTS

Using the information produced by the scanner, a computer constructs cross-sectional images of the tissue under examination. These images, displayed on a TV screen, reveal soft tissues (including tumors) more clearly than normal X-ray pictures. The images are particularly valuable in brain scans due to their sharp definition of ventricles (fluid-filled spaces). The images can be manipulated

C

PERFORMING A CT SCAN

CT scanning combines the use of a computer and X rays passed through the body at different angles to produce clear cross-sectional images of areas of body tissue. Before the scan is carried out, a contrast medium may be injected to make blood vessels, organs, or abnormalities show up more clearly; a drink of contrast medium may be given to highlight loops of intestine.

1 The patient lies on a table that can be moved up or down to allow easy transfer and accurate positioning within the machine.

A central sliding cradle in the table moves the patient, at a controllable rate, into the machine

The machine can be tilted in either direction to allow precise areas to be X-rayed

Right kidney

Spinal cord

Spine

Rib

Abnormal left kidney

Cysts

Cysts

Gas in stomach   Liver

2 A great number of X-ray beams, each of low dosage and lasting only a fraction of a second, are passed through the body at different angles as the scanner rotates around the patient.

3 The amount of X rays absorbed by different tissues is recorded by detectors in the scanner and transformed by a computer into an image, which is interpreted by a radiologist.

electronically to provide the best view of the area of interest, and adjacent two-dimensional "slices" can be reconstructed to produce three-dimensional representations as well as images in different planes.

Culture

A growth of bacteria or other microorganisms, cells, or tissues cultivated artificially in the laboratory.

WHY IT IS DONE

Microorganisms are collected and cultivated to enable the cause of an infection to be accurately diagnosed. Cultivation produces larger numbers of microorganisms in a form suitable for further tests.

Healthy cells are cultured to diagnose various disorders prenatally and for studying chromosomes. Human tissues, such as skin, may be cultured to produce larger amounts for use in grafting. Other tissues, notably human *amnion* (embryonic tissue) and monkey kidney, are cultivated to provide a medium in which viruses can be grown and identified in the laboratory; viruses will multiply only within living cells.

HOW IT IS DONE

MICROORGANISMS The type of specimen collected from the patient depends on the suspected site of infection. For example, a throat swab is made if a streptococcal throat infection is suspected, a urine specimen is collected if urinary tract infection is thought likely, a sputum sample if respiratory infection is suspected, or a feces sample if gastrointestinal infection is suspected. Likewise, a blood sample is cultured (blood culture) if the bloodstream is thought to be infected. Bacteria, fungi, and, occasionally, viruses may be cultured directly from the blood.

The specimen is collected in a sterile container and is incubated at body temperature in a carefully chosen culture medium. Liquid or solid culture media, usually agar gel or meat-based broth, are used for culturing bacteria. These media contain various nutrients chosen for the particular needs of the organism suspected of causing the infection; the media may also contain ingredients to discourage the growth of other organisms.

Any bacteria present will multiply to form visible colonies. The type of bacteria can be identified by noting the appearance of the colony, by chemical tests, and by examining the bacteria under the microscope. Bacterial cultures can be tested with various antibiotics to determine which antibiotic may be the most effective against a particular infection.

CELLS AND TISSUES For the diagnosis of prenatal abnormalities, cells are collected by *amniocentesis* or *chorionic villus sampling*. Cells for studying chromosomes (see *Chromosome analysis*) are cultured from white blood cells or cells gathered from the inside of the cheek. Cells and tissues to be used for analysis, for growing viruses, or to be used for grafting are cultured in a small amount of fluid containing nutrients essential for their growth.

Cupping

An ancient form of treatment used to draw blood to the surface of the skin. Cupping is still used in folk healing in some countries, particularly in China and Turkey.

A small vessel—commonly a glass jar, animal horn, ceramic vessel, or a closed-ended bamboo tube—is heated and applied to the skin. When it cools and the air inside contracts, a partial vacuum is created, causing the skin to be sucked into the vessel, producing a rounded area of inflammation. Believers in this form of treatment think the inflammatory response is therapeutic.

Heated glass applied to skin

Uses of cupping
Conditions treated by this technique include bronchitis, asthma, and musculo-skeletal pains.

Curare

An extract from the bark and juices of various trees that has been used for centuries by South American Indians as an arrow poison. The principal active ingredient is tubocurarine, a drug that inhibits muscle contractions by interfering with the action of *acetylcholine*, a *neurotransmitter* (chemical released from nerve endings).

Cure

To treat successfully; that is, to restore to normal health after an illness. The term usually means the complete disappearance of a disease rather than just a halt in its progress. Any medication or therapy used in the treatment of an illness may also be called a cure.

In general, infections may be cured, as may some tumors. By contrast, chronic conditions, such as *osteoarthritis*, or endocrine deficiency diseases, such as *hypothyroidism* (underactivity of the thyroid gland), are never cured but undergo remission or are controlled with long-term hormone treatment.

Curet

A spoon-shaped surgical instrument for scraping away material or tissue from an organ, cavity, or surface.

Curettage

The use of a sharp-edged, spoon-shaped surgical instrument called a curet to scrape abnormal tissue, or tissue for analysis, from the lining of a body cavity or from the skin. Curettage is commonly used to remove infected material from an abscess, to scrape tissue from the lining of the uterus as part of a *D and C* (dilatation and curettage) operation, and to remove small growths from the skin. (See also *Curettage, dental*.)

Curettage, dental

The scraping of the wall of a cavity with a dental *curet* (a narrow, spoon-shaped, scaling instrument). It is one method used in the treatment of simple periodontal pockets occurring in *periodontitis*. The curet is used to remove the lining and diseased tissue from the lateral walls of the root. This enables the healthy, underlying tissue to reattach itself to the root surface, which is cleared of calculus deposits before curettage.

Curling's ulcer

A type of *stress ulcer* (a disruption in the lining of the stomach or duodenum following any severe injury, infection, or shock) that occurs specifically in people who have suffered extensive skin burns. Ulcers develop about 24 hours after the burns and are usually small and multiple. Diagnosis and treatment are as for other types of stress ulcer.

Cushing's syndrome

A hormonal disorder caused by an abnormally high circulating level of corticosteroid hormones, produced naturally by the *adrenal glands*.

CAUSES AND INCIDENCE
Cushing's syndrome may be produced directly by an adrenal gland tumor, causing excessive secretion of corticosteroids, by prolonged administration of *corticosteroid drugs*, or by enlargement of both adrenal glands due to a pituitary tumor. Corticosteroid drugs are widely used for inflammatory conditions such as rheumatoid arthritis, inflammatory bowel disease, and asthma.

The pituitary gland controls the activity of the adrenal gland by producing a hormone known as *ACTH* (adrenocorticotropic hormone), which stimulates the cortex (outer portion) of the adrenal gland to grow. Overactivity or a tumor of the pituitary can thus lead to overproduction of ACTH, overgrowth of the adrenal glands, and excess secretion of corticosteroids. Some lung cancers and various other tumors may also secrete ACTH, with similar results.

Cushing's syndrome can occur at any age, but is most common in middle age. Most cases today are caused by excessive, prolonged use of corticosteroid drugs, but these cases are usually mild. The patient is often described as having cushingoid features rather than full-blown Cushing's syndrome. Cases caused by pituitary overactivity (sometimes called Cushing's disease) are much more common in women, and those caused by lung tumors are more common in men.

SYMPTOMS
People with Cushing's syndrome have a characteristic appearance. The face appears round ("moon-faced") and red, the trunk tends to become obese with a humped upper back, and the limbs become wasted. Acne develops and purple stretch marks may appear on the abdomen, thighs, and breasts. The skin is thin and bruises easily. The bones become weakened and are at increased risk of fracturing (see *Osteoporosis*). Women may become increasingly hairy. Affected people are more susceptible to infection and may suffer from stomach or duodenal ulcers.

Mental changes often occur, including *depression*, *paranoia*, or sometimes *euphoria*. Insomnia may be a problem. Patients may develop *hypertension* (increased blood pressure) and *edema* (fluid collection in the tissues). About one fifth of patients develop *diabetes mellitus*. In children, Cushing's syndrome may suppress growth.

DIAGNOSIS
Anyone suspected of having Cushing's syndrome should be examined by an endocrinologist. Obese or depressed patients may have many of the clinical features of Cushing's syndrome, making diagnosis difficult. Diagnosis requires measurement of ACTH levels in the blood and corticosteroid levels in the blood and urine. *CT scanning* of the adrenal and pituitary glands is performed to look for abnormalities.

TREATMENT
If the cause is overtreatment with corticosteroid drugs, the condition is usually reversible with gradual withdrawal of drug treatment.

If the cause is shown to be a tumor or overgrowth of an adrenal gland, the gland is removed surgically. If the tumor lies in the pituitary gland, it is removed by surgery or shrunk by irradiation and medication. Patients subsequently need hormone replacement therapy; without it, they would be left completely deficient in adrenal or pituitary hormones.

Cusp, dental
One of the small, protruding areas occurring on the grinding surface of a tooth (see *Teeth*).

Cuspid
A name for a canine tooth (see *Teeth*).

Cutaneous
Pertaining to the skin. For example, a subcutaneous injection is an injection given beneath the skin.

Cutdown
The creation of a small incision in the skin over a vein to gain access to the vein. A cutdown may be necessary when it is essential to take blood or give intravenous fluid, and a vein cannot be identified through the skin.

CVS
See *Chorionic villus sampling*.

Cyanide
Any of a group of mostly highly toxic substances that contains the cyanogen chemical group. Chemicals in this group consist of a carbon atom linked to a nitrogen atom.

The poisonous effects of cyanides are due to their ability to block a specific *enzyme* (cytochrome oxidase) that plays an essential role in the uptake of oxygen by cells. This blocking action deprives cells of oxygen, which, in turn, produces a rapid progression of symptoms from breathlessness, through paralysis and unconsciousness, to death.

Because of their toxicity, cyanides have few applications. Hydrogen cyanide is used to kill rodents and fumigate buildings. It has also been used in gas chambers. Certain other cyanides are powerful eye irritants and are used in some tear gases.

Cyanocobalamin
A name for *vitamin B$_{12}$*.

Cyanosis
Bluish coloration of the skin and mucous membranes (such as the lining of the mouth) due to too much deoxygenated *hemoglobin* in the blood. Cyanosis is generally most obvious in the beds of the fingernails and toenails and on the lips and tongue.

Cyanosis occurs most frequently because of slow blood flow through the skin as a result of low temperatures (the familiar sign of turning blue with cold). In such cases, where no other symptoms are present, it does not indicate a serious underlying disease process.

In other cases, however, cyanosis may be a serious sign and requires medical investigation. Cyanosis may indicate poor peripheral blood circulation in which the fingers and toes turn blue even in relatively warm conditions. It may also be a sign of a heart or lung disorder, such as *heart failure*, lung damage, or pulmonary *edema* (fluid in the lungs). More rarely, cyanosis may be present at birth, when it may be a sign of a congenital heart disease in which some of the blood is not pumped to the lungs (where oxygen, and thereby a bright red color, is obtained). Instead, the blood goes directly to the rest of the body (see *Heart disease, congenital*).

Cyclacillin
A penicillin-type antibiotic commonly used to treat acute otitis media (acute infection of the middle ear), sinusitis, and cystitis. (See *Penicillins*.)

Cyclobenzaprine
A *muscle-relaxant drug* mainly used in the short-term treatment of painful muscle spasm caused by injury.

Cyclophosphamide
An *anticancer drug* used mainly in the treatment of Hodgkin's disease and leukemia, often in combination with other anticancer drugs. It is also useful as an *immunosuppressant drug*, helping prevent rejection of a transplanted organ by modifying the body's natural defense against abnormal or foreign cells. Cyclophosphamide has also been used to treat connective tissue diseases such as severe systemic *lupus erythematosus*.

Cycloplegia
Paralysis of the ciliary muscle, which controls the shape of the lens in the eye. With the ciliary muscle out of action, the process of *accommodation* is not able to work properly. Accommodation occurs when light rays from near objects are focused onto the retina (visual receptive layer) at the back of the eye.

Cyclosporine

IMMUNOSUPPRESSANT

Injection

Prescription needed

Not available as generic

An *immunosuppressant drug* that suppresses the body's natural defense against abnormal cells; it was introduced in 1984.

WHY IT IS USED
Cyclosporine's immunosuppressant action is of particular use following *transplant surgery*, when the body may start to reject the transplanted organ unless the immune system is damped down. Cyclosporine is now widely used following many different types of transplant surgery, including heart, kidney, bone marrow, liver, and pancreas transplants. Its use has considerably reduced the risk of tissue rejection and also the need for large doses of *corticosteroid drugs*. Cyclosporine may need to be taken in oral form for an indefinite period following surgery.

POSSIBLE ADVERSE EFFECTS
Because cyclosporine reduces the effectiveness of the immune system, people being treated with this drug have an increased susceptibility to infection. Any flulike illness or localized infection requires immediate treatment by a physician.

Cyclosporine has also been found to cause kidney damage in some people. Regular monitoring of kidney function is therefore necessary for people being given this drug. If signs of kidney damage, such as protein in the urine, are detected, the dose of cyclosporine may need to be reduced or another drug substituted. Another adverse effect related to kidney damage is *hypertension*. A fairly common adverse effect of cyclosporine is swelling of the gums.

Cyclothymia
A type of personality characteristic that is associated with marked changes of mood. From being cheerful, energetic, and sociable people, these individuals may, for no apparent reason, quickly become withdrawn, gloomy, and listless. These swings of mood may be regular, may last for days or months, and may be separated by relatively "normal" periods of behavior. Sometimes an obvious *manic-depressive illness* results, or there may be a family history of

C

such illness. There may be an associated pyknic (rounded and stout) body build. People with cyclothymia who are mainly "up" or "manic" often have very successful careers; others may resort episodically to heavy drinking or difficult behavior.

Cyst

An abnormal lump or swelling, filled with fluid or semisolid material, in any body organ or tissue.

The causes of cysts are numerous. They may result from blockage of the duct leading from a fluid-forming gland—*sebaceous cysts* in the skin, for example. Alternatively, there may be abnormal activity or growth of a fluid-forming tissue, with no means of the fluid escaping—in an *ovarian cyst*, for example. Finally, cysts may form

Sebaceous cysts under the ear
These cysts result from blockage of ducts leading from sebaceous glands in the skin. The cysts are benign; if they become unsightly, they can be surgically removed.

around parasites in organs such as the liver, brain, or intestinal wall in diseases such as *hydatid disease*, *cysticercosis*, and *amebiasis*.

Other types of cyst include *Baker's cyst* (behind the knee) and *dermoid cyst* (a type of skin cyst that may contain particles of hair follicles, sweat glands, nerves, and teeth).

Cysts are usually harmless in themselves, but they may disrupt the function of the organ or tissues in which they grow. Those in the skin are unsightly, but, if accessible, can be surgically removed.

Cyst-/cysto-

Prefixes that denote the bladder, as in *cystitis* (inflammation of the bladder) and *cystoscopy* (endoscopic examination of the bladder).

Cystectomy

Surgical removal of the bladder, after which urine is passed from the body via a specially constructed channel emerging in a *stoma* (mouthlike opening) on the lower abdomen.

WHY IT IS DONE

Cystectomy is performed either as a curative or palliative procedure for a widespread cancer of the bladder (see *Bladder tumors*). Once a cancer begins to invade the bladder muscle, treatment may be by surgery, radiation therapy, chemotherapy, or a combination of the treatments.

RISKS AND OUTLOOK

A cystectomy is likely to cause a major disturbance in life-style. In men, the operation in most cases causes impotence (due to damage to nerve tracts involved in penile erection) and in women it leads to infertility (although the majority of women who undergo the operation are past childbearing age). In addition, the patient needs to adapt to wearing an external pouch to collect urine and to learn about care of the stoma. Before undergoing surgery, cystectomy patients are thus advised to discuss their concerns about the operation and its consequences with the physician, surgeon, and enterostomy (stoma care) therapist. Many patients, however, are able to return to a fully active and healthy life. In recent years, the use of continent *urinary diversions*, with no external pouch, has been investigated. The newer pouches permit the patient to control the drainage of urine by emptying the pouch with a catheter. Results are encouraging, although they are still considered experimental.

HOW CYSTECTOMY IS DONE

The operation is a major procedure performed using general anesthesia. An incision is made in the abdomen, and the ureters are cut and tied. The bladder and other organs are removed (see below) and the stoma formed. After the operation, the patient is given intravenous infusions of fluids, salt, and glucose until the intestines function normally again.

Ureters usually cut here

Line of incision

In men, the prostate gland and the bladder are removed

Bladder

Prostate gland

In women, the uterus, fallopian tubes, ovaries, and part of the vagina (as well as the bladder) are removed

Uterus

Large intestine

Piece of small intestine with blood supply intact

Formation of the stoma
The two ureters are joined to a short section of small intestine that has been detached from the remainder of the intestines. One end of this loop of intestine is formed into a stoma by insertion through the abdominal wall.

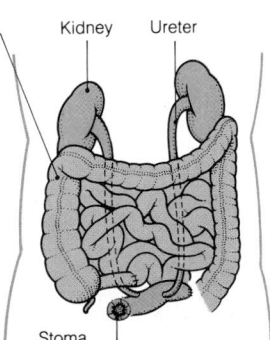

Kidney   Ureter

Stoma

Urine expulsion
Urine produced by the kidneys is channeled via the ureters and intestinal loop out of the body through the stoma.

Cysticercosis

An infection characterized by the presence, in tissues such as the muscle and brain, of cysts formed by the larval (immature) stage of the pork *tapeworm*.

Cysticercosis is an extremely rare disease in the US and most other developed countries, although cases occur in Latin America, Africa, parts of Asia, and Eastern Europe.

Cystic fibrosis

An inherited disease, present from birth, characterized by a tendency to chronic lung infections and an inability to absorb fats and other nutrients from food.

When cystic fibrosis (CF) was first identified in the 1930s, before effective antibiotics were available, almost all sufferers died in early childhood. More recently, however, and particularly since 1975, the outlook has changed dramatically. With more advanced methods of diagnosis and treatment, including the use of a wide range of antibiotics, over two thirds of CF sufferers now survive into adult life, although few of them are in perfect health. CF remains, however, a serious and potentially fatal disorder.

CAUSES AND INCIDENCE

CF (or mucoviscidosis, as it is sometimes called) is caused by a defective *gene*. The defect is of the recessive type, which means that a person must inherit it in a double dose (one gene from each parent) before any outward abnormality is apparent (see *Genetic disorders*). People who inherit the defective gene in a single dose (from one parent only) are called "carriers"; they are normally unaware of the fact and have no symptoms.

Among whites in the US and elsewhere, about one person in 22 is such a "carrier." The chance that any (random) procreating white couple are both carriers is roughly one in 500. In this event, each of their children has a one in four chance of inheriting the defective gene from both parents and of being born with CF. The incidence of the disease among whites is thus about one per 2,000 live births. In nonwhites, however (for example, among black Africans), the disease is very rare (perhaps only one person in 90,000 is affected).

The mechanism by which the gene defect leads to the features of CF is unknown. It is known, however, that certain glands do not function properly. Most seriously, the glands in the lining of the bronchial tubes produce excessive amounts of thick mucus, which predisposes the person to chronic lung infections. A further serious malfunction is failure of the pancreas to produce enzymes involved in the breakdown of fats and their absorption from the intestines; this deficiency causes malnutrition. Sweat glands are also affected.

SYMPTOMS AND SIGNS

The pattern of development of the disease, and the severity of its features, varies considerably among individuals. Hence, although the disease is sometimes obvious soon after birth, in other cases it escapes detection for months or years.

In a typical, or classical, case, the child passes feces that are pale, greasy-looking, and foul-smelling, and in some cases he or she may fail to thrive. The child also suffers from persistent chest infections, causing constant coughing and breathlessness. Pneumonia, bronchiectasis, and bronchitis commonly develop, and the lungs become damaged.

Sterility (not impotence) occurs in the majority of male sufferers but not in affected females; some otherwise healthy adult males have attended infertility clinics and been diagnosed subsequently as having CF. Other features of the disease include stunted growth in many cases, and also abnormally salty sweat, which may require salt replacement in hot climates, but is otherwise harmless.

DIAGNOSIS AND TREATMENT

Suspicious symptoms should be reported to a physician as soon as they are noticed, since the earlier treatment with antibiotics is started, the less lung damage will be caused by chest infections. Once the diagnosis is considered, it is easily confirmed or refuted by simple laboratory tests, including a sweat test. In some areas, screening of all newborn infants for CF is available.

Confirmation of the diagnosis and supervision of treatment is best carried out from a special center staffed by physicians, nurses, and physiotherapists who have a particular knowledge of the disease.

To enable food to be properly digested, replacement pancreatic enzyme preparations must be taken with meals. The diet needs to be rich in calories and proteins, and a vitamin supplement is often prescribed as an extra precaution. These measures bring about weight increase and more normal feces.

AFFECTED FAMILIES

The parents of a child with CF must assume that any subsequent child has a one in four chance of being born with the disease. Unaffected siblings of affected people have a two in three chance of being "carriers," creating problems if they plan to have children with someone who also has CF in the family. Advice can be obtained through *genetic counseling*.

Recent research has succeeded in establishing the location (on *chromosome* number 7 in a person's cells) of the gene involved in CF and has identified biochemical "markers" on the gene that are present when it is defective. It is now possible, therefore, to identify carriers of the defective gene, and also to detect CF before birth.

This service can sometimes be offered to parents who already have a CF child and are contemplating a second pregnancy. First, the presence of the markers for the defective gene is established in both parents. Between eight and 10 weeks into pregnancy, fetal cells obtained by *chorionic villus sampling* are analyzed to see if the markers of CF are present; alternatively, chemical tests on cells obtained by *amniocentesis* (at 17 or 18 weeks of pregnancy) can confirm whether or not the child will have CF. In either case, the parents may choose to terminate the pregnancy if the fetus is affected.

OUTLOOK

The highly specialized treatment given to CF sufferers today provides them with a much better quality of life than was formerly possible. Even so, most suffer permanent lung damage and have a considerably shortened life expectancy. Some people have been treated by heart and lung transplantation, while others have had a lung transplantation only; the results seem very encouraging.

Cystitis

Inflammation of the inner lining of the bladder, caused by an infection that is usually due to bacteria. Anything that obstructs the voiding of urine from the bladder, or leads to incomplete voiding of urine, tends to encourage infection; stagnant urine in the bladder or urethra (the tube leading from the bladder to the exterior) provides a good breeding ground for bacteria.

INCIDENCE AND CAUSES

In women, cystitis is common because the urethra is short, making it easier for infectious agents to pass from the mucous membrane around the urethral opening up into the bladder. The bacteria may come from the vagina or from the intestine via the anus. Most women have cystitis at some time. A *calculus* (stone) in the bladder, a *bladder tumor*, or a *urethral stricture* increases the risk of infection due to obstruction of urine flow.

In men, cystitis is rare (because of the longer urethra) and usually occurs only in the presence of an obstruction, which in most cases is due to an enlarged prostate gland compressing the urethra where it leaves the bladder. Rarely, the obstruction is due to a urethral stricture.

In children, cystitis is often due to a structural abnormality of the ureters (tubes that carry urine from the kidneys to the bladder) at the point at which they enter the bladder, allowing reflux (backward flow) of urine into the ureters when the bladder muscle contracts. This leads to incomplete voiding of urine and to subsequent infection.

Another possible source of infection is the introduction of a catheter (flexible tube) into the bladder—a procedure used to drain urine in a variety of circumstances (see *Catheterization, urinary*), including the treatment of incontinence and urinary retention. Diabetics are particularly susceptible to urinary tract infections.

SYMPTOMS
The main symptom of cystitis in both sexes is a frequent urge to pass urine, with only a small amount of urine passed each time. Passing urine is accompanied by pain, which is usually of a burning or stinging nature. Occasionally, the urine is foul smelling or contains blood. There may be a fever and occasionally chills and continuous discomfort in the lower abdomen. In children, there may be no urinary symptoms, only fever, or the child may cry when passing urine.

DIAGNOSIS
The diagnosis of a urinary infection can be confirmed by examining a sample of urine under the microscope, looking for pus cells, and in certain instances trying to grow the bacteria in a *culture*. When no infection is found in someone with symptoms of cystitis, the diagnosis may be *urethritis* (inflammation of the urethra), a bacterial prostatitis, or, in women only, the *urethral syndrome*, in which the cause is thought to be trauma to the urethra from sexual activity.

TREATMENT
Women with the symptoms of cystitis should drink large quantities of fluid,

AVOIDING CYSTITIS
A few simple measures can help women prone to cystitis reduce the chances of recurrence. In particular, women should drink a lot of fluid, especially cranberry juice, to encourage acidity of the urine.

Fluid consumption
Drink plenty of fluids—so that the urine is consistently pale—and ensure that the bladder is completely emptied at each visit to the toilet.

Rectum
Bladder
Urethra
Anus

Hygiene
Women prone to cystitis should wipe from front to back after a bowel movement and empty the bladder soon after intercourse.

including cranberry juice, which encourages acidity of the urine.

If an infection is present, antibiotics are prescribed to destroy the bacteria and prevent the infection from spreading to cause *pyelonephritis* (infection of the kidneys).

In many cases, the physician will have the patient start a course of antibiotics, especially when pus cells are in the urine, before waiting for the result of the urine culture. The physician will then check the results of the culture to confirm the presence of an infection. Cultures are more frequently performed when there have been recurrent urinary tract infections. Sensitivity of the bacteria to various antibiotics is ascertained from a culture.

In men, antibiotics are prescribed to treat the symptoms of cystitis, but more tests are arranged to look for any obstruction to urinary flow. In children, antibiotics are prescribed and usually more tests are performed to check for a disorder such as reflux of urine into the ureters.

OUTLOOK
Prompt treatment of cystitis with antibiotics usually settles the infection within 24 hours, with no complications. Occasionally, damage to the kidneys due to pyelonephritis occurs, usually because the infection has spread before significant symptoms have appeared.

More tests are performed when there are recurrent infections in women, any infection in men, and usually after one infection in children.

Cystocele
A swelling at the front and top of the vagina formed where the bladder pushes against weakened tissues in the vaginal wall. Weakened tissues may be associated with descent of the uterus from its normal position down into the vagina (see *Uterus, prolapse of*). A cystocele may not cause symptoms, but occasionally the urethra (through which urine drains from the bladder) is pulled out of position. This may cause stress *incontinence* (leakage of urine on coughing, lifting, or sneezing) or the bladder may not empty completely when urine is passed. The urine remaining in the bladder may then become infected, causing frequent and very painful urination (see *Cystitis*).

Exercises to strengthen the pelvic floor muscles (which support the bladder, uterus, and other pelvic organs) may help relieve the symptoms (see *Pelvic floor exercises*). In severe cases, surgery is needed to lift and to tighten the tissues at the front of the vagina.

Cystometry
A procedure carried out to provide information about normal bladder function and about abnormalities either of the nerves supplying the bladder or of the bladder muscle itself. The procedure measures pressure changes in the bladder as it fills, and also the total bladder capacity and the presence of any residual urine after the bladder has fully contracted.

WHY IT IS DONE
Cystometry is used to investigate urinary *incontinence* or poor bladder emptying caused by damage to the bladder muscles (following childbirth or pelvic surgery, for example) or to disruption of the nerve control of these muscles (as in *Parkinson's disease* or *diabetes mellitus*).

C

HOW IT IS DONE

The examination, which takes about 20 minutes, is performed by a urologist or a trained urological technician. It is usually done on an outpatient basis and no anesthetic is required. A catheter (flexible tube) and pressure measuring probe are inserted into the bladder and sometimes the rectum. The bladder is gradually filled with water or carbon dioxide and a series of pressure readings is taken. They indicate the point at which reflex bladder emptying occurs.

Cystoscopy

The examination of the urethra and bladder cavity using a cystoscope (viewing tube inserted up the urethra). Modern cystoscopes have a metal sheath with interchangeable fiberoptic telescopes, allowing a viewing angle ranging from zero to 120 degrees. The zero-angle lens is best for examination of the urethra and prostate; the 70- and 120-degree angles are used to inspect the bladder wall.

WHY IT IS DONE

Cystoscopes have both diagnostic and therapeutic uses. Diagnostic uses include inspection of the bladder cavity for calculi (stones), *bladder tumors*, and sites of bleeding and infection, as well as the obtaining of urine samples from each kidney individually to look for infection or tumor cells. In addition, by means of radiopaque dye injected into the ureters via the cystoscope, X rays can be taken to investigate the site of any obstruction to the flow of urine (see retrograde *pyelography*).

Many diseases of the urethra and bladder lend themselves to treatment via the cystoscope. Bladder tumors can be both biopsied and treated with diathermy or laser, calculi can be crushed or removed with basket forceps from the bladder or ureter, and stents (narrow tubes) can be inserted into the ureter to relieve any obstruction.

Cystostomy

The surgical creation of a hole in the bladder. A cystostomy is usually performed to drain urine when the introduction of a *catheter* (flexible tube) into the bladder via the urethra is inadvisable or impossible.

Cystourethrogram, voiding

An X-ray procedure for studying a person's bladder while he or she is urinating. The technique is most commonly used on young children who have had urinary infections to detect reflux of urine—that is, urine being forced back up the ureters (the tubes leading from the kidneys) as the bladder contracts. If severe, reflux leads to repeated infection, which can damage the kidneys.

-cyte

The suffix that denotes a cell. A *leukocyte* is a white blood cell; an *erythrocyte* is a red blood cell.

Cyto-

The prefix used to describe a relationship to a cell, as in cytomegalic, which means "giant cell."

Cytologist

A technician skilled in differentiating the appearance of normal from malignant cells.

Cytology

The study of individual cells, as distinct from *histology* (the study of groups of cells forming a tissue). The main application of cytology in medicine is to detect abnormal cells; it is thus used extensively to diagnose cancer. Cytology is becoming more important in *prenatal screening* for certain fetal abnormalities.

APPLICATIONS

The best known use of cytology is screening for cancer of the cervix, a procedure known as the *cervical smear test* (Pap test). A scraping of cells from the cervix and vagina is examined under a microscope; if they show precancerous changes, the woman's condition can be observed and she can be treated before cancer develops.

Cytology is also used to confirm (or exclude) the diagnosis of other cancers. Coughing up blood may be due to lung cancer, but a cytological examination of cells in a sample of sputum (phlegm) will help determine whether or not cancer actually is the cause. Similarly, cytology is valuable in detecting recurrent tumors in people who have already been treated for cancer. It is used particularly in cases of bladder cancer, in which tumors tend to recur after the original cancer has been successfully treated. Regular urinary cytology can detect any recurrent tumors at an early stage. Cytology may be helpful in determining the cause of conditions such as *pleural effusion* (fluid in the pleural cavity around the lungs) and *ascites* (fluid in the abdomen). Examination of cells in a sample of fluid usually indicates whether the condition is caused by cancer or an infection.

Fine needle aspiration *biopsy* of internal organs is growing as a method of diagnosis that utilizes cytology. A needle is guided to the organ (usually with the help of *ultrasound* or *CT scanning*) and a sample taken for examination. The procedure may eliminate the need for surgical biopsy or a major operation.

The other principal application of cytology is in various screening techniques for the early detection of fetal

---

PROCEDURE FOR CYSTOSCOPY

Cystoscopy allows inspection and treatment of the bladder using local anesthesia. There is no risk of damage to the genital organs or urinary tract, although the patient may feel some discomfort when passing urine for a few days afterward.

View through cystoscope

The cystoscope

Eyepiece ⌐ Viewing light and forceps

C

abnormalities such as Down's syndrome. The most widely used of these techniques is *amniocentesis*, in which a sample of the fluid that surrounds the fetus is removed and the cells in the fluid examined for abnormalities. *Chorionic villus sampling* is used earlier in the pregnancy. Usually, the cells must be cultured before a determination is made.

MODERN DEVELOPMENTS Various techniques are being developed to improve the ability to detect abnormal cells. Cells aspirated from various organs or tissues, as well as cells from cervical smears, can be studied further by the technique of *flow cytometry* (which uses a laser beam to scan cells and produce an image of the cells' DNA contents, thus differentiating between cells that are benign and those that are malignant).

The use of monoclonal antibodies—highly specific proteins that react with only one particular type of protein on the surface of a cell (see *Antibody, monoclonal*)—makes it easier to detect small numbers of abnormal cells in the midst of many normal ones, thereby improving the sensitivity of cytological tests for cancer. A refinement of this technique involves labeling the monoclonal antibodies with fluorescent stains, which makes them stand out against a dark background.

Other modern techniques have made it possible to detect abnormalities in *chromosomes* and even in individual *genes*. Such procedures have a potentially wide application for prenatal screening for congenital abnormalities, but many of them are still in the developmental stages and are not yet generally available.

Cytomegalovirus

One of the family of *herpes* viruses. It has the unique effect of causing the cells it infects to take on a characteristic enlarged appearance.

Infection with the cytomegalovirus (CMV) is extremely common. Approximately 80 percent of adults have *antibodies* to it in their blood (an indication of previous infection). In most cases, however, it produces no symptoms.

More serious CMV infections can occur in people with impaired immunity, such as the elderly and those with *AIDS*. A pregnant woman can transmit the virus to her unborn child; this could cause malformations and brain damage in the child.

Cytopathologist

A specialist in the microscopic appearances of cells in health and disease; also called a cellular pathologist. (See also *Cytology*.)

Cytotoxic drugs

A group of drugs that kills or damages cells; a type of *anticancer drug*. Cytotoxics primarily affect abnormal cells but they can damage or kill healthy cells, especially those that are multiplying rapidly. For example, they may affect noncancerous cells in bone marrow, causing anemia and increasing susceptibility to infection.

CYTOLOGY METHODS

Cells for cytological examination are obtained in several ways, depending on the part of the body being investigated. Recent improvements in imaging techniques have made it possible to collect cells from previously inaccessible sites. If the cytologist can make a definite diagnosis from a cell sample removed from a tumor using a very fine needle, the patient may be spared an exploratory operation.

Cells from the cervix
These are scraped away with a spatula.

Cells from the respiratory tract, esophagus, or stomach
These are usually obtained by using an *endoscope* and small brush or suction tube.

Cells from body fluids
These are obtained either by passing the fluid through a filter or by centrifugation.

Aspiration biopsy
A very fine needle can be accurately passed into a suspected tumor and a biopsy sample of cells removed.

EXAMINATION UNDER THE MICROSCOPE

The cells are smeared on a microscope slide and stained with dyes. The cytologist then examines them, looking for abnormalities of size or shape in the cells or their nuclei. The smears are then graded—as normal, as displaying abnormalities, or as showing malignant cells.

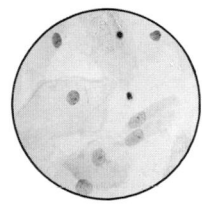

Normal cells in cervical smear

Smear showing abnormal cells

Smear showing malignant cells

Dacryocystitis

Inflammation of the tear sac, which lies between the inside corner of the eyelids and the nose.

CAUSES

The inflammation usually results from blockage of the duct, which carries the tears from the tear sac to the nose. Inflammation may be followed by bacterial infection of fluid trapped in the tear sac. In infants, the tear duct may fail to develop an opening. In adults, the cause of the duct blockage is usually unknown. Rarely, it follows an injury; more often, it follows inflammation in the nasal region.

Mechanism of dacryocystitis
Inflammation of the tear sac occurs when the duct that carries tears from the tear sac becomes blocked.

SYMPTOMS

Usually only one eye is affected. There may be pain, redness, and swelling in the area between the inner corner of the eyelids and nose. Occasionally, pus discharges from the inner canthus (corner). Prior to infection in the tear sac, the only symptom may be a watery eye and tearing due to obstruction of the duct.

TREATMENT

Irrigation can sometimes clear the obstruction. A *cannula* (fine tube) is introduced into one of the drainage openings into the tear duct and saline flushed through it. Antibiotic drops or ointment are prescribed to treat infection. In infants, massage of the tear sac can empty the sac and sometimes clear a blockage.

If irrigation and antibiotics fail to clear up the symptoms, a dacryocystorhinostomy (surgery to drain the tear sac into the nose) can be performed. In the infirm elderly, if recurrent infection is the main problem, the tear sac may be removed.

Danazol

ANDROGEN HORMONE	
Capsule	
Prescription needed	
Not available as generic	

An antiestrogenic drug used in the treatment of *endometriosis* (a condition in which fragments of the lining of the uterus occur elsewhere in the pelvic cavity), fibrocystic breast disease (breast tenderness and lumpiness that worsen before menstruation), and *menorrhagia* (heavy periods).

HOW IT WORKS

Danazol suppresses the release of *gonadotropin hormones* (pituitary hormones that stimulate activity in the ovaries and testes). This reduces the production and release of estrogen from the ovaries. The change in hormone levels usually prevents ovulation, which results in irregularity or absence of menstruation.

Danazol is usually administered in courses lasting a few months. The disorder may recur once treatment has been discontinued.

POSSIBLE ADVERSE EFFECTS

Side effects may include nausea, dizziness, rash, back pain, weight gain, and flushing. Pregnancy should be avoided while taking (and shortly after taking) danazol because the drug can cause masculine characteristics in a female fetus.

D and C

A gynecological procedure in which the endometrium (lining of the uterus) laid down after each menstrual period is scraped away. Short for dilatation and curettage, D and C is commonly used in the diagnosis and treatment of *menorrhagia* (heavy menstrual bleed-

ing) and other disorders of the *uterus*. It is also used as a means of terminating a pregnancy (see *Abortion, elective*) and may sometimes be carried out following a *miscarriage*.

HOW IT IS DONE

D and C is usually carried out under general anesthesia. The cervix is dilated (stretched open) so that a *curet* (a spoon-shaped surgical instrument) can be inserted into the uterus to scrape away the endometrium. The scrapings may then be examined under the microscope to assess the condition of the uterus.

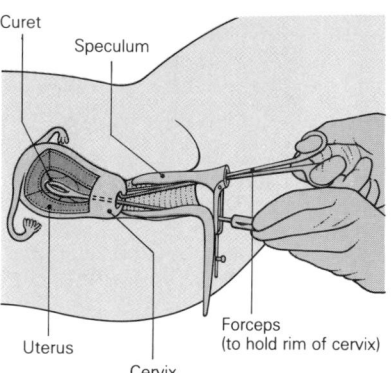

Procedure for D and C
The vagina is dilated with a speculum, the cervix is dilated, and a curet is inserted into the uterus to scrape away the endometrium.

RESULTS

Removal of the endometrium causes no side effects and it may be beneficial if the lining has thickened, causing heavy periods. The endometrium soon grows again normally as part of the menstrual cycle (see *Menstruation*).

Dander

 Minute scales shed from an animal's skin, hair, or feathers. Both humans and pets produce such scales, which float in the air or settle on a surface, making up a large proportion of household dust. Human *dandruff* is a type of dander, except that the scales produced by the scalp are relatively large and easily visible.

Some people are allergic to animal dander and develop the symptoms of allergic *rhinitis* (hay fever) or *asthma* if they breathe in the scales.

Dandruff

A common, harmless, but irritating condition in which dead skin is shed from the scalp, often producing unsightly white flakes in the hair and on the collar and shoulders of clothes.

The usual cause of the condition is seborrheic *dermatitis*, an itchy, scaly rash on the scalp, which may also occur on the face, chest, and back.

TREATMENT
Shampoo frequently with an anti-dandruff shampoo. If this fails, a physician may prescribe a *corticosteroid* cream or lotion to apply to the scalp or an *antifungal* cream (even though dandruff is not a fungal infection), which sometimes helps. Whatever the treatment, dandruff usually requires constant control.

Dantrolene

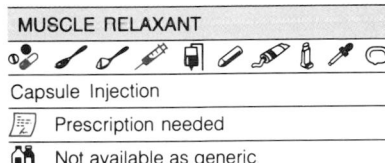

MUSCLE RELAXANT	
Capsule Injection	
📄 Prescription needed	
🔒 Not available as generic	

Used to relieve muscle spasm caused by *spinal injury, stroke,* or neurological disorders such as *cerebral palsy* or *multiple sclerosis*. It does not cure the underlying disorder, but often leads to a gradual improvement in mobility. Dantrolene is occasionally used to treat abnormal urine retention (see *Urine retention*).

POSSIBLE ADVERSE EFFECTS
Dantrolene acts predominantly on the muscles rather than the nervous system; consequently, it causes less sedation than many other muscle-relaxant drugs. Alcohol should be avoided during treatment, however, because it increases the sedative effect. Dantrolene may cause diarrhea, muscle weakness, and, rarely, kidney damage. In rare cases, dantrolene may also cause a skin rash on exposure to sunlight. Exposure to sun should therefore be avoided during treatment.

Dapsone

An antibiotic used in the treatment of *leprosy* and *dermatitis herpetiformis*, a rare skin condition.

POSSIBLE ADVERSE EFFECTS
Dapsone may cause nausea, vomiting, and, rarely, damage to the liver, red blood cells, and nerves. During long-term treatment, blood tests are carried out regularly to monitor liver function and the number of red cells in the blood.

Daydreaming

Conjuring up pleasant or exciting images or situations in one's mind during waking hours. Everyone daydreams to some extent, but it may be more common during unhappy or stressful periods in a person's life.

Children and teenagers may spend a considerable amount of time daydreaming. In general, this is not a cause for concern unless schoolwork and relationships suffer, at which time professional help may be needed.

DDT

The generally used abbreviation for the insecticide dichloro-diphenyl-trichloro-ethane. Developed in Switzerland in the early 1940s, DDT was much more effective than previous insecticides and it became an important weapon against insect-transmitted diseases, particularly in hot climates. A disadvantage of DDT is that some insects have adapted genetically to it so that their offspring become resistant to its toxic effects. (See also *Pesticides*.)

Deafness

Complete or partial inability to hear. Total deafness is rare and is usually congenital (present from birth). Partial deafness, ranging from mild to severe, is most commonly the result of an ear disease, injury, or degeneration of the hearing mechanism with age.

All deafness is either conductive or sensorineural. Conductive deafness is faulty transportation of sound from the outer to the inner ear, usually due to damage to the eardrum or the three connected bones in the middle ear— the malleus, incus, and stapes. In sensorineural deafness, sounds that reach the inner ear fail to be transmitted to the brain because of damage to the structures within the inner ear or to the acoustic nerve, which connects the inner ear to the brain.

CAUSES
CONDUCTIVE DEAFNESS In an adult, the most common cause of conductive deafness is *earwax* blocking the outer ear canal. Less commonly, *otosclerosis* (in which the stapes loses its normal mobility) may be responsible. In a child, *otitis media* (middle-ear infection) with effusion (a collection of fluid in the middle ear that is often sticky like glue) is by far the most common cause of this type of deafness.

Rarely, conductive deafness can be caused by *barotrauma* (damage to the eardrum or middle ear due to sudden pressure changes in an aircraft or under water) or by a perforated eardrum (see *Eardrum, perforated*) as the result of injury, a middle-ear infection, or surgery on the ear.

SENSORINEURAL DEAFNESS Defects of the inner ear are sometimes congenital, due to an inherited fault in a chromosome, to *birth injury*, or to damage to the developing fetus—for example, as the result of the mother having had *rubella* (German measles) during pregnancy. Damage to the inner ear may also occur soon after birth as the result of severe *jaundice*.

Sensorineural deafness that develops in later life can be caused by prolonged exposure to loud noise, by *Meniere's disease* (increased fluid pressure in the labyrinth), by certain drugs (such as streptomycin), or by some viral infections. All damage to the cochlea and/or labyrinth. These structures also degenerate naturally with old age (*presbycusis*).

Damage to the acoustic nerve may be the result of an *acoustic neuroma* (a benign tumor on the nerve). As the acoustic neuroma enlarges, it causes increasing deafness.

INCIDENCE
Deafness at birth—which is sensorineural and incurable—is rare, occurring in only one in 1,000 babies. But deafness that develops in young children—usually conductive and curable—is common. As many as one fourth of the 5 year olds starting school have some degree of hearing loss as the result of previous middle-ear infections.

The hearing mechanism gradually degenerates with age, and about one fourth of the population over 65 need a hearing aid.

SYMPTOMS, SIGNS, AND DIAGNOSIS
A baby suffering from congenital deafness fails to respond to sounds, and, although crying is often normal, he or she does not babble or make the other baby noises that precede speech. This condition is usually first noticed by a parent, but the deafness is almost always diagnosed during one of the child's regular visits to a pediatrician.

Routine *hearing tests* are performed on children to detect any hearing loss, which is usually due to otitis media with effusion.

In an adult who has started to become deaf, sounds heard are not only quieter than before but are also distorted and less clear, high tones are less audible than low ones, the sounds "s," "f," and "z" are not heard, and speech may be difficult to understand if there is background noise. Deafness in one ear may be noticed only when that ear alone is used (for example, when the sufferer uses the affected ear when on the telephone).

D

Earwax | Perforated eardrum | Meniere's disease | Drug toxicity | Acoustic neuroma | Occupational deafness | Otosclerosis | Barotrauma | Middle-ear effusion

Some possible causes of deafness
The affected part is shown in each case.
Some problems (e.g., earwax) cause conductive deafness; others (e.g., drug toxicity) cause sensorineural deafness.

Deafness may be accompanied by *tinnitus* (noises in the ear) and *vertigo* (dizziness and loss of balance). It sometimes causes confusion, *paranoia*, and auditory *hallucinations*, and can lead to withdrawal and depression.

Examination of the ear with an *otoscope* (a viewing instrument with a light attached) can show if the outer ear canal is obstructed by wax or if the eardrum is inflamed or there is fluid behind it. To determine whether deafness is conductive or sensorineural, hearing tests are used.

TREATMENT
Children born deaf need special instruction if they are to learn to speak. The process is a long and

difficult one, but eventually many children can communicate effectively, often with sign language.

Conductive deafness in children due to otitis media with effusion is treated by an operation to drain the fluid from the middle ear through a hole in the eardrum (see *Myringotomy*). While awaiting surgery the child should sit at the front of the classroom to hear as much as possible.

When conductive deafness is caused by wax in the ear, the wax is removed by syringing the ear with warm water.

A perforated eardrum is usually allowed to heal of its own accord, but, if it has not done so after two or three

months, a surgical repair, called *tympanoplasty*, is often carried out.

Conductive deafness due to otosclerosis is usually treated by *stapedectomy*, an operation in which the overgrown stapes is replaced with an artificial substitute.

Hearing aids are sometimes used to lessen deafness caused by otosclerosis, in which case the hearing aid takes the form of a bone-conducting device that transmits sound to the inner ear through a vibrating pad touching the bone behind the ear. The main use of hearing aids, however, is in treating sensorineural deafness, which cannot be cured because the structures of the inner ear are too delicate to allow surgery to be performed on them. These hearing aids increase the volume of sound reaching the inner ear by means of an amplifier and an earphone that fits into the outer ear.

A new development in the treatment of sensorineural deafness is the *cochlear implant*, in which electrodes that can receive sound signals are implanted in the inner ear. The single channel device has been replaced by one with multiple channels. Up to now, however, it has achieved only limited success.

Lipreading is an invaluable aid for all deaf people, whatever the type and severity of their deafness. People addressing a deaf person should remember to face him or her and not shout, which only distorts sounds.

Various household aids, such as an amplifier for the earpiece of a telephone, are available.

Death

Permanent cessation of all vital functions; the end of life. The classic indicators of death are the permanent cessation of the function of the heart and lungs; in most cases these remain the criteria by which a physician diagnoses and certifies death.

During the 1960s, however, medical technology advanced to allow the artificial (machine-assisted) maintenance of breathing and heart beat in cases where the lungs and heart would otherwise have stopped due to gross structural brain damage. This prompted a reexamination of the concepts of death and, in the late 1970s, state legislatures, at the urging of the medical profession, began recognizing an alternative criterion of death. This alternative is *brain death*, defined as the irreversible cessation of all func-

tions of the entire brain, including the brain stem.

An individual can thus now be certified legally dead if there is either irreversible cessation of circulatory and respiratory functions or if the criteria for brain death are satisfied.

DIAGNOSIS OF DEATH
The determination of death is considered a medical diagnosis. Physicians are expected to exercise their medical judgment within a defined legal framework.

The diagnosis of death under normal circumstances, when the individual is not on a *ventilator* (breathing machine), is based on absence of spontaneous breathing, absence of heart beat, and on the pupils being dilated and unresponsive to light.

The legal criteria for diagnosing brain death are based on the deter-

mination of the irreversible cessation of brain function. The guidelines state there must be clear evidence of irreversible damage to the brain; persistent deep coma; no attempts at breathing when the patient is taken off the ventilator; and absence of brainstem function (such as the response of the pupils to light, grimacing in response to pain, and the involuntary blink when the surface of the eye is touched). The guidelines warn that this assessment might not be reliable if the patient is intoxicated, has an extremely low body temperature, or is in shock.

An *EEG* showing absence of electrical activity in the brain's cerebrum is not required, but sometimes provides useful confirmatory evidence of brain death diagnosed by the above criteria. (See also *Mortality*.)

SUDDEN DEATH

In infants (mainly up to 1 year of age), death that occurs without warning is called *sudden infant death syndrome* (SIDS) or crib death. The causes of SIDS are unknown, although there are several theories.

In adults, common causes of sudden death include injury, *myocardial infarction* (heart attack), *brain hemorrhage*, and *pneumonia*. Less common causes include *anaphylactic shock*, *asthma*, and *suicide*.

Cases of sudden death must be reported to the coroner or medical examiner, who decides if a postmortem examination (see *Autopsy*) should be performed.

Debility

Generalized weakness and lack of ambition and energy. Debility may be caused by a physical disorder (such as *anemia*) or a psychological disorder (such as *depression*).

Debridement

Surgical removal of foreign material and/or dead, damaged, or infected tissue from a wound or burn to expose healthy tissue. Such treatment promotes healthy healing of badly damaged skin, muscle, bone, and other tissue.

Decalcification, dental

The dissolving of minerals in a tooth. The first stage of decay, it is caused by the bacteria in *plaque* acting on refined carbohydrates (mainly sugar) in food to produce acid. After prolonged or numerous exposures, the acid causes changes on the surface of the tooth. The decalcified area can be seen as a chalky white patch when the plaque is brushed away. At this stage, the process is partly reversible if a mineralizing solution is applied.

If the decalcification penetrates the enamel, it spreads along the junction between the enamel and dentin, and then into the dentin. Lack of professional treatment at this point will permit bacteria to enter the pulp. Further destruction of dentin will then be caused by bacterial enzymes, and the pulp, once infected, may die. (See also *Caries, dental*.)

Decay, dental

See *Caries, dental*.

Decerebrate

The state of being without a functioning *cerebrum* (the cerebral hemispheres and associated structures), which is the main controlling part of the brain. This situation occurs when the *brain stem* (the upward extension of the spinal cord) is severed, which effectively isolates the cerebrum.

Deciduous teeth

See *Primary teeth*.

Decompression sickness

A hazard of scuba divers, also known as the "bends" and formerly known as caisson disease. Decompression sickness results from the formation of gas bubbles in the diver's tissues during ascent from depth.

CAUSES AND INCIDENCE

The amount of gas that can be held dissolved in a tissue (such as blood or body fat) increases with pressure (such as at great depth underwater) and decreases when the pressure is released. At depth, divers accumulate large quantities of inert gas in their tissues from the high-pressure gas mixture they breathe (see *Scuba-diving medicine*); if air is being breathed (as is usual for amateur divers), the main inert gas is nitrogen.

When the diver ascends, pressure falls and the gas can no longer be held within the tissues; if the pressure reduction is rapid, the gas may form bubbles—just as bubbles form in a bottle of beer when the cap is flipped off. The bubbles may block blood vessels, causing various symptoms.

Trained divers avoid problems by allowing the excess gas built up in their tissues to escape slowly via their blood into their lungs during controlled, very slow ascent.

SYMPTOMS

Symptoms may appear any time within 24 hours after a dive. Common symptoms include skin itching and mottling, and severe pains in and around the larger joints, particularly the shoulders and knees. Symptoms of nervous system impairment (such as leg weakness, visual disturbances, or problems with balance) are particularly serious, as is a painful, tight feeling across the chest, which may indicate the presence of bubbles in the vessels feeding the heart and in the circulation to the lungs.

TREATMENT

Any diver with the symptoms described should be transported immediately to a decompression chamber. Pressure within the chamber is raised by pumping in air; this causes the bubbles within the diver's tissues to redissolve, and symptoms to disappear. Subsequently, the

Pressure increased (descent)

Inert gas dissolved in tissue fluids and blood

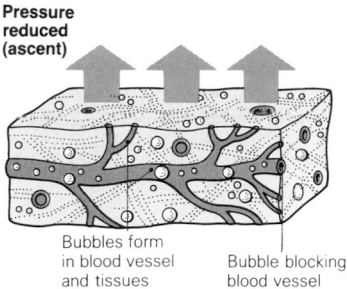

Pressure reduced (ascent)

Bubbles form in blood vessel and tissues

Bubble blocking blood vessel

How decompression occurs
On ascent, pressure is reduced rapidly and the gas may form bubbles that may, in turn, cause symptoms. Divers avoid this by ascending slowly.

pressure is slowly reduced, allowing the excess gas to escape safely via the blood and lungs.

OUTLOOK

If treated promptly by decompression, most divers with the bends make a full recovery. However, in serious, untreated cases, there may be long-term complications such as partial paralysis. Repeated episodes lead to degenerative disorders of the bones and joints.

Decompression, spinal canal

A surgical procedure to relieve pressure on the spinal cord or on a nerve root emerging from the cord.

WHY IT IS DONE

Pressure on the spinal cord may be due to a *disk prolapse*, to a tumor (in most cases benign) of the membranes surrounding the cord or of the cord itself, to a narrow spinal canal (spinal *stenosis*), which may be present from birth or caused by *osteoarthritis*, or to fracture of the vertebrae after an accident. Any of these conditions can cause weakness or paralysis of the limbs and also loss of bladder and bowel control.

HOW IT IS DONE

To treat major disk prolapses and tumors, a *laminectomy* (removal of the bony arches of one or more vertebrae) to expose the affected part of the cord or nerve roots must be performed.

D

Severely prolapsed disks are cut away and affected nerve roots are freed from surrounding tissues.

It is sometimes preferable to treat compressive conditions by using an anterior approach in which the spinal column is entered from the front.

When pressure is being caused by a tumor or abscess in a vertebra, the affected section of bone is removed. If a large portion of bone is removed, bone grafting is carried out at the end of the operation.

RECOVERY PERIOD
Confinement to bed in a flat position is necessary initially, with measures taken to prevent bedsores and physical therapy given to keep the leg muscles strong. Usually a patient can get up within a few days. Heavy lifting and carrying must be avoided for several weeks.

OUTLOOK
Recovery of movement, sensation, and bladder control, and achievement of pain relief after treatment, depend on the severity and duration of the pressure before the operation, the success of the surgery in relieving the pressure, and whether damage was sustained by the cord and nerves during the operation.

Decongestant drugs

COMMON DRUGS

Ephedrine Oxymetazoline
Phenylpropanolamine Pseudoephedrine
Xylometazoline

> **WARNING**
> Symptoms worsen when, after several days of treatment, decongestants are suddenly withdrawn. Use only in low doses for a short time.

Drugs used to relieve nasal congestion. Small amounts of these drugs are present in many over-the-counter cold remedies, which are available in tablet or nose-drop form. Decongestant drugs are commonly used in the treatment of upper *respiratory tract infections*, especially in patients susceptible to *otitis media* (middle-ear infection) or *sinusitis* (sinus infection).

POSSIBLE ADVERSE EFFECTS
Taken by mouth, decongestant drugs may cause tremor and palpitations; they are therefore not usually prescribed if a person has heart disease. In the form of nose drops, only small amounts are absorbed into the bloodstream and adverse effects are unlikely.

THE ACTION OF DECONGESTANTS
Decongestants work by narrowing blood vessels in the membranes that line the nose. This action reduces swelling, inflammation, and the amount of mucus produced by the nasal lining.

Congested nasal lining
When blood vessels enlarge in response to infection or irritation, increased amounts of fluid pass into the lining, which swells and produces more mucus.

Effect of decongestants
Chemicals stimulate constriction of the blood vessels in the nasal lining, which reduces swelling, mucus production, and nasal congestion.

If decongestant nose drops are taken for several days and then stopped, congestion frequently recurs ("rebounds") and may be worse than that for which the drug was taken. For this reason, decongestants should be taken for as short a time as possible.

Deductible
A provision in many health insurance policies that makes the patient responsible for a certain dollar amount of medical charges before the benefits of the insurance policy begin to apply. (See also *Coinsurance*.)

Defecation
The expulsion of feces from the body via the anus.

Defense mechanisms
Techniques used by the mind as a means of coping with unpleasant or unwelcome events, experiences, impulses, or emotions.

For example, death of a relative normally provokes grief and/or anger. One defense against these emotions may be repression—refusal to recognize these feelings and appearing to be unaffected by the event. Another reaction is denial—carrying on as though the relative is still alive.

A person who feels guilty about hating his or her father may transfer this hate to another person or turn the bad feelings toward himself or herself.

Disturbing impulses may take the opposite form in conscious thought. For instance, a person with strong sexual feelings may be excessively prudish or inhibited.

The body's defense mechanisms against infection are described under *immune system*.

Defensive medicine
The practice of ordering medical tests or procedures primarily to protect against any charge of malpractice.

Defibrillation
A technique in which a brief electric shock is administered to the heart, usually via two metal plates placed on the wall of the chest. Also called cardioversion, defibrillation is performed to treat some types of *arrhythmia* (irregular or rapid heart beat). The sudden burst of electricity through the heart converts *fibrillation* (rapid, uncoordinated heart beat) or *tachycardia* (rapid heart beat) back into a normal, regular heart beat. Occasionally a drug, such as lidocaine, is injected into a vein before the procedure to try to stabilize the heart rhythm.

Defibrillation can be carried out as an emergency procedure to treat *ventricular fibrillation*, which most commonly starts after a *myocardial infarction* (heart attack). It may also be used to treat an arrhythmia that has lasted several hours or days.

Defoliant poisoning

Defoliants are applied to plants to cause their leaves to drop off and the plants to die. Commonly used as weedkillers, defoliants are poisonous if swallowed. They should therefore always be kept in clearly labeled containers and stored out of the reach of children. The most widely used defoliant weedkillers are sodium chlorate, potassium chlorate (see *Chlorate poisoning*), and *paraquat*.

Another familiar defoliant is dioxin, which was used by US forces in Vietnam and has also occasionally been released into the atmosphere as a result of industrial accidents. Allegations have been made that this toxic substance caused nerve and other disorders in many Vietnam veterans and in others who have been exposed to it (as well as causing birth defects in their children). There is no convincing scientific evidence to support these allegations.

Deformity

Any malformation or distortion of part of the body. Deformities may be *congenital* (present at birth) or they may be acquired as a result of injury, disease, disorder, or disuse.

Most congenital deformities are relatively rare. Among the more common are clubfoot (*talipes*) and *cleft lip and palate*. The last two may occur separately or together.

Injuries that can cause deformity include burns, torn muscles, broken bones, and dislocated joints. Among the various diseases and disorders that may cause deformity are infections (such as *tuberculosis* and *leprosy*), damage to or disorders of nerves (such as paralysis of the facial nerves), some deficiency diseases (such as *rickets*), and a condition of unknown cause called *Paget's disease* of the bone. Disuse of a part of the body—as a result of being bedridden or confined to a wheelchair, for example—can lead to deformity through stiffening and *contracture* (shortening) of unused muscles or tendons.

Many deformities can be corrected by *reconstructive surgery*, various orthopedic techniques (including surgery), exercise, or by a combination of these methods. For example, cleft lip and cleft palate are now routinely treated during childhood by reconstructive surgery, with good results in most cases.

It is often possible to prevent the development of a deformity due to disuse by regular exercise.

Degeneration

Physical and/or chemical changes in cells, tissues, or organs that reduce their efficiency. Its true cause is unknown, but may be due to a disease process; degeneration is also a feature of aging. Other known causes include injury, reduced blood supply, poisoning (by alcohol, for example), or a diet deficient in a specific vitamin. (See also *Degenerative disorders*.)

Degenerative disorders

A blanket term covering a wide range of conditions in which there is progressive impairment of both the structure and function of part of the body. This definition excludes diseases caused by infection, inflammation, altered immune responses, chemical or physical damage, or malignant change. Many of the features of aging, such as wrinkling of the skin, are due to degenerative changes in body tissues, but, in degenerative disorders, the changes come on earlier in life, are more rapid, and typically affect some organs and not others.

Microscopic examination of an organ affected by degenerative disease often shows that the number of specialized cells or structures is reduced and that their place has been taken by connective or scar tissue.

Some diseases that were once thought to be degenerative disorders later proved to be due to slow viruses (such as *Creutzfeldt-Jakob syndrome*). Other degenerative disorders, such as *Parkinsonism*, may be traceable to poisoning—with carbon monoxide or with MPTP, an impurity formed during the illegal manufacture of one of the many *designer drugs*. Future research may identify specific infective or environmental causes for other degenerative disorders that are at present thought to be degenerative.

NERVOUS SYSTEM

Among degenerative disorders affecting the nervous system the most common is *Alzheimer's disease*, the main cause of presenile and senile dementia. In *Huntington's chorea*, dementia is combined with disorders of movement. Susceptibility to the degenerative changes in the brain is due to an abnormality in a single gene; the disease is transmitted from one generation to the next in a dominant pattern of inheritance (see *Genetic disorders*). In *Parkinson's disease* and in degenerative disorders that affect the *cerebellum*, abnormalities of movement are the main features. In *motor neuron diseases*, such as *Werdnig-Hoffmann*

disease and other diseases in their infantile forms, the prime symptom is muscular weakness.

EYES

Blindness in early adult life can be caused by a condition called Leber's *optic atrophy*, which is due to loss of nerve cells in the retina. *Retinitis pigmentosa*, another retinal degeneration, can cause blindness in childhood, but some vision may be preserved until late middle age. Both disorders have a genetic basis. By contrast, senile *macular degeneration* is not an inherited condition and rarely develops before the seventh decade.

JOINTS

The most familiar degenerative disorder is *osteoarthritis*, sometimes known as degenerative joint disease. Susceptibility to the condition seems to run in families; it also develops in sports enthusiasts and manual workers who have repeatedly damaged their joints. The prime features of osteoarthritis are thinning and destruction of the cartilage covering the surfaces of the joints and overgrowth and distortion of the bone around affected joints.

ARTERIES

Some hardening of the arteries seems to be a feature of aging. In some individuals, however, the degenerative changes in the muscle coat of these blood vessels are unusually severe and calcium deposits may be seen on X-ray films (as in Monckeberg's sclerosis, a type of *arteriosclerosis*).

MUSCLES

The *muscular dystrophies* are a group of genetic disorders that cause distinctive patterns of muscular weakness, sometimes associated with increased muscle bulk. *Myopathies*, by contrast, are muscle disorders for which an external cause, such as a chemical toxin, can usually be identified. Myopathies are not classed as degenerative disorders.

Deglutition

The medical term for *swallowing*.

Dehiscence

The splitting open of a partly healed wound, most commonly the splitting open of a surgical incision that has been closed with sutures or clips.

Dehydration

A condition in which a person's water content has fallen to a dangerously low level. Water accounts for about 60 percent of a man's weight and 50 percent of a woman's, and the total water

D

D

content must be kept within fairly narrow limits for healthy functioning of cells and tissues (see *Water*).

The concentration in the body's fluids of mineral salts and other dissolved substances also must be kept within a narrow range. In many cases of dehydration, salt will have been lost as well as water.

CAUSES

Normally, dehydration is prevented by the sensation of thirst, which encourages a person to drink when the body is short of water. This mechanism may fail because water is not available or because of high losses of water from the body.

Even in a temperate climate, a minimum of three pints of water continues to be lost every 24 hours through the skin via perspiration, from the lungs into the air, and in the urine to rid the body of waste products. Severe dehydration is likely to develop within a few days if no water is taken. Large amounts of water may be lost in vomit or diarrhea, particularly if the diarrhea is profuse and watery (as in *cholera*) or in the urine of anyone with uncontrolled *diabetes mellitus*, *diabetes insipidus*, and some types of *renal failure*. In all these cases, the thirst sensation may not encourage sufficient water intake to balance the losses.

SYMPTOMS AND SIGNS

Symptoms and signs of water depletion include severe thirst, dry lips and tongue, an increase in heart rate and breathing, dizziness, confusion, and eventual coma. The skin looks dry and loses its elasticity. Any urine passed is small in quantity and dark-colored. If there is salt depletion (usually as a result of heavy sweating, vomiting, or diarrhea), there may be lethargy, headaches, cramps, and pallor.

PREVENTION

When living in a hot climate, or when suffering from a fever, vomiting, or diarrhea, the simplest rule is to drink enough water to produce urine that is consistently pale. This often means drinking well beyond the point of thirst (possibly a pint of water every hour during the heat of the day).

Salt losses from heavy sweating need to be replaced either in the diet or by adding a quarter of a teaspoon of table salt to each pint of drinking water. Bottled mineral water can help maintain the intake of salts. For vomiting and diarrhea, special salt and glucose rehydration mixtures for adding to water may be purchased from drugstores.

TREATMENT

Once dehydration has developed, fluid and salt replacement may be required at a far faster rate than that required to simply prevent dehydration. Sometimes, fluids must be given intravenously and the water/salt balance requires careful monitoring with blood tests and adjustment.

Déjà vu

French for "already seen." A sense of having already experienced an event that is happening at the moment. Déjà vu is a common phenomenon that has never been properly explained. Some people believe that it is due to an unconscious emotional response caused by similarities between the current event and some past experience. Others believe that a neurological "short circuit" results in the experience registering in the memory before reaching consciousness. Frequent occurrence of déjà vu may sometimes be a symptom of temporal lobe *epilepsy*.

Delinquency

Behavior in a juvenile that in an adult would be considered a crime. The term is often extended to include noncriminal behavior, such as being truant, running away from home, drinking alcohol, or using drugs.

Juvenile delinquency is probably caused by a combination of factors—social, psychological, and biological—but relatively few offenders suffer from a definite mental disorder or mental retardation.

Child guidance or *family therapy* may be recommended for delinquents and their families. Persistent offenders are sometimes sent to special schools and may be taken into care or made wards of the court.

Delirium

A state of acute mental confusion, commonly brought on by physical illness. The symptoms are those of disordered brain function, and vary according to personality, environment, and the severity of illness. Failure to understand events or remember what has been happening, increased anxiety, physical restlessness, and sudden swings of mood occur as delirium worsens. At its most severe, the patient may hallucinate, suffer from *illusions* (for example, seeing nurses as threatening monsters), lapse into terrified panic, and resort to shouting and violence. Usually the symptoms are worse at night, because of sleep disturbance and the fact that darkness and quiet make visual illusions more likely.

CAUSES

While any severe illness may underlie this state, high fever and disturbances of body chemistry are often present. Children and older people are most liable, particularly after major surgery or when there is a preexisting brain disturbance such as *dementia*. Drugs, various poisons, and alcohol are common precipitants.

TREATMENT

Treatment is of the underlying physical disorder, with appropriate nursing management to reduce anxiety. Suitable lighting, calm and clear communication, appropriate seclusion, and known, trusted attendants are all important. Particular attention must be paid to fluids and nutrition, but tranquilizers (e.g., chlorpromazine, haloperidol, or thioridazine) are often necessary for sedation of the physical restlessness. The control of infection by antibiotics has probably made this condition much rarer than it was 50 years ago.

Delirium tremens

A state of confusion accompanied by trembling and vivid *hallucinations*. It usually arises in chronic alcoholics after withdrawal or abstinence from alcohol, and often occurs following admission to the hospital with an injury or for a surgical operation.

SYMPTOMS, SIGNS, AND TREATMENT

In the early stages, symptoms include restlessness, agitation, trembling, and sleeplessness. Overactivity of sympathetic nerve pathways causes a rapid heart beat, fever, dilation (widening) of the pupils, and profuse sweating that may lead to dehydration. Confusion follows with visual and sometimes auditory hallucinations, and the patient appears terrified. Convulsions may also occur.

The symptoms usually subside within three days. Treatment consists of rest, rehydration, and sedation in a hospital. Sedative drugs used include chlorpromazine or chlordiazepoxide. Injections of vitamins, particularly thiamine (vitamin B), may be given, since some of the features of delirium tremens seem to be linked with thiamine deficiency (see *Wernicke-Korsakoff syndrome*).

Delivery

Expulsion or extraction of a baby from the mother's uterus. In most cases the baby lies lengthwise in the uterus with its head facing downward and is delivered head first through the vaginal opening by a combination of uterine contractions and maternal effort at the end of the second stage of labor (see *Childbirth*).

If the baby is lying in an abnormal position (see *Breech delivery; Malpresentation*), if uterine contractions are weak, or if there is disproportion between the size of the baby's head and the mother's pelvis, a *forceps delivery* or *vacuum extraction* may be required; these are called operative deliveries. In some cases, vaginal delivery is impossible or potentially dangerous to the mother or the baby, and *cesarean section* is necessary.

Deltoid

The triangular muscle of the shoulder region that forms the rounded flesh of the outer part of the upper arm, and passes up and over the shoulder joint. The wide end of the muscle is attached to the scapula (shoulder blade) and clavicle (collarbone). The muscle fibers converge to form the apex of the triangle, which is attached to the humerus (upper-arm bone) about halfway down its length.

The central, strongest part of the muscle raises the arm sideways. The front and back parts of the muscle twist the arm.

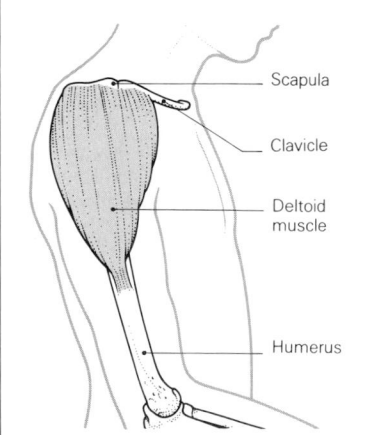

LOCATION OF THE DELTOID
Muscle of the shoulder region, forming the rounded, outer part of the upper arm, and attached to the scapula and clavicle.

Scapula

Clavicle

Deltoid muscle

Humerus

Delusion

A fixed, irrational idea not shared by others and not responding to reasoned argument. The central idea

in a paranoid delusion involves persecution or jealousy. For instance, a person may believe that he or she is being poisoned or that a partner is persistently unfaithful (see *Paranoia*). A person suffering from delusions of grandeur believes, for example, that he or she is related to royalty.

Persistent delusions are a sign of serious mental illness, notably *schizophrenia* and *dementia*. (See also *Hallucination; Illusion*.)

Dementia

A general decline in all areas of mental ability. Dementia is usually due to brain disease and is progressive, the most obvious feature being increasing intellectual impairment.

INCIDENCE
Dementia is the great health problem of modern developed societies, since long life is creating an increasing proportion of elderly citizens. Some 10 percent of those over 65 years and 20 percent of those over 75 years are affected to some degree by dementia.

CAUSES
Traditionally, dementing illnesses were divided into presenile (under 65 years of age at onset) and senile (over 65 years). This is now regarded as an artificial division, although treatable causes are more common in the younger age group. Causes include head injury, pernicious anemia, encephalitis, myxedema, syphilis, brain tumor, and alcoholism.

Such "reversible" illnesses account only for some 10 percent of dementias. The great majority of them result from *cerebrovascular disease* (including *strokes*) and from *Alzheimer's disease*. While the former can sometimes be helped by treatment of *hypertension* (high blood pressure) or heart disease, the recurrent loss of blood supply to the brain is often due to narrowed or blocked arteries within the brain, and a gradual deterioration occurs. Alzheimer's disease is at present completely irreversible, consisting as it does of gradual loss of brain cells and shrinkage of the brain substance.

SYMPTOMS
The person with dementia may not remember recent events, may become easily lost in a familiar neighborhood, may fail to grasp what is going on, and may become confused over days and dates. These symptoms tend to come on gradually and may not be noticed right away. People also tend to cover up their problems by *confabulation* (making up stories to fill the gaps in their memories). Sudden emotional

outbursts or embarrassing behavior (such as urinating in public) may be the first obvious signs of the illness.

Commonly the person's failures in judgment result in the magnification of his or her unpleasant personality traits; families may have to endure unreasonable demands, accusations, pilfering, and even physical assault. Paranoid and depressive illnesses (see *Paranoia; Depression*) with psychotic *delusions* may occur as dementia worsens. Irritability or anxiety, with the patient retaining some awareness of his or her emotional state, alters to a shallow indifference toward all feelings. Personal habits deteriorate, clothes and possessions become soiled and dirty, and speech becomes incoherent. Demented individuals lapse into "second childhood" and require total nursing care of their feeding, toilet, and physical activities.

TREATMENT
While appropriate treatment of certain illnesses is effective in arresting decline (such as surgery for a brain tumor or thyroid replacement for myxedema), management of the most common, Alzheimer-type illness is based mostly on the treatment of symptoms. The patient should be kept clean and well nourished in comfortable surroundings with good nursing care, and sedatives should be given for obvious restlessness or paranoid beliefs. These measures can help ease the distress for both patient and family. Timing of a transfer to suitable hospital or custodial care must be sensitively organized.

Research into medication to alleviate memory loss and intellectual decline has shown some promise, but no truly effective treatment is yet available commercially.

Dementia praecox

An outdated term for severe *schizophrenia*, especially that developing in adolescence or early adulthood. It means literally "prematurely out of one's mind."

De Morgan's spots

Harmless red or purple raised spots in the skin, about one tenth of an inch across, that usually affect middle-aged or elderly people. De Morgan's spots are also called cherry spots or cherry angiomas and consist of a cluster of minute blood vessels. With increasing age they become more numerous but do not increase in size.

The spots are of no significance but may bleed if injured.

Demyelination

Breakdown of the fatty sheaths that surround and electrically insulate nerve fibers. The sheaths provide nutrients to the nerve fibers and are vital to the passage of electrical impulses along them. Demyelination "short-circuits" the functioning of the nerve, causing loss of sensation, coordination, and power in specific areas of the body. The affected nerves may be within the central nervous system (CNS, comprising the brain and spinal cord) or may be part of the peripheral nervous system, which links the CNS to the body's sense receptors, muscles, glands, and organs.

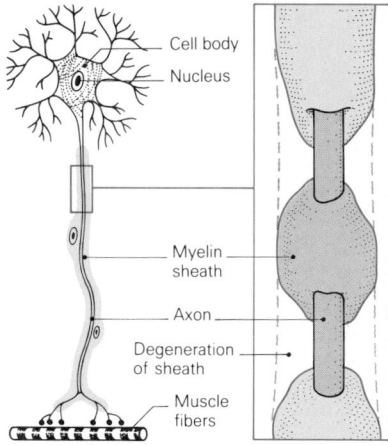

Mechanism of demyelination
The fatty myelin sheaths that surround and insulate nerve fibers break down, causing the affected nerves to "short-circuit."

Patches of demyelination are the prime feature of *multiple sclerosis*, a disease with symptoms that include blurred vision, muscle weakness, and loss of coordination. The cause of the demyelination is not known. In many cases, attacks of demyelination alternate with periods of partial or complete recovery of nerve function.

Encephalomyelitis is a rare disorder caused by inflammation of nerve cells within the CNS and sometimes areas of demyelination. It may be due to a viral infection or very rarely an allergiclike reaction following immunization. Symptoms vary from headache to brain damage.

Dendritic ulcer

A type of *corneal ulcer* characterized by threadlike extensions that branch out in various directions from the center. The ulcer is commonly caused by infection of the cornea by the virus that causes *herpes simplex*.

Dengue

A tropical disease caused by a virus spread by the mosquito *AEDES AEGYPTI*. It occurs in Southeast Asia, the Pacific region, parts of Africa, South and Central America, and the Caribbean. There have been occasional outbreaks in Mexico, Puerto Rico, and the US Virgin Islands in recent years, and a few cases have occurred along the Gulf coast.

Symptoms and signs appear five to eight days after a bite by an infected mosquito and include fever, rash, severe joint and muscle pains, and headache. These symptoms often subside after about three days, recur a few days later, and then subside again. Serious complications are uncommon. Full recovery may take several weeks. The symptoms of severe muscle and bone pain have led to dengue being called breakbone fever.

No specific treatment is available for dengue, though analgesics (painkillers) may relieve symptoms. No vaccine is available at present, so avoidance involves personal protection against mosquito bites in areas where the disease is prevalent (see *Insect bites*).

Densitometry

The measurement of bone density, as determined by the concentration of calcified material.

WHY IT IS DONE

Densitometry is used to confirm the presence of *osteoporosis* (wasting away of bone substance) or to diagnose *rickets* in young children. It is also useful in assessing the response of these conditions to treatment.

HOW IT IS DONE

The most accurate way to measure bone density is by analyzing the weight and content of a bone *biopsy* sample. However, this technique is time-consuming and requires an operation to remove the sample.

CT scanning provides more detailed pictures of the internal bone structure that enable smaller changes in bone density to be seen.

A relatively new and expensive technique is single or dual photon absorption, in which the pattern of absorption of a beam (or beams) of radiation as it passes through the bone is analyzed on an electronic counter. The dual photon method is used to evaluate the mineral content of the type of bone found in the vertebrae and most other bones where fractures from osteoporosis occur.

Density

The "heaviness" of a substance per unit volume. Density is a measure of how much a given volume of a substance weighs. For instance, a cubic inch of lead is considerably heavier than a cubic inch of wood; lead is therefore denser than wood.

In radiology, the term density relates to the amount of radiation absorbed by the structure being X rayed. Bone, which absorbs much radiation, appears white on X-ray film. By contrast, a lung, which contains mostly air, absorbs very little radiation and appears dark on film. The same holds true in *CT scanning*.

Dental assistant

A person who is trained to help a *dentist* at chairside and in the office.

The dental assistant is responsible for maintaining the cleanliness of the dentist's office and equipment, and for sterilizing and setting out instruments for each patient. During treatment of a patient, he or she passes instruments to the dentist and mixes any materials that are needed, such as cement for fillings. Other duties include record-keeping, processing X-ray films, and giving patients instructions on *oral hygiene*.

Dental emergencies

Injuries or disorders of the teeth and gums that require immediate treatment because of severe pain and/or because delay could lead to poor healing or complications.

A tooth that has become avulsed (completely dislodged from its socket) in an accident will be gently washed, reimplanted as rapidly as possible (see *Reimplantation*), and then immobilized with a splint. The success rate is about 90 percent if the tooth is out of its socket for 30 minutes or less, but falls to about 70 percent if the tooth is not reimplanted for 90 minutes. An extruded tooth (one that is partially dislodged from its socket) should be manipulated back into the socket within a few minutes of the injury.

A direct blow to a tooth may cause a fracture (see *Fracture, dental*). If the root is fractured so that the tooth is split in two, the halves will be brought closely together and splinted in position, usually for several months (see *Splinting, dental*). If the crown is fractured, but only the enamel and dentin are affected, a tooth-colored, composite filling will prevent pain from the exposed dentin, stop bacteria from entering the tooth, and restore

D

appearance. If the fracture of the crown involves the pulp of a mature tooth, a root canal filling is needed (see *Root canal treatment*). In a young tooth, a dressing of calcium hydroxide placed over the pulp soon after the accident may allow a hard tissue barrier to form and prevent the pulp of the tooth from dying.

Sometimes a blow hard enough to fracture teeth may also fracture the jaw; the fractured parts may need to be wired together to allow them to heal (see *Wiring of the jaws*).

Toothache may be so severe that eating and sleeping are disturbed. Temporary pain relief can be gained by placing a sedative dressing in the tooth until the cause of the pain can be treated. The most severe dental pain is usually caused by an abscess (infection). This is treated either by antibiotics to reduce the swelling, or by draining the abscess (see *Abscess, dental*), followed by endodontic treatment. Swelling, pain, and inflammation also may occur around an impacted wisdom tooth, and the jaw may become stiff and difficult to open. This requires immediate treatment to prevent the infection from spreading (see *Impaction, dental*).

Acute necrotizing ulcerative *gingivitis* comes on suddenly and causes pain, inflammation, ulceration, and bleeding of the gums. It is a destructive condition, and professional treatment should be sought as quickly as possible.

Dental examination

Examination of the mouth, gums, and teeth by a dentist. A dental examination may be performed as a routine check at least once a year or as part of the assessment of the condition of a person complaining of a symptom.

WHY IT IS DONE

Routine examinations enable caries (cavities) and diseases of the gums and mouth to be detected and treated at an early stage before they cause serious damage. The examinations also allow the efficiency of *oral hygiene* to be checked.

It is particularly important for children to have their teeth examined by a dentist regularly so that the dentist can monitor replacement of the primary teeth by permanent teeth. If any problems occur, such as crowding, the dentist can refer the child for orthodontic treatment at the correct stage.

HOW IT IS DONE

Before the examination, the dentist or dental hygienist usually asks about the patient's general health, especially if it is the person's first visit to a dentist or the first visit after a long time. Understanding the person's general health is important since it can affect the type of treatment that is recommended. A person with a heart valve disorder, for example, may be under increased risk of contracting bacterial *endocarditis* after extraction of a tooth or any other dental treatment. Particular care also is needed when treating diabetics and people who have had *hepatitis*. People with allergies may react dangerously to penicillin; people taking certain drugs can react badly to anesthesia. If the person feels pain, the dentist will ask him or her questions, such as when the pain was first noticed and whether it is continuous or intermittent.

The dentist begins by noting the general appearance of the patient and by examining the face and neck externally. The face is inspected for puffiness that might indicate a dental *abscess* and the neck is felt for swollen lymph glands, which may be caused by an infection of the mouth or teeth. The dentist also feels the temporomandibular joint (jaw joint) for any abnormal movements (see *Temporomandibular joint syndrome*).

Next the dentist examines the patient's bite and the teeth as a whole, noting any tilted, rotated, overlapping, or missing teeth and observing points of contact between teeth, and the presence of any excessive movement in a tooth when the patient makes chewing movements.

Using a mirror to see the backs of the teeth and into the back of the mouth, the dentist then examines individual teeth, using a metal instrument to probe for cavities or chips. Fillings and crowns are inspected for fit, jagged edges, and signs of erosion or cracks. If teeth are missing, the alveolus (bone that surrounds and supports the teeth) is examined for signs of abnormality, especially if the patient is to be fitted with a prosthodontic appliance, such as a bridge. If the patient wears a denture, it is checked to ensure it still fits.

SCOPE OF DENTAL EXAMINATION

A dental examination includes an assessment of the condition of the teeth, of the gums, of the mouth, and of the bone that surrounds the teeth.

Dental assistant

X-ray viewing screen

Light

Dentist

Rinsing bowl

Constructing a dental record
During the main part of the dental examination, the dentist checks for the presence or absence of individual teeth. Any abnormalities and all fillings are recorded by the assistant.

Instruments used
The dentist uses a mirror to see the backs of the teeth and into the back of the mouth; a metal instrument is used to probe for cavities or chips.
Mirror
Probe

D

The gums and inside of the mouth are examined for signs of disease. Gums that are red, puffy, or receding or that bleed easily when touched with the probe may indicate *gingivitis* or *periodontitis*. White discoloration of the inside of the mouth may signify *candidiasis* or *leukoplakia*.

Finally, the dentist assesses the accumulation of plaque and calculus on the teeth; this indicates the efficiency of the patient's oral hygiene. Inspection of the teeth and gums is sometimes followed by *dental X rays*.

Dental hygienist

See *Hygienist, dental.*

Dental X ray

An image of the teeth and jaws that provides information essential for detecting, diagnosing, and treating conditions that can threaten oral and general health. The part to be imaged is placed between a tube emitting *X rays* and a photographic film. Because X rays are unable to pass easily through hard tissue, a shadow of the teeth and bone is seen on the film.

WHY IT IS DONE

X rays can reveal disorders of the teeth and surrounding tissues that a dentist would not see during a normal visual examination of the mouth. Small caries (cavities), abscesses, cysts, tumors, and other disorders can be detected and treated before obvious signs and symptoms have developed, avoiding serious long-term damage. Early identification of dental problems, such as impacted teeth, allows treatment to be carefully planned and carried out at an early stage.

RISKS

The amount of radiation received from dental X rays is extremely small, and the risk of any harmful effects is negligible. However, a woman who is, or suspects she may be, pregnant should tell her dentist, who may recommend the use of a leaded apron during the examination or postpone X rays until after the pregnancy.

Dentifrice

A paste, powder, or gel used with a toothbrush to clean the teeth. Although brushing without a dentifrice removes food debris and some plaque (see *Plaque, dental*), a slightly abrasive dentifrice is needed to remove the remaining plaque and the salivary pellicle (a thin protein film).

A dentifrice contains the following: an abrasive—usually an insoluble, organic salt, such as dicalcium phosphate, which ideally does not scratch the teeth; a synthetic detergent for foaming action; humectants to bind the ingredients together and keep them moist; thickening agents; flavorings; and colorings.

Fluoride has been added to dentifrices for many years, and the dramatic drop in caries has been partly attributed to its presence in the majority of preparations.

A variety of desensitizing dentifrices is available for teeth that are sensitive due to exposed dentin near the gum margin.

Dentin

Hard tissue surrounding the pulp of a tooth (see *Teeth*).

Dentist

The equivalent of the family practitioner for teeth. Dentists perform regular checkups, clean teeth, fill cavities, extract teeth (if absolutely necessary), correct problems with tooth alignment, and provide and fit bridges and/or dentures to replace missing teeth. They also check for cancer of the mouth, perform cosmetic procedures (such as bonding) and give general advice on how to care for the teeth and gums. Most dentists refer patients with complicated problems to dental specialists in different branches of *dentistry*.

Dentistry

The science or profession concerned with the teeth and associated structures of the mouth. Dentistry involves the prevention, diagnosis, and treatment of disease, injury, or malformation of the teeth, gums, and jaws. The majority of *dentists* work in

---

TYPES OF DENTAL X RAY

There are three different types of X ray. Each is useful for revealing particular problems.

Bite-wing X rays
These X rays show the crowns of the teeth. They are useful for detecting areas of decay between teeth and changes in bone caused by periodontal (gum) disease. The film is in a holder with a central tab onto which the patient bites.

Periapical X rays
These X rays give detailed pictures of whole teeth and the surrounding gums and bone. They show unerupted or impacted teeth, root fractures, abscesses, cysts, tumors, and the characteristic bone patterns of some skeletal diseases. The film, in a protective casing, is placed in the patient's mouth and is held in position behind the teeth to be X rayed.

Panoramic X rays
These X rays show all the teeth and surrounding structures on one large film. They are invaluable for finding unerupted or impacted teeth, cysts, jaw fractures, or tumors. Pictures are recorded continuously onto film as the camera swings around from one side of the jaw to the other.

general dental practice (77 percent in the US). They are qualified to undertake all aspects of dental care, including cleaning teeth, filling cavities, extracting teeth, and fitting crowns, bridges, and dentures. Although they are qualified to diagnose and treat complicated problems, dentists may refer patients to a practitioner in one of the specialized branches of the dental profession.

Orthodontics concerns the moving of improperly aligned teeth to improve function and appearance. *Prosthodontics* concerns the provision of bridgework and dentures to replace missing teeth and the provision of substitutes for missing oral tissues.

Two branches specialize in the treatment of diseases: *endodontics* involves the treatment of diseases of the pulp, while *periodontics* involves the treatment of disorders that damage the supporting structures of the teeth, such as the gums.

Dentition

The characteristics of a person's *teeth*, including the number and arrangement in the jaw. The term is also used to describe the *eruption of teeth*.

Denture

An appliance that replaces missing natural teeth. A denture consists of an acrylic (tough plastic) and/or metal base mounted with acrylic or porcelain teeth. A natural appearance is achieved by choosing artificial teeth of the size, color, and shape that closely resemble the original teeth and that blend well with the contours of the person's face.

FITTING

The dentist takes impressions of the upper and lower gums. The impressions are removed from the mouth and allowed to harden. Models are then made by pouring plaster of Paris into the hardened impressions. Denture baseplates created from these models will fit the mouth accurately, but, to ensure that the bite will be correct when the artificial teeth are positioned, the dentist must also record the relationship of the upper and lower jaw. This is done by having the patient bite onto wax-rimmed plates (bite blocks) that can be trimmed to indicate the correct relative positions of the teeth.

Using the bite blocks as a guide, a temporary denture with the teeth waxed into position is then produced. The patient tries it on so the dentist can make adjustments to the position or choice of teeth. When the dentist and patient are satisfied with the bite and appearance, the wax is replaced by acrylic or metal, and the finished, polished dentures are fitted at the patient's next visit. Additional visits may be needed to modify any part of the base that is uncomfortable.

Dentures fitted immediately after tooth extraction usually require extra visits so that adjustments to the fit can be made as the tissues heal. Often a new acrylic lining is fused to the existing baseplate. Sometimes a soft lining (made of slow-setting impression material) is inserted temporarily to minimize pain.

Deodorant

A substance that removes bad smelling odors, especially body odors. Deodorants may contain *antiseptics* to destroy bacteria, perfume to mask odors, and *antiperspirants* (drugs that reduce the production of sweat).

Deodorant preparations are a useful aid against body odor caused by decomposition of sweat by bacteria on the skin. Deodorant liquids are also available to put into a *colostomy* or *ileostomy* bag. Deodorant drugs, such as bismuth, can be taken by mouth to reduce ostomy odor.

Deoxyribonucleic acid

See *DNA*; *Nucleic acids*.

Dependence

Psychological or physical reliance on persons or drugs. An infant is naturally dependent on parents, but, as he or she grows, dependency normally wanes. Some adults never become fully independent, continuing to demand excessive love, admiration, and help from others.

Alcohol and drugs (such as opiates, amphetamines, and tranquilizers) may induce a state of physical or emotional dependence in heavy, regular users. A person who is dependent may develop physical symptoms (sweating and abdominal pains) or emotional distress if deprived of the drug. The pattern of dependence varies with the drug and with the personality of the individual. (See also *Alcohol dependence*; *Drug dependence*.)

Depersonalization

A state of feeling unreal. The sufferer often describes feeling "like a robot" or "as though a glass screen came down." The sensation usually comes on suddenly, though it may be momentary or last for hours. It is often accompanied by *derealization* (experiencing the world as unreal).

An otherwise healthy person may experience depersonalization as an isolated event, especially if he or she is tired or worried. Although frightening, it is rarely serious. More often, people who have *anxiety disorders* experience depersonalization during *panic attacks*, especially if *hyperventilation* (rapid, shallow breathing) occurs. Other causes include drugs (e.g., LSD, antidepressants, or cannabis), migraine, and temporal lobe *epilepsy*.

TYPES OF DENTURES

Partial dentures	Partial dentures are used when only some teeth are missing. They fill unsightly gaps, make chewing easier, maintain clear speech, and keep the remaining teeth in position. Teeth on either side of a gap may tip (making cleaning more difficult) or drift (placing unnatural stress on the	tissues of the mouth). Partial dentures are held in place by metal clasps that grip adjacent teeth or by clasps combined with metal rests (extensions of the denture plate that rest on the tooth surface).
Full dentures	Full dentures are needed when there are no teeth left in the mouth. They stay in place by resting on the gum ridges and, in the case of upper dentures, by	suction. Fitting is usually delayed for several months after extraction of teeth to allow the gums to shrink and change shape as they heal.
Immediate dentures	Immediate dentures are fitted immediately after extraction of teeth. They protect the gum and control bleeding from extraction sites. Since a toothless period is avoided, they are particularly useful	for replacing front teeth. However, they can be expensive and require follow-up visits for refitting or relining so that they fit comfortably.

D

Depilatory

A chemical hair remover, such as barium sulfide, in the form of a cream or paste. Depilatories are used for cosmetic reasons and in the treatment of *hirsutism* (excessive hairiness).

HOW THEY WORK

Depilatories dissolve hair at the surface of the skin. They do not affect the hair root and therefore do not permanently remove the hair.

POSSIBLE ADVERSE EFFECTS

Depilatories may cause an allergic reaction, with inflammation and swelling. It is advisable to test them first on a small area of skin (they are not usually recommended for use on the face). Depilatories should not be used after a hot bath or shower. Heat increases blood flow to the skin and opens skin pores, thus increasing the amount of chemical that is absorbed into the body.

Depot injection

An intramuscular (into a muscle) injection of a drug specially formulated to give a slow, steady absorption of its active chemicals into the bloodstream.

Depot injections usually contain a much higher dose than that normally given by injection. Absorption of the drug is slowed by the inclusion of substances such as oil or wax. The release of the active drug can be made to last for hours, days, or weeks, depending on the formulation.

A depot injection is useful for patients who may not take their medication correctly. A depot injection also prevents the necessity of giving a series of injections over a short period. Examples of drugs given by depot injection include *corticosteroid drugs* and *antipsychotic drugs*.

Disadvantages of this type of injection include side effects caused by the uneven release of the drug into the bloodstream and prolonged adverse reactions caused by the long-acting nature of the treatment.

Patients who are receiving regular depot injections usually carry a warning card in case emergency treatment is required from another physician.

Depression

Feelings of sadness, hopelessness, pessimism, and a general loss of interest in life, combined with a sense of reduced emotional well-being. Most people experience these feelings occasionally, often as a normal response to a particular event. For example, it is natural to feel sad when a close relative dies. However, if the depression occurs without any apparent cause, deepens, and persists, it may be a symptom of a wide range of psychiatric illnesses. When a person's behavior and physical state are also affected, it then becomes part of a true depressive illness.

SYMPTOMS

Symptoms vary with the severity of the illness. In a person with mild depression, the main symptoms are anxiety and a variable mood. Sometimes he or she has fits of crying that occur for no apparent reason. A person with more serious depression may suffer from loss of appetite, difficulty sleeping, loss of interest and enjoyment in social activities, feelings of tiredness, and loss of concentration. Movement and thinking may become slowed; in some cases, the opposite occurs, and the person becomes extremely anxious and agitated. Severely depressed people may have thoughts of death and/or *suicide*, and feelings of guilt or worthlessness. In extreme cases, they may have *hallucinations* or *delusions* (believing, for example, that someone is poisoning them).

Intensity of symptoms often varies with the time of day. Most depressed people feel slightly better as the day progresses, but in some people the symptoms are worse at night. As a depressive illness progresses, the symptoms become more and more prominent. Finally, the person may become totally withdrawn and spend most of the time huddled in bed.

CAUSES

Usually, a true depressive illness has no single obvious cause. It may be triggered by certain physical illnesses (such as *stroke* or *hepatitis*), by hormonal disorders (such as *hypothyroidism*), or by the hormonal changes that occur after childbirth (see *Postpartum depression*). Some drugs, including the birth-control pill and sleeping pills, are contributing factors. If the depression is a part of a *manic-depressive illness*, inheritance may play a part, since this illness tends to run in families.

Aside from these biological causes, social and psychological factors may play a part. Lack of a satisfactory mother-child relationship may lead to depression in later life (see *Bonding*), especially when combined with difficult social circumstances. For example, a woman whose mother died early in her life may be particularly vulnerable if she has to cope with bringing up a child on her own.

Depression may also be related to the number of disturbing events or changes in a person's life.

INCIDENCE

Depression is the most common serious psychiatric illness. Some 10 to 15 percent of people suffer from it at some time in their lives, especially the milder forms. The more severe manic-depressive type affects only about 1 to 2 percent of depressed people, but the incidence of all forms of the illness increases with age. This may be due to social isolation, failing mental powers, and physical illness.

Depression appears to be more common in women, with about one in six seeking help for depression at some time in their lives (as opposed to only one in nine men). This may be a true difference or may result from the fact that women are more prepared to visit physicians for their depressive symptoms while men may be more likely to resort to alcohol, violence, or other expressions of discontent.

TREATMENT

There are three main forms of treatment for depression, depending on the type and severity of the illness.

Psychotherapy, whether individual or in a group, is most useful for those people whose personality and life experiences are the main causes of their illness. Many different types of therapy are available, ranging from an informal, purely practical approach to problem-solving, to the more structured approaches of *cognitive-behavioral therapy* and *psychoanalysis*.

Drug treatment is used for people who have predominantly physical symptoms. *Antidepressant drugs* are usually effective in over two thirds of these patients, provided the drugs are taken in a sufficient dosage over a long enough period of time.

Electroconvulsive therapy (*ECT*), which is given under a general anesthetic, is usually reserved for treating severely depressed people, especially if they are suffering from delusions or have failed to respond to treatment. ECT is effective and safe, and may be lifesaving; the only side effect may be a mild, temporary memory impairment. Trials have shown that ECT relieves severe depression faster than drugs.

OUTLOOK

Although depressive illness is a common cause of distress and social problems, the outlook is good for most sufferers, provided they are given appropriate treatment and advice. The main risk is suicide. In affluent societies the rate of suicide is about 20 per 100,000 population; at least 80 percent of these deaths are related to depression. The rate is highest in elderly men who are socially isolated and physically ill or in pain, but the rate is increasing in younger people.

Many people suffering from depression do not require hospitalization and make a good recovery. People with severe and prolonged depression (especially the elderly) may require continuous treatment and may be socially handicapped. However, spontaneous recovery is possible after many years of illness.

Derangement

An outdated term for severe mental disorder. It was first used in the nineteenth century to describe the idea of an orderly mind that had become "disarranged." Today it is usually applied to wild, disturbed behavior rather than a specific mental state.

The term derangement also applies to disorders of the ligaments in the knee joint (i.e., internal derangement of the knee).

Derealization

Feeling that the world has become unreal. It usually occurs with *depersonalization* and shares the sudden onset, symptoms, and causes of that condition. Sufferers commonly describe feeling that they are "looking at the world through a glass screen." Derealization may be caused by excessive tiredness, hallucinogenic drugs, or disordered brain function.

Dermabrasion

The removal of the surface layer of the skin by high-speed sanding to reduce the pitted scars of acne, to improve the appearance of unsightly raised scars, or to remove tattoos. The skin is numbed with a local anesthetic and the surface layer removed by a fast-revolving abrasive wheel. Healing takes about two weeks and the full effect of the treatment is apparent after two months.

Dermatitis

Inflammation of the skin, sometimes due to an allergy but in many cases occurring without any known cause. Many types of dermatitis are better known as *eczema* (for example, atopic, discoid, infantile, and hand eczema).

Apart from eczemas, the three main forms of skin inflammation are seborrheic dermatitis, contact dermatitis, and photodermatitis.

SEBORRHEIC DERMATITIS

This is a red, scaly, itchy rash that develops on the face (particularly the nose and eyebrows), scalp, chest, and back. On the scalp it is the most common cause of *dandruff*. The rash often develops during times of stress, but its exact cause is unknown. Generally, the treatment of dermatitis must be tailored to each case. Applying topical corticosteroids and/or antimicrobials is often helpful. Also, gentle handling of the involved skin is imperative (i.e., avoidance of scratching and irritating substances—like detergents).

CONTACT DERMATITIS

In this type, the rash is a reaction to some substance that comes in contact with the skin. The reaction may result from a direct toxic effect of the substance or may be an allergic response.

Among the more common causes of the reaction are detergents (including traces left in washed clothes), nickel (in watch straps, bracelets, necklaces, and the fastenings of underclothes), chemicals in rubber gloves and condoms, certain cosmetics, plants (such as poison ivy), and medications (among them the antibiotic neomycin in cream or droplet form).

The type of rash varies considerably according to the substance causing it, but it is often itchy, and may flake or blister; its distribution corresponds to the skin area in contact with the causative substance.

When it is not clear what substance is responsible, suspected chemicals are placed in contact with the skin of the back and are kept in place there with tapes for a few days to see whether any produces a patch of dermatitis. Once the offending substance is identified, it can then be avoided, if possible. A corticosteroid medication may be used for the treatment of an existing rash.

Contact dermatitis
Reaction to the nickel in a watch strap produced the itchy, blistering rash on the inside of the wrist shown above.

Dermatitis artefacta

Any self-induced skin condition. It may range from a mild scratch self-inflicted by someone under stress to severe and extensive mutilation by a psychologically disturbed patient.

The skin damage may take any form—ulcers, blisters, or scratches. The damage often has a symmetrical or bizarre pattern and, to the trained eye, does not resemble that seen in any skin disease.

Dermatitis herpetiformis

A chronic skin disease in which clusters of tiny, red, intensely itchy blisters occur in a symmetrical pattern on various parts of the body, most commonly the back, elbows, knees, buttocks, and scalp.

The disease usually develops in adult life and is believed to be related to *celiac sprue*, a condition in which the small intestine is allergic to gluten, a constituent of wheat and other cereals. One of the symptoms of celiac sprue is chronic diarrhea, which also occurs in some people with dermatitis herpetiformis. Both conditions often improve after treatment with a gluten-free diet.

Dermatographia

Sensitivity of the skin to mechanical irritation, to the extent that firm stroking leads to the appearance of itchy wheals (raised areas), which are slightly darker than the surrounding skin. The term dermatographia literally means "writing on the skin," and in fact it is sometimes possible with a few finger strokes actually to write visible words on the skin of a sufferer's back.

Dermatographia (also called dermographism) is a form of *urticaria* (hives) and is most common among fair-skinned people with a tendency to allergic conditions such as *eczema*.

Dermatologist

A physician who has been trained to treat problems relating to the skin, hair, and nails. Problems include everything from wrinkles, warts, and hair loss to acne, athlete's foot, and skin cancer. Treatment methods include medication (topical and/or oral), surgery, or the destruction of unwanted growths by freezing, burning, lasers, and radiation.

Dermatology

The study of *skin* diseases. Dermatology is involved with the study of the physiology and pathology of the skin and its appendages (e.g., hair, sweat glands, and oil glands). In the study of disease it includes investigation (such as examining skin scrapings under a microscope), diagnosis, and treatment, which principally consists of applying the appropriate creams, lotions, or ointments.

Dermatopathology is the study of the microscopic appearance of diseased skin tissue.

Skin diseases are relatively common, accounting for about 15 percent of all illnesses. In many instances no cause can be found or permanent cure provided. This is true for many cases of *psoriasis* and *eczema*, two of the most common skin conditions.

Dermatome

An area of skin supplied with nerves from one spinal root (see *Nervous system*). The entire surface of the body is an interlocking mosaic of dermatomes, the pattern of which is very similar from one person to another.

Loss of sensation in a dermatome signifies damage to a particular nerve root, the most usual cause of which is a *disk prolapse*.

Dermatome also refers to an instrument for cutting variable thicknesses of skin for use in skin grafting.

Dermatomyositis

A rare, sometimes fatal, disease in which the muscles and skin become inflamed, causing weakness of the muscles and a skin rash.

CAUSES AND INCIDENCE

The disorder belongs to a group of illnesses called the *autoimmune disorders*, in which, for reasons that are not fully understood, the body's defense system against disease starts attacking the body's own tissues. The condition is sometimes associated with underlying cancer of an internal organ. Two thirds of people suffering from dermatomyositis are middle-aged women.

SYMPTOMS

The first sign is often a red rash on the bridge of the nose and cheeks, followed by a purple discoloration on the eyelids and sometimes a red rash on the knees, knuckles, and elbows. Muscles then start to become weak, stiff, and painful, particularly those in the shoulders and pelvis where the limbs join the trunk. The skin over them feels thicker than normal. Sometimes the muscle pains precede the rash. The sufferer may also experience bouts of nausea, a loss of weight, and fever.

DIAGNOSIS AND TREATMENT

The diagnosis is confirmed by blood tests, electromyography (to detect the electrical activity of muscles; see *EMG*), and a *biopsy* (removal of a small piece of tissue for microscopic analysis) of skin or muscle.

Treatment is with *corticosteroid* and/or *immunosuppressant drugs* (to reduce the inflammation) and *physical therapy* (to prevent muscles from scarring and shrinking as they heal).

OUTLOOK

In about 50 percent of cases, full recovery occurs after a few years. In about 30 percent, the disease is persistent, causing muscle weakness. In the remaining 20 percent, it is progressive and affects the lungs and other organs and may be fatal.

Dermatophyte infections

A group of common fungal infections of the skin, hair, and nails, also called tineal infections (some are also called ringworm). Dermatophyte fungi can be spread from one person to another or from an animal such as a cat or dog to a person. The infections they cause usually have both a Latin name incorporating the term "tinea" and a common name—for example, tinea pedis (athlete's foot) and tinea capitis (ringworm of the scalp). (See *Tinea*.)

Dermoid cyst

A benign tumor with a cell structure similar to that of skin and containing hairs, sweat glands, and sebaceous glands. Fragments of cartilage, bone, and even teeth are also often found within such tumors.

About 10 percent of ovarian tumors are dermoid cysts. They are often readily diagnosed because the bony material within them is opaque to X rays. They very rarely become malignant (cancerous), but can enlarge up to several inches in diameter to cause discomfort and abdominal swelling. As with any enlarging ovarian tumor, surgery is recommended.

Appearance of dermoid cyst on head
The growth is firm, painless, and has an inner cavity that contains a fatty substance and sometimes hair, teeth, and bony material.

A dermoid cyst also sometimes develops in the skin of the head and neck, causing a small painless swelling, which may be removed for cosmetic reasons. This type of dermoid cyst is usually congenital and contains only skin structures.

Dermoid tumor

See *Dermoid cyst*.

DES

The abbreviation for the synthetic estrogen drug *diethylstilbestrol*.

Desensitization

A technique, used in *behavior therapy* for treating *phobias*, in which the patient is gradually exposed to the cause of the fear.

Desensitization, allergy

See *Immunotherapy*.

Designer drugs

> **WARNING**
> Designer drugs carry a high risk of *drug dependence*, with severe withdrawal reactions, and of *drug poisoning*, causing effects such as brain damage.

A group of illegally produced chemicals that mimics the effects of specific drugs of abuse. Made in illicit laboratories, these drugs are cheap to produce and thus undercut the street prices of drugs such as *LSD* and *amphetamine drugs*. Designer drugs are often made in such a way that their structures are subtly different from the drugs they imitate. As a result, these drugs escape the federal laws that control the manufacture and distribution of drugs listed under the Controlled Substance Act (CSA).

TYPES

Designer drugs can be divided into three major groups: those derived from narcotic *analgesics* (painkillers) such as meperidine and fentanyl; drugs that mimic amphetamine drugs (stimulants); and variants of phencyclidine (PCP), a drug originally used in animal anesthesia that causes hallucinations.

POSSIBLE ADVERSE EFFECTS

Designer drugs are highly potent. Some derivatives of fentanyl, for example, are between 20 to 2,000 times more powerful than *morphine*; this has led to a high incidence of death due to *drug poisoning*.

Amphetamine derivatives cause brain damage at doses only slightly higher than those required for a stimulant effect. Although they have been abused as aphrodisiacs, amphetamine derivatives commonly impair orgasm in both men and women and may prevent erection.

Many designer drugs contain impurities. For example, a substance known as MPTP, contained within an analogue (derivative) of meperidine, has caused permanent brain damage that has resulted in symptoms and signs of Parkinson's disease. Phencyclidine analogues often cause seizures and psychosis.

OUTLOOK

New laws are being introduced in many states to control the use of designer drugs. The Analogue Enforcement Act, if approved by Congress, will restrict the use of all such substances.

Desipramine

An *antidepressant drug*. It takes about 10 to 14 days before desipramine improves the condition of the person who is depressed. It has less of a sedative effect than some other antidepressants, and is therefore useful in treating patients for whom sedation is undesirable. Possible adverse effects include a dry mouth, and, rarely, constipation and blurred vision.

Desmoid tumor

A growth, usually in the abdominal wall. The tumor is hard, with a well-defined edge.

Desmoid tumors occur most frequently in women who have had children. Stretching or bruising of the abdominal muscle fibers during pregnancy may be a factor in their development. Desmoid tumors may also arise at the sites of old surgical incisions in the abdomen or elsewhere in the body, and they are often regarded as overgrowths of scar tissue.

Surgical excision is the usual treatment, although recurrence of the growth at the same site is common. *Radiation therapy* may arrest the growth of desmoid tumors.

Detergent poisoning

If swallowed, the cleaning agents in shampoos, laundry powders, and cleaning liquids cause vomiting, diarrhea, and a swollen abdomen. The treatment is to dilute the detergent by giving the victim plenty to drink. The same types of detergents can irritate the skin by removing its natural oils; people who constantly use them should protect their hands.

Developmental delay

A term used when a baby or young child has not achieved new abilities within the normal time range and has a pattern of behavior that is not appropriate for his or her age.

Development is an increase in the abilities—physical, intellectual, and social—and is a well-orchestrated process, with new abilities and new patterns of behavior appearing at given ages, while existing patterns of behavior change and sometimes disappear (see *Child development*).

Delays may be of varying severity and may affect any or all of the major areas of human achievement (i.e., development of the ability to walk upright, of fine hand-eye coordination, of listening, language, and speech, and of social interaction). Developmental delay is not a term used for slow increase in physical size (see *Growth*; *Short stature*) or for late appearance of sexual characteristics (see *Puberty*). The term developmental delay is not usually applied to children over the age of 5.

In general, the child who is slow in one or two aspects of development and of average or perhaps advanced ability in others needs to be distinguished from the child who is delayed in most aspects. When there is a significant delay in a few aspects, there may be a specific (although often not obvious) disability such as a visual or hearing impairment, which, if adequately treated, may allow the child to catch up. Children who are developmentally delayed in most aspects usually have a more generalized problem—for example, lack of adequate stimulation and teaching at home or a slowness to learn because of limited intellectual abilities.

CAUSES

Some important causes of generalized developmental delay are shown in the accompanying table. It is important to remember that a child born prematurely will reach most developmental milestones later than other children. Parents will want to recognize how old the baby would be if born at term rather than prematurely. Causes of delay in specific areas of development are outlined below.

WALKING AND MOVEMENT SKILLS There is an enormous time range within which most children learn to walk; children are not considered delayed unless they are not walking by themselves by 18 months.

In most late walkers, no serious cause is found. Late walking is an

CAUSES OF GENERALIZED
DEVELOPMENTAL DELAY

Unsatisfactory parental interaction (e.g., lack of affection, stimulation, or teaching, or lack of consistent and constant guidelines of acceptable behavior).

Severe visual impairment. Vision is vitally important for normal development in all areas. Children learn to recognize objects by sight before learning their names, they learn about sounds by seeing which objects make which sounds, and they become motivated to crawl and walk by the desire to explore the surroundings they see. (See *Vision, disorders of*; *Blindness*.)

Severe hearing impairment. (See *Deafness*.)

Limited intellectual abilities. (See *Mental retardation*.)

Damage to the brain before, during, or after birth, or in infancy. The results of damage depend on which parts of the brain are damaged and on severity. (See *Brain damage*; *Cerebral palsy*.)

Severe disease of other organs and systems of the body. (See *Nutritional disorders*; *Heart*, *Bone*, *Muscles*, and *Kidney* disorders boxes.)

inherited feature in some families and is probably due to delayed maturation of the nervous system. Such children learn to walk a few months later than other children, and from then on usually develop new skills at a normal rate. Other children develop slightly unusual patterns of locomotion—for example, creeping on their abdomens or shuffling on their bottoms. These traits also tend to run in families. Such children may miss out on the crawling stage. They eventually stand and walk and from then on follow the normal developmental sequence in all other developmental aspects.

A more specific reason for delayed walking and other skills is weakness of the leg muscles and other muscles. This can occur in boys with pseudohypertrophic *muscular dystrophy* and in children with *spina bifida*. *Cerebral palsy* is a disorder affecting all aspects of motor development; it may

D

cause slowness and difficulty in gaining control of the head and neck muscles during the first months of life as well as delay in sitting and walking.

HAND-EYE COORDINATION Any defect of vision or of the nerves and muscles used to control fine finger movements may be a cause of delayed manipulative skills. However, the most common cause is not a specific abnormality but lack of experience—stimulation and encouragement are extremely important in the acquisition of these skills. If a child has only large toys to play with and is not encouraged to use the small finger muscles, skills involving the muscles will be delayed. Similarly, if a child is left lying down for most of the time instead of in a sitting position, the hands will not be in the correct position to acquire certain skills.

RESPONSE TO SOUND If a child is unresponsive to sound it may be due to deafness. However, children who are not talked to may show a lack of interest in the human voice, although they may respond normally to other sounds. Children exposed continually to a great deal of noise may show a general lack of interest in sound.

A rare cause of unresponsiveness to the human voice is the psychiatric condition of *autism*. An affected child can hear normally but shows little interest in human contact of any kind. Although unresponsive to human voices, autistic children often become obsessively interested in particular sound-producing toys.

SPEECH AND LANGUAGE The most important cause of delayed speech is deafness of any degree. Other common causes are lack of stimulation (when parents do not talk to the child sufficiently) and a familial pattern of delayed speech, which is more common in boys than girls. Twins are often late talkers, perhaps because they may receive less individual parental attention. Twins sometimes develop a private language that includes idiosyncratic words and nonverbal communication.

Children exposed to two or more languages may show signs of speech delay and may confuse the languages. However, many children become naturally bilingual or trilingual with no difficulties.

Any generalized difficulty with muscle control can affect speech production; muscle control can be a particular difficulty in children with cerebral palsy. Damage to, or structural defects of, the speech muscles,

larynx, or mouth may also cause speech difficulties, as may any disorder affecting the speech area of the brain (see *Dysarthria; Dysphonia; Aphasia; Speech disorders*).

BLADDER AND BOWEL CONTROL Children vary enormously in the age at which confident control of bowel and bladder function is acquired. Usually bowel function is acquired first. Delay in bladder control is much more common than delayed bowel control. There are many possible causes. (See *Incontinence, urinary; Enuresis; Incontinence, fecal; Encopresis.*)

ASSESSMENT AND TREATMENT
In many instances, the parents will be the first to notice that their child is not acquiring new skills at the same rate as his or her peers. A physician should be consulted. Problems are sometimes detected during one of the developmental checks that are carried out routinely in the US and other developed countries. These checks are performed by physicians or other health professionals at varying ages, but usually at birth, 6 weeks, 6 to 8 months, 12 to 15 months, 2 years, 3 years, and 5 years.

If a developmental delay is discovered, the first step is to establish the cause by undertaking a full assessment. This examination usually includes hearing and vision testing, a full physical examination, and thorough developmental assessment. Further investigation is arranged as necessary. It may include referral to a pediatrician, neurologist, psychologist, speech therapist, occupational therapist, or physical therapist.

Once the severity of the delay, and the probable cause, has been discovered, appropriate treatment can be arranged. In many cases, the parents can be reassured that there is no serious abnormality and that their child can be expected to develop normally without any specific treatment. Sometimes advice is given regarding suitable toys and other stimulation.

Specific treatment may include provision of glasses or a hearing aid; treatment may also include a lengthy course of speech therapy or psychiatric counseling for the whole family. In some cases it is felt that the child's best interests are served by admission to a special school for children with specific difficulties—for example, a language unit or a school for physically handicapped children.

Whatever the cause, children can be helped to achieve their full potential by provision of appropriate therapy.

Professionals are usually involved in assessing the abilities of a child and deciding on the appropriate help. Parents are often of prime importance in providing this help.

Deviation, sexual

A form of sexual behavior in which intercourse between adults is not the final aim. Instead, the man (deviation is rare in women) achieves erection and orgasm in other ways, such as by being whipped or wearing women's clothes. Forms of sexual deviation include *exhibitionism, transvestism, fetishism, frottage, necrophilia, pedophilia, sadism,* and *masochism.*

Dexamethasone

CORTICOSTEROID			
Tablet	Injection	Nasal spray	Eye drops

Prescription needed

Available as generic

Dexamethasone is a *corticosteroid drug* prescribed as a nasal spray to relieve nasal congestion caused by allergic *rhinitis* (hay fever) and as eye drops in the treatment of *iritis* (inflammation of the iris). It is given in tablet form to treat severe cases of *asthma* and to reduce inflammation of the brain due to *head injury, stroke,* or a *brain tumor.* Occasionally, dexamethasone is injected into an inflamed joint to ease pain and stiffness caused, for example, by osteoarthritis.

POSSIBLE ADVERSE EFFECTS
Taken as a nasal spray or in eye-drop form, minor local side effects, such as a nosebleed or eye irritation, may occur. When prescribed as a tablet, either for a prolonged period or in high doses, adverse effects common to other corticosteroids may occur.

Dextroamphetamine

A central nervous system stimulant (see *Stimulants*). Dextroamphetamine is prescribed for *narcolepsy* (a rare condition characterized by excessive sleepiness). Paradoxically, it is also used to treat children with *hyperactivity,* although the reason it helps in this condition is not known.

Dextroamphetamine is no longer recommended as an *appetite suppressant* for people who are attempting to lose weight.

ABUSE
Because of its stimulant properties, dextroamphetamine has become a drug of abuse. It is one of a group of

drugs commonly referred to as "uppers." If use is prolonged, the stimulant effects lessen and a higher dose must be taken to produce the desired effect. In an overdose, dextroamphetamine can cause seizures and hypertension.

Dextrocardia

A rare condition, present from birth, in which the heart is situated in, and points toward, the right-hand side of the chest instead of the left. The heart may also, but not necessarily, be malformed. Sometimes, the position of the abdominal organs is also reversed, so that the liver is on the left-hand side and the stomach on the right. When all organs are on the opposite side of the body from where they are customarily found, it is known as *situs inversus*.

The cause of dextrocardia is unknown. No treatment is necessary unless the heart is malformed, in which case surgery may be necessary (see *Heart disease, congenital*).

Abnormal position   Normal position

Heart positions
In dextrocardia, the heart is situated in, and points toward, the right-hand side of the chest instead of the left.

Dextrose

Another name for *glucose*, one of the monosaccharide sugars. Dextrose is absorbed from digested *carbohydrates* through the intestinal wall into the bloodstream. It is also available in the form of tablets, as an injection used in the emergency treatment of *hypoglycemia* (low blood sugar), and as a component of feedings given by infusion (see *Feeding, artificial*).

Diabetes, bronze

Another name for *hemochromatosis*, a rare disease in which excessive amounts of iron are deposited in tissues such as the liver, pancreas, and skin. Its name comes from the bronze skin coloration and *diabetes mellitus* that usually develop in people who suffer from this disorder.

Diabetes insipidus

A rare condition characterized by the passing of enormous quantities of dilute urine (polyuria) and excessive thirst (polydipsia). These symptoms also occur, in a milder form, early in *diabetes mellitus*, a much more common disease that in all other respects is different from diabetes insipidus.

CAUSES

Diabetes insipidus usually results from a failure of the *pituitary gland* to secrete antidiuretic hormone (*ADH*). Normally, this hormone diminishes the amount of water passed by the kidneys into the urine to maintain a constant dilution of the blood. Diseases of the pituitary, including damage from injury or a tumor, can cause failure of secretion.

In rare cases, the disease (called nephrogenic diabetes insipidus) is due to failure of the kidneys to respond to normal levels of ADH. This type is usually congenital (present from birth), but may result from a kidney disease called *pyelonephritis*.

SYMPTOMS, DIAGNOSIS, AND TREATMENT

A person with diabetes insipidus may pass between 10 and 40 pints of urine every 24 hours—provided this output is matched by a similar intake of water. If water is unobtainable or withheld, the signs and symptoms of *dehydration* will appear, leading to confusion, stupor, and coma.

Treatment is normally by administration of a synthetic variety of antidiuretic hormone. This, however, is ineffective in treating people with the nephrogenic variety of the disease. These people must be placed on a low-sodium diet and treated with a drug that slows the development of thirst symptoms.

Diabetes mellitus

A disorder in which the pancreas produces insufficient or no *insulin*, the hormone responsible for the absorption of glucose into cells for their energy needs and into the liver and fat cells for storage. As a result, the level of glucose in the blood becomes abnormally high, causing excessive urination and constant thirst and hunger. The body's inability to store or use glucose causes weight loss and fatigue. Diabetes mellitus also results in disordered *lipid* metabolism and accelerated degeneration of small blood vessels.

Apart from the symptoms of thirst and excessive urination, the disease has nothing in common with the much rarer disorder *diabetes insipidus*.

There are two main types of diabetes mellitus. Insulin-dependent (type I) diabetes, the more severe form, usually first appears in people under the age of 35 and most commonly in people between the ages of 10 and 16. It develops rapidly. The insulin-secreting cells in the pancreas are destroyed, probably as a result of an *immune response* after a virus infection, and insulin production ceases almost completely. Without regular injections of insulin, the sufferer lapses into a coma and dies.

The other main type, non-insulin-dependent (type II) diabetes, is usually of gradual onset and occurs mainly in people over 40. In many cases is discovered only during a routine medical examination. Insulin is produced, but not enough to meet the body's needs, especially when the person is overweight. Often the body is resistant to the effects of insulin. In most cases, insulin-replacement injections are not required; the combination of dietary measures, weight reduction, and oral medication keeps the condition under control.

CAUSES AND INCIDENCE

Diabetes mellitus tends to run in families. However, of those who inherit the genes responsible for the insulin-dependent form, only a very small proportion eventually develop the disease. In these cases the disorder possibly occurs as the delayed result of a viral infection that had damaged the pancreas several years earlier.

In the case of non-insulin-dependent diabetes, the greater proportion of people predisposed to the disease by heredity (primarily those who are overweight) go on to acquire it.

Although obesity is the primary cause of unmasking latent diabetes, other causes that can unmask or aggravate diabetes are certain illnesses (among them *pancreatitis* and *thyrotoxicosis*), certain drugs (including some corticosteroids and some diuretics), infections, and pregnancy (see *Diabetic pregnancy*).

In the US about two persons per 1,000 have insulin-dependent diabetes by the age of 20; overall, the insulin-dependent form affects about 150 to 200 persons per 100,000. Non-insulin-dependent diabetes is more common, with as many as 2,000 persons per 100,000 affected.

DIAGNOSIS

A physician who suspects diabetes in a patient can often obtain confirmation from testing a sample of urine for its glucose level. Further confirmation

D

D

LIVING WITH DIABETES MELLITUS

As the level of glucose in the blood rises, the volume of urine required to carry it out of the body is increased, causing not only a continuous need to urinate but also constant thirst. The high levels of sugar in the blood and urine impair the body's ability to fight infection, leading to urinary tract infections (such as *cystitis* and *pyelonephritis*), vaginal yeast infections (*candidiasis*), and recurrent skin infections.

Because the body's cells are starved of glucose, the sufferer feels weak and fatigued. The cells are able to obtain some energy from the breakdown of stored fat, resulting in weight loss. However, the chemical processes involved in this breakdown of fat are defective (especially in insulin-dependent diabetics), leading to the production of acids and substances called ketones, which can cause coma and sometimes death.

Other possible symptoms of undiagnosed diabetes include blurred vision, boils, increased appetite, and tingling and numbness in the hands and feet.

Symptoms develop in all untreated insulin-dependent diabetics, but symptoms develop in only one third of those with the non-insulin-dependent type. There are many people suffering from a mild form of the disease who are unaware of it. The disease often is diagnosed only after complications of the diabetes have been detected.

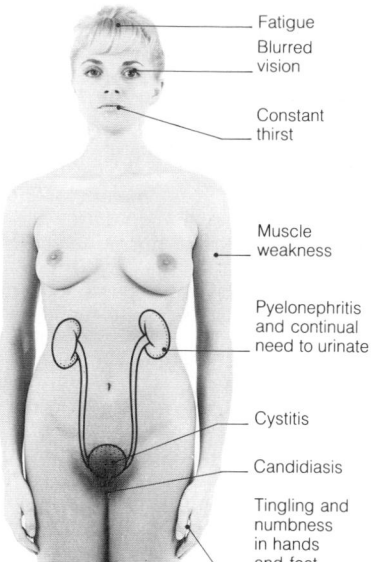

- Fatigue
- Blurred vision
- Constant thirst
- Muscle weakness
- Pyelonephritis and continual need to urinate
- Cystitis
- Candidiasis
- Tingling and numbness in hands and feet

Testing urine for glucose
Urine can be tested for glucose by means of a chemically impregnated strip dipped into a sample of urine. The resulting color change in the strip is compared with a chart to indicate the glucose level.

Direct testing of blood glucose
A pricking device is used to obtain blood, which is spread on a chemically coated strip. The strip is inserted into an instrument that reads the blood glucose.

DEVICES FOR INJECTING INSULIN

Insulin can be injected using a disposable syringe and needle or a pen with refill cartridges (below), or it may be infused continuously from a portable pump (right).

- Insulin pen
- Spare needles
- Refill cartridge

- Cannula
- Pump

Insulin pen
This device is useful if multiple daily injections are needed.

Portable pump
The pump infuses insulin via a cannula inserted through the skin.

---

is secured when significantly high glucose levels are obtained from blood samples following an overnight fast or from samples taken two hours after a meal. Glucose-tolerance tests are not usually required.

TREATMENT

The aims of treatment are to prolong life, relieve symptoms, and prevent long-term complications. Success depends on keeping the level of blood glucose as near normal as possible through maintenance of normal weight, regular physical activity, and careful dietary management.

In people with insulin-dependent diabetes, treatment consists of regular self-injections, one to four times a day, with insulin (either obtained from animals or of a human type synthesized by *genetic engineering*). In addition, the person must follow a diet in which carbohydrate intake is regulated and spread out over the day according to a consistent timetable. In this way, marked fluctuations in the glucose levels in the blood can be avoided.

Disturbances in the careful balance between insulin and glucose intake can result in *hyperglycemia* (too much glucose in the blood), causing the symptoms of the untreated disease, or *hypoglycemia* (too little glucose), which can lead to weakness, confusion, dizziness, sweating, and even unconsciousness and seizures. To help prevent this, diabetics (of both types) are advised to regularly moni-

tor their blood and urine glucose levels with do-it-yourself testing kits.

For difficult-to-control diabetes, an insulin pump is an alternative treatment for those who are willing to monitor their blood glucose levels carefully. Insulin is continuously infused from a refillable pump through a needle implanted in the skin. Control is often no better than that for multiple daily injections.

As a precaution against an attack of hypoglycemia, insulin-dependent diabetics need to carry some sugar or glucose with them at all times. Because of the disabling effects of hypoglycemia, insulin-dependent diabetics who drive must declare their disorder to insurance companies and car-licensing authorities. Those with poorly controlled insulin-dependent diabetes are sometimes advised against doing jobs that involve working at a height or operating a public conveyance, and against engaging in activities like race-car driving or flying, where they may be a danger to themselves and others.

Because the pancreas does produce some insulin in non-insulin-dependent diabetics, the disorder can often be controlled by dietary means alone (regulating the carbohydrate intake with meals spaced out over the day). This not only lowers the blood glucose level, but also reduces weight. If diet fails to lower the glucose level sufficiently, *hypoglycemic* tablets (oral antidiabetic drugs that stimulate the pancreas to produce more insulin) may be prescribed, though these are ineffective unless dietary restrictions are observed.

All people with mild diabetes need regular advice from their physicians so that any complications can be detected and treated at an early stage. Diabetics should wear or carry information identifying them as diabetics in case of an emergency.

COMPLICATIONS

Complications eventually develop in a large number of diabetics. These complications tend to be more likely if the diabetes has not been well controlled, but they can occur even if there has been good control. Complications include *retinopathy* (damage to the retina, the light-sensitive area at the back of the eye, and the blood vessels serving it), peripheral *neuropathy* (damage to nerve fibers), and *nephropathy* (kidney damage). Ulcers on the feet, which in severe cases can develop into gangrene, are another risk, but with good foot care they can usually be prevented.

Diabetics also have a higher-than-average risk of *atherosclerosis* (narrowing of the arteries), *hypertension* (high blood pressure), other *cardiovascular disorders*, and *cataracts* (opacities of the lens of the eye).

There are, however, people who have lived full and active lives with diabetes mellitus for 50 years or more with few complications.

OUTLOOK

With modern treatment and sensible self-monitoring, almost all diabetics can look forward to a normal life. The life expectancy of people who have well-regulated, insulin-dependent diabetes is little different than that of nondiabetics. Those with the non-insulin-dependent illness have a slightly reduced life expectancy because of circulatory and heart disorders, which often are present when the diabetes is diagnosed.

Diabetic pregnancy

A small number of women acquire *diabetes mellitus* during pregnancy—a phenomenon called gestational diabetes. Diabetes mellitus may also have been present and under treatment before pregnancy. In both cases, special precautions are necessary.

PREEXISTING DIABETES

Nearly all women with established diabetes mellitus can have a normal pregnancy, provided the diabetes is well controlled throughout. It is important to plan the pregnancy and to make sure that the blood glucose level is under particularly good control before and at the time of conception; otherwise there is a slightly increased chance of the baby being malformed. If control is poor during the pregnancy, there may be an increase in the amount of glucose reaching the baby (which makes the baby grow faster than normal) and this may cause difficulties at birth. Also, the growth of infants of diabetic mothers may be stunted; these babies may have complications in the days immediately after birth.

GESTATIONAL DIABETES

Gestational diabetes is most often detected in the second half of pregnancy, when increased glucose appears in the urine or the baby is found to be bigger than expected when a physician examines the mother's abdomen (though these findings do not always mean the mother is diabetic). Apparently, not enough insulin is produced to keep the blood glucose levels normal during the pregnancy. Obstetricians now screen for diabetes at 26 weeks. Gestational diabetes usually disappears with the delivery of the baby, but can be a sign of future diabetes in up to three fourths of these mothers.

CARE

When feasible, diabetic pregnancies are treated at high-risk obstetrical centers (many of which offer prepregnancy clinics for those with established diabetes to help achieve good control before conception) and at antenatal clinics to supervise all aspects of the pregnancy.

The chances that the baby of a diabetic parent will become diabetic are about one in 100 and, if both parents are diabetic, about one in 20. If only the father is diabetic, no special precautions need to be taken at conception or during the pregnancy.

Diacetylmorphine

A synthetic drug similar to *morphine*, usually referred to by its popular name, *heroin*.

Diagnosis

The determination by a physician of the cause of a person's problem. Usually this entails identifying both the disease process—pneumonia or cirrhosis of the liver, for example—and the agent responsible, such as pneumonia due to legionnaires' disease, or cirrhosis due to alcohol. Diagnosis is part science and part art; an experienced physician relies not only on his or her scientific knowledge and experience, but also on intuition to recognize the pattern of an illness and establish a diagnosis.

THE MEDICAL HISTORY

The patient's own account of his or her illness is perhaps the most important part of the diagnostic procedure. This history provides vital clues, which can then be augmented by questions from the physician in an exchange that may last some 20 to 30 minutes in a complex case or if the physician has not previously seen the patient. What the physician is looking for is a pattern of symptoms that is strongly suggestive of a single disease. For example, the features of a migraine headache, duodenal ulcer, enlarged prostate gland, or angina pectoris are often unmistakable.

In some circumstances the physician may not attempt to reach a final diagnosis. If a patient has had only a sore throat for 48 hours, the physician may be content to treat the condition symptomatically, attempting to relieve the symptoms while awaiting the results of a throat culture or other laboratory tests.

However, when symptoms have been more prolonged, the physician will want to reach at least a provisional diagnosis before beginning treatment, partly because any treatment is likely to affect the symptoms and thus make diagnosis more difficult.

EXAMINATION AND TESTS

Tests may be ordered after a physical examination and the formation of a provisional diagnosis.

However, confirmation is obtained in a variety of ways, including tissue biopsy, culture of microorganisms, or finding the cause at surgery. If specific treatment (either with drugs or by

D

D

STEPS IN DIAGNOSING A CONDITION

A physician may go through several steps to ascertain the cause of a person's problem. The history, physical examination, and tests may provide vital clues. A physician usually makes at least a provisional diagnosis before beginning any treatment because treatment can mask symptoms, making the physician's job of establishing an exact diagnosis more difficult.

Taking the medical history

Perhaps the most important part of the diagnostic procedure is the patient's own account of his or her illness – the medical history. "Listen to the patients, they are telling you their diagnosis" is the traditional teaching given to medical students. Many physicians believe that the medical history provides the strongest basis for ascertaining a diagnosis. The added information derived from the physical examination is small, but at times, critical.

Conducting a physical examination

After the medical history has been obtained, the physician has in mind a short list of probable diagnoses. A physical examination helps shorten the list. The physician is then left with a differential diagnosis. A differential diagnosis is a group of possible diseases that could account for the patterns of symptoms and signs (i.e., physical findings, such as enlargements of lymph glands or tenderness in a specific region of the abdomen).

Ordering special tests

Next, based on his or her working diagnosis, the physician may order a series of laboratory tests on the blood (and sometimes the urine) and may also arrange for diagnostic imaging of suspect organs by techniques such as *ultrasound scanning, X rays,* *CT scanning, MRI,* or *radionuclide scanning.* The results of these tests either confirm the physician's working diagnosis or narrow the possibilities so the physician may be confident that he or she has found the correct diagnosis.

Using a computer

Physicians today also use computer systems and algorithms to help reach a diagnosis. Both approaches rely on analysis of large numbers of patient records to quantify probabilities and to devise an orderly series of questions – a decision tree. The main purpose of computer assistance is to remind the physician of the full range of possible diagnoses for a particular set of symptoms, thereby making it less likely that any possibility will be overlooked. It remains the task of the physician to integrate the facts and decide upon a diagnosis.

surgery) relieves the symptoms and cures the patient, the diagnosis is likely to have been correct—although it is also possible that the patient may have recovered spontaneously and the treatment may simply have coincided with the time of recovery. Alternatively, if the patient dies, a pathologist can usually, but not always, determine by postmortem examination (see *Autopsy*) what the disease process had been.

Diagnosis-related group

A system of payment for medical service to patients getting care from certain provider organizations and to *Medicare* patients. The system was established by amendments to the Social Security Act in 1983.

Under the diagnosis-related group (DRG) system, hospitalized patients are classified into one of 467 diagnosis-related groups; hospitals are then reimbursed at a set rate for each of the diagnosis categories. If the costs of a patient's care exceed the fixed rate, the hospital must absorb the cost. But, if the hospital's costs are less than the set rate, it may retain the difference. By determining costs prospectively, hospitals presumably have an incentive to manage patient care efficiently. Under the former system of retrospective payments, hospitals had little incentive to monitor costs.

Dialysis

A technique used to remove waste products from the blood and excess fluid from the body as a treatment for *renal failure* (kidney failure).

WHY IT IS DONE

The main function of the kidneys is the maintenance of *electrolyte* and water balance and the excretion of waste products. Fully one fifth of the blood pumped by the heart goes to the kidneys; the kidneys filter approximately 150 liters of blood daily. From this volume of blood, the kidney reabsorbs important elements, such as sodium, potassium, calcium, amino acids, glucose, and water. The kidneys excrete, as urine, the protein breakdown product nitrogen in the form of urea, as well as other excess minerals, toxins, and drugs.

In people whose kidneys have been damaged, this process may fail—either suddenly (in acute renal failure) or gradually (in the chronic form of the disease). Wastes start to accumulate in the blood, with harmful, sometimes life-threatening effects. In severe cases, the function of the kidneys must be taken over by the artificial means of dialysis. In cases of acute kidney failure, dialysis continues until the kidneys recover and start functioning normally again. However, in chronic kidney failure, patients may need to undergo dialysis for the rest of their lives or until they can be given a *kidney transplant.* Dialysis therapy may not always be chosen by the patient and physician when kidney failure is simply a part of an otherwise rapidly fatal disorder.

D

PROCEDURE FOR DIALYSIS

There are two methods of removing wastes from the blood and excess fluid from the body when the kidneys have failed. The first, hemodialysis, may also be used as emergency treatment in some cases of poisoning or drug overdose. It makes use of an artificial kidney (or "kidney machine") and can be carried out at home. Peritoneal dialysis, also done in the home, requires an abdominal incision (which is done in the hospital).

HOW HEMODIALYSIS IS DONE

1 Access to the bloodstream for rapid removal and return of blood is obtained by a shunt connecting an artery to a vein.

Vein   Artery   Shunt sewn into blood vessel

2 A needle connected to plastic tubing passes blood to the artificial kidney and back to the patient. The artificial kidney consists of many layers of special membrane.

Artificial kidney (dialyzer)

Blood out of dialyzer

Machine that prepares dialysate

Blood into dialyzer

Dialysate to and from dialyzer

4 The dialysate is discarded and the purified blood is returned to the patient. Each session lasts two to six hours.

Shunt

WHY IT IS DONE

In people with damaged kidneys, the process of maintaining the balance of electrolytes and water, and of excreting waste products, may fail, causing harmful, if not life-threatening, effects. Dialysis can take over the function of the kidneys until they start working normally again. Or dialysis can function for the kidneys for the rest of a seriously affected person's life if a kidney transplant is not performed.

Diseased kidney
The kidney at right was removed from a person with adult polycystic kidney disease—one of many disorders that may damage kidney function to the extent that dialysis is needed.

3 The membrane separates the patient's blood from a special fluid called dialysate. Wastes, toxic molecules, and excess fluid pass from the blood into the dialysate.

Blood cell

Artificial membrane

Dialysate

Waste chemicals

HOW PERITONEAL DIALYSIS IS DONE

1 A small abdominal incision is made (using a local anesthetic); a catheter is inserted through it into the peritoneal cavity. Dialysate from a bag attached to the catheter passes into the cavity, where it is left for several hours.

Spinal column

Catheter

Fluid

Bag   Bladder

Blood cell

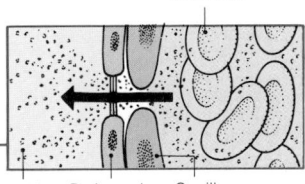

Fluid   Peritoneal membrane   Capillary wall

2 Waste products and excess water from the blood vessels lining the peritoneal cavity seep through the peritoneal membrane into the cavity and mix with the dialysate. The fluid is then allowed to drain out (by the release of a clamp) through the catheter and into the empty dialysate bag.

3 The bag is discarded and replaced with a bag containing fresh dialysate. The process, which takes about an hour, is repeated during the day or overnight.

D

HOW IT IS DONE

There are two methods of dialysis. Hemodialysis, which removes wastes by passing blood through an artificial kidney machine, was pioneered early in the 1940s. Peritoneal dialysis, which makes use of a natural filtering membrane within the body's abdomen, was developed in the early 1970s.

In most cases, hemodialysis is performed in outpatient dialysis centers by trained staff nurses, but, in the US, 5 percent of patients undergoing dialysis carry it out themselves with a kidney machine installed in the home.

Peritoneal dialysis may be performed in a hospital, but an increasing number of patients are now able, once the catheter has been inserted into the abdomen, to carry out the dialysis themselves at home, a procedure known as continuous ambulatory peritoneal dialysis.

For patients with chronic kidney failure, hemodialysis needs to be carried out several times a week. In the treatment of acute kidney failure, the process is carried out more intensively over a period of days or weeks until the kidneys are working normally again. Complications of hemodialysis may include weakening of the bones (see *Osteomalacia; Osteodystrophy*), anemia, infections, and pericarditis. Complications of peritoneal dialysis are the same as for hemodialysis along with peritonitis.

OUTLOOK

Long-term dialysis enables people who would once have died from chronic kidney failure to live relatively normal lives. Their diet and fluid intake must be restricted somewhat and they may not feel completely well. However, many do return to full or part-time employment. Since the patient's health is invariably affected in the long run, many physicians feel that dialysis should be replaced with a kidney transplant, which, if successful, can bring about a dramatic restoration of general health.

Diaper rash

A common condition affecting babies with otherwise healthy skin. Diaper rash results from skin irritation by substances contained in the feces or urine. Friction from rough diapers and prolonged wetting also play a part. Babies vary in their susceptibility to diaper rash. Occasionally, skin inflammation is severe. In some babies, diaper rash may be the first indication of sensitive skin and future skin problems, such as *eczema*.

Symptoms of diaper rash
The skin over the buttocks, genitals, and inner thighs becomes red and sore at first, and may progress to blistering.

TREATMENT AND OUTLOOK

Prevention is better than cure. The aim is to keep the baby's skin dry for as long as possible. A newborn breast-fed baby passes urine about 20 times each day and has a bowel movement after each feeding, so this presents a major practical problem. Change diapers frequently and, after each change, apply a water-repellent emollient. Ideally, the diaper should be left off for an hour or so each day.

Cloth diapers should be well rinsed and kept soft. Sometimes an ointment containing a mild *corticosteroid drug* needs to be prescribed to suppress the inflammation. It is often prescribed in combination with an antifungal drug to kill any thrush organisms that are present (see *Candidiasis*).

Diaphragm, contraceptive

The most commonly used female barrier method of contraception, in the form of a hemispherical dome of thin rubber with a coiled metal spring in the rim. The diaphragm is individually fitted to each woman. (See *Contraception, barrier methods*.)

Diaphragm muscle

The dome-shaped sheet of muscle that separates the thorax (chest) from the abdomen. The diaphragm is attached to the spine, ribs, and sternum.

The diaphragm plays a vital role in breathing. For air to be drawn into the lungs, the muscle fibers of the diaphragm contract, thereby pulling the central tendon downward. This action enlarges the chest, and air passes into the lungs to fill the increased space. (See also *Breathing*.)

ANATOMY OF THE DIAPHRAGM

The diaphragm is attached to the spine, the lower pairs of ribs, and the lower end of the sternum (breastbone). The muscle fibers of the diaphragm converge on the central tendon, a thick, flat plate of dense fibers. There are openings in the diaphragm for the esophagus, phrenic nerve (which controls diaphragm movements and hence breathing), and the aorta and vena cava blood vessels.

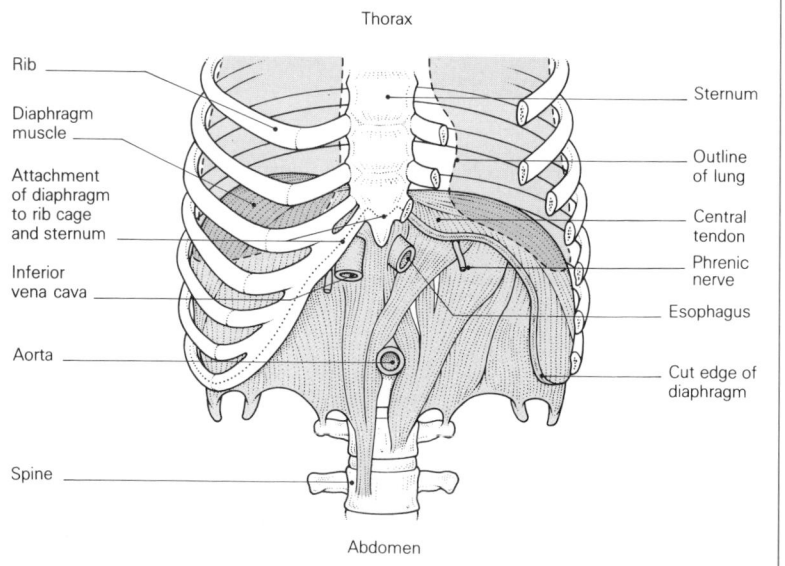

D

DIARRHEA Frequent passing of unusually loose bowel movements.

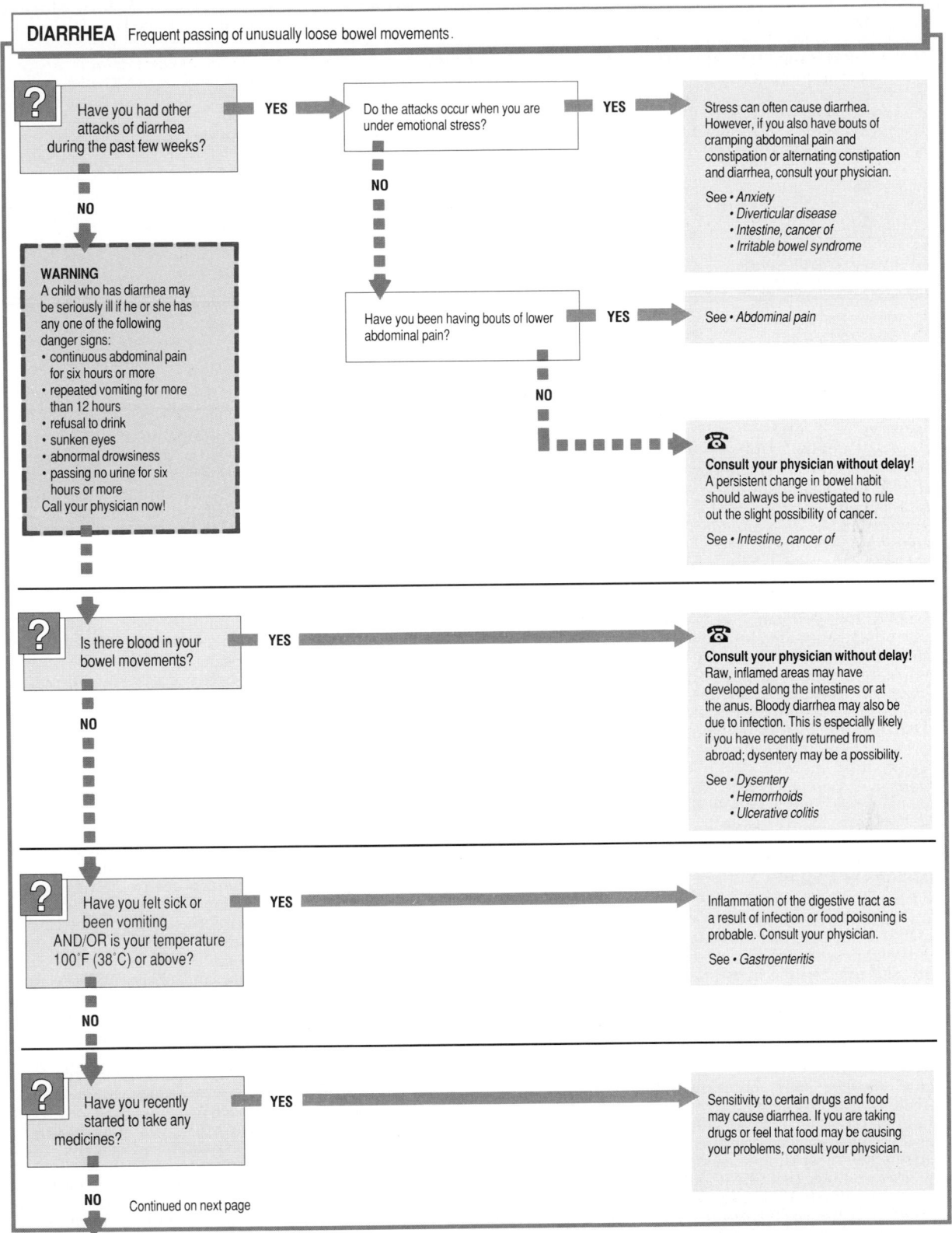

? Have you had other attacks of diarrhea during the past few weeks?

YES → Do the attacks occur when you are under emotional stress?

YES → Stress can often cause diarrhea. However, if you also have bouts of cramping abdominal pain and constipation or alternating constipation and diarrhea, consult your physician.

See • Anxiety
• Diverticular disease
• Intestine, cancer of
• Irritable bowel syndrome

NO (from emotional stress) →

Have you been having bouts of lower abdominal pain?

YES → See • Abdominal pain

NO →

☎ **Consult your physician without delay!**
A persistent change in bowel habit should always be investigated to rule out the slight possibility of cancer.

See • Intestine, cancer of

NO (from first question) →

WARNING
A child who has diarrhea may be seriously ill if he or she has any one of the following danger signs:
• continuous abdominal pain for six hours or more
• repeated vomiting for more than 12 hours
• refusal to drink
• sunken eyes
• abnormal drowsiness
• passing no urine for six hours or more
Call your physician now!

? Is there blood in your bowel movements?

YES → ☎ **Consult your physician without delay!**
Raw, inflamed areas may have developed along the intestines or at the anus. Bloody diarrhea may also be due to infection. This is especially likely if you have recently returned from abroad; dysentery may be a possibility.

See • Dysentery
• Hemorrhoids
• Ulcerative colitis

NO →

? Have you felt sick or been vomiting AND/OR is your temperature 100˚F (38˚C) or above?

YES → Inflammation of the digestive tract as a result of infection or food poisoning is probable. Consult your physician.

See • Gastroenteritis

NO →

? Have you recently started to take any medicines?

YES → Sensitivity to certain drugs and food may cause diarrhea. If you are taking drugs or feel that food may be causing your problems, consult your physician.

NO Continued on next page

D

? Have you eaten anything in the past 24 hours that might have gone bad OR to which you may be allergic?

YES → You may have food poisoning, especially if others who shared the meal with you have the same symptoms.

See • *Food poisoning*

NO

↓

If you are unable to make a diagnosis from this chart and your diarrhea persists for more than 48 hours or recurs, consult your physician.

Persistent diarrhea
If your diarrhea is severe, you may lose a dangerous amount of body fluid. Drink plenty of fluids and consult your physician without delay.

See • *Rehydration therapy*

Diarrhea

Increased fluidity, frequency, or volume of bowel movements, as compared to the usual pattern for a particular person. Diarrhea itself is not a disorder but is a symptom of an underlying problem.

Acute diarrhea affects almost everybody from time to time—usually as the result of eating contaminated food or drinking contaminated water. These attacks normally clear up within a day or two with or without treatment. Chronic diarrhea may be due to a serious intestinal disorder and requires investigation by a physician.

Diarrhea in infants is generally more serious than diarrhea in adults because it is more likely to cause severe, even potentially fatal, *dehydration*. However, elderly people also do not tolerate diarrhea well, and possible dehydration must be anticipated and treated immediately.

DIARRHEA IN ADULTS

In normal bowel activity the colon (large intestine) absorbs much of the water from the food residues (in liquid form) that pass through it, producing semisolid feces. If the intestinal contents pass through the colon too quickly, or if the small intestine is inflamed and secretes fluid into the fecal material, diarrhea may result.

CAUSES

Acute diarrhea starts abruptly and usually lasts from a few hours to two or three days. The most common cause is *food poisoning*. Diarrhea that starts within six hours of eating usually indicates that the food has been contaminated by toxins from *STAPHYLOCOCCUS* or *CLOSTRIDIUM* bac-

teria. If diarrhea develops 12 to 48 hours after eating, it is probably due to contamination by bacteria such as *SALMONELLA* or *CAMPYLOBACTER*, or by a virus such as the rotavirus or Norwalk virus. Infective *gastroenteritis* may also be acquired as a result of droplet infection, with adenoviruses or echoviruses, for example. Acute diarrhea may be caused by interference with the intestinal flora (harmless bacteria in the intestine) as a result of travel to a country where these bacteria are of a different type.

Other causes of acute diarrhea include anxiety and, less commonly, *shigellosis, typhoid* and *paratyphoid*, drug toxicity, *food allergy*, and *food intolerance*. In the case of shigellosis and *amebic dysentery*, there may be blood in the feces.

Chronic diarrhea generally takes the form of repeated attacks of acute diarrhea. Causes include *Crohn's disease, ulcerative colitis, diverticular disease*, cancer of the large intestine (see *Intestine, cancer of*), *thyrotoxicosis*, and *irritable bowel syndrome*. In all of these conditions, except thyrotoxicosis and irritable bowel syndrome, there may be blood in the bowel movements.

TREATMENT

The water and electrolytes (salts) lost during a severe attack of diarrhea need to be replaced to prevent dehydration. An effective means of doing this is to drink water to which salt and sugar have been added. To make up such an oral rehydration solution, dissolve one teaspoon of salt and four teaspoons of sugar (which helps the intestine absorb the water

and salt) in one quart (0.95 liter) of water. It is important to be accurate with the measurements as too much salt may cause further dehydration. Alternatively, it is possible to buy ready-prepared electrolyte mixtures that also contain small amounts of potassium replacement that need only to be added to a specific amount of water. A pint of the oral rehydration liquid should be drunk every hour, and no solid food eaten, until the diarrhea subsides.

Antidiarrheal drugs should not be taken to treat attacks of diarrhea resulting from infection because they may prolong the illness.

Diarrhea that recurs, persists for more than a week, or is accompanied by blood in the bowel movements requires investigation to discover the underlying cause. In addition to taking the patient's case history, the physician will probably arrange for a stool *culture* to determine whether or not infection is the underlying cause. If it is not, other tests may be carried out, such as a barium enema or meal (see *Barium X-ray examinations*), *sigmoidoscopy*, and a *biopsy* of the rectum. These tests enable the physician to discover the underlying cause; treatment will be for that cause.

DIARRHEA IN INFANTS

Most cases of diarrhea in infants are of the acute form, which carries the risk of rapid dehydration (especially when accompanied by vomiting); it can be fatal unless countered quickly.

CAUSES

The most common cause is gastroenteritis resulting from a viral infection. Babies who are entirely breast-fed are

D

less likely to contract the illness than those who have been bottle-fed. Viral gastroenteritis can damage the lining of the small intestine, thereby impairing its ability to absorb nutrients, and can cause a temporary deficiency of the enzyme lactase. The latter may lead to lactose intolerance (inability to absorb sugar from milk), which may produce secondary diarrhea that can last for several weeks.

TREATMENT

An infant who shows signs of dehydration (drowsiness, unresponsiveness, prolonged crying, loose skin, glazed eyes, a depressed fontanelle at the front of the head, and a dry, sticky mouth and tongue) needs urgent medical attention. In other cases, the baby should not be fed milk, and an electrolyte mixture (obtainable from a pharmacist) should be given to replace lost water and salts.

If the diarrhea persists for more than 48 hours, a physician should be consulted. However, if the diarrhea clears up within this period, milk can be gradually reintroduced over a 24-hour period. The first feeding should consist of one part milk to three parts water, the second of equal parts of milk and water, the third of three parts milk to one part water, and the fourth of undiluted milk.

Diastole

The resting period of the heart muscle; it alternates with the period of muscular contraction (*systole*).

Diathermy

The production of heat in a part of the body using high-frequency electric currents, microwaves, or ultrasound. The heat generated can be used to increase blood flow and to reduce deep-seated pain in rheumatic and arthritic conditions. By using large currents, enough heat can be produced to bloodlessly destroy tumors and diseased parts. A diathermy knife is used by surgeons to coagulate bleeding vessels or to separate tissues without causing them to bleed (see *Electrocoagulation*).

Diathesis

A condition of the body that makes the tissues react in a specific way to an outside stimulus. For example, a bleeding diathesis is present when a *bleeding disorder* (such as hemophilia) makes a person susceptible to prolonged bleeding after an injury. A diathesis may be inherited or acquired as a result of an illness.

Diazepam

| BENZODIAZEPINE ANTICONVULSANT MUSCLE RELAXANT | | |

| Tablet Capsule Injection Rectal suppository |
| Prescription needed |
| Available as generic |

One of the best known and most widely used *benzodiazepine* drugs. Diazepam is used mainly to treat anxiety and insomnia. It is also prescribed as a *muscle-relaxant drug* (for example, to treat spasm of the back muscles), and as an *anticonvulsant drug* in the emergency treatment of epileptic seizures. Diazepam is also commonly used to treat the symptoms of alcohol withdrawal.

POSSIBLE ADVERSE EFFECTS

Diazepam may cause drowsiness, dizziness, and confusion; driving and hazardous work should therefore be avoided. Alcohol increases the sedative effect of diazepam and should therefore be avoided during treatment with this drug.

Like other drugs in this group, diazepam can be habit-forming if taken regularly, and its effect may diminish with prolonged use. Individuals who have taken diazepam regularly for more than two weeks should never stop their treatment suddenly. Instead, they should gradually decrease the dose under medical supervision to avoid withdrawal symptoms. Withdrawal symptoms include severe anxiety, sweating, and, in rare circumstances following large doses, seizures.

Dicumarol

An *anticoagulant drug* used to treat venous *thrombosis* and *pulmonary embolism* (blood clot in the lungs). It is also prescribed to prevent formation of an embolism in patients with a heart valve disorder or *arrhythmia* (irregular heart beat), or after heart surgery.

Dicumarol takes three to five days to have its full effect; a faster acting anticoagulant, such as *heparin*, is usually also given during the first few days of treatment. Frequent *blood-clotting tests* (prothrombin times) are usually given during treatment with dicumarol.

POSSIBLE ADVERSE EFFECTS

Adverse effects include flatulence, diarrhea, nausea, and, occasionally, bleeding in some part of the body, which may produce a nosebleed, bruising, or *hematuria*.

Dicyclomine

An *antispasmodic drug* used to relieve abdominal pain in *irritable bowel syndrome* and infantile *colic*. It is also used in the treatment of urinary incontinence caused by *irritable bladder*. Dicyclomine may cause dry mouth, blurred vision, and constipation.

Dideoxycytidine

Originally developed for use as an *anticancer drug*, dideoxycytidine (DDC) has been found to slow the multiplication of the *HIV* virus and is currently under investigation as a treatment for *AIDS*.

Dienestrol

An *estrogen drug* used as a cream to treat atrophic *vaginitis* (dryness of the vagina), which commonly occurs after the *menopause*.

Diet

See *Nutrition*.

Diet and disease

Until comparatively recently, medical concern about diet in Western countries was focused on dietary deficiencies in the poor. Today, however, deficiency diseases are very rare in developed countries (except in alcoholics, in people with malabsorptive intestinal disorders, and in people on extremely restricted diets) but are a major problem in many developing countries. In these countries, starvation or malnutrition may result in *marasmus* or *kwashiorkor*. Specific vitamin deficiencies in childhood may cause *rickets* or blindness due to *keratomalacia*; lack of certain vitamins in adult life may lead to *beriberi*, *pellagra*, or *scurvy*.

In the West, the pendulum has swung the other way, and many common disorders are due partly to overconsumption of certain types of food.

FATS

Virtually all people in developed countries have some degree of *atherosclerosis* (narrowing of arteries by deposits of fatty material), which can lead to cardiovascular diseases (such as *coronary heart disease*, *stroke*, and *peripheral vascular disease*). Most nutritionists believe that a major cause of atherosclerosis is a high level of the chemical *cholesterol* in the blood due to a high intake of saturated *fats*, which are found in meat, eggs, and dairy products. The disease is much less common in countries (such as Japan) in which fat in the diet is minimal and mostly polyunsaturated.

D

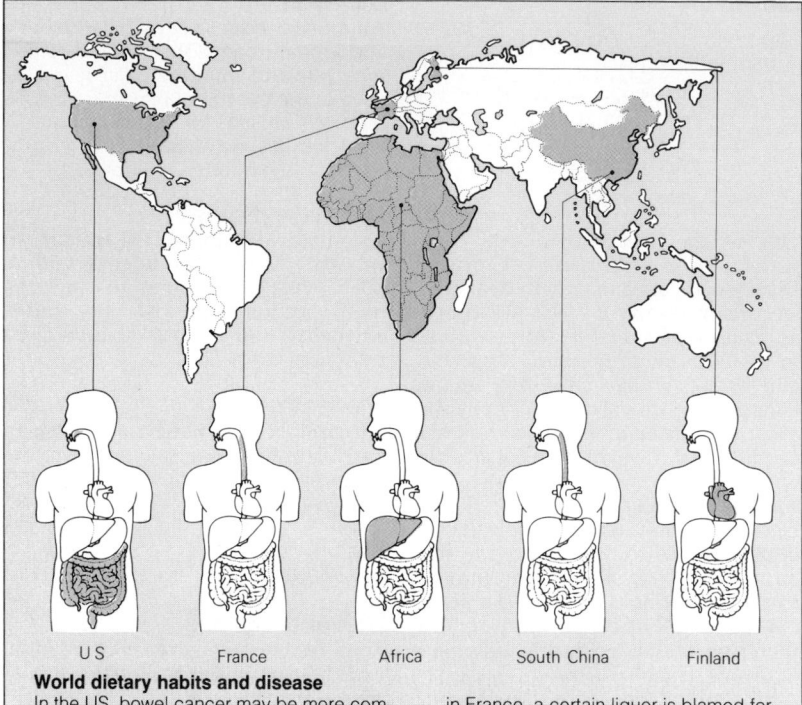

World dietary habits and disease
In the US, bowel cancer may be more common because of high fat, low fiber consumption; dental caries are caused by high sugar intake. Coronary heart disease is common among Finns because of their fatty diets; in France, a certain liquor is blamed for the frequency of esophageal cancer; in South China, certain fungi in food cause esophageal cancer; and in Africa, aflatoxins may cause liver cancer.

U S   France   Africa   South China   Finland

CALORIES

Obesity places a person at greater risk of acquiring serious disorders, such as *diabetes mellitus*, coronary heart disease, stroke, and *osteoarthritis*. Americans are among the most overweight of populations; the cause is simply an excess intake of *calories* (units of energy), mostly in the form of refined carbohydrates (such as are found in white bread, cakes, cookies, candy, and soft drinks), fatty meat and meat products, dairy products, and alcohol.

ALCOHOL

Apart from causing obesity, overconsumption of alcohol can lead to *cirrhosis* of the liver, brain damage (see *Wernicke-Korsakoff syndrome*), peripheral *neuritis*, and *cardiomyopathy*, and has been linked with *pancreatitis*, esophageal cancer (see *Esophagus, cancer of*), and many other disorders.

FIBER

The part played by diet in digestive disorders is less clear than the part played by diet in cardiovascular disease or obesity, but there is evidence suggesting that fiber may be an important factor in some illnesses.

Fiber—found in foods such as wholegrain bread and vegetables—provides bulk to enable the large intestine to work effectively and also helps regulate the absorption of nutrients in the small intestine. Lack of dietary fiber has been implicated in intestinal disorders such as *diverticular disease*, chronic *constipation*, and *hemorrhoids*.

SALT

In Western countries, *hypertension* (high blood pressure) is far more prevalent than in primitive societies. Many nutritionists believe the main reason is the much higher intake of salt in the West. However, it is unlikely that some people would accept the large cut in salt from their diet that would be necessary to have any substantial effect on blood pressure.

DIET AND CANCER

Comparisons of the patterns of cancer in different countries suggest that diet may be as important a factor as tobacco in the cause of cancers. A high intake of fat (and possibly of meat) has been linked with cancer of the bowel (see *Intestines, cancer of*) and the breast (see *Breast cancer*). Moldy foods are known to cause cancer of the

esophagus and liver (see *Liver cancer*), and research groups are examining many other associations.

FOOD ALLERGIES

It is fashionable to ascribe a great deal of illness to food allergy, but in fact the numbers of people in whom disease can definitely be traced to this factor are small. They include those who suffer from *celiac sprue*, as the result of an intolerance to gluten, a protein in cereals; some *migraine* sufferers, in whom foods such as chocolate, cheese, or red wine produce an attack; and people who develop a rash after eating shellfish or soft fruit (see *Urticaria*). In addition, some attacks of *asthma* and *eczema* may be due to an allergy to eggs and dairy products; and an allergy to food additives, such as artificial flavorings and colorings, may be a factor in eczema and *irritable bowel syndrome*. Some physicians believe that allergy to food additives is a major cause of behavioral disorders, such as *hyperactivity* in children, but research evidence suggests that this association is rare. Treatment for self-diagnosed food allergy should always be supervised by a physician.

A PRUDENT DIET

Although the connection between certain types of food and disease has not been proved in all cases, enough evidence exists to indicate that it is wise to make sure your diet is low in fats and refined carbohydrates, high in fiber, and free of artificial additives. (See also *Nutritional disorders*.)

GOOD DIETARY HABITS

Eat fresh rather than preserved, packaged, or convenience foods.

Eat plenty of vegetables and fruit. When raw or lightly cooked, they retain a higher nutritional value.

Eat whole-grain products including whole-grain bread.

Cut down consumption of red meat, instead, eat fish, poultry, and legumes.

Keep the fat content of your diet low and use polyunsaturated fats and vegetable oils rather than saturated fats.

Cut down on sugar in all foods.

When choosing filling foods, eat potatoes in their skins, pasta, or rice.

D

Dietetics

The study of *nutrition* and the application of nutritional science to people both sick and healthy. Dietetics involves not only a detailed knowledge of the composition of foods, the effects of cooking and processing, and dietary requirements, but also psychological aspects, such as eating habits.

Diethylstilbestrol

ESTROGEN		
Tablet Injection Vaginal suppository		
Prescription needed		
Available as generic		

A drug that mimics the natural estrogen hormone *estradiol*; it may be used to replace or supplement estrogen when natural hormone production is abnormal.

WHY IT IS USED

Diethylstilbestrol (DES) is used to treat the symptoms of *hypogonadism* (underdeveloped ovaries), symptoms of the *menopause* (such as hot flashes and sweating), and atrophic *vaginitis* (dryness of the vagina), which is common after the *menopause*.

DES is sometimes prescribed in high doses as a postcoital contraceptive (see *Contraception, postcoital*). It is also useful in the treatment of prostate cancer. It was formerly used as a treatment for threatened miscarriage, but this use has been abandoned as a result of evidence that vaginal cancer may develop many years later in daughters of women who took DES.

POSSIBLE ADVERSE EFFECTS

Side effects are as for other estrogen drugs. DES should not be taken during pregnancy.

Differentiation

The process by which the cells of the early *embryo*, which are almost identical and have not yet taken on any particular function, gradually diversify to form the distinct tissues and organs of the more developed embryo.

In cancer terminology, the word means the degree to which the microscopic appearance of the tissue resembles normal tissue.

Diffusion

The spread of a substance (by movement of its molecules) in a fluid from an area of high concentration to one of lower concentration, thus producing a uniform concentration throughout.

Diflunisal

A *nonsteroidal anti-inflammatory drug* (NSAID) used to relieve joint pain and stiffness in *osteoarthritis, rheumatoid arthritis*, and other types of arthritis. It is also prescribed to treat back pain, sprains, and strains. Occasionally, it is prescribed to ease pain after a minor operation or dental treatment. Diflunisal may cause nausea, indigestion, diarrhea, and a rash.

Digestive system

The group of organs that breaks down food into chemical components that the body can absorb and use for energy and for building and repairing cells and tissues.

The digestive system consists of the digestive tract (also known as the alimentary tract or alimentary canal) and various associated organs. The digestive tract is basically a tube through which food passes; it consists of the *mouth, pharynx* (throat), *esophagus, stomach, intestines* (the small intestine, comprising the *duodenum, jejunum*, and *ileum*, and large intestine, comprising the *cecum, colon*, and *rectum*), and the *anus*. The associated digestive organs—such as the *salivary glands, liver*, and *pancreas*—secrete digestive juices that break down food as it passes through the tract.

Food and digestion products are moved through the intestine, from the throat to the rectum, by *peristalsis* (waves of muscular contractions of the intestinal wall).

THE DIGESTIVE PROCESS

The human diet is made up of foods consisting of nutrients (*vitamins, minerals, carbohydrates, proteins*, and *fats*), residues (mainly vegetable *fiber*), and water. Most vitamins and minerals are absorbed into the bloodstream without change. However, before other nutrients can be absorbed, they must be broken down by digestive agents into simpler substances with smaller molecules.

Part of food breakdown is physical, performed by the teeth, which cut and chew food, and the stomach, which churns it. The rest of the process is chemical, performed by the action of *enzymes*, acids, and salts.

Carbohydrates, which are provided mainly by starchy and sugary foods, are the body's principal source of energy. The digestive process eventually converts all carbohydrates to three simple forms of sugar: glucose, fructose, and galactose.

Proteins, which are found in abundance in meat, fish, eggs, cheese, peas, beans, and lentils, are essential for the replacement and repair of cells. They are broken down into *polypeptides, peptides*, and *amino acids*.

Fats (also known as lipids), which are found not only in meat and dairy products, but also in oily plant foods such as peanuts, provide energy and some of the materials for cell building and maintenance. Fats also carry the fat-soluble vitamins A, D, E, and K. When fats are digested by lipases (enzymes that are secreted by the pancreas and intestine), they are broken down into *glycerol*, glycerides, and *fatty acids*.

The digestive process begins in the mouth, where the teeth chop food and the salivary glands secrete saliva, which lubricates the food and contains enzymes that begin to break down carbohydrates. The mouth also contains sensory nerves in the taste buds on the tongue. The tongue manipulates food in the mouth and forms it into small balls for easy swallowing.

From the mouth, food passes into the pharynx, which then pushes it into the esophagus. The esophagus does not contribute to the breakdown or absorption of food products; its sole function is to squeeze food down into the stomach. In the stomach, food is mixed with acids and digestive juices produced in the stomach lining; these help break down proteins. The stomach also breaks down food mechanically by its continual churning action. When the food has been converted to a semiliquid consistency, it passes into the duodenum.

The liver produces bile salts and acids, which are stored in the gallbladder and then released into the duodenum. These salts and acids help break down fats. The pancreas also releases digestive juices into the duodenum, and these juices contain enzymes that further break down carbohydrates, fats, and proteins. The final breakdown stages are completed in the small intestine, carried out by enzymes produced by glands in the lining of the intestine.

As the breakdown products of digestion pass through the small intestine, they are absorbed by its thin lining and pass into the bloodstream or the lymphatic system.

Finally food passes into the large intestine, where most of the water it contains is absorbed by the lining of the colon. Undigested matter and sloughed lining cells from the digestive tract are then expelled via the rectum and anus as feces.

D

THE DIGESTIVE PROCESS

Digestion starts when food enters the mouth. It continues as the food is propelled through the digestive tract by waves of muscular contractions (peristalsis). The digestive process also involves other organs (the salivary glands, liver, gallbladder, and pancreas), which produce enzymes and acids that help break down the food.

ACTION OF DIGESTIVE AGENTS

Agent or enzyme (where produced)	Digestive action
Amylase (mouth and pancreas)	Converts starch (a form of carbohydrate) to maltose
Sucrase, maltase, and lactase (pancreas and small intestine)	Break down vegetable and milk sugars into glucose, fructose, and galactose
Hydrochloric acid (stomach) Pepsin (stomach) Trypsin (pancreas) Peptidase (small intestine)	Assist in the breakdown of proteins into polypeptides, peptides, and amino acids
Lipase (pancreas) Bile salts and acids (liver—stored in the gallbladder)	Break down fats into glycerol, glycerides, and fatty acids

TIME SCALE

The approximate period food spends in each part of the digestive system is shown below.

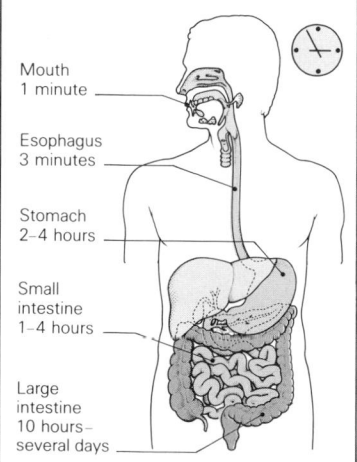

Mouth
1 minute

Esophagus
3 minutes

Stomach
2–4 hours

Small intestine
1–4 hours

Large intestine
10 hours–several days

Bolus

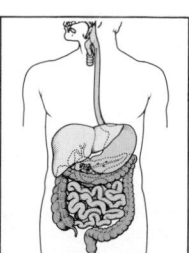

Swallowing

In the mouth, food is cut and ground by the teeth and mixed with saliva, which softens food and breaks down certain carbohydrates. After swallowing, the food mass (bolus) enters the esophagus.

Esophagus
Food is carried down the esophagus by peristaltic action and enters the stomach.

Stomach
Food is broken down further by churning and by the action of hydrochloric acid and digestive enzymes secreted by the stomach lining. Food remains in the stomach until it is reduced to a semiliquid consistency (chyme), when it passes into the duodenum.

Gallbladder

Bile duct

Pancreas

Duodenum
As food travels along the duodenum, it is broken down further by digestive enzymes from the liver, gallbladder, and pancreas. The duodenum leads directly into the small intestine.

Small intestine
Additional enzymes secreted by glands in the lining of the small intestine complete the digestive process. Nutrients are absorbed through the intestinal lining into the network of blood vessels and lymph vessels supplying the intestine. Undigested matter passes into the large intestine (the colon).

Colon
Water in the undigested matter leaving the small intestine is absorbed through the lining of the colon. The residue passes into the rectum.

Rectum
Undigested matter enters this final part of the large intestine and is expelled.

Anus

DISORDERS

Digestive system disorders include a large number of conditions that disrupt the digestive process, either because they obstruct or prevent the passage of food along the digestive tract, or because they interfere with the breakdown or absorption of nutrients. Other conditions may have little effect on digestion but produce distressing symptoms such as difficulty swallowing, heartburn, flatulence, abdominal pain, diarrhea, constipation, or rectal bleeding.

The disease processes causing such disorders range from congenital abnormalities and inherited biochemical defects to inflammatory and autoimmune disorders, tumors, viral, bacterial, and parasitic infections, and chronic allergic conditions. (See also disorder boxes for *Mouth, Esophagus, Stomach, Liver, Gallbladder, Pancreas,* and *Intestines.*)

Digitalis drugs

A group of drugs extracted from the leaves of plants belonging to the foxglove family. They are used to treat various heart conditions. The most commonly used drugs in this group are *digoxin* and *digitoxin*.

Digital subtraction angiography

See *Angiography*.

Digitoxin

A *digitalis drug*, digitoxin is used to treat *heart failure* (reduced pumping efficiency) and certain types of *arrhythmia* (irregular heart beat). Digitoxin is usually prescribed as an alternative to *digoxin* for patients with kidney disease.

Digoxin

DIGITALIS
Tablet Capsule Liquid
Prescription needed
Available as generic

The most widely used of the *digitalis drugs*, digoxin is used in the treatment of *heart failure* (reduced pumping efficiency) and certain types of *arrhythmia* (irregular heart beat), such as *atrial fibrillation* (a rapid, irregular beating of the heart muscle).

HOW IT WORKS

Digoxin increases the force of heart muscle contractions, making the heart work more efficiently. It also slows down abnormally rapid nerve impulses as they pass between the atria (upper chambers of the heart) to the ventricles (main chambers of the heart), which allows the ventricles time to fill up with blood and empty normally with each contraction.

POSSIBLE ADVERSE EFFECTS

If digoxin is to be effective, the dose must be just below that of a toxic dose. The patient must therefore be given regular blood tests to ascertain the digoxin level. An excessive dose may cause loss of appetite, nausea, vomiting, and headache. Digoxin occasionally interferes with the normal heart beat, causing *heart block* (an abnormally slow rate of contraction).

Adverse effects are more likely if the potassium level in the body is low. Patients who are also taking *diuretic drugs* (and therefore are more likely to become deficient in potassium) are given regular blood tests to monitor potassium levels.

Because digoxin is removed from the body mainly in the urine, patients with kidney disease are usually given *digitoxin* as an alternative drug because of the risk of a buildup of toxic levels of digoxin.

Dilatation

A condition in which a body cavity, tube, or opening is enlarged or stretched as a result of normal physiological processes (as in dilatation of the pupil), or because of disease (as in dilatation of the heart). Dilatation also refers to the process of achieving such enlargement, as in surgical procedures such as *D and C* (dilatation and curettage) of the cervix. Also called dilation.

Dilatation and curettage

See *D and C*.

Dilator

An instrument for stretching and enlarging a narrowed body cavity, tube, or opening.

Diltiazem

A *calcium channel blocker drug* used in the treatment of *hypertension* (high blood pressure) and *angina pectoris* (chest pain due to impaired blood supply to heart muscle). Taken regularly, diltiazem often reduces the frequency of angina attacks, but does not act quickly enough to relieve pain in an acute attack.

Diltiazem may cause headache, appetite loss, nausea, constipation, and ankle swelling.

Dimenhydrinate

An *antihistamine drug* used as an *antiemetic drug* to relieve nausea and vomiting caused by a number of disorders. Dimenhydrinate is especially effective when these symptoms occur with vertigo (dizziness with loss of balance)—for example, in *motion sickness*. It may also be used to relieve nausea and vomiting in early pregnancy. Like other antihistamine drugs, dimenhydrinate has a sedative effect that can be dangerous when operating machinery or driving.

Dioxin

A toxic defoliant chemical (see *Defoliant poisoning*).

Diphenhydramine

An *antihistamine drug* used to treat allergic disorders such as *urticaria* (hives) and allergic *rhinitis* (hay fever). It is given by injection to treat *anaphylactic shock* (a severe allergic reaction), which may occur, for example, as a result of an insect sting.

Diphenhydramine is also prescribed as an *antiemetic drug* to relieve nausea and vomiting in pregnancy and to prevent *motion sickness*. It is used as an ingredient in some *cough remedies* because of its cough suppressant effect. It has also been used to control abnormal movements in *Parkinson's disease*.

POSSIBLE ADVERSE EFFECTS

Diphenhydramine often causes drowsiness and, because of its sedative effect, has occasionally been used to treat insomnia. Driving and hazardous work should be avoided if the drug is causing sedation. Other possible side effects include dry mouth and blurred vision.

Diphenoxylate

An *antidiarrheal drug* (used to relieve diarrhea) chemically related to the narcotic *analgesics* (morphinelike painkillers). Diphenoxylate works by reducing the contractions of the muscles in the walls of the intestine, thus slowing down the frequency of bowel movements.

POSSIBLE ADVERSE EFFECTS

In normal doses, drowsiness and abdominal pain occur in rare instances. When taken in high doses, diphenoxylate produces euphoria due to its narcotic ingredient. Adding *atropine* to the preparation prevents abuse; a dose high enough to produce euphoria causes unpleasant side effects, such as dry mouth, flushing, blurred vision, and vomiting.

D

Diphtheria

An acute bacterial illness that causes a sore throat and a fever, and sometimes causes more serious or even fatal complications. Diphtheria was one of the most important causes of childhood death worldwide until the 1930s, but, since then, mass immunization has made it extremely rare in the US and other developed countries. However, diphtheria is still a hazard for people living in poor developing countries and is a particular risk for nonimmunized people who travel to such countries.

CAUSES AND INCIDENCE

Diphtheria is caused by the bacillus *CORYNEBACTERIUM DIPHTHERIAE*. It may live in the skin or in the nose of a person immune to the disease or, during an infection, may multiply in the throat or skin. Serious complications are caused by a toxin released by the bacterium into the bloodstream.

The few cases that occur in the US are invariably among immigrants from poor developing countries. In these countries, the disease is usually caught from a healthy "carrier" of diphtheria bacilli, who harbors the organisms in his or her nose or skin and spreads them through the air or by touch. These carriers have acquired immunity to the illness, having in the past recovered from a relatively mild infection.

SYMPTOMS

When a nonimmune person is infected by the bacterium spread from a carrier, the bacterium usually multiplies in the throat, giving rise to a membrane that appears over the tonsils and may spread over the palate or downward to the larynx (voice box) and trachea (windpipe). This may cause breathing difficulties and a husky voice. Other symptoms include enlarged lymph glands in the neck, an increased heart rate, and mild fever. Sometimes, an infection is confined to the skin, where it may cause no more than a few yellow spots or sores with an appearance similar to *impetigo*.

Life-threatening symptoms develop only in nonimmune people and are caused by the bacterial toxin. Occasionally, victims collapse and die within a day or so of getting the throat infection. More often they are recovering from this condition when heart failure or paralysis of the throat or limbs develops. These later complications can occur up to seven weeks after onset of infection in the throat. If victims survive the disease they make a complete recovery.

PREVENTION

In the US and other developed countries, the triple vaccine, also known as the *DPT vaccine* (against diphtheria, pertussis, and tetanus), is given routinely to children in the first year of life. The practice of immunizing against diphtheria must continue, despite the extreme rarity of the disease in these countries, because carriers can arrive from developing countries at any time; if large numbers of children were not immune, there could be a disastrous epidemic.

Those traveling to poor, developing countries who are in doubt as to whether they were immunized against diphtheria as children should have their immune status checked or simply be vaccinated.

Spread of effective immunization programs to all countries could eventually eradicate diphtheria (as smallpox has been eradicated), although this possibility is not envisaged at present.

TREATMENT

Penicillin kills diphtheria organisms in the throat, but is ineffective against the toxin in the blood. If the disease is suspected, an *antitoxin* (derived from the blood of immunized horses) must be given as soon as possible in addition to penicillin. If severe breathing difficulties develop in a patient, a *tracheostomy* (surgical introduction of a breathing tube into the windpipe) may be necessary.

Victims are kept in isolation until no diphtheria bacilli can be detected in the nose and throat (by swabs taken on six consecutive days).

Diplopia

The medical term for *double vision*.

Dipsomania

A form of *alcohol dependence* in which periods of excessive drinking and craving for drink alternate with periods of relative sobriety.

Dipyridamole

A drug that reduces the stickiness of platelets (cells in the blood that aid blood clotting) and, as a result, helps prevent the formation of abnormal blood clotting within the arteries. Possible adverse effects include headache, flushing, and dizziness.

Disability

Temporary loss or permanent impairment of a faculty, such as weakness of a limb or loss of sight. The distinction between disability and *handicap* is vague, and in practice the two terms are often used interchangeably. However, disability is sometimes defined as the physical disorder, and handicap as the extent to which a disorder impairs normal functioning. Thus two people with the same disability—blindness, for example—may suffer different degrees of handicap because one person manages to cope with everyday living better than the other. (See also illustrated box showing aids for the disabled; *Rehabilitation*.)

Discharge

Visible emission of fluid from a body cavity, such as the nose. Discharge may be part of the cavity's normal function, as in some types of *vaginal discharge*—during pregnancy, for instance. Alternatively, it may be due to infection or inflammation of the lining of the cavity, as in *rhinitis* (inflammation of the lining of the nose), *urethritis* (infection of the urethra, the tube that carries urine from the bladder to outside the body), *proctitis* (infection of the rectum), or *vaginitis* (infection of the vagina).

Disclosing agents

Dyes that make the plaque deposits on teeth more visible so that they can be seen and removed. As part of oral hygiene advice, the dentist or hygienist may apply a disclosing solution to the teeth to show the presence of harmful dental *plaque* and pellicle (a thin protein film), and to demonstrate an effective method of tooth cleaning.

Plaque revealed by disclosing agent
The plaque appears here as the dark areas on the teeth near the gums. Plaque consists of bacteria, mucus, and food debris; it builds up quickly if the teeth are not brushed and flossed regularly.

D

AIDS FOR THE DISABLED

There are a variety of articles that are specially designed or adapted to assist disabled people in performing everyday activities. Aids include prostheses, supports, and mobility aids that enable people to function more efficiently, as well as equipment designed to help them perform specific tasks more easily.

Devices that help vision, hearing, and movement improve the ability of disabled people to cope with all aspects of everyday life. Such devices include walkers, glasses, hearing aids, artificial limbs, corsets, and wheelchairs. Ventilators, home dialysis, and enteral and parenteral feeding devices are life-sustaining aids.

There are various household aids available that can help people cook, feed and dress themselves, wash and use the toilet, and get in and out of beds and chairs. Specially designed furniture and devices can help disabled parents care for their children; sexual aids can facilitate an active sexual life.

Faucet turner
Helps grip and turn faucet.

Tongs
Extending grippers to pick up dropped items. Closes up to fit in pocket or purse.

Bottle opener
A small hand-held device designed to grip and open small bottle tops.

Cutlery
A range of knives, forks, and spoons with thick, molded handles for easy manipulating.

Toothpaste extruder
A wall-mounted device that dispenses toothpaste with minimal finger pressure.

Scissors
Self-opening scissors with easy-grip handles.

"A" frame
A lightweight walker that doubles as a seat and can be folded flat.

Discolored teeth

Teeth tend naturally to darken with age. The red pulp tissue in the center of the tooth, which makes young teeth look bright, gradually recedes while at the same time more dentin is laid down around it, resulting in the tooth's dull yellow color.

Both the tooth's surface and its internal structures are liable to be stained by a variety of substances brought to the mouth or carried by the blood supply. Extrinsic stains, those found on the tooth's surface, are common, but are easily removed by polishing and can be prevented by regular tooth-cleaning. Intrinsic stains, those within the tooth's substance, are permanent. Many stains, both extrinsic and intrinsic, can be covered or diminished with the newer cosmetic dental procedures that are available in the dentist's office.

EXTRINSIC STAINS

BROWNISH-BLACK DEPOSIT or TOBACCO STAIN Usually found on the inside surfaces of the teeth, this staining is due to the accumulation of tars and resins.

BLACK STAIN A firmly attached, black or brown line, close to and following the contour of the gum, usually on the inside surfaces of the upper back teeth. More common in children, it is thought to be due to pigment-producing bacteria.

GREEN STAIN A heavy, "furry," grayish-green stain, firmly attached close to the gum, usually on the front surfaces of the upper front teeth. It is most commonly found in children and may be due to staining of remnants of developmental membrane by color-producing bacteria.

DULL YELLOW STAIN May be due to discoloration of *plaque* by dyes in foodstuffs; it is easily removed.

BROWN STAIN A thin, dark line near the gum, formed from little dots of pigmented plaque usually colored by iron salts taken internally or that come into contact with the mouth.

ORANGE-RED STAIN May be caused by pigment-producing bacteria; it is easily removed.

STAINED DENTIN With advancing age the full thickness of enamel may be worn away in parts and the dentin becomes stained by dyes in foods.

METALLIC STAINING May follow the use of medicines containing metallic salts. Iron-containing liquids stain the teeth brown. Inhalation of metallic dust by metal workers (prior to stringent safety measures) caused accumulation of metals in the plaque. Brass, copper, lead, bronze, and other copper alloys caused a bluish-green stain, iron produced brown staining, and mercury led to black staining.

D

INTRINSIC STAINS

BLACK TEETH Teeth may darken following the death of the pulp or the removal of the pulp during root canal treatment. This is caused by the decomposition of red blood cells that pass from damaged blood vessels in the pulp into the dentin.

TETRACYCLINE STAINING This antibiotic is absorbed by developing teeth and causes discoloration of primary or permanent teeth. Which teeth are affected depends on the stage of tooth development at the time it is absorbed, the amount taken, and the type of tetracycline prescribed. Tetracycline given to a pregnant woman often causes discoloration of her child's teeth. If mildly affected, the teeth will appear yellow but, if severely affected, they will be brown or blue-violet.

After the age of 7 years, discoloration is not such a problem, because all the cosmetically important teeth are already formed.

FLUOROSIS A mottling of the tooth enamel occurs if excessive amounts of fluoride are taken during development of the enamel (see *Fluorosis*).

Disinfectants

Substances that kill microorganisms and thus prevent infection. The term is usually applied to strong chemicals that are harmful to human tissue and so are used to decontaminate inanimate objects, such as pieces of equipment. Decontaminants that are safe for human tissue are called *antiseptics*.

Disk, intervertebral

A flat, circular, platelike structure containing *cartilage* that lines the surfaces of the ends of bones in the joints between adjacent vertebrae throughout the length of the spine.

Each of the intervertebral disks is composed of a hard, outer layer and a soft, jellylike core. The material acts as a shock absorber to cushion the vertebrae during movements of the spine, and to minimize jarring when jumping or running. With increasing age, intervertebral disks can wear out, becoming less supple and more susceptible to damage from injury. One of the most common forms of damage is a *disk prolapse*, in which part of the disk's soft center bulges out through a weak area in the hard, outer layer. This may compress a spinal nerve root and produce symptoms (such as interference with muscle strength and/or pain in the back and leg) along the course of the nerve.

Diskography

A diagnostic technique in which a dye visible on *X-ray* films is injected into an invertebral disk, one of the shock-absorbing structures between the vertebrae (bones of the spine).

WHY IT IS DONE

The technique is one of the methods used to diagnose *disk prolapse*. Ordinary X-ray films fail to reveal disks, which show on the film only as spaces between the vertebrae.

HOW IT IS DONE

After a local anesthetic has been given, a long thin needle is passed through the skin into the disk under X-ray control, dye is injected into the disk, and X-ray pictures are taken. Occasionally the site of the injection is sore afterward, but the pain usually clears up quickly.

RESULTS

The image obtained provides only a rough outline of the disk, but reveals clearly any leakage of dye, proving that the disk is ruptured. In some people the rupture may be due to small tears in the disk rather than a prolapse. However, if the procedure itself causes pain in the spine, and sciatica (pain down the back of a leg) or arm pain, it indicates a strong possibility of prolapse.

Because of its relative imprecision, diskography is of more limited use than *CT scanning* or *myelography*.

Disk prolapse

A common, painful disorder of the spine in which an intervertebral disk ruptures and part of its pulpy core protrudes. Disk prolapse causes a painful and at times disabling pressure on a nerve.

About 95 percent of disk prolapses occur in the lower back, but they can affect any part of the back or the neck.

CAUSES AND INCIDENCE

Although a prolapsed disk may sometimes be caused by a sudden strenuous action (such as lifting a heavy weight or twisting violently), it usually develops gradually as the result of disks degenerating with age.

People between the ages of 30 and 40 are the most likely to suffer from the disorder. Over the age of 30, disks start to dehydrate and become less resilient but, after 40, extra fibrous tissue forms around them, increasing their stability.

Disk prolapses are slightly more common in men than women, and their incidence is higher in people who spend long periods sitting without a break.

DIAGNOSIS

Many other disorders may cause back and leg pain or neck and arm pain, and various tests may be needed to arrive at a firm diagnosis. After the physician has examined the spine and tested movement and reflexes in the affected arm or leg, he or she may arrange for tests, including the following: *X rays, CT scanning, myelography* (the injection into the fluid around the spinal cord of a dye visible on X rays), *diskography* (the injection of the same dye into a disk), and electromyography (tests of electrical activity in muscles; see *EMG*).

If a certain nerve root is suspected of being compressed, a local anesthetic may be injected into its lining; if this relieves the pain, the location of the trouble is confirmed.

OUTLOOK

In most cases treatment without surgery clears the pain, but the pain tends to recur. An operation is performed when muscle function is impaired.

Dislocation, joint

Complete displacement of the two bones in a joint so that they are no longer in contact, usually as a result of injury. (Displacement that leaves the bones in partial contact is called *subluxation*.) Dislocation is usually accompanied by tearing of the joint ligaments and damage to the joint capsule (the membrane that encases the joint); it is the tearing that makes the injury so painful. Injury severe enough to cause dislocation often also causes fracture of one or both of the bones involved.

SYMPTOMS AND COMPLICATIONS

Dislocation restricts or prevents the movement of the joint and is usually accompanied by severe pain. The joint looks misshapen and soon swells. In some cases, dislocation is followed by complications. For example, dislocation of the spinal vertebrae resulting from a severe back injury can damage the spinal cord, sometimes causing paralysis below the point of injury. Dislocation of the shoulder or hip joint can damage major nerves in the arm or leg, again sometimes resulting in paralysis.

Rarely, the tissue around a dislocated joint, usually the shoulder, becomes so weakened that after the joint has mended only minimal pressure causes another dislocation.

TREATMENT

SELF-HELP A medically unqualified person should not attempt to manipulate the joint back into position because of

SYMPTOMS AND TREATMENT OF DISK PROLAPSE

A prolapsed disk in the lower back causes low back pain and, if the sciatic nerve root is compressed, *sciatica* (pain running down the back of the leg from the buttock to the ankle), sometimes accompanied by numbness and tingling. Low back pain and sciatica are usually aggravated by coughing, sneezing, bending, and sitting for long periods. Prolonged pressure on the sciatic nerve can lead to weakness in the muscles of the leg.

A prolapsed disk in the neck causes neck pain, stiffness, and, if the root of a nerve that is in the arm is compressed, tingling and weakness in that arm and hand.

In rare cases, pressure is exerted on the spinal cord itself, sometimes leading to paralysis of the legs and loss of bladder or bowel control.

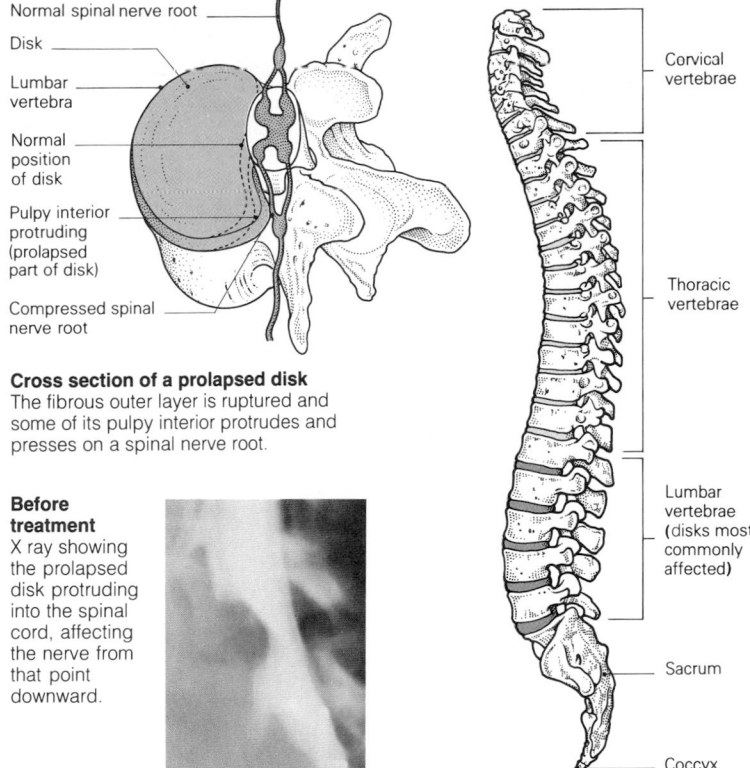

Normal spinal nerve root
Disk
Lumbar vertebra
Normal position of disk
Pulpy interior protruding (prolapsed part of disk)
Compressed spinal nerve root

Cervical vertebrae
Thoracic vertebrae
Lumbar vertebrae (disks most commonly affected)
Sacrum
Coccyx

Cross section of a prolapsed disk
The fibrous outer layer is ruptured and some of its pulpy interior protrudes and presses on a spinal nerve root.

Before treatment
X ray showing the prolapsed disk protruding into the spinal cord, affecting the nerve from that point downward.

TREATMENT
Disk prolapse often responds to bed rest (lying flat on the back on a firm mattress for a few weeks) and analgesics; later, a supportive collar or corset and special exercises are helpful. If these measures fail and the nerve root compression is producing muscle weakness, an operation may relieve the pressure (see *Decompression, spinal canal*).

Shoulders, hips, and ankles should be aligned to ease pressure on spine

the risk of seriously damaging nerves around the joint or making an accompanying fracture worse. Movement of the joint should be prevented by means of a *splint* or, in the case of a dislocated shoulder, a *sling* on the arm. No food or drink should be taken, because a general anesthetic is usually required to reset the bones.

PROFESSIONAL The joint is usually X-rayed first to see whether a fracture is present. Then the bones are manipulated back into their proper position as quickly as possible, or, when manipulation is not feasible, an operation may be performed to reset them. After either procedure, the joint is usually immobilized by means of a splint or plaster cast to allow it to heal without disturbance. Recurrent dislocation is treated by surgery to shorten and tighten the ligaments of the joint, thus strengthening it.

Disopyramide

An *antiarrhythmic drug* used to treat abnormally rapid heart beats (for example, following *myocardial infarction*). Disopyramide reduces the force of heart muscle contraction and, as a result, may occasionally aggravate preexisting heart failure. This drug may also cause dry mouth, constipation, and blurred vision.

Disorientation

Confusion over time, place, or personal identity. The experience is similar to being awakened from a deep sleep. Disorientation is usually caused by head injury, intoxication, or a chronic brain disorder such as *dementia*.

The disoriented person's speech and behavior tend to be muddled, and he or she is often unable to answer simple questions about time, date, present whereabouts, or name and address. Although *hysteria* or inattention may cause such symptoms, if disorientation comes on suddenly, the cause is almost always an organic brain disease. (See also *Delirium*.)

Displacement activity

The transference of feelings from one object or person to another. This is usually a conscious act, performed to obtain emotional relief in a manner that will not cause harm to oneself or to another person. For example, a person who is angry may hit a wall or throw something rather than risk harming someone else.

Psychoanalysts regard displacement as an unconscious *defense mechanism*. Disturbing or unwelcome

D

feelings are prevented from entering consciousness by being transferred onto another person or object. An understanding of this unconscious process is an important part of the interpretation of a patient's dreams during psychoanalysis.

Dissociative disorders

A group of psychological illnesses in which a particular mental function becomes cut off from the mind as a whole. While the process of dissociation is common in everyday life (for example, not hearing what is said because of intense concentration on another task), when taken to extremes it can lead to serious problems.

A common type of dissociative disorder is hysterical amnesia. The affected person is unable to remember his or her name or personal history, but can still speak, read, and learn new material (see *Hysteria*). Other forms of this disorder are *fugue*, *depersonalization*, and *multiple personality*. (See also *Conversion disorder*.)

Distal

Describing a part of the body that is farther away from a central point of reference, such as the trunk of the body. For example, the fingers are distal to the arm with the trunk as the point of reference. The opposite of distal is *proximal*.

Disulfiram

A drug that acts as a deterrent to drinking alcohol, disulfiram is prescribed for people who request help for an alcohol problem. Treatment with disulfiram is usually combined with a counseling program (see *Alcohol dependence*).

HOW IT WORKS
Alcohol is normally converted in the liver to acetaldehyde, which in turn is broken down to form acetic acid. Disulfiram reduces the breakdown of acetaldehyde, resulting in an increased level of this toxic substance and causing flushing, headache, nausea, dizziness, and palpitations.

These unpleasant symptoms generally start within an hour of drinking alcohol after taking disulfiram and can last for several hours.

POSSIBLE ADVERSE EFFECTS
Drowsiness and a metallic or garlic taste in the mouth frequently occur. These symptoms usually disappear within a few days as the body adapts to the drug.

Occasionally, large amounts of alcohol taken during treatment can cause unconsciousness, so a warning card indicating the person is taking disulfiram should be carried.

Diuretic drugs

COMMON DRUGS
Thiazide
Chlorothiazide Hydrochlorothiazide Metolazone
Loop
Bumetanide Furosemide
Potassium-sparing
Amiloride Spironolactone Triamterene

A group of drugs that helps remove excess water from the body by increasing the amount lost in the urine.

TYPES
The different types of diuretic drug vary markedly in their speed and mode of action.

THIAZIDE DIURETICS These diuretics cause moderate diuresis (increased urine production) and are suitable for prolonged use.

LOOP DIURETICS So called because they act on the region of the kidneys called Henle's loop, these are fast-acting, powerful drugs, especially when given by injection. Loop diuretics are particularly useful as an emergency treatment for heart failure.

POTASSIUM-SPARING DIURETICS These drugs are often used with thiazide and loop diuretics, both of which may cause potassium deficiency.

CARBONIC ANHYDRASE INHIBITORS Drugs that block the action of carbonic anhydrase (an enzyme that affects the amount of bicarbonate ions in the blood); these diuretics cause a moderate diuresis, but are effective only for short periods.

OSMOTIC DIURETICS These powerful diuretics are used to maintain urine production after serious injury or major surgery.

WHY THEY ARE USED
By increasing the production of urine, diuretic drugs reduce the amount of water in the circulation and thus reduce the *edema* (fluid retention) that causes breathlessness and ankle swelling in *heart failure*, *nephrotic syndrome* (a kidney disorder), *cirrhosis* of the liver, and bloating and breast tenderness before *menstruation*.

Diuretic drugs also lower the blood pressure and thus are used in the treatment of *hypertension* (high blood

HOW DIURETICS WORK

The normal filtration process of the kidneys (which takes place in the tubules) removes water, salts (mainly potassium and sodium), and waste products from the bloodstream. Most of the salts and water are returned to the bloodstream, but certain amounts are expelled from the body along with the waste products in the urine.

Diuretic drugs interfere with this normal kidney action. Osmotic, loop, and thiazide diuretics reduce the amount of sodium and water taken back into the blood, thus increasing urine volume. Other diuretics increase blood flow through the kidneys and thus the amount of water they filter and expel in the urine.

Osmotic diuretics
Act on the first part of the tubules to reduce water reabsorption.

Loop diuretics
Take effect on the middle part of the tubules and block sodium and chloride reabsorption.

Thiazide diuretics
Act on the last part of the tubules to reduce the loss of sodium into the bloodstream.

pressure). Carbonic anhydrase inhibitors are sometimes used to treat *glaucoma* (increased fluid pressure in the eyeball).

POSSIBLE ADVERSE EFFECTS

Diuretic drugs may cause chemical imbalances in the blood, most commonly hypokalemia (low blood potassium). Symptoms of this condition include weakness, confusion, and palpitations. Treatment usually consists of a course of potassium supplements or a potassium-sparing diuretic drug. A diet rich in potassium (containing plenty of fruits and vegetables) may be helpful.

Some diuretic drugs may increase the level of uric acid in the blood, and thus the risk of *gout*. Certain types of diuretics increase the blood sugar level, an effect that can cause or aggravate *diabetes mellitus*.

Diverticular disease

The presence of diverticula (small sacs caused by the protrusions of the inner lining of the intestine or other hollow organs) and any symptoms or complications caused by their presence.

Diverticula may form in any part of the intestines but usually affect the lower part of the colon (the main section of the large intestine). The cause is not conclusively established, but diverticula are thought to arise when pressure forces the lining of the colon through areas of weakness in the intestinal wall. Diverticulosis merely signifies the presence of diverticula in the colon. Diverticulitis is a complication produced by inflammation due to obstruction and, occasionally, perforation (formation of a hole) in one or more diverticula.

DIVERTICULOSIS

Diverticulosis is rare in developing countries, but in Western Europe and the US it affects more than half the population by the age of 80. Its incidence increases progressively with age, being rare before the age of 20. Lack of adequate dietary fiber or roughage is believed to play an important role in its development.

SYMPTOMS

Symptoms occur in only 20 percent of patients with diverticulosis and usually result from spasm or cramp of the intestinal muscle near diverticula. Many patients have symptoms of *irritable bowel syndrome*, which may coexist with diverticulosis. In such patients, symptoms include a bloated sensation, episodes of pain in the lower abdomen, and changes in bowel habits, such as constipation, diarrhea,

or alternating attacks of both. Complications, which are uncommon, include hemorrhage (indicated by bleeding from the rectum), diverticulitis, and stricture formation (narrowing of the intestine). A physician should rule out the possibility of cancer in patients with symptoms of diverticulosis; tumors developing in areas affected by diverticulosis may be difficult to diagnose.

DIAGNOSIS

Diverticula are easily diagnosed by *barium X-ray examination* of the colon or by *colonoscopy* (visual examination via a flexible, fiberoptic instrument).

X ray showing diverticulosis
In this X ray taken after a barium meal, the bright, winding tube is the patient's colon. The knobs on its outer surface are diverticula.

TREATMENT

In patients with muscle spasms that cause cramps, a high-fiber diet, fiber supplements, and *antispasmodic drugs* may abolish symptoms. A high-fiber diet has also been shown to reduce the incidence of complications. Bleeding from diverticula usually subsides without treatment, but occasionally requires surgical treatment such as that for diverticulitis. Otherwise, surgery is rarely necessary.

DIVERTICULITIS

Inflammation and perforation of diverticula cause fever, pain, tenderness, and rigidity of the abdomen over the area of the intestine involved. Rarely, a large abscess can form in the tissues around the colon; it may be felt as a tender lump when a physician examines the abdomen. In exceptional circumstances, perforation may lead to *peritonitis* (inflammation of the lining of the abdomen). Complications of diverticulitis may also include the development of a stricture (narrowing of the intestine) at the site of the inflammation or of a fistula (narrow channel) connecting one part of the intestine to another.

TREATMENT

Diverticulitis usually subsides with bed rest and antibiotics. If the symptoms are severe, treatment may also include a liquid diet or intravenous fluids when oral feeding must be temporarily stopped. Surgical treatment may be needed if perforation causes a large abscess or peritonitis, if a tight stricture develops, or if hemorrhage cannot be controlled. In most cases requiring surgery, the diseased section of the intestine is removed and the remaining sections joined together. In some patients, a temporary *colostomy* (an operation to bring part of the large intestine to the body surface to form an artificial anus) is required.

Diving medicine

See *Scuba-diving medicine*.

Dizziness

A sensation of unsteadiness and lightheadedness. It may be a mild, brief symptom that occurs by itself, or it may be part of a more severe, prolonged attack of *vertigo* (characterized by a sensation of spinning, either of oneself or the surroundings) accompanied by nausea, vomiting, sweating, or fainting.

CAUSES

Most attacks of dizziness are harmless and are caused by a momentary fall in the pressure of blood to the brain, as can occur, for example, when getting up quickly from a sitting or lying position (a phenomenon called *postural hypotension*). Postural hypotension is more common in the elderly and in people taking drugs to treat *hypertension* (high blood pressure). Similar symptoms may result from a temporary, partial blockage in the arteries that supply the brain—a *transient ischemic attack*.

Other causes of dizziness include tiredness, stress, fever, *anemia*, *heart block* (impairment of the conduction of excitatory impulses through the heart muscle, causing slow, uncoordinated beating of the individual chambers), *hypoglycemia* (low blood sugar level), and *subdural hemorrhage* and *hematoma* (bleeding between the outer two membranes that cover the brain).

Dizziness as part of vertigo is usually due to a disorder of the inner ear, *acoustic nerve*, or *brain stem*.

The principal disorders of the inner ear that can cause dizziness and vertigo are *labyrinthitis* and *Meniere's disease*. In labyrinthitis, the labyrinth (the fluid-filled canals within the inner

367

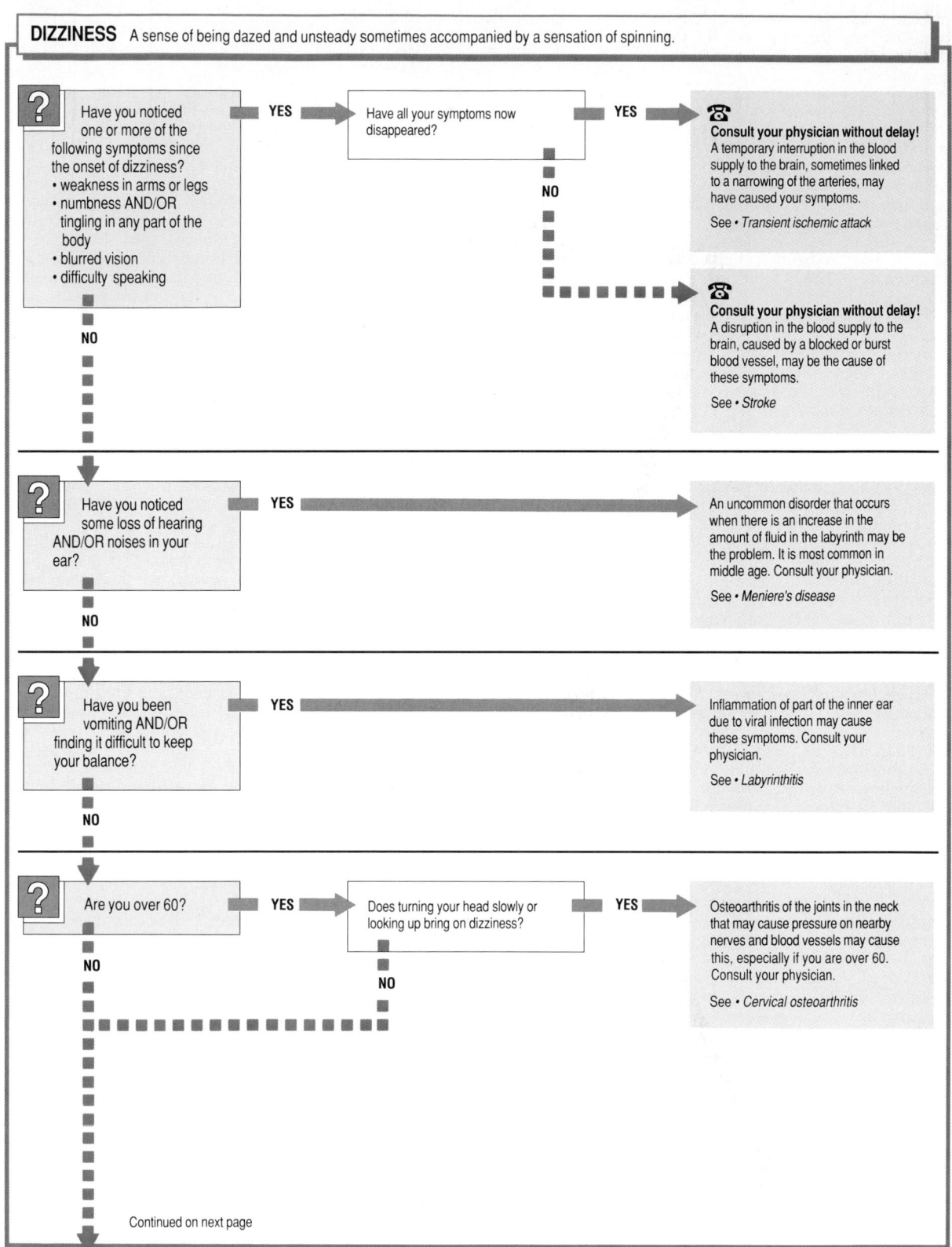

DIZZINESS A sense of being dazed and unsteady sometimes accompanied by a sensation of spinning.

Have you noticed one or more of the following symptoms since the onset of dizziness?
• weakness in arms or legs
• numbness AND/OR tingling in any part of the body
• blurred vision
• difficulty speaking

NO

YES → Have all your symptoms now disappeared?

YES →

☎ **Consult your physician without delay!** A temporary interruption in the blood supply to the brain, sometimes linked to a narrowing of the arteries, may have caused your symptoms.

See • *Transient ischemic attack*

NO

☎ **Consult your physician without delay!** A disruption in the blood supply to the brain, caused by a blocked or burst blood vessel, may be the cause of these symptoms.

See • *Stroke*

Have you noticed some loss of hearing AND/OR noises in your ear?

NO

YES → An uncommon disorder that occurs when there is an increase in the amount of fluid in the labyrinth may be the problem. It is most common in middle age. Consult your physician.

See • *Meniere's disease*

Have you been vomiting AND/OR finding it difficult to keep your balance?

NO

YES → Inflammation of part of the inner ear due to viral infection may cause these symptoms. Consult your physician.

See • *Labyrinthitis*

Are you over 60?

NO

YES → Does turning your head slowly or looking up bring on dizziness?

NO

YES → Osteoarthritis of the joints in the neck that may cause pressure on nearby nerves and blood vessels may cause this, especially if you are over 60. Consult your physician.

See • *Cervical osteoarthritis*

Continued on next page

D

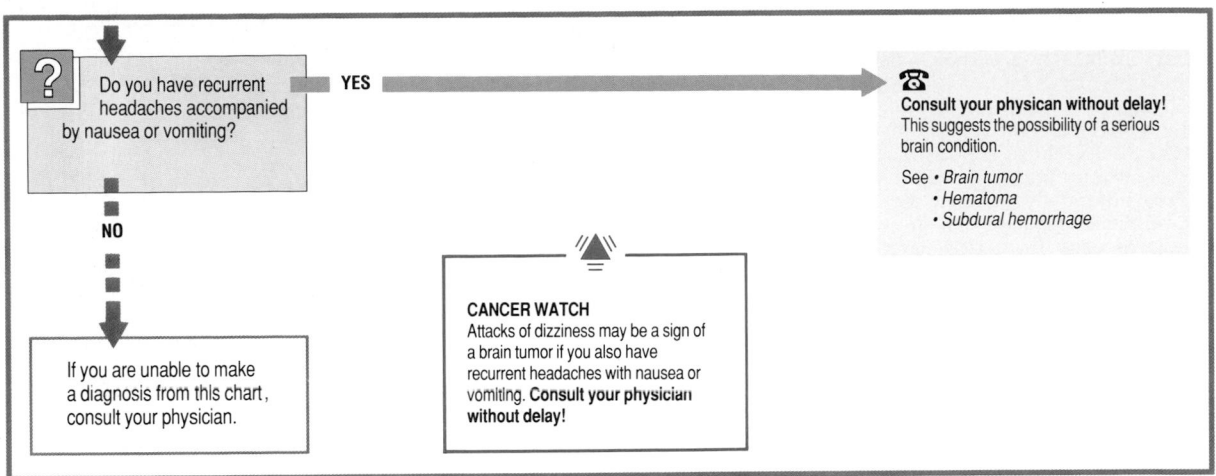

Do you have recurrent headaches accompanied by nausea or vomiting?

YES → ☎ **Consult your physican without delay!** This suggests the possibility of a serious brain condition.

See • *Brain tumor*
• *Hematoma*
• *Subdural hemorrhage*

NO

If you are unable to make a diagnosis from this chart, consult your physician.

CANCER WATCH
Attacks of dizziness may be a sign of a brain tumor if you also have recurrent headaches with nausea or vomiting. **Consult your physician without delay!**

D

---

ear that play a vital role in balance) becomes inflamed, usually as a result of a viral infection. In severe cases, any movement of the head can cause vomiting and fainting. In Meniere's disease, a degenerative disease of the ear, the dizziness and vertigo are often associated with hearing loss and *tinnitus*.

Disorders of the acoustic nerve are relatively rare causes of dizziness and vertigo. They include *acoustic neuroma* and cases of *meningitis* in which the acoustic nerve is affected.

Disorders of the brain stem (specifically the part of the brain stem that connects with the acoustic nerve) that can cause dizziness and vertigo include narrowing of the blood vessels that supply this part of the brain stem (a condition called *vertebrobasilar insufficiency*); cases of migraine that involve blood vessels in the brain stem; and brain tumors that press on the brain stem. Vertebrobasilar insufficiency is itself often due to *cervical osteoarthritis* (arthritis of the neck region of the spine); it produces pain and dizziness on turning the head or moving the neck.

TREATMENT

Brief episodes of mild dizziness usually clear up after taking a few deep breaths, or, if this fails, after resting for a short time. Severe, prolonged, or recurrent dizziness should be investigated by a physician, who will try to determine the cause from a description of symptoms, examination of the ears, and, in some cases, further diagnostic tests.

In certain cases of dizziness and vertigo due to a disorder of the inner ear, the physician may prescribe *antiemetic* or *antihistamine drugs*.

DNA

The commonly used abbreviation for deoxyribonucleic acid, the principal carrier of genetic information in almost all organisms (the exceptions are certain viruses that use *RNA*, ribonucleic acid, to carry genetic information). DNA is found in the *chromosomes* of cells; its double-helix structure allows the chromosomes to be copied exactly during the process of cell division. (See also *Nucleic acids*.)

Dogs, diseases from

Infectious or parasitic diseases, acquired from contact with dogs, that may be caused by viruses, bacteria, fungi, protozoa, worms, insects, or mites living in or on the dog.

People and dogs have been sharing living quarters for more than three million years, so it is not surprising that they share some parasites. Many of these parasites show a marked preference for dogs, but may accidentally be transferred to humans who stroke a dog's fur or touch contaminated dog feces.

Overall, diseases contracted from dogs are uncommon—especially the more serious ones—and must be viewed in light of the tremendous psychological benefits and pleasure that owners derive from their pets.

Fleas and ticks
Ticks may transfer from a dog's fur; fleas inhabit the pet's resting places and can cause irritating bites.

Worms and eggs
Worm eggs in dog feces are a more serious danger than adult worms.

Dander
Tiny scales from dog fur (known as dander) may cause an allergy if they are inhaled.

Transmission of infection
Transmission from feces occurs when a person (often a child) directly handles a dog's feces or anus (or contaminates his or her fingers with fecal material from the soil or from the dog's fur) and transfers infective organisms to his or her mouth. Infection can also occur from eating food that has been contaminated with dog feces. Other means of transferring infection are through saliva and direct contact.

SPECIFIC DISEASES

The most serious disease that can be caught from a dog is *rabies*, usually transmitted by a bite. Any dog bite, particularly if the dog is a stray, should be treated with suspicion. Dog bites can also cause serious bleeding and shock and may become infected.

Two potentially serious, although rare, diseases caused by the ingestion of worm eggs from dogs are *toxocariasis* and *hydatid disease*. Toxocariasis is mainly an infection of children; the passage of worm larvae through the body can cause allergic symptoms such as asthma, and, rarely, a larva may lodge in an eye and cause blindness. Hydatid disease can lead to the development of cysts in the liver, lungs, brain, or elsewhere. Usually sheep, not people, pick up the infection and then reinfect dogs; the disease is most common in sheep-rearing areas.

In the tropics, walking barefoot on sand or soil previously contaminated with dog feces can lead to infection with dog *hookworms*.

Bites from dog *fleas* are an occasional nuisance. The fleas inhabit places in a house where the dog habitually rests and, if the dog is absent, may jump onto humans for a meal. *Ticks* and *mites* from dogs, including a canine version of the *scabies* mite, are other common problems. The fungi that cause *tinea* (ringworm) infections may come from dogs, although the disease is usually evident in the dog because it causes progressive hair loss.

Finally, some people become allergic to animal *dander* (tiny scales derived from fur or skin and present in household dust) and have such symptoms as *asthma* or *urticaria* when a dog is in the house. (See also *Cats, diseases from*; *Zoonoses*.)

Donor

A person who provides blood for transfusion, tissues or organs for transplantation, or semen for artificial insemination.

Many individuals carry donor cards to indicate that they have bequeathed all or parts of their bodies to be used, should they die unexpectedly, for the treatment of others. The bequest may also be made by the next-of-kin at the time of death.

Donors should be between the ages of 1 and 55 years, should be free of cancer (except primary brain cancer), should be free of serious infection (such as hepatitis B), and should not carry HIV (the AIDS virus).

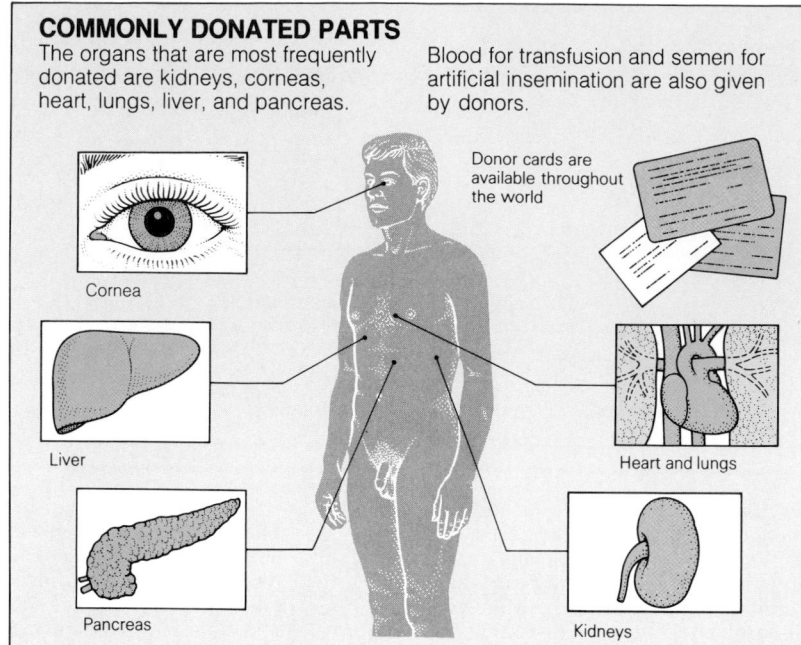

COMMONLY DONATED PARTS

The organs that are most frequently donated are kidneys, corneas, heart, lungs, liver, and pancreas.

Blood for transfusion and semen for artificial insemination are also given by donors.

Donor cards are available throughout the world

Cornea

Liver

Pancreas

Heart and lungs

Kidneys

In general, organs for transplantation must be removed within a few hours of *brain death*, and before or immediately after the heart beat has stopped. An organ is used only if it is completely healthy.

In about one third of kidney transplants, the kidney is provided by a living donor. The living volunteer is usually a sibling or parent whose body tissues match well on the basis of *tissue typing*. Tests are performed to make sure that both kidneys are healthy before one is removed for transplantation. A healthy donor's life is not shortened because the remaining kidney grows to compensate for the kidney that has been removed.

Suitable related donors whose tissue types match may also provide bone marrow for transplantation and sometimes skin for grafting. (See also *Artificial insemination*; *Blood donation*; *Bone marrow transplantation*; *Organ donation*; *Transplant surgery*.)

Do not resuscitate

The term used to request that hospital staff do not attempt heroic measures to save or restore life in patients with severe, progressive disease.

Doppler effect

A change in the frequency with which waves from a given source reach an observer when the source is in rapid motion with respect to the observer.

When a fast-moving train blows its whistle as it passes through a station, a person standing on the platform hears an apparent increase in pitch (frequency) as the train approaches and then a lowering of pitch once the train has passed and is moving away. In fact, the whistle gives off a constant pitch, but it seems to rise and then fall to the person on the platform because the train is moving. This change in the observed frequency of sound as a result of movement is called the Doppler effect or Doppler shift.

The Doppler effect is utilized in various medical *ultrasound scanning* techniques. In these techniques, an emitter sends out pulses of ultrasound (inaudible high-frequency sound) of a specific frequency. When these pulses bounce off a moving object—blood flowing through a blood vessel or the beating heart of a fetus in the uterus, for example—the frequency of the echoes is changed from that of the emitted sound (the Doppler effect in action). A special sensor detects the frequency change and, for the examples above, converts this data into information about how fast the blood is flowing or the rate at which the fetal heart is beating.

Doppler ultrasound techniques are used to measure blood pressure in superficial blood vessels and to detect air bubbles in *dialysis* and in *heart-lung machines*.

Dorsal

Relating to the back, located on or near the back, or describing the uppermost part of a body structure when a person is lying facedown. For example, dorsalgia is pain in the back, and the dorsal part of the tongue is the back of the tongue. In human anatomy, the term dorsal means the same as posterior. The opposite of dorsal is *ventral* (anterior or front).

Dose

A term used to refer to the amount of a drug taken at a particular time, or to the amount of radiation an individual is exposed to during one session of *radiation therapy*.

DRUG DOSE

The dose of a drug can be expressed in several ways: in terms of the weight of its active substance, usually in milligrams; in terms of the volume of liquid to be drunk, usually in milliliters; or in terms of its biological activity potential (its effects on body tissues as calculated in a laboratory). This last value is usually expressed in units or international units.

It is not possible to compare the effects of two different drugs from the same group on the body simply by comparing the size of the doses. Some are "stronger" (more potent) than others, just as different alcoholic drinks vary in their alcohol content.

RADIATION DOSE

The dose of radiation received during a session of radiation therapy is expressed in rads or grays (see box on *Radiation* units). These units are a measure of the amount of radiation absorbed by body tissues. Different types of body tissue are able to absorb different amounts of energy from the same beam of radiation.

Double-blind

A type of *controlled trial*—the aim of which is to test the effectiveness of a treatment or to compare the benefits of different treatments. Double-blind trials differ from other types of controlled trials in that neither the patients taking part nor the physicians who assess the treatments know which patients are receiving which treatment. This eliminates any conscious or unconscious expectations about which treatment will be most effective, thus affecting the results of the trial.

For example, a new drug and an older, standard treatment might be compared by placing the two drugs into identical capsules (by a person who otherwise takes no part in the trial) and giving them to different groups of patients on a random selection (chance) basis. The patients are later examined by one or more physicians. Only after all assessments have been made is the identity of the drug that was given to each patient revealed—usually by the person who originally prepared the capsules.

Double vision

The seeing of two instead of one visual image of a single object, also known as diplopia. It should not be confused with *blurred vision*.

Example of double vision
Two images, rather than a single image, are seen. Prompt investigation by a physician is required.

CAUSES

Double vision is usually a symptom of *strabismus* (deviation or malalignment of the two eyes), although not all strabismus produces double vision. Paralytic strabismus is a type of strabismus that commonly causes double vision. In this condition movement of the eye in a particular direction is impaired due to paralysis of one or more of the muscles. Tilting or turning the head can sometimes overcome the double vision.

A growth in the eyelid pressing on the front of the eyeball can also cause temporary image separation by distorting the shape of the front of the eye and by causing a slight displacement in the path of light rays entering that eye (and thus variation in the points at which they are focused on the retina). Double vision may be caused by a tumor or blood clot behind the eye that prevents the normal motion of the eyeball.

In endocrine-related *exophthalmos*, protrusion of the eyeballs is the result of an underlying hormonal disorder and double vision results from swelling and scarring in the eye muscles, causing abnormal alignment and motion of the eyes.

Rarely, double vision arises because of an abnormality within the eye. For example, a dislocation of the *lens* in the eye may result in some light rays passing through the lens and others around it, so that separate images fall on the retina of one eye.

COMPLICATIONS AND TREATMENT

The brain of a young child with strabismus (congenital, accommodative, or paralytic) learns to suppress the second, unwanted image seen by the misaligned, strabismic eye so as not to see double. Continued misalignment of the child's eyes may eventually lead to poor vision in the affected eye. This poor vision is called *amblyopia*, or lazy eye. Patching of the better-seeing eye may improve the vision in the poorly seeing, deviated eye. The strabismus may need to be corrected early (by means of glasses and/or surgery) in children to prevent amblyopia from developing; otherwise, it may become permanent. A young child with strabismus should be seen by a physician to find the cause and to begin treatment.

The onset of double vision in adult life needs immediate investigation to exclude the possibility of a tumor, aneurysm, and/or neurologic abnormality. The double vision could be a symptom of a very serious underlying disorder that requires prompt attention and treatment.

Douche

Introduction of water and/or a cleansing agent into the vagina using equipment consisting of a bag and tubing with a nozzle attached. Intended to clean the vagina, a douche is unnecessary; the vagina is normally slightly acidic and cleans itself.

In the past, douches were widely used after sexual intercourse to cleanse the vagina and as a means of contraception. They were also used by women who were worried about having excessive or offensive vaginal discharge. Douches were sometimes recommended to treat vaginal infections and were also used after vaginal repair operations.

Today it is recognized that a douche carries the risk of introducing infection into the vagina, especially if the nozzle is not cleaned properly before use. A douche also may spread an existing vaginal infection into the uterus or fallopian tubes. A douche is completely ineffective as a contraceptive method. Today gynecologists rarely, if ever, recommend douches for any reason.

D

Down's syndrome

A *chromosomal abnormality* resulting in mental handicap and a characteristic physical appearance. Down's syndrome was originally named "mongolism" because it was thought that the facial features of affected children resembled those of Mongolians. The term is no longer used by the medical profession.

CAUSES

The cause of Down's syndrome remained a mystery until 1959, when researchers discovered that each of the body cells of people with Down's syndrome has one too many chromosomes—47 instead of the normal 46. Because in most cases the extra chromosome is number 21, the disorder is also called trisomy 21.

There are several possible reasons for the chromosomal abnormality. In most cases it is the result of a failure of the two chromosomes numbered 21 in a parent cell to go into separate daughter cells during the first stage of sperm or egg cell formation (see *Chromosomes*). Some eggs or sperm are therefore formed with an extra number 21 chromosome and, if one of these takes part in fertilization, the resulting baby will also have the extra chromosome. This type of abnormality is particularly likely if the mother is over 35, suggesting that defective egg formation, rather than sperm formation, is usually at fault.

A less common cause is a chromosomal abnormality in either parent, known as a *translocation*, in which part of one of the parent's own number 21 chromosomes has joined with another chromosome. The parent is not affected except for the risk of having a child with Down's syndrome.

INCIDENCE

About one in 650 babies born is affected by Down's syndrome. The incidence of affected fetuses rises steeply with increased maternal age to about one in 40 among mothers over 40. Pregnant women over 35, and

Typical features
The eyes slope upward at the outer corners and the inner corners are covered, the facial features are small, and the tongue is large and tends to stick out. The back of the head is usually flat.

Inward-curving finger

Single transverse crease

Down's syndrome

Normal

those with a family history of Down's syndrome or other factors putting them at risk, are usually offered *chromosome analysis* of the fetus' cells after these have been obtained by *amniocentesis* or *chorionic villus sampling*. If the fetus is found to be affected, termination of the pregnancy may be one of the options.

SYMPTOMS

Most people with Down's syndrome have eyes that slope up at the outer corners and folds of skin on either side of the nose that cover the inner corners of the eye. The face and features are small, the tongue is large and tends to protrude, the head has a flattened back, and the hands are typically short and broad. The degree of mental handicap varies. A Down's syndrome child's IQ may be anywhere from 30 to 80. Virtually all affected children are capable of a limited amount of learning, including

in some cases the ability to read. Down's syndrome children are usually affectionate, friendly, and cheerful, and they get along well with other family members.

About one fourth of Down's syndrome children have a heart defect at birth (see *Heart disease, congenital*). They also have a higher-than-average incidence of intestinal *atresia* (narrowing at some point in the intestines), congenital *hearing* defects, and acute *leukemia*, and they are especially susceptible to repeated ear infections. For unknown reasons, *atherosclerosis* (narrowing of the arteries), which leads to an increased risk of heart disease, tends to develop in adults affected by Down's syndrome.

DIAGNOSIS

Because of the distinctive physical features, Down's syndrome is usually recognized soon after birth. The diagnosis is confirmed by a count of the chromosomes in white blood cells taken from a blood sample (see *Chromosome analysis*).

TREATMENT

There is no cure for the mental handicap, but Down's syndrome children can make the most of their capabilities through constant educational and environmental stimulation. Institutional care is sometimes necessary, but affected children are generally happiest in a sympathetic home environment. It is possible to alter the facial appearance by plastic surgery.

OUTLOOK

Until recently (less than a generation ago) most Down's syndrome children did not survive beyond their teens because of the high incidence of defects present from birth as well as their susceptibility to infection. Advances in medical and surgical techniques, together with improved long-term care facilities, have extended the life expectancy of Down's syndrome sufferers, but they still tend not to survive beyond early middle age.

Doxepin

An *antidepressant drug*, doxepin has a strong sedative effect and is useful in the treatment of depression accompanied by anxiety or insomnia.

Possible adverse effects include dry mouth, blurred vision, dizziness, drowsiness, and attacks of flushing, which may disappear if the dosage is reduced. This drug usually takes between two to six weeks to become fully effective.

Doxorubicin

An *anticancer drug* given by injection, usually in combination with other anticancer drugs of this group. Doxorubicin is used to treat a variety of cancers, including *leukemia, Hodgkin's disease*, and lung cancer.

Doxycycline

A *tetracycline* antibiotic drug. Doxycycline has been found to be more effective than most other tetracyclines

in the treatment of chronic *prostatitis* (prostate gland infection), *pelvic inflammatory disease*, and attacks of chest infection in chronic bronchitis.

Doxycycline is also used to treat severe attacks of traveler's diarrhea and is occasionally prescribed to prevent this condition before traveling to foreign countries.

Because its action lasts longer than that of some other tetracyclines, doxycycline must be taken only once or twice a day. It is also useful in treating people with kidney disease because it is broken down by the liver rather than excreted in the urine. Possible adverse effects, such as nausea and indigestion, can be reduced by taking doxycycline with food; absorption of doxycycline, unlike many other tetracyclines, is not impaired if the drug is taken with food.

DPT vaccination

A series of injections that provides immunity against *diphtheria, pertussis* (whooping cough), and *tetanus.*

HOW IT IS DONE

DPT vaccine is given initially as a course of three injections at the ages of 2, 4, and 6 months. More doses are given at 15 to 18 months and before school at the age of 4 to 6 years.

WHY IT IS DONE

DPT vaccination causes the body to produce antibodies to fend off diphtheria, pertussis, and tetanus infections. The vaccine does not provide complete immunity to diphtheria, but it does protect against the dangers of infection. Since DPT was not routinely administered in the US until the late 1940s, any adult exposed to diphtheria should be checked for immunity. If a blood sample shows no antibodies against the disease, diphtheria vaccine will then be administered.

The pertussis vaccine also does not provide absolute protection, but children who have been immunized get only a mild version of the disease and are unlikely to become seriously ill. The protection against pertussis gradually wanes, so adults can get the infection. In adults, the disease is mild, but adults can infect unimmunized children. The disease can be fatal in children.

Protection against tetanus is not permanent; it needs to be "boosted" with another shot every 10 years or at the time of any dirty, penetrating injury if vaccination has not been done within the last five years.

RISKS

In the cases of diphtheria and tetanus, the life-threatening feature of the infection is a toxin (poison) produced by the bacteria. The vaccine contains toxoids—modified versions of the diphtheria and tetanus toxins—that stimulate the formation of antibodies. Because the toxoids are chemicals and not organisms, physical reactions to them are rare.

Pertussis vaccine consists of killed bacteria, which stimulate antibodies (but are more likely to provoke a reac-

tion). The pertussis component commonly causes a slight fever and some irritability for a couple of days after the vaccination. More serious reactions, including signs of irritation of the brain and nervous system, including convulsions, occur in less than one in 100,000 vaccinations. Permanent damage from the vaccine is even more rare. Nevertheless, many babies are being given vaccine without the pertussis component. In England, when pertussis vaccinations were refused by many parents, an epidemic of pertussis occurred. It is estimated that, between 1977 and 1983, close to 500 children died as a result of pertussis infection; some cases of permanent brain damage or lung damage occurred as well. The benefits outweigh the minimal risk from the vaccine. Vaccine without pertussis is given to children who have reacted severely to DPT vaccine or who suffer from, or have a history of, brain abnormalities or seizures.

REASONS TO QUESTION THE ADMINISTRATION OF THE PERTUSSIS VACCINE TO YOUR CHILD

1. If your child is an infant with a neurologic disorder that is characterized by progressive developmental delay or seizures.
2. If your child's prior DPT immunization has caused any of the following:
- Encephalopathy (severe alterations in consciousness and focal neurologic signs) within seven days (usually seen within three days) after receiving the vaccination.
- Convulsions with or without fever within three days after receiving the vaccination.
- Persistent, inconsolable screaming or crying (or an unusual, high-pitched cry) for three or more hours within 48 hours after receiving the vaccine.
- Collapse or shocklike state within 48 hours after receiving the vaccine.
- Temperature of 104.9°F (40.5°C) or more that is unexplained by any other cause within 48 hours after receiving the vaccine.
- Allergic reaction to vaccine (such as anaphylaxis) after receiving the vaccine; this is extremely rare.

Drain, surgical

An appliance inserted by the physician into a body cavity or wound to release and permit drainage of fluid or air from it.

TYPES

The simplest drains are soft rubber tubes that pass from a body cavity into a dressing. More sophisticated drains are wide-bore tubes that connect to a

TYPES OF DRAINS

Wide-bore drain

Corrugated drain

Perforated drain

T-shaped drain

D

collection bag or bottle. A valve prevents fluid from refluxing back into the body. Another type, corrugated drains, have a series of curved ridges to help collect fluid from a wound. Suction drains consist of a thin tube with many small holes to help collect fluid, which is drawn into a vacuum bottle. Suction can also be applied to a drain by means of a vacuum pump.

A drain that removes bile from the biliary system (gallbladder and bile ducts) after surgery in that area is T-shaped to hold it in place.

Dream analysis

The interpretation of a person's dreams as part of *psychoanalysis* or *psychotherapy.* First developed by Sigmund Freud, the technique relies on the idea that a person's repressed feelings and thoughts are revealed in dreams, but in a disguised manner. The therapist unravels the significance of the dream by using a knowledge of the patient's character to interpret symbols, and by asking the patient for any associations suggested by the dream.

Dreaming

Mental activity that takes place during *sleep.* The evidence suggests strongly that dreaming occurs only during periods of REM (rapid eye movement) sleep, which last for about 20 minutes and occur four or five times a night.

D

Although there are still arguments about the exact function of dreams, their physiological aspects are well understood. Using an electroencephalograph (a machine that records the electrical activity of the brain, see *EEG*), it is possible to describe various phases of sleep in terms of their different electrical patterns. Compared to other phases, the REM phase is active, as if the sleeper were awake but drowsy. At the same time, blood flow and brain temperature increase, and there are sudden changes in heart rate and blood pressure. All this may indicate that the brain is restoring itself for further activity.

Dreaming can be seen as a parallel process in which the mental impressions, feelings, and ideas that have been taken in during the day are sorted out. The content of dreams therefore closely represents the day's preoccupations—with the ideas and memories distorted by the lack of a conscious and awake mind.

People roused during periods of REM sleep report especially vivid dreams, but those who wake normally after normal dream activity has ended may not remember dreaming at all.

SIGNIFICANCE
As a proportion of total sleep, REM sleep is much greater in young babies and after head injury. This indicates that it may have an important role in promoting brain activity. Whether or not dreams have an important psychological role is more controversial. Depriving people of their dreams by constantly waking them during REM phases was once thought to cause severe psychological disorders, but this is now less generally accepted. Certain hypnotic drugs suppress REM sleep without causing any obvious psychological harm.

Dressings

Protective coverings for wounds. Dressings may be used to control bleeding, absorb secretions, or prevent contamination by bacteria. They are placed directly onto wounds and are large enough to cover them completely. They should be sterile so as not to introduce bacteria that could cause infection. A dressing should also be absorbent; if sweat cannot evaporate, the skin around the wound becomes moist and soft and the dressing sodden, thus encouraging the growth of bacteria and further infection. Unless a wound must be regularly cleaned, dressings should be

FIRST AID: DRESSINGS

1 Remove outer protective wrapping, being careful not to touch the gauze. If possible, wash your hands before touching the unwrapped dressing. Then hold the dressing, gauze-side down, over the wound.

Assorted dressings
In addition to sterile dressings, plain gauze and a variety of adhesive-strip bandages can be used.

2 Wind the short end of the bandage once around the arm and dressing. Bandage firmly (not tightly) and cover pad.

3 Secure the bandage by tying the two ends over the gauze pad using a square knot (left end over right end and under; right end over left end and under).

left undisturbed. A wound should be covered for the minimum length of time. (See also *Compress*.)

TYPES
ADHESIVE BANDAGES Available in a range of sizes, these consist of absorbent pads held in place by waterproof adhesive backings. They are commonly used to protect small wounds, such as cuts and abrasions, but may also be used to cover surgical wounds.
GAUZE Usually applied in layers, gauze is made of woven or nonwoven cotton or a synthetic material and is used to cover larger wounds. It is held in place by a bandage or a length of adhesive strapping. The gauze is usually applied dry, but ribbon gauze, soaked in a substance to promote granulation of the tissue, may be used to pack a deep wound. Sterile, unmedicated dressings consist of layers of fine gauze and a pad of absorbent cotton attached to a roller bandage.

NONSTICK DRESSINGS Of recent development, these dressings consist of a nonadherent contact layer of perforated polyethylene or viscose with an impregnated gauze pad backing. Such dressings do not adhere to wounds and can be removed without disturbing newly formed tissue.
IMPROVISED DRESSINGS In emergency first-aid treatment, any clean, dry, and absorbent material may be used to cover a wound (for example, a handkerchief or piece of sheeting) if a sterile dressing is not available. Absorbent cotton or woolly fibrous materials should not be used because the fibers may become embedded in the wound.
APPLYING A DRESSING
See illustrated box.

Dressler's syndrome

An uncommon condition, also called postinfarction syndrome, that may occur after a *myocardial infarction* (heart attack) or heart surgery. The condition is characterized by fever, chest pain, *pericarditis* (inflammation of the outer covering membrane of the heart), and *pleurisy* (inflammation of the outer lining of the lungs).

Dressler's syndrome is thought to be an *autoimmune disorder*. The body's immune system produces antibodies (proteins with a defensive role) that are directed against the damaged areas of heart muscle.

The features of the condition first appear any time between a few days and several weeks after a myocardial infarction or heart surgery. The diagnosis is confirmed by detecting specific antibodies in the blood. Treatment with aspirin usually clears the condition, although, in some more severe cases, treatment with *corticosteroid drugs* is needed.

DRG

The abbreviation for *diagnosis-related group*.

Dribbling

A term commonly used to denote involuntary leakage of urine (see *Incontinence, urinary*).

Drip

See *Intravenous infusion*.

Drooling

The involuntary leakage of saliva from the mouth—normal behavior in infants up to the age of about 12 months. Drooling in an adult may simply be due to poorly fitting dentures or may be the result of facial paralysis, *dementia*, or a serious underlying disorder, most commonly *Parkinson's disease*.

Drop attack

A brief disturbance affecting the nervous system, causing a person to fall suddenly to the ground without warning; the legs just seem to buckle. Unlike *fainting*, the person may not lose consciousness, but injuries can occur to the hands, face, or knees as a result of the fall.

CAUSES AND INCIDENCE

Although drop attacks can affect all age groups, elderly women are the most commonly affected. The causes are not fully understood, although in some cases there may be a fall in blood flow to nerve centers in the *brain stem*.

Occasionally, elderly men may experience a drop attack while passing urine or while standing. Lowered blood pressure or an abrupt alteration in the heart's rhythm may be involved; it is advisable for these people to sit down while urinating.

Other rare causes of drop attacks include a block in the flow of cerebrospinal fluid around the brain—usually in patients with a type of *hydrocephalus*. One uncommon form of epileptic convulsion, an akinetic seizure, is sometimes also described as a drop attack. During this seizure, the sufferer falls suddenly to the ground and briefly loses consciousness, but does not convulse.

TREATMENT

Drop attacks in the elderly cannot be treated but usually disappear in time. Akinetic seizures respond to anticonvulsant drug treatment.

Dropsy

An outmoded term for generalized *edema* (fluid collection in body tissues). In the past, many people were certified as dead "due to dropsy."

Dropsy is not itself a disease, but merely a sign of malfunction in the body (especially congestive *heart failure* or kidney disease).

Drowning

Death caused by suffocation and *hypoxia* (lack of oxygen) associated with immersion in a fluid.

In about four fifths of cases the person has inhaled liquid into the lungs; in the other fifth, no liquid has entered the lungs—a condition called dry drowning (see *Drowning, dry*). People who are resuscitated after prolonged immersion are said to be victims of "near drowning."

INCIDENCE AND CAUSES

Drowning is the third most common cause of accidental death in the US (after motor vehicle accidents and falls). About one person in 280 in the US dies from drowning (or more than 7,000 people every year). Many more are victims of near drowning. Worldwide, possibly as many as 200,000 people drown annually.

Many victims are competent swimmers who have failed to take into account factors such as tidal currents (or undertow) and have tired and panicked. A relatively small number are nonswimmers. Other drowning circumstances include floods, sinkings, immersion in freezing cold water after falling through ice, and infant drownings, which can occur in as little as six inches of water.

Over one third of drowning victims have a significant amount of alcohol in their blood upon postmortem examination. Alcohol intoxication impairs judgment and at the same time reduces physical coordination—an extremely dangerous combination before swimming.

Some methods of minimizing the risks of a drowning accident are shown in the table, next page.

MECHANISM OF DROWNING

When a person panics at the surface of the water, the thrashing movements are incapable of keeping the body afloat, and the person begins taking in small amounts of water. Initially, automatic contraction of a muscle at the entrance to the windpipe—a mechanism called the laryngeal reflex—prevents water from entering the lungs and instead it enters the esophagus and stomach. However, the laryngeal reflex impairs breathing, which can quickly lead to *hypoxia* and to loss of consciousness.

If the person is buoyant at this point and floats face-up, his or her chances of survival are reasonable because the laryngeal reflex begins to relax and normal breathing may recommence. On the other hand, the person may float face-down or may sink.

D

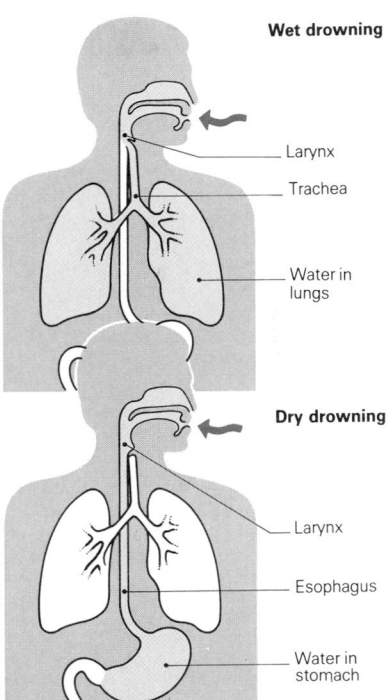

Wet drowning

- Larynx
- Trachea
- Water in lungs

Dry drowning

- Larynx
- Esophagus
- Water in stomach

Types of drowning
In four fifths of deaths due to drowning, the victim has inhaled liquid into his or her lungs. In the other fifth, no liquid is present in the lungs (dry drowning). In both cases, death is the result of suffocation.

FIRST AID AND TREATMENT

If a person is panicking at the surface of the water, he or she should be thrown any large item that will float. Ideally, the person should be approached in a boat and reached. If approached by swimming, an attempt should be made to calm the person before contact is made, otherwise he or she may struggle, possibly causing the rescuer to drown as well.

The victim should be supported with the head above water and towed to the nearest boat or shore. An ambulance should be called and the person's medical condition assessed. If breathing and/or the pulse (felt in the neck) is absent, resuscitative measures should be started (see *Cardiopulmonary resuscitation*). They should be continued until an ambulance or physician has arrived.

Often, a victim of near drowning will make an apparently remarkable recovery after being resuscitated. The person should nevertheless be sent to a hospital for investigation and observation. Water may have passed from the lungs into the blood, and the lining of the lungs may have been damaged. In either case, symptoms may develop some hours after rescue and may be life threatening.

Drowning, dry

A form of drowning in which no fluid enters the lungs.

About one fifth of fatal drowning cases are "dry"—illustrating the fact that death from drowning results mainly from lack of oxygen, whether or not water has entered the lungs (see *Drowning*). Victims of dry drowning have a particularly strong laryngeal reflex, which diverts water into the stomach instead of the lungs, but at the same time impairs breathing.

Drowsiness

A state of consciousness between full wakefulness and sleep or unconsciousness. It is medically significant if it is abnormal.

Abnormal drowsiness may be the result of a head injury, high fever, *meningitis* (inflammation of the membranes that surround the brain and spinal cord), a metabolic disorder such as *uremia* (excessive metabolic products in the blood), or liver failure. Alcohol or drugs may also produce this effect. In a diabetic, drowsiness may be due to *hypoglycemia* (low blood sugar), usually as a result of taking too much insulin, or to *hyperglycemia* (high blood sugar) due to inadequate control of the disorder.

If a person who is drowsy fails to awaken after being shaken, pinched, and shouted at—or wakes and then relapses into drowsiness—treat the situation as a medical emergency and call for professional help immediately. (See *Unconsciousness*.)

Drug

Any chemical substance that alters the function of one or more body organs or changes the process of a disease. Drugs include prescribed medicines, over-the-counter remedies, and the recreational, social, and illicit use of drugs, such as cocaine. Many foods and drinks contain small quantities of substances classed as drugs—tea, coffee, and cola drinks, for example, all contain *caffeine*, which is both a *stimulant* and a *diuretic drug*.

Each drug normally has three names: a detailed, descriptive chemical name; a shorter, generic name (see *Generic drug*) that has been officially approved; and a specific brand name chosen by the company that manufactures it. Drugs are either licensed for prescription by a physician only or are over-the-counter preparations available at a drugstore or supermarket.

SOURCES

Originally, all drugs were naturally occurring substances extracted from animals, plants, and minerals. Today, most drugs are produced artificially in the laboratory, ensuring a purer preparation with a predictable potency (strength) that is safer for medical use. Some drugs, such as *insulin* and *growth hormone*, are now sometimes synthesized using *genetic engineering* procedures.

New drugs are discovered in a number of ways: by screening a substance

---

DROWNING: RESCUE METHODS

Throwing the victim something to hold on to is useful if he or she is still conscious and has not panicked.

Otherwise, go to the person in a boat or, if no boat is available, reach him or her by swimming.

Throwing a buoy or line
If no life buoy is available, use any large object that floats. It should preferably have a rope attached to pull the person to safety (a rope alone may be sufficient).

Rescuing from a boat
After grasping the person's arms, it may be necessary to "bounce" him or her in the water to gain momentum for a lift into the boat. With two rescuers, one can enter the water to assist.

Towing
A panicky victim may need to be calmed before making contact; otherwise, he or she may struggle. During the tow ashore, it is important to keep the person's face above water.

MEASURES THAT MAY HELP PREVENT DROWNING ACCIDENTS

1 Never jump into deep water without ensuring that there is an easy and obvious method of exit.

2 Wear a life jacket or buoyancy device for all water sports (such as sailing and windsurfing).

3 Swim only in pools or from public beaches designated as safe and patrolled by lifeguards.

4 Do not drink alcohol before swimming or water sports of any kind.

5 Children should always be supervised when swimming and when they are taking baths.

6 Never walk on an iced-over pond or river unless the ice has first been tested by an adult.

for different types of activity against a disease; by making alterations to the structure of an established drug; or, occasionally, by finding a new application for a drug that is being used for another condition.

CLASSIFICATION

A drug is classified in one of the following ways: 1) according to its chemical make up (a *corticosteroid drug*, for example); 2) according to the disorder it treats (an *antihypertensive drug*, for example, is used to treat high blood pressure); or 3) according to its specific effect on the body (a diuretic drug, for example, increases the volume of urine).

EVALUATION

All new drugs are tested for their efficiency and safety. Tests usually go through three stages: laboratory trials on animals; laboratory trials on human volunteers; and, finally, clinical trials on patients.

The Food and Drug Administration (FDA) will issue a license if studies provide evidence of the drug's efficacy and safety according to strictly defined standards. The FDA also establishes standards of quality, purity of the preparation, and adequate labeling.

Evaluation continues even after a drug has become widely prescribed. A drug's license may be withdrawn if toxic effects are reported frequently or if even a few patients develop serious illness attributable to the drug.

WHY DRUGS ARE USED

Drugs can be used in the treatment, prevention, or diagnosis of a disease. They are prescribed to relieve physical or mental symptoms, to replace a deficient natural substance (such as a *hormone*), or to stop the excessive production of a hormone or other body chemical. Some drugs are given to destroy foreign organisms, such as bacteria or viruses. Others, known as *vaccines*, are given to stimulate the body's *immune system* (natural defenses) to form antibodies.

Antibiotic drugs, diuretics, *analgesics* (painkillers), and *tranquilizers* are among the most frequently prescribed drugs. The most frequently used over-the-counter remedies include analgesics, cough and cold remedies, vitamins, and tonics.

HOW DRUGS WORK

Drugs act on cells in the body or the infecting organism by stimulating or blocking chemical reactions. In many cases, this action occurs because the drug impersonates a chemical that occurs naturally in the body.

METHODS OF ADMINISTERING DRUGS

How taken		Action
By mouth		Drugs are digested and absorbed from the intestine in the same way as nutrients. How quickly the tablet or liquid works depends on how rapidly it is absorbed. This, in turn, depends on such factors as the drug's composition, how quickly the drug dissolves, and the effect of digestive juices on it.
By injection		Drugs given by injection have a very rapid effect. Injection is also used if digestive juices would destroy a drug.
As a cream, anal or vaginal suppository, pessary, nasal spray, or by inhaler		These drugs have a local effect on the parts of the body that are exposed to them as well as a systemic (generalized) effect if some of the drug is absorbed into the bloodstream from the site of application.

Some drugs act by binding (becoming attached) to a drug receptor (a specific site on the cell's surface that matches the chemical structure of the drug). This triggers a change in chemical activity within the cell. Other drugs work by being absorbed into the cell, where they affect the chemical processes directly.

Drugs may also have a placebo effect, which occurs because of the individual's positive or negative expectations of the drug's action.

METHODS OF ADMINISTRATION

Drugs are given in different forms and in different ways (see table). These methods depend on many factors, including the severity of the illness, the part of the body being treated, the properties of the drug, and the speed and duration of action required.

ELIMINATION

Drugs taken by mouth that are not absorbed in the intestine are excreted in the stools. Drugs that have entered the bloodstream are eliminated through the kidneys in the urine. Some drugs are broken down into inactive forms in the liver by *enzymes* before elimination.

COMPLIANCE

If drug treatment is to be beneficial, the full course must be taken as instructed by a physician. It is estimated that as many as two out of every five people who are prescribed a drug do not take it properly, if at all. Reasons for noncompliance include failure to understand instructions for taking the drug, fear of possible reactions, or simply not bothering to take the drug.

DRUG INTERACTIONS

Taking drugs together or in combination with food or alcohol may produce effects on the body that differ from those occurring when a drug is taken on its own. Such drug interactions occur if chemicals in the different substances act on the same receptors or if one chemical alters the absorption, breakdown, or elimination of another chemical.

Physicians often make use of interactions to increase the effectiveness of a treatment; combinations of drugs are often prescribed to treat infection, cancer, or hypertension (high blood pressure). Many interactions, however, are unplanned; they may reduce the benefit from a drug or increase its level in the blood and cause adverse effects.

Patients undergoing long-term drug treatment may be advised to carry warning cards to avoid dangerous interactions from any treatment received during an emergency. Patients should tell their physicians about any other drugs they are taking to prevent interactions with drugs the physician may prescribe.

ADVERSE EFFECTS

Most drugs can produce adverse effects—harmful or unpleasant reactions that result from a normal dose of the drug. These adverse effects can be divided into predictable adverse reactions, which result from the effects of the chemical structure of the drug, and bizarre (unpredictable) reactions, which are unrelated to the drug's normal chemical effects on cells. Predictable adverse reactions are

D

due to the difficulty experienced by the drug manufacturer in targeting the action of a drug to a single tissue or organ. For example, *anticholinergic drugs* prescribed to relieve spasm in the intestine also cause blurred vision and dryness of the mouth. Symptoms may wear off as the body adapts to the drug; otherwise, they usually are relieved by reducing the dose or increasing the interval between doses.

Any change in the absorption, breakdown, or elimination of a drug (caused, for example, by gastro-intestinal, liver, or kidney disease) that increases its concentration in the blood will increase the risk of predictable adverse effects.

Bizarre drug reactions may be due to a genetic disorder (for example, lack of a specific enzyme that usually inactivates the drug), an allergic reaction, or the formation of *antibodies* that damage tissue. Common side effects of this type include a rash, facial swelling, or jaundice. Occasionally, *anaphylactic shock* (a severe allergic reaction), characterized by breathing difficulty or collapse, may occur. All bizarre drug reactions usually necessitate withdrawal of the drug.

Many drugs cross the placenta and some adversely affect growth and development of the fetus. Most drugs pass into the breast milk of a nursing mother; some have adverse effects on the baby.

A drug is useful only if its overall benefit to the patient outweighs the risk and severity of any adverse effects. Research on new drugs partly aims to discover preparations that act selectively on target organs to avoid unwanted effects on other tissues.

Drug abuse

COMMON DRUGS
Stimulants
Amphetamines
Depressants
Alcohol Barbiturates
Psychedelics
LSD
Narcotics
Cocaine Heroin
Anabolic steroids

The use of a drug for a purpose other than that for which it is normally prescribed or recommended. The reasons for drug abuse include the desire to escape from reality or achieve a mystical experience, curiosity about its effects, and the search for self-awareness. Certain types of drugs (for example, anabolic steroids) are sometimes abused to improve performance in sports.

Problems resulting from drug abuse may arise from the adverse effects of the drug, from accidents during intoxication, and from the habit-forming potential of many drugs, which may lead to *drug dependence*.

Drug addiction
Physical or psychological dependence on a drug. (See *Drug dependence*.)

Drug dependence
The compulsion to continue taking a drug, either to produce the desired effects that result from taking it, or to prevent the ill effects that occur when it is not taken.

TYPES
Drug dependence takes two forms: psychological and physical. A person is psychologically dependent if he or she experiences craving or emotional distress when the drug is withdrawn. In physical dependence the body has adapted to the presence of the drug, causing the symptoms and signs of a withdrawal syndrome when the drug is withdrawn. Withdrawal is usually associated with severe physical and mental distress.

CAUSES AND INCIDENCE
Drug dependence develops as a result of regular and/or excessive use of a drug. Several million people in the US are dependent on nicotine, on the caffeine in coffee and tea, and on alcohol. Many thousands are dependent on tranquilizers.

Dependence occurs most frequently with drugs that alter the individual's mood or behavior. Narcotic *analgesics* used briefly to treat a disorder (for example, the use of *morphine* to treat a heart attack) hardly ever lead to dependence. Intravenous drug abuse carries a high risk of dependence; the rapidity with which the drug produces its effects reinforces the habit of injecting the drug.

Some people seem to be more susceptible to dependency than others. Factors that usually play a part include pressure from friends and associates, and environmental factors, such as poverty, unemployment, disrupted family life, and the availability of drugs.

SYMPTOMS AND SIGNS
A mild withdrawal reaction may cause yawning, sneezing, a runny nose, watering eyes, and sweating. More severe reactions include diarrhea, vomiting, trembling, cramps, confusion, and, rarely, seizures and coma. These symptoms are usually relieved if the drug is taken again.

Withdrawal symptoms probably occur because the body has become adapted to the continuous presence of the drug, which reduces the release of certain natural chemicals (for example, nicotine affects production of *epinephrine* and similar substances). When the drug is no longer taken or is withheld, the chemical deficiency is exposed.

COMPLICATIONS
Drug dependence may cause physical problems, such as lung and heart disease from tobacco smoking and liver disease from drinking excessive amounts of alcohol. Mental problems, such as anxiety and depression, are common during withdrawal. Dependence may also be associated with drug tolerance, in which an increasingly higher dose of the substance is needed to produce the desired effect.

Complications may occur as an indirect result of dependence. For example, people who inject a narcotic drug may get sick and die as a result of an infection, such as *hepatitis* or *AIDS*, introduced into the bloodstream on a dirty needle. In other cases, the abusers may suffer from an overdose because of confusion about the dosage or because they take a purer, more potent preparation than they are used to. In severe cases, social problems result from the disruption of family life and from criminal acts carried out to pay for drugs.

TREATMENT
Controlled withdrawal programs are available in special centers and larger hospitals. These programs usually offer supervised reductions in dose. Alternative, less harmful drugs may be given, as well as treatment for withdrawal symptoms. Social service agencies and support groups may provide follow-up care.

OUTLOOK
Successful treatment requires motivation on the part of the addict. Problems frequently recur when addicts return to the circumstances that originally gave rise to drug abuse and dependence.

Druggist
A *pharmacist*. A person who is licensed to dispense drugs and to make up prescriptions.

Drug overdose

The taking of an excessive amount of a drug, which may cause toxic effects. (See *Drug poisoning*.)

Drug poisoning

The harmful effects on various organs of the body as a result of taking an excessive dose of a drug.

CAUSES AND INCIDENCE

Drug poisoning may be accidental or deliberate. Accidental poisoning is most common in young children under the age of 5 years who swallow colored tablets thinking they are candies. Child-resistant drug packaging has helped reduce this risk. In adults, accidental poisoning usually occurs in the elderly because they are confused about their treatment and dosage requirements. Accidental poisoning may also occur during *drug abuse*.

Deliberate poisoning is usually unsuccessful and is done as a cry for help (see *Suicide; Suicide, attempted*). The drugs taken in overdose are usually *benzodiazepine drugs, antidepressant drugs, acetaminophen*, or *aspirin*. Homicide and suicide may involve administration of a drug by another person.

TREATMENT

In dealing with a drug overdose, first-aid measures depend on the condition of the patient. If the patient is unconscious, ensure that the *airway* is clear and that there is normal breathing and a pulse before rolling the patient into the *recovery position* and summoning emergency help. If the person is not breathing, *artificial respiration* should be started.

Any individual who has taken a drug overdose and any child who has swallowed tablets belonging to someone else should be seen by a physician. It is important to identify which drugs have been taken. Empty bottles may provide vital clues; save any you find. Contact the poison control center, hospital emergency room, or a physician for advice. If the victim is fully conscious, you may be advised to induce vomiting by sticking a finger down the throat or giving *ipecac* if this is available.

Some drugs taken in excess may cause *hypothermia*; if this occurs, keep the victim warm with blankets.

Treatment in the hospital may involve gastric *lavage* (emptying the stomach using several pints of water passed down a tube through the mouth and esophagus). This procedure usually is effective only if the drug has been taken within the pre-

vious four hours or a few hours longer for drugs (such as aspirin and antidepressants) that slow down normal stomach emptying.

Charcoal may be given in some cases to reduce the *absorption* of the drug from the intestine into the bloodstream. Diuresis (increased production of urine) may be induced using an *intravenous infusion* to speed up the elimination of the drug from the bloodstream.

Antidotes are available only for specific drugs. They include naloxone (given to reverse breathing difficulty caused by morphine), methionine (given to reduce the formation of toxic substances in the liver from acetaminophen), and *chelating agents* with deferoxamine (given to absorb and inactivate iron).

COMPLICATIONS

Drug poisoning may cause drowsiness and breathing difficulty (due to effects on the brain), irregular heart beat, and, rarely, cardiac arrest, seizures, and kidney and liver damage. *ECG* monitoring (electrical recording of the heart) is usually done for the first 24 to 48 hours after poisoning with a drug that is known to have effects on the heart. *Antiarrhythmic drugs* are prescribed to treat any heart beat irregularity as it develops. Seizures are treated with *anticonvulsant drugs*. In some serious cases, the patient requires artificial *ventilation* because of severe drug-induced breathing difficulty.

Blood tests to monitor liver function and careful monitoring of urine output are carried out if the drug is known to have any toxic effect on associated organs.

Dry eye

See *Keratoconjunctivitis sicca*.

Dry ice

Frozen *carbon dioxide*, also known as carbon dioxide snow. Unlike most substances, carbon dioxide changes directly from a gas to a solid when it is cooled, without first passing through a liquid phase. In practice, dry ice is produced by allowing carbon dioxide gas stored under pressure to escape through a small nozzle. This rapid expansion cools the carbon dioxide to about $-95°F$ ($-70°C$), and dry ice is formed as a powder. This powder is then compressed into cakes.

Dry ice is sometimes applied to the skin to destroy *warts* and *nevi*, which it does by virtue of its low temperature. (See also *Cryosurgery*.)

Dry socket

Infection at the site of a recent tooth extraction, causing pain, bad breath, and an unpleasant taste. A complication of about 2 percent of extractions, dry socket occurs most commonly when a blood clot fails to form in the tooth socket after a difficult extraction, such as removal of an impacted wisdom tooth. Infection may also develop following a normal extraction if the blood clot becomes dislodged (for instance, because of excessive rinsing of the mouth). In some cases, the clot itself may become infected, or infection may have been present before the extraction. The inflamed socket appears dry, and exposed bone, which may be dead and fragmented, is often visible.

TREATMENT

The socket is gently irrigated to remove debris, and then may be coated with a soothing, anti-inflammatory paste, such as zinc oxide or eugenol (oil of clove). Antibiotics may also be prescribed if drainage of the socket is incomplete. The infection usually begins to clear up within a few days.

DSM III

The third, and most recent, edition of the "Diagnostic and Statistical Manual of Mental Disorders," published by the American Psychiatric Association in 1980. DSM III provides criteria for classifying psychiatric illnesses for use by physicians when making diagnoses and by those compiling statistics and insurance forms.

Dual personality

See *Multiple personality*.

Duct

A tube or a tubelike passage leading from a gland to allow the flow of fluids—for example, tears through the tear ducts.

Dumbness

See *Mutism*.

Dumping syndrome

Symptoms including sweating, faintness, and palpitations resulting from the rapid passage of food from the stomach into the upper intestine. It mainly affects people who have had a partial or total *gastrectomy* (surgical removal of the stomach). Symptoms may occur within 30 minutes of eating (early dumping, usually associated with a lowered blood volume) or after 90 to 120 minutes (late dumping,

D

usually due to low blood sugar and potassium). Some tense people may have symptoms of dumping with an intact stomach.

CAUSES

Gastric surgery interferes with the normal mechanism by which food is emptied from the stomach. If a meal that is rich in carbohydrates is "dumped" too quickly from the stomach, it may cause the upper intestine to swell. In addition, certain hormones are released in excess into the bloodstream. These hormones, with the intestinal swelling, cause the symptoms of early dumping.

As sugars are absorbed from the intestine, they rapidly increase the blood glucose level, causing an excess amount of *insulin* to be released, which in turn may later lower the blood sugar level below normal, causing the symptoms of late dumping. A person who has had a gastrectomy can avoid symptoms by eating frequent, small, dry meals that do not contain refined carbohydrates such as white sugar. Symptoms may also be prevented by lying down after a large meal. Drug treatment is not often successful, but adding guar gum to food to slow the emptying of the stomach and the absorption of sugars is sometimes effective.

Duodenal ulcer

A raw area in the wall of the duodenum, caused by erosion of its inner surface lining. Duodenal and gastric ulcers (similar raw areas in the lining of the stomach) are also called *peptic ulcers* and have similar causes, symptoms, and treatment.

Duodenitis

Inflammation of the duodenum of uncertain cause, vague symptoms, and no physical signs. Treatment (which has never conclusively proved to be effective) is similar to treatment for a duodenal ulcer (see *Peptic ulcer*).

The diagnosis of duodenitis is made by *gastroscopy* (examination of the walls of the duodenum with a gastroscope, a fiberoptic viewing tube passed through the esophagus, stomach, and pylorus). Instead of an ulcer there is a diffuse area of inflammation, with redness and swelling of cells in the duodenal lining and often bleeding after contact with the tip of the gastroscope. A direct correlation between the gastroscope findings and any symptoms that could be considered duodenitis has yet to be made from clinical studies.

LOCATION OF THE DUODENUM
The duodenum is about 10 inches (25 cm) long and shaped like a C on its side; it forms a loop around the head of the pancreas.

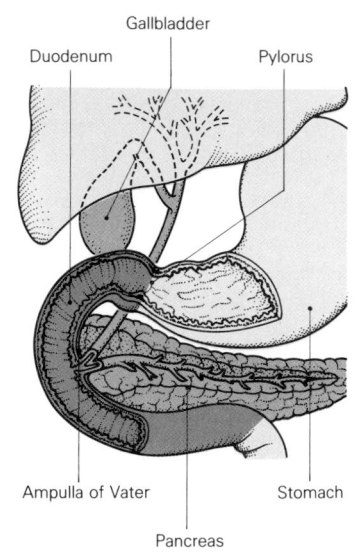

Gallbladder

Duodenum

Pylorus

Ampulla of Vater

Stomach

Pancreas

Duodenum

The first part of the small intestine, extending from the pylorus (the muscular valve at the lower end of the stomach) to the ligament of Treitz, which marks the boundary between the duodenum and the jejunum (the second part of the small intestine).

Ducts from the pancreas, liver, and gallbladder feed into the duodenum through a small opening called the ampulla of Vater, which is surrounded by the sphincter of Oddi. Digestive enzymes (proteins that break down food) contained in bile and the pancreatic secretions are released into the duodenum through this opening.

Dupuytren's contracture

A disorder of the hand in which the ring and little fingers become fixed in a bent position and can be straightened only by an operation. In about half the cases, both hands are affected. The disorder is named after the French surgeon who first described it, Baron Guillaume Dupuytren (1777-1835).

CAUSES AND INCIDENCE

The cause of the disorder is unclear. In most cases there is no apparent or

known cause, although the condition is slightly more common in certain groups—for example, in people whose work involves gripping tools, especially those that vibrate. The condition is a common feature in people with alcoholic liver *cirrhosis*. There is a slight tendency for the condition to run in families, though this does not necessarily mean it is inherited genetically. Men over 40 are the most commonly affected.

SYMPTOMS AND SIGNS

The tissues under the skin in the palm of the hand become thickened and shortened, with tethering of the tendons that run into the fingers. A small, hard nodule forms on the palm of the hand and it spreads to form a band of hard tissue under the skin, with puckering of the skin itself. The affected fingers start to bend more and more over a period of months or years and cannot be pulled back straight.

TREATMENT

The only treatment is surgical and is performed when the deformity has become unsightly or has started to impede hand function. During surgery the bands of thickened tissue under the skin are cut and separated to free the tendons.

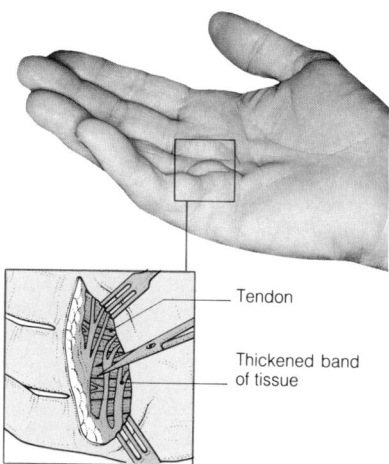

Tendon

Thickened band of tissue

Surgery for Dupuytren's contracture
Bands of tissue under the skin that have become thickened are cut and separated so that the tendons are freed.

Dust diseases

A group of lung disorders caused by inhalation, usually over several years at work, of dust particles that are absorbed into the lung tissues. There they cause *fibrosis* (formation of scar tissue) and progressive lung damage with crippling symptoms.

The main symptoms are a cough (with dark sputum) and breathing difficulty. It usually takes at least 10 years of exposure to dusts containing coal, silica, talc, or aluminum before serious lung damage develops (see *Pneumoconiosis*). Inhalation of asbestos dust can cause damage in much less time (see *Asbestosis*).

Workers in relevant industries show considerable variation in their susceptibility to dust disease. These people should have regular medical checkups to ensure that any signs of disease are detected early and serious damage is thus prevented.

Dwarfism

See *Short stature*.

Dying, care of the

People who are near death should be provided with physical and psychological care so that their final period of life is as free from pain, discomfort, and emotional distress as possible. Today, with good quality medical care, many deaths, even those from cancer, are pain-free and are associated with little physical discomfort. Emotional distress can be minimized by perception, understanding, and sensitive communication on the part of all those caring for the dying person. Usually, these people include physicians and other medical professionals, counselors, social workers, clergy, family, and friends. Family and friends should realize that they may undergo great emotional strain and may sometimes experience guilt for not being able to do more for the dying person. They, too, may benefit from counseling.

WHEN AND WHAT TO TELL THE DYING PERSON

Over the last 20 years it has become more common for physicians to tell dying people, particularly cancer patients, the facts related to their diagnoses. Generally, if a person can discuss the likely outcome of his or her illness and can prepare for death, then dying itself is eased. However, there are people who prefer not to know or block out the knowledge. The wishes of the patient should be paramount; these wishes may not always be clear and those caring for the patient need considerable perception and understanding. Careful probing should be attempted before any blunt statements are made.

Sometimes, even though the dying person has made it clear that he or she would prefer to talk about death, family members feel unable to do so, and this can cause the patient much isolation and suffering. Sometimes, the dying person may find it easier to talk to someone who is not a relative. In both cases, specially trained people, counselors, and members of the clergy may be able to help promote communication between the patient and the family.

PHYSICAL CARE

For most dying people, pain is often the most feared problem. Today, however, virtually all pain can be relieved by the use of analgesics (painkillers). Regular, low doses of the drugs are given so that pain never builds up and the patient remains alert. Powerful analgesics, such as morphine and other opiates, are commonly given to relieve severe pain.

When analgesic drugs are not adequate, other methods may be needed. These include nerve blocks (in which a nerve carrying pain from the body to the brain is interrupted by an injection or surgery), cordotomy (also called rhizotomy, or severing of nerve fibers in the spinal cord), or *TENS* (nerve stimulation with small electric currents), which is less likely to be effective once narcotic analgesics have been used.

Physical symptoms other than pain may also cause great distress. Nausea and vomiting may be a problem when the kidney and liver have ceased to function adequately. A combination of two or three drugs may occasionally control the symptom. An obstruction in the esophagus can cause vomiting or difficulty swallowing and may need to be relieved by an operation or by laser treatments through an esophagoscope. Another common problem is breathlessness, which usually responds to morphine.

The patient may develop aches or become stiff from being in bed. Comfort can be improved by keeping the patient as active as possible.

Toward the end, the dying person may become restless and breathing may become difficult, either because the lungs become waterlogged as the heart fails or because of a constant trickle of saliva into the windpipe. These symptoms can be relieved by medication and by placing the patient in a more comfortable position.

PSYCHOLOGICAL CARE

Emotional care is every bit as important (if not more so) as the relief of pain. Many people feel anger or depression at the thought of dying; feelings of guilt or regret over the past are also common. Ultimately, however, given loving, caring support from family, friends, and others, most terminally ill people come to terms with the thought of death. Sometimes antidepressant drugs are prescribed to relieve severe depression.

A great cause of anxiety and worry may be fear of a painful end. Patients should be reassured that adequate pain relief will be maintained at all times and that even when death is very close they need not fear suffering. Most people sink into unconsciousness just before the end and die "in their sleep." Fear of dependency and loss of dignity may also cause worry. The dying person should be allowed to participate as much as possible in family discussions and decisions regarding the future.

Preparing for death may include practical matters, such as writing a will, or other less tangible things such as saying "I'm sorry," "thank you," or "goodbye." Confession and reassurance from a priest or spiritual counselor are also important for some people. Perhaps the most pressing need for the terminally ill person is communication. Relatives, friends, and caregivers must be willing to share the dying person's concerns.

HOME OR HOSPITAL?

The treatment of most types of cancer requires hospital facilities at one time or another. However, once an illness has a foreseeable end, many people prefer and many families choose to care for a dying relative at home. Few terminally ill patients require complicated nursing for a prolonged period, and the sort of loving understanding and emotional care needed may be best provided at home. At home, too, the dying person can maintain some dignity and independence, avoid isolation, and participate in family life. By contrast, a hospital is better equipped to deal with acute illness.

HOSPICES

Hospices are small units, sometimes linked to a general hospital, that have been established specifically to care for the dying and their families. Their numbers have grown considerably during the last few years. Hospital routine is generally absent; instead, the efforts of the hospice staff, which includes nurses specially trained in terminal care, are directed toward the relief of physical and emotional pain. Basic to the hospice philosophy is the idea that dying people and their families need help, care, and understanding. It has been argued that a dying person might find the sight of other people dying depressing, but it has been found that most people who die in a hospice are reassured because death occurs peacefully.

Dys-

A prefix meaning abnormal, difficult, painful, or faulty, as in dysuria (pain on passing urine).

Dysarthria

A speech disability caused by disease or damage to the physical apparatus of speech, or to nerve pathways controlling this apparatus.

Dysarthria differs from *aphasia* (another type of speech disorder) in that dysarthric patients have nothing wrong with the speech center in the brain. They are able to formulate, select, and write out words and sentences grammatically; it is only vocal expression that causes problems. *Dysphonia* is a speech disability with a more restricted meaning than dysarthria, referring only to defects of sound production caused by some disease or damage to the larynx.

CAUSES

Dysarthria is a common feature of many degenerative conditions affecting the nervous system, such as *multiple sclerosis*, *Parkinson's disease*, and *Huntington's chorea*. It also affects some children who have *cerebral palsy*. Dysarthria may result from a *stroke*, *brain tumor*, or an isolated defect or damage to a particular nerve (such as the hypoglossal nerve that controls tongue movements). Structural defects of the mouth, as occur in *cleft lip and palate*, or even ill-fitting false teeth may also affect speech.

TREATMENT

There is no specific treatment for dysarthria. In some cases, drug or surgical treatment of the underlying disease or structural defect may restore the ability to speak clearly. In other instances, patients may benefit from *speech therapy*. (See also *Speech*.)

Dyschondroplasia

A rare disorder, present from birth, characterized by the presence of multiple tumors of cartilaginous tissue within bones. Dyschondroplasia is caused by a failure of normal bone development from cartilage. Usually only the bones in one limb are affected; the bones and limb are shortened, with resultant deformity.

Dysentery

A severe infection of the intestines, causing diarrhea (often mixed with

Key

High prevalence

Moderate prevalence

Areas of amebic dysentery
Amebic dysentery is most prevalent in countries where standards of hygiene are low. The photograph shows a magnified sample of *ENTAMOEBA HISTOLYTICA*.

blood, pus, and mucus) and abdominal pain. The person may spend hours straining on the toilet, producing little but blood-stained watery mucus.

There are two distinct forms of dysentery. *Shigellosis*, also called bacillary dysentery, is caused by infection with any of a group of bacteria called shigella. The diarrhea starts suddenly and is watery; sometimes toxemia (the presence of bacterial toxins in the blood) develops.

Amebic dysentery is caused by the protozoan (single-celled) parasite *ENTAMOEBA HISTOLYTICA*. It starts more gradually and often runs a chronic course.

The main risk with acute dysentery is *dehydration* from loss of fluid in the diarrhea. (See also *Colitis*.)

Dyskinesia

Abnormal muscular movements caused by a brain disorder. Uncontrollable twitching, jerking, or writhing movements occur that cannot be suppressed and may impair the performance of voluntary (willed) movements. The disorder may involve the whole body or may be restricted to a group of muscles, such as those around the eye.

Different types of dyskinesia include *chorea* (mainly jerking movements), *athetosis* (writhing movements), *choreoathetosis* (a combined form), *tics* (repetitive fidgets), *tremors*, and *myoclonus* (muscle spasms).

Dyskinesias may result from brain damage at birth or it may be a side effect of certain drugs, particularly

some drugs used to treat psychiatric illnesses and the antiemetic drug metoclopramide. The affected brain region is a group of linked nerve centers called the *extrapyramidal system*, which includes the *basal ganglia*.

Dyskinesias due to drugs often resolve when drug use is stopped. Otherwise they are difficult to treat. Drugs such as tetrabenazine may help reduce choreic movements, but often the physician must prescribe several drugs in turn before one (if any) is effective. (See also *Parkinsonism*).

Dyslexia

A specific reading disability characterized by difficulty in coping with written symbols. The term is not used to describe other types of reading difficulty, such as problems arising from brain damage or mental handicap, or from speech or visual defects. In addition, dyslexia does not include reading problems caused by educational or social neglect.

CAUSES AND INCIDENCE

Emotional disturbance, minor visual defects, and failure to "train" the brain have all been suggested as possible causes of dyslexia, but there is now good evidence that a specific, sometimes inherited, neurological disorder underlies true dyslexia. Some 90 percent of dyslexics are male.

SYMPTOMS

The key feature of dyslexia is that in other respects the child has entirely normal intelligence. Thus, his or her attainment of reading skills lags far behind other scholastic abilities and

D

overall IQ. Usually, the child can read numbers or musical notes much more easily than words.

Furthermore, while many first- and second-grade children tend to reverse letters and words (for example, writing or reading p for q, b for d, was for saw, no for on), the majority soon correct such errors. Dyslexic children continue to confuse these symbols. Letters are transposed (as in pest for step) and spelling errors are common. These children may even be unable to read words they can spell correctly. Writing from dictation may be difficult even though most dyslexics can copy sentences.

TREATMENT
It is important to recognize the problem early to avoid any added frustrations. Specific remedial teaching can help the child develop "tricks" to overcome the deficit, and avoidance of pressure from parents combined with praise for what the child can do is equally important. Given the right support and training, sufferers can usually overcome their difficulties. Many dyslexics have developed notable careers while still retaining some features of dyslexia.

Dysmenorrhea
Pain or discomfort during or just before a menstrual period. Most teenage girls and young women suffer to some degree from what is called primary dysmenorrhea. It usually starts two or three years after the first period, once ovulation is established; often it diminishes after the age of about 25, and it is rare after childbirth.

Dysmenorrhea is known to be associated with the hormonal changes that occur during a period, but the exact mechanism of the link between them remains uncertain. One possibility is that dysmenorrhea is due to excessive production of, or undue sensitivity to, prostaglandin, the hormone that stimulates muscular spasm of the uterus.

Secondary dysmenorrhea is, by definition, due to an underlying disorder (such as *endometriosis* or *pelvic inflammatory disease*).

Either type of dysmenorrhea may or may not be accompanied by *premenstrual syndrome*, a bloated feeling and irritability, depression, and other changes that commonly occur in the days preceding *menstruation*.

SYMPTOMS
Dysmenorrhea is typically felt as cramplike pain or discomfort in the lower abdomen, which may come and go in waves. There may also be dull lower backache and, in some women, nausea and vomiting. In primary dysmenorrhea the pain starts shortly before a period and usually lasts for less than 12 hours. About 10 percent of women have symptoms severe enough to interfere with their work or leisure activities. In secondary dysmenorrhea the pain begins several days before a period and lasts throughout it.

Mild primary dysmenorrhea is often relieved by analgesics (such as aspirin) or prostaglandin inhibitors (drugs that block the action of prostaglandin) such as naproxen. Rest in bed with a heating pad or hot-water bottle is a traditional and sometimes effective remedy. If symptoms are severe, they can usually be relieved by suppressing ovulation, either with the birth-control pill or with non-contraceptive hormones.

Treatment of secondary dysmenorrhea depends on the cause.

Dyspareunia
The medical term for painful sexual intercourse. (See *Intercourse, painful*.)

Dyspepsia
The medical term for *indigestion*.

Dysphagia
The medical term for *swallowing difficulty*.

Dysphasia
A term sometimes used to describe a disturbance in the ability to select the words with which we speak and write (and/or to comprehend and read) caused by damage to regions of the brain concerned with speech and comprehension. (See *Aphasia*.)

Dysphonia
Defective production of vocal sounds in speech, caused by disease or damage to the larynx (the voice box at the top of the windpipe) or to the nerve supply to the laryngeal muscles. Dysphonia should be distinguished from *dysarthria*, in which speech is defective because of damage or disease involving the controlling nerve pathways or muscles of other speech apparatus (e.g., respiratory muscles, throat, tongue, or lips); it is also to be distinguished from expressive *aphasia*, in which the ability to speak may be profoundly disturbed by damage to the speech center in the brain. (See also *Larynx* disorders box; *Speech*; *Speech disorders*.)

Dysplasia
Any abnormality of growth. The term applies to misshapen structures such as the skull (cranial dysplasia) and to abnormalities of single cells (cellular dysplasia). Abnormal cell features include the size, shape, and rate of multiplication of cells.

Dyspnea
The term for difficult or labored breathing. (See *Breathing difficulty*.)

Dysrhythmia, cardiac
The medical term, sometimes used as an alternative to *arrhythmia*, meaning disturbance of heart rhythm.

Dystonia
Abnormal muscle rigidity, causing painful muscle spasms, unusually fixed postures, or strange movement patterns. Dystonia may affect a localized area of the body, or it may be more generalized.

The most common types of localized dystonia are *torticollis* (painful neck spasm) and *scoliosis* (abnormal curvature of the spine) caused by an injury to the back that produces muscle spasm.

More generalized dystonia occurs as a result of various neurological disorders, including *Parkinson's disease* and *stroke*, and may also be a feature of *schizophrenia*. Dystonia may be a side effect of *antipsychotic drugs*.

Dystrophy
Any disorder in which the structure and normal activity of cells within a tissue have been disrupted by inadequate nutrition. The usual cause is poor circulation of blood through the tissue, but dystrophy can also be due to damage to nerves or to lack of catalytic protein (a specific enzyme) in that tissue.

In *muscular dystrophies*, muscle cells fail to develop normally, causing weakness and paralysis. In the leukodystrophies, there is *demyelination* (loss of the sheath surrounding nerves) within the brain, causing a variety of disturbances of sensation, movement, and intellect.

Corneal dystrophies are a rare, usually inherited, cause of blindness. In this condition, cells lining the cornea are damaged and the eye's surface becomes opaque.

Dysuria
The medical term for pain, discomfort, or difficulty in passing urine. (See *Urination, painful*.)

E

Ear

The organ of hearing and balance. The ear consists of three parts: the outer ear, the middle ear, and the inner ear. The outer and middle ear are concerned primarily with the collection and transmission of sound. The inner ear is responsible for analyzing sound waves; it also contains the mechanism by which the body keeps its balance.

OUTER EAR

The outer ear consists of the pinna (also called the auricle), which is the visible part of the ear, composed of folds of skin and cartilage. The pinna leads into the ear canal (also called the meatus), which is 1 inch (2.5 cm) long in adults and closed at its inner end by the tympanic membrane (eardrum). The part of the canal nearest the outside is made of cartilage. The cartilage is covered with skin that produces wax, which, along with hair, traps dust and small foreign bodies.

The eardrum separates the outer ear from the middle ear. The eardrum is a thin, fibrous, circular membrane covered with a thin layer of skin. It vibrates in response to the changes in air pressure that constitute sound and works in conjunction with the other components of the middle ear.

MIDDLE EAR

The middle ear is a small cavity between the eardrum and the inner ear. It conducts sound to the inner ear by means of a chain of three tiny, linked, movable bones called ossicles. They link the eardrum to an oval window in the bony wall on the opposite inner side of the middle-ear cavity. The bones are named because of their shapes. The malleus (hammer) is joined to the inside of the eardrum. The incus (anvil) has one broad joint with the malleus (which lies almost parallel to it) and a delicate joint to the third bone, the stapes (stirrup). The base of the stapes fills the oval window, which leads to the inner ear.

The middle ear is cut off from the outside by the eardrum, but it is not completely airtight; a ventilation passage, called the eustachian tube,

ANATOMY OF THE EAR

The outer ear comprises the pinna and ear canal; the middle ear—the eardrum, hammer, anvil, stirrup, and eustachian tube; and the inner ear—the vestibule, semicircular canals, and cochlea. Sensory impulses from the inner ear pass to the brain via the vestibulocochlear nerve.

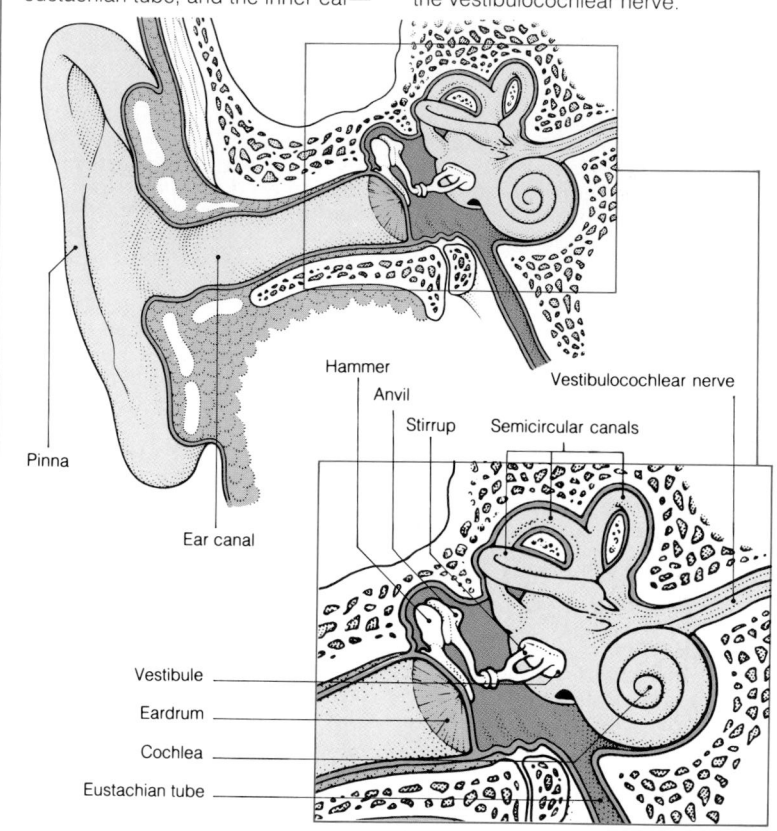

Pinna
Ear canal
Hammer
Anvil
Stirrup
Semicircular canals
Vestibulocochlear nerve
Vestibule
Eardrum
Cochlea
Eustachian tube

runs forward and down into the back of the nose. The eustachian tube is normally closed, but it opens by muscular contraction with yawning and swallowing.

The middle ear acts as a transformer, passing the vibrations of sound from the air outside (which is a thin medium) to the fluid in the inner ear (which is a thicker medium).

INNER EAR

The inner ear is an extremely intricate series of structures contained deep within the bones of the skull. It consists of a maze of winding passages, collectively known as the labyrinth. The front part, the cochlea, is a tube resembling a snail's shell and is concerned with hearing. (For a detailed discussion of how this system works, see *Hearing*.) The rear part (three semicircular canals and two other organs) is concerned with balance. The semicircular canals are set at right angles to each other and are connected to a cavity known as the vestibule. The canals contain hair cells bathed in fluid. Some of these cells are sensitive to gravity and acceleration; others respond to positions and movements of the head (i.e., side to side, up and down, or tilted). The information concerning posture or direction is registered by the relevant cells and conveyed by nerve fibers to the brain. (See also *Ear* disorders box.)

Earache

The most common cause of earache is acute *otitis media* (infection of the middle ear), most commonly occurring in young children. The pain is likely to be severe and stabbing; there may also be loss of hearing and a raised temperature. If the eardrum bursts, there is a discharge of fluid and immediate relief from the pressure and therefore the accompanying pain.

DISORDERS OF THE EAR

The ear is susceptible to a large variety of disorders, some of which can lead to *deafness. Vertigo* (dizziness associated with a disturbance of balance) as a result of ear disease is not common, but it occurs in some disorders of the inner ear.

CONGENITAL DEFECTS

Very rarely, a baby is born with an absent or extremely narrowed external ear canal, and sometimes the small bones of the middle ear are deformed or absent.

Occasionally, the pinna (external ear) is missing or distorted. *Rubella* (German measles) affecting a woman during the first three months of pregnancy can cause severe damage to the baby's hearing apparatus, leading to deafness.

INFECTION

Infection is the most common cause of ear disorders. Infection may occur in the ear canal, leading to *otitis externa,* or may affect the middle ear, causing *otitis media,* which often leads to perforation of the eardrum (see *Eardrum, perforated*). Persistent *middle-ear effusion* (buildup of fluid within the middle ear), often due to infection, is the most common cause of hearing difficulties in children.

Middle-ear infection can spread to cause *mastoiditis* (infection of the mastoid process, the bone behind the ear) or brain abscess, but these complications have become extremely rare since the introduction of antibiotics.

Virus infection of the inner ear may cause *labyrinthitis* with severe vertigo and/or sudden hearing loss.

INJURY

Cauliflower ear is the result of repeated injury to the pinna. Injury to the external ear canal and perforation of the eardrum can result from poking objects into the ear or, rarely, from careless syringing. A sudden blow, especially a slap, to the ear or a very loud noise may also perforate the eardrum. Prolonged exposure to loud noise or close proximity to a loud explosion can cause *tinnitus* (noises within the ear) and/or deafness. Pressure changes associated with flying or scuba diving can also cause minor damage and pain (see *Barotrauma*).

TUMORS

Tumors in the ear are rare, but occasionally a *basal cell carcinoma* (rodent ulcer) or a *squamous cell carcinoma* affects the pinna. The latter may also involve the ear canal. Cancers of the middle and inner ears are extremely rare. *Acoustic neuroma* is a benign (nonmalignant), slow-growing tumor of the acoustic nerve that may press on structures within the ear to cause deafness, tinnitus, and imbalance. *Cholesteatoma,* a growing collection of skin cells and debris, is not a tumor, but may be equally dangerous.

OBSTRUCTION

Ear canal obstruction is most often caused by dried *earwax,* but may also result from otitis externa. In children, a frequent cause is putting a foreign body into the ear (see *Ear, foreign body in*).

DEGENERATION

Deafness in many elderly people is due to *presbycusis,* deterioration of the hair cells in the cochlea.

POISONING/DRUGS

The inner ear is especially sensitive to damage by certain classes of drugs. The most important—the aminoglycoside *antibiotic drugs*—include such drugs as streptomycin and gentamicin. These drugs can cause damage to the cochlear hair cells, especially if used in high concentration and particularly in the presence of kidney disease, which can delay the excretion of the drugs from the body.

There are other drugs that can damage ear function, including quinine, aspirin, and the *diuretic drugs* furosemide, ethacrynic acid, and bumetanide.

OTHER DISORDERS

In *otosclerosis,* a hereditary condition, the base of one of the small bones in the middle ear becomes fixed, causing deafness. *Meniere's disease* is an uncommon disorder in which deafness, vertigo, and tinnitus result from the accumulation of fluid within the labyrinth in the inner ear.

INVESTIGATION

The function of hearing is investigated by various tuning-fork and audiometric *hearing tests,* which reveal different types and levels of hearing loss. The external ear canal and the eardrum may be examined with an *otoscope* and mirror; an otoscopic microscope may also be used.

The function of the balancing mechanism of the inner ear is investigated by observing *nystagmus* (jerky eye movements) when the head is placed in different positions or the whole body rotated, and when the ear is gently syringed with hot or cold water (*caloric tests*). These tests may be refined and recorded by *electronystagmography.*

E

Another common cause of earache is *otitis externa* (inflammation of the outer ear canal), which is often caused by infection. Infection may be localized or affect the whole canal, sometimes taking the form of a boil or abscess. The earache may be accompanied by irritation or itching in the ear, a discharge, and mild deafness.

A much rarer cause of earache is *herpes zoster* infection, which causes blisters in the ear canal. The earache may persist for weeks or months after the infection has cleared.

Intermittent earache may also occur in people with dental problems, tonsillitis, throat cancer, pain in the lower jaw or neck muscles, and other disorders affecting areas near the ear. Earache in this case is caused because the ear and many nearby areas are supplied by the same nerves; in these cases the pain is said to be "referred" to the ear.

INVESTIGATION

The physician inspects the outer ear manually and then examines the ear canal and drum with an *otoscope* and, if necessary, a binocular microscope; he or she may arrange for X rays and other tests to be carried out (see *Ear, examination of*). The mouth, throat, and teeth are also examined.

TREATMENT

Analgesics (painkillers) may be given and the underlying cause of the

E

earache treated. Antibiotic drugs are prescribed for an infection. Pus in the outer ear may need to be aspirated (sucked out), usually as an office procedure. Pus in the middle ear may require draining through a hole made in the eardrum; this operation is known as *myringotomy*.

Ear, cauliflower

See *Cauliflower ear*.

Ear, discharge from

Fluid emitted from the ear, usually as the result of an infection of the outer ear (see *Otitis externa*) or middle ear (see *Otitis media*).

In very rare cases following fracture of the skull, cerebrospinal fluid or blood may be discharged from the ear.

INVESTIGATION AND TREATMENT

Any discharge from the ear should be reported to your physician. Tests may include performing *hearing tests* and taking a swab of the discharge to produce a *culture* for laboratory analysis. It may be necessary to clean and carefully inspect the ear using a special microscope and/or take special X rays to rule out *cholesteatoma* (a benign condition associated with chronic drainage from the ear).

Eardrum, perforated

Rupture or erosion of the eardrum, usually as the result of acute *otitis media* (infection of the middle ear).

CAUSES

In acute otitis media, pus builds up in the middle-ear cavity and, unless the infection is treated, the pressure may burst the eardrum. A hole may also be eroded in the eardrum as the result of chronic otitis media. Less common causes of rupture are inserting a sharp object into the ear to relieve irritation, a blow on the ear (usually a hard slap), a nearby explosion, fracture of the base of the skull, *barotrauma* (caused by air pressure change during flying or diving), or, very rarely, a tumor of the middle ear. The physician may puncture the eardrum to drain the middle ear and prevent rupture in a more critical area.

TREATMENT AND OUTLOOK

Anyone who suspects a perforated eardrum should first cover the ear with a clean, dry pad to prevent infection from entering the middle ear; next, consult a physician. An analgesic (painkiller) may be taken.

The physician will prescribe *antibiotic drugs* to treat any infection. Except in chronic otitis media that has damaged the sound-transmitting

bones in the middle ear, no other treatment is usually required, since the eardrum generally heals on its own. Normal hearing is restored within a month.

If a perforation fails to heal or close sufficiently within six months, a *myringoplasty* (an operation in which the eardrum is repaired with a tissue graft from elsewhere in the body) may be performed. Many perforations can be healed with an office treatment that "freshens" the edges of the perforation so that it has another chance to heal on its own.

Ear, examination of

The ear requires examination any time the following symptoms develop: earache, discharge from the ear, loss of hearing, a feeling of fullness in the ear, disturbance of balance, tinnitus (noises in the ear), or swollen or tender lymph nodes below or in front of the ear.

The physician can inspect only the pinna (the visible outer ear), the ear canal, and the eardrum. To investigate the middle and inner ears, more specialized tests are required.

HOW IT IS DONE

The physician inspects the pinna manually for any evidence of swelling, tenderness, ulceration, or deformity and examines the skin above and behind the ear for signs of previous surgery. To inspect the ear canal and eardrum, the physician usually uses an *otoscope* (a viewing instrument for examining the ear). If necessary, a more magnified, three-dimensional image can be obtained by using a binocular microscope.

To obtain images of the middle and inner ears, the physician may arrange for plain X rays, *tomography*, *CT scanning*, or *MRI* to be carried out. Hearing and balance may require assessment by means of *hearing tests*, *caloric tests*, and *electronystagmography*.

Ear, foreign body in

The external ear canal is a common location for foreign bodies. Children often insert small objects, such as beads, peas, or stones, into their ears. It is also possible for insects to fly or crawl into the ear.

TREATMENT

SMALL OBJECTS These must always be removed by a physician. Under no circumstances should removal be attempted by poking with cotton swabs, hair pins, or similar objects; these efforts usually drive the object farther into the ear canal.

FIRST AID: FOREIGN BODY IN EAR

DO NOT
■ attempt to dislodge the object by probing. Small objects must be removed by a physician
■ pour liquid into the ear unless you are certain the object is an insect

TO REMOVE AN INSECT

Tilt the victim's head so that the affected ear is facing upward. Pour lukewarm water into the ear and the insect may float to the surface. If this fails, call your physician.

The physican will remove the object either by syringing or by grasping it with a pair of fine-toothed forceps. A brief general anesthetic may be required if the object is impacted, as often occurs with organic foreign bodies, such as beans, which swell when moistened by ear secretions.

INSECTS An insect can sometimes be removed from the ear by having the person tilt his or her head so that the affected side is uppermost and then pouring oil or lukewarm water into the ear. If this is not successful, a physician will need to syringe the ear after killing the insect with chloroform or drowning it with oil. It is impossible for insects to penetrate the brain from the ear.

Ear piercing

Making a hole in the earlobe or, occasionally, another part of the external ear, to accommodate an earring. Ear piercing was once performed with a needle, but the risk of transmitting diseases through the use of unsterile needles caused this method to be replaced by a special ear-piercing gun.

HOW IT IS DONE

A local anesthetic is not necessary, since the procedure causes only minor discomfort. The ear lobe is pierced by a post or stud (sometimes called a sleeper), fired into it by the gun, which does not come into contact with the ear. The posts are of gold or gold-plate (cheaper metals can cause contact *dermatitis*), are kept sealed in a sterile pack before use, and are not handled during the procedure.

For six weeks after insertion, the posts must be cleaned regularly with hydrogen peroxide or rubbing alcohol to prevent infection; the posts are kept in the ears and turned twice daily to prevent the hole from closing.

Ears, pinning back of

See *Otoplasty*.

Ear tube

A small tube that can be inserted through the eardrum at *myringotomy* (a surgical incision made in the eardrum) to treat persistent *middle-ear* *effusion* in children. The tube equalizes the pressure on both sides of the eardrum, permitting drainage. Tubes are usually allowed to fall out on their own, which generally occurs between six and 12 months after insertion. Children should not swim unless they wear special earplugs.

Earwax

A deep yellow or brown secretion, medically known as cerumen, produced by glands in the outer-ear canal. In most people, wax is produced in only small amounts, falls out on its own, and causes no trouble; in other people, so much wax forms that it regularly obstructs the canal, sometimes as often as every few months.

Excess earwax may produce a sensation of fullness in the ear and, if the canal is blocked completely, partial deafness. These symptoms are made worse if water enters the ear and makes the wax swell. Prolonged blockage may also inflame the skin of the canal, causing irritation.

Wax completely blocking the ear should always be removed. A firm plug of wax can be removed by a physician with a ring probe, right-angle hook, or *forceps*. If the wax is too soft for this, it can be softened further with oil and then flushed out with an ear syringe containing warm water. If there is a possibility that the eardrum is damaged, the physician uses suction instead of syringing.

A person can remove his or her own earwax with mineral oil drops (for hard wax) or hydrogen peroxide drops (for soft wax) or with commercially available preparations. Cotton swabs should not be used. They can push wax deep into the canal, making the problem worse.

Ecchymosis

The medical term for a *bruise*.

ECG

Also sometimes called EKG, the abbreviation for electrocardiogram, a record of the electrical impulses that

---

THE ELECTROCARDIOGRAM (ECG)

Electrocardiography causes no discomfort. Electrodes connected to a recording machine are applied to the chest, wrists, and ankles. The machine displays the electrical activity in the heart as a trace on a moving graph or on a screen. Any abnormality is thus revealed to the physician. At below right are shown normal and abnormal recordings.

An ECG can be taken at home, in the physician's office, or in the hospital; a 24-hour record can be obtained from a tape recorder worn by the patient.

Lead positions
Recordings are taken with a lead attached to these positions.

Modern electrocardiograph
A modern, lightweight, portable ECG machine. Leads from the machine are attached to the chest, wrists, and ankles using conducting jelly.

Printout

Normal ECG
This tracing shows the electrical activity preceding one normal heart beat. The vertical axis shows the current flowing toward the recording lead. The rise at P occurs just before the atria (upper heart chambers) begin to contract, the QRS "spike" occurs just before the ventricles (lower chambers) begin to contract, and the rise at T occurs as the electrical potential returns to zero.

Normal rhythm
The heart chambers are contracting with complete regularity.

Ventricular fibrillation
Here, the contractions of the lower heart chambers are extremely irregular.

Complete heart block
The upper and lower heart chambers are beating independently.

Atrial fibrillation
Caused by the upper heart chambers beating fast and irregularly.

E

immediately precede contraction of the heart muscle. The waves produced are known as the P,Q,R,S, and T waves. An ECG is a useful means of diagnosing disorders of the heart, many of which produce deviations from normal electrical patterns. Among these disorders are *coronary heart disease, coronary thrombosis, pericarditis* (inflammation of the membrane surrounding the heart), *cardiomyopathy* (heart muscle disorders), *myocarditis* (inflammation of the heart muscle), and arrhythmia (see *Arrhythmia, cardiac*).

Echocardiography

A method of obtaining an image of the structure of the heart using *ultrasound* (inaudible, high-frequency, sound waves). The sound is reflected differently by each part of the heart and a complex series of echoes results.

WHY IT IS DONE

Echocardiography is a major diagnostic technique used to detect structural, and some functional, abnormalities of the heart wall, the heart valves, and the heart's large blood vessels. Blood flow across valves is also measured.

The procedure is especially valuable for studying disorders of the heart valves. Abnormal opening and closing of the valves can be detected because they deviate from normal patterns of valve movement. Other diagnostic uses include detection of congenital heart disease (such as ventricular *septal defect*, a hole in the wall between the two lower chambers of the heart), various abnormalities of the large blood vessels, *cardiomyopathy* (enlargement or damage of the heart muscle), *aneurysms* (swellings caused by weakening of the heart wall or the walls of blood vessels), the presence of a blood clot within the chambers of the heart, and *pericarditis*.

HOW IT IS DONE

Echocardiography is harmless and the patient feels nothing; it has the added advantage of producing recordings without having to place an instrument inside the patient's body.

The transducer (the instrument that sends out and receives sound signals) is placed on the chest in a position that allows its sound waves to reach the structures under investigation. The echoes are detected, amplified, and then displayed visually as a series of lines on an oscilloscope screen or a paper tape. This information is interpreted by cardiologists as a picture of the heart and its valves and the way they are working.

Echocardiography has become more sophisticated and methods have been developed that incorporate a moving transducer, or a set of transducers, attached to a computer. This allows a series of different views of the heart to be obtained, and a two-dimensional scan can thus be produced. When recorded on videotape, an easily recognizable picture of the activity of the interior of the heart can be seen. Another recently developed feature is Doppler echocardiography. This technique can indirectly measure the flow velocity of blood as it passes through the heart. It can be useful in assessing malfunctioning valves (e.g., in *aortic stenosis* or *mitral insufficiency*) and in assessing patients with congenital heart disease.

Echolalia

The compulsive repetition of what is spoken by another person. The tone and accent of the speaker are copied as well as the actual words. It is an unusual symptom of catatonic *schizophrenia* and sometimes also occurs in people suffering from *autism* and some forms of *mental retardation*. Echolalia may be accompanied by echopraxia (imitating the behavior of another person).

Eclampsia

A rare, serious condition of late pregnancy, labor, and the period following delivery. Eclampsia is characterized by seizures (convulsions) in the woman, sometimes followed by coma and death; eclampsia also threatens the life of the baby. The disorder occurs as a complication of moderate or severe (but not mild) *preeclampsia*, a common condition of late pregnancy that is marked by *hypertension* (high blood pressure), *proteinuria* (protein in the urine), and *edema* (an excessive accumulation of fluid in the tissues).

CAUSES

Both preeclampsia and eclampsia are believed to be caused by a substance or toxin produced by the placenta, the organ in the uterus that sustains the unborn child. To date, however, extensive investigations have failed to identify the cause.

Eclampsia occurs more commonly in women who have had little or no *prenatal care*. Preeclampsia develops in these women without it being recognized and treated.

INCIDENCE

About half of all cases develop in late pregnancy, one third during labor, and the rest after delivery.

SYMPTOMS AND SIGNS

In eclampsia the symptoms that characterize severe preeclampsia are present. In addition, before the onset of seizures, the woman may suffer from headache, confusion, blurred vision, and abdominal pain. The seizures consist of violent, rhythmic, jerking movements of the limbs caused by involuntary contraction of the muscles; there may also be breathing difficulty caused by constriction of the muscles of the larynx. The seizures may sometimes be followed by coma.

TREATMENT

The seizures are treated by ensuring that the woman can breathe properly (sometimes by inserting an endotracheal tube down her throat) and by giving *anticonvulsant drugs*, which prevent further seizures.

The baby's condition is monitored throughout. Rapid delivery (often by emergency *cesarean section*) is usually performed, since the condition often clears once the baby is born.

OUTLOOK

About one third to one half of babies fail to survive eclampsia, usually because of lack of oxygen in the uterus. Of these deaths, half occur before delivery, the others soon after.

After delivery, the mother's blood pressure usually returns to normal within a week and proteinuria clears within six weeks. In about 5 to 10 percent of cases, however, serious complications develop in the woman before, during, or after delivery. These may include failure of the heart and lungs, kidney, or liver, *intracerebral hemorrhage, pneumonia*, or pulmonary *edema*.

Econazole

An *antifungal drug* used in the form of a cream to treat fungal skin infections (see *Athlete's foot; Tinea*). Econazole is also prescribed to treat *candidiasis*.

Econazole is a fast-working antifungal drug (usually beginning to act within two days). Skin irritation is a rare adverse effect.

ECT

The abbreviation for electroconvulsive therapy, which uses an electric shock to induce a *seizure* as a form of psychiatric treatment. Muscle-relaxant drugs are used to minimize movements of the body and the effects of ECT are limited primarily to the brain.

WHY IT IS USED

ECT is used almost exclusively to treat severe depressive illness that is causing symptoms such as weight loss or apathy. It is used less widely to treat *postpartum depression*, catatonic *schizophrenia*, and some cases of *mania* that have not responded to other treatments. ECT is not used to treat people with severe physical illness or those who have had a recent myocardial infarction (heart attack).

HOW IT IS DONE
The patient is given an anesthetic and a muscle relaxant before two padded electrodes are applied to the temples, one on each side or both on the same side. A controlled electric pulse is delivered to the electrodes from a small machine until the patient experiences a brain seizure. The seizure is indicated by brief muscular rigidity, followed by twitching of the limbs and eyelids. Afterward, patients experience only a mild discomfort similar to the discomfort felt after a minor dental operation.

Treatment usually consists of six to 12 seizures (two or three per week).

OUTLOOK
If a true brain seizure has been induced at each session, the patient's condition usually begins to improve

by the third treatment, often dramatically. Temporary *amnesia* is a possible side effect.

Ectasia
A medical term for widening or distention, usually used to refer to a disorder affecting a duct that carries secretions from a gland or organ. For example, mammary duct ectasia—a rare disorder that affects mainly menopausal women—is widening of the ducts that carry secretions from the tissues of the breast to the nipple (see *Breast*).

-ectomy
A suffix denoting surgical removal. Tonsillectomy is surgical removal of the tonsils.

Ectoparasite
 A parasite that lives in or on its host's skin and derives nourishment from the skin or by sucking the host's blood. Various *lice*, ticks, mites, and some types of *fungi* are occasional ectoparasites of humans. By contrast, endoparasites live inside the body.

Ectopic
A medical term used to describe a structure that occurs in an abnormal location or position or an activity that occurs at an abnormal time.

Ectopic heart beat
A contraction of the heart muscle that is out of the normal timed sequence. An ectopic heart beat occurs shortly after a normal beat and is followed by a longer than usual interval.

Ectopic beats can occur in a heart that is otherwise functioning normally and may cause no symptoms. Multiple ectopic beats can sometimes cause *palpitations*.

After a *myocardial infarction* (heart attack), the occurrence of multiple ectopic beats is a sign of damage to the conduction system of the heart muscle. Multiple ectopic beats may lead to ventricular *fibrillation*, a rapid uncoordinated heart beat that can cause collapse and death.

Multiple ectopic beats that are causing palpitations, or that occur after a myocardial infarction, are often treated with an *antiarrhythmic drug*. (See also *Arrhythmia, cardiac*.)

Ectopic pregnancy
A pregnancy that develops outside the uterus, most commonly in the fallopian tube, but sometimes in the ovary or, rarely, in the abdominal cavity or cervix. It is a cause of acute abdomen (see *Abdomen, acute*).

INCIDENCE AND CAUSE
About one in every 100 pregnancies is ectopic. The fertilized ovum (egg) may become "stuck" in the fallopian tube if the tube is damaged or abnormal in any way. Ectopic pregnancies are more common if there is some congenital abnormality of the fallopian tubes, if the tubes have been previously operated on or infected, or if the woman has an *IUD*. They are also more likely if the woman has been taking the progesterone-only birth-control pill, has ingested postcoital hormonal contraception, or has undergone a (failed) sterilization, especially if the fallopian tubes have been cauterized.

SYMPTOMS AND SIGNS
Most ectopic pregnancies are discovered in the first two months, often before the woman realizes she is pregnant. In most cases a menstrual period is missed, but, in about 20 percent of the women, menstruation occurs. Symptoms of ectopic pregnancy usually include severe abdomi-

nal pain and vaginal spotting. After rupture or internal hemorrhage, the symptoms of internal bleeding appear—pallor, sweating, weakness, and faintness.

COMPLICATIONS
An ectopic pregnancy may cause the woman to go into *shock* due to severe loss of blood when the developing fetus damages the surrounding struc-

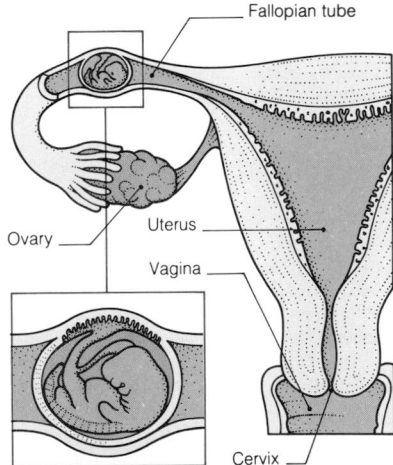

Location of an ectopic pregnancy
The pregnancy usually develops in the fallopian tube; occasionally it develops in the ovary, abdominal cavity, or cervix.

tures. Ectopic pregnancies are life-threatening and are responsible for about 10 percent of maternal deaths (deaths as a result of pregnancy or its complications). In the US approximately 50 women die each year as a result of ectopic pregnancy.

DIAGNOSIS
The physician usually performs a *pregnancy test* on any sexually active woman of childbearing age who has persistent, unexplained lower abdominal pain. *Ultrasound scanning* and a *laparoscopy* (examination of the abdominal cavity with a viewing instrument) may also be performed.

TREATMENT
Once an ectopic pregnancy is confirmed, an operation is performed to remove the developing fetus, the placenta, and any damaged tissue at the site of the pregnancy. Any torn blood vessels are repaired and, if the fallopian tube cannot be repaired, it is removed. If blood loss has been severe, transfusions are needed.

OUTLOOK
It is still possible to have a normal pregnancy even if one fallopian tube has been removed, although the chances of conception are slightly reduced. Women with two damaged tubes may require *in vitro fertilization* to achieve an intrauterine pregnancy.

Ectropion

A turning outward of the eyelid so that the inner surface is exposed.

INCIDENCE AND CAUSE

Ectropion most commonly occurs in elderly people because of weakness of the muscle surrounding the eye; it usually affects the lower lid. It may also be caused by the contraction of scar tissue (from wounds, burns, or surgical treatment) in the skin near the lids. In these cases, the upper lid may be affected. Ectropion often follows *facial palsy*, in which the muscles surrounding the eye (and other facial muscles on that side) are paralyzed.

The appearance of ectropion
An example of ectropion affecting the lower eyelid of one eye. The lid is turned outward to reveal the lining of its inner surface.

SYMPTOMS AND SIGNS

Even slight ectropion interferes with normal drainage of tears by distorting the opening of the tear duct. Chronic *conjunctivitis* may result, with redness, discomfort, and overflow of tears so that the skin becomes damp and inflamed. Constant wiping tends to pull the lid farther from the eye.

TREATMENT

Lid-tightening surgery (the removal of a wedge of tissue from the lid) is simple and effective in the early stages of ectropion. Even plastic surgery with skin grafting is liable to fail if the condition is long-standing.

Eczema

An inflammation of the skin, usually causing itching and sometimes accompanied by scaling or blisters. Some forms of eczema are better known as *dermatitis* (such as seborrheic dermatitis, contact dermatitis, and photodermatitis). Eczema is sometimes caused by an *allergy*, but often occurs for no known reason.

TYPES

ATOPIC ECZEMA This chronic, superficial inflammation occurs in people who have an inherited tendency toward allergy. They, or members of their family, may also have other allergies, such as *asthma* or allergic *rhinitis*.

Atopic eczema is common in babies and often appears between the ages of 2 and 18 months. A mild but intensely itchy rash occurs, usually on the face, in the inner creases of the elbows, and behind the knees. The skin often scales in these areas, and small red pimples may appear. As the baby scratches, the pimples begin to "weep" (leak) and join to form large weeping areas. Infection may occur, particularly in the diaper area.

For mild cases, treatment consists of applying emollients, such as petroleum jelly, which help keep the skin in the infected area soft. In severe cases, corticosteroid ointments may be prescribed, and *antibiotic drugs* may be given for infection. *Antihistamine drugs* may be prescribed to reduce itching, particularly if it keeps the baby awake at night. It is important to prevent the baby from becoming too hot (e.g., by wearing too many clothes), which aggravates the condition. Only cotton clothing, which is nonirritating and absorbent, should be in direct contact with the skin.

Atopic eczema
An example of atopic eczema on the creases of the inner wrist, showing the characteristic pimples and raw, scaling skin. Because the rash is intensely itchy, scratching is usually inevitable and aggravates the condition.

Atopic eczema often clears of its own accord as the child grows older, although it may come and go for several years before disappearing finally. Most children outgrow the condition by the time they reach puberty.

NUMMULAR ECZEMA This type usually occurs in adults. The cause is unknown. Nummular eczema takes the form of circular, itchy, scaling patches anywhere on the skin, similar to those of the fungal infection *tinea* (ringworm), from which the eczema needs to be distinguished.

Corticosteroid ointments may be applied to the affected skin to help reduce inflammation, although the disorder is persistent and often resistant to treatment.

HAND ECZEMA This type is usually a result of irritation by substances such as detergents, household cleansers, and dishwashing liquid, but may occur for no ascertainable reason. Itchy blisters, up to about 1 inch (2.5 cm) across, develop, usually on the palms, and the hand may be covered with scales and cracks. Tests are performed to check for allergy.

Hand eczema usually improves if rubber gloves are worn over white cotton gloves when in contact with any irritants. The hands should be thoroughly patted dry after washing. An unscented hand cream should be applied several times a day. If severe, corticosteroids may be prescribed for the inflammation and antibiotics may be given for infection.

STASIS DERMATITIS In people with varicose veins, the skin on the legs may become irritated, inflamed, and discolored. The most important factor is swelling of the legs, which may be controlled with compression bandages or special stockings. Mild corticosteroid ointments may give temporary relief.

GENERAL TREATMENT

To reduce irritation and the likelihood of scratching, a soothing ointment should be applied to the affected areas, which should then be covered by a dressing to prevent scratching. Absorbent, nonirritating materials such as cotton should be worn next to the skin; irritating fabrics such as wool, silk, and rough synthetics should be avoided.

Edema

An abnormal accumulation of serum-like fluid in the body tissues. It may or may not be visible (as a swelling) and can be either local (as following an injury) or general (as in *heart failure*). Generalized edema (also called anasarca) was once popularly known as dropsy.

WATER BALANCE IN THE BODY

Water accounts for roughly three fifths of body weight and it is constantly exchanged between blood and tissues. Water is forced out of the capillaries and into the tissues by the pressure of blood being pumped around the body. By a reverse process, which depends on the water-drawing power of the proteins in the blood (see *Osmosis*), it is reabsorbed into the capillaries from the tissues. These two mechanisms normally are in balance, keeping the levels of water in the blood and the tissues more or less constant.

Another factor involved in maintaining this balance is the action of the kidneys, which pass excess salt from the blood into the urine to be excreted from the body.

CAUSES OF EDEMA

Various disorders can interfere with these processes. Heart failure leads to blood congestion in the veins, creating backward pressure in the capillaries. This backward pressure overcomes osmotic pressure in the capillaries and thus causes more fluid than normal to be forced into the tissues at various places throughout the body. Backward pressure can also be created by a tumor pressing on veins. The edema produced is confined to the area drained by the obstructed vein.

In the *nephrotic syndrome*, there is an abnormal loss of protein from the blood, which reduces its osmotic pressure and prevents enough fluid from being drawn from the tissues into the blood. *Renal failure* prevents salt from being excreted from the body, allowing it to accumulate in the tissues and attract water to it.

Other disorders that can cause edema include *cirrhosis* of the liver, which leads to blood congestion in the veins of the liver, lowers blood protein (and therefore osmotic pressure), and causes salt retention. A deficiency of protein in the diet, as may occur in alcoholics, can also reduce osmotic pressure; edema in alcoholics may also be due to deficiency of thiamine (vitamin B_1), leading to *beriberi*.

Injury may cause edema by damaging capillaries and thus allowing fluid to leak out of them. *Lymphedema* may result from blocked lymphatics.

Finally, certain drugs may cause edema. These include *corticosteroid* and *androgen drugs*, and high-estrogen *oral contraceptives*, which act on the kidneys, causing a certain amount of salt retention. Antidiuretic hormone (see *ADH*) increases water retention by the kidneys.

SYMPTOMS AND SIGNS

Until the excess fluid in the body increases by more than about 15 percent, edema may show itself only as an increase in weight. After that it is evident as a swelling, often in the lower part of the body, commonly in the lower back and around the ankles.

In severe cases, fluid accumulates in one or more of the large body cavities. For example, in *ascites*, fluid collects in the peritoneal cavity of the abdomen,

Chronic edema
An example of chronic edema, showing the characteristic swelling and stretched, shiny skin. In this patient, the skin of the left leg is also ulcerated.

causing abdominal swelling. In *pleural effusion*, fluid fills the pleural cavity of the lungs, resulting in compression of the lungs and breathing difficulty. In pulmonary edema, the air sacs of the lungs become waterlogged, again causing breathing difficulty.

If a finger is pressed into skin swollen by edema, it makes an indentation that slowly flattens out as the fluid seeps back.

TREATMENT

The aim is always to remedy the underlying cause of the edema. In many cases, however, the underlying cause is not remediable and the only treatment is to make the body excrete the excess fluid by increasing the output of urine by the kidneys. This is done by restricting dietary sodium and taking *diuretic drugs*, which the patient may need indefinitely.

Edentulous

Without teeth, either because they have not yet grown or because they have fallen out or been removed.

EEG

The abbreviation for electroencephalogram. An EEG records the minute electrical impulses produced by the activity of the brain. The technique of electroencephalography was first

---

HOW ELECTROENCEPHALOGRAPHY IS DONE

A number of small electrodes are attached to the scalp. Shaving of the scalp is unnecessary. The electrodes are connected to an instrument that measures the brain's impulses in microvolts and amplifies them for recording purposes. The technique is painless, produces no side effects, and takes about 45 minutes. Recordings are taken with the subject at rest, with eyes open and then shut, during and after *hyperventilation*, and while looking at a flashing light. It is also helpful, especially when epilepsy is suspected, to record activity as the patient goes to sleep.

EEG wave patterns

Alpha waves
The prominent pattern of an awake, relaxed adult whose eyes are closed.

Beta waves
The lower, faster oscillation of a person who is concentrating on an external stimulus.

Delta waves
The typical pattern of sleep, but also found in young infants; rarely, they are caused by a brain tumor.

Theta waves
The dominant waves of children aged 2 to 5; also produced by frustration and found occasionally in psychopaths.

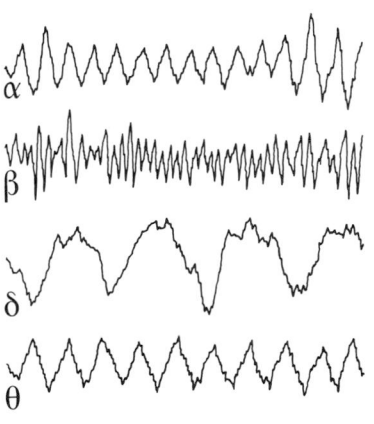

used in medicine in 1928, although it was known since the nineteenth century that electrical impulses could be recorded from animal brains.

WHY IT IS DONE

An EEG indicates, by the frequency of the recorded activity, the mental state of the subject—that is, whether he or she is alert, awake, or asleep. Also, by revealing characteristic wave patterns, the EEG can help in diagnosing certain conditions, especially *epilepsy* and certain types of *encephalitis*, *dementia*, and tumors.

Electroencephalography can also be used to monitor the conditions of patients during surgery and to assess the depth of anesthesia on the brain and spinal cord. It is also used as a test for *brain death*, but it is not required to make the determination.

Effusion

The escape of fluid through the walls of a blood vessel into a tissue or body cavity, often as a result of a vessel being inflamed or congested. For example, *pleural effusion*, a symptom of *heart failure*, occurs when raised blood pressure in the veins leads to fluid being forced out of the blood and through the walls of capillaries into the pleural cavity that surrounds the lungs.

Effusion, joint

Accumulation of fluid within a joint space, causing swelling and sometimes pain and tenderness. A joint is enclosed by a capsule lined with a membrane called the synovium. This membrane normally secretes small amounts of fluid to lubricate the joint, but if it is damaged or inflamed (by arthritis, for example) it produces excessive amounts of fluid.

Location of knee joint effusion
Excessive production and accumulation of fluid within a knee joint may be caused by injury or inflammation.

TREATMENT

Analgesics (painkillers), anti-inflammatory drugs, and corticosteroid injections help relieve pain and inflammation. The swelling can be reduced by rest, firm wrapping with a bandage, ice packs, and, when possible, keeping the affected joint raised. In some cases, the fluid may need to be aspirated (drawn out) with a hypodermic needle and syringe. Antibiotics may also be given if the cause is infective arthritis (also called septic arthritis). *Physical therapy* may be necessary later to restore full movement to the joint.

Egg

See *Ovum*.

Ego

The conscious sense of oneself, equivalent to "I." In Freudian *psychoanalytic theory*, this part of the personality maintains a balance between the primitive, unconscious instincts of the id, the controls of the superego (or conscience), and the demands of the outside world.

Egomania

An unhealthy overconcern with oneself. People described as egomaniacs talk constantly about themselves or their own activities, to the exclusion of everything else. Egomania is not regarded as a mental disorder, but such extreme self-conceit is sometimes said to indicate underlying mental instability.

Ehlers-Danlos syndrome

An inherited disorder of collagen, the most important structural protein in the body. Affected individuals have abnormally stretchy, thin skin that bruises very easily. Wounds are slow to heal and leave paper-thin scars. Sufferers tend to bleed easily from the gums and gastrointestinal tract. The joints are exceptionally loose and are prone to recurrent dislocation.

Ehlers-Danlos syndrome is usually (although not always) inherited in an autosomal dominant pattern (see *Genetic disorders*). This means that many affected individuals have an affected parent; each of an affected person's children has a 50 percent chance of being affected.

There is no known specific treatment for Ehlers-Danlos syndrome, although unnecessary accidental injury, as may occur in contact sports, should be avoided. The outlook for a normal life expectancy is good.

Eisenmenger complex

A complication of ventricular *septal defect* (a hole in the heart between the two pumping chambers). Normally, the ventricles are separate and no blood flows between them. The pressure of blood flow from the left ventricle is normally much higher than from the right; when a ventricular septal defect exists, the shunt of blood from the left to the right ventricle raises the pressure of blood flow to the lungs, and there is a gradual rise in blood pressure in the pulmonary (lung) arteries.

If the defect is not corrected surgically within the first few years of life, the prolonged pulmonary hypertension damages small blood vessels in the lung tissue and increases the resistance to blood flow, making it harder and harder to pump the blood through the lungs. As the pressure increases, it reverses the flow of blood through the septal defect so that blood then flows from the right ventricle to the left. At first this reversal is intermittent, often associated with exercise. Deoxygenated blood (blood that is on its way to the lungs to receive oxygen) instead of going to the lungs to get oxygen, gets passed directly into the body.

SYMPTOMS AND SIGNS

Eisenmenger complex causes breathing difficulty, fainting during exercise, and *cyanosis* (blue skin) due to *hypoxia* (lack of oxygen in the blood). The diagnosis is confirmed by cardiac *catheterization* (the insertion of a thin tube into the heart via a blood vessel under X-ray control).

TREATMENT AND OUTLOOK

Once permanent changes have developed, surgical correction of the ventricular septal defect does not help because the lung damage has already occurred. Most affected people die in their 30s or 40s. The only treatment in a severely disabled individual is a *heart-lung transplant*. (See also *Heart disease, congenital*.)

Ejaculation

The emission of semen from the penis at *orgasm*. Ejaculation is a reflex action that depends on regular and rhythmic pressure on the penis, usually during intercourse or masturbation. This stimulation acts on spinal nerves and triggers ejaculation.

Shortly before ejaculation the muscles around the epididymides (ducts where sperm are stored), the *prostate gland*, and the seminal vesicles contract rhythmically, forcing the

EJACULATORY DISORDERS

Premature ejaculation	Premature ejaculation is the most common sexual problem in men and is especially common in adolescents. Most adult men occasionally experience premature ejaculation, often because of overstimulation or	anxiety about sexual performance. If premature ejaculation occurs frequently, the cause may be psychological. Sexual counseling and techniques for delaying ejaculation may help (see *Sex therapy*).
Inhibited ejaculation	Inhibited ejaculation is a rare condition in which erection is normal, or even prolonged, but ejaculation does not occur. It may be psychological in origin, in which case sexual counseling may help, or it may be a	complication of other disorders, such as *diabetes mellitus*. Inhibited ejaculation may also occur during treatment with certain drugs, such as some antihypertensives.
Retrograde ejaculation	In this disorder, the valve at the base of the bladder fails to close during ejaculation. This forces the ejaculate backward into the bladder. Retrograde ejaculation can occur as a result of a neurological disease, after	surgery on the neck of the bladder, after prostatectomy, or after extensive pelvic surgery. There is no treatment, but intercourse with a full bladder can sometimes lead to normal ejaculation.

sperm from the epididymides to move forward and mix with the secretions from the seminal vesicles and prostate. At ejaculation, this fluid is propelled through the *urethra* and out of the body.

Because both semen and urine leave the body by the same route, a valve at the base of the bladder closes during ejaculation. This not only prevents ejaculate from going into the bladder but also stops urine from contaminating the semen.

Ejaculation, disorders of
Conditions in which ejaculation occurs before or very soon after penetration, ejaculation does not occur at all, or in which the ejaculate is forced backward into the bladder (see box, above).

EKG
See *ECG*.

Elbow
The joint between the lower end of the humerus (upper arm bone) and the upper ends of the radius and ulna (forearm bones). The joint is stabilized by ligaments at the front, back, and sides. The elbow enables the arm to be bent and straightened, and the forearm to be rotated through almost 180 degrees around its long axis without movement of the upper arm.
DISORDERS
Disorders include arthritis and injuries to the joint and its surrounding muscles, tendons, and ligaments.

ANATOMY OF THE ELBOW
The elbow is a hinge joint between the lower end of the humerus and the upper ends of the radius and ulna. The biceps muscle bends and rotates the arm at the elbow.

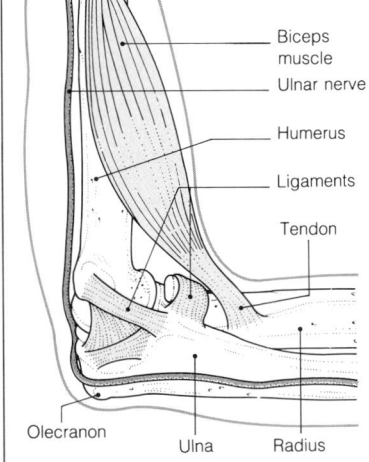

Biceps muscle
Ulnar nerve
Humerus
Ligaments
Tendon
Olecranon
Ulna
Radius

SOFT TISSUE INJURY AND INFLAMMATION
Repetitive strain on the tendons of the forearm muscles at the points at which they attach to the elbow (at the bony outgrowths called epicondyles) can lead to an inflammation at these points called *epicondylitis*. The two main types of epicondylitis are *tennis elbow* and *golfers' elbow*. Alternatively, a *sprain* of the joint ligaments can occur, especially in children.

Olecranon *bursitis* occurs over the tip of the elbow in response to local irritation. Repeated overstraightening of the joint can cause *baseball elbow*. Strain on the joint produces an *effusion* or traumatic *synovitis*.

A sharp blow on the olecranon process (the bony tip of the elbow, also called the "funny bone") may impinge on the ulnar nerve as it passes in a groove in this area, causing temporary discomfort—a pins and needles sensation and lancing pains that shoot down the forearm into the fourth and fifth fingers.
FRACTURES A fall onto an outstretched hand or onto the tip of the elbow can lead to any of various types of fracture around or at the lower end of the humerus. Children may alternatively sustain an injury to the epiphyses (growing areas) at the ends of the humerus, radius, or ulna. Dislocation of the elbow can occur at any age as a result of falling onto an outstretched hand; dislocations and fractures of the elbow frequently occur together.
ARTHRITIS Osteoarthritis, *rheumatoid arthritis*, and infective arthritis can affect the elbow joint.

Elderly, care of the
As people age they become prone to an increasing number of physical disorders and are more likely to suffer from loneliness and isolation. Efforts to stress personal pride and independence (along with appropriate medical care) can minimize physical and mental deterioration. Sensitive attention to psychological needs can help the elderly enjoy old age and can encourage them to feel that they are useful members of society rather than a burden.
PHYSICAL CARE
Elderly people often ignore symptoms of illness, either because they do not want to be a nuisance to those caring for them or because they are afraid of being "put away" in a home. Some conditions, such as *hypothyroidism* (underactive thyroid gland) and *anemia* (often due to a poor diet) cause a very gradual deterioration, which may incorrectly be assumed to be a natural effect of old age; as a result, these conditions tend not to be diagnosed and treated.

Failing vision and hearing are frequently regarded as inevitable features of old age, but in many cases surgical removal of a cataract or provision of a hearing aid can enable the individual to lead a more independent and active life.

THE ELDERLY AS A PERCENTAGE OF THE POPULATION (1984)

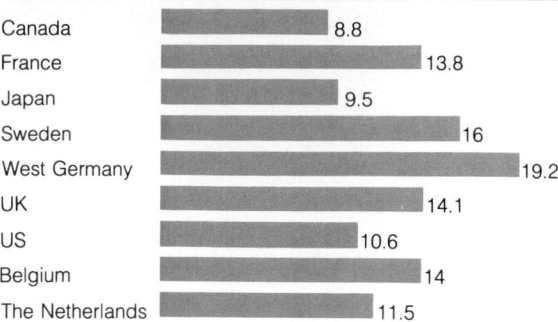

Canada	8.8
France	13.8
Japan	9.5
Sweden	16
West Germany	19.2
UK	14.1
US	10.6
Belgium	14
The Netherlands	11.5

National comparisons
People over 65 now make up more than 10 percent of the total population in most Western countries. This population pattern results from lower birth rates and increases in life expectancy due to improved medical care.

To ensure that medical problems are detected early and treated, it is important that caregivers remain alert to the symptoms and signs of illness. In addition, all people over age 65 should have regular checkups by a physician.

PSYCHOLOGICAL CARE
Common causes of depression in the elderly are isolation, inactivity, and a feeling of not being wanted. Elderly people can be helped by making them part of family activities. Attending a day-care center or senior citizen club can provide contact with other people and the opportunity to develop new interests. *Dementia* (loss of normal brain function) becomes more common as a person ages; it increases the level of supervision required.

DAY-TO-DAY CARE
Many elderly people prefer to live with their families, ideally in a separate section of the house, where they can have some degree of independence. If this is not possible, they may be able to live near relatives so that help can be provided with daily activities, such as shopping, cooking, and laundry. Assistance with personal care, such as bathing or getting in and out of bed, may also be required.

While this type of arrangement may be ideal for the elderly person, the responsibility can be a great strain on other members of the family. Voluntary agencies can sometimes help by providing a daily meal or occasional domestic help.

The elderly person's home, or that part of the house set aside for his or her use, should be well-heated in winter and cooled in summer to prevent *hypothermia* or *hyperthermia*; a high level of artificial illumination should be provided to make activities such as reading and sewing easier. The risk of falls can be reduced by ensuring that there are no loose rugs or slippery surfaces (see *Falls in the elderly*) and the

person living alone can be provided with an alarm that enables him or her to summon help in an emergency.

Sheltered housing is becoming a popular choice for many elderly people. It allows independence while providing discreet supervision and assistance when needed.

Elective

A term used to describe the degree of urgency and thus the timing of any procedure that a patient may be advised to undergo. When there is no need for urgency, the patient—in consultation with his or her physician—can select the most convenient time. A second surgical opinion is recommended for elective procedures that may be unnecessary.

Elective surgery

Surgery of a nonemergency nature. It includes correction of conditions such as hemorrhoids or a hernia as well as some cosmetic procedures.

Electrical injury

Damage caused by the passage of an electric current through the body and by its associated heat release.

INCIDENCE AND CAUSES
More than 1,000 people die from electrical accidents in the US each year and many others are injured, some seriously. Most fatal cases occur in the electrical generating and construction industries as the result of workers coming into contact with high voltages, but hundreds of people also die at home each year through handling frayed electric cords or by using electrical appliances near water. In addition, lightning causes about 300 deaths in the US annually.

The internal tissues of the body, being moist and salty, are good conductors of electricity; the main limitation to current flow is the electrical

resistance of the skin. Dry skin provides a high resistance (several tens of thousands of ohms), but moist skin has a resistance of only a few thousand ohms and thus allows a substantial current to flow. In these circumstances, voltage levels in the home are high enough to prove fatal. This is particularly so if the person is "well-grounded"—that is, if he or she is sitting or standing on a good conductor of electricity. Thus, a person in a bathtub of water is likely to suffer a fatal shock, whereas someone in a dry environment, and especially someone wearing shoes soled with rubber (which is a poor conductor of electricity), is less likely to be harmed by exposure to the same hazard.

EFFECTS
All except the mildest electric shocks are liable to cause unconsciousness. The extent of tissue damage depends on the size and type of the current flowing through the body. Alternating current (AC) is more dangerous than direct current (DC), because it causes sustained muscle contractions, which, by preventing hand movement, may prevent the victim from releasing his or her grip on the source of the current.

A current as small as one tenth of an amp passing through the heart can bring about a fatal *arrhythmia* (disturbance of the heart beat). This quantity is about the size of current passing through the filament of a very low-power bulb. The same current passing

Check that the power is off before attempting repairs on any electrical appliance.

Wear rubber-soled shoes.

Electrical injury in the home
A small electric current may cause death through heart damage. Shoes with rubber soles reduce the effect of an electric shock.

FIRST AID: ELECTRICAL INJURY

DO NOT
- attempt first aid until contact with the electrical current has been broken
- touch the victim with anything wet

1 Pull the electric plug out. If this is impossible, stand on a dry object and push the victim away from the source using a dry broomstick.

2 If the victim is unconscious and not breathing, start *cardiopulmonary resuscitation*.

3 If the victim is breathing, place in the *recovery position*. Follow first-aid advice for *burns* and *shock* until an ambulance arrives.

through the brain stem may cause the heart to stop beating and breathing to cease. Larger currents, generated by high voltages, may also char tissues, especially at points where resistance is highest, usually where the current enters and exits the body.

Electric shock treatment
See *ECT* (electroconvulsive therapy).

Electrocardiography
See *ECG*.

Electrocautery
See *Electrocoagulation*.

Electrocoagulation
The use of high-frequency electric current to seal blood vessels by heat and thus stop bleeding. Electrocoagulation may be used during all forms of surgery to close freshly cut blood vessels. It is also used to destroy

spider nevi and other kinds of abnormal blood vessel formations and to stop nosebleeds. The current is applied through a fine needle or, in surgery, may be delivered through a knife, enabling the surgeon to make bloodless incisions.

Electroconvulsive therapy
See *ECT*.

Electrodesiccation
The use of high-frequency electric current to destroy tissue by heat. Electrodesiccation is used to treat small *skin cancers*, *cervical erosion*, early *cervical cancer*, *warts*, and precancerous changes in the soft, moist tissue in the mouth. It is also used to destroy small tumors spread from other areas.

The procedure, which may be performed using a local anesthetic, consists of applying an electric probe to the tissue for one or two seconds.

Electroencephalography
See *EEG*.

Electrolysis
Permanent removal of unwanted hair by means of short-wave electric current, which destroys the hairs' roots.

WHY IT IS DONE
Hair on the face and body can be removed temporarily by shaving or plucking, or by the use of depilatory creams, abrasives, or wax preparations. Electrolysis is the only means of permanent removal.

Unskilled electrologists abound. Before embarking on treatment a person should first ensure that the operator is fully trained; damage from incompetent treatment can cause permanent disfigurement.

AREAS THAT CAN BE TREATED
With a few exceptions, electrolysis can be safely used on any part of the body where excessive hair is regarded as unsightly. Its use should be avoided on the lower margins of the eyebrows, where the skin above the eyelids is delicate and easily damaged, and it is questionable whether it should be used on the armpits because of a risk of bacterial infection. Electrolysis has no harmful effect on the breasts (where hair sometimes grows around the areola, the dark area surrounding the nipple) or on the ability of mother or infant to breast-feed.

The legs are not well suited for electrolysis; treatment of large areas requires so many sessions that it is too time-consuming and expensive for most people.

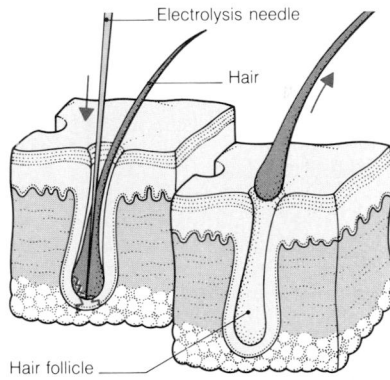

How electrolysis is done
To remove each hair, a fine needle is inserted into the follicle and a small electric current is passed through it. The current destroys the root of the hair, which is then pulled out. The procedure may cause some pain, but, in skilled hands, it is harmless. If the treatment is successful, there should be no more hair growth from that follicle.

E

Electrolyte

A substance whose molecules dissociate (split) into its constituent *ions* (electrically charged particles) when dissolved or melted. For example, sodium chloride (table salt) dissociates into positive sodium ions and negative chloride ions when dissolved in water. Ions that play an important role in regulating body processes include sodium, potassium, hydrogen, magnesium, calcium, bicarbonate, phosphate, and chloride.

Electromyography

See *EMG*.

Electronystagmography

A method of recording the various types of *nystagmus* (uncontrollable eye movements) to investigate their cause. Electrical changes caused by eye movement are picked up by electrodes placed near the eyes and recorded on a graph for analysis.

Electrophoresis

The movement of electrically charged particles suspended in a *colloid* solution under the influence of an electric current. The direction, distance, and rate of movement vary according to factors such as the size, shape, and electrical charge of the particle. Because of this, electrophoresis can be used to analyze mixtures of substances, particularly to identify different proteins in a mixture. For example, it can be used to identify and quantify the various proteins in blood; furthermore, by comparing the results from a particular blood sample with normal values, it is possible to diagnose disorders such as *myeloma*, a tumor of the bone marrow that produces abnormally high levels of a specific *immunoglobulin* in the blood.

Elephantiasis

A disease encountered in the tropics, characterized by massive swellings of the legs, arms, and scrotum, with thickening and darkening of the overlying skin so that it resembles the skin of an elephant. Most elephantiasis is due to chronic lymphatic obstruction occurring as a feature of *filariasis* (a worm infestation).

ELISA test

A laboratory blood test commonly used in the diagnosis of infectious diseases. ELISA stands for enzyme-linked immunosorbent assay. (See also *Immunoassay*.)

Elixir

A clear, sweetened liquid, often containing alcohol, that forms the basis for many liquid medicines, such as cough medicines.

Embolectomy

Surgical removal of an embolus, a fragment of material—usually a blood clot—that has been swept into an artery after formation elsewhere in the bloodstream; an embolus can threaten life if it blocks blood flow through a vital artery (see *Embolism*).

Embolism

Blockage of an artery by a clump of material traveling in the bloodstream. The particle causing the blockage is called an embolus and may be a blood clot, a bubble of air or other gas, a piece of tissue or tumor, a clump of bacteria, bone marrow, cholesterol, or fat, or any of various other substances.

TYPES

Blood clots are the most common type of embolus; they have usually broken off from a larger clot that has formed elsewhere in the blood circulation. Pulmonary embolism is usually the result of a fragment from a deep vein *thrombosis* (a blood clot formed deep in a vein, usually in a leg) breaking off and being carried via the heart to block an artery supplying the lungs; this is a common cause of sudden, unexpected death. Similar blood clots may form in the lining of the heart after a *myocardial infarction* (heart attack); they may travel as emboli toward the vital arteries of the brain and cause a cerebral embolism, leading to a *stroke*.

Fat embolism is a blockage of blood vessels caused by fat globules, particularly after fractures of the arm or leg. Amniotic fluid embolism is when some of the fluid that surrounds the baby in the uterus is forced into the mother's circulation toward the end of a normal pregnancy.

SYMPTOMS

Factors that determine symptoms include the extent of blockage, the size and type of embolus, and the size, nature, and location of the affected blood vessel. In pulmonary embolism the sufferer feels faint and breathless, and has chest pains. If the embolus causes a stroke, the symptoms depend on which part of the brain is affected; it may, for example, cause inability to speak, inability to move a part of the body, loss of consciousness, or a disturbance of vision. In the small number of serious cases of fat embolism, 48 hours after the major fracture occurs the patient's heart rate and rate of breathing rise dramatically; this is accompanied by restlessness, confusion, drowsiness, and *cyanosis*.

TYPES OF EMBOLISM

Embolisms are named after the part of the circulation affected or the embolus involved (e.g., a fat embolism is caused by fat globules released from a bone fracture). When an embolus is released, it is carried through branches of an artery until it becomes lodged. Blood is prevented from reaching parts of the body beyond the blockage.

Arm embolism
This X ray of the upper arm was taken after the injection of a radiopaque dye into the blood vessel. It shows, near the top, an embolus obstructing the normal flow of blood through one of the main arteries.

Cerebral embolism
A blockage of one of the arteries that supplies blood to the brain; it is one of the most common causes of a stroke.

Pulmonary embolism
A blockage of one of the arteries that supplies blood to the lungs. This may cause chest pain, breathlessness, and sudden death.

Amniotic fluid embolism
The escape of some of the fluid that surrounds the baby in the uterus into the mother's circulation. This may cause blockage of an artery in one of her lungs.

Leg embolism
An embolism that blocks one of the arteries that supplies blood to the leg. Gangrene may occur below the blockage.

TREATMENT

If a pulmonary or other severe type of embolism causes the person to collapse, emergency lifesaving procedures are carried out to keep breathing and circulation going. If the person survives, *embolectomy* (surgery to remove the blockage) may be possible. Under general anesthesia, an incision is made in the artery and the embolus is aspirated (sucked out). The incision is closed with stitches. If surgery is not possible, *thrombolytic drugs* (to dissolve blood clots) and *anticoagulant drugs* (to prevent clot formation) may be given.

OUTLOOK

In all severe types of embolism, survival depends on the success of resuscitation attempts, the importance of the vessel obstructed, and the speed with which blood flow is reestablished. If the source of the embolus is treated, the long-term prospects for the patient are good.

Embolism, therapeutic

Also called embolization, the deliberate obstruction of a blood vessel to stop internal bleeding or cut off blood flow to a tumor.

WHY IT IS DONE

Therapeutic embolism is increasingly being performed to stop otherwise uncontrollable bleeding, particularly when the patient is too sick to undergo surgery. Among its uses are the control of bleeding from small vessels in the lining of the intestines, often due to a malformation of blood vessels (similar to a birthmark in the skin).

Using the technique to deprive a tumor of its blood supply has several effects. It can relieve the pain caused by the growth; it can cause the tumor to shrivel, making it easier to remove surgically; or it may stop the tumor from spreading. Therapeutic embolism may be used to treat tumors that would be difficult to remove surgically, such as tumors in the liver. It is also used to treat certain vascular tumors on the face, such as *hemangiomas*, in preference to surgery that might leave unsightly scars.

HOW IT IS DONE

The procedure is usually carried out by a radiologist with the patient under a general anesthetic. The first step is to obtain an image of the blood vessel to be blocked and those leading to it. This image is obtained by means of *angiography*, an X-ray procedure in which an opaque dye is introduced into the blood vessels through a *catheter* (a flexible tube).

The catheter is then guided, by means of television monitoring, as close as possible to the vessel to be blocked, and the embolus that will block the blood vessel is released. Emboli are made of many materials, such as blood-clotting agents (such as fibrin), metal coils, silicone balloons, wool, and medicinal glue.

RISKS

There is always a risk that an embolus may lodge in the wrong place; an embolus that blocks a vessel in the brain may cause a *stroke*. The procedure is still being refined.

Embolus

A clump of material that is present (usually as a result of an accident or a disease of the heart and blood vessels) in the blood circulation, where it travels eventually to cause an arterial obstruction. (See *Embolism*.)

Embryo

The unborn child during the first eight weeks of its development following conception; for the rest of the pregnancy it is known as a *fetus*.

Development of the embryo is governed internally by genes inherited from the parents, and externally by factors such as the woman's diet and any medication taken during pregnancy. (See box, overleaf.)

THE FIRST TWO WEEKS

The embryo develops from an egg, fertilized by a sperm (see *Fertilization*). It starts as a single cell—just large enough to be seen by the naked eye. As the fertilized egg travels along the tube to the uterus, the cell divides in two. These cells divide further, eventually forming a spherical mass of cells; a hollow depression develops in the center of the sphere. The cells form into two groups: one makes up the wall lining the sphere; the other expands to form the embryo itself.

On about the sixth day the sphere of cells becomes attached to and then embedded in the lining of the uterus. At the site of attachment the outer layer of cells obtains nourishment from the woman's blood; the outer layer later will become the placenta.

Two bubbles form side by side within the cell mass. Between the bubbles a flat disk forms, consisting of layers of cells from which all the baby's tissues and organs will form. The amniotic sac develops around the growing embryo.

THE THIRD WEEK

Early in the third week the disk of cells becomes pear-shaped. The head of the embryo forms at the rounded end and the lower spine at the pointed end. A group of cells develops along the back of the embryo to form the notochord, a rod of cells that constitutes the basis for the spine. From this time on, the embryo has two recognizable halves that develop more or less symmetrically. The notochord then furrows and the edges grow toward each other. They fuse to form the neural tube, which later will develop into the brain and spinal cord.

THE FOURTH WEEK

During the fourth week the embryo becomes recognizable as a mammal. The back grows more rapidly than the front, giving the embryo a C-shape, and a tail becomes visible. Within the embryo, buds of tissue form that will later develop into the lungs, pancreas, liver, and gallbladder.

The neural tube extends toward the head of the embryo, where a broad fold becomes visible that eventually will grow into the brain. The developing ears first appear as pits. Rudimentary eyes develop in the form of stalks. The outer layers begin to form the limb buds and the branchial arches (folds of tissue) that will become the jaws and other structures in the neck.

Paired bulges appear on the sides of the neural tube that will become the cartilage, bone, and muscle of the back. On the front of the embryo, just beneath the head, a rudimentary heart develops in the form of a straight tube. As the branchial arches develop, the heart is pushed down into the chest. It is during this period that the embryo is at the greatest risk of birth defects caused by abnormal genetic or external factors (see *Birth defects*).

THE FIFTH WEEK

The external ears become visible, pits mark the position of the developing nose, the upper and lower jaws form, and the limb buds extend, becoming flattened at the end where the hands and feet will develop.

The two folds of tissue meet at the front of the embryo and fuse to form the front wall of the chest and abdomen. The umbilical cord develops.

THE SIXTH TO EIGHTH WEEKS

The face becomes recognizably human, the neck forms, the trunk becomes less curved and the head more erect, the tail between the buttocks disappears, the limbs become jointed, and fingers and toes appear.

After eight weeks the embryo is 1 inch (2.5 cm) long. Most of the internal organs have formed and all the external features are present.

THE DEVELOPING EMBRYO

From the time of conception until the eighth week, the developing baby is known as an embryo. At conception, the fertilized egg consists of a single cell, the zygote, which contains genetic material from the sperm and the egg. The zygote divides several times to form a ball of cells, which then implants into the lining of the uterus. At the point of attachment, the outer layer of cells forms the placenta, while a group of cells within one area of the cell ball develops into the embryo. A sac filled with amniotic fluid forms around the embryo to protect it. As the embryo grows, it begins to form features and, by the fifth week, it has developed a recognizable head and limb buds.

Embryo at about six weeks
The embryo is floating in the amniotic sac. The smaller sac at left (the yolk sac) provides nourishment for the early embryo.

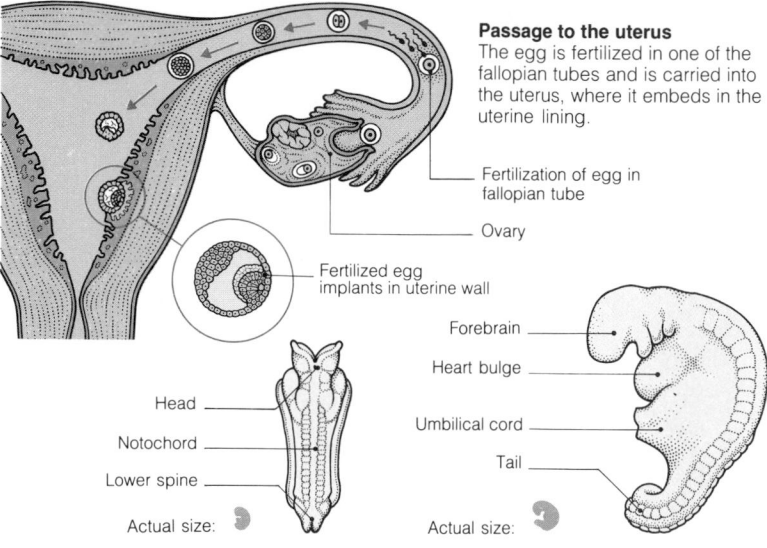

Passage to the uterus
The egg is fertilized in one of the fallopian tubes and is carried into the uterus, where it embeds in the uterine lining.

Fertilization of egg in fallopian tube

Ovary

Fertilized egg implants in uterine wall

Forebrain
Heart bulge
Umbilical cord
Tail
Actual size:

Head
Notochord
Lower spine
Actual size:

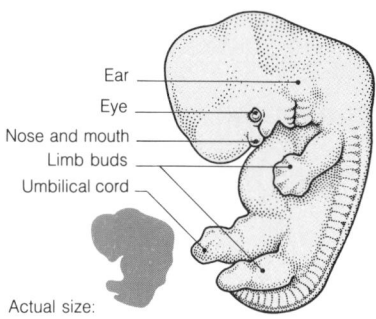

Ear
Eye
Nose and mouth
Limb buds
Umbilical cord
Actual size:

Three weeks
The embryo becomes pear-shaped, with a rounded head, pointed lower spine, and notochord running along its back.

Four weeks
The embryo becomes C-shaped and a tail is visible. The umbilical cord forms and the forebrain enlarges.

Six weeks
Eyes are visible and the mouth, nose, and ears are forming. The limbs grow rapidly from initial tiny buds.

INTERNAL ORGANS AT FIVE WEEKS

All the internal organs (such as the liver, pancreas, stomach, heart, lungs, kidneys, and sex organs) have begun to form by the fifth week. During this critical stage of development, the embryo is highly vulnerable to harmful substances consumed by the mother (such as alcohol and medication), which may cause birth defects.

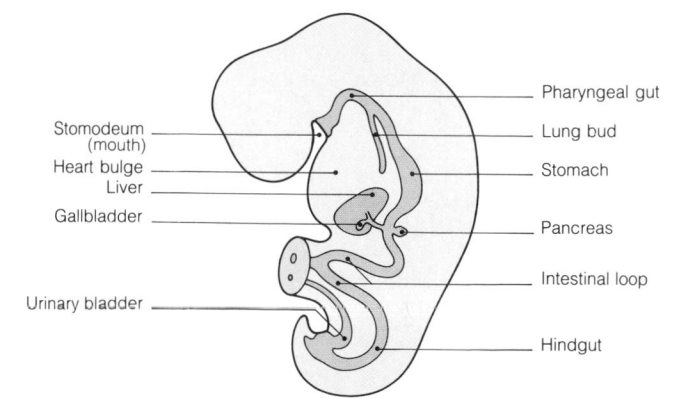

Stomodeum (mouth)
Heart bulge
Liver
Gallbladder
Urinary bladder

Pharyngeal gut
Lung bud
Stomach
Pancreas
Intestinal loop
Hindgut

Actual size:

Eight weeks
The face is more "human," the head is more upright, and the tail has gone. Limbs become jointed and digits appear.

Embryology

The study of the development and growth of the *embryo* and then the *fetus* from conception until birth.

Embryology is an essential part of the medical student's training, since it leads to a greater understanding of adult anatomy and of the ways structural defects in the body arise. For example, the occurrence of congenital heart defects (such as "holes in the heart" and transposition of the main blood vessels) is easier to understand when the stages of fetal heart development have been explained.

Until recently, embryology was based on the study of animal embryos and dead human embryos at different stages of development. More details about the nature of physical and chemical processes involved in embryo development have been established by examination of live embryos grown in the laboratory (see *Embryo, research on*).

Embryo, research on

Human embryos are regularly grown in laboratories as part of the treatment of infertility (see *In vitro fertilization*). Physicians usually fertilize more eggs than they need, since they do not know how many will "take" (begin the process of cell division and growth); the unwanted embryos may then be frozen for use in later attempts at achieving a pregnancy. Surplus embryos are being used for research aimed at improving the results of in vitro fertilization, at finding better methods of contraception, and at detecting genetic disorders at an early stage in pregnancy.

In several countries, such research has been prohibited or the physicians concerned have agreed not to perform it for ethical reasons. As yet there is no consensus on the circumstances under which research on embryos is ethically acceptable.

Emergency

Any condition that requires urgent medical treatment, such as cardiac arrest, or any procedure that must be performed immediately, such as *cardiopulmonary resuscitation*.

Emergency physician

A physician who has been specially trained to deal with a broad range of life-threatening conditions, ranging from acute asthma attacks to bullet wounds. The first concern of the emergency-care physician is to save the life of the patient and then to stabilize the condition as much as possible before transferring the patient to an appropriate hospital unit for further care.

Emesis

The medical term for *vomiting*.

Emetic

A substance that causes vomiting, used to treat some types of poisoning and drug overdose. Emetics work by stimulating the part of the brain that controls vomiting and/or by irritating the lining of the stomach.

The most widely used emetic is *ipecac*. Emetics should not be given to a person who is drowsy because he or she may inhale the vomit.

EMG

The abbreviation for electromyogram, a test in which the electrical activity in muscle is analyzed after being amplified, displayed, and recorded.

WHY IT IS DONE

An EMG can reveal the presence of muscle disorders, such as *muscular dystrophy*, or disorders in which the nerve supply to muscle is impaired, such as *neuropathy* or *radiculopathy*. In cases of nerve injury, the actual site of nerve damage can often be located.

HOW IT IS DONE

The technique for obtaining an EMG (called electromyography) is harmless and takes 30 to 60 minutes to perform, depending on the number of muscles to be tested. There are no side effects. Impulses are recorded by attaching small disk electrodes to the skin surface over the muscle or by inserting needle electrodes into the muscle. The electrical activity is evaluated during muscle contraction and at rest. Impulses are seen on an oscilloscope screen or heard over a loudspeaker. Changes in the electrical wave forms and sounds associated with them allow the electromyographer to determine whether nerve or muscle disorders are present.

Emollient

A substance such as olive oil, lanolin, or petroleum jelly that has a soothing, softening effect when applied to the skin, eyes, or mucous membranes (for example, the lining of the nose and mouth). By forming an oily film, emollients prevent the loss of water from these surfaces and therefore have a moisturizing effect. Emollients are used in creams, ointments, nasal sprays, and suppositories.

Emotional deprivation

Lack of sufficient loving attention and warm, trusting relationships during a child's early years, leading to difficulty in normal emotional development. Emotional deprivation may result if *bonding* does not occur in the early months of life, if a child is frequently separated from his or her parents for long periods during the first five years, or if parents cannot meet the child's emotional needs.

Emotionally deprived children are often impulsive, crave attention, cannot cope with frustration, and may even be mildly mentally retarded.

Emotional problems

A common term for a wide range of psychological difficulties. The problems may be due to upbringing, relationships, or psychiatric illness, but external feelings of *anxiety* and *depression* generally predominate. Age, sex, and social and cultural factors influence the most suitable methods of coping with emotional problems.

Empathy

The ability to partake in and understand the thoughts and feelings of others. It is possible to share an emotion with another person by comparing it with our own experiences.

In *psychoanalysis* the therapist relies on empathy to establish a relationship with a patient. Empathy can also help in making a diagnosis.

Emphysema

A disease in which the alveoli (tiny air sacs) in the lungs become damaged. The disorder causes shortness of breath and in severe cases can lead to respiratory and/or heart failure.

CAUSES

In almost all cases, emphysema is caused by cigarette smoking. Atmospheric pollution is sometimes a predisposing factor. Rarely, a predisposition to emphysema is inherited due to a deficiency of a chemical called alpha$_1$-antitrypsin in the lungs; the disease appears early in life, but its development is hastened and intensified by smoking.

The alveoli, of which there are many millions in each lung, are groups of air sacs at the end of bronchioles (tiny air passages). Through their thin walls, inhaled oxygen is passed into the bloodstream and carbon dioxide is removed from the capillaries to be breathed out. Tobacco smoke and other air pollutants are believed to cause emphysema by provoking the

E

E

release of chemicals within the alveoli that damage the alveolar walls. Alpha$_1$- antitrypsin is thought to protect against this chemical damage; hence, people with a deficiency of this substance are particularly badly affected. The damage is slight at first, but in heavy smokers it becomes progressively worse, with the alveoli bursting and blending to form fewer, larger sacs with less surface area, and with consequent impairment of oxygen and carbon dioxide exchange. Over the years the lungs become less and less elastic, which further reduces their efficiency.

Eventually—sometimes after many years—the level of oxygen in the blood starts to fall, with one of two effects. In some cases *pulmonary hypertension* (raised blood pressure in the pulmonary artery) develops, leading to *cor pulmonale* (enlargement and strain on the right side of the heart) and, subsequently, *edema* (accumulation of fluid in the tissues), particularly in the lower legs. Other sufferers are able to compensate for oxygen deficiency to some extent by breathing faster. Why individuals react in these different ways is not known.

Emphysema is often accompanied by chronic *bronchitis*, also brought on by air pollutants and smoking. Emphysema and chronic bronchitis together are sometimes called chronic obstructive lung (or airways) disease.

INCIDENCE
Several hundred people per 100,000 in the US suffer from some degree of emphysema. About 30 people per 100,000 in the US each year die from chronic obstructive lung disease; of these, about six deaths are ascribed to emphysema alone.

SYMPTOMS AND SIGNS
Initially, and for a considerable time in mild cases, there may be no symptoms, but as the disease progresses it results in increasing shortness of breath. At first this may be noticed only when climbing stairs or steep inclines, but gradually it becomes more severe until eventually it occurs after only mild exercise or is present even at rest.

A sign of emphysema is a barrel-shaped chest associated with air being trapped in the outer part of the lungs. There may also be a chronic cough (caused by accompanying bronchitis) and a slight wheeze.

As the disease progresses, sufferers in whom cor pulmonale develops start to turn purple-blue due to oxygen deficiency in the blood and their legs

swell because of edema; these people are known as blue bloaters. Those who breathe rapidly and retain normal coloring are called pink puffers. Many people, however, show signs somewhere in between these two extremes. As respiratory and/or heart failure develops, sufferers find it increasingly difficult to breathe.

DIAGNOSIS
The diagnosis is made from the patient's symptoms and signs, from a chest examination, and from various tests. Tests include taking a blood sample from an artery to measure the concentration of the blood gases (e.g., oxygen and carbon dioxide) and sometimes a sample from a vein (to determine whether the disease is due to alpha$_1$-antitrypsin deficiency). Chest X rays are taken to exclude the possibility of another lung disease being responsible for the symptoms and to determine how great an area of the lungs has been affected. *Pulmonary function tests* are carried out to assess breathing capacity and the efficiency of the alveoli in exchanging gases.

TREATMENT
Because emphysema is incurable—lung tissue that has been damaged cannot be replaced—treatment can only control the disease. This means preventing more damage to the lungs by a total and lifelong ban on smoking, and improving the efficiency of remaining lung tissue, which is done in various ways. *Bronchodilator drugs* are given to widen the bronchi (the airways linking the windpipe to the lungs) and the bronchioles. These drugs can be taken by means of a hand-held aerosol inhaler or an electrically operated *nebulizer* that produces a fine spray. Occasionally, *corticosteroid drugs*, taken by inhaler to reduce inflammation in the lungs, are also beneficial.

To treat edema, a sodium-restricted diet and *diuretic drugs* may be given to reduce the volume of fluid within the body by promoting output through increased urine production.

If the oxygen level of the blood falls considerably, oxygen may need to be given by mask or *cannula*. The patient may be given oxygen equipment to use at home.

OUTLOOK
The course of the disease depends on how far it has progressed before the patient gives up smoking. If extensive areas of lung have been damaged or if cor pulmonale has developed, death occurs sooner or later from respiratory and/or heart failure.

Emphysema, surgical
The abnormal presence of air in tissues underlying the skin. It most often occurs as a complication of *pneumothorax* (the abnormal presence of air in the pleural cavity between the lung and chest wall). This can itself result from injury, chest surgery, or as a result of a diving accident.

Empirical treatment
Treatment undertaken when a precise diagnosis cannot be made. In the case of a fever of undetermined origin, for example, a physician might prescribe antibiotics on the basis of experience with similar cases.

Empyema
An accumulation of pus in a body cavity or in certain organs.

Pleural empyema occurs as a rare complication of a lung infection such as pneumonia or pleurisy; it may also develop after a severe injury to the chest that penetrates the pleural space. The main symptoms are chest pain, breathlessness, and fever.

The diagnosis is confirmed by taking X rays of the chest and aspirating some of the pus for smear and culture. Treatment is an operation to open the infected cavity and drain the pus; antibiotic therapy is also used.

Empyema of the gallbladder may occur as a complication of *cholecystitis*, when it usually causes abdominal pain, fever, and sometimes jaundice. It is treated by *cholecystectomy* (surgical removal of the gallbladder).

Enalapril
An *ACE inhibitor drug* used in the treatment of *hypertension* (high blood pressure) and *heart failure* (reduced pumping efficiency). It may be given in conjunction with a *diuretic drug*. Enalapril was introduced in 1986.

Enamel, dental
The hard outer layer of a tooth that covers and protects the inner structures (see *Teeth*).

Encephalitis
Inflammation of the brain, usually caused by a viral infection. In many cases the *meninges* (the membranes that cover and enclose the brain) are also affected. An attack may be so mild that it is barely noticeable, but in most cases it is a serious condition.

CAUSES AND INCIDENCE
The virus most commonly responsible for encephalitis is the *herpes simplex* virus type 1, which also causes cold

sores. In the US, another cause is a virus transmitted to humans by mosquito bites, which causes an illness known as St. Louis encephalitis. In addition, an increasing number of cases are caused by infection with HIV (human immunodeficiency virus), the organism responsible for *AIDS*. Rarely, the condition may be a complication of certain other viral infections, including measles and mumps.

SYMPTOMS AND SIGNS

Encephalitis has variable effects but often starts with headache, fever, and prostration, and progresses to hallucinations, confusion, paralysis of one side of the body, and disturbed behavior, speech, memory, and eye movement. There is a gradual loss of consciousness and sometimes coma. Epileptic seizures may also occur.

If the meninges as well as the brain are inflamed, the neck usually becomes stiff and the eyes become abnormally sensitive to light.

DIAGNOSIS

Diagnosis is based on symptoms, signs, and the results of *CT scanning* of the brain, an *EEG* (which records the electrical activity of the brain), and a *lumbar puncture* (taking a sample of cerebrospinal fluid from the spinal canal for analysis). Blood tests and, rarely, a brain *biopsy* (removal of a small sample of tissue for analysis) may also be required to confirm the diagnosis, which permits lifesaving treatment of some patients.

TREATMENT AND OUTLOOK

The antiviral drug acyclovir, administered by an intravenous drip, has proved an effective treatment for encephalitis caused by the herpes simplex virus. When the disease results from other viral infections, there is no known effective treatment. Depending on the infecting agent, some patients die and some of those who recover are left with brain damage, resulting in mental impairment, behavioral disturbances, and persistent epilepsy.

Encephalitis lethargica

An epidemic form of encephalitis (inflammation of the brain). There have been no major outbreaks since the 1920s, although rare sporadic cases still occur.

The symptoms are as for encephalitis, with additional lethargy and drowsiness—hence the illness's popular name of "sleeping sickness."

About 40 percent of sufferers died during the major epidemics; of those who survived, many later developed postencephalitic *parkinsonism*, a movement disorder marked by symptoms such as tremor, rigidity, immobility, and disturbed eye movements.

A small number of survivors from the post-World War I epidemics were still alive in the 1970s, when administration of a new antiparkinsonian drug, levodopa, brought a remarkable improvement in their conditions. However, after half a century of almost complete immobility, most sufferers were seemingly unable to cope with this "awakening," and lapsed back into their torpid state.

Encephalomyelitis

Inflammation of the brain and spinal cord, resulting in damage to the nervous system. The condition occurs as a complication of about one in 1,000 cases of measles, developing a few days after the rash appears. Rarely, it may occur after other viral infections, such as chickenpox, rubella (German measles), or infectious mononucleosis (glandular fever), or it may follow vaccination against rabies.

SYMPTOMS

Symptoms include fever, headache, drowsiness, confusion, epileptic seizures, partial paralysis or loss of sensation, and sometimes coma.

DIAGNOSIS AND TREATMENT

Diagnosis is as for *encephalitis*. Critically ill patients require careful nursing in a hospital. There is no cure for the disease, but *corticosteroid drugs* are given to reduce inflammation and *anticonvulsant drugs* are given to control epileptic seizures.

OUTLOOK

About 10 to 20 percent of patients die; those that recover may suffer permanent damage to the nervous system, causing mental retardation, epilepsy, paralysis, pituitary insufficiency, loss of sensation, or incontinence.

Encephalopathy

Any disease or disorder affecting the brain, especially chronic degenerative conditions (see *Brain* disorders box).

Wernicke's encephalopathy is a degenerative condition of the brain caused by a deficiency of thiamine (vitamin B_1) and is most common in alcoholics. Hepatic encephalopathy is caused by the effect on the brain of toxic substances having accumulated in the blood as a result of liver disease and liver failure, and is characterized by symptoms such as impaired consciousness, memory loss, personality change, tremors, seizures, stupor, and coma.

Encopresis

A type of *soiling* in which children pass normal feces in unacceptable places after the age at which bowel control is normally achieved (usually 2 to 3 years). These children have no specific physical problem, but often refuse to use a potty or toilet; they defecate in their clothes or in other, secretive, places, such as behind furniture, usually during the day. The problem almost invariably improves with time and is rare after the age of 10.

Endarterectomy

An operation to remove the lining of an artery narrowed by *atherosclerosis*, the buildup of fatty tissue. Removing the diseased lining restores normal blood flow to the part of the body supplied by the artery.

WHY IT IS DONE

Endarterectomy is performed to treat *cerebrovascular disease* (in which there is a serious reduction of blood supply to the brain) or to treat *peripheral vascular disease* (in which blood supply to the legs is impaired).

HOW IT IS DONE

Before surgery, the site of narrowing is located by means of an X-ray procedure called *angiography*, which requires a local anesthetic. For the operation itself the patient is given a general anesthetic.

Endarterectomy is a delicate procedure that may take several hours to perform. The artery is exposed, clamps are applied, an incision is made, and the diseased lining is removed along with any thrombus (blood clot) that has formed. The incision is closed with stitches.

RESULTS

New lining grows in the artery within a few weeks of surgery. The operation often brings about a considerable improvement in symptoms (for example, it can greatly reduce pain in the legs in peripheral vascular disease), but its long-term effect is more limited, since narrowing of an artery is rarely confined to one site. When narrowing is widespread, *arterial reconstructive surgery* may have to be carried out.

Endemic

A medical term applied to a disease or disorder that is constantly present in a particular region or specific group of people, in contrast to an *epidemic*, which is not generally present but occasionally affects a large number of people. *AIDS*, for example, has become endemic in central Africa and

E

has also spread to many other parts of the world. The lung disease *pneumoconiosis* was formerly endemic in coal miners before safety regulations enforced controls over coal dust, the causative agent.

Endocarditis

Inflammation of the endocardium (internal lining of the heart), particularly the heart valves, usually due to infection. It may occur alone or as a complication of another disease. The various types of endocarditis include acute bacterial, subacute bacterial, fungal, and nonbacterial.

CAUSES AND INCIDENCE

In both types of bacterial endocarditis, causative microorganisms enter the bloodstream and infect the lining of the heart and valves, eventually causing damage. This process is encouraged if the endocardium is already damaged (by congenital *heart disease* or *rheumatic fever*, for example) because clots form on the injured surface and then trap the microorganisms, which multiply rapidly at the site of damage.

Bacteria may be introduced into the bloodstream during cardiac surgery, particularly in places where foreign bodies such as stitches, monitoring tubes, or an artificial heart valve are inserted. Large numbers of microorganisms pass into the bloodstream when people undergo major dental treatment, especially tooth extraction. Surgical and investigative procedures of the gastrointestinal and genitourinary systems—for example, *cystoscopy* (passing a viewing tube through the urethra to inspect the bladder)—carry the same risks.

Drug addicts are susceptible to endocarditis (even if their hearts are healthy) because of the possibility of introducing bacteria and fungi from a dirty syringe and because of the risk of transmitting infection from unclean skin at the site of injection.

Fungal endocarditis may occur in people with previously damaged tissue and in people who have low resistance to infection, especially those on *immunosuppressant drugs*.

Endocarditis that is nonbacterial is a rare feature of some cancers as well as *autoimmune disorders* such as systemic *lupus erythematosus*.

SYMPTOMS

In the subacute form, the disease smolders undetected, sometimes for many months, during which time it causes serious damage to a heart valve. Symptoms are general and nonspecific; the sufferer may complain of fatigue and weakness, feverishness, night sweats, and vague aches and pains. On examination the only evident abnormality may be a heart murmur that changes from time to time.

Acute bacterial endocarditis, which occurs less frequently, comes on suddenly. The patient suffers from severe chills, high fever, shortness of breath, and rapid or irregular heart beat. The infection progresses quickly and may destroy the heart valves, leading to rapidly progressive heart failure (reduced pumping efficiency).

Apart from the inflammation and its effects on the heart, the clots attached to the valves tend to break up and fragments of infected tissue are carried in the blood. This may cause an *embolism* (blockage of an artery) and may carry the infection to other parts of the body.

DIAGNOSIS AND TREATMENT

Any patient suspected of having endocarditis is given a thorough physical examination. Blood samples are examined for bacteria or fungi and, if possible, the organisms are grown in culture so that their sensitivity to antibiotics can be determined. Tests on the heart may include the *ECG*, *echocardiography*, and *angiography*.

Once the diagnosis is confirmed by blood tests, patients are treated with high doses of *antibiotic drugs*. The drugs are usually given intravenously; treatment is started in the hospital, may be continued at home, and may last for as long as 6 weeks.

If a valve has been extensively damaged by erosion due to infection it may have to be replaced surgically with an artificial one. Artificial valves often become infected, in which case they must be replaced. Heart valve replacement may need to be done as an emergency procedure.

PREVENTION AND OUTLOOK

People who are known to have heart valve defects are prescribed antibiotics before undergoing any procedure that runs a significant risk of introducing bacteria into the bloodstream. People with heart valve defects should also be aware of the warning signs of endocarditis and call the physician should they appear.

Before the introduction of antibiotics, endocarditis was practically incurable and the bloodstream infection and valve damage resulted in death in 95 percent of patients; today, 65 to 80 percent recover. The disease is usually fatal if not treated.

Endocrine gland

A gland that secretes chemicals directly (that is, not through a duct) into the bloodstream. Examples include the thyroid gland, ovaries, and adrenals, which release thyroxine, estrogens, and hydrocortisone, respectively. The endocrine glands in the body make up the *endocrine system*. (See also *Exocrine gland*.)

Endocrine system

A collection of glands that produces hormones (chemical substances necessary for normal body functioning) that regulate the body's rate of metabolism, growth, and sexual development and functioning. Unlike *exocrine glands*, the secretions of which pass through ducts to local areas, endocrine glands are ductless and release their hormones directly into the bloodstream to be transported to organs and tissues throughout the body. (See also box, opposite.)

Endocrinologist

An internist who specializes in diseases and disorders of the *endocrine system*. Patients include people with *thyroid* disorders or *diabetes mellitus*.

Endocrinology

The study of the endocrine glands and the hormones they secrete, including the investigation and treatment of their disorders.

The hormones produced by the endocrine glands are responsible for numerous body processes, including growth, metabolism, sexual activity, temperature regulation, and response to stress. Any increase or decrease in the production of a specific hormone interferes with the process it controls.

One example of overproduction is *Graves' disease*, in which the thyroid gland produces too much thyroxine.

The symptoms and signs of an endocrine disorder may lead a family physician to suspect such a disease, but confirmation usually requires referral to an endocrinologist for specialized tests, including measurement of the amounts of various hormones in the blood and urine.

Endodontics

The specialized branch of dentistry concerned with the causes, prevention, diagnosis, and treatment of disease and injury affecting the nerves and pulp in teeth and the periapical (surrounding) tissues in the gum. Endodontics includes *pulpotomy* and *root-canal treatment*.

ENDOCRINE SYSTEM

The system consists of a collection of hormone-producing glands, many regulated by trophic (stimulating) hormones secreted by the pituitary. The pituitary is itself influenced by hormones secreted by the hypothalamus in the brain. Shown are the principal glands, with a note on the hormones they produce.

Pancreas
Secretes insulin and glucagon, which control the body's utilization of glucose.

Adrenal cortex
When stimulated by ACTH, produces hydrocortisone, which has widespread effects on metabolism; also produces androgen hormones and aldosterone, which maintains blood pressure and the body's salt balance.

Ovaries
Produce the hormones estrogen and progesterone, which influence multiple aspects of female physiology. These processes are controlled by gonadotropic hormones secreted by the pituitary.

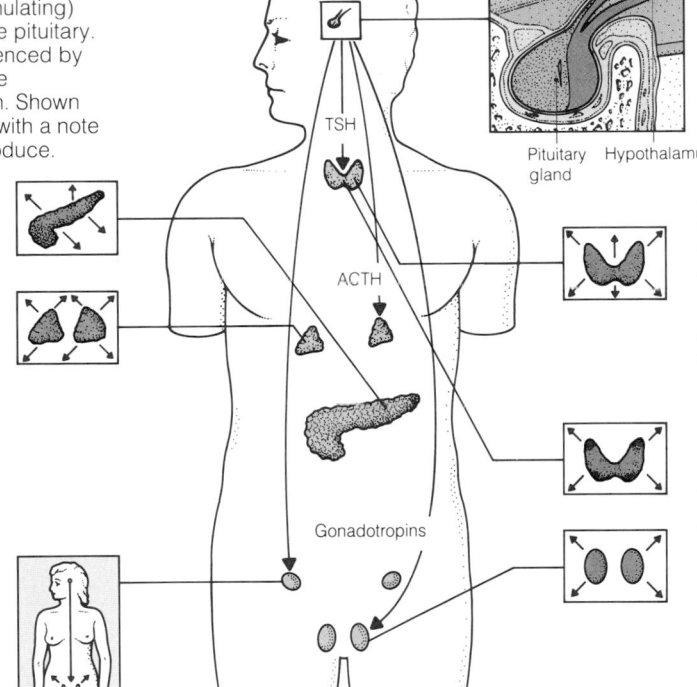

Pituitary gland
Secretes hormones that stimulate the adrenals, thyroid, pigmentation-producing skin cells, and gonads; also secretes growth hormone, antidiuretic hormone, prolactin, and oxytocin.

Pituitary gland   Hypothalamus

Thyroid gland
Produces the hormones thyroxine, triiodothyronine, and calcitonin, which stimulate metabolism, body heat production, and bone growth. Thyroid activity is controlled by TSH, secreted by the pituitary.

Parathyroid glands
Secrete parathyroid hormone, which maintains the calcium level in the blood.

Testes
Produce testosterone in response to gonadotropins secreted by the pituitary. A combination of gonadotropins and testosterone stimulates sperm production and the development of other male characteristics.

CONTROL OF HORMONE PRODUCTION

Production of too much or too little hormone by a gland is prevented by feedback mechanisms. Variations in the blood level of the hormone are detected by the part of the brain known as the hypothalamus, which prompts the pituitary to modify its production of trophic (gland-stimulating) hormone accordingly.

1 The production of hormone by the target gland (in this illustration, the thyroid gland) and of trophic hormone by the pituitary gland is normal.

2 If hormone production by the target gland rises too high, the feedback effect causes less trophic hormone to be produced, which tends to return the situation to normal.

3 If hormone production by the target gland drops too low, the feedback lessens and more trophic hormone is produced, which tends to return the situation to normal.

ENDOCRINE DISORDERS

In all endocrine disorders, there is either deficient or excess production of a hormone by a gland. Common causes of abnormal hormone production include a tumor or an autoimmune disease affecting a gland, or a disorder of the pituitary or the hypothalamus, which control many other glands. Abnormal hormone production often has a feedback effect on the secretion of trophic (stimulating) hormones by the pituitary and the hypothalamus – as in two of the examples shown. The blood levels of different hormones may need to be measured to pinpoint the cause of a disorder.

Thyrotoxicosis
This disorder is usually due to an autoimmune disease of the thyroid. Excess hormones cause the symptoms; the output of TSH and its hypothalamic releasing hormone is reduced, but the thyroid continues to overproduce.

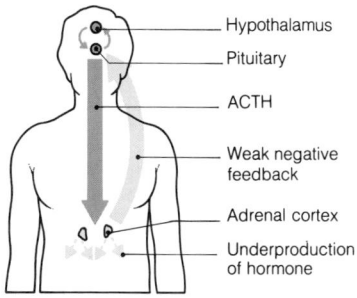

Addison's disease
Symptoms are caused by reduced hormone production by the defective adrenal cortices. Feedback is weak, so the pituitary pours out adrenocorticotropic hormone (ACTH), but it fails to stimulate the adrenals.

Cushing's syndrome
This disorder is caused by excess ACTH secretion by a pituitary tumor. This stimulates the adrenal cortices to make excess hydrocortisone, leading to the symptoms of the syndrome. Feedback fails to suppress ACTH secretion.

Endodontist

A dentist who is specially trained to treat the nerves and pulp in teeth and the periapical (surrounding) tissues in the gum. *Root-canal treatment* is a common endodontic procedure.

Endogenous

Arising from causes within the body. For example, an endogenous infection may occur if bacteria from around the anus invade the urinary tract.

The term endogenous depression was formerly used to describe depression with no discoverable external cause that was thought to be due to a chemical imbalance in the brain.

Most disorders, however, are exogenous (caused by external infections, poisoning, or injury).

Endometrial cancer

See *Uterus, cancer of*.

Endometriosis

A condition in which fragments of the *endometrium* (lining of the uterus) are found in other parts of (or on organs within) the pelvic cavity.

INCIDENCE AND CAUSE

Endometriosis is most prevalent between 25 and 40 and is a common cause of *infertility*. About 10 to 15 percent of infertility patients have endometriosis and about 30 to 40 percent of women suffering from endometriosis are infertile.

The exact cause of endometriosis is uncertain, but in some cases it is thought to occur because fragments of

SITES OF ENDOMETRIOSIS

Fragments of the *endometrium* may travel from the uterus into the pelvic cavity via the fallopian tubes. They then implant on parts of the pelvic organs (such as the uterus, ovaries, vagina, cervix, bladder, and

rectum). The patches of endometrium continue to respond to the menstrual cycle and bleed every month, causing the formation of painful cysts, which can be very small or as large as a grapefruit.

Severe endometriosis
The uterus, fallopian tubes, and ovaries shown above had large cysts growing around them due to endometriosis. As the patient was nearing the menopause, the affected organs were surgically removed.

the endometrium that are shed during *menstruation* do not leave the body with the menstrual flow. Instead, they travel up the fallopian tubes and into the pelvic cavity. There, they may adhere to and grow on any of the pelvic organs.

These displaced patches of endometrium continue to respond to the menstrual cycle as if they were still inside the uterus, so each month they bleed. This blood cannot escape, however, and causes the formation of slowly growing cysts from the size of a pinhead to the size of a grapefruit. The growth and swelling of the cysts are responsible for much of the pain associated with endometriosis.

SYMPTOMS AND SIGNS

The symptoms of endometriosis vary widely, with abnormal or heavy menstrual bleeding being most common. There may be severe abdominal and/or lower back pain during menstruation, which is often most severe toward the end of a period. Other possible symptoms include dyspareunia (see *Intercourse, painful*) and digestive tract symptoms such as diarrhea, constipation, or painful defecation. Rectal bleeding that happens only at the time of the menses may occur. In some cases, however, endometriosis causes no symptoms.

DIAGNOSIS AND TREATMENT

Laparoscopy (examination of the abdominal cavity with a viewing instrument) confirms the diagnosis.

Treatment depends on many factors, including the age and health of the patient, the severity of the condition, and the desire of the woman to have children. Some cases are mild and require no treatment. Drugs to prevent menstruation (including danazol, progesterone, or the combined birth-control pill) may be given. In some cases, pregnancy can suppress endometriosis.

In severe cases, surgical removal of the cysts may be necessary in addition to drug therapy. This may relieve symptoms and aid fertility. If the woman is planning to have no children or she is nearing the menopause, a *hysterectomy* may be considered.

Endometritis

Inflammation of the *endometrium* (uterine lining) due to infection.

Endometritis is a feature of *pelvic inflammatory disease* (PID). It may also occur as a complication of abortion or childbirth, after the insertion of an *IUD*, or as the result of a sexually transmitted infection.

Symptoms include fever, vaginal discharge, and lower abdominal pain. Treatment includes removing any foreign body (such as an IUD or retained placental tissue) and the administration of antibiotics.

Endometrium

The membrane that lines the inside of the *uterus*. It increases in thickness during the menstrual cycle until ovulation occurs. The surface layers are shed during *menstruation* if conception does not take place.

Endorphins

A group of substances formed within the body that relieves pain. Endorphins have a similar chemical structure to *morphine* (it is because of this similarity that morphine has an analgesic effect).

In 1973 morphine was found to act at specific sites (called opiate receptors) in the brain, spinal cord, and at other nerve endings. This discovery led to the identification of small protein molecules produced by cells in the body that also act at opiate receptors; these morphinelike proteins were named endorphins (short for endogenous morphines).

Two other small proteins produced within the brain were originally considered to be examples of endorphins, but they have now been reclassified as *enkephalins* because they are released from different nerve endings.

FUNCTIONS

Since their discovery, endorphins have been found at several sites in the body apart from the nervous system, including the pancreas and testes. Research is being performed to elucidate their full range of functions.

In addition to their analgesic effect, endorphins are thought to be involved in controlling the body's response to stress, regulating contractions of the intestinal wall, and determining mood. They may also regulate the release of hormones from the pituitary gland, notably growth hormone and the *gonadotropin hormones* (which act on the ovaries or testes).

Addiction and *tolerance* to narcotic analgesics, such as morphine, are thought to be due to suppression of the body's production of endorphins; the withdrawal symptoms that occur when the effects of morphine wear off may be due to a lack of these natural analgesics. Conversely, acupuncture is thought to produce analgesia partly by stimulating the release of endorphins and enkephalins.

Endoscope

A lighted viewing instrument that is inserted into a body cavity for the purpose of investigating and treating disorders. (See also box, overleaf.)

Endoscopy

Examination of a body cavity by means of an *endoscope*, a tubelike instrument with lenses and a light source attached. The procedure is safe and in only some cases is a general anesthetic required. Endoscopes may be used with a camera or video recorder, which enable permanent records of the appearance of the internal organs of the body to be obtained and used for reference.

HISTORY

Attempts to view the interior of the body through a rigid, lighted, telescopelike tube were made in the early 1900s, but endoscopy really began in the 1930s with the invention of a semiflexible gastroscope for viewing the stomach. In the late 1950s, a second revolution came with the introduction of *fiberoptics* (flexible bundles of glass or plastic fibers along which light is transmitted). This enabled more versatile instruments to be developed and led to the acceptance of endoscopy as a routine part of hospital medicine.

USES

There are two main uses of endoscopy—diagnostic and therapeutic. For patients suspected of having a tumor or other disorder in the stomach, bladder, lungs, or other organs, endoscopy enables the physician to study the relevant organ and to take a *biopsy* sample (small piece of suspicious tissue for testing), procedures that once required a major operation. Since endoscopy is safe and can be repeated at frequent intervals, it is also useful in assessing how well an ulcer of the stomach or duodenum is healing.

Endoscopy is valuable in the treatment of acute emergencies such as bleeding from the stomach. It allows the cause and site of the bleeding to be identified and, in some cases, to be treated with electrocautery or a *laser*.

Many minor disorders of the knee joint that formerly required a major operation can now be treated quickly and easily. Other uses include removal of polyps (small growths) and swallowed foreign bodies, local application of drugs, and sterilization operations for women. (See also *Arthroscopy; Bronchoscopy; Colonoscopy; Cystoscopy; ERCP; Gastroscopy; Laparoscopy; Laryngoscopy.*)

ENDOSCOPES

A typical flexible fiberoptic endo-scope consists of a bundle of light-transmitting fibers (see *Fiberoptics*). At one end is the head (featuring a viewing lens and steering device) and a power source. The tip has a light, a lens, and an outlet for air or water. Side channels enable attach-ments to be passed through to the tip of the endoscope.

A rigid endoscope is a straight, narrow viewing tube that is not flexi-ble. Attached to it is a light source, which is usually fiberoptic.

COMMON TYPES OF ENDOSCOPES

Instruments	Region	Nature
Cystoscope	Bladder	Rigid
Bronchoscope	Bronchi (main airways of the lungs)	Flexible or rigid
Gastroscope	Esophagus, stomach, and duodenum	Flexible
Colonoscope	Colon (large intestine)	Flexible
Laparoscope	Abdominal cavity	Rigid
Arthroscope	Knee joint	Rigid

Rigid endoscope

Light cable · Viewer · Handle · Power source · Water tubing · Tip · Handle

Flexible endoscope

Power source · Instrument attachment · Viewer · Steering mechanism · Tip

Endoscopic examination
The physician looks through the viewing lens and uses the handles to manipu-late the attachments.

ATTACHMENTS

Various specialized attachments are available for use with the endo-scope. They enable the physician to perform diagnostic and therapeutic procedures such as taking a biopsy specimen (a small piece of tissue for analysis).

Snare attachment · Grasping attachment · Lens · Light cable

Grasping forceps
Sharp-toothed for-ceps that allow foreign bodies to be grasped firmly and removed.

Biopsy forceps
Used for taking small samples of tissue for microscopic analysis.

Scissors
Tiny surgical scissors are used for cutting through tissue and remov-ing small growths.

Brushes
Small brush attachments are used to obtain cells for cytologic examination.

Snare
A thin wire loop, used to remove polyps, through which an electric current is passed.

Basket
A wire basket is sometimes used to trap and remove stones from the bile duct.

Endothelium

The layer of cells that lines the heart, blood vessels, and lymphatic ducts. The cells are squamous (thin and flat), providing a smooth surface that aids the flow of blood and lymph and helps prevent the formation of thrombi (blood clots). See also *Epithelium*.

Endotoxin

 A poison produced by certain bacteria but not released until after the death of the bacteria; until then the toxin remains in the cell wall of the bacteria. Released endotoxins produce two major effects. First, they cause a fever by acting on the temperature-regulating center in the brain. Second, they make the walls of blood capillaries more permeable. This causes fluid to leak into the surrounding tissue, sometimes resulting in a serious drop in blood pressure, a condition called endotoxic shock. (See also *Enterotoxin*; *Exotoxin*.)

Endotracheal tube

A narrow plastic tube passed through the mouth or nose into the trachea (windpipe) by an anesthesiologist. The tube is held in place by an inflatable cuff at its lower end, giving an airtight fit. Endotracheal intubation is performed to deliver oxygen to the lungs if a patient is not breathing adequately and needs mechanical *ventilation*. It may be necessary in a comatose or anesthetized patient, or in a person with respiratory disease.

Enema

A procedure in which fluid is passed into the rectum through a tube inserted into the anus, either as treatment or for diagnostic reasons.

WHY IT IS DONE

An enema is performed for one of three reasons. It can be used to clear the intestine of feces to relieve constipation or to make the tract suitably clean for surgery of the abdominal cavity. Traditionally, this enema was performed by passing soap and water into the rectum. The soap irritated the wall of the intestine, causing contractions and thus stimulating defecation. Soap and water has now largely been replaced by prepacked, small volume enemas containing medication that has the same effect.

Another use of the enema is to administer medicine, such as corticosteroids dissolved in small volumes of fluids to relieve bleeding and inflammation in ulcerative colitis,

or, less commonly, electrolyte solutions to treat severe dehydration.

A third use is in *barium X-ray examinations* to investigate the large intestine for the presence of disease. Barium sulfate, a metallic chemical impervious to X rays, is introduced by enema and outlines the intestine on X-ray pictures.

HOW IT IS DONE

No anesthetic is needed, although the procedure may cause slight discomfort as the fluid distends the intestine. The patient lies on his or her side with hips raised on a pillow. A catheter (flexible tube) with a soft, well-lubricated tip, is gently inserted into the rectum and the fluid for the enema, warmed to prevent sudden contraction of the intestine, is slowly introduced through it.

Energy

The capacity to do work or effect a physical change; nutritionists now also refer to the fuel content of a food as its energy content.

There are many different forms of energy—including light, sound, heat, chemical, electrical, and kinetic (the energy possessed by an object by virtue of its motion)—and most of them play a role in the body. For instance, the retina converts light energy to electrical nerve impulses, thereby making vision possible. Muscles use chemical energy—obtained from food—to produce kinetic energy (movement) and heat.

Energy is measured in units called calories (symbol c), which are becoming obsolete, or joules (symbol J). One calorie is defined as the amount of energy needed to raise the temperature of 1 gram (about 0.033 ounce) of water by 1°C (about 0.6°F); 1 calorie is equivalent to about 4.2 joules (therefore, 1 joule equals approximately 0.24 calories). However, these units are too small for many practical purposes. In medicine, especially in nutrition, the most commonly used units of energy are the kilocalorie (1,000 calories, often called simply a Calorie and represented by a capital C) and the kilojoule (1,000 joules, or 1 kJ).

METABOLIC ENERGY

The most important forms of energy in the body are chemical and heat. The body's *metabolism* comprises thousands of different chemical reactions, some of which liberate energy and some of which use it. Overall, there is a balance between the amount liberated and the amount consumed (see *Energy requirements*).

In general, the energy liberated from the breakdown of nutrients such as glucose and fats (protein is broken down for energy only in extreme situations) is stored as chemical energy in the form of ATP (adenosine triphosphate) molecules. The energy in the molecules is then available to power processes that consume energy, such as muscle contraction or the building up of complex substances needed for repair and maintenance of body structures. Some body processes (muscle contraction, for instance) produce energy in the form of heat. A certain amount of this energy is needed to maintain body temperature, but any excess cannot be used and must leave the body by mechanisms such as radiation of heat from the skin or sweating.

Energy requirements

The amount of *energy* needed by a person for cell metabolism, muscular activity, and growth. This energy is provided by nutrients in the diet, primarily carbohydrate, fat, and protein, and from stored nutrients in the liver and muscles.

ENERGY EXPENDITURE

Energy is needed to keep the heart beating and the lungs functioning and to maintain body temperature. The rate at which these processes use energy is known as the basal metabolic rate (BMR). The BMR accounts for three quarters of the total daily expenditure of energy of the average sedentary person. Any form of movement increases energy expenditure above the BMR. The greater the muscular effort required, the more energy is expended.

Additional energy is needed during growth to provide for extra body tissue. During pregnancy and lactation the mother's energy requirement increases because she must meet the needs of the baby as well as her own. (See also *Nutrition*; *Obesity*.)

Engagement

The arrival of the head of the fetus into the mother's pelvis. In a woman's first pregnancy, engagement usually occurs by the 37th week but, in subsequent pregnancies, it may not occur until labor begins. Rarely, engagement may fail to occur—if, for example, the baby's position in the uterus is abnormal, the baby's head is too big for the mother's pelvis, or if there is *placenta previa* (abnormal position of the placenta across the opening of the uterus).

Enkephalins

A group of small protein molecules that are produced in the brain and by nerve endings elsewhere in the body (in the digestive system and adrenal glands, for example) that have an analgesic effect. In addition, they are thought to produce sedation, to affect mood, and to stimulate motivation.

Enkephalins were initially considered to be *endorphins* (endogenous morphines), but it has since been discovered that they are released by different nerve endings and that they differ slightly chemically.

Enophthalmos

A sinking inward of the eyeball. The most common cause is fracture of the floor of the orbit (bony cavity making up the eye socket).

Enteric-coated tablet

A form of drug preparation whose surface is covered with a substance that is resistant to the action of stomach juices. Enteric-coated tablets pass undissolved through the stomach into the small intestine, where the covering dissolves and the contents are absorbed.

Such tablets are used either when the drug might harm the stomach lining (as may occur with certain corticosteroids, such as prednisone) or when the stomach juices may destroy the efficacy of the drug, as can happen with sulfasalazine.

The drawback of some enteric-coated tablets is that they may pass through the gastrointestinal tract without dissolving.

Enteric fever

An alternative name for either *typhoid fever* or *paratyphoid fever*.

Enteritis

Inflammation of the small intestine. Enteritis may result from infection, particularly *giardiasis* and *tuberculosis*, or from *Crohn's disease*, which is sometimes called regional enteritis. Enteritis usually causes diarrhea. (See also *Gastroenteritis; Colitis*.)

Enteritis, regional

Another name for *Crohn's disease*.

Enterobiasis

An infestation of the intestines by a small roundworm, ENTEROBIUS VERMICULARIS. (See *Pinworm infestation*.)

Enterostomy

An operation in which a portion of small or large intestine is joined to another part of the gastrointestinal tract or to the abdominal wall. When part of the colon (large intestine) is brought through an incision in the abdominal wall to allow the discharge of feces into a bag attached to the skin, the operation is called a *colostomy*. When the ileum (last section of the small intestine) is used for the opening, it is called an *ileostomy*.

Enterotoxin

A type of *toxin* (poison released by certain bacteria) that inflames the lining of the intestine, causing vomiting and diarrhea. Staphylococcal *food poisoning* is due to eating food contaminated with an enterotoxin that is produced by staphylococci bacteria; the toxin is resistant to heat and thus is not destroyed by cooking. The severe intestinal purging that occurs in *cholera* is also caused by an enterotoxin, but by one that is actually produced in the intestine by the cholera bacteria. (See also *Endotoxin*.)

Entropion

A turning in of the margins of the eyelids so that the lashes rub against the cornea and the conjunctiva.

CAUSES

Entropion is sometimes congenital, especially in fat babies. It is common in the elderly, when weakness of the muscles surrounding the lower part of the eye allows the lower lid plate to turn inward. Entropion of the upper or lower lid may be caused by scarring on the inner surface of the lid—for example, due to *trachoma* (a bacterial eye infection).

SYMPTOMS AND SIGNS

Entropion is easily recognized by the sufferer or his or her family. The lid margin is rolled inward so that the lashes are concealed, which sometimes irritates the conjunctiva. When gentle pressure is applied with the fingertip over the lid, the margin pops out, revealing the lashes again.

COMPLICATIONS

In babies, entropion rarely causes any complications because the lashes are very soft and unlikely to damage the cornea. In later life, entropion can cause irritation, conjunctivitis, or corneal ulceration. Persistent entropion may permanently damage the cornea and cause problems with vision and, in some people, blindness.

TREATMENT

Entropion that affects babies usually disappears spontaneously within a few months and seldom requires treatment. In the elderly or in sufferers from trachoma, surgery to correct the entropion prevents damage to the cornea.

ENT surgeon

See *Otolaryngologist, head and neck surgeon*.

Enuresis

The medical term for bed-wetting. Enuresis is a common phenomenon; about 10 percent of children still wet the bed at the age of 5 years, and many of these continue to do so until the age of 8 or 9. A slightly higher number of boys than girls are bed-wetters, and the problem tends to run in families.

CAUSES

In most cases, bed-wetting is due to slow maturation of nervous system functions concerned with control of the bladder. Occasionally it results from psychological stress. In a small number of bed-wetters, there is a specific physical cause—for example, a structural abnormality of the urinary tract present from birth, *diabetes mellitus*, infection of the urinary tract, or a nervous system defect, such as *spina bifida* or spinal cord damage. In each of these cases, the child also has difficulty with daytime bladder control (see *Incontinence, urinary*).

INVESTIGATION

The physician tries to discover, by a full physical examination, urine testing, and other procedures, whether the problem is due to psychological stress or to a nervous system or other physical disorder. If these diagnoses are excluded, tests may be needed to assess bladder function (see *Cystometry*). However, these tests are usually performed only on older children. They involve inserting a catheter into the bladder, which is difficult for a young child to tolerate.

TREATMENT

In the absence of an ascertainable cause, or until the problem can be more fully investigated, treatment starts with training the child to pass urine regularly during the day. This helps the child recognize when the bladder is full, even during sleep. Systems such as rewarding the child with a star on a chart for each dry night are often successful.

If such simple measures fail to work, a nighttime alarm system may be recommended by the physician. The system consists of a pad, placed in the child's bed between the lower sheet and the mattress, that is sensitive to moisture and that triggers a loud alarm when urine is passed. This awakens the child, who can then use the toilet. Eventually, the child wakes whenever urine is about to be passed. Alarms are said to help over two thirds of bed-wetting children over 7 years old.

Other measures that can help include encouraging the child not to drink for two or three hours before sleep, getting him or her to go to the toilet each night immediately before bed, and waking the child to use the toilet two or three hours after going to bed. Antidepressant drugs have also been used successfully in the treatment of bed-wetting.

Parents should not punish a child for bed-wetting or focus undue attention on it, as this may only make the child more anxious and make the problem worse. The vast majority of bed-wetting children eventually become dry at night.

Environmental medicine

The study of the effects on health inherent in different naturally occurring phenomena, such as climate, altitude, sunlight, and the presence of various minerals. The effects of working environments, such as in coal mining, is a separate study (see *Occupational medicine*).

CLIMATE

Certain regions, such as the south of France and the Canary Islands, have long been considered generally beneficial to health; more recently, these sites have been joined by Florida and California.

There is also convincing evidence that particular types of illness respond well to certain climates. For example, sufferers from chest disorders, such as chronic bronchitis and asthma, usually obtain some relief from their symptoms in warm, dry climates. In the US and Europe, where most respiratory complaints are more common in winter, sufferers benefit from spending their winters in a warm environment. Until the introduction of chemotherapy in the 1940s, the prime treatment for pulmonary tuberculosis was to move the patient to a mountain sanatorium to enjoy cool, clean, dry air.

ALTITUDE

Although mountainous regions have much less atmospheric pollution, they are not necessarily beneficial to health because air becomes thinner as altitude increases. Anyone with a chest disease who ascends quickly from sea level to 5,000 feet (about 1,500 meters)—the altitude of Denver, Colorado—may find that his or her breathing difficulty becomes worse. Above 10,000 feet (about 3,000 meters), breathing becomes difficult even for healthy people. Rapid ascent from sea level to 12,000 feet (3,600 meters) or higher carries the risk of altitude sickness, which can produce symptoms ranging from nausea and sleeplessness to coma or death. Only a few communities in the high Andes of South America live permanently above that level.

Sustained living seems to be impossible above 20,000 feet (about 6,000 meters) since at that level the blood cells increase to compensate for lack of oxygen. This strains the heart and causes a predisposition to thrombosis (blood clotting).

SUNLIGHT

White people who live in sunny climates may more easily suffer ill effects from repeated exposure to sunlight, including wrinkling of the skin and an increased risk of skin cancers, such as *basal cell carcinoma* and malignant *melanoma*, and the precancerous condition actinic *keratosis*.

MINERALS

Variations in the distribution of certain *minerals* in the environment are known to have an effect on health. For example, it has recently been discovered that, in areas where the radioactive gas radon is emitted (from rocks of the granite type), there is a higher-than-average incidence of cancers. In contrast, communities that are located in regions where the water has a high fluoride content have a lower-than-average incidence of dental caries.

E

THE GROWING IMPORTANCE OF ENVIRONMENTAL MEDICINE

Large areas of the world are naturally hostile to humans and were, in the past, avoided. Today, exploitation of natural resources has lured people into these regions and has highlighted the importance of environmental medicine.

Key

Desert regions

Cold regions with average winter temperature below −10°F (−23°C)

Mountain regions above 10,000 feet (3,000 m)

Enzyme

A protein that regulates the rate of a chemical reaction in the body. There are thousands of enzymes, each with a different chemical structure. It is this structure that determines the specific reaction regulated by an enzyme. To function properly, many enzymes need an additional component called a coenzyme, which is often derived from a vitamin or mineral.

Every cell in the body produces various enzymes; different sets of enzymes occur in different tissues, reflecting their specialized functions. For example, the pancreas produces the digestive enzymes lipase, protease, and amylase; among the numerous enzymes produced by the liver are some that metabolize drugs.

INDUCTION AND INHIBITION

Enzyme activity is influenced by many factors. Liver enzyme activity is increased by certain drugs, such as barbiturates, which affect the rate at which other drugs are metabolized by the liver. This effect, known as enzyme induction, is responsible for many important *drug* interactions.

Conversely, many drugs inhibit or block enzyme action. Some antibiotics destroy bacteria by blocking bacterial enzymes while leaving human ones unaffected. Similarly, some anticancer drugs work by blocking enzymes in tumor cells, affecting normal body cells to a lesser degree.

ENZYMES AND DISEASE

Measuring enzyme levels in the blood can be useful for diagnosing disorders of certain organs or tissues. For example, the level of heart enzymes is raised after a *myocardial infarction* (heart attack) because the damaged heart muscle cells release enzymes into the bloodstream; muscle enzyme levels are raised in *muscular dystrophy*; and liver enzymes—measured in *liver function tests*—may be raised as a result of certain liver disorders.

Many inherited metabolic disorders, such as *phenylketonuria*, *galactosemia*, and *G6PD deficiency*, are caused by defects in, or deficiencies of, specific enzymes.

ENZYMES AND TREATMENT

Enzymes can play a valuable role in treating certain diseases and disorders. Pancreatic enzymes may be given as digestive aids to patients with *malabsorption* related to pancreatic disease; enzymes that loosen phlegm in the airways may be given to people with chronic lung disease who find it difficult to cough up the phlegm; enzymes such as streptokinase from bacteria and activated tissue plasminogen are used to treat acute *thrombosis* (especially in the coronary arteries) and arterial *embolism* (especially pulmonary embolism). Papain from the papaw fruit can be used in the dressing of wounds and ulcers because it dissolves dead tissue and coagulated blood and may also reduce bruising and swelling.

HOW ENZYMES WORK

An enzyme is a type of protein that acts as a catalyst for a chemical change in the body – that is, it greatly speeds up the rate at which the change occurs. The change may be a small modification to the structure of a substrate (chemical) in a body tissue, the splitting of a substrate, or the joining of two substrates.

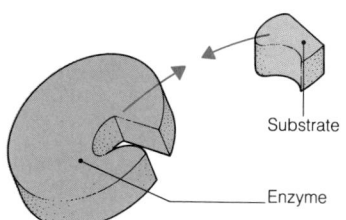

Substrate

Enzyme

1 The shape of an enzyme determines its activity. It will combine only with a specific substrate that has molecules of a complementary shape.

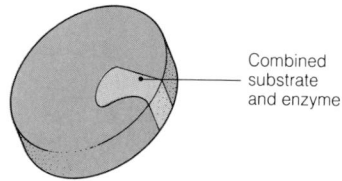

Combined substrate and enzyme

2 When enzyme and substrate combine, their interaction causes a chemical change within the substrate – in this case, splitting it into two products.

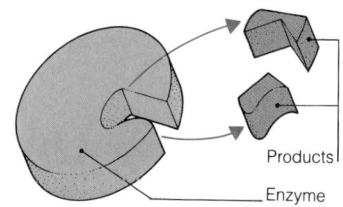

Products

Enzyme

3 After the reaction, the enzyme molecule is unchanged and can move on to combine with another substrate molecule and repeat the process.

Ependymoma

A type of *brain tumor* that occurs commonly in children. It is a *glioma*, a tumor arising from the glial (supporting) cells within the nervous system.

Although ependymomas are one of the more common types of tumor in childhood, in overall terms they are rare. In the US, there are about two to three cases annually per million people. The cause is unknown.

Symptoms, diagnosis, and treatment of ependymomas are as for other types of brain tumor.

Ephedrine

A drug that stimulates the release of *norepinephrine* (a chemical *neurotransmitter* released from nerve endings).

Ephedrine is used in eye drops to narrow dilated blood vessels and to relieve redness of the eyes caused by minor irritation, such as smoke.

Other uses occasionally include the relief of motion sickness, bed-wetting in children, and delayed ejaculation. Ephedrine is prescribed as a *decongestant drug* and as a *bronchodilator drug*.

Epicanthic fold

A vertical fold of skin extending from the upper eyelid to the side of the nose. It is a normal feature in Orientals. In other races, it is rare except in babies; the folds usually disappear as the nose develops.

Epicondylitis

A painful inflammation of an epicondyle, one of the bony prominences of the elbow at the lower end of the humerus (upper arm bone). Various forearm muscles that bend or straighten the wrist or fingers are attached by tendons to the epicondyles. Overuse of these muscles can lead to epicondylitis due to repeated tugging of the tendons at their point of attachment to the bone.

Epicondylitis affecting the prominence on the outer side of the elbow, caused by overuse of the muscles that straighten the fingers and wrist, is called *tennis elbow*. When the prominence on the inner side of the elbow is affected, caused by overuse of muscles that bend the fingers and wrist, it is called *golfers' elbow*.

Epidemic

A medical term applied to a disease that for most of the time is rare in a community, but which suddenly spreads rapidly to affect a large number of people. Epidemics of new strains of influenza are probably the most common, occurring periodically when the influenza virus changes to a form to which the population has no resistance. (See also *Endemic*.)

Epidemiology
The study of disease as it affects groups of people, as opposed to individuals. Originally, as its name suggests, epidemiology dealt mainly with epidemics of infectious diseases (such as cholera, plague, and influenza) and outbreaks of infections (such as gastroenteritis) associated with food poisoning. More recently, it has been applied to widespread noninfectious diseases, such as cancer and heart disease.

Members of a population (or, in comparative studies, populations) under study are carefully counted and defined in terms of each person's race, sex, age, occupation, social class, marital status, and the like. Then the incidence of the disorder (the number of new cases per week, month, or year) and its prevalence (the number of people with the disorder at any given time) are determined. These observations may be repeated at regular intervals to detect changes occurring over time. The result is an exact statistical record that often yields many valuable findings.

Groups that spend all their lives in one defined area often provide more useful information than highly mobile populations whose environments change considerably over the course of their lives. For example, a high incidence of cancer of the esophagus has been studied among the inhabitants of one region of China and among other inhabitants of Iran. This incidence has been compared to similar groups in other regions of the countries; certain foods have been implicated.

COMPARATIVE EPIDEMIOLOGY
In the attempt to conquer cancer, heart disease, and other widespread diseases that afflict people in the West today, comparative epidemiology is proving to be one of the most potent weapons. Two or more groups are chosen—one having, the other not having, a characteristic that may affect the frequency of a disease. For example, in a study of the link between smoking and lung cancer, one group may consist of smokers and the other of nonsmokers; the proportion with cancer in each group is then calculated. In such cases, the epidemiologist is careful to make the two groups as nearly identical as possible in other respects, carefully

matching such factors as age, sex, weight, and socioeconomic status.

Another approach is to compare a group of people that has a certain disease, such as hypertension, with a control group (people without the condition but similar in other respects); the aim is to isolate identifying factors, such as obesity, that differ between the two groups.

The links discovered by comparative epidemiology—such as the correlation of a high level of fish oils in the diet and low prevalence of heart disease—do not demonstrate cause and effect. For example, epidemiologists have discovered that the prevalence of heart disease is high in countries in which most people have an automobile. This association obviously does not mean that owning an automobile causes heart disease, but, since such ownership suggests a more sedentary life-style, the link does reinforce the belief that lack of exercise increases the risk of heart disease. The study thus justifies more research on the subject.

Epidermolysis bullosa

A rare, inherited condition in which blisters appear on the skin after minor damage. The disorder mainly affects young children and has a wide range of severity, from the type in which blisters form on the feet in hot weather, to a form with widespread blistering and scarring.

CAUSES AND OUTLOOK
The condition is caused by a genetic defect that may show either an autosomal dominant or autosomal recessive pattern of inheritance (see *Genetic disorders*). It is diagnosed by skin *biopsy* (removal of a small amount of skin for microscopic analysis).

No special treatment for the condition is available, although injury to the skin should be avoided and simple protective measures should be taken to prevent rubbing of affected areas when blisters appear.

The outlook varies from a gradual improvement in mild cases of epidermolysis bullosa to progressive serious disease in the most severe cases.

Parents of affected children should obtain *genetic counseling* so that the risks of any future children being affected can be calculated.

Epididymal cyst
A harmless swelling, usually painless, that may develop in the upper rear part of a testicle. Small cysts are very

common in men over the age of 40 and need no treatment. Rarely, they may become tender or may enlarge and become uncomfortable, in which case it may be necessary to remove the cysts surgically.

Epididymis
A long, coiled tube connecting the vasa efferentia (small tubes leading from the testicle) to the vas deferens (the sperm duct leading to the urethra). Sperm cells produced in the testicle pass slowly along the epididymis, maturing there until they are capable of fertilizing an egg. They are then stored in the seminal vesicles until *ejaculation*.

Disorders affecting the epididymis include *epididymo-orchitis* (inflammation of the epididymis and testicle) and *epididymal cysts* (fluid-filled swellings). Infection or injury can block the epididymis; if this occurs in both testicles, it can cause infertility.

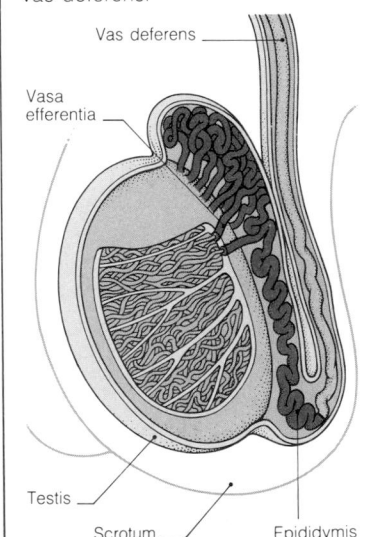

LOCATION OF THE EPIDIDYMIS
The epididymis runs along the back of the testis and links the vasa efferentia to the vas deferens.

Vas deferens
Vasa efferentia
Testis
Scrotum
Epididymis

Epididymitis
See *Epididymo-orchitis*.

Epididymo-orchitis
Acute inflammation of a testicle and its associated epididymis (the coiled tube that carries sperm away from it) characterized by severe pain and

swelling at the back of the testicle and accompanied by swelling and redness of the scrotum in severe cases.

The inflammation is caused by infection. Often there is no obvious source of infection, but sometimes the cause is a bacterial infection spread from the urinary tract via the vas deferens (sperm duct). Rarely, epididymo-orchitis occurs through spread of a tuberculosis infection.

DIAGNOSIS AND TREATMENT

The symptoms of severe pain and swelling are similar to those of torsion of the testicle, in which the testicle cord becomes twisted and blocks its own blood supply (see *Testis, torsion of*). An exploratory operation may be necessary to make a firm diagnosis and save the testicle. In some cases testicular scans may be helpful.

Treatment is with antibiotics and rest. If there is an underlying urinary tract infection, its cause is investigated. The tuberculous form of the disease usually responds to treatment given for tuberculosis elsewhere in the body. In all cases it may take several months for the testicle to return to its normal size. Sometimes normal size is never attained. (See also *Orchitis*.)

Epidural anesthesia

A method of pain relief for surgery in which local anesthetic is injected into the epidural space in the middle and lower back to numb the nerves leading to the chest and the lower half of the body. Epidural anesthesia may be combined with a light general anesthesia. Usually a catheter (a flexible, fine tube) is introduced into the

Vertebra

Epidural space

Spinal cord

Hollow needle

Administering an epidural anesthetic
The anesthetic is injected into the epidural space (the region surrounding the spinal cord within the spinal canal).

epidural space to allow further anesthetic doses to be given as necessary without more needle puncture.

Epidural *analgesia* is pain relief achieved by injecting narcotics or dilute local anesthetic solutions into the epidural space. Its applications include postoperative analgesia, pain relief during childbirth, and the control of cancer pain that is unresponsive to all other measures.

Epiglottiditis

A rare but serious and sometimes fatal infection that mainly affects children between 2 and 6. Caused by the bacterium HEMOPHILUS INFLUENZAE, it results in sudden inflammation and swelling of the epiglottis (the flap of cartilage at the back of the tongue that closes off the windpipe during swallowing). The swollen epiglottis obstructs breathing. If the condition is not recognized and treated promptly, it can cause death by suffocation.

SYMPTOMS

The illness comes on suddenly. The child becomes feverish, breathing becomes noisy (stridor), swallowing is painful, and the child drools because he or she cannot swallow saliva. Breathing becomes increasingly difficult and the child prefers to sit upright in an attempt to make breathing easier. Within a few hours of the onset of the illness, the child may become semiconscious and cyanotic (bluish) due to lack of oxygen.

DIAGNOSIS AND TREATMENT

The symptoms and signs of epiglottiditis resemble those of *croup* (inflammation of the airways); expert assessment by an experienced pediatrician may be necessary to distinguish between them. For this reason, any child who becomes feverish and in whom noisy breathing develops should be seen by a physician as soon as possible. If he or she suspects epiglottiditis, the child will be admitted to a hospital. In the hospital, neck X rays are usually taken to help confirm the diagnosis. A tube is almost always passed through the nose or mouth and into the trachea so breathing can be maintained; often a ventilator is needed. Intravenous antibiotics (usually ampicillin and/or chloramphenicol) are needed to cure the infection. With prompt treatment the prognosis is good; recovery usually takes place within two weeks.

The bacterium H. INFLUENZAE is highly contagious; family members should be screened or treated with antibiotics to prevent its spread.

Epiglottis

The flap of cartilage lying behind the tongue and in front of the entrance to the larynx (voice box). At rest, the epiglottis is upright and allows air to pass through the larynx and into the rest of the respiratory system. During swallowing it folds back to cover the entrance to the larynx, preventing food and drink from being inhaled.

Epilepsy

A tendency to recurrent seizures or temporary alteration in one or more brain functions.

Seizures are defined as transient neurological abnormalities caused by abnormal electrical activity in the brain. Human activities, thoughts, perceptions, and emotions are normally the result of the regulated and orderly electrical excitation of nerve cells in the brain. During a seizure, a chaotic and unregulated electrical discharge occurs. In some cases, a stimulus such as a flashing light sets off this abnormal sequence, but often seizures appear spontaneously.

CAUSES

Seizures are a symptom of brain dysfunction and, like symptoms in other parts of the body, can result from a wide variety of disease or injury. Seizures may occur in association with *head injury*, birth trauma, brain infection (such as *meningitis* or *encephalitis*), *brain tumor*, *stroke*, drug intoxication, drug or alcohol withdrawal states, or metabolic imbalance in the body. A tendency to seizures may develop for no obvious reason or there may be an inherited predisposition.

INCIDENCE

About one person in 200 suffers from epilepsy. The number of epileptics in the US is estimated to be close to 1 million. The disorder usually starts in childhood or adolescence. Many people outgrow epilepsy and do not require medication.

TYPES AND SYMPTOMS

Epileptic seizures can be classified into two broad groups—generalized and partial seizures. The form a seizure takes depends on the part of the brain in which it arises and on how widely and rapidly it fans out from its point of origin. Generalized seizures, which cause loss of consciousness, affect the whole body and may arise over a wide area of the brain. *Temporal lobe epilepsy* is a type of partial seizure. Partial seizures, in which consciousness may be retained, are usually caused by damage to a more limited area of the brain. Though partial seizures begin in a limited area, the electrical disturbance may spread and affect the whole brain, causing a generalized seizure.

Many people with epilepsy lead normal lives and have no symptoms between seizures. Some can tell when an attack is imminent by experiencing an aura (a restless, irritable, or uncomfortable feeling).

GENERALIZED SEIZURES

There are two main types of generalized seizure—grand mal and petit mal (absence) seizures.

GRAND MAL During a grand mal seizure the person falls down unconscious and the entire body stiffens and then twitches or jerks uncontrollably. There may be an initial cry; breathing is then absent or very irregular during the seizure. Following the seizure, the muscles relax, and bowel and bladder control may be lost. The person may feel confused and disoriented and perhaps have a headache; often he or she will want to sleep. These effects usually clear in several hours. The person usually has no memory of the event. Prolonged seizures, referred to as status epilepticus, can be fatal without emergency treatment.

ABSENCE SEIZURES These seizures, in which there is a momentary loss of consciousness without abnormal movements, occur mainly in children. There is a blank period lasting from a few seconds to up to half a minute or so, during which the sufferer is unaware of anything. To the onlooker, it may appear that the person is simply daydreaming or inattentive, and the attack may even pass unnoticed. Absence seizures may occur hundreds of times daily and can markedly impair school performance.

PARTIAL SEIZURES

Partial seizures are divided into simple seizures (in which consciousness is maintained) and complex seizures (in which it is lost). In simple partial seizures an abnormal twitching movement, tingling sensation, or even hallucination of smell, vision, or taste, occurs without warning and lasts several minutes. When the twitching occurs and spreads slowly from one part of the body to another on the same side, it is referred to as jacksonian epilepsy. Sufferers retain awareness during the event and can recall the details.

During complex partial seizures, the person becomes dazed and may not respond if addressed. Sometimes involuntary actions, such as fumbling with buttons or lip smacking, occur.

These actions are called automatisms and can (rarely) take more bizarre forms. The person typically remembers little, if any, of the event.

Both types of partial seizure can sometimes spread to involve the entire brain, in which case generalization is said to have occurred. The symptoms then become the same as those of a grand mal seizure.

PREVENTION

Many epileptics experience seizures at times of extreme fatigue or stress. Infectious illnesses, especially if fever is present, also lower the seizure threshold. By avoiding these situations and taking prescribed medication regularly, epileptics can reduce seizure frequency. Occasionally, epileptics discover a distracting technique that can abort a seizure once the aura has begun.

DIAGNOSIS

In making the diagnosis, the physician seeks as much information as possible about the attacks. Since patients frequently do not have recall, information may be obtained from witnesses. After a complete neurological examination, the physician usually orders an *EEG* to help with the diagnosis. It is important to realize that the EEG cannot always absolutely confirm or refute the diagnosis of seizures, and that the results must be weighed in light of other clinical findings. Sometimes tests of heart function (such as an *ECG* or *Holter monitor*) are obtained to exclude cardiac irregularities as a cause of loss of consciousness in an adult. Patients thought to have seizures are usually given *CT scanning* of the brain and *blood tests* to check for the conditions associated with epilepsy. Opinion is divided on whether a single seizure should be treated; physicians agree that people with recurrent seizures should take *anticonvulsant drugs*.

TREATMENT

Anticonvulsant drugs are the first line of treatment for epilepsy, and, in almost all cases, they lessen the frequency of seizures. The drugs may have unpleasant side effects, including drowsiness and impaired concentration. The physician will attempt to find the one drug that works best, but, with very severe epilepsy, a combination may be needed to control seizures. If no seizures occur for two to three years (depending on their cause), the physician may suggest reducing or stopping drug treatment.

Rarely, surgery may be considered if it is thought that a single area of

brain damage (usually in the temporal lobe) is causing the seizures and medication is ineffective.

OUTLOOK

If epilepsy develops during childhood and there is a strong family history of the disease, the chances are good that the problem will decrease after adolescence; it may even disappear altogether. However, seizure control is likely to be more difficult in temporal lobe epilepsy or if the disorder has been brought about by severe brain damage.

One third of those in whom epilepsy develops eventually grow out of the condition and experience no further seizures. Another third find that the seizures become less frequent in response to drug treatment. The conditions of the remaining third remain the same.

Sufferers from epilepsy usually are able to work, but the disorder may limit their choice of jobs. There are restrictions on obtaining a driver's license (generally an applicant is required to have been seizure-free for several years). It is advisable, unless the seizures are very well controlled, to avoid high-risk jobs involving heights or dangerous machinery and sports such as skiing.

Many epileptics carry a special card, tag, or bracelet that states they have epilepsy. Epileptics are recommended to advise colleagues on what to do if a seizure occurs.

DEALING WITH AN EPILEPTIC SEIZURE

Most major epileptic seizures last only a minute or two and demand little of the bystander. All that is necessary is to let the attack run its course and to ensure that the person is in no physical danger and can breathe while he or she is unconscious.

E

The person should not be held down, nor should his or her movements be restrained. Any tight clothing around the neck should be loosened and something soft should be placed beneath the head. The mouth should not be forced open and no object should be wedged between the teeth. Once the convulsions have ceased, the victim should be put into the *recovery position*.

An ambulance should be called if the seizure continues for more than five minutes, if another seizure immediately follows the first one, or if consciousness is not regained a few minutes after the epileptic seizure has come to end.

Epiloia
See *Tuberous sclerosis*.

Epinephrine

ALLERGY BRONCHODILATOR
GLAUCOMA DECONGESTANT

Injection Inhaler Eye drops Nose drops

	Prescription needed
	Available as generic

A naturally occurring hormone, also called adrenaline. Epinephrine has been produced synthetically as a drug since 1900.

Epinephrine is one of two chemicals (the other is *norepinephrine*) released by the adrenal gland in response to signals from the sympathetic division of the *autonomic nervous system*. These signals are triggered by stress, exercise, or by an emotion such as fear.

Epinephrine increases the speed and force of the heart beat and thereby the work that can be done by the heart. It dilates the airways to improve breathing and narrows blood vessels in the skin and intestine so that an increased flow of blood reaches the muscles, allowing them to cope with the demands of exercise.

USE AS A DRUG
Epinephrine is sometimes given by injection as an emergency treatment for *cardiac arrest* (stopped heart beat) and is used to treat *anaphylactic shock* (a severe allergic reaction) and acute *asthma* attacks.

During surgery, it is injected into tissues to reduce bleeding. When combined with a local anesthetic, epinephrine prolongs the effect by slowing down the rate at which the anesthetic spreads into the surrounding tissues.

Epinephrine eye drops are used to treat *glaucoma* and they are used during eye surgery because they reduce pressure in the eyeball. Epinephrine is also used to stop nosebleeds and reduce *nasal congestion*.

POSSIBLE ADVERSE EFFECTS
Regular use of epinephrine as eye drops may cause a burning pain and, occasionally, blurred vision or pigment deposits on the eye's surface.

In nose-drop form, epinephrine may cause palpitations, restlessness, and nervousness; newer *decongestant drugs* are now usually preferred.

Epiphora
See *Watering eye*.

Epiphysis
Either of the two growing ends of the long bones (femur, tibia, humerus, ulna, radius, and fibula) of the limbs. The epiphysis is separated from the diaphysis (shaft of the bone) by a layer of cartilage, called the epiphyseal plate or growth plate.

During childhood and adolescence, bones grow as the result of *ossification*, a process in which cartilage cells multiply and absorb calcium to develop into bone. In this way, the cartilage in the epiphyseal plate is gradually replaced by new bone.

LOCATION OF THE EPIPHYSIS
Each epiphysis is situated at the ends of the long bones of the body and is separated from the shaft of the bone by an epiphyseal plate.

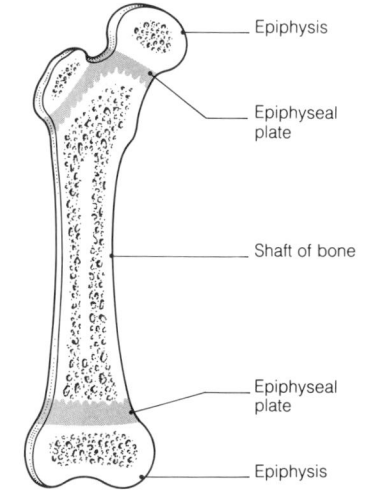

Epiphysis

Epiphyseal plate

Shaft of bone

Epiphyseal plate

Epiphysis

Epiphysis, slipped
See *Femoral epiphysis, slipped*.

Episcleritis
A localized patch of inflammation affecting the outermost layers of the sclera (the white of the eye) immediately under the conjunctiva (outer covering layer of the eye).

Episcleritis usually occurs for no known reason and usually affects middle-aged men. It may be a complication of rheumatoid arthritis. The purplish patch of inflammation is oval, slightly raised, and only a fraction of an inch across. It may cause a deep, dull, aching pain that tends to be worse at night. During the day there may be photophobia.

The condition usually disappears by itself within a week or two but may recur. Symptoms may be relieved by corticosteroid eye drops or ointment.

Episiotomy
A surgical procedure in which an incision is made in the perineum (the tissue between the vagina and the anus) to facilitate the delivery of a baby. After delivery, the cut tissues are stitched back together.

WHY IT IS DONE
Episiotomy is used to enlarge the vaginal opening. Some medical practitioners advocate its use almost routinely on the theory that a surgical cut will heal better than a tear, and that women who have had episiotomies will experience less "vaginal relaxation" (stretching of the vagina) later in life. Other practitioners rarely perform episiotomies on the theory that the naturally elastic vagina should not have to be cut to allow a normal delivery, and that small tears cause less damage and pain than does an episiotomy.

If the perineum fails to stretch up over the baby's head and/or a large perineal tear looks likely, an episiotomy is advisable. It prevents a ragged tear that is more painful, more difficult to repair, and more easily leads to complications. When the woman has had a previous vaginal repair (for *prolapse* of the uterus or urinary incontinence), an episiotomy prevents damage to the repair by increasing the size of the vaginal opening. Episiotomy is usually necessary in forceps deliveries because the instruments occupy additional space in the vaginal opening; it is likewise necessary in a breech delivery, when there is little opportunity for gradual stretching of the perineal tissues to occur.

Indications for episiotomy that concern the baby directly include *fetal distress* (when the baby is not receiving enough oxygen during labor), because episiotomy also speeds delivery. An episiotomy also reduces pressure on the head of a premature baby.

HOW IT IS DONE
As the baby's head descends through the maternal pelvis and begins to distend the perineum, local anesthetic is injected into the area (unless the woman has already been given an epidural or another anesthetic).

Scissors or a scalpel are used to make a cut extending from the back wall of the vagina through the perineal skin and muscles. This cut may be directed to the side of the anus (mediolateral) or in a direct vertical line with the anus (midline).

HOW IT IS REPAIRED
An episiotomy is usually repaired shortly after delivery of the baby. The woman lies on her back with her feet in stirrups. The perineum is thoroughly cleaned and more local anesthetic is injected if necessary. The vagina is then inspected to assess the size of the incision and to see whether further tears have occurred. The wound is repaired in layers, usually with absorbable sutures.

RECOVERY PERIOD
The woman can walk as soon as she wishes. Perineal washes and/or showers are advised. Occasionally, ice packs and analgesics are required. Care is taken to avoid constipation. The sutures dissolve after about 10 days (if catgut is used) and thus do not require removal. In most cases, healing is straightforward. Discomfort in the scar is sometimes noted for up to three months.

Epispadias
A rare congenital abnormality in which the opening of the urethra is not in the glans (head) of the penis, but on the upper surface of the penis. The penis may also curve upward.

Surgery is carried out in infancy, using tissue from the foreskin to reconstruct the urethra and to create a penis that will allow satisfactory sexual intercourse in adult life. Sometimes more than one operation is needed to correct the condition.

Epistaxis
The medical term for a *nosebleed*.

Epithelium
The cells, occurring in one or more layers, that cover the entire surface of the body and that line most of the hollow structures within it. (The blood vessels, lymph vessels, and the inside of the heart are lined with *endothelium*, and the chest and abdominal cavities are lined with mesothelium.)

Epithelium varies in cell type and thickness of layer according to the function it performs. There are three basic cell shapes: squamous (thin and flat), cuboidal, and columnar. These structures may vary further. In the respiratory tract, for example, epithelial cells bear whiplike filaments called cilia that propel dust particles from inhaled air back up the tracheobronchial tree.

Most internal organs lined with epithelium are covered with only one layer of cells, but the skin, which is subjected to more trauma, consists of many layers with a dead outer layer of cells that is constantly being shed.

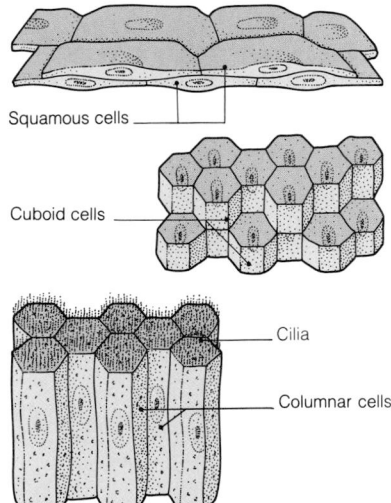

Types of epithelium
The cells of the epithelium vary in shape and size according to function. The three basic types are squamous, cuboidal, and columnar.

Epstein-Barr virus
A virus that causes infectious *mononucleosis* and is associated with *Burkitt's lymphoma* and nasopharyngeal cancer.

ERCP
The abbreviation for endoscopic retrograde cholangiopancreatography, an X-ray procedure for examining the biliary system and the pancreatic duct. It is used mainly when *ultrasound scanning* or *CT scanning* fails to provide a sufficiently detailed image.

HOW IT IS DONE
ERCP is usually an outpatient procedure and takes 20 to 40 minutes. No food or drink is taken for eight hours before the examination. A sedative and a local anesthetic of the throat are usually given.

An *endoscope* (a flexible viewing tube with a lens and light attached) is passed down the esophagus, through the stomach, and into the duodenum (the upper part of the small intestine). After identifying the ampulla of Vater (the entrance within the duodenum to both the common bile duct and the pancreatic duct), the endoscope operator passes a catheter (fine, flexible tube) through the endoscope and into the ampulla. He or she then passes a radiopaque dye (one that shows up on X-ray film) through the catheter to fill the pancreatic duct and all the ducts of the biliary system. X-ray pictures are then taken to show any abnormalities in the ducts.

If disease is detected, it can sometimes be treated at the same time. For example, stones obstructing the lower end of the common bile duct can be removed by using an attachment on the endoscope to widen the duct. If there is a suspected tumor at the ampulla, the endoscope can be used to perform a *biopsy* (removal of a small sample of tissue for analysis) and/or brushing of cells for cytologic examination (see *Cytology*).

Erection
Hardness, swelling, and elevation of the *penis*. Usually caused by sexual arousal or physical stimulation, it also occurs regularly during sleep and may occur for no obvious reason in very young boys.

The penis contains three cylinders of erectile tissue with a network of blood vessels controlled by the spinal nerves. During an erection, the penis becomes filled with blood as the vessels dilate (widen) to allow increased blood flow. Muscles around the vessels contract and prevent blood from leaving to maintain the erection.

Erection, disorders of
Conditions in which there is total or partial failure to attain or maintain erection (see *Impotence*), persistent erection without any sexual desire (see *Priapism*), or a painfully bowed erection (see *Chordee*).

Ergocalciferol
An alternative name for vitamin D_2 (see *Vitamin D*), also called calciferol.

Ergometer

A machine that measures the amount of physical work done and the body's response to a controlled amount of exercise. It makes continuous recordings, during and immediately after activity, of heart rate and rhythm (using an *ECG*), blood pressure, the rate of breathing, and the volume of oxygen that is taken up from the surrounding air.

The physician-supervised exercise is done on a fixed bicycle, rowing machine, or treadmill, and the effort required is adjusted to suit the particular test being performed. In *fitness testing*, the exercise is vigorous enough to require maximum effort; in a *cardiac stress test*, the exercise is adjusted to a level sufficient to produce a certain predetermined level of heart rate. Symptoms that occur during the exercise, such as chest pain, breathing difficulty, or a fall in blood pressure, terminate the test.

Ergonovine

A drug that is injected after childbirth or termination of pregnancy to control the loss of blood from the uterus. Ergonovine works by causing the muscles of the uterus to contract, which compresses the blood vessels and thus reduces bleeding.

If blood loss remains heavy after the injection and there is no underlying cause (such as a retained placenta or infection) requiring treatment, ergonovine may be prescribed as a tablet for one or two days to help control bleeding.

Ergot

A product of CLAVICEPS PURPUREA, a fungus that grows on rye and other grains. Ergot contains several *alkaloids* (nitrogen-containing substances) with medicinal and poisonous effects.

The most important drugs produced from ergot are *ergotamine*, used to treat migraine, and *ergonovine*, used to control blood loss from the uterus following childbirth or an abortion.

Before it was known that ergot was a poison, bread made with contaminated rye caused outbreaks of ergot poisoning. The effects included gangrene of the toes and fingers, seizures, mental disorders, and, in some cases, death.

Ergotamine

A drug used in the prevention and treatment of *migraine*. It works by con-stricting the dilated blood vessels surrounding the brain and is used as an alternative to *analgesics* (painkillers).

Ergotamine is most effective if taken during the very early warning stages of a migraine attack. Once the headache and nausea of migraine are present, it is less likely to be effective and may even increase the nausea.

Erosion, dental

Loss of enamel from the surface of a tooth as a result of attack by chemicals or acids, such as from gastric juices brought through the mouth in vomiting or from tobacco juice. The first sign of enamel loss is a dull, frosted appearance. As the condition progresses, smooth, shiny, shallow cavities form.

Erosion affecting the outer surfaces of the front teeth is most often caused by excessive consumption of citrus fruits, fruit juices, or carbonated drinks; it also sometimes occurs in workers using acid in industrial processes (such as battery construction). Erosion that mainly affects the inner surfaces of the molar teeth may be caused by frequent regurgitation of acidic fluid from the stomach—for example, in people suffering from *acid reflux* or *bulimia*.

Erosion may be combined with, and also accelerate, *abrasion* (mechanical wearing away of teeth) and attrition (wearing down of the chewing surfaces), leading to extensive damage to many teeth.

Eroticism

A state of sexual excitement. People are usually most easily stimulated by thoughts, but this stimulation may be augmented by touching of the erogenous zones—the breasts, genitals, mouth, and anus. Sexual arousal can also be produced by a variety of other sensations and stimuli (i.e., the look and feel of certain clothes, the scent of a perfume, or the sound of a piece of music).

In *psychoanalytic theory*, eroticism (named for Eros, the Greek god of physical love) is contrasted with *narcissism* (self love). Eroticism is a mature love that can be fulfilled only when the loved one is also satisfied. Narcissism is typical of immature personalities and is a love that merely wishes to satisfy itself.

Eruption

Breaking out or appearing, as in the development of a skin rash or the appearance of a new tooth.

Eruption of teeth

The process by which developing *teeth* move through the bone of the jaws and the covering gum to project into the mouth.

DECIDUOUS DENTITION

Deciduous (primary) teeth (the milk teeth) usually begin to appear at around 6 months of age, with the lower front teeth erupting first, but the timing may vary. Occasionally a baby is born with one or two of these teeth already visible, while in other babies no teeth appear until about 9 months of age. All 20 deciduous teeth usually erupt by age 3. Infants may suffer a mild general upset at the time of eruption (see *Teething*).

PERMANENT DENTITION

Permanent teeth (the secondary teeth) generally begin erupting at 6 years. The first permanent molars erupt toward the back of the mouth, behind the existing deciduous teeth rather than replacing any of them. Children and parents are often unaware that these are permanent teeth. The later eruption of permanent teeth nearer the front of the mouth is preceded by reabsorption of the roots of the deciduous teeth, which become loose and detach. The succeeding permanent tooth emerges a few weeks after its deciduous predecessor falls out. Wisdom teeth (the last molar teeth) usually erupt between the ages of 17 and 21, but in some people never appear. Frequently, wisdom teeth are impacted (blocked from erupting) because of lack of available space in the jawbone (see *Impaction, dental*).

Erysipelas

An infection of the face caused by streptococcal bacteria, which are thought to enter the skin through a small wound or sore. Young children and elderly people are the groups mainly affected.

SYMPTOMS AND TREATMENT

The disorder starts abruptly with malaise, fever, headaches, and vomiting. Itchy, red patches appear on the face and spread across the cheeks and bridge of the nose to form an inflamed area with raised edges. Within this area, pimples develop that first blister, then burst, and then crust over.

Treatment is with penicillin, which usually clears the condition within a week. (See also *Cellulitis*.)

Erythema

Redness of the skin. Disorders of which skin redness is one symptom include *erythema multiforme*, *erythema*

TOOTH ERUPTION

The top diagrams show the approximate ages at which particular deciduous teeth usually appear. The ages at which specific types of permanent teeth usually appear are shown in the lower diagrams. Red denotes erupting teeth; gray denotes erupted deciduous teeth; white denotes erupted permanent teeth.

6 to 10 months: lower central incisors

8 to 12 months: upper central incisors

9 to 16 months: lateral incisors

13 to 19 months: first molars

16 to 23 months: canines

23 to 33 months: second molars

Deciduous teeth
The full deciduous set (left) consists of eight incisors, four canines, and eight molars. They usually start erupting at 6 months.

Permanent teeth
The full set of permanent teeth (below) consists of eight incisors, four canines, eight premolars, and 12 molars

6 to 7 years: first molars

6 to 8 years: central incisors

7 to 9 years: lateral incisors

10 to 12 years: first premolars

10 to 12 years: second premolars

9 to 12 years: canines

11 to 13 years: second molars

17 to 21 years: third molars

E

---

nodosum, *lupus erythematosus*, and erythema infectiosum (*fifth disease*).

Facial erythema can have many causes, including *blushing*, *hot flashes*, *sunburn*, raised temperature, and skin conditions such as *acne*, *dermatitis*, *eczema*, *erysipelas*, *rosacea*, and *urticaria* (hives).

Erythema ab igne
Red skin that may also be dry and itchy, caused by exposure to strong direct heat. It occurs most commonly in elderly women—on the shins, as the result of sitting too close to a fireplace in cold weather, or on the abdomen, due to hugging a heating pad or a hot-water bottle.

Dryness and itching of the skin can often be relieved by an *emollient* (soothing cream). The redness usually fades in time, although it rarely disappears completely.

Erythema infectiosum
See *Fifth disease*.

Erythema multiforme
An acute inflammation of the skin, and sometimes of the internal mucous membranes (the thin moist tissue that lines bodily cavities). Erythema multiforme is sometimes accompanied by generalized illness. Erythema multiforme means literally "skin redness of many varieties."

CAUSES AND INCIDENCE
The disease can occur as a reaction to certain drugs (including penicillin, sulfonamides, salicylates, and barbiturates), or may accompany certain viral infections (including cold sores) or bacterial infections (such as streptococcal throat infection). Pregnancy, vaccination, and radiation therapy are other possible causes. However, half of all cases occur for no apparent reason. The disease is most common in children and young women.

SYMPTOMS
A symmetrical rash of red, often itchy spots, similar to the rash of measles, erupts on the limbs and sometimes on

The rash of erythema multiforme
The spots of this rash are usually itchy and have a bull's-eye appearance, with concentric rings of different shades of red around a pale center.

the face and the rest of the body. The spots may blister or may progress to urticaria (hives), in which there are raised, red, pale-centered wheals. Those affected may have fever, sore throat, headache, and/or diarrhea.

In a severe form of erythema multiforme, called Stevens-Johnson syndrome, the mucous membranes of the mouth, eyes, and genitals become inflamed and ulcerated.

TREATMENT
If treatment for some other disorder is believed to be the cause of the erythema, the treatment will be withdrawn. Similarly, any possible causative illness will be treated. Corticosteroid drugs are sometimes given to reduce inflammation and irritation. Patients suffering from Stevens-Johnson syndrome are given analgesics (painkillers), plenty of fluids (sometimes intravenously), sedatives, and sometimes corticosteroid drugs.

Erythema multiforme usually clears within five to six weeks, although it may recur. The Stevens-Johnson syndrome normally responds to treatment, but in some cases the patient may become seriously ill as a result of shock or of inflammation spreading within the body.

Erythema nodosum
A condition characterized by an eruption of red-purple swellings on the

legs in association with another illness. It is most common between the ages of 20 and 50 and affects women more than men.

CAUSES AND INCIDENCE

The most common cause of erythema nodosum is a throat infection with streptococcal bacteria, but it is also associated with other diseases, most commonly *tuberculosis* and *sarcoidosis*, and may occur as a reaction to certain drugs, including sulfonamides, penicillin, and salicylates. In about one third of cases of erythema nodosum no cause can be discovered.

SYMPTOMS AND TREATMENT

The swellings, which range from 0.5 to 4 inches in diameter, are shiny and tender and occur on the shins, thighs, and, less commonly, the arms. They are usually accompanied by fever and joint and muscle pains.

Effective treatment of any underlying condition clears the swellings. Otherwise, the only treatment that is necessary is bed rest, analgesics (painkillers), and, occasionally, *corticosteroid drugs* to reduce inflammation. The condition usually subsides within a month.

Erythrocyte

The medical name for a red blood cell. See *Blood cells*.

Erythroderma

See *Exfoliative dermatitis*.

Erythromycin

ANTIBIOTIC

Tablet Capsule Liquid Injection Ointment
💊 Prescription needed
🏷 Available as generic

A drug used to treat infections of the skin, chest, throat, and ears. Erythromycin is particularly useful in the treatment of *pertussis* (whooping cough) and *legionnaires' disease*. In children under 8 years old, this drug is a useful alternative to tetracycline, an antibiotic that can cause permanent staining of developing teeth.

Erythromycin is destroyed by the acid in the stomach. To overcome this problem, the drug is prepared as a specially coated tablet or as compounds, such as erythromycin estolate and erythromycin stearate, which are more resistant to acid.

POSSIBLE ADVERSE EFFECTS

Adverse effects include nausea, vomiting, abdominal pain, diarrhea,

and an itchy rash. Certain brands of erythromycin can be taken with food to reduce the likelihood of irritation of the stomach.

Eschar

A scab on the surface of the skin formed to cover damage caused by a burn, abrasion, severe scratching, or some skin diseases and infections.

Esmarch's bandage

A broad, rubber bandage wrapped around the elevated limb of a patient to force blood out of the blood vessels toward the heart; this enables surgery to be performed more easily in a blood-free area. The Esmarch's bandage is wrapped from the toes or fingers upward, and a pneumatic (inflatable) tourniquet is then applied to the thigh or upper arm to stop blood from returning to the limb. The Esmarch's bandage is removed, leaving the inflated tourniquet in position during surgery.

Esophageal atresia

A rare birth defect caused by a failure of the esophagus to form correctly during embryonic development. A short section of the esophagus is absent, so that its upper part comes to a dead end, and the upward projection of the esophagus from the stomach is also blind-ending. In most cases, there is also an abnormal channel (known as a *tracheoesophageal fistula*) between one of these sections of esophagus and the trachea (windpipe). This abnormality occurs in about one live-born baby in 3,500.

SYMPTOMS, DIAGNOSIS, AND TREATMENT

The infant cannot swallow saliva or milk, and continuous regurgitation from the mouth occurs. If there is an upper tracheoesophageal fistula, milk may be sucked into the lungs; as a result, attempts at feeding provoke attacks of coughing and cyanosis (a blue-purple skin coloration).

A soft tube inserted into the nose can normally be passed down the esophagus; in cases of esophageal atresia, it cannot be passed. The diagnosis is confirmed by a chest X ray.

Immediate surgery is necessary. Using a general anesthetic, the baby's chest is opened, the blind ends of the esophagus are joined, and any tracheoesophageal fistula is closed.

Complications can be prevented by skilled nursing care. Some affected babies do not survive, but usually the operation is successful and the baby is able to lead a normal, healthy life.

Esophageal dilatation

Stretching of the esophagus after it has become narrowed by disease (see *Esophageal stricture*), which prevents normal swallowing. The usual cause of the narrowing is swelling and scarring from *esophagitis* (inflammation of the esophagus), but the narrowing may also be due to cancer (see *Esophagus, cancer of*) or *achalasia* (inability of the muscles in the lower esophagus to relax).

HOW IT IS DONE

The patient must not eat for at least eight hours before the esophageal dilatation, which is usually carried out under sedation.

First, an *endoscope* (a fine, flexible viewing tube) is passed through the mouth and down the esophagus to permit identification of the obstruction. The patient then swallows a length of thread, which anchors in the intestine, and a metal guide is passed over the string.

The next step is to pass a series of *bougies* (cylindrical rods with olive-shaped tips) of increasing size down over the guide wire to stretch the narrowed area. Bougies are being replaced by the *balloon catheter* (a fine tube with a balloon at the end). After being inflated, the balloon is kept in position for three minutes, then deflated and withdrawn; the same procedure is repeated later with a larger balloon. Guide wires are not always used with balloons.

Esophageal diverticulum

A saclike outward protrusion of part of the wall of the esophagus.

TYPES

There are two types of esophageal diverticulum—a pharyngeal pouch (Zenker's or pulsion diverticulum) and a mid-esophageal diverticulum (traction diverticulum).

PHARYNGEAL POUCH This type lies at the top of the esophagus, at its entrance from the pharynx (throat). It usually projects backward. The cause is a failure of the sphincter (circular muscle) at the entrance to the esophagus to relax during the act of swallowing, due to muscular incoordination. Instead, the sphincter resists the passage of food. As the powerful throat muscles used for swallowing work against this resistance, part of the lining of the esophagus is forced through the esophageal wall, thus forming the diverticulum.

Once the diverticulum is formed, it gradually enlarges, and food becomes trapped in it, causing irritation,

Location of esophageal diverticulum
The pharyngeal pouch forms at the top of the esophagus as a reaction to the sphincter's failure to relax during swallowing. The usually symptomless mid-esophageal diverticulum is a pouch that forms further down the esophagus.

difficulty swallowing, *halitosis* (bad breath), and regurgitation. The diagnosis is made by an *esophagogram* and the diverticulum is treated by removal after the surgeon has made an incision in the neck. The sphincter muscle is partly cut at the same time to weaken it and prevent recurrence.

MID-ESOPHAGEAL DIVERTICULUM This disorder consists of a pouch formed further down the esophagus. It rarely causes symptoms and usually requires no treatment.

Esophageal spasm

Uncoordinated contractions of the muscles in the esophagus that fail to propel food effectively down into the stomach. The contractions may be caused by some other esophageal disorder, such as reflux *esophagitis*, but in many cases they occur for no apparent reason. Women are affected more often than men. Pain is felt in the chest or upper abdomen and there is difficulty swallowing, but symptoms are intermittent and do not worsen.

An *esophagogram* will show the irregular contractions of the esophagus and, along with *endoscopy* (passage of a viewing tube down the esophagus) and esophageal *manometry*, can rule out the possibility of a more serious condition, such as a cancer. There is no treatment unless an underlying cause, such as esophagitis, can be treated.

Esophageal stricture

Narrowing of the esophagus, which may cause swallowing difficulty.

CAUSES AND SYMPTOMS
Narrowing may be due to a cancer (see *Esophagus, cancer of*) or to any of numerous noncancerous causes. These include persistent reflux *esophagitis*, in which constant irritation from gastric acid causes inflammation and swelling followed by the formation of fibrous scar tissue and narrowing. Prolonged use of a *nasogastric tube* may inflame the esophagus, leading to a stricture, as may the accidental swallowing of a corrosive liquid.

The symptoms of a stricture are difficulty swallowing, pain, weight loss, and regurgitation of food.

DIAGNOSIS AND TREATMENT
A barium swallow (see *Barium X-ray examinations*) shows a smooth narrowing of the esophagus. *Endoscopy* (passage of a viewing tube down the esophagus) is used to look at the narrowed area, and a *biopsy* (removal of a small piece of tissue for analysis) is performed to exclude cancer.

In most cases, the narrowed area is widened by *esophageal dilatation*. In cases of very severe narrowing over a long segment of the esophagus (usually due to swallowing corrosives), the affected area may require surgical removal. A loop of colon may be substituted for the removed section, or the ends of the esophagus may be joined and the stomach brought up into the chest. These operations are rarely required.

Patients too old or frail for surgery may be treated by the insertion of a soft, pliable, plastic tube through the stricture or by a feeding *gastrostomy*.

Esophageal varices

Dilated, incompetent veins in the walls of the lower part of the esophagus and, at times, the upper part of the stomach. They arise as a consequence of *portal hypertension* (increased blood pressure in the portal vein due to liver disease). Blood passing from the intestines to the liver via the portal vein meets increased resistance and is instead diverted through the veins in the walls of the esophagus and stomach, where the pressure causes the veins to balloon outward.

SYMPTOMS, DIAGNOSIS, AND TREATMENT
The affected veins are thin-walled and contain blood at high pressure; they may rupture, causing recurrent episodes of torrential hematemesis (vomiting of blood) and melena (tarry, black feces). Most patients also have other symptoms of chronic liver disease.

Endoscopy (passage of a viewing tube down the esophagus) or a barium swallow (see *Barium X-ray examinations*) shows the affected veins bulging from the esophageal walls.

Acute bleeding may be controlled by means of a specially designed *balloon catheter*, which is passed into the esophagus and stomach; the balloon is blown up to press on the bleeding varices. Later, the varices may be treated with intravenous pitressin and/or by injection of a sclerosant—a solution that clots the blood and permanently hardens and seals off the affected veins. Surgery may be performed to lower the pressure in the blood supply to the liver. Recurrent bleeding can also sometimes be controlled by drugs such as propranolol.

Esophagitis

Inflammation of the esophagus.

TYPES
There are two main types—corrosive esophagitis, caused by the swallowing of caustic chemicals (acid or lye) accidentally or in a suicide attempt, and reflux esophagitis, caused by regurgitation of the stomach contents into the esophagus.

CORROSIVE ESOPHAGITIS The severity of the inflammation depends on the amount, concentration, and type of caustic chemical swallowed. Chemicals likely to cause very severe corrosive esophagitis include cleaning or disinfectant solutions.

Immediately after swallowing such a chemical, there is severe pain with *shock* and *edema* (swelling) in the throat and mouth. Antidotes are of limited value and gastric lavage (washing out the stomach) must be avoided as this may only increase the damage. Treatment consists mainly of reducing pain and providing nursing care until the esophagus heals. Sometimes a severe *esophageal stricture* (narrowing of the esophagus) develops, requiring prolonged dilatation and/or extensive surgery later.

REFLUX ESOPHAGITIS This is a very common condition. The cause is poor function of the musculature of the lower esophageal segment, which permits reflux of the stomach's con-

E

tents. Poor lower esophageal segment function may be associated with a *hiatal hernia*, in which the top part of the stomach slides back and forth between the chest and the abdomen. Symptoms may be worsened by alcohol, smoking, and obesity.

The stomach content is usually acid but, after certain operations, such as partial *gastrectomy*, the stomach contains bile. If this bile flows backward into the esophagus, it causes an alkaline type of esophagitis, which tends to be more severe and difficult to treat. Severe, chronic esophagitis can cause an esophageal stricture.

The main symptom of reflux esophagitis is heartburn—a burning pain in the chest—which worsens on bending over.

Barrett's esophagus is a complication of reflux esophagitis in which stomach lining is found in the esophagus. It may lead to cancer.

DIAGNOSIS AND TREATMENT
A barium swallow (see *Barium X-ray examinations*) will show reflux of stomach contents, and *endoscopy* (passage of a viewing tube down the esophagus) will show inflammation. In doubtful cases, special tests may be required. A small tube may be swallowed and a probe positioned in the lower esophagus to record the acidity over a 24-hour period; alternatively, a dilute acid solution may be introduced into the stomach to see if it reproduces the symptoms.

The treatment for most cases of persistent esophagitis is for the sufferer to change his or her life-style—to reduce weight and alcohol consumption, stop smoking, and avoid heavy meals. *Antacid drugs* may be given to reduce the acidity of the stomach contents. Elevation of the head of the bed with blocks may be employed. Sometimes, surgical treatment may be needed for a hiatal hernia.

Esophagogastroscopy
See *Gastroscopy*.

Esophagogram
A type of barium swallow of the esophagus (see *Barium X-ray examinations*) that is documented by still or motion X-ray films. The films show alterations in function and motility (muscular activity) of the esophagus. In addition, the pictures can reveal structural anatomic disorders such as a tumor, stricture, ulcer, diverticulum, or hernia. (See also *Esophagus, cancer of*; *Hiatal hernia*; *Esophageal diverticulum*.)

Esophagoscopy
Examination of the esophagus by means of an *endoscope*, a thin, flexible viewing instrument with a light and lenses attached. (See *Gastroscopy*.)

Esophagus
The muscular tube that carries food from the throat to the stomach.

STRUCTURE
The top end of the esophagus is the narrowest part of the entire digestive tract and is encircled by a sphincter (circular muscle) that is normally closed but can open to allow the passage of food. There is a similar sphincter at the point where the esophagus enters the stomach. The walls of the esophagus consist of strong muscle fibers arranged in bundles, some circular and others longitudinal. The inner lining of the esophagus consists of smooth, squamous epithelium (flattened cells).

FUNCTION
The esophagus acts as a conduit by which liquids and food (once it has

---

ANATOMY OF THE ESOPHAGUS
A muscular tube that propels food to the stomach from the throat. The upper and lower ends are bounded by sphincters – muscular valves that open to allow food to pass through.

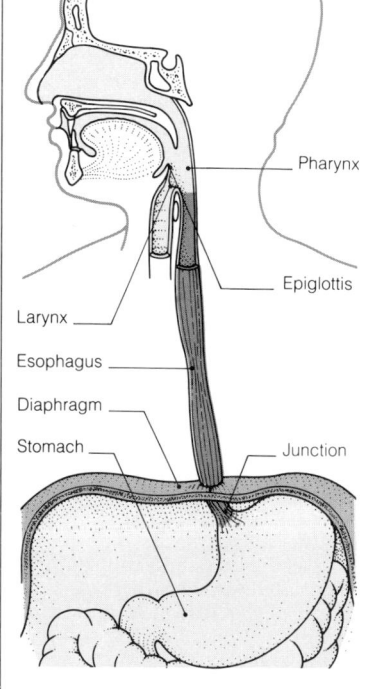

Pharynx

Epiglottis

Larynx

Esophagus

Diaphragm

Stomach

Junction

---

been chewed) are conveyed to the stomach and intestines for digestion. Food is propelled downward toward the stomach by a peristaltic action, powerful waves of contractions passing through the muscles in the esophageal wall. Gravity plays little part in getting food into the stomach—making it possible to drink while upside down. (See also *Swallowing*.)

Esophagus, cancer of
A malignant tumor of the esophagus, which ultimately causes difficulty in swallowing. Most esophageal cancers develop in the middle or lower sections of the esophagus.

CAUSES AND INCIDENCE
The causes of esophageal cancer are mainly unknown, but a high alcohol consumption and smoking are thought to play a role.

The incidence varies throughout the world, but there are about seven to 10 new cases diagnosed per 100,000 population in the US each year, mainly in people over 50. The cancer is more common in men than women and more common in blacks than whites. There is a particularly high incidence in parts of the Far East and Iran, where the cancer is linked to chemicals in certain foods.

SYMPTOMS
Difficulty in swallowing is noticed first with solids and later with fluids (even saliva) and becomes progressively worse. If food cannot pass it is immediately regurgitated. Rapid weight loss occurs, but no pain develops until the cancer is well advanced. Respiratory infections are common, because regurgitated fluid spills over into the trachea.

DIAGNOSIS
A barium swallow (see *Barium X-ray examinations*) can indicate the site and often the nature of the obstruction of the esophagus. Definite diagnosis is provided by examination of a *biopsy* sample (small piece of tissue) obtained through an *endoscope* (viewing tube with a tissue-collecting attachment).

TREATMENT AND OUTLOOK
Esophagectomy (removal of the esophagus) provides the best hope of cure but is a major undertaking. Incisions are made in the abdomen, chest, and sometimes in the neck. Most of the esophagus is then removed and the stomach or sometimes a portion of the colon is pulled up into the chest and joined to the upper esophagus.

For older patients who might not survive this operation, *radiation therapy*, sometimes combined with

DISORDERS OF THE ESOPHAGUS

Despite its apparently simple structure, the esophagus is prone to a number of disorders, most of which lead to difficulty, or completely prevent, swallowing and/or cause a pain in the chest.

CONGENITAL DEFECTS

Esophageal atresia is an absence from birth of a section of the esophagus, with the remaining sections ending in dead ends. It requires urgent surgical correction. Rarely, babies arc born with weblike constrictions of the esophagus. These are rarely serious enough to require treatment, but may, if necessary, be broken down with a rubber dilator.

INFECTION AND INFLAMMATION

Infections of the esophagus are uncommon, but can occur in severely immunosuppressed patients whose defenses against infection are weakened. The most common infections are *herpes simplex* infection or *candidiasis* (thrush) extending downward from the mouth. Both cause pain on swallowing.

Esophagitis (inflammation of the esophagus) is usually due to reflux of the contents of the stomach, causing heartburn (a burning sensation in the chest). A more severe form—corrosive esophagitis—can occur as a result of swallowing caustic chemicals. Either of these types of esophagitis may lead to formation of an *esophageal stricture* (narrowing of the esophagus).

INJURY

Apart from the damaging effects of swallowing corrosive chemicals, the most common cause of injury to the esophagus is severe vomiting and retching, which occasionally tear the esophageal lining (and result in bleeding) or in extreme cases lead to rupture. A hard, swallowed *foreign body* can also cause injury and sometimes perforation if it lodges in the esophageal wall.

TUMORS

Tumors of the esophagus are not rare. About 90 percent are malignant (see *Esophagus, cancer of*); the remainder are benign. With both types, the initial symptom is usually difficulty swallowing.

OTHER DISORDERS

An *esophageal diverticulum* is an outwardly protruding sac, formed usually at the top end of the esophagus, in which food may collect and cause halitosis (bad breath) and sometimes difficulty swallowing. *Esophageal spasm* consists of uncoordinated and uncontrollable contractions of the esophagus, which may make swallowing difficult. In *achalasia,* the sphincter muscle at the junction between esophagus and stomach fails to relax to allow the passage of food, causing pain on swallowing and sometimes regurgitation of food. (See also *Swallowing difficulty*.)

> ### INVESTIGATION
> Esophageal disorders are investigated by barium swallow (see *Barium X-ray examinations*) and by *endoscopy*. Occasionally, a *biopsy* (tissue sample) may be taken for pathologic examination.

E

chemotherapy (particularly cisplatin), can sometimes provide a significant regression of the cancer, relief from symptoms, and even an occasional cure. Some relief from starvation can also be achieved by intubation—the insertion of a rigid tube through the tumor to allow swallowing of liquid or semiliquid food.

The overall outlook is poor, with only about 5 percent of patients surviving for five years; if the cancer is diagnosed early, the outlook is better.

Esotropia

Convergent squint, or "cross-eye," in which only one eye looks directly at the object while the other turns inward. (See also *Strabismus*.)

ESR

The abbreviation for erythrocyte sedimentation rate, measurement of the rate at which red blood cells sink toward the bottom of a test tube. Because the ESR is increased in certain disorders, it is a useful aid to diagnosis and can also be used to monitor the effect of treatment.

HOW IT IS DONE

Whole blood from the patient is mixed with anticoagulant (which prevents the blood from clotting) in a test tube and left undisturbed at a constant temperature for one hour.

The red blood cells, which can be seen as a dark red clump, settle toward the bottom of the tube, leaving the clear, straw-colored plasma at the top. The ESR is the number of millimeters the red cells fall in one hour.

RESULTS

The ESR is high when the red cells are sticky due to abnormal levels of fibrinogen or *globulins* (types of protein) in the blood. Globulins are usually produced in response to serious infection, inflammation of blood vessels (as in *temporal arteritis*), and some types of cancer, such as *myeloma*. Fibrinogen is produced in response to inflammation.

Estradiol

ESTROGEN		
Tablet	Injection	Cream
📋 Prescription needed		
🔖 Available as generic		

The most important of the *estrogen hormones* (female sex hormones). They

are essential for the healthy functioning of the reproductive system and for breast development.

In its synthetic form, estradiol is prescribed as a tablet to treat symptoms of the *menopause* (see *Hormone replacement therapy*), to treat *osteoporosis*, and to stimulate sexual development in *hypogonadism* (underdeveloped ovaries). Estradiol is also prescribed as a cream to treat atrophic *vaginitis* (dryness of the vagina).

Estriol

One of the *estrogen hormones* (female sex hormones).

Estrogen drugs

COMMON DRUGS

Conjugated estrogens Diethylstilbestrol Dienestrol Estradiol Estrone Ethinyl estradiol

> ### WARNING
> *Tobacco smoking* while taking estrogen drugs significantly increases the risk of abnormal blood clotting, which may cause myocardial infarction, pulmonary embolism, or stroke.

421

E

A group of drugs produced synthetically for use in the birth-control pill (see *Oral contraceptives*) and to supplement or replace the naturally occurring estrogen hormones in the body (see *Ovary*). Estrogen drugs are often used in conjunction with *progesterone drugs*.

Estrogens suppress the production of *gonadotropin hormones* (hormones that stimulate cell activity in the ovaries). High doses of estrogens may be given as postcoital contraception (see *Contraception, postcoital*).

Synthetic estrogens are used to treat, and in some cases to prevent, symptoms and disorders related to the *menopause*, including atrophic *vaginitis* (dryness of the vagina) and *osteoporosis* (a bone disorder).

Estrogens may also be used to treat certain forms of infertility, *hypogonadism* (underdeveloped ovaries), menstrual disorders in which there is abnormal bleeding from the uterus, prostate cancer, and certain types of breast cancer.

POSSIBLE ADVERSE EFFECTS
Estrogen drugs may cause breast tenderness and enlargement, bloating, weight gain, nausea, reduced sex drive, depression, migraine, and bleeding between periods. Side effects often settle after two or three months, but, if they persist or are troublesome, a different estrogen drug may be prescribed. Vaginal creams containing estrogen should be used sparingly and usually only for a short time to reduce the risk of adverse effects throughout the body.

Estrogen drugs increase the risk of abnormal blood clotting and are therefore not recommended for people with a history (or family history) of *stroke*, *pulmonary embolism*, or deep-vein *thrombosis*, or for people about to undergo surgery. Estrogen drugs may increase a person's susceptibility to *hypertension* (high blood pressure) and are not usually prescribed if a person has suffered from this disorder in the past. Estrogens should not be taken during pregnancy as they may adversely affect the fetus.

Estrogen hormones

A group of hormones essential for normal female sexual development and for the healthy functioning of the reproductive system. In women, they are produced mainly in the ovaries. Estrogen hormones are also formed in the placenta during pregnancy and, in both men and women, in small amounts in the adrenal glands. In men, estrogens have no known specific function. (See also *Ovary*.)

Estrone

One of the *estrogen hormones*. Estrone is also prepared synthetically and given by injection or as a tablet in the treatment of symptoms of the menopause (see *Hormone replacement therapy*) and osteoporosis. It is also prescribed as a cream for the treatment of atrophic *vaginitis* (dryness of the vagina).

ESWL

Extracorporeal shock wave lithotripsy. See *Lithotripsy*.

Ethambutol

A drug used in conjunction with other drugs in the treatment of *tuberculosis*. Ethambutol rarely causes side effects, although occasionally it may cause inflammation of the optic nerve, resulting in blurred vision.

Ethanol

The chemical name for the *alcohol* in alcoholic drinks; it is also sometimes called ethyl alcohol.

Ether

The first general anesthetic. Ether was commonly used for surgery until the 1930s, but has now largely been replaced by other anesthetic agents. Ether (full name, diethyl ether) is a colorless liquid administered on a gauze mask placed over the patient's nose and mouth. When inhaled, ether fumes produce unconsciousness.

Ether is among the safest of all anesthetics, but it is so flammable that even static electricity can cause it to explode. Ether has therefore been superseded by other agents (see *Anesthesia, general*), although these require more skill to administer.

Ethical drug

A drug that requires a physician's prescription for purchase.

Ethics, medical

A code of behavior that addresses the relationships between the patient and physician, and among physicians.

The characteristic that distinguishes a profession, such as medicine, from a trade, such as repairing automobiles, is that the members establish and maintain standards of training, competence, and professional behavior. These standards are enforced by professional organizations, such as the American Medical Association, which has a Council on Ethical and Judicial Affairs.

Traditionally, medical ethics covers a wide range of behavior, including the physician's involvement with patients and their families, and his or her competence, public image, and commercial behavior.

Physicians must not abuse the relationship of trust they develop with patients. In particular, they must not enter into sexual relationships with patients and they must maintain in confidence information learned from patients. They must give clear priority to their patients' interests.

Physicians are expected to maintain their skills and to update their knowledge to the standard of their colleagues. They should not refer patients to unlicensed practitioners of alternative medicine. Fees should conform to recognized schedules; all forms of fee splitting or rebates are unacceptable. In addition, it is against ethical standards for a physician to be dependent on alcohol or drugs.

The physician should ensure that the patient not only consents to all procedures, investigations, and treatments, but that this consent is based on an unbiased and full explanation of any risks, drawbacks, and alternatives that might be considered.

Any time a patient is asked to enroll in a research study, the investigator should see that consent is full and free, and that patients do not feel pressured to agree because of a sense of gratitude owed to the physician for previous treatment. Research on children or on patients with mental handicap should, in general, be considered only when there is a reasonable prospect that the person concerned will benefit from the investigation and that the risks and any discomfort inherent in the research are minimal.

Ethical considerations are also important in the care of the dying, in termination of pregnancy, in the care of children born with major physical and mental handicaps, and in the care of patients with mental disorders.

Ethinyl estradiol

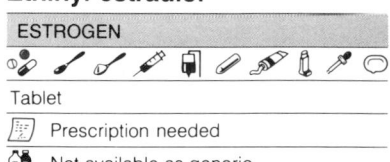

ESTROGEN		
Tablet		
Prescription needed		
Not available as generic		

A synthetic form of the female sex hormone estradiol. It is most commonly used in *oral contraceptives*, where it is combined with a *progesterone drug*.

Ethinyl estradiol is also prescribed to stimulate sexual development in female *hypogonadism* (underdeveloped ovaries) and in the treatment of symptoms caused by the *menopause*, such as hot flashes and sweating (see *Hormone replacement therapy*). It is also used to treat menstrual disorders.

Ethosuximide

An *anticonvulsant drug* used to treat petit mal (a form of *epilepsy*). Ethosuximide is often prescribed in preference to other anticonvulsant drugs because, unlike some of them, it rarely causes drowsiness or liver damage. Ethosuximide may, however, cause nausea and vomiting and in rare cases affects the production of blood cells in the bone marrow and causes aplastic anemia (see *Anemia, aplastic*).

Ethyl alcohol

Another name for ethanol, the *alcohol* in alcoholic drinks.

Ethyl chloride

A colorless, flammable liquid once used as a general anesthetic and now as a local anesthetic.

WHY IT IS USED

Applied to the skin as a spray, ethyl chloride quickly evaporates and, as a result, makes the skin feel so cold that any pain or irritation is reduced. It may be used to numb an area of skin before a minor surgical procedure, such as lancing a boil, and is sometimes used to alleviate the pain that arises from sprained or strained muscles or ligaments.

Ethyl chloride is also used in the treatment of *larva migrans*, a hookworm infection acquired from cats and dogs. (See also *Anesthetics, local*.)

Etiology

The study of the causes of disease. In some cases a specific cause may be found. For example, the cause of *meningitis* may be identified as tuberculosis bacillus after examining a sample of cerebrospinal fluid under a microscope. Many disorders have a multifactorial etiology. The causative factors of degenerative arthritis, for example, include genetic susceptibility, being overweight, and repeated joint injuries. Many disorders, such as osteoarthritis and cancer of the intestine, are of unknown etiology.

Eunuch

A man whose testicles have been removed or destroyed so that he is sterile. The term was used especially to describe boys who were castrated before puberty to preserve their high-pitched singing voices or to make them suitable for guarding harems. A male castrated before puberty has eunuchoid body proportions (i.e., undeveloped male secondary sexual characteristics with a small penis, sparse body hair, broad hips, narrow shoulders, and a feminine distribution of body hair).

Euphoria

A state of confident well-being. A normal reaction to personal success, it can also be induced by drugs.

Feelings of euphoria with no rational cause may indicate the presence of brain disease or damage caused by *head injury* (particularly damage to the frontal lobes), *dementia*, *brain tumors*, or *multiple sclerosis*. In these cases, the euphoria results from the victim's general lack of awareness.

Eustachian tube

The passage that connects the middle ear and the back of the nose. It acts as a drainage passage from the middle ear and maintains hearing by opening periodically to regulate air pressure.

STRUCTURE

The tube is about 1.33 inches (36 mm) long in an adult. From the middle ear it runs forward, downward, and in toward the middle of the head; it ends in the space at the back of the nose just above the soft *palate* (part of the roof of the mouth). A smooth, wet, mucous membrane lines the tube.

FUNCTION

The lower end of the eustachian tube opens during swallowing and yawning, thus allowing air to flow up to the middle ear and equalizing air pressure on both sides of the eardrum. If a change in external pressure is large and rapid, pressure may build up on one side of the eardrum, pushing it inward or outward; this is uncomfortable and dulls hearing. Most people have experienced this sensation when taking off in a plane (reduced pressure) or going into a tunnel in a car or train (increased pressure). Symptoms can usually be relieved by swallowing hard to open the tube.

A person with a blocked eustachian tube who is subjected to rapid changes in pressure may suffer from *barotrauma* (pressure damage to the eardrum or other structures).

When a head cold blocks the eustachian tube, equalization cannot occur, which may cause severe pain. Because the displaced eardrum cannot vibrate properly, hearing may be temporarily impaired.

DISORDERS

Persistent *middle-ear effusion* (chronic accumulation of secretions in the middle ear) or chronic *otitis media* (middle-ear infection) may occur if the eustachian tube becomes blocked, preventing adequate drainage from the middle ear. These conditions, which often cause partial hearing loss, are more common in children because their adenoids are larger and more likely to block the tube if they become infected. Children's eustachian tubes are shorter, making it easier for bacteria to travel from infected areas in the throat to the middle ear.

E

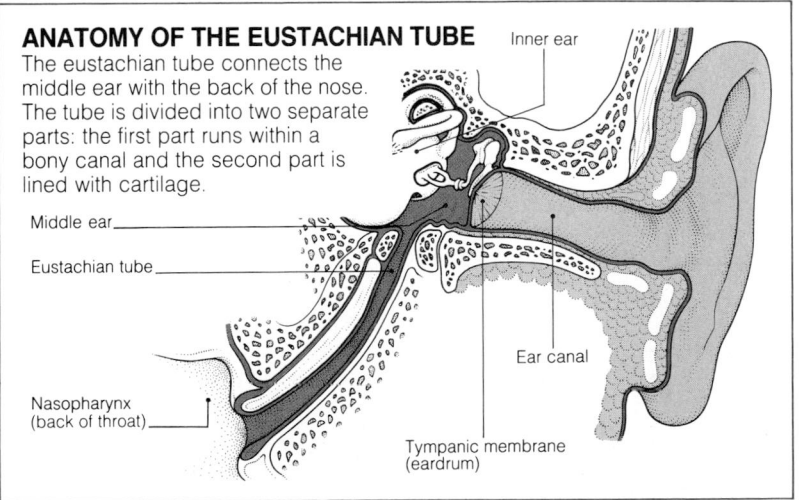

ANATOMY OF THE EUSTACHIAN TUBE
The eustachian tube connects the middle ear with the back of the nose. The tube is divided into two separate parts: the first part runs within a bony canal and the second part is lined with cartilage.

Inner ear

Middle ear

Eustachian tube

Nasopharynx (back of throat)

Ear canal

Tympanic membrane (eardrum)

Euthanasia

The act of killing a person painlessly to relieve suffering. Even when it is requested by a patient with incurable disease, euthanasia (the literal meaning is "easy death") is against the law in most Western countries. There are groups attempting to change the law to allow patients to ask physicians to give a fatal dose of drugs.

Euthanasia is distinct from nonintervention, which is the physician's recognition that, if a patient has an advanced or incurable disease, he or she has a right to refuse medical treatment that would simply prolong the process of dying.

Euthyroid

The term used to describe a person whose *thyroid gland* is functioning normally, or to describe a person who has been successfully treated for *hypothyroidism* (underactive thyroid) or *hyperthyroidism* (overactive thyroid) so that the gland functions normally.

Eversion

A turning outward. The term is commonly applied to a type of ankle injury or deformity in which the foot is turned outward.

Evoked responses

The tracing of electrical activity in the brain in response to a specific external stimulus. The responses are much smaller than the impulses recorded by electroencephalography (see *EEG*) and are a refinement of that technique. Evoked responses were first demonstrated in 1947. Today, with the increased sophistication of computerized electronic technology, it is a widely used diagnostic tool.

WHY IT IS DONE
The functioning of various sensory systems—for example, sight, hearing, and touch—can be checked by this technique. The information obtained can be used to reveal abnormalities in the system caused by inflammation, pressure from a tumor, or other pathological changes, and to confirm the diagnosis of *multiple sclerosis*. The test is extremely sensitive and can often pinpoint the location of a fault.

HOW IT IS DONE
The method for testing each sensory system is similar, painless, and takes 30 to 60 minutes, depending on whether more than one system is being assessed.

A set of small disk electrodes is attached to the scalp in the same way as in electroencephalography. The electrodes are attached to different parts of the scalp, depending on which sensory system is being tested. The output from the brain is linked to a computer, which produces a printout after a specific period of stimulation (e.g., 100 flashes from a light).

Analysis is based on the time lapse between stimulus and response; the computer is used to extract this information from the background brain activity that shows up on an EEG.

For testing the visual system, a series of flashes from a stroboscopic light may be used. An example of a more demanding stimulus for the brain, which gives more consistent results, is a board made up of black and white squares constructed so that the colors alternate every second.

To test hearing, the ears are subjected to different sounds. To test touch and pain sensations, small electrical stimuli are applied, for example, to a nerve at the wrist.

RESULTS
This test does not necessarily give an unequivocal diagnosis and is used as a supplement to other tests of the nervous system (e.g., EEG or *EMG*), other investigations, and radiological tests such as *CT scanning*.

Ewing's sarcoma

A rare malignant tumor of bone. The sarcoma (cancer of connective tissue) arises in a large bone, most commonly the femur (thigh bone), tibia (shin), humerus (upper arm bone), or one of the pelvic bones, and spreads to other parts of the body at an early stage.

The condition is most common in children between 10 and 15; it affects twice as many boys as girls and is rarely seen in black children.

SYMPTOMS
The affected bone is painful and tender and part of it may swell. It may also become weakened and fracture easily (called a pathologic fracture). Other possible symptoms include weight loss, fever, and anemia.

DIAGNOSIS
The sarcoma is diagnosed by X rays and a bone *biopsy* (removal of a small piece of bone for analysis). If cancer is found, the complete skeleton is examined by X rays and *radionuclide scanning*, and the lungs by *CT scanning*, to determine if, and how far, the cancer has spread. Spreading by the time of diagnosis is found in 15 to 20 percent of cases.

TREATMENT
Treatment is by *radiation therapy* and *chemotherapy*. Before the introduction of chemotherapy, death usually occurred within two to three years of diagnosis. Today, the chances of survival have improved considerably; 65 percent of those affected are still alive five years after diagnosis and most of those remain well.

Examination, physical

The inspection, palpation, percussion, and auscultation of the various body parts and organs. Physical examination is the second stage of most medical consultations; it follows history-taking, in which the physician listens to the patient's complaints and then asks questions. Aside from history-taking, the physical examination is the physician's most important means of making a diagnosis or of finding the clues that aid him or her in selecting the appropriate diagnostic studies. If there are generalized symptoms, such as loss of energy, the physician examines the patient's entire body. The physician also performs a complete physical examination during the patient's initial visit and usually annually thereafter. Examination may be limited to a certain part of the body (such as when a patient has a localized injury).

Excision

Surgical cutting out of diseased tissue from surrounding healthy tissue, such as the removal of a breast lump or gangrenous skin.

Excoriation

Injury to the surface of the skin or of a mucous membrane (the thin, moist tissue that lines parts of the body, such as the mouth) caused by physical abrasion (such as scratching) or chemical action. The loss of surface cells causes a raw area to develop. (See also *Ulcer*.)

Excretion

The discharge of waste material from the body. To maintain health, the body must dispose of the by-products of digestion (such as food residues and an excess of salt or other substances), waste products from the repair of body tissues, medication or its breakdown products, poisonous substances, and water (to maintain the correct volume of fluid and to remove solid wastes in solution).

ORGANS OF EXCRETION
The *kidneys* excrete excess nitrogen in the urine in the form of urea, along with excess water, salts, some acids, and most prescribed drugs.

TYPES OF PHYSICAL EXAMINATION

Examination may include looking for skin changes and feeling organs for size, consistency, and shape. Assessment is made of muscle strength, coordination, joint mobility, and skin sensation. The state of the eyes, ears, mouth, throat, and teeth is checked.

Percussion
The chest is tapped and the vibration felt and heard. A loss of resonance suggests a lung disorder.

Auscultation
The physician uses a stethoscope to listen to lung and heart sounds. Abnormal sounds suggest disease.

Tendon reflexes
One test of the nervous system is to tap a stretched tendon. If the reflex is normal, the muscle should contract.

The *liver* excretes bile, which, as well as containing salts that help emulsify fats in the small intestine, consists of waste products and bile pigments formed from the breakdown of red blood cells. Part of the bile is passed from the body in the feces, which it colors brown.

The large *intestine* excretes undigested food, some salts, and some excess water in the form of feces.

The *lungs* discharge carbon dioxide and water vapor into the atmosphere.

Sweat glands excrete salt and water onto the surface of the skin as a method of regulating the body's temperature.

Exenteration

The surgical removal of all organs and soft tissue in a body cavity in the hope of arresting a cancerous process. Exenteration is an operation that is occasionally performed for cancer in the orbit (the bony structure surrounding the eye) or the pelvis.

Exercise

The performance of any physical activity that improves health or that is used for recreation or correction of physical injury or deformity (see *Physical therapy*). Different types of exercise affect the body in one or more of the following ways: some improve flexibility, some improve muscular strength, some improve physical endurance, and some improve the efficiency of the cardiovascular and respiratory systems. (See illustrated box, next page.)

BENEFITS OF EXERCISE

There is an established association between high levels of aerobic exercise and low incidence of *coronary heart disease*. Regular exercise usually leads to a reduction in blood pressure. It also increases the amount of high-density lipoprotein in the blood, which is thought to help protect against *atherosclerosis* (fat deposits in arteries) and *myocardial infarction* (heart attack). Exercise has also been shown to be valuable in relieving the symptoms of peripheral vascular disease and of some psychological disorders such as depression.

Vigorous work with a muscle or a group of muscles, even if it is of short duration, leads to an increase in the size, strength, and possibly the number of the muscle cells, and an increase in the strength of their ligamentous attachment to bones. Improving the strength of muscles in the back and abdomen can help prevent or ease

lower back pain. The increased strength of the muscles and tendons is also an insurance against damage due to an unexpected strain.

Elderly people are especially inclined to become inactive and lose joint mobility. Regular, gentle, rhythmic movements can help maintain the range of movement of important joints. Coordination and balance deteriorate with age; exercise helps maintain muscle strength and reduce the risk of falls. (See also *Aerobics; Fitness; Fitness testing*.)

Exfoliation

Flaking off, shedding, or peeling from a surface in scales or thin layers, as in *exfoliative dermatitis*.

Exfoliative dermatitis

Inflammation, marked redness, and scaling of the skin of most of the body, also called erythroderma.

Exfoliative dermatitis may be the result of a drug reaction (an allergic response to a particular drug) or may be caused by the worsening of a skin condition, such as *psoriasis* or *eczema*. Sometimes, exfoliative dermatitis occurs in *lymphoma* and *leukemia*.

There is a widespread rash with severe flaking of the skin. The loss of surface skin, with exposure of its deeper layers, results in increased loss of water and protein from the body surface. Water loss may result in a rise in body temperature; protein loss may cause *edema* (a buildup of fluid in tissues) and muscle wasting. Further complications are infection and *heart failure* (reduced pumping efficiency of the heart).

The treatment and outlook depend on the cause. About 60 percent of sufferers recover within two to three months, but about 30 percent die as a result of complications; in the remainder the disease takes a chronic form unresponsive to treatment.

Exhibitionism

The habit of deliberately exposing the genitals to strangers.

This form of behavior is almost always confined to men. The exhibitionist displays his penis to a female passerby, usually in a secluded spot (such as a side street) or from a car or house window with the aim of surprising or frightening the victim.

In 80 percent of cases, a single court appearance puts an end to the exhibitionist's behavior. *Psychotherapy* can help those who relapse; the outlook is poor for persistent offenders.

E

THE EFFECTS OF EXERCISE

There are many changes in different body organs during exercise. Muscles require an increase in blood flow because of their greater energy requirements; the heart and lungs work faster and more efficiently. These changes are controlled by the release of the chemicals epinephrine and norepinephrine from the sympathetic nervous system.

The lungs
The rate and depth of breathing increase to ensure sufficient flow of oxygen from the lungs into the blood. This also aids in the removal of additional carbon dioxide produced by muscle cells during exercise.

The joints
Regular exercise helps maintain the mobility of joints. Increased strength in the muscles and tendons around joints makes them more resistant to injury.

The muscles
There is a rise in the chemical activity within muscle cells. The rate of consumption of oxygen and glucose increases.

Flexed muscles

Relaxed muscles

The heart and circulation
The heart beats more rapidly and more powerfully to provide an increased flow of blood to the working muscles. Blood vessels in the stomach and beneath the skin are narrowed to compensate for the increased requirements of the muscles.

ECG printouts
Resting heart rate (above) and during exercise (below).

COMMON TYPES OF EXERCISE

Aerobic	Isometric	Isotonic	Isokinetic
Exercise in which the body continuously needs to take in additional oxygen to meet the muscles' increased demands. Regular aerobic exercise improves the performance of the cardiovascular and respiratory systems. Jogging, swimming, and cycling are examples of aerobic exercise.	Exercise without movement in which one group of muscles exerts pressure against an immovable object or an opposing group of muscles. It is an effective means of increasing muscle strength, but does not exercise the cardiovascular system or aid in muscular endurance.	Exercise with movement in which muscle tension remains more or less constant and the body works against its own weight or against external weights. Isotonic exercise includes weight training and calisthenics (repetitious movements with little or no equipment). Isotonic exercise increases muscle strength, size, and endurance.	Isokinetic exercise involves both isotonic and isometric exercise. The muscles move reasonably heavy loads, but are also put through their full range of movement. Isokinetics combines strength training with some aerobic exercise, but requires special equipment.

Exocrine gland

A gland that secretes substances through a duct onto the inner surface of an organ or onto the outer surface of the body. Examples include the *salivary glands*, which release saliva into the mouth, *lacrimal* glands, which release tears, and *sweat glands*. The release of exocrine secretions can be triggered by a hormone or by a neurotransmitter, released by nerve endings. (See also *Endocrine gland*.)

Exomphalos

A rare birth defect in which a part of the intestines, covered by a thin membrane, protrudes through the umbilicus (navel). In mild cases only one or two loops of intestine protrude, but in severe cases most of the abdominal organs are exposed.

Also called omphalocele, exomphalos is associated with other birth defects, especially *anencephaly*. Many babies with the condition are stillborn or die soon after birth. Exomphalos is treated by surgery.

Exophthalmos

Protrusion of one or both eyeballs caused by a swelling of the soft tissue in the bony orbit (eye socket). The eyeball is pressed forward, exposing an abnormally large amount of the front of the eye, forcing the eyelids apart and causing a staring appearance.

CAUSE

The most common cause of exophthalmos is *thyrotoxicosis* (overactive thyroid gland). Other causes include an *eye tumor*, an *aneurysm* (swelling of an artery) behind the eye, or inflammation of eye tissues; in these cases only one eye is affected.

SYMPTOMS AND SIGNS

Exophthalmos may restrict eye movement and cause double vision. In severe cases, the pressure in the orbit

Appearance of exophthalmos
An affected eye protrudes markedly compared with a normal eye. In most cases, both eyes are affected.

may be so high that the blood supply to the optic nerve may be restricted; blindness results. The lids may be prevented from closing, and vision may become seriously blurred due to drying of the cornea.

TREATMENT AND OUTLOOK

In thyroid exophthalmos, treatment of the thyroid disorder may sometimes relieve the exophthalmos, but often it does not. Early treatment usually returns the vision to normal. Surgery to decompress the orbit may be required to relieve pressure on the optic nerve.

Exostosis

A type of benign *bone tumor* in which there is an outgrowth of bone. It occurs most commonly at the end of the femur (thigh bone) or tibia (shin).

Exostoses account for 90 percent of all bone tumors; they affect twice as many men as women. In about 65 percent of cases the condition is due to hereditary factors; another cause is prolonged pressure on a bone.

SYMPTOMS AND TREATMENT

In most cases, exostosis produces no symptoms and goes unnoticed. Often it is recognized (as a hard swelling) only after an injury. Occasionally the bony outgrowth presses on a nerve, causing pain or weakness in the affected area (usually when it is beneath a fingernail or toenail).

A preliminary diagnosis of the condition is confirmed by X ray. Treatment may be surgical removal of the growth, but usually surgery is performed only if the exostosis causes symptoms or is unsightly.

Exotoxin

 A poison released by some types of bacteria into the bloodstream, from where it causes widespread effects throughout the body. Exotoxins are among the most poisonous

substances known. They are produced by bacteria such as tetanus bacilli, which enter the body through a wound and produce an exotoxin that affects the nervous system to cause muscle spasms (lockjaw) and paralysis, and diphtheria bacilli, which initially infect the throat, but release an exotoxin that damages the heart and nervous system.

Immunization with vaccines consisting of detoxified exotoxins can prevent dangerous symptoms from bacterial diseases that are potentially fatal due to the effects of exotoxins. If such an infection occurs, treatment usually includes antibiotics and an antitoxin to neutralize the exotoxin. (See also *Endotoxin*; *Enterotoxin*.)

Exotropia

Divergent squint, in which one eye is used for detailed vision; the other is directed outward. (See *Strabismus*.)

Expectorants

A group of *cough remedies* used to promote the coughing up of phlegm.

Expectoration

The coughing up and spitting out of sputum (phlegm). See also *Cough*.

Expiration

The act of breathing out air from the lungs. See *Breathing*.

Exploratory surgery

Any operation to investigate or thoroughly examine part of the body to discover the extent of known disease or to establish a diagnosis. Exploratory thoracotomy is performed on the chest and exploratory laparotomy on the abdomen.

Explosive disorder

A mental condition characterized by uncontrolled violent behavior that is completely out of proportion to any known cause. There may be several separate acts of aggression or a single violent outburst; in any case, the resulting damage to people or property may be very serious.

Similar behavior may occur in people with *epilepsy*, *brain damage*, *schizophrenia*, or an *antisocial personality disorder*, but in these cases there are also other symptoms.

Exposure

The effects on the body from being subjected to very low temperatures, or to a combination of cold, wet, and high winds. The primary danger

comes from the lowering of body temperature in these conditions (see *Hypothermia*). The term also applies to being subjected to radiation or a variety of environmental pollutants.

Expressing milk

A technique used by breast-feeding women for removing milk from the

 E

EXPRESSING MILK BY HAND
Wash your hands thoroughly before starting, then follow the method below. Repeat the sequence twice on each breast, alternating between breasts. If the breasts are engorged, bathe them in hot water first to help milk flow.

1 Cup the breast in both hands, thumbs on top and fingers underneath. Squeeze the outer part of the breast firmly. Repeat 10 times, moving around the breast.

2 Move hands closer to the nipple area and repeat the squeezing movement 10 more times.

3 Hold the breast in one hand. With the thumb and forefinger of the other hand, squeeze the edge of the areola in and up so that milk squirts out. Move your hand around the areola, squeezing gently and rhythmically for about five minutes.

---

breasts. Expressing milk may be necessary when the breasts are engorged (overfull), which often happens several days after delivery when the milk supply arrives quickly and forcibly. Not only is engorgement painful for the mother, but the tightly swollen nipples are impossible for the baby to suckle.

A woman may also want to express milk from her breasts so that the milk can be given to the baby in her absence. In this case, the milk should be expressed into a sterilized container and sealed and stored in the refrigerator; it will keep for 48 hours. When properly prepared, milk may be frozen and stored in a freezer. Milk may be kept up to six months in the back or bottom of a deep freeze unit. Most women find it easier to express milk by hand, but a *breast pump* can also be used.

Exstrophy of the bladder
A rare birth defect in which the bladder is turned inside out and is open to the outside of the body through a space in the lower abdominal wall.

Usually, there are also other defects, such as *epispadias* (emergence of the urethra through a hole in the shaft of the penis) in males, and failure of the pubic bones to join at the front.

Untreated, an affected child constantly leaks urine. Surgical treatment consists of reconstructing the bladder and closing the abdominal wall.

Extraction, dental
The removal of one or more teeth.
WHY IT IS DONE
Extraction may be performed when a tooth is severely decayed, when an abscess has formed, or when a tooth is too badly broken to be repaired by crowning or root-canal treatment. Teeth that are causing crowding or malocclusion (incorrect bite), teeth that are loose because of advanced gum disease, or teeth that are preventing another tooth from erupting may also require extraction.
HOW IT IS DONE
For most extractions, local anesthesia is used. General anesthesia may be used to extract badly impacted wisdom teeth, to extract several teeth at once, or for extremely anxious patients or young children.

Most teeth are extracted with dental forceps, which are designed to grasp the root of the tooth. When gentle but firm pressure is applied, the blades cut through the periodontal ligaments (the tough fibrous membranes sup-

porting the tooth in its socket), the socket is gradually expanded, and the tooth is removed. Occasionally the root of the tooth fractures during this procedure, especially if the bone is dense (as in older people) and may need to be removed separately.

If the tooth is especially difficult to remove—for example, if it is impacted, the crown is missing, or the roots are very curved—it may be necessary to cut a small flap into the gum and remove a small amount of bone nearby. The tooth is then extracted and the gum sewn up.
COMPLICATIONS
Most extractions take place without complications. Occasionally, if a blood clot fails to form in the empty tooth socket, or if the blood clot is dislodged, *dry socket* (infection in the tooth socket) develops. Dislodging a clot can also cause bleeding from the wound to begin again; this can be eased by placing a tightly folded handkerchief or a gauze pad on the wound and biting on it gently for about 30 minutes. If bleeding continues, suturing of the tissue around the socket may be necessary.

Extradural hemorrhage
Bleeding into the space between the inner surface of the skull and the external surface of the dura mater, the outer layer of the meninges (protective covering of the brain).
CAUSES AND SYMPTOMS
An extradural hemorrhage usually results from a blow to the side of the head that fractures the skull and ruptures an artery running over the surface of the dura mater. The person may momentarily lose consciousness and then apparently recover.

A hematoma (collection of clotted blood) forms and rapidly enlarges, increasing pressure within the skull (which is the main cause of symptoms occurring a few hours to days after the injury). A headache that gradually increases in severity develops in the affected person; other symptoms include drowsiness, vomiting, seizures, and paralysis on one side of the body. The patient eventually lapses into a coma and, without treatment, may die.
DIAGNOSIS AND TREATMENT
CT scanning confirms the diagnosis. Surgical treatment consists of drilling burr holes in the skull (see *Craniotomy*), draining the blood clot, and clipping the ruptured blood vessel. If the bleeding is diagnosed early (before serious symptoms develop), the

outlook is excellent; hence the importance of seeking medical advice and investigation following even a moderate blow to the head (see *Head injury*).

Extrapyramidal system
A network of nerve pathways that links nerve nuclei in the surface of the *cerebrum* (the main mass of the brain), the *basal ganglia* deep within the brain, and parts of the *brain stem*. The system influences and modifies electrical impulses that are sent from the brain to the skeletal muscles.

Damage or degeneration of components in the extrapyramidal system can cause a disturbance in the execution of voluntary (willed) movements and in muscle tone, and can also cause the appearance of involuntary (unwanted) movements such as tremors, jerks, or writhing movements. Such disturbances are seen in *Huntington's chorea*, *Parkinson's disease*, some types of *cerebral palsy*, and can also occur as a side effect of taking phenothiazine drugs, which are used to treat some psychiatric disorders.

Extrovert
A person whose interests are constantly directed outward, to other people and the environment. Extroverts are active, energetic, sociable, easy to talk to, and have many outside interests and concerns. (See also *Personality*.)

Exudation
The discharge of fluid from blood vessels into a tissue or onto the tissue's surface. An exuded fluid (called an exudate) contains cells, pus, and/or a large amount of protein (or a combination of these) and is usually produced as a result of *inflammation*. When tissue is inflamed, its small blood vessels become wider and the tiny pores in the vessel walls become enlarged, which allows fluid and cells (mainly white blood cells) to escape.

Eye
The organ of sight. It consists of structures that focus an image onto the retina at the back of the eye and a network of nerves that convert this image into electrical impulses recorded in a region of the brain.

The two eyes work in conjunction under the control of the brain, aligning themselves on an object so that a clear image is formed on each *retina*. If necessary, the eyes sharpen images by altering focus in an automatic process known as *accommodation*.

ANATOMY OF THE EYE

The eye is a complex organ that focuses light rays to form an image on the retina, which then converts this image into a pattern of nerve impulses that are transmitted to the brain. The cornea and lens focus the light, the pupil controls the amount of light entering the eye, the ciliary body alters the shape of the lens to adjust the focus, and the retina contains millions of nerve cells that respond to light.

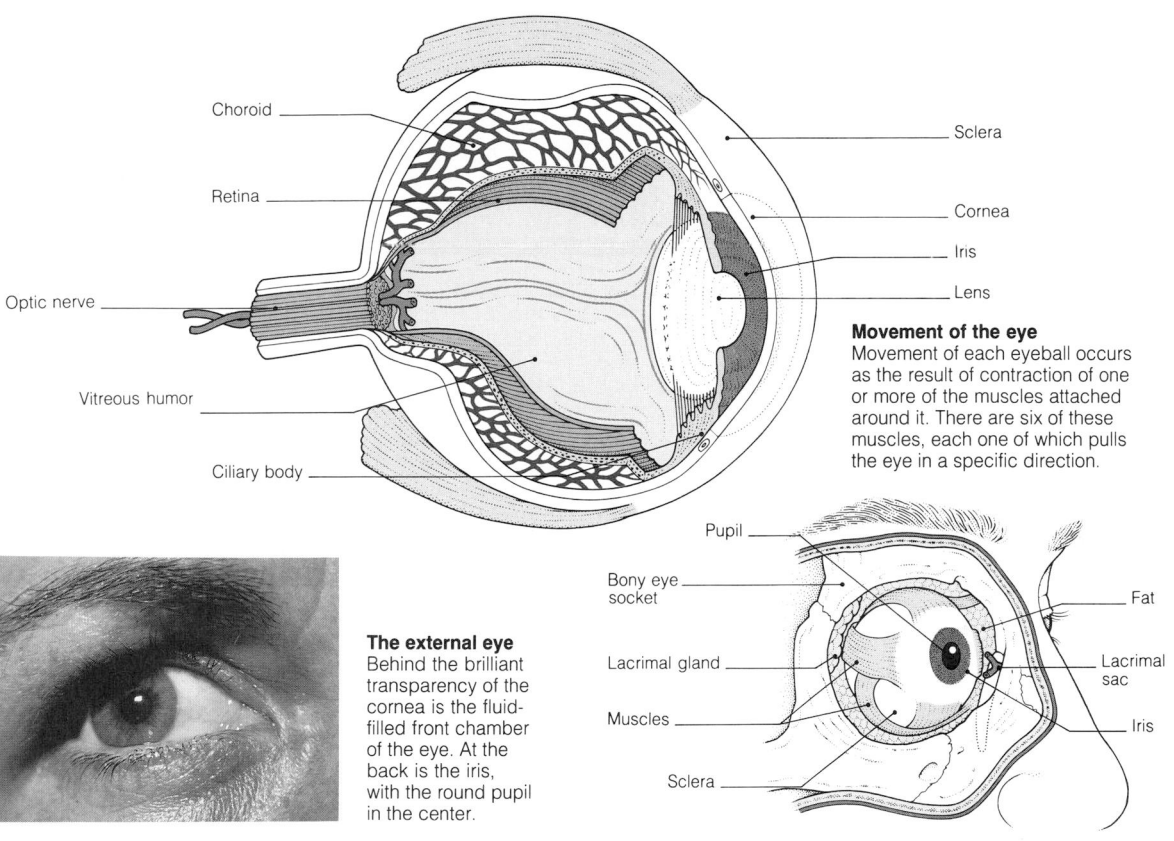

Choroid

Retina

Optic nerve

Vitreous humor

Ciliary body

Sclera

Cornea

Iris

Lens

Movement of the eye
Movement of each eyeball occurs as the result of contraction of one or more of the muscles attached around it. There are six of these muscles, each one of which pulls the eye in a specific direction.

Pupil

Bony eye socket

Lacrimal gland

Muscles

Sclera

Fat

Lacrimal sac

Iris

The external eye
Behind the brilliant transparency of the cornea is the fluid-filled front chamber of the eye. At the back is the iris, with the round pupil in the center.

The pattern of light falling on the retina stimulates a complex flow of impulses along the optic nerves to the brain. The two optic nerves pass into the skull, meet, partially cross over, and run back, at first on the underside of the brain, and then through its substance to the visual cortex—the area of the back surface of the brain concerned with vision.

STRUCTURE

EYEBALL The eyeball lies in pads of fat within the orbit, the bony eye socket that provides protection from injury. Each eyeball is moved by six delicate muscles, the action of these muscles for both eyes being coordinated by a nerve network in the brain stem.

The eyeball has a tough outer coat, the *sclera* (the white of the eye). The front, circular part of the outer coat, the *cornea*, is transparent and protrudes slightly. The cornea is the main lens of the eye and performs most of the focusing. Behind the cornea is a shallow chamber full of aqueous humor (watery fluid), at the back of which is the *iris* (colored part) with its *pupil* (central hole). The pupil appears black and its size is altered with changes in light intensity to control the amount of light entering it.

Immediately behind the iris, and in contact with it, is the crystalline *lens*, suspended by delicate fibers from a circular muscle ring called the ciliary body. Contraction of the ciliary body alters the shape of the lens to allow focusing power. Behind the lens is the main cavity of the eyeball, filled with a clear gel called the vitreous humor.

On the inside of the back of the eye is the retina, a complex structure of nerve tissue on which the image formed by the cornea and the crystalline lens falls. The retina requires a constant supply of oxygen and sugar. To meet this need, a thin network of branching blood vessels, the choroid plexus, lies immediately under it. The *choroid* is continuous at the front with the ciliary body and the iris. These three parts constitute the uveal tract.

CONJUNCTIVA The eyeball is sealed off from the outside by a flexible membrane called the *conjunctiva*, which is firmly secured around the margin of the cornea but lies freely on the sclera over the front third of the globe. It is attached to the skin at the corners of the eye and forms the inner lining of the lids, with a deep cul-de-sac above and below. This arrangement provides a permanent seal while allowing free mobility of the eyeball.

The conjunctiva contains many tiny tear-secreting and mucus-producing glands. They, along with an oily secre-

E

tion from the meibomian glands in the eyelids, provide the important, three-layer tear film that must constantly cover the cornea and conjunctiva to protect them from damage due to drying out of the cells.

EYELIDS Each lid contains about 30 meibomian glands, with their openings along the lid margin just behind the roots of the lashes. The glands secrete an oil that prevents lid margin adhesion during sleep and forms the outer layer of the tear film—a layer that retards evaporation and helps maintain the continuity of the tear film. The blink reflex is protective and helps to spread the tear film evenly over the cornea. This is essential for clear vision. Should the tear film dry out, corneal abrasion is more likely.

Just under the skin of the lid is a flat but powerful muscle that can, in an emergency, contract to push the globe back into the orbit and interpose a bunched-up mass of tissue to protect the eye; this occurs as a rapid, reflex response to danger. (See also *Vision.*)

Eye, artificial

A prosthesis to replace an eye that has been removed. It is worn for cosmetic and psychological reasons.

Often wrongly called a "glass eye," the ocular prosthesis is actually a slim plastic shell. The artificial iris behind the transparent artificial cornea may be produced by hand painting or by a photograph.

The eye fits neatly behind the eyelids within the cavity left when the natural eye has been removed. Movement is achieved by attaching the eye-moving muscles to the conjunctiva, or by using a buried magnetic implant.

Eye drops

Medication in solution for the treatment of eye disorders or to aid in diagnosis. To use eye drops, the lower lid is held away from the eye and the drop allowed to fall behind it. Care should be taken to avoid touching the skin or eye with the dropper to reduce the risk of contamination.

Common examples of drugs given in this form are antibiotics, corticosteroids, antihistamines, drugs to control glaucoma (raised pressure in the eye), and drugs to dilate or constrict the pupil.

Eye, examination of

An inspection of the external and internal appearance of the eyes either as part of a standard vision test or to make a diagnosis.

WHY IT IS DONE

Eye examinations are performed to determine the cause of vision disturbance or other symptoms relating to the eye, and to assess whether or not glasses or contact lenses are necessary. Some serious eye disorders, such as glaucoma, are symptomless in the early stages and can be detected only by an eye examination.

HOW IT IS DONE

The examination begins with an inspection of the external appearance of the eyes, the lids, and the surrounding skin. A check of eye movements is usually performed. The examiner looks for *strabismus*, using the cover test to demonstrate that a squinting eye will move to align itself when the other eye is covered. A check of the visual acuity (sharpness of vision) in each eye using a Snellen's chart (the standard eye testing wall chart) follows. Refraction testing (using lenses of different strengths) may be done to determine the requirement for glasses or contact lenses.

A test of the visual fields (extent of the peripheral vision) may also be performed, especially in suspected glaucoma or neurological conditions. Color vision may also be checked because it is disturbed in certain conditions affecting the retina.

To check for abrasions or ulcers, the cornea and conjunctiva may be stained with fluorescein (a yellow dye); any abrasions or ulcers are then revealed as green areas under light.

Applanation tonometry (measurement of the pressure within the eye) is an essential test for glaucoma. It is done using a slit lamp microscope.

EQUIPMENT

The retina can be examined with an *ophthalmoscope*. The slit lamp microscope, with its brilliant illumination and lens magnification, allows meticulous examination of the conjunctiva, cornea, front chamber of the eye, iris, and crystalline lens.

By means of special corneal contact lenses, the magnified view may be extended to include the vitreous gel behind the lens and the retina. These contact lenses incorporate mirrors to allow examination of structures at the base of the iris and the front edge of the retina. For a full view of the crystalline lens and the structures behind it, the pupil must be widely dilated with drops, such as tropicamide or phenylephrine.

CONDUCTING AN EYE EXAMINATION

During an eye examination, the physician checks external appearance, eye movement, visual acuity, visual field, and color vision. The eyes are checked for the presence of strabismus, abrasions, and ulcers. Applanation tonometry and a refraction test are also done.

View of retina through ophthalmoscope
The retina (inner back surface of the eye) is examined to assess conditions such as hypertensive *retinopathy*, as seen here.

Applanation tonometry
Measurement of the pressure within the eye is a routine test for glaucoma.

Snellen's chart
The chart is used to check visual acuity of each eye; the patient's ability to read letters of different sizes from the same distance is assessed.

DISORDERS OF THE EYE

Many eye disorders are minor, but some lead to serious complications unless treated. (See also *Cornea* disorders box; *Retina* disorders box; *Eye, painful red*.)

CONGENITAL DEFECTS

Strabismus (squint or malalignment of the eyes) is often congenital (present at birth). *Cataracts* (opacity of the lens of the eye) can occur in infants, when the cause may be maternal *rubella* infection early in pregnancy. Very rarely, babies are born with microphthalmos (abnormally small eye) on one or both sides. Vision in a microphthalmic eye is usually very poor. *Nystagmus* (rapid, uncontrollable movement in the eyes) can be congenital.

Retinoblastoma is a malignant tumor of the retina that appears in early life and may occur in one or both eyes. Other congenital disorders affecting the eye include *albinism* (absence of pigment) and abnormalities of development of the cornea and retina.

INFECTION

Conjunctivitis, the most common infection, rarely affects vision. In the late stages of neglected conjunctival infection, such as *trachoma* or severe bacterial conjunctivitis, vision can be impaired.

Corneal infections are more serious and can lead to blurred vision or corneal perforation if not treated early. Endophthalmitis (infection within the eye), which may make it necessary to remove the eye surgically, can occur after a penetrating injury, after severe ulceration, in rare cases after major eye surgery, or from infections elsewhere in the body.

IMPAIRED BLOOD SUPPLY

Narrowing, blockage, inflammation, or other abnormalities of the blood vessels of the retina may cause partial or total loss of vision.

TUMORS

Malignant *melanoma* of the choroid (middle layer of the eye) is the most common primary malignant eye tumor. It can be found in the eyes of people who do not have symptoms (during routine examinations) or it can cause a decrease in vision.

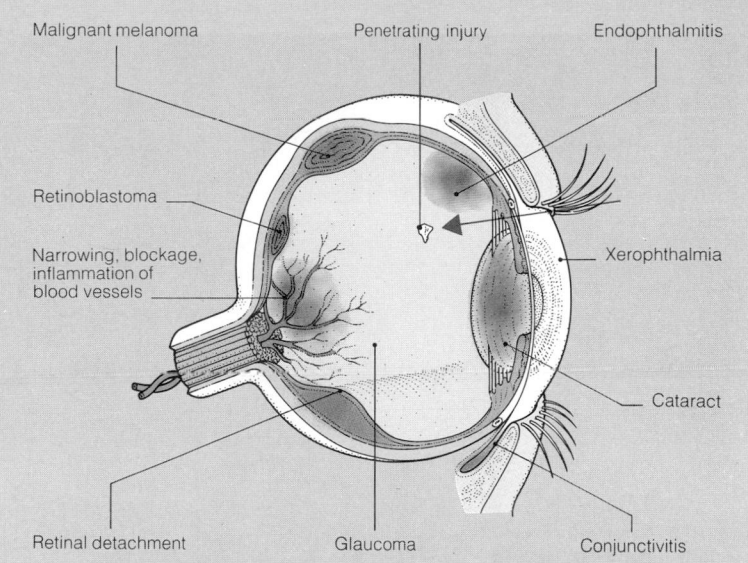

Malignant melanoma — Penetrating injury — Endophthalmitis — Retinoblastoma — Narrowing, blockage, inflammation of blood vessels — Xerophthalmia — Cataract — Retinal detachment — Glaucoma — Conjunctivitis

NUTRITIONAL DISORDERS

Various vitamin deficiencies (particularly vitamin A deficiency) can affect the eye. This may lead to xerophthalmia (dryness of the cornea and conjunctiva), night blindness, or, ultimately, *keratomalacia* (corneal softening and destruction) and total loss of vision.

AUTOIMMUNE DISORDERS

Uveitis (inflammation of the uveal tissues—iris, choroid, and/or ciliary body), when not caused by an infectious agent, may have an autoimmune basis (when the defense mechanisms of the body attack its own tissues). It is commonly encountered in people with *ankylosing spondylitis* (crippling and deforming arthritis of the spine) and *sarcoidosis.*

DEGENERATION

Macular degeneration of the retina is common in the elderly. It causes loss of fine, detailed vision, although peripheral vision remains.

Cataract is also common in elderly people; although the exact cause of the condition is unknown, the process is thought to be degenerative.

OTHER DISORDERS

Glaucoma (a condition in which the pressure in the fluid that maintains the normal shape of the eye is raised) may take various forms. If untreated, glaucoma can lead to permanent loss of vision.

In *retinal detachment*, the retina lifts away from the underlying layer of the eye; this may have various causes.

Ametropia is a general term that means the eye has a refractive error (an error in focusing), such as *myopia* (nearsightedness), *hyperopia* (farsightedness), *astigmatism*, or *anisometropia*. None of these is a disease in the ordinary sense of the word; they are caused simply by variations of shape and focusing ability of the eye. *Presbyopia* is the progressive loss of accommodation (ability to focus at near range) with age. *Amblyopia* (poor vision in one eye without any obvious structural abnormality) is often due to strabismus.

INVESTIGATION

Because of the transparency of its structures, the eye is particularly accessible for examination. Many of the disease processes affecting it can be viewed directly by use of the *ophthalmoscope* and *slit lamp*. Photography of the retina and *fluorescein* angiography are also used. (See also *Eye, examination of*.)

E

FIRST AID: FOREIGN BODY IN THE EYE

WARNING
Never attempt to remove a particle embedded in the eyeball. Do not remove a foreign body if it is resting on the iris (colored part of the eye).

LOWER LID

1 Wash your hands. Ask the victim to look up while you separate the lids and examine the eye.

2 First try floating an object out with water; then try lifting it out with the moistened corner of a cloth.

UPPER LID

1 Grasp the lashes and carefully draw the upper lid outward and downward. If this does not dislodge the object, try floating it off by having the victim blink under water.

2 If these measures fail, ask the victim to look down while you place a matchstick across the upper lid and fold the lid up over it. Then pick off the object with a clean cloth.

CORROSIVES IN THE EYE

Flush with continuously running water – some alkalis penetrate deeply and take longer to wash out.

Eye, foreign body in

Any material on the surface of the eye or under the eyelid, or an object that penetrates the eyeball.

INCIDENCE AND CAUSES

Most people get something in their eye at least once in their lives. Usually it is a particle of dust; occasionally it is a metal, plastic, or wood fragment that has been deflected into the eye while doing some home or car maintenance. Rarely, an object traveling at high speed actually penetrates the eyeball—for example, a piece of metal in an industrial accident.

SYMPTOMS

A foreign body under the eyelid or on the cornea or conjunctiva irritates the eye, causing pain, redness, and tearing. It usually causes blepharospasm (uncontrollable eyelid contractions). These symptoms may improve even if the foreign body remains. Occasionally, there will not be any symptoms, especially if the eye has been penetrated.

COMPLICATIONS

Some foreign bodies left within the eyeball may dissolve to release pigment into the substance of the eye, causing blindness. Other foreign bodies may remain whole but cause infection, again leading to blindness.

DIAGNOSIS

If a foreign body is suspected, a physician should be consulted. He or she will examine the eye and both eyelids. Fluorescein (a yellow stain) is used to show up abrasions or sites of penetration. Imaging procedures are used if a penetrating injury is suspected.

TREATMENT

Superficial foreign bodies may be removed at home. Use the corner of a clean cloth, or pull the upper lid down over the lower lid or irrigate the eye using an eyecup.

Objects on the iris or pupil or embedded in the eye should be removed by a physician. A sharp spatula is often used after the surface of the eye has been anesthetized with local anesthetic eye drops. The eye is then stained with fluorescein to assess the area of damage to the cornea. Antibiotics as drops or ointment will be prescribed and the eye is then protected with a patch (see also *Corneal abrasion*). Metallic objects that have penetrated the eye can sometimes be extracted using a powerful magnet.

Eye injuries

The greatest danger to the eye arises from objects of relatively small size traveling at high speed, such as BB gun pellets, slingshot missiles, or small stones sometimes thrown up by rotary lawnmowers. Many industrial activities, such as drilling, sawing, hammering, or grinding, can cause objects from high-speed machinery to penetrate the eye. Penetrating injuries also can occur from windshield glass in automobile accidents. Foreign bodies within the eye can cause serious problems.

The serious injuries are generally those that damage both the cornea and the crystalline lens. Central corneal wounds impair vision by causing scarring (see *Corneal abrasion*). Damage to the lens may cause a *cataract* to form, with resultant loss of vision in that eye. The most serious injuries also extend to the back of the eye to include the retina and posterior sclera (outer lining).

Blunt trauma to the eyeball, such as a blow from a stick, may cause tearing of the iris or may cause rupture of the sclera, with collapse of the eyeball and permanent blindness. Lesser degrees of injury that do not cause penetration may lead to a vitreous hemorrhage (bleeding behind the lens), *hyphema* (bleeding into the front chamber of the eye), retinal detachment, or injury to the trabeculum (fluid outflow drain of the eye), which can lead to glaucoma. Hyphema affects vision until the blood absorbs, unless other vision-threatening damage occurred with it. (See also *Eye, foreign body in*.)

Eyelashes, disorders of

Eyelashes are arranged in two rows at the front edge of each lid and curve outward. Growth in an abnormal direction may be due to injury to the lid or, more commonly, infection. Occasionally, lashes grow in an abnormal direction for no obvious reason. With age, the lashes become finer.

Severe *blepharitis* (eyelid infection) may cause the lid margins to be so damaged that lash roots are destroyed. *Trachoma*, an eye infection in which the lid is distorted by scarring, may lead to trichiasis, a condition in which the lashes turn inward. They may rub against the cornea, causing corneal abrasion.

Eye, lazy

A popular term for *amblyopia*, in which normal vision has failed to develop, usually in one eye.

Eyelid

One of a pair of complex structures that lies on the upper and lower edges of the eye socket. The eyelids are held in position by ligaments attached to the socket's bony edges. They consist of thin fibrous tissue, called the tarsal plate, covered by muscle and a very thin layer of skin. The inner layer is covered by part of the *conjunctiva*.

Along the edge of the eyelid are two rows of eyelashes, which are strong, curved hairs. Immediately behind the eyelashes are the openings of the ducts leading from the meibomian glands, which secrete the oily part of the tear film from within the tarsal plate (see also *Tears*).

The eyelids act as protective shutters, closing very rapidly as a reflex action in response to anything approaching the eye. A squeezing action of the eyelids pushes the eyeball back into the socket as an additional protective measure. The eyelids also act as wipers to smear the tear film across the cornea.

DISORDERS

Disorders include a *chalazion* (a swelling of a meibomian gland), *blepharitis* (inflammation of the edge of the eyelid), and a *stye* (an abscess at the root of one of the eyelashes).

The shape and position of the eyelids are abnormal in a number of disorders, including *entropion* (the eyelid margin turning inward), *ectropion* (the eyelid margin turning outward), *ptosis* (a drooping eyelid covering all or part of the eye), and baggy eyelids due to dermatochalasis (excess lid skin) or blepharochalasis (excess fat under the lid skin).

Myokymia (twitching of the eyelid) is a common phenomenon usually due to fatigue. *Blepharospasm* (rapid contractions of the eyelid) is usually caused by a foreign body in the eye.

The skin of the eyelid is a common site for a *basal cell carcinoma*.

Eyelid, drooping

See *Ptosis*.

Eyelid surgery

See *Blepharoplasty*.

Eye, painful red

A very common combination of eye symptoms that can be due to several different eye disorders. The presence of pain and redness in one or both eyes requires examination and treatment by a physician.

The most common eye disorder that causes pain and redness is *conjunctivitis*. The redness is due to dilation of the superficial (conjunctival) blood vessels. The pain is similar to that caused by grit in the eye. Conjunctivitis can be due to viral or bacterial infections, irritants (such as chemicals), or allergies. Viral conjunctivitis usually eventually affects both eyes and precautions should be taken to prevent infecting others.

Uveitis (inflammation of all or a portion of the uvea, such as the iris) is another common cause. The dull, aching pain may be due to swelling within the front of the eye and spasm in muscles around the iris. The redness is caused by widening of blood vessels around the iris.

A serious cause of pain and redness in one eye is acute closed-angle *glaucoma* (sudden, highly increased pressure within the eyeball). The pain is severe and may be accompanied by nausea, vomiting, halos, and blurred vision. There is redness of the white of the eye due to increased blood flow in the surrounding vessels.

Other important causes of painful, red eye include a *corneal ulcer, keratitis* (inflammation of the outer protective layer of the eye), or the presence of a foreign body on the surface of the eye or under one of the eyelids.

Eyestrain

A term often used to describe aching or discomfort in the eye. Eyestrain is not a medical term, and physicians do not accept the popular belief that the eyes can be damaged by being used.

Eye teeth

A common name for canine *teeth*.

Eye tumors

Tumors of the eye are rare. When eye tumors do occur, they are usually malignant and painless.

TYPES AND TREATMENT

RETINOBLASTOMA This is a *congenital malignant tumor* of the retina that occurs in one or both eyes. If the central vision in only one eye is affected, the child may have strabismus (squint). If the tumor is not discovered in its early growth, it may be seen as a white or yellowish reflection in one pupil. Retinoblastoma may sometimes be treated by *radiation therapy, laser treatment*, or freezing, but the eye may require removal to prevent spread of the tumor.

MALIGNANT MELANOMA A form of skin cancer, this is a tumor of the choroid layer that usually affects the middle-aged and elderly. It is the most common eye tumor. Often there are no early symptoms, but the tumor eventually causes detachment of the retina and distortion of vision. Small malignant melanomas can be destroyed by laser treatment, but removal of the eye is often advised to avoid spread of the tumor to the brain or elsewhere.

SECONDARY EYE TUMORS These occur when cancer in another part of the body spreads to the eye, where it produces effects similar to those of the primary tumor. If the secondary tumors grow behind the eyeball, they may cause bulging of the eye. Their effect on vision varies, depending on the location and growth rate. Secondary tumors may sometimes be controlled by radiation therapy; separate treatment is necessary for the primary tumor.

BASAL CELL CARCINOMA This is the most common eyelid tumor. Like other basal cell carcinomas, it is related to excessive exposure to sunlight. The tumor usually has a small crusty central crater and a hard rolled edge. Although it may grow large, it very rarely spreads to other parts of the body. In the early stages, basal cell carcinoma of the lids may be treated by surgery, radiation therapy, or freezing. Extensive plastic surgery or removal of the eye may be necessary.

F

Face-lift

A cosmetic operation to smooth out wrinkles and lift sagging skin on an aging face to make it look younger. A face-lift is usually performed as an outpatient procedure using a local anesthetic. The two sides of the face are treated during the same operation.

OUTLOOK

Some bruising of the face is common, but there is usually no pain. The stitches are removed three to five days after the operation. In most cases, the scars, which fade within a year, are hidden by natural crease lines or by the hair. The effect of a face-lift usually lasts about five years.

Occasionally, satisfactory healing does not occur as a result of *hematoma* (bleeding under the skin) or infection, leading to severe scarring; in the worst cases, a *skin graft* may be necessary.

Facial nerve

The seventh *cranial nerve*. It arises from the pons and medulla oblongata (parts of the brain stem) and sends branches to the face, neck, salivary glands, and outer ear.

LOCATION OF THE FACIAL NERVE

Arising from the brain stem, the facial nerve has branches that connect to the outer ear, tongue, salivary glands, and muscles of the neck and face.

Brain

Facial nerve

Salivary glands

FACE-LIFT

A face-lift is really a skin-lift. It is a serious surgical operation and its effects are not always permanent. There is some discomfort after a face-lift and the cosmetic effects are not immediately apparent. Care should be taken in choosing a highly reputable surgeon.

Before and after treatment
The results of most face-lifts are excellent. However, it should be realized that the outcome may not be exactly as expected, and there is always some risk associated with any operation.

Skin removed

Line of incision

How it is done
An incision is made where shown. The skin is undercut as far as the crease running from the nose to the corner of the mouth. It is then pulled upward and backward, and its margins are sewn near the hairline.

The facial nerve performs both motor and sensory functions. It controls the muscles of the neck and of facial expression (including muscles in the forehead); it also stimulates secretion by the submandibular and sublingual salivary glands. In addition, the facial nerve conveys taste sensations from the front two thirds of the tongue and carries sensations from the outer ear.

Damage to the facial nerve causes weakness of the facial muscles (see *Facial palsy*) and, in some cases, loss of taste. Such damage is most commonly due to a virus infection. It may also be a feature of a *stroke*; more rarely, it may occur as a result of surgery (typically for a tumor) to the parotid gland (one of the salivary glands).

Facial pain

Pain in the face may be caused by injury, infection, or a nerve disorder, may be referred from elsewhere in the body (see *Referred pain*), or may occur for no known reason.

INJURY

In addition to pain in the face from a direct injury, pain may be caused indirectly by *teething* problems in a baby, wisdom tooth problems in an adult (see *Impaction, dental*), or partial dislocation of the jaw.

INFECTION

Sinusitis (inflammation of the air spaces around the nose) can cause pain around the eyes and in the cheek bones. The onset of *mumps* also can cause pain in the cheeks before any swelling appears in front of and/or below the ears. Pain from a boil in the nose or ear may radiate to the face, as may pain from a tooth abscess (see *Abscess, dental*) or dental *caries*.

NERVE DISORDERS

Damage to a nerve that supplies the face can result in severe pain. Examples include the knifelike pain that precedes the one-sided rash in *herpes zoster* (shingles), and the intermittent shooting pain of *trigeminal neuralgia* (tic douloureux), which usually affects only one side of the face and is often brought on by touching the face or chewing.

REFERRED PAIN

In *angina pectoris* (pain in the chest due to lack of oxygen to the heart), pain may be felt in the jaw. With *migraine* headaches, pain may occur on one side of the face. When facial pain or headache occurs for no reason, it may be a symptom of *depression*.

TREATMENT

Analgesics (painkillers) can provide temporary relief, but, if the pain is severe or persistent, a physician or dentist should be consulted.

Facial palsy

Also known as Bell's palsy (for the Scottish surgeon Sir Charles Bell), paralysis of the facial muscles, usually one-sided and temporary, due to inflammation of a facial nerve. Facial palsy is common and usually comes on suddenly. The cause is unknown, although, rarely, it may be associated with *herpes zoster* (shingles).

SYMPTOMS
The eyelid and corner of the mouth droop on one side of the face and there may be pain in the ear on that side. It may be impossible to wrinkle the brow or to close the eye, and smiling is distorted. Depending on which branches of the nerve are affected, taste may be impaired or sounds may seem unnaturally loud.

TREATMENT
Corticosteroid drugs or *ACTH* is sometimes given to reduce inflammation of the nerve, along with analgesics (painkillers) if the ear is painful. Exercising the facial muscles may facilitate recovery. Electrostimulation of the nerve is of unproved value. It may be necessary to tape the eyelid shut at bedtime to avoid corneal abrasion. In most cases, the condition clears up with or without treatment.

Facial spasm
An uncommon disorder in which there is frequent twitching of facial muscles supplied by the *facial nerve*. (This condition is often called a tic, but, in fact, tic is a general term that can refer to spasmodic twitching in any part of the body.) The disorder, which affects mainly middle-aged women, is of unknown cause.

Facies
A medical term for the appearance of the face, as in adenoid facies, the dull, open-mouthed expression seen in many children whose nasal passages are blocked due to enlarged adenoids.

Factitious disorders
A group of disorders in which symptoms mimic a true illness, but actually have been invented and are under the control of the patient. This is done willingly and for no apparent reason other than the wish to receive the attention given to a patient.

The most common type of factitious disorder is characterized by real physical symptoms and is known as *Munchausen's syndrome*. In a second form, called *Ganser's syndrome*, there is a psychological disturbance.

These disorders differ from malingering, in which the person claims to be ill for a particular purpose, such as obtaining time off from work or claiming compensation.

Factor VIII
One of the blood proteins (coagulation factors) that takes part in the "coagulation cascade"—an important process in *blood clotting*. Some people with the inherited condition *hemophilia* have a reduced level of factor VIII in their blood and, consequently, have a tendency to abnormal bleeding and prolonged bleeding when injured.

Freeze-dried concentrates of factor VIII are given to hemophiliacs by regular intravenous injection (some hemophiliacs administer the treatment themselves at home), which reduces the bleeding tendency and improves the quality of life.

Fahrenheit scale
A temperature scale in which the melting point of ice is 32° and the boiling point of water is 212°. On this scale, normal body temperature is 98.6°F (37°C). The scale is named for the German physicist Gabriel Fahrenheit.

To convert Fahrenheit to Celsius, subtract 32 and then multiply by 0.56 (or 5/9). To convert a Celsius temperature to a Fahrenheit temperature, multiply by 1.8 (or 9/5) and then add 32. (See also *Celsius scale*.)

Failure to thrive
Lack of expected growth in an infant, usually assessed by comparing the rate at which a baby gains weight with a standardized growth chart. Babies who fail to thrive are not growing enough in relation to birth weight.

The undernourishment may be due to some problem at home, often an unsatisfactory relationship between parent and child. In some cases, the child is actually neglected. Deprived children often have delayed emotional and intellectual development as well as failure to thrive.

If a baby fails to gain weight despite receiving an adequate diet and having a stable family background, other conditions may be responsible. Failure to thrive can indicate a serious problem, such as congenital *heart disease*, *renal failure*, or *malabsorption*.

A baby who fails to thrive is often observed (along with a parent) for a week or two to see how the parent feeds and handles the baby. The baby's diet and weight are carefully monitored. If there are social problems, support for the family can be initiated. (See also *Short stature*.)

Fainting
Temporary loss of consciousness due to insufficient oxygen reaching the brain. A fainting attack, known medically as syncope, is often preceded by dizziness, nausea, or a feeling of extreme weakness.

CAUSES
One common cause of fainting is a vasovagal attack, overstimulation of the *vagus nerve* (which helps control breathing and blood circulation). Usually such an attack is due to severe pain, stress, or fear; more rarely it may be caused by prolonged coughing, or by straining to defecate, urinate, or blow a wind instrument. In such cases, unconsciousness is usually accompanied by profuse sweating or

FIRST AID: FAINTING

1 Anyone who feels faint should sit down and lean forward, head between the knees.

2 If a fainting victim is unconscious and breathing normally, lay the person down and raise his or her legs above chest level.

F

F

paleness of the skin. A common cause of fainting is being in a stuffy atmosphere that has little oxygen.

Standing still for a long time, or standing up suddenly, can cause fainting. This is due to blood pooling in veins in the legs and reducing the amount available for the heart to pump to the brain, with a resultant drop in blood pressure (postural *hypotension*). It is common in the elderly, in sufferers from *diabetes mellitus*, and in people taking *antihypertensive* or *vasodilator drugs*.

In some people, episodes of fainting may be associated with temporary difficulty in speaking or weakness in the limbs; this may indicate a disorder called *vertebrobasilar insufficiency*, in which there is an obstruction to the blood flow in vessels that pass through the neck to the brain. This is one form of a *transient ischemic attack*.

Fainting may be a symptom of *Stokes-Adams syndrome*, in which the blood flow to the brain temporarily is inadequate due to an *arrhythmia* (irregularity of the heart beat) usually associated with a form of *heart block* (interruption of electrical impulses in the heart).

TREATMENT
Recovery from syncope takes place when normal blood flow to the brain is restored. This usually happens within minutes because falling to the ground places the head at the same level as the heart. To ensure another attack does not occur, the person should remain lying down for 10 to 15 minutes after regaining consciousness.

A person who experiences warning signs of a faint can sometimes prevent fainting by sitting with the head between the knees or, if possible, lying flat with the legs raised.

If a person fails to regain consciousness within a minute or two of fainting, medical help should be obtained promptly and appropriate first aid given (see *Unconsciousness*) until help arrives. Repeated attacks require investigation by a physician.

Faith healing
The supposed ability of certain people to cure disease by their possession of a healing force inexplicable to science. The healer usually transmits this supposed force to the sufferer by direct contact, placing his or her hands on the body ("laying on of hands"). Often the healer and patient have a deep religious faith and believe the force to be divine, but in many cases no religious faith is involved—only a firm

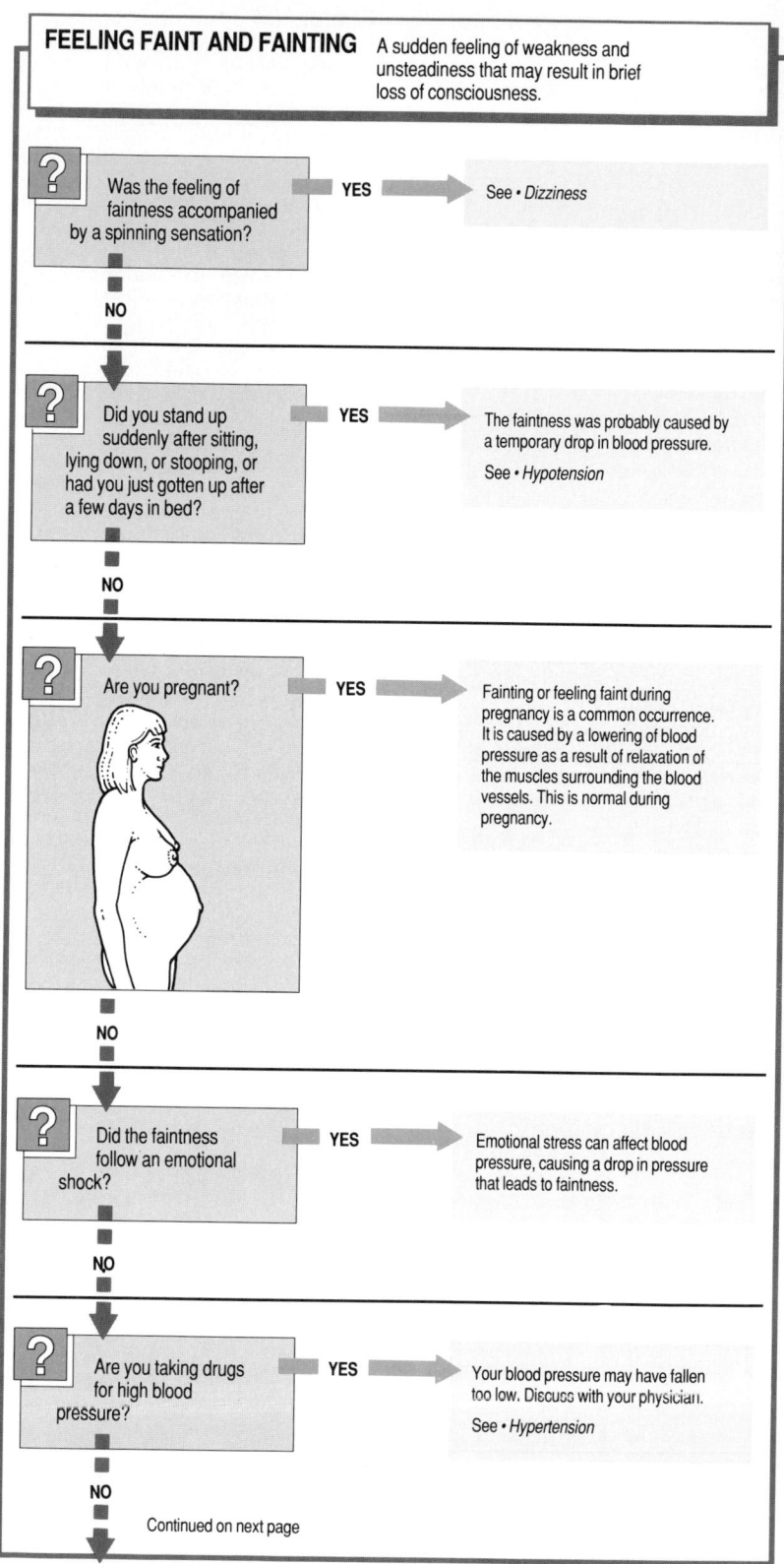

FEELING FAINT AND FAINTING A sudden feeling of weakness and unsteadiness that may result in brief loss of consciousness.

? Was the feeling of faintness accompanied by a spinning sensation? — **YES** → See • *Dizziness*

NO

? Did you stand up suddenly after sitting, lying down, or stooping, or had you just gotten up after a few days in bed? — **YES** → The faintness was probably caused by a temporary drop in blood pressure. See • *Hypotension*

NO

? Are you pregnant? — **YES** → Fainting or feeling faint during pregnancy is a common occurrence. It is caused by a lowering of blood pressure as a result of relaxation of the muscles surrounding the blood vessels. This is normal during pregnancy.

NO

? Did the faintness follow an emotional shock? — **YES** → Emotional stress can affect blood pressure, causing a drop in pressure that leads to faintness.

NO

? Are you taking drugs for high blood pressure? — **YES** → Your blood pressure may have fallen too low. Discuss with your physician. See • *Hypertension*

NO

F

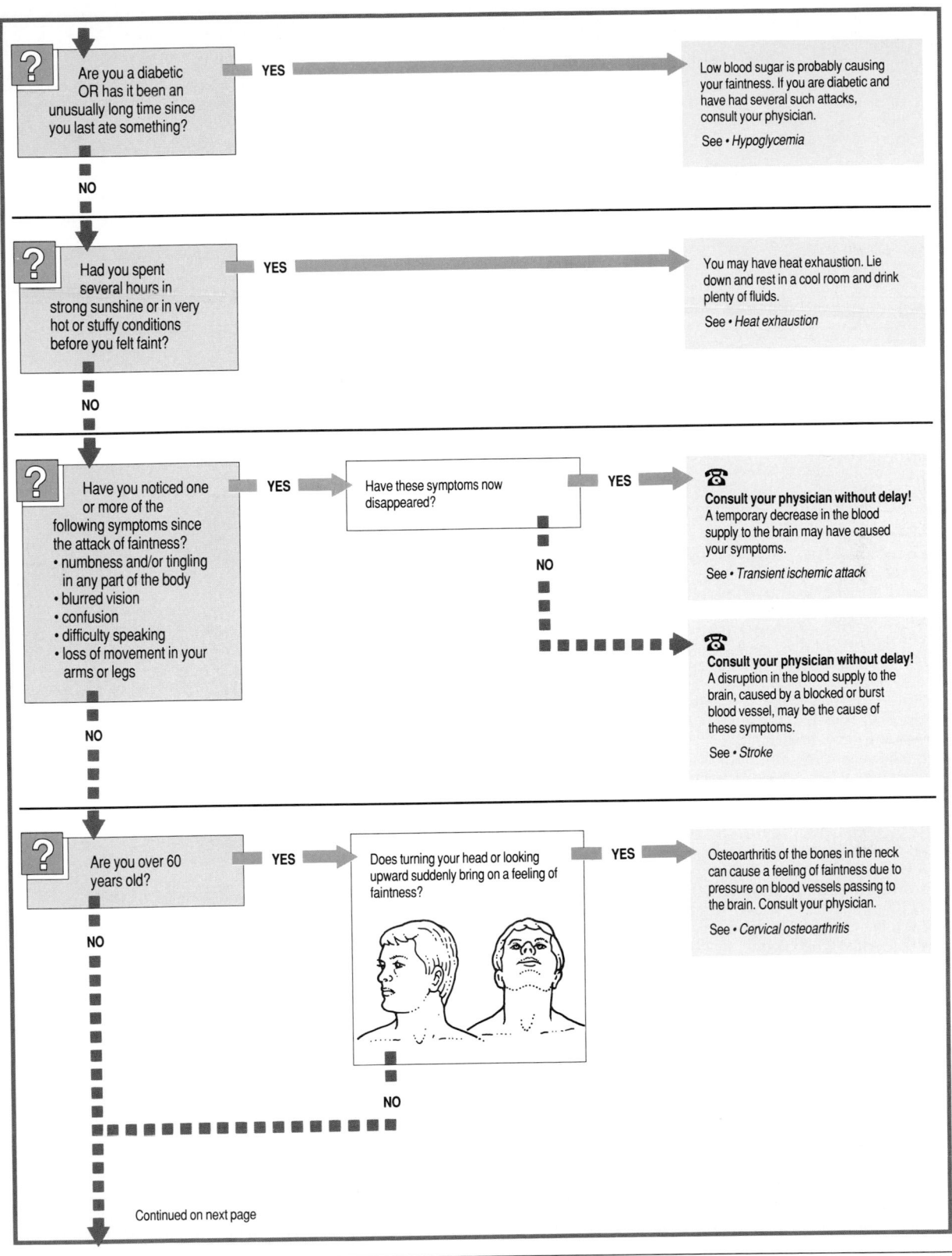

Are you a diabetic OR has it been an unusually long time since you last ate something?

YES → Low blood sugar is probably causing your faintness. If you are diabetic and have had several such attacks, consult your physician.

See • *Hypoglycemia*

NO

Had you spent several hours in strong sunshine or in very hot or stuffy conditions before you felt faint?

YES → You may have heat exhaustion. Lie down and rest in a cool room and drink plenty of fluids.

See • *Heat exhaustion*

NO

Have you noticed one or more of the following symptoms since the attack of faintness?
• numbness and/or tingling in any part of the body
• blurred vision
• confusion
• difficulty speaking
• loss of movement in your arms or legs

YES → Have these symptoms now disappeared?

YES → ☎ **Consult your physician without delay!** A temporary decrease in the blood supply to the brain may have caused your symptoms.

See • *Transient ischemic attack*

NO → ☎ **Consult your physician without delay!** A disruption in the blood supply to the brain, caused by a blocked or burst blood vessel, may be the cause of these symptoms.

See • *Stroke*

NO

Are you over 60 years old?

YES → Does turning your head or looking upward suddenly bring on a feeling of faintness?

YES → Osteoarthritis of the bones in the neck can cause a feeling of faintness due to pressure on blood vessels passing to the brain. Consult your physician.

See • *Cervical osteoarthritis*

NO

Continued on next page

F

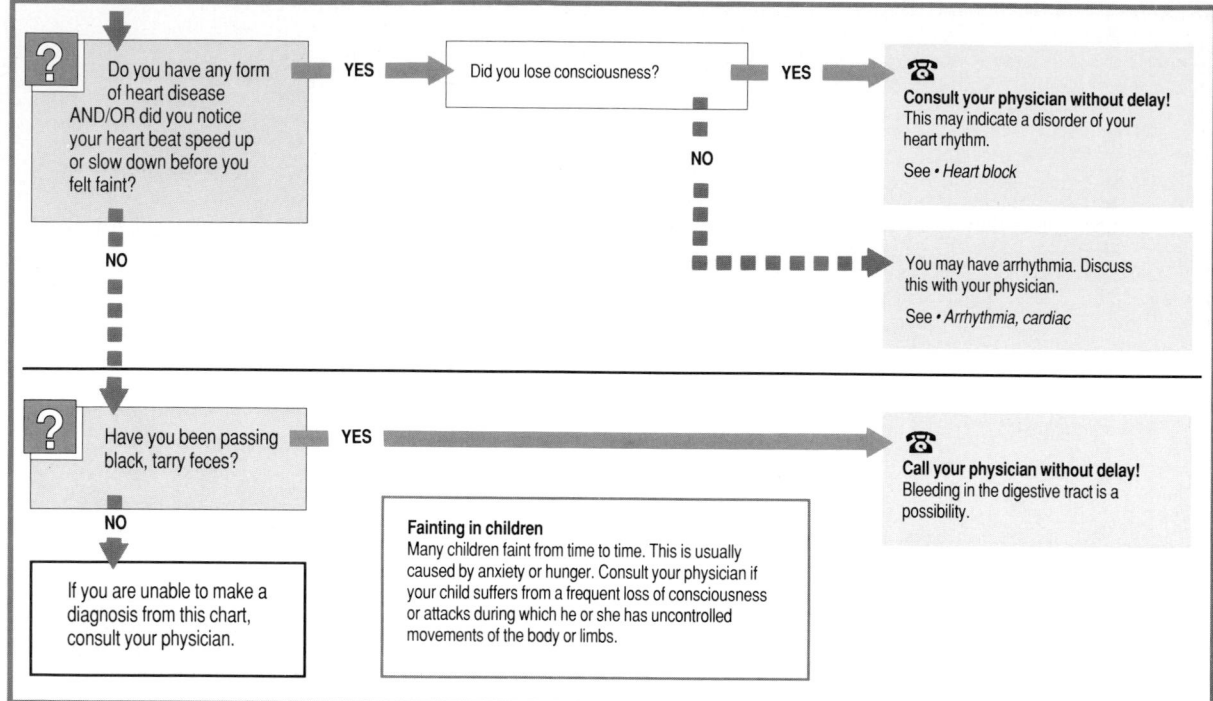

? Do you have any form of heart disease AND/OR did you notice your heart beat speed up or slow down before you felt faint?

YES → Did you lose consciousness? **YES** →

☎ **Consult your physician without delay!** This may indicate a disorder of your heart rhythm.

See • *Heart block*

NO

You may have arrhythmia. Discuss this with your physician.

See • *Arrhythmia, cardiac*

NO

? Have you been passing black, tarry feces?

YES →

☎ **Call your physician without delay!** Bleeding in the digestive tract is a possibility.

NO

If you are unable to make a diagnosis from this chart, consult your physician.

Fainting in children
Many children faint from time to time. This is usually caused by anxiety or hunger. Consult your physician if your child suffers from a frequent loss of consciousness or attacks during which he or she has uncontrolled movements of the body or limbs.

---

belief, by healer and sufferer alike, in the healer's powers.

The existence of cures by faith healing is not in doubt—they have been demonstrated many times to the satisfaction of medical observers; in addition, the cures do not involve any of the risks that may accompany medical or surgical treatment. However, the medical profession tends to argue that most such cures are due not to a divine or otherwise inexplicable force, but to the fact that the disorders were hysterical in origin (see *Hysteria*) and therefore susceptible to *autosuggestion*. Physicians also believe that people who turn to faith healing rather than seek medical advice are depriving themselves of effective treatment of the underlying problem.

Fallen arches
A cause of *flatfoot*, which can develop as a result of weakness of the muscles that support the arches of the foot.

Fallopian tube
The tube that extends from the *uterus* to the *ovary*. The fallopian tube transports eggs and sperm and is where *fertilization* takes place.
STRUCTURE
The funnel-shaped tube is about 3 inches long. The narrow end opens into the uterus and the free, expanded end, divided into fimbriae (fingerlike projections), lies close to the ovary. Its muscular wall is lined by cells with cilia (hairlike projections).

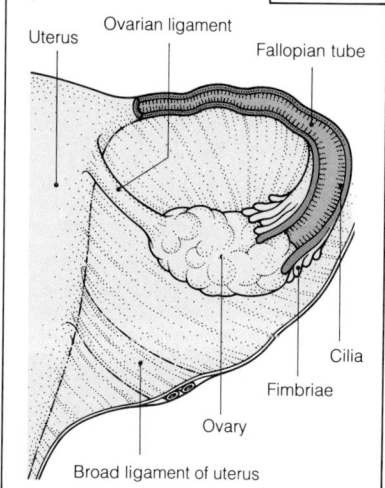

LOCATION OF THE FALLOPIAN TUBES Situated in the pelvic portion of the abdominal cavity, each tube extends from an ovary and becomes the upper part of the uterus.

Uterus — Ovarian ligament — Fallopian tube — Cilia — Fimbriae — Ovary — Broad ligament of uterus

FUNCTION
The fimbriae sweep up the egg after it is expelled from the ovary. The beating cilia and waves of muscular contractions propel the egg toward the uterus. After intercourse, sperm swim up the fallopian tube from the uterus. The lining of the tube and its secretions sustain the egg and sperm. They also encourage fertilization and nourish the egg until it reaches the uterus.
DISORDERS
Salpingitis is inflammation of the fallopian tube, usually following bacterial infection. It accounts for almost 15 percent of cases of *infertility*.

Ectopic pregnancy (development of an embryo outside the uterus) usually occurs in the fallopian tube. A delay in the transport of the fertilized egg along the tube results in implantation within the tube wall, which is too thin to sustain growth. The tube then ruptures and may hemorrhage.

Fallot's tetralogy
See *Tetralogy of Fallot*.

Fallout
See *Radiation hazards*.

Falls in the elderly
The tendency to fall increases steadily with age. Although the majority of

falls produce no permanent injury, a significant number of the injuries that do result are ultimately fatal.

CAUSES AND INCIDENCE

Reflex actions in the elderly are much slower than in the young, and an elderly person who trips or stumbles is often too slow to prevent a fall.

Half of all falls are accidental and half have a medical cause. Poor sight, walking disorders, arrhythmias (see *Arrhythmia, cardiac*), *hypotension* (reduced blood pressure), dizziness for various reasons, and the effect of drugs are causes. Falls sometimes herald the onset of serious illness such as pneumonia, stroke, myocardial infarction (heart attack), or internal hemorrhage. Epilepsy, Parkinson's disease, alcohol consumption, the hangover effects of some sleeping tablets, and use of daytime tranquilizers may also increase the likelihood of a fall.

RISKS AND COMPLICATIONS

Broken bones as a result of falls are particularly common in the elderly. Women are more vulnerable to broken bones than men. Not only do women have more falls, they are also more likely to suffer fractures because their bone strength is reduced as a result of calcium loss after the menopause (see

Osteoporosis). The incidence of fractures of the neck of the femur (thigh bone) doubles approximately every seven years after the age of 65, and, by the age of 90, one woman in four has suffered this type of fracture.

Apart from injuries, there may be serious indirect consequences of the fall. The outlook is particularly grave for those who fall and lie on the floor for more than an hour, particularly if it is cold. This may lead to *hypothermia* (low body temperature) or pneumonia. In this group, 50 percent die within three months of the fall.

A serious fall, or fear of such a fall and the helplessness and dependence it could bring, can have bad psychological effects on an elderly person, sometimes causing a previously active person to become demoralized and housebound.

ACTION AFTER A FALL

Immediate medical help should be obtained if the person is unconscious, is in severe pain, is bleeding profusely, is burned, has suspected broken bones, or is showing signs of shock. First-aid measures (for bleeding, burns, or fractures) and *cardiopulmonary resuscitation* (if the heart and/or breathing have stopped) may be necessary.

PREVENTION AND OUTLOOK

These measures can be taken to guard against falls: ensure that handles in bathrooms and on stairs are secure, good lighting is available, suitable footwear is worn, floor coverings and wiring are safe, and that there is minimal clutter on the floor. Elderly people who live alone can arrange for an alarm system to be installed or for a regular visit by a neighbor. It is also helpful to teach the elderly person several different ways of getting up from the floor.

False teeth
See *Denture*.

Familial
A term applied to a characteristic or disorder that runs in families (that is, it occurs in more members of a particular family than would be expected from the occurrence in the population as a whole). An example of a familial characteristic is male pattern baldness (see *Alopecia*); an example of a familial disorder is *hyperlipidemia* (abnormally high levels of fat in the blood).

Familial Mediterranean fever
An inherited condition that affects certain Sephardic Jewish, Armenian, and

PREVENTING FALLS

Half of all falls are accidental, caused by hazards in the home such as poor lighting, worn carpets, rickety stair rails, trailing wires, loose rugs and mats, ill-fitting shoes, and inaccessible cabinets. Snow and ice on walks outside are also a major hazard. The illustration shows some of the main hazards in a typical living room, and ways to remedy them.

Worn areas of carpet
Make safe by tacking down loose edges.

Trailing wires
Secure to a wall or molding.

Loose rugs and mats
All should have nonslip backing; they should never be used to cover a slippery floor.

Uncovered floor areas
Do not polish to a slippery finish. Carpet edges should be firmly fixed to the floor.

Furniture with protruding legs
Do not place in frequently used areas of a room.

Shoes and other clutter
Floors should be free of all clutter.

Arab families. Its cause is unknown. Symptoms usually begin between the ages of 5 and 15 years. The main symptoms are recurrent episodes of fever, abdominal pain, arthritis, and chest pain. Red swellings in the skin sometimes occur, and affected people may also suffer psychiatric problems.

Attacks usually last between 24 and 48 hours, but may last longer. Between attacks there are usually no symptoms. There is no specific treatment, but known sufferers are able to reduce the incidence of attacks by taking colchicine, a drug usually used to treat gout. Death may eventually occur from *amyloidosis*, which is a complication of the condition.

Family planning

Limitation of the number or spacing of children through choices made by sexually active people. In some countries, financial and taxation incentives are used by the state to encourage couples to have more or fewer children; in other countries, penalties are imposed on those who do not conform to government recommendations.

In most countries the factors governing family size are economic and social. In many developing countries few older people have pensions, and those too frail to work rely on support from their adult children. Under these circumstances, having many children is seen as a provision for care in old age. In the past 20 years, however, most nations have experienced the economic ill effects of rapid population growth and large families are no longer encouraged.

The number of children born to a couple may be limited by social factors—late marriage for both men and women reduces the reproductive period, and economic barriers to marriage may restrict childbearing to a fraction of the population.

Strategies for restricting family size include contraceptive techniques (see *Contraception*) and elective abortion (see *Abortion, elective*).

Family practitioner

A physician who provides comprehensive medical services for individuals, regardless of sex or age, on a continuing basis. The family practitioner (FP) often cares for all members of a family.

Emphasis is placed on treatment of all problems experienced by the person and on coordination of care, with referrals to specialists as necessary. Care by an FP may range from stitches

and sniffles to management of long-term conditions (e.g., terminal cancer, congestive heart failure, or diabetes mellitus), including the delivery of a baby and care afterward. Family practitioners have replaced the former general practitioner (GP), but the training for the FP is broader.

Family therapy

Treatment of the family as a whole rather than individual treatment of one or more members. Family therapy is based on the belief that a troubled or mentally ill person cannot be seen in isolation from the family unit. Disturbed children may merely reflect parental conflicts. This approach has become popular in recent years for dealing with the problems of children and adolescents.

Usually the therapist arranges regular meetings with the family to find out what feelings lie behind the way parents and children deal with each other. Through discussion and confrontation, these feelings can gradually be changed, leading to greater harmony and understanding.

Famotidine

A recently released (1986) *ulcer-healing drug* related to the *antihistamine drugs*. Famotidine reduces the secretion of acid in the stomach and, by doing so, promotes healing of *peptic ulcers* and reduces *esophagitis* (inflammation of the esophagus).

Fanconi's anemia

A rare type of aplastic *anemia*, characterized by a severely reduced production of all types of blood cells by the bone marrow.

Fanconi's syndrome

A rare kidney disorder, occurring mainly in childhood, in which various important nutrients and chemicals such as amino acids, phosphate, calcium, and potassium are lost in the urine; this leads to failure to thrive, stunting of growth, and bone disorders such as *rickets*.

Fanconi's syndrome has a wide variety of possible causes, including a number of rare inherited abnormalities of body chemistry; it may also occur as a side effect of some drugs, such as the ingestion of outdated tetracycline. In some cases there is no obvious cause.

The child may resume normal growth if an underlying chemical abnormality can be corrected. Alternatively, he or she may benefit from a

kidney transplant. In some cases, neither of these measures is possible or beneficial and kidney function progressively worsens, leading to death in childhood or early adolescence. Fanconi's syndrome in adults has a much brighter outlook.

Fantasy

The process of imagining events or objects that are not actually occurring or present. The term also refers to the mental image itself. Fantasy can give the illusion that wishes have been met. In this sense, it provides satisfaction and can be a means of helping people to cope when reality becomes too unpleasant. Fantasy can also be creative, stimulating ideas and activities by presenting mental images in new combinations.

Psychoanalysts believe that some fantasies are unconscious and represent certain primitive instincts; these fantasies are always presented to the conscious mind in symbols. For example, the fantasy of returning to the womb might be represented by the image of a cave deep within the earth.

Farmers' lung

An occupational disease affecting the lungs of farm workers in whom *hypersensitivity* (an excessive allergic reaction) develops when exposed to certain molds or fungi that grow on hay, grain, or straw.

CAUSES AND INCIDENCE

Farmers' lung is an example of an allergic *alveolitis*—a reaction of the lungs to inhaled dust containing fungal spores. The causative fungi grow on hay or grain that has been stored in warm, damp conditions. Outbreaks of farmers' lung often occur toward the end of a winter following a wet summer in areas with a high rainfall.

SYMPTOMS

Typical symptoms develop about six hours after exposure to dust containing fungal spores. The symptoms may include shortness of breath and flulike symptoms of fever, headache, and muscle aches. In single acute attacks, the symptoms persist for one or two days. Repeated exposure to the molds or fungi that provoked the attack may lead to a chronic form of the disease, causing permanent scarring of the lung tissues.

DIAGNOSIS AND TREATMENT

The physician takes a full occupational history and listens through a stethoscope for crackles. A chest X ray may show abnormalities; *pulmonary func-*

tion tests show that the efficiency of the lungs is reduced. Specific blood tests, indicating that the patient has antibodies to the fungus, can confirm the diagnosis.

The sufferer should avoid further exposure to moldy hay or grain; if symptoms persist, *corticosteroid drugs* may be prescribed. Complete recovery can be expected, provided the disease is diagnosed before permanent lung damage has occurred.

PREVENTION
Farmers can reduce their own and their workers' chances of developing the condition by reducing the water content of hay and grain before storage and by ensuring that storage conditions are cool and dry (to discourage growth of fungi). Well-ventilated work areas help prevent a buildup of fungal spores in the air; wearing protective masks may help.

Farsightedness
See *Hyperopia*.

Fascia
Fibrous *connective tissue* that surrounds many structures in the body. One layer of the tissue, known as the superficial fascia, envelopes the entire body just beneath the skin. Another layer, the deep fascia, encloses muscles, forming a sheath for individual muscles and separating them into groups. The deep fascia also holds in place soft organs, such as the kidneys. Thick fascia in the palm of the hand and sole of the foot have a cushioning, protective function.

Fasciculation
Spontaneous, irregular, and usually continual contractions of a muscle apparently at rest. Unlike *fibrillation*, a similar condition, fasciculation is visible under the skin and is described as fine or coarse.

A minor degree of fasciculation is common and is no cause for concern. However, persistent fasciculation with weakness in the affected muscle indicates damage to (or disease of) nerve cells in the spine that control the muscle or nerve fibers that connect the spinal nerves to the muscle; *motor neuron disease* is one such disorder.

Fasciitis
Inflammation of a layer of *fascia* (fibrous connective tissue), causing pain and tenderness. Fasciitis is usually the result of straining or injuring the fascia surrounding a muscle; it most commonly affects the sole of the foot (a condition called plantar fasciitis). It may occur in people who suffer from *ankylosing spondylitis* (rheumatism of the spine) or *Reiter's syndrome* (inflammation of the urethra with conjunctivitis and arthritis).

Treatment consists of resting the affected area and protecting it from pressure (i.e., by wearing cushioned pads in the shoes if the foot is affected). In some cases, injections of *corticosteroid drugs* have been given in an attempt to relieve pain.

Fasciotomy
An operation to relieve pressure on muscles by making an incision in the fascia (connective tissue) that surrounds them.

WHY IT IS DONE
Fasciotomy is usually performed to treat *compartment syndrome*, a painful condition in which a group of muscles is constricted with consequent obstruction of their blood flow. The condition can result in damage to, or even the death of, affected muscles. Fasciotomy gives the muscles space in which to expand.

The operation is also sometimes performed as a surgical emergency to treat a crush injury in which the muscle group has swollen or there is bleeding into the muscle compartment, raising the pressure within it.

HOW IT IS DONE
Fasciotomy is performed using a general anesthetic. An incision is made in the skin over the affected muscle group and then in the underlying fascia to allow the muscles to bulge through. For compartment syndrome, only a small incision is usually required; in an emergency procedure, a much larger incision may be needed.

Once the muscles have expanded through the opening, the wound is sewn up. In some cases, the muscle bulges out so much that a *skin graft* is required to repair the incision.

Fasting
Abstaining from all food and drinking only water. In temperate conditions and at moderate levels of physical activity, a person can survive on water alone for more than two months; without food or drink, death usually occurs within about 10 days (survival times are shorter in hot or cold conditions and at high levels of activity).

EFFECTS ON THE BODY
Without food, the energy needed to maintain essential body processes, such as *metabolism*, is supplied by substances stored in the body.

About six hours after the last meal, the body starts to use glycogen (a carbohydrate stored in the liver and muscles). This continues for about 24 hours, after which, while the body adapts to obtaining energy from stored fat, protein from the breakdown of muscles is also used as an energy source.

After a few days, most energy is obtained from fat, although some continues to come from muscle breakdown. If fasting continues, the body's metabolism slows to conserve energy. As a result of this slowdown, the fat and protein from muscles is consumed more slowly.

In the initial stages of fasting, weight loss is rapid. Later it slows, not only because metabolism slows down, but also because the body starts to conserve its salt supply, which causes water retention. Water that would normally be excreted in the urine is absorbed by the tissues. The accumulated fluid causes edema (swelling), mainly of the legs and abdomen.

In prolonged fasting, the ability to digest food may be impaired or lost entirely because the stomach gradually stops secreting digestive juices. If this occurs, medical supervision may be necessary when eating resumes. Prolonged fasting also halts the production of sex hormones, causing *amenorrhea* (absence of periods) in women. In addition, the body's ability to fight infection deteriorates, which, along with degeneration of the heart muscle, may be fatal.

FASTING TO REDUCE WEIGHT
Omitting a main meal each day for a limited period, or occasionally not eating anything for up to 24 hours, may be an effective means of losing weight. However, nobody should go without any food for more than a day without consulting a physician.

Fatigue
See *Tiredness*.

Fats and oils
Nutrients that provide the body with its most concentrated form of *energy*; 1 gram of fat provides nine Calories, whereas 1 gram of carbohydrate produces only four to five Calories.

Fats are compounds containing *carbon* and hydrogen with very little *oxygen*. Chemically, they consist mostly of *fatty acids* combined with an oily alcohol, *glycerol*. They are divided into two main groups, saturated and unsaturated, depending on the proportion of hydrogen atoms. If the fatty acids contain the maximum quantity possible of hydrogen, they are said to be saturated. If there are some sites on the carbon atom unoccupied by hydrogen, they are unsaturated; when many sites are vacant, they are polyunsaturated. Animal fats, such as those found in meat and dairy products, are highly saturated with hydrogen, while vegetable fats tend to be unsaturated to varying degrees.

There is no difference between fats and oils except in consistency. Saturated fats are solid at room temperature (but liquid when heated); oils are liquid at room temperature.

TYPES

Dietary fats are sources of the fat-soluble vitamins A, D, E, and K and of essential fatty acids. They are mainly triglycerides (combinations of glycerol and three fatty acids) but also contain other types of fats. Sources in the diet include not only the visible fats (such as butter, margarine, and vegetable oils) but also the so-called invisible fats found in meat, fish, poultry, and dairy products. The oils of certain cold-water ocean fish are being investigated for their potential ability to protect against coronary heart disease.

Structural fats (referred to as lipids) include triglycerides, phospholipids, and sterols. Triglycerides are the main form of fat found in stores of body fat. These stores act as an energy reserve as well as providing insulation and a protective layer for delicate organs. Phospholipids are structural fats found in cell membranes. Sterols, such as *cholesterol*, are found in animal and plant tissues; they have a variety of functions within the body, often being converted by chemical actions into hormones or vitamins.

FAT METABOLISM

Dietary fats are first dissolved by the action of bile salts and then broken down into fatty acids and glycerol by lipase, a pancreatic enzyme. They are absorbed via the lymphatic system before entering the bloodstream.

The lipids are carried in the blood bound to a protein, when they become known as lipoproteins. There are four classes of lipoprotein—chylomicrons, very low-density lipoproteins (VLDLs), high-density lipoproteins (HDLs), and low-density lipoproteins (LDLs). LDLs and VLDLs contain large amounts of cholesterol, which they carry through the bloodstream and deposit in cells. The HDLs pick up cholesterol and carry it back to the liver for processing and excretion. (See also *Nutrition*.)

Fatty acids

Organic acids, containing *carbon*, hydrogen, and *oxygen*, that are constituents of fats. There are over 40 different fatty acids found in nature, distinguished by their number of carbon atoms.

Certain fatty acids cannot be synthesized by the body and must be provided by the diet. These fatty acids are linoleic, linolenic, and arachidonic acids, sometimes referred to collectively as the essential fatty acids. (See also *Nutrition*.)

Favism

A disorder characterized by an extreme sensitivity to the broad bean *VICIA FABA* (fava). If an affected person eats these beans, a chemical in the bean causes rapid destruction of his or her red blood cells, leading to a severe type of anemia (see *Anemia, hemolytic*).

Favism is uncommon except in some areas of the Mediterranean, especially lowland Greece, where up to 10 percent of the population is affected. Favism is an inherited condition caused by a sex-linked *genetic disorder*. Affected people have a defect in a chemical pathway within their red blood cells that helps to protect the cells from injury. This defect is called glucose-6-phosphate dehydrogenase deficiency or *G6PD deficiency*.

Children in any family with a history of favism should be screened for the condition at an early age. If the disorder is found, they must avoid broad beans and certain drugs (including some antimalarials and antibiotics) that can have a similar destructive effect on their red blood cells. A list of drugs to avoid can be obtained from a physician when the disorder is diagnosed. With these precautions, affected people are able to remain in good health.

FDA

See *Food and Drug Administration*.

Febrile

Feverish or related to *fever*, as in febrile seizures—convulsions that occur mainly in young children who have high temperatures.

Fecal impaction

A large mass of hard feces that cannot be evacuated from the rectum. The condition usually is associated with long-standing *constipation*, along with dehydrated feces. Fecal impaction is most common in very young children and the elderly, especially those who are bedridden.

The main symptoms are an intense desire to have a bowel movement, pain in the rectum, anus, and center of the abdomen, and, in some instances, watery feces (which may be mistaken for diarrhea) that are passed around the impacted mass.

To diagnose the condition, the physician inserts a gloved finger into the rectum. Treatment consists of giving enemas (see *Enema*). If this is ineffective, the fecal mass may require removal manually.

Fecalith

A small, hard, almost stonelike piece of impacted feces that occasionally forms in a diverticulum (an outpouching, usually in the large intestine). A fecalith is harmless unless it blocks the entrance to the appendix, causing *appendicitis*, or a diverticulum, causing diverticulitis (see *Diverticular disease*).

Feces

Waste material from the digestive tract that is expelled through the anus. Solidified in the large intestine, feces consists of indigestible food residue (roughage, or dietary *fiber*), dead bacteria (which may account for as much as half the weight of the feces), dead cells shed from the intestinal lining, secretions from the intestine (such as mucus), bile from the liver (which colors the feces brown), and water.

Examination of the feces—for color, odor, consistency, or the presence of blood, pus, fat, parasites, or unusual microorganisms—is important in the diagnosis of digestive tract disorders. (See also *Feces, abnormal*.)

Feces, abnormal

Feces that differ from normal in color, odor, consistency, or content. The changes may be the result of a harmless condition, but in some cases they are due to a disorder of the digestive tract or a disorder of a related organ, such as the liver.

Liquid or very loose feces, passed frequently (see *Diarrhea*), may be due simply to anxiety but may also be caused by an intestinal infection (see *Gastroenteritis*); by an intestinal disorder such as *ulcerative colitis* or *Crohn's disease*; or by the *irritable bowel syndrome*. Loose stools may also reflect various states of *malabsorption*. At the other extreme, feces may be very hard and infrequently passed (see *Constipation*). Constipation is usually harmless but may be associated with rumbling and gurgling (*borborygmi*), bloating, and abdominal discomfort attributable to an irritable colon.

Pale feces may be due to diarrhea, to a lack of bile in the intestine as a result of *bile duct obstruction*, or to a disease that causes malabsorption (such as *celiac sprue*). In malabsorption, the paleness of the feces is due to the high fat content. Such feces may be oily, frothy, foul-smelling, and difficult to flush away.

Dark feces may simply be the result of unusually large amounts of iron or red wine in the diet. However, if feces are black, there may be bleeding in the stomach, duodenum, small intestine, or cecum.

Slimy feces, which contain excessive mucus, may be passed normally, but are sometimes associated with constipation or the irritable bowel syndrome. *Enteritis*, *dysentery*, or a tumor of the intestine (see *Intestine, tumors of*) may also cause slimy feces, often accompanied by blood.

Blood in the feces varies in appearance according to the site of bleeding. When blood is in the stomach or duodenum, it usually shows only as black, tarry feces; blood from a disease of the colon, such as ulcerative colitis or a tumor, is red and can usually be seen separate from the feces. Bleeding from the rectum, which occurs with *hemorrhoids* or rectal tumors, often streaks the feces, is visible only on toilet paper, or drips into the toilet bowl. This blood is usually bright red.

INVESTIGATION

Blood in the feces and any other persistent abnormality should be reported immediately to a physician, who may ask for a sample of the feces. (See also *Rectal bleeding*.)

Feces, blood in the

See *Feces, abnormal*; *Rectal bleeding*.

Feeding, artificial

Administration of nutrients other than by mouth, usually through a tube inserted into the stomach or small intestine. Occasionally, a tube is inserted directly into the stomach or jejunum (upper part of the small intestine) by surgical means. This is called enteral nutrition. If the gastrointestinal tract is not functioning, food must be sent into the bloodstream by *intravenous infusion*. This technique is known as total parenteral nutrition.

WHY IT IS DONE

Tube feeding may be necessary for people with disorders of the gastro-

intestinal tract, *malabsorption*, or neurological or renal disorders. Premature babies often require tube feeding if their sucking reflexes are undeveloped, as do burn or fever patients because of their increased nutritional requirements.

Intravenous feeding is usually necessary when there has been damage to the small intestine as a result of disease or surgical removal of large areas of the absorbing surface.

HOW IT IS DONE

TUBE FEEDING Suitable food mixtures or preparations of predetermined levels of nutrients are administered via a narrow plastic tube. The tube is passed through the patient's nose (guided via the nasopharynx to the esophagus) and into either the stomach or the duodenum.

If tube feeding is the sole means of nutrition, it must provide all of the essential nutrients (and adequate fluids) to meet the person's daily needs, which can vary markedly. There are two alternative methods of tube feeding—bolus feeding and continuous drip feeding.

Bolus feeding involves the rapid administration of a set amount of nutrients at intermittent periods throughout the day. Continuous drip feeding is, however, more widely preferred because it is tolerated better by the patient. In both methods the rate of flow can be controlled by a pump. The tube is left in place for adults and older children, but, for infants and young children, it is removed and reinserted for each feeding.

INTRAVENOUS FEEDING This method is generally used only when tube feeding is impractical or ineffective; its main drawback is the risk of introducing infection directly into the bloodstream or of blocking a blood vessel. Some problems with the liver or gallbladder have occurred.

The nutrient preparations are given directly into a large central vein near the heart via a catheter (thin, flexible tube) inserted using an anesthetic and strict *aseptic techniques*. Intravenous feeding is sometimes used to supplement feeding by mouth, but can if necessary provide all the nutrients needed to meet a patient's requirements. Essential vitamins and minerals are included.

Feeding, infant

During a baby's first year, it grows more rapidly than at any other time in its life. A good diet is essential for healthy growth.

BREAST- OR BOTTLE-FEEDING

NUTRITIONAL REQUIREMENTS During the first four to six months, most babies' nutritional requirements are met by milk alone, whether by *breast-feeding* or *bottle-feeding*. Both human milk and artificial milk (modified dried cow's milk) contain carbohydrate, protein, fat, vitamins, and minerals in similar proportions (see *Milk* for components), but human milk is the food of choice because it provides these nutrients in the perfect blend as well as containing antibodies and white blood cells that protect the baby against infections.

After the baby is 6 months old, vitamin D supplements should be given to breast-fed babies and to bottle-fed babies whose locations or backgrounds pose a risk of rickets. At 6 months a baby can safely be taken off artificial milk and fed with natural cow's milk. Supplementary vitamin D should be given until the baby is established on a mixed diet. Drops containing vitamins A, C, and D, although often given, are usually not required by most infants.

If a baby seems unable to tolerate milk of any kind (see *Food allergy*; *Food intolerance*), the pediatrician should be consulted; he or she may recommend a preparation based on soybeans, vegetable oils, sucrose, corn sugar, modified meat protein, and other substances. Babies should not be fed skim milk, which has relatively too much protein and minerals and insufficient calories compared with whole milk.

EMOTIONAL REQUIREMENTS For healthy emotional development, a baby requires warmth, security, and contentment; the act of feeding plays an important part in meeting these needs. Breast-feeding is again preferable in this respect because it establishes an intimate bond between mother and child, but bottle-feeding is a perfectly satisfactory alternative if the baby is cuddled and talked to while he or she is fed.

INTRODUCING SOLIDS

Solid foods, initially in the form of purees and cereals, should be introduced into an infant's diet at some time between the ages of 3 and 6 months, depending on the baby's birth weight and rate of growth. By 6 months the baby should be eating some true solids, such as chopped up meat and vegetables. The accompanying chart gives the optimum times for the introduction of solids, but a baby's general contentment also provides some guide. A rapidly growing baby

F

F

who is unable to drink enough milk to satisfy his or her hunger needs the more concentrated calories found in solid food.

Many parents prefer to give their infants home-prepared purees rather than prepared foods. In this case, salt and other additives should not be used, since an overconcentration of salt and other minerals can dangerously overburden a baby's kidneys. Sugar, too, should be kept to a minimum in the diet; a baby easily learns to have a "sweet tooth," which will lead to future dental decay; for the same reason, babies should not be given bottles of sweetened drinks to comfort them.

A baby can live healthily on a vegetarian diet (one that contains no meat or fish) provided eggs are included, but a baby fed on a vegan diet (one that also excludes all animal products, such as dairy produce and eggs) runs the risk of severe malnutrition. A vegan diet makes it very hard to obtain enough calories, essential fatty acids, vitamins (especially B_{12}), and protein. Overall, it is a very bad diet for infants and growing children whose nutrient requirements are much greater than adults.

FEEDING PROBLEMS
Any difficulties associated with milk usually appear within the first month.

Some babies have an intolerance to certain foods; reactions can include vomiting, diarrhea, or allergic rashes. For this reason, solids should be introduced one by one so that any that cause problems can be identified.

Prolonged crying after feedings may mean that the baby needs help bringing up gas, that artificial milk is not being digested properly, or that the baby has colic (see *Colic, infantile*). See also *Nutritional disorders.*

Fee for service
The traditional financial arrangement between patient and physician. The patient is charged for each service he or she receives; the physician is compensated for each service he or she provides. (See also *Health maintenance organization.*)

Femoral epiphysis, slipped
Displacement of the upper *epiphysis* (growing end) of the femur (thigh bone). Such displacement is rare, usually affects those between the ages of 11 and 13, and occurs more often in boys, in obese children with delayed sexual and physical development, and in children who grow rapidly.

APPROXIMATE AGES FOR INTRODUCING SOLIDS

4 months	At second breast- or bottle-feeding offer one or two	teaspoons of vegetable or fruit puree or cereal.
4½ months	At second breast- or bottle-feeding offer two teaspoons of cereal. At third breast- or bottle-	feeding offer two teaspoons of vegetable or fruit puree.
5 to 6 months	*Early morning* Breast- or bottle-feeding. *Breakfast* Two teaspoons of cereal and lightly boiled egg yolk, followed by breast- or bottle-feeding. *Lunch* One teaspoon of meat or fish puree with three teaspoons	of strained vegetables. Offer water or well-diluted fruit juice instead of milk. *Mid-afternoon* Mashed banana or other soft fruit followed by usual milk feeding. *Dinner* Breast- or bottle-feeding if the baby is still hungry.
6 to 7 months	*Early morning* Breast- or bottle-feeding. *Breakfast* Two teaspoons of cereal with lightly scrambled egg. Offer cow's milk from a cup.	*Lunch* Offer minced or mashed food instead of pureed. Give meat or fish with some vegetables, then offer yogurt and fruit. Give a drink of water or well-diluted fruit juice.
7 to 8 months	*Early morning* Offer a drink of water or diluted juice instead of the milk. *Breakfast* Cereal and boiled egg with whole-grain bread and butter. A drink of cow's milk. *Lunch* Cheese, fish, or minced	meat with mashed vegetables. Pudding or fresh fruit. A drink of water or well-diluted fruit juice. *Late afternoon/dinner* Whole-grain bread and butter with peanut butter or cheese. Fresh fruit and a drink of cow's milk.
9 to 12 months	*Early morning* A drink of water or well-diluted fruit juice. *Breakfast* Cereal, then egg or fish with whole-grain toast and butter. A drink of cow's milk. *Lunch* Chopped meat or fish, or	cheese, with vegetables. Pudding or fresh fruit. A drink of water or well-diluted fruit juice. *Late afternoon/dinner* Meat or cheese sandwiches. A drink of cow's milk.

While the bone is still growing, the epiphysis is separated from the shaft of the bone by a plate of cartilage. This constitutes a zone of relative weakness in the bone, so that a fall or other injury, even a minor one, can cause the epiphysis to slip out of position.

SYMPTOMS
A limp develops and the child feels pain in the knee rather than in the hip. The leg tends to turn outward and hip movements are restricted.

TREATMENT
An operation is performed using general anesthetic to manipulate the displaced parts of bone and fix them together with metal pins. To prevent possible damage to the other thigh, it, too, may be strengthened with pins during the same operation.

OUTLOOK
Surgery usually provides an effective repair and prevents further accidents of the same type. However, after the injury, the hip tends to be more susceptible than normal to *osteoarthritis*. In rare cases, the hip becomes stiff and painful, sometimes permanently so.

Femoral nerve
One of the primary nerves of the leg. It is made up of fibers from nerves in the second, third, and fourth segments of the lumbar spinal cord. The nerves emerge from the lower back region of the spine and run down into the thigh, where they branch to supply the skin and muscles of the front of the thigh. The nerve branches that supply the skin convey sensation; the branches that supply the muscles stimulate contraction of the *quadriceps muscle* of the thigh, causing the knee to straighten.

Damage to the femoral nerve (which impairs the ability of the knee to straighten) is usually caused by a slipped disk in the lumbar region of the spine (see *Disk prolapse*). Damage may also occur as the result of a backward dislocation of the hip or, rarely, as a result of a *neuropathy*.

Femur

The medical name for the thigh bone, the longest bone in the body. The lower end hinges with the tibia (shin) to form the knee joint. The upper end is rounded into a ball (head of the femur) that fits into a socket in the pelvis to form the hip joint. The head of the femur is joined to the bone shaft by a narrow piece of bone called the neck of the femur. While it gives the hip joint a wide range of movement, the neck of the femur is a point of structural weakness and a common fracture site (see *Femur, fracture of*).

The femur can be felt through the skin at two sites. At the lower end, the bone is enlarged to form two lumps (the condyles) that distribute the weight-bearing load on the knee joint. On the outer side of the upper end of the femur is a protuberance (called the greater trochanter).

The shaft of the femur is surrounded by powerful muscles whose principal functions are to move the hip and knee joints. The shaft is also well supplied with blood vessels; because of this, a fracture can result in considerable blood loss.

LOCATION OF THE FEMUR

The femur extends from the hip joint, down the thigh, to the knee joint.

Greater trochanter

Neck of femur

Femur

Condyles

Tibia

Femur, fracture of

The nature, symptoms, treatment, and possible complications of a fractured femur (thigh bone) depend on whether the bone has broken across its neck (the short section between the top of the shaft and the hip joint) or across the shaft.

NECK OF FEMUR

This type of fracture is very common in elderly people suffering from *osteoporosis* (thinning of the bone) and is usually associated with a fall. The broken ends of the bone are often considerably displaced; in such cases there is usually severe pain in the hip and groin (made worse by movement) and the leg cannot bear any weight. Occasionally, the broken ends of bone become impacted (wedged together). In this case there is less pain and walking is often still possible, which may delay reporting of the injury and detection of the fracture.

DIAGNOSIS AND TREATMENT Diagnosis of a suspected fracture is confirmed by X ray. If the bone ends are displaced, an operation using general anesthesia is necessary, either to realign the bone ends (a procedure called reduction) and to fasten them together with metal screws, plates, or nails, or to replace the entire head and neck of the femur with a metal or plastic substitute (see *Hip joint replacement*). Both procedures produce a stable repair, and hip and knee movement can be resumed immediately.

If the bone ends are impacted, the person is kept in bed for a few weeks to prevent any jarring movement that might dislodge the bones. The fracture heals naturally without surgery, but supervised exercise is necessary to maintain hip and knee mobility. X rays are taken periodically to determine how well the fracture is healing.

With either type of repair, walking is started with the aid of crutches, progresses to walking with a walker, walking with a cane, and, finally, walking without aid.

COMPLICATIONS These depend on the site of the fracture. A break at the union of the neck and shaft may result in hip deformity (see *Coxa vara*). A fracture across the neck itself may damage the blood supply to the head of the femur, causing the head to crumble (osteonecrosis). As a result, the bone ends may fail to fuse, or *osteoarthritis* may develop. In either case, more surgery (usually hip joint replacement) is required. Osteoarthritis may also develop even if avascular necrosis does not occur.

SHAFT OF FEMUR

This type of fracture usually occurs when the femur is subjected to extreme force, such as in an automobile accident. In most cases, the bone ends are considerably displaced, causing severe pain, tenderness, and swelling.

DIAGNOSIS AND TREATMENT Diagnosis of this injury is confirmed by X rays. With a fractured femoral shaft there is often substantial blood loss from the bone. In most cases, the fracture is repaired by an operation (using general anesthesia) in which the two ends of the bone are realigned and fastened together with a long metal pin. However, sometimes the bone ends can be realigned by manipulation, and surgery is not necessary. After realignment of the bones, the leg is supported with a *splint* and put in *traction* to hold the bone together while it heals.

Following both types of treatment, supervised exercise and massage of the knee, ankle, and foot is started to prevent the joints from becoming stiff. The progress of healing is checked regularly by X rays; when it is complete, weight bearing and walking is started gradually.

COMPLICATIONS These include failure of the bone ends to unite or successful fusion of the broken ends at the wrong angle, infection of the bone, or damage to a nerve or artery. All of these complications usually require more surgery. A fracture of the lower end of the shaft can result in permanent stiffness of the knee.

Fenoprofen

A *nonsteroidal anti-inflammatory drug* (NSAID). Fenoprofen is used to relieve pain and stiffness caused, for example, by *rheumatoid arthritis*, *osteoarthritis*, and *gout*. Fenoprofen is also used in the treatment of muscle and ligament sprains; it reduces pain and helps speed recovery.

Ferrous sulfate

An alternative name for iron sulfate (see *Iron*).

Fertility

The ability to reproduce children without undue difficulty.

MALE FERTILITY

A man's fertility depends on the production of normal quantities of healthy *sperm* in the testes, and on the ability to achieve *erection* and to ejaculate *semen* into the vagina during *sexual intercourse*.

F

THE PROCESS OF FERTILIZATION

Fertilization occurs when the head of a sperm penetrates a mature ovum in a fallopian tube. After penetration, the nuclei (which contain the genetic material) of the sperm and ovum fuse, and the body and tail of the sperm drop off. The newly fertilized ovum, called a zygote, then forms an outer layer that is impenetrable to other sperm. The zygote undergoes repeated cell divisions as it passes down the fallopian tube, so that, by the time it reaches the uterus, it has grown into a solid ball of cells called a morula. It then develops an inner cavity with a small cluster of cells to one side; this is called a blastula.

FERTILE PERIOD

Ovulation occurs about halfway through the menstrual cycle (14 to 16 days before the start of a period), after which the released ovum is available for fertilization for about two days. Sperm can also live for approximately two days, so the actual fertile period is about four days.

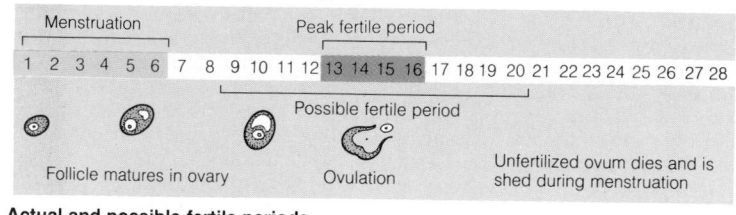

Actual and possible fertile periods
Although the actual fertile period is about four days, the possible fertile period may last seven to 12 days, due to variations in how long the ovum and sperm can survive and the timing of ovulation. The illustration shows the actual and maximum possible fertile periods in a 28-day cycle.

Sperm and ovum
A single sperm penetrates the ovum, thereby fertilizing it. To achieve this, the sperm releases enzymes that dissolve a path through the ovum's outer layers.

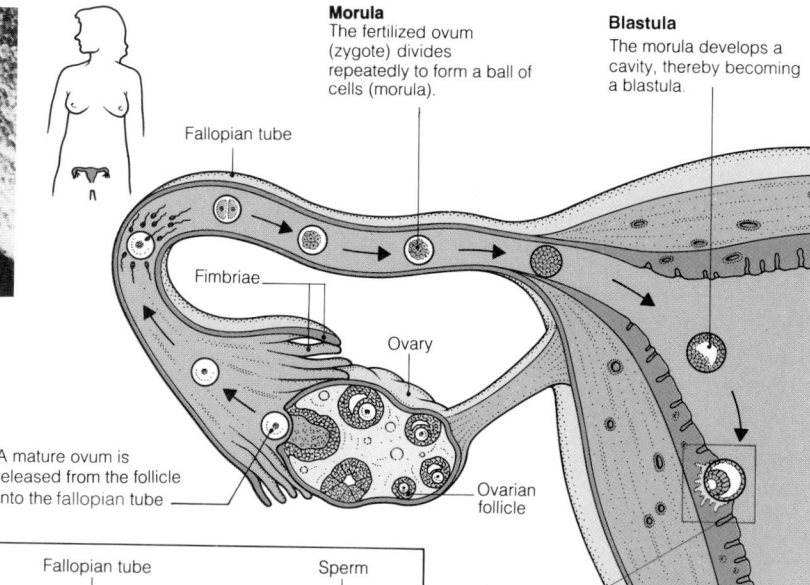

Morula
The fertilized ovum (zygote) divides repeatedly to form a ball of cells (morula).

Blastula
The morula develops a cavity, thereby becoming a blastula.

Fallopian tube

Fimbriae

Ovary

A mature ovum is released from the follicle into the fallopian tube

Ovarian follicle

Uterus

Blastula

Uterine wall

Blastula
The blastula embeds in the uterine wall (implantation), where it develops into an embryo and also forms the placenta.

JOURNEY OF THE SPERM

When semen is ejaculated into the vagina, as many as 500 million sperm are released, most of which are capable of fertilizing an ovum. But, as they travel upward (propelled by their whiplike tails), more than half are killed by acidic vaginal secretions; many more die during the journey up through the cervix and uterus and into the fallopian tubes. The journey can take from one to five hours, and, in the end, only a few thousand sperm have survived.

Fallopian tube

Sperm

Ovum

Ovary

Uterus

Cervix

Vagina

Penis

Life span of sperm
A sperm can live in a fallopian tube for up to 48 hours, during which time it is capable of fertilizing an ovum.

The testes—under the influence of *gonadotropin hormones* from the pituitary gland—produce hundreds of millions of sperm. The large output is necessary for normal fertility because only about one in 80,000 sperm ejaculated into the vagina reaches a fallopian tube (see *Fertilization*).

Normal fertility also requires a large proportion of the sperm to be healthy. After ejaculation, the sperm must be able to pass through the hostile environment of acid secretions in the vagina, penetrate a barrier of mucus around the cervix, and swim upward into the fallopian tubes.

Men become fertile at puberty and usually remain so (although to a lesser degree) well into old age.

FEMALE FERTILITY
The ability of a woman to conceive depends on normal *ovulation* (the monthly production of a healthy *ovum* by one of the ovaries) and the egg's unimpeded passage down a fallopian tube toward the uterus, on thinning of the mucus surrounding the mouth of the cervix to enable sperm to penetrate more easily, and on changes in the lining of the uterus that prepare it for the implantation of a fertilized ovum. These processes are in turn dependent on normal production of gonadotropins by the pituitary, and on production of the sex hormones *estrogen* and *progesterone* by the ovaries.

Women become fertile at puberty and remain so until *menopause*, which usually occurs during a woman's 40s or 50s. (See also illustrated box, left; *Fertility drugs*; *Infertility*.)

Fertility drugs
A diverse group of hormonal or hormone-related drugs used to treat female and male *infertility*. In women, fertility drugs may be prescribed when abnormal hormone production by the pituitary gland or ovaries disrupts *ovulation* or causes mucus around the cervix to become so thick that sperm cannot penetrate it. In men, fertility drugs may be used when abnormal hormone production by the pituitary gland or the testes interferes with normal sperm production. (See also *Clomiphene*; *Gonadotropin hormones*; *Infertility*.)

Fertilization

The union of a *sperm* and an *ovum*. In natural fertilization, this occurs after *sexual intercourse* (see box). Fertilization may also occur as a result of semen being artificially intro-duced into the cervix (see *Artificial insemination*), or may take place in the laboratory (see *In vitro fertilization*).

Fetal alcohol syndrome
A combination of birth defects resulting from high alcohol consumption by the mother during pregnancy.

Even small amounts of alcohol may be harmful in pregnancy, since (like tobacco) alcohol seems to affect fetal growth. The risks of miscarriage and congenital physical defects may also be increased. Fetal alcohol syndrome, however, normally occurs only if there is persistent alcohol consumption during pregnancy. Fetal alcohol syndrome has been reported in babies of women who consistently drank 30 milliliters of alcohol per day (equal to two mixed drinks or two to three bottles of beer or glasses of wine). While there is no evidence that an occasional glass of wine or beer is dangerous, it is best to abstain completely from alcohol during pregnancy.

The affected baby is abnormally short, has small eyes with epicanthic folds (vertical folds of skin extending from the upper eyelid to the side of the nose), and a small jaw. He or she may have a small brain, a cleft palate, heart defects, a dislocated hip, and other joint deformities. As a newborn, the baby sucks poorly, sleeps badly, and is irritable. In effect, he or she is suffering from alcohol withdrawal.

Almost one fifth of affected babies die during the first few weeks of life; many who survive are physically and mentally retarded to some degree. (See also *Alcohol dependence*.)

Fetal circulation
Blood circulates differently in the fetus than it does after birth (see *Circulatory system*). The fetus neither breathes nor eats, so oxygen and nutrients are obtained—via the *placenta* and *umbilical cord*—from the mother's blood. The other fundamental difference in circulation is that blood bypasses the lungs in the fetus.

Oxygen and nutrients enter the fetal blood in the placenta, an organ embedded in the inner lining and wall of the uterus and connected to the fetus by the umbilical cord. The oxygenated blood flows to the fetus along a vein in the umbilical cord, then enters the right atrium (right upper chamber) of the heart, after which, instead of flowing to the lungs, it bypasses them. It does this by passing into the left atrium through a hole called the foramen ovale.

The blood then passes to the left ventricle (left lower chamber), from where it is pumped to the upper parts of the body to provide the tissues with oxygen. It then returns to the heart, flowing into the right atrium and from there into the right ventricle. (After birth, blood pumped from this ventricle passes via the pulmonary artery to the lungs for reoxygenation and elimination of carbon dioxide and other wastes.) However, in the fetus, the blood is only partly deoxygenated at this stage and has more tissues to supply with oxygen. Bypassing the lungs again, it flows from the pulmonary artery into the aorta; it does this through a channel called the ductus arteriosus which, like the foramen ovale, closes after birth.

Before birth

To upper body
Foramen ovale
Ductus arteriosus
Right atrium
Left atrium
Right ventricle
Left ventricle
From placenta
To lower body/ placenta

After birth

To upper body
To lungs
Ductus arteriosus closed
Foramen ovale closed
From lungs
From lower body
To lower body

Fetal heart circulation
In the fetus, blood passes from the right atrium of the heart to the left atrium through the foramen ovale. Another channel, the ductus arteriosus, allows blood to pass from the pulmonary artery to the aorta. Both channels close after birth.

The aorta carries the blood to the lower parts of the body, from where, completely deoxygenated, it is carried by two arteries in the umbilical cord to the placenta. There, carbon dioxide and other waste products diffuse into, and are carried away by, the mother's blood and are excreted by the mother.

In rare cases, the foramen ovale or ductus arteriosus fails to close after birth, causing a congenital heart disorder (see *Heart disease, congenital*).

F

Fetal distress

Physical stress experienced by a fetus during labor as the result of not receiving enough oxygen. The most stressful period of labor for a baby is during a contraction, when the uterus tightens to squeeze it out and thus reduces its supply of oxygen from the placenta. If, in addition, there are problems with the labor, such as the mother losing blood or having a pelvis too small for the size of the baby's head, the amount of oxygen reaching the baby may be inadequate.

MONITORING

Fetal distress causes the baby's heart rate to slow, which can be seen as a dip on a cardiotocograph (see *Fetal heart monitoring*). Alternatively, a distressed baby may show no variability in heart rate. This is in contrast to a healthy baby, whose heart rate varies within a normal range of from 120 to 160 beats per minute. The obstetrician keeps a close watch on the heart rate and, if necessary, may obtain a blood sample from the baby's scalp for analysis. High acidity indicates that the baby is not getting enough oxygen. In addition, the fluid around the baby is examined for signs of meconium (fetal feces), which a distressed baby often passes.

DELIVERY

A fetus in distress needs to be delivered promptly—by *cesarean section* if oxygen shortage occurs during the first stage of labor, and by *forceps delivery* or *vacuum extraction* during the second stage.

Fetal heart monitoring

Use of an instrument to record and/or listen to an unborn baby's heart beat during pregnancy and labor. Some form of monitoring of fetal well-being is performed during labor in all hospitals. In its simplest form the nurse or obstetrician uses a special fetal stethoscope to listen to the baby's heart beat. A more sophisticated version is the electronic fetal heart monitor, which is used to make a continuous paper or sound recording of the heart beat.

WHY IT IS DONE

In pregnancy, monitoring is carried out at intervals if tests indicate that the placenta is not functioning normally or if the baby's growth has been slow. Uterine contractions or other stimuli, such as the baby kicking, increases the heart rate in a healthy fetus; the obstetrician can detect this using a fetal heart monitor.

During labor, monitoring can detect *fetal distress*, caused by the baby not receiving enough oxygen. A fetus deprived of oxygen has an abnormal heart rate. Fetal monitoring can detect this abnormality and, at an early stage, allows the attending physician to take appropriate action.

HOW IT IS DONE

An electronic fetal monitor is used to make a continuous recording of the baby's heart beat. The beat is picked up either externally by an ultrasound transmitter strapped to the mother's abdomen or, as an alternative during labor, internally by an electrode attached to the baby's head and linked to the recording device by a wire inserted through the mother's vagina. The fetal heart beat is amplified and heard as a beeping noise or printed as a paper trace. Electronic monitors also have a pressure gauge for measuring and recording contractions. Contractions of the uterus can also be measured by an external gauge that is strapped to the mother's abdomen or by an internal plastic tube that is inserted through the vagina into the amniotic fluid.

ADVANTAGES AND DISADVANTAGES

Electronic fetal monitoring has the advantage of giving the physician a minute-by-minute assessment of the baby's condition. Many obstetricians are convinced that babies are less likely to become hypoxic (deprived of oxygen) during labor with continuous monitoring and therefore feel that the monitoring results in healthier babies.

However, routine electronic fetal monitoring has been controversial for a number of reasons. Critics have claimed that it limits maternal mobility during labor and that it leads to overdiagnosis of fetal distress and therefore to unnecessary cesarean sections. Critics also claim that external monitoring unnecessarily exposes the healthy baby to ultrasound and that internal monitoring may increase the risk of infection during labor without resulting in improvement in the outcome of low-risk pregnancies.

Fetishism

Reliance on special objects for achieving sexual arousal. Fetishism is thought to be rare and restricted to men; because of the nature of the practice, there are no reliable statistics.

The objects need not have an obvious sexual meaning; they include shoes, gloves, rubber or leather garments, and parts of the body such as the feet or ears. It seems that once a particular fetish has led to successful orgasm, it becomes increasingly difficult to obtain sexual satisfaction without it. Nevertheless, many fetishists are able to have a stable sexual relationship, provided their partners join in the practice.

CAUSES

Fetishism usually has no obvious cause, although it may, rarely, result from certain forms of brain damage. According to psychoanalysts, the origin may be a childhood *fixation* of sexual interest upon some aspect of the mother's body or appearance.

TREATMENT

As long as fetishism does not impair sexual or social life, there is no reason for any form of medical interference. Treatment is needed only if the behavior is causing distress or if there are persistent criminal acts, such as stealing underwear.

Fetoscopy

A procedure for directly observing a fetus inside the uterus by means of a fetoscope, a type of *endoscope* (flexible viewing tube). The fetoscope can also be used to take samples of fetal blood and tissue for *biopsy* and to permit treatment of some fetal disorders.

WHY IT IS DONE

Fetoscopy is used to diagnose various congenital abnormalities and genetic defects before the baby is born. Because the technique carries some risks, it is attempted only if there is a higher-than-normal chance that the baby will have some abnormality (for example, if the mother has already had an abnormal baby or if there is a family history of genetic defects).

Fetoscopy allows a close-up look at the developing fetus, particularly the face, limbs, genitals, and spine, and can detect abnormalities, such as spinal column defects, facial clefts, and limb defects. By attaching additional instruments, the fetoscope can also be used to surgically correct some defects, such as certain urinary system disorders. (See also *Amniocentesis; Chorionic villus sampling*.)

Fetus

The unborn child from the end of the eighth week after fertilization until birth. For the first eight weeks, the unborn child is called an *embryo*.

The fetus develops in the mother's uterus in a sac filled with *amniotic fluid*, which cushions it against injury. The oxygen and nutrients the fetus needs are supplied through the *placenta*, an organ embedded in the inner wall of the uterus and attached to the fetus by the umbilical cord (see box).

DEVELOPMENT OF THE FETUS

By the 32nd week of pregnancy, the internal organs of the fetus are almost fully mature and it is perfectly formed. In most cases, the fetus has turned to lie head-down in the pelvis.

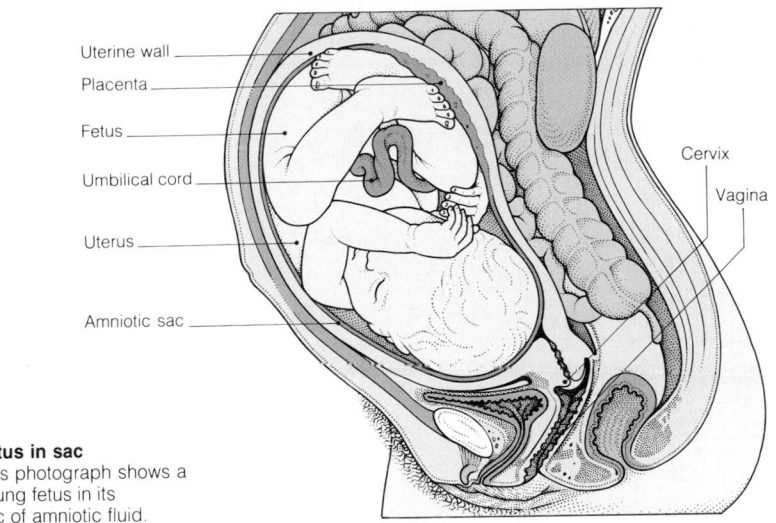

Uterine wall
Placenta
Fetus
Umbilical cord
Uterus
Amniotic sac
Cervix
Vagina

Fetus in sac
This photograph shows a young fetus in its sac of amniotic fluid.

GROWTH OF THE FETUS FROM 8 TO 40 WEEKS

Between the eighth week and term (40th week), the length of the fetus increases twentyfold; its weight increases about 1,700 times.

Week	8	12	16	20	24	28	32	36	40
Length	1.0 in.	3.0 in.	6.5 in.	10.0 in.	13.0 in.	14.5 in.	16.0 in.	18.0 in.	20.0 in.
Weight	0.07 oz.	0.6 oz.	5.0 oz.	12.0 oz.	1.3 lbs.	2.0 lbs.	3.5 lbs.	5.5 lbs.	7.5 lbs.

Fever

Known medically as pyrexia, a fever is defined as a body temperature above 98.6°F, measured in the mouth, or 99.8°F, measured in the rectum.

A fever may be accompanied by other symptoms, such as shivering, headache, sweating, thirst, a flushed face, hot skin, and faster than normal breathing. In some cases there may be rigors (attacks of severe shivering followed by drenching sweats and a sudden fall in body temperature). Confusion or delirium sometimes occurs with fever, especially in the elderly; a very high fever may also cause seizures or coma.

CAUSES

Most fevers are caused by bacterial or viral infections, such as typhoid, tonsillitis, influenza, or measles. In these cases, proteins called pyrogens are released when the white blood cells of the body's defense system fight the microorganisms responsible for the illness. These pyrogens act on the temperature-controlling center in the brain, causing it to raise body temperature in an attempt to destroy the invading microorganisms.

Fever may also occur in noninfectious conditions, such as dehydration, thyrotoxicosis (a condition that results from overactivity of the thyroid gland), myocardial infarction (heart attack), and tumors of the lymphatic system. Its function is not understood in such cases. (See also *Fever* chart, next page.)

TREATMENT

A physician should be consulted if a fever lasts longer than three days or if there are atypical accompanying symptoms, such as severe headache with stiff neck, abdominal pain, or painful urination. Medical advice is also necessary if the sufferer is a baby less than 6 months old, a child with a history of febrile seizures (see *Seizures, febrile*), or an elderly person.

Antipyretic (temperature-lowering) drugs may be given to treat fevers due to infections; such drugs also help relieve any aches and pains accompanying the fever. Otherwise, treatment is directed toward the underlying cause (for example, giving the appropriate antibiotics for a bacterial infection).

Febrile seizures can often be prevented by cooling the entire body as soon as the fever starts, either in a lukewarm bath or by sponging with lukewarm water.

Fever blister

Also known as a cold sore, a blister caused by the *herpes simplex* virus, usually on the face. The term dates from the preantibiotic era, when such blisters would often appear during feverish infectious illnesses.

FEVER Temperature of about 100°F (38°C) or above. Consult your physician if your temperature remains raised for longer than 48 hours or rises above 104°F (40°C) .

Do you have a cough? → YES →

Are you short of breath even when resting AND/OR have you been coughing up brownish sputum (phlegm)? → YES →

☎
Call your physician without delay!
A chest infection such as pneumonia is a possibility. This may be serious, especially in the elderly and those in poor health.

See • *Pneumonia*

NO ↓

Have you been coughing up gray-yellow sputum (phlegm) AND/OR have you been wheezing? → YES →

Infection of the airways in the lung is a possibility. Consult your physician.

See • *Bronchitis*

NO ↓

Do you have one or more of the following symptoms?
• headache
• aching limbs
• runny nose
• sore throat
→ YES →

A generalized viral infection such as the flu is a strong possibility. Take analgesics (painkillers) as required and drink plenty of fluids.

NO

Do you have a severe headache? → YES →

Do you have two or more of the following symptoms?
• pain when you bend your head forward
• nausea or vomiting
• dislike of bright light
• drowsiness or confusion
→ YES →

☎
Call your physician without delay!
Inflammation of the membranes surrounding the brain due to infection may be the cause of such symptoms.

See • *Meningitis*

NO ↓

Do you have one or more of the following symptoms?
• aching limbs
• runny nose
• sore throat
→ YES →

A generalized viral infection such as the flu is a strong possibility. Take analgesics (painkillers) as required and drink plenty of fluids.

NO

Do you have a sore throat? → YES →

You may have a throat infection. Consult your physician.

See • *Pharyngitis*
    • *Strep throat*
    • *Tonsillitis*

NO

Continued on next page

F

F

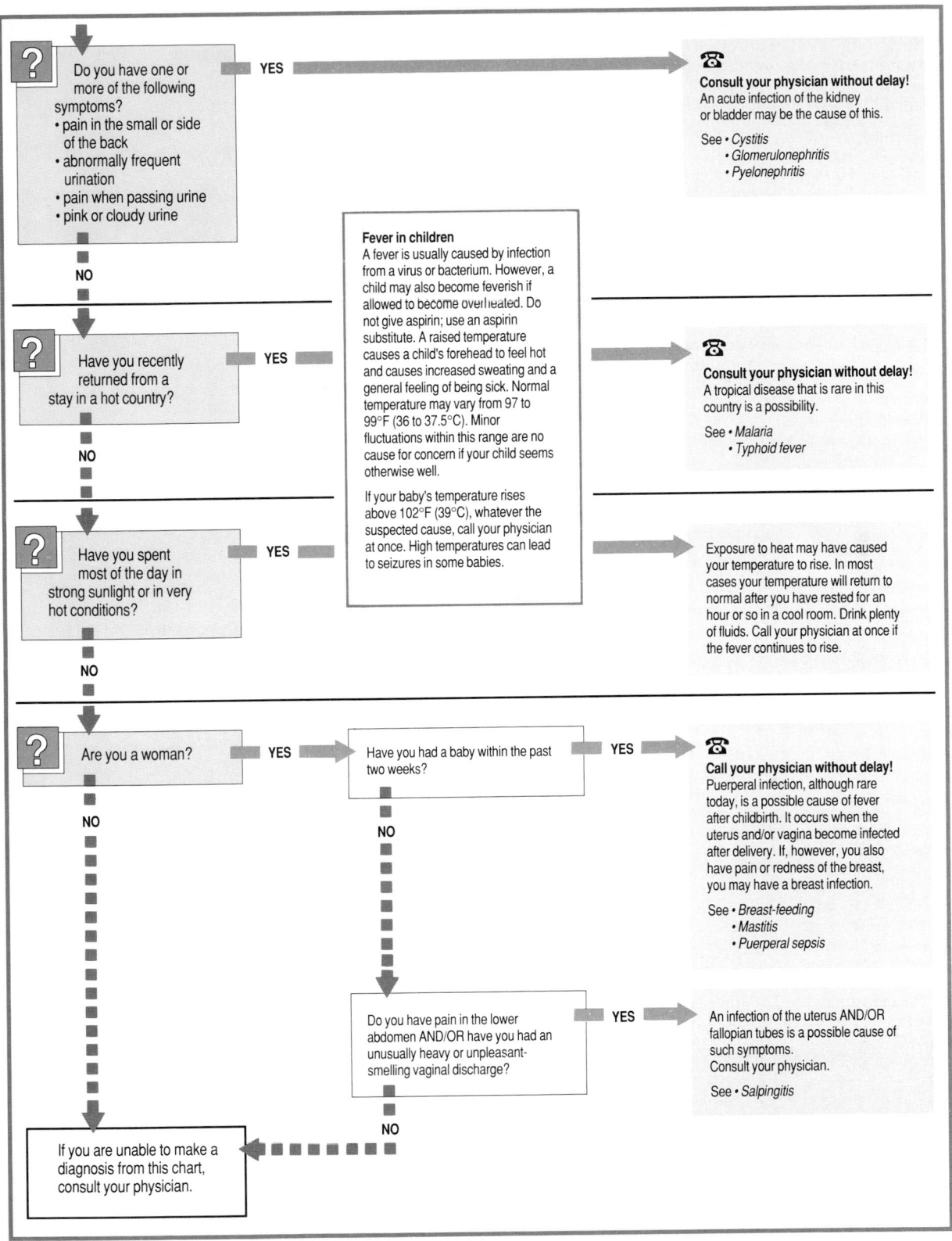

? Do you have one or more of the following symptoms?
- pain in the small or side of the back
- abnormally frequent urination
- pain when passing urine
- pink or cloudy urine

YES →

☎
Consult your physician without delay!
An acute infection of the kidney or bladder may be the cause of this.

See • *Cystitis*
    • *Glomerulonephritis*
    • *Pyelonephritis*

NO ↓

? Have you recently returned from a stay in a hot country?

YES →

☎
Consult your physician without delay!
A tropical disease that is rare in this country is a possibility.

See • *Malaria*
    • *Typhoid fever*

NO ↓

? Have you spent most of the day in strong sunlight or in very hot conditions?

YES →

Exposure to heat may have caused your temperature to rise. In most cases your temperature will return to normal after you have rested for an hour or so in a cool room. Drink plenty of fluids. Call your physician at once if the fever continues to rise.

NO ↓

Fever in children
A fever is usually caused by infection from a virus or bacterium. However, a child may also become feverish if allowed to become overheated. Do not give aspirin; use an aspirin substitute. A raised temperature causes a child's forehead to feel hot and causes increased sweating and a general feeling of being sick. Normal temperature may vary from 97 to 99°F (36 to 37.5°C). Minor fluctuations within this range are no cause for concern if your child seems otherwise well.

If your baby's temperature rises above 102°F (39°C), whatever the suspected cause, call your physician at once. High temperatures can lead to seizures in some babies.

? Are you a woman?

YES →

Have you had a baby within the past two weeks?

YES →

☎
Call your physician without delay!
Puerperal infection, although rare today, is a possible cause of fever after childbirth. It occurs when the uterus and/or vagina become infected after delivery. If, however, you also have pain or redness of the breast, you may have a breast infection.

See • *Breast-feeding*
    • *Mastitis*
    • *Puerperal sepsis*

NO ↓

Do you have pain in the lower abdomen AND/OR have you had an unusually heavy or unpleasant-smelling vaginal discharge?

YES →

An infection of the uterus AND/OR fallopian tubes is a possible cause of such symptoms.
Consult your physician.

See • *Salpingitis*

NO ↓

NO ↓

If you are unable to make a diagnosis from this chart, consult your physician.

Fiber, dietary

The indigestible components of plants, some of which are fibrous. Dietary fiber includes certain types of polysaccharides, cellulose, hemicelluloses, gums, and pectins, and also lignin (see *Carbohydrates*).

STRUCTURE

Cellulose, hemicelluloses, and lignin form the main structural components of plant cell walls. Pectins and gums are viscous substances in plant sap. Together, these five substances provide the plant with a structure that is stable and partially rigid. Humans do not possess the necessary enzymes to digest these substances. They pass through the digestive system virtually unchanged and are unable to be used as a source of energy. Some of them are fermented by bacteria in the large intestine to produce acids and gas.

FUNCTION

Some components of dietary fiber have the capacity to bind water and add bulk to the feces, which then pass through the intestines more easily, aiding normal bowel function. For this reason, dietary fiber can be effective in treating *constipation* and such disorders as *diverticular disease*. It may also be valuable in the treatment of *irritable bowel syndrome*.

The easiest way to increase the amount of fiber in the diet is to increase the intake of unrefined carbohydrate foods such as whole-grain bread, cereals, and grains, root vegetables, and fruits. (See also *Nutrition*.)

Fiberoptics

The transmission of images through bundles of thin, flexible, glass or plastic threads that propagate light by total internal reflection. This means that all the light from a powerful external source travels the full length of the fiber without losing its intensity.

Fiberoptics has led to the development of *endoscopes*, instruments that enable structures deep within the body to be viewed directly. One bundle of fibers carries light to the far end of the instrument and another bundle transmits the image to the viewer's eye or to a still or video camera. The flexibility of the fibers allows them to be passed through the loops of the large intestine or down through the curve of the stomach and into the duodenum without distorting the image. (See also *Endoscopy*.)

Fibrillation

Localized, spontaneous, rapid contractions of individual muscle fibers.

GOOD SOURCES OF FIBER (per 100-gram portion)

Recommended daily intake 25 to 30 grams	
Whole-grain flour	9.6
Dried apricots	24
Peanuts	8.1
Celery	4.9
Peas	12
Raisins	6.4
Green beans	7.4
Prunes	16.1
Bran	44

Essential for the efficient working of the digestive system, fiber is usually eaten as fruit or grains. Among the best sources are bran, apricots, prunes, and whole-grain bread. Eating sufficient fiber in food can reduce constipation.

Unlike *fasciculation* (a similar muscular "quivering"), fibrillation cannot be seen under the skin. It is detected by tests such as an electromyogram (*EMG*) or electrocardiogram (*ECG*).

Fibrillation usually occurs after a nerve that supplies a muscle is destroyed, in which case the affected muscle becomes weak and wastes away. Fibrillation of the heart muscle is caused by disruption of the spread of nerve impulses through the muscle wall of a heart chamber. As a result, the chamber no longer contracts as a single unit; instead, it produces a rapid, irregular rhythm (see *Atrial fibrillation*; *Ventricular fibrillation*).

Fibrinolysis

The breakdown or dissolution of fibrin, the principal component of any blood clot. Fibrin is a stringy protein that is formed in blood from a precursor substance, fibrinogen, as the end product of coagulation. Along with platelets and red blood cells, fibrin forms the final clot that plugs and seals a damaged blood vessel (see *Blood clotting*).

In addition to the coagulation system, blood contains a fibrinolytic system, the end product of which is an enzyme called plasmin, formed from a precursor called plasminogen. Plasmin acts directly to break up fibrin filaments and thus dissolve clots.

The fibrinolytic system is activated in parallel with the coagulation system when a blood vessel is damaged. It helps restrain clot formation in blood vessels (thus helping to prevent clots from blocking blood vessels) and eventually dissolves a clot once a broken blood vessel wall has healed. *Thrombosis* (i.e., the formation of undesirable, persistent blood clots) occurs only if there is a disturbance in the balance between mechanisms that encourage clot formation, such as sluggish blood flow, and those, such as fibrinolysis, that restrain clot formation or dissolve clots.

Fibrinolytic drugs

Drugs used to dissolve blood clots. (See *Thrombolytic drugs*.)

Fibroadenoma

A benign, fibrous tumor found commonly in the breast. Fibroadenomas of the breast are painless, firm, round lumps, usually 0.5 to 2 inches (1 to 5 cm) in diameter, and movable. Fibroadenomas occur most often in women under 30 and are more common in black women. Multiple fibroadenomas may develop in one or both breasts.

Removal is accomplished using either a local or a general anesthetic. After removal, the lump is examined by a pathologist to rule out the small chance of breast cancer.

Fibrocystic breast disease

See *Breast lump*.

Fibrocystic disease

A term that may refer either to the inherited disorder *cystic fibrosis*, characterized by the secretion of abnormal mucus by various glands and by recurrent respiratory infection, or to the presence of single or multiple benign tumors or cysts in the breast (see *Breast lump*; *Mastitis*).

Fibroid

A benign tumor of the uterus. Fibroids consist of smooth muscle bundles and connective tissue that grow slowly within the uterine wall. As the fibroid enlarges, it may grow within the muscle so that the uterine cavity is distorted, or it may protrude from the uterine wall into the uterine cavity but remain attached by a stalk. Fibroids vary from the size of a pea to that of a grapefruit, and several of them may develop simultaneously.

Uterus

Fibroids

Uterine wall

Location of fibroids

INCIDENCE AND CAUSE

Fibroids are one of the most common tumors, occurring in about 20 percent of women over 30. They appear most often in women aged 35 to 45 and seldom before age 20.

The cause of fibroids is unknown, but it is thought to be related to an abnormal response to estrogens. Pregnancy and estrogen hormone replacement therapy can cause fibroids to enlarge; decreased estrogen production after the menopause usually causes them to shrink.

SYMPTOMS

In many cases there are no symptoms, especially if the fibroid is small. If the fibroid grows and erodes the lining of the uterine cavity, it may cause heavy or prolonged menstrual periods; if severe, the bleeding can lead to iron-deficiency *anemia*. Large fibroids may exert pressure on the bladder, causing discomfort or urinary frequency, or on the bowel, causing backache or constipation. Occasionally, a fibroid attached to the uterine wall becomes twisted and causes a sudden pain in the lower abdomen. Fibroids that distort the uterine cavity may cause recurrent miscarriage or infertility.

DIAGNOSIS

Symptomless fibroids are often discovered during a routine pelvic examination. When fibroids are thought to be the cause of menstrual disturbances or responsible for other symptoms, *ultrasound scanning* can confirm the diagnosis.

TREATMENT

Small, symptomless fibroids usually require no treatment, but regular examinations may be necessary to determine if they are growing. Surgery is required for fibroids causing serious symptoms or complications. A *hysterectomy* (removal of the uterus) is sometimes considered if there are large numbers of fibroids. Myomectomy (shelling out the fibroid from its capsule) saves the uterus and is another alternative. Fibroids tend to shrink after the menopause.

Fibroma

A benign tumor of the cells that make up connective tissues (tissues that surround and support specialized structures). For example, a neurofibroma is a tumor of the cells that surround nerve fibers (see *Neurofibromatosis*). An ovarian fibroma is a tumor of the cells that surround the follicles from which ova (eggs) develop. If the tumor is not causing symptoms, treatment is not required.

Fibrosarcoma

A rare, malignant (cancerous) tumor of the cells that make up connective tissue (any tissue that surrounds and supports specialized structures). A fibrosarcoma may develop from a fibroma (a benign tumor) or it may be malignant from the start.

A fibrosarcoma is usually found in the tissues around the muscles in a limb but it can also affect a bone or the cells around nerve fibers. It can spread to damage nearby structures.

A fibrosarcoma causes a localized swelling, which may not be noticed at first, depending on its site and how deep it is. Occasionally, widened veins appear on the skin over the growth; the fibrosarcoma may feel warm or may pulsate.

Treatment is by surgical removal or *radiation therapy*; this may be only temporarily successful if cells from the tumor have spread via the blood to start growths elsewhere.

Fibrosis

An overgrowth of scar or connective tissue (any tissue that surrounds and supports specialized structures). Fibrous tissue may be formed as an exaggerated healing response to injury, infection, or inflammation. It can also result from a lack of oxygen in a tissue, usually due to inadequate blood flow through it—for example, in heart muscle damaged by myocardial infarction (heart attack).

As fibrous tissue replaces specialized structures (such as kidney cells or muscle cells) the function of the organ concerned is impaired and its structure modified.

An overgrowth of fibrous tissue can compress and thus block hollow structures. An example is *retroperitoneal fibrosis*, in which the tubes draining urine from the kidneys (ureters) into the bladder become blocked.

Fibrous tissue formed within a muscle after a tear shortens the muscle and disrupts the normal contraction of fibers. This increases the likelihood of further tears unless the muscle is stretched and exercised.

Fibrositis

Pain and stiffness in the muscles around joints and sometimes in the back. Fibrositis is not a medical term, and some physicians refuse to recognize the condition because investigation usually fails to reveal any inflammation of the muscles. In addition, there is no other detectable reason for the pain in most cases.

Tension and bad posture may cause the condition. It seems to occur more often in anxious people and in those who spend time sitting in a cramped position. Sometimes, an attack occurs after an infection or new exercise. Fibrositis is most common in middle-aged and elderly people.

SYMPTOMS

Pain and stiffness may be felt in the neck, shoulders, chest, buttocks, and knees, as well as in the back. There is usually no restriction of movement. Trigger zones may be felt in the affected muscles and are tender to the touch. In some cases, attacks (which are generally worse in cold, damp weather) are accompanied by exhaustion and disturbed sleep.

TREATMENT

Analgesics (painkillers), hot baths, massage, and relaxation exercises can usually relieve the pain and stiffness.

It is likely that exercises to improve posture, starting with a gradual program to tone the muscles, can help prevent attacks. (See also *Back pain*.)

Fibula

The outer and thinner of the two long bones of the lower leg. The fibula is much narrower than the other bone, the *tibia* (shin), to which it runs parallel and to which it is attached at both ends by ligaments. The top end of the fibula does not reach the knee, but the lower end extends below the tibia and forms part of the ankle.

F

LOCATION OF THE FIBULA
The fibula lies beside the tibia on the outside of each lower leg.

- Femur
- Knee joint
- Tibia
- Fibula
- Ankle joint

The main function of the fibula is to provide an attachment for muscles. It provides little supportive strength to the lower leg, which is why bone can safely be taken from it for grafting elsewhere in the body.

FRACTURE
The fibula is one of the most commonly broken bones. The usual site of fracture is just above the ankle as the result of a violent twisting movement, which can occur in a severe ankle sprain. Rarely, such a fracture of the fibula occurs with dislocation of the ankle, with or without fracture of the tibia (see *Pott's fracture*).

A suspected fracture of the fibula is X rayed; if the diagnosis is confirmed, the lower leg is immobilized in a plaster cast to allow the bone to heal, but, if the fracture occurs in the middle portion of the fibula, no immobilization is necessary for healing. With a severe fracture (especially accompanied by dislocation), surgery may be necessary to fasten together broken pieces of bone with metal pins.

A fractured fibula may take up to six weeks to heal, depending on the severity of the break and the age of the person.

Fifth disease

An infectious childhood disease characterized by a widespread rash. It is also known as slapped cheeks' disease (because it often starts as a dramatic rash on the cheeks) or as erythema infectiosum. Fifth disease is the least well known of five common childhood infections, the other four being *measles, mumps, chickenpox,* and *rubella* (German measles).

Fifth disease affects young children, usually occurring in small outbreaks in the spring. The cause is a virus known as parvovirus.

SYMPTOMS AND TREATMENT
The rash starts on the cheeks as separate, rose-red, raised spots, which subsequently converge. Within a few days the rash spreads in a lacy pattern over the trunk, buttocks, and limbs. It is often accompanied by mild fever.

The only treatment required is bed rest, plenty of clear fluids, and acetaminophen to reduce any fever. The rash usually clears within 10 days.

Fight or flight response

The physical response when the sympathetic division of the *autonomic nervous system* is aroused. The features are common to all animals, including man, and are a reaction to sensing a threat of any kind. Epinephrine, norepinephrine, and other hormones are released from the adrenal glands and the nervous system, leading to a raised heart rate, dilation of the pupils, the hair standing on end, and increased flow of blood to the muscles. All these responses make the body more efficient in either fleeing or fighting the apparent danger. These physiological changes occur in fear and also in *anxiety* and its disorders.

Filariasis

A group of tropical diseases caused by various parasitic worms or their larvae, which are transmitted to man by insect bites. Adult females, which vary in length from three quarters of an inch (2 cm) to 20 inches (50 cm), produce thousands of microfilariae (larvae) that are carried throughout the body in the bloodstream. Blood-sucking insects (primarily certain species of mosquito, fly, and midge) ingest the microfilariae while feeding on blood from infected people and transmit them by biting others.

Filariasis is prevalent in tropical Africa, Indonesia, the South Pacific, coastal Asia, southern Arabia, southern Mexico, and Guatemala.

TYPES AND SYMPTOMS
Some species of worm live in the lymphatic vessels, which they block. This results in localized *edema* (an accumulation of fluid in the tissues, causing swelling). Following repeated infections, the affected area—commonly a limb or the scrotum—becomes enormously enlarged and the skin becomes thick, coarse, and fissured, leading to a condition known as *elephantiasis*.

The larvae of another type of worm invade the eye, causing blindness (see *Onchocerciasis*). A third type, which may sometimes be seen and felt moving just beneath the skin, produces irritating, sometimes painful areas of edema called Calabar swellings.

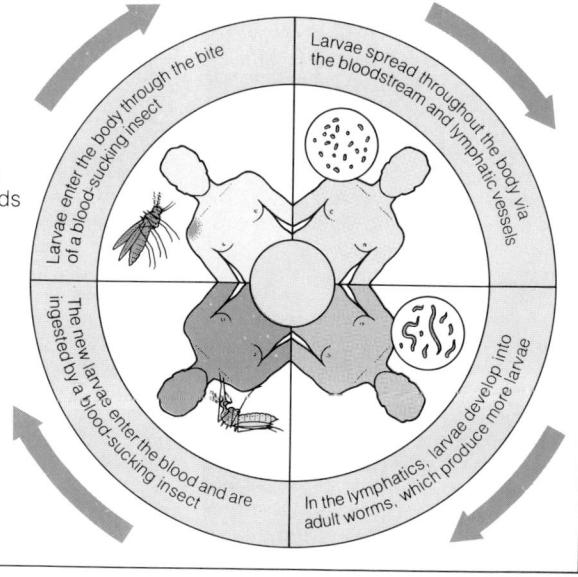

THE CYCLE OF FILARIASIS
Filariasis is caused by parasitic worms and/or their larvae. There are several stages in the development of this infection as it spreads through the body.

Larvae enter the body through the bite of a blood-sucking insect

Larvae spread throughout the body via the bloodstream and lymphatic vessels

In the lymphatics, larvae develop into adult worms, which produce more larvae

The new larvae enter the blood and are ingested by a blood-sucking insect

The diagnosis of filariasis is confirmed by microscopic examination of blood or lymph fluid for the presence of microfilariae.

A three-week course of the drug diethylcarbamazine usually cures the infection, but may cause a reaction marked by fever, sickness, and muscle and joint pains.

PREVENTION
Where resources are available, filariasis can be controlled by all persons taking diethylcarbamazine preventively and by the use of insecticides, repellents, nets, and protective clothing to help avoid insect bites. (See also *Roundworms; Guinea worm disease; Insects and disease*.)

Filling, dental

The process of replacing a chipped or decayed area of a tooth with an inactive material. The term is also used to describe the restorative (filling) material itself. Amalgam, a hardwearing mixture of silver, mercury, and other metals, is generally used for back teeth, where the filling will not show. Tooth-colored plastic material, porcelain, or acrylic is more likely to be used for front teeth. Other substances, such as gold, also are used.

WHY IT IS DONE
When enamel is damaged, bacteria can invade the dentin beneath and eventually attack the pulp (blood vessels and nerves), causing the tooth to die. It is therefore preferable to repair teeth at as early a stage as possible—ideally when only the enamel is affected. Filling also restores a tooth to its original shape, which is important not only for appearance but for maintaining a correct bite.

HOW IT IS DONE
If the filling required is large or in a sensitive area, the dentist will numb the surrounding gum with a local anesthetic. Any soft, decayed material is scooped out with sharp instruments. A high-speed drill is used to remove harder material and to shape a hole that will hold the filling securely. While the dentist works, a suction tube placed in the patient's mouth draws away saliva; the cavity is kept as dry as possible with occasional bursts of compressed air.

If the pulp is exposed, the bottom of the cavity is lined with a sedative paste to protect the sensitive pulp from pressure and temperature changes. If one or more of the walls of the tooth is missing because of extensive decay, a matrix (steel band) may be placed around the tooth to support the filling. The dentist then mixes the amalgam (or other filling material), which at first has a gummy consistency, and packs it into the cavity, contouring the surface so that it is smooth. The filling sets sufficiently to allow the matrix to be removed after a few minutes. The amalgam hardens completely over the next 24 hours.

If a front tooth is chipped, the dentist may use a *bonding* technique in which the surface of the tooth is etched with a mild acid solution and plastic or porcelain tooth-colored material is then attached to the roughened surface, shaped, polished, and finished.

OUTLOOK
Amalgam fillings have a limited longevity and may need to be replaced after about 10 years. Occasionally, a filling needs to be replaced earlier—for example, if decay has continued to spread underneath the filling, either because of leakage at the filling margins or due to recurrent decay. Occasionally, fillings are dislodged, usually by chewing on sticky candy, or they fracture as a result of biting.

Film badge

A device that enables hospital staff members to monitor their exposure to radiation. Film badges are worn by those who perform X-ray procedures and radiation therapy to keep their exposure within safe levels.

The badge consists of a piece of photographic film in a holder that is worn on the clothing. The film has a fast (sensitive) emulsion on one side and a slow emulsion on the other. Small doses of radiation blacken the fast emulsion only; higher dosages start to blacken the slow emulsion and make the fast emulsion opaque.

Finger

One of the digits of the hand. Each finger has three phalanges (bones), except for the thumb, which has two. The phalanges join at hinge joints moved by muscle tendons that flex (bend) or extend (straighten) the finger. The tendons are covered by synovial sheaths that contain fluid, to enable the muscles to work without friction. A small artery, vein, and nerve run down each side of the finger. The entire structure is enclosed in skin with a nail at the tip.

DISORDERS
Congenital disorders include *polydactyly* (extra fingers), *syndactyly* (fused

STRUCTURE OF A FINGER
The phalanges (bones) are joined at hinge joints and are moved by tendons.

Nail — Tip
Tendons
Phalanges
Synovial sheath
Artery

fingers), or missing fingers. Sometimes the skin membrane between the fingers is very long and deep, giving an appearance of *webbing*.

Injuries to the finger are common, particularly *lacerations, fractures*, and tendon ruptures. *Baseball finger* occurs when the extensor tendon that runs along the back of the finger is pulled from its attachment following a blow to the fingertip.

Inflammation due to *rheumatoid arthritis* or *osteoarthritis* may affect the finger joints, causing stiffness, pain, swelling, and deformity. The flexor tendons, which run along the front of the fingers, may become inflamed and stuck in the tendon sheath, causing *trigger finger*.

Infections commonly occur in the finger pulp at the tip; *paronychia* (infection of the tissue around the nail) usually follows a minor cut.

Altered control of the muscles in the walls of the vessels and impaired blood supply to the hands and fingers may cause *Raynaud's disease*.

Dactylitis is a term for a spindle-shaped swelling of the fingers that occurs in *sickle cell anemia*. Dactylitis is also an uncommon feature of tuberculosis and syphilis.

Clubbing of the fingers may occur as a sign of chronic lung disease, lung cancer, and some forms of congenital heart disease, especially *tetralogy of Fallot*.

F

Tumors of the finger are rare but may be due to chondromas, which are benign cartilage tumors. (See also *Hand; Nail.*)

Finger joint replacement

A surgical procedure in which artificial joints made of metal, plastic, or silicone rubber are used to replace finger joints destroyed by disease.

WHY IT IS DONE

The main use of the operation is to relieve pain and restore some degree of movement to hands that have been crippled by *rheumatoid arthritis*, which destroys the cartilage, bone, and lining of finger (and other) joints, leaving them weak and unstable.

Less commonly, surgery is performed to relieve pain and improve mobility in joints in which *osteoarthritis* has destroyed the cartilage and created new bone.

HOW IT IS DONE

The operation is performed using an anesthetic. Several joints are usually treated simultaneously.

An incision is made to expose the joint; the ends of the two diseased bones in the joint are cut away, along with diseased cartilage. An artificial joint is then inserted into the bone ends. The tissue covering the joint and the overlying skin are sewn up and the finger is immobilized in a splint until the wound has healed.

RECOVERY PERIOD

The hand is bandaged and held high in a sling to prevent swelling. The stitches are removed after about 10 days, after which the patient is encouraged to move the fingers and return to normal activities. Exercises for the fingers may be required later to maintain function in them.

RESULTS

The procedure is usually successful in relieving pain and enabling the patient to use his or her hands again. However, it can rarely restore normal movement to the hand because joint diseases affect not only bones and cartilage in the joints, but also surrounding tissue that contributes to the flexibility of joints.

Fingerprint

An impression left on a surface by the pattern of fine curved ridges on the skin of the fingertips. The impression is made by minute amounts of sweat from pores in the skin or by ink or some other substance applied to the fingertips. The ridges occur in four main patterns—loops, arches, whorls, and compounds (combinations of the other three). It is on these ridges that fingerprint classification is based.

In law, fingerprints are accepted as a means of identification, since no two people—not even identical twins—have the same fingerprints.

First aid

The treatment of any injury or sudden illness given before professional medical care can be provided.

MINOR INJURIES

Most first aid consists of treating minor injuries, such as small *wounds*, *sprains*, foreign bodies in the eye (see *Eye, foreign body in*), minor *burns*, and *fractures*. Coping with these injuries requires proficiency with *bandages* and *splints*, and in applying *dressings*.

EMERGENCY FIRST AID

The aims of first-aid treatment in an emergency are to preserve life, to prevent the condition from worsening and protect the individual from further harm, to aid recovery, to provide reassurance to victim and family, and to make the ill or injured person as comfortable as possible.

The role of the person giving first aid is to assess the situation, to give immediate and appropriate treatment, and to arrange for the ill or injured person to be seen by a physician or taken to the hospital without delay. Additionally, the person administering first aid should find out as much as possible about the events surrounding the accident or injury from the victim or from bystanders.

If the person is unconscious or losing consciousness, the person giving first aid must first ensure that the airway is clear, that breathing is satisfactory (by checking respiratory rate), and that the circulation is good (by checking pulse and skin color). Airway, breathing, and circulation are easily remembered by the letters ABC.

The *recovery position* helps maintain an open airway in an unconscious person who is breathing. *Artificial respiration* is necessary if a patient is not breathing. *Cardiopulmonary resuscitation* is essential if the person is not breathing and has no heart beat. Any significant *bleeding* must be controlled by the rescuer applying pressure at the appropriate *pressure point*.

No severely injured or ill person should be moved without trained help

FIRST AID: FIRST-AID KIT

1 Adhesive bandages	**7** Roll of sterile cotton	**14** Antiseptic cream
2 Aspirin or aspirin substitute	**8** Adhesive tape	**15** Antiseptic wipes
3 Absorbent gauze bandages	**9** Flashlight	**16** Hydrogen peroxide (3% solution) or rubbing alcohol
4 Foil or "space" blanket	**10** Elastic bandages	**17** Syrup of ipecac
5 Triangular bandage	**11** Round-ended tweezers	
6 Calamine lotion	**12** Safety pins	
	13 Snub-nosed scissors	

unless life is in immediate danger. This especially applies to anyone with a suspected *spinal injury*. The person should be covered to keep him or her warm, and any tight or constricting clothing should be loosened.

If there are many people injured, the person giving first aid must establish an order of priority for their care. Highest priority is for those who have no pulse, are breathing with difficulty or not at all, are unconscious, or bleeding severely. Such people may die unless immediate treatment is given.

First-aid training is provided by various organizations, which award certificates to those who have attended courses and passed an examination. (See also *Childbirth* emergency box; *Choking*; *Drowning*; *Frostbite*; *Heat stroke*; *Hypothermia*; *Poisoning*. First-aid treatment for specific conditions appears under the appropriate heading—for example, *Epilepsy*; *Nosebleeds*.)

Fistula

An abnormal passage from an internal organ to the body surface or between two organs.

Fistulas may be congenital (present from birth) or may be acquired as a result of tissue damage. Congenital types include *tracheoesophageal fistulas*, branchial fistulas (see *Branchial disorders*), and thyroglossal fistulas (see *Thyroglossal disorders*). Acquired fistulas may result from injury, infection, or cancer. Some types of arteriovenous fistula (between an artery and a vein) are constructed artificially to provide ready access to the blood circulation, which may be necessary in *dialysis* patients.

Fistulas of the urinary tract, which open from the urethra or bladder to the perineum (the area between the anus and the genitals) usually occur as a complication of radiation therapy to the pelvis or damage caused by a difficult childbirth. Such fistulas may cause urinary *incontinence* or infection.

Fistulas between the intestine and the skin may occur in people with *Crohn's disease* and may also occur as complications of abdominal surgery. The intestinal contents may escape through an opening to the skin or through a surgical wound.

Some types of fistula close spontaneously, but most need to be cut and repaired surgically.

Fitness

Having the capacity for physical work so that normal daily activities can be performed without exhaustion. Fitness depends on strength (the ability to exert force for pushing, pulling, lifting, and other bodily functions), flexibility (the ability to bend, stretch, and twist through a full range of movements), and endurance (the ability to maintain a certain amount of effort for a certain period of time).

HOW FITNESS IS ACHIEVED

Because cardiovascular fitness is the precondition for all other forms of fitness, aerobic exercise, which increases the efficiency of the body's use of oxygen, is the basis for any fitness program. Exercises to develop flexibility and strength should be combined with aerobic exercise for a total fitness program. Although fitness training has cumulative effects that build up over many months (providing there is a sustained increase in activity levels), the effects are specific to the muscles used and the ways in which they are used. A variety of activities is necessary to achieve a general training effect.

BENEFITS OF FITNESS

A person who is fit has a better chance of avoiding *coronary heart disease* and preventing the effects of age and chronic disease. When the body is fit, the maximum work capacity is increased, endurance is increased, and a particular task utilizes a smaller proportion of the work capacity.

The strength, endurance, and efficiency of the heart is also increased by exercise. A fit heart pumps 25 percent more blood per minute when at rest and over 50 percent more blood per minute during physical exertion than an unfit heart. A fit person's heart normally beats 60 to 70 times a minute; an unfit person's heart beats 80 to 100 times per minute. The heart of a fit person works more efficiently than that of an unfit person and is therefore less subject to strain. (See also *Aerobics*; *Exercise*.)

Fitness testing

A series of exercises designed to determine an individual's level of fitness, primarily cardiovascular fitness and muscle performance.

WHY IT IS DONE

Fitness testing is usually performed to determine a person's level of fitness before starting an exercise program. It also determines whether or not a person will be at risk when starting to exercise, particularly following a heart attack. Fitness testing is also done periodically to assess and monitor progress during an exercise program.

HOW IT IS DONE

The tests are usually carried out by a physician in his or her office or in the outpatient department of a hospital. A physical examination is usually performed, including taking measurements of height, weight, and body fat. Blood and urine tests may be done, including an analysis of blood cholesterol and high-density and low-density lipoprotein content, since high cholesterol levels are related to *atherosclerosis*.

One test involves measuring the performance of the heart during physical work. The heart's efficiency at pumping blood is measured using the pulse rate (number of heart beats) per minute. The more efficient the heart, the slower it works during exercise and the quicker it returns to normal afterward. The pulse is taken at rest, and then the heart performance is measured during exercise at one or more intensities. This exercise may include step climbing, riding a stationary bicycle, or walking or running on a treadmill. After a specific period, the exercise is stopped and the pulse is taken to determine how hard the heart is working at its maximum level. The pulse is usually taken again after a minute to determine how long it takes for the heart beat to return to normal. The blood pressure response to exercise also provides useful information to the physician and patient.

Another type of exercise test involves measuring the overall performance in a standard exercise. This is most suitable for monitoring progress through an exercise program and for setting goals. The test may be based on measuring the distance covered in a fixed time or on the time needed to cover a fixed distance. (See also *Aerobics*; *Exercise*; *Fitness*.)

Fixation

A term used by Sigmund Freud to describe the attachment of a person's libido (sexual drive or interest) to real or imagined events during early childhood. Freud suggested that young children go through various stages related to certain parts of the body. In modern psychoanalysis, the stages are viewed within the context of the child's early relationships, starting with the mother. The major stages Freud called the oral, anal, and phallic, because putting things in the mouth, concern about feces, and playing with the penis or clitoris seemed to be prominent forms of behavior (because they are zones of pleasure).

F

EFFECTS

Fixations are unconscious and exist to some extent in all human beings; experiences from childhood are seen as permanently affecting the adult's thoughts and feelings. However, when the fixations are very powerful, resulting from especially traumatic relationships or series of events (experiences), they lead to the sort of repetitive behavior that would be expected from an immature child. Regression (going back) to one of these early stages is thus regarded by some analysts as the underlying cause of certain emotional disorders.

The type and severity depend on the stage regressed to. For example, fixation at the anal stage may be associated with concerns about control (*obsessive-compulsive behavior*), whereas fixation at the phallic stage may be associated with other deviations. Because these fixations are unconsciously repressed, the task of *psychoanalysis* is to uncover them so that patients become aware of the reason for their feelings and reactions.

Flail chest

A type of chest injury, usually resulting from a traffic accident or from violence. In flail chest, multiple rib fractures, usually at the front and side of the chest, produce an isolated portion of the chest wall. This portion moves in when the victim breathes in and moves out when he or she breathes out; this motion is opposite to the normal direction.

The injury may severely impair the efficiency of breathing and result in collapse due to *respiratory failure* and *shock*. It makes breathing and coughing very painful, which can predispose to chest infection and collapse of the lung (see *Atelectasis*).

Emergency treatment consists of turning the person onto the affected side or supporting the flail segment by firm strapping. In the most severe cases, the patient may need immediate admission to an intensive-care unit, where artificial *ventilation* will be performed. This treatment is continued for about 10 days until the ribs are sufficiently healed.

Flatfoot

Lack of an arch in the foot, resulting in the sole resting flat on the ground. The condition, known medically as pes planus, usually affects both feet.

CAUSES

Almost everyone is born with flatfeet. The arches, which then begin to develop from the formation of supportive ligaments and muscles in the soles of the feet, are not fully formed until the age of 6. In some people, however, the ligaments and muscles are weak and the feet remain flat (for unknown reasons). Less commonly, the arches do not form because of a hereditary defect in the structure of the small bones of the foot.

Flatfeet can also be acquired in adult life due to fallen arches, sometimes as a result of a rapid increase in weight. Flatfeet may also be caused by a weakening of the muscles and ligaments that support the arch, which sometimes occurs in a neurological or muscular disease such as *poliomyelitis*.

SYMPTOMS AND TREATMENT

Most flatfeet—due to ligaments and muscles never having developed fully—are usually painless and require no treatment. When the condition is caused by a defect in the foot bones or develops in adult life, the feet may ache when walking or standing. Affected children infrequently require an operation to correct the bones in the feet. In adults, treatment consists of wearing arch supports in the shoes and performing exercises to strengthen the weakened ligaments and muscles.

Flatulence

Expulsion of *flatus* (intestinal gas formed by swallowed air or fermentation) through the anus, sometimes accompanied by abdominal discomfort, which is relieved by the passage of flatus.

In an upright position, most swallowed air passes back up the esophagus to be expelled through the mouth. However, when in a prone position, the air may pass through the intestine and anus instead. Gas formed in the intestine is always passed through the anus.

Flatus

Gas or air in the intestines. Gas is formed in the large intestine as a result of the action of bacteria on carbohydrates and amino acids in digested food; the gas consists of hydrogen, carbon dioxide, and methane. Air in the stomach or intestine is swallowed usually while eating, but also (in anxious people) in times of stress.

Large amounts of flatus do not, as many believe, cause abdominal discomfort; such discomfort is usually due to intestinal sensitivity to normal amounts of flatus (see *Irritable bowel syndrome*; *Flatulence*).

Flatworm

Any species of worm that has a flattened shape—as opposed to a *roundworm* or nematode, which has a cylindrical shape. Flatworms are also sometimes called platyhelminths.

Two types of flatworm are parasites of humans—cestodes (tapeworms) and trematodes (flukes and schistosomes). (See also *Tapeworm infestation*; *Liver fluke*; *Schistosomiasis*.)

Flavoxate

ANTICHOLINERGIC ANTISPASMODIC

Tablet

	Prescription needed

	Not available as generic

A drug used to treat the urinary symptoms of *cystitis*, *prostatitis*, and *urethritis*. The underlying disorder is treated with other drugs, usually *antibiotic drugs*.

HOW IT WORKS

Flavoxate works by suppressing muscular activity in the bladder by blocking the action of acetylcholine. As a result, the muscles that control urination relax and the volume of urine that can be held by the bladder increases. The drug also has an analgesic (painkilling) effect.

POSSIBLE ADVERSE EFFECTS

Adverse effects are rare, but may include dry mouth, blurred vision, and constipation.

Flea bites

See *Insect bites*.

Flies

See *Insects and disease*.

Floaters

Semitransparent bodies perceived to be floating in the field of vision. Floaters move rapidly with eye movement but drift slightly when the eyes are still. They do not affect vision.

Most floaters are shadows cast on the retina by microscopic structures in the *vitreous humor*, a jellylike substance that lies behind the lens. In older people, the vitreous humor tends to shrink slightly and detach from the retina, often causing conspicuous floaters, which usually decrease with time.

The sudden appearance of a cloud of dark floaters, especially if accompanied by bright light flashes, suggests *retinal detachment*. A large red floater that obscures vision is usually due to a *vitreous hemorrhage*.

Floppy infant syndrome
A condition in which a baby's muscles lack normal tension or tone. (See *Hypotonia in infants*.)

Floppy valve syndrome
See *Mitral valve prolapse*.

Floss, dental
Soft nylon or silk thread, waxed or unwaxed, used to remove plaque and food particles from between the teeth and around the gum line.

Flow cytometry
An automated test that reveals the arrangement and amount of deoxyribonucleic acid (DNA), or genetic material, within cells as a means of diagnosing malignancy. The pattern of DNA in cancer cells is different from that of normal cells.

The test is helpful in distinguishing benign from malignant cells, and also in monitoring the effects of *anticancer drug* treatment. (See also *Cytology*.)

Flu
See *Influenza*.

Fluctuant
A medical term for the sensation of fluid moving within a swelling as it is palpated (examined by touch). It is a sign that the swelling contains liquid (such as pus in an abscess).

Fluke

A type of flattened worm, also called a trematode, that may infest humans or animals. The two main diseases caused by flukes are *liver fluke* infestation, which occurs worldwide, and *schistosomiasis*, a common and debilitating disease in the tropics.

Fluocinolone
A *corticosteroid drug*. Fluocinolone is prescribed as an ointment to relieve symptoms of skin inflammation, such as itching and redness, caused by *eczema* or another skin disorder.

Fluorescein
A harmless orange-red dye used mostly in ophthalmology. Fluorescein drops are useful for showing up corneal ulcers, which stain bright green. The dye is also used in fluorescein *angiography*, a method of highlighting the details of blood circulation in the

HOW TO USE DENTAL FLOSS
Floss should be used as an adjunct to toothbrushing to remove plaque and food particles from gaps between teeth and around gums. Care should be taken to avoid damaging the gum margins.

1 Break off a generous length of floss (about 18 inches) and wrap the ends around one finger of each hand. Do not use the same length of floss twice.

2 Holding the floss taut, guide it gently into the gap between the teeth until it reaches the gum line. Then rub the sides of each tooth with the floss using an up-and-down motion.

inside of the back of the eye. For this procedure, a sterile solution of fluorescein is injected into a vein. While the dye is passing through the eye in the bloodstream, photographs are taken of the retina (the innermost layer of the eye) using blue light and a green filter on the camera.

Fluoridation
The addition of fluoride to the water supply as a means of reducing the incidence of dental *caries* (tooth decay). Fluoridation began in the US in the 1940s; since then, water supplies serving 60 percent of the population have been fluoridated.

WHY IT IS DONE
Fluoride has been shown to be effective in helping to prevent dental caries, particularly if the fluoride is ingested while the teeth are forming. Children drinking fluoridated water from birth have up to 65 percent fewer

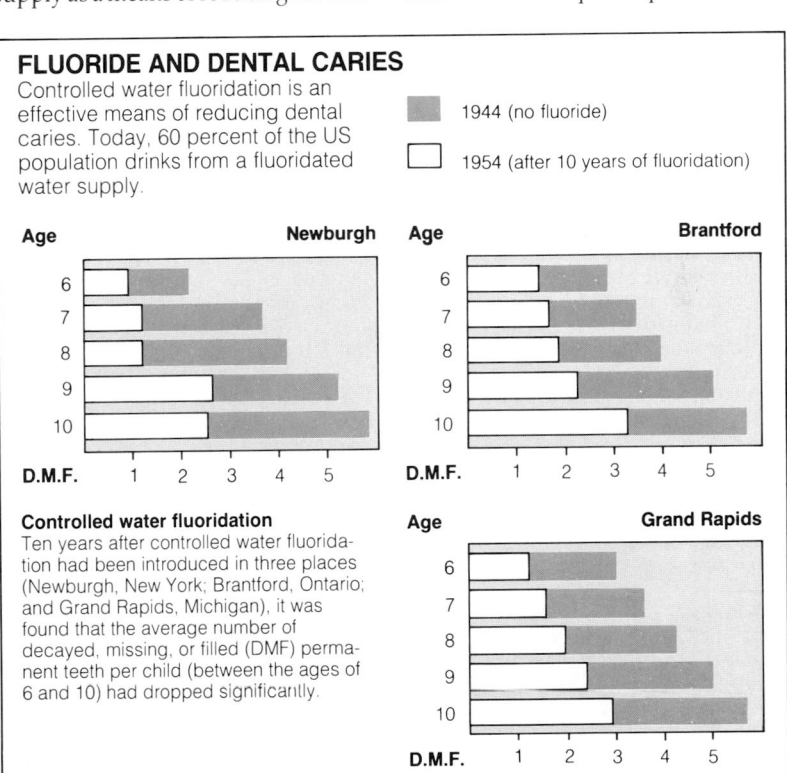

FLUORIDE AND DENTAL CARIES
Controlled water fluoridation is an effective means of reducing dental caries. Today, 60 percent of the US population drinks from a fluoridated water supply.

1944 (no fluoride)
1954 (after 10 years of fluoridation)

Controlled water fluoridation
Ten years after controlled water fluoridation had been introduced in three places (Newburgh, New York; Brantford, Ontario; and Grand Rapids, Michigan), it was found that the average number of decayed, missing, or filled (DMF) permanent teeth per child (between the ages of 6 and 10) had dropped significantly.

cavities and 90 percent fewer extractions during childhood than their counterparts who have drunk water with less than the recommended fluoride level.

Some areas have naturally high levels of fluoride in the drinking water; in other areas fluoride is added to bring levels up to the recommended standard of 0.7 to 1.2 parts per million, depending on the climate.

SAFETY

Although considerable controversy has surrounded fluoridation programs, there is no evidence that fluoridation at the recommended level has any harmful effects.

Fluoride

A mineral that is useful in helping prevent dental caries (tooth decay). Fluoride is thought to work by strengthening the mineral composition of the tooth enamel, making it more resistant to acid attacks; it may also affect plaque directly, reducing the acid-producing ability of the organisms plaque contains.

Fluoride is most effective when ingested during the formation of teeth, when it becomes incorporated into the tooth substance. It is most beneficial when taken from birth and has a lifelong effect. The water supply may naturally provide adequate amounts of fluoride (the recommended level is 0.7 to 1.2 parts per million) or provide fluoride as a result of *fluoridation*. If the level is inadequate, children can be given fluoride drops or tablets.

Fluoride is also beneficial to both children and adults when applied directly to the teeth. The dentist may treat children's teeth by painting on a fluoride solution or by holding a fitted tray filled with fluoride gel against the teeth for a few minutes. Fluoride mouthwashes and toothpastes are available for daily use at home.

Ingestion of excess fluoride during tooth formation may lead to *fluorosis*, mottling of the teeth that sometimes causes brown discoloration.

Sodium fluoride has been used without FDA approval to treat certain cases of osteoporosis.

Fluorosis

Mottling of the tooth enamel caused by ingestion of excess fluoride during tooth formation. In the most severe cases, mottling is so great that the enamel develops unsightly brown stains. Severe cases usually occur only in people living in areas where the natural level of fluoride in water is many times greater than the recommended level of 0.7 to 1.2 parts per million. Fluorosis can occur in other areas if excessive additional fluoride is consumed—for instance, via the unsupervised use of fluoride tablets.

Mild white mottling of the teeth may occur in a small percentage of children ingesting water at the recommended level, but this form of fluorosis does not cause discoloration or impair appearance.

Fluorouracil

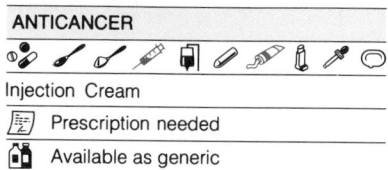

ANTICANCER
Injection Cream
📋 Prescription needed
🔲 Available as generic

An anticancer drug used in the treatment of cancers of the breast, bladder, ovary, stomach, and intestine.

Fluorouracil in cream form is used to treat some types of skin tumor, such as *keratosis* and *basal cell carcinoma*. It is used especially when several tumors occur together, making surgical removal difficult.

POSSIBLE ADVERSE EFFECTS

Fluorouracil may cause nausea, vomiting, diarrhea, hair loss, and impaired production of blood cells. Applied as a cream, it can cause inflammation of the skin.

Fluphenazine

One of the phenothiazine group of *antipsychotic drugs* used to relieve the symptoms of disorders such as *schizophrenia*, *mania*, and *dementia*. Fluphenazine (given as a tablet, liquid, or by injection) suppresses confused or abnormal behavior and has a tranquilizing effect.

Flurazepam

A *benzodiazepine drug* used in the treatment of *insomnia*.

Flush

See *Blushing*.

Foam, contraceptive

See *Spermicide*.

Folic acid

A vitamin essential to the production of red blood cells by the bone marrow. Folic acid is contained in a variety of foods, particularly liver and raw vegetables; adequate amounts are usually obtained from a well-balanced diet.

During pregnancy, folic acid plays an important part in fetal growth—in the development of the nervous system and in the formation of blood cells. During the last three months of pregnancy, folic acid tablets may be necessary to supplement the diet.

Folic acid deficiency is a cause of megaloblastic *anemia*, which causes symptoms such as fatigue, depression, and pallor.

Folk medicine

Any form of medical treatment based on the beliefs of a particular society. Examples include the charming of warts, the use of copper bracelets for the treatment of rheumatism, and the piercing of ears to improve the eyesight. What these remedies have in common is their support by belief within the culture and their lack of reliance on a practitioner. By contrast, the diagnostic and healing techniques used by a witch doctor are known as traditional medicine; those used by a chiropractor or a homeopathist are known as *alternative medicine*.

Follicle

A small cavity in the body. One example is a hair follicle, a pit on the surface of the skin from which a hair grows. Another is an ovarian follicle, one of the many fluid-filled cavities in the female ovary from which an ovum (egg) develops.

Follicle-stimulating hormone

A *gonadotropin hormone* (one that stimulates the gonads—the ovaries and testes) produced by the anterior part of the pituitary gland; also known by its initials, FSH.

Folliculitis

Inflammation of one or more hair follicles as a result of infection with STAPHYLOCOCCUS bacteria. Folliculitis may occur almost anywhere on the skin. It commonly is found on the neck, thighs, buttocks, or armpits, causing a boil, or it may affect the bearded area of the face, which leads to the development of pustules (see *Sycosis vulgaris*).

Treatment is with antibiotics. The infection often spreads from an infected person to the rest of the family. To prevent this or to control an outbreak, each person should shower frequently and use a separate washcloth and towel; clothes worn next to the skin should be washed daily in boiling water.

Fomites

Inanimate objects, such as clothing, books, bed linen, or a telephone receiver, that are not harmful in themselves, but which may be capable of harboring bacteria, viruses, parasites, or other harmful organisms and thus may convey an infection from one person to another.

Fomites mainly transmit respiratory infections, such as influenza.

Fontanelle

One of the two soft areas on a baby's scalp, a membrane-covered gap between the bones of the skull. At birth the skull bones are not yet fully fused and there are spaces between them. The only gaps of any size are the anterior (front) fontanelle, which is diamond-shaped, about 1 inch (2.5 cm) across, and usually closes up by the age of 18 months, and the posterior (rear) fontanelle, which is triangular, about 0.25 inch (0.6 cm) across, and closes within about two months of birth.

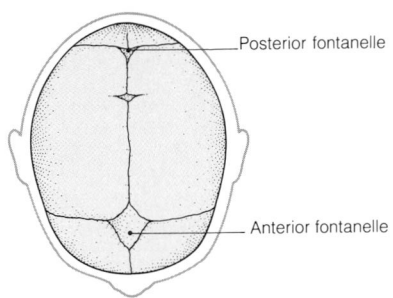

Posterior fontanelle

Anterior fontanelle

Location of the fontanelles
Two soft areas on the baby's skull—the anterior fontanelle is diamond-shaped, the posterior fontanelle is triangular.

DISORDERS

It is normal for the fontanelles to bulge and become tense when a baby cries. However, persistent tension at other times may indicate an abnormality, particularly *hydrocephalus* (an accumulation of fluid within the baby's skull). A sunken fontanelle may be a sign of *dehydration*. If a fontanelle is abnormally large or takes a long time to close, it may be due to *rickets* or a brain abnormality. Early closure of the fontanelles results in a deformity called *craniosynostosis*.

Occasionally, a third fontanelle is present between the other two; this occurs most commonly in *Down's syndrome*. Some babies have extra bones in the anterior fontanelle; this is normal. The extra bones fuse into the skull when the gap closes.

Food additives

Any substance that is added to food to perform a technological function. Contrary to popular belief, not all additives are artificial; sugar and salt are probably the most common.

Before any additive is accepted for use in food processing, the need for the additive must be proved and its safety assessed by the *Food and Drug Administration* (FDA).

TYPES AND USES

Additives fall into four main groups: those that preserve food and affect its "keeping" quality, those that affect texture, those that affect appearance and taste, and miscellaneous additives, such as rising and glazing agents, flour "improvers," and antifoaming agents.

Preservatives, such as sodium nitrate, are added to food to control the growth of bacteria, molds, and yeasts, especially those that might contaminate the food after it has left the manufacturer. Other additives, such as antioxidants, improve the keeping quality of the food by preventing undesirable changes (such as by stopping rancidity in foods containing fat).

Additives that improve food texture include emulsifiers, stabilizers, thickeners, and gelling agents. They alter the "mouth feel" and consistency of food. Lecithin, which occurs naturally in all animal and plant cells, is an emulsifier added to margarine to prevent separation.

Appearance and taste are often improved by the use of colorings, flavorings, sweeteners, and flavor enhancers. Colors and flavors are used mainly to compensate for losses during processing, to strengthen existing colors or flavors, and to ensure standardization in products. *Artificial sweeteners*, such as saccharin and aspartame, are used in place of sugar, especially in products designed for diabetics and weight control.

RISKS

All food additives are carefully monitored and regulated; there is no evidence that any additives in general use can harm the population as a whole. However, even though an additive may be harmless to most people, it may produce an allergic reaction in others. The best known flavor enhancer, *monosodium glutamate* (MSG), often causes *Chinese restaurant syndrome*, with reactions similar to a migraine. Tartrazine, a widely used yellow food coloring, produces an allergic reaction in a significant number of people.

Additives are often blamed for causing hyperactivity in children, but most physicians believe that, although this is true for a very small number of children, the majority of hyperactive children are not allergic to food additives. Foods containing nitrites and nitrates have been alleged to be involved with causing certain cancers (e.g., stomach cancer).

Food allergy

An inappropriate or exaggerated reaction of the *immune system* to a food. Sensitivity to cow's milk protein is a common food allergy in young children. Other foods most commonly implicated in food allergy include wheat, fish, shellfish, and eggs.

Food allergy is more common in people who suffer other forms of allergy or hypersensitivity, such as asthma, allergic rhinitis (hay fever), and dermatitis.

Immediate reactions, occurring within an hour or sometimes minutes of eating the trigger food, include lip swelling, tingling in the mouth or throat, vomiting, abdominal distention, *borborygmi* (audible bowel sounds), and diarrhea.

The only effective treatment of food allergy is to strictly avoid eating the offending food.

Food and Drug Administration

Part of the US Department of Health and Human Services, the Food and Drug Administration (FDA) monitors the safety of foods and cosmetics, and the radiation hazards of TV sets and microwave ovens. Most important, it determines, before general distribution, the safety and effectiveness of drugs and medical devices (such as insulin pumps).

Food-borne infection

Any infectious illness caused by eating food that has been contaminated with viruses, bacteria, worms, or other organisms.

CAUSES

There are two main mechanisms by which food can become infected.

First, many animals that are kept or caught for food may harbor disease organisms in their tissues or internal organs. If meat or milk from such an animal is eaten without being thoroughly cooked or pasteurized, the organisms may cause illness in their human host. In the US, the only common infection of this type is *food poisoning* from improperly cooked poultry, meat, fish, or shellfish.

F

Second, food may be contaminated with disease organisms spread from an infected person or animal—usually from their excrement (such as by flies moving from feces to food).

PREVENTION

In developed countries, food-borne infections are controlled or prevented by adequate sanitation and sewage treatment; by multiple laws and regulations that govern animal husbandry, the production of food in farms and factories, and its subsequent storage and distribution; and by generally high standards of personal hygiene with regard to handling and eating of food.

In some less affluent parts of the world, many of these controls do not exist and the chances of a food-borne infection are thus much higher. When visiting such countries, it is wise to avoid certain foods, particularly salads, any meat or fish that looks suspect or not thoroughly cooked, shellfish, milk, butter, cream, and ice cream. Raw fruits and vegetables are generally safe once the exterior peel or skin has been removed.

Immunization is available against certain food-borne and water-borne infections, such as typhoid and cholera, but it usually provides only partial protection and is no substitute for good food hygiene. (See also *Water-borne infection*.)

Food fad

A like or dislike of a particular food or foods that is carried to extremes. It may lead to an undue reliance on, or avoidance of, a particular foodstuff.

Fads are particularly common in toddlers and adolescents and in those under stress. For most people, food fads are not serious since they are either short-lived or restricted to a limited number of foods. However, when food fadism or food aversion has an obsessional quality about it, or is persistent, it may be indicative of a more serious eating disorder. (See also *Anorexia nervosa*; *Bulimia*.)

Food intolerance

A reproducible, adverse reaction to a food or food ingredient that is not caused either psychologically or by *food poisoning*.

CAUSES AND INCIDENCE

Food intolerance is mainly of unknown cause, but is sometimes due to various unknown irritants, toxins,

INFECTED ANIMAL PRODUCTS

Some animals harbor disease organisms (e.g., bacteria, worms, and parasites) in their tissues and these may cause infection if meat or milk is consumed raw or improperly cooked. Beef, pork, and fish tapeworm infestations, salmonella poisoning, and (rarely) brucellosis can be transmitted in this way.

1 Cows, pigs, poultry, fish, and particularly shellfish are sources of bacterial, viral, or worm infection or infestation.

2 Adequate milk pasteurization and inspection of meat and fish before sale prevents most infections and infestations of this type.

3 Thorough thawing, preparation, and cooking of meats, fish, shellfish, and poultry further reduces the risk of infection.

FOOD CONTAMINATION

Intestinal infections may be spread from person to person if organisms in feces contaminate food, directly or indirectly. This can occur if vegetable crops are sprayed with sewage, if flies settle on feces and then on food, or if food is handled by a person who has not washed his or her hands.

Contaminating organism
The photograph (left) taken through an electron microscope shows a typical *SALMONELLA* bacterium. The organism uses its many flagellae (whiplike structures) to move. *SALMONELLA* is a common contaminant of poultry, eggs, and egg products and causes severe food poisoning.

Infective organisms pass to a person via contaminated meat, fruit, shellfish, etc.

The organisms multiply in the intestines and elsewhere, causing illness, and pass out in the feces.

The organisms may pass to food via hands, flies, or via sewage contaminating shellfish, crops, etc.

If standards of hygiene and sanitation are low, organisms in feces may contaminate people's hands or may be picked up by flies.

or *food additives*. It may be associated with an adverse reaction to foods such as green peppers, fried foods, or onions. Food intolerance can be caused by an inborn or acquired biochemical defect, such as *lactase deficiency* (an inability to digest milk sugar found more commonly in blacks, Asians, Indians, and people of Mediterranean origin).

Food poisoning

A term used for any illness of sudden onset, usually with stomach pain, vomiting, and diarrhea, suspected of being caused by food eaten within the previous 48 hours. Most cases are the result of contamination of food by bacteria or viruses.

Food poisoning is usually suspected when, for example, several members of a household (or customers at a restaurant) become ill after eating the same food.

TYPES AND CAUSES

Food poisoning can be classified, according to cause, into infective and noninfective types. Some foods can cause poisoning of either type. For example, shellfish such as mussels, clams, and oysters can become contaminated by viruses or bacteria, by toxins acquired from poisonous plankton (tiny marine animals and plants), or by chemical pollutants in the water.

BACTERIAL CAUSES

The bacteria most commonly responsible for food poisoning belong to a group called salmonella, certain strains of which are able to multiply rapidly in the intestines to cause widespread inflammation. Some farm animals, especially poultry, commonly harbor such bacteria. If frozen poultry is not completely thawed before being cooked, it is liable to cause poisoning.

Salmonella bacteria may also be transferred to food from the excrement of infected animals or people, either by flies or by the handling of food by an infected person—especially if the hands have not been washed after using the toilet. If contaminated food is left for any time in warm conditions, a large colony of bacteria may develop without obvious food spoilage.

Other bacteria cause the formation of toxins that may be difficult to destroy even with thorough cooking. Toxin-forming strains of staphylococcal bacteria, for example, may spread to food from a septic abscess on a foodhandler's skin. *Botulism* is a rare, life-threatening form of food poisoning

caused by a bacterial toxin and associated with home preservation of food.

VIRAL CAUSES

The viruses that most commonly cause food poisoning are Norwalk virus (a common contaminant of shellfish) and rotavirus. They cause food poisoning when raw or partly cooked foodstuffs have been in contact with water contaminated by human excrement.

NONINFECTIVE CAUSES

include poisonous mushrooms and toadstools (see *Mushroom poisoning*), and fresh fruit and vegetables that have been accidentally contaminated with high doses of insecticide. Chemical poisoning can also occur if food has been stored in an unsuitable container—for example, if a container that has previously held a poison is used to store food, or if acidic fruit juice is kept in a metal container made partly of zinc.

Various exotic foods (for example, the puffer fish, considered a delicacy in Japan, or cassava, a staple food in many tropical countries) can also cause moderate to lethal poisoning if improperly prepared and cooked.

SYMPTOMS

The onset of symptoms varies according to the cause of poisoning. The symptoms usually develop within 30 minutes in the case of chemical poisoning, between one and 12 hours in the case of bacterial toxins, and between 12 and 48 hours with virus and salmonella infections. Symptoms vary considerably according to how heavily the food was contaminated, but usually include nausea, vomiting, diarrhea, stomach pain, and, in severe cases, *shock* and collapse.

The symptoms of botulism are markedly different, with nervous system symptoms such as difficulty speaking, visual disturbances, muscle paralysis, and vomiting.

DIAGNOSIS

The diagnosis of bacterial food poisoning can usually be made from a culture of a sample of the person's vomit or feces. Chemical food poisoning can often be diagnosed from a description of what the person has eaten within the previous few hours, and from analysis of a sample of the suspect food, if available.

FIRST AID AND TREATMENT

If severe vomiting and diarrhea suddenly develop (or if a person collapses), medical assistance should be sought. Samples of any food left from a recent meal should be kept; they may help pinpoint the cause and possibly prevent a widespread outbreak of food poisoning.

If poisoning by a chemical or bacterial toxin is suspected, gastric *lavage* (washing out the stomach) may be carried out. Otherwise, treatment in a hospital is directed primarily toward preventing dehydration by replacing fluids intravenously.

Milder cases can be treated at home. The affected person should eat no solid food but should drink plenty of fluids, which should include some salt and sugar to replace what is being lost (see *Rehydration therapy*).

Except for botulism and some cases of mushroom poisoning, most food poisoning is not serious. Recovery generally occurs within three days.

PREVENTION

Some simple measures can virtually eliminate the chances of food poisoning. Hands should always be washed before handling food, and fresh vegetables and fruit rinsed in clean water. Cutting boards and implements used on raw meat should also be rinsed before they are used on other food. Frozen poultry should always be completely thawed before cooking and then should be well cooked.

Ask for advice on the preparation of any food unfamiliar to you at the point of sale. Suspect items—such as mussels that do not open when boiled, bulging tin cans, or any food that smells or looks obviously spoiled—should be rejected. Finally, people who preserve food at home should take care to sterilize food thoroughly by heating it in a pressure cooker at 250°F (120°C) for 30 minutes.

Foot

The foot has two vital functions—to support the weight of the body in standing or walking and to act as a lever to propel the body forward.

STRUCTURE

One of the bones of the foot is the calcaneus (heel bone); it is jointed with the talus, the second largest bone of the ankle. In front of the talus and calcaneus is a series of smaller bones—the navicular, cuboid, and cuneiform. These in turn are jointed with five long bones called the metatarsals. The phalanges are the bones of the toes; the big toe has two phalanges, all the other toes have three.

Tendons passing around the ankle connect the muscles that act on the various bones of the foot and toes. The main blood vessels and nerves pass in front of and behind the inside of the ankle joint to supply the foot. The undersurface of the normal foot forms a natural arch that is supported by

F

SKELETON OF THE FOOT

The calcaneus is attached to the talus above. In front are the navicular, cuboid, and cuneiform bones, which are attached to the metatarsals. Phalanges form the toes. An adult has 26 bones in each foot—one eighth of the total number in the entire skeleton.

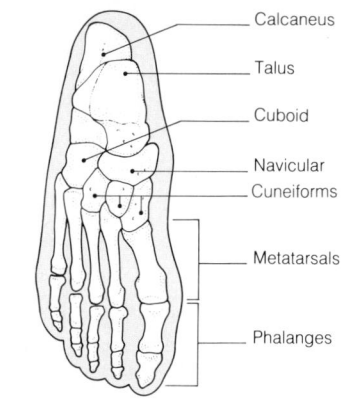

Calcaneus

Talus

Cuboid

Navicular

Cuneiforms

Metatarsals

Phalanges

ligaments and muscles. Fascia (fibrous tissue) and fat form the sole of the foot, which is covered by tough skin.

DISORDERS

Injuries to the foot commonly result in *fracture* of the metatarsals and phalanges. The calcaneus may fracture following a fall from a height onto a hard surface.

Deformities of the foot are fairly common and include *talipes* (clubfoot), *flatfoot*, and *clawfoot*. Another common deformity is a *bunion*, which is a *bursa* (fluid-filled pad) overlying the joint at the base of the big toe.

A number of disorders can affect the skin of the foot. *Corns*, small areas of thickened skin on a toe, are usually caused by tight-fitting shoes. *Plantar warts* appear on the skin on the sole, while *athlete's foot*, a fungal infection, mainly affects the skin between the toes, causing it to become itchy, sore, and cracked.

Gout, a fairly common type of arthritis, often affects the joint at the base of the big toe or one of the joints in the foot. *Ingrown toenail* commonly affects the nail of the big toe, causing inflammation of the surrounding tissue and *paronychia* (infection of these tissues). *Footdrop*, the inability to raise the foot properly, is due to damage to the muscles in the leg that perform this movement or the nerves that supply these muscles.

Footdrop

A condition in which the foot cannot be raised properly. It hangs limp from the ankle joint, causing it to catch on the ground when walking.

CAUSES

Neuritis (inflammation of a nerve) affecting the nerves that supply muscles that move the foot is a common cause of footdrop; it may be due to *diabetes mellitus, multiple sclerosis,* or certain neuropathies (see *Neuropathy*). Pressure on a nerve root as it leaves the spinal cord due to *disk prolapse* or, rarely, a tumor can also cause weakness in the foot muscles.

TREATMENT

The underlying cause is treated, but in many people the weakness persists. A footdrop splint (see *Brace, orthopedic*) can keep the foot fixed in position when walking.

Foramen

A natural hole or passage in a bone or other body structure, usually to allow the passage of nerves or blood vessels. The foramen magnum is the large opening in the base of the skull through which the spinal cord passes.

Forceps

A tweezerlike instrument used for handling tissues or equipment during surgical procedures. Various types of forceps are designed for specific purposes. For example, forceps used for holding or removing wound dressings have scissor handles to make manipulation easier. Tissue forceps have fine teeth at the tip of each blade so that tissues can be handled delicately during operations. (See also *Forceps delivery; Forceps, obstetric*.)

TYPES OF FORCEPS

Dressing forceps

Long jaw for grasping

Artery forceps

Locking handles

Forceps delivery

The use of forceps (see *Forceps, obstetric*) by an obstetrician to ease out the baby's head during a difficult birth (see also *Childbirth*). *Vacuum extraction* may be used as an alternative.

WHY IT IS DONE

Forceps delivery is used if the mother is overtired or unable to push out her baby unaided, or if the baby is showing signs of *fetal distress*. (If fetal or maternal distress occurs before the second stage of labor begins, a *cesarean section* rather than a forceps delivery is necessary.)

Forceps are used to control the head in *breech delivery* (with the baby's buttocks first) to prevent a too-rapid delivery. Forceps are also used if the baby's head is stuck in the middle of the mother's pelvis and needs to be rotated before delivery is possible. Called a midforceps delivery, this requires extreme skill on the part of the obstetrician; a cesarean section may be performed instead.

HOW IT IS DONE

The mother is given an analgesic (painkiller) and either local or *epidural anesthesia*. She then lies on her back, with her legs raised in stirrups, and her bladder is emptied with a catheter. The obstetrician then examines the mother. Forceps can be applied only if the cervix (neck of the uterus) is fully dilated and the baby's head is engaged in the pelvis. An *episiotomy* (making of a small cut in the perineum) is usually performed before a forceps delivery.

The forceps blades are placed on either side of the infant's head, just in front of the ears. If the baby's chin points downward, gentle traction is applied to the forceps and the baby delivered. If the chin is pointing sideways or upward, rotation of the head is necessary before traction can be applied; in such cases, rotation forceps are used.

RECOVERY PERIOD

After a forceps delivery, care is similar to that following a spontaneous (unassisted) vaginal delivery. Sometimes there is greater bruising of the perineum, but this usually heals rapidly and can be eased by the application of ice packs. After a forceps delivery, the baby may have forceps marks on the face. They disappear after a few days. The length of stay in the hospital is usually the same as after a delivery without forceps.

Forceps, obstetric

Surgical instruments used to deliver the head of a baby in a difficult labor.

OBSTETRIC FORCEPS

The two wide, blunt blades are designed to fit around the baby's head. The handles lock together so that the blades are held apart.

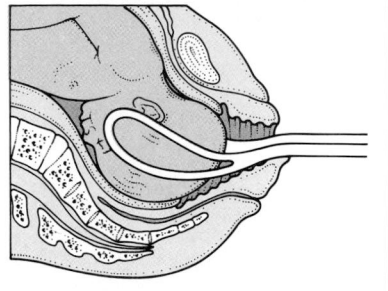

Positioning
The forceps blades lie along the sides of the baby's head, just in front of the ears.

The first obstetric forceps were invented about 300 years ago by the obstetrician Peter Chamberlen. They were kept as a family secret for use on private patients, and were not in common use until about 100 years later.

Obstetric forceps consist of two blades that cup the baby's head. Each blade is joined to a separate handle and the two handles are fitted together; when assembled, the blades are separated by a fixed distance (see illustrated box).

Foreign body

Any object in an organ, opening, or passage of the body that should not be there. It may enter accidentally (by inhalation or swallowing, for example) or it may be deliberately introduced. Common sites include the airways (see *Choking*), ear (see *Ear,*

foreign body in), eye (see *Eye, foreign body in*), rectum, urethra, and vagina. A metallic, glass, or wood splinter that embeds in the subcutaneous tissue is also a foreign body.

Foreign medical graduate

Graduates of non-US medical schools, even if US citizens. Foreign medical graduates (FMGs) may qualify for training in US residency programs and for subsequent licensing after successfully passing a test of language and medical skills.

Forensic medicine

The branch of medicine concerned with the law, especially criminal law. The forensic pathologist is a physician who specializes in the examination of bodies when circumstances suggest death was unnatural (i.e., suicide, homicide, or an accident). The examination usually includes an assessment of the time of death (from data such as the temperature of the corpse and its state of decomposition), deduction of the likely nature of any weapon used (from study of the injuries), and matching of blood, hair,

COMMON FOREIGN BODIES IN CHILDREN

Children constantly experiment with objects in the environment. They frequently place small objects into their mouths, noses, or ears. As a result, a swallowed or stuck foreign body is a common occurrence. It is wise to keep all small objects well out of reach of children.

Ear and nose
Attempting to remove a foreign body from the ear can be dangerous because of the risk of pushing the object further in. The physician uses a syringe, suction, or forceps. A foreign body in the nose may be taken out with tweezers by the physician; an older child may be able to blow it out while the other nostril is blocked.

Lungs
Inhaled objects such as peanuts or teeth may become lodged in the bronchi and cause obstruction of air flow, resulting in pneumonia or lung collapse. Symptoms may include choking, coughing, and breathing difficulty. The child should *not* be inverted, slapped on the back, or made to vomit, but should be taken to the hospital immediately.

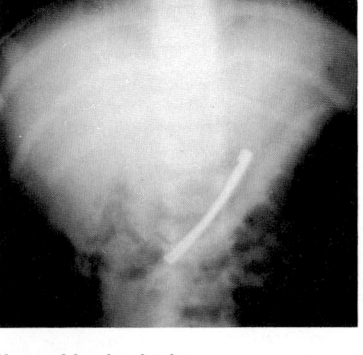

X ray of foreign body
This X ray shows that the child has swallowed a closed hair barrette.

Stomach
Foreign bodies in the stomach include coins, batteries, marbles, and buttons. Most small, smooth objects pass safely out of the body in feces, but an object that has failed to pass through the body after seven to ten days usually requires removal. Batteries should be removed surgically because they release acid that seriously damages the digestive tract.

and skin from the victim with those on any weapons, on the clothing of suspects, or on parts of an automobile.

Forensic pathologists may also be asked to examine victims of alleged sexual assault or child abuse. They also consult in cases of attempted poisoning and possible drug deaths.

Forensic scientists use laboratory methods to study body fluids (such as blood, semen, and saliva) found on or near the victim and compare the fluids with those from suspects. They are also trained in ballistics and the identification of fibers from clothing.

In addition, forensic scientists may advise on blood grouping (see *Blood groups*) in cases of disputed paternity.

Foreskin

The popular name for the prepuce, the loose fold of skin that covers the glans (head) of the penis when it is flaccid and which retracts during erection.

At birth, the foreskin is attached to the glans, but, after the age of 6 months, it gradually separates from the glans. In some boys, the foreskin remains tight until the age of 3 or 4, making retraction difficult or impossible. However, unless this causes recurrent infection (by preventing adequate cleaning of the glans) or prevents normal urination, there is no need to consult a physician and no attempt should be made to force the foreskin back.

In some societies, the foreskin is routinely removed from newborn boys, an operation called *circumcision*, usually for religious or hygienic reasons. Circumcision may be performed at any age as a treatment for disorders of the foreskin.

DISORDERS

In *phimosis*, the foreskin remains persistently tight after the age of 5, causing difficulty in urination and ballooning of the foreskin. There may be recurrent *balanitis* (infection and inflammation of the glans and foreskin). Erection is often painful, which is why the condition is frequently discovered only at puberty.

In the related disorder *paraphimosis*, the foreskin becomes stuck in the retracted position, causing painful swelling of the glans.

Forgetfulness

See *Memory*.

Formaldehyde

A colorless, pungent, irritant gas. In medicine, a solution of formaldehyde and a small amount of alcohol in water—a preparation known as formalin—is used to preserve tissue specimens or to harden them (a procedure called fixation) before they are stained and examined. Formalin is also used as a *disinfectant*.

Formication

An unpleasant sensation, as if ants were crawling over the skin. It is an uncommon symptom, most often resulting from abuse of cocaine or similar drugs. Formication should be distinguished from a paranoid *delusion* in which people falsely believe they are infested by ants or worms. In either case, a rash may result from excessive scratching and lead in rare cases to a misleading diagnosis of a skin disease.

Formula, chemical

A way of expressing the constituents of a chemical in symbols and numbers. Every known chemical substance has a formula. Water, for example, has the formula H_2O, indicating that it is composed of two hydrogen atoms (H_2) and one oxygen atom (O).

Fracture

A break in a bone, most commonly caused by a fall. A bone is usually broken directly across its width, but can also be fractured lengthwise, obliquely, or spirally.

TYPES OF FRACTURE

Fractures are divided into two main types: closed (or simple) and open (or compound). In a closed fracture the broken bone ends remain beneath the skin and little or no surrounding tissues are damaged; in an open fracture one or both bone ends project through the skin.

Fractures may also be classified according to the shape or pattern of the break (see box).

If the two bone ends have moved apart, the fracture is termed displaced; in an undisplaced fracture the ends remain in alignment and there is simply a crack in the bone.

CAUSES AND INCIDENCE

Most fractures are caused by a sudden injury that exerts more force on the bone than it can withstand. The force may be direct, as when a finger is hit by a hammer, or indirect, as when twisting the foot exerts severe stress on the tibia (shin).

Some diseases, such as *osteoporosis* and certain forms of cancer, weaken bone so much that it takes only a minor injury—or none at all—for the bone to break. This type of fracture is termed pathological.

Common sites of fracture include the hand, the wrist (see *Colles' fracture*), the *ankle joint*, the *clavicle* (collarbone), and the neck of the *femur* (thigh bone), usually as the result of a fall.

Elderly people are the most prone to fractures because they fall more and because their bones are fragile.

SYMPTOMS AND SIGNS

There is usually swelling and tenderness at the site of the fracture and, in some cases, deformity or projecting bone ends. The pain is often severe and is usually made worse by any movement of the area.

FIRST-AID TREATMENT

Anyone suffering a suspected or known fracture should be taken to the hospital; if the injured person cannot walk, medical help should be summoned. Do not try to force back a displaced bone yourself.

Treat severe bleeding (see *Bleeding, treatment of*), covering any open wounds with a clean dressing. Move the patient as little as possible. *Splinting* is usually necessary, especially if the injured person needs to be moved or if there is a long delay before help arrives. If an injured arm can be bent comfortably across the chest, splint it first and then apply a *sling*. If *spinal injury* is suspected, do not move the person at all unless his or her life is in immediate danger or he or she is choking on vomit.

Do not give the injured person any food or liquid in case an operation requiring a general anesthetic must be carried out.

PROFESSIONAL TREATMENT

X rays are taken to confirm the diagnosis and to provide a clear picture of the type of fracture and the degree of displacement or malalignment.

Bone begins to heal immediately after it has broken. The first aim of treatment is therefore to ensure that the bone ends abut each other and are in alignment so that, when the fracture heals, the bone will retain its previous shape. Bone ends that have been displaced are maneuvered back into position—a procedure known as reduction. The bone may be manipulated through the skin (closed reduction) using a local or general anesthetic. Alternatively, the bone may be repositioned by means of an operation using anesthetic in which the site is opened (open reduction).

Once the fracture has been reduced, the bone is immobilized to allow the broken pieces to reunite firmly.

FRACTURES: TYPES AND TREATMENT

There are two main types of fractures: simple (closed) and compound (open). Within these two categories are several other types, three of which are illustrated here.

Compound fracture
A sharp piece of bone punctures the skin and is therefore exposed to organisms. There is a high risk of infection.

Transverse fracture
The result of a sharp, direct blow or a stress fracture caused, for example, by prolonged running.

Greenstick fracture
This type usually occurs in children. Sudden force causes only the outer side of the bent bone to break.

Comminuted fracture
The bone shatters into more than two pieces. This fracture usually is caused by severe force, such as in a car accident.

Simple fracture
The broken bone does not break the skin. Because organisms do not come into contact with the fracture, infection is rare.

REPAIR OF FRACTURES

There are various ways of repairing fractures, depending on the particular bone, the severity of the fracture, and the age of the patient.

Internal fixation
The photograph at left shows immobilization of an unstable hip fracture by the insertion of metal screws across the bone ends.

External fixation
Immobilization may be achieved by means of a plaster cast (above) or, in cases such as an unstable fracture of the tibia (left and above left), through the use of metal pins inserted into the bone on either side of the break and locked into position on an external metal frame.

THE BONE HEALING PROCESS

After a fracture, the bone starts to heal immediately. Any displacement of the bone ends must therefore be corrected without delay to minimize deformity.

2 Macrophages invade the fracture site to remove wound debris. Fibroblasts then create a mesh to form a base for new tissue.

4 Remodeling takes place, with more dense, stronger bone laid down.

1 A blood clot forms between the bone ends, sealing off the ends of the damaged vessels.

3 New bone (callus) is laid down between the bone ends and over the fracture line.

5 Over a period of weeks, the bone returns to its former shape.

F

In some cases the ends of the fractured bone may be fixed together by metal pins inserted through the skin and into the bone and kept in position by attachment to an external frame (external fixation); once the fracture has healed, the pins and frame are removed. In other cases an operation is done to open up the injury site and fasten together the bone pieces with metal screws, nails, plates, rods, or wires (internal fixation).

RECOVERY PERIOD

The time taken for fractures to heal varies considerably and depends on many factors. Fractures mend much more easily in children than in adults, and in babies they can heal in as little as two weeks. In an adult a weight-bearing bone, such as the tibia, may take up to six months to knit together completely; bones that do not bear weight, such as the radius and clavicle (collarbone), generally take no longer than eight weeks.

COMPLICATIONS

Most fractures heal without problem. Healing is sometimes delayed because the blood supply to the affected bone is inadequate (as a result of damaged vessels) or because the bone ends are not close enough together. If the fracture fails to unite, internal fixation or a *bone graft* may be required.

Occasionally, bone ends reunite at the wrong angle. If this causes deformity, an operation may be necessary to refracture the bone, set it correctly, and fix it with nails. *Osteomyelitis* is a danger of open fractures and may be difficult to eradicate.

REHABILITATION

Complete immobility of a bone for a prolonged period can cause loss of muscle bulk, stiffness in nearby joints, and *edema* (accumulation of fluid in the tissues) with the risk, especially in the elderly, of permanent disability. For this reason the patient is encouraged to begin gradually using the affected part as soon as is safely possible and is given exercises to perform to restore flexibility to the joints and strength to the muscles (see *Physical therapy*).

Fracture, dental

A break in a tooth. Although tooth enamel is hard, it is also brittle and can easily be fractured by suddenly striking a hard surface, as may occur in a sports injury or a fall.

If the fracture is confined to the tooth's enamel or to the enamel and dentin, it can usually be repaired by bonding, in which the surface of the tooth is etched with a mild acid solu-

tion and a plastic resin material is attached to the roughened surface. If the pulp is affected, *root-canal treatment* may be necessary. Fractures of the root are most damaging if they occur in the lower two thirds of the tooth because the remaining fragment does not offer sufficient support for a replacement crown. A tooth fractured vertically usually cannot be saved.

Front teeth that project more than normal are vulnerable to accidental fracture. They should be repositioned by orthodontic treatment. (See also *Orthodontics*; *Bonding, dental*.)

Fragile X syndrome

An inherited defect of the X *chromosome* that causes mental retardation. Fragile X syndrome is the most common cause of mental retardation in males after *Down's syndrome*.

The disorder occurs within families according to an X-linked recessive pattern of inheritance (see *Genetic disorders*). Although males are mainly affected, women are able to carry the genetic defect responsible for the disorder and pass it on to some of their sons, who are affected, and some of their daughters, who in turn become carriers of the defect.

Approximately one in 1,500 men is affected by the condition; one in 1,000 women is a carrier. In addition to being mentally retarded, affected males are generally tall, physically strong, have a prominent nose and jaw, increased ear length, large testicles, and are prone to epileptic seizures. About one third of female carriers show some degree of intellectual impairment.

There is no treatment for the condition. If a woman has a history of the syndrome in her family, it is useful to seek *genetic counseling* regarding the risk of a child being affected.

Freckle

A tiny patch of pigmented skin, often round or oval in shape. Freckles occur on sun-exposed areas of skin and tend to become more numerous as a result of continued exposure. The tendency to freckling is inherited and most often occurs in fair and red-haired people.

Freckles are harmless, but people with highly freckled complexions should avoid excess sunlight and should use sunscreens.

Free-floating anxiety

Vague feelings of apprehension and tension associated with *generalized anxiety disorder*.

Frequency

See *Urination, frequent*.

Freudian slip

Also known as a slip of the tongue, a minor error in speech or action that turns out to be what the person really wanted to say or do. The term, also called a parapraxia, is derived from Sigmund Freud's book "The Psychopathology of Everyday Life." As the error tends to be laughed off, Freud saw the process as a compromise between the fulfillment of an unconscious wish and the conscious effort to repress it.

Freudian theory

A discipline of psychology developed by Sigmund Freud (1856-1939), a Viennese neurologist. The theory developed out of his treatment of neurotic patients using hypnosis and formed the basis of his technique of *psychoanalysis*. Freud believed that feelings, thoughts, and behavior were controlled by unconscious wishes and conflicts and that problems occurred when these desires were not fulfilled or the conflicts remained unresolved.

According to Freud, the conflicts originated in childhood and persisted into adulthood. The essence of his theory concerns early psychological development, particularly sexual development, which now is seen to encompass much more than just the "sexual" to include the early relationship with the parent. Freud defined a number of stages—oral, anal, and genital (representing the areas of the body on which an infant's attention becomes fixed at different ages)—and three components of personality—the id, ego, and superego (based on pleasure, reality, and moral and social constraints, respectively). The classic Freudian model sees all behavior as having its roots in unconscious instincts, but ultimately being determined by the interplay between the id, ego, and superego.

Psychoanalysis aims to treat mental disorders by encouraging the patient to allow thoughts to flow in any conscious direction without censorship. Freud believed that important information would emerge from the unconscious mind. (See also *Psychoanalytic theory*; *Psychotherapy*.)

Friedreich's ataxia

A very rare inherited disease in which degeneration of nerve fibers in the spinal cord causes *ataxia* (loss of coordinated movement and balance). The disease is the result of a genetic defect, usually of the autosomal recessive type (see *Genetic disorders*). It affects about two people per 100,000.

SYMPTOMS

Symptoms first appear in late childhood or adolescence. The main symptoms are unsteadiness when walking, clumsy hand movements, slurred speech, and rapid, involuntary eye movements. In many cases there are also abnormalities of bone structure and alignment.

TREATMENT AND OUTLOOK

There is as yet no cure for the disease. Once it has developed, it becomes progressively more severe, and, within 10 years of onset, more than half the sufferers are confined to wheelchairs. If *cardiomyopathy* (heart muscle disease) develops, it may contribute to an early death. People who have blood relatives with Friedreich's ataxia should seek *genetic counseling* before starting a family.

Frigidity

A term used to describe the inability to want or enjoy sexual intercourse (see *Sexual desire, inhibited*). The term has been used almost exclusively with reference to women and is now being discouraged because of its negative connotations—blaming a woman for something that may exist only in the mind of her partner.

In the past, the term frigid was also used to describe a woman who does not achieve orgasm. This condition is now called inhibited sexual excitement; the terms anorgasmia, and foreorgasmy are also sometimes used (see *Orgasm, lack of*).

Frostbite

Damage to tissues caused by extremely cold temperatures—below 32°F (0°C). Frostbite can affect any part of the body that is not properly covered, but the nose, ears, fingers, and toes are most susceptible. If only the skin and underlying tissues are damaged, recovery may be complete. If blood vessels are affected, the damage is permanent and *gangrene* can follow, which may necessitate amputation of the affected part.

The lower the temperature, the shorter the time required to cause damage; wind and blizzard conditions also cause damage more quickly.

The first symptoms are a pins and needles sensation, followed by complete numbness. The skin appears white, cold, and hard, and then becomes red and swollen. After the

FIRST AID: FROSTBITE

DO NOT
- rub the affected parts
- attempt to burst blisters
- warm the affected area with direct heat
- allow the victim to walk on a frostbitten foot

WARNING
Frostbite is often accompanied by hypothermia, which must be treated first. Proper medical attention should be sought promptly, but first aid should be given immediately.

1 Shelter the victim from the cold and remove clothing from the affected part. Remove anything that constricts, such as rings or a watch.

2 Rewarm the affected area by covering it with warm hands or clothing. Frostbitten hands can be warmed in the victim's armpits; feet can be warmed in the rescuer's armpits.

3 If warm water (no hotter than 110°F) is available, immerse the affected part. The area should then be covered with a sterile dressing.

tissue has thawed, blisters form and some areas of skin are black, indicating that the tissue is dead.

Frostbite must be treated promptly. The person should be sheltered from the cold and the affected parts warmed as quickly as possible by immersing them in lukewarm water at 110°F (44°C). Movement of the affected parts should be avoided; massage is not helpful.

Frottage

The act of rubbing against another person to achieve sexual arousal. Also called frotteurism, it is usually carried out in a densely packed crowd where a man rubs his (clothed) genitals against a woman's buttocks or thigh. Such men commonly indulge in other sexual deviations, may have a fetishist interest in buttocks, and are unable to form successful sexual relationships.

Frozen section

A rapid technique for preparing *biopsy* specimens (small pieces of tissue) for microscopic examination.

WHY IT IS DONE

Frozen section is carried out during surgical procedures to determine whether tissue is malignant, so that the surgeon knows whether to remove more tissue before completing the operation. It is primarily used in diagnosing a breast lump as benign or malignant, but can also be useful in excluding malignancy as a diagnosis in growths of the thyroid or intestine or in diagnosing a lymphoma.

In many instances, diagnosis is made before surgery, obviating the need for frozen section. Diagnosis may be by percutaneous (through the skin) needle biopsy.

HOW IT IS DONE

A small piece of tissue is removed by the surgeon and sent to the histology laboratory. After being frozen quickly in liquid nitrogen, the specimen is cut into very thin sections, placed on a glass slide, and stained so that the cells can be examined under the microscope. The entire process takes about 20 minutes.

Frozen shoulder

Stiffness and pain in the shoulder, making normal movement of the joint impossible. In severe cases, the shoulder may be completely rigid and pain may be extremely intense.

Frozen shoulder is caused by inflammation and thickening of the lining of the capsule in which the joint is contained. The problem usually develops for no known reason, but in some cases it follows a minor injury to the shoulder, a *stroke*, chronic *bronchitis*, or *angina pectoris*.

The condition mainly affects middle-aged people, and there is a higher-than-average incidence among people with *diabetes mellitus*.

TREATMENT

Moderate symptoms can be eased by taking analgesics (painkillers) and anti-inflammatory drugs, and by applying ice packs to the shoulder or using a heat lamp on it. A severe case may require injections of *corticosteroid drugs* into the joint to relieve pain and exercises to restore movement. Manipulation of the joint using a general anesthetic can also restore mobility, but carries the risk of initially increasing pain in the joint.

Whatever the severity and treatment of the condition, recovery is usually slow and may be prolonged.

Frustration

A deep feeling of discontent and tension because of unresolved problems, unfulfilled needs, or because the path to a goal is blocked. In a person who is mentally healthy, frustration can be dealt with in a socially acceptable way. In less well-adapted people, it may lead to *regression* (going back to childlike behavior) and, in particular, *aggression* or *depression*.

There has been much research into the relationship between frustration and violent and criminal behavior. Some people believe that all aggressive acts are related to exposure to violence while growing up or are an indication of prior frustration.

FSH

Abbreviation for *follicle-stimulating hormone*, a *gonadotropin hormone* (one that stimulates the gonads—the ovaries and testes) produced by the anterior part of the pituitary gland.

Fugue

An episode of altered consciousness that causes the sufferer to wander (e.g., from home or work). It may last hours or days and the subject does not remember it afterward.

In a fugue of long duration, behavior may appear normal but certain symptoms (e.g., hallucinations, feeling unreal, or an unstable mood) may accompany it. In a fugue that

lasts only for a matter of hours, the patient may be confused and agitated. A fugue is not common, but causes great alarm among relatives and friends because of its sudden onset and strange quality.

Causes include *dissociative disorders*, the *automatism* of certain types of *epilepsy* (especially temporal lobe or psychomotor epilepsy), *depression*, *head injury*, and *dementia*.

Fulminant

A medical term used to describe a disorder that develops and progresses suddenly and with great severity. The term is usually applied to an infection that has spread rapidly through the bloodstream to affect several organs and cause a high fever.

The term may also be applied to types of arthritis in which many joints are painful and stiff and deformities appear soon after the onset of symptoms, or to a cancer that has spread rapidly to cause dramatic weight loss and debility.

Fumes

See *Pollution*.

Functional disorders

A term for illnesses in which there is no evidence of organic disturbance even though performance is impaired.

Fungal infections

Diseases of the skin or other organs caused by the multiplication and spread of fungal organisms. Infections range from mild and unnoticed to severe and sometimes fatal. Fungal infections are also called mycoses. Fungi can also cause *asthma* and allergic *alveolitis* but these are allergic disorders not infections.

CAUSES

Some fungi are harmlessly present all the time in areas of the body such as the mouth, skin, intestines, and vagina, but are prevented from multiplying through competition from bacteria. Other fungi are dealt with by the body's *immune system* (defenses against infection).

Fungal infections are more common and serious in people who are taking long-term antibiotics (which destroy the bacterial competition) and in those who are taking *corticosteroid drugs* or *immunosuppressant drugs* (used to suppress the immune system). These infections more commonly involve people with an immune deficiency disorder, such as *AIDS*. Fungal infections are described as opportunistic

because they take advantage of the victim's lowered defenses.

Some fungal infections are also more common in people with *diabetes mellitus*. A warm, moist atmosphere encourages the development of fungal skin infections.

TYPES

Fungal infections can be broadly classified into superficial infections (those that affect the skin, hair, nails, genital organs, and the inside of the mouth); subcutaneous infections (those beneath the skin); and "deep" infections (those affecting internal organs, such as the lungs or, more rarely, the liver, bones, lymph nodes, brain, heart, or urinary tract).

SUPERFICIAL INFECTIONS The main superficial fungal infections are *candidiasis* (thrush) and *tinea* (including ringworm and athlete's foot), both of which are very common. Candidiasis is caused by the yeast CANDIDA ALBICANS and usually affects the genitals or inside of the mouth. Tinea affects external areas of the body.

SUBCUTANEOUS INFECTIONS These are rare. The most common is called *sporotrichosis* and may follow contamination of a scratch. Most other conditions of this type occur mainly in tropical countries. The most important example of this type is *mycetoma*, or Madura foot.

DEEP INFECTIONS These are rare or uncommon (although becoming more common), but can be a serious threat to people who have an immune deficiency disorder or are taking immunosuppressive drugs. In the US, fungal infections of this sort include *aspergillosis*, *histoplasmosis*, *cryptococcosis*, and *blastomycosis*, all caused by different fungi. The fungal spores enter the body by inhalation into the lungs. Candidiasis can also spread from its usual sites to infect the esophagus, urinary tract, and numerous other internal sites.

Fungi

Simple parasitic life-forms including molds, mildews, yeasts, mushrooms, and toadstools. There are more than 100,000 different species of fungi worldwide. Of these, most are either harmless or positively beneficial to human health, including various yeasts used in baking and brewing, some molds that are the source of certain *antibiotic drugs*, and various edible mushrooms and truffles that are considered gastronomic delicacies in many parts of the world. There are,

FUNGAL DISEASES

The skin, scalp, genitals, and nails are the most common sites of fungal infection. Examples of types include *tinea* (ringworm) and *candidiasis* (thrush). Fungi also (rarely) infect the lungs and other internal organs to cause a more serious disease. They may also cause allergic lung disease, such as farmers' lung.

Fungal nail infection
This condition most often affects people whose hands are frequently immersed in water. It is liable to last for years. Antifungal medications benefit some people.

Colony of fungal cells
The microscope photograph at left shows a colony of yeast cells in a skin fragment.

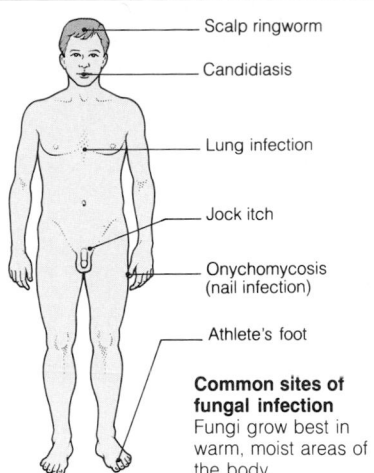

Scalp ringworm
Candidiasis
Lung infection
Jock itch
Onychomycosis (nail infection)
Athlete's foot

Common sites of fungal infection
Fungi grow best in warm, moist areas of the body.

FUNGAL GROWTH

Spore

Hyphae

Spores

1 Many fungal colonies originate from spores that have been carried in the air and have settled at a suitable site for growth.

2 If nutrients are available and other conditions (such as temperature) are favorable, a spore starts to divide.

3 The cells of many fungi divide to form a network consisting of branched chains of tubular filaments called hyphae.

4 Eventually a colony may start forming its own spores. They may be carried to new sites to set up new growths.

however, also a number of types of fungi that can cause illness and sometimes fatal disease in humans. The study of fungi and fungal diseases is known as *mycology*.

Some fungi, notably the yeasts, occur as colonies of individual cells. In others, the cells divide to form chains of tubular filaments called hyphae, which are organized into a complex network called a mycelium. With some soil-living fungi, parts of the mycelium form into large fruiting bodies, seen as mushrooms or toadstools. Many fungi form minute bodies called spores, which are like seeds. These spores can be carried in the air and, if they settle in a suitable location with nutrients available, they divide to form a new mycelium; the molds that eventually form on exposed food are a type of mycelium. Fungal spores are ever-present in the air and soil.

FUNGI AND DISEASE

Fungi can cause illness and disease in a variety of ways.

First, the fruiting bodies of some soil-living fungi contain toxins that can produce direct poisoning if eaten (see *Mushroom poisoning*).

Second, certain fungi that infect food crops produce dangerous toxins that can cause a type of food poisoning if contaminated food is eaten. The best known of these are a fungus that infects rye and other cereals and produces a toxin called *ergot*, and another that grows on groundnuts and produces the poison *aflatoxin*. Ergot poisoning is rare today, but chronic aflatoxin poisoning from eating moldy groundnuts is a suspected cause of liver cancer in some regions of Asia and Africa.

Third, the inhaled spores of some fungi can cause a persistent allergic reaction in the lungs, known as allergic *alveolitis*. Farmers' lung, caused by spores from moldy hay, is an example of such a reaction. Fungal spores are also sometimes responsible for other allergic disorders such as *asthma* and allergic *rhinitis* (hay fever).

Fourth, some fungi are able to invade and form colonies or mycelia within the lungs, in the skin, beneath the skin, or sometimes in various tissues throughout the body, leading to conditions ranging from mild skin irritation to severe, or even fatal, widespread infection and illness (see *Fungal infections*).

Fungicidal
See *Antifungal drugs*.

Funny bone
Popular term for the small area at the back of the *elbow* where the ulnar nerve passes over a prominence of the humerus (upper arm bone). A blow to the nerve causes acute pain and sometimes numbness of the forearm.

Furosemide
A *diuretic drug* commonly used to treat *edema* (fluid retention) and *hypertension* (high blood pressure). When given by injection, furosemide has a rapid effect. It is therefore often used in emergencies to treat pulmonary *edema* (fluid in the lungs).

Furuncle
Another name for a *boil* that usually involves a hair follicle.

G6PD deficiency

An inherited disorder that affects the chemistry of red blood cells, making them prone to damage during an infectious illness or from certain drugs or foods.

CAUSES AND INCIDENCE

G6PD deficiency is caused by the production within red blood cells of abnormal molecules of an enzyme (a type of protein) called glucose-6-phosphate dehydrogenase. Because the molecules of this substance are defective, they cannot carry out their normal function, which is to help in a chemical process that protects the cells from damage.

The disorder is the result of an abnormality in the affected person's genetic material and is inherited in an X-linked recessive pattern (see *Genetic disorders*). This means that most of those affected are male, but women may carry the defective gene in a hidden form and pass it on to some of their sons.

The disorder is much more common among blacks than whites, affecting about 15 percent of black males in the US. A variant of the disorder, called *favism*, affects a small number of whites of Mediterranean origin.

The particular drugs that can precipitate hemolysis (red cell destruction) in affected people are shown below. Individuals with favism are, in addition, extremely sensitive to a chemical in broad beans, which they must avoid eating.

SYMPTOMS

A few days after taking an incriminated drug or food, or during the course of an infectious illness, symptoms of hemolytic *anemia* (such as jaundice, fatigue, headaches, shortness of breath on exertion, and sometimes darkening of the urine due to the destruction of red blood cells) may develop in affected people.

DIAGNOSIS AND TREATMENT

The presence of G6PD deficiency can be established by a blood screening test. The deficiency cannot be treated but any episode of hemolytic anemia caused by a drug can be halted by stopping use of the drug. Full recovery then takes place within a few days.

Anyone with a history of G6PD deficiency in the family should ask for a screening test before taking any of the incriminated drugs. If the test result is positive, these drugs should be avoided. Anyone known to have the condition should also seek prompt treatment for any infectious illness to prevent a hemolytic crisis.

GABA

Common abbreviation for gamma-aminobutyric acid, a *neurotransmitter* (chemical released from nerve endings). GABA controls the flow of nerve impulses by blocking the release of other neurotransmitters (e.g., *norepinephrine* and dopamine) that stimulate nerve activity. The activity of GABA is increased by *benzodiazepine drugs* and by *anticonvulsant drugs*.

It has been suggested that people with *Huntington's chorea* (a hereditary disease characterized by mental retardation and involuntary movement) have insufficient GABA-producing nerve cells in the brain centers that coordinate movement.

Gait

The style or manner of *walking*. Some neuromuscular disorders are evaluated on the basis of altered gait.

Galactorrhea

Spontaneous, persistent production of milk by a woman who is not pregnant or lactating (producing milk after childbirth), or, very rarely, production of milk by a man.

CAUSES

Lactation is initiated by a rise in the level of prolactin (a hormone produced by the pituitary gland). Galactorrhea is caused by an excessive amount of prolactin being secreted as a result of a *pituitary tumor*, or due to other endocrine diseases, such as *hypothyroidism*. Certain *antipsychotic drugs* (such as chlorpromazine) and some brain diseases (for example, *meningitis*) may be associated with increased prolactin production. However, in about 50 percent of cases, no cause can be found.

SYMPTOMS AND SIGNS

The breast secretion is obviously milklike. If it is of any other color or bloodstained, another cause (such as a breast tumor) should be suspected. Excessive levels of prolactin may also adversely affect the ovaries, causing *amenorrhea* (absence of menstrual periods) or *infertility*. If the underlying cause is a pituitary tumor, the symptoms may include headache and visual disturbances.

TREATMENT

Surgery or *radiation therapy* may be required if there is a pituitary tumor, but the symptoms are often controlled and the size of the tumor is decreased by treatment with *bromocriptine*.

In addition to treating the underlying cause, hormone or drug therapy may be used to suppress prolactin and prevent milk production. Bromocriptine, which suppresses prolactin production, can successfully treat galactorrhea when the cause is unknown, and also may regulate periods and fertility.

Galactosemia

An extremely rare inability of the body's biochemical system to break down galactose (a sugar derived from the milk sugar lactose) into glucose because of the absence of an enzyme in the liver. Galactosemia is caused by an autosomal recessive genetic defect (see *Genetic disorders*).

SYMPTOMS

Galactosemia causes no symptoms at birth, but jaundice, diarrhea, and vomiting soon develop and the baby fails to gain weight. If untreated, the condition results in liver disease, *cataract* (opacity in the lens of the eye), and *mental retardation*.

DRUGS TO BE AVOIDED BY PEOPLE WITH G6PD DEFICIENCY

Class	Drugs to avoid
Antimalarial drugs	Primaquine, chloroquine, quinine, dapsone
Antibacterial and antibiotic drugs	Nitrofurantoin, sulfonamides (such as sulfisoxazole and sulfacetamide), chloramphenicol,* nalidixic acid
Analgesics (painkillers)	Aspirin*
Miscellaneous	Vitamin K (water-soluble form), probenecid, quinidine*

*These drugs do not usually cause problems in the type of G6PD deficiency that affects blacks in the US.

DIAGNOSIS AND TREATMENT

The diagnosis is confirmed from urine and blood tests. Feeding with a special lactose-free milk leads to dramatic improvement; normal milk must be avoided throughout life.

Gallbladder

A small, pear-shaped sac situated underneath the liver, to which it is attached by fibrous tissue. Bile produced by the liver passes to the gallbladder by means of a small tube, the cystic duct. This duct branches off from the bile duct, which carries bile from the liver to the duodenum.

Within the gallbladder, bile is stored and concentrated (by absorption of its water content through the gallbladder walls). When food passes from the stomach to the duodenum, secretin and cholecystokinin (gastrointestinal hormones) cause the gallbladder to contract and expel its content of bile into the duodenum, where the bile emulsifies fats contained in the food. (See also *Biliary system*.)

ANATOMY OF THE GALLBLADDER

A small, muscular sac that lies under the liver. The gallbladder expels bile via the common bile duct into the duodenum.

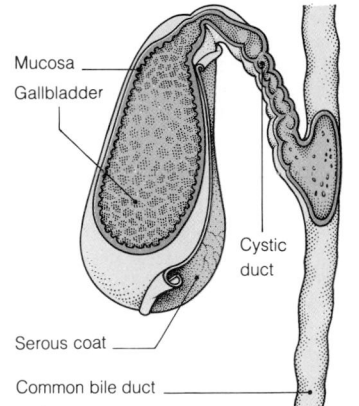

Mucosa

Gallbladder

Cystic duct

Serous coat

Common bile duct

Gallbladder cancer

A rare cancer of unknown cause, occurring mainly in old age. It usually occurs in gallbladders with *gallstones*, but affects only a minute number of gallstone sufferers. The incidence of this cancer is less than three new cases per 100,000 population per year.

The cancer may cause *jaundice* and tenderness in the upper right abdomen but is sometimes symptomless. It is diagnosed by *ultrasound scanning*; occasionally, the cancer is discovered during surgery on the gallbladder.

Cancer of the gallbladder is treated by removal of as much of the tumor as possible. The cancer often has invaded the liver by the time it is detected, making the outlook poor.

Gallium

A metallic element whose radioactive form is used in *radionuclide scanning* (a technique for obtaining images of internal organs). Gallium is injected into the bloodstream and, about 72 hours later, scanning is performed.

G

DISORDERS OF THE GALLBLADDER

The gallbladder rarely causes problems in childhood or early adulthood but, from middle age onward, the increasing occurrence of gallstones can sometimes give rise to symptoms.

Because the digestive system can function normally without a gallbladder, its removal has little known long-term effect.

CONGENITAL AND GENETIC DEFECTS

Abnormalities present from birth may include no gallbladder, an oversized gallbladder, or two gallbladders; these defects rarely cause problems.

METABOLIC DISORDERS

The principal disorder of the gallbladder, with which most other problems are associated, is the formation of *gallstones*. Gallstones are common, but only about 20 percent of people with gallstones have symptoms requiring *cholecystectomy* (surgical removal of the gallbladder). Attempts by the gallbladder to expel the stone or stones can cause severe *biliary colic* (abdominal pain). There are three main types of gallstones: cholesterol gallstones, pigment gallstones, and mixed gallstones. The great majority are cholesterol or

mixed gallstones, and women are affected four times as often as men. Every year about 1 million Americans develop gallstones. Many people carry "silent" gallstones, which produce no symptoms.

INFECTION AND INFLAMMATION

If a gallstone becomes stuck in the outlet from the gallbladder, the trapped bile may irritate and inflame the gallbladder walls and the bile itself may become infected. This is called acute *cholecystitis*. The first symptom may be biliary colic, which is followed by fever and abdominal tenderness.

Repeated attacks of biliary colic and acute cholecystitis can lead to chronic cholecystitis, in which the gallbladder becomes shrunken and thick-walled and ceases to function. Rarely, the gallbladder may become inflamed without the presence of gallstones—a condition that is called acalculous cholecystitis.

Occasionally, cholecystitis proceeds to a condition in which the gallbladder fills with pus, called *empyema* of the gallbladder. This can cause a high fever and severe abdominal pain.

TUMORS

Gallbladders harboring *gallbladder cancer* usually contain gallstones. However, this cancer is extremely

uncommon compared to the high prevalence of gallstones.

OTHER DISORDERS

In rare cases where a gallbladder is empty when a stone obstructs its outlet, it may fill with mucus secreted by the gallbladder walls, resulting in a distended, mucus-filled gallbladder known as a *mucocele*.

INVESTIGATION

Gallbladder problems are investigated by physical examination and techniques such as *ultrasound scanning*, *radionuclide scanning*, or *cholecystography* (X rays of the gallbladder after it has been filled with a contrast medium). Blood tests may also be carried out.

G

Gallium tends to accumulate in tumors and pus cells; its main uses in scanning are to detect malignant diseases, such as *Hodgkin's disease*, and abscesses or areas of *osteomyelitis*.

Gallstones

Round or oval, smooth or faceted lumps of solid matter found in the gallbladder (the sac under the liver where bile is stored and concentrated). Gallstones are sometimes found in the bile ducts (which connect the gallbladder and liver to the duodenum). In these cases, the symptoms can be severe. There may be between one and 10, or sometimes more, stones varying in size from about 0.05 inch to 1 inch (1 to 25 mm) across. Gallstones composed principally of cholesterol are the most common type, but some contain a high content of bile pigments and other substances, such as chalk.

CAUSES AND INCIDENCE
Gallstones develop when an upset occurs in the chemical composition of bile. When the liver makes bile, it can put too much cholesterol into it (which occurs in obesity) or it may fail to put in enough of the detergent substances that normally keep cholesterol, a fatty substance, in solution.

Once the bile is overloaded with cholesterol, a tiny particle can form that gradually grows as more material solidifies around it, eventually forming a stone. Something else in the bile (its nature is unknown) actually triggers this process. Fasting for long periods may help gallstones develop by causing bile to stagnate in the gallbladder.

Gallstones are rare in childhood and become progressively more common with age. Two to three times more women than men are affected (autopsies show that 20 percent of all women have gallstones when they die).

Risk groups include overweight people and women who have had many children. Use of the birth-control pill may cause gallstones to form earlier than they would otherwise.

PREVENTION
People should avoid becoming overweight and should eat as little sugar and fat as possible. Some experts believe a high intake of fiber helps and that drinking one alcoholic drink a day has a protective value.

SYMPTOMS
Only about 20 percent of gallstones cause symptoms or complications. Symptoms commonly begin only when a gallstone gets stuck in the duct leading from the gallbladder. This causes *biliary colic* (intense pain in the upper right side of the abdomen or between the shoulder blades) and may make the sufferer feel sick and possibly vomit. Indigestion made worse by fatty foods often seems to be associated with gallstones. Other potential complications include *cholecystitis* (inflammation of the gallbladder) and *bile duct obstruction* leading to jaundice.

DIAGNOSIS AND TREATMENT
Ultrasound scanning can detect 95 percent of gallstones and is therefore the first test to be performed. An older and slightly less sensitive method is X-ray *cholecystography*, which utilizes an iodinated dye that is taken either by mouth or injected into a vein. Blood tests may also be performed. If the physician suspects the stones have escaped into the bile ducts, *cholangiography* may be carried out.

Stones that do not cause symptoms can safely be left alone, as they are unlikely to cause trouble. When symptoms are severe, *cholecystectomy* (surgical removal of the gallbladder) is carried out; this cures the problem in 95 percent of cases.

In some cases drug treatment may be used, especially if the stones are small and noncalcified. Tablets containing chenodiol or ursodeoxycholic acid can dissolve stones over several months. X rays or ultrasound scans of the gallbladder are done to check progress. Stones recur in about half the cases when the drug is stopped, so ultrasound scans are carried out over the following few years.

OUTLOOK
New treatments are being developed. Extracorporeal shock-wave *lithotripsy* uses shock waves to shatter the stones. In another technique a tube is inserted into the gallbladder and a strong solution that dissolves cholesterol is flushed through. The safety and long-term value of these treatments is still being investigated.

Gambling, pathological
Chronic inability to resist impulses to gamble, resulting in personal or social problems. Most gamblers can stop at a given point; pathological or "compulsive" gamblers seem unable to control the amount they spend and are unable to stop even when they continue to lose. The urge to gamble is so great that tension can be relieved only by more gambling. Family problems, bankruptcy, and crime may follow.

Gamma globulin
A substance prepared from human blood that contains *antibodies* against most common infections. (See *Immune serum globulin*.)

Ganglion
A cystic swelling associated with the sheath of a tendon. It is a common condition and usually occurs on the wrist, although a finger or foot may sometimes be affected. The cyst, which contains thick fluid derived from the synovial fluid that lubricates tendons and joints, can vary from the size of a small pea to, rarely, the size of a golf ball.

A ganglion may disappear spontaneously; if it does not, treatment is usually necessary only if it is painful or unsightly. The fluid may be sucked out with a needle and syringe. The cyst commonly recurs after such treatments, however. The best approach is to remove the cyst surgically, after which recurrence is rare.

Gangrene
Death of tissue, usually as a result of loss of blood supply. It may affect a small area of skin, a finger, or a substantial portion of a limb.

SYMPTOMS
Pain is felt in the dying tissues, but once they are dead they become numb. The affected skin and underlying tissue turn black. Bacterial infection may develop, causing the gangrene to spread and give off an unpleasant smell. There may be redness, swelling, and oozing pus around the blackened area.

There are two types of gangrene (dry and wet). In dry gangrene there is usually no bacterial infection; the deprived area dies because its blood supply is blocked. This type of gangrene does not spread to other tissues. It may be caused by *arteriosclerosis*, *diabetes mellitus*, *thrombosis*, an *embolism*, or *frostbite*.

Gangrene of the foot
This photograph shows a foot with an extensive area of dead tissue, with blackening of the overlying skin.

Wet gangrene develops when dry gangrene or a wound becomes infected by bacteria. A particularly virulent type—known as gas gangrene—is caused by a dangerous strain of bacteria that destroys muscles and produces a foul-smelling gas. Gas gangrene has caused millions of deaths in war.

TREATMENT

Treatment of dry gangrene consists of improving circulation to the affected body part before it is too late. If the tissue becomes infected, the patient is given antibiotics to prevent wet gangrene from setting in.

If wet gangrene is diagnosed, *amputation* of the affected part is unavoidable. Usually, some of the adjacent living tissue must be removed as well.

Ganser's syndrome

A rare, *factitious disorder* in which a person seeks, consciously or unconsciously, to mislead others regarding his or her mental state. Ganser's syndrome occurs most often in prisoners. A characteristic of the disorder is the giving of "approximate answers" (for example, 2x2=5); the choice of an answer near the correct one suggests that the person knows the real response. The sufferer also displays symptoms that simulate *psychosis*, such as episodes of intense agitation or stupor.

Gardnerella vaginalis

A bacterium found in increasing numbers in the vaginal discharge of women with *vaginitis* (inflammation of the vagina).

Gargle

A liquid preparation to wash and freshen the mouth and throat, usually not meant to be swallowed. Gargles may contain mouth fresheners, flavorings, *antiseptics*, or local anesthetics (see *Anesthesia, local*). Those containing antiseptics and local anesthetics relieve the irritation associated with sore throats, but do not cure the underlying cause. The home remedy of gargling with salt water is equally effective in most circumstances.

Gastrectomy

Removal of the whole stomach (total gastrectomy) or, more commonly, a part of the stomach (partial gastrectomy). Gastrectomy is a major operation requiring hospitalization and extensive postoperative care.

WHY IT IS DONE

Total gastrectomy is a rare operation used to treat some stomach cancers. Partial gastrectomy is fairly common; it is usually performed to deal with a *peptic ulcer* (gastric ulcer or duodenal ulcer), ulcers that have failed to heal after changes in diet or drug treatment, ulcers that bleed very badly or perforate (break through the stomach

or duodenal wall), and some cancers located closer to the stomach's outlet. In treating duodenal ulcers, removal of part of the stomach may be combined with *vagotomy* (cutting of the nerves to the acid-secreting part of the stomach) to prevent more ulcers.

HOW IT IS DONE

A general anesthetic is given and the stomach emptied by means of a *nasogastric tube* (a tube passed through the nose down the esophagus into the stomach). The entire stomach is removed in a total gastrectomy; the risk of complications or death from this procedure is high. Smaller portions of stomach are removed with less danger.

RECOVERY PERIOD

After the operation, the nasogastric tube is left in position to allow digestive system secretions to drain. When the volume of these secretions diminishes and normal *peristalsis* (the rhythmic contractions that force food through the digestive system) returns, the patient is given small amounts of water. If these do not cause abdominal pain or nausea, the nasogastric tube is removed. Intake of fluids is gradually increased and, within a few days, a light diet can be started.

COMPLICATIONS

Because removal of the stomach disturbs normal digestion, post-gastrectomy syndromes (side effects after gastric surgery) can develop

G

TYPES OF GASTRECTOMY

There are several different types of gastrectomy operations. In total gastrectomy, the whole stomach is removed; in partial gastrectomy, between one half and two thirds of the stomach is removed. There are two common types of partial gastrectomy operation—the Billroth I and the Billroth II.

Esophagus
Duodenum
Stomach
Jejunum

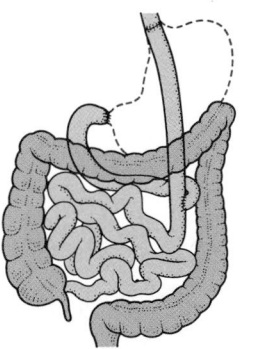

Total gastrectomy
The whole stomach is removed and the esophagus is joined directly to the jejunum (the middle section of the small intestine).

Billroth I gastrectomy
The remaining part of the stomach is joined to the duodenum (the first part of the small intestine).

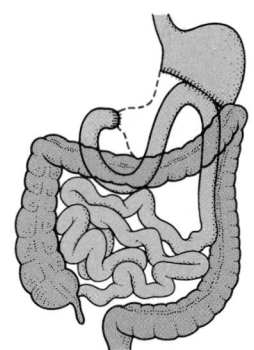

Billroth II gastrectomy
The surgeon performs a *gastrojejunostomy* (a procedure in which the stomach is joined to the jejunum) and seals the end of the duodenum to form a blind loop.

G

in some patients. The most troublesome are fullness and discomfort after meals; formation of an ulcer at the new junction between stomach and small intestine; regurgitation of bile, which may lead to *gastritis* (inflammation of the stomach), *esophagitis* (inflammation of the esophagus), and vomiting of bile; diarrhea; and the *dumping syndrome* (sweating, nausea, dizziness, and weakness felt soon after eating a meal because food leaves the stomach too quickly). These side effects usually disappear in time, but diet and drug treatment or another operation may be necessary.

Other complications include *malabsorption* (a reduced ability to absorb food, minerals, and vitamins), which may lead to *anemia* or *osteoporosis* (thinned bones). After total gastrectomy, patients cannot absorb vitamin B_{12} and are therefore given monthly injections for the rest of their lives.

OUTLOOK
Only about 10 percent of patients suffer complications requiring further treatment. Ulcer recurrence is infrequent, but there is a small risk of cancer of the stomach developing after partial gastrectomy.

Gastric bubble
A balloon, about 2 inches (5 cm) in diameter and 3.5 inches (9 cm) long, that is inserted through the mouth and into the stomach as a means of weight control in people who are dangerously obese.

The gastric bubble was approved in 1985 by the US Food and Drug Administration (FDA) only for people who are 100 percent overweight. The procedure is not without risk. In addition, no studies have been performed to evaluate whether or not weight is regained after removal of the balloon.

Gastric erosion
A break in the innermost layer (mucosa) of the membrane that lines the stomach. If a break extends deeper than this layer, it is called a gastric ulcer (see *Peptic ulcer*). Gastric erosion occurs in some cases of *gastritis* (inflammation of the stomach lining).

The causes of gastric erosions are not clear, but many cases are the result of the ingestion of alcohol, iron tablets, aspirin, or other nonsteroidal anti-inflammatory drugs (NSAIDs), such as phenylbutazone or indomethacin. The stress of serious illness, such as septicemia (blood poisoning), burns, or renal failure, may also bring on a gastric erosion.

Often there are no symptoms, although erosions may bleed, resulting in hematemesis (see *Vomiting blood*) or melena (black feces containing blood). The blood loss, on the other hand, may be small but persistent, eventually causing *anemia*. The condition is diagnosed by *gastroscopy* (direct examination of the stomach through a flexible viewing tube), which reveals the small bleeding points in the stomach lining.

Gastric erosions usually heal completely in a few days when treated with *antacid drugs* and *ulcer-healing drugs*, such as cimetidine, ranitidine, or famotidine.

Gastric ulcer
A raw area in the wall of the stomach caused by a breach of its inner surface lining. (See *Peptic ulcer*.)

Gastritis
Inflammation of the mucous membrane that lines the stomach. The illness may be acute, occurring as a sudden attack, or chronic, developing gradually over a long period.

CAUSES
Gastritis may be caused by irritation of the stomach lining by a drug, most commonly aspirin or alcohol; by infection of the stomach by CAMPYLOBAC-TER bacteria; or, in some people, by extreme physical stress such as head injury, severe burns, or the development of liver failure.

Chronic gastritis may be caused by prolonged irritation of the stomach by alcohol, tobacco smoke, or bile; damage of the lining by an *autoimmune disorder*, as in pernicious anemia (see *Anemia, megaloblastic*); or degeneration of the lining with age.

Acute gastritis may cause erosions in the lining that bleed easily. In the chronic form, blood may ooze continually from the lining.

SYMPTOMS
Gastritis produces many of the same symptoms as a gastric ulcer, with which it may be confused. Symptoms include discomfort in the upper abdomen (often aggravated by eating), nausea, and vomiting. In acute erosive gastritis, the feces may be black with blood lost from the stomach; in the chronic condition, slow blood loss may cause anemia (see *Anemia, iron-deficiency*), resulting in pallor, tiredness, and breathlessness.

DIAGNOSIS
The diagnosis is made by examining the stomach lining through a gastroscope, a viewing tube passed down

the esophagus to the stomach (see *Gastroscopy*). A *biopsy* (removal of a tiny sample of tissue for analysis) may be performed at the same time, using an attachment at the end of the gastroscope. Microscopic examination of the sample indicates the type of inflammation. The correlation between the microscopic findings and the symptoms is not always clear.

TREATMENT
A person with gastritis should take acetaminophen rather than aspirin for pain relief, avoid alcohol, and not smoke. *Ulcer-healing drugs* may help heal the inflamed lining.

Gastroenteritis
Inflammation of the stomach and intestines, often causing sudden and sometimes violent upsets. The illness does not usually last for more than two or three days and the sufferer tends to recover without any specific treatment other than replacement of lost fluid and salt. *Dysentery, typhoid fever, cholera, food poisoning*, and travelers' diarrhea—as well as many milder stomach upsets—are all forms of gastroenteritis.

CAUSES AND INCIDENCE
Gastroenteritis is an extremely common cause of mild illness in developed countries and a major cause of death in some developing ones.

The illness may be caused by any of a variety of viruses, bacteria, and other small organisms that have contaminated food or water supplies. There are also a number of noninfectious causes of gastroenteritis—for example, *food intolerance*, very spicy foods, certain drugs, toxic substances, and excessive intake of alcohol. In many people, *antibiotic drugs* cause symptoms similar to those of gastroenteritis because the drugs can upset the balance of bacteria that occur naturally in the intestines.

SYMPTOMS
The onset and severity of symptoms depends on the type and concentrations of the microorganisms, food, or toxic substance causing the illness. Appetite loss, nausea, vomiting, cramps, and diarrhea are the symptoms; these may come on gradually, but more often appear suddenly. The combination of symptoms may be so mild that they cause little disruption to daily routine, or the attack may be so severe and persistent that it is disabling, causing dehydration, *shock*, and collapse. In babies and the very old, this may warrant intravenous fluid treatment.

DIAGNOSIS

In mild attacks, the symptoms alone are sufficient to make a diagnosis, but in more serious cases the physician may ask about contact with infected people, food that has been eaten recently, and recent travel abroad.

TREATMENT AND OUTLOOK

Mild cases are treated at home. The affected person should rest, preferably in bed, and take plenty of fluids, which should include salt and sugar if much fluid is being lost by vomiting and diarrhea—4 level teaspoons of sugar and a quarter of a teaspoon of salt for each pint of liquid (see *Rehydration therapy*). No solid food should be eaten until symptoms subside.

In severe cases where shock and collapse occur, the person will be taken to the hospital. Patients are given intravenous fluids to replace the vital body salts lost by vomiting and diarrhea. After the acute phase, water and then other clear fluids are given; if these fluids do not cause further upset, a bland diet is introduced. Antibiotic treatment is reserved for specific bacterial infections such as typhoid.

In most cases the illness subsides gradually without any special measures; recovery is usually complete with no complications.

PREVENTION

Care taken in food preparation and hygiene can substantially reduce the chances of gastroenteritis (see *Food poisoning; Food-borne infection*). Some protection against typhoid and cholera can be acquired by vaccination before traveling to countries where these diseases are still common. Avoidance of substances known to cause upset helps minimize noninfectious attacks of gastroenteritis.

Those caring for a person with the symptoms of gastroenteritis should be scrupulous about personal hygiene to prevent the illness from spreading.

Gastroenterologist

A physician specially trained in the management of disorders of the digestive system. His or her work is concerned with the treatment of *peptic ulcers* of the stomach and duodenum, conditions affecting the gastrointestinal tract from mouth to anus, and diseases of the liver and gallbladder.

The work of the gastroenterologist has been revolutionized in recent years by the development of fiberoptic *endoscopes*. Much of the gastrointestinal tract can now be visualized directly by these instruments and samples can be taken for laboratory examination.

HORMONES IN THE DIGESTIVE TRACT

Hormones released from endocrine cells in the stomach, pancreas, and intestine aid digestion by stimulating the release of bile from the gallbladder and enzymes from the pancreas into the duodenum.

Cholecystokinin
Released by the duodenum in response to fats and acid. It causes the gallbladder to squeeze bile into the duodenum and stimulates the production of pancreatic enzymes, which pass into the duodenum through the pancreatic duct.

Secretin
Secreted by the lining of the duodenum in response to acid entering from the stomach. It acts on the pancreas to increase the output of bicarbonate, which neutralizes acid from the stomach. It also increases the release of enzymes from the pancreas.

Gastrin
Secreted mainly by cells in the stomach in response to eating food (especially protein). It causes the stomach to produce more acid and stimulates contraction of muscle in the wall of part of the stomach, ileum, and colon. This contraction propels food through the digestive tract.

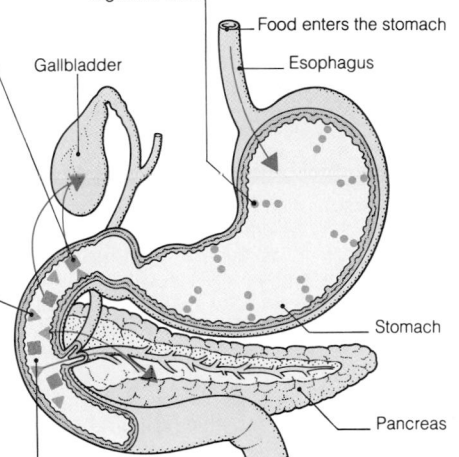

Food enters the stomach
Esophagus
Gallbladder
Stomach
Pancreas
Duodenum

The gastroenterologist, whenever possible, treats patients by advising on diet and life-style and/or by prescribing medication; if necessary, the gastroenterologist refers patients for surgical treatment.

Gastroenterology

The study of the digestive system and the diseases and disorders affecting it. The major organs involved include the mouth, esophagus, stomach, duodenum, small intestine, colon, and rectum. Diseases of the liver, gallbladder, and pancreas are also included in this specialty.

Gastrointestinal hormones

A group of hormones released from specialized endocrine cells in the stomach, pancreas, and intestine that controls various functions of the digestive organs. Gastrin, secretin, and cholecystokinin are probably the best documented of these hormones. (See illustrated box, above.)

Various other gastrointestinal hormones released by the intestine include motilin, neurotensin, and enteroglucagon; their precise functions are still being studied.

DISORDERS

Disorders that are produced by gastrointestinal hormones are relatively rare. The most notable example is a tumor of gastrin-secreting cells in the pancreas or the wall of the intestine, a condition called *Zollinger-Ellison syndrome*.

Gastrointestinal tract

The part of the *digestive system* that consists of the *mouth, esophagus, stomach,* and *intestine*; it excludes the liver, gallbladder, and pancreas.

Gastrojejunostomy

A surgically created connection between the stomach and the jejunum (the middle two thirds of the small intestine). It is sometimes combined with partial *gastrectomy* (removal of the lower part of the stomach).

WHY IT IS DONE

The operation is performed as part of the treatment of a duodenal ulcer (see *Peptic ulcer*). The purpose of the procedure is to allow food to pass directly from the stomach to the small intestine, thereby avoiding the faulty emptying encountered when *vagotomy* alone is performed, and permitting a bypass around a scarred, obstructed duodenum.

HOW IT IS DONE

The preparation of the patient is the same as for gastrectomy. If the gastrojejunostomy is to be combined with partial gastrectomy, some of the lower part of the stomach is removed. The surgeon then pulls up the first part of the jejunum and stitches it to the lower part or remnant of the stomach; a new opening is made through which food will pass.

RECOVERY PERIOD AND OUTLOOK

Complications, recovery, and outlook are the same as for gastrectomy.

Gastroscopy

Examination of the lining of the esophagus, stomach, and duodenum (first part of the small intestine) by means of a long, flexible viewing tube, called an esophagogastroduodeno-scope, inserted through the mouth (see *Endoscope*).

WHY IT IS DONE

Gastroscopy is used to investigate symptoms (such as severe pain or bleeding in the upper abdomen) and to look for disorders of the esophagus, stomach, and duodenum. The procedure may also be used to assess how these disorders are responding to treatment. Gastroscopy is used to identify the source of bleeding and sometimes to treat bleeding sites in the stomach and duodenum.

Attachments at the end of the instrument enable the physician to remove *biopsy* samples (small amounts of tissue for inspection).

Other procedures may be carried out using a gastroscope, such as injecting *esophageal varices* (abnormally enlarged veins in the esophagus) or dilatation (opening up) of an *esophageal stricture*. The gastroscope is also used to facilitate passage of a gastric feeding tube through the skin (percutaneous gastrostomy).

HOW IT IS DONE

The stomach should be empty for gastroscopy, so patients are asked to fast for at least six hours beforehand.

The procedure is usually performed using a local anesthetic sprayed onto the back of the throat and a sedative to relax the patient. A general anesthetic is used if elaborate investigations or treatments are required or if the patient is particularly anxious.

A diagnostic examination usually lasts for between five and 20 minutes. Some discomfort may be felt as the tube passes down the throat; there may be a sore throat afterward.

Complications from gastroscopy are rare. Most are caused by inhalation of vomit or reactions to the sedatives.

Gastrostomy

A surgically produced opening in the stomach, usually connecting the stomach to the outside so that a feed-ing tube can be placed into the stomach or passed into the small intestine. (*Gastroscopy* utilizes a flexible viewing tube to examine the lining of the stomach and other organs.)

People who are starving because of cancer of the esophagus (see *Esophagus, cancer of*) or who are unable to chew and swallow due to stroke or other neurologic disease may be candidates for gastrostomy. (See also *Feeding, artificial*.)

Gauze

An absorbent, open-weave fabric, usually made of cotton. For medical purposes it is usually sterilized and sealed in a package.

Gauze is often used as a *dressing* for wounds. It can be applied dry or can be immersed in an antiseptic fluid or cream; a bandage is used to hold it in place. The gauze absorbs blood and other fluids oozing from the wound. Gauze is usually not used to dress skin ulcers because it tends to stick to moist surfaces and, when removed, dis-lodges new tissue.

Surgeons sometimes insert pieces of gauze into wounds during surgery to keep the operative site relatively free of blood, which otherwise might obscure structures.

Gavage

The process of feeding liquids through a *nasogastric tube* (one passed into the stomach through the nose). See *Feeding, artificial*.

Gavage also refers to hyperalimen-tation (treatment of a patient by excessive feeding beyond the requirements of appetite).

Gay bowel syndrome

A group of conditions affecting the anus, rectum, and colon that occurs most frequently, but not exclusively, in male homosexuals.

Most of the conditions in gay bowel syndrome result from various forms of sexual contact, including penile-anal contact, oral-anal contact, and fisting (insertion of the fist into the rectum). If carried out regularly, these activities are likely to cause structural abnor-malities (such as *hemorrhoids*, *anal fistulas*, and rectal ulcers) or inflamma-tory anal-rectal conditions (such as *proctitis*). They may also cause the spread of *AIDS*, *hepatitis*, and intesti-nal infections (such as *shigellosis* and *amebiasis*) or other infections (such as genital *warts*, *gonorrhea*, *syphilis*, and *lymphogranuloma venereum*) that can also be spread by vaginal intercourse.

Gemfibrozil

A *lipid-lowering drug* used in the treat-ment of certain types of *hyperlipidemia* (raised levels of fats such as cholesterol in the blood). Gemfibrozil works mainly by reducing the produc-tion of lipoproteins (fats combined with protein) in the liver.

Gender identity

The inner feeling of maleness or femaleness. Gender identity is not necessarily the same as biological sex. Gender identity is fixed within the first two to three years of life and is reinforced during puberty; once estab-lished, it usually cannot be changed. Gender role is the public declaration of gender identity—that is, the image people present outwardly that con-firms their inner feelings about their gender.

Gender identity problems occur when a person has persistent feelings of discomfort about his or her sexual identity. *Transsexualism* is the most common example of this problem.

Gene

A unit of the material of heredity. In physical terms, a gene consists of a short section of the sub-stance deoxyribonucleic acid (DNA) contained within the nucleus of a cell (see *Nucleic acids*). In functional terms, a particular gene has a specific influence on the workings of a cell; the activities of the same gene in many different cells specifies a particular physical or biochemical feature of the whole body (for example, hair color or a chemical step in the digestion of food).

Every human cell holds, within its nucleus, more than 50,000 different genes. Through the sum of their effects, genes influence and direct the development and functioning of all organs and systems within the entire body. In short, they provide an instruction manual or program for growth, survival, reproduction, and possibly also for aging and death.

Each of a person's cells (with the exception of egg and sperm cells) con-tains an identical set of genes. This is because all the cells are derived, by a process of division, from a single fer-tilized egg, and with each division the genes are copied to each offspring cell. Within any cell, however, some genes are active and others are idle, accord-ing to the specialized nature of the cell (e.g., different sets of genes are active within liver cells and nerve cells).

WHERE DO YOUR GENES COME FROM?

A person's genes are inherited from his or her parents. Half come from the mother and half from the father via the egg and sperm cells. Each parent provides a different selection, or "mix," of his or her genes to each child; this accounts for the marked differences in appearance, health, and personality among most brothers and sisters. Everyone holds a copy of his or her genes within each body cell.

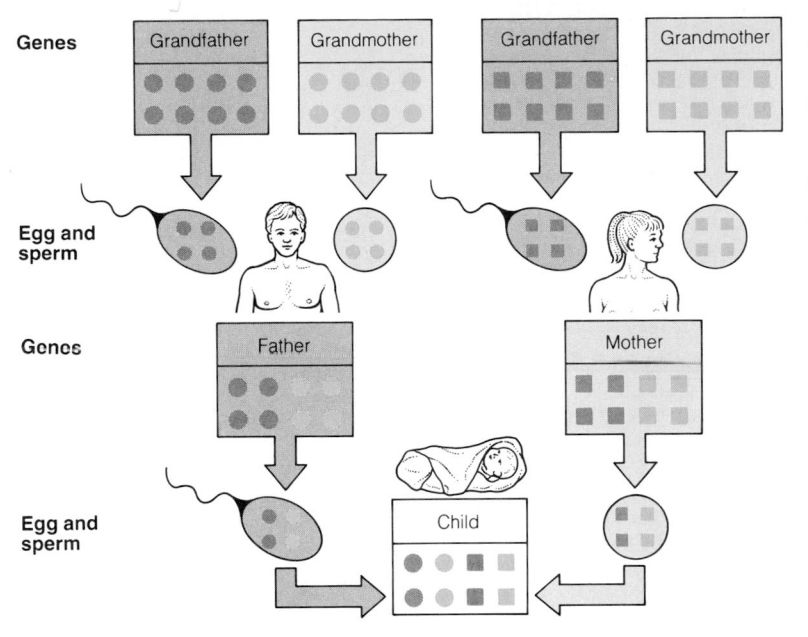

Gene transmission
In this diagram, only eight genes are shown—in reality, each cell in the body contains about 50,000 genes. Half of them come from the mother and half from the father—thus a quarter of the genes originate from each of the four grandparents.

G

If the genes from any two people (other than identical twins) are compared, they always show a number of differences. These differences account for all or much of the variation among people in such aspects as gender, height, skin, hair and eye color, and body shape, and in susceptibility to certain diseases and disorders (see *Inheritance; Genetic disorders*). Genes also influence intelligence, personality, physical and mental talents, and behavior, although the extent of their contribution here is less clear-cut because environment and learning also play an important role.

GENE STRUCTURE AND FUNCTION

The physical material of inheritance, DNA, is an extremely long, chainlike structure. Along with some protein, it is what makes up the 23 pairs of *chromosomes* in the nuclei of all cells. A gene corresponds to a small section of DNA within a chromosome.

All genes fulfill their function, or exert an influence in cells or in the body at large, by directing the manufacture of particular proteins. (See illustrated box, next page.)

Although many proteins have a particular structural or catalytic role in the body, others are synthesized solely for the purpose of influencing the activity of other genes, which they are able to switch "on" or "off." The genes responsible for making these proteins are termed "control" genes. The whole process of development and growth can be thought of as being programmed by the sequential switching "on" or "off" of particular genes; this control program is exceedingly complex.

The activities of control genes help differentiate, for example, between nerve and liver cells, where quite different sets of genes are active or idle. If the control genes are disrupted, cells may lose their specialist abilities and begin to multiply out of control; this is the probable mechanism by which cancers and other tumors are started (see *Carcinogenesis; Oncogenes*).

MUTANT GENES

Whenever a cell divides, copies of all of its genetic material are made for the two daughter cells by the process of DNA replication (see *Nucleic acids*) and chromosomal division. However, the copying process is not perfect, and very occasionally a fault occurs, leading to a small change (mutation) in the nucleic acid sequence; this, in turn, alters the structure of the DNA in one of the daughter cells—and thus leads to a change in one of its genes. This mutant gene is then passed on each time the cell subsequently divides. If a gene mutation occurs during the formation of an egg or sperm cell that later takes part in fertilization, the person who develops from the fertilized egg will have the mutant gene in each of his or her cells.

Carrying a mutant gene can have various effects. In some cases, it affects the structure of the protein whose manufacture the gene directs. Depending on the importance of the protein and the change in its structure, this usually has a disadvantageous effect, ranging from mild to lethal. Moreover, the mutant gene may be passed on to some of the person's own children. Diseases or disorders that result from such mutant genes are known as *genetic disorders*. Very rarely, genetic mutations occur that have a positively beneficial effect (see *Mutation*).

ALLELES, DOMINANCE, AND RECESSIVENESS

The consequences of inheriting a mutant gene are influenced by further factors. For every protein in the body, there are normally two genes capable of directing the manufacture of that protein—one inherited from the mother and one from the father. These may or may not be identical. The two genes are carried at the same location on each of a pair of chromosomes. If one of the genes mutates, leading to production of an altered protein, it can often be "masked" by the presence of a normal gene on the other chromosome of the pair.

In fact, the gene at any particular location on a chromosome can exist in any of various forms, called alleles, consisting usually of a normal form and one or more mutant forms, which

479

WHAT GENES ARE AND WHAT THEY DO

Genes are units of hereditary material contained in a person's cells. They hold information for all aspects of bodily growth and development, exerting their effects by directing the manufacture of proteins. All of a person's genes come from his or her parents. The physical differences between people, such as in eye, hair, and skin color, arise from slight differences in gene structure.

DNA PRINTOUT
Through painstaking laboratory research, the exact structure of many genes is now known.

```
TTC-GAG-CAT-CTG-GGG-ATG-
TCA-TGT-CCT-TCA-TCG-TTT-
TGA-TTA-CCG-ACC-CCA-TCG-
TAT-GAC-ACG-CAA-GTT-CCG-
CGG-TCA-CGC-ACG-TCA-TGT-
GGG-GAC-TCG-TAA-TCA-CGT-
CAA-GCG-AGT-TTA-AAT-AGA-
CGA-CGC-AGC-TTT-GAA-TTC-
TAT-AAC-TAC-TAA-CTG-TTA-
TTG-TTA-TGT-GAT-GGG-TTA-
ATG-AGC-GGA-GTG-CAT-TAT-
```

This printout shows a small part of the DNA base sequence in the gene that codes for the protein trypsin, a digestive enzyme.

Chromosomes
Genes are contained in the chromosomes within the nuclei of a person's cells. Each chromosome contains a long strand of the hereditary substance deoxyribonucleic acid (DNA).

Basic body cell

Nucleus

Cytoplasm

DNA

Genes

DNA and genes
DNA has a long, threadlike molecule made up of two intertwined strands, "the double helix." Genes are segments of DNA within chromosomes. Each gene has a function (to direct the manufacture of one type of protein); the instructions for this function are encoded within the structure of its segment of DNA.

DNA double helix

Sugar-phosphate side chain

Sequence of bases
Each strand of DNA is a string of "nucleotide bases," linked by sugar and phosphate side chains. There are four types of base—adenine, cytosine, guanine, and thymine (A, C, G, and T). The sequence of bases in a gene (segment of DNA) is the code for protein manufacture.

Guanine

Thymine

Adenine

Cytosine

Decoding apparatus
To decode a gene, a negative copy of it is made, using the gene as a template; this copy (called messenger RNA) then passes to the cytoplasm of the cell for decoding (see *Protein synthesis*).

Protein molecule

Protein molecule
The information in a gene is decoded to make a protein molecule, which is folded and consists of a string of amino acids.

Structural proteins
Some proteins are used as structural components of cells, tissues, and organs.

Enzymes
Other proteins are enzymes, which promote important chemical processes vital to bodily growth and functioning.

cause the production of altered proteins. If the effects of a particular allele mask or override those of the allele carried at the same location on its partner chromosome, it is said to be dominant. The masked allele is said to be recessive.

Dominant genetic traits, such as brown eyes and blood group A, are those in which the allele producing the trait needs to be present only in a single dose for it to have an outwardly apparent effect. Recessive traits, such as blue eyes and blood group O, are those in which an allele for the trait must usually be present in a double dose for it to have an outward effect.

The patterns by which various traits and disorders are passed on from parents to children, including the further complication of sex-linked and multifactorial inheritance and disorders, are discussed under *Inheritance* and *Genetic disorders*. Medical advice on genetic matters—for example, to parents on the chances of an intended child being affected by a particular genetic disorder—is the province of *genetic counseling*.

Generalized anxiety disorder

A neurotic illness in which the main symptoms are chronic and persistent apprehension and tension about nothing in particular ("free-floating anxiety"). There may also be many unspecific physical reactions such as trembling, jitteriness, sweating, lightheadedness, and irritability.

Symptoms may be so severe that they interfere with everyday living and require medical attention. *Psychotherapy* and drugs are the treatment, although sedatives and tranquilizers are kept to a minimum because dependence can result.

General paralysis of the insane

The common term for the mental and physical deterioration that occurs in the late stage of untreated *syphilis* when it affects the brain substance.

Generic drug

A medicinal drug marketed under its official, chemical name (its generic name) rather than under a patented brand name. Generic names are chosen by appointed drug experts and approved by governmental agencies.

Genetic code

The inherited instructions, contained in chemical form within the nuclei of cells, that specify the activities of cells and thus the development and functioning of the whole body. The term "genetic code" is also used more widely to include the system by which the instructions are copied from a cell to its offspring, the chemical basis by which the instructions are encoded, and the "key" by which the coded instructions are translated.

The basis of the genetic code is contained within molecules of the long, chainlike substance deoxyribonucleic acid (DNA). DNA, along with some protein, makes up the *chromosomes* present in the nuclei of cells. A particular *gene*, or unit of inheritance, corresponds to a section of DNA within a chromosome. Each gene contains the coded instructions for a cell to manufacture a particular protein, which may be an *enzyme* with a vital role in the cell's activities or may have some other function or structural use in the body. Most activity in the body stems from the manufacture of proteins under the guidance of genes.

Little was known about how bits of DNA could specify the manufacture of proteins until the chemical structure of DNA was worked out in 1953. It was found that DNA consists of two long intertwined strands (the "double helix"), each consisting of a sequence of simple chemicals called nucleotide bases. Four different types of base, labeled A, C, G, and T, occur in DNA. The sequence of these bases along particular sections of one of the strands provides the instructions for protein manufacture.

The bases A, C, G, and T can be thought of as the letters of the code. Their sequence along a section of DNA (for example, CGGATCCTAGT-TGATCATGAC) would be completely meaningless without the key to the code, employed by the cell's decoding apparatus. This decoder reads the bases three at a time, and each triplet of bases codes for a particular amino acid, the chemical unit from which proteins are made. For example, the base sequence ACG in a section of DNA codes for the amino acid cysteine and the sequence TGA codes for threonine. As triplets of nucleotide bases are read in turn, the corresponding amino acids are brought together and linked, and, as a complete sequence of bases is read, a chain of amino acids (a polypeptide chain) is formed. This may be a protein molecule itself or may form part of a larger protein structure. Certain base triplets, found at the end of gene sequences, code for termination of protein synthesis.

A complication of the system is that the decoding apparatus does not read directly from DNA but from an intermediary substance, messenger ribonucleic acid (RNA). The DNA acts as a template for RNA manufacture (see *Protein synthesis*). See *Nucleic acids* for the process by which DNA is copied and passed on from each cell to its offspring (and via egg and sperm cells to a new individual).

Genetic counseling

Guidance given to a person or persons (usually by a physician who has experience in genetics) who are considering having a child but are concerned because there is a blood relative (including perhaps a previous child) with an inheritable disorder, or because they are at risk for some other reason of bearing a child with such a disorder.

In most cases, genetic counseling entails predicting the chances of recurrence of a condition that has already affected one or more members of a family. Such counseling depends first on a precise diagnosis of the disorder; the counselor must be able to explain why the disorder occurred and how it is inherited.

Genetic counseling may also include discussion of the prognosis (outlook) for an affected child, advising couples about contraception if, after counseling, they decide not to have children or more children, and sometimes discussing the alternative routes to parenthood.

WHO IS COUNSELED?

Counseling is important for parents of a child with a *genetic disorder*, such as cystic fibrosis or hemophilia, or a *chromosomal abnormality*, such as Down's or Turner's syndrome. It may be useful if a child is born with *birth defects*, such as a cleft lip or congenital heart disease, and may be helpful in many other conditions, such as epilepsy, mental retardation, or abnormal sexual development. It may also be useful for prospective parents if there is a history of any of these conditions in a blood relative.

Genetic counseling may also help in relation to first-cousin marriages and advanced maternal age.

HOW IT IS DONE

Genetic counseling may be provided by a clinical geneticist, by a pediatrician, or by the family practitioner.

The counselor makes a pedigree (family tree) of the family. This includes details of any diseases in the family, any blood relationship between partners, or any history of miscarriages. Information from death certificates or postmortem reports of relatives may also be needed.

When a couple has already had a child with abnormalities, the counselor will ask if there was any exposure to radiation or drugs during pregnancy, or if there was any injury to the child at birth, as these can cause abnormalities in otherwise healthy families. The counselor also examines the affected child (and his or her parents) and arranges for any necessary tests, such as *chromosome analysis*, to be done. The parents' chromosomes may sometimes need to be studied as well, because certain conditions, such as Down's syndrome, sometimes result from abnormalities in the parents' chromosomes.

For many genetic disorders, it is now possible to establish with some certainty whether or not the parents of an affected child are "carriers" of a defective gene, which can significantly affect the chances of recurrence. Although the actual genes are not identified, DNA markers (fragments of genetic material known to be close to the defective gene on a chromosome) have been identified, and these can be looked for on the parents' chromosomes by advanced laboratory techniques (see *Genetic probe*). Such techniques are becoming more readily available.

Virtually every case investigated by a genetic counselor is unique. Several factors may influence the chances of a disorder recurring and, in some cases, complex mathematical calculations must be carried out to estimate the risk for a couple.

WHAT IT CAN OFFER
When a couple has had a child with abnormalities, an important aspect of counseling is the explanation of how it occurred and how the child will fare, including the chances of the child having children and whether they, too, will be affected.

Otherwise, advice consists mainly of an estimate of the risk of occurrence or recurrence of the disorder in question. The couple's decision to have children or more children of their own depends partly on the risk estimate, but also on other factors, such as the severity of the disorder, the burden an affected child would place on the family, and the availability of alternative routes to parenthood.

The decision on the best course of action is left to the parents after they have had detailed discussions with the counselor and feel satisfied that they understand the condition in question and its implications.

When there is a significant risk of producing an abnormal child, the parents may choose to try for a healthy child (but may allow the pregnancy to continue to term only if no abnormality is found during prenatal testing). This applies only to certain conditions, such as spina bifida, Down's syndrome, hemophilia, and muscular dystrophy, in which prenatal diagnosis by *amniocentesis* or *chorionic villus sampling* is able to reveal (with reasonable accuracy) an abnormality early in pregnancy. In such cases, an elective abortion may be chosen if an abnormality is found.

If a couple decides against having children, options for parenthood include adoption and *artificial insemination* by donor (the mother's egg is fertilized by a donor sperm). The latter is worth considering if both parents are carriers of a rare inherited condition or if the father has a dominant or X-linked genetic disorder.

Test-tube fertilizaton of a donor egg by the father's sperm, in cases where the mother carries an abnormal gene, is not yet widely available but is a possibility for the future.

Genetic disorders
Any disorder caused, wholly or in part, by a fault or faults in the inherited, genetic material within a person's cells—that is, in the *genes* formed from the substance deoxyribonucleic acid (DNA), which make up the *chromosomes* in a person's cells. A large number of diseases have, wholly or in part, a genetic cause.

Many genetic disorders are apparent at birth and are thus also *congenital*. However, the terms genetic and congenital are not synonymous; many genetic defects do not become apparent until many years after birth, and many congenital abnormalities are not genetic in origin.

Most people with a genetic disorder have one or more relatives affected by the same disorder—that is, the disorder is also *familial*. However, there are also occasions when a child is born unexpectedly with a genetic disorder (that is, with no previous family history). There are a number of mechanisms by which this can occur.

CAUSES AND TYPES
The reason abnormal genetic material can lead to disorders or disease is that genes control the manufacture in cells of *enzymes* and other proteins that play roles of varying importance in cells and in the body as a whole. If the genetic material is defective, abnormal proteins (or abnormal amounts of proteins) may be produced, causing disturbances in body chemistry that lead to disease.

For a person to exhibit a genetic disorder, the abnormality in the genetic material must usually be present in each of his or her cells, which means that it must also have been present in either the egg or the sperm cell (or both) from which the individual was derived. There are two ways in which this can happen. The first is that one or both parents carried a defect in their own genetic material; the second is that a *mutation* (a change in the genetic material) occurred during the formation of egg or sperm cell. Mutations are one of the mechanisms by which a child affected by a genetic disorder can be born into a family that has never had a known history of genetic disorders. With some of the more common genetic disorders, such as hemophilia, about one third of cases are due to new mutations.

Genetic disorders fall into three broad classes: chromosome abnormalities, unifactorial defects, and multifactorial defects. In the first, a child is born with an abnormal number of whole chromosomes, or extra or missing bits of chromosomes, in the cells. Since chromosomes contain many genes, this can lead to multiple disturbances and disorders. (See *Chromosomal abnormalities*.)

Unifactorial disorders are caused by a single defective gene or pair of genes; these disorders are distributed among the members of an affected family according to relatively simple laws of inheritance. Multifactorial disorders are caused by the additive effects of several genes, along with environmental factors; the pattern of inheritance is less straightforward.

UNIFACTORIAL DISORDERS
These disorders are rare, but there are many, and in total they cause a considerable amount of disability.

All unifactorial genetic disorders are the result of defects in a gene, or in a pair of genes, controlling the production of a particular protein. They can be divided into two groups—called sex-linked and autosomal disorders— according to whether the affected gene or genes are located on the sex chromosomes (nearly always the X chromosome) or on any of the other 22 pairs of chromosomes, which are called autosomes (see *Chromosomes*).

UNIFACTORIAL GENETIC DISORDERS

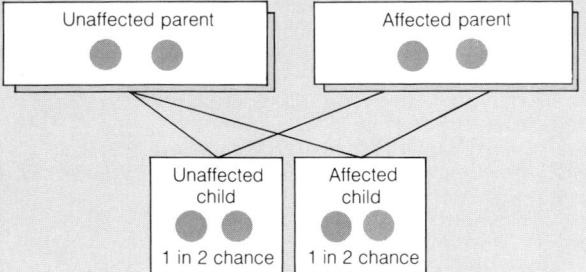

Autosomal dominant
In these disorders, the defective gene must be present in only a single dose to cause outward abnormality. Each child of an affected person usually has a 1 in 2 chance of inheriting the defective gene and of being affected and a 1 in 2 chance of being unaffected.

Unaffected parent

Affected parent

Unaffected child — 1 in 2 chance

Affected child — 1 in 2 chance

Examples
Achondroplasia
Hereditary spherocytosis
Huntington's chorea
Marfan's syndrome
Neurofibromatosis
Polycystic kidney (adult type)
Polyposis coli
Tuberous sclerosis

Key
Defective gene
Normal gene

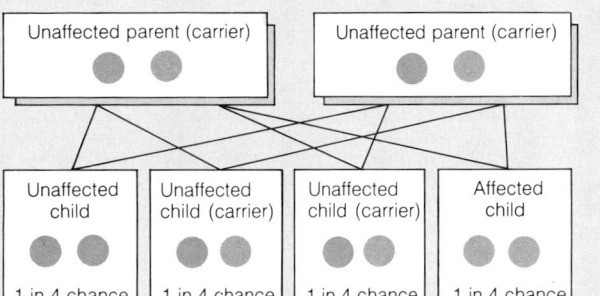

Autosomal recessive
Here, a defective gene must be inherited in a double dose to cause abnormality. Usually both parents of an affected person are unaffected carriers of the defective gene. Each of their children has a 1 in 4 chance of being affected and a 2 in 4 chance of being a carrier.

Unaffected parent (carrier)

Unaffected parent (carrier)

Unaffected child — 1 in 4 chance

Unaffected child (carrier) — 1 in 4 chance

Unaffected child (carrier) — 1 in 4 chance

Affected child — 1 in 4 chance

Examples
Albinism (oculocutaneous)
Cystic fibrosis
Friedreich's ataxia
Galactosemia
Hurler's syndrome
Phenylketonuria
Sickle cell anemia
Tay-Sachs disease

Key
Defective gene
Normal gene

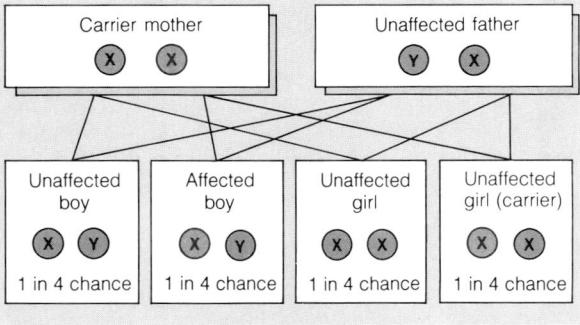

X-linked recessive
These conditions are caused by defects on the X chromosome usually leading to outward abnormality in males only, where the defect cannot be masked by a second, normal, X chromosome. Women can be carriers of the defect and half their sons may be affected.

Carrier mother

Unaffected father

Unaffected boy — 1 in 4 chance

Affected boy — 1 in 4 chance

Unaffected girl — 1 in 4 chance

Unaffected girl (carrier) — 1 in 4 chance

Examples
Christmas disease
Color blindness (most types)
Fragile X syndrome
G6PD deficiency
Hemophilia
Muscular dystrophy (Duchenne)

Key
Defective X chromosome
Normal X chromosome
Y chromosome

Autosomal disorders generally affect both sexes equally and are further divided into two groups, called autosomal dominant and autosomal recessive, according to whether the defective gene need be present in a single or double dose to cause an outward abnormality.

The sex-linked disorders show a bias in their incidence among the sexes. Most are of one type—called X-linked recessive disorders—and primarily males are affected.

Some examples of these three varieties of unifactorial disorder are shown in the table.

AUTOSOMAL DOMINANT DISORDERS With these disorders, a person need carry the defective gene in only a single dose for it to have an outwardly apparent effect. Such individuals are termed *heterozygotes* with respect to the gene, which means they carry one normal copy and one defective copy of the gene. Because the defective gene is dominant—that is, it overrides the normal gene—its presence usually leads to an outward abnormality (but not always a severe one).

Some affected people have inherited the defective gene from one of their parents. In other cases there is no family history of the condition; the defect has usually arisen as a result of a mutation.

If an affected individual has children, each one has a 50 percent chance of inheriting the defective gene and thus also the chance of being affected. Often these disorders appear in each of several generations, finally disappearing only when the affected individuals in a generation have no affected children or no children at all.

AUTOSOMAL RECESSIVE DISORDERS People who manifest these disorders have always acquired the particular gene defect in a double dose—they are said to be *homozygotes* with respect to the defective gene. In most cases, both parents of an affected person are heterozygotes—they carry the defective gene in a single dose along with a normal gene. But, because the defective gene is recessive and "masked" by the normal gene, they display no outward abnormality.

G

G

With all autosomal recessive defects, the number of such carriers in the population always outnumbers those who are actually affected. For example, with *cystic fibrosis* (the most common disorder of this type), one in 22 of the population is a carrier of the defective gene, but only one person in 2,000 is born with the condition. The majority of carriers are unaware of the fact and have no family history of the condition—the defective gene has been passed on to them silently over many generations. When two carriers have children and one is born with an autosomal recessive condition, the manifestation of the defect thus usually comes as a complete surprise.

If both parents are carriers, any subsequent child will have a one in four chance of also being affected.

X-LINKED RECESSIVE DISORDERS In these conditions, the defective gene is on the X chromosome. Women have two X chromosomes in their cells; men have only one, which they inherit from their mothers and pass on to their daughters.

When a woman inherits the defective gene in a single dose, because it is recessive, it is masked by the normal gene on her other X chromosome, so she displays no outward abnormality. She is a heterozygote carrier of the defective gene. However, when a male inherits the defective gene, there is no normal gene on a second X chromosome to mask it, and he will display the abnormality.

The familial pattern of these disorders is as follows. Affected males far outnumber affected females and in all cases have inherited the genetic defect from their mother (who is a carrier). They pass the defective gene to none of their sons but to all of their daughters, who become carriers in turn. Carrier females transmit the defective gene on average to half their sons, who are affected, and to half their daughters, who become carriers in turn. Thus, the pattern is for some of the males in an affected family to have the disorder, while the females in the family are either known or possible carriers.

MULTIFACTORIAL DISORDERS
A large number of disorders fall into this category—including *asthma,* insulin-dependent *diabetes mellitus, schizophrenia,* and a number of conditions present at birth, such as clubfoot and *cleft lip and palate.*

In each case, susceptibility to the disorder is thought to be determined by a number of different genes that,

along with environmental influences, have an additive effect. The degree to which susceptibility to each of these various disorders is determined by genes has been estimated and is termed its *heritability.*

AFFECTED FAMILIES
The underlying cause of genetic disorders (defects in genes) cannot be treated. However, there are a number of methods by which the chances of a child being born with a genetically based disorder can be reduced.

If a couple is considering having children and any parents or close blood relatives (or they themselves) have a genetically based disorder, they would be wise to obtain *genetic counseling.* This is especially important if the couple has had a child with a genetically based condition.

Once a pregnancy is established, study of the genetic material in fetal cells obtained by techniques such as *chorionic villus sampling* and *amniocentesis* can establish whether or not certain genetic disorders are present. In cases where a serious disorder is found, a termination of the pregnancy may be chosen.

Genetic engineering

A branch of *genetics* concerned, in its broadest sense, with the alteration of the inherited, genetic material carried by a living organism to produce some desired change in the characteristics of the organism.

In practice, the main application of genetic engineering to date has been to mass-produce a variety of substances—all proteins of various sorts—that have uses in medical treatment and diagnosis. The function of any *gene* is to control the production of a particular protein in a living cell. If the gene responsible for synthesizing a useful protein can be identified, and if such a gene can be inserted into another cell that can be made to reproduce rapidly, then a colony of cells containing the gene can be grown. The colony will then produce the protein in large amounts.

WHY IT IS DONE
Genetic engineering has been used for producing some human hormones (notably *insulin* and *growth hormone*), some proteins for use in vaccines (against hepatitis, for example), and *interferon,* a substance with potential for treating viral infections. Other valuable aids to treatment are genetically engineered *factor VIII* (a protein used for the treatment of hemophilia), TPA (*tissue plasminogen*

activator), a substance that dissolves blood clots, and many other medically useful substances.

HOW IT IS DONE
The main technique for mass-producing useful proteins by genetic engineering is called recombinant deoxyribonucleic acid (DNA) technology. DNA is the substance in cells that consists of strings of genes, which control the manufacture of different proteins.

The first step is to identify the gene in the DNA of a cell that controls the manufacture of a particularly useful protein. This involves a number of highly sophisticated laboratory techniques. The next step is either to extract the gene from the cell or, if the exact chemical structure of the gene can be worked out, to synthesize it.

The final step is to introduce the gene into the DNA of a suitable recipient cell. By the use of *enzymes* that can split a molecule of the recipient cell's DNA at certain sites, a gap can be produced into which the additional gene can be spliced (hence the term recombinant DNA).

The types of cells or organisms suitable for such genetic alteration are those that can subsequently be made to reproduce rapidly and indefinitely. The most popular organisms to date have been the common intestinal bacterium *ESCHERICHIA COLI* and various yeasts, but cells of other organisms, including human cancer cells, have also been used with success.

OUTLOOK
In view of the ease with which some of the bacteria and other organisms used for genetic engineering can reproduce, and the possibility of accidentally creating and liberating highly dangerous microorganisms, doubts have frequently been expressed about the dangers of "tampering with nature" in this way. These dangers are real but are well recognized by researchers in the field, who have produced stringent codes of practice and regulations to ensure safety.

In the future, it may be possible to extend genetic engineering to the manipulation of human genetic material for purposes of treating *genetic disorders.*

Genetic probe

A specific fragment of deoxyribonucleic acid (*DNA*) used to determine whether particular defects or genetic "markers" are present in a person's or a fetus's genetic material—that is, in the DNA that, along with some protein, makes up the *chromosomes* in his or her cells.

Genetic probes are used primarily in the prenatal diagnosis of certain genetic disorders and to determine whether or not certain people are "carriers" of gene defects. Often, there is no technique for detecting the defective gene itself. However, for certain gene defects (e.g., the one responsible for *cystic fibrosis*) markers (sections of DNA with a specific base sequence) have been identified that very commonly occur on particular chromosomes in association with the defect. Hence, if the marker can be found, it provides strong evidence that the gene defect is also present. This has particular implications for *genetic counseling*.

In one technique, the chromosome under test (obtained from a cell of the person or the fetus under investigation) is first broken up using *enzymes* (the probe) in a test tube; the fragments are then fixed onto a filter. A radioactively labeled sequence of DNA that will bind to the "marker" sequence of DNA in the chromosome (if present) is then added, and sophisticated techniques are performed to see whether such binding has occurred.

Genetics

The study of *inheritance*—that is, how the characteristics of living organisms are passed from one generation to another, the chemical basis by which such characteristics are determined, and the causes of the similarities and differences among individuals of one species (for example, the human species) or among different species. More particularly, genetics includes the study of deoxyribonucleic acid (*DNA*), the substance in cells that determines the characteristics of an organism, and of *genes*, which are units of inheritance corresponding to specific bits of DNA.

Particular branches of human genetics include population genetics, which studies the relative frequency of various genes in different human races; molecular genetics, which is concerned with the structure, function, and copying of DNA from one cell to another, and also how *mutations* (changes) occur in DNA; and medical or clinical genetics, which is concerned with the study and prevention of *genetic disorders*.

Genital herpes

See *Herpes, genital*.

Genitalia

The reproductive organs, especially the external ones. The male genitalia include the *penis*, *testes* (within the *scrotum*), *prostate gland*, seminal vesicles, and associated ducts, such as the *epididymis* and *vas deferens*. The female genitalia include the *ovaries*, *fallopian tubes*, *uterus*, *vagina*, *clitoris*, *vulva*, and *Bartholin's glands*.

Genital ulceration

An eroded area of skin on the *genitalia*. In men the ulcer may be on the skin of the penis or scrotum; in women it may be on the vulva or within the vagina.

CAUSES

The most common cause of genital ulceration is a *sexually transmitted disease*. The early stages of *syphilis* are characterized by a hard *chancre*, a painless ulcer where the bacteria penetrated the skin. This may be followed by shallow, elongated ulcers once the chancre has healed. The *herpes simplex* virus causes painful, fluid-filled blisters to develop on the genitalia; if these blisters become infected by bacteria they may ulcerate. Both *chancroid* and *granuloma inguinale* are bacterial infections that cause genital ulcers; they are common in tropical countries. In the former the ulcers are painful, in the latter they are painless. *Lymphogranuloma venereum* is a viral infection in which the resulting blisters occasionally ulcerate.

Other causes of genital ulceration include *herpes zoster*, *tuberculosis*, or a tumor of the testis, which can erode the scrotum to cause an ulcer.

Genital ulceration may also be a side effect of drugs. It can be caused by solutions applied to genital warts in high concentrations. It can also be a reaction to a drug taken by mouth; sulfonamide antibacterial drugs, for example, can cause mouth and genital ulcers (see *Stevens-Johnson syndrome*).

Behçet's syndrome is a rare condition that causes tender, recurrent ulcers in the mouth and on the genitals. Cancer of the penis or vulva may cause a single, painless ulcer with raised, rolled edges that turn outward.

DIAGNOSIS

The diagnosis of the underlying cause is made from the appearance of the ulcer and the presence of other signs, such as enlarged lymph glands or a skin rash. Swabs from the ulcer are taken and the material examined and cultured to look for a specific bacterium or virus. Blood tests to detect antibodies to a specific type of infection may be performed.

Genital warts

See *Warts, genital*.

Gentamicin

ANTIBIOTIC
Injection Ointment Cream Eye drops
📄 Prescription needed
🔲 Available as generic

A drug given by injection, sometimes in combination with another antibiotic, to treat serious infections. For example, gentamicin is used to treat *meningitis*, *septicemia* (blood poisoning), and *endocarditis* (inflammation of the heart lining). Gentamicin cannot be given by mouth because it is inactivated during digestion.

During treatment, blood tests are taken to determine gentamicin levels to monitor dosage and thus reduce the risk of toxic damage to the kidneys or inner ear.

The drug is used in eye drops to treat *conjunctivitis* caused by infection.

Gentian violet

A purple dye used mainly by biologists to make bacteria visible under the microscope. Gentian violet also has antiseptic properties and can be applied to the skin to treat burns, boils, carbuncles, and fungal infections. It is occasionally used to relieve soreness in the mouth caused by *candidiasis* (thrush).

Genu valgum

The medical term for *knock-knee*.

Genu varum

The medical term for *bowleg*.

Geriatrician

A physician who specializes in treating elderly patients and the special conditions related to aging.

Geriatric medicine

The medical specialty concerned with care of the elderly. Many diseases and disorders that affect the elderly may occur in patients of all ages, but older people tend to respond differently to sickness and treatment. For example, *aging* is associated with a progressive decline in the functioning of major organs—the heart, lungs, kidneys, liver, and brain. Consequently, an infection in one of these organs or elsewhere in the body that would cause only minor illness in a young adult might be life-threatening in an

G

older person. Any illness in an elderly person may cause a temporary but marked slowing of thought processes, and may even lead to confusion and other features that may be mistaken for dementia. This is due to the added stress placed on the brain during the illness. Furthermore, many medicinal drugs are eliminated from the body by the liver or kidneys and, if these organs are affected by aging, dosages of drugs used in treatment may need to be modified to avoid dangerous side effects.

A physician who specializes in geriatrics is expert at assessing the health of patients and in assessing the complex features of their disease. He or she takes particular care not to give excessive doses of drugs and tries also to avoid moving the patient away from familiar surroundings unless hospital admission is essential. Geriatricians are also skilled at rehabilitation; they usually make the contacts (with social services and voluntary agencies) that are necessary to arrange a comprehensive rehabilitation program.

Germ

 The popular term for any microorganism that causes disease. Examples include a *virus* or bacterium (see *Bacteria*). In medicine, the term is used to describe simple, undifferentiated cells that are capable of developing into specialized tissues, such as the cells of the early embryo.

German measles
Another name for *rubella*.

Germ cell tumor
A localized proliferation of cells that are the immature forms of either sperm in the male testis or ova (eggs) in the female ovary. (See *Seminoma*.)

Gerontology
The study of *aging* in all its aspects (developmental, biological, medical, sociological, and psychological). The specialty that treats the medical problems of the elderly is called geriatrics (see *Geriatric medicine*).

Gestalt theory
Ideas based on the notion that the whole is more than the sum of its parts; a school of psychology based on the idea that a sense of wholeness is more important than the individual bits and pieces of perception and behavior. It was founded in Germany

early this century by a group that adopted the name gestalt, meaning "form," "pattern," or "configuration." In studying emotional states and social issues, Gestalt theory emphasizes viewing things as a whole rather than breaking them down into collections of stimuli and responses. Gestalt therapy became popular as a means of coping with personal problems and is still practiced today by some therapists; this type of therapy aims to increase self-awareness by looking at all aspects of an individual within his or her environment.

Gestation
The period from conception to birth, during which the developing fetus is carried in the uterus.

Gestation normally lasts around 270 days, about nine months. Because of the difficulty in determining the precise date of conception, physicians time pregnancies from the first day of the last normal menstrual period, giving a gestation period of 284 days.

Giardiasis

 An infection of the small intestine, caused by the protozoan (single-celled) parasite *GIARDIA LAMBLIA*. Giardiasis is most common in tropical areas and in travelers to the tropics. Recently it has become more common in developed countries, affecting especially homosexual men, people living in institutions, and preschool children. The infection is particularly

common where large numbers of young children gather together—for example, in day-care centers and preschools. The disease is spread by contaminated food or water or by direct personal contact (e.g., by hand-to-mouth contact).

SYMPTOMS
About two thirds of those infected have no symptoms. When symptoms do occur they begin one to three days after the parasite has entered the body. The person has violent attacks of diarrhea accompanied by flatus (gas); the feces are foul-smelling, may be greasy, and tend to float in the toilet bowl. Abdominal discomfort, cramps, or swelling, loss of appetite, and nausea may also occur. In some cases, the infection becomes chronic.

DIAGNOSIS AND TREATMENT
The infection is diagnosed from microscopic examination of a sample of feces for the presence of the parasites. If there is any doubt, a jejunal *biopsy* (removal of a small sample of tissue for microscopic analysis) may be carried out.

Acute giardiasis usually clears up without treatment. However, treatment incorporating the antibiotic metronidazole or quinacrine relieves symptoms quickly and prevents the spread of infection.

PREVENTION
Infection can be prevented by thorough hand washing before handling food and by avoiding eating food or drinking water that could possibly be contaminated.

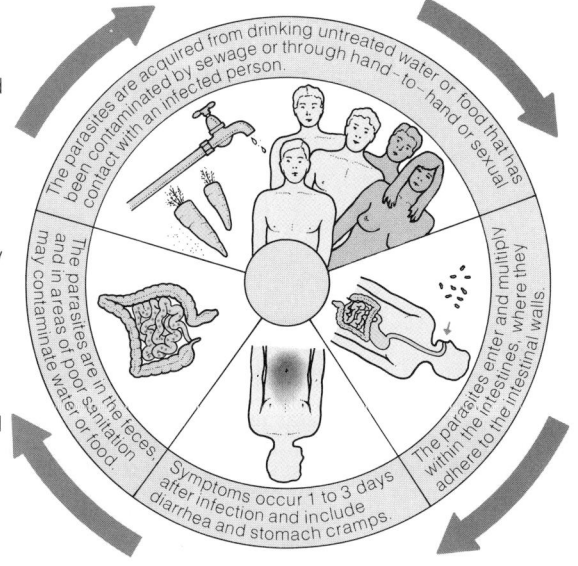

HOW GIARDIASIS IS SPREAD
Giardiasis is spread by contaminated water or food, or by personal contact. This parasitic infection is most common in the tropics, but recently it has become a more frequent occurrence in developed countries, especially among groups of preschool children.

The parasites are acquired from drinking untreated water or food that has been contaminated by sewage or through hand-to-hand or sexual contact with an infected person.

The parasites are in the feces, and in areas of poor sanitation may contaminate water or food.

Symptoms occur 1 to 3 days after infection and include diarrhea and stomach cramps.

The parasites enter and multiply within the intestines, where they adhere to the intestinal walls.

Giddiness
See *Dizziness*.

Gigantism
Excessive growth (especially height) resulting from overproduction, during childhood or adolescence, of growth hormone by a tumor of the pituitary gland. Untreated, the tumor eventually destroys the pituitary gland and results in death during early adult life. If the tumor develops after growth has stopped, the result is *acromegaly* rather than gigantism.

Oversecretion of growth hormone from early life can result in an individual attaining an immense height. The tallest documented giant in medical history, Robert Wadlow, reached a height of 8 feet 11 inches and a weight of 475 pounds before he died at age 22. Such instances are rare, however. By far the most common reason for a child being tall is that his or her parents are tall. Other rare causes of excessive height in childhood are *Marfan's syndrome* and *thyrotoxicosis*.

DIAGNOSIS AND TREATMENT
The diagnosis of gigantism is made when *brain imaging* and blood tests confirm the presence of a pituitary tumor and excessive growth hormone. The condition may be treated with bromocriptine, a drug that blocks the release of growth hormone, or by surgery or radiation therapy to destroy or remove the tumor.

Gilbert's disease
An inherited disorder that affects the way bilirubin is processed by the liver and that may cause mild jaundice. Sufferers are otherwise healthy.

Gilbert's disease is common, affecting about 2 percent of the population. Usually there are no symptoms. When there are symptoms, they may include malaise, anorexia, upper abdominal pain, and mild jaundice.

Usually no treatment is necessary, but the drug phenobarbital can relieve jaundice and other symptoms.

Gilles de la Tourette's syndrome
A rare disorder of movement, named for the French neurologist who first described it in 1885. It starts in childhood with repetitive grimaces and tics, usually of the head and neck, sometimes of the arms, legs, and trunk. Involuntary barks, grunts, or other noises may appear as the disease progresses. In about half the cases, the sufferer has episodes of coprolalia (using foul language).

The syndrome is more common in males, partially inherited, and is probably underdiagnosed because of its strange symptoms. It is usually of lifelong duration but *antipsychotic drugs*, such as haloperidol, can often provide effective relief.

Gingiva
The Latin name for the *gum* that surrounds the base of the teeth.

Gingivectomy
Surgical removal of part of the gum margin. Gingivectomy may be used to treat severe cases of gingival *hyperplasia* (thickening of the gums), a condition usually caused by anticonvulsant treatment with phenytoin. Gingivectomy also is used to remove pockets of infected gums formed during advanced stages of gum disease (*periodontitis*).

Gingivectomy is performed in the dentist's office using local anesthetic. After surgery, the newly exposed area around the base of the teeth may initially be sensitive; the exposure also gives the teeth a longer appearance. There are no complications as long as scrupulous *oral hygiene* is maintained after surgery.

Gingivitis
Inflammation of the gingiva (gums), often due to infection. Gingivitis is a reversible stage of gum disease.

CAUSES
Gingivitis is usually caused by the buildup of plaque (a sticky deposit of bacteria, mucus, food particles, and other irritants) around the base of the teeth. It is thought that toxins produced by bacteria within the plaque irritate the gums, causing the gums to become infected, tender, and swollen. Gingivitis can result from injury to the gums, usually from overvigorous toothbrushing or careless flossing.

INCIDENCE
Mild gingivitis is very common in young adults. Pregnant women and diabetics are susceptible because of changes in their hormone levels.

SYMPTOMS
Healthy gums are pink or brown and firm; in people with gingivitis, they become red-purple, soft, shiny, and swollen. The gums bleed easily, especially during toothbrushing, and are often tender.

PREVENTION AND TREATMENT
Good *oral hygiene* is the main means of preventing and treating gingivitis. Teeth should be thoroughly brushed with a fluoride dentifrice (toothpaste)

Example of gingivitis
The gums around the bases of the upper teeth are puffy, shiny, and tender. They overhang the teeth margins. Affected gums often bleed when brushed.

at least once a day and after meals, if possible; dental floss should be used at least once a day. It is also important to visit your dentist at least once a year (or more often if he or she recommends) so that teeth can be cleaned to remove calculus (mineralized plaque) and accumulated plaque through a procedure known as scaling. The dentist may prescribe an antibacterial mouthwash for use at home.

COMPLICATIONS
Untreated gingivitis may damage gum tissue around the base of the teeth, leading to the formation of pockets in which plaque and calculus can collect. Bacteria within the plaque may cause inflammation to spread, eventually leading to *periodontitis*, an advanced stage of gum disease in which the supporting tissues of the teeth and the surrounding bone become eroded, loosening the teeth.

Acute necrotizing ulcerative gingivitis may develop due to invasion of tissue by *anaerobic* bacteria in people with chronic gingivitis, especially those with lowered resistance to infection. Also called trench mouth or Vincent's disease, acute necrotizing ulcerative gingivitis is a serious condition resulting in destruction of gum tissue; it requires a course of antibiotic treatment.

Gland
A group of specialized cells that manufactures and releases chemical substances, such as hormones and *enzymes*, for use in the body.

There are two main types of glands: endocrine and exocrine. *Endocrine glands* do not have ducts and thus release their secretions directly into the bloodstream; examples include the pituitary, thyroid, and adrenal glands. Target organs may be quite distant from the endocrine glands.

Exocrine glands have ducts and release their secretions either onto the surface of the skin or into a hollow structure such as the mouth or digestive tract; examples include the sebaceous glands, which secrete sebum onto the skin, and the salivary glands.

Collections of cells in the *lymphatic system*, the lymph nodes, are sometimes referred to as glands. Strictly speaking, this is incorrect usage because they do not secrete chemical substances. However, they do release white blood cells, which play an important role in fighting infections and allergic reactions.

Glanders

An infection of horses and donkeys that is rarely transmitted to humans. It occurs in Asia, Africa, and South America and is caused by the bacterium *PSEUDOMONAS MALLEI*, which enters the body through a cut or abrasion or by being breathed in.

Initially, symptoms (mild fever, headache, general aches and pains, and possibly some generalized swelling of the lymph nodes) are vague. If bacterial entry was through a wound, ulcers or abscesses may then appear at the site; if entry was through the lungs, *pneumonia* may develop. In severe cases, *septicemia* (blood poisoning) may then follow.

DIAGNOSIS AND TREATMENT

The disease is diagnosed by identifying the bacteria in a sample of pus or sputum (phlegm) or by detecting antibodies to the bacteria in a blood sample. Early treatment with an appropriate antibiotic usually clears the infection.

Glands, swollen

Known medically as lymphadenopathy, enlargement of the lymph nodes (glands) as a result of inflammation and/or proliferation of white blood cells within them.

CAUSES

Swollen glands are a very common symptom and are usually due to an infection or allergic reaction (see *Allergy*). Children are especially prone to swollen glands as a result of infection, partly because the lymphatic system plays a more important part in combating infections in childhood than in adult life.

Rarer causes of swollen glands include *lymphoma, Hodgkin's disease, leukemia* (cancer of the white blood cells), or a *metastasis* (secondary cancer that has spread from elsewhere in the body).

When the underlying cause is localized, swollen glands also tend to be confined to a limited area; for example, a throat infection may result in swelling only of the lymph glands in the neck.

Swollen glands near the surface of the skin—in the groin or neck, for example—are usually felt as tender, slightly warm lumps. However, swelling of deeper glands, such as those in the lungs or abdomen, is almost invariably unnoticeable.

INVESTIGATION AND TREATMENT

In many cases, the cause of swollen glands is obvious from the presence of a localized infection or a bee sting that has caused an allergic reaction. In other cases, the accompanying symptoms usually indicate the cause; for example, swollen glands with a sore throat, fever, and tiredness suggest infectious *mononucleosis* (glandular fever).

If swollen glands persist or there is no obvious cause, tests may be necessary. These may include a blood count, chest X rays to look for swollen glands in the lungs, or a *biopsy* (removal of tissue for microscopic analysis) of an affected gland.

Treatment depends on the underlying cause. Antibiotics may be given for a bacterial infection, antihistamines for an allergy, or *radiation therapy* or *chemotherapy* (or both) may be used to treat a tumor.

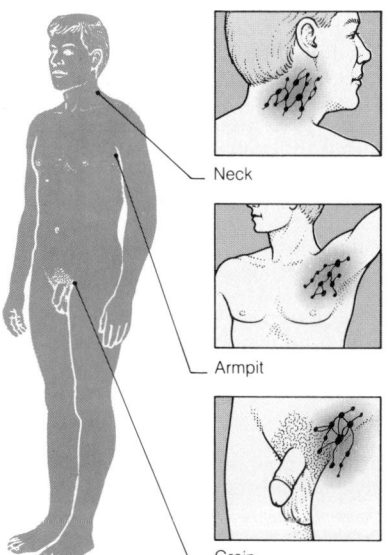

Neck

Armpit

Groin

Common sites of swollen glands
The three most common sites where swollen glands can be felt are in the neck, armpit, and groin.

Glandular fever

See *Mononucleosis, infectious.*

Glasses

Simple optical devices used to correct focusing errors in the eyes so that clear vision is achieved. The lenses are made of glass or plastic and the shape and thickness are chosen during an eye test (see *Vision tests*).

TYPES OF LENSES

Lenses may be convex (outwardly curved), concave (inwardly curved), or cylindrical. Most are single-vision lenses, but bifocal or trifocal lenses, with smaller areas differing in power from the main lens, are common. Varifocal lenses, with power increasing gradually from the center to one edge, are becoming popular. Lenses may have a permanent tint or may incorporate chemicals that produce darkening on exposure to light.

Glass eye

See *Eye, artificial.*

Glaucoma

A condition in which the pressure of the fluid in the eye is so abnormally high that it causes damage. A minimal pressure is required to maintain the shape of the eyeball, but excessive pressure may result in the compression and obstruction of the small internal blood vessels and/or the fibers of the optic nerve. The result is nerve fiber destruction and partial or complete loss of vision.

TYPES AND CAUSES

The most common form is chronic open-angle glaucoma, which rarely occurs before the age of 40 and often causes no symptoms until blindness is advanced. It is due to a gradual blockage of the outflow of aqueous humor (fluid in the front compartment of the eye) over a period of years, causing a slow rise in pressure. This type tends to run in families.

In acute closed-angle glaucoma, there is a sudden obstruction to the outflow of aqueous humor from the eye and the pressure rises suddenly. Subacute angle-closure glaucoma is similar to acute glaucoma, but develops more slowly or occurs intermittently.

Congenital glaucoma is due to a structural abnormality in the drainage angles of the eyes.

Glaucoma can also be caused by injury to the eye, or by a serious eye disease such as *uveitis*, dislocation of the lens, or adhesions between the iris and the cornea.

WHY GLASSES ARE USED

For *hyperopia* (farsightedness), convex (or plus) lenses are needed. Sufferers of *presbyopia* also need plus (magnifying) lenses. Myopia (nearsightedness) requires concave (or minus) lenses.

FARSIGHTEDNESS

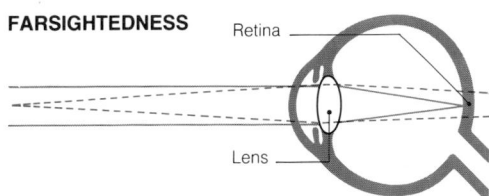

Retina

Lens

Before correction
Farsightedness is caused when focusing power is inadequate. Light from a distant object is focused on the retina, but light from a close object is focused behind it.

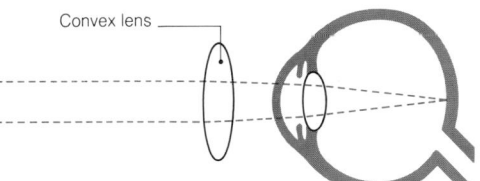

Convex lens

After correction
Convex magnifying (or plus) lenses cause the light from the close object to focus on the retina.

NEARSIGHTEDNESS

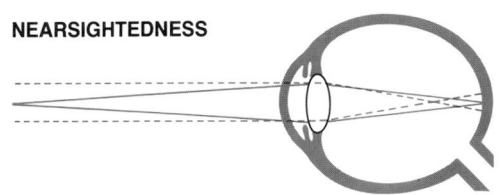

Before correction
Distant objects are blurred, because the focusing power of the eye is too great. Light from the distant object is focused in front of the retina.

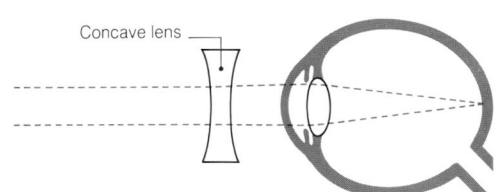

Concave lens

After correction
Concave weakening (or minus) lenses are used to cause the light from the distant object to focus onto the retina.

ASTIGMATISM

The surrounding surfaces of the cornea are steeper in one direction than in the other. The correcting lenses are designed with additional curvature in one meridian. The lenses are then set accurately in the frame of the glasses so that the steepest curves correspond to the flattest meridian of the cornea. Both concave lenses for myopia and convex lenses for hyperopia and presbyopia can be designed in this way to correct astigmatism.

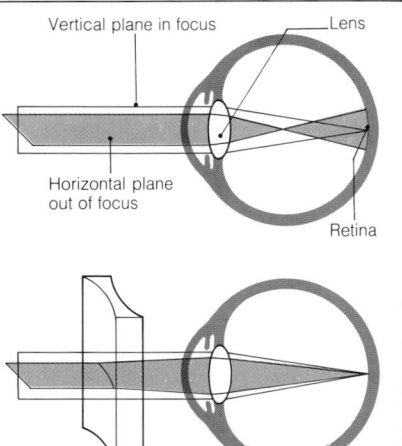

Vertical plane in focus
Lens

Horizontal plane out of focus

Retina

INCIDENCE

Glaucoma is one of the most common major eye disorders in people over 60; it is responsible for 15 percent of blindness in adults in the US. Nearly 2 percent of people over the age of 40 have chronic glaucoma. The incidence rises with age and about 10 percent of people over 70 have abnormally raised pressure within the eye.

SYMPTOMS AND SIGNS

Chronic glaucoma often causes no symptoms because the gradual loss of peripheral vision is not apparent to the affected person. Only late in the disease, when there is severe, irreversible damage, may the person be aware of some visual loss.

Ciliary body

Blocked drainage channel

Cornea

Iris

Aqueous humor

Lens

Acute closed-angle glaucoma
This type of glaucoma is caused by an unduly narrow angle between the iris and the back of the peripheral cornea. Dilation of the pupil may therefore lead to a sudden complete blockage of the outflow, causing a rapid increase in pressure in the eyeball.

The symptoms of acute glaucoma include a dull, severe, aching pain in and above the eye, some fogginess of vision, and the perception of rainbow rings around lights at night (halos). Nausea and vomiting can occur and the eye can become red and have a partly dilated pupil and a hazy cornea. Subacute glaucoma can cause similar mild, brief episodes.

DIAGNOSIS

Chronic glaucoma often causes no symptoms and is usually detected only by regular, routine eye examina-

G

tions. Applanation tonometry (by which eye pressure is measured) is an essential check for glaucoma (see *Eye, examination of*), especially if there is a family history of the disorder. Use of an *ophthalmoscope* to examine the back of the eye may show an abnormal optic nerve. Visual field testing and gonioscopy (examination of the drainage angle) can also be important.

TREATMENT

Chronic open-angle glaucoma can usually be controlled with eye drops, which reduce the pressure in the eye. Repeated tonometry and visual field testing may be carried out to ensure that the pressure is being controlled; if necessary, other eye drops will be given. If drops fail to control the pressure, tablets or long-acting capsules may also be prescribed. The medications for treatment of chronic glaucoma usually are prescribed for life since, if stopped, the pressure generally rises. If medications fail to reduce the pressure in chronic glaucoma, and if there is a continuing loss of visual field or vision, laser surgery or cutting surgery may be necessary to open up the drainage channel or to create an artificial channel for the aqueous humor.

Acute closed-angle glaucoma is a medical emergency calling for urgent treatment. Various treatments (i.e., eye drops, pills, liquids, and/or intravenous fluids) are given to try to reduce the very high eye pressure. Usually, after the pressure is controlled, laser surgery or cutting surgery is necessary for the treatment of acute glaucoma and subacute glaucoma to try to prevent a recurrent attack. Usually a peripheral *iridectomy* is done. A small opening is made in the periphery of the iris so that aqueous humor can drain more easily. The iridectomy is often curative but, if the drainage angle was damaged by the attack, medications may be needed to control the pressure after surgery. If the iris is scarred at the drainage angle, other types of surgery, such as creating an artificial drainage channel, may be necessary.

OUTLOOK

The pressure rise of glaucoma can be prevented by treatment, but early diagnosis and treatment are needed to prevent any impairment of vision. Regular eye examinations are important for early detection.

Glioblastoma multiforme

A fast-growing and highly malignant type of *brain tumor*. Glioblastoma multiforme is a type of *glioma*, a tumor arising from glial (supporting) cells within the brain. Most glioblastomas develop within the cerebrum (the main mass of the brain).

There are about five to 10 new cases of glioblastoma multiforme per million population per year in the US. The cause is unknown.

Symptoms, diagnosis, and treatment are as for other types of brain tumor. Despite treatment, the outlook is poor, with few patients surviving beyond two years.

Glioma

A type of *brain tumor* arising from the supporting glial cells within the brain.

Gliomas make up about 60 percent of all primary brain tumors (growths originating from the brain itself rather than spread from elsewhere). There are about two to four new cases of glioma per 100,000 people annually in the US.

Cross section of a brain
This photograph (taken from an autopsy specimen) shows a large area of brain infiltrated by a glioma (dark color).

Types of glioma include *astrocytoma*, *glioblastoma multiforme* (a highly malignant variety of astrocytoma), *ependymoma* and *medulloblastoma* (more common in children), and *oligodendroglioma*. Symptoms, diagnosis, and treatment are as for other types of brain tumor.

Glipizide

An oral *hypoglycemic drug* used in the treatment of non-insulin-dependent *diabetes mellitus*. Glipizide stimulates the pancreas to produce *insulin*, which promotes glucose uptake into muscle and fat, thereby lowering the blood glucose level.

Globulin

Any of a group of proteins characterized by being insoluble in water but soluble in dilute salt solutions; *antibodies* (also known as *immunoglobulins*) are an example.

TYPES

Globulins can be divided into three main groups, known as alpha-, beta-, and gamma-globulins.

Alpha-globulins include alpha$_1$-antitrypsin and haptoglobin. The former is an enzyme produced by the lungs and liver; deficiency is associated with *hepatitis* in children and *emphysema* (a lung disorder) in young adults. Haptoglobin is found in the blood, where it binds together *hemoglobin* (the oxygen-carrying protein in red blood cells) and prevents it from being excreted in the urine by the kidneys. Various other alpha-globulins are produced as a result of inflammation, tissue damage, *autoimmune disorders* (when the immune system attacks the body's own tissues), or certain cancers.

Beta-globulins consist mainly of low-density lipoproteins (LDLs), substances involved in the transport of fats in the blood circulation, and transferrin, which carries iron in the blood. The amount of beta-globulins is increased in certain types of *hyperlipidemia* (abnormally high levels of fats in the blood).

All of the gamma-globulins are antibodies, proteins produced by the immune system in response to infection, during allergic reactions, and after organ transplants. Gamma-globulins may also be produced in any disorder that causes persistent inflammation of an organ, such as *rheumatoid arthritis* or *cirrhosis* of the liver. In addition, certain conditions, such as *multiple myeloma*, result in the production of large amounts of a specific gamma-globulin.

Globus hystericus

A form of hysteria in which there is an uncomfortable feeling of a "lump in the throat." This lump is felt to interfere with swallowing and breathing, sometimes so much so that the sufferer is convinced that he or she cannot breathe. Respiration comes in sighs or gasps, anxiety increases, and *hyperventilation* (rapid breathing) and symptoms of a *panic attack* often ensue. Some patients insist that their Adam's apple has become larger or displaced in some way.

There is no true physical basis for these attacks, which occur in anxious or depressed people. The condition is not life-threatening. Breathing in and out of a small paper bag fitted tightly around the nose and mouth will alleviate the symptoms brought on by hyperventilation. Treatment is by

G

reassurance, breath-control training, and, in some instances, psychotherapy. Use of *antianxiety drugs* or *antidepressant drugs* to treat the condition is rarely helpful.

Glomerulonephritis

Inflammation of the glomeruli (filtering units of the kidney). Both kidneys are affected, although not all the glomeruli are affected simultaneously. Damage to the glomeruli hampers the removal of waste products, salt, and water from the bloodstream, which may cause serious complications.

CAUSES AND INCIDENCE

The incidence of glomerulonephritis varies markedly among different parts of the world, mainly because some common tropical diseases (such as malaria and schistosomiasis) are important causes. Although these diseases rarely are responsible for glomerulonephritis in developed countries, glomerulonephritis is still the most common cause of chronic *renal failure* (loss of kidney function) in the US and Europe.

Some types of the disease are caused by the patient's *immune system* making antibodies to eliminate microorganisms—usually the bacteria responsible for a minor infection, such as streptococcal sore throat infections. Particles called immune complexes, formed from antibodies and bacterial antigens, circulate in the bloodstream and become trapped in the glomeruli; this triggers an inflammatory process that may damage the glomeruli and prevent them from working normally. Glomerulonephritis also occurs in some *autoimmune disorders*, systemic *lupus erythematosus* (a chronic disease of connective tissues), and the immunoglobulin A (IgA) glomerulonephritis known as Berger's disease.

SYMPTOMS

Mild forms of glomerulonephritis may produce no symptoms and the disease may be noted only when a urine sample is tested for some other reason. Sometimes a mild puffiness of the soft tissues surrounding the eyeballs (periorbital edema) may be apparent. Other times it comes to light only when renal failure has reached an advanced stage and symptoms arise because of the accumulation of waste products and fluid that are usually eliminated in the urine.

High blood pressure may develop and some sufferers experience a dull ache in the loins. Damaged glomeruli may allow the escape of red blood cells

into the urine, which can become blood-stained. When protein is continually lost in the urine, the result is *edema* (swelling of parts of the body; see illustration). The combination of proteinuria (large amounts of protein in the urine), low albumin (protein) in the blood, and edema is called the *nephrotic syndrome*.

In some cases, glomerulonephritis is severe and sudden, so that kidney failure develops over a few days; patients often notice that they are passing very small quantities of urine.

DIAGNOSIS

There are numerous types of glomerulonephritis; one cause may produce a different type in different individuals. Urinalysis and examination of the urine sediment (after centrifugation) is helpful in diagnosis. Kidney *biopsy* (removal of a small amount of tissue for laboratory analysis) is also important for diagnosis. Other tests that may be performed are blood and urine sampling to measure how well the kidney is removing waste products and to measure how much protein is being lost in the urine. These tests may be repeated during treatment to see how the kidneys are responding.

TREATMENT AND OUTLOOK

Treatment depends on the type and severity of the disease, as revealed by biopsy. Affected children usually have mild forms characterized by the nephrotic syndrome; they usually recover completely after treatment. Children who experience acute glomerulonephritis after a streptococcal infection usually recover even without specific treatment of the glomerulonephritis.

Adults tend to respond less well to treatment, but drugs may be prescribed to control hypertension and a special diet given to reduce the kidneys' load. This may prevent or delay eventual renal failure. A minority of people with severe glomerulonephritis may be given *immunosuppressant drugs* (to dampen the body's defense system), or *plasmapheresis* to remove substances and particles from the bloodstream that trigger the inflammation (i.e., substances released as a result of the immune response).

Glomerulosclerosis

Scarring that occurs as a result of damage within the glomeruli (filtering units) of the kidney.

G

THE EFFECTS OF GLOMERULONEPHRITIS

The glomeruli are damaged as a result of inflammation. Red blood cells and protein leak into the urine.

Protein loss from the circulation causes fluid to accumulate in body tissues, causing edema.

Kidney

Kidney tubule

Damaged glomerulus

Red blood cells

Protein

Urine travels toward the bladder

Cross section of a damaged glomerulus
Damage to the glomerulus causes red blood cells and protein to pass into the urine, which may be blood-stained.

Normal tissue

Water

Blood

Protein

Swollen tissue

Water

Blood

Protein

Healthy tissue
Through osmotic pressure, protein molecules in the blood draw back water lost to surrounding tissues.

Edema
If protein is lost into the urine, there is a fall in osmotic pressure and more water escapes into surrounding tissues, causing swelling.

Mild glomerulosclerosis occurs normally with age; a 10 percent decrease in renal function is common each decade after age 30. However, even a 75 percent reduction in renal function is compatible with a normal life.

Glomerulosclerosis may occur in some severe types of *glomerulonephritis* that are difficult to treat and in which damage progresses to destroy the kidneys. Typically, sufferers develop heavy *proteinuria* (the presence of protein in the urine) and severe *edema* (swelling of parts of the body due to fluid collection).

Glomerulosclerosis is also found in some people with *diabetes mellitus*. It is seen in reflux nephropathy (backflow of urine from bladder to kidney sometimes associated with infection) and in some people with hypertension. Intravenous drug abuse may cause glomerulosclerosis. The condition has also been found in some people who have AIDS.

Glomus tumor

A small, painful, bluish swelling in the skin, usually on a finger or toe near or under the nail, that is tender to touch and more painful if the limb is hot or cold. The tumors result from an overgrowth of glomus bodies, structures with numerous nerve endings that normally control blood flow and temperature in the skin. Glomus tumors are surgically removed.

Glossectomy

Removal of all or part of the tongue. Glossectomy may be performed in the treatment of cancer of the tongue, but more usually such cancers are treated by radiation therapy. If a large part of the tongue is removed, speech is impaired and eating is difficult. A liquid diet is then necessary.

Glossitis

Inflammation of the tongue. The tongue feels sore and swollen and looks red and smooth; adjacent parts of the mouth may also be inflamed.

Glossitis occurs in iron deficiency anemia, in pernicious and megaloblastic anemias, and in other vitamin B deficiencies. Other causes include infection (especially *herpes simplex*) of the mouth, irritation by dentures, and excessive use of alcohol, tobacco, or spices. A congenital form of glossitis affects the middle portion of the back of the tongue.

Treatment is for the underlying cause. Self-help measures include maintaining good oral hygiene, not smoking, and avoiding acidic or spicy foods that aggravate the soreness. Regular rinsing of the mouth with a salt solution may help.

Glossolalia

Speaking in jargon or an imaginary language that has no actual meaning or syntax. Today it occurs almost exclusively at religious meetings. Some Christians regard glossolalia as a sign of possession by the Holy Spirit; scientists tend to view it as a form of *hypnosis* or *hysteria*.

Glossopharyngeal nerve

The ninth *cranial nerve*, the glossopharyngeal nerve performs both sensory and motor functions. It conveys sensations, especially taste, from the back of the tongue, regulates secretion of saliva by the parotid gland, and controls movement of the throat muscles.

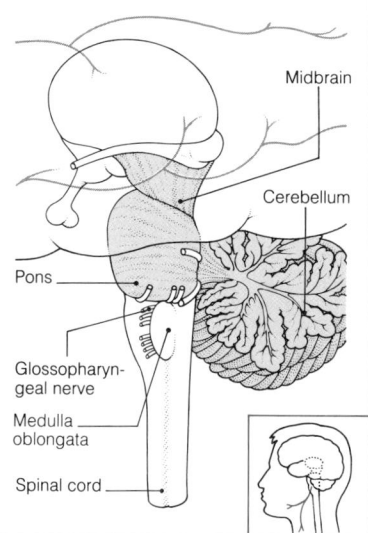

LOCATION OF THE GLOSSOPHARYNGEAL NERVE
The nerve arises from the medulla oblongata and branches to the tongue, parotid gland, and pharynx.

Midbrain

Cerebellum

Pons

Glossopharyngeal nerve

Medulla oblongata

Spinal cord

Glottis

The part of the *larynx* (voice box) that consists of the vocal cords and the slitlike opening between them.

Glucagon

A hormone produced by the pancreas. Glucagon stimulates the breakdown of glycogen (a carbohydrate stored in the liver and muscles) into glucose (sugar). The glucose is then released into the bloodstream, where it is available as a source of energy for cells anywhere in the body. Glucagon therefore regulates the level of glucose in the blood; when the level falls, glucagon is released from the pancreas. Glucagon opposes the action of *insulin*.

USE AS A DRUG
Glucagon is extracted from the pancreas of pigs or cows for use as a drug. It is given by subcutaneous (under the skin) injection in the emergency treatment of sufferers of *diabetes mellitus* who are unconscious as a result of hypoglycemia (low blood sugar). Glucagon produces recovery within 15 to 20 minutes; the patient is then given glucose by mouth to prevent a relapse. Nausea and vomiting are occasional adverse effects.

Glucocorticoids

Hormones produced by the cortex (outer layer) of the adrenal glands that affect carbohydrate metabolism by increasing the blood sugar level and the amount of glycogen in the liver. The principal glucocorticoid is *hydrocortisone* (also called cortisol), which also has a milder *mineralocorticoid* (affecting sodium and potassium balance) effect.

Glucose

The body's chief source of energy for cell *metabolism*. A monosaccharide (simple sugar) *carbohydrate*, it comes principally from the digestion of other carbohydrates, although a small amount is also produced in cells by the metabolism of fats and proteins.

BLOOD SUGAR LEVELS
Despite wide variation in carbohydrate intake (and, therefore, large fluctuations in the amount of glucose in the body), the concentration of glucose in the blood—the blood sugar level—is normally kept within narrow limits. This is achieved by the actions of several hormones, notably *insulin*, *glucagon*, *epinephrine*, *corticosteroids*, and *growth hormone*. If the blood sugar level is abnormally high (known as *hyperglycemia*), it may cause *glycosuria* (glucose in the urine). An abnormally low blood sugar level is called *hypoglycemia*.

Insulin, released by the pancreas in response to increased blood sugar levels, lowers the level by stimulating the uptake of glucose by cells. Inside the cells, glucose may be "burned" to produce energy, converted to *glycogen* for storage (mainly in the liver and muscles), or used in the production of triglycerides and fats.

Glucagon is released by the pancreas when the blood sugar level is low. It stimulates the breakdown of stored glycogen to glucose, which is then released into the bloodstream.

Epinephrine (released by the adrenal glands at times of stress) and corticosteroids (also released by the adrenals in response to factors such as infection) have the same basic effect as glucagon. That is, they stimulate the release of glucose to increase the blood sugar level.

Glue sniffing
See *Solvent abuse*.

Gluten

One of the proteins of wheat and certain other grains that gives dough its tough, elastic character. *Celiac sprue*, a sensitivity to gluten, is thought to affect between 0.1 and 0.2 percent of the population.

Gluten enteropathy
See *Celiac sprue*.

Gluten intolerance
See *Celiac sprue*.

Gluteus maximus
The large, powerful muscle in each of the buttocks that helps give them their rounded shape. The gluteus maximus is responsible for moving the thigh sideways and backward.

Glyburide
An oral *hypoglycemic drug* used to treat non-insulin-dependent *diabetes mellitus*. Glyburide stimulates the pancreas to produce insulin, which promotes the uptake of glucose (sugar) into muscle and fat tissue, thereby lowering the level of glucose in the blood.

Glycerin
A colorless syrup made from *glycerol* (an essential constituent of fats) and used in several drug preparations. Glycerin has a high water content, evaporates slowly, is easily absorbed, and has a softening effect.

WHY IT IS USED
Glycerin is used in moisturizing creams to help prevent dryness and cracking of the skin (for example, it is used to protect the nipples during breast-feeding).

Glycerin is used in ear drops to help soften *earwax* prior to syringing of the ears, and in *cough remedies* to help soothe a dry, irritating cough. Taken as a suppository or an enema, glycerin relieves constipation by softening hard feces.

Glycerol
An essential constituent of fats. Glycerol is released during digestion and absorbed either alone or in combination with fatty acids. When one molecule of glycerol combines with three molecules of fatty acids, the result is a type of fat known as a triglyceride.

Most of the glycerol is deposited in the body's fat stores; the remainder is taken up by the liver, where it may be converted into *glucose* (sugar) to provide energy.

Glycogen
The principal *carbohydrate* storage material in the body. It is a polysaccharide, consisting of many saccharide (sugar) molecules linked to form a long chain, and is found mainly in the liver and muscles.

Glycogen plays an important role in controlling blood sugar levels. When there is too much sugar (glucose) in the blood, the excess is converted to glycogen. This conversion (controlled by *insulin* and *corticosteroid hormones*) takes place chiefly in the liver and muscles. When the blood sugar level is low, glycogen is converted back to glucose (a process regulated by the hormones *glucagon* and *epinephrine*) and released into the bloodstream.

Glycosuria
The presence of glucose (a type of sugar) in the urine.

CAUSES
Glucose is normally filtered from the bloodstream by the kidneys (along with many other normal blood constituents and unwanted waste products). The filtered fluid passes down the many tubules of the kidneys, where all except the unwanted substances are reabsorbed and returned to the bloodstream (see *Kidney*). Glucose is one of the substances that the tubules almost completely reabsorb.

The kidney may fail to reabsorb all the glucose because of *hyperglycemia* (a high level of glucose in the blood) or if the tubules have been damaged and are unable to reabsorb even normal amounts of glucose. Hyperglycemia occurs in *diabetes mellitus*. Damage to the kidney tubules may be a result of rare metabolic disorders present from birth or be a consequence of drug or heavy metal poisoning.

Glycosuria can also sometimes occur in people with healthy kidneys that are unable to reabsorb all of the glucose filtered out of the bloodstream. This condition tends to run in families. Glycosuria often occurs during pregnancy because of hormonal changes, a condition that is usually not serious if it is not accompanied by other symptoms and if the blood glucose level is normal.

DIAGNOSIS AND TREATMENT
Glycosuria by itself does not necessarily indicate a serious condition. It may be found during a routine examination or if the physician is performing specific tests because diabetes mellitus is suspected. Urine can be tested for glucose by using a chemically impregnated strip that changes color when it comes in contact with glucose. Treatment depends on the underlying cause.

Gnat bites
See *Insect bites*.

Goiter
Enlargement of the thyroid gland, visible as a swelling on the neck.

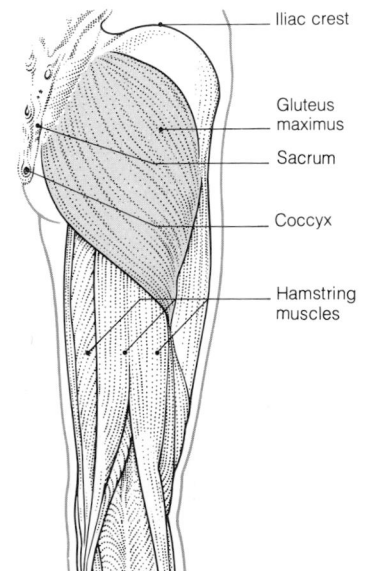

LOCATION OF THE GLUTEUS MAXIMUS
The top is attached to the sacrum, coccyx, and pelvis. The lower part is attached to the femur (thigh bone).

Iliac crest

Gluteus maximus

Sacrum

Coccyx

Hamstring muscles

CAUSES

The thyroid gland may enlarge (without any disturbance of its function) at puberty, during pregnancy, or as a result of taking the birth-control pill. In many parts of the world the main cause of a goiter is lack of sufficient iodine in the diet. The thyroid requires this mineral to produce the hormone thyroxine; a deficiency causes the gland to swell.

A toxic goiter is one that develops in *Graves' disease* or with other types of overactivity of the thyroid gland in which there is excessive production of thyroid hormones. This leads to *thyrotoxicosis*, characterized by symptoms such as increased appetite, warm, dry skin, weight loss, tremor, insomnia, and occasional muscle weakness and agitation. A goiter also usually is found in *Hashimoto's thyroiditis*, an autoimmune disorder, and de Quervain's *thyroiditis*, an inflammatory condition, both of which damage the gland; it may also be caused by a tumor or nodule in the gland and, in rare cases, by cancer (see *Thyroid cancer*). A goiter can also be caused by taking antithyroid drugs for overactivity of the thyroid gland.

Appearance of goiter
The thyroid may become enlarged for any of various reasons, including dietary deficiency of iodine, inflammation, or an autoimmune disorder affecting the gland.

SYMPTOMS

A goiter can range in size from a barely noticeable lump to an enormous swelling, depending on the cause. Large swellings may press on the esophagus or the trachea, making swallowing or breathing difficult. Any accompanying symptoms must be verified with X-ray pictures.

DIAGNOSIS AND TREATMENT

Diagnosis is based on the nature of the swelling, along with accompanying symptoms and the results of blood tests or *radionuclide scanning* carried out to determine the activity of the thyroid gland.

A goiter not caused by disease may eventually disappear naturally or may be so small that it does not require treatment. However, a large or unsightly goiter, or one that is causing difficulties with swallowing or with breathing may require total or partial removal (see *Thyroidectomy*).

If iodine deficiency is identified as the cause, the patient will be advised to eat more fish and iodized salt, which are rich in the mineral. When a goiter is the result of disease, treatment will be for the underlying disorder. If a drug is the cause, the goiter usually disappears once the course of treatment is over.

Gold

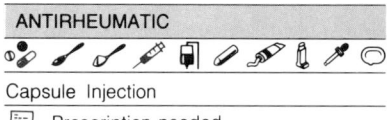

ANTIRHEUMATIC		
Capsule Injection		
📋 Prescription needed		
🔒 Not available as generic		

Gold is used to treat *rheumatoid arthritis* and arthritis arising as a complication of *psoriasis*. It is usually prescribed in severe active cases when a *nonsteroidal anti-inflammatory drug* (NSAID) has been ineffective.

HOW IT WORKS

Gold has an anti-inflammatory action that relieves joint pain and stiffness and can prevent more damage.

POSSIBLE ADVERSE EFFECTS

A common adverse effect of gold is *dermatitis* (inflammation of the skin); if itching occurs, the drug is usually withdrawn. Gold may damage the kidneys, liver, and bone marrow. Tests are performed during treatment to check the function of these organs.

Gold may cause loss of appetite, nausea, diarrhea, abdominal pain, and, occasionally, *anaphylactic shock* (a serious allergic reaction that requires emergency treatment).

Golfers' elbow

A condition caused by inflammation of the bony prominence (epicondyle) on the inner side of the elbow, to which certain forearm muscles are attached. It is caused by overuse of these muscles, which act to bend the wrist and fingers. Activities that can cause the condition include gripping and twisting (such as using a screwdriver) or playing golf with a faulty grip or swing.

SYMPTOMS AND TREATMENT

The inflammation causes pain and tenderness at the inner side of the elbow and sometimes in the forearm. Treatment consists of resting the elbow, applying ice packs, and taking analgesics (painkillers) and/or anti-inflammatory tablets. If the pain is severe or persistent, injection of a *corticosteroid drug* may be helpful.

If the pain has occurred after participation in a sport, it is wise to take a break from the sport for a week or two to prevent recurrence and to seek advice about playing technique.

Gonadotropin hormones

Hormones that stimulate cell activity in the gonads (ovaries and testes). Gonadotropins are essential for female and male fertility. The most important gonadotropins, follicle-stimulating hormone (FSH) and *luteinizing hormone* (LH), are secreted by the *pituitary gland*. Another gonadotropin, HCG (see *Gonadotropin, human chorionic*), is produced by the placenta.

GONADOTROPIN HORMONE THERAPY

Synthetic HCG is used in the treatment of recurrent *miscarriage* and certain types of female and male *infertility*. Menotropin (a gonadotropin extracted from the urine of women past the menopause) contains both FSH and LH and is used in the treatment of female infertility due to a failure to ovulate.

Gonadotropinlike substances are currently being evaluated as contraceptives and as a treatment for cancer of the prostate gland.

Gonadotropin, human chorionic

A hormone produced by the placenta in early pregnancy. Human chorionic gonadotropin (HCG) stimulates the ovaries to produce *estrogen* and *progesterone*, hormones needed to maintain a healthy pregnancy.

HCG is excreted in the urine; its measurement forms the basis of most pregnancy tests (a high level confirming pregnancy).

HCG THERAPY

HCG extracted from the urine of pregnant women is given by injection to treat certain types of *infertility*. Along with clomiphene tablets it may induce ovulation in women who have not been ovulating. In men, it may be used to increase sperm production.

HCG is occasionally given to prevent *miscarriage* in women whose production of progesterone is deficient.

HCG is also prescribed for the treatment of cryptorchidism (see *Testis, undescended*) in young boys, although surgical correction is usually required.

Gonads

The sex glands—the *testes* in men and the *ovaries* in women. The testes, situated in the scrotum, produce sperm and secrete the hormone *testosterone*. The ovaries, situated in the abdomen, release usually one ovum (egg) between them each month and secrete the hormones *estrogen* and *progesterone*. The activities of the gonads—both male and female—are regulated by *gonadotropin hormones* released by the pituitary gland.

Gonorrhea

A sexually transmitted disease, commonly known as "the clap." It is one of the most common infectious diseases in the world.

CAUSES AND INCIDENCE

Gonorrhea, caused by the bacterium *NEISSERIA GONORRHOEAE*, is most frequently transmitted during sexual intercourse, including oral or anal sex. An infected woman may also transmit the disease to her newborn baby during childbirth.

Gonorrhea is the second most common sexually transmitted disease, after *nonspecific urethritis*, and is most prevalent among young adults who have had multiple sexual partners. There are approximately 1 million cases of gonorrhea reported annually in the US. Since many cases are not reported, the true annual incidence may be closer to 3 million cases.

SYMPTOMS AND SIGNS

Gonorrhea has a short incubation period of two to 10 days. In men, symptoms usually include a urethral discharge and pain on urination. About 60 percent of infected women have no symptoms; if symptoms are present, they usually consist of a vaginal discharge or a burning sensation when urinating.

Infection acquired through anal sex causes gonococcal *proctitis* (inflammation of the rectum and anus). It causes pain and anal discharge in only about 10 percent of infected people. Oral sex with an infected person may lead to gonococcal *pharyngitis*, causing soreness in the throat but, again, most people have no symptoms. A baby exposed to infection in the mother's reproductive tract during childbirth may acquire gonococcal *ophthalmia*, a severe inflammation affecting one or both eyes.

COMPLICATIONS

Untreated gonorrhea may spread to other parts of the body. In men, it may cause *prostatitis* (inflammation of the prostate) or *epididymo-orchitis* (inflammation of the testes), affecting fertility. In women, untreated gonorrhea involves the fallopian tubes, causing *pelvic inflammatory disease* (PID). If the fallopian tubes are damaged, the woman is very likely to become infertile as a result.

Gonococcal bacteria may spread through the bloodstream to cause gonococcal *arthritis*, with pain and swelling of joints around the body. Multiplication of bacteria in the bloodstream causes *septicemia*, with generalized symptoms and signs, including fever and malaise; it can even spread to the brain or heart and cause death.

DIAGNOSIS

Many disorders can cause urethral or vaginal discharge. To confirm a diagnosis of gonorrhea, laboratory tests are necessary. Tests are carried out on a sample of the discharge or on swabs taken from the urethra or cervix.

TREATMENT

Gonorrhea is treated with antibiotics, usually *penicillin* or ampicillin. If the infection is caused by penicillin-resistant *NEISSERIA GONORRHOEAE* or if the infected person is allergic to penicillin, other antibiotics, such as tetracycline, ceftriaxone, or spectinomycin, may be used. Tests are performed to ensure that the infection has been cured.

OUTLOOK

Treatment for gonorrhea is effective but does not protect against reinfection. Sexual partners must be told that they might have gonorrhea even if they have no symptoms; many clinics have counselors (known as contact tracers) who identify and inform all people who might have been infected by the patient.

Goodpasture's syndrome

A rare condition characterized by *glomerulonephritis* (inflammation of the filtering units of the kidney), *coughing up blood* (hemoptysis), and *anemia*. Goodpasture's syndrome is a serious disease; unless treated at an early stage, it may lead to life-threatening bleeding into the lungs and progressive *renal failure*.

Goodpasture's syndrome is an *autoimmune disorder* (one in which the body's *immune system* attacks its own tissues). Antibodies are formed that attack the capillaries (tiny blood vessels) in the lungs and kidneys, eventually resulting in inflammation and disruption of the normal functioning of the lungs and kidneys.

The disease usually affects young men, but can develop at any age. Mild forms may be treated with *immunosuppressant drugs* (drugs that hamper the normal working of the body's immune system) and plasma exchange (*plasmapheresis*). The outlook is not good for people with severe and repeated attacks; they are treated by *dialysis* (a technique for removing waste products from the blood) and, eventually, *kidney transplant*.

Good Samaritan laws

Statutes (in most states) that legally protect a physician who voluntarily aids an injured or unconscious person at the scene of an accident.

Gout

A metabolic disorder that causes attacks of *arthritis*, usually in a single joint. Gout may be associated with kidney stones and ultimately may lead to kidney failure.

SYMPTOMS AND SIGNS

An acute attack of gout usually affects a single joint, most commonly the joint at the base of the big toe, but it can affect other joints, including the knee, ankle, wrist, foot, and small joints of the hand.

The affected joint is red, swollen, and extremely tender; the pain reaches a peak level of intensity within 24 to 36 hours. The redness and swelling may spread and be confused with *cellulitis* (inflammation of the connective tissue). The intensity of the pain is such that the person may not be able to stand on an affected foot or even tolerate the pressure of bedclothes on it. Sometimes there is a mild fever.

The first attack usually involves only one joint and lasts a few days. Some people never have another attack, but most have a second attack between six months and two years after the first. After the second attack, more and more joints may be involved, and there may be constant pain due to damage to the joint from chronic inflammation.

TREATMENT

Pain and inflammation in gout can be controlled with large doses of a *nonsteroidal anti-inflammatory drug* (NSAID). If use of an NSAID is contraindicated, *colchicine* may be prescribed. For maximal benefit, treatment should start as soon as an attack begins; patients prone to recurrent attacks should carry their gout

G

medication. As the inflammation subsides, usually within two to three days, the dose of medication is reduced and finally stopped. If an attack of gout is not responding to treatment with NSAIDs or colchicine, a *corticosteroid drug* may be injected into the affected joint.

Increased levels of purine (a product of DNA) can raise the level of uric acid in the blood. Although a strict low-purine diet is not necessary, people with gout should avoid foods that are high in purine, such as liver and other organ meats, legumes, and poultry. Excess alcohol consumption should also be avoided because it may precipitate an acute attack in a susceptible individual.

Many people never have more than a few attacks of gout, and further treatment is usually unnecessary. If attacks are recurrent, the frequency can be reduced by lowering the urate levels with drugs that either inhibit the formation of uric acid (such as allopurinol) or increase the excretion of uric acid by the kidneys with uricosuric drugs (such as probenecid and sulfinpyrazone). If the serum urate is very high, these drugs will need to be taken for life, as untreated hyperuricemia may lead to hypertension or kidney disease.

Grafting

The process of transplanting healthy tissue from one part of the body to another (autografting), from one person to another (allografting or homografting), or from an animal to a person (xenografting).

Grafting is used to repair or replace diseased or otherwise defective tissue. The primary tissues transplanted are skin (see *Skin graft*); bone (see *Bone graft*); bone marrow (see *Bone marrow transplantation*); the cornea of the eye (see *Corneal graft*); the kidney, the heart, and the liver (see *Kidney transplant; Heart transplant; Liver transplant; Transplant surgery*); heart valves (see *Heart valve surgery*); and blood vessels and nerves (see *Microsurgery*).

COMPLICATIONS
With autografting, the grafted tissue is usually assimilated at the new site without any trouble and soon grows into the surrounding tissue to provide a good repair.

Problems occur, however, with allografting (homografting) and xenografting, both of which are usually carried out to replace rather than repair tissue. Xenografting is not performed clinically except for the use of porcine (pig) heart valves. The major drawback to allografting is that the recipient's defense system automatically attempts to reject the foreign cells of the donor's tissue and to destroy them in the same way that it would invading microorganisms. The only exceptions are in the case of identical twins (because their tissue matches exactly) and in that of corneal grafting, since the cornea has no blood supply (and therefore no white blood cells and antibodies to act as a defense system).

To overcome rejection, as close a match as possible between the tissues of the recipient and donor is sought (see *Tissue-typing*). *Immunosuppressant drugs* (especially *cyclosporine*) are given to suppress the body's defense system—though this can cause other problems, such as decreased kidney function. Cyclosporine, the immunosuppressant drug introduced in 1984, has been particularly effective in the control of organ rejection and *graft-versus-host disease*.

GOUT

Gout is a common joint disease, affecting 10 times more men than women. In men it occurs at any time after puberty; in women it usually occurs only after the menopause. There is often a family history of the disorder. Hyperuricemia (excess uric acid in the blood) leads to formation of uric acid crystals in joints; crystals may also be deposited in soft tissues in the ears and around tendons.

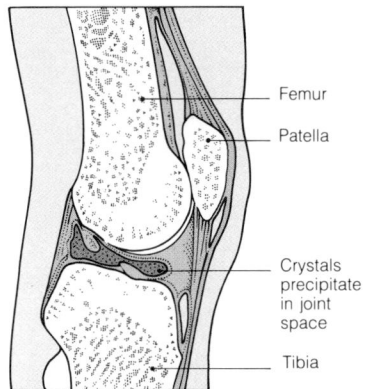

Crystal precipitation
Crystals of uric acid precipitate into the joint space and surrounding tissues of the knee, causing intense inflammation and extreme pain.

Appearance of gout
Deposition of uric acid crystals in the joint space have caused inflammation and obvious swelling of the affected right knee.

DIAGNOSIS
Gout is considered as a diagnosis whenever an attack of arthritis affects a single joint. A blood test is usually performed; a high level of uric acid suggests gout.

Aspiration
Fluid is aspirated (removed through a needle into a syringe) from the swollen knee joint and examined under a microscope.

Microscopic evidence
The presence of uric acid crystals confirms the diagnosis.

G

G

Growth hormone
A substance produced by the *pituitary gland* that stimulates normal body growth and development by altering chemical activity in cells. Growth hormone stimulates the production of protein in muscle cells and the release of energy from the breakdown of fats.

GROWTH HORMONE THERAPY
In the past, growth hormone was extracted from human corpses; it is now prepared synthetically. Growth hormone therapy is used to treat *short stature* when the underlying cause is a pituitary gland disorder. Treatment is usually started in early childhood. Growth hormone is sometimes given with an anabolic *steroid*, which also promotes tissue growth.

POSSIBLE ADVERSE EFFECTS
There is a slight risk that *diabetes mellitus* may develop during treatment. Some people produce *antibodies* to growth hormone, but this does not seem to reduce its effectiveness.

Guanethidine
An *antihypertensive drug* used to treat severe *hypertension* (high blood pressure) that has not responded to other drugs. Adverse effects of guanethidine include dizziness or fainting, diarrhea, and impotence.

Guanethidine is currently under investigation as a treatment for *glaucoma* (raised pressure in the eyeball) in combination with *epinephrine*, in the form of eye drops.

Guar gum
A high-fiber plant substance used to help control the blood glucose (sugar) level in people with *diabetes mellitus*. Guar gum granules are either sprinkled on food or dissolved in water to form a thick gel for drinking.

HOW IT WORKS
Guar gum forms a sticky solution in the stomach and slows the movement of nutrients from there into the small intestine. This action slows the rate at which glucose is absorbed from the small intestine into the bloodstream, thus preventing a sudden rise in blood glucose after a meal.

POSSIBLE ADVERSE EFFECTS
Guar gum has an unpleasant taste and may cause flatulence, nausea, and abdominal discomfort.

Guillain-Barré syndrome
A rare form of damage to the peripheral nerves (see *Peripheral nervous system*) that causes weakness of the limbs. The nerves become inflamed, particularly where their roots leave the spine, impairing both movement and sensation. The disease is also known as acute polyneuritis and ascending paralysis.

CAUSES AND INCIDENCE
The cause of the disease is believed to be an allergic reaction to an infection, usually viral; the nerves are inflamed by antibodies produced by the reaction. In most cases the disease develops two or three weeks after the onset of an infection, usually an infection of the upper respiratory tract, such as a sore throat or influenza, or a gastrointestinal upset. In 1976, an epidemic occurred in the US following mass vaccination against swine flu. The incidence is about 15 cases per million population per year in the US.

SYMPTOMS
Weakness, often accompanied by numbness and tingling, usually starts in the legs and spreads to the arms. It becomes progressively worse and may develop into paralysis. The muscles of the face and those that control speech, swallowing, and breathing may also be affected, causing difficulty with all three activities.

DIAGNOSIS
The diagnosis is made from the patient's symptoms and signs, from the results of electrical tests to measure how fast nerve impulses are being conducted, and from a *lumbar puncture*, in which a sample of cerebrospinal fluid is taken from the spinal canal for analysis.

TREATMENT AND OUTLOOK
Patients are treated in the hospital, where their condition (particularly any breathing difficulty) can be closely monitored. If it becomes severe, *intubation* (inserting a breathing tube down the throat) and mechanical *ventilation* are carried out. *Plasmapheresis* (in which blood plasma is withdrawn from the patient, treated to remove antibodies, and replaced) may be employed in severe cases.

Most people recover completely without specific treatment, but some are left with permanent weakness in affected areas and/or suffer from further attacks of the disease.

Guilt
A painful feeling that arises from the awareness of having broken a moral or legal code. Guilt is self-inflicted, unlike shame, which depends on others knowing about the transgression. Some psychoanalysts see guilt as a result of the prohibitions of the *superego* (conscience) instilled by parental authority in early life. Others see guilt as a conditioned response to actions that in the past have led to punishment.

Feeling guilty from time to time is normal. However, feeling very guilty for no reason or experiencing guilt at an imagined crime is one of the main symptoms of psychotic *depression*.

Guinea worm disease

A tropical disease caused by a female parasitic worm more than 3 feet (1 meter) long. Infection is the result of drinking water containing the crustacean water flea *CYCLOPS*, which harbors larvae of the worm. The larvae pass through the intestinal wall of the infected person and mature in connective tissue. After about a year, the adult female worm, now pregnant, approaches the surface of the skin, and creates an inflamed blister that bursts, exposing the end of the worm.

The disease occurs in Africa, South America, the Caribbean, the Middle East, and India.

SYMPTOMS AND TREATMENT
Urticaria (hives), nausea, vomiting, and diarrhea often develop while the blister is forming.

The traditional remedy is to wind the worm gently from the skin onto a small stick. Once the worm is out, the condition usually clears up.

The drugs niridazole and thiabendazole are given to reduce inflammation and make extraction of the worm safer, antibiotics are given to control secondary infection, and the patient is immunized against tetanus.

Gum
Also called the gingiva, the soft tissue surrounding the teeth that protects underlying structures and helps keep the teeth tightly in position in the jaw. The gingival margin, a cuff of gum about 2 mm thick, fits tightly around the base of the teeth and is anchored within the bony socket by the periodontal ligaments.

Normal, healthy gums are pink or brown and firm. Careful *oral hygiene*, including daily brushing and flossing, is needed to avoid gum disease, especially on reaching middle age.

DISORDERS
Gingivitis (an early, reversible stage of gum disease characterized by inflammation of the gums) may occur if plaque, which contains bacteria, is allowed to collect around the base of the teeth. Bleeding gums are nearly always a symptom of gingivitis; rarely, they are due to *leukemia* (blood

cell cancer) or *scurvy* (vitamin C deficiency). Bruised gums are more likely to be caused by a *bleeding disorder*. Gingival *hyperplasia* (fleshy thickening of the gums) is most commonly a side effect of *anticonvulsant drug* treatment with phenytoin.

Untreated gingivitis may lead to *periodontitis*, the advanced stage of gum disease, in which infected pockets form between the gums and the teeth.

Gumma

A soft tumor that is characteristic of the late stages of untreated *syphilis*.

Gut

Popular name for the *intestine*.

Guthrie test

A blood test performed routinely on babies between the eighth and fourteenth day after birth to check for *phenylketonuria*. This is an inherited disorder in which the amino acid phenylalanine accumulates in the blood and tissues, usually leading to severe brain damage unless treated. The Guthrie test measures the amount of phenylalanine in the blood.

Carrying out a Guthrie test
A few drops of blood are taken from the baby's heel and sent to the laboratory to be tested for phenylalanine content.

HOW IT IS DONE
The baby's heel is pricked with a needle and a few drops of blood are soaked onto a piece of absorbent filter paper. The paper is then placed onto a nutrient medium containing bacteria whose growth is activated by phenylalanine. The size of the area of bacterial growth that appears is directly related to the concentration of phenylalanine in the blood.

RESULTS
A concentration of phenylalanine above 20 mg/ml indicates that phenylketonuria may be present; other, more accurate tests are performed to confirm the diagnosis.

Gynecologist

A physician who specializes in diagnosing and treating problems of the female reproductive tract, including disorders relating to *menstruation* and *menopause* and sexual dysfunctions that may have a physical cause. A gynecologist also offers advice on *contraception* and treats *infertility*.

From the time a woman starts menstruating, she should see a gynecologist every one to three years for a *pelvic examination* and a *cervical smear* (Pap test). These tests are often performed on a preventive basis, because cervical smears can detect cancer of the cervix at an early stage. A gynecologist also investigates and treats menstrual disorders, such as *amenorrhea* (lack of menstruation), *menorrhagia* (excessive menstrual bleeding), *dysmenorrhea* (painful menstruation), and *premenstrual syndrome* as well as structural disorders, including uterine *fibroids*, cervical *polyps*, and ovarian *cysts*.

Although an *obstetrician* deals with the management of pregnancy, the gynecologist treats disorders of early pregnancy, including recurrent *miscarriage*. Many gynecologists are also obstetricians.

Gynecology

The study of the female *reproductive system* and the diagnosis and treatment of disorders affecting it. Gynecology involves both medical treatment, using drugs including hormones, and surgical procedures, such as *D and C* (dilatation and curettage) and *hysterectomy* (removal of the uterus). The specialty also involves the investigation and treatment of *infertility*, including *artificial insemination* and *in vitro fertilization*, and advice on *contraception*, including *sterilization*. (See also *Gynecologist*.)

Gynecomastia

Enlargement of one or both breasts in the male, almost always due to an excess of the female sex hormone *estrogen* in the blood.

CAUSES
Estrogen, which is responsible for female secondary sexual characteristics, is produced in large quantities in women, but is also produced in small amounts in all men (just as all women produce small amounts of male sex hormones). In some males, however, an abnormal amount of estrogen is produced, usually for reasons that are not fully understood, but sometimes because of disease.

Gynecomastia is quite common at puberty, taking the form of a slight swelling in one or both breasts, often accompanied by some tenderness. A young boy with gynecomastia is likely to be worried and embarrassed; he should be reassured that his masculinity is not threatened and that the problem will soon pass. Gynecomastia of this mild, temporary kind can also occur at birth.

If the condition develops later—most commonly when a man is over the age of 50—the enlargement may be greater, especially in an already obese man. Such cases are usually not serious, but investigation is necessary to rule out the possibility of an underlying disease. This disease could be *cirrhosis* of the liver, in which the liver is unable to break down estrogen; a tumor of the testis (see *Testis, cancer of*), which can raise the level of estrogen in the blood; or, if only one breast is affected, *breast cancer*, in which case the swelling is caused by a tumor.

Adult gynecomastia can also occur when any one of a number of drugs changes the balance of sex hormones in the blood.

DIAGNOSIS
The physician may arrange for blood tests. If cancer is suspected, a *biopsy* (removal of the entire nodule or a piece of tissue for analysis) will be performed; early treatment is essential for breast cancer.

TREATMENT
The treatment depends on the underlying cause. If a drug is responsible, an alternative drug will be prescribed if possible; otherwise, the gynecomastia must be weighed against the effects of withdrawing drug treatment.

If there is no underlying disease, the swelling usually subsides without treatment, although it may take a few years. A man who is embarrassed by enlarged breasts may prefer to have cosmetic surgery.

If the swelling is moderate or bothersome, an operation can be performed that leaves only a small, unnoticeable scar around part of the areola (the dark skin surrounding the nipple). In many cases, this operation can be carried out as an office procedure using a local anesthetic. *Mammoplasty*, an operation more frequently performed on women, is used when breast enlargement is severe. This operation takes longer, requires a general anesthetic, and leaves extensive and obvious scarring.

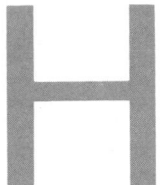

H-2 receptor antagonists
See *Histamine-2 receptor antagonists*.

Habituation
The effect of becoming accustomed to an experience. In general, the more a person is exposed to a stimulus, the less he or she is aroused by it. Experiments have shown that frightening pictures make the pulse rate rise less the more they are seen. Likewise, people can become habituated to drugs (see *Tolerance*).

Habsburg jaw
An inherited prominence of the lower jaw named for the European royal house of Habsburg.

Hair
A threadlike structure composed of dead cells filled with *keratin*, the protein that makes up nails and the outer skin layer.

STRUCTURE
The root of each hair is embedded in a tiny pit in the skin called a hair follicle. Each shaft of hair consists of a spongy semihollow core (the medulla), a surrounding layer of long, thin fibers (the cortex), and, on the outside, several layers of overlapping cells (the cuticle). During the growing phase of a hair the root is firmly enclosed by live tissue called a bulb, which supplies the hair with keratin; the bulb is the pale swelling that sometimes can be seen when a hair is pulled out. The upgrowth of dead cells and keratin from the root forms the hair.

TYPES
There are three types of human hair. From the fourth month of gestation, the fetus is covered with downy hair called lanugo, which is shed during the ninth month. After birth and until puberty, vellus hair, which is fine, short, and colorless, covers most of the body. The third type, terminal hair, is thicker, longer, and often pigmented; it grows on the scalp, the eyebrows, and the eyelashes. At puberty, terminal hair replaces vellus in the pubic area and the armpits. In

THE STRUCTURE OF A HAIR
The hair shaft contains dead cells and keratin (a type of protein). The root is embedded in the skin.

Cuticle
Medulla
Cortex
Hair shaft
Sebaceous gland

Follicle   Root   Bulb   Erector pili muscle

Cross section through hairs
The central medulla, cortex, and outer cuticle can all be clearly differentiated in this microscope photograph.

most men and some women the process continues on the face, limbs, and trunk (see *Hirsutism*).

COLOR AND TEXTURE
Hair color is determined by the amount of pigment called *melanin* in the hair shaft. Melanin is produced by special pigment-producing cells called melanocytes at the base of the hair follicle. Red melanin is responsible for red and auburn hair, black melanin for all other colors. If cells receive no pigment, the cortex of each hair becomes transparent and the resulting hair appears white.

The degree of curliness of a hair depends on the shape of its follicle (see box, overleaf).

DISORDERS
Many hair disorders appear to be purely cosmetic, but they can also be a symptom of a more serious underlying disorder.

Brittle hair, which breaks easily and splits at the ends, is usually due to excessive shampooing, combing, or blow-drying. Occasionally, it can be a sign of severe vitamin or mineral deficiency, or may indicate *hypothyroidism*. Very dry hair is often the result of excessive use of hot rollers or curling irons, or frequent perming, tinting, or bleaching; it can also be caused by malnutrition.

Ingrown hairs occur primarily in blacks or people with very curly hair. The free-growing end of the hair penetrates the skin near the follicle, often causing severe inflammation.

Hairball
A ball of hair in the stomach. Also known as a trichobezoar, it is found in people who nervously pull, suck, or chew their hair. (See *Bezoar*.)

Hairiness, excessive
See *Hirsutism*; *Hypertrichosis*.

Hair removal
Hair is usually removed from different parts of the body for cosmetic reasons. It may also be shaved from around an incision site to allow thorough cleansing before surgical operations.

HOW IT IS DONE
The method used depends on the part of the body involved and the degree of permanency required.

Shaving removes hair at skin level and is suitable for the legs, for armpit and pubic hair, and for the facial beard in men. Shaving is quick and safe, but the hair soon grows back.

Depilatory creams dissolve the hair just below the skin surface, creating a smoother effect than shaving. However, depilatories may irritate sensitive areas and their use is generally best restricted to the legs.

Waxing, a method often used in beauty salons, is suitable for the legs and face. The wax is applied to the area and peeled off, pulling out the hair with it. Plucking with tweezers is suitable for small areas. After each of these methods, hair takes several weeks to regrow.

Permanent removal of hair requires *electrolysis*, in which an electric current is used to destroy the growing part of

H

HAIR GROWTH

Hair on the scalp grows about half an inch per month. There are about 300,000 hairs on the scalp at any given time, though there is considerable individual variation. The exact number of hairs depends on the number of hair follicles, which is established before birth. Each hair goes through alternating periods of growth and rest. On average, each person sheds 100 to 150 hairs a day from the scalp.

Growth phase
At the start of a growth phase (which, on the scalp, lasts about three years for each hair), the hair root stimulates the growth of a bulb and then a shaft.

Rest phase
During the rest phase (which lasts about three months on the scalp), the bulb retracts from the root and eventually the hair falls out. A new hair begins to grow in the same follicle.

Hair shaft

Root

Bulb

Old hair falls out

New hair forms

TYPES OF HAIR
There are three types of hair—straight, curly, and wavy.

Straight hair
Grows from a more or less round follicle and is round in cross section.

Curly hair
Oval in cross section and grows from a highly curved follicle.

Wavy hair
Kidney-shaped in cross section; the extent of the curl depends on the curve of the follicle.

the hair. Electrolysis requires expertise, is very time-consuming, and is expensive, so it is usually used only for small areas.

Hair transplant
A cosmetic operation in which hairy sections of scalp are removed and transplanted to hairless areas as a treatment of baldness.

HOW IT IS DONE
One or a combination of the following techniques may be employed.

PUNCH GRAFTING This is the most common method of hair transplantation; it is performed using a local anesthetic and is an outpatient procedure. A punch is used to remove small areas of bald scalp, about 0.25 inch (0.6 cm) across, which are replaced with areas of hairy scalp. The grafts are taped into position until the natural healing process takes effect.

STRIP GRAFTING This requires a general anesthetic and is carried out in the hospital. Strips of bald skin are cut from the top of the head; strips of hairy scalp are then stitched in position to replace them.

FLAP GRAFTING This is often used to form a new hairline. It is similar to strip grafting, except that flaps of hairy skin are lifted, swiveled, and stitched to replace areas of bald skin.

MALE PATTERN BALDNESS REDUCTION This relatively new technique consists of cutting out areas of bald skin and then stretching surrounding areas of hair-bearing scalp to replace the bald areas.

RESULTS
The success of hair transplantation varies. The hair in punch grafts often falls out after transplantation, leaving unsightly patches for several months until new hair grows. Also, hair does not always grow properly in the areas from which graft skin is taken. Even successful transplants do not last indefinitely; as time passes, the transplanted areas also become bald.

Half-life
The time taken for the activity of a substance to reduce to half its original level. The term is usually used to refer to the time taken for the level of radiation emitted by a radioactive substance to decay to half its original value. This is useful in *radiation therapy* to assess the length of time radioactive material will remain in the body.

The term half-life is also used in pharmacology to refer to the time the body takes to eliminate enough of a drug so that the amount remaining in the bloodstream is halved.

Halitosis
The medical term for bad breath. Halitosis is occasionally a sign of illness, but is usually simply a result of smoking, drinking alcohol, eating garlic or onions, or poor oral and dental hygiene. Contrary to popular belief, neither constipation nor indigestion is a cause.

If bad breath is persistent and is not due to any of the above causes, it may be a symptom of a mouth infection, *sinusitis*, or certain lung disorders, such as *bronchiectasis*.

Hallucination
A perception that occurs when there is no external stimulus (for example, hearing voices or seeing faces when there is no one there). Hallucination differs from an *illusion*, in which a real stimulus is present but has been misinterpreted (thinking that the ticking of a clock is a bomb, for example).

TYPES AND CAUSES
Auditory hallucinations (the hearing of voices) are the most common type. They are a major symptom of *schizophrenia*, but may also be caused by *manic-depressive illness* and certain brain disorders. Visual hallucinations (seeing visions) are most often found in states of *delirium* brought on either by a physical illness (such as pneumonia) or by alcohol withdrawal (see *Delirium tremens*). *Hallucinogenic drugs*, such as mescaline, are another common cause. Hallucinations of smell are often a sign of *temporal lobe epilepsy*, especially when the epilepsy is caused by a tumor. Hallucinations of touch and taste are uncommon; they probably occur primarily in people with schizophrenia.

There is evidence that people subjected to *sensory deprivation* or to overwhelming physical stress hallucinate temporarily.

Hallucinogenic drug
A drug that causes a *hallucination*. Hallucinogens include drugs of abuse, also called psychedelic drugs, such as

LSD, *marijuana*, *mescaline*, and *psilocybin*. Alcohol may also have a hallucinogenic effect if taken in large amounts; hallucinations also occur during alcohol withdrawal. Certain prescription drugs, including *anticholinergic drugs*, *levodopa*, and *timolol*, may cause takers to have hallucinations in rare instances.

Hallux

The medical name for the big toe.

Hallux rigidus

Loss of movement in the large joint at the base of the big toe due to *osteoarthritis*. The condition often follows an injury and is aggravated by sports that involve running and jumping. The joint is usually tender and swollen, and pain is worse during walking or running.

Hallux rigidus, which may be mistaken for *gout*, is diagnosed if X rays reveal degeneration of the joint. Treatment consists of resting the toe and wearing an insert in the shoe to support the front of the foot and to reduce movements of the toe during walking. If severe symptoms persist, surgery may be required.

Hallux valgus

A deformity of the big toe in which the joint at the base projects outward and the top of the toe turns inward. The condition (which is more common in women) is usually caused by wearing narrow, pointed shoes with high heels, but is sometimes caused by an inherited weakness in the joint. A hallux valgus often results in a *bunion* (a firm, fluid-filled, sometimes painful swelling over the joint) or *osteoarthritis* in the joint.

Treatment is required only if the bunion becomes very large or persistently inflamed or if the osteoarthritis causes pain and limits foot movement. In these cases, the toe may be straightened by means of *osteotomy* (removing part of a bone and realigning its ends) or *arthrodesis* (fusing the bones of a joint).

Haloperidol

An *antipsychotic drug* used in the treatment of mental illnesses such as *schizophrenia* and *mania*. Haloperidol is also given to control the symptoms of *Gilles de la Tourette's syndrome* (a rare neurological disorder) and is used to sedate aggressive or hostile people with *dementia*. Because haloperidol has a powerful *antiemetic* effect, it is sometimes used to relieve nausea and vomiting caused by *narcotic drugs*, *anesthesia*, *anticancer drugs*, and *radiation therapy*.

POSSIBLE ADVERSE EFFECTS
Adverse effects include drowsiness, lethargy, weight gain, dizziness, and, more seriously, *parkinsonism* (a neurological disorder that causes symptoms such as abnormal involuntary movements and stiffness of the face and limbs).

Halothane

A colorless liquid inhaled as a vapor to induce and help maintain general anesthesia (see *Anesthesia, general*). In rare cases it may cause *arrhythmia* (irregular heart beat) or liver damage.

Hamartoma

A benign, tumorlike mass consisting of an overgrowth of tissues that are normally found in the affected part of the body. Hamartomas are most frequent in the skin (the most common is a *hemangioma*, an overgrowth of blood vessels in the skin), but also occur in the lungs, heart, or kidneys.

Hammer toe

A deformity of the toe (usually the second toe) in which the main toe joint is bent upward like a claw. There is often a painful *corn* on this joint due to pressure from the overlying shoe. The deformity is caused by an abnormality of the tendons in the toe.

A protective felt pad usually eases pressure on the joint and thus relieves pain. If pain persists, the deformity may require surgical correction.

Hamstring muscles

A group of muscles at the back of the thigh that bends the knee and swings the leg backward from the thigh.

DISORDERS
Tearing of the muscles is common in sports, particularly in sprinting. The injury happens suddenly and is very painful. Bruising over the area develops several days later. Repeated strenuous exercise may cause a sprain of the muscles, with pain coming on gradually (see *Overuse injury*). Both types of injury can often be prevented by warm-up exercises.

Sciatica (pain down the back of the leg caused by pressure on the sciatic nerve) may be particularly severe in the hamstring muscles. Painful spasms of the muscles may also occur as a protective response to a knee injury. By restricting movement of the damaged knee joint, the spasms limit further injury.

Hand

The most flexible part of the skeleton, the hand allows humans (and other primates) to hold and manipulate objects. This movement is primarily due to the ability of the thumb and fingers to move independently of, and oppose, each other (see *Grip*).

STRUCTURE
The hand is made up of the wrist, palm, and fingers (see next page).

Movements of the hand are achieved mainly by tendons that attach the muscles of the forearm to the bones of the hand. These tendons are surrounded by synovial sheaths containing a lubricating fluid to prevent friction. Other movements are controlled by short muscles in the palm of the hand, some of which make up the prominent areas along the sides of the hand from the bases of the thumb and little fingers to the wrist.

Blood is supplied to the hand by two arteries (the radial on the thumb side of the wrist and the ulnar on the little finger side) and is carried away by veins prominent on the back of the hand. Sensation and movement in the hand are controlled by the radial, ulnar, and median nerves.

DISORDERS
Because they are so frequently used, the hands are susceptible to injury, including cuts, burns, bites, fractures,

H

ANATOMY OF THE HAMSTRING MUSCLES

The upper ends of these muscles are attached by tendons to the pelvis, and the lower ends by tendons called hamstrings to the tibia and fibula.

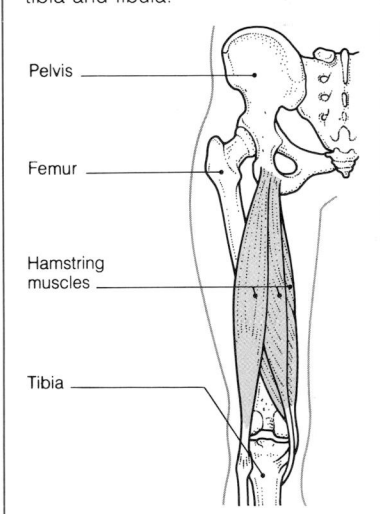

Pelvis

Femur

Hamstring muscles

Tibia

H

and, occasionally, tendon injuries. *Dermatitis* is also common, since the hands are exposed to a variety of irritating agents.

The hand may be affected by contracture, a deformity caused by shrinkage of tissues in the palm of the hand (see *Dupuytren's contracture*) or damage to muscles in the forearm (see *Volkmann's contracture*). Degeneration of a synovial sheath on the upper side of the wrist may cause a harmless swelling known as a *ganglion*.

Osteoarthritis commonly attacks the joint at the base of the thumb, rendering it painful and immobile. *Rheumatoid arthritis* may cause deformity by attacking the joints at the base of the fingers and rupturing tendons.

Handedness

Preference for using the right or left hand. Some 90 percent of healthy adults use the right hand for writing; two thirds favor the right hand for most activities requiring coordination and skill. The remainder are either left-handed or ambidextrous (able to use both hands equally) to a varying degree. There is no male-female difference in these proportions.

It is uncertain why all humans are not simply ambidextrous. Up to the age of about 12, it is possible to switch handedness if a person's dominant hemisphere of the brain is damaged.

CAUSES
Inheritance is probably the most important factor in determining handedness. Studies have shown a greater number of nerves going to one side of the brain even in the newborn. A child made to use the right hand despite natural preference, however, may "become" right-handed. In earlier times, left-handed people were considered to be unlucky or evil (the word sinister is derived from the Latin word for left), so children were trained to be right-handed. Even today, so many people are naturally right-handed that the pressure to conform is high, especially in some cultures where the left hand is reserved for wiping the anus after defecation. Some left-handed people have been known to rebel subconsciously when forced to use the right hand.

Handedness is related to the division of the human brain into two hemispheres, each of which controls movement and sensation on the opposite side of the body. In most right-handed people, the speech center is in the left hemisphere, so that a *stroke* affecting this side of the brain

THE SKELETAL STRUCTURE OF THE HAND AND WRIST

Four of the eight wrist bones (carpals) articulate with the radius and ulna. The rest are connected to the five bones of the palm (metacarpals), each of which is joined to a phalanx.

Trapezium bone
Trapezoid bone
Capitate bone
Hamate bone
Scaphoid bone — Carpals
Pisiform bone
Lunate bone
Triquetral bone

Radius

Ulna

Phalanges   Metacarpals

causes *aphasia* (speech impairment) as well as paralysis and weakness of the right arm and leg. In 70 percent of left-handed people, the speech center is on the right, and left hemisphere damage does not cause aphasia.

EFFECTS OF HANDEDNESS
It is not clear whether handedness is related to special abilities. Left-handed tennis players or "southpaw" pitchers seem to succeed because their shots or balls come from an unusual angle. While the left brain is related to verbal ability and logical reasoning, and the right to emotional and spatial awareness, there is no evidence that more artists are left-handed or more philosophers are right-handed.

Hand-foot-and-mouth disease

A common infectious disease of toddlers, caused by a type of virus called coxsackievirus. Hand-foot-and-mouth disease often occurs in small epidemics in nursery schools, usually in the summer months.

The illness is usually mild and lasts only a few days. Symptoms include blistering of the palms, soles, and inside of the mouth, reluctance to eat, and a slight fever.

There is no treatment other than mild *analgesics* (painkillers) to relieve the discomfort of the blisters. The illness is unrelated to foot-and-mouth disease in cattle.

Handicap

The extent to which a physical or mental *disability* (loss or permanent impairment of a faculty) prevents a person from performing everyday activities such as walking or dressing.

The management and treatment of a handicap involves assessment of the specific disability, the provision of suitable aids, and, in severe cases, institutional care.

Hangnail

A strip of skin torn away from the side or base of a fingernail, exposing a raw, painful area. It usually occurs after frequent immersion in water has dried the skin on the fingers. Biting the nails is another common cause. The raw area may become infected and develop into a *paronychia*.

A hangnail should be trimmed with scissors and covered until it heals. The condition may be prevented by applying a moisturizing cream.

Hangover

The unpleasant effects sometimes experienced on waking after overindulgence in *alcohol*. Characterized by headache, nausea, vertigo, and depression, the severity of a hangover is determined by the amount and type of alcohol consumed. Brandy, bourbon, and red wine have high concentrations of congeners (secondary products of alcohol fermentation) and usually produce bad hangovers.

Alcohol has a diuretic effect and some of the symptoms of a hangover are due to mild dehydration; drinking a large quantity of water before going to sleep may help. Recovery from a hangover is usually just a matter of time, but, in alcoholics (see *Alcohol dependence*) there may be withdrawal symptoms or the hangover may be more severe and persistent. (See also *Alcohol intoxication*.)

Hansen's disease
See *Leprosy*.

Hardening of the arteries
The popular term for *arteriosclerosis*, the most common form of which is *atherosclerosis*.

Hare lip
A common term for the congenital defect in which there is a split in the upper lip due to failure of the two halves to fuse during fetal development. Also called cleft lip, it is often associated with a similar failure of the two halves of the palate to join. (See *Cleft lip and palate*.)

Hashimoto's thyroiditis
An *autoimmune disorder* in which the body's immune system develops antibodies against its own thyroid gland cells. As a result, the thyroid gland becomes unable to produce enough hormones, a condition called *hypothyroidism*.

The principal symptoms are tiredness, muscle weakness, and weight gain. Enlargement of the thyroid gland (goiter) is present.

The condition is diagnosed by blood tests to measure the level of thyroid hormones and detect the presence of thyroid antibodies. Treatment consists of thyroid hormone replacement therapy, which is continued for life. It does not always cure the goiter, which may require surgery.

Hay fever
The popular name for allergic *rhinitis*.

Headache
One of the most common types of pain; a headache is very rarely a sign of some underlying, serious disorder. The pain of a headache comes from outside the brain (the brain tissue itself does not contain sensory nerves). Pain arises from the *meninges* (the outer linings of the brain) and from the scalp and its blood vessels and muscles. It is produced by tension in, or stretching of, these structures.

The pain may be felt all over the head or may occur in one part only—for example, in the back of the neck, the forehead, or one side of the head. Sometimes the pain moves to another part of the head during the course of the headache. The pain may be superficial or deep, throbbing or sharp, and there may be accompanying or preliminary symptoms, such as nausea, vomiting, and visual or sensory disturbances.

TYPES
Many headaches are simply the body's response to some adverse stimulus, such as hunger or a change in the weather. These headaches usually clear up in a few hours and leave no aftereffects.

Tension headaches, caused by tightening in the muscles of the face, neck, and scalp as a result of stress or poor posture, are also common. They may last for days or weeks and can cause variable degrees of discomfort.

Some types of headaches are especially painful and persistent, but, despite these symptoms, do not indicate any progressive disorder. *Migraine* is a severe, incapacitating headache preceded or accompanied by visual and/or stomach disturbances. Cluster headaches cause intense pain behind one eye and may wake the sufferer nightly for periods of weeks or months.

CAUSES
Common causes of headache include *hangover*, irregular meals, prolonged travel, poor posture, a noisy or stuffy work environment, excitement, and excessive sleep. Recent research has shown that certain foods (such as cheese, chocolate, and red wine) trigger migraine attacks in susceptible people. *Food additives* may also cause headache. Other causes include *sinusitis*, toothache, ear infection, head injury, and *cervical osteoarthritis*. (See also chart, overleaf.)

Among the rare causes of headache are *brain tumor*, *hypertension* (high blood pressure), *temporal arteritis* (inflammation of the arteries of the brain and scalp), *aneurysm* (localized swelling of a blood vessel), and increased pressure within the skull.

INVESTIGATION
If headaches are persistent, without obvious cause, and do not respond to self-help treatment, medical advice should be sought. The physician will ask about the nature and site of the pain and at what intervals the headaches occur. A careful general physical and neurological examination will be performed. *CT scanning* or *MRI* (magnetic resonance imaging) may be carried out if a neurological cause is suspected.

TREATMENT
Prevention is more important than treatment; many of the known causes can easily be avoided, particularly if the sufferer knows what triggers the headaches. Once a headache has started, however (if it is not a migraine or cluster headache), one or more of the following measures should ease the pain: relaxing in a hot bath, lying down, avoidance of aggravating factors (such as excessive noise or a stuffy room), stretching and massaging the muscles in the shoulders, neck, face, and scalp, taking a mild analgesic, such as acetaminophen, and, if convenient, sleeping for a few hours.

Head injury
Injury to the head may occur as the result of traffic accidents, sports injuries, falls, assault, accidents at work and at home, or bullet wounds. Most people have a head injury at least once in their lives, but very few of the injuries are severe enough to require treatment by a neurosurgeon. One percent of all deaths are caused by head injury, half of them as a result of traffic accidents.

A head injury can damage the scalp, skull, or brain in any combination. Minor injuries cause no damage to the underlying brain. Even when there is a *skull fracture*, or the scalp is split, the brain may not be damaged. However, a blow may severely shake the brain, sometimes causing *brain damage*, even when there are no signs of external injury (closed head injury).

A blow often bruises the brain tissue, causing death of some of the brain cells in the injured area. When an object actually penetrates the skull, foreign material and dirt may be implanted into the brain and lead to infection. A blow or a penetrating injury may tear blood vessels and cause *brain hemorrhage* (bleeding in or around the brain). Head injury may cause edema (swelling) of the brain; this is particularly notable after bullet wounds because their high velocity causes extensive damage. If the skull is fractured, bone may be driven into the underlying brain.

SYMPTOMS AND SIGNS
If the head injury is mild, there may be no symptoms other than a slight headache. In some cases there is *concussion*, which may cause confusion, dizziness, and blurred vision (sometimes persisting for several days). More severe head injuries, particularly blows to the head, may result in unconsciousness that lasts longer than a few minutes, or *coma*, which may be fatal.

Postconcussive *amnesia* (loss of memory of events that occurred after an accident) may occur, especially if the skull has been fractured. It usually lasts more than an hour after consciousness is regained. There may also

HEADACHE Pain in the head that may be anything from mild to severe and incapacitating.

? Is your temperature 100°F (38°C) or above?

→ **YES** → Many feverish illnesses may cause a headache.

See • *Fever*

NO ↓

? Have you injured your head within the past few days?

→ **YES** → Are you feeling unusually drowsy AND/OR have you felt nauseated or been vomiting?

→ **YES** → ☎ **EMERGENCY! GET MEDICAL HELP NOW!** This suggests the possibility of a brain injury.

See • *Extradural hemorrhage*

NO ↓

NO ⋯→ A persistent headache is common following a head injury.

See • *Head injury*

? Have you felt nauseated or been vomiting?

→ **YES** → Do you have severe pain in and around one eye AND is your vision in that eye blurred?

→ **YES** → ☎ **Call your physician without delay!** This suggests the possibility of raised pressure inside the eye.

See • *Glaucoma*

NO ↓

Do you have two or more of the following symptoms?
• pain when you touch your chin to your chest
• dislike of bright light
• drowsiness or confusion

→ **YES** → ☎ **EMERGENCY! GET MEDICAL HELP NOW!** These symptoms suggest the possibility of a brain injury or irritation of the meninges.

See • *Subarachnoid hemorrhage*

NO ↓

Have you suddenly begun to have a severe throbbing pain in one or both temples?

→ **YES** → ☎ **Consult your physician without delay!** Inflammation of the arteries in the head is a possibility, especially if you are over 50.

See • *Temporal arteritis*

NO ↓

Was the pain one-sided, preceded by disturbed vision, AND/OR accompanied by vomiting?

→ **YES** → You may have a migraine

See • *Migraine*

NO

NO ↓

Continued on next page

508

Have you had a similar headache on waking several days or more out of the past week?

→ **YES** → Do the headaches only occur when you have drunk a lot of alcohol the night before?

→ **YES** → You probably have a hangover.

See • *Hangover*

NO ▼

NO ┈┈► **Consult your physician without delay!** Such headaches may be a symptom of tension (when felt at the back of the head) or high blood pressure but, in very rare cases, may indicate a brain tumor.

See • *Brain tumor*
• *Hypertension*

Have you recently had OR do you now have a runny or stuffy nose?

→ **YES** → Do you have a dull pain and tenderness around the eyes and cheekbones that worsens when you bend forward?

→ **YES** → You may have an infection of the sinuses.

See • *Sinusitis*

NO ▼

NO ┈┈► You may have a common cold.

See • *Cold, common*

Are you feeling tense or under stress AND/OR are you sleeping poorly?

→ **YES** → Anxiety often causes tension headaches.

See • *Anxiety*
• *Headache*

NO ▼

Did the headache occur after you had been reading or doing close work such as sewing?

→ **YES** → Strain on your neck muscles may have caused the headache.

See • *Headache*

CANCER WATCH
A recurrent headache that is present on waking AND is accompanied by nausea or vomiting may, in rare cases, indicate a brain tumor.
Consult your physician without delay!

NO ▼

Continued on next page

H

Did any of the following apply in the 12 hours before the headache started?
- you were exposed to strong sunlight
- you were in stuffy, smoky, or noisy surroundings
- you drank more alcohol than usual
- you missed a meal

YES → Headaches are often brought on by such circumstances and are usually no cause for concern.

NO

Are you currently taking any medicines AND/OR are you taking the birth-control pill?

YES → Certain drugs can cause headaches as a side effect. Discuss promptly with your physician.

NO

If you are unable to make a diagnosis from this chart and the headache persists overnight or if you have other symptoms, consult your physician.

Head lag

The backward flopping of the head that occurs when an infant is placed in a sitting position. Head lag is notable in the newborn because the neck muscles are still weak, but, by 4 months of age, the baby can hold the head upright in line with the trunk. The disappearance of head lag is a measure of motor development (see *Child development*); good control of the head is essential before a baby can learn to sit.

Healing

The process by which the body repairs bone, tissue, or organ damage caused by injury, infection, or disease. In popular usage, the term means simply "restoring to health."

THE HEALING PROCESS

The initial stages of healing are the same for all parts of the body. After injury, the blood clots in damaged areas of tissue, and white blood cells and various chemicals (including *histamine, enzymes*, and proteins from which new cells can be made) accumulate at the site of damage. Fibrous tissue is laid down within the blood clot to form a supportive structure; any dead cells are broken down and absorbed by the white blood cells.

Some tissues, such as bone, are then able to regenerate by proliferation of the cells that remain around the damaged area. In such cases, the original structure and function are fully restored. In other cases, however, the cells may be unable to proliferate (nerve cells, for example) or there may be an inadequate blood supply or persistent infection that prevents tissue regeneration. If this occurs, the fibrous tissue that forms in the blood clot may develop into tough scar tissue that keeps the tissue structure intact, but may impair its function (e.g., the restriction of movement that may occur after a muscle tear).

WOUND HEALING

There are two processes by which the body repairs skin wounds—healing by first intention and healing by second intention.

Healing by first intention occurs when the edges of the wound are close together and there has been minimal loss of tissue. If the wound is deep, the edges of the skin may need to be held together with stitches or a butterfly bandage. The blood that seeps from the edges of the wound forms a clot that becomes the base on which scar tissue is laid down. When healing is complete, only a fine scar remains.

be preconcussive amnesia (loss of memory of events that occurred before the accident). The longer the period of unconsciousness and the longer the period of amnesia, the more serious the injury to the brain.

After severe brain injury the person may have some muscular weakness or paralysis and loss of sensation.

Symptoms such as persistent vomiting, pupils of unequal size, double vision, or a deteriorating level of consciousness suggest progressive brain damage. The symptoms may begin immediately after the injury or after apparent recovery.

INVESTIGATION

Any person suffering loss of consciousness, however brief, should see a physician. The person may be hospitalized for observation; skull X rays are performed to identify any fracture. If brain hemorrhage is suspected, *CT scanning* is carried out.

TREATMENT

Cuts to the scalp may require stitching using local anesthesia. People whose consciousness is deteriorating may be kept in a neurosurgical unit for close observation. If a blood clot forms inside the skull, the clot may be life-threatening and requires surgical removal; severe skull fractures may also require surgery.

OUTLOOK

Recovery from a minor head injury may be delayed due to persistent symptoms of concussion, but these symptoms usually improve within a few days. Survival following a major head injury has improved due to advances in nursing and medical care, but permanent physical or mental disability (including changes in personality) has been observed if there has been permanent damage to the brain. Epileptic seizures sometimes occur after severe head injury (usually after penetrating injuries, a severe skull fracture, or serious brain hemorrhage). Recovery from a major head injury is very slow, and victims may continue to show signs of progressive recovery for as long as five years.

H

Healing by second intention occurs when the edges of the wound are not brought together. In this slower type of healing, pink *granulation tissue* grows from the exposed tissue. It is eventually covered by skin that grows over the wound from the cut edges. By the time healing is complete, the granulation tissue has developed into tough scar tissue.

Health

At its simplest, health is the absence of physical and mental disease. However, the wider concept promoted by the World Health Organization is that all people should have the opportunity to fulfill their genetic potential. This includes the ability to grow and develop physically and mentally without the impediments of inadequate nutrition or environmental contamination, and to be protected as much as possible against infectious diseases. (See also *Diet and disease; Health hazards.*)

Health food

 A term applied to products that are meant to promote health, including unprocessed and whole grains, organically grown fruits and vegetables, and dietary supplements. The term is misleading because it suggests that only "health foods" are good for people. In fact, a healthy diet is based on sound *nutrition.*

Health hazards

Environmental factors that are known or suspected to cause disease. Some health hazards are obvious, such as contamination of water supplies with sewage or other effluents, and pollution of the air with smoke or poisonous chemicals. Others are less apparent—for example, radioactivity (which is detectable only with special instruments) and sunlight.

TYPES

For people in developing countries (the majority of the world's population), the main hazards come from lack of access to safe, pure water, from inadequate means of disposal of sewage and domestic refuse, and from insufficient or contaminated food. Foods contaminated with microorganisms (such as bacteria and molds) present far greater health hazards than those associated with the additives that are used in developed countries to combat such contamination (see *Food additives; Food-borne infection; Food poisoning*).

There are four other main types of health hazard, all of which are present worldwide. First, there are many *infectious diseases* transmitted by contact or by insects or other animals. (See *Bacteria; Fungal infections; Insects and disease; Viruses; Zoonoses.*)

The second type comprises work-related hazards (such as industrial accidents) and the wide variety of occupational disorders—for example, *asbestosis, pneumoconiosis, lead poisoning,* and cancers associated with exposure to chemicals. (See *Accidents; Occupational disease and injury.*)

The third category of hazards includes those associated with domestic and social life, such as *accidents* in the home or on the road, and injuries and other hazards (such as drowning) from sports activities. In many developed countries, domestic and traffic accidents are the most important risks to health in early adult life. Alcohol and tobacco are other primary hazards to health.

Finally, there are many types of global environmental hazards, ranging from sunlight and cosmic radiation to air *pollution* and background radioactivity. (See *Radiation hazards.*)

Health Maintenance Organization

A form of prepaid hospital and medical insurance that first received attention in about 1970. A person or family enrolling in a Health Maintenance Organization (HMO) pays the same monthly premium regardless of the amount of services needed. Care may be provided by HMO staff physicians (closed panel) or by members of an outside group (independent practice association).

According to original theory, HMOs would limit costs by encouraging preventive medicine. Since the HMO's financial performance would depend on premium income exceeding the cost of services, the HMO theoretically would have a financial incentive to keep patients healthy through periodic checkups and screenings. Recent studies indicate that HMOs do reduce medical costs. But the reason appears to be reduced rates of hospitalization rather than preventive care.

Hearing

The sense that enables sound to be perceived. The *ear* (the organ of hearing) transforms the sound waves it receives into nerve impulses that pass to the brain.

MECHANISM OF HEARING

Almost all sound is heard by a mechanism known as air conduction (see box, next page). This process, in which sound waves are channeled down the ear, is supplemented by a secondary form of hearing called bone conduction. Some sound waves set up vibrations in the skull bones that pass directly to the inner ear. This form of hearing affects the way a person hears his or her own voice.

HEARING DISORDERS

Problems with hearing (from minor sound distortions to total deafness) result when any part of the sound-transmitting and analyzing mechanism is damaged. (See also *Deafness.*)

Hearing aids

Electronic devices that improve hearing in people with certain types of *deafness.* A hearing aid consists of a tiny microphone (to pick up sounds), an amplifier (to increase their volume), and a tiny speaker (to transmit sounds to the ear).

HOW IT WORKS

A tiny microphone collects sound and transforms it into electric current. The amplifier increases the strength of the current and feeds it along a tube to an earpiece, which fits into the outer-ear canal and converts the current back to (now amplified) sound.

A volume control on the aid, usually operated by turning a tiny wheel, enables the level of incoming sound to be adjusted. The aid is designed at the factory to amplify those pitches for which the user has the most loss. Further modifications of this sort may be made by the hearing aid dispenser.

TYPES

The most common types of hearing aids are inconspicuous. The mechanical parts, along with a battery to power them, are contained in a small plastic case that fits comfortably behind the ear, in the side piece of an eyeglass frame, or entirely within the ear canal. Aids that fit entirely in the ear are most popular today.

More powerful aids that amplify sound to a greater degree are also available, but rarely used anymore. In these aids, the microphone, amplifier, and battery are contained in a larger case worn on the body; the current is carried to the earpiece by a thin wire.

Most modern hearing aids include switches that enable normal reception of sound by the microphone to be replaced by a process known as electromagnetic induction. This process picks up transmitted speech in

HEARING

The ears are the organs of hearing. Each ear has three separate regions—the outer ear, middle ear, and inner ear. Sound waves are channeled into the ear canal to the middle ear, where a complex system of membranes and tiny bones conveys the vibrations to the inner ear. A part of the auditory nerve converts the vibrations to nerve impulses, which are then transmitted to the brain.

To function properly, the eardrum must have equal air pressure on each side so that it can vibrate freely. Pressure is equalized via the eustachian tube, which runs from the back of the throat to the middle ear.

ROUTE TO THE BRAIN
Auditory sensations are picked up by nerve fibers in the cochlea and travel along the auditory nerve to the medulla. From there, they pass via the thalamus to the superior temporal gyrus—the part of the cerebral cortex involved in receiving and perceiving sound.

Thalamus

Cerebral cortex

Auditory nerve

Medulla

Function of cochlea
Inside the cochlea (shown uncoiled), the first part of the basilar membrane responds most to high-frequency vibrations; the far end registers only lower frequencies.

Outer ear
The pinna (the visible part of the ear) channels sound waves into the outer-ear canal (auditory canal) toward the eardrum. Hairs and waxy cerumen line the canal.

Eardrum
The tympanic membrane (eardrum) is a taut membrane between the outer and middle ears. Sound waves of different frequencies cause the eardrum to vibrate at different speeds.

Malleus (hammer) and incus (anvil)
The malleus, attached to the eardrum, transmits vibration to the incus.

Stapes (stirrup) and oval window
The incus in turn transmits vibration to the stapes and the oval window membrane.

Cochlea
The cochlea consists of a hollow spiral passage in the temporal bone. The cochlear duct, a fluid-filled membranous tube, virtually divides the cochlea lengthwise; it is full of microscopic hairs that stimulate nerve cells in response to sound vibrations, transmitted through the oval window.

Cochlea

Oval window

Basilar membrane

Nerve fibers

COMPARISON OF FREQUENCY RANGES
Different animals are able to hear different ranges of sound frequencies. The diagram shows the normal ranges of sound, in hertz (cycles per second), that can be heard by a human, a bat, a dolphin, and a dog.

10 Hz   100 Hz   1,000 Hz   10,000 Hz   100,000 Hz

Lowest note on piano   Highest note on piano

Electron micrograph of inner ear
The section shows four rows of hair cells, which convert sound waves into electrical impulses to be sent to the brain.

Hearing aid

Outer ear canal

Battery

Volume control

Microphone

Hearing aids
Hearing aids amplify sound waves for people who are hearing impaired. Many hearing aids include an earpiece, a microphone, an amplifier, volume control, and a battery.

telephones and in many public buildings that have been equipped for the purpose. The greatest advantage of electromagnetic induction is that it obscures amplified background noise.

Other devices are available for the hard-of-hearing. They include amplified telephone receivers, flashing lights instead of doorbells and telephones that ring, vibrators that respond to sound, headphones for television sets, and teletypewriters. Exciting developments include the *cochlear implant* and *temporal bone implant*, which aid nerve and bone conduction deafness, respectively.

Hearing loss
See *Deafness.*

Hearing tests
Tests performed to determine whether a person has a hearing loss, how bad the hearing loss is, and what part of the ear may be causing the loss. The tests may be done routinely as part of a general assessment of *child development* or during a general medical examination. The tests may be used for a person who complains of impaired hearing or in whom hearing loss is suspected (such as a child with poor speech development or an elderly person suffering from apparent *dementia*). Hearing tests may be carried out regularly as a safeguard for people who are exposed to high noise levels in their work. A hearing test can also help determine the cause of *tinnitus* and dizziness.

The physician attempts to establish the extent and pattern of any hearing deficit by testing the ability to hear sounds of different frequencies and volumes; the physician also tries to ascertain whether any hearing loss is conductive or sensorineural.

Conductive hearing loss is caused by a defect in sound conduction through the outer-ear canal or middle ear. Sensorineural loss is caused by damage to the inner ear, acoustic nerve, or hearing centers in the brain; the inner ear is isolated for testing by placing a speaker directly on the mastoid bone behind the ear.

The lowest level at which a person can hear and repeat words (the speech reception threshold) is tested, as is the ability to hear words clearly (speech discrimination).

The results of hearing tests (see box, below) enable the physician and patient to decide on treatment, usually a *hearing aid* or surgery.

TYPES OF HEARING TEST

Tests	Function	
Tuning fork tests	These tests are used to determine whether hearing loss is conductive or sensorineural. In the Rinne test, the patient is asked whether the sound is louder with the vibrating tines held near the opening of the ear canal (air conduction) or with the base of the fork held against the mastoid bone (bone conduction). In a normal ear or in one with sensorineural loss,	air conduction is greater than bone conduction. In conductive loss, bone conduction is greater than or equal to air conduction. Weber's test, in which the base of the fork is placed on the forehead, is useful for diagnosing unilateral hearing loss. If hearing loss is conductive, the patient hears the tuning fork better in the ear with the poorer hearing.
Pure-tone audiometry	This is a test in which an audiometer is used to generate sounds of varying frequency and intensity. The audiometer is an electrical instrument that measures a person's ability to hear sounds of different frequencies and intensities. Hearing is first assessed by transmitting the sounds through one earphone while the other ear is prevented from hearing them. The sound frequencies range from 250 to 8,000 hertz (cycles per second); for each	frequency, the sound is decreased in intensity until it can no longer be heard. The person whose hearing is being tested gives a signal at the moment when he or she detects each sound, and the results are recorded on a graph called an audiogram. Bone conduction hearing is then assessed using a rubber rod connected to the audiometer (the rod is placed against the mastoid bone behind the ear and kept in place by a headband).
Auditory evoked response	In this form of testing, the brain's response to sound stimulation by the audiometer is analyzed by means of electrodes placed on the scalp. This test attempts to evaluate the presence of hearing in a person who is unable to cooperate with other	tests (because of mental handicap, for example). Auditory evoked response is commonly used to assess hearing in very young babies. The test can also help rule out acoustic neuroma (a benign tumor within the auditory canal).
Impedance audiometry	This test is used to determine the type of middle-ear damage occurring in cases of conductive deafness. A probe is fitted tightly into the entrance to the outer-ear canal, sealing it off from outside air pressure and sound. The probe emits a continuous sound. Air is pumped through the probe at varying pressures and, at the same time, a microphone in the probe registers the differing	reflections of sounds from the eardrum as pressure changes in the ear canal. The reflections are recorded on a graph known as a tympanogram. The pattern of differing reflections reveals the extent of elasticity in the eardrum and middle-ear bones, thus indicating the type of disease that is causing the deafness. This device can also measure the air pressure in an air-filled middle ear.

H

THE HEART

The heart is positioned centrally in the chest, with its right margin directly underneath the right side of the sternum (breastbone). The rest of the heart points to the left, with its lowest point (the apex) located directly underneath the left nipple.

The heart acts as a dual pump. Deoxygenated blood from the body arrives, via the vena cava, in the right atrium (upper heart chamber), is transferred to the right ventricle (lower chamber), and is then pumped via the pulmonary artery to the lungs. There it is reoxygenated and returns, via the pulmonary veins, to the left side of the heart. It enters the left atrium, is transferred to the left ventricle, and is then pumped, via a large vessel (the aorta) to all parts of the body.

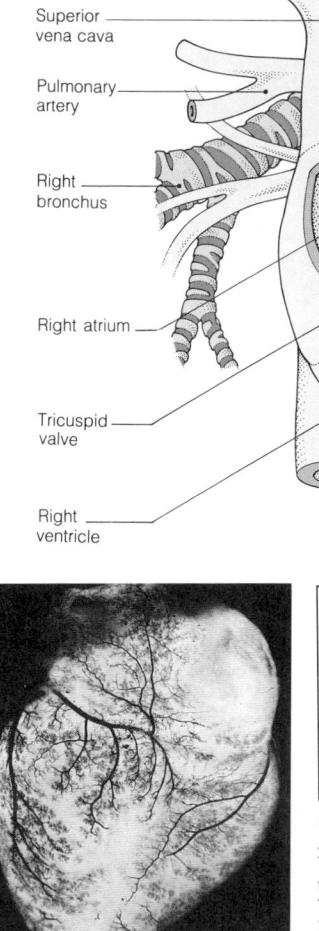

Trachea

Superior vena cava

Pulmonary artery

Right bronchus

Right atrium

Tricuspid valve

Right ventricle

Aorta

Left atrium

Pulmonary valve

Mitral valve

Left ventricle

Septum

Inferior vena cava

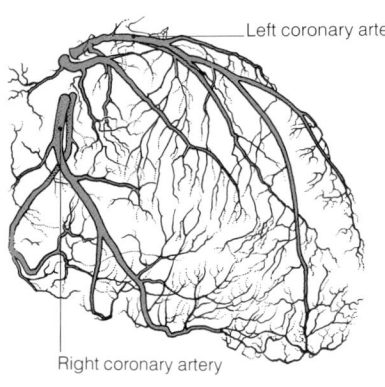

Left coronary artery

Right coronary artery

Blood supply
Although the heart muscle is continually pumping blood, it cannot obtain much oxygen from this flow, so it needs its own blood supply. This is furnished by the two coronary arteries, which arise from the aorta. With their branches, these arteries supply the entire heart muscle.

Right atrium

Left coronary artery

Circumflex branch of left coronary artery

Right coronary artery

Right ventricle

Left ventricle
Angiogram of coronary arteries
The image at left gives a view of the heart from the rear and shows clearly the coronary arteries. The image was achieved by angiography—an X ray of the heart was taken after injecting the coronary arteries with a contrast medium.

Heart

The muscular pump in the chest that, throughout life, beats continuously and rhythmically to send blood to the lungs and to the rest of the body. During an average lifetime, the heart contracts more than 2.5 billion times.

STRUCTURE

Much of the heart consists of a special type of muscle, called myocardium. The myocardium, given sufficient oxygen and nutrients, contracts rhythmically and automatically without any other stimulation.

The interior of the heart consists of four distinct chambers. A thick central muscular wall (the septum) divides the cavity into right and left halves. Each half consists of an upper chamber (atrium) and a larger lower chamber (ventricle). Various large blood vessels emerge from the top and sides of the heart; they deliver blood to the atria or carry blood pumped out by the ventricles.

The internal surface of the heart is lined with a smooth membrane (the endocardium) and the entire heart is enclosed in a tough, membranous bag (the pericardium).

FUNCTION

The two sides of the heart have distinct, although interdependent, functions. The right side receives deoxygenated blood from the entire body via two large veins called the vena cava. This blood arrives in the right atrium and, after transfer to the right ventricle, is pumped to the lungs via the pulmonary artery to be oxygenated (receive oxygen from the *alveoli*) and to lose carbon dioxide. The left side receives oxygenated blood from the lungs (via the pulmonary veins, which drain into the left atrium); this blood is first transferred to the left ventricle and then pumped to all tissues in the body. The heart can thus be viewed as a dual pump.

Nonreturn (one-way) valves situated at the exits from each heart chamber guarantee that blood can flow through the circuit in one direction only (see *Heart valves*).

THE CARDIAC CYCLE

The pumping action of the heart consists of three phases, which together make up a cycle corresponding to one heart beat. These phases are called diastole, atrial systole, and ventricular systole (see illustration).

To work efficiently, the different parts of the heart must contract in a precise sequence. This sequence is brought about by electrical impulses that emanate from the sinoatrial node, the heart's own pacemaker situated at the top of the right atrium. The electrical impulses are carried partly by the heart muscle itself and partly by specialized nerve fibers.

To avoid bottlenecks developing in the blood circulation, the volume pumped at each stroke by the two sides of the heart must exactly balance each other. However, resistance to blood flow through the general circulation is much greater than resistance to flow through the lungs; this means that the left side of the heart must contract much more forcibly than the right side. Hence, the muscular bulk of the left side of the heart is considerably greater than that of the right side.

FACTORS AFFECTING HEART RATE AND OUTPUT

The rate at which the heart beats, and the amount of blood it puts out with each contraction, can vary considerably according to the demands of the body's muscles for oxygen, and thus blood. At rest, the heart contracts at 60 to 80 beats per minute and puts out about one sixth of a pint of blood at each stroke, thus pumping about 12 pints per minute. However, during extreme exercise, the heart rate may increase to 200 contractions per minute and the output may increase to almost half a pint per beat, thereby increasing the total output to 100 pints per minute.

Such changes in heart rate and output are brought about in two ways. First, the heart muscle is able to respond automatically to any increase in the amount of blood returned to it from active muscles by increasing its output. This occurs because the more the ventricles are filled with blood during the filling phase of the heart's cycle, the more forcibly they contract during ventricular systole to expel the blood. Second, the heart rate is under external control of the *autonomic nervous system* (the part of the nervous

HEART CYCLE

The pumping action of the heart has three main phases for each heart beat. Each beat is brought about by electrical waves that emanate from the heart's own pacemaker, the sinoatrial node. The electrocardiogram tracing also shows the phases of the cycle.

Diastole
During this resting phase, the heart fills with blood. Deoxygenated blood flows into the right side of the heart; at the same time, oxygenated blood flows into the left side.

Atrial systole
In this second phase, the two atria (upper chambers of the heart) contract simultaneously, squeezing more blood into the two ventricles, which become fully filled.

Ventricular systole
The ventricles contract to pump deoxygenated blood into the pulmonary artery and oxygenated blood into the aorta. When the heart is emptied, diastole begins again.

In diastole, the heart muscle is at rest. Toward the end of this phase of the heart cycle, an electrical impulse begins to emanate from the sinoatrial node.

Atrial systole is brought about by the impulse from the sinoatrial node spreading over the atria. The impulse soon reaches another node, the atrioventricular node.

Ventricular systole is brought about by waves of electrical activity carried from the atrioventricular node to all parts of the ventricles by means of special fibers.

system concerned with automatic control of body functions). The parts of the autonomic nervous system concerned with heart action are a nucleus of nerve cells called the cardiac center in the brain stem, and two sets of nerves (parasympathetic and sympathetic) whose activities, controlled by the cardiac center, exert opposite effects on the heart.

At rest it is the parasympathetic nerves—particularly the *vagus nerve*—that are active. Signals carried along the vagus nerve act on the sinoatrial node to slow the heart rate from its inherent rate of about 140 impulses per minute to a rate closer to 70 per

minute. This phenomenon is called vagal inhibition. During or in anticipation of muscular activity, the vagal inhibition lessens, the heart rate speeds up, and may speed up even more when the sympathetic nerves come into action. The nerves release norepinephrine, which increases the heart rate and the force of contraction.

The switch from parasympathetic to sympathetic activity is triggered by any influence on the cardiac center that signals an extra need for increased blood output from the heart. Such influences may include fear or anger, low blood pressure, or a reduction of oxygen in the blood.

Heart, artificial

An implantable mechanical device that takes over the heart's action in pumping blood to maintain the circulation. First used in humans in 1985 after years of research in animals, the presently available artificial heart is now seen as a temporary measure to keep a patient alive from a few days to weeks until heart transplant surgery can be performed.

HOW IT WORKS

The type of artificial heart used most frequently, but not exclusively, to date (the Jarvik 7) is a metal and plastic device installed in the patient's chest in place of the diseased heart. During installation, the device is sewn to parts of the two atria (upper chambers) remaining from the original heart and to the pulmonary artery and aorta (main blood vessels carrying blood out of the heart).

The device is powered by an external machine connected to the device by air lines passing through the chest wall. Pulses of pressure sent through these lines operate the device's pumping action. The patient's movements are restricted by the need to be continuously connected to the machine.

LIMITATIONS AND RISKS

As a temporary measure, the artificial heart has a place in the treatment of life-threatening heart disease, but medical opinion is, at present, strongly against attempts to employ it on a permanent basis. The complications of its use have included *renal failure*, infection, internal bleeding, mental confusion, and *stroke* from blood clots being formed in the heart and carried to the brain. Up to early 1987, all four US patients in whom an artificial heart had been installed on a permanent basis had died. Several of these people experienced strokes and serious infection, which contributed to their deaths.

ALTERNATIVES

A device known as the intra-aortic balloon pump has been in use since the middle 1970s; it has been found helpful as an alternative method of maintaining the circulation when the heart is grossly diseased. The balloon is inflated automatically between each heart beat to provide extra force to the circulation. It has the extra advantage of increasing the pressure in the arteries that supply blood to the heart muscle and of relieving the strain on the heart.

Heart attack

See *Myocardial infarction*.

Heart beat

A contraction of the heart to pump blood to the lungs and rest of the body. The heart beat is readily felt on the left side of the chest, where the apex of the left ventricle (lower heart chamber) lies close beneath the skin (see *Heart*). The rate at which contractions occur is called the *heart rate*. The term *pulse* refers to the character and rate of the heart beat when felt (at the wrist, for example).

Heart block

A disorder of the heart beat that may lead to episodes of dizziness, fainting attacks, or strokes. Heart block is caused by an interruption to the passage of impulses through the specialized conducting system of the heart. Consequently, although the atria beat normally, the ventricles lag behind or contract less often than the atria. This is a completely different problem from the blockage of vessels associated with atherosclerosis.

TYPES

There are several grades of heart block. In the least severe form, the delay between the contractions of the atria and ventricles is just slightly longer than normal (called a prolonged P-R interval from its appearance on an *ECG*). Sometimes the delay lengthens with successive beats, until eventually a ventricular beat is dropped. In more severe cases, only a half, a third, or a quarter of the atrial beats is conducted to the ventricles. In complete heart block, the atria and ventricles beat independently. Thus, while the rate of atrial contraction varies according to the patient's activity, the ventricles contract at a fairly constant rate of about 40 beats per minute.

CAUSES AND INCIDENCE

Heart block may occur as a result of *coronary heart disease*, in active *myocarditis* (inflammation of heart muscle), with an overdose of a *digitalis drug*, in *rheumatic fever*, or in syphilitic *aortitis*. In about half the cases, the patient has no history of heart disease.

Heart block is a common disorder. It develops in about 30 persons per 100,000 annually in the US.

SYMPTOMS

A prolonged P-R interval causes no symptoms even though it can be detected on an *ECG*. Dropped beats may also be symptomless.

In other cases, the rate of the ventricular beat is slower than normal; in complete heart block, the rate does not increase in response to exercise. Sometimes the ventricles are able to compensate by expelling more blood with each contraction. In other cases, the blood output from the ventricles is inadequate, and the patient may become breathless due to *heart failure*, may develop the chest pains of *angina pectoris*, or may faint.

If the ventricular beat becomes very slow, or stops altogether for a few seconds, the patient may black out and have a seizure due to insufficient blood reaching the brain. However, the ventricular beat usually restarts within a few seconds. If the delay is prolonged and cerebral *atherosclerosis* exists, *stroke* may result.

DIAGNOSIS

Heart block may be diagnosed by a physician who finds a slow regular heart beat (below 50 beats per minute) that does not accelerate during exercise and is confirmed by an ECG.

TREATMENT

Some cases of heart block do not require treatment (e.g., when there are no symptoms or in the case of an elderly person whose only symptom is slight uneasiness). If the heart block is causing fainting attacks, it usually is treated by fitting an artificial *pacemaker*, which overrides the natural pacemaker and faulty electrical conducting system in the heart.

Less commonly, the condition may be treated with drugs (such as isoproterenol), although usually only in emergencies or as a temporary measure until an artificial pacemaker can be fitted.

Heartburn

A burning pain in the center of the chest that may travel from the tip of the breastbone to the throat.

Heartburn may be caused by overeating, eating rich or spicy food, or drinking alcohol. Recurrent heartburn is a symptom of *esophagitis*, which is usually caused by *acid reflux* (backflow of stomach acid). This backflow of acid is associated with the inability of the lower esophageal segment to close completely (sometimes accompanied by a *hiatal hernia*). Heartburn is often brought on by lying down or bending forward.

Occasionally, heartburn may cause chest pain that is mistaken for the pain of heart disease.

H

DISORDERS OF THE HEART

Heart disorders are by far the most common cause of death in developed countries. They also impair the quality of life of millions of people, restricting activity by causing pain, breathlessness, fatigue, fainting spells, and anxiety. A wide range of conditions can affect the heart by ultimately interfering with the pumping action of the heart.

GENETIC DISORDERS
In general, inherited or genetic factors do not play a large part in the causation of heart disorders. However, they do contribute to the *hyperlipidemias* that predispose a person to *atherosclerosis* and *coronary heart disease*.

CONGENITAL DEFECTS
Structural abnormalities in the heart are among the most common birth defects, but are usually treatable. They result from errors of development in the fetus and include such conditions as *septal defects* ("holes in the heart") and some types of abnormal *heart valves*. (See *Heart disease, congenital*.)

INFECTION
Endocarditis is an infection of the heart valves, usually occurring in people whose hearts have already been damaged by *rheumatic fever* or are abnormal because of some congenital or degenerative disorder. It may also affect drug addicts who inject themselves intravenously with nonsterile needles. The infection may cause deformity and malfunctioning of any of the heart valves, leading to, for example, *mitral insufficiency* or *aortic insufficiency* (although heart valve disease can also have other causes). Some types of cardiomyopathy are triggered by viral infection.

TUMORS
Tumors arising from the heart tissues are rare, the most common being the benign *myxoma* (which grows inside one of the chambers of the heart and may interfere with blood flow or valve action). Occasionally a malignant *sarcoma* develops. Secondary tumors, spreading from cancer elsewhere in the body (such as the breast or lung) are several times more common than primary tumors.

These *metastases* usually grow within the heart muscle or the pericardium (sac that surrounds the heart), but seldom affect the valves. The tumors may produce electrocardiographic (see *ECG*) abnormalities and, if extensive, result in congestive *heart failure*.

MUSCLE DISORDERS
Cardiomyopathy is a general term for disease of the heart muscle itself. One type of cardiomyopathy is inherited; others may be caused by vitamin deficiency or alcohol poisoning, or may be triggered by a viral infection.

Myocarditis is inflammation of the heart muscle. It may be caused by a viral infection or by toxins released during a bacterial infection. Rarely, it results from drugs or radiation therapy.

INJURY
Blunt injury to the heart usually occurs in car accidents through impact with the steering wheel. The heart is compressed between the sternum (breastbone) and the spine and may suffer injury ranging from mild bruising to complete rupture. In immediately fatal car accidents, up to two thirds of the victims have suffered rupture of a heart chamber. Seat belt use could probably prevent some of these deaths.

Stab wounds to the heart are often fatal within minutes, but, of patients who reach the hospital, the great majority survive. Bullet wounds are more serious; about 10 percent of people shot in the heart reach the hospital alive.

NUTRITIONAL DISORDERS
The heart muscle is sensitive to severe nutritional deficiency and may become thin and flabby from simple lack of protein and calories. Thiamine (vitamin B_1) deficiency, which is common in chronic alcoholics, causes *beriberi* with congestive heart failure. *Obesity* is another important factor in causing heart disease, probably through its effect on other risk factors such as *hypertension*, *diabetes*, and *cholesterol*.

IMPAIRED BLOOD SUPPLY
The major cause of heart disease in developed countries is impaired blood supply. The coronary arteries (which supply blood to the heart) become narrowed due to *atherosclerosis* and parts of the heart muscle are deprived of oxygen. The result of coronary heart disease may be *angina pectoris* or, eventually, a *myocardial infarction*.

POISONING
The most common toxic substance affecting the heart is alcohol. A large intake for many years may cause a type of cardiomyopathy in which the heart becomes enlarged and heart failure develops. If alcohol intake is stopped, recovery is possible.

DRUGS
Certain drugs may disturb the heart beat or even cause permanent damage to the heart muscle. These drugs include the anticancer drug doxorubicin, the tricyclic antidepressants, and even many drugs used to treat heart disease.

OTHER DISORDERS
Many common and important heart disorders may result from some other underlying condition, such as coronary heart disease, cardiomyopathy, or a congenital defect. Such disorders include cardiac *arrhythmia* (a disturbance in the rhythm of the heart beat), some cases of *heart block* (in which contractions of the upper and lower parts of the heart are not synchronized), and heart failure (inability of the heart to keep up with its work load). *Cor pulmonale* is a failure of the right side of the heart; it is a consequence of lung diseases (such as *emphysema*), which increase resistance to blood flow.

H

INVESTIGATION
Heart disease and disorders are investigated by such techniques as auscultation (listening to the heart sounds) and *ECG* (electrocardiography); heart *imaging techniques* such as chest X ray, echocardiography, coronary angiography, *CT scanning*, and *MRI*; cardiac catheterization; blood tests; and, in rare cases, by a *biopsy* of the heart muscle (removal of a small sample of tissue for analysis).

H

TYPES OF CONGENITAL HEART DISEASE

The major malformations are *septal defects, coarctation of the aorta, transposition of the great vessels, patent ductus arteriosus, tetralogy of Fallot, hypoplastic left heart syndrome, pulmonary stenosis,* and *aortic stenosis.* The bars (right) show the incidence of each type of malformation among affected babies.

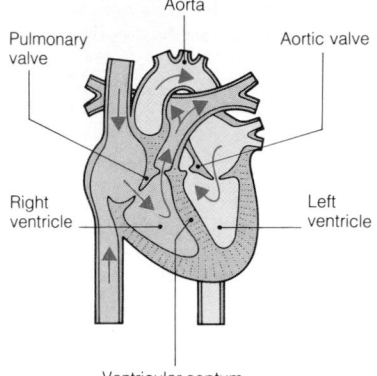

Aorta
Pulmonary valve
Aortic valve
Right ventricle
Left ventricle
Ventricular septum

How blood circulates
Deoxygenated blood (gray) is pumped from the right ventricle into the lungs, where it exchanges carbon dioxide for oxygen. The newly oxygenated blood (pink) enters the left side of the heart and is then pumped out of the left ventricle to all body tissues.

5%

Pulmonary stenosis
Narrowing of the pulmonary valve, or (rarely) of the upper right ventricle, which reduces blood flow to the lungs.

10%

Coarctation of the aorta
In this disorder, localized narrowing of the aorta reduces the supply of blood to the lower part of the body.

8%

Patent ductus arteriosus
The ductus arteriosus fails to close after birth and blood from the aorta continues to flow through it into the pulmonary artery.

20%

Ventricular septal defect
A hole in the ventricular septum, causing blood to flow from the left ventricle to the right and into the lungs.

7%

Tetralogy of Fallot
A hole in the ventricular septum, displacement of the aorta, pulmonary stenosis, and thickening of the right ventricle.

14%

Transposition of the great vessels
Oxygenated blood passes back to the lungs, instead of through the aorta to the tissues.

Heart disease, congenital

Any heart abnormality that has been present from birth. Congenital heart defects are the most common major malformations compatible with life.

CAUSES AND INCIDENCE
About 700 babies per 100,000 are born with a congenital heart defect. The errors of development leading to defects arise early in the life of the embryo. In most cases, there is no known cause. Of known causes, the most significant is *rubella* in the mother during the first three months of pregnancy. This can be prevented by vaccination. About one third of babies with *Down's syndrome* have a congenital heart defect, and congenital heart disease often accompanies other birth defects.

Hereditary factors do not seem to play a significant role. If a couple has an affected child, there is little increased risk of a second child being affected. People born with heart defects have little increased risk of having an affected child.

SYMPTOMS AND COMPLICATIONS
The symptoms of congenital heart disease arise from insufficient or excessive circulation of blood to the lungs or to the body. The defects in heart anatomy can also mean that some deoxygenated blood is pumped to the body instead of to the lungs or some oxygenated blood to the lungs instead of to the body. These anomalies can result in *cyanosis* (blueness caused by a reduced oxygen level in the general blood circulation), breathlessness, or both.

Symptoms may first appear at any time over a wide range of ages, according to the defect. Similarly, recognition of a defect may occur any time from before birth to adulthood.

Apart from cyanosis and breathlessness, an untreated heart defect can cause stunted growth and underdeveloped limbs and muscles. Colds repeatedly lead to pneumonia. With prolonged cyanosis, *clubbing* (thickening and broadening) of the tips of fingers and toes may develop. If there

is insufficient capacity of the heart to increase blood flow during exercise, the child may rapidly tire and be unable to take part in physical exercise. In some untreated cases, a serious complication called *Eisenmenger complex* (in which there is increased resistance of the lungs to blood flow) develops.

DIAGNOSIS
A heart defect may be diagnosed by procedures such as *chest X rays, ECG, echocardiography,* and, less commonly, cardiac *catheterization.*

TREATMENT
Rest, oxygen, and various drugs to assist the circulation and lung function may improve matters for a limited time or sometimes indefinitely. Some conditions, such as small septal defects, may get smaller or disappear on their own. Other defects are likely to worsen, and surgical correction often is a consideration.

Today, surgical correction is available for most affected children; the risk of death from unsuccessful surgery lessens every year. One condition—hypoplastic left heart syndrome (in which the left side of the heart is severely underdeveloped)—can be treated only by performing a *heart transplant* operation.

Narrowed heart valves can now frequently be treated by balloon *valvuloplasty*, in which a special catheter is introduced into the heart to widen the narrowed valve.

In other cases, *open heart surgery* is necessary. Sometimes, any of a range of *prostheses* (artificial spare parts), such as replacement heart valves or blood vessels, may be used. In some cases, a heart transplant or *heart-lung transplant* may be necessary.

OUTLOOK

Following successful heart surgery, recovery to good health with resumption of growth, increased activity, and better appetite follow rapidly, and the child usually has a near-normal life expectancy. Full activities, including sports, are generally possible after three to six months.

Children with heart defects (corrected or uncorrected) are at an increased risk of bacterial *endocarditis*, a potentially dangerous infection of the lining of the heart. Preventive antibiotics may be prescribed.

Heart disease, ischemic

The most common form of heart disease, in which there is a reduced blood supply resulting from narrowing or obstruction of the coronary arteries. (See *Coronary heart disease*.)

Heart failure

A medical term that describes an inability of the heart to keep up its work load of pumping blood to the lungs and to the rest of the body. Although it sounds life-threatening, heart failure is usually a treatable condition and compatible with survival for many years.

TYPES AND CAUSES

Failure of the heart is conventionally divided into left- or right-sided failure.

LEFT-SIDED FAILURE Left-sided heart failure may be due to *hypertension, anemia,* or *hyperthyroidism,* to a heart valve defect (such as *aortic stenosis* or *aortic insufficiency*), or to a congenital heart defect (such as *coarctation of the aorta*). In all these conditions, the left side of the heart must work harder to pump the same amount of blood. Sometimes, the extra load can be compensated for by an increase in the size of the left side of the heart and in the thickness of its muscular walls, or by an increase in heart rate. Compensation is only temporary, however, and heart failure follows.

Other causes of left-sided heart failure include heart *arrhythmias, myocardial infarction* (death of part of the heart muscle due to interruption of its blood supply), and *cardiomyopathy* (intrinsic muscle disease). In cardiomyopathy, the pumping power of the heart is reduced and it can no longer deal with its normal load.

Whatever the cause, the left side of the heart fails to empty completely with each contraction or has difficulty accepting blood returning from the lungs. The retained blood creates a back pressure that causes the lungs to become congested with blood. This in turn leads to pulmonary *edema* (excess fluid in the lungs), of which the main symptom is shortness of breath.

RIGHT-SIDED FAILURE Right-sided failure most often results from *pulmonary hypertension* (raised pressure and resistance to blood flow through the lungs)—itself caused by left-sided failure or by lung disease (such as chronic *bronchitis* or *emphysema*). Right-sided failure can also be due to a valve defect (such as *tricuspid insufficiency*) or a congenital heart defect (such as a *septal defect, pulmonary stenosis,* or *tetralogy of Fallot*).

In all types of right-sided failure, there is a back pressure in the blood circulation from the heart into the venous system, causing distended neck veins, enlarged liver, and *edema* (fluid in the tissues).

SYMPTOMS

Fatigue is an early symptom of heart failure. Breathing difficulty is the most frequent symptom of left-sided heart failure caused by fluid in the lungs. Breathlessness may first be noticed only during or after exercise, but worsens and is eventually apparent even at rest. The patient may be able to breathe easily only when well propped up in bed. Sometimes he or she may awaken at night with an attack of breathlessness, wheezing, and sweating. Such paroxysms may subside on their own or may require urgent, lifesaving treatment.

Right-sided heart failure produces less breathlessness and more swelling of the ankles and legs, often with enlargement of the liver and congestion of the intestines, causing discomfort and indigestion.

TREATMENT

Immediate treatment of the heart failure is followed by treatment of its underlying cause.

Immediate treatment consists of bed rest, with the patient sitting up. The patient is given *diuretic drugs* (which increase the output of urine from the kidneys), thus ridding the body of excess fluid and reducing blood volume. In some cases, *vasodilator drugs* (which ease the work load of the heart) or digitalis (which strengthens the contractions of the heart beat) may also be given. Morphine is sometimes given as an emergency treatment in acute left-sided failure. These measures usually bring about a significant improvement within a few days.

Once the heart failure is treated, attention is directed to treating the underlying cause. If a defective heart valve is responsible, it may be treated by *heart valve surgery* (although, ideally, defective heart valves should be corrected surgically before severe heart failure develops).

Many other causes of heart failure are also treatable; hypertension and arrhythmias are treated through drug treatment and congenital septal defects are treated by open heart surgery. However, when the cause is a long-standing disease of the heart muscle (a cardiomyopathy) or chronic lung disease, the outlook is generally not as good.

Heart imaging

Techniques that provide images of the heart and its structure. Imaging is performed to detect structural abnormality, disease, or impaired function.

TYPES

A *chest X ray* is the simplest and most widely used method of obtaining an image of the heart. It can show the heart size and shape, and whether or not abnormal calcification is present in the valves, major blood vessels, or the pericardium. Pulmonary *edema* (accumulation of fluid in the lungs) and engorgement of the vessels connecting the heart and lungs are usually detectable on a chest X ray, which may indicate the presence of *heart failure*. Pacemakers and artificial heart valves show up clearly on X ray and can be checked for position.

Angiography may be performed to show the heart chambers. Children with complex forms of congenital heart disease (such as *tetralogy of Fallot*) may benefit from this procedure. Angiography is also performed to evaluate the state of the coronary arteries in patients with *coronary heart disease* and helps with decisions about valve replacement.

H

H

Echocardiography (cardiac ultrasound) is most useful as the first step in investigating congenital heart abnormalities or in evaluating valvular or heart wall abnormalities. *Doppler* techniques enable the physician to measure blood flow across valves. *Radionuclide scanning* produces images that give less anatomical detail but some information about heart function. For example, radionuclide scanning can show how well the heart wall moves and how effectively it empties.

A new generation of extremely fast CT scanners has been developed with heart imaging in mind; previous scanners were too slow to "freeze" a heart beat (see *CT scanning*).

Magnetic resonance imaging (*MRI*) techniques are also capable of producing high quality cardiac images. These techniques are sometimes used to test graft efficiency after a *coronary artery bypass*. They eliminate the need for angiography and for other techniques used previously to investigate congenital heart disease.

Heart-lung machine

A machine that temporarily takes over the function of the heart and lungs to facilitate certain operations in the chest. A heart-lung machine consists principally of a pump (to replace the heart) and an oxygenator (to replace the lungs). The machine is sometimes called a cardiopulmonary bypass or pump oxygenator.

Once the machine is connected and working, the patient's heart and lungs are effectively bypassed and the heart can be stopped. The surgeon can then operate unhurriedly in a blood-free surgical field to perform *open heart surgery*, a *heart transplant*, or a *heart-lung transplant*.

HOW IT WORKS
Blood is taken via cannulas (tubes) inserted into the inferior and superior venae cavae (the main veins draining blood into the heart) and pumped through the oxygenator, which acts as an artificial lung, putting oxygen into the blood and removing carbon dioxide from it. The freshly oxygenated blood is then returned to the arterial circulation via a cannula inserted into the aorta (the main artery carrying blood from the heart) or the femoral artery (a large artery in the leg).

There are two main types of oxygenator. In one type, the blood is passed up a column, through which a gas mixture with a high oxygen content is bubbled. This adds oxygen and removes carbon dioxide. The blood is

then treated with a defoaming agent and held in a reservoir until it is returned to the patient. In the second type, called a membrane oxygenator, the blood and gas flow on either side of a thin, semipermeable membrane, through which oxygen passes from gas into blood; carbon dioxide passes in the opposing direction. This method more closely mimics the function of the lungs.

A heat exchanger is another component of the machine. Generally, it is used to rewarm blood before returning it to the patient (otherwise, blood cools in the machine); sometimes the blood is intentionally cooled to cause a drop in the patient's temperature (see *Hypothermia, surgical*), giving surgeons more time for the operation.

PRECAUTIONS AND LIMITATIONS
The main difficulty with heart-lung machines is they tend to damage red blood cells and cause the blood to clot. To minimize these problems, the patient is given the anticoagulant drug heparin before the bypass is started. During operation of the machine, the supply of blood to the patient's vital organs is less efficient than normal. A patient can thus be kept on a heart-lung machine only for a few hours.

Heart-lung transplant

A radical procedure in which both the heart and lungs of a person are removed and replaced with organs from a donor who has been declared brain dead. (See illustrated box for how and why the operation is done.)

RISKS AND COMPLICATIONS
The early attempts at heart-lung transplant were unsuccessful. In the early 1980s the risk of donor organ rejection was reduced by the introduction of the drug cyclosporine. Some centers are now obtaining very good results. Nevertheless, the operation carries substantial risks. Problems may arise from airway obstruction and other lung complications (including *bronchiolitis*) in addition to the risks of organ rejection. Patients face the long-term problems associated with receiving any form of organ transplant (see *Transplant surgery*).

Heart rate

The rate at which the heart beats—that is, contracts to pump blood around the body.

Most people have a heart rate of between 60 and 100 beats per minute at rest. This rate remains fairly constant throughout life, although it tends to be faster in childhood and to

slow slightly with age. Some athletes have a resting rate below 60 beats per minute. Their hearts are very well developed and can pump blood around the body as efficiently at a slow rate as the normal heart can pump it at a faster rate.

Exercise or stress causes an increase in heart rate. In either case, the increase is due to the release of the hormones epinephrine and norepinephrine by the adrenal glands and of norepinephrine by the sympathetic nerves around the sinoatrial node, the heart's own pacemaker. A small decrease in heart rate occurs during total relaxation and sleep.

Many people have a harmless irregularity of heart rhythm in which the rate is more rapid during breathing in than breathing out.

MEASURING HEART RATE
A physician uses one of two methods to measure heart rate and rhythm (the regularity of the beat). One is to feel the pulse (the expansion of an artery in response to contractions of the heart). The other method, which can be more accurate, is to listen with a stethoscope placed just below the left nipple (see *Heart sounds*).

An even more accurate record is provided by an *ECG* (electrocardiogram), which registers the pattern of electrical activity from the heart muscle that precedes each beat.

DISORDERS OF HEART RATE
A resting heart rate above 100 beats per minute is termed a *tachycardia* and a rate below 60 beats per minute a *bradycardia*. Tachycardias and bradycardias are considered abnormal when the cause is a condition affecting nerve conduction pathways through the heart or the activity of the sinoatrial node, rather than a response of the heart to exercise or relaxation. Irregularities may also occur in the rhythm of the heart's contractions. (See also *Arrhythmia, cardiac*.)

Heart sounds

The sounds made by the heart with each beat. The two main sounds can be heard simply by putting an ear to someone's chest. Classically, the sounds are said to sound like "lubb" followed by a higher-pitched "dupp." A pause follows each lubb-dupp. These sounds are caused by the slamming shut of the heart valves in each heart cycle, and are sometimes called the first and second heart sounds.

Using a stethoscope, a physician can hear the heart sounds much more clearly (and may sometimes hear

HEART-LUNG TRANSPLANT

In this procedure, both the heart and lungs of a patient are removed and replaced with organs taken from a brain-dead donor. The removed heart can sometimes be given to another patient.

HOW IT IS DONE

Heart and lungs must be removed from both donor and patient; the donor organs then are inserted into the patient.

1 The donor heart and lungs must be healthy, and the lungs must match the size of the patient's chest, as measured by chest X rays.

2 In both donor and patient, the heart and lungs are reached via an incision made in the breastbone, and the chest is opened up.

Site of incision

H

3 The patient is connected to a heart-lung machine. It takes over the function of heart and lungs, oxygenating blood taken from the venae cavae and pumping it back to the body via the aorta.

— Trachea

— Aorta

— Right atrium/Vena cava

4 In both patient and donor, heart and lungs are removed through cuts in the trachea, aorta, and where the heart connects to the venae cavae. The blood vessels linking donor heart and lungs are left intact.

WHY IT IS DONE

Subject to availability of a donor, a heart-lung transplant can offer hope to someone who is dying of an end-stage chronic lung disease, whether or not he or she is also suffering from heart disease. Diseases treated include *emphysema*, *cystic fibrosis*, *sarcoidosis*, or *interstitial pulmonary fibrosis*. The heart-lung transplant operation has a better success record than that of lung transplant alone.

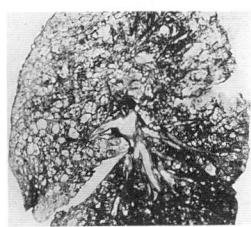

These sections were taken from a healthy lung (at left) and an emphysematous lung; transplanting of heart and lungs may give an emphysema patient new hope.

— Tracheal reconnection

— Aortic reconnection

— Right atrium/Vena cava reconnection

5 Insertion of the donor organs into the patient is, in some respects, easier than in the heart transplant, since fewer reconnections have to be made. The main reconnections are between the patient's and donor's tracheas and aortas and between the right atrium of the donor heart and the patient's venae cavae.

abnormal additional sounds or an abnormality of one of the two main sounds). Interpretation of these sounds can be important in the diagnosis of heart valve disorders and other heart abnormalities.

FIRST AND SECOND SOUNDS

The first sound (lubb) results from the closure of the tricuspid and mitral valves at the exits from the upper chambers of the heart. This occurs when the ventricles (lower chambers) begin contracting to pump blood out of the heart. The second heart sound (dupp) is caused by closure of the pulmonary and aortic valves at the exits from the ventricles when they have finished contracting.

Through a stethoscope, the second heart sound is heard to consist of a double sound, especially in children and young adults. This is due to a slight time gap between the closure of the aortic and pulmonary valves, and is normal.

ADDITIONAL SOUNDS

In children and young adults, there is often a normal low-pitched third heart sound after the second sound. It is thought to be caused by vibration of muscle fibers in the ventricles as they begin to refill. In people over age 40, this sound is abnormal and a sign of heart failure.

A fourth sound, preceding the first sound and also low-pitched, is occasionally heard; it always indicates an abnormality of heart muscle. The sound is often present after a *myocardial infarction* (heart attack) or in someone with a *cardiomyopathy*.

An opening "snap" is an abnormal sound that may occur during opening of the mitral valve. It is high pitched, heard shortly after the second heart sound, may be accompanied by a presystolic *murmur*, and is associated with *mitral stenosis*.

Ejection sounds or "clicks" are high-pitched sounds caused by the abrupt halting of valve opening. They can occur in *hypertension* (high blood pressure) or in the heart valve defects *mitral valve prolapse, aortic stenosis*, or *pulmonary stenosis*.

Heart *murmurs* are abnormal sounds caused by turbulent blood flow. They may occur as a result of any of various heart valve defects or types of congenital heart disease.

Heart surgery

Any operation performed on the heart. Heart surgery was a rare and hazardous undertaking until the early 1950s, when an operation called mitral valvotomy, performed to correct a narrowed heart valve (by means of a finger passed into the beating heart to stretch open the tight valve), became a standard and successful procedure.

Such "closed" operations on the heart are still occasionally performed, but have largely been superseded in developed countries by *open heart surgery*, in which the heart beat is deliberately stopped and the heart opened to make repairs. Open heart surgery became possible through developments such as controlled surgical *hypothermia* (cooling of the patient before surgery) and the *heart-lung machine*, introduced in the middle 1950s. The machine allows the circulation of oxygenated blood to the brain and other tissues to be maintained with the heart stopped, considerably prolonging the time during which the surgeons can work.

Open heart surgery allows the treatment of many previously serious or fatal conditions, including most types of congenital *heart disease* (heart defects present at birth) and various disorders of the heart valves (see *Heart valve surgery*). *Coronary artery bypass* (for the treatment of obstructed arteries supplying the heart muscle) was first performed in 1967, and, within five years, was being done all over the world. In the same year, the first *heart transplant* was performed in South Africa; the results have since improved largely because of advances in preventing organ rejection.

Another significant development was the introduction in 1979 of balloon *angioplasty*. In this procedure, a fine catheter with an inflatable segment is carefully passed along a narrowed coronary artery and then inflated to stretch the constriction. The results are excellent and many lives have been saved because of it. Angioplasty balloons are also being used to open up narrowed heart valves.

Balloon angioplasty is not without risk; the vessel may fracture or the fatty plaque narrowing the vessel may rupture, permitting cholesterol-rich material to travel down the vessel, thus plugging it. The procedure is most safely performed at centers where facilities for emergency open heart surgery are available.

Experimental work using lasers to open up more stubborn narrowing in arteries is also being done.

Heart transplant

Replacement of a person's damaged or diseased heart by a healthy human heart taken from a donor in whom *brain death* has been certified.

HISTORY

Heart transplantation was first achieved in animals in 1959, but it was not until 1967 that Professor Christiaan Barnard in South Africa carried out the first human heart transplant. Early results were disappointing, with few patients surviving beyond a month or two, but, in 1969, the Stanford University team led by Professor Norman Shumway began its program, which, in 1984, showed that as many as 85 percent of patients could be expected to survive for at least a year after surgery.

WHY IT IS DONE

Heart transplantation is considered for the treatment of patients with progressive, irremediable heart disease, but who are otherwise in good health. Many such patients have advanced *coronary heart disease*; most of the others have *cardiomyopathy* (disease of the heart muscle). If the heart disorder is associated with lung disease, a *heart-lung transplant* may be performed.

HOW IT IS DONE

Heart transplantation poses some special problems compared with the more common procedure of kidney transplantation. First, there can be a problem of timing. Whereas the condition of a patient with kidney failure can be maintained in health by *dialysis* until a donor kidney becomes available, there is no equivalent method for maintaining the condition of someone with a nonfunctioning heart for a prolonged period. Hence, heart transplantation is possible only when a suitable donor heart is available at the right time. Furthermore, heart transplantation has no "fall back" system; if the heart is rejected (attacked by the body's *immune system*), the only hope for the patient is another transplant.

The mechanical, artificial heart is a possible solution to these problems, though in practice the best it seems able to offer is a temporary respite for a patient until the desperately needed new heart becomes available (see *Heart, artificial*).

A further limitation of heart transplantation is that the heart must be removed from the donor while it is still beating for the operation to have the best chance of success. One reason for the success of the Stanford heart transplant program was that California was the first state to allow physicians to certify death with the heart still beating (provided the brain was irreversibly destroyed by disease or accident). Certification of brain death in a patient connected to an artificial ventilator is now permitted in most developed countries, allowing the heart to be removed in optimum condition. The donor heart can then be chilled in saline at 40°F (4°C) and transported many miles by air before being implanted in the recipient.

The actual heart transplant operation is no more or less difficult than other major heart surgery. The first step is to connect the patient's major blood vessels to a *heart-lung machine*, which pumps oxygenated blood to the brain and other vital organs while the surgeon operates. Once the bypass is working, the surgeon removes the diseased heart, leaving the back walls of the atria (upper heart chambers) in place, and then inserts the donor heart, which is kept cooled in saline after its removal. The major blood vessels are reconnected and the new heart is ready to function. The nerves that help control the heart rate are severed during the procedure, but the heart functions without them.

OUTLOOK

Once the immediate postoperative period is over, the outlook is good, with better than 80 percent of patients surviving the first year at certain centers; there is a death rate of around 5 percent per year thereafter. These results are much better than for the surgical treatment of lung or stomach cancer. The main problems are rejection (countered by *immunosuppressant drugs* such as cyclosporine, prednisone, and cyclophosphamide) and infection, which is always a hazard for people taking immunosuppressives, since these drugs weaken the body's natural defenses.

Heart valve

A structure at the exit of a heart chamber that allows blood to flow out of the chamber, but which prevents back-wash. There are four heart valves (one at the exit of each heart chamber). Their correct functioning is vital to the efficiency of the heart as a pump. (See *Heart* illustration.)

e opening and, more particularly, the closing of heart valves during the cycle of a heart beat are responsible for *heart sounds*.

DISORDERS

Any of the four heart valves may be affected either by stenosis (narrowing)—so that it takes more work for the heart to force blood through the

HEART VALVE REPLACEMENT

Any one of the four heart valves (aortic, pulmonary, mitral, or tricuspid) may require replacing (see diagram below right). Replacement of the aortic heart valve is described in the steps below.

Sternum
Line of incision
Heart

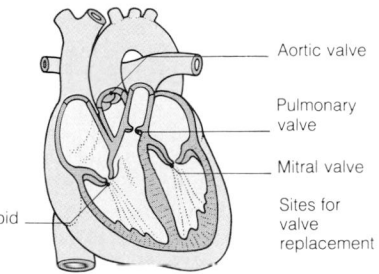

Aortic valve
Pulmonary valve
Mitral valve
Sites for valve replacement
Tricuspid valve

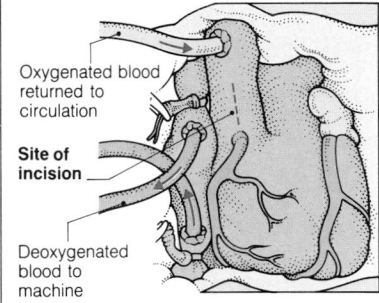

Oxygenated blood returned to circulation
Site of incision
Deoxygenated blood to machine

1 In nearly all surgery on the heart valves, the incision into the chest cavity is made through the sternum (breastbone). The patient is put on a *heart-lung machine*, the beating of the heart is stopped, and the heart is opened.

2 The valve is first examined to determine whether it can be repaired or whether it requires replacement. If the latter is necessary (as here), the valve is excised (dotted line indicates where the incision is made).

3 A prosthesis is sutured into position and the aorta is closed. The patient is disconnected from the machine and the chest wall is sewn up. The operation takes between two and four hours.

Artificial heart valve in place
This chest X ray shows the metal components of an artificial heart valve. A ball-and-socket valve has been used to replace the patient's diseased valve.

valve—or by insufficiency or incompetence (inability to prevent backwash of blood). With these valve defects, characteristic murmurs are heard by the physician.

Valve defects may be present at birth, either alone or with other defects (see *Heart disease, congenital*), or may be acquired later in life. The most common congenital valve defects are *aortic stenosis* and *pulmonary stenosis*.

Acquired heart valve disease is usually the result of degenerative changes or ischemia (diminished blood supply) affecting part of the heart and leading to aortic stenosis or *mitral insufficiency*.

Rheumatic fever was once the main cause of *mitral stenosis* and insuffi-

H

ciency, aortic valve defects, and, less commonly, *tricuspid stenosis* and *tricuspid insufficiency*. Rheumatic fever is now rare in developed countries, but still prevalent in poorer countries.

Valves are also destroyed by bacterial *endocarditis*, seen often among intravenous drug users. Bacterial endocarditis is, however, a possible complication of any valve disorder.

The symptoms and signs of valve disorders vary, but generally they lead to *heart failure*, rhythm irregularities, or symptoms resulting from reduced blood supply to body tissues.

Valve defects may be diagnosed by *auscultation* (listening to the heart sounds), *chest X ray, ECG, echocardiography, Doppler* echocardiography, and cardiac *catheterization*. They may be corrected by *heart valve surgery*.

Heart valve surgery

An operation to correct a *heart valve* defect or, in many cases, to remove the diseased or damaged valve. The valve is replaced by a mechanical valve (made from metal and plastic), a valve fashioned from human or bovine tissue, a pig valve, or a human valve taken from a corpse.

WHY IT IS DONE

A heart valve may need to be corrected or replaced either because it is stenotic (narrowed) or insufficient (leaky). The mitral and aortic valves (on the left side of the heart) are the ones that most often need correction or replacement, followed by the tricuspid; pulmonary valve surgery is performed only rarely in adults.

In general, heart valve surgery is considered only when the potential effects of the malfunctioning valve on the heart and on general health are so severe that they will soon be a threat to the patient.

The timing of the operation is crucial; it is based on the patient's symptoms and on the results of tests (such as *ECG, chest X rays, echocardiography*, and cardiac *catheterization*).

HOW IT IS DONE

The illustration on the previous page shows how an aortic valve is replaced.

Valvuloplasty, a new technique, uses a balloon catheter that is inserted into the circulatory system through the skin without opening the chest. It can be used in the treatment of some cases of stenotic valves.

RECOVERY AND OUTLOOK

After the operation, the patient is usually kept in an intensive-care unit for 24 hours, followed by a few days in the hospital. However, a longer hospital stay may result if complications develop or if the patient had been suffering from severe heart failure before the operation.

Symptoms such as breathlessness may take many weeks to improve and may require continuing medication to maintain the improvement. Some people (those with a mechanical replacement valve and those with heart rhythm abnormalities, for example) require long-term treatment

---

TYPES OF REPLACEMENT HEART VALVES

The three main types
There are three main types of replacement valve—biological, mechanical, and homograft. Biological valves are taken from pigs or made from bovine tissue or the patient's own tissue; examples include the Carpentier-Edwards and Ionescu-Shiley valves. Mechanical valves are made from metal, plastic, and carbon fiber. There are two main types—ball-and-cage valves (such as the Starr-Edwards valve) and those with one or more tilting disks (such as the Bjork-Shiley and St. Jude valves). Homografts are human valves that have been removed from people who have died of a disease that does not affect the heart.

	Biological	Mechanical	Homograft
Examples	Carpentier-Edwards; Ionescu-Shiley	Starr-Edwards (ball-and-cage); Bjork-Shiley (tilting disk); St. Jude (two tilting disks)	Taken from cadaver
Availability	Readily available	Readily available	Some centers only
Ease of insertion	Routine	Routine	Specialized
Suitable age group	Over 35	All ages	All ages
Duration	About seven years	More than 12 years	More than 12 years
Postoperative drug therapy	Short-term anticoagulants	Lifelong anticoagulants	None necessary
Possible complications	Infection; stroke; damage to blood cells	Infection; stroke; calcification	Infection; calcification

with anticoagulant drugs. This treatment prevents blood clots from forming around the new valve, prevents them from becoming detached, and prevents them from being carried to the brain or other organs. All patients need long-term follow-up examinations to ensure that the corrected or replaced valve is working well. In addition, most need to take antibiotics before any dental and certain other operative procedures to reduce the risk of the valve becoming infected.

Most heart valve surgery is successful; the death rate is low and is continuing to decline. If a replacement valve malfunctions, it is often possible to insert a new one.

Heat cramps

Painful spasms in a muscle caused by excessive salt loss due to profuse sweating. Heat cramps are usually brought on by strenuous physical activity in extreme heat. The condition may occur by itself or as a symptom of *heat exhaustion* or *heat stroke*.

Treatment (and prevention) consists of the use of salt tablets or drinking enough of a weak salt solution (0.25 level teaspoon of salt to a pint of cold water) to keep the urine pale.

Heat disorders

The body functions most efficiently at a temperature of 98.6°F (37°C); any major deviation disrupts the body processes. Malfunctioning or overload of the body's mechanisms for keeping its temperature constant may lead to a heat disorder. For example, poor adaptation to heat may lead to *heat cramps*, *heat exhaustion*, or *heat stroke*; excessive environmental heat may result in *prickly heat*. In addition, excessive heat production by the body due to a very high fever-producing infection may be damaging.

HEAT REGULATION

The mechanisms by which the body loses unwanted heat to maintain the optimum internal temperature are controlled by the *hypothalamus* (part of the brain). When the hypothalamus is disrupted (for example, by drugs or a fever) the body may overheat progressively, which may lead to fatal heat stroke if emergency treatment is not given.

When the temperature of the blood rises, the hypothalamus sends nerve impulses to stimulate the sweat glands and dilate blood vessels in the skin. Sweating itself does not cool the body; the cooling effect is caused by the evaporation of sweat from the

skin. However, excessive sweating can result in an imbalance of salts and fluids in the body, which can lead to heat cramps or heat exhaustion. Dilation of the blood vessels increases the blood flow near the surface of the skin, thereby increasing the amount of heat that is lost by convection and radiation.

ACCLIMATION

Most heat disorders can be prevented by gradual acclimation to hot conditions. Full acclimation takes one to three weeks. It involves spending gradually longer periods in the heat, alternating with rest periods in cool conditions. Strenuous exercise should be avoided. Frequent cool baths or showers should be taken and salt tablets or dilute salt solution used (0.25 level teaspoon of salt dissolved in a pint of cold water) to replace salt lost by sweating. It is also helpful to eat a light diet, avoid alcohol, and wear loose, lightweight clothes.

Heat exhaustion

Fatigue, sometimes culminating in collapse, caused by overexposure to heat. It is most common in people unaccustomed to working in a hot environment. Unless treated, heat exhaustion may develop into *heat stroke*, which is a life-threatening condition.

CAUSES

There are three principal causes of heat exhaustion—insufficient water intake, insufficient salt intake, and a deficiency in the production of sweat, the evaporation of which helps to cool the body (see *Heat disorders*).

SYMPTOMS AND SIGNS

Heat exhaustion causes fatigue, faintness, dizziness, nausea, restlessness, headache, and, when salt loss is heavy, *heat cramps* in the legs, arms, back, or abdomen. The skin is usually

pale and clammy, breathing is fast and shallow, and the pulse is rapid and weak. There may also be vomiting, and the victim may faint.

TREATMENT

The victim should lie down in a cool place and, if conscious, should take 1 to 2 grams of sodium chloride (salt) tablets or continual sips of weak salt solution made up of 0.25 level teaspoon of salt to a pint of cold water. If the victim is unconscious, he or she should be placed in the *recovery position* until consciousness returns, when salt can be administered.

With rest and replacement of lost water and salt, a full recovery usually takes place. However, the victim should consult a physician because of the risk of heat stroke.

Heat stroke

A life-threatening condition in which overexposure to extreme heat and a consequent breakdown of the body's heat-regulating mechanisms cause the body to become overheated to a dangerous degree. In some cases, body temperature may reach 107°F (41.5°C) or more. Without emergency treatment, the victim lapses into a coma and death soon follows.

CAUSES

Heat stroke is most commonly brought on by prolonged, unaccustomed exposure to the sun in a hot climate. It is more likely to occur in humid conditions, which reduce the body's ability to cool itself by the evaporation of sweat.

Heat stroke can also be caused by working in an extremely hot environment or, very rarely, by a severe fever. Susceptibility is greater in those with a disorder of the skin or sweat glands, those taking *anticholinergic drugs* (which reduce sweating), and in older people in poor health. Overstrenuous

H

H

FIRST AID: HEAT STROKE

1 Move the victim to a cool, shady place and remove clothing. Place him or her in a half-sitting position and support the head and shoulders (for example, using pillows).

2 Cover the victim with a wet sheet and keep it wet. Fan him or her with a magazine or use an electric fan until the temperature drops to 101°F. Seek medical help immediately.

activity, unsuitable clothing, overeating, and drinking too much alcohol are sometimes contributory factors.

SYMPTOMS AND SIGNS

Heat stroke is often preceded by *heat exhaustion*, with fatigue, weakness, faintness, and profuse sweating. However, with the onset of heat stroke itself, sweating diminishes markedly and often stops completely. The skin becomes hot, dry, and flushed, breathing is shallow, and the pulse is rapid and weak. As the condition progresses, body temperature rises dramatically, and, without treatment, the victim may quickly lose consciousness and die.

TREATMENT

Emergency medical help should be summoned as soon as possible. The victim should be wrapped naked in a cold, wet sheet; the material should be kept continuously wet. Alternatively, the victim should be constantly sponged with cold water. Cooling should be increased by fanning. If the victim is unconscious, he or she should be placed in the *recovery position* while being cooled.

The above treatment should be continued until the victim's rectal temperature falls to 101°F (38.3°C) or until the body feels cool to the touch. If the victim is conscious, he or she may be given sodium chloride (salt) tablets or a weak salt solution to sip (0.25 level teaspoon of salt dissolved in a pint of water).

If heat stroke is treated early, the victim usually recovers fully.

PREVENTION

The key to preventing heat stroke is acclimation (see *Heat disorders*).

Heat treatment

The use of heat to treat disease or aid recovery from injury.

Moist heat may be administered by soaking the affected part in a warm bath or by applying a hot *compress* or *poultice*. Dry heat may take the form of a heating pad, hot-water bottle, or heat lamp that produces *infrared* rays. More precise methods of administering heat to tissues deeper in the body include *ultrasound treatment* and shortwave *diathermy*.

WHY IT IS USED

Heat is used to aid recovery from injury, such as a muscle tear or ligament sprain; by stimulating blood flow, it is thought to help tissues heal more rapidly. Heat is also useful in relieving pain and stiffness in joints and muscles caused by excessive exercise or by rheumatic disorders, such as osteoarthritis. A hot compress is effective in encouraging the formation and drainage of pus from skin infections.

To avoid the risk of internal bleeding and swelling, heat usually should not be used within 48 hours after an injury. This allows time for the blood vessels to heal.

Heel

The part of the foot below the ankle and behind the arch. The heel consists of the *calcaneus* (heel bone), an underlying pad of fat (which acts as a protective cushion), and a layer of skin that usually has thickened (especially on the ball of the heel) as a result of pressure from walking.

Heimlich maneuver

A first-aid treatment for *choking*.

Heliotherapy

Treatment by exposure to sunlight; a form of *phototherapy*.

Helminth infestation

An infestation by any species of parasitic worm (see *Worm infestation*).

Hem-

A prefix indicating blood, as in *hemoglobin* (an important protein in red blood cells).

Hemangioblastoma

A rare type of brain tumor that consists of blood-vessel cells. It usually develops in the form of cysts in the *cerebellum* and affects mainly children and young adults. The principal symptoms include headache, vomiting, *ataxia* (incoordination), and *nystagmus* (rapid, involuntary eye movements).

The tumor, which is slow-growing, is normally clearly differentiated from the surrounding brain tissue so it can usually be removed surgically. In most cases, such treatment completely cures the condition.

Hemangioma

A red-purple birthmark caused by an abnormal distribution of blood vessels in the skin.

TYPES

There are two types of hemangioma—flat and raised. Large, flat, purple-red marks are known as port-wine stains. They are permanent and can be unsightly. In rare cases, they are associated with abnormalities in the blood vessels of the brain (see *Sturge-Weber syndrome*). Small, flat marks are common in newborn babies, particularly on the back of the neck (where they are called stork bites); they fade about three weeks after birth.

Raised marks may be bright red and protuberant (when they are known as strawberry marks) or may be tinged with blue, caused by the presence of blood from a vein. They usually enlarge rapidly for the first few weeks after birth. After the age of about 6 months, the redness gradually fades and the lump subsides. By the age of about 7 years, the mark may have disappeared altogether.

COMPLICATIONS AND TREATMENT

Hemangiomas do not usually require treatment unless they are causing a particular problem. If a hemangioma starts to bleed, medical advice should be sought; meanwhile, the bleeding can be controlled by firm pressure with a clean handkerchief.

A hemangioma that bleeds persistently may require removal, especially if it is on the lip or tongue, where it may easily be bitten, or if it is on the vulva (external female genitalia) or anus, where it is subject to repeated pressure. It may also be necessary to remove a hemangioma from the eyelid because it interferes with vision and threatens blindness in the affected eye. A hemangioma on the face may need to be removed if it is causing psychological distress.

Removal is carried out by *laser treatment* (most successful in young people), *cryosurgery* (destroying tissue by extreme cold), or plastic surgery. If removal is not possible, the marks can be disguised with cosmetics.

Hemarthrosis

Bleeding into a joint, causing the capsule that encloses the joint to swell.

CAUSES

Hemarthrosis is usually the result of severe damage to a joint, such as a torn capsule, torn ligaments, or fracture of a bone forming part of the joint. The most common cause is a sports injury to the knee.

A rarer cause is a *bleeding disorder*, such as *hemophilia* (in which failure of the blood-clotting mechanism causes all bleeding to persist). Any joint may be affected and bleeding into the joint may occur spontaneously or be caused by even the slightest knock. Overuse of *anticoagulant drugs* can cause hemarthrosis.

SYMPTOMS AND SIGNS

Hemarthrosis causes a joint to swell immediately after injury; swelling that occurs 12 to 24 hours later is probably caused by *synovitis* (inflammation of the lining of the joint). In addition to swelling and pain, hemarthrosis may cause the joint to stiffen into a fixed position as a result of spasm in surrounding muscles.

DIAGNOSIS AND TREATMENT

As a first-aid measure, *ice packs* may be used to reduce swelling and pain. After a sports injury, *aspiration* (withdrawing fluid from the joint through a needle) is used to diagnose the condition and to relieve pain; X rays may be necessary if fracture is suspected. Hemophiliacs are given *factor VIII* to promote blood clotting.

To prevent further bleeding, the physician will bandage the joint and advise resting it in an elevated position; cells in the joint capsule gradually absorb any remaining blood. Surgery (such as *ligament* repair) is sometimes necessary.

Repeated hemarthrosis may damage the surfaces of the joint, causing *osteoarthritis* (characterized by persistent pain and stiffness).

Hematemesis

The medical term for *vomiting blood*.

Hematologist

A physician who specializes in diagnosing and treating disorders of the *blood* and blood-forming organs.

Hematology

The study of *blood* and disorders of the blood. Measurements of blood constituents are used in the diagnosis of a wide range of disorders, not only those of the blood. Microscopic examination and the counting of blood and bone marrow cells are essential procedures in diagnosing different types of blood disorders, such as *anemia* or *leukemia*.

Hematoma

A localized collection of blood (usually clotted) caused by bleeding from a ruptured blood vessel. A hematoma may occur almost anywhere in the body and, depending on the site and amount of accumulated blood, may vary in seriousness from a minor to a potentially fatal disorder.

TYPES

Less serious types include subungual hematoma (under a fingernail or toenail), hematoma auris (in the tissues of the outer ear, better known as *cauliflower ear*), and perianal hematoma (under the skin around the anus). The accumulated blood presses on the surrounding tissues, which may cause considerable pain. In such cases, a physician may lance and drain the hematoma to relieve the pressure and alleviate the pain. Most hematomas disappear on their own within a few days.

Among the more serious types are those that press on the brain, notably extradural and subdural hematomas (see *Extradural hemorrhage*; *Subdural hemorrhage*). They usually are due to an injury that ruptures a blood vessel just under the skull and may be fatal unless treated promptly. (See also *Intracerebral hemorrhage.*)

Hematoma auris

The medical term for *cauliflower ear*.

Hematuria

Red blood cells in the urine. Blood in the urine may be readily visible or small amounts may give the urine a smoky appearance. However, sometimes the blood is not visible to the naked eye. Hematuria can be caused by blood entering the urine at any point along the urinary tract, from the kidney to the urethral opening.

CAUSES

Almost any disorder of the urinary tract can cause hematuria. Infection (including *cystitis*, *urethritis*, and *pyelonephritis*) is one of the most common causes; *prostatitis* often causes hematuria in men. Cysts, tumors, and kidney or bladder stones may cause blood in the sufferer's urine, as can *glomerulonephritis*, in which the glomeruli (the filtering units of the kidney) become inflamed. *Bleeding disorders* may also cause hematuria.

INVESTIGATION

If the blood is not visible to the naked eye, it may be discovered during a urine test when the urinary sediment is examined under the microscope. Urine dip sticks have a small patch that is impregnated with a dye at one end; when dipped in urine containing blood, the patch turns blue.

To determine the cause of blood in the urine, it may be necessary to obtain images of the urinary tract by *ultrasound scanning*, *CT scanning*, or intravenous *pyelography*. These tests usually detect conditions such as cysts, stones, and tumors. If bladder disease is thought to be the cause, a *cystoscopy* (direct examination of the bladder through a viewing tube passed through the urethra) is performed. If a kidney tumor seems likely, *angiography* may be performed to show the blood vessels of the affected kidney.

Hemianopia

Loss of one half of the field of vision in each eye. Hemianopia may be homonymous (affecting the same side of each eye) or heteronymous (affecting opposite sides of each eye). In either case the visual loss may be temporary or permanent.

Hemianopia is not caused by any disorder of the eyes themselves; it is caused by damage to the nerve tracts or brain. Transient homonymous hemianopia in young people is usually caused by *migraine*. In older people it occurs in *transient ischemic attacks* (symptoms of *stroke* lasting less than 24 hours). Permanent homonymous hemianopia is usually caused by stroke, but may be caused by damage to the back of the brain from tumor, injury, or infection. Hemianopia may also be caused by a

H

Hemiballismus

Irregular, uncontrollable, flinging movements of the arm and leg on one side of the body, caused by disease of the *basal ganglia* (part of the brain). The movements are unpredictable in timing and strength, and may be so severe that they cause injury to the afflicted person or others. (See also *Athetosis; Chorea.*)

Hemicolectomy

Surgical removal of half or a major portion of the *colon*. The surgeon may remove either the portion between the beginning of the colon and a point two thirds of the way across the transverse colon, or the portion between this point of the colon and the end, including (or excluding) the rectum. (See also *Colectomy.*)

Hemiparesis

Muscular weakness or partial paralysis affecting one side of the body only. (See *Paralysis.*)

Hemiplegia

Paralysis or weakness in the arm, leg, trunk, and sometimes the face on one side of the body only. One or more sites may be involved at the same time. When the affected muscles are stiff, the disorder is known as spastic hemiplegia; when the muscles are limp and wasted, the term flaccid hemiplegia is used.

CAUSES AND SYMPTOMS

A common cause of hemiplegia is a *stroke* (associated with *hypertension* or *diabetes mellitus*). Others are *head injuries, brain tumor, brain hemorrhage, encephalitis* (inflammation of the brain), *multiple sclerosis*, complications of *meningitis*, or a *conversion disorder* (a type of psychological illness).

TREATMENT AND OUTLOOK

Treatment is directed at the underlying cause and is carried out in conjunction with *physical therapy* to exercise the unused muscles. The prospects for a person with hemiplegia depend on how successfully the underlying cause can be treated and on how motivated the person is to recover.

Hemochromatosis

An inherited disease (also known as "bronze diabetes") in which too much dietary iron is absorbed. Over the years the excess iron accumulates in the liver, pancreas, heart, testes, and, to a lesser extent, in other organs.

CAUSES

The disease is confined almost entirely to men. Women are very rarely affected because they regularly lose iron in their menstrual blood. Although the disease is known to be genetic in origin, the exact mode of inheritance is unclear. Male relatives of an affected person are at risk.

SYMPTOMS, COMPLICATIONS, AND DIAGNOSIS

Hemochromatosis rarely causes problems until middle age. A loss of sexual drive and a reduction in the size of the testes are often the first signs. Eventually the iron overload causes liver enlargement and *cirrhosis* (chronic liver damage), deficient insulin production by the pancreas leading to *diabetes mellitus*, bronzed skin coloration due to iron pigment deposition under the skin (hence the alternative name), cardiac *arrhythmia* and other heart disorders, and, during the late stages of the disease, *liver failure* and *liver cancer*.

The diagnosis is based on *blood tests* that reveal a high level of iron in the blood and a *liver biopsy* (removal of a small sample of tissue for analysis).

TREATMENT

The disease is treated by *venesection* (removing blood) in the same way that blood is removed during blood donation. Initially, venesection is performed once or twice a week. Once the iron level has returned to normal, the procedure is required only three or four times a year.

For young men, treatment can prevent the development of complications; for those who have the fully developed disease, regular venesection can prolong life. *Chelating agents* (such as deferoxamine) have been investigated as an alternative to venesection. (See also *Hemosiderosis.*)

Hemodialysis

One of the two means of *dialysis* (purification of the blood by means of blood filtration to treat *renal failure*).

Hemoglobin

The oxygen-carrying pigment found in red blood cells. Hemoglobin binds with oxygen to form oxyhemoglobin, a compound that gives oxygenated blood its bright red color. There are 350 million hemoglobin molecules in the average blood cell, and each can carry four molecules of oxygen.

STRUCTURE

Hemoglobin is a large molecule made in the bone marrow from two components, heme and globin.

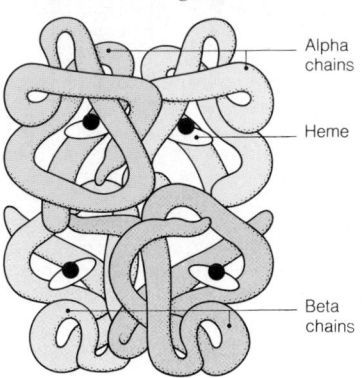

Alpha chains

Heme

Beta chains

Structure of hemoglobin
Each molecule contains four globin chains—two alpha and two beta. Each chain carries a heme component capable of binding oxygen.

The composition of the globin chains can vary, giving rise to several different normal and abnormal forms of hemoglobin. Hemoglobin F is the normal form in fetal life and infancy. It is replaced by the normal adult forms, hemoglobin A and A_2.

FUNCTION

The principal function of hemoglobin is to combine with and transport oxygen from the lungs and deliver it to all body tissues, where it is required to provide energy for the chemical reactions of all living cells. Carbon dioxide, which is produced as the waste product of these reactions, is transported to the lungs for excretion during breathing out.

Defects in hemoglobin production may be either genetic in origin (for example, *sickle cell anemia*) or acquired (see *Anemia, iron-deficiency; Anemia, megaloblastic*). The genetic defects are subdivided into errors of heme production known as *porphyria* and those of globin production known collectively as the *hemoglobinopathies*.

Hemoglobinopathy

A term used to describe a variety of genetic (inherited) disorders in which there are errors in the production of globin chains (one of the main components of *hemoglobin*, the oxygen-carrying substance in the blood).

There are two primary categories of hemoglobinopathy. In the first category, abnormal globin chains are produced, giving rise to abnormal hemoglobin molecules. This is the underlying defect in *sickle cell anemia*.

In the second category, normal globin chains are produced in abnormal amounts (known as the *thalassemias*). Combined forms also occur.

The hemoglobinopathies cause anemia and chronic sickness in millions of people in Asia, Africa, and the Caribbean, and in many blacks and Hispanics in the US.

Hemoglobinuria

The presence of hemoglobin in the urine. *Hemoglobin* (the oxygen-carrying pigment in the blood) is mainly contained within red blood cells, although a small amount is free in plasma. Excessive *hemolysis* (breakdown of red cells), which may be caused by heavy exercise, cold weather, falciparum *malaria* (blackwater fever), and hemolytic *anemia*, increases the concentration of hemoglobin in the plasma.

Hemolysis

The destruction of red blood cells, a process that releases iron (which is repackaged into new red cells), bilirubin (which is excreted by the liver in bile), and other breakdown products of the red cell.

Hemolysis is usually a normal process, occurring when red cells age and lose their elasticity; it takes place mainly in the spleen. When red cells are destroyed prematurely, the hemolysis is considered abnormal and may cause anemia and jaundice (see *Anemia, hemolytic*).

Hemolytic anemia

See *Anemia, hemolytic*.

Hemolytic disease of the newborn

Excessive destruction of red blood cells (hemolysis) in the fetus and newborn infant by antibodies produced by the mother. Hemolytic disease of the newborn is typically caused by *Rh incompatibility* factor (a blood group incompatibility between mother and baby, named after the Rhesus monkey in which the Rh factor was discovered), although a milder form of the disease may result from ABO and more rare blood group incompatibilities.

CAUSE
Hemolytic disease may occur if the woman's blood is Rh negative, if she is carrying a baby whose blood is Rh positive, and if she has previously had a baby whose blood was Rh positive. A previous miscarriage, elective abortion, or *amniocentesis* in which the

fetus's blood was Rh positive can also sensitize the woman. In each of these situations, blood has passed at some stage from the fetus to the woman. This causes the woman to produce Rh antibodies (directed against the Rh-positive blood cells) because her *immune system* recognizes the fetal blood cells as "foreign." The Rh antibodies have not formed sufficiently to harm the first baby, but, during a subsequent pregnancy, they cross the placenta and attack the fetal blood cells. A mismatched *blood transfusion* (giving Rh-positive blood to a woman who is Rh negative) also sensitizes the woman so that she produces Rh antibodies.

DIAGNOSIS
All pregnant women have their blood groups tested at the first prenatal check. Rh-negative women are tested for Rh antibodies at this visit and again at 32 and 38 weeks' gestation. They are tested more frequently if there has been a previous pregnancy.

If the pregnant woman shows rising levels of Rh antibodies, amniocentesis is performed at intervals to measure *bilirubin* levels in the *amniotic fluid*. Bilirubin is a breakdown product of red blood cells, so the bilirubin level indicates the severity of blood cell destruction in the fetus.

SYMPTOMS AND SIGNS
In mild cases, the newborn baby becomes mildly jaundiced during the first 24 hours of life (due to excess bilirubin in the blood) and slightly anemic. In more severe cases, the blood level of bilirubin may increase to a dangerous level, risking a form of brain damage known as *kernicterus*. The most severely affected babies have marked anemia in the uterus, become very swollen (hydrops fetalis), and are often stillborn.

TREATMENT
If the condition is very mild, no treatment is required. In other cases, the aim is to deliver the baby before anemia becomes very severe. This usually means *induction of labor* between 35 and 39 weeks' gestation. If the baby is severely affected before he or she is mature enough to be delivered safely (about 30 weeks' gestation), fetal blood transfusions may be necessary. Rh-negative blood is injected into the fetal abdominal cavity at 30 to 32 weeks' gestation, with the procedure being monitored by *ultrasound scanning*.

After the baby is born, frequent blood tests are performed to assess jaundice and anemia. *Phototherapy*

(light treatment that breaks down bilirubin in the skin) and plenty of fluids help reduce the jaundice. However, if the bilirubin level becomes dangerously high, exchange transfusion is performed (blood is removed from the baby and replaced by Rh-negative blood).

PREVENTION AND OUTLOOK
The disorder is far less common since the introduction and use of $Rh_o(D)$ *immune globulin* (anti-D serum) in the early 1970s. It is given by injection to any Rh-negative woman within 72 hours of childbirth, miscarriage, or elective abortion, destroying Rh-positive blood cells from the fetus before they have had time to sensitize the woman's immune system.

Improved general obstetric and pediatric care have also resulted in a reduction in the severity of the cases that still occur.

Hemolytic-uremic syndrome

A rare disease in which red blood cells are destroyed prematurely and the kidneys are severely damaged, causing *renal failure*. Hemolytic-uremic syndrome occurs mostly in infants and young children.

CAUSES
The precise cause of the disorder is unknown. It is thought that the lining of small blood vessels in the kidneys becomes damaged, causing small clots to form. These clots cause *hemolysis* (breakdown of red cells) as blood flows past them, leading to anemia. The resultant damage to the kidneys causes them to fail; this often occurs in epidemics and appears to be triggered by a bacterial or viral infection.

SYMPTOMS AND SIGNS
The onset of the disease is sudden, with headache, fatigue, shortness of breath, and sometimes jaundice. Little urine is passed and what is passed may contain blood. Severe *hypertension* (high blood pressure) is common and may cause *seizures*.

DIAGNOSIS AND TREATMENT
Blood and urine tests are performed to determine the degree of kidney damage. *Dialysis* (artificial removal of waste products from the blood) is necessary until the kidneys have recovered. *Antihypertensive drugs* are given to lower the blood pressure and transfusions of red blood cells may be given to control the anemia. In severe cases, transfusion of plasma (the fluid in which blood cells are suspended) may be required to prevent continual blood clotting and red cell breakdown. Most children make a full recovery.

Hemophilia

An inherited *bleeding disorder* caused by a deficiency of a particular blood protein. Hemophiliacs (who are almost exclusively male) suffer recurrent bleeding, most often into their joints. Bleeding may occur spontaneously and/or after injury. In recent years, the problems of hemophiliacs have been compounded by the very high incidence of *AIDS* among their numbers as a direct result of the treatment of their condition.

INCIDENCE AND CAUSES
About one male in 10,000 is born with hemophilia. The blood protein lacking is called *factor VIII*; it is one of a series of proteins essential to the process of *blood clotting*.

The lack of factor VIII is due to a defective gene, which shows a sex-linked pattern of inheritance (see *Genetic disorders*). Affected males pass the defective gene on to none of their sons but to all of their daughters, who are carriers of the condition. Some of the sons of carrier females may be affected, and some of the daughters of carriers may themselves be carriers. Many hemophiliacs have an uncle, brother, or grandfather who is affected, but, in about one third of the cases, there is no family history.

SYMPTOMS
The severity of the disorder varies markedly among affected individuals. Hemorrhage into joints and muscles makes up the majority of the bleeding episodes. The episodes often start when an affected child reaches weight-bearing age as a toddler. The bleeding episodes are painful and, unless treated promptly, can lead to crippling deformities of the knees, ankles, and joints.

Injury and even minor operations such as tooth extraction may lead to profuse bleeding. Internal bleeding can give rise to symptoms such as *hematuria* (blood in the urine) or extensive bruises.

DIAGNOSIS AND TREATMENT
Hemophilia is diagnosed by *blood-clotting tests* that reveal factor VIII activity is abnormally low.

Fifty years ago, most hemophiliacs did not survive to adulthood; today, bleeding episodes can be controlled by infusions of concentrates of factor VIII. Infusions must be given as soon as possible after the start of bleeding. Alternatively, the person can take regular doses of factor VIII as a preventive treatment. Patients can be trained to administer the treatment themselves. However, for more serious or unusual bleeding, the patient may require hospitalization.

Although the use of factor VIII concentrates has considerably improved the quality of life for many hemophiliacs, in recent years problems have arisen because of the AIDS virus. Factor VIII must be made from large pools of donor blood (2,000 to 5,000 individual donations). During the first few years of the AIDS epidemic (before its cause was recognized) large numbers of hemophiliacs became infected with HIV (the virus responsible for AIDS) through factor VIII infusions. Consequently, a percentage of hemophiliacs (and their sexual partners) have been exposed to the virus and some have died of AIDS.

Blood donations are now screened for evidence of the AIDS virus to prevent transmission of the virus by transfusion. Work is also under way to produce a genetically engineered factor VIII, which would prevent all problems of blood-borne transmission for hemophiliacs.

OUTLOOK
A child with hemophilia should avoid activities that expose him or her to a risk of injury, including contact sports such as judo and football; activities such as swimming and walking should be encouraged.

Hemophiliacs who test positive for the HIV antibody should take the usual precautions against transmitting the virus (see *AIDS*) and are advised not to have children.

Hemophiliacs who do not test positive for the HIV antibody (as well as the female relatives of hemophiliacs) should obtain *genetic counseling* before starting a family to discuss concerns about children or grandchildren being affected. Any female relative is a possible carrier of the condition; carrier status can now be ascertained with high accuracy by means of a blood test. The diagnosis can sometimes be determined prenatally.

Hemoptysis
The medical term for *coughing up blood*.

Hemorrhage
The medical term for *bleeding*.

Hemorrhoidectomy
The surgical removal of hemorrhoids.

WHY IT IS DONE
Hemorrhoidectomy is carried out if other, simpler methods of treatment (see *Hemorrhoids*) fail to resolve the problem. The procedure therefore tends to be reserved for people who have large, prolapsing, bleeding hemorrhoids.

HOW IT IS DONE
Stages in a hemorrhoidectomy are shown in the illustrated box.

RECOVERY PERIOD
Laxatives such as mineral oil are given after the operation to soften the stools and make them easier to pass. Nonnarcotic analgesics (painkillers) and warm baths ease discomfort. Complete healing occurs after three to six weeks. Avoidance of constipation can frequently prevent recurrences.

COMPLICATIONS
Bleeding is a possible complication. There may be a slight loss of sensation in the anal area that may impair the ability to control release of gas.

Hemorrhoids
Distended veins in the lining of the anus. Hemorrhoids may be near the beginning of the anal canal (internal hemorrhoids) or at the anal opening (external hemorrhoids). Hemorrhoids sometimes protrude outside the anus (prolapsing hemorrhoids).

CAUSES AND INCIDENCE
Hemorrhoids are very common, particularly during pregnancy and immediately after childbirth. Some people have a congenital weakness of the veins in the anus that makes them more likely to develop hemorrhoids. Hemorrhoids occur because of increased pressure in the veins of the anus, usually due to straining during attempts to move hard feces that are difficult to pass. Modern diets consisting of too many highly refined foods fail to provide enough fiber and bulk, which is what produces normal stools.

SYMPTOMS
Rectal bleeding and increasing discomfort, even pain, on defecation are the most common features. Prolapsed hemorrhoids often produce a mucous discharge and itching around the anal opening. A complication of prolapse is thrombosis and strangulation (in which a clot forms in the vein, the vein does not spring back into position in the anus, and its blood supply is reduced); this can cause extreme pain. Iron deficiency *anemia* may result from prolonged bleeding.

DIAGNOSIS AND TREATMENT
Proctoscopy (examination of the rectum through a viewing tube) is usually performed to exclude cancer.

REMOVING HEMORRHOIDS
In both procedures shown below, the patient is first usually given a laxative so that the lower bowel is clear of feces. General or epidural anesthesia is given before a hemorrhoidectomy is performed.

BANDING HEMORRHOIDS

1 This common, simple, and effective procedure is usually painless (causing no more than a mild ache afterward) and no anesthesia is required. The patient lies on his or her side, the proctoscope is positioned and the hemorrhoid is grasped with the forceps.

2 Gentle traction is applied to draw the mass into the drum and the banding instrument is pressed into the anal wall.

3 The trigger mechanism of the banding instrument is fired and the bands are squeezed off onto the neck of the hemorrhoid. The proctoscope is withdrawn, leaving the hemorrhoid with its base tightly constricted by the bands. The hemorrhoid then withers and drops off painlessly.

HEMORRHOIDECTOMY

Using general or epidural anesthesia, the patient is examined with a proctosigmoidoscope to exclude a diagnosis of tumor. The patient is then placed in the *lithotomy position*. The hemorrhoid is clamped, placed under traction, secured with a suture, and then removed with a knife.

Mild cases are controlled by drinking fluids, eating a high-fiber diet, and having regular toilet habits. Rectal suppositories and creams containing *corticosteroid drugs* and local anesthetics help reduce swelling and pain.

Internal hemorrhoids can be treated during proctoscopy on an outpatient basis. If the hemorrhoids are very distended, tiny, tight rubber bands may be slipped onto the end of each vein, causing them to wither within a few days. Alternatively, *cryosurgery* may be used to shrink the veins.

Prolapsing hemorrhoids require a *hemorrhoidectomy*.

Hemosiderosis
A general increase in iron stores. It may occur after repeated blood transfusions or, more rarely, as a result of excessive ingestion of iron. Hemosiderosis does not usually cause organ dysfunction.

Hemospermia
The medical term for blood in the semen (see *Semen, blood in the*).

Hemostasis
The arrest of bleeding. There are three main natural mechanisms by which bleeding is stopped after injury. First, small blood vessels constrict when damaged, thus lessening the "gaps" through which blood can flow. Second, blood cells called platelets aggregate (clump) and plug the bleeding points. Third, the blood plasma coagulates, forming filaments of a substance called fibrin. These filaments enmesh blood cells at the bleeding points and contract to form a solid clot that seals the damaged blood vessel (see *Blood clotting*). Defects in any of the three natural mechanisms of hemostasis can cause a *bleeding disorder*. (See also *Bleeding, treatment of*.)

Hemostatic drugs
A group of drugs used in the treatment of *bleeding disorders*.

Preparations of coagulation factors are an important type of hemostatic drug. Coagulation factors are present naturally in the body to aid *blood clotting* but are deficient in certain disorders. Preparations of factor VIII, for example, are used to treat *hemophilia*; factor IX is used in the treatment of *Christmas disease*. The coagulation factor is injected after abnormal bleeding to allow clotting, or before surgery to reduce the risk of excessive bleeding.

Other commonly prescribed hemostatic drugs include *vitamin K* preparations (used to treat an overdose of certain *anticoagulant drugs*) and aminocaproic acid, which disrupts *fibrinolysis* (the body's mechanism for dissolving blood clots).

Hemostatic preparations of gelatin and cellulose may be applied to the skin or gums to stop bleeding (e.g., following tooth extraction).

Hemothorax
A collection of blood in the pleural cavity (the space between the chest wall and the lung). Hemothorax is most commonly caused by chest injury, but it may arise spontaneously in people with defects of blood coagulation or, occasionally, as the result of cancer.

Symptoms include pain in the affected side of the chest and the upper abdomen, breathlessness, and an increased pulse. If extensive, hemothorax may compress the lung and cause it to partially collapse. Blood in the pleural space tends to remain in a fluid state and can be drawn off by a needle.

Heparin
An *anticoagulant drug* used to prevent and treat abnormal *blood clotting*. Heparin is given by injection and is

H

531

particularly useful as an immediate treatment for deep-vein *thrombosis* or pulmonary *embolism*.

POSSIBLE ADVERSE EFFECTS

Bruising around the injection site is common. Other adverse effects include rash, aching bones, and abnormal bleeding in different parts of the body. Long-term use may cause *osteoporosis* (a bone disorder).

Hepatectomy, partial

Surgical removal of part of the liver. The liver has remarkable powers of regeneration; up to three quarters of the organ can be removed before it ceases to function.

WHY IT IS DONE

Severe injury to the liver sometimes occurs in automobile accidents, causing serious bleeding of and death to the damaged area. Treatment is to remove the dead tissue.

Benign liver tumors and sometimes *hydatid disease* require partial hepatectomy; rarely, *liver cancer* is also treated in this way.

Hepatectomy, total

Surgical removal of the liver. Hepatectomy is performed as the first stage in a *liver transplant* operation.

Hepatic

Related to the liver. For example, the hepatic vein is the vessel that drains blood from the liver.

Hepatitis

An inflammation of the liver, with accompanying liver cell damage or death, caused most frequently by viral infection, but also by certain drugs, chemicals, or poisons. Hepatitis may be either acute (of limited duration) or chronic (continuing).

ACUTE HEPATITIS

This form is a common condition, with about 20 to 30 cases per 100,000 population per year in the US. The most frequent cause is infection with a virus, such as viral hepatitis, type A or type B or non-A, non-B virus (see *Hepatitis, viral*). Other causes include overdose with drugs (such as acetaminophen), exposure to certain chemicals (such as dry-cleaning agents), or, rarely, a reaction to certain drugs in normal dosage. Acute hepatitis may also affect heavy drinkers who have progressive liver disease (see *Liver disease, alcoholic*).

SYMPTOMS

The most obvious sign of acute hepatitis is *jaundice*. In many cases, it is preceded by a flulike illness, accompanied by nausea, vomiting, loss of appetite, tenderness in the right upper abdomen, aching muscles, and sometimes joint pain.

In uncommon, severe cases, jaundice may be intense and *liver failure* may develop, with possible effects on other organs (including the brain), resulting in coma.

DIAGNOSIS AND TREATMENT

A physician may strongly suspect acute hepatitis from the symptoms alone, particularly if the patient is in a risk group for exposure to one of the causative viruses, chemicals, or drugs. *Ultrasound scanning* of the liver may help rule out bile duct obstruction (another cause of jaundice), and *liver function tests* can aid in diagnosis.

There is no specific treatment of acute hepatitis. However, if drug or chemical poisoning is suspected, the physician must determine the causative substance and stop the patient's exposure to it (for example, by withdrawing a drug). Sometimes, detoxification may be possible using an antidote to the substance. In all cases, rest and a nourishing diet are usually recommended; recovery usually occurs after a few weeks. Abstinence from alcohol after the illness aids in liver regeneration.

In severe cases leading to liver failure, intensive care is required. Acute hepatitis causes several hundred deaths in the US each year.

CHRONIC HEPATITIS

Occasionally, a person may fail to recover fully from an episode of acute hepatitis, leading to continued liver cell damage and inflammation. This occurs most commonly, but not exclusively, with certain types of viral hepatitis. Chronic hepatitis may also develop insidiously over a number of years without any acute episodes. Heavy alcohol consumption may again be responsible. In some cases the cause is an *autoimmune disorder* (in which the body's defenses attack its own tissues), a reaction to a medication, or a metabolic disorder affecting the liver.

Several types of chronic hepatitis are recognized, although generally they can be distinguished only by taking a *liver biopsy* (tissue sample) and looking at the liver cells under a microscope. In the type affecting heavy drinkers, damaged liver cells with areas of inflammation around them are scattered throughout the liver, and fat droplets can be seen within the cells. In another type, called chronic active hepatitis, there is obvious liver cell destruction and scarring that can lead to liver *cirrhosis* if untreated. In a third type, called chronic persistent hepatitis, there is a lesser degree of inflammation and little risk of progression to cirrhosis.

SYMPTOMS AND DIAGNOSIS

The symptoms of chronic hepatitis are usually no worse than a vague feeling of being sick. Often the disease remains undetected until the patient has a medical examination and the liver is found to be enlarged, a causative virus or specific antibody is found in the blood, or the results of *liver function tests* are abnormal. Liver biopsy helps the physician establish the type of chronic hepatitis.

TREATMENT

For hepatitis caused by alcohol consumption, total abstinence is the only cure. If strictly observed, it allows complete restoration of liver function. For chronic persistent hepatitis, treatment is not usually needed. For the chronic active form, therapy depends on the precise cause of the disease (see *Hepatitis, chronic active*).

Hepatitis A

See *Hepatitis, viral*.

Hepatitis B

See *Hepatitis, viral*.

Hepatitis, chronic active

A type of chronic *hepatitis* in which there is intense and progressive inflammation and destruction of cells surrounding certain structures within the liver. Scar tissue forms and leads to liver *cirrhosis*.

CAUSES

Chronic active hepatitis may be caused in any of four ways—as a result of an autoimmune reaction (immune system disturbance), a viral infection, a reaction to a medication (rare), or to a metabolic disorder (rare).

In the autoimmune type, antibodies (proteins with a defense role) that inappropriately attack liver cells are formed. This is the most common cause of hepatitis in Northern Europe and one of the most common causes in the US. Women are affected more often than men. Primary biliary cirrhosis may fall into this category.

Viral infection is the most common cause in the US, most often due to viral hepatitis, type B, or non-A, non-B virus (see *Hepatitis, viral*). Men are affected more often than women.

Medications are a rare cause of chronic active hepatitis. Drugs that have been implicated include

MAIN TYPES OF VIRAL HEPATITIS

	Viral hepatitis type A (infectious hepatitis)	Viral hepatitis type B (serum hepatitis)
Transmission of infection	Virus is present in feces of infected people and transmitted to others by fecal contamination of food (e.g., through infected people handling food). Feces are infective from two to three weeks before until eight days after onset of jaundice. Local epidemics can occur.	Virus is present in blood and other body fluids of infected people. In the US, virus is spread mainly sexually and by needle-sharing among drug abusers. Health workers are at risk from infected blood. In Africa and Asia, spread from mother to baby is common.
Incidence	Worldwide. In the US, about 40 percent of young adults have been exposed to the virus. In some parts of the world where hygiene is poor, almost everyone has been exposed to this type of hepatitis.	Worldwide. In parts of Africa and Asia, up to 20 percent of the population has been carrying the virus without symptoms for years. In the US, carrier rate is much lower (less than 1 percent).
Groups at particular risk	Travelers to areas where hygiene standards are poor and prevalence of the virus is high (i.e., parts of Asia, Africa, or South America).	Homosexuals, people with multiple sexual partners, intravenous drug abusers, health care personnel, or children born to carrier mothers.
Incubation period	Three to six weeks after virus has entered the body.	A few weeks to several months after infection.
Illness	In many cases there is no illness. Otherwise, typical acute hepatitis (flulike illness with jaundice), usually mild and never progressing to chronic hepatitis.	Typical acute hepatitis, often more severe than with type A virus. Progression to chronic hepatitis and other liver disease may occur. Sometimes, no illness.
Prevention	For nonimmune travelers at risk, passive immunization with immunoglobulin plus good hygiene and care in selection of food and drink. A vaccine has also recently been developed.	Observance of *"safe" sex* with possibly infected sexual partners and avoidance of blood exchange. Vaccine and/or passive immunization for groups at high risk.

oxyphenisatin, nitrofurantoin, and isoniazid. Metabolic disorders that may cause the disease include *hemochromatosis* and *Wilson's disease*.

SYMPTOMS, DIAGNOSIS, AND TREATMENT
The disease may cause vague feelings of tiredness, or no symptoms at all. It is diagnosed by *liver biopsy*.

The autoimmune type is treated with *corticosteroid drugs*, which usually bring some improvement. Antiviral agents have been tried unsuccessfully against viral infections. In the drug-induced type, withdrawal of the medication can lead to recovery. For metabolic disturbances, treatment depends on the underlying disorder.

Hepatitis, viral
Any type of *hepatitis* (inflammation of the liver) caused by a viral infection.
TYPES AND CAUSES
A number of viruses may secondarily infect the liver, but, for certain viruses, the liver is a primary target. These are called hepatotropic viruses and include hepatitis viruses type A, type B, and delta viruses. Tests are available for detecting any of these in the blood or tissues. Sometimes, a person has obvious symptoms of viral hepatitis, but the type A, type B, and delta viruses cannot be detected; in such cases the illness is called non-A, non-B hepatitis. A few viruses may cause this type, which is a common form among people who contract hepatitis from blood transfusions.

The different viruses have varying incidences in different parts of the world and different modes of transmission (see table).

Hepatitis, type A (formerly called infectious hepatitis), is thought to be spread by virus from an infected person's feces directly or indirectly contaminating food, drinking water, or someone else's fingers. In most parts of the world, a high proportion of the population has been infected with the virus, often without symptoms, and is immune to further attack. Many cases occur among travelers who have recently returned from an area where the virus is prevalent and standards of hygiene are low.

Viral hepatitis, type B, used to be spread mainly by blood transfusions and blood products (and was referred to as serum hepatitis), but the development of tests for the virus has removed this risk. Today hepatitis B is mainly sexually transmitted (being particularly common among male homosexuals) or spread by mechanisms in which an infected person's blood is inoculated into someone else (i.e., by needle sharing among drug abusers, razor sharing, or ear piercing). These are precisely the same mechanisms by which *HIV* (the virus responsible for *AIDS*) is spread.

Viral hepatitis, type B, is in many respects more serious than viral hepatitis, type A. In a proportion of cases, the virus persists for years after the initial infection and may lead to a chronic form of hepatitis (see *Hepatitis, chronic active*) and eventually to liver *cirrhosis* and/or *liver cancer*. Carriers of the virus may have few or no symptoms during this time, but can infect others. The non-A, non-B hepatitis virus is the cause of most transfusion-associated hepatitis cases.

Hepatitis delta virus can exist only in someone who is already carrying or has recently been infected with hepatitis, type B. In the US, it seems to be spread mainly by needle sharing among drug abusers.
SYMPTOMS, DIAGNOSIS, AND TREATMENT
Infection with any of the causative viruses may be symptomless or may cause a typical acute *hepatitis* with a flulike illness followed by jaundice. About 10 percent of patients infected with the hepatitis, type B; delta; or non-A, non-B viruses go on to acquire chronic hepatitis. This rarely, if ever, happens with hepatitis, type A.

H

H

Diagnosis is made by identification of the virus (or by identification of antibodies to the virus) in the blood or, in the case of non-A, non-B hepatitis, by exclusion of the other types. Treatment is as for other causes of hepatitis.

PREVENTION

Vaccines are available against viral hepatitis, type B. However, vaccination is generally offered or recommended only to those who are at high risk of infection. For viral hepatitis, type B, it includes health care workers, children born to carrier mothers, male homosexuals, and drug addicts.

Passive immunization with immunoglobulins (antibodies) directed against viral hepatitis, type A and type B, is also available and can provide some protection. It is recommended for people who will be traveling to high incidence areas on vacation or on short business trips. Hepatitis, type B, immunoglobulin is also given immediately after birth to babies who had carrier mothers, to prevent infection while the vaccine (given at the same time) is beginning to build up.

Avoidance of viral hepatitis, type A, is further helped by observing good hygiene, especially food hygiene, in parts of the world where sanitary standards are low (see *Food-borne infection*). The chances of getting viral hepatitis, type B, can be reduced through use of a condom, by not sharing needles, and by avoiding activities such as ear piercing or tattooing unless the equipment used is sterile. These precautions are broadly the same as for the avoidance of *AIDS*.

Hepatoma

The most common form of malignant tumor arising within the liver. (See *Liver cancer*.)

Hepatomegaly

Enlargement of the liver, which may occur as a result of virtually any type of liver disorder. Enlargement of the liver may cause tenderness just beneath the ribs and can be detected by a physician during the course of a physical examination. (See *Liver* disorders box.)

Herbal medicine

 Systems of medicine in which various parts of different plants are used to treat symptoms and promote health. Herbal medicine was the most common medical treatment in most cultures for many centuries.

Heredity

 The transmission of traits and/or disorders through genetic mechanisms. Each person inherits a combination of *genes* (units of inheritance)—half paternal, half maternal—via the sperm and egg cells from which he or she is derived. The interaction of these genes determines the person's inherited characteristics, including, in some cases, disorders or susceptibility to disorders. Half of an individual's genes are passed on, in turn, to each of his or her children. (See also *Genetic disorders; Inheritance*.)

Heritability

A measure of the extent to which a disease or disorder is the result of inherited (genetic) factors as opposed to environmental influences, such as diet and climate.

Certain disorders (such as *hemophilia* or *cystic fibrosis*) are known to be caused entirely by hereditary factors. Others (such as occupational disorders) are caused entirely by environmental factors. Between these two extremes lies a large number of disorders in which both inheritance and environment probably play a part.

Pinpointing hereditary factors is notoriously difficult. A rough estimate of heritability can be obtained from the known incidence of a disorder in the first-degree relatives (i.e., parents, siblings, and offspring) of affected people and by comparing it to the incidence in a population exposed to similar environmental influences. Other estimates of heritability are obtained from studies of identical twins who have been reared apart.

Such studies suggest a relatively high heritability for *schizophrenia*, *asthma*, *coronary heart disease*, non-insulin-dependent *diabetes mellitus*, *ankylosing spondylitis*, and some birth defects, such as *cleft lip and palate*, *pyloric stenosis*, and *talipes* (clubfoot). The heritability for congenital *heart disease* and *peptic ulcer* is low.

Estimates of heritability are useful in *genetic counseling*. (See also *Genetic disorders; Histocompatibility antigens*.)

Hermaphroditism

A congenital disorder in which both male and female gonads (testes and ovaries) are present and the external genitalia are not clearly male or female. True hermaphroditism is extremely rare and its cause unknown. The majority of affected children are raised as males because

the external genitalia usually appear more male than female.

A more common condition is pseudohermaphroditism, in which the external genitalia may be ambiguous, but the gonads of only one sex are present. Pseudohermaphroditism is caused by a hormonal imbalance (such as in congenital *adrenal hyperplasia*) and can usually be treated by plastic surgery and hormone therapy.

Hernia

The protrusion of an organ or tissue through a weak area in the muscle or other tissue that normally contains it. The term is usually applied to a protrusion of the intestine through a weak area in the abdominal wall. In *hiatal hernia*, the stomach protrudes through the diaphragm into the chest. Very rarely, other organs or tissue (e.g., the brain) may herniate.

CAUSES

Abdominal hernias are usually caused by a *congenital* weakness in the abdominal wall. They may appear following surgery or after damage caused by lifting heavy objects, substantial weight gain, persistent coughing, or straining to defecate.

SYMPTOMS

The first symptom of a hernia is usually a bulge in the abdominal wall. There may also be abdominal discomfort. In some people, the protruding intestine can be pushed back through the abdominal wall.

Severe pain occurs when the hernia bulges out and cannot be replaced. If the blood supply to a twisted, trapped intestine becomes impaired (a condition known as a strangulated hernia), the bowel may become gangrenous. This requires urgent treatment.

DIAGNOSIS AND TREATMENT

Hernias are diagnosed by physical examination. If the hernia is causing only slight discomfort and is readily pushed back, a supportive garment, or truss, may be recommended. Hernias that are painful or impossible to push back are usually treated surgically (see *Hernia repair*).

Hernia repair

Surgical correction of a *hernia*. The procedure is performed to treat a hernia of the abdominal wall that is painful or cannot be pushed back. A strangulated hernia requires an emergency operation.

HOW IT IS DONE

Many hernias are repaired on an outpatient basis unless an underlying

MAIN TYPES OF ABDOMINAL HERNIA

Inguinal hernia

At least 2 percent of adult males in the US suffer from this kind of hernia, in which part of the intestine bulges through the inguinal canal (the passage through which the testes descend into the scrotum). The hernia is detected as a bulge in the groin or scrotum; untreated, the hernia may become stuck, so early surgery is generally recommended.

Femoral hernia

This type of hernia occurs most commonly in obese women; part of the intestine emerges where the femoral vein and artery pass from the abdomen to the thigh. A femoral hernia is noticed as a swelling of the top front of the thigh. Although the hernia itself may be large, its neck is narrow, and the condition can only be corrected by surgery.

Epigastric hernia

Also called a ventral hernia, an epigastric hernia is caused by a weakness in the muscles of the central upper abdomen; the intestine bulges out at a point between the navel and the breastbone. This form of hernia is three times more common in men than in women and is most likely to occur in people between 20 and 50 years old.

Umbilical hernia

This occurs when part of the intestine protrudes through the abdominal wall near the navel. Babies are the most common sufferers; the hernia can be repaired surgically or it may disappear naturally by about age 5. A similar problem, a parumbilical hernia, occurs mostly in obese, middle-aged women who have had several children.

Incisional hernia

An area of weakness may occasionally develop following a surgical incision in the wall of the abdomen. This area may then develop into an incisional hernia. The defect may become so severe that a large amount of intestine bulges through the abdominal wall; if this happens, a repair using a piece of mesh may be necessary.

HERNIA REPAIR

During surgery the hernia is removed or repositioned and the weakened abdominal wall is reinforced with stitching or mesh.

1 The protruding sac of intestine is pushed back into the abdomen or, in some cases (e.g., strangulation), the sac is removed surgically.

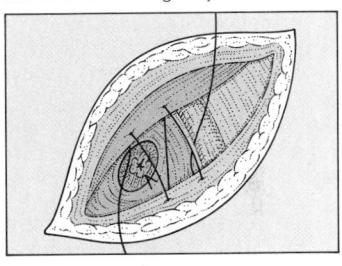

2 The wall of the abdomen may then be repaired by overlapping the edges of the weakened area and securing with rows of stitching.

LARGE HERNIAS

For repair of some large hernias, two mesh leaves are secured by rows of stitching, then joined at the center.

H

medical condition necessitates hospitalization. A local, epidural, or general anesthetic may be used. The surgeon's aim is to push the protruding intestine back into place and then strengthen the weakened muscle wall (see illustrated box).

RECOVERY AND OUTLOOK
The speed of recovery depends on the patient's underlying medical condition and on the type of hernia repaired. Lifting heavy objects should be avoided for three to six months.

The risk of a recurrence of the condition varies with the type of hernia treated. Inguinal and incisional hernias both recur quite commonly; femoral and epigastric hernias recur only rarely.

Herniated disk
See *Disk prolapse.*

Herniorrhaphy
Surgical correction of a hernia. (See *Hernia repair.*)

Heroin

A *narcotic drug* derived from *morphine,* a substance extracted from the pods of the opium poppy. Heroin is a white or brownish powder that can be smoked, sniffed, or dissolved in water and injected. Its chemical name is diacetylmorphine.

Heroin abuse is a major health problem in many countries. It has many adverse effects on the user and is a sociological and economic problem of immense proportions.

EFFECTS

In addition to having an analgesic (painkilling) effect, heroin produces sensations of warmth, calmness, drowsiness, and a loss of concern for outside events.

Long-term use causes *tolerance* (the need for greater amounts of the drug to have the same effects) and psychological and physical dependence (see *Drug dependence*). Sudden withdrawal of the drug produces symptoms such as shivering, abdominal cramps, diarrhea, vomiting, sleeplessness, and restlessness.

Other common problems of heroin addiction include injection scars, skin abscesses, weight loss, and impotence. Infections, such as *hepatitis B* and *AIDS*, are spread by sharing needles. Death commonly occurs from accidental overdose.

Herpangina

A throat infection caused by a type of virus called coxsackievirus. Herpangina most commonly affects young children, although it occurs in adults. The virus is usually transmitted via infected droplets coughed or sneezed into the air. Many people harbor the virus but do not experience any symptoms.

SYMPTOMS

After an incubation period of two to seven days, there is a sudden onset of fever, loss of appetite, and sore throat. There may also be headache, abdominal discomfort, and vague muscular aches and pains. The throat becomes red and a few small blisters appear, which enlarge and burst, forming shallow ulcers. The condition usually clears up within a week.

TREATMENT

Usually no treatment is required other than simple *analgesics* (painkillers). There is no specific antiviral therapy available. Antibiotics are generally of no therapeutic value unless a bacterial infection develops as a secondary complication. Recurrent attacks of herpangina may result from infection with different strains of the virus.

Herpes

Any of a variety of conditions characterized by an eruption of small, usually painful, blisters on the skin.

When a person is said to be suffering from herpes, it usually refers to an infection with the *herpes simplex* virus. Forms of the virus are responsible for *cold sores* (painful blisters around the lips) and for the sexually transmitted infection genital herpes, which is characterized by blisters on the sex organs (see *Herpes, genital*). The virus can also cause a number of other conditions affecting the skin, mouth, eyes, brain, or, in rare cases, the whole body.

A closely related virus, the varicella-zoster virus, is responsible for two more conditions in which skin blisters are a feature—*chickenpox* (also known as varicella) and *herpes zoster* (also known as shingles). Like the herpes simplex virus, the varicella-zoster virus can affect the eyes or, rarely, may infect the brain or cause an infection throughout the body.

Herpes gestationis and *dermatitis herpetiformis* are among various other conditions in which "herpetiform" (herpeslike) groups of blisters may appear on the skin, but neither is related to herpes simplex or varicella-zoster virus infections.

Herpes, genital

A sexually transmitted disease that produces a painful rash on the genitals. Caused by the *herpes simplex* virus (*HERPESVIRUS HOMINIS*, type 2), genital herpes is transmitted by sexual intercourse with an infected person.

SYMPTOMS AND SIGNS

After an incubation period of about a week, the virus produces itching, burning, soreness, and small blisters in the genital area. The blisters burst to leave small, painful ulcers, which heal within 10 to 21 days. The lymph nodes in the groin may become enlarged and painful, and the affected person may feel sick, with headache and fever. Women with genital herpes may find urination very painful if the urine comes into contact with the sores. Occasionally, there may be cold sores around the mouth.

TREATMENT

Genital herpes cannot be cured, but the earlier treatment is given, the more likely the treatment will prevent or reduce the severity of an attack. An antiviral medication (such as acyclovir) helps make the ulcers less painful and encourages them to heal more quickly. Additional soothing measures include taking analgesics (painkillers) and warm baths with a tablespoon of salt added.

Subsequent attacks tend to occur after sexual intercourse, after sunbathing, or when the affected person is run down; these recurrent attacks often clear up quickly with or without treatment. Sexual activity should be avoided until the symptoms have disappeared. If a pregnant woman has an attack of genital herpes when the baby is due, a cesarean section is performed to prevent the baby from being infected during delivery.

OUTLOOK

Once the virus enters the body, it stays there for the rest of the person's life. About 40 percent of those affected never have another attack after the first. Others, however, suffer four or five attacks annually for several years. Gradually, the attacks become less severe and the intervals between recurrences become longer.

The herpes virus may have a role in the development of cervical cancer (see *Cervix, cancer of*); it is important for any woman who has had herpes to have a *cervical smear test* (Pap test) every one to two years.

Herpes gestationis

A rare skin disorder, characterized by crops of blisters on the legs and abdomen, that occurs only in pregnancy. The cause is not known and, despite its name, herpes gestationis is not related to any of the disorders caused by the *herpes simplex* viruses.

Severe herpes gestationis is treated with *corticosteroid drugs* in tablet form and may require hospital admission because of the risk of *miscarriage*. The disorder usually clears up completely after the birth of the baby, but tends to recur in subsequent pregnancies.

Herpes simplex

A common and troublesome viral disease. Although most herpes simplex infections are symptomless, mild, or merely irritating, others can be extremely distressing (notably infections affecting the genitals) and even life-threatening.

TYPES

The virus exists in two forms, known as HSV1 (herpes simplex virus, type 1) and HSV2 (type 2). HSV1 is usually associated with infections of the lips, mouth, and face. HSV2 is often associated with infections of the genitals and infections acquired by babies at birth. However, there is a considerable amount of overlap. Some conditions usually caused by HSV1 are sometimes caused by HSV2 and vice versa. Both virus types are contagious. Infection is spread by direct contact with the lesions themselves or by the fluid contained therein.

TYPE 1 VIRUS Most people have been infected with HSV1 by the time they reach adulthood; most of the remainder are infected during adulthood. The initial infection may cause no symptoms or may cause a sometimes severe flulike illness with mouth ulcers. Thereafter, the virus remains in the nerve cells within the facial area. In many people, however, the virus is occasionally reactivated, causing recurrent *cold sores* that always erupt in the same site (usually around the lips), but are not serious. They often recur at times when there is an elevated temperature at the affected site (such as with fever or prolonged sun exposure).

Rarely, the virus may infect the fingers, causing an eruption of very painful blisters known as a herpetic *whitlow*. Sometimes it may cause an extensive rash of blisters (known as eczema herpeticum) in someone with a preexisting skin condition such as dermatitis.

If a person with an *immunodeficiency disorder* (such as *AIDS*) or someone who is taking *immunosuppressant drugs* is infected with the virus, it may cause a severe, generalized infection that is occasionally fatal.

If the virus gets into an eye, it may cause *conjunctivitis* (which usually lasts only a few days) or, more seriously, a *corneal ulcer*.

Very rarely, the type 1 virus may spread to the brain, leading to a serious *encephalitis*.

TYPE 2 VIRUS This form of the virus is the usual cause of sexually transmitted genital herpes, in which painful blisters erupt on the sex organs (see *Herpes, genital*). As with cold sores, the blisters recur in some people.

TREATMENT
Treatment of herpes simplex depends on its type, site, and severity. Antiviral drugs, such as acyclovir, are sometimes helpful. Lesions may also become infected with bacteria. If so, antibiotics (topical or oral) and tepid soaks may be helpful.

Herpes zoster
The medical term for shingles. Herpes zoster is an infection of the nerves that supply certain areas of the skin. It causes a painful rash of small, crusting blisters. After the rash heals, pain may persist for months or, rarely, years.

TYPES
Herpes zoster often affects a strip of skin over the ribs on one side or, less commonly, a strip on one side of the neck and arm or the lower part of the body. Sometimes it involves the upper half of the face on one side; in this case, the eye may also be affected. Shingles in this area is known as herpes zoster ophthalmicus.

CAUSES
Herpes zoster is caused by the varicella-zoster virus, which also causes *chickenpox*. During an attack of chickenpox, most of the viral organisms are destroyed, but some survive and lie dormant in certain sensory nerves, remaining there for many years. In some people, a decline in the efficiency of the *immune system* (the body's defenses against infection) allows the viruses to reemerge and cause shingles.

The competence of the immune system declines with age; this decline is probably accelerated by stress and by the use of *corticosteroid drugs*. Herpes zoster commonly follows a stressful episode.

INCIDENCE
Herpes zoster is a common disease. Every year in the US, a few hundred people per 100,000 suffer an attack. It mainly affects people over 50 and the incidence rises with age. Herpes zoster is very common in people whose immune systems have been weakened either by diseases such as *lymphoma* or *Hodgkin's disease*, or by treatment with *immunosuppressant* or *anticancer drugs*.

SYMPTOMS AND SIGNS
The first indication is excessive sensitivity in the area of skin to be affected; this is soon followed by pain, which is sometimes severe and which may, until the rash appears, be mistaken for pleurisy or appendicitis.

After about five days, the rash appears, starting as small, slightly raised, red spots that quickly turn to tense blisters, teeming with viruses. Within three days the blisters have turned yellowish and soon dry, flat-

Example of herpes zoster
An extensive rash of crusting blisters over one side of the neck that spreads over the shoulder and onto the front of the chest.

ten, and crust over. During the next two weeks or so these crusts drop off, often leaving small pitted scars.

The most serious feature of herpes zoster is pain following the attack. The pain is a consequence of damage to the nerves, causing strong nerve impulses to be constantly produced and passed upward to the brain. The pain, which affects about one third of sufferers, may be severe and may last for months or years. The older the patient and the more pronounced the rash, the more likely the pain will be severe and persistent.

Ophthalmic herpes zoster may be confined to the skin of the lids and the forehead and need not affect the eye, but, if it does, it may cause a *corneal ulcer* or *uveitis*, both of which are potentially serious.

TREATMENT
Once the rash is fully established, little can be done to influence the course of the disease or the likelihood of postherpetic pain. Only palliative measures and *analgesics* (painkillers) are of value. It is, however, possible to reduce the severity of the active stage and to minimize nerve damage by the prompt use of *antiviral drugs* (such as acyclovir).

Many different measures have been advocated, in addition to analgesics, for the relief of postherpetic pain. They include skin stimulation by intermittent rubbing, the passage of alternating electric currents through the skin, local heat, cold spraying, injection of local anesthetics, and even surgical cutting of the nerves. None of these measures has been shown to be consistently effective.

Heterosexuality
Sexual attraction to members of the opposite sex. (See also *Bisexuality; Homosexuality, male; Lesbianism*.)

Heterozygote

A term used to describe a person whose cells contain two different *genes* controlling a specified inherited trait, in contrast to a *homozygote* who has identical genes controlling that trait. (See also *Inheritance; Genetic disorders*.)

Hiatal hernia
A condition in which part of the stomach protrudes upward into the chest through a hiatus (opening) in the diaphragm (the sheet of muscle involved in respiration that separates the chest from the abdomen).

H

CAUSES AND INCIDENCE

The underlying cause of this common condition is unknown, but it tends to occur more frequently in obese people (and especially in upper middle-aged women) and in those who smoke. In some cases it is present at birth.

SYMPTOMS

Many people have no symptoms, but in some people hiatal hernia affects the efficiency of the muscle at the end of the esophagus (esophagogastric junction), permitting *acid reflux* (regurgitation of acidic juices from the stomach into the esophagus). This reflux may in turn cause *heartburn*, which is often made worse by bending over or lying down, and peptic *esophagitis* (inflammation of the esophagus). The pain of esophagitis or esophagospasm may mimic the pain of *coronary heart disease*.

DIAGNOSIS

Esophagoscopy (passage of a viewing tube down the throat into the esophagus) may be performed to determine the severity of esophagitis and to check for stricture (narrowing) of the esophagus (see *Esophageal stricture*). If there is any suspicion of esophageal cancer, a *biopsy* (removal of a small sample of tissue for examination) is carried out. Manometric studies (pressure measurements, see *Manometry*) can confirm the reduced pressure at the esophagogastric junction. A barium swallow (see *Barium X-ray examinations*) is performed with the patient tilted headdown. If the barium is seen on X ray to cause reflux into the esophagus, it indicates incompetence at the esophagogastric junction.

TREATMENT

To alleviate symptoms, the patient should avoid eating large, heavy meals and should never lie down or bend over immediately after a meal. The head of the bed should be raised to prevent reflux during the night. People who are obese need to lose weight and smokers should stop smoking. *Antacids* may be given to reduce stomach acidity and to protect the esophagus against acid juices.

In severe cases, an operation may be required to return the protruding part of the stomach to the abdomen and to prevent further reflux of acid gastric contents into the esophagus.

Hiccup

A sudden, involuntary contraction of the diaphragm followed by rapid closure of the vocal cords (which causes the characteristic sound); also called hiccough. Hiccups usually occur at brief intervals and attacks last for only a few minutes.

CAUSES AND TREATMENT

Attacks of hiccups are extremely common; in almost all cases, they occur without obvious cause and are not medically significant. Such minor attacks often stop of their own accord. There are also numerous popular remedies, the effectiveness of which varies from one person to another.

Rarely, hiccups may be due to a condition that causes irritation of the diaphragm or of the phrenic nerves that supply it. Known causes include pleurisy, pneumonia, certain disorders of the stomach or esophagus, pancreatitis, alcoholism, and hepatitis. Most bouts are of unknown cause.

Frequent, prolonged attacks of hiccups, which are extremely rare, may lead to severe exhaustion. In such cases, when medication has failed, surgery may be recommended. It may involve either crushing or injecting a drug around one of the phrenic nerves to paralyze half the diaphragm; this measure is sometimes unsuccessful.

Hip

The joint between the pelvis and the upper end of the femur (thigh bone). The hip is an extremely stable ball-and-socket joint; the smooth, rounded head of the femur fits securely into the acetabulum, a deep, cuplike cavity in

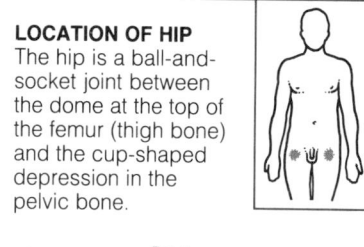

LOCATION OF HIP
The hip is a ball-and-socket joint between the dome at the top of the femur (thigh bone) and the cup-shaped depression in the pelvic bone.

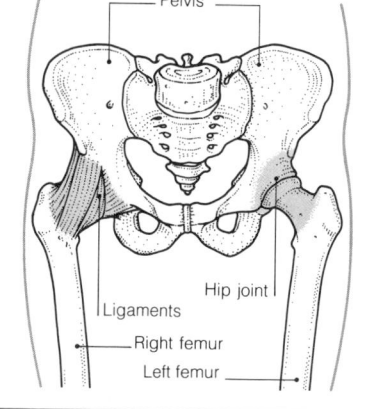

Pelvis

Hip joint

Ligaments

Right femur

Left femur

the pelvis. Tough ligaments attach the femur to the pelvis, further stabilizing the joint and providing it with the necessary strength to support the weight of the upper body and to take the strain of running, jumping, and other vigorous leg movements. In addition, the ball-and-socket structure of the joint allows the leg a considerable range of movement that is available only because of the unique design of this joint.

DISORDERS

ARTHRITIS *Osteoarthritis* of the hip, one of the most common of all disorders, causes stiffness and pain in the joint, particularly during movement. Occasionally, *ankylosing spondylitis* and *rheumatoid arthritis* of the hip cause similar problems.

FRACTURE What is commonly called fracture of the hip (most common in elderly people as the result of a fall) is in fact fracture of the head or neck of the femur (see *Femur, fracture of*).

DISLOCATION Congenital dislocation of the hip usually clears up of its own accord or is remediable (see *Hip, congenital dislocation of*). Dislocation of the hip by injury is rare and usually results only from extreme force, such as that from an automobile accident. Such dislocation may cut off the blood supply to the head of the femur, causing the bone to die (aseptic necrosis), or may injure the sciatic nerve, leading to weakness in the leg.

Hip, congenital dislocation of

A disorder present at birth in which the ball-like head of the femur (thigh bone) fails to fit into the cuplike socket in the pelvis to form a joint but instead lies outside. One or both of the hips may be affected.

CAUSES AND INCIDENCE

The cause of congenital dislocation of the hip is not known, but it is more common in babies born by *breech delivery* and following pregnancies in which there was *oligohydramnios* (an abnormally small amount of amniotic fluid in the uterus).

About 400 in every 100,000 babies born are affected; in most cases the condition soon corrects itself. Only about 125 in 100,000 suffer from persistent dislocation. The disorder runs in families and affects many more girls than boys.

DIAGNOSIS

Shortly after birth and at intervals until walking starts, all babies are given a routine physical examination of the hip to check its stability and range of motion. If the condition is not

X ray showing congenital dislocation
The left femur (thigh bone) is displaced upward and backward from its socket.

detected in infancy it may be diagnosed when a limp develops when the child is learning to walk.

TREATMENT

If the condition is found in early infancy, light splints are applied to the thigh to maneuver the ball of the joint into the socket and keep it in position. The splints are worn for two to four months and usually aid in correcting the problem.

If the condition is not discovered until later in infancy, traction is used. The head of the femur is moved into the correct position and kept there by a system of weights and pulleys attached to the leg.

If the dislocation is not detected until childhood, surgery using a general anesthetic may be required to correct it. The child usually must stay in the hospital for several weeks and wear a plaster cast for a few months.

OUTLOOK

Provided the disorder is treated in infancy, the child usually walks normally and there are no aftereffects. When treatment is delayed until childhood, there may be lifelong problems with walking. If the condition remains untreated, the dislocation often leads to shortening of the leg, limping, and early *osteoarthritis* in the joint.

Hippocratic oath

A part of the writings attributed to Hippocrates, a fifth century BC Greek physician. The oath has served as a widely used ethical guide for the medical profession ever since. It pledges the physician to work for the good of the patient, to do him or her no harm, to prescribe no deadly drugs, to give no advice that could cause death, and to keep confidential medical information regarding the patient. The oath is often administered as a part of the graduation ceremonies at medical schools.

Hip replacement

A surgical procedure to replace all or part of a diseased hip joint with an artificial substitute.

WHY IT IS DONE

Hip replacement is most often carried out in older people whose joints are stiff and painful as a result of *osteoarthritis*. It may also be needed if *rheumatoid arthritis* has spread to the hip joint, making walking difficult, or if the top end of the femur is badly fractured (see *Femur, fracture of*).

The operation is not usually advised for young patients, since their greater activity puts more strain on the joints and it is unknown how long any artificial replacement is likely to last.

PERFORMING A HIP REPLACEMENT

In this operation, the surgeon pushes aside or cuts through the surrounding muscles to expose the hip joint. The femur (thigh bone) is cut and the pelvis is drilled to make room for the two components of the artificial joint. These parts are secured in place, the femur is repaired, and the muscles and tendons are replaced and repaired.

Sites of incision

Pelvis

Trochanter

Femur

1 The trochanter at the top of the femur is detached, and the hip joint is dislocated to separate the femur and the pelvis. The ball at the top of the femur is then cut away.

2 An instrument known as a reamer is used to make the hollow in the pelvis large enough to make room for the cup-shaped socket (one of the two components of the artificial hip joint).

3 A coarse file is used to cut a shaft in the femur, and the ball part of the artificial joint is inserted. The components are fixed in place with a special cement, which binds them to the bone.

4 The ball is placed in the socket and the trochanter is reattached to the femur with wires. The muscles and tendons are replaced and repaired, and the incision is then closed.

Before
This X ray shows a hip joint that has been badly damaged by arthritis.

Ball

Socket

Shaft

Components
The ball and shaft are made of metal; the socket may be metal or plastic.

After
This X ray shows the artificial hip joint in position after surgery.

H

RECOVERY PERIOD

The joint remains unstable for a week or two after the operation, and patients must take care not to dislocate the new joint during this time. Patients are advised to sleep on their backs and not to cross their legs, and are taught how to get in and out of a bathtub without disturbing the joint.

OUTLOOK

Hip joint replacement is a remarkably successful operation that has transformed the lives of many people who suffered from severe pain and stiffness. However, with time, a substantial proportion of artificial joints show signs on X ray of loosening at the cemented union between bone and metal. Surgeons and engineers are continuing to develop newer joint designs that do not rely on cement to hold them in place.

Hip, snapping

A fairly common condition in adults in which a characteristic clicking is heard and felt during certain movements of the joint. Snapping hip is generally harmless and does not indicate disease of the hip joint.

The noise and sensation are caused by a tendon slipping over the bony prominence on the outside of the femur when the hip is bent upward.

Snapping hip should not be confused with a hip that clicks when a newborn baby is being examined, which is a sign that there may be congenital dislocation of the hip (see *Hip, congenital dislocation of*).

Hirschsprung's disease

Also known as congenital megacolon, a congenital disorder in which a segment of intestine (sometimes near the anus) lacks the ganglion cells that control the rhythmic motion of the bowel. This segment becomes narrowed and blocks the movement of fecal material. The bowel above becomes dilated and tortuous (twisted). Hirschsprung's disease is uncommon and tends to run in families. It occurs about four times more often in boys than girls.

SYMPTOMS

Symptoms usually appear in infancy or early childhood; they include marked constipation and bloating. The child usually has a poor appetite and may fail to grow properly.

DIAGNOSIS

A barium enema (see *Barium X-ray examinations*) can show the narrowed rectal segment of the intestine. A *biopsy* sample taken from the involved area during *proctoscopy* or surgical biopsy confirms the lack of ganglion cells and establishes the diagnosis.

TREATMENT

Treatment involves removing the narrowed intestinal segment and rejoining the normal colon to the normal colonic or rectal segments. Before surgery, a temporary *colostomy* (making an artificial outlet for the colon on the abdominal wall) may be necessary if the child is considerably underweight or to facilitate treatment for severe anemia.

Hirsutism

Excessive hairiness, particularly in women. The additional hair is coarse, like a man's, and grows in a male pattern on the face, trunk, and limbs.

CAUSES AND INCIDENCE

Hirsutism occurs in some conditions in which the level of male hormones in the blood is abnormally high (e.g., in *polycystic ovary* syndrome and congenital *adrenal hyperplasia*).

Much more commonly, hirsutism is not a sign of any underlying disorder; it occurs in many normal women, especially after the menopause. The condition tends to run in families. Dark-haired women, particularly those of Hispanic or Indian extraction, are particularly likely to be hirsute.

TREATMENT

Hair can be bleached or removed in various ways (see *Hair removal*); the only method of permanent removal is by *electrolysis* (destruction of hair roots by an electric current). See also *Hypertrichosis*.

Histamine

A chemical present in cells (mainly *mast cells*) throughout the body that is released during an allergic reaction (see *Allergy*); histamine is one of the substances responsible for the symptoms of *inflammation*. It also stimulates production of acid by the stomach and narrows the bronchi (airways) in the lungs.

The effects of histamine can be counteracted by *antihistamine drugs*; its action on the gastric acid-forming glands is blocked by *histamine-2 receptor antagonists*.

Histamine-2 receptor antagonists

A group of *ulcer-healing drugs* related to the *antihistamine drug* group. Histamine-2 (or H-2) receptor antagonists work by blocking the action of the chemical histamine at specific *receptors* (sites on a cell's surface), preventing release of acid in the stomach. Acid reduction promotes the healing of *peptic ulcers* and relieves symptoms of *esophagitis*. (See also *Cimetidine*; *Ranitidine*; *Famotidine*.)

Histiocytosis X

A rare childhood disease in which there is an overgrowth of a type of tissue cell called a histiocyte. The cause is unknown, but it probably results from a disturbance of the *immune system*.

In the mildest form of the disease, rapid cell growth occurs in one bone only, usually affecting the skull, clavicle, or a rib or vertebra, causing swelling and pain. The chances of recovery are good in these cases.

The most severe, and least common, form of the disease affects infants. This form of the disease behaves like advanced *leukemia*, leading rapidly to death.

Histocompatibility antigens

A group of proteins that is naturally present within tissues and has a role in the *immune system* (body's defenses against infection). The main group of histocompatibility antigens is known as the HLA (human leukocyte antigen) system. The particular set or types of HLAs in a person's tissues (called his or her tissue type) is inherited. These antigens have an influence on the outcome of organ transplantation (see *Transplant surgery*) and also seem to affect susceptibility to certain diseases. However, these are probably just side effects of the primary immunologic (defense) function of the antigens.

TYPES AND STRUCTURE

Like all proteins, histocompatibility antigens are synthesized in cells under the control of genes. The genes controlling their production are called the major histocompatibility complex; they give rise to several series of antigens called HLA-A, HLA-B, HLA-C, HLA-D, and HLA-DR.

Each histocompatibility antigen is composed of two parts, a constant region (which is the same for all people) and a variable region (which differs among people). The structure of this region is genetically determined (inherited from one of the parents) and can take any of several forms, which have been given numbers. Thus, a particular antigen has a letter (the series it belongs to) and a number corresponding to the form within the series—for example, HLA-A3, HLA-B13, or HLA-C5 types. The number of possible combinations of antigens from the different series is vast, and, apart from identical twins, each person has a unique combination. By a technique called *tissue-typing*, every person can be immunologically "fingerprinted."

IMMUNOLOGICAL FUNCTION
Histocompatibility antigens within the series HLA-A, B, and C are present on virtually all living cells in the body. They are essential for the function of certain *lymphocytes* (white blood cells with an immunological function) called killer T cells. The antigens act as a guide for killer T cells to recognize and kill abnormal cells (i.e., virus-infected and tumor cells).

Histocompatibility antigens within the HLA-D series are present on the surfaces of various other cells with a defense role; they influence the interactions of these cells in fighting infection and tumors.

EFFECT IN TRANSPLANTATION
When an organ is transplanted from one person to another, the histocompatibility antigens in the donor organ are generally recognized as foreign and are attacked by the recipient's immune system, leading to rejection. However, if a donor can be found whose HLA types are very similar to those of the recipient (often a blood relative and ideally an identical twin), the chances of rejection occurring are minimized.

DISEASE ASSOCIATION
Certain HLA types occur more frequently in patients with particular diseases than in the rest of the population. For example, *multiple sclerosis* is associated with HLA-A3, *celiac sprue* with HLA-B8, and *ankylosing spondylitis* with HLA-B27.

It is suspected that susceptibility to these diseases is influenced by the HLA types, presumably as a result of their immunologic actions. The associations are of interest because they allow identification of individuals at risk and can help in the confirmation of disease.

LEGAL USES
An individual's HLA types are inherited (half from the father and half from the mother); blood relatives in general have similar types. Study of HLA types is thus sometimes of use in *paternity testing* and other situations in which there is a dispute as to whether two people are related. For example, if two people both have a highly unusual combination of HLA types, it may provide very strong evidence (although it can never be proven absolutely) that they are related.

Histologist
A specialist in *histology*, the study of the microscopic appearance of tissues.

Histology
The study of tissues, including their cellular structure and function. Its main practical use in medicine is in the diagnosis of disease. This often involves obtaining a tissue sample by *biopsy* and examining it for abnormalities. The histologist's skill lies in his or her familiarity with the range of normal appearances of tissues and the recognition of the abnormal appearances in different diseases.

Histopathology
The branch of *histology* (the study of tissues) concerned with the effects of disease on the microscopic structure of tissues.

Histoplasmosis
An infection caused by inhaling the spores of HISTOPLASMA CAPSULATUM, a fungus found in soil, particularly areas contaminated with droppings from birds or bats. Histoplasmosis occurs in the central and southern US and in parts of South America, the Far East, and Africa.

Most people who inhale the spores are not affected by them. The rare cases of infection occur either in people who are exposed to large quantities of the spores (such as pigeon handlers) or in people whose resistance to infection has been lowered—for example, by an *immunodeficiency disorder*, such as *AIDS*.

SYMPTOMS AND TREATMENT
The most common form of histoplasmosis is an acute illness (marked by breathlessness, cough, and joint pains) that usually clears up on its own. However, in some people (mainly in those with a low resistance to infection) the disease takes a chronic form and spreads throughout the body, resulting in fever, loss of weight, mouth ulcers, enlargement of the spleen, liver, and lymph nodes, failure of the adrenal glands, and anemia. Treatment with the antifungal drugs amphotericin B or ketoconazole is usually effective. In severe, untreated cases, the disease may be fatal (it causes about 50 to 100 deaths in the US each year).

History-taking
The process by which a physician learns from patients the symptoms of their illnesses and any previous disorders. (See *Diagnosis*.)

HIV
Human immunodeficiency virus. HIV belongs to the class of retroviruses (see *Virus*) and is the cause of *AIDS* and *AIDS-related complex*.

HIV gains access to the body by entering the bloodstream via blood transfusions, nonsterile needles, or sexual intercourse. A fetus can be infected by its mother. HIV has an affinity for the T-*lymphocytes* (part of the *immune system*), in which the virus multiplies and, in some cases, destroys function. HIV also attacks the brain and may cause severe damage with *dementia*; most infected people are likely to succumb to AIDS before this happens.

HIV is an organism of low infectivity; infected people present no threat to the health of their contacts at work or home, except for sexual partners and needle sharers.

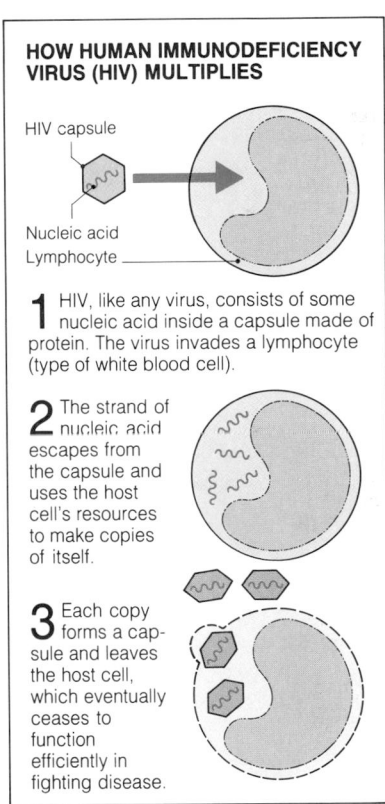

HOW HUMAN IMMUNODEFICIENCY VIRUS (HIV) MULTIPLIES

HIV capsule

Nucleic acid
Lymphocyte

1 HIV, like any virus, consists of some nucleic acid inside a capsule made of protein. The virus invades a lymphocyte (type of white blood cell).

2 The strand of nucleic acid escapes from the capsule and uses the host cell's resources to make copies of itself.

3 Each copy forms a capsule and leaves the host cell, which eventually ceases to function efficiently in fighting disease.

Hives
The popular name for *urticaria*.

HLA types
See *Histocompatibility antigens*.

HMO
See *Health Maintenance Organization*.

HOARSENESS OR LOSS OF VOICE

Any abnormal huskiness in the voice that may be so severe that you can make little or no sound.

H

 Has the hoarseness started within the past three days?

YES → Do you have or have you just had a cold, cough, or sore throat?

YES → You probably have inflammation of the vocal cords.

See • *Laryngitis*

NO ↓

Had you been using your voice more than usual just before the hoarseness or loss of voice developed?

YES → Overuse can irritate the vocal cords.

See • *Laryngitis*

NO ↓

Have you recently become tense, nervous, or depressed?

YES → Anxiety can sometimes cause a sudden loss of voice.

See • *Anxiety*

NO

NO ↓

 Are you over 40 years old and has your voice deepened?

YES → Have you noticed two or more of the following symptoms?
- feeling the cold more than you used to
- dry skin or hair
- weight increase without overeating
- unexplained tiredness

YES → An underactive thyroid gland is a possibility. This is an uncommon problem that is most likely to occur in middle-aged women. Consult your physician.

See • *Hypothyroidism*

NO

NO ↓

 Do you smoke?

YES → Smoking can lead to inflammation of the vocal cords.

See • *Laryngitis*

NO ↓

 Have you been drinking alcohol recently?

YES → Drinking alcohol can lead to inflammation of the vocal cords.

See • *Laryngitis*

NO ↓

Self-help
Hoarseness usually clears up after a few days with simple measures such as resting the voice and abstaining from smoking and alcohol.

Continued on next page

542

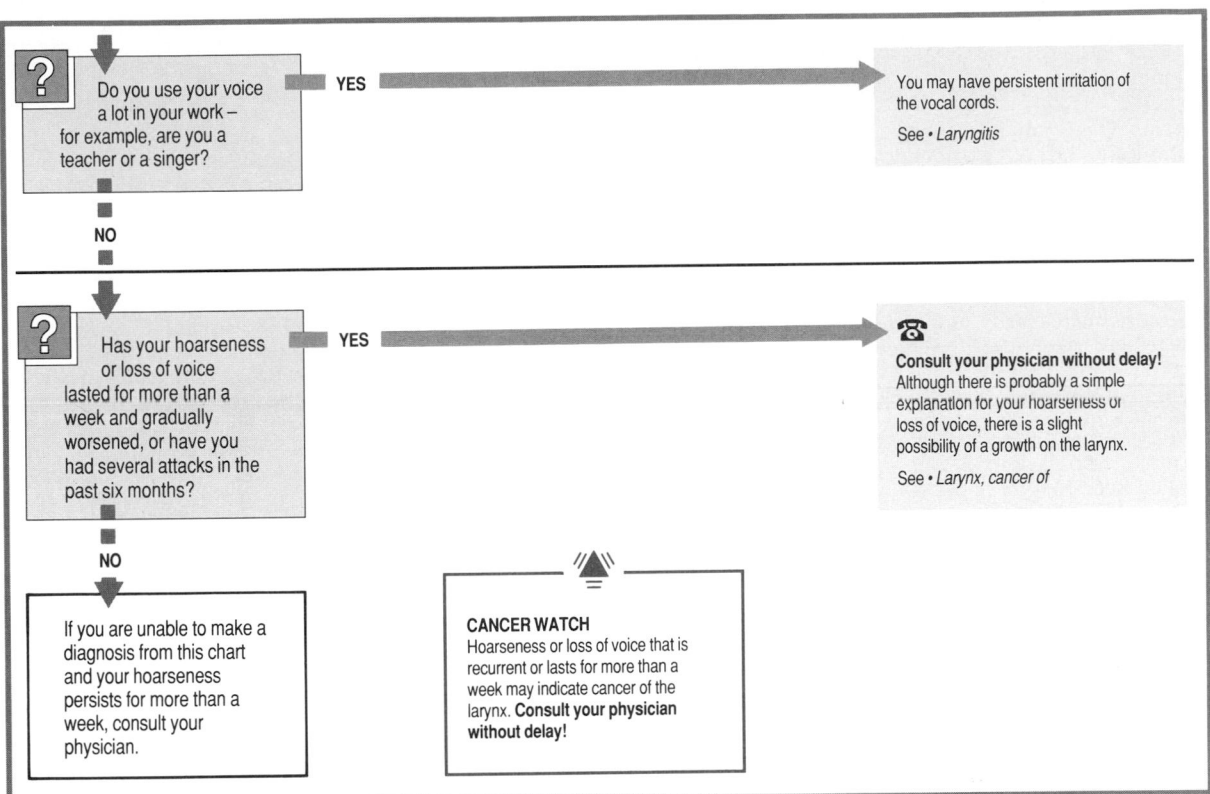

The flowchart reads:

? Do you use your voice a lot in your work – for example, are you a teacher or a singer?

YES → You may have persistent irritation of the vocal cords.

See • *Laryngitis*

NO

? Has your hoarseness or loss of voice lasted for more than a week and gradually worsened, or have you had several attacks in the past six months?

YES → ☎ **Consult your physician without delay!** Although there is probably a simple explanation for your hoarseness or loss of voice, there is a slight possibility of a growth on the larynx.

See • *Larynx, cancer of*

NO

If you are unable to make a diagnosis from this chart and your hoarseness persists for more than a week, consult your physician.

CANCER WATCH
Hoarseness or loss of voice that is recurrent or lasts for more than a week may indicate cancer of the larynx. **Consult your physician without delay!**

Hoarseness

A rough, husky, or croaking voice, usually caused by interference with the normal working of the vocal cords in the *larynx* (voice box). Most attacks do not last long and clear up of their own accord, but persistent hoarseness needs investigation to exclude the possibility of serious disease.

CAUSES

Hoarseness of limited duration is often due to overuse of the voice (for example, in teachers or singers), which strains small muscles in the larynx. It is also commonly caused by inflammation of the vocal cords as part of acute *laryngitis*, which is usually due to an upper respiratory tract infection such as a cold or sore throat.

Persistent hoarseness has many possible causes. It may be due to chronic irritation of the larynx (which can be caused by smoking or excessive consumption of alcohol) or chronic *bronchitis*. Irritation can also be caused by mucus constantly dripping on the larynx, as may occur in nasal *polyps* (harmless growths in the nose), allergic *rhinitis* (hay fever), *sinusitis*, or a deviated *nasal septum* (crookedness of the cartilage wall that separates the two nostrils).

Polyps on the vocal cords may also cause hoarseness, as may any accidental damage to them as the result of thyroid gland surgery. In *hypothyroidism* (underactivity of the thyroid gland), hoarseness can result from tissue forming on the vocal cords.

In young children, hoarseness is one of the symptoms of *croup* (inflammation and narrowing of the airways).

Occasionally, persistent hoarseness in adults has a more serious cause—including cancer of the larynx (see *Larynx, cancer of*). Less commonly, persistent hoarseness is caused by *thyroid cancer*.

SELF-HELP

Anyone suffering from hoarseness believed to be brought on by straining the voice should rest his or her voice until it has returned to normal; otherwise, permanent damage may eventually occur in the vocal cords. Voice training may reduce the chance of recurrence. Resting the voice, along with not smoking or drinking alcohol, also helps clear up laryngitis.

INVESTIGATION

If hoarseness persists for more than two weeks in anyone over the age of 40, it is essential to consult a physician. The physician will perform a *laryngoscopy* (examination of the larynx with a viewing tube) to exclude the possibility of cancer, which can be completely cured if diagnosed early.

Hodgkin's disease

Also known as Hodgkin's lymphoma, a malignant disorder of lymphoid tissue (found mainly in the *lymph nodes* and *spleen*) in which there is proliferation of its constituent cells and a resultant enlargement of the lymph nodes. The lymphoid tissues constitute an important part of the immune system and frequently do not function normally. The cause of Hodgkin's disease is unknown.

INCIDENCE

Hodgkin's disease is rare; about three new cases per 100,000 are diagnosed annually in the US. It is more common in men than women, and occurs with a peak incidence in people in their 20s and in people between 55 and 70 years of age.

SYMPTOMS AND SIGNS

The most common symptom is painless enlargement of a group of lymph nodes, typically those in the neck or armpits. Most other symptoms are caused by the presence of the enlarged nodes, invasion of other organs by proliferating lymphoid tissue, or impairment of the body's immune system. Thus, there may be a general feeling of illness, with fever, loss of appetite, weight loss, and night sweats. There may also be generalized itching and, rarely, pain after drinking alcohol. Involvement of other organs may cause a diverse range of symptoms (such as breathlessness if the lungs are involved or paralysis if the spine is affected). As the disease progresses, the immune system becomes increasingly impaired and the patient may suffer life-threatening complications from an infection that would be trivial in a healthy person.

DIAGNOSIS

For a positive diagnosis of Hodgkin's disease, it is necessary to identify cells (called Reed-Sternberg cells) having a characteristic appearance in a sample of tissue (obtained by *biopsy*) from an enlarged lymph node or from another organ affected by the Hodgkin's disease. In addition, the relative proportions of other surrounding cells—including plasma cells, eosinophils, lymphocytes, and granulocytes (all types of white blood cell)—are usually determined. This enables the disease to be classified according to its histological type, which is one factor that affects the chances of a cure.

The extent of the disease (known as its *stage*) is also assessed in terms of the number of groups of lymph nodes affected and in terms of any other organs that are involved. This process, called staging, is important for the planning of treatment. Typically, this assessment includes a *chest X ray*, *CT scanning* of the abdomen, and a *bone marrow biopsy*. Other tests may include *laparotomy* (surgical exploration of the abdomen) sometimes with node biopsies, liver biopsy, *splenectomy*, or *lymphangiography* (X-ray imaging of the lymphatic system) of the abdomen.

TREATMENT AND OUTLOOK

Treatment varies according to the stage of the disease. In an early stage, *radiation therapy* is usually curative. If the disease has progressed to involve many organs, however, *chemotherapy* with *anticancer drugs* is usually recommended; this treatment may need to be continued for several months. In some cases, both radiation therapy and chemotherapy are used to increase the chances of a cure.

The outlook depends on the stage to which the disease has progressed and on the histological type. However, after treatment, some 70 to 80 percent

of patients survive for at least five years. The condition is apparently cured in most people who receive treatment at an early stage. (See also *Lymphoma, non-Hodgkin's.*)

Hole in the heart

The common name for a *septal defect*.

Holistic medicine

A form of therapy aimed at treating the whole person—body and mind—not just the part or parts in which symptoms occur. A holistic approach is claimed to be emphasized by practitioners of *alternative medicine*, such as homeopathists, acupuncturists, and herbalists.

Holter monitor

A portable (worn by the patient), 24-hour electrocardiographic (see *ECG*) monitoring device used to detect paroxysmal *arrhythmias* (intermittent, irregular heart beats or palpitations). See also *Monitor*.

Shoulder strap

Electrodes

Tape recorder
containing
cassette

The Holter monitor
The patient wears the Holter monitor over one shoulder; electrodes attached to the chest transmit the heart rhythms to a slow-running cassette tape in the monitor.

Homatropine

An *anticholinergic drug* that is similar to, but less powerful than, *atropine*.

Homeopathy

A system of *alternative medicine* that seeks to treat patients by administering small doses of medicines that would bring on symptoms similar to those of the patient in a healthy person. For example, the homeopathic treatment for diarrhea would be a miniscule amount of a laxative.

Homeostasis

The dynamic processes by which an organism maintains a constant inter-

nal environment despite external changes. It is a major function of most organs. Examples of homeostatic mechanisms include the regulation of blood pressure, body temperature, and blood sugar levels.

Homeostasis plays a vital role in the body because tissues and organs can function efficiently only within a narrow range of conditions such as temperature and acidity. The homeostatic mechanisms regulate such conditions by negative feedback. When a certain factor varies from its optimum set point, automatic regulatory mechanisms act to counterbalance the disturbance and reestablish the internal equilibrium. For example, when the body overheats, sweating is stimulated until the temperature returns to normal. Similarly, when the level of oxygen in the blood is low, breathing is stimulated; when blood pressure falls, the heart rate increases.

Homeostatic mechanisms sometimes malfunction. For example, in malignant *hyperthermia*, the body's thermostat is somehow reset to a higher temperature than normal. In *diabetes mellitus*, blood sugar levels can no longer be regulated because of a malfunction of insulin production.

Homocystinuria

A rare, inherited condition caused by an *enzyme* deficiency. Homocystinuria is a type of inborn error of *metabolism* in which there is an abnormal presence of a particular *amino acid* (homocystine) in the blood and urine. Affected people resemble those with *Marfan's syndrome*—very tall and long-limbed with long, spindly fingers, and sometimes skeletal deformities (such as curvature of the spine).

The disease cannot be cured, but can be improved by vitamin B_6 and a special diet.

Homosexuality, female

See *Lesbianism*.

Homosexuality, male

Sexual attraction to other men. According to Alfred Kinsey's studies of sexuality carried out in the 1940s, about 5 to 10 percent of men are completely homosexual; up to one third of men have had sexual contact with another man at some time.

CHARACTERISTICS

Homosexuals are no more effeminate than heterosexuals, despite the popular stereotype. Each partner may adopt a particular role in the relationship (either active or passive) that may be reflected in styles of dress and behavior; more often, however, roles are interchangeable. Homosexuals achieve orgasm in various ways, including oral sex, mutual masturbation, and anal penetration.

Some male homosexuals have monogamous relationships. Others have multiple partners, high rates of sexual activity, and are consequently at high risk of venereal disease. It was in male homosexuals that the *AIDS* virus was first identified.

Homosexuality is more openly considered than it once was, but some homosexuals feel guilty about their sexual orientation. This may cause them to mask their feelings behind a cloak of apparent heterosexuality or to seek a medical cure.

CAUSES

Various theories have been put forward to explain homosexuality. Some studies have shown an increased incidence of homosexuality among men who had absent or weak fathers and who formed close emotional relationships with their mothers. Evidence for either a genetic tendency or a hormone imbalance is lacking.

The prevalence of homosexuality appears to be much the same in all cultures, with no change over thousands of years—suggesting that homosexuality is a consistent variation in behavior. (See also *Bisexuality*.)

Homozygote

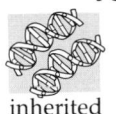
A term used to describe a person whose cells contain two identical *genes* controlling a specified inherited trait, in contrast to a *heterozygote*, whose cells contain two different genes controlling that trait. (See also *Inheritance*; *Genetic disorders*.)

Homunculus

From the Latin for "a little man." It may refer to a perfectly proportioned person of *short stature*; a fetus, by extension of the archaic theory that human germ cells contained minute human beings; a small model of a person, particularly one created by magic or alchemy; and, in psychiatry, a little man created by the imagination.

Hookworm infestation

An infestation of the small intestine by small, round, blood-sucking worms of the species NECATOR AMERICANUS or ANCYLOSTOMA DUODENALE. The worms are about half an inch long and have hooklike teeth.

HOOKWORM LIFE CYCLE

Infestation begins with larvae that penetrate the skin or are ingested and enter the bloodstream. They migrate throughout the body, particularly to the small intestine. Adult worms develop and lay eggs, which leave the body in feces and eventually hatch into larvae.

Head of hookworm
The hookworm uses its sharp, curved, toothlike structures to cling to the bowel.

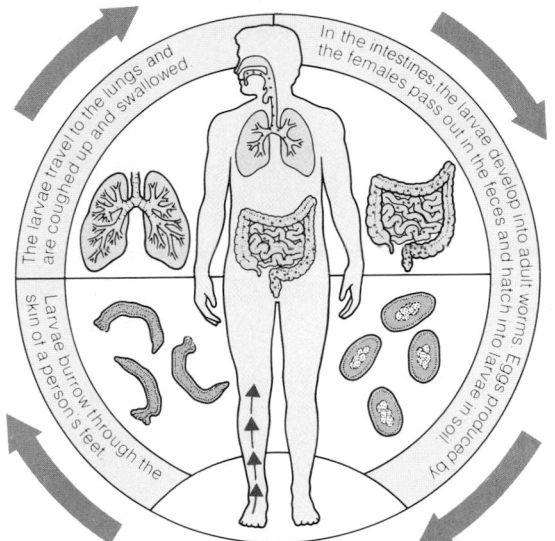

INCIDENCE AND CAUSES

Hookworms infest about 700 million people worldwide, mainly those living in poor countries in the tropics. There is very little risk of contracting a hookworm infestation in the US.

The illustration above shows how hookworms can enter and multiply in the body. In a heavy infestation, there may be several hundred worms in the intestine, consuming up to one tenth of a pint of blood every day.

SYMPTOMS AND COMPLICATIONS

When the larvae penetrate the skin, a red and intensely itchy rash may develop on the feet. This is called ground itch and may last for several days. In light infestations, no symptoms may be felt. In heavier infestations, migration of the larvae through the lungs may produce cough and pneumonia; the presence of adult worms in the intestines may cause vague abdominal discomfort.

By far the most important problem caused by a heavy infestation is iron-deficiency *anemia* due to loss of blood.

DIAGNOSIS AND TREATMENT

Diagnosis is made by microscopic examination of feces, which can reveal hookworm eggs. *Antihelmintic drugs*, such as mebendazole, kill the worms. Treatment also involves improving nutrition with a high-protein diet and correcting anemia with iron tablets or

blood transfusion, if necessary. Elimination of the disease from a community depends on efficient sanitation. (See also *Larva migrans*.)

Hormonal disorders

See *Endocrine system*.

Hormonal methods of contraception

See *Contraception, hormonal methods*.

Hormone antagonist

A drug that blocks the action of a hormone. *Tamoxifen*, for example, blocks the effects of *estrogen hormones* and is used in the treatment of some types of breast cancer.

Hormone replacement therapy

The use of a synthetic or natural hormone to treat a hormone deficiency. In its broadest sense, the term describes the replacement of any deficient hormone, such as giving thyroxine to treat *hypothyroidism* or *insulin* to treat *diabetes mellitus*. More commonly, however, the term hormone replacement therapy refers to the use of *estrogen hormones* to treat symptoms accompanying the *menopause*.

WHY IT IS DONE

Estrogen replacement therapy is given to relieve menopausal symptoms such as hot flashes and excessive sweating at night. Estrogen hormones help prevent atrophic *vaginitis* (dryness of the vagina) and shrinkage of the genitals, which may make sexual intercourse painful and difficult. Estrogen hormones also help prevent the develop-

ment of *osteoporosis* (a bone disorder) and *atherosclerosis* (narrowing of the arteries causing impaired blood flow).

HOW IT IS DONE

In hormone replacement therapy, estrogen drugs are usually prescribed

in combination with a *progesterone drug* (which can result in monthly spotting in place of menstruation) because estrogen drugs given alone may increase a woman's susceptibility to cancer of the uterus.

H

THE SOURCES AND MAIN EFFECTS OF SELECTED HORMONES

Section of body	Hormone secreted	Effects
Hypothalamus	Releasing hormones	Stimulate hormone secretion by pituitary gland
Pituitary gland	Growth hormone	Stimulates growth and metabolism
	Prolactin	Stimulates milk production after childbirth
	ACTH (adrenocorticotropic hormone)	Stimulates hormone production by adrenal glands.
	TSH (thyroid-stimulating hormone)	Stimulates hormone production by thyroid gland
	FSH (follicle-stimulating hormone); LH (luteinizing hormone)	Stimulate gonads (ovaries or testes)
	ADH (antidiuretic hormone)	Acts on kidneys to reduce urine production.
	Oxytocin	Stimulates contractions of uterus during labor and ejection of milk during breast-feeding
	MSH (melanocyte-stimulating hormone)	Acts on the skin to promote production of skin pigment (melanin)
Brain	Endorphins; enkephalins	Alleviate pain
Thyroid gland	Thyroid hormone	Increases metabolic rate; affects growth
	Calcitonin	Controls level of calcium in blood
Parathyroid glands	Parathyroid hormone	Controls level of calcium in blood
Thymus	Thymic hormone	Stimulates lymphocyte development
Adrenal glands	Epinephrine; norepinephrine	Prepare body for stress
	Hydrocortisone	Affects metabolism
	Aldosterone	Regulates sodium and potassium excretion by kidneys
	Androgens	Affect growth and, in women, sex drive
Kidneys	Renin	Regulates blood pressure
	Erythropoietin	Stimulates erythrocyte production
	Vitamin D	Controls calcium and phosphorus metabolism
Pancreas	Insulin; glucagon	Regulate blood sugar level
Placenta	Chorionic gonadotropin; estrogens; progesterone	Maintain pregnancy
Gastrointestinal tract	Gastrin; secretin; cholecystokinin	Regulate secretion of some digestive enzymes
Testes	Testosterone	Affects development of male secondary sexual characteristics and genital organs
Ovaries	Estrogens; progesterone	Affect development of female secondary sexual characteristics and genital organs; control menstrual cycle; maintain pregnancy

The various glands that make up the hormonal system constitute a control and communications network that is complementary to the nervous system. However, instead of using nerve impulses, the glands secrete chemical messengers (hormones) to affect other glands and tissues in various parts of the body. Hormones are carried in the bloodstream to their targets, where they exert their specific effects. This table lists the hormones secreted by different parts of the body and gives a description of their wide-ranging actions.

The drugs are usually taken orally in a three-stage cycle repeated each month—estrogen for the first 11 to 14 days, estrogen and progesterone for the next seven to 10 days, and no drugs for the last seven days.

Alternatively, an implant containing estrogen is placed under the skin of the abdomen. The estrogen is released slowly and progesterone is taken in tablet form.

Therapy is usually continued for between two and five years. Regular tests, including weight and blood pressure checks, breast and pelvic examinations, and cervical smears, are carried out to monitor the effects of the therapy. Occasionally, a *biopsy* of the lining of the uterus may be carried out to test for cancer.

POSSIBLE ADVERSE EFFECTS
Minor adverse effects include nausea, breast tenderness, fluid retention, and leg cramps. In some women, estrogen replacement therapy may increase the risk of abnormal blood clotting. It is therefore not usually given to women who smoke heavily or have suffered from *thrombosis*, *stroke*, liver disease, or severe *hypertension* (raised blood pressure). Women who have had cancer of the breast or uterus are also not usually given hormone replacement therapy because estrogen may increase the risk of recurrence.

Hormones
A group of chemicals (such as *cortisol*, *estrogen*, *insulin*, and *epinephrine*), each of which is released into the bloodstream by a particular gland or tissue to have a specific effect on tissues elsewhere in the body. Hormones control numerous body functions, including the *metabolism* (chemical activity) of cells, growth, sexual development, and the body's response to stress or illness.

Glands that primarily produce hormones make up the *endocrine system*, which comprises the *adrenal glands*, gonads (*ovaries* or *testes*), *pancreas*, *parathyroid glands*, *pituitary gland*, *placenta* (in pregnant women), and *thyroid gland*. Hormones are also secreted by other organs, including the kidneys, intestines, and brain.

Horn, cutaneous
A hard, noncancerous protrusion occasionally found on the skin (usually the face) of elderly people. Horns are slow growing and vary in color from yellow to brown to black. They may develop where there was previously a wart on normal skin.

Appearance of cutaneous horn
The horny protuberance that has developed under the arm results from an overgrowth of keratin (a skin protein).

Left untreated, they can grow to a considerable size and may protrude as much as 0.75 inch (2 cm). Surgical removal is usually recommended.

Horner's syndrome
A group of physical signs that affects one side of the face and indicates damage to part of the sympathetic nervous system (see *Autonomic nervous system*). The signs are narrowing of the pupil of the eye (miosis), drooping of the lid (ptosis), and absence of sweating (anhidrosis). They are caused by damage to or destruction of sympathetic nerve fibers, usually in the lower part of the neck, and may be the first sign of disease in the area.

Hornet stings
See *Insect stings*.

Horseshoe kidney
A congenital abnormality in which the two kidneys are joined at the base, forming a horseshoe shape, rather than being separate. Horseshoe kidney affects about one person in 600; it is twice as common in men.

The joined kidneys usually function normally and cause no problems.

Hospice
A hospital or part of a hospital devoted to the care of patients who are dying, often from one specified cause. One hospice may thus care only for AIDS patients, another for cancer patients, and another for those dying of old age (see *Dying, care of the*).

Hospitals, types of
The roughly 7,000 hospitals in the US, which maintain about 1.3 million beds, can be classified in many ways. There are government hospitals—federal, state, county, and municipal.

Many hospitals are owned and run by religious orders. Though graduate medical education is conducted in many hospitals, teaching hospitals generally have a close affiliation with universities and medical schools. A growing number of hospitals are owned by for-profit corporations. Far more are community hospitals that depend on community-generated contributions. By far the largest number of hospitals are classified as short-term acute care general hospitals.

Hot flashes
Reddening of the face, neck, and upper trunk usually facilitated by decreased *estrogen hormone* production by the ovaries during or after the *menopause*. A hot flash typically lasts one to two minutes and is accompanied by a sensation of heat; it is often followed by sweating. Hot flashes are aggravated when the sufferer is under stress.

Hot flashes may also occur after a total *hysterectomy*, in which the uterus and the ovaries are removed. Occasionally, men experience hot flashes after *orchiectomy* (removal of a testis), which causes a reduction in testosterone levels. If hot flashes are severe, they can usually be alleviated by *hormone replacement therapy*.

Housemaid's knee
Inflammation of the *bursa* that acts as a cushion over the kneecap. The inflammation is usually caused by prolonged kneeling, but may develop after a sharp blow to the front of the knee. (See also *Bursitis*.)

HTLV III
Human T-cell lymphotropic virus, strain III, a name once used for the virus that causes *AIDS*. The organism is now called *HIV*.

Human chorionic gonadotropin
See *Gonadotropin, human chorionic*.

Humerus
The bone of the upper arm. The smooth, dome-shaped head of the bone lies at an angle to the shaft and fits into a shallow socket in the scapula (shoulder blade) to form the shoulder joint. Below the head, the bone narrows to form a cylindrical shaft. It flattens and widens at its lower end, forming a prominence on each side called an epicondyle. At its base, the humerus articulates with the ulna and radius (the bones of the lower arm) to form the elbow.

H

LOCATION OF HUMERUS
The humerus is the bone of the upper arm, located between the shoulder and elbow joints.

Shoulder

Clavicle

Scapula

Humerus

Elbow

Ulna

Radius

A spiral groove in the shaft of the humerus carries the *radial nerve*, the major nerve of the arm.

Humerus, fracture of

The most usual site of fracture of the humerus (the bone of the upper arm), especially in the elderly, is at the neck of the bone, just below the head. Fracture of the lower end of the bone (a supracondylar fracture) occurs most commonly in children. The fracture may be accompanied by damage to the brachial artery. If injury to this artery goes undetected, it may impair circulation to the arm, resulting in *Volkmann's contracture*, a deformity of the forearm and hand due to muscle damage caused by *ischemia* (insufficient blood supply).

Any suspected fracture of the humerus is first X rayed. If the neck of the bone is found to be fractured, it usually requires only a sling to keep the bone immobilized; a supracondylar fracture usually needs to be put in a plaster cast.

A fractured humerus normally takes six to eight weeks to heal. However, supracondylar fractures sometimes fail to mend properly, resulting in deformity of the elbow.

Humors

Liquid or jellylike substances in the body. The term usually refers to the aqueous humor (the watery fluid in the front chamber of the *eye*) and vitreous humor (the jellylike substance in the rear chamber of the eye).

According to early medical theory, there were four humors—blood, phlegm, black bile, and yellow bile—that permeated the entire body and determined its state of health. This theory was generally discarded in the 17th century.

Hump back

See *Kyphosis*.

Hunch back

See *Kyphosis*.

Hunger

A disagreeable feeling caused by the need for food (as opposed to *appetite*, a pleasant sensation felt in anticipation of a meal).

Hunger occurs when the stomach is empty and when the blood sugar level is low. In response to these stimuli, the hypothalamus in the brain indirectly causes the muscular wall of the stomach to contract rhythmically, signaling the need for food; if pronounced, these contractions produce hunger pains.

Hunger caused by a low blood sugar level is usually the result of strenuous exercise. However, it can also occur in certain diseases (notably *thyrotoxicosis*, which is marked by a speeding-up of body processes) and insulin-dependent *diabetes mellitus* if an incorrect balance between insulin and carbohydrate intake causes *hypoglycemia*.

Huntington's chorea

An uncommon disease in which degeneration of the basal ganglia (paired nerve cell clusters in the brain) results in *chorea* (rapid, jerky, involuntary movements) and *dementia* (progressive mental impairment). Symptoms do not usually appear until the age of 35 to 50; in rare cases the condition is apparent in childhood.

Huntington's chorea is a *genetic disorder* with an autosomal pattern of inheritance. Because the age of onset of symptoms is generally so late, an affected person may bear children before realizing that he or she has the disease. Each child has a 50 percent chance of the condition developing. The disease develops in about 5 persons per 100,000 in the US.

SYMPTOMS
The chorea usually affects the face, arms, and trunk, resulting in random grimaces and twitches and general clumsiness. Dementia takes the form of personality and behavior changes, irritability, difficulty making decisions, memory loss, and apathy.

When the disease starts in childhood, it may be marked by loss of movement and muscle rigidity.

DIAGNOSIS
Until recently there was no way of detecting whether a child of a person with Huntington's chorea had inherited the abnormal gene responsible for the condition. As a result of recent advances in genetics, young adults with parents who have the condition can now learn, with 95 percent accuracy, whether or not they have the abnormal gene and thus have the disorder. This may affect their decisions on whether to have children themselves (see *Genetic counseling*).

TREATMENT AND OUTLOOK
There is no known cure. Treatment is aimed at lessening the chorea with drugs, such as chlorpromazine (which was investigational in 1987), and alleviating the effects of dementia with good nursing care.

Most sufferers survive for about 15 years after the onset of symptoms; some live for up to 30 years afterward.

Hurler's syndrome

A rare, inherited condition caused by an *enzyme* defect. Hurler's syndrome is a type of inborn error of *metabolism* in which there is an abnormal accumulation of substances called mucopolysaccharides in the tissues.

Affected children may appear normal at birth, but, between 6 and 12 months of age, cardiac abnormalities, umbilical hernia, skeletal deformities, and enlargement of the tongue, liver, and spleen develop. Physical growth is limited and mental development slows, leaving the child mentally retarded. The strange features of affected children gave the condition its former name of gargoylism.

Hydatid disease

 A rare infestation caused by the larval stage of the small tapeworm *ECHINOCOCCUS GRANULOSUS*. The larvae settle in the liver, lungs, or the brain or other organs and cause the development of slowly growing cysts.

CAUSE AND INCIDENCE
The illustration on the next page shows how eggs or larvae can enter the body.

Hydatid disease is prevalent only in areas of the world where sheep are reared with the aid of dogs, including some parts of California and Utah. About 200 cases of hydatid disease are diagnosed in the US each year.

SYMPTOMS AND TREATMENT

Although the infestation is usually acquired in childhood, the cysts grow very slowly, so symptoms, if any, occur mainly in adults. In many cases there are no symptoms. However, a cyst in the liver may cause a tender, localized lump or lead to *bile duct obstruction* and jaundice. In the lungs, a cyst may press on an airway, causing *bronchitis*. Rupture of a cyst can cause chest pain, hemoptysis (coughing up blood), wheezing (if present in the lung), or *anaphylactic shock* (a severe allergic reaction). Cysts in the brain can cause seizures or other symptoms similar to those of a brain tumor.

Hydatid cysts are diagnosed by *CT scanning*. Treatment of cysts that are causing symptoms consists of surgical removal, or sterilization followed by drainage. Newer antiparasite drugs are under investigation.

Hydatidiform mole

An uncommon benign tumor that develops from placental tissue during an early pregnancy in which the embryo has failed to develop normally. A hydatidiform mole, which resembles a bunch of small grapes, is caused by degeneration of the chorionic villi, minute fingerlike projections in the placenta. The cause of the degeneration is unknown.

INCIDENCE

A hydatidiform mole is the most common form of *trophoblastic* disease. It occurs in about one in 2,000 pregnancies in developed countries; the incidence is much higher in developing areas. In about 3 percent of affected pregnancies the growth develops into a *choriocarcinoma*, a malignant tumor that can invade the walls of the uterus if left untreated.

SYMPTOMS AND DIAGNOSIS

There is usually vaginal bleeding and excessive morning sickness. The diagnosis is made by *ultrasound scanning* and from urine and blood tests. The mole produces excessive amounts of the hormone human chorionic *gonadotropin* (HCG), which can be detected in urine and blood.

TREATMENT

The tumor can be removed either by suctioning out the contents of the uterus or by a *D and C*. A *hysterectomy* may be considered.

OUTLOOK

There is a small risk that a malignant tumor may develop later; for this

ORIGINS OF HYDATID DISEASE

The infestation is generally confined to dogs and sheep, but occasionally a child swallows eggs from dog feces. These hatch into larvae, which migrate through the body, especially to the liver or lungs, to form slow-growing cysts. Symptoms may not appear until years later.

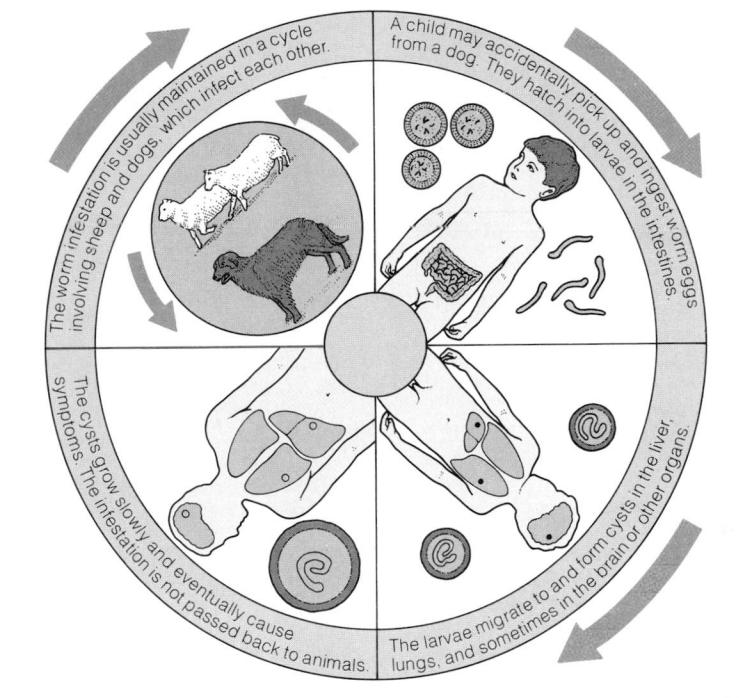

reason, tests are performed regularly for several years to determine the levels of HCG in the blood and urine.

A woman should not become pregnant again until her HCG levels have returned to normal for at least a year. There is a one in 75 risk of the growth recurring in a future pregnancy.

Hydralazine

An *antihypertensive drug* that is particularly useful as an emergency treatment for *hypertension*. Hydralazine is often also used when the combination of *diuretic* and *beta-blocker drugs* fails to control high blood pressure.

Hydralazine may cause nausea, vomiting, headache, dizziness, and irregular heart beat. Less common adverse effects include loss of appetite, rash, and joint pain. When prescribed in high doses over a prolonged period, hydralazine may cause *lupus erythematosus*.

Hydramnios

Excess *amniotic fluid* in the uterus during pregnancy. Hydramnios occurs in about one in 250 pregnancies.

CAUSES

In many cases, there is no known cause for hydramnios. It sometimes occurs if the fetus has a malformation (particularly *anencephaly* or *esophageal atresia*) that makes normal swallowing impossible. Hydramnios may also occur if the pregnant woman has *diabetes mellitus*. It occurs in about 10 percent of multiple pregnancies.

SYMPTOMS AND SIGNS

An excess of amniotic fluid usually accumulates slowly during the second half of the pregnancy, producing symptoms from about week 32. The main symptom is abdominal discomfort. Other possible symptoms are breathlessness and edema of the legs. The uterus is larger than usual for the duration of the pregnancy.

Less commonly, the fluid accumulates rapidly, causing abdominal pain, breathlessness, nausea, and vomiting. The abdomen becomes tense, the overlying skin is stretched and shiny, and the legs swell. Hydramnios may cause premature labor and the baby may not be in the usual delivery position (see *Malpresentation*).

DIAGNOSIS

Hydramnios is usually evident from the patient's history and a physical examination. *Ultrasound scanning* is needed to detect fetal abnormality or multiple pregnancy.

TREATMENT

In the case of severe fetal abnormality, a therapeutic *abortion* may be performed. Mild cases without fetal abnormality require no treatment other than extra rest. Withdrawal of amniotic fluid via a needle inserted through the abdominal wall can provide relief in severe cases although the procedure may cause premature labor. If the pregnant woman has diabetes mellitus, careful attention must be paid to her diabetic control. If symptoms occur in late pregnancy, *induction of labor* may be performed to deliver the baby early.

Hydrocele

A soft, painless swelling in the scrotum caused by the space around the testis filling with fluid. A hydrocele is sometimes caused by inflammation, infection, or injury to the testis. Occasionally, a tumor may cause fluid to accumulate, but in most cases there is no apparent cause. Hydroceles occur very commonly in middle-aged men.

Treatment is rarely necessary. If the swelling is large enough to be uncomfortable or painful, the fluid may be aspirated (drawn off through a hollow needle) using local anesthetic. The most common surgical method of dealing with recurrent swelling is to remove the lining around the testis.

Hydrocephalus

An excessive amount of *cerebrospinal fluid*, usually under increased pressure, within the skull. The term "water on the brain" is sometimes used to describe the condition. Hydrocephalus is often associated with other congenital abnormalities, particularly *spina bifida*.

CAUSES

The condition may be *congenital* (present at birth) or may develop as a result of major head injury, brain hemorrhage, infection (*meningitis*, for example), or a tumor.

Hydrocephalus is caused by excessive formation of cerebrospinal fluid, by a block in the circulation of this fluid, or both.

SYMPTOMS

When the condition is congenital, the main feature is an enlarged head that continues to grow at an abnormally

Infant with hydrocephalus
Skull enlargement is due to pressure from excess fluid within the cavities of the brain. To prevent brain damage, the fluid must be drained by means of a tube inserted through a hole made in the skull.

fast rate because the bones are not rigid and expand to accommodate the fluid. Other features are rigidity of the legs, *epilepsy*, irritability, lethargy, vomiting, and the absence of normal reflex actions. If the condition is not treated, it progresses to extreme drowsiness, severe brain damage, and seizures, which may lead to the baby's death within a matter of weeks.

When the condition occurs later in childhood or in adulthood, the skull is no longer flexible and symptoms are caused by raised pressure within the skull. Symptoms include headache, vomiting, loss of coordination, and deterioration of mental function.

DIAGNOSIS AND TREATMENT

CT scanning or *MRI* show the location and nature of any obstruction.

In most cases, treatment aims to drain excess fluid away from the brain to another part of the body, such as the lining of the abdomen or chest wall, where it can be absorbed. Drainage is achieved by means of a *shunt* (tube), which is inserted into the brain through a hole made in the skull. In some cases, the shunt must be left in position indefinitely. In older children and adults, treatment is sometimes for the underlying cause only.

Hydrochloric acid

A strong acid released by the stomach lining. It forms part of the stomach juices and is important in the digestion of proteins. Excessive acid production, which may be stimulated by stress or tobacco smoking, is an important factor in the development of *peptic ulcers*. *Acid reflux* (regurgitation of stomach acid into the esophagus) resulting in *esophagitis* and heartburn is another problem created by hydrochloric acid secretion. (See also *Digestive system*.)

Hydrochlorothiazide

A thiazide *diuretic drug* used to reduce *edema* (fluid retention) in people with *heart failure* (reduced pumping efficiency), *nephrotic syndrome* (a kidney disorder), *cirrhosis* of the liver, and breast tenderness before menstruation. Hydrochlorothiazide is also given to treat *hypertension* (high blood pressure), and is occasionally used to prevent the recurrence of certain types of kidney stones.

POSSIBLE ADVERSE EFFECTS

Adverse effects include leg cramps, lethargy, dizziness, rash, and impotence. Hydrochlorothiazide may (rarely) cause *gout* and may aggravate *diabetes mellitus*.

Hydrocortisone

CORTICOSTEROID		
Tablet Injection Rectal suppository Cream Eye drops		
📇	Prescription sometimes needed	
🔳	Available as generic	

A *corticosteroid drug* sometimes used to treat inflammatory and allergic disorders, such as *dermatitis*, *uveitis*, *ulcerative colitis*, types of *arthritis*, and *asthma*. Hydrocortisone is chemically identical to *cortisol*, a hormone produced by the adrenal glands. Hydrocortisone is therefore given to replace this hormone when the amount produced by the body is insufficient, as in *Addison's disease*.

POSSIBLE ADVERSE EFFECTS

Hydrocortisone creams used in excess may cause thinning of the skin. Taken by mouth over a prolonged period, high doses of hydrocortisone may cause *diabetes mellitus*, *glaucoma*, *osteoporosis*, *peptic ulcer*, fluid retention, weight gain, acne, muscle weakness, mood changes, and retarded growth in children.

Hydrogen peroxide

An *antiseptic* solution used to treat infections of the skin or mouth and to bleach hair. Hydrogen peroxide combines with catalase, an enzyme present in the skin and mouth, to release oxygen. This effect kills bacteria and cleanses infected areas. Hydrogen peroxide occasionally causes soreness and irritation.

Hydronephrosis

A condition in which the kidney becomes distended with urine due to a blockage or narrowing of the *ureter*. If left untreated, hydronephrosis can severely damage the kidney and, if bilateral, cause *renal failure*.

CAUSES
Obstruction of a ureter is usually caused by a stone (see *Calculus, urinary tract*), a *kidney tumor*, or sometimes by a blood clot. Alternatively, the urine in the bladder may be under pressure caused by obstruction of its outflow from an enlarged prostate gland. In some cases, constriction of the ureter is present from birth.

SYMPTOMS AND SIGNS
Acute hydronephrosis, with sudden blockage of the ureter, results in severe pain in the small of the back. Chronic hydronephrosis, in which the obstruction develops slowly, may, however, cause no symptoms until the ureter has become completely blocked and renal failure occurs. There is also a risk that the kidney may become infected, resulting in pyonephrosis (pus-filled kidney).

DIAGNOSIS AND TREATMENT
Ultrasound scanning can provide an image of the kidneys and ureter. If it reveals obstruction and the kidney is still relatively healthy, the blockage is removed or relieved by surgery; the kidney soon resumes normal functioning. Occasionally, however, the kidney is so badly damaged that it requires removal (see *Nephrectomy*). In this case, the remaining kidney compensates for the loss of the other.

Hydrophobia
A popular term—now almost obsolete—for *rabies*. Meaning "fear of water," hydrophobia refers to the inability to drink that is one of the characteristic symptoms of rabies.

Hydrops
An abnormal accumulation of fluid in the body tissues or in a sac (such as the gallbladder). Hydrops fetalis is marked generalized *edema* (fluid collection causing tissue swelling) affecting the fetus. It may occur in pregnancy as a result of severe *hemolytic disease of the newborn*.

Hydrotherapy
 The external use of water to treat patients recovering from injury or suffering from lack of mobility. It includes the use of exercise pools, whirlpool baths, and showers.

People who are unable to bear full weight on a limb (because of arthritis or after a fracture, for example) often can exercise more fully and effectively in a hydrotherapy pool. The buoyant effect of the water allows a greater range of movement and permits fuller use of the limb with little discomfort.

Warm whirlpool baths provide a gentle massage to stimulate areas of the body and relieve stiffness. Cold baths or showers can reduce blood flow, swelling, and bruising after injury and minimize tissue damage. (See also *Heat treatment*; *Ice packs*.)

Hydroxocobalamin
A long-acting synthetic preparation of *vitamin B₁₂*.

Hydroxyprogesterone
A *progesterone drug* given by injection to treat cancer of the uterus (see *Uterus, cancer of*) and certain types of *breast cancer*.

Hydroxyzine
An *antihistamine drug* commonly used in the treatment of *urticaria* (hives) and other allergic rashes. Hydroxyzine is also used as a *premedication* before surgery, in the management of alcohol withdrawal, and, occasionally, in the short-term treatment of mild anxiety. It is also used to relieve nausea and vomiting in *motion sickness*, *vertigo*, and following a general anesthetic.

Possible adverse effects include drowsiness, dry mouth, and tremor.

Hygiene
The science and practice of preserving health. Today the word is commonly equated with cleanliness. However, in the early years of this century the term hygiene was widely used as an equivalent to *public health*—the scientific study of environmental influences on health (especially the provision of pure water supplies, safe sanitation, good housing, and safe conditions in the workplace).

Hygiene, oral
See *Oral hygiene*.

Hygienist, dental
A licensed professional who is qualified to carry out *scaling* (the removal of calculus from the teeth) and to demonstrate methods of keeping the teeth and gums healthy (see *Oral hygiene*). Keeping the teeth and gums healthy is especially important in preventing or controlling gum disorders occurring in middle life, such as *gingivitis* and *periodontitis*.

Hygroma, cystic
A type of *lymphangioma*.

Hymen
The thin fold of membrane surrounding the vaginal opening. The hymen has a central perforation that is usually stretched or torn by the use of tampons or during first sexual intercourse. Once torn, the hymen becomes an irregular ring of tissue around the vaginal opening.

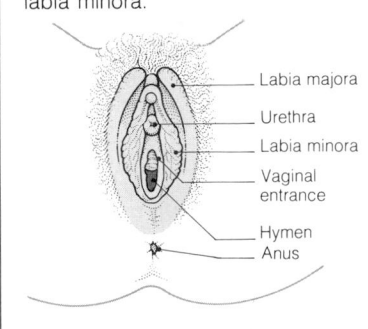

LOCATION OF HYMEN
The membrane that forms the hymen surrounds the opening to the vagina, inside the woman's labia minora.

- Labia majora
- Urethra
- Labia minora
- Vaginal entrance
- Hymen
- Anus

Imperforate hymen is a rare condition in which the hymen has no perforation; at the onset of menstruation, menstrual blood collects in the vagina, causing lower abdominal pain. It is corrected by minor surgery.

Hyoid
A small, U-shaped bone situated deep in the muscles at the back of the tongue. It is not joined to any other bone but is suspended by ligaments

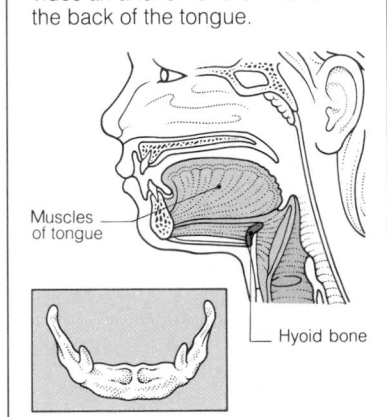

LOCATION OF HYOID BONE
The U-shaped hyoid bone provides an anchor for the muscles at the back of the tongue.

Muscles of tongue

Hyoid bone

H

from the base of the skull. Its function is to provide an anchor point for the muscles of the tongue and for those in the upper part of the front of the neck.

The hyoid is commonly fractured in homicidal strangulation.

Hyoscyamine

An *anticholinergic drug* used to treat the spasm of the bladder muscle that occurs with an *irritable bladder* and the spasm of the intestinal wall that accompanies *irritable bowel syndrome*.

Hyper-

A prefix meaning above, excessive, or greater than normal, as in *hypertension* (raised blood pressure) and *hyperthyroidism* (overactivity of the thyroid gland).

Hyperacidity

A condition in which an excessive amount of acid is produced by the stomach. Hyperacidity is commonly confused with *acid reflux* (which causes a burning sensation in the upper abdomen or lower chest) or a sudden filling of the person's mouth with a fluid (water brash). Most people with a duodenal ulcer (see *Peptic ulcer*) produce more acid than normal, and those with *Zollinger-Ellison syndrome* produce vast amounts.

Hyperactivity

A behavior pattern of certain children who are constantly overactive and have difficulty concentrating on one activity. Also known as hyperkinetic syndrome, the condition may affect as many as 5 to 10 percent of children in the US. It is four to five times more common in boys than girls.

CAUSES

It has been suggested that some hyperactive children, especially those who are clumsy, may have a subtle form of "minimal" brain damage. However, there is no definite, conclusive evidence. Hyperactive children seem more likely to have fathers who were hyperactive, so the condition may be partly inherited. Children with *mental retardation*, *cerebral palsy*, or *temporal lobe epilepsy* are also more likely to be hyperactive.

SYMPTOMS

The main feature of hyperactivity is continual overactivity, which is often worse in the classroom or in a group situation; it may not be evident during an interview by a physician. Hyperactive children are always on the go, full of energy, fidgety, and seem to sleep less than their peers. In addition, they tend to be impulsive and reckless, with no sense of danger, and are usually irritable, emotionally immature, and aggressive. Their attention span is short and, as a result, they do not conform to orderly routine.

Hyperactivity often leads to antisocial acts and difficulty learning, although IQ is normal. It is uncertain whether this behavior is a part of the disorder or simply a result of an affected child's poor attention span and disruptive activity.

DIAGNOSIS

Overactivity in itself does not indicate that hyperactivity is present, since overactivity can be caused by a stressful home environment or physical illness. In addition, many of the behavioral problems mentioned are, to some degree, common to all young children. However, when other causes have been eliminated and the behavior continues past the age of 4 years, is intense, and is different from that of "normal" children, then it is reasonable to regard the child as being hyperactive.

TREATMENT

Paradoxically, *stimulant drugs* (amphetamine or methylphenidate) seem to be the most effective treatment. This suggests that hyperactivity results from "underarousal" of the midbrain, which causes no damping down or control of movements and sensations. Stimulant drugs seem to work by stimulating the midbrain enough to suppress the extra activity. Behavior therapy and counseling of the child and parents are also useful.

Diets that exclude certain artificial food colorings, additives, or foods are popular and heavily promoted, but research has shown that these diets benefit very few children.

Hyperactive children should have formal educational and psychological assessment; many need help at school with reading and spelling.

OUTLOOK

In many cases, hyperactivity disappears completely at puberty. In others, the overactivity subsides and is replaced by sluggishness, depression, and moodiness; these teenagers often fail at school and resort to antisocial and criminal behavior. Sometimes all the symptoms of hyperactivity continue into adult life.

Hyperacusis

An exceptionally developed sense of hearing. It may cause the sensation of pain or discomfort in the ears on exposure to loud noises.

Hyperaldosteronism

An alternative name for *aldosteronism*, or Conn's syndrome, a metabolic disorder caused by overproduction of the hormone aldosterone (secreted by the cortex of the adrenal gland).

Hyperalimentation

Administration of nutrients to patients unable to take food by mouth. (See *Feeding, artificial*.)

Hyperbaric oxygen treatment

A method of increasing the amount of oxygen in the tissues by exposing a person to oxygen at a much higher than normal atmospheric pressure.

WHY IT IS DONE

The technique is occasionally used to treat poisoning from *carbon monoxide*, in which the tissues are starved of oxygen because *hemoglobin* (the oxygen-carrying component of red blood cells) is prevented from taking up oxygen. Hyperbaric oxygen treatment is also used in cases of gas *gangrene*; the bacteria that infect gangrenous tissue cannot survive if they are oxygenated.

HOW IT IS DONE

The patient is placed in a chamber into which oxygen is pumped at up to three times normal atmospheric pressure for no more than three hours. The oxygen is inhaled and dissolves in the blood.

Hyperbilirubinemia

A raised blood level of bilirubin (a waste product formed from the destruction of red blood cells). Hyperbilirubinemia may be undetectable except by a blood test, but *jaundice* becomes apparent if the blood bilirubin level rises to two times the normal level. Both have similar causes and implications.

Hypercalcemia

An abnormally high level of calcium in the blood. Normally the blood carries (in the plasma) less than 0.1 percent of the body's total amount of calcium—the optimum amount for the efficient functioning of cells throughout the body. A raised level or a lowered one (hypocalcemia) may seriously disrupt cell function, particularly in muscles and nerves.

CAUSES

The most common cause of hypercalcemia is secondary *bone cancer*, which releases calcium from an affected bone into the blood. Other causes include *hyperparathyroidism* (overproduction of parathyroid hormone, which helps control the blood calcium level); certain inflammatory disorders, such as *sarcoidosis*; taking too much vitamin D, which helps regulate the absorption of calcium from the diet; a diet too rich in foods containing calcium; or, infrequently, taking large amounts of calcium-containing antacids.

SYMPTOMS

Mild hypercalcemia causes nausea, vomiting, lethargy, and excessive urination. Higher levels of calcium in the blood produce confusion, extreme fatigue, and muscle weakness. If the disorder is untreated and the blood calcium level continues to increase, arrhythmia (irregular heart beat), coma, and even death may result. Long-standing mild hypercalcemia may cause kidney calcifications, or stones, to form.

DIAGNOSIS

The condition is diagnosed by tests that measure the blood calcium level. If the diagnosis is confirmed, more tests are performed to discover and treat the underlying cause.

Hypercapnia

Excessive carbon dioxide in the blood. Carbon dioxide is a waste product of the metabolic processes that produce energy in body cells; dissolved in body fluids, it forms carbonic acid. The blood circulation carries the acid to the lungs, where it is eliminated from the body as carbon dioxide during exhalation. The amount of carbonic acid in the blood is normally maintained within narrow limits by mechanisms such as the breathing rate. However, if these mechanisms fail to remove enough carbon dioxide from the body (which may occur as a result of impaired breathing), carbonic acid accumulates and the blood becomes too acidic, a condition called *acidosis*.

Hyperemesis

The medical term for excessive *vomiting*, as in hyperemesis gravidarum (vomiting during pregnancy that causes dehydration and weight loss).

Hyperglycemia

An abnormally high level of glucose (sugar) in the blood. The condition occurs in people suffering from untreated or inadequately controlled *diabetes mellitus*; it may also occur in diabetics as a result of an infection, stress, or surgery.

The symptoms of hyperglycemia are the same as those of diabetes: thirst, the passing of large amounts of urine, *glycosuria* (glucose in the urine), and *ketosis* (an accumulation of ketones in the body). In severe cases, hyperglycemia may lead to confusion and coma, which require emergency medical treatment with insulin and an intravenous infusion of fluids.

Hypergonadism

Overproduction of estrogen or androgen *hormones* by the *ovaries* or *testes*, causing precocious sexual development and excessive growth.

Hyperhidrosis

A disorder marked by excessive sweating that occurs at times other than in hot conditions or during or just after exercise. It usually begins at puberty and worsens in the summer, affecting the palms, soles, armpits, or all three. Hyperhidrosis may cause the sufferer distress. The constantly moist hands that result may rule out certain occupations and activities, and excessively sweaty armpits or feet may produce an unpleasant *body odor*, which can cause social embarrassment. In many sufferers, the condition improves on its own in the middle 20s or early 30s.

TREATMENT

Treatment includes taking *anticholinergic drugs* and applying aluminum chloride paint to the affected areas to block the sweat pores. Wearing clothing and shoes made of natural, absorbent materials (such as cotton and leather) can be helpful.

Hyperkeratosis

Thickening of the outer layer of the skin due to an increased amount of *keratin* (a tough protein that is the major component of the outer layer of skin). The most common forms of hyperkeratosis are *corns* and *calluses*, caused by prolonged pressure or friction, and *plantar warts*. Hyperkeratosis also occurs in *lichen planus*.

The term is also used to describe thickening of the nails in people with a fungal nail infection or in people with *psoriasis* (a skin condition).

Hyperkinetic syndrome

Another name for *hyperactivity*.

Hyperlipidemias

A group of metabolic disorders characterized by high levels of lipids in the blood. Hyperlipidemias are the most common of the lipid disorders and are an important factor in the health disorders of middle-aged, sedentary people.

TYPES

There are six types of hyperlipidemia, differentiated principally by the extent to which the blood levels of various fatty substances are higher than normal. The characteristics of each type of hyperlipidemia, along with their symptoms and treatment, are given in the table on the next page. Many of the types produce similar symptoms; diagnosis usually depends on blood tests to measure the levels of lipids.

Lipids are carried in the blood in several forms, chiefly cholesterol, triglycerides, and lipoproteins. Lipoproteins consist of fat and cholesterol molecules linked to protein molecules. There are different types: very low-density lipoproteins (VLDLs), low-density lipoproteins (LDLs), and intermediate-density lipoproteins (IDLs). There are also high-density lipoproteins (HDLs), but they are not involved in the hyperlipidemias. Lipoproteins are differentiated according to their relative proportions of cholesterol and protein. The higher the proportion of cholesterol, the lower the density of the lipoprotein. Chylomicrons (microscopic droplets in the blood containing triglycerides, cholesterol, and protein) are usually also classed as lipoproteins.

CAUSES

Each type of hyperlipidemia may be inherited or may be secondary to another disorder. The main secondary causes for each type are: Type I—systemic lupus erythematosus (SLE), Types IIa and IIb—hypothyroidism, nephrotic syndrome, Cushing's syndrome, and corticosteroid therapy; Type III—hypothyroidism and SLE; Types IV and V—diabetes mellitus, obesity, alcoholism, nephrotic syndrome, renal failure, and corticosteroid therapy or estrogen therapy.

RISKS

There is some evidence that the hyperlipidemias are associated with a number of serious disorders, notably *atherosclerosis* and *coronary heart disease*. For this reason, if a close relative has or had either of these disorders, particularly if he or she has had a heart attack at an early age (under 50), other members of the family should be tested. Treatment is given to reduce the blood lipid levels and thus lower the risk of atherosclerosis.

Hypermetropia

See *Hyperopia*.

TYPES OF HYPERLIPIDEMIA

Type	Lipoprotein elevated	Blood cholesterol level	Blood triglyceride level	Symptoms and signs in addition to risk of heart disease	Treatment
I	Chylomicrons	Small elevation	Large elevation	Fatty nodules in skin; abdominal pain; inflammation of pancreas	Diet very low in fats
IIa	Low-density lipoproteins	Small to medium elevation	Normal	Fatty nodules around tendons (especially Achilles tendon and hand tendons) and over joints; white line around rim of cornea	Diet low in saturated fats and cholesterol; cholestyramine, colestipol, lovastatin, or clofibrate may be prescribed
IIb	Low-density and very low-density lipoproteins	Small to medium elevation	Small elevation	Fatty nodules on eyelids; white line around rim of cornea	Diet low in saturated fats, cholesterol, and carbohydrates; cholestyramine, lovastatin, or colestipol may be prescribed
III	Intermediate-density lipoproteins	Small to medium elevation	Small to medium elevation	Fat deposits in palms and sometimes over joints	Diet low in fats and carbohydrates; clofibrate, niacin, gemfibrozil, or lovastatin may be prescribed
IV	Very low-density lipoproteins	Normal	Small to medium elevation	Fatty nodules in skin; patient is often obese	Diet low in carbohydrates; weight reduction; clofibrate and sometimes niacin and gemfibrozil may be prescribed
V	Chylomicrons and very low-density lipoproteins	Small elevation	Small to medium elevation	Fatty nodules in skin; abdominal pain; inflammation of pancreas; patient may be obese	Diet low in fats and carbohydrates; weight reduction; gemfibrozil and niacin may be prescribed

Hypernephroma

An alternative name for renal cell carcinoma, a type of *kidney cancer*.

Hyperopia

Commonly called farsightedness, an error of *refraction* that initially causes difficulty in seeing near objects and then affects distance vision. Hyperopia tends to run in families.

Hyperopia is caused by the eye being too short from front to back, so that images are not clearly focused on the retina. Mild or moderate hyperopia in the young is overcome by *accommodation* (the action of the ciliary muscles to change the shape of the lens), which brings the point of focus forward to produce a clear image.

SYMPTOMS AND SIGNS

The error is present from early childhood, but symptoms generally do not appear until later life. The more severe the hyperopia, the lower the age at which the problem appears. People with hyperopia experience varying degrees of difficulty viewing close objects because the power of accommodation declines with age. In time, distant objects are also blurred.

Hyperopia may lead to *eyestrain*. Neither blurred images nor eyestrain permanently affects vision.

TREATMENT

When blurred vision occurs, an ophthalmologist may prescribe *glasses* or *contact lenses* with convex lenses to reinforce focusing power.

Hyperparathyroidism

Overactivity of the *parathyroid glands*. These pea-sized glands are embedded in the thyroid gland in the neck and produce parathyroid hormone. This hormone, together with vitamin D and calcitonin (a hormone produced by the thyroid gland), controls the level of calcium in the body. Overproduction of parathyroid hormone raises the level of calcium in the blood (a condition called *hypercalcemia*) by removing the mineral from bones, leading to *osteoporosis* and *osteomalacia* (weakening of the bones).

In an attempt to normalize the high blood calcium level, the kidneys excrete large amounts of calcium in the urine, which can result in the formation of kidney stones (see *Calculus, urinary tract*).

CAUSES AND INCIDENCE

Hyperparathyroidism is most often caused by a small benign tumor of one or more of the parathyroid glands. However, sometimes it is due to an enlargement of the glands, the cause of which is unknown.

About 40 persons per 100,000 suffer from the disorder. It usually develops after the age of 40 and is twice as common in women as men.

SYMPTOMS

Hyperparathyroidism may cause generalized aches and pains, depression, and abdominal pain. Often, the only symptoms are those of kidney stones, but if the hypercalcemia is severe, it may cause nausea, vomiting, tiredness, excessive urination, confusion, and muscle weakness.

DIAGNOSIS AND TREATMENT

The condition is diagnosed by X rays of certain bones and by tests to measure the level of calcium, phosphorus, and parathyroid hormone in the blood.

Surgical removal of all abnormal parathyroid tissue usually cures the condition; sometimes all but part of one gland requires removal. In this case, the remaining parathyroid tissue may not produce enough hormone. The affected person may then require treatment for *hypoparathyroidism* (underactivity of the glands).

Hyperplasia

Enlargement of an organ or tissue due to an increase in the number of its constituent cells. The new cells are normal, unlike those of a tumor.

Hyperplasia is usually the result of hormonal stimulation. It may be a normal occurrence (such as in the enlargement of breast tissue and uterine muscle that occurs during pregnancy) or it may indicate a disorder (such as in hyperplasia of the thyroid or adrenal glands, which may be due to oversecretion of certain pituitary hormones). See also *Hypertrophy*.

Hyperplasia, gingival

Swelling of the gums. The condition may be a feature of *gingivitis* (inflammation of the gums), especially when it occurs during pregnancy; it can also develop around the front teeth as a result of persistent breathing through the mouth. Hyperplasia can also be caused by phenytoin, the anticonvulsant drug used to treat *epilepsy*.

Ill-fitting dentures can cause rolls of fibrous tissue to form beyond the edges of the dentures. This can be irritating and may require surgical treatment. Whatever the cause, gingival hyperplasia should be checked by a dentist.

Hyperpyrexia

A medical term for extremely high body temperature; it is synonymous with hyperthermia. Heat hyperpyrexia is a term for *heat stroke*.

Hypersensitivity

An overreaction of the *immune system* (defense against infection) to an *antigen* (protein recognized as foreign). Hypersensitivity reactions occur only on second or subsequent exposures to particular antigens, after the first exposure has sensitized the immune system. Such reactions have the same mechanisms as those of protective *immunity*. However, while the latter protect against disease, hypersensitivity reactions lead to tissue damage and disease.

Hypersensitivity is closely related to *allergy*, except that only one of the four main types of hypersensitivity reaction (type I) is closely associated with allergic illnesses.

TYPES
The four main types of hypersensitivity reaction are as follows.

TYPE I This type is also called immediate or anaphylactic hypersensitivity. After a first exposure to an antigen (which may be a harmless substance such as grass pollen), *antibodies* (substances that can recognize and bind to the antigen) are formed; these antibodies coat cells called mast cells in various tissues. On second exposure, the antigen and antibodies combine, causing the mast cells to disintegrate and release various chemicals that cause the symptoms of *asthma*, allergic *rhinitis* (hay fever), *urticaria* (hives), *anaphylactic shock*, or other illnesses of an allergic nature.

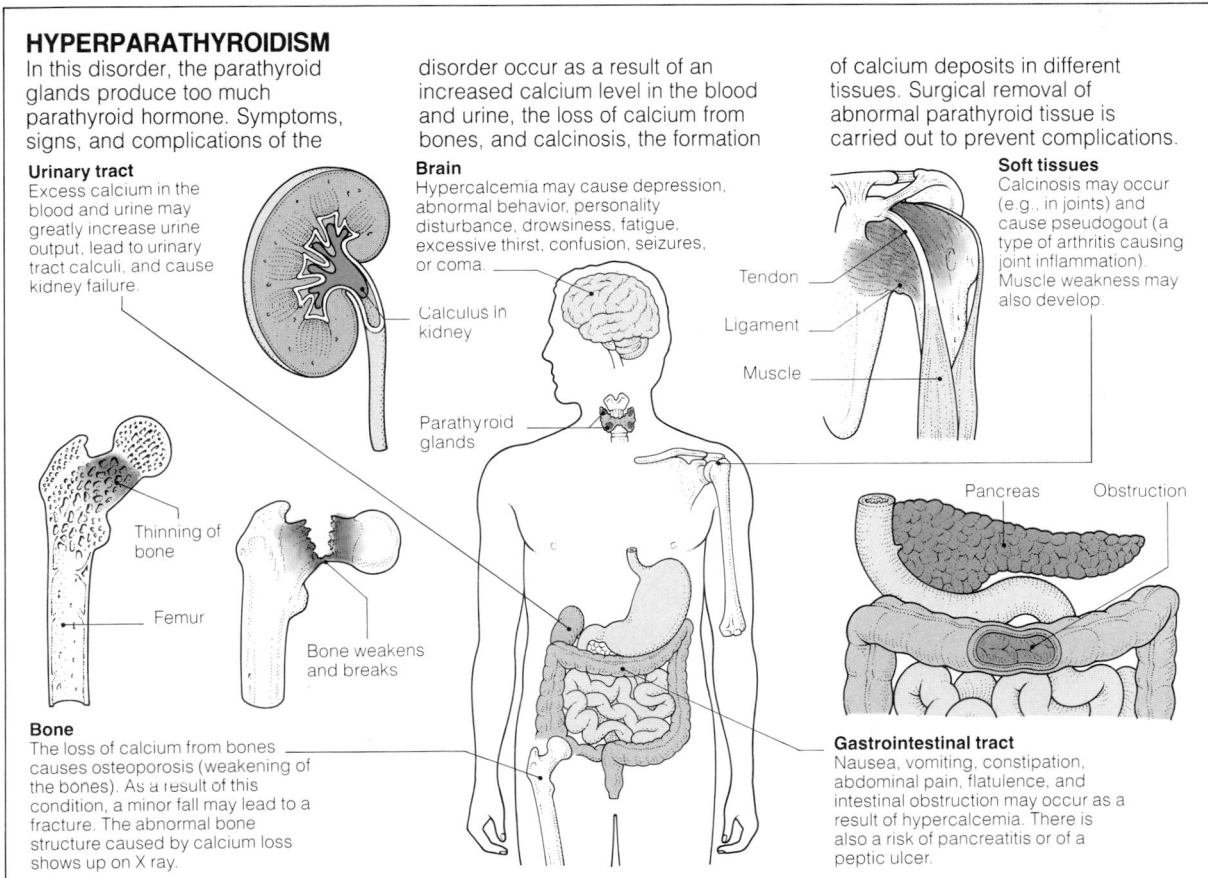

HYPERPARATHYROIDISM

In this disorder, the parathyroid glands produce too much parathyroid hormone. Symptoms, signs, and complications of the disorder occur as a result of an increased calcium level in the blood and urine, the loss of calcium from bones, and calcinosis, the formation of calcium deposits in different tissues. Surgical removal of abnormal parathyroid tissue is carried out to prevent complications.

Urinary tract
Excess calcium in the blood and urine may greatly increase urine output, lead to urinary tract calculi, and cause kidney failure.

Calculus in kidney

Parathyroid glands

Thinning of bone

Femur

Bone weakens and breaks

Bone
The loss of calcium from bones causes osteoporosis (weakening of the bones). As a result of this condition, a minor fall may lead to a fracture. The abnormal bone structure caused by calcium loss shows up on X ray.

Brain
Hypercalcemia may cause depression, abnormal behavior, personality disturbance, drowsiness, fatigue, excessive thirst, confusion, seizures, or coma.

Tendon

Ligament

Muscle

Soft tissues
Calcinosis may occur (e.g., in joints) and cause pseudogout (a type of arthritis causing joint inflammation). Muscle weakness may also develop.

Pancreas   Obstruction

Gastrointestinal tract
Nausea, vomiting, constipation, abdominal pain, flatulence, and intestinal obstruction may occur as a result of hypercalcemia. There is also a risk of pancreatitis or of a peptic ulcer.

HYPERTENSION

Hypertension is a common condition, affecting up to 10 percent of adults in the US. It is diagnosed if a person's resting blood pressure is persistently raised. Blood pressure is expressed by two values—the systolic and diastolic pressures (see bottom right) and measured in millimeters of mercury.

Although hypertension rarely causes symptoms, it is an important condition. Left untreated, it increases the risk of stroke and other disorders. In many cases, there is no obvious cause, but, in some, there is a specific cause, such as a kidney disorder, pregnancy, or use of oral contraceptives. Hypertension is linked to obesity and, in some people, to a high salt intake. Smoking appears to aggravate the effects of hypertension.

Atheroma
Hypertension and atherosclerosis, in which arteries are narrowed (left), are closely linked both to each other and to obesity.

Fatty deposits

Contracted muscle

Constriction
Factors such as nicotine in tobacco cause artery constriction (left) and a short-term rise in blood pressure that may worsen hypertension.

Artery wall

Stress

Nerve signals

Stress and hypertension
Stress acts on the nervous system, causing blood vessels to constrict and the heart to work harder. Both lead to a temporary rise in blood pressure. Hence, pressure should be measured when a person is relaxed. It is possible (but unproven) that frequent stress may eventually cause hypertension.

Variation in blood pressure
In any population, blood pressure varies over a wide range in the same way as height. Many people are considered to be hypertensive because they are at the top end of this range (see above). In obese people, the range is similarly wide but shifted toward the top end; hence, more obese people are hypertensive.

MEASURING BLOOD PRESSURE

During one heart beat, pressure varies between the (higher) systolic and the (lower) diastolic pressures.

Diastolic

Systolic

Systolic pressure
The systolic pressure is the maximum pressure attained as blood surges into the arteries.

Diastolic pressure
The diastolic pressure is the lowest value to which the pressure drops.

COMMON FACTORS AND PREVENTIVE MEASURES

Factors associated with essential hypertension	Age (incidence higher in the elderly)	Family history	Race (incidence higher in blacks than in whites)		
Factors that may aggravate hypertension	Smoking	Obesity	Excess alcohol intake	Diabetes mellitus	Stress
Self-help and treatment	1. Regular screening of blood pressure is important for early diagnosis and can help prevent complications. 2. Sufferers from essential hypertension should: Reduce weight Not smoke Reduce or stop alcohol intake Reduce salt intake Learn relaxation methods to combat stress 3. Antihypertensive drugs, prescribed by a physician, can usually keep high blood pressure under control.				

TYPE II In this type, antibodies are formed that bind to antigens bound to cell surfaces, leading to possible destruction of the cells. Type II reactions may be responsible for certain *autoimmune disorders* (in which antibodies attack the body's own tissues) and for some cases of red blood cell destruction (*hemolysis*) triggered by certain drugs.

TYPE III Antibodies combine with antigens to form particles called immunocomplexes, which can lodge in various tissues and activate further immune system responses, leading to tissue damage. This type of hypersensitivity reaction is responsible for *serum sickness*, for allergic *alveolitis* (a lung disease caused by exposure to the spores of certain fungi), and for the large swellings that sometimes form after booster vaccinations.

TYPE IV This type is also called delayed hypersensitivity. In type IV, sensitized T-*lymphocytes* (a class of white blood cell and an important component of the immune system) bind to antigens and subsequently release chemicals called lymphokines, which promote an inflammatory reaction. Type IV reactions are responsible for contact *dermatitis* and the rash of *measles*; they are important in the body's defense against *tuberculosis* and may also play a part in some "allergic" reactions to drugs.

TREATMENT
Effective treatment of a hypersensitivity reaction depends on its type, cause, and severity. When possible, exposure to the offending antigen should be avoided.

Hypersplenism
Overactivity of the spleen, resulting in and associated with blood disease. One of the functions of the spleen is to break down blood cells as they age and wear out. An overactive spleen may begin to destroy cells indiscriminately, causing a deficiency of any of the types of blood cell. In most cases of hypersplenism, the spleen is also enlarged.

Hypersplenism may be primary, occurring for no known reason, but more commonly it is secondary to another disorder in which the spleen has become enlarged, such as *Hodgkin's disease* or *malaria*.

SYMPTOMS AND TREATMENT
A person with hypersplenism is likely to have the symptoms of *anemia* (due to destruction of red blood cells) or of *thrombocytopenia* (platelet deficiency), and there is sometimes a decrease in

resistance to infection due to lack of white cells. There may also be symptoms of an underlying disorder, such as malaria.

Treatment of secondary hypersplenism aims to control the underlying cause. Primary hypersplenism requires *splenectomy*.

Hypertension
Abnormally high *blood pressure* (the pressure of blood in the main arteries). Blood pressure goes up as a normal response to stress and physical activity. However, a person with hypertension has a high blood pressure at rest.

Hypertension is usually defined as a resting blood pressure greater than 140 mm Hg (systolic)/90 mm Hg (diastolic). However, an elderly person normally has blood pressure readings above these values because blood pressure increases with age. Young children usually have blood pressure readings well below these values.

CAUSES
The majority of people have no obvious cause for their elevated blood pressure; in such cases it is called essential hypertension. However, in about 10 percent of patients, a definite cause can be found, including various disorders of the *kidney*, certain disorders of the *adrenal glands*, and *coarctation of the aorta*.

Tobacco smoking and *obesity* significantly increase the risk of hypertension. Hypertension sometimes develops in women who are taking the birth-control pill.

SYMPTOMS AND COMPLICATIONS
Hypertension usually causes no symptoms and generally goes undiscovered until detected by a physician during the course of a routine physical examination.

Possible complications of untreated hypertension include *stroke*, *heart failure*, kidney damage, and *retinopathy* (damage to the retina at the back of the eye). Severe hypertension may cause confusion and seizures.

TREATMENT
Mild hypertension may respond to weight reduction and a reduction in personal stress. Smokers should stop smoking and heavy drinkers should drastically reduce their consumption of alcohol. Restriction of salt intake is sometimes recommended.

If these measures have no effect, *antihypertensive drugs* may be prescribed. Occasionally, in severe cases, admission to the hospital for investigation of the cause, emergency treatment, and bed rest are required.

Hyperthermia
A medical term for extremely high body temperature. Hyperthermia has been used to treat advanced cancer. (See also *Heat stroke*.)

Hyperthermia, malignant
A rapid rise in body temperature to a dangerously high level brought on by general anesthesia. The condition is rare, occurring in only about one in 50,000 operations, and, in most cases, susceptibility to it is inherited. People suffering from certain muscle disorders may also be at risk.

The patient's temperature rises soon after the anesthetic is given. At the same time, large amounts of *lactic acid* pass from the muscles into the blood, causing *acidosis*. The muscles then stiffen and the patient turns blue; this may be followed rapidly by seizures and death if emergency treatment is not delivered.

Malignant hyperthermia may be suspected if the patient does not relax normally during the early, induction stage of anesthesia, or if he or she shows signs of abnormal muscle contractions after being given succinylcholine (a chemical used to relax muscles during operations).

TREATMENT
If malignant hyperthermia occurs, the anesthetic is stopped immediately and the patient is cooled with ice packs. Pure oxygen and intravenous injections of bicarbonate may also be given to counteract acidosis.

Hyperthyroidism
Overactivity of the *thyroid gland* and, therefore, simultaneous overproduction of thyroid hormones.

CAUSES AND INCIDENCE
The most common form of hyperthyroidism is *Graves' disease*, an *autoimmune disorder* in which the body develops antibodies that stimulate the production of excessive amounts of thyroid hormones. This condition affects about 1 percent of the adult population and is most common in young to middle-aged women. More rarely, hyperthyroidism may be associated with the development of enlarged nodules on the thyroid.

SYMPTOMS AND SIGNS
See illustration, next page.

DIAGNOSIS AND TREATMENT
The diagnosis of hyperthyroidism is confirmed by tests to measure the level of thyroid hormones in the blood. The condition may be treated with drugs that inhibit the production of thyroid hormones or by surgical

H

H

SYMPTOMS AND SIGNS OF HYPERTHYROIDISM

Oversecretion of thyroid hormones produces symptoms associated with overactivity of the body's metabolism. Weight loss, increased appetite, intolerance to heat, and increased sweating are early signs; there may also be tremors and a rapid heart rate. In more severe cases, the thyroid gland is often enlarged and there tends to be physical and mental hyperactivity and wasting of the muscles.

Thyroid gland enlargement
This symptom (known as goiter) may be due to hyperthyroidism. However, it may also be associated with hypothyroidism (underactivity of the thyroid).

Muscle wasting
Severe hyperthyroidism may cause wasting of both skeletal and heart muscle; the latter may lead to irregularities of heart rhythm.

Increased appetite
This symptom is a result of the metabolic overactivity that hyperthyroidism causes. Despite increased appetite, there is often weight loss.

Protruding eyes
This symptom (known as exophthalmos) affects some 30 to 50 percent of people with Graves' disease.

Hyperthyroid heart rate
Excessive thyroid hormones may result in the heart beating too rapidly or irregularly.

Healthy rhythm
A healthy hear beat, as shown in this ECG tracing, has a regular rhythm and a normal rate of beating.

Hyperthyroid rhythm
The hyperthyroid heart beat shown in this tracing is irregular and abnormally rapid.

Appearance of exophthalmos
Hyperthyroidism can cause swelling of tissues around the eyes, resulting in a staring appearance.

removal of part of the thyroid gland. In older patients, an alternative is a single dose of radioactive iodine, which is taken up by the thyroid and destroys some of its tissue.

Hypertonia

Increased rigidity in a muscle. It may be caused by damage to its nerve supply or by cell changes within the muscle itself. Hypertonia causes episodes of continuous muscle spasm (e.g., in the bladder wall when the outflow of urine is being obstructed by an enlarged prostate gland).

Persistent hypertonia in limb muscles following a *stroke* or major *head injury* causes *spasticity*.

A variable increase in muscle tension associated with abnormal patterns of movement and posture is referred to as *dystonia*.

Hypertrichosis

Growth of excessive hair, often in places not normally covered with hair. Hypertrichosis is often a result of taking certain drugs (including cyclosporine, minoxidil, and diazoxide).

The disorder is not the same as *hirsutism*, which is excessive hairiness in women due to abnormal levels of male hormones.

Hypertrichosis is also the term used to describe hair growth in a colored, fleshy mole.

Hypertrophy

Enlargement of an organ or tissue due to an increase in the size, rather than number, of its constituent cells. For example, skeletal muscles increase in size in response to increased physical demands. (See also *Hyperplasia*.)

Hyperuricemia

An abnormally high level of *uric acid* in the blood. Hyperuricemia may lead to the development of *gout* due to the deposit of crystals of uric acid in the joints; it may also cause kidney stones (see *Calculus, urinary tract*) and tophi (crystals in the tissues).

CAUSES

Hyperuricemia may be caused by an inborn error of *metabolism*, by rapid destruction of cells as part of a disease such as *leukemia*, or by medication

(such as *diuretic drugs*) that reduces the excretion of uric acid by the kidneys. Increased amounts of purine in the diet may raise the level of uric acid in the blood, precipitating gout.

TREATMENT

Drugs such as allopurinol (which reduces uric acid production in cells) and probenecid or sulfinpyrazone (which increase the excretion of uric acid by the kidneys) may be prescribed for life to prevent complications. Foods high in purine (e.g., liver, poultry, and dried peas and beans) need to be avoided.

Hyperventilation

Abnormally deep or rapid breathing, usually caused by *anxiety*. Hyperventilation may also occur as a result of uncontrolled *diabetes mellitus*, oxygen deficiency, *renal failure*, and some lung disorders (such as pulmonary *edema* and *emphysema*).

Hyperventilation causes an abnormal loss of carbon dioxide from the blood, which can lead to *alkalosis* (increase in blood alkalinity). Symptoms include numbness of the extremities, faintness, and *tetany* (painful spasms and twitches of the muscles in the hands and feet), and a sense of an inability to take a full breath. The effects of alkalosis often add to the already existing feelings of anxiety, and may give rise to the "hyperventilation syndrome," in which the sufferer experiences a feeling of impending doom.

Breathing into a plastic or paper bag during an attack may help reduce the loss of carbon dioxide and avoid the risk of alkalosis.

Hyperventilation associated with uncontrolled diabetes or uremia represents a compensatory effort by the body to eliminate excess carbon dioxide in dealing with *acidosis*. In this case, the hyperventilation syndrome does not develop.

Hyphema

Blood in the front chamber of the eye, almost always caused by an injury that ruptures a small blood vessel in the iris or the ciliary body.

Vision is markedly affected while the blood remains mixed with the aqueous humor, but it clears as the red cells sink. Usually the blood disappears completely within a few days and vision is fully restored, but there is a risk of delayed bleeding three to five days after the injury. Drug treatment or surgical evacuation of the blood is sometimes necessary.

Appearance of hyphema
Blood that has collected in the front chamber of the eye is clearly visible in front of the iris; hyphema is usually caused by an injury.

Hypnosis

A trancelike state of altered awareness that is characterized by extreme suggestibility. Hypnosis was once believed to be a form of sleep. However, the *EEG* (electrical tracing of brain-wave activity) of a hypnotized person does not show any of the normal sleep patterns.

HISTORY

A form of hypnotism was first practiced by the Austrian physician Franz Mesmer in the eighteenth century. Mesmerism (renamed hypnotism after the Greek god of sleep) began to receive attention from many leading members of the medical community in the nineteenth century. The celebrated Parisian physician Charcot gave public demonstrations, and Freud used hypnosis in his early treatment of hysteria. Hypnotism continues to attract much popular interest, both theoretical and medical, but its clinical use is still much debated. Likewise, its use to stimulate the memory of witnesses for courtroom testimony is controversial. Hypnosis for this purpose is acceptable in some jurisdictions and not in others.

HOW IT IS DONE

For hypnosis to succeed, the subject must first want to be hypnotized. The second requirement is relaxation, so a comfortable chair and a quiet, dimly lit room are usually necessary. The subject is usually asked to fix his or her attention on a particular object while the therapist quietly repeats phrases such as "Be still and listen to my voice" or "Empty your mind of all thoughts." The person gradually becomes more and more relaxed, eventually losing touch with the environment and hearing only the therapist's voice. At the end of the session, the subject "wakes up" when told to do so.

With training, it is possible for people to practice autohypnosis (self-hypnosis) by repeating certain phrases to themselves or imagining relaxing scenes.

Some people are more easily hypnotized than others, usually those with an intense imaginative life. The ability seems to be related to early childhood experiences and may be partly inherited.

CHARACTERISTICS

Hypnotized subjects wait passively to be told what to do by the therapist and are very suggestible—they touch or hold imaginary objects and act out suggested roles. They do not, however, obey commands to behave in a manner they would normally regard as dangerous or improper.

Attention usually becomes highly selective, so that only one person at a time is heard. Subjects frequently will obey orders to forget everything that has happened during hypnosis, or, alternatively, to remember or repeat behavior learned while hypnotized (posthypnotic suggestion).

THERAPEUTIC USES

Some psychoanalysts use hypnosis as a means of helping patients remember and come to terms with disturbing events or feelings that have been repressed from consciousness. More often, hypnosis is used as a means of helping patients relax. It may be useful in people suffering from *anxiety*, *panic attacks*, or *phobias*, and is sometimes successful in treating addictive habits, such as smoking. Scientific studies are lacking, however, and claims of fantastic cures should be treated with skepticism.

Hypnotic drugs

Drugs that induce sleep, such as *antianxiety* and *barbiturate drugs*.

Hypo-

A prefix meaning under, below, or less than normal, as in hypodermic (under the skin), hypoglycemia (abnormally low blood sugar level), and hypotension (lower than normal blood pressure).

Hypoaldosteronism

A deficiency of *aldosterone* in the body. This hormone, along with other *corticosteroid hormones* (notably hydrocortisone), is produced by the adrenal cortex (outer part of the adrenal glands). Removal of, or damage to, the cortex results in a deficiency of these hormones, which, in turn, causes *Addison's disease*.

Hypochondriasis

The unrealistic belief or fear that one is suffering from a serious illness, despite medical reassurance.

SYMPTOMS

Hypochondriacs worry constantly about their bodily health and interpret any physical symptom, however trivial, as evidence of a serious disorder. The feared disease may involve many parts of the body or may center on a particular organ and a single disease, as in *cardiac neurosis* (fear of heart disease). Hypochondriacs constantly seek medical advice and undergo numerous tests and treatments. Rarely, an obscure physical disorder is discovered, but it does not justify the symptoms described.

CAUSES

Hypochondriasis is usually a complication of other psychological disorders, including *obsessive-compulsive behavior*, *phobia*, *generalized anxiety disorder*, *schizophrenia*, *depression*, and brain diseases, such as *dementia* and *brain tumors*.

H

The cause of hypochondriasis in the absence of an underlying disorder is uncertain. However, it seems to be more common in people who suffered from a true organic illness during childhood or were constantly exposed to sick relatives. The reason for this may be that the hypochondriac becomes programmed to overreact to every bodily feeling, though there may also be an inherited sensitivity to pain. Other factors that may predispose a person to hypochondriasis include social stresses and personality type (usually obstinate).

TREATMENT
When there is an underlying mental disorder, it is treated as required. Hypochondriasis alone is more difficult to treat. An understanding and patient physician can often help relieve distress.

Hypoglossal nerve
The nerve that controls movements of the tongue. The hypoglossal nerve is rarely damaged. If damage does occur (e.g., as a result of a stroke), one side of the tongue becomes paralyzed.

LOCATION OF HYPOGLOSSAL NERVE
The hypoglossal nerve arises in the medulla oblongata (part of the brain stem), passes through the base of the skull, and runs around the throat to the tongue.

Skull

Brain stem

Tongue muscles

Hypoglossal nerve

Hypoglycemia
An abnormally low level of glucose (sugar) in the blood. Almost all cases occur in sufferers from insulin-dependent *diabetes mellitus*. In this disease, the pancreas fails to produce enough *insulin* (a hormone that regulates the level of glucose in the blood), resulting in an abnormally high level of glucose. To lower it, diabetics take either *hypoglycemic* drugs by mouth or insulin by injection. Too high a dose of either can reduce the blood sugar to too low a level, thus starving the body cells of energy. Hypoglycemia can also occur if a diabetic person misses a meal, fails to eat enough carbohydrates, or exercises too much.

Rarely, hypoglycemia can result from drinking a large amount of alcohol or from an *insulinoma* (an insulin-producing tumor of the pancreas); it also occurs for no known reason in some children, but is usually only temporary.

Hypoglycemia is a serious condition. The brain needs glucose for its metabolism and to function properly, and prolonged lack of it may lead to permanent intellectual impairment in an affected person.

SYMPTOMS
The principal symptoms include sweating, weakness, hunger, dizziness, trembling, headache, palpitations, confusion, and sometimes double vision. Behavior is often irrational and aggressive and movements are uncoordinated; this state may be mistaken for drunkenness. The victim may lapse into a coma due to extremely low blood sugar.

TREATMENT
Insulin-dependent diabetics should always carry sugar with them (in a convenient form such as sugar lumps or glucose tablets) to take at the first sign of an attack of hypoglycemia. If it is suspected that an unconscious person has suffered a hypoglycemic attack, medical help should be summoned immediately. The physician will give an injection of either glucose solution or the hormone glucagon; the latter counteracts the effects of insulin and raises the blood sugar level by stimulating the conversion of glycogen to glucose.

Hypoglycemics, oral

COMMON DRUGS
Acetohexamide Chlorpropamide Glipizide Glyburide Tolazamide Tolbutamide

WARNING
Consult your physician if you regularly experience symptoms, such as dizziness, nausea, and sweating, that are relieved only by food or a sugary drink.

A group of drugs that are used to treat non-insulin-dependent *diabetes mellitus* when *hyperglycemia* (raised blood glucose level) cannot be controlled simply by diet.

HOW THEY WORK
Oral hypoglycemics lower blood glucose levels by increasing the production by the pancreas of *insulin*, a hormone that increases the amount of glucose that is absorbed from the bloodstream into body cells. Insulin rather than oral hypoglycemics may need to be prescribed temporarily to control the blood glucose level (e.g., during surgery, pregnancy, or a severe illness). Oral hypoglycemics are of no use in treating insulin-dependent diabetes because in these cases the pancreas is unable to produce any insulin.

POSSIBLE ADVERSE EFFECTS
Oral hypoglycemic drugs may cause *hypoglycemia* (abnormally low blood glucose) if the dosage is too high or if the person has not had enough to eat.

Hypogonadism
Underactivity of the gonads (testes or ovaries). Hypogonadism may be caused by disorders of the *testis* or *ovary* or by a *pituitary gland* disorder resulting in deficient production of *gonadotropin hormone*. In affected males, hypogonadism causes the symptoms and signs of *androgen hormone* deficiency. In females, it causes the symptoms and signs of *estrogen hormone* deficiency.

Hypohidrosis
Reduced activity of the sweat glands. It is a feature of hypohidrotic ectodermal dysplasia, a rare, inherited, incurable condition characterized by reduced production of sweat usually accompanied by dry, wrinkled skin, sparse, dry hair, small, brittle nails, and conical teeth. Other causes include exfoliative *dermatitis* and some *anticholinergic drugs*.

Hypomania
A moderate form of *mania*.

Hypoparathyroidism
Insufficient production of parathyroid hormone produced by the *parathyroid glands*, which lie behind the thyroid gland in the neck. Parathyroid hormone, along with vitamin D and calcitonin (a hormone produced by the thyroid gland), regulates the level of calcium in the body. A deficiency of the hormone results in low levels of calcium in the blood and tissue fluids.

HYPOPLASTIC LEFT HEART SYNDROME

The heart defects associated with this syndrome are shown (at right) and compared with those of the normal heart (at left). Neither the left ventricle (pumping chamber) nor the aorta is properly formed.

Aorta
Pulmonary artery
Left ventricle
Right ventricle

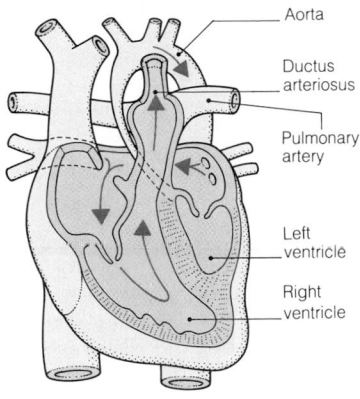

Aorta
Ductus arteriosus
Pulmonary artery
Left ventricle
Right ventricle

In a normal heart, blood is pumped by the left ventricle to the body via the aorta. If the left ventricle is poorly formed, blood can reach the body only via the ductus arteriosus, which closes soon after birth.

CAUSES
The most common cause of hypoparathyroidism is the accidental removal of the parathyroid glands during surgery on the thyroid gland. It may also result from surgery to remove a portion of the parathyroid glands themselves in the treatment of *hyperparathyroidism* (overproduction of parathyroid hormone). Occasionally, the parathyroid glands are absent from birth, or they may cease to function for no apparent reason.

SYMPTOMS
The main effect of a low level of calcium in the body is *tetany*, an increased excitability of the nerves that causes uncontrollable, painful, cramplike spasms of the face, hands, arms, and sometimes the feet. Rarely, general seizures similar to those of an epileptic attack may occur.

DIAGNOSIS AND TREATMENT
The condition is diagnosed by tests to measure the level of parathyroid hormone in the blood.

If the patient is suffering from an attack of tetany, calcium may be injected slowly into a vein to provide quick relief. To maintain the blood calcium at a normal level, a lifelong course of calcium and vitamin D tablets is necessary (the vitamin D is needed to increase absorption of calcium from the diet). Regular checkups are also necessary.

Hypophysectomy
Surgical removal of the pituitary gland or destruction of the gland by radioactive *implants*.

WHY IT IS DONE
Hypophysectomy is sometimes performed to remove a *pituitary tumor* that may be the cause of a number of endocrine diseases, such as *acromegaly* and *Cushing's syndrome*.

The operation may also be performed to treat some types of breast, ovary, or prostate gland cancer, the growth of which is stimulated by hormones secreted by the pituitary gland.

HOW IT IS DONE
A general anesthetic is given. Usually the gland is removed via the nose. However, if the tumor is very large, a *craniotomy* (incision into the skull) is performed just above the hairline, and a flap of bone temporarily removed to give access to the gland.

Hypoplasia
Failure of an organ or tissue to develop fully and reach its normal adult size.

Hypoplasia, enamel
A defect in tooth enamel. It is usually due to *amelogenesis imperfecta* (a hereditary condition), but may also be caused by vitamin deficiency, injury, or infection of a primary tooth that interferes with maturation of enamel.

Hypoplastic left heart syndrome
A serious and usually fatal form of congenital *heart disease* that affects about one to two newborn babies in every 10,000 live births. The baby is born with a poorly formed ventricle (pumping chamber) on the left side of the heart and other heart defects. The aorta (main artery carrying blood from the heart to the body) is malformed and blood can reach it only via a duct (the ductus arteriosus) that links the aorta to the pulmonary artery (blood vessel that transports blood to the lungs).

At birth the baby may seem healthy, but within a day or two the ductus arteriosus closes off and the baby collapses, becoming pallid and breathless. There is no effective surgical treatment for the condition and most affected babies die within a week. The risk of parents having another affected child is small.

Hypospadias
A congenital defect, occurring in about one in 300 male babies, in which the opening of the *urethra* is situated on the underside of the glans (head) or shaft of the penis. Sometimes the penis curves downward, a condition known as *chordee*.

In an extreme form of hypospadias the urethral opening lies between the genitals and the anus, the scrotum is small, and the testes are undescended. In such cases the genitals may resemble those of a female and the true sex of the child may be in doubt.

TREATMENT
Single-stage operations to correct hypospadias are available today. The penis is straightened and a tube of skin (or occasionally bladder lining) is used to create a new urethra that extends to the tip of the penis. The operation is usually performed before the boy is two years old. Surgery is usually successful, allowing the boy to pass urine normally and, later, to have satisfactory sexual intercourse.

Hypotension
The proper medical term for low blood pressure.

Some healthy people with a normal heart and blood vessels have blood pressure well below average for their age. The term hypotension is usually used only when blood pressure has fallen to the extent that blood flow to the brain is reduced, causing dizziness and fainting.

In postural hypotension (the most common type), symptoms occur after abruptly standing or sitting up. Usually, blood pressure increases slightly with these changes in posture; in people with postural hypotension, this increase fails to occur. Postural hypotension may be an adverse effect of *antidepressant drugs* or *antihypertensive drugs* (drugs used to treat high

H

blood pressure). It also occurs in diabetics because of nerve damage disrupting the reflexes that control blood pressure.

Acute hypotension (of sudden onset) may be caused by injuries involving heavy blood loss or serious burns leading to *hypovolemia* (reduced blood volume) and physiological *shock*, or by any crisis, such as *myocardial infarction* (heart attack) or *adrenal failure*, that leads to shock.

Treatment of hypotension depends on the underlying cause (diabetes mellitus, for example). For many people with postural hypotension, adjustment of medication may resolve the condition.

Hypothalamus

A region of the brain, roughly the size of a cherry, situated behind the eyes and beneath another brain region called the thalamus. It has nerve connections to most other regions of the nervous system.

LOCATION OF HYPOTHALAMUS
This small area of the forebrain lies under the thalamus and above the pituitary gland.

Cerebrum   Hypothalamus

Pituitary

Brain stem

FUNCTION

The hypothalamus exerts overall control over the sympathetic nervous system (part of the *autonomic nervous system*, which controls the internal body organs). When we are suddenly alarmed or excited, signals are sent from higher regions of the brain to the hypothalamus, which initiates sympathetic nervous system activity. This causes a faster heart beat, increased breathing, widening of the pupils of

the eyes, and increased blood flow to muscles (known as the "fight or flight" response).

Other groups of nerve cells in the hypothalamus are concerned with the control of body temperature. Some are sensitive to heat and cold so that, when blood flowing to the brain is hotter or cooler than normal, the hypothalamus switches on temperature-regulating mechanisms (among them sweating or shivering). The hypothalamus receives information from internal sense organs regarding the level of glucose in the blood and the body's water content; if they are too low, it stimulates appetite for food and drink. The hypothalamus is also involved in regulating sleep, in motivating sexual behavior, and in determining mood and the experience of emotions.

Another role of the hypothalmus is coordination of the function of the nervous and endocrine (hormonal) systems of the entire body. The hypothalamus connects with the pituitary gland through a short stalk of nerve fibers and controls hormonal secretions from this gland. It does this in two ways—through direct nerve connections and through specialized nerve cells, which secrete hormones called releasing factors into the blood to flow directly to the pituitary. In this way, the hypothalamus can convert nerve signals into hormonal signals. Thus, the hypothalamus indirectly controls many of the endocrine organs, including the pituitary, thyroid, adrenal cortex, and gonads.

DISORDERS

Disorders of the hypothalamus are usually caused by a brain hemorrhage within the hypothalamic region (see *Intracerebral hemorrhage*) or by an expanding pituitary tumor. Loss of hypothalamic function can have diverse effects, ranging from hormonal disorders (see *Endocrine system*) to disturbed temperature regulation, and increased or decreased appetite for food, sex, and sleep.

Hypothermia

A fall in body temperature to below 95°F (35°C). It causes drowsiness, lowers breathing and heart rates, and may lead to unconsciousness or death. Most victims are elderly people who are unable to keep sufficiently warm in winter.

The term hypothermia is also used to describe the deliberate lowering of body temperature during some forms of surgery (see *Hypothermia, surgical*).

CAUSES

Hypothermia can be caused by prolonged exposure to extremely cold weather, swimming in the sea, or wearing damp clothing in cold conditions. However, most cases occur in elderly people living in poorly heated homes. As the body ages, it gradually loses its sensitivity to cold; an elderly person's body temperature may drop without the individual being aware of it. In addition, the aging body also becomes increasingly less able to reverse a fall in temperature. This reduced ability is also present in the very young; aside from the elderly, babies are the most common victims of hypothermia.

The risk of hypothermia is increased if an elderly person is also suffering from a disorder that reduces the body's heat production (such as *hypothyroidism*), impairs mental function (such as senile *dementia*), or reduces mobility (such as *arthritis*).

Certain drugs may also contribute to the onset of hypothermia. For example, *tranquilizers* (such as chlorpromazine) may lower the level of consciousness and reduce the ability to shiver (shivering has a protective function against cold).

SIGNS

A person suffering from hypothermia is usually pale, puffy-faced, and listless. The heart rate is slow and the victim is often drowsy and confused. Areas of the body that are normally warm (such as the armpits and the groin) are cold.

In severe hypothermia, breathing becomes slow and shallow, the muscles are often stiff, the victim may become unconscious, and the heart may beat only faintly and irregularly or—especially if the body temperature falls below 90°F (32.2°C)—it may stop beating altogether.

DIAGNOSIS

The condition is usually obvious from the above signs and the victim's circumstances. To determine how cold the body has become, the physician takes a rectal temperature with a special low-reading thermometer. Alternatively, the temperature of the urine may be measured.

TREATMENT

Hypothermia is a medical emergency and anyone suspected of suffering from it requires immediate medical attention. Mild hypothermia usually responds to giving the victim warm drinks and covering the head (from which as much as 20 percent of the body's heat loss takes place).

FIRST AID: HYPOTHERMIA

DO NOT
- let the victim walk
- warm the victim by rubbing his or her skin
- give the victim any alcohol
- warm the victim by applying direct heat

IN BABIES

Medical help should be sought immediately. Hypothermia is often difficult to detect. The baby may look pink and healthy, but he or she may be unusually limp and drowsy. Rewarm the baby by keeping him or her well wrapped.

IN ADULTS

1 Seek medical help. If the victim is unconscious and breathing, place in the *recovery position*. If not breathing, begin *artificial respiration*.

2 Move the victim to a warm place. Take off wet clothing and replace with dry, or dry off and cover with waterproof material.

3 If the victim is conscious, give a warm (not hot) drink. Hold the mug if necessary.

4 If the victim is otherwise healthy, place in a warm (not hot) bath.

When the condition is more severe, treatment varies according to the age of the victim. A young person is usually warmed in a hot bath. However, this causes a rush of blood to the surface of the body, reducing the supply to the heart and brain, which could be fatal to an elderly person. For this reason, warming is carried out gradually in the elderly (at a rate of about 1°F (0.6°C per hour) by placing the person in a room with a temperature of 78°F (25°C) and covering him or her with layers of heat-reflecting material known as space blankets. Rectal temperature is monitored every half hour until the temperature and vital signs show improvement.

When hypothermia is severe enough to be life-threatening, the victim is admitted to an intensive-care unit and warmed rapidly by safe means; part of the circulating blood is bypassed outside the body, where it is warmed, or warm fluid is run into the abdominal cavity.

PREVENTION

It is recommended that an elderly person's living quarters be heated at a temperature of at least 65°F (18°C). Relatives or neighbors of elderly people living by themselves should check regularly throughout winter that these people have additional means of keeping warm, including suitable clothing, warm blankets, and nutritious food.

Elderly people should also be made aware of the need to eat hot food and drink warm fluids several times a day and wear a warm hat at all times.

People walking or climbing in cold weather should carry survival bags, lined with space blankets, which they can crawl into while waiting for help in the event of an accident.

Hypothermia, surgical

The deliberate reduction of body temperature to prolong the period for which the vital organs can safely be deprived (partially or totally) of their normal blood supply during *open heart surgery*. Cold reduces the rate of metabolism in cells and tissues; hence, lack of oxygen is better tolerated as the temperature is lowered.

In the early days of heart surgery, induced hypothermia allowed sur-geons to perform quick (eight to 10 minutes) operations on the heart while blood circulation throughout the body was completely stopped.

Today, open heart surgery is usually performed with the general blood circulation maintained by means of a *heart-lung machine*. Nevertheless, mild hypothermia—with the body temperature reduced from 98.6°F (37°C) to about 82 to 88°F (28 to 31°C)—is still generally induced as a safety measure. It can allow heart operations to proceed for several hours. A heat exchanger, installed into the machine circuit, can be used to cool the blood before return to the body, thus inducing hypothermia.

The blood supply to the heart muscle itself is interrupted during open heart surgery, so the heart also must be vigorously cooled by continuously instilling cold saline into the open chest cavity at a temperature of about 40°F (4°C). By this method, damage to the heart muscle from lack of oxygen is minimal, even after an operation lasting several hours.

At the end of the operation, rewarming of the patient is carefully synchronized with restarting the heart and the switch back from use of the heart-lung machine.

Hypothyroidism

Underactivity of the *thyroid gland* and, therefore, underproduction of thyroid hormones.

CAUSES AND INCIDENCE

Most cases of hypothyroidism are caused by the body developing antibodies against its own thyroid gland (an example of an *autoimmune disorder*) with a resultant reduction in thyroid hormone production. *Hashimoto's thyroiditis* is an example of this phenomenon. More rarely, hypothyroidism may result from surgery to remove part of the thyroid gland as a treatment for *hyperthyroidism* (overactivity of the thyroid).

Hypothyroidism affects about 1 percent of the adult population. It is most common in elderly women, though it occurs at all ages and in both sexes.

SYMPTOMS AND SIGNS

Thyroid hormones stimulate energy production, so a deficiency of them causes generalized tiredness and lethargy. There may also be muscle weakness, cramps, a slow heart rate, dry and flaky skin, hair loss, and a deep and husky voice. In addition, the skin and other body tissues may thicken and there may be weight gain—a syndrome known as *myx-*

H

edema. In some cases, a goiter (enlargement of the thyroid gland) develops, although not all goiters are due to hypothyroidism.

The severity of the symptoms depends on the degree of thyroid deficiency. Mild deficiency may cause no symptoms; severe deficiency may produce all of the above symptoms.

If hypothyroidism occurs in childhood and remains untreated, it may retard growth, delay sexual maturation, and inhibit normal development of the brain.

DIAGNOSIS AND TREATMENT
The disorder is diagnosed by tests to measure the level of thyroid hormones in the blood.

Treatment consists of replacement therapy with the thyroid hormone thyroxine; in most cases, hormone therapy must be continued for life. Such treatment may not cure a goiter, which may require surgery.

Hypotonia

Abnormal muscle slackness. Normally, a muscle that is not being used has a certain built-in tension. In a number of disorders affecting the nervous system (such as *Huntington's chorea*) this natural tension or tone is moderately or markedly reduced.

Hypotonia in infants

Excessive limpness in infants, also called floppy infant syndrome.
FEATURES
Hypotonic babies cannot hold their limbs up against gravity and thus tend to lie flat with their arms and legs splayed. Their limbs and joints seem slack when moved by someone else. Floppy babies move around less than normal babies and their mothers may report that they did not feel the baby move much during pregnancy. When held horizontally by the trunk, face downward, they hang limply.
CAUSES
Premature infants are naturally more floppy than full-term infants, but, as they mature, their muscles attain the normal tension.

Hypotonia is often a feature of chromosomal disorders, such as *Down's syndrome*. Illnesses that affect general health (e.g., malnutrition, congenital *heart disease*, and *hypothyroidism*) may also cause hypotonia.

More specifically, disorders of the brain (particularly *cerebral palsy*) and of the spinal cord (such as *Werdnig-Hoffmann disease*) are characterized by hypotonia. Treatment depends on the cause.

Hypovolemia

An abnormally low volume of blood circulating in the body. It usually follows severe blood loss, which may occur as a result of injury, internal bleeding, or surgery. Hypovolemia also occurs in various other conditions, such as serious burns, severe dehydration, or, rarely, adrenal crisis (see *Addison's disease*).

Hypovolemia is a dangerous condition because, untreated, it can lead to *shock*, which is potentially fatal.

Hypoxia

An inadequate supply of oxygen to the tissues.
CAUSES
Temporary hypoxia may occur as a result of strenuous exercise in which the normal supply of oxygen cannot meet the additional requirements of the tissues. In such cases, the condi-

---

PERFORMING A HYSTERECTOMY

Hysterectomy may be performed through the abdomen or the vagina. For an abdominal hysterectomy, the incision is made in the lower abdomen (see below). In vaginal hysterectomy, the uterus is removed through an incision at the top of the vagina.

Site of incision for abdominal hysterectomy
The incision is made in the lower abdomen (in this case horizontally) level with the top of the pubic hair.

Abdominal hysterectomy
The uterine vessels are clamped. Traction is placed on the top of the uterus and the vessels are tied and then divided. In some cases, the fallopian tubes are cut and the tubes and ovaries left in place.

Vaginal hysterectomy
After a vaginal incision is made, the uterus and cervix are removed (the ovaries cannot be removed in a vaginal hysterectomy). The upper end of the vagina is repaired by stitching.

POSTOPERATIVE PROBLEMS

Many women worry that their sex lives will be affected by hysterectomy. Physically, there should be no noticeable change in the woman's sex life. Counseling before the procedure can help dispel any misconceptions or fears. Depression is not uncommon in women who are inadequately counseled.

tion disappears once exercise has stopped and breathing has reoxygenated the tissues.

More serious causes include impaired breathing (see *Respiratory failure*), usually as a result of a lung disorder; *ischemia* (reduced blood flow to a tissue), which may be due to an artery disorder or a heart disorder; and severe *anemia*, in which the oxygen-carrying capacity of the blood is reduced. Another, rare, cause is *carbon monoxide* poisoning, which prevents the blood from being adequately oxygenated. In severe cases, any of these more serious causes may lead to *anoxia* (complete absence of oxygen in a tissue), which, if prolonged, may cause tissue death.

SYMPTOMS AND SIGNS

Hypoxia in muscles forces the muscle cells to produce energy by *anaerobic* metabolism, which produces lactic acid as a by-product. The accumulation of lactic acid causes cramps. Hypoxia in heart muscle may cause the chest pain of *angina pectoris*. Hypoxia of the brain initially causes confusion, dizziness, and incoordination, progressing to unconsciousness and death if the condition persists.

TREATMENT

Severe, potentially life-threatening hypoxia may require treatment by *oxygen therapy* or artificial *ventilation*. Otherwise, the treatment depends on the underlying cause.

Hysterectomy

Removal of the uterus. Hysterectomy is one of the most frequently performed operations in the US.

WHY IT IS DONE

Hysterectomy is most often performed to treat *fibroids* (benign tumors of the uterus) that are causing symptoms. It is also performed to treat cancer of the uterus or cervix (see *Uterus, cancer of*; *Cervix, cancer of*). Occasionally, a hysterectomy is performed to relieve *menorrhagia* (heavy menstrual bleeding) or *endometriosis* (a condition in which fragments of the uterine lining occur elsewhere in the pelvis) that has not responded to a *D and C* or hormone treatment. A hysterectomy may also be performed to remove a severely prolapsed uterus (see *Uterus, prolapse of*).

TYPES

The most common type of hysterectomy is a simple hysterectomy, in which the uterus and cervix only are removed. In a total hysterectomy, the fallopian tubes and ovaries are removed as well. If cancer is advanced, a radical hysterectomy (in which the pelvic lymph nodes are also removed) is necessary.

RECOVERY PERIOD

After the operation a drainage tube may be inserted at the site of the incision. For a few days there may be some vaginal bleeding and discharge and considerable tenderness and pain. The stay in the hospital depends on the age and health of the woman and whether there are postoperative problems. Full recovery requires another three to six weeks; sexual intercourse can be resumed about a month after the surgery.

OUTLOOK

After hysterectomy the woman is unable to bear children; she does not menstruate and needs no contraception. If the ovaries have also been removed from a woman before or around the *menopause, hormone replacement therapy* should be considered.

Hysteria

A term encompassing a wide range of physical or mental symptoms that are attributed to mental stress in someone who is not psychotic.

Derived from the Greek word for uterus, hysteria was originally thought to be a physical disorder confined to women. By the nineteenth century, hysteria was believed to have a psychological origin and was used to describe many seemingly bizarre states (including hallucination, sleepwalking, and trances).

Today, many psychiatrists feel that the term hysteria is no longer helpful in diagnosis. In modern classifications, therefore, the symptoms formerly grouped under this term are now included in the more specific diagnostic categories of *conversion disorder*; *dissociative disorders*; *somatization disorder*; and *factitious disorders*.

Physicians still sometimes use the term loosely to describe any difficult, unusual, or exotic behavior that does not seem consistent with the symptoms or situation of the patient. Mass hysteria describes the spread of psychologically produced symptoms (such as fainting) from person to person. It usually occurs in schools or institutions of young women in response to group tensions or worries and is often triggered by a person with a charismatic personality.

Hysterosalpingography

An X-ray procedure performed to examine the inside of the uterus and fallopian tubes.

WHY IT IS DONE

The examination is performed as part of the investigation of *infertility*. Dye injected during *laparoscopy* indicates whether the tubes are blocked, but hysterosalpingography is needed to determine the site of the blockage, which is most often due to scar tissue caused by a previous infection. Hysterosalpingography also outlines any distortion in the uterus, such as a congenital abnormality or a *fibroid*.

A normal hysterosalpingogram
The X-ray image shows radiopaque dye filling the uterus and passing through the fallopian tubes into the pelvic cavity.

HOW IT IS DONE

The test is an outpatient procedure performed by a radiologist and/or a gynecologist. Because the procedure may be uncomfortable (often producing a cramplike pain), the patient is usually mildly sedated.

A plastic or metal *cannula* is inserted into the cervix (neck of the uterus), a radiopaque dye (one that shows up on X-ray film) is passed through it into the uterus and the fallopian tubes, and X-ray pictures are taken to reveal any abnormalities. The procedure takes 10 to 30 minutes.

RISKS

In a woman who has just become pregnant, the dye may wash the fertilized egg out of the fallopian tube; if this does not happen, the embryo may be damaged by radiation from the X rays. To avoid these risks, the test is carried out only in the second half of the menstrual cycle, when it is certain the woman is not pregnant.

Hysterotomy

A method of late *abortion* in which the abdomen and uterus are surgically opened to remove the fetus. Hysterotomy is the most complicated method of abortion and carries the highest risk. It is rarely used today; instead, *prostaglandin drugs* are used to terminate pregnancy by inducing labor.

Damaged tissue

- Inflamed tissue
- Bleeding
- Enlarged blood vessels
- Nerve

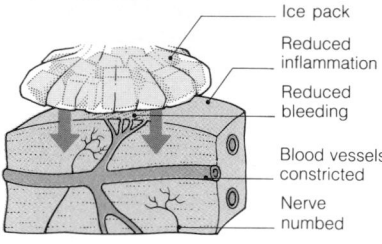

Ice pack application

- Ice pack
- Reduced inflammation
- Reduced bleeding
- Blood vessels constricted
- Nerve numbed

Use of an ice pack
Applying an ice pack to an area of damaged tissue helps relieve pain, reduce inflammation and further tissue damage, and minimize bleeding and swelling.

Iatrogenic

Meaning literally "physician produced," the term iatrogenic can be applied to any medical condition, disease, or other adverse occurrence that results from medical treatment. The development of an iatrogenic condition does not necessarily imply a lack of care or knowledge on the part of the physician. Effective forms of treatment are seldom, if ever, entirely free of possible unwanted effects. The drowsiness produced by some groups of antiallergy drugs is one example.

Ibuprofen

A *nonsteroidal anti-inflammatory drug* (NSAID) used as an *analgesic* (painkiller) in the treatment of headache, menstrual pain, and painful injury to soft tissues (such as muscles and ligaments). The anti-inflammatory effect of ibuprofen helps reduce joint pain and stiffness occurring in some types of arthritis, such as *rheumatoid arthritis* and *osteoarthritis*.

Ibuprofen may cause abdominal pain, diarrhea, nausea, heartburn, and, rarely, dizziness. It may also cause a *peptic ulcer*, but is less likely to do so than some other NSAIDs.

Ice packs

Means of applying ice (in a towel or other material) to the skin to relieve pain, stem bleeding, or reduce inflammation. Cold causes the blood vessels to contract, reducing blood flow.

WHY IT IS DONE

Ice treatment is used to relieve pain in a variety of disorders, including severe *headache*, *hemorrhoids*, and pain in the throat after a *tonsillectomy*. Another common use is after sports injuries to minimize swelling, bruising, and further tissue damage. In sports injuries, ice is usually combined with the application of a pressure bandage and the raising of the injured part. Ice may also be used to stop bleeding from small vessels, as in a nosebleed.

HOW IT IS DONE

Ice is wrapped in a wet cloth (to prevent it from burning the skin) and applied to the skin's surface. Chemical packs are also available; striking or shaking the pack mixes the chemicals within, producing a liquid with a very low temperature.

Ichthyosis

A rare, inherited condition in which the skin is dry, thickened, scaly, and darker than normal due to an abnormality in the production of *keratin* (a protein that is the main component of skin). The name ichthyosis is taken from the Greek word "ichthus" (meaning fish); the condition is commonly called fish skin disease.

Ichthyosis usually appears at or shortly after birth and generally improves during childhood. The areas most commonly affected are the thighs, arms, and backs of the hands.

There is no special treatment, although lubricants and emulsifying ointments help the dryness and bath oils moisten the skin. Washing with soap makes ichthyosis worse and should be avoided. The condition improves in a warm, humid atmosphere. Ichthyosis is at its worst in cold weather (when the sufferer should wear additional layers of protective, warm clothing).

Icterus

Another term for *jaundice*.

Id

One of the three parts of the personality (with the *ego* and *superego*) described by Sigmund Freud. The id is the primitive, unconscious store of energy from which come the instincts for food, love, sex, and other basic needs. The id seeks simply to gain pleasure and to avoid pain. (See also *Psychoanalytic theory*.)

Idiocy

An outdated term for severe *mental retardation*. Idiots were defined as having an IQ of under 35.

Idiopathic

Of unknown cause. For example, epilepsy in which no specific cause can be found is referred to as idiopathic epilepsy. The word idiopathic comes from the Greek "idio-" meaning "one's own" and "pathos" meaning disease.

Idoxuridine

An *antiviral drug*. Idoxuridine is used to treat *herpes simplex* infections affecting the eyelids or cornea of the eye. It is occasionally given to prevent a recurrence of herpes simplex infection in people receiving *corticosteroid drug* treatment for a different eye disorder.

Idoxuridine may cause irritation of the eye and, in rare cases, photophobia (abnormal sensitivity to light), swollen eyelids, or blurred vision.

Ileostomy

An operation in which the ileum (lower part of the small intestine) is brought through an incision in the abdominal wall and formed into an artificial outlet for the bowel to allow the discharge of feces into a bag attached to the skin. An ileostomy is usually permanent.

WHY IT IS DONE

Permanent ileostomy is usually performed for people with *ulcerative colitis* or *Crohn's disease* whose health, despite drug treatment, continues to deteriorate because of chronic inflammation of the colon. For these people, the only means of restoring health is to perform a *colectomy* (an operation to remove the colon and rectum) followed by an ileostomy.

Temporary ileostomy is sometimes required at the time of partial colectomy (removal of part of the colon) to allow the repair of the colon to heal before waste material passes through it. Temporary ileostomy may also be carried out as an emergency measure in a person who is very ill due to an

PROCEDURE FOR ILEOSTOMY

Two incisions are made in the abdominal wall (usually on the right side)—a small circular cut for the stoma (most often located about 2 inches below the waist and away from the hipbone and groin crease) and a vertical cut to give access to the intestine and *mesentery*.

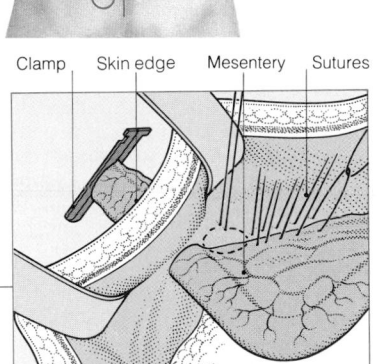

Sites of incisions

Clamp   Skin edge   Mesentery   Sutures

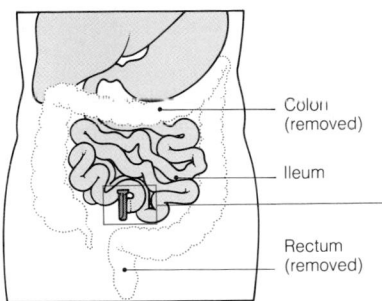

Colon (removed)

Ileum

Rectum (removed)

1 After removal of the colon, the cut end of the ileum is clamped and part of the mesentery is cut to free a short length of ileum for the stoma.

2 The free end of the ileum is pushed out through the circular incision in the abdomen; the mesentery is then stitched to the inner abdominal wall.

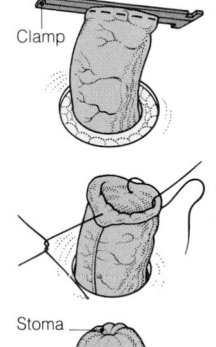

Clamp

Stoma

3 The main vertical incision is closed, and the clamp is removed from the protruding end of the ileum (top). The end of the ileum is then turned back and attached to the abdomen with sutures (middle). When completed, this creates a small protruding stoma (bottom). A temporary ileostomy appliance is usually fitted immediately.

4 After the intestine begins to function normally, an ileostomy bag is fitted around the stoma. The bag attaches closely to the skin with adhesive seals.

obstruction high in the large intestine that is preventing the normal passage of feces. The ileostomy is made above the obstruction and, by allowing waste material to discharge, enables the patient to recover sufficiently to undergo a partial colectomy to remove the obstruction. Temporary ileostomies are closed when the rejoined colon has healed.

HOW IT IS DONE

When the whole of the colon and rectum has been removed, the cut end of the ileum is brought to the surface of the skin through an incision in the abdominal wall. In the case of a temporary ileostomy, a loop of bowel is brought to the surface and opened so that waste material can pass through. The edges of this opening are then stitched to the skin at the edge of the abdominal incision to create a stoma (an artificial opening). The stoma is usually located on the right side about 2 inches (5 cm) below the natural waist and away from the hipbone.

POSTOPERATIVE CARE

For a few days, patients may need to be fed by *intravenous infusion*. After that, the intestine starts to function normally again; liquid waste is discharged through the stoma into a bag that is closely attached to the skin by adhesive seals.

During the convalescent period, patients with permanent ileostomies are given counseling to help them come to terms with an altered body image and the appearance of the stoma. They are also taught the practical aspects of stoma care. There is no muscle control over evacuation of body wastes through the stoma. These wastes are semiliquid and contain enzymes that can damage the skin around the stoma. For these reasons, it is usually necessary for the bag to be worn at all times. The nursing staff (ideally a stoma-care nurse clinician) teaches the patient how to empty, change, and dispose of the bag, and how to maintain a good seal between bag and body to protect the skin and prevent leaks.

Full recovery from the operation takes about six weeks, during which time patients should avoid vigorous physical activity.

OUTLOOK

The condition of patients who are given ileostomies after removal of a chronically inflamed colon usually improves dramatically. Because their ability to be active is enhanced, many of these people say they wish they had had the operation years earlier.

Following convalescence, patients should be able to return to their usual employment, life-style, and family and social activities. After an ileostomy it is necessary to drink increased amounts of water and to ensure that the intake of salt is adequate, thus compensating for the lack of a colon (the main functions of which are the absorption of water and salt). Apart from this recommendation, it is generally possible to eat a normal diet.

Only an occasional medical checkup is needed to make sure that the stoma is in good condition, although the physician should always be informed of any change in the function or appearance of the stoma. Occasionally, the channel of the stoma becomes narrowed or prolapses (protrudes too far from the abdomen), requiring surgical correction.

Various attempts have been made to devise ileostomies that require emptying only once or twice a day at fixed times and do not require an external appliance. These devices include internal reservoirs made from loops of small intestine, magnetic closures, and carbon filter systems for gas. However, none has yet proved consistently reliable, and most patients are still offered a conventional ileostomy.

Ileum

The final, longest, and narrowest section of the small intestine. It is joined at its upper end to the *jejunum* and at its lower end to the large intestine.

The function of the ileum is to absorb nutrients from food that has been digested in the stomach and first two sections of the small intestine. The millions of *villi* (minute fingerlike projections) that line the ileum considerably increase its surface area and thus its powers of absorption.

LOCATION OF THE ILEUM
The ileum (the final part of the small intestine) joins the jejunum and cecum (the first part of the large intestine).

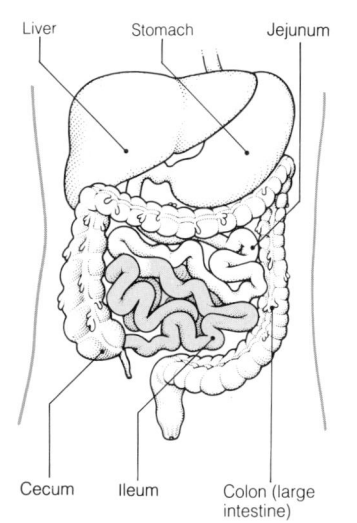

Liver Stomach Jejunum

Cecum Ileum Colon (large intestine)

DISORDERS

Occasionally, the ileum becomes obstructed—by pushing through a weakness in the abdominal wall (see *Hernia*) or by becoming caught up with scar tissue following abdominal surgery, for example.

Other disorders of the ileum include *Meckel's diverticulum* (a pouch in the ileum wall that may become ulcerated), *Crohn's disease*, and diseases in which absorption of nutrients is impaired, such as *celiac sprue*, tropical *sprue*, and *lymphoma*.

Ileus, paralytic

A failure, usually temporary, of the normal contractility of the muscles of the intestine. As a result, intestinal contents can no longer pass out of the body and the bowel becomes obstructed. This condition commonly follows abdominal surgery and may also be induced by severe abdominal injury, *peritonitis* (inflammation of the membrane lining the abdomen), internal extraintestinal bleeding, acute *pancreatitis* (inflammation of the pancreas), or interference with the blood or nerve supply to the intestine.

Symptoms include a distended abdomen, vomiting, and failure to pass stools. The condition is usually successfully treated by sucking out the intestinal contents through a tube passed through the nose or mouth into the stomach or intestine and by maintaining body fluid levels by *intravenous infusion* (drip).

Illness

Perception by a person that he or she is not well. Illness is a subjective sensation and may have physical or psychological causes; illness is not synonymous with disease or disorder.

Illusion

A distorted sensation. An illusion is based on misinterpretation of a real stimulus (for example, a pen is seen as a dagger or the sound of a screeching brake is heard as a scream). This is not the same as a *hallucination*, in which a perception occurs with no stimulus.

Usually, illusions are brief and can be understood when explained. They may be due to tiredness or anxiety, to drugs of many sorts, or to certain forms of brain damage. *Delirium tremens* is a classic inducer of illusions.

Imaging techniques

Techniques that produce images of structures within the body that cannot otherwise be seen. Imaging techniques are an invaluable aid in diagnosing abnormalities and disease.

X RAYS

In 1895 the discovery of *X rays* revolutionized medical diagnosis by making it possible for the first time to visualize bone, organs, and other internal tissue without opening up the body. The rays are electromagnetic waves of short wavelength. Some are absorbed and others pass through tissues; the shadow that is cast is projected onto a fluorescent screen or a film.

CONTRAST MEDIA X-ray images of bones are distinct, but soft tissues show up less clearly. To overcome this, radiologists from the 1920s onward began using substances opaque to radiation as part of certain X-ray procedures.

When such substances (known as contrast media) are introduced into internal organs, blood vessels, or ducts, they produce (on the X-ray screen or film) an outline of the cavities they fill.

A contrast medium can be introduced into the body in various ways. In *cholecystography* (carried out to examine the gallbladder and common bile duct) and in some *barium X-ray examinations* of the esophagus, the stomach, and the small bowel, the medium is swallowed in tablet or liquid form. In *bronchography* (used to diagnose various chest disorders) the contrast medium is placed into the airways (bronchi) connecting the windpipe to the lungs. In *angiography* and *venography*, it is injected into an artery or vein, respectively, to provide images of the blood vessels. In intravenous *pyelography*, contrast medium injected into a vein in the arm travels to the kidneys and urinary tract. In *ERCP* (by which the pancreatic duct and biliary system are examined), the medium is passed into the ducts by means of a catheter (tube) passed through a channel in an endoscope (a flexible viewing instrument).

SCANNING TECHNIQUES

Since the 1970s many X-ray imaging techniques have been superseded by newer procedures that are simpler to perform and are safer and more comfortable for the patient. *Ultrasound scanning* consists of passing high-frequency sound waves through the body with a transducer placed against the skin. The waves are reflected to varying degrees by structures of different density, and the pattern of the echoes is electronically recorded on a screen. Ultrasound scanning is the first choice for diagnostic imaging of the gallbladder, female genital tract, and fetus. It also provides remarkably clear pictures of the kidney.

COMPUTERS Many scanning techniques use a computer to provide images. In *CT scanning* (computerized tomography scanning), X rays are passed through the body at different angles. The computer produces cross-sectional images ("slices") of the tissues being examined. In *MRI* (magnetic resonance imaging), the patient is placed in a strong magnetic field and radio-frequency waves are passed through the body. A computer analyzes changes in the magnetic alignment of the hydrogen protons of the cells to give an image of the tissues.

CT scanning and MRI are particularly valuable in the diagnosis of brain disorders. So, too, is a more recent

IMAGING THE BODY

Over the past decade, many new methods of imaging the body have been developed. These new imaging techniques have made it possible to visualize internal structures in a variety of different ways. Today, in addition to conventional X rays (which show primarily bones), techniques such as CT scanning, radionuclide scanning, ultrasound scanning, MRI, and PET scanning are used to provide detailed diagnostic pictures of soft tissues and organs. The examples given here show some of the different ways in which the kidneys can be imaged. Annotated diagrams and explanatory text will help you interpret the images.

X RAYS

Radiopaque contrast media may be utilized to give distinct X-ray images of soft tissues, as in intravenous pyelography, which is used to clearly visualize the kidneys and urinary tracts.

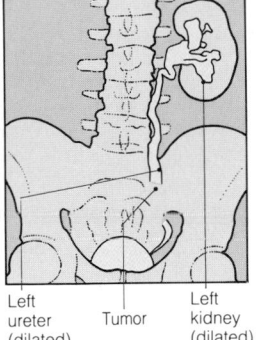

Left ureter (dilated)   Tumor   Left kidney (dilated)

Intravenous pyelogram

The intravenous pyelogram (far left) shows the left kidney and ureter, which are visible because they are filled with contrast medium that has been retained due to a tumor obstructing the ureter (see left).

SCANNING TECHNIQUES

Many new techniques have been developed for imaging the body, particularly the soft tissues. Some of these techniques, such as CT scanning, rely on computers to process the raw imaging data and produce the actual image. Others, such as ultrasound scanning and radionuclide scanning, can produce images without a computer, although one may be used for image enhancement.

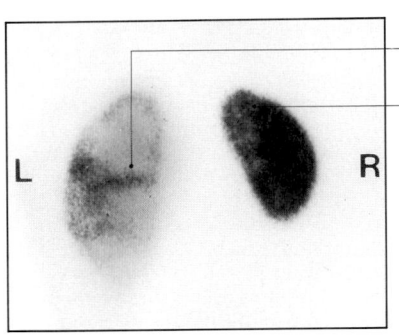

Damaged left kidney

Normal right kidney

L   R

Radionuclide scanning

A radioactive substance is introduced into the body, and the radiation emitted is detected by a gamma camera, which converts it into an image. In the scan of the kidneys (left), the left one has taken up little of the radioactive substance (and thus appears faint), which indicates that it is damaged.

Ultrasound scanning

Ultrahigh frequency sound waves reflected from tissues in the body are converted into an image by special electronic equipment. The scan (below left) shows a section through a diseased kidney; the inner tissues (calyx and pelvis) are greatly dilated, and the outer cortex is abnormally thin (see diagram, below right).

CT scanning

A CT scanner produces cross-sectional images (slices) of the body. The CT scan (right) shows a greatly dilated right kidney (see diagram, below right).

Back   Thin cortex

Renal calyx (dilated)   Renal pelvis (dilated)

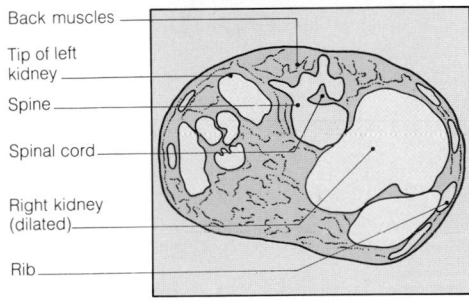

Back muscles

Tip of left kidney

Spine

Spinal cord

Right kidney (dilated)

Rib

technique called *PET* (positron emission tomography) *scanning*, in which very short-lived radioisotopes are introduced into tissues; the paths of gamma rays emitted are analyzed by a computer, giving information about brain function and structure.

In *radionuclide scanning*, a gamma camera records, and a computer transforms into images, radiation emitted from tissues into which a radioactive substance has been introduced. The computer may be used to obtain more information.

Imipramine

A tricyclic *antidepressant drug*. Imipramine is most commonly used as a long-term treatment for *depression*, but may take up to six weeks to have a beneficial effect.

Possible adverse effects include excessive sweating, blurred vision, dry mouth, dizziness, constipation, nausea, and difficulty passing urine in older men. Overdose, particularly in a child, can be fatal.

Immersion foot

A condition that occurs in shipwreck survivors and soldiers (in whom it is known as trench foot) resulting from the feet being wet and cold for a long time. Initially, the feet turn pale and have no detectable pulse; later, they become red, swollen, and painful, and have a strong pulse.

TREATMENT

If the feet are at the pale stage, they should be gradually and carefully rewarmed; overheating may lead to *gangrene* (tissue death). Conversely, if they are red and swollen, they should be gradually cooled.

If the condition is ignored and becomes severe, muscle weakness, skin ulcers, or gangrene may develop. Even with mild cases, the feet may be painful and sensitive to cold for several years afterward.

Immobility

Reduced physical activity and movement. Immobility is particularly harmful in the elderly because it causes muscle wasting and progressive loss of function.

CAUSES

Total immobility is rare; it occurs in coma, which is sometimes the result of *stroke*, *brain tumor*, or major *head injury*. *Catatonia* is associated with varying degrees of immobility.

Temporary loss of mobility, lasting a few days, occurs during recovery from any serious illness, such as a

myocardial infarction, or from a major surgical procedure.

Fractures in a lower limb may be treated by *traction*, which requires several weeks in bed, or by use of a *cast*, which also hinders mobility.

Loss of mobility may be caused by the symptoms of a specific medical disorder, such as *asthma* or *angina pectoris* (chest pain due to reduced blood supply to the heart muscle). Both these conditions may, in severe cases, be aggravated by exercise. *Arthritis* (inflammation of joints) limits mobility if the hips, knees, ankles, or feet are affected by pain and stiffness. Nervous system disorders that restrict mobility include *hemiplegia* (paralysis on one side of the body), *Parkinson's disease*, and *multiple sclerosis*.

A person may find it difficult to move around because of deteriorating eyesight, or may lack motivation due to *depression* or the effects of alcohol or other drugs (such as tranquilizers).

COMPLICATIONS

Total immobility can cause *bedsores*, *pneumonia* caused by secretions building up in the lungs, or *contractures*.

A common complication of partial immobility is *edema* (abnormal retention of fluid in body tissues), which causes swelling of the legs as a result of the calf muscles not working to pump the fluid back to the heart in the circulation. Rarely, a *thrombosis* (blood clot) forms in one of the veins in the leg because of this lack of blood flow.

Obesity is more likely to occur in people who do not exercise. Stiffness tends to develop in any joint not being used properly. Muscle wasting and *osteoporosis* are common problems caused by immobility in the elderly.

TREATMENT

Regular *physical therapy* and adequate nursing care are important for any person who is totally immobile. Regular turning and the use of a special mattress and bed reduce the risk of bed sores. Stretching exercises may prevent contractures.

Early mobilization after serious illness or major surgery is usually encouraged to avoid the problems of prolonged bed rest. After a lower limb fracture, walking with the aid of crutches is started as soon as possible.

Aids for the disabled (see *Disability*) can increase mobility that is impaired by leg weakness, stiffness, loss of balance, or poor coordination. If the person is unable to walk despite assistance, exercises may be done in a chair or in bed to keep the muscles and joints in reasonable working order.

Immobilization

An orthopedic term for techniques used to prevent movement of joints or displacement of fractured bones so that the bones can unite properly. (See also *Fracture*.)

Immune response

A defensive reaction of the body to invading microorganisms, cancer cells, transplanted tissue, and other substances or materials that are recognized as antigenic or "foreign" (that is, different from normal body components). The response consists of the production of substances called *antibodies* or *immunoglobulins*, sensitized cells called *lymphocytes*, and other substances and cells that act to destroy the antigenic material. (See also *Immune system*.)

Immune serum globulin

A preparation of *antibodies*, also known as immune globulin and gamma globulin, used to prevent and sometimes treat infectious diseases.

Its main use is in the prevention of viral *hepatitis* (e.g., before traveling to a country where the disease is common). It is also given to prevent *measles* and *rubella* in people who are exposed to these infections and are not already immune to them from previous infection or *immunization*.

Immune serum globulin is also given to people with *immunodeficiency disorders* (impaired natural defenses).

HOW IT WORKS

Immune serum globulin provides immunity to a range of common infectious diseases. It works by passing on antibodies obtained from the blood of large numbers of people who have previously been exposed to these diseases and thus have developed antibodies to them.

POSSIBLE ADVERSE EFFECTS

Immune serum globulin may cause rash, fever, and pain and tenderness at the injection site.

Immune system

A collection of cells and proteins that works to protect the body from potentially harmful, infectious microorganisms (microscopic life-forms), such as bacteria, viruses, and fungi. The immune system also plays a role in the control of cancer and is responsible for the phenomena of *allergy*, *hypersensitivity*, and rejection problems when organs or tissue are transplanted.

Some of the main components of the body's immune system are described in the illustrated boxes.

A newborn child is, to some extent, protected against infection by barriers (such as the skin), by substances in the mouth, in the urinary tract, or on the eye surface that destroy microorganisms, and by *antibodies* or *immunoglobulins* (protective proteins) that have been passed to the child from the mother (including those received in breast milk).

This natural, or innate, immunity cannot guard against all disease-causing organisms. As the child grows, he or she encounters organisms that overcome the innate defenses and thus cause disease. The second line of immune defense, called the adaptive immune system, then comes into play. As the name implies, this system adapts its response specifically to fight the invading organism. In addition, it retains a memory of the invader so that defenses can be rallied instantly in the future. The person is then said to have acquired immunity to the infection. If these microorganisms invade again, they are quickly recognized and dealt with (which explains why diseases such as measles and diphtheria rarely affect the same person twice).

The acquisition of immunity in response to an infection can take a few days or weeks to develop; in the interim, a child or adult can become very ill or even die. In the past, many did die. Today, our chance of surviving, recovering, or totally avoiding infectious diseases is much improved, partly as a result of better general health and nutrition (which bolsters the immune system) and partly through *immunization* against specific disease-causing microorganisms.

INNATE IMMUNITY
The skin provides an impenetrable barrier to the vast majority of infectious agents, most of which can gain entry only via the mucous membranes (e.g., in the mouth, throat, eyes, intestines, vagina, or urinary tract). These areas are protected by the movement of mucus and other fluids (such as tears) and the presence of enzymes (such as lysozyme) that destroy bacteria.

If microorganisms are able to penetrate the outer layer of the skin or a mucous membrane, they soon encounter white blood cells called phagocytes (literally, "engulfing" cells), which attempt to destroy them, and other types of white cells, such as natural killer (cytotoxic) cells. Microorganisms may also meet naturally produced substances (such

as *interferon*) or a system of blood proteins known as the complement system, which act to destroy the invading microorganisms.

ADAPTIVE IMMUNITY
The adaptive part of the immune system is extremely complex and only partly understood. Its function is to produce specific defenses against a range of different invading organisms or tumor cells. Broadly, however, it first must recognize part of an invading organism or tumor cell as an *antigen* (a protein that is foreign or different from any natural body protein).

A response (either humoral or cellular) is then mounted against the antigen. The humoral response consists of the production of soluble proteins, called antibodies or immunoglobulins, manufactured by cells called B-lymphocytes. Cellular responses center around the activities of the cells called T-lymphocytes.

HUMORAL IMMUNITY
This type of immunity is particularly important in the defense against bacteria. After a complex recognition process, certain B-lymphocytes are stimulated to multiply. These cells then begin to produce vast numbers of antibodies that are able to bind to the antigens. Once this has occurred, the organisms bearing the antigens are easy prey to phagocytic ("engulfing") white cells. Binding of antibody and antigen may also activate the complement system, which increases the efficiency with which phagocytes engulf and destroy the invading organisms.

CELLULAR IMMUNITY
This is particularly important in the defense against viruses, some types of parasites that hide within cells, and, possibly, cancer cells. The T-lymphocytes at the center of cellular immunity are of two types, called helper cells and killer cells. The helper cells play a role in the recognition of antigens. Along with various other functions, they activate the killer cells. Killer lymphocytes lock onto cells that have been invaded by viruses or other parasites that have left recognizable antigens on the cell surfaces. The killer lymphocytes then destroy these parasitized cells. They may act in a similar way against tumor cells and against the cells in transplanted tissue.

The memory of the immune system (which provides acquired immunity to certain diseases) relies on the long-term survival of lymphocytes that were activated or sensitized to antigens when these antigens were first encountered.

IMMUNE SYSTEM DEFECTS
The immune system is an essential asset for the protection of the body from infectious agents and probably cancer. In certain circumstances, however, it may itself be a cause of disease or other undesirable consequences. In some cases, the body's own proteins are misidentified as antigens, and an immunological attack is mounted against them, causing *autoimmune disorders*. In other cases, the immune system mounts an inappropriate response to what are usually innocuous antigens, such as pollen, causing *hypersensitivity* or *allergy*.

SUPPRESSION OF THE IMMUNE SYSTEM
In certain circumstances, such as after transplantation of tissues (see *Transplant surgery*) and in people with an autoimmune disorder, it is advantageous to suppress the immune system (especially the adaptive part of the immune system) through use of drugs. This prevents the rejection of the donor organ by lymphocytes and other cells that recognize proteins in the transplanted tissue as antigens. Immunosuppression can also occur as an inherited disorder or after infection with certain viruses, including HIV, the virus that causes *AIDS* (see *Immunodeficiency disorders*).

Immunity
A state of protection against a disease or diseases through the activities of the *immune system*. Natural, or innate, immunity is present from birth and is the first line of defense against the vast majority of infectious agents. Acquired immunity is the second line of defense. It develops either through exposure to invading microorganisms (after they have broken through the innate immune defenses) or as a result of *immunization*.

Immunization
The process of inducing *immunity* as a preventive measure against certain infectious diseases. The incidence of a number of diseases (*diphtheria* and *measles*, for example) has declined dramatically since the introduction of effective immunization programs; one disease (*smallpox*) has been eradicated worldwide.

Although diseases such as diphtheria, measles, *mumps*, rubella (German measles), *poliomyelitis*, and *pertussis* (whooping cough) are today rare in the US, routine immunization against them must continue. If a large proportion of the population were nonimmunized, there would be a risk

THE INNATE IMMUNE SYSTEM

Each of us has many inborn defenses against infection, including external barriers (below), the inflammatory response (right), and phagocyte action (below right). Others include chemicals called complement (which is activated by and attacks bacteria) and *interferon* (which has antiviral effects).

All these defenses are nonspecific and quick-acting. By contrast, the adaptive immune system (next page) mounts specific attacks against particular microbes. These cells are most effective on second exposure to the organisms.

The two parts of the immune system work together; antibodies produced by the adaptive immune system assist phagocyte action.

THE INFLAMMATORY RESPONSE

If microbes break through the body's outermost barriers, inflammation is the second line of defense. Chemicals (such as histamine) are released, prompting the effects shown below, including the attraction of phagocytes to the microbes. The symptoms of inflammation are redness, pain, swelling, and heat.

Following tissue injury (here caused by a splinter) and entry of bacteria or other microbes, blood vessels in the area widen and there is increased leakage of fluid from the blood into the tissues. This allows easier access for immune system components that fight the invaders, including phagocytes and soluble factors (such as the group of chemicals known as complement).

Physical and chemical barriers

These barriers, summarized below, provide the first line of defense against harmful microbes (bacteria, viruses, and fungi).

Eyes

Tears produced by the lacrimal apparatus help wash away microorganisms; tears contain an enzyme (lysozyme) that can destroy bacteria.

Mouth

Lysozyme present in saliva destroys bacteria.

Breast-feeding

Antibodies (proteins with a protective role) formed by the mother against certain microbes are transferred to the baby in breast milk. This action provides some extra immunity until the baby can form his or her own specific antibodies.

Nose

Hairs in the nose help prevent entry of microorganisms on dust particles. This process is assisted by the sneeze reflex.

Respiratory tract

Mucus secreted by cells lining the throat, windpipe, and bronchi traps microbes, which are then swept away by cilia (hairs on cells in the lining) or engulfed by phagocytes (types of white cells). The cough reflex also helps to expel microbes.

Stomach and intestines

Stomach acid destroys the vast majority of microorganisms. The intestines contain harmless bacteria (commensals) that compete with and control the harmful organisms.

Genitourinary system

The vagina and urethra also contain commensals and are protected by mucus. Spermine in semen may exert some antimicrobial action.

Skin

Intact skin provides an effective barrier against most microbes. The sebaceous glands secrete chemicals that are highly toxic to many bacteria.

ACTION OF PHAGOCYTES

These white blood cells are attracted to infection sites, where they engulf and digest microorganisms and debris.

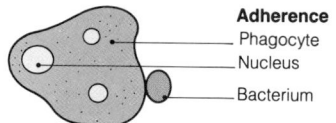

Adherence
Phagocyte
Nucleus
Bacterium

1 The phagocyte must first contact and recognize a microbe as foreign. This process is assisted by chemicals released during inflammation.

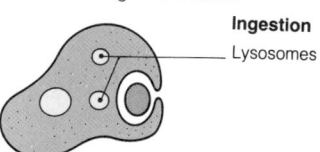

Ingestion
Lysosomes

2 The phagocyte engulfs the microbe in a pouch formed in its membrane. Fluid-filled particles called lysosomes move toward the microbe.

Digestion
Enzymes released

3 Enzymes within the lysosome are released into the pouch to help digest the microbe. Debris from this process is later ejected.

THE ADAPTIVE IMMUNE SYSTEM

This system is based on cells called lymphocytes. It has two parts. Humoral immunity relies on the production, by B-lymphocytes, of antibodies, which circulate and attack specific microbes. In cellular immunity, cells called T-lymphocytes are activated and attack specific microbes or abnormal cells (such as virally infected or tumor cells).

HUMORAL IMMUNITY

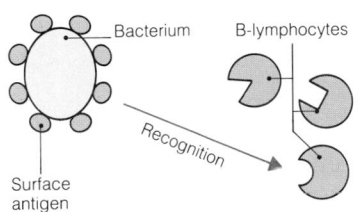

1 A humoral response is started when an antigen (foreign protein)—here on the surface of a bacterium—activates one type of B-lymphocyte.

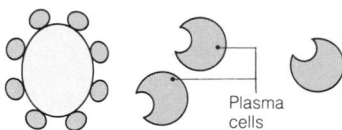

2 The particular type of B-lymphocyte multiplies, forming cells called plasma cells, which make antibodies designed specifically to attack the bacterium.

3 After a few days, the antibodies are released and travel to and attach to the antigen. This triggers more reactions, which ultimately destroy the bacterium.

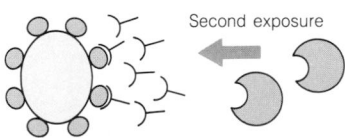

4 Some B-lymphocytes remain in the body as memory cells; if the bacterium enters the body again, they rapidly produce antibodies to halt the infection.

CELLULAR IMMUNITY

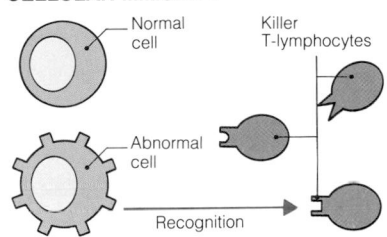

1 An antigen, here on the surface of an abnormal cell (such as a virus-infected or tumor cell), is identified by, and activates, specific killer (cytotoxic) T-lymphocytes.

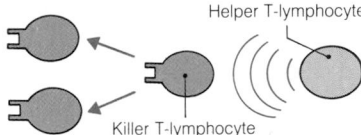

2 With the assistance of helper T cells (another type of T-lymphocyte), the killer T-lymphocytes begin to multiply.

 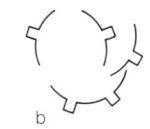

3 The killer T-lymphocytes travel to, and attach to, the abnormal cells (a), leading to their destruction (b). The T-lymphocytes survive and may go on to kill more targets.

4 Some of the killer T-lymphocytes remain as memory cells, and quickly attack abnormal cells should they reappear (e.g., after reinfection with a virus).

Lymphocyte
Lymphocytes are found in the blood and lymphoid organs (lymph nodes, spleen, and thymus). The two main types—B- and T-lymphocytes—have different functions but look identical under the microscope.

AIDS AND CELLULAR IMMUNITY

HIV—the virus responsible for AIDS—causes illness by disrupting the cellular part of the adaptive immune system.

1 HIV invades and destroys the helper T-lymphocytes, thus preventing the assistance they normally give to killer T-lymphocytes.

2 As a result, the killer T-lymphocytes fail to multiply and attack in response to abnormal cells or invading microorganisms.

3 Opportunistic viruses and other microbes or tumor cells may thus proliferate unchecked, causing the features of AIDS.

EXAMPLES OF INFECTIOUS ORGANISMS COMBATTED

Humoral immunity particularly important against:

| Some viruses (e.g., measles) |
| Many bacteria (e.g., cholera) |
| Some parasites (e.g., malaria) |

Cell-mediated immunity particularly important against:

| Many viruses (e.g., herpes simplex) |
| Some bacteria (e.g., tuberculosis) |
| Some fungi (e.g., candidiasis) |

of a new epidemic because there is still a steady flow of cases of infectious diseases (many imported).

IMMUNIZATION AND VACCINATION

Immunization may be active or passive (see diagram). The terms vaccination and active immunization are used interchangeably. The word vaccination is derived from the vaccinia virus (which is similar to the smallpox virus), which was used for vaccination against smallpox.

WHO SHOULD BE IMMUNIZED

Some types of immunization, such as against polio and DPT (diphtheria, pertussis, and *tetanus*), are aimed at the general population, primarily young children. Others are intended for specific people, such as those exposed to dangerous infections during local outbreaks or those who are at risk of contracting unusual infections through occupational exposure (e.g., laboratory workers or veterinarians).

Immunization before foreign travel may be necessary for entry into certain countries (today, this usually applies only to immunization against *yellow fever*) and to protect the traveler against infection. The traveler should determine a few months before departure which immunizations are necessary or recommended.

The accompanying table gives details of a typical immunization schedule during childhood. (See also *Travel immunization*.)

HOW IMMUNIZATION IS DONE

Most immunizations are given by injection, either into the muscle or into the tissues under the skin in the upper arm. If the injection contains a large volume of fluid, it may be given in the buttock. Polio vaccine is almost always given orally.

ADVERSE REACTIONS

Usually there are no aftereffects following immunization. Some vaccines cause pain and swelling at the injection site and may produce a slight fever and a feeling of irritability and malaise. Acetaminophen should be given to young children in whom fever develops after being immunized. Some vaccines, such as the measles vaccine, may produce a mild form of the disease.

In very rare cases, severe reactions (such as seizures) occur following immunization. This has led to controversy about the advisability of some types of vaccination, notably against pertussis (whooping cough). However, for most people, the risks of vaccination are much smaller than the risk of damage through the disease.

TYPICAL CHILDHOOD IMMUNIZATION SCHEDULE

Age	Disease	
2 months	Diphtheria, pertussis (whooping cough), tetanus*	Poliomyelitis†
4 months	Diphtheria, pertussis, tetanus*	Poliomyelitis†
6 months	Diphtheria, pertussis, tetanus*	
15 months	Measles, mumps, rubella (German measles)*	
18 months	Diphtheria, pertussis, tetanus*	Poliomyelitis†
4 to 6 years	Diphtheria, pertussis, tetanus*	Poliomyelitis†
	* Combined injection	† Oral

Although most modern vaccines provide a reliable method of preventing disease, they do not all provide 100 percent protection. *Cholera* and *typhoid fever* vaccinations, in particular, give only partial protection, so other precautions (principally food and water hygiene) must be observed during travel to areas where there is a risk of these diseases.

WHO SHOULD NOT BE IMMUNIZED

Immunization should not be given to any person who suffers from an *immunodeficiency disorder* or a cancer

TYPES OF IMMUNIZATION

There are two main types. In passive immunization, antibodies (protective proteins) are injected and provide immediate, but short-lived, protection against specific disease-causing bacteria, viruses, or toxins. Active immunization primes the body to make its own antibodies against such microorganisms and confers longer-lasting immunity.

PASSIVE IMMUNIZATION

1 Blood is taken from a person or, rarely, an animal previously exposed to a specific microorganism. The blood contains antibodies against that organism.

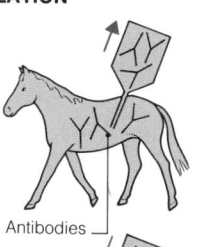

Antibodies

2 An extract of the blood containing the antibodies (called immune serum or antiserum) is injected into the person to be protected.

Serum

Bloodstream

3 The antibodies help destroy the microorganism if it is present in the blood or enters it over the following few days.

Microorganism

ACTIVE IMMUNIZATION

Vaccine

1 The person to be protected is inoculated with a killed or modified microorganism (vaccine) that does not cause disease.

2 The immune system is provoked to make antibodies against the modified microorganism; it also retains a "memory" of the organism.

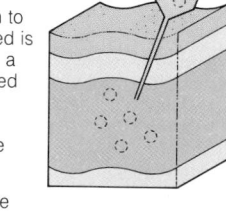

Antibodies

3 If the real microorganism then enters the blood, antibodies are produced in large numbers to halt the infection.

Disease-causing microorganism

that has spread. Any person who is taking *corticosteroid drugs* or who has previously had a severe reaction to the same vaccine should not be vaccinated. Some vaccines, such as those for typhoid and yellow fever, should not be given to very young children. Vaccination should be deferred if the person has a fever or infection. A number of vaccines, particularly the rubella vaccine, should not be given during pregnancy due to the risk of affecting the fetus.

Immunoassay

A group of laboratory techniques that includes ELISA (enzyme-linked immunosorbent assay) and radioimmunoassay. Both are used in the diagnosis of infectious diseases; variants of radioimmunoassay, such as the radioallergosorbent test (RAST) and the radioimmunosorbent test (RIST), are also used in the diagnosis of allergies and in the measurement of blood hormone concentrations.

Either technique can determine the presence or absence in a person's blood of a specific protein—such as an *antigen* (a protein on the surface of a microorganism or an allergen), a specific *antibody* (a protein formed by the body's immune system to protect against a particular type of microorganism or allergen), or other protein, such as a hormone.

The principle underlying these techniques is that, for any specific antibody, there is a specific antigen. If molecules of these two proteins come in close contact, they will bind strongly to each other. Any specific antibody will bind only to its own antigen, and vice versa.

HOW IT IS DONE

First, the surface of a plate or the inside of a test tube is prepared with a covering of the specific protein (antigen or antibody) that will bind to the antibody or antigen whose presence in the blood is to be tested. For example, in the ELISA test for antibody to *HIV* (the virus responsible for *AIDS*), the inside of a test tube is lined with small amounts of antigen from HIV.

This surface is then exposed to plasma of the blood; if the antibody (or antigen) under test is present, it will stick strongly to the surface. The surface is then washed and a chemical added that will bind to the bound protein. This chemical is itself linked either to an enzyme called peroxidase (in the ELISA test) or to a radioactive isotope (in radioimmunoassay).

Any excess chemical is washed away, and, if the antibody or antigen was present, either peroxidase or radioactivity is left on the surface. Peroxidase can be detected by adding another chemical that changes color in its presence; radioactivity can be measured by a gamma counter.

The RIST differs from other types of radioimmunoassay in that the blood serum containing the substance being tested is first mixed with a solution containing the same substance, which has been radioactively labeled. The radioactive and the test versions compete to bind to the test plate. The result is that, after washing, the less radioactivity found on the test plate, the more test substance must have been present in the blood serum.

Immunodeficiency disorders

Disorders in which there is a failure of the *immune system's* defenses to fight infection and tumors. Immunodeficiency may be the result of an inherited or congenital defect that interferes with the normal development of the immune system or the result of acquired disease that damages the system's function. The result, in either case, is the appearance of persistent or recurrent infection by organisms that would not ordinarily cause disease, incomplete recovery from illness with poor response to customarily effective treatment, and an undue susceptibility to certain forms of cancer.

The infections seen in people with immunodeficiency disorders sometimes are called *opportunistic infections* because the microorganisms take advantage of the person's lowered defenses. Infections of this type include pneumonia caused by *PNEUMOCYSTIS CARINII*, widespread *herpes simplex* infections, and many *fungal infections.*

INHERITED IMMUNODEFICIENCY

The adaptive part of the immune system (which mounts specific defenses against particular microorganisms or tumor cells) has two major prongs. One of these, the humoral system, relies on the production of antibodies, or immunoglobulins, manufactured by B-*lymphocytes*. The other prong is called the cellular system and relies on the activity of T-lymphocytes. Congenital or inherited deficiencies can occur in either of these systems.

Deficiencies of the humoral system include hypogammaglobulinemia (in which the production of one or more types of immunoglobulin is interfered

with) and agammaglobulinemia (in which there is an almost complete absence of B-lymphocytes and immunoglobulins). The most common type of hypogammaglobulinemia affects about one person in 600 and may cause no more than repeated mild attacks of respiratory infection. Agammaglobulinemia is a rare, grave condition that often has a fatal outcome in infancy or childhood.

Congenital deficiencies of the T-lymphocytes may lead to problems such as persistent and widespread *candidiasis* (thrush) affecting the skin, mouth, throat, and vagina. Problems of this type are caused by the inability of the immune system to fight fungi.

A combined deficiency of both prongs of the immune system is also known. It is called severe combined immunodeficiency. Infants with this combined deficiency usually die within the first year of life.

ACQUIRED IMMUNODEFICIENCY

Acquired deficiency of the immune system may occur in either of two ways—by damage to the immune system as a result of its suppression with drugs or by disease processes.

Deliberate suppression of the immune system with *immunosuppressant drugs* and *corticosteroid drugs* is usually carried out as part of the treatment of *autoimmune disorders* and after transplantation to minimize the risk of organ rejection.

Diseases that cause immunodeficiency include infection with *HIV* (human immunodeficiency virus), which leads to *AIDS* (acquired immunodeficiency syndrome). Severe malnutrition, especially with protein deficiency, and many types of cancer can also cause immunodeficiency.

IMMUNODEFICIENCY IN THE ELDERLY

A degree of immunodeficiency arises simply as a consequence of age. The thymus, which plays an important part in the production of T-lymphocytes, reaches peak size in puberty and steadily shrinks thereafter. This results in a decline in the number and activity of T-lymphocytes with age; there is also a decline in the numbers of B-lymphocytes.

Immunoglobulins

Proteins found in the blood serum and in tissue fluids, also known as *antibodies*. Immunoglobulins are produced by cells of the *immune system* called B-lymphocytes. Their function is to bind to substances in the body that are recognized as foreign antigens (often proteins on the surface of bacteria and viruses). This binding is a crucial event in the destruction of the microorganisms that bear the antigens. Immunoglobulins also play a central role in *allergies* and *hypersensitivity* reactions. In this case they bind to antigens that are not necessarily a threat to health, which may provoke an inflammatory reaction.

There are five classes of immunoglobulins; of these, immunoglobulin G (IgG) is the major immunoglobulin in human blood serum. The IgG molecule consists of two parts, one of which binds to antigen; the other binds to other cells of the immune system. These other cells are principally white cells called phagocytes, which then engulf the microorganisms bearing the antigen. The antigen-binding site of the IgG molecule is variable in its structure, the different versions of the molecule being capable of binding to an almost infinite number of antigens.

Immunoglobulins can be extracted from blood of recovering patients and used for passive *immunization* against certain infectious diseases.

Immunologist

A specialist in the functioning of the *immune system* who may also devise ways in which the immune system can be stimulated to provide immunity (principally through the use of *vaccines*) and who investigates and treats problems related to the immune system. The latter include *allergies*, *autoimmune disorders*, and *immunodeficiency disorders* such as *AIDS*.

Immunologists also play an important part in *transplant surgery*, looking preoperatively for a good immunological match between recipient and donor organ, and suppressing the recipient's immune system after transplantation to minimize the chances of organ rejection.

Immunology

The study of the functioning and disorders of the *immune system*.

Immunostimulant drugs

A group of drugs that increases the efficiency of the body's *immune system* (natural defenses against infection and abnormal cells). Immunostimulant drugs include *vaccines*, which protect against specific infectious diseases (see *Immunization*). Two drugs belonging to this group are *interferon* (used to treat viral infections and certain types of cancer) and *zidovudine* (used to treat *AIDS*).

Some immunostimulant drugs enhance the ability of a vaccine to stimulate the immune system and are added to the vaccine for this reason. Aluminum phosphate, for example, increases the effectiveness of the *tetanus* vaccine.

Immunosuppressant drugs

COMMON DRUGS
Anticancer drugs
Azathioprine Chlorambucil
Cyclophosphamide Methotrexate
Corticosteroid drugs
Dexamethasone Prednisone
Others
Cyclosporine

A group of drugs that reduces the activity of the body's *immune system* (natural defenses against infection and abnormal cells).

Immunosuppressant drugs are prescribed after *transplant surgery* to prevent the rejection of foreign tissues. They are also given to halt the progress of *autoimmune disorders* (in which the body's immune system attacks its own tissues) when other treatments are ineffective. They are unable, however, to restore tissue that has already been damaged.

HOW THEY WORK

Immunosuppressant drugs work by suppressing the production and activity of *lymphocytes*, a type of white blood cell that plays an important part in fighting infection and in eliminating abnormal cells that may form a malignant tumor.

POSSIBLE ADVERSE EFFECTS

Apart from the individual effects of each type, these drugs increase the risk of infection and of the development of certain cancers.

Immunotherapy

A preventive treatment of allergy to substances such as grass pollens, house-dust mites, and wasp and bee venom. Immunotherapy involves giving gradually increasing doses of the substance, or allergen, to which the person is allergic. This works by making the *immune system* less sensitive to that substance, probably by causing production of a particular "blocking" *antibody*, which reduces the symptoms of allergy when the substance is encountered in the future.

Before starting treatment, the physician and patient try to identify trigger factors for allergic symptoms. Skin or sometimes blood tests are per-

formed to confirm the specific allergens to which the person has antibodies. Immunotherapy is usually recommended only if the person seems to be selectively sensitive to several allergens (such as grass).

HOW IT IS DONE

A purified extract of a small amount of the allergen is injected into the skin of the arm. An injection is given once a week for about 30 weeks, after which injections can be administered every two weeks. Eventually, injections can be given every four weeks; the duration of therapy is three to four years.

RISKS

There is a danger of *anaphylactic shock* (a severe allergic reaction) shortly after an injection. Therefore, immunotherapy requires medical supervision and is not done at times of exposure to the substance causing the allergy.

IMMUNOTHERAPY IN CANCER TREATMEMT

Another use of the term immunotherapy refers to stimulation of the immune system to treat cancer. It is still largely experimental, but it may prove a useful adjunct to other therapies, such as *chemotherapy*, in the treatment of *leukemia*, *lymphoma*, and some other cancers.

One type of immunotherapy relies on the use of immunostimulants, substances that cause general stimulation of the immune system.

Another technique is to inoculate the patient with tumor cells or cellular extracts, rendered harmless by irradiation, that have been taken from another person suffering from the same disease. The patient's immune system then produces its own *antibodies*, which attack the tumor cells. Alternatively, immunoglobulins (ready-made antibodies) from another person with the same type of tumor can be given to the patient. More recently, monoclonal antibodies (see *Antibodies, monoclonal*) to be directed against tumors have been produced artificially by *genetic engineering*. *Interferon* or chemical poisons can be linked to these antibodies to increase their ability to destroy tumor cells.

One drawback to the administration of some of these anticancer treatments is that they, too, may be recognized as foreign by the person's immune system, causing either allergic reactions (serum sickness) or new antibody production, which interferes with the activity against cancer.

Impaction, dental

Failure of a tooth to emerge fully or at all from the gum when, because of

Impacted wisdom teeth
This X ray shows impacted wisdom teeth lying horizontally in the lower jaw. The impacted teeth are wedged against the adjacent molars and are not able to erupt normally.

mechanical impediment, it is embedded in bone or soft tissue beyond its normal eruption time.

Impaction is caused by overcrowding of the teeth in places where little room is left for the teeth that erupt last (the wisdom teeth and the upper canines). It is also caused by the tooth traveling in the wrong direction and by dense bone that impedes the tooth's progress.

IMPACTED WISDOM TEETH

These are common, but usually cause no trouble unless they partially penetrate the gum, leaving a flap of tissue over most of the crown. Plaque bacteria and food debris then collect between the tooth and the gum, which often becomes inflamed and painful. There may also be swollen lymph nodes in the upper neck and difficulty opening the mouth.

Rinsing the area with warm, salt water and taking *analgesics* (painkillers) can relieve some symptoms of the condition, but, if it is severe, *antibiotic drugs* are required to clear up the infection. A dentist may decide that the tooth requires extraction to prevent more trouble.

IMPACTED UPPER CANINES

These teeth play a much more important part than do wisdom teeth in biting and chewing. If they are impacted, they are not usually removed, but instead are trained into the correct position by means of an *orthodontic appliance*.

Impetigo

A highly contagious skin infection, common in children, that usually occurs around the nose and mouth.

CAUSES AND INCIDENCE

Impetigo is caused by bacteria entering the skin through a broken area, such as a cut, cold sore, or an area affected by *eczema*. The infection is more common in warm weather. Impetigo was once extremely common, but occurs less frequently now because of improved standards of personal hygiene. Small epidemics occasionally occur in schools.

SYMPTOMS AND SIGNS

The skin reddens and small, fluid-filled blisters appear on the surface. The blisters tend to burst, leaving moist, weeping areas underneath; the released fluid dries to leave honey-colored crusts on the skin. The infected area may spread at the edges or another patch may develop nearby.

In severe cases there may be swelling of the *lymph nodes* in the face or neck, accompanied by a fever. Very occasionally, complications such as *septicemia* (blood poisoning) or *glomerulonephritis* (inflammation of the kidneys) develop.

TREATMENT

Because impetigo spreads rapidly, it is advisable to consult a physician. *Antibiotic drugs* in tablet or ointment form usually clear up the problem in about

---

TYPES OF IMPLANTS

Implants may be inserted into various parts of the body. They can be used to replace a diseased structure, to improve appearance, to maintain proper functioning of an internal organ, to treat certain disorders, or to deliver drugs or hormones.

Hormonal
Some hormonal drugs (particularly hormonal contraceptives) can be placed in implants that are inserted under the skin to release the drug slowly over time. Alternatively, such drugs can be incorporated in some IUDs (intrauterine contraceptive devices).

Breast
Silicone implants can be used to restore breast shape after mastectomy (breast removal) for cancer or to increase breast size for cosmetic purposes (augmentation mammoplasty).

Therapeutic
Radioactive materials in sealed containers can be inserted into tissue to treat malignant tumors, for example, a cancer of the cervix.

Eye
An implant can be used to replace the lens of the eye after cataract removal, or the entire eyeball if it requires removal because of injury or disease.

Face
Pieces of bone taken from another part of the body, or shaped pieces of silicone, can be implanted on the face to make a receding chin more prominent or to improve the contour at a fracture site.

Heart
Cardiac pacemakers (battery-powered electronic devices connected by wires to the heart muscle) can be implanted in the chest to regulate the heart beat; diseased heart valves may be replaced with artificial or natural substitutes.

Joints
Diseased joints can be replaced with artificial substitutes to help restore full function. The elbow, the hip, the knee, the finger joints, and the shoulder can all now be treated in this way.

Artery
Diseased sections of artery, such as the lower aorta and upper iliac arteries (shown here), can be replaced or bypassed with artificial tubular materials made from woven or knitted synthetic fibers.

The appearance of impetigo
Fluid-filled blisters appear on the skin (in this case, on the neck and chest). The blisters often burst, releasing fluid that dries to leave pale-brown crusts.

five days. Any loose crusts should be gently washed off with soap and water and the area dabbed dry.

To prevent spreading, pillowcases, towels, and washcloths should not be shared and should be boiled after use. Children should not touch affected skin and should stay out of school until the infection clears.

Implant
Any material, natural or artificial, inserted into the body (see box on the previous page).

Implantation, egg

Attachment of a fertilized ovum to the wall of the uterus. About six days after fertilization, the developing *embryo* comes into contact with the wall of the uterus and attaches to it. As the cells of the embryo divide, the outer cell layer grows into the lining of the uterus to obtain oxygen and nutrients from the mother's blood; later, this layer develops into the *placenta*.

The embryo usually implants in the upper part of the uterus; if it implants low down near the cervix, *placenta previa* may develop. Rarely, the embryo does not reach the uterus and implants in a fallopian tube, resulting in an *ectopic pregnancy*.

Impotence
The inability to achieve or maintain an *erection*. Impotence is the most common male sexual disorder, affecting most men at some time in their lives.
CAUSES
In the majority of men, impotence is caused by psychological factors. They may be temporary (caused by stress or fatigue) or long-standing (caused by anxiety and guilt that originated in childhood). Impotence may be a symptom of *depression*.

Approximately 10 percent of impotence is caused by a physical disorder (including *diabetes mellitus* or hormonal imbalance) or by a neurological disorder (such as spinal cord damage or chronic alcohol abuse). Impotence may be caused by taking various drugs—particularly antipsychotics, antidepressants, antihypertensives, and diuretics. Impotence is also more common as men get older, possibly because of altered circulation or, less often, lowered levels of the male sex hormone *testosterone*.
DIAGNOSIS AND TREATMENT
If the cause is psychological, counseling or *sex therapy* (preferably with the person's partner) is successful in more than half the cases of long-term impotence. To eliminate the possibility of any physical disorder, tests may be performed. The physician may stop medication or alter the dose to aid in diagnosis; attempts are also made to treat any depression or alcohol abuse. *Penile implants* help some men whose impotence is caused by disease.

Impression, dental
A mold taken of the teeth, gums, and sometimes the palate. A quick-setting material, such as alginate or a rubber compound, is placed in a shaped tray that is eased over the area of which a replica is to be made and left in position until the material has set. After the mold has been removed, plaster of Paris is poured into it to obtain a model of the area. This is then used as a base on which to build a *denture*, *bridge*, *inlay*, or *onlay*.

Impressions are also used in *orthodontics* to study the position of the teeth and the structure of the mouth, and to make any orthodontic appliances to correct the irregularities.

Impulse control disorders
A group of psychiatric disorders characterized by the inability to resist an impulse or temptation to do some-

INCIDENCE OF RELATIVELY SHORT-LIVED CONDITIONS* IN THE US

Incidence (new cases per 100,000 people per year)	Categorization	Examples
More than 10,000	Extremely common	Common cold
1,000 to 10,000	Very common	Sexually transmitted infection (all types)
100 to 1,000	Common	Basal cell carcinoma, gonorrhea, lung cancer, myocardial infarction, shingles, stroke
20 to 100	Fairly common	Breast cancer, viral hepatitis, intestinal cancer, symptomatic kidney stones
5 to 20	Uncommon	AIDS, brain tumor, acute leukemia, malignant melanoma, syphilis (primary and secondary), tuberculosis
0.5 to 5	Rare	Amebiasis, gallbladder cancer, Guillain-Barré syndrome, Hodgkin's disease, measles, motor neuron disease, pertussis
0.005 to 0.5	Very rare	Botulism, leptospirosis, lymphogranuloma venereum, malaria
Less than 0.005	Extremely rare	Cholera, diphtheria, rabies

* conditions that are self-resolving, curable, or fatal

thing that ultimately proves harmful to oneself. The group includes pathological *gambling*, *kleptomania*, *pyromania*, and *explosive disorders*.

Incest

Legally defined as sexual intercourse between close relatives (parent-child or brother-sister intercourse is regarded as first degree; with a grandparent, aunt, or uncle, it is regarded as second degree; with a cousin it is regarded as third degree).

Marriage between close kin is forbidden by law in certain jurisdictions and religions, but permitted in others. Incest prohibitions are widespread and are probably based on concerns over the higher risk of certain congenital problems due to inbreeding.

The actual prevalence of incest is unknown. Recent estimates state that 5 to 10 percent of girls experienced sexual contact with a brother, father, or other male relative, as did 1 to 2 percent of boys with either a male or a female relative.

The 1978 Federal Child Abuse Laws mandate reporting to child protection authorities "any sexual act" (not just intercourse) between an adult and a child inside or outside the family; this aberrant and psychologically damaging behavior is regarded as criminal.

Incest was customary in the royal families of ancient Egypt and contemporary Hawaii. It is more common in isolated mountain and rural communities, where incest-accepting families remain unaware of the law. Education and individual and family therapy are useful.

Incidence

One of the two principal measures (the other is prevalence) of how common a disease is in a defined population. The incidence of a disease is the number of new cases that occurs during a given period (e.g., 17 cases per 100,000 people per year). Prevalence is the total number of cases of a disease in existence at any one time; it includes both new and old cases. Thus, in 100,000 people, there may be an incidence of, say, 400 cases of a specific type of cancer per year, but a prevalence of 4,000 cases, because the disease lasts an average of 10 years before being cured or causing death.

Incision

A cut made into the tissues of the body by a scalpel (surgical knife). Most incisions are made to gain access to tissue inside the body (usually to repair or

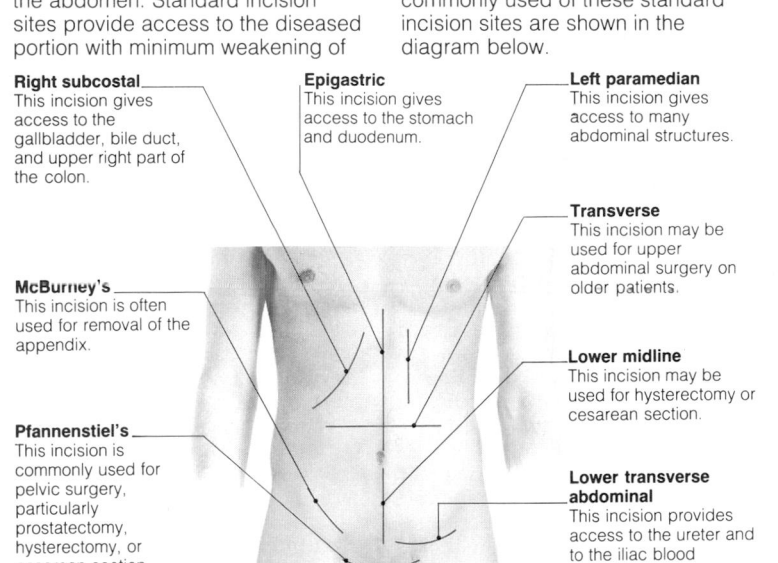

ABDOMINAL INCISIONS

Surgery is frequently performed on the abdomen. Standard incision sites provide access to the diseased portion with minimum weakening of the abdominal wall. The most commonly used of these standard incision sites are shown in the diagram below.

Right subcostal
This incision gives access to the gallbladder, bile duct, and upper right part of the colon.

Epigastric
This incision gives access to the stomach and duodenum.

Left paramedian
This incision gives access to many abdominal structures.

Transverse
This incision may be used for upper abdominal surgery on older patients.

McBurney's
This incision is often used for removal of the appendix.

Lower midline
This incision may be used for hysterectomy or cesarean section.

Pfannenstiel's
This incision is commonly used for pelvic surgery, particularly prostatectomy, hysterectomy, or cesarean section.

Lower transverse abdominal
This incision provides access to the ureter and to the iliac blood vessels.

remove a diseased organ) or to relieve pressure (e.g., from pus in an abscess). Standard incision sites for abdominal surgery are shown in the illustrated box.

Incisor

One of the eight front teeth (four in the upper jaw and four in the lower) used for incising (cutting through) food. (See *Teeth*.)

Incompetent cervix

See *Cervical incompetence*.

Incontinence, fecal

Inability to retain feces in the rectum.
CAUSES
The most common cause of fecal incontinence in the elderly and in children who have been toilet trained is *fecal impaction*. The feces lodged in the rectum irritate and inflame its lining and, as a result, fecal fluid and small pieces of feces are passed involuntarily. Temporary loss of continence may occur at any age with severe *diarrhea* when the need to evacuate the bowel becomes too great to contain.

Less common causes include injury to the anal muscles (for example, during childbirth or surgery), *paraplegia* (paralysis of the legs and lower trunk), mental handicap, and *dementia*.

TREATMENT
Impaction, often caused by constipation, may be prevented by a high-fiber diet. Glycerin suppositories taken daily (or laxative suppositories taken occasionally) may be used if the constipation has persisted for several days. Incontinence due to dementia or nerve injury can be avoided by regularly using enemas or suppositories to empty the rectum.

Incontinence, urinary

Uncontrollable, involuntary urination, often due to injury or disease of the *urinary tract*. This disorder often affects the elderly because the efficiency of the sphincter muscles surrounding the *urethra* declines with age. Women are affected more often than men.
TYPES AND SYMPTOMS
STRESS INCONTINENCE This refers to the involuntary escape of a small amount of urine when a person coughs, laughs, picks up a heavy package, or moves excessively (such as during athletic activity). Stress incontinence is very common in women, particularly after childbirth when the urethral sphincter muscles are stretched.
URGE INCONTINENCE In this type, an urgent desire to urinate is accompanied by inability to control the bladder. Urge incontinence may occur when walking or sitting, but is fre-

quently triggered by a sudden change in position. Once urination starts, it continues until the bladder is empty.

TOTAL INCONTINENCE This refers to a complete lack of bladder control resulting from the total absence of sphincter activity. In rare cases, total incontinence occurs because the urine bypasses the sphincter, as in a vesicovaginal fistula (a hole between the bladder and vagina) or an ectopic ureter (in which the ureter enters the urethra rather than the bladder).

OVERFLOW INCONTINENCE This occurs in chronic *urine retention*, a condition in which the sufferer is unable to empty the bladder normally, often because of an obstruction such as an enlarged *prostate gland*. The bladder is always full, leading to constant dribbling of the overflow. Relief of the obstruction restores continence.

CAUSES
Incontinence may be caused by localized disorders of the urinary tract (including infections, bladder stones, or tumors) or by *prolapse* of the uterus or vagina. Incontinence due to lack of control by the brain commonly occurs in the young (see *Enuresis*), the elderly, and those with mental impairment. Damage to the brain or spinal cord by injury or disease also affects bladder control, as does stress, anger, and anxiety. Weak pelvic muscles, a fractured pelvis, or cancer of the prostate can cause incontinence. *Irritable bladder*, in which the bladder muscle twitches intermittently, raises the pressure in the bladder to push some urine out of the urethra; this causes an intense desire to urinate.

DIAGNOSIS
Urinalysis (examination of the urine) is performed to eliminate the possibility of infection, inflammation, diabetes, or protein loss. *Ultrasound scanning*, intravenous *pyelography* (X rays of the kidney and ureters after injection of a dye), and a voiding *cystourethrogram* (X rays taken while the patient is urinating) are used to investigate the possibility of an obstruction. *Cystometry*, which measures the pressure within the bladder, can determine if the bladder is functioning normally or if there is any abnormality of the nerves supplying the bladder. *Cystoscopy* (examination of the urethra and bladder through a rigid or flexible viewing tube) is performed to look for the presence of bladder *calculi*, tumors, or cysts.

TREATMENT
If weak pelvic muscles are causing stress incontinence, *pelvic floor exercises* may help to restore sphincter function. Sometimes an operation is performed to tighten the urethra. In severe cases, an inflatable artificial plastic sphincter may be placed around the urethra; when urination is required, a trigger is pressed to deflate the mechanism to allow urine to flow.

Anticholinergic drugs are sometimes used to relax the spastic bladder muscle if irritable bladder is the cause.

If normal bladder function cannot be restored, special incontinence underpants (with an internal pad to absorb the urine) can alleviate discomfort. Men can wear a sheath over the penis; the sheath leads into a tube connected to a portable urine bag. Some people are able to pass a catheter into the bladder four or five times a day to empty it and avoid incontinence.

If these measures are unsuccessful and the condition is severe, a *urinary diversion* operation to bypass the bladder may be necessary.

Incoordination

Loss of the ability to produce smooth, harmonious muscular movements, leading to clumsiness and unsteady balance. Incoordination can also mean the failure of a group of organs to work together successfully. (See *Ataxia*.)

Incubation period

The time during which any infectious disease develops, from the point when the infecting organism enters the body until the appearance of symptoms. Different infections have characteristic incubation periods—for example, 14 to 21 days for chickenpox and seven to 14 days for measles. The incubation period for cholera may be as short as several hours. (See also *Infectious disease* table.)

Incubator

A transparent plastic container in which oxygen, temperature, and humidity levels are controlled to provide premature or sick infants with ideal conditions for survival. An incubator also provides some protection from airborne infection.

Incubators have portholes to allow handling of the baby and smaller holes through which monitoring cables and intravenous and respiratory tubing can pass. The air temperature within the incubator is carefully regulated.

Indian medicine

In contrast to Chinese medicine, traditional East Indian medicine was based on empirical observation and practice rather than on philosophy. The earliest Indian literature, the Vedas, which date from about 1500 BC, contain detailed descriptions of numerous disorders and their treatments. Ayurvedism, as Vedic medicine is known, was based largely on herbal treatment, although early Vedic physicians also used simple surgical techniques and invented artificial limbs and eyes.

The Vedic era ended in about 800 BC, but the medical traditions of ayurvedism survived and were further developed (especially the surgical aspect) under the Brahmans, the caste of wise men. As a result, by about 500 AD, Indian medicine had become a scientifically based system with a wide range of surgical techniques available (such as operations for cataracts and kidney stones) along with the herbal tradition. The Brahmans, however, cloaked their medical knowledge in theology and superstition and traditional Indian medicine stagnated. Today, most Indian medicine follows Western practices.

Indigestion

A term covering a variety of symptoms brought on by eating, including *heartburn*, *abdominal pain*, *nausea*, and *flatulence* (excessive gas in the stomach or intestine, causing belching or discomfort).

Indigestion refers to a burning discomfort in the upper abdomen, often brought on by eating too much, too quickly, or by eating very rich, spicy, or fatty foods. Nervous indigestion is a common effect of stress. Occasionally, persistent or recurrent indigestion is associated with a *peptic ulcer*, *gallstones*, or *esophagitis* (inflammation of the esophagus).

TREATMENT
Self-help treatment includes avoiding foods and situations that bring on symptoms and finding time to eat

Premature infant in an incubator
Portholes make it possible to handle the infant without disturbing the special conditions provided by the incubator.

three or four times a day, at regular times, without rushing. Taking *antacid drugs* or drinking milk may make symptoms subside.

Anyone who takes antacid drugs regularly should see a physician so that the underlying cause of the problem can be investigated. If abdominal pain persists for more than six hours, or if there are other symptoms, such as prolonged vomiting, vomiting blood (which may appear brown), passing very dark or black feces, or feeling weak or faint, a physician should be consulted immediately.

Indomethacin

A *nonsteroidal anti-inflammatory drug* (NSAID) used to relieve pain, stiffness, and inflammation in disorders such as *osteoarthritis, rheumatoid arthritis, gout, ankylosing spondylitis,* and *tendinitis*. Indomethacin is also prescribed to relieve pain caused by injury to soft tissues, such as muscles and ligaments.

Treatment with indomethacin may cause abdominal pain, nausea, heartburn, headache, dizziness, and an increased risk of *peptic ulcer*.

Induction of labor

Use of artificial means to initiate the process of childbirth. Labor is induced if the health of the mother or baby would be endangered by allowing the pregnancy to continue. If the pregnancy is not at full term, the risks of induction are weighed against the risks of a premature delivery.

WHY IT IS DONE
The primary reason for inducing labor is that the pregnancy has continued past the estimated delivery date, which increases the chance of both maternal and fetal complications during childbirth. Most obstetricians induce labor if the delivery is more than two weeks overdue.

Labor is induced early if the mother is suffering from *eclampsia* or *preeclampsia*, or if she has chronic *hypertension*. Labor may also be induced if there is Rh incompatibility between the mother and baby (because of the risk of *hemolytic disease of the newborn*) or if there are indications of *intrauterine growth retardation*.

HOW IT IS DONE
The most common technique of inducing labor is to rupture the membrane around the baby to release some of the amniotic fluid. This is usually sufficient to start labor. If not, vaginal suppositories containing prostaglandin (a hormone that stimulates the uterus to contract) may be inserted high in the vagina. If this is unsuccessful, an intravenous infusion of *oxytocin* (another hormone that stimulates uterine contractions) may be necessary. If the uterus fails to respond to any of these treatments, the baby may be delivered by cesarean section.

COMPLICATIONS
The conditions of both the mother and baby are monitored closely during an induced labor because of the danger that *hypoxia* (reduced oxygen supply) may develop in the baby. Special care facilities are needed if the baby is born prematurely.

Industrial diseases

See *Occupational disease and injury*.

Infant

A baby up to the age of 12 months; sometimes this description also includes the period up to 24 months.

Infantile spasms

A rare type of recurrent seizure that affects babies. Infantile spasms are a form of *epilepsy* in which the baby suddenly stiffens, bending the trunk, limbs, and neck. There may be several hundred such spasms per day, each lasting a few seconds and sometimes preceded by a cry. In most cases the seizures are a sign of brain damage and affected babies grow up with severe mental retardation.

Infant mortality

The number of infants who die during the first year of life per 1,000 live births. About two thirds of all infant deaths occur during the neonatal period (the first month of life). Most of those who die are very premature (born before the 30th week of pregnancy) or have severe birth defects.

Infant mortality varies greatly among different countries and among different racial and social groups. For example, in Sweden (in the early 1980s), the mortality was low, at eight deaths per 1,000 live births, whereas, in certain African countries, it was as high as 150 per 1,000. In the US, the mortality was 19 per 1,000 live births for black infants, compared with 10 per 1,000 for white infants.

In most developed countries, there has been an overall decline in infant mortality since about the turn of the century. This is largely due to improvements in nutrition and in social conditions and to medical advances, particularly in *prenatal care* and neonatal intensive care.

Infarction

Death of an area of tissue caused by *ischemia* (lack of blood supply). Common examples include *myocardial infarction* (heart attack) and pulmonary infarction, which is lung damage caused by a *pulmonary embolism* (a blood clot that has moved into a vessel in the lung and is obstructing the flow of blood). See also *Necrosis*.

Infection

 The establishment of a colony of disease-causing microorganisms (such as bacteria, viruses, or fungi) in the body. The organisms actively reproduce and cause disease directly by damage to cells or indirectly by toxins they release. Infection normally provokes a response from the *immune system*, which accounts for many of the features of the infection.

Toxic symptoms, such as fever, weakness, and joint aches, are expressions of *infectious disease*. In such cases, the microorganisms are often spread throughout the body (this is called "systemic" infection). Infection may also be localized within a particular tissue or area, often through spread of organisms from parts of the body where they are harmless to parts where they are harmful (e.g., through leakage from the intestines into the abdomen to cause *peritonitis*).

Entry of microorganisms from soil into wounds or during the course of surgical operations and procedures is another common cause of localized infection. In the early days of surgery, infection of internal body cavities was the major (and frequently fatal) risk to the patient. Antiseptic surgical techniques have largely eliminated this problem.

AVOIDANCE
Localized infections (as opposed to infectious diseases) can be avoided by standard hygienic measures, such as keeping the hands clean, not picking at blemishes, washing and covering cuts and grazes, having wounds attended to by a physician, and seeking regular dental treatment.

SYMPTOMS, DIAGNOSIS, AND TREATMENT
Localized infection is generally followed by *inflammation*, which increases the flow of blood to the infected area, bringing white blood cells and other components of the immune system. Symptoms and signs usually include pain, redness, swelling, formation of a pus-filled abscess at the site of infection, and sometimes a rise in temperature.

Any suspected infection should be brought to the attention of a physician. Once the nature of the causative microorganism has been discovered, treatment consists of an antimicrobial drug, such as an *antibiotic*.

Infection, congenital

Any infection present at birth that was acquired by the infant either in the uterus or during passage through the birth canal.

INFECTIONS ACQUIRED IN THE UTERUS

Many viruses, bacteria, and other microorganisms can pass from the mother's blood through the placenta and into the circulation of the growing fetus. Particularly serious are organisms responsible for *rubella* (German measles), *syphilis*, and *toxoplasmosis*, and the *cytomegalovirus*. Any of these infections may cause *intrauterine growth retardation*. Further effects depend on the stage of pregnancy at which the infection was acquired. Thus, rubella occurring at around nine to 10 weeks (the stage at which various organs are beginning to develop) may cause *deafness*, congenital *heart disease*, and other damage. If infection occurs much later in pregnancy, it may cause no serious harm.

A woman who is infected with the HIV virus (responsible for *AIDS*) risks passing the infection on to her baby during pregnancy. AIDS usually develops within the first two years of life in infants infected with HIV.

INFECTIONS ACQUIRED DURING BIRTH

These infections are almost always acquired from the mother's vaginal secretions or uterine fluid that has become infected with microorganisms. If the membranes rupture prematurely, the baby is at risk of infection from organisms ascending into the uterus from the birth canal.

Conditions acquired in this way include *conjunctivitis* (caused by infection with the organisms responsible for *gonorrhea*), genital *herpes*, a *chlamydial infection*, and infantile *diarrhea* (caused by salmonella or other bacteria). *Meningitis*, *hepatitis B*, *listeriosis*, and staphylococcal and streptococcal bacterial infections may also be acquired in this way. Babies who inhale infected maternal secretions may develop *pneumonia*.

PREVENTION

The risk of a baby acquiring an infection in the uterus is minimized by all girls being immunized against rubella in childhood and by pregnant women avoiding sexually transmitted disease (or by having any such disease treated promptly).

If a woman has an active genital herpes infection close to the time of delivery, cesarean section is usually performed, because infection of the newborn baby with herpes simplex virus is particularly serious and commonly fatal.

TREATMENT

If a baby is diagnosed as having an infection at birth, treatment against the infecting agent is started. Any stunting of growth that has occurred due to infection in the uterus cannot usually be reversed. Some types of birth defects caused by infection (e.g., heart defects) are treatable; others (such as deafness) usually are not.

Infectious disease

Any illness that is caused by a specific microorganism.

INCIDENCE

Infectious diseases are a large and important group of conditions and, until recently, were the major cause of illness and death throughout the world. (In many developing countries, they remain a major cause of death.) Over the last century or so, this situation has changed in the more developed countries as a result of four important advances. First, better methods are employed for controlling the spread of disease organisms— including better sanitation, water purification, housing, pest control, personal hygiene, and quarantining procedures (see *Public health*). Second, many effective antimicrobial drugs have been developed. Third, vaccines and other preparations have been developed to provide immunity to certain infectious diseases (see *Immunization*). Fourth, better general health and nutrition have bolstered immunity and improved survival.

In developed countries, such measures have brought about a dramatic decline in the incidence of some serious diseases (such as *poliomyelitis*, *smallpox*, *diphtheria*, and *tuberculosis*). In poorer countries, however, infectious diseases remain a huge problem, for reasons that include lack of resources, ignorance, low standards of public and personal hygiene, the presence of insect transmitters of disease, and, perhaps most importantly, malnutrition. Diseases such as measles have a mortality of 20 percent or more in malnourished children.

HOW INFECTIOUS DISEASES ARE TRANSMITTED

In developed countries, infectious diseases are usually spread by sexual transmission, airborne transmission, blood-borne transmission, or direct skin contact. In poorer countries, insect-borne, food-borne, and waterborne infection are other important mechanisms of transmission. Certain infections can also pass from a pregnant woman's blood across the placenta into the blood of the fetus.

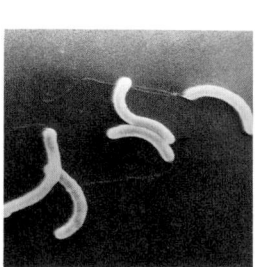

Cholera bacteria
The comma-shaped bacteria that cause the dangerous infectious disease cholera are spread by contamination of water.

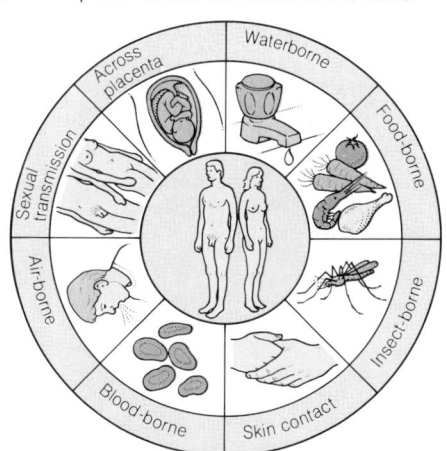

CAUSES

Disease-causing organisms fall into a number of well-defined groups. Among the most important are the *viruses*, *bacteria*, and *fungi*, along with three smaller groups, the rickettsiae, chlamydiae, and mycoplasmas. All are relatively simple organisms that can readily multiply in a host's tissues when defenses are low. Other groups include the *protozoa* (single-celled animal parasites), *worms*, and *flukes*. These more complex parasites may spend only part of their life cycle in human tissues; the rest of their lives is spent in another animal or in soil. Colonization of the body by worms and flukes (along with external parasites, such as *scabies* and *lice*) is generally referred to as an *infestation* rather than an infection.

See table, below, for examples of transmission mechanisms.

AVOIDANCE

Serious infectious diseases can largely be avoided by measures such as *immunization*, good hygiene with respect to food and drink and washing the

SOME IMPORTANT INFECTIOUS DISEASES

VIRAL INFECTIONS

Infective agent	Transmission	Incubation period	Symptoms	Treatment
AIDS virus infection				
Human immuno-deficiency virus (HIV)	Sexual contact; sharing hypodermic needles; mother to child; blood product infusion before March 1985	Variable, usually several years	Fever; weight loss; fatigue; diarrhea; swollen lymph nodes; shortness of breath	Treatment of complicating infections; zidovudine can prolong life expectancy
Chickenpox				
Varicella-zoster virus (herpes zoster virus)	Airborne droplets; direct contact	11 to 21 days	Slight fever; malaise; characteristic rash	Relief of symptoms; acyclovir beneficial in adults
Common cold				
Numerous rhino-viruses; corona-viruses	Airborne droplets; hand-to-hand contact	1 to 3 days	Sneezing; chills; muscle aches; runny nose; cough	Relief of symptoms
Hepatitis, viral				
Hepatitis virus types A and B; others	Infected food or water (type A); sexual contact; blood-borne transmission; sharing hypodermic needles (type B)	3 to 6 weeks (type A); a few weeks to several months (type B)	Influenzalike illness; jaundice; many people are asymptomatic	Relief of symptoms; interferon may be beneficial in some cases
Influenza				
Influenza viruses types A, B, or C	Airborne droplets	1 to 3 days	Fever; chills; aches; headache; sore throat; cough; runny nose	Relief of symptoms; fluids
Measles				
Measles virus (a paramyxovirus)	Airborne droplets	7 to 14 days	Fever; coldlike symptoms; characteristic rash; conjunctivitis	Relief of symptoms
Meningitis, viral				
Various viruses	Various methods, including via rodents	Variable	Fever; headache; drowsiness; confusion	Relief of symptoms; acyclovir in some cases
Mononucleosis, infectious				
Epstein-Barr virus	Possibly via saliva	1 to 6 weeks	Swollen glands; fever; sore throat; headache; malaise; lethargy	Relief of symptoms; rest; fluids
Poliomyelitis				
3 polioviruses	From feces to mouth via hands; airborne droplets	Minor illlness— 3 to 5 days. Major illness— 7 to 14 days	Minor illness—sore throat; headache; vomiting. Major illness— fever; stiff neck and back; muscle aches; paralysis	Relief of symptoms
Rabies				
Rabies virus (a rhabdovirus)	Bite from infected animal	10 days to 8 months	Fever; general malaise; irrationality; throat spasms; hydrophobia	No effective treatment
Rubella				
Rubella virus	Airborne droplets; mother to child	2 to 3 weeks	Low fever; characteristic rash	Relief of symptoms

CHLAMYDIAL INFECTIONS

Infective agent	Transmission	Incubation period	Symptoms	Treatment
Nonspecific urethritis				
Chlamydia trachomatis	Sexual contact	1 to 4 weeks	Pain on passing urine; watery, mucus discharge	Antibiotics
Psittacosis				
Chlamydia psittaci	Inhalation of dust containing feces from infected birds	1 to 3 weeks	Flulike and feverish symptoms, shortness of breath	Antibiotics

RICKETTSIAL INFECTIONS

Infective agent	Transmission	Incubation period	Symptoms	Treatment
Q fever				
Coxiella burnetti	Inhalation of infected dust	7 to 14 days	Sudden onset of fever and sweating; cough; chest pains; headache	Antibiotics
Rocky Mountain spotted fever				
Rickettsia rickettsii	Bite from infected tick	2 to 7 days	Severe headache; high fever; muscle aches; weakness; rash	Antibiotics

BACTERIAL INFECTIONS

Infective agent	Transmission	Incubation period	Symptoms	Treatment
Gonorrhea				
Neisseria gonorrhoeae	Sexual contact; mother to baby	2 to 6 days	Pain on passing urine; discharge; pain in abdomen	Penicillin; ampicillin; other antibiotics for resistant forms
Meningitis, bacterial				
Neisseria meningitidis (meningococcus); *Streptococcus pneumoniae*; others	Mother to baby via vagina; infection reaching bloodstream from another organ	Less than 3 weeks, could be less than 24 hours	High fever; stiff neck; nausea; confusion	Antibiotic treatment
Pertussis (whooping cough)				
Bordetella pertussis	Airborne droplets	1 to 2 weeks	Runny nose and moderate fever; slight cough leading to characteristic cough spasms	Erythromycin in early stage; small children may require hospitalization
Pneumonia				
Streptococcus pneumoniae; Legionella pneumophila; others	Airborne droplets	1 to 3 weeks	Cough; fever; chest pain; shortness of breath	Antibiotics
Tuberculosis				
Mycobacterium tuberculosis	Airborne transmission; cow's milk	Several weeks to several years	Malaise; weight loss; cough; shortness of breath; chest pain	Various antibiotics; possibly surgery
Typhoid fever				
Salmonella typhosa	Food or water contaminated with infected feces	1 to 2 weeks, sometimes longer	Headache; lethargy, intestinal upsets; very high, prolonged fever	Several effective drugs, but fever takes a long time to control

FUNGAL INFECTIONS

Infective agent	Transmission	Incubation period	Symptoms	Treatment
Histoplasmosis				
Histoplasma capsulatum	Inhalation of fungus from soil; bird or bat droppings, mostly in Ohio river valley region	2 to 3 weeks	Headache; chills; fever; cough; possible chest pain	Antifungal drugs
Meningitis, fungal				
Cryptococcus neoformans	Inhalation of fungus from pigeon droppings	Unknown	Headache; stiff neck; photophobia	Antifungal drugs

PROTOZOAL INFECTIONS

Infective agent	Transmission	Incubation period	Symptoms	Treatment
Amebiasis				
Entamoeba histolytica	Food or water contaminated by feces	A few weeks to many years	Severe diarrhea	Antiprotozoal drugs (e.g., metronidazole)
Giardiasis				
Giardia lamblia	Food or water contaminated by feces; sexual contact	3 to 40 days	Diarrhea; abdominal discomfort; bloating	Antiprotozoal drugs (e.g., metronidazole)
Malaria				
Plasmodium falciparum; Plasmodium vivax; others	Bite from infected mosquito	10 to 40 days	Chills; high fever; sweating; headache; fatigue	Various drugs (e.g., chloroquine)

hands after using the toilet, avoiding contact with animal feces and secretions, and prudence in choice of sexual partners (or precautions, such as the use of condoms). For travel outside of the US, Canada, Northern Europe, Australia, and New Zealand, extra immunizations, and, in some cases, antimalarial tablets and protective measures against insects, may be recommended by your travel agent and confirmed by your physician.

SYMPTOMS AND DIAGNOSIS

The symptoms of an infectious disease are caused in part by microorganisms damaging cells and tissues, releasing toxins, and drawing on their host's reserves of nutrients; symptoms are also caused by the efforts of the body's defenses (including the *immune system*) to destroy the microorganisms. The outcome depends on whether the microorganisms or the defenses (sometimes aided by drug therapy) gain the upper hand. The strength of a person's immune system, which reflects his or her general health, strongly influences this outcome.

Fever is a feature in many infectious diseases; symptoms generally are related to the system or organ attacked—for example, cough, diarrhea, or skin rash.

Apart from diseases in which the symptoms and signs are usually easily recognizable (such as *chickenpox*), diagnosis relies on identifying the causative microorganism; testing may be by direct microscope examination of a specimen of infected tissue or body fluid, by *culture* techniques, or by detecting antibodies (proteins manufactured by the body to defend against a particular organism) in blood serum (see *Immunoassay*).

A particular problem with infectious diseases is that there is always a time gap (the incubation period) between entry of the microorganisms into the body and the first appearance of symptoms. The incubation period may last from a few hours to several years; during this time, the infected person is likely to pass the microorganism to other people. Moreover, symptoms may never develop in some infected people, but they nonetheless continue to carry the disease organisms and unwittingly transmit them to others.

As a result, an epidemic can be well established before it is recognized and control measures introduced. This can be particularly devastating when the disease is a new one and has a long incubation period and a high mortality (*AIDS* is a classic example).

TREATMENT

The mainstay of treatment is the use of *antibiotic* and other antimicrobial drugs. Drug treatment must be carefully selected through culture and identification of organisms because certain microorganisms are susceptible only to certain antibiotics. For many viruses, no effective antiviral drug is available and treatment relies on supportive measures, such as reducing temperature, maintaining food and fluid intake, and so on.

OUTLOOK

Although great strides have been made in the fight against infectious diseases, many problems remain, even in developed countries. The spread of certain diseases (such as sexually transmitted infections) is difficult to control except by modifying human behavior. For many infections, no effective vaccine has been developed. The majority of viral illnesses cannot be effectively combated with drugs, and some bacteria have developed *resistance* to the drugs available. When a new infectious disease appears, it may be years before an effective vaccine or drug treatment can be devised. In the meantime, large numbers of people may die (AIDS again provides the most recent example).

Infectious mononucleosis

See *Mononucleosis, infectious.*

Inferiority complex

A neurotic state of mind that develops because of repeated hurts or failures in the past. Inferiority complex arises from a conflict between the positive wish to be recognized as someone worthwhile and the haunting fear of frustration and failure. Attempts to compensate for the sense of worthlessness may take the form of aggression and violence, or of overzealous involvement in activities. (See also *Superiority complex.*)

Infertility

The inability of a couple to conceive. Conception depends on the production of healthy sperm by the man, healthy eggs by the woman, and sexual intercourse so that the sperm reach the woman's fallopian tubes. There must not be a mechanical obstruction to prevent the sperm from reaching the egg, and the sperm must be able to fertilize the egg when they meet (see *Fertilization*). Next, the fertilized egg must be able to become implanted in the uterus (see *Implantation, egg*). Finally, the developing embryo must be healthy and its hormonal environment must be adequate for further development so that the pregnancy can continue to full term. Infertility may result from a disturbance of one or more of these factors.

INCIDENCE

Infertility is a common problem. As many as one in six couples requires help from a specialist. Infertility increases with age; the older a couple is when trying to conceive, the more difficult it may be.

INFERTILITY FACTORS

Male factors	
Female factors	
Joint factors	
Percentage	0 10 20 30 40 50

Factors responsible for infertility
In rough terms, about 30 percent of infertility cases are due to factors that affect the man; another 30 percent are due to factors that affect the woman. In the remaining 40 percent of cases, infertility is due to factors that affect both partners.

CAUSES

MALE INFERTILITY The major cause of male infertility is failure to produce enough healthy sperm. *Azoospermia* (in which there is no sperm) and *oligospermia* (in which few sperm are produced) both cause infertility.

In some cases the sperm are malformed or their life span after ejaculation is too short for them to travel far enough to reach the egg. Defects in the sperm may be due to a blockage of the spermatic tubes or damage to the spermatic ducts, usually due to a sexually transmitted disease, such as *gonorrhea*. A *varicocele* (varicose veins in the scrotum) may also be a factor. Abnormal development of the testes due to an endocrine disorder (see *Hypogonadism*) or damage to the testes by *orchitis* (inflammation of the testes) may also cause defective sperm. Toxins such as alcohol, cigarettes, or various drugs can lower the sperm count.

Infertility in men may also be caused by a failure to deliver the sperm into the vagina, as occurs in *impotence* or in disorders affecting ejaculation, such as inhibited ejaculation or retrograde ejaculation (see *Ejaculation, disorders of*).

In rare cases, there may be a chromosomal abnormality (such as *Klinefelter's syndrome*) or a genetic disease (such as *cystic fibrosis*) that causes infertility in men.

FEMALE INFERTILITY Anovulation (failure to ovulate) is the most common cause of female infertility. Failure to ovulate often occurs for no obvious reason. It can be caused by a hormonal imbalance, stress, or a disorder of the *ovary*, such as a tumor or cyst.

Blocked *fallopian tubes*, which frequently occur after *pelvic inflammatory disease*, may prevent the sperm from reaching the egg. The woman may have one tube or no tubes because of a congenital defect or because they were removed during surgery for *ectopic pregnancy*. Disorders of the uterus (such as *fibroids*) often cause infertility, as can *endometriosis*.

Infertility also occurs if the woman's cervical mucus provides a hostile environment for her partner's sperm by producing antibodies that kill or immobilize them.

Rarely, a chromosomal abnormality or allergy to her partner's sperm may cause a woman's infertility.

DIAGNOSIS

If pregnancy has not resulted after a year of unprotected intercourse (about 90 percent of women trying to get pregnant do so within a year), the couple may seek professional help.

A physical examination of both the man and the woman will be performed to determine the general state of their health, and to eliminate untreated physical disorders that may be causing the infertility. The couple is also interviewed, separately and together, regarding their sexual habits to determine if intercourse is taking place correctly for conception. If the cause of infertility remains undiagnosed after these examinations, special tests may be performed (see illustrated box).

TREATMENT

When no specific cause can be found, improving the general state of health may help. The physician may suggest changes in diet, such as reducing alcohol intake, and may suggest relaxing and eliminating stress.

Treatment of male infertility is limited. When azoospermia exists, the couple must accept their childless state or consider adoption or *artificial insemination* by donor. If the sperm count is low, artificial insemination by the husband may be tried, although its success rate varies. In some cases of male infertility due to an endocrine imbalance, drugs such as *clomiphene* or *gonadotropin hormone* therapy may prove useful.

For female infertility, failure to ovulate requires ovarian stimulation with a drug such as clomiphene with or without a gonadotropin hormone. Microsurgery can sometimes repair damage to the fallopian tubes if it is not too severe. If surgery on the fallopian tubes is unsuccessful, *in vitro fertilization* is the only way that pregnancy will be possible. Uterine abnormalities or disorders, such as fibroids, may require treatment. If the cervical mucus has proved hostile, artificial insemination of the husband's semen directly into the cervix can prevent the sperm from coming into contact with the mucus.

OUTLOOK

Only about half the couples professionally treated for infertility achieve a pregnancy, but the chances vary according to cause.

Infestation

The presence of animal parasites (such as mites, ticks, or lice) in the skin or hair or of worms (such as tapeworms) inside the body.

Infiltrate

Accumulation of substances or cells within a tissue that are either not normally found in it or are usually present only in smaller amounts. Infiltrate

INVESTIGATING INFERTILITY

If no cause for infertility is found after a general checkup and/or a personal interview regarding sexual behavior, more specialized tests may be performed. Both partners may require testing because infertility can be attributed to one person, to both of them, or to mutual incompatibility.

CAUSES OF INFERTILITY

Conception is a complicated process; the organs involved can be affected in numerous ways, resulting in infertility. Some of the principal underlying causes of infertility—in men and women—are illustrated at right.

Vas deferens
Blockage or structural abnormality may impede passage of sperm.

Fallopian tubes
Blockage may prevent sperm from reaching egg; one or both tubes may be absent or damaged.

Penis
Failure to achieve or maintain erection; abnormality of ejaculation.

Ovaries
Eggs may fail to mature or may not be released.

Uterus
Abnormality or disorder may prevent implantation of fertilized egg.

Testes
Too few sperm produced; sperm are abnormally shaped, too short-lived, or have impaired motility.

Cervix
Cervical mucus may damage or destroy sperm.

FEMALE INFERTILITY

Investigations to discover the cause of a woman's infertility may include taking a menstrual history, a study of body temperature during the menstrual cycle (below) and/or blood and urine tests to discover whether ovulation is normal, hysterosalpingography (right), or laparoscopy (below right).

Hysterosalpingography
This X-ray technique is used to visualize the uterus and/or fallopian tubes. The image (left) shows a blockage of the left fallopian tube.

MALE INFERTILITY

The first test for investigating male infertility is a semen analysis (below). If it reveals a low sperm count, more tests may be needed to investigate the underlying cause.

Day of cycle

	10	11	12	13	14	15	16	17	18

°F

Body temperature and ovulation
Charting a woman's body temperature during her menstrual cycle can indicate abnormalities of ovulation. The chart above shows typical temperature fluctuations during a normal cycle (black line) and those associated with failure to ovulate (red line).

Laparoscopy
In this technique, a laparoscope (a type of viewing tube) is inserted through the abdominal wall to examine the woman's reproductive organs and determine whether an abnormality, such as a cyst or tumor, is present. The laparoscope view (above) shows a tumor in the left ovary.

Semen analysis
Semen produced by masturbation is examined as soon as possible for the number, shape, and degree of motility of the sperm. A postcoital semen test may also be performed.

Abnormal sperm
The presence in the semen of large numbers of abnormally shaped sperm, such as the two-headed one (left), may reduce a man's fertility.

may refer to a drug (such as a local anesthetic) that has been injected into a tissue or to the buildup of a substance within an organ (such as of fat in the liver caused by excessive alcohol consumption). Radiologists use the term to refer to the presence of a tumor or pneumonia within a tissue (such as lung cancer or bronchopneumonia as seen on a chest X ray).

Inflammation

Redness, swelling, heat, and pain in a tissue due to chemical or physical injury, or to infection.

When body tissues are damaged, specialized *mast cells* release a chemical called *histamine* (other substances are also involved in the inflammatory response, but histamine is believed to be responsible for most of the effects). Histamine increases blood flow to the damaged tissue, which causes the redness and heat. It also makes the blood capillaries more leaky, resulting in fluid oozing out of them and into the tissues, which causes localized swelling. The pain of inflammation is due to stimulation of nerve endings by the inflammatory chemicals.

Inflammation is usually accompanied by an accumulation of white blood cells, which are attracted by the inflammatory chemicals. These white cells help destroy invading microorganisms and are involved in repairing the damaged tissue. Thus, inflammation is an essential part of the body's response to injury and infection.

If inflammation is inappropriate (as in *rheumatoid arthritis* and some other *autoimmune disorders*), it may be suppressed by *corticosteroid drugs* or *nonsteroidal anti-inflammatory drugs*.

Inflammatory bowel disease

A general term for a pair of chronic inflammatory disorders affecting the small and/or large intestine. The cause is unknown. Specific conditions within this group are *Crohn's disease* and nonspecific *ulcerative colitis*.

Influenza

A viral infection of the respiratory tract (air passages) that causes fever, headache, muscle ache, and weakness. Popularly known as "the flu," it is spread by virus-infected droplets coughed or sneezed into the air. Influenza usually occurs in small outbreaks, or every few years in epidemics. Outbreaks tend to occur in winter; they spread particularly rapidly through schools and institutions for the elderly.

CAUSES

There are three main types of influenza virus, called A, B, and C. A person who has had an attack with the type C virus acquires antibodies (proteins made by the *immune system*) that provide immunity against the type C virus for life. Anyone who has been infected with a certain strain of the type A or B viruses acquires immunity to that strain. Both the A- and B-type viruses occasionally alter to produce new strains that may be able to dodge or overcome immunity built up from a previous attack, thus leading to a new infection.

The type B virus is fairly stable, but it occasionally alters sufficiently to overcome resistance. The new strain often causes small outbreaks of infection. The type A virus is highly unstable; new strains arise constantly throughout the world. These are the strains that caused the influenza *pandemics* of this century, most notably Spanish flu in 1918, Asian flu in 1957, and Hong Kong flu in 1968.

SYMPTOMS

The classic symptoms of flu (chills, fever, headache, muscular aches, loss of appetite, and fatigue) are brought on by types A and B. Type C causes only a mild illness that is indistinguishable from a common cold. In general, type A is more debilitating than type B.

The general symptoms described, which are more common in adults than in children, are usually followed by a cough (often accompanied by chest pain), a sore throat, and a runny nose. After two days, fever and other symptoms start to subside and, after five days, these symptoms have usually disappeared. Respiratory symptoms persist, however; the sufferer may feel weak and sometimes depressed. The illness usually clears up completely within seven to ten days. In rare cases, however, it takes a severe form, causing acute pneumonia that may be fatal within a day or two even in healthy young adults. The Spanish flu epidemic of 1918 killed millions of young adults in all countries of the world.

Type B infections in children sometimes mimic *appendicitis* and have been implicated in *Reye's syndrome*. In babies, the type A virus can cause febrile *seizures*.

Secondary bacterial infection is common, particularly in the elderly and in those with lung or heart disease; it may cause fatal *bronchitis*, *bronchiolitis*, or *pneumonia*.

PREVENTION

Anti-influenza vaccines, containing killed strains of types A and B virus currently in circulation, are available, but have only a 60 to 70 percent success rate in preventing infection. In addition, any immunity provided is short-lived. Vaccination must be repeated each year just before the start of the influenza season. It is recommended that older people and sufferers of respiratory or circulatory disease be vaccinated, especially those living in institutions.

TREATMENT

In all but the mildest cases, a person with influenza should rest in bed in a warm, well-ventilated room. Analgesics (painkillers) should be taken to relieve aches and pains and to reduce fever. Warm fluids soothe a sore throat and inhaling steam has a soothing effect on the lungs.

In the case of an elderly person or someone with a lung or heart disease, a physician should be called as soon as symptoms develop. The drug amantadine, which can reduce the severity of an attack if given within 24 hours of onset of symptoms, may be given. Antibiotics may also be used to combat secondary bacterial infection.

Once the fever has abated, the patient can get out of bed, but still needs rest. When he or she has started to regain strength, the return to normal activities should be gradual.

Informed consent

Before a medical diagnostic procedure (or a surgical operation) a careful explanation is provided and the patient is asked to state that he or she understands the procedure and the risks involved, and that he or she consents to it. In most hospitals, the patient signs a consent form before an operation. (See also *Consent*.)

Infrared

A term denoting the part of the electromagnetic spectrum immediately beyond the red end of the visible light spectrum. Directed onto the skin, infrared radiation heats the skin and the tissues immediately below it.

The infrared wave band includes heat waves; an infrared lamp is one means of giving *heat treatment*.

Infusion, intravenous

See *Intravenous infusion*.

Ingestion

The act of taking any substance (i.e., food, drink, or medications) into the body through the mouth. The term also refers to the process by which certain cells (e.g., some white blood cells) surround and engulf small particles.

Ingrown toenail

A painful condition of the big toe in which one or both edges of the nail press into the adjacent skin, leading to infection and inflammation.

Infection is usually caused by poor personal hygiene, wearing tight-fitting shoes, or cutting the nail incorrectly. The nail should be cut straight across (not down the sides) to avoid exposing tender skin that easily becomes infected if a splinter of nail from the cut edge grows into it.

TREATMENT

While waiting for medical treatment, pain can be relieved by bathing the foot in a strong, warm, salt solution once or twice a day and covering the nail with a dry gauze dressing.

The condition is usually treated by giving antibiotics to control infection and, if necessary, by removing the edge of the affected nail after applying a local anesthetic.

Unless preventive measures are taken, the problem is likely to recur.

Preventing ingrown toenails
Cutting the toenails straight does not damage the skin at the corners of the nail and helps to prevent ingrown toenails.

Inguinal

Relating to the groin (the area between the abdomen and thigh), as in inguinal *hernia*, the protrusion of part of the intestine into the muscles of the groin.

Inhalation

The act of breathing in air (see *Breathing*). An inhalation is also a substance in gas, vapor, powder, or aerosol form to be breathed in.

Inhaler

A device used for administering a drug in powder or vapor form. Inhalers are used principally in the treatment of various respiratory dis-

---

HOW TO USE AN INHALER

With each type, the user puts the nozzle of the inhaler in the mouth, presses the end to release the drug, and simultaneously breathes in through the mouth. If the device is used correctly, the drug is dispersed to the bronchi. A *nebulizer* is a special type of inhaler that delivers the drug as a fine mist through a face mask.

Canister of liquid drug

Press

Drug delivered as aerosol spray

Mouthpiece

Aerosol inhaler
This type of inhaler delivers the drug as an aerosol spray when the user presses the top of the canister.

Capsule of powdered drug

Press

Prongs to break capsule

Mouthpiece

Drug delivered as fine powder

Turbo-inhaler
Here, a drug capsule is placed in the end chamber, the top of which is pressed to pierce the capsule and release the drug.

---

orders, including *asthma*, chronic *bronchitis*, and *alveolitis*. Among the medications administered in this way are *bronchodilator drugs* (to widen the airways) and *corticosteroid drugs* (to reduce inflammation).

Inheritance

 The transmission of traits, characteristics, and disorders from parents to their children through the influence of *genes*. Genes are the units of DNA (deoxyribonucleic acid) in a person's cells; DNA controls all growth and body functioning. Half of a person's genes come from the mother, half from the father.

Children tend to resemble their parents, particularly in their physical characteristics. However, this resemblance may also apply to mental abilities, mannerisms, personality, and behavior. In addition, many disorders show a moderate to very notable tendency to "run in families."

Although there is a temptation to ascribe similarities in a family to inheritance, there are equally plausible alternative explanations for many family traits. For example, all the members of a family may be fat not

through the influence of genes, but because they all eat the same fattening food and rarely exercise. Children may behave like their mother not because of inheritance, but because they imitate her. Certain abilities and behaviors (e.g., the language a person speaks) are clearly not inherited. Nevertheless, it is accepted that most physical characteristics, many disorders, and some mental abilities and aspects of personality are inherited.

MECHANISMS OF INHERITANCE

Each of a person's cells contains exactly the same genes, which come originally from the egg and sperm cells from which he or she is derived.

The genes in a cell are organized into long strands of DNA called *chromosomes*. The genes controlling most characteristics come in pairs—one gene originating from the father, the other from the mother. Everyone has 22 pairs of chromosomes (called autosomes) bearing these paired genes. In addition, every individual has two more chromosomes called sex chromosomes. Women have two X chromosomes; men have an X chromosome and a Y chromosome.

The inheritance of normal traits and disorders can be divided into those

INHERITANCE OF EYE COLOR

Eye color is determined by two main alleles (forms of a gene), one coding for brown eyes and the other for blue eyes. The brown allele is dominant to the blue one (which is therefore recessive).

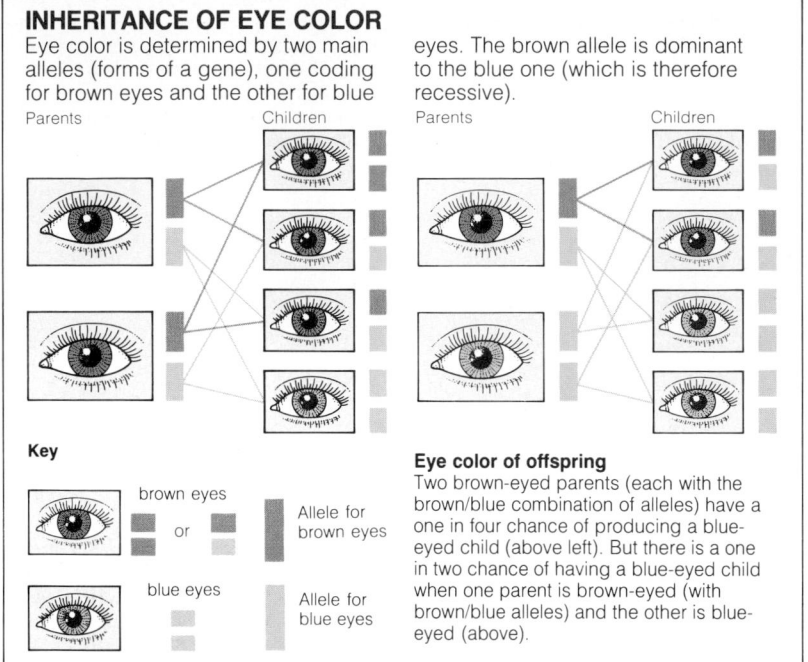

Key

brown eyes

or

blue eyes

Allele for brown eyes

Allele for blue eyes

Eye color of offspring
Two brown-eyed parents (each with the brown/blue combination of alleles) have a one in four chance of producing a blue-eyed child (above left). But there is a one in two chance of having a blue-eyed child when one parent is brown-eyed (with brown/blue alleles) and the other is blue-eyed (above).

---

controlled by a single pair of genes on the autosomal chromosomes (unifactorial inheritance); those controlled by genes on the sex chromosomes (sex-linked inheritance); and those controlled by the combination of many genes (multifactorial inheritance).

UNIFACTORIAL INHERITANCE

A large number of variable traits, such as eye color, blood groups, and the ability to taste certain substances, is thought to be controlled by a single pair of genes. The ways in which these traits are inherited conform to laws first elucidated in the 19th century by the Austrian monk Gregor Mendel. Since then, they have been referred to as the laws of Mendelian inheritance.

Either of the pair of genes controlling a trait may take any of several forms, which are known as alleles. For example, the genes controlling eye color exist as two main alleles, coding for blue and brown eye color. Thus, an individual's gene pair for eye color may be blue/blue (giving blue eyes), brown/brown (giving brown eyes) or brown/blue (also giving brown eyes, because the brown allele is dominant, or "masks," the blue allele, which is called recessive to the brown allele).

When a couple has a child, only one of the pair of genes controlling a trait is passed to the child. For example, someone with the brown/blue combination for eye color has a 50 percent chance of passing the blue gene, and a 50 percent chance of passing on the brown gene, to any child. This factor is combined with the gene coming from the other parent, according to dominant or recessive relationships, to determine the child's eye color. According to the combination of the parental genes, the numbers of brown- and blue-eyed offspring of a particular couple tend to conform to a certain ratio, in accordance with Mendelian laws (see illustration).

Similar laws and ratios apply to the inheritance of other traits controlled by single gene pairs, and also to the inheritance of certain *genetic disorders* (e.g., *cystic fibrosis* and *achondroplasia*).

SEX-LINKED INHERITANCE

The most obvious example of sex-linked inheritance is gender itself. Male gender is caused by the existence in males of the genes on the Y chromosome, which is present only in males and is inherited by boys from their fathers. The genes on the Y chromosome almost certainly direct the development of the male primary sex organs (the testicles) and all male characteristics derive from the secretion of hormones by these organs.

The X chromosome, on the other hand, is less closely associated with the female sex because it is present in both males (in a single dose) and in females (in a double dose). It seems that female gender is the natural course of development in the absence of the Y chromosome, does not require any extra genes to direct it, and that the X chromosome is concerned with general development.

Any faults in a male's genes on the X chromosome tend to be expressed outwardly, because such a fault cannot (as it can in females) be masked by the presence of a normal gene on a second X chromosome. Faults in the genes of the X chromosome include those responsible for *color vision deficiency*, *hemophilia*, and other sex-linked inherited disorders, which almost exclusively affect males.

MULTIFACTORIAL INHERITANCE

A number of traits (such as height and build) are believed to be controlled by the combined effects of many genes, along with environmental effects. Using height as an example, a simple model proposes that there are several genes determining a person's stature, some of which are "tall" genes and others "short." A person's height depends on the relative number of tall to short genes.

When two people have children, a child may, in rare cases, inherit all the tall or all the short genes from both parents, and thus be exceptionally tall or short. The laws of chance dictate, however, that, in most cases, a child will inherit a mixture of tall and short genes and thus be in the range of average stature. Nevertheless, the child of tall parents tends to inherit more tall genes than the child of short parents. Dietary and other factors also affect growth so that a person with many short genes may still attain an average stature through good diet.

Multifactorial inheritance, along with the effects of environment, may also play a part in causing disorders, such as *diabetes mellitus* and *spina bifida* (see *Genetic disorders*).

Inhibition

The process of preventing any mental or physical activity. Inhibition in the brain and spinal cord is carried out by special *neurons*, which damp down the action of other nerve cells to keep the brain's activity in balance.

In a psychological sense, certain mental activities can be described as inhibiting other thoughts or reflexes.

In *psychoanalysis*, an inhibition refers to the unconscious restraint of instinctual impulses. Such inhibition may cause symptoms, such as being temporarily unable to write because writing arouses forbidden ideas.

Injection

Introduction of a drug or vaccine into the body from a syringe through a needle. An injection may be intravenous (into a vein), intramuscular (into a muscle), subcutaneous (under the skin), or intra-articular (into a joint).

Injury

Harm to any part of the body. Injury may arise from a wide variety of causes, including physical influences (such as force, heat, cold, electricity, vibration, and radiation), chemical causes (such as poisons and caustic substances), animal or human bites, or oxygen deprivation.

(See *Accidents*; *Bite, animal*; *Bite, human*; *Bleeding*; *Burns*; *Cold injury*; *Dislocation, joint*; *Electrical injury*; *First aid*; *Fractures*; *Head injury*; *Heat stroke*; *Insect bites*; *Poisoning*; *Radiation sickness*; *Snakebites*; *Soft-tissue injury*; *Spinal injury*; *Sports injuries*; *Sprains*; *Venomous bites and stings*; *Wounds*.)

Ink blot test

A psychological test in which the subject is asked to interpret a number of ink blots. The most widely used example is the *Rorschach test*.

Inlay, dental

A filling of porcelain or gold made outside the mouth and used to restore a badly decayed tooth. An inlay may be needed for back teeth or to provide protection for a weakened tooth.

The dentist first makes an angular cavity in the tooth to accept the inlay. A replica of the cavity is then made, generally using a wax *impression*; the inlay is constructed on the replica and cemented in place in the tooth.

Inoculation

The act of introducing a small quantity of a foreign substance into the body, usually by injection, for the purpose of stimulating the *immune system* to produce *antibodies* (protective proteins) against the substance. Inoculation is usually done to protect against future infection by particular bacteria or viruses. (See *Immunization*.)

Inoperable

A term applied to any condition that cannot be alleviated or cured by surgery, such as a very advanced cancer that has spread to many parts of the body or a brain tumor that is not surgically accessible.

Inorganic

A term used to refer to any of the large group of substances that do not contain carbon (excepting certain simple carbon compounds such as *carbon dioxide* and *carbon monoxide*). Common examples of inorganic substances include table salt (sodium chloride) and bicarbonate of soda (sodium bicarbonate). See also *Organic*.

Inpatient treatment

Medical care given to a patient who has been admitted to a hospital.

Insanity

The common term for serious mental disorder. Today it has no technical meaning for psychiatrists, but is used in law to indicate a mental state that renders a person not legally responsible for his or her own actions. The "insanity defense" was introduced to ensure that people committing criminal acts as a result of mental illness or deficiency would not be imprisoned or given the death penalty, but would instead receive proper treatment. *Psychosis* now covers serious illnesses formerly denoted by insanity.

Insect bites

Tiny puncture wounds in the skin inflicted by blood-sucking insects, such as mosquitoes, lice, midges, gnats, horseflies, sand flies, fleas, and bedbugs. Some small arachnids (eight-legged animals similar to insects), such as ticks and mites, can cause similar injuries.

Most bites cause only temporary pain (or itching for a day or two) although some people have severe skin reactions. In the tropics and subtropics, insect bites are potentially more serious because certain biting species can transmit disease (see *Insects and disease*).

CAUSES

Insects that bite do so to obtain a blood meal. The mouthparts of biting insects are specially adapted for piercing skin and sucking blood. Insect bites are most common on exposed parts of the head, hands, arms, or legs.

Although mosquitoes (which attack mainly after dark) may be the most troublesome biting insects, many bites blamed on mosquitoes are in fact caused by cat or dog fleas. These fleas inhabit various domestic locations where the pet habitually rests (e.g., carpets, sleeping baskets, or sofas); when their normal host is absent, they may jump onto humans to feed.

Of the more easily visible insects, horseflies can produce a particularly painful bite, while gnats can be a menace if encountered in a swarm.

SYMPTOMS

All insect bites provoke a reaction in the skin that is primarily an allergic response to substances in the insect's saliva or its feces, which are often deposited at or near the site of the bite and rubbed in by scratching. Reactions vary from innocuous red pimples to painful swellings (which may weep) or an intensely itching rash. People vary in their reactions to the same biting insect; in some people the reaction is extremely severe.

AVOIDANCE

Avoiding insect bites can be particularly important for campers and hikers, anyone living in a mosquito-infested area, and travelers or residents in tropical countries.

Bites outdoors can be reduced by wearing trousers, socks, and long-sleeved shirts (especially after dark, when mosquitoes are most active), and by using insect repellents.

Indoors, bites can be reduced by using insect screens over open windows and by spraying bedrooms with aerosols containing pyrethroid insecticides before going to bed. If this fails, it may be necessary to use mosquito nets and slow-burning antimosquito coils that give off pyrethroids.

TREATMENT

Bites or bitten areas should be thoroughly washed with soap and water, and a soothing ointment, such as calamine lotion, should be applied. Scratching should be avoided. If there is a severe reaction, a physician should be called; a cream containing an antihistamine may be required.

Severe itching on the scalp or in the pubic hair suggests the possibility of a louse infestation, which is treated with insecticidal lotions (see *Lice*). In the case of flea bites, the entire residence (not just the pet) may require treatment with insecticide to kill the flea population. (See also *Spider bites*; *Mites and disease*; *Ticks and disease*.)

Insects and disease

Insects are six-legged animals with a pair of antennae, a firm exterior skeleton, and, in many cases, wings. They include such animals as ants, bees, cockroaches, fleas, flies, lice, and mosquitoes, but not mites, ticks, or spiders, which belong to another animal group, the arachnids. The insects and arachnids belong to a larger animal group, the arthropods.

INSECT-BORNE DISEASES
Malaria is by far the most prevalent of the insect-borne diseases, affecting an estimated 200 to 300 million people worldwide.

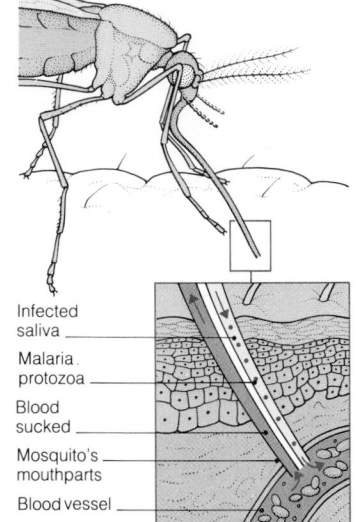

Infected saliva

Malaria protozoa

Blood sucked

Mosquito's mouthparts

Blood vessel

Transmission of malaria
When an infected ANOPHELES mosquito feeds on a person's blood, it injects saliva through its mouthparts; the protozoa that cause malaria enter the blood via the insect's saliva.

DISEASE CAUSED BY INSECTS
There are about 1 million known species of insects; most are either harmless or positively beneficial to humans. The majority of the harmful species cause sickness by attacking crops or stored food, thus contributing to malnutrition and famine.

Other insects are a more direct cause of illness or disease. Certain insects directly parasitize humans, living underneath the skin or on the body surface (see *Lice*; *Chigoe*; *Myiasis*). Still others will sting if provoked, causing moderate discomfort (in most cases) to a severe life-threatening reaction (see *Insect stings*).

The most troublesome insects are flies and various biting insects. Many types of flies settle first on human or animal excrement and then on food to lay eggs or to feed. They can transmit disease organisms from excrement to food via their feet and legs. This is probably important in the spread of intestinal infections such as *typhoid fever* and *shigellosis*.

Insect bites are irritating in themselves, but the much more serious risk is of an insect spreading infectious organisms as a result of its bite. Serious diseases spread by biting insects include *malaria* and *filariasis* (transmitted by mosquitoes), *sleeping sickness* (tsetse flies), *leishmaniasis* (sand flies), epidemic *typhus* (lice), and *plague* (rat fleas). Also, various mosquitoes, sand flies, and ticks spread a group of viral illnesses called the arthropod-borne or arboviruses. They include *yellow fever*, *dengue*, and some types of viral *encephalitis*.

In each case, organisms picked up when an insect ingests blood from an infected animal or person are able to survive or multiply in the insect. Later, the organisms are either injected into a new human host via the insect's saliva or deposited in the feces at or near the site of the bite and later rubbed in by the victim.

Most of these diseases (of which malaria is by far the most important) are confined to the tropics and subtropics. However, some cases of plague and arthropod-borne encephalitis occur each year in the US. Leishmaniasis can be contracted by sand-fly bites in the Mediterranean.

AVOIDANCE
The avoidance of insect-borne disease is largely a matter of keeping flies off food, discouraging insect bites by the use of suitable clothing and insect repellents, and, in areas of the world where malaria is present, the use of mosquito nets and screens, *pesticides*, and antimalarial tablets.

Insect stings

A fairly small number of insects (bees, wasps, hornets, and yellow jackets) are capable of stings. Insect venom contains inflammatory substances that cause local pain, redness, and swelling for about 48 hours. Normally, a very large number of stings (hundreds in the case of an adult) must be received for them to be life-threatening. However, about one person in 200 is allergic to insect venom. This means that, after the person's *immune system* has been sensitized by the venom from a sting, one subsequent sting (possibly months or years later) can provoke a severe allergic reaction leading to *anaphylactic shock*. The symptoms may include a severe itchy rash (hives), dizziness, facial and throat swellings, wheezing, vomiting, breathing difficulties, and collapse. About 50 to 100 people die of this cause annually in the US (more deaths than from snake bites).

Immunotherapy—a technique for reducing sensitivity to bee or wasp venom (and some other types of allergy)—is recommended for those known to suffer hypersensitivity.

TREATMENT
A bee often leaves its sting sac in the wound. The sac should be gently scraped out with a knife blade or fingernail, not by grasping with fingers or tweezers (which injects more venom). The stung area should be washed with soap and water, a cold compress applied, and analgesics taken to ease the discomfort.

If the symptoms of anaphylactic shock develop, obtain medical help immediately for emergency treatment, which initially consists of an injection of *epinephrine*. Any person known to be hypersensitive to bee or wasp venom should obtain and carry an emergency kit for self-injecting epinephrine. In severe cases, the victims of insect stings require *cardiopulmonary resuscitation*.

A sting in the mouth or throat may also be dangerous because swelling may obstruct breathing. Again, seek medical help immediately and give the victim ice cubes to suck. (See also *Scorpion stings*.)

Insecurity
Lack of self-confidence and uncertainty about one's abilities, aims, and relationships with others. Repeated changes of environment (such as frequent moves of home or school) can lead to a sense of insecurity, especially in childhood. A feeling of insecurity may be a feature of *anxiety* and other neurotic mental disorders.

Insight
Being aware of one's own mental state. In a general sense, this means knowing one's own strengths, weaknesses, and abilities.

The term insight also has the specific psychiatric meaning of knowing that one's symptoms are an illness. Some psychiatrists thus regard loss of insight as a sign of a *psychosis*, since it indicates being out of touch with reality. Others, however, point out that many people with psychotic illness know when they are ill and seek treatment, while those with neurotic and personality disorders often deny they are ill and fail to see the causes or results of their behavior.

In *psychoanalysis*, insight refers to a deep emotional understanding of one's inner feelings; it is regarded as essential to successful treatment.

FIRST AID: INSECT STINGS AND BITES

INSECT STING

1 Use a needle to remove the stinger and poison bag by dragging the stinger out of the skin's surface. Do not use tweezers because you may squeeze more poison into the wound.

2 Apply some hydrocortisone cream or a weak solution of ammonia to the wound. An ice pack held on the wound will help reduce swelling.

TICK BITE

1 If the tick is still clinging to the skin, dislodge it by holding the glowing end of a cigarette or an extinguished match to its body. Do not attempt to pull it off.

2 Use soap and warm water to wash the area thoroughly. Then rinse well and dry gently. Apply hydrocortisone cream.

In situ

A Latin term meaning "in place." The phrase "carcinoma in situ" is used to describe tissue (particularly of the skin or cervix) that is cancerous only in its surface cells and is completely surrounded by normal cells without any signs of spread to deeper layers.

Insomnia

Trouble sleeping. Insomnia is a common problem. A national survey has shown that one in every three US adults has some trouble sleeping and that hypnotic drugs are among the most widely used of all medicines. People with insomnia have difficulty falling asleep or staying asleep. Most insomnia sufferers also complain of increased daytime fatigue, irritability, and difficulty coping.

CAUSES
The most common cause of insomnia is worry about a problem (such as bad news received during the day or a difficult task to cope with the following morning), but other causes are implicated in about half of all cases.

Causes include physical disorders such as *sleep apnea* (a breathing problem), *restless legs*, environmental factors (such as noise and light), life-style factors (such as too much coffee in the evening, lack of exercise during the day, or keeping erratic hours), or misuse of hypnotic drugs (see *Anti-anxiety drugs; Barbiturate drugs*).

Insomnia also can be a symptom of a psychiatric illness. People with *anxiety* and/or *depression* may have difficulty getting to sleep; those suffering from depression typically wake early in the morning. Sleeping much less than usual is common in *mania*, in which the person is so full of drive and energy that he or she does not need much sleep. *Schizophrenia* often causes people to pace at night, aroused by "voices" or delusions. People with *dementia* or other brain disorders may be afraid in the dark and become restless and noisy, confused by the shadows and sounds of the night.

Withdrawal syndrome from hypnotic drugs, antidepressants, tranquilizers, and illicit drugs (such as heroin) may cause many weeks of insomnia.

People sometimes believe they have insomnia because of a misconception about the amount of sleep they need. In fact, sleep needs vary greatly, with some people requiring less than four hours and others needing more than 10. Some people who think they have insomnia are in fact "out of phase," lying awake for hours after going to bed, but sleeping normally if allowed to sleep late in the morning.

INVESTIGATION AND TREATMENT
If there is an obvious physical or psychological cause for insomnia, it is treated. For long-term insomnia with no obvious cause, *EEG* recordings of brain-wave patterns and an assessment of breathing, muscle activity, and other bodily functions during sleep may be useful in discovering the extent and pattern of the problem. Keeping a log of sleep patterns may also be helpful.

Studies have shown that many insomniacs sleep much more than they think they do. However, they also tend to wake more frequently than normal sleepers. It is the quality, more than the quantity, of sleep that is the problem in insomnia. People with insomnia should ensure they are active during the day and should establish a regular time and routine for going to bed each night and a regular time for waking in the morning. *Sleeping drugs* should be used only with a physician's advice.

Instinct

An innate primitive urge. The needs for warmth, food, love, and sex are forms of instinct, although the instinct for survival is probably the most powerful. An instinct is distinguished from a reflex, which is an involuntary response to a stimulus (such as withdrawing one's hand from a fire).

In animals, instincts often take the form of specific inherited patterns of behavior. For example, ducks follow their mothers, birds fly, and beavers build dams—activities that do not appear to have been learned.

Humans have few of these set behaviors, and instincts may be more appropriately regarded as motivators of behavior. This idea was first developed as a central part of *Freudian theory*. Freud believed that instincts arose from energy aroused in the unconscious. The aim of the instinct was to calm the aroused state by directing the energy onto some outside object (e.g., sexual arousal leads to intercourse and orgasm).

Freud also described two "primal" (most important) instincts—Eros, the life instinct (which is positive, creative, and aimed at preserving life), and Thanatos, the death instinct (which is negative and destructive). Life was seen as a continual struggle between these two instincts.

Institutionalization

The loss of personal independence that stems from living for long periods in a mental hospital, prison, or other large institution. Apathy, obeying orders unquestioningly, accepting a standard routine, and loss of interests are the main features. They are thought to be caused by a lack of rights and personal responsibility, the attitudes of controlling staff, and the effects of drugs.

Care of the long-term sick within the community (as an alternative to hospitalization) is designed to combat the institutionalization process.

Insulin

A hormone produced by the *pancreas* in varying amounts depending on the level of blood glucose (sugar). Carbohydrate is absorbed as glucose, increasing the blood glucose level and stimulating the pancreas to produce insulin. Insulin promotes the absorption of glucose into the liver and into muscle cells (where it is converted into energy). In the liver, glucose is stored as glycogen, which is reconverted to glucose in response to stress or exercise. Insulin thus prevents a buildup of blood glucose and ensures that various tissues have sufficient amounts of glucose.

Diabetes mellitus occurs when the pancreas produces little or no insulin, causing *hyperglycemia* (abnormally high blood glucose). An *insulinoma* is a rare benign tumor that causes excessive production of insulin.

INSULIN THERAPY

Insulin supplements have been used in the treatment of diabetes mellitus since 1922. Insulin preparations are produced from pig or ox pancreas (and now by *genetic engineering*). A variety of short-, intermediate-, or long-acting preparations is available.

Insulin is used in all cases of insulin-dependent diabetes mellitus (total absence of insulin production) and, occasionally, when oral *hypoglycemic* drugs are unable to control non-insulin-dependent diabetes mellitus (deficient production of insulin), such as during serious illness, surgery, or pregnancy. Insulin therapy is used to prevent hyperglycemia (high blood glucose) and *ketosis* (a buildup of certain acids in the blood), which, in severe cases, may cause coma.

Insulin is given to mimic the body's production of the natural hormone. Insulin may be self-injected before meals to act on the increase in blood glucose that occurs after eating. Alternatively, an insulin pump (see *Pump, insulin*) may be used to deliver insulin over 24 hours; the dose is increased before each meal.

Adjustment of the dose is often needed when there are variations in diet and exercise, and during illness (especially when there has been vomiting). Regular self-monitoring of the blood glucose level, either by blood or urine tests, is necessary to ensure adequate control.

POSSIBLE ADVERSE EFFECTS

Insulin injections may cause irritation or dimpling of the skin. Too high a dose causes hypoglycemia with symptoms (such as dizziness, sweating, irritability, and a feeling of weakness) that are relieved by consuming food or a sugary drink. Severe hypoglycemia may cause coma, for which emergency treatment with an injection of glucose or *glucagon* (a hormone that opposes the effects of insulin) is necessary.

Allergic reactions to insulin, causing rash or breathing difficulty, are rare. Pig or ox insulin may make the body produce *antibodies* that reduce the effectiveness of the insulin preparation. If this occurs, an alternative preparation is taken.

Insulinoma

A rare benign tumor of the insulin-producing cells of the pancreas. Such a tumor can produce abnormal quantities of *insulin* so that the amount of glucose in the blood (which is reduced by insulin) can fall to dangerously low levels. This is called *hypoglycemia* and, unless sugar is given immediately, can cause *coma* and death.

Blood insulin levels are normally low during fasting; insulinoma can be diagnosed by finding high levels after a period of fasting. A drug (diazoxide) is administered to prevent hypoglycemia until surgery can be performed to remove the tumor.

Intelligence

The ability to understand concepts and reason them out. There is much confusion about the precise definition of intelligence. Many people use the word to mean a special degree of knowledge. The widespread use of *intelligence tests* has led to the idea that intelligence is a single quality.

Many scientists prefer to divide intelligence into various factors. Some see it as having three basic parts—speed of thought, learning, and problem-solving. Others argue that a general factor of intelligence exists, made up of seven special abilities—understanding the meaning of words, fluency with words, working with numbers, visualizing things in space, memory, speed of perception, and reasoning ability. Other researchers go further, dividing intelligence into more than 100 different factors.

Intelligence can also be considered as having three entirely separate forms—abstract intelligence (understanding ideas and symbols); practical intelligence (aptitude in dealing with practical problems, such as repairing machinery); and social intelligence (coping reasonably and wisely with human relationships). Personality plays an important role in this last type of intelligence.

AGE AND INTELLIGENCE

Intelligence, however it is defined, increases up to the age of about 6 years and then stabilizes. Intelligence quotient (IQ), as measured by intelligence tests, continues to increase to about age 26, stays the same until about age 40, and then gradually declines (the drop occurring later in a person with an intellectually demanding job).

HEREDITY AND INTELLIGENCE

The role of heredity in intelligence is much argued, but there is no doubt that intelligence is inherited in a fashion similar to height. Environment also plays a major part, as does physical health and personality. Intelligent parents tend to have intelligent children, but, even within one family, some children may be brighter than others. Adopted children from deprived social backgrounds, although having IQs closer to their biological than their adopted parents, often score higher than would be expected had they been reared by their biological parents.

Whether or not some races are more intelligent than others is unknown since so many factors having to do with culture, health, and environment must be taken into account. People from different countries seem to excel at different sports, artistic activities, and occupations, but the reasons for these differences are unknown.

There are extremes of intelligence, as seen in *mental retardation* (defined by a low IQ) and the very gifted (defined by scores over 140). The latter are often very successful, but not always. Personality and social adjustment are equally important.

Intelligence tests

Tests designed to provide an estimate of a person's mental abilities.

TYPES

WECHSLER TESTS These are the most widely used of all tests today. There are two basic versions—the Wechsler Adult Intelligence Scale (WAIS) and the Wechsler Intelligence Scale for Children (WISC). Each is divided into verbal and performance sections, which can be used separately or combined to produce an overall score. The verbal sections are concerned with language skills and include measures of vocabulary, general knowledge, verbal reasoning, and verbal memory. The performance sections include measures of constructional ability and visual-spatial and perceptual ability (interpretation of shapes).

The performance sections of the test may be used separately for people with language problems. In this sense they can measure basic intellectual ability; verbal tests tend to be more culture-bound since they test skills that reflect social background.

STANFORD-BINET TEST This is a revised version of one of the oldest intelligence tests, devised by the Frenchman Alfred Binet (1857-1911). It is still widely used, mainly as a measure of scholastic ability.

OTHER TESTS Numerous tests that concentrate on testing one particular aspect of intelligence have been devised. The Goodenough-Harris test assesses performance by asking a child to make a picture of a man; scoring counts such items as details of the body, proportions, and clothing.

SCORING

In most intelligence tests, scoring is based on the notion of mental age (MA) in relation to actual chronological age (CA), since intelligence normally increases with maturity. The intelligence quotient (IQ) is therefore MA divided by CA, multiplied by 100 to simplify the results. The tests are devised to ensure that three quarters of people have an IQ between 80 and 120. They are also standardized so that the score indicates the same relative ability at different age levels. Regardless of age group, an IQ of 65 indicates that a person is in the lower 1 percent of his or her age group; an IQ of 135 indicates the person is in the upper 1 percent of his or her age group.

USES

Intelligence tests are useful in predicting whether a person has the ability to cope with certain jobs or pass certain exams; they may be used to assess school or job aptitude. However, intelligence tests have been criticized for their alleged bias regarding gender and race. The tests are also used to define the legal notion of *mental retardation* and to assess the effects of brain disease or dementia. In particular, a large difference in verbal and performance scores helps in assessing the degree of brain disease. Children with a particular difficulty (such as delayed reading) may be tested to assess the severity and nature of the problem so remedial teaching can be planned.

Intensive care

The constant, close monitoring of seriously ill patients, which enables immediate treatment to be given if the patient's condition deteriorates. The intensive-care unit of a hospital contains electronic monitoring equipment

A TYPICAL INTENSIVE-CARE UNIT

A modern intensive-care unit has a wide variety of sophisticated equipment so that the condition of seriously ill patients can be continuously monitored and any deterioration treated immediately.

Automatic sphygmomanometer This unit monitors the patient's blood pressure.

Communication unit This unit relays the patient's condition to a central control station.

ECG machine An ECG monitors the patient's heart beat.

Intravenous drip The intravenous drip maintains the patient's body fluids and blood sugar level within optimum limits.

Defibrillator This device is used to reestablish an effective heart rhythm.

Ventilator A ventilator is used to maintain the patient's breathing.

that allows continuous assessment of vital body functions, such as blood pressure and heart and respiratory rate. Medical and nursing staff are in a high ratio to patients and are specially trained in the techniques of resuscitation. Most intensive-care units are under the supervision of hospital-employed specialists.

Intensive care is most often needed for patients who are on artificial *ventilation*; they may be unconscious and not breathing or may be suffering from a respiratory illness. Close monitoring in an intensive-care unit is also required for people recovering from a myocardial infarction or after

major surgery, for patients in *shock* who are not responding to emergency treatment, and for those with acute *renal failure* who require *dialysis*. (See also *Coronary care unit*.)

Inter-
A prefix that means between, as in intercostal (between the ribs). See also *Intra-*.

Intercostal
The medical term for between the ribs, as in the intercostal muscles, thin sheets of muscle between each rib that help expand and contract the chest during breathing.

Intercourse, painful
Known as dyspareunia, pain during intercourse can affect both men and women. The pain may be superficial, occurring around the external genitals, or it may be experienced deep within the pelvis.

CAUSES
Superficial pain is usually due to the condition of the external genitals. *Sexually transmitted diseases* (such as genital *herpes*, *gonorrhea*, or *chlamydial infections*) cause dyspareunia, with the pain being felt on the penis or around the vulval area. *Spermicides* sometimes cause a burning sensation in both men and women.

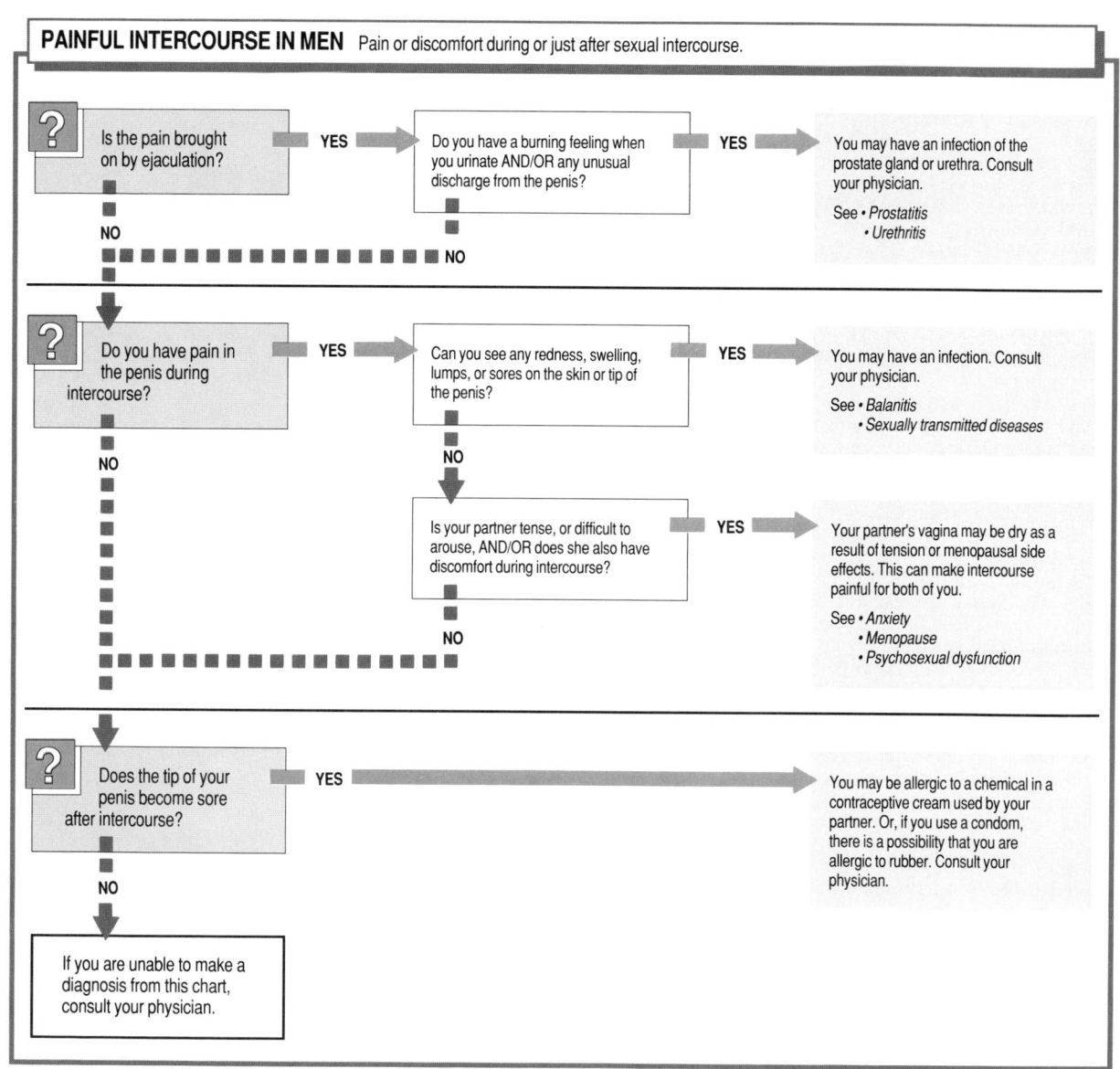

PAINFUL INTERCOURSE IN MEN Pain or discomfort during or just after sexual intercourse.

? Is the pain brought on by ejaculation? — **YES** → Do you have a burning feeling when you urinate AND/OR any unusual discharge from the penis? — **YES** → You may have an infection of the prostate gland or urethra. Consult your physician.

See • *Prostatitis*
• *Urethritis*

NO ... **NO**

? Do you have pain in the penis during intercourse? — **YES** → Can you see any redness, swelling, lumps, or sores on the skin or tip of the penis? — **YES** → You may have an infection. Consult your physician.

See • *Balanitis*
• *Sexually transmitted diseases*

NO

Is your partner tense, or difficult to arouse, AND/OR does she also have discomfort during intercourse? — **YES** → Your partner's vagina may be dry as a result of tension or menopausal side effects. This can make intercourse painful for both of you.

See • *Anxiety*
• *Menopause*
• *Psychosexual dysfunction*

NO

? Does the tip of your penis become sore after intercourse? — **YES** → You may be allergic to a chemical in a contraceptive cream used by your partner. Or, if you use a condom, there is a possibility that you are allergic to rubber. Consult your physician.

NO

If you are unable to make a diagnosis from this chart, consult your physician.

PAINFUL INTERCOURSE IN WOMEN Pain or discomfort during or just after sexual intercourse.

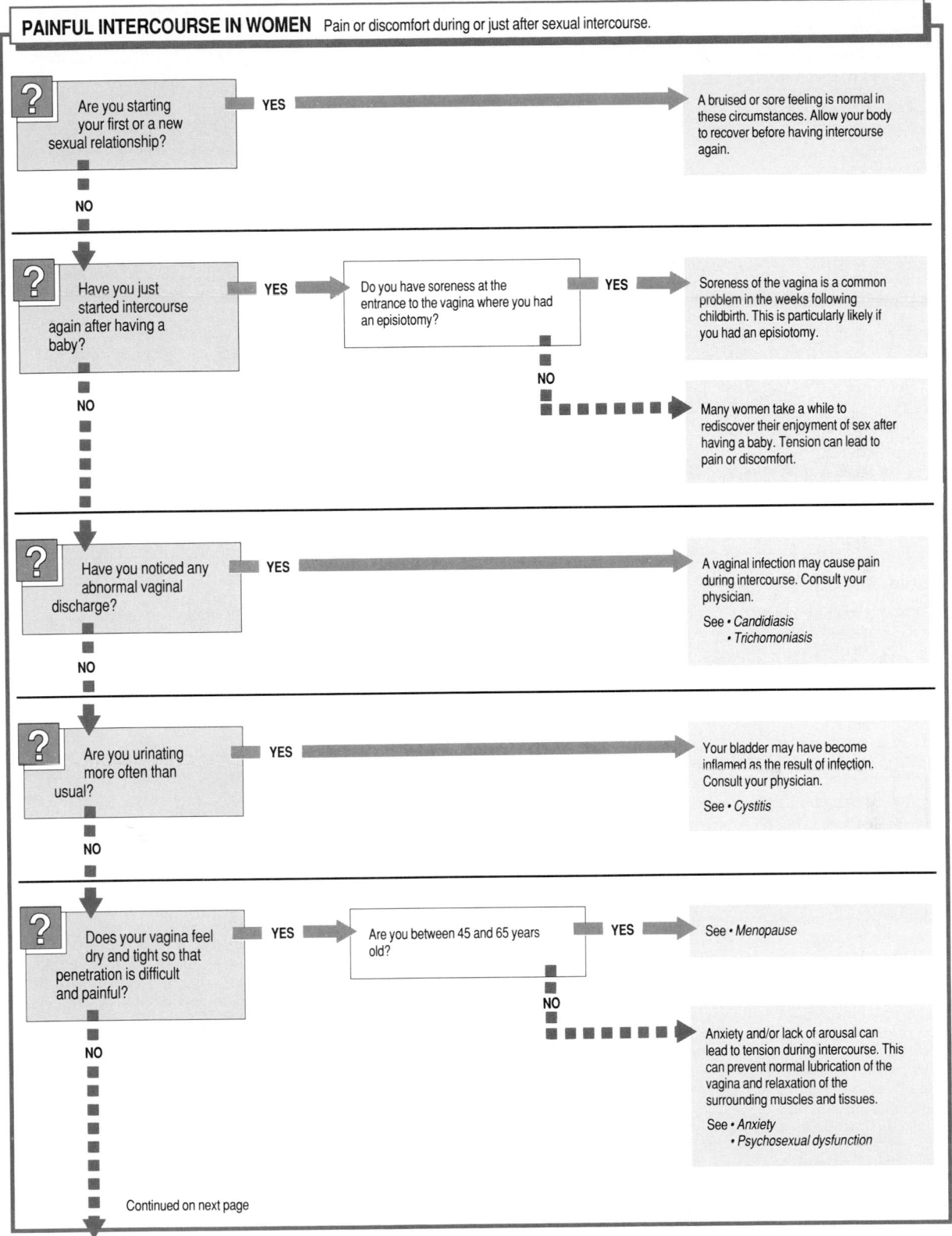

Are you starting your first or a new sexual relationship?

YES → A bruised or sore feeling is normal in these circumstances. Allow your body to recover before having intercourse again.

NO ↓

Have you just started intercourse again after having a baby?

YES → **Do you have soreness at the entrance to the vagina where you had an episiotomy?**

YES → Soreness of the vagina is a common problem in the weeks following childbirth. This is particularly likely if you had an episiotomy.

NO → Many women take a while to rediscover their enjoyment of sex after having a baby. Tension can lead to pain or discomfort.

NO ↓

Have you noticed any abnormal vaginal discharge?

YES → A vaginal infection may cause pain during intercourse. Consult your physician.

See • *Candidiasis*
• *Trichomoniasis*

NO ↓

Are you urinating more often than usual?

YES → Your bladder may have become inflamed as the result of infection. Consult your physician.

See • *Cystitis*

NO ↓

Does your vagina feel dry and tight so that penetration is difficult and painful?

YES → **Are you between 45 and 65 years old?**

YES → See • *Menopause*

NO → Anxiety and/or lack of arousal can lead to tension during intercourse. This can prevent normal lubrication of the vagina and relaxation of the surrounding muscles and tissues.

See • *Anxiety*
• *Psychosexual dysfunction*

NO ↓

Continued on next page

597

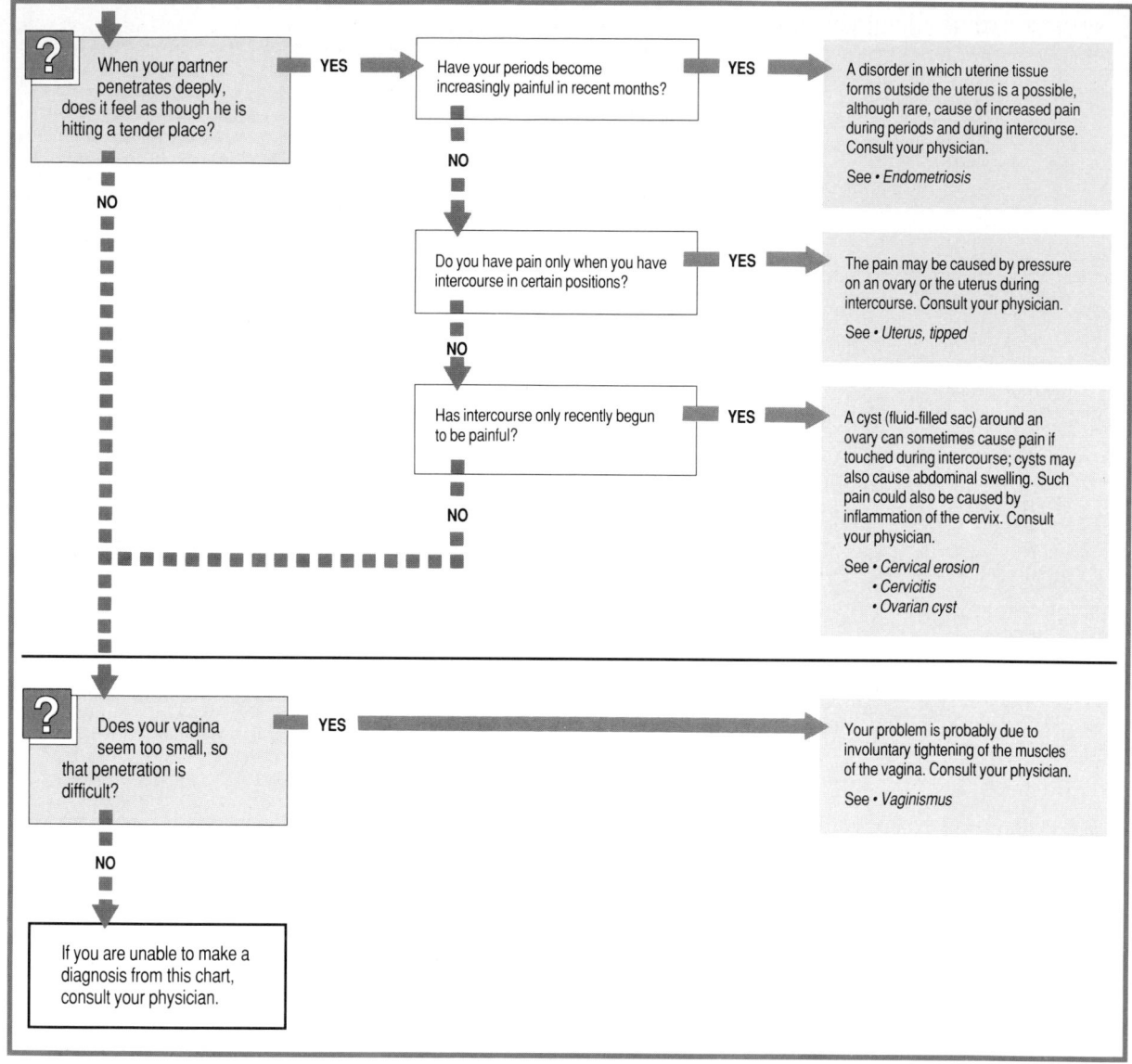

When your partner penetrates deeply, does it feel as though he is hitting a tender place?

YES → Have your periods become increasingly painful in recent months?

YES → A disorder in which uterine tissue forms outside the uterus is a possible, although rare, cause of increased pain during periods and during intercourse. Consult your physician.

See • *Endometriosis*

NO → Do you have pain only when you have intercourse in certain positions?

YES → The pain may be caused by pressure on an ovary or the uterus during intercourse. Consult your physician.

See • *Uterus, tipped*

NO → Has intercourse only recently begun to be painful?

YES → A cyst (fluid-filled sac) around an ovary can sometimes cause pain if touched during intercourse; cysts may also cause abdominal swelling. Such pain could also be caused by inflammation of the cervix. Consult your physician.

See • *Cervical erosion*
• *Cervicitis*
• *Ovarian cyst*

NO

Does your vagina seem too small, so that penetration is difficult?

YES → Your problem is probably due to involuntary tightening of the muscles of the vagina. Consult your physician.

See • *Vaginismus*

NO → If you are unable to make a diagnosis from this chart, consult your physician.

In men, superficial pain during intercourse may be caused by anatomical abnormalities, such as *chordee* (bowed erection) or *phimosis* (tight foreskin). *Prostatitis* may cause a sharp, stabbing pain from the penis tip; there may also be a widespread pelvic ache or a burning sensation.

In some women, scarring (after tears from delivery or a poorly healed *episiotomy* repair, for example) may cause dyspareunia. Insufficient vaginal lubrication, especially after the menopause, is another cause of painful intercourse in women.

Deep dyspareunia in women is often caused by pelvic disorders (such as *fibroids*, *ectopic pregnancy*, or *pelvic inflammatory disease*) or by disorders of the *ovary* (such as ovarian cysts or tumors). *Endometriosis* can cause thickening behind the uterus, resulting in deep pain during intercourse. Varicose veins in the pelvis and cervical disorders (such as tumors or infections) can also cause deep pain during intercourse. *Cystitis* commonly causes pain, primarily in women, as do other urinary tract infections.

Psychosexual problems may also cause painful intercourse. *Vaginismus*, in which the muscles of the vagina go into spasm, preventing insertion of the penis, is usually psychological.

TREATMENT
Treatment is directed at the underlying cause of the pain (for example, antibiotics for an infection or a lubricant for vaginal dryness). Analgesics (painkillers) may be helpful. If the discomfort is psychological in origin, special counseling may be required (see *Sex therapy*).

Interferon
The name given to a group of proteins produced naturally by body cells in response to viral infections and other stimuli. Interferon inhibits viral multiplication (see illustration) and increases the activity of natural killer

HOW INTERFERON FIGHTS VIRAL INFECTIONS

Interferon is part of the body's immune system, providing a defense against many different types of virally infected or tumor cells. It is produced naturally in the body during viral infections, but can also be given as a drug to enhance its natural actions.

VIRAL MULTIPLICATION

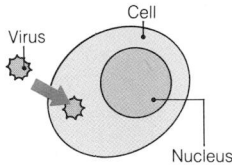

1 A virus can multiply only by first invading one of its host's cells.

2 The virus takes over the cell's chemical machinery to make copies of itself.

3 The copies of the virus escape to invade more of the host's cells.

HOW INTERFERON WORKS

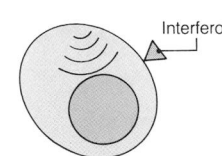

1 Interferon attaches to the membrane of host cells and stimulates them against viral attack.

2 If a virus invades a cell primed by interferon, enzymes are produced that impair viral copying.

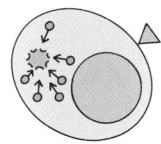

3 Unable to copy itself, the virus is nullified, and the infection is stopped or shortened.

1 Interferon also causes natural killer cells to attack virally infected cells or tumor cells.

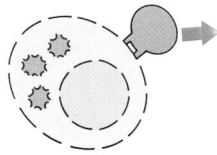

2 A natural killer cell attaches to the abnormal host cell and makes it disintegrate.

3 The effect of this process is to help limit a viral infection or to slow tumor growth.

---

cells—types of *lymphocytes* that form part of the body's *immune system* (natural defenses).

USE AS DRUG

Interferon has been approved for use in the treatment of hairy cell *leukemia*. It is currently under investigation for use in the treatment of various types of cancer, especially *Kaposi's sarcoma* (a skin cancer common in people with *AIDS*). Interferon is also being assessed as a treatment for life-threatening viral infections, particularly in people who have *immunodeficiency disorders*.

Interferon is produced from a culture of human cells exposed to a specific virus or is synthesized in the laboratory from specific nucleic acids (genetic material). It is given by injection or taken as a nasal spray. Possible adverse reactions include fever, headache, aching muscles, fatigue, nausea and vomiting, hair loss, and abnormal bleeding.

Intern

A term for a medical graduate in the first year of hospital training.

Internist

A specialist in the diagnosis and treatment of diseases in adults, particularly those related to the internal organs. Internists often provide a person's primary care.

Intersex

A group of abnormalities in which the affected person has ambiguous genitalia (abnormal external sex organs that could be of either sex) or in which the external genitalia have the opposite appearance to the chromosomal sex of the individual. (See also *Sex determination*.)

Interstitial pulmonary fibrosis

Scarring and thickening of the deep lung tissues, leading to shortness of breath; it is also known as IPF.

TYPES AND CAUSES

The most important form of the disorder is known as idiopathic or diffuse interstitial pulmonary fibrosis, or fibrosing alveolitis. It is of unknown cause, but is probably an *autoimmune disorder* (caused by the body's *immune system* attacking its own tissues).

Less common causes include occupational exposure to mineral dusts and chemical fumes, radiation therapy, reactions to certain drugs, *lung cancer*, and allergic *alveolitis*.

SYMPTOMS AND DIAGNOSIS

The symptoms are progressive shortness of breath, cough, chest pain, and finger clubbing, as well as symptoms of any underlying disease. The diagnosis is based on the patient's history and physical examination and is confirmed by *chest X ray* and lung *biopsy*.

TREATMENT AND OUTLOOK

Treatment of idiopathic IPF often includes azathioprine and *corticosteroid drugs*, which suppress the immune system. In other cases, treatment of the disorder is directed to the underlying cause.

The outlook for recovery is generally poor for occupational dust diseases and idiopathic IPF, in which the lungs progressively stiffen. Progression of the disease may lead to heart failure and bronchopneumonia.

When IPF is caused by allergic alveolitis, the condition is more easily treated or reversible and the outlook may not be as gloomy.

Interstitial radiation therapy

Treatment of a malignant tumor by inserting radioactive material into the growth (also called brachytherapy) or into neighboring tissue. With this method, radiation can be directed more accurately than is possible with X rays to the diseased area; there is also less risk of radiation harming healthy tissue.

HOW IT IS DONE

The patient is given a general anesthetic. Radioactive material (usually artificial isotopes) contained in wires or small tubes is then implanted into or near the diseased tissue. If the tumor is in an easily accessible area (such as the mouth), the containers may be pushed in by means of a special needle; for a tumor deep in the body, a surgical procedure is necessary. The material is left in place for variable amounts of time (and sometimes permanently), depending on the radioactive substance and the tumor being treated. (See also *Intracavitary therapy*; *Radiation therapy*.)

DISORDERS OF THE INTESTINE

The intestine is subject to various structural abnormalities and to the effects of many infective organisms and parasites; it may also be affected by tumors, impaired blood supply, and other disorders.

CONGENITAL DEFECTS

Babies are sometimes born with an obstruction to the flow of the intestinal contents. This may be due to *atresia* (congenital closure), *stenosis* (narrowing), *volvulus* (twisting of loops of bowel), or blockage by meconium (fetal intestinal contents). Early surgery may be required.

INFECTION AND INFLAMMATION

The general term for inflammation of the stomach and intestines is *gastroenteritis*. This is caused most commonly by viral or bacterial infections, which can range from the trivial to the life-threatening. They encompass many cases of *food poisoning* and travelers' diarrhea as well as serious diseases such as *typhoid fever* and *cholera*. Protozoal infections (caused by simple, single-celled parasites) include *giardiasis* and *amebiasis*.

Intestinal worm infestations are exceedingly common worldwide (see *Roundworms; Tapeworms*), although, in the US, only a few species of worms—including the *pinworm*—are prevalent.

Two important inflammatory conditions of the intestine, not caused by infection, are *ulcerative colitis* (mainly affecting the colon) and *Crohn's disease* (which may affect any part of the digestive tract but usually the small intestine). Sometimes, inflammation is confined to a localized area, such as in *appendicitis* and *diverticular disease*.

TUMORS

Tumors of the small intestine are rare, but *lymphomas*, carcinoid tumors (producing *carcinoid syndrome*), and benign growths occur.

By contrast, tumors of the large intestine are very common (see *Intestine, cancer of*). Certain forms of familial *polyposis* (a disorder in which benign polyplike tumors grow in the colon) may progress to cancer.

IMPAIRED BLOOD SUPPLY

Like other organs, the intestine is dependent on an adequate blood

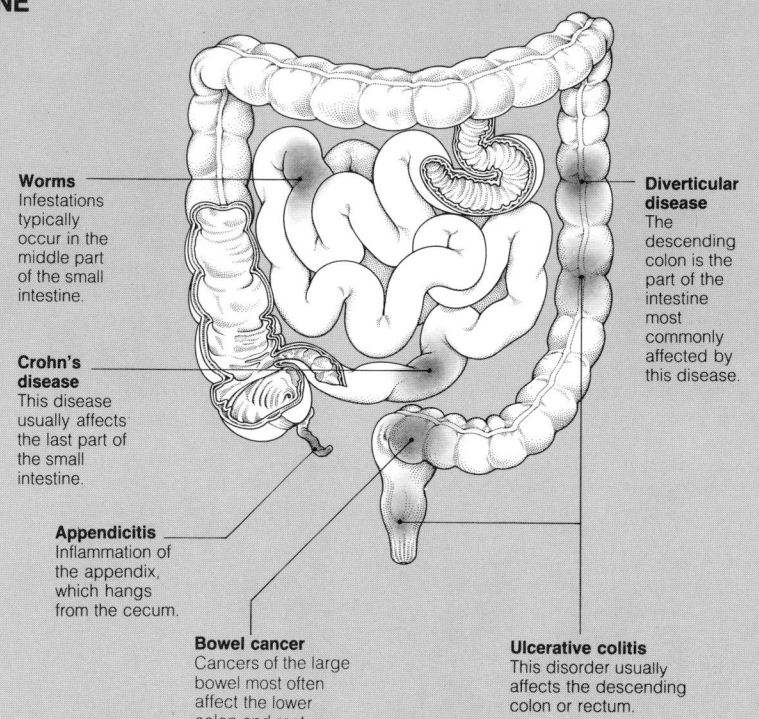

Worms
Infestations typically occur in the middle part of the small intestine.

Crohn's disease
This disease usually affects the last part of the small intestine.

Appendicitis
Inflammation of the appendix, which hangs from the cecum.

Bowel cancer
Cancers of the large bowel most often affect the lower colon and rectum.

Diverticular disease
The descending colon is the part of the intestine most commonly affected by this disease.

Ulcerative colitis
This disorder usually affects the descending colon or rectum.

supply. *Ischemia* (lack of blood) may result from several causes. Causes include partial or complete obstruction of the arteries in the abdominal wall (from disease such as *atherosclerosis, thrombosis,* or *embolism*) or from the blood vessels being compressed or trapped, as in *volvulus, intussusception,* or *hernias* (protrusion of intestines through the abdominal wall). Loss of blood supply to a segment of intestine may cause *gangrene* (tissue death) requiring immediate surgery.

OBSTRUCTION

Intestinal obstruction may be caused by pressure from the outside, disease of the intestinal wall (such as cancer, Crohn's disease, or diverticular disease), or internal blockage (such as from *gallstones* or intussusception). One of the most common causes is paralytic *ileus,* in which intestinal contractions cease and the intestinal contents are no longer transported.

OTHER DISORDERS

Peptic ulcer of the duodenum is a very common disorder, thought to affect 10 percent of the population. Ulceration of the small intestine occurs in typhoid and Crohn's

disease and may cause bleeding into the intestine or even perforation (hole formation). Ulceration of the large intestine occurs in amebiasis and in ulcerative colitis.

Diverticula are small outpouchings from the inside of the bowel. They are usually harmless, but, in diverticular disease, become inflamed. *Malabsorption* and *celiac sprue* result from changes to the intestinal lining. Finally, *irritable bowel syndrome* is associated with persistent abdominal pain and either constipation or diarrhea (or both) and is the most common intestinal disorder in Western societies.

INVESTIGATION

Intestinal disorders are investigated by physical examination, and by techniques such as *barium X-ray examination, sigmoidoscopy,* or possibly *colonoscopy,* and by laboratory examination of the feces or of a *biopsy* specimen taken from the intestinal lining.

Intertrigo

Inflammation of the skin caused by two surfaces rubbing together. Intertrigo is most common in obese people and usually occurs on the inner thighs, in the armpits, on the underside of the breasts, in folds of the abdomen, and between fingers and toes. The affected skin is red, moist, and may have an odor; there may be scales or blisters. The condition is made worse by sweating. It is sometimes accompanied by seborrheic *dermatitis* or *candidiasis* (thrush).

Treatment consists of weight reduction, keeping affected areas as clean and dry as possible, and, if dermatitis or candidiasis is present, applying a *corticosteroid* or *antifungal* cream.

Intestinal imaging

See *Barium X-ray examinations.*

Intestinal lipodystrophy

See *Whipple's disease.*

Intestine

The major part of the digestive tract, extending from the exit of the stomach to the anus. The intestine forms a long tube divided into two main sections—the small intestine and the large intestine. The function of the intestine is to break down and absorb food and water into the bloodstream and carry away the waste products of digestion to be passed as feces.

STRUCTURE

The small intestine is about 21 feet (6.5 m) in length and 1.5 inches (35 mm) in diameter. It has three sections—the duodenum (a short, curved segment fixed to the back wall of the abdomen) and the jejunum and ileum (two larger, coiled, and mobile segments). The bile and pancreatic ducts enter the duodenum (see *Biliary system*).

The walls of the intestine consist of circular and longitudinal muscles with an internal lining (the mucosa) and an external covering (the serosa). *Peristalsis* (the rhythmic contraction of the muscles) forces partially digested food along the intestine. The mucosa consists of many *villi* (small, fingerlike projections) covered with millions of fronds that create a large surface area to help the absorption of substances into the blood.

The large intestine is about 6 feet (1.8 m) in length and 2 inches (50 mm) in diameter; it frames the loops of the small intestine. Unlike the small intestine, much of it is fixed in position, the muscles run in bands rather than forming a continuous sheet along

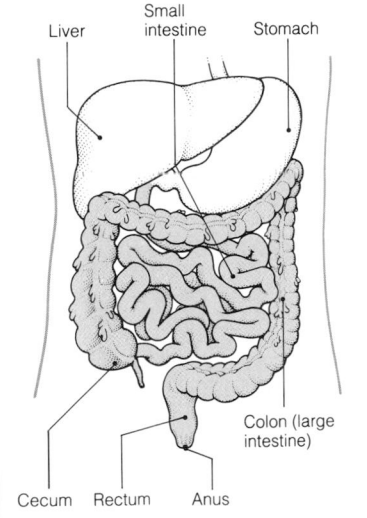

LOCATION OF THE INTESTINE
Situated below the stomach and liver, the intestine occupies much of the central and lower parts of the abdomen.

Liver — Small intestine — Stomach

Colon (large intestine)

Cecum   Rectum   Anus

its length, and there are no internal villi. The main section, the colon, is divided into an ascending, a transverse, a descending, and a pelvic portion (the sigmoid colon) that hangs down into the pelvis. The appendix hangs from a pouch (the cecum) between the small intestine and the colon. The final section of intestine, before the anus, is the rectum.

FUNCTION

The small intestine is concerned with the digestion of food and the absorption of food into the bloodstream. Some digestion occurs in the stomach, but more digestive enzymes and bile are added to the partly digested food in the duodenum. Glands within the walls of each section of the small intestine produce mucus and more enzymes, all of which help to break down the food into easily absorbable chemical units. The numerous blood vessels in the intestinal walls then carry the digested food to the liver for distribution to the rest of the body.

Unabsorbed material leaves the small intestine in the form of liquid and fiber. As they pass through the large intestine, water, vitamins, and mineral salts are absorbed into the bloodstream, leaving feces made up of undigested food residue, small

amounts of fat, secretions from the stomach, liver, pancreas, and bowel wall, and various bacteria. The feces are gradually compressed and pass into the rectum. Distention of the rectum usually produces the desire to empty the bowel.

Intestine, cancer of

Cancerous tumors in the small intestine are extremely rare, but the large intestine is overall the second most common cancer site (after the lung). Colorectal cancer accounts for about 20 percent of all cancer deaths in the US.

Types found in both the small and large intestine include carcinoid tumors and lymphomas. Carcinoid tumors are very slow growing and usually symptomless (however, they may spread to the liver, leading to *carcinoid syndrome*). Lymphomas, which damage the wall of the intestine and nearby lymph nodes, cause malabsorption of food.

CAUSES

Although there is no single cause of intestinal cancer, there are a number of possible contributory factors.

The higher incidence of cancer of the colon (by far the most common type of intestinal cancer) in Western countries suggests an environmental, probably dietary, factor. It is believed that a high-meat, high-fat, and low-fiber diet encourages the production and concentration of *carcinogens*.

There is also thought to be a genetic factor. Brothers, sisters, and children of people suffering from cancer of the colon are more likely than average to acquire the disease later in life.

Cancer of the colon frequently occurs in association with other diseases of the colon, such as *ulcerative colitis* and familial *polyposis*.

SYMPTOMS

An inexplicable change in bowel movements (either constipation or diarrhea) lasting for 10 days or so may be one of the first symptoms of cancer of the large intestine.

Blood mixed in the feces (as opposed to the blood from *hemorrhoids*, which usually coats the feces) is another important warning signal, although, if the growth is high up in the colon, the blood can be detected only by chemical tests.

There may be pain and tenderness in the lower abdomen. Sometimes, however, there are no symptoms at all until the tumor grows so big that it causes an obstruction in the intestine or causes the intestine to rupture.

DIAGNOSIS AND TREATMENT

Tests on feces, *barium X-ray examinations*, *sigmoidoscopy*, and *colonoscopy* may be carried out.

Treatment depends on the stage of development of the cancer, but, in most cases, a partial *colectomy* is performed. The diseased tissue and a small amount of surrounding normal tissue are removed and the cut ends are sewn together to reestablish the channel. If the disease is extensive, surgery may not be possible.

OUTLOOK

The long-term prospects vary according to the stage the disease has reached when it is discovered. More than 50 percent of patients survive in good health for at least five years after a colectomy. Nonsurgical treatments merely arrest the growth and spread of the cancer and are not curative. The earlier the tumor is detected, the greater the chances of a full recovery after treatment. Anyone over the age of 50 who suddenly experiences a change in bowel movements should see a physician without delay. (See also *Rectum, cancer of*.)

Intestine, obstruction of

A partial or complete blockage of the small or large intestine. Without treatment, complete obstruction of the intestine is usually fatal.

CAUSES

The most common cause of intestinal obstruction is paralytic *ileus*, in which (for no medical reason) *peristalsis* (the rhythmic muscle contractions of the intestine) stops, the bowel dilates, and the intestinal contents are no longer moved along the digestive tract.

Other common causes, which have a mechanical basis, are strangulated *hernia*, *atresia* (congenital closure), *stenosis* (narrowing of the intestinal canal), adhesions (postoperative bands of scar tissue that bridge across the outer surface of segments of bowel, sometimes trapping another loop), *volvulus* (twisting or knotting of the bowel), and *intussusception*.

Intestinal obstruction also occurs in diseases (such as *Crohn's disease, diverticular disease*, and tumors) that affect the intestinal wall. Less commonly, internal blockage of the intestinal canal is caused by impacted food, feces, gallstones, or by some accidentally swallowed object.

SYMPTOMS

The location and type of obstruction (partial or complete) dictate the symptoms. A blockage in the small intestine usually causes intermittent cramplike middle abdominal pain, which tends to be more severe the higher the obstruction. This is accompanied by increasingly frequent bouts of vomiting and by failure to pass gas or stools.

The symptoms of obstruction in the large intestine, particularly the colon, are pain, distention (swelling) of the abdomen, and failure to pass stools; the blockage may be so complete that even gas cannot be passed. Partial obstruction may be accompanied by diarrhea when the obstruction is intermittent. There is temporary relief when the liquid stool is able to pass through the remaining gap and the symptoms abate for a while.

DIAGNOSIS AND TREATMENT

A careful history and physical examination are usually all the physician requires to make a diagnosis. Abdominal *X rays* are confirmatory. Most of the gas and intestinal contents are removed through a flexible tube inserted down the throat. Complete mechanical obstruction must be corrected by surgery, but the actual type of operation depends on the nature and site of the blockage to the flow of intestinal contents.

OUTLOOK

The prospects for a full recovery after surgery are excellent, particularly if the underlying problem is a hernia, congenital atresia, or intussusception. However, if the problem is a tumor in the colon of an elderly patient, the risks of the operation are greater.

Intestine, tumors of

Tumors of the intestine may be cancerous or benign (noncancerous). Cancers of the intestine include carcinoid tumors, lymphomas, cancer of the colon (see *Intestine, cancer of*), and cancer of the rectum (see *Rectum, cancer of*).

Noncancerous tumors are rare, but *polyps* in the colon, and *adenomas, leiomyomas, lipomas*, and *angiomas* in the small intestine are occasionally found. These tumors are usually symptomless and are often discovered only accidentally when *barium X-ray examinations* are being carried out for some other reason.

Very occasionally polyps undergo transformation and become cancerous, which is why they are usually removed at an early stage.

Intoxication

A general term for a condition resulting from *poisoning*; it customarily refers to the effects of excessive drinking (see *Alcohol intoxication*), but also includes *drug poisoning* or poisoning from accumulation of metabolic substances in the body.

Intra-

A prefix that means within, as in intramuscular (within a muscle). See also *Inter-*.

Intracavitary therapy

Treatment of a malignant tumor in a body cavity by placing radioactive material within the cavity. The treatment is used mainly for cancer of the uterus, cervix (neck of the uterus), vagina, or rectum.

HOW IT IS DONE

The radioactive material (usually in the form of artificial isotopes embedded in wires or small tubes) is introduced into the cavity and left there for a period of time, using a general or local anesthetic.

Sometimes *anticancer drugs* are introduced directly into the abdominal cavity or pleural cavity (the space around the lungs) to treat a malignant effusion (a fluid containing cancerous cells). A needle, sometimes with a catheter (fine tube) attached, is passed through the wall of the abdomen or chest into the cavity, using a local anesthetic. The needle is used to draw off the effusion and then to inject the drug. (See also *Interstitial radiation therapy; Radiation therapy*.)

Intracerebral hemorrhage

Bleeding into the brain from a ruptured vessel. Intracerebral hemorrhage is one of the three main mechanisms by which a *stroke* can occur.

INCIDENCE AND CAUSES

Each year in the US, about one person in 2,500 suffers an intracerebral hemorrhage. Most victims are middle-aged or elderly people with untreated *hypertension* (high blood pressure) or *atherosclerosis* (fatty deposits causing narrowing of the arteries) in the brain. Unlike most cases of *subdural* and *extradural hemorrhage* (bleeding between the surface of the brain and the skull), an intracerebral hemorrhage can occur without any injury or blow to the head.

The ruptured artery is usually in the cerebrum (the main mass of the brain), although sometimes it is in other brain structures (such as the cerebellum or the brain stem). The escaped blood seeps outward, forming a circular or oval mass up to a few inches in diameter, disrupting brain tissue in its path as bleeding continues and its volume increases. Adjacent brain tissues are displaced and compressed.

SYMPTOMS
The symptoms are sudden headache, weakness, and confusion, and often loss of consciousness. Usually the victim falls unconscious to the ground with no warning. Signs resulting from disruption of brain tissue (speech loss, facial paralysis, or one-sided weakness) may develop over periods of minutes or hours.

DIAGNOSIS, TREATMENT, AND OUTLOOK
Diagnosis is by *CT scanning*. Surgical treatment is usually impossible due to the inaccessibility of the rupture, so treatment is aimed at life-support and reduction of blood pressure.

Large hemorrhages are usually fatal, and, overall, only about 25 percent of patients survive. Recurrent bleeding from the same site is uncommon. For the survivor of an intracerebral hemorrhage, rehabilitation and outlook are as for stroke.

Intractable
Any condition that does not respond to treatment.

Intramuscular
A medical term meaning within a muscle, as in an intramuscular injection, in which a drug is injected deep within a muscle. Such injections are usually given into the upper, outer part of the buttock. The drug is absorbed from the muscle into the bloodstream, which distributes it throughout the body.

Intraocular pressure
The balance between the rate of production and removal of aqueous humor within the eye, which maintains the shape of the eyeball. Aqueous humor enters the eye from the ciliary body, which constantly produces the fluid, and exits from the drainage angle (a network of tissue between the iris and cornea).

If drainage is impeded, intraocular pressure builds up and leads to *glaucoma*. Intraocular pressure is usually measured by *tonometry* during a routine eye examination.

Intrauterine contraceptive device
See *IUD*.

Intrauterine growth retardation
Poor fetal growth, usually due to a fetal defect or to failure of the placenta to provide adequate nutrients. Intrauterine growth retardation causes

the fetus to be smaller than expected for the length of gestation.

CAUSES
Intrauterine growth retardation may be due to a chromosomal defect, such as *Down's syndrome*, which causes the fetus to be "small for dates." A maternal infection, such as *rubella* (German measles), in which the virus passes through the placenta, can also cause poor fetal growth.

Maternal factors may also be responsible, especially when the fetus is otherwise normal. Conditions such as *preeclampsia, hypertension*, or chronic *renal failure* can affect fetal growth, as can the mother's diet. Cigarette smoking is a major cause of intrauterine growth retardation, as are malnutrition and alcoholism.

DIAGNOSIS AND TREATMENT
The physician can check whether the uterus is smaller than expected during a prenatal examination; *ultrasound scanning* may be performed to estimate the fetal growth. The mother may be required to rest, and tests of placental function may be needed, including blood tests or electrical monitoring of the baby's heart.

If intrauterine growth retardation is diagnosed, the pregnancy is carefully monitored and the underlying cause of the placental insufficiency treated, if possible. If the baby's growth is slowing, *induction of labor* or a *cesarean section* may be necessary.

OUTLOOK
Because babies suffering intrauterine growth retardation have been chronically undernourished in the uterus, they are usually underweight and may be premature if labor has been induced. Because they are prone to low blood sugar, *hypothermia*, and infection, they are usually transferred to an *incubator* immediately after birth to provide them with special care.

Intravenous
A term meaning within a vein, as in *intravenous infusion* (slow introduction of a substance into a vein) and intravenous *injection* (rapid introduction of a substance into a vein).

Intravenous infusion
The slow introduction of a volume of fluid into the bloodstream. The fluid passes down from a plastic or glass container through tubing into a cannula (thin plastic tube) inserted into a vein, usually in the patient's forearm. The rate at which the fluid drips into the circulation is controlled by an adjustable valve.

An intravenous infusion, commonly known as a drip, is used to give blood (or plasma) to replace that lost in a serious accident or during an operation (see *Blood transfusion*). It is also used to replace or maintain body fluids in patients who are unable to drink or eat. In this case, the fluid is usually a mixture of glucose (sugar) and saline (salt solution). Other uses include providing more varied and concentrated nutrients to people unable to digest food normally (see *Feeding, artificial*) and administering certain drugs.

Intravenous pyelography
See *Pyelography*.

Introitus
A general term for the entrance to a body cavity or space, most commonly the vagina.

Introvert
A person more concerned with his or her inner world. Introverts prefer to work alone, are shy, quiet, and withdrawn when under stress. (See also *Extrovert*; *Personality*.)

Intubation
The process of passing an *endotracheal tube* (breathing tube) into the trachea (windpipe). Intubation is performed if a person needs mechanical ventilation to deliver oxygen to the lungs—for example, because he or she is in a coma, is anesthetized, or has severe respiratory disease.

Endotracheal tube — Laryngoscope

Endotracheal intubation
Guided by an anesthesiologist, the endotracheal tube is passed through the patient's mouth and down the throat into the trachea.

HOW IT IS DONE
The anesthesiologist looks at the patient's throat with a laryngoscope (a viewing instrument) to identify the vocal cords. An endotracheal tube is passed through the patient's mouth and down the throat between the vocal cords into the trachea. Alter-

natively, the tube is passed through the nose. The external end of the tube is then secured by tape; an inflatable cuff may be used to hold the tube in place within the trachea.

Intubation also refers to the placement of a gastric or intestinal tube for purposes of suction or the giving of nutrients (see *Feeding, artificial*).

Intussusception

A condition in which part of the intestine telescopes in on itself, forming a tube within a tube (like pulling a shirt sleeve partially inside out), usually resulting in intestinal obstruction (see *Intestine, obstruction of*). Intussusception occurs primarily in young children.

CAUSES AND INCIDENCE

It is not known exactly why this condition occurs, but in some cases there is a definite association with a recent infection. In other instances it may start at the site of a *polyp* or *Meckel's diverticulum* (a small, pouchlike projection from the end section of the small intestine). An intussusception is the most common cause of intestinal obstruction in children under 2 years, affecting approximately two babies per 1,000.

SYMPTOMS

Severe abdominal colic usually develops in the child, causing intermittent screaming attacks. Vomiting is a common feature, and blood and mucus are often found in the feces. In severe cases, the blood supply to the intestine becomes blocked and *peritonitis* (inflammation of the membrane covering the organs in the abdomen), *perforation* (formation of a hole in the intestine wall), or *gangrene* (tissue death) may follow.

Intussusception
This disorder is characterized by part of the intestine telescoping in on itself. It usually affects parts of the small intestine and is most common in infants.

PROCEDURE FOR IN VITRO FERTILIZATION

Fertilization of eggs outside a woman's body can be used to treat some types of infertility. The main stages involved in the procedure of in vitro fertilization are illustrated below.

1 to 8 days During the first eight days of a woman's menstrual cycle, she is given fertility drugs to stimulate the ripening of several eggs.

9 to 13 days During the ninth to 13th days, the woman undergoes a series of ultrasound scans to monitor ripening of the eggs in her ovaries.

16 to 17 days After about 40 hours, the eggs are examined to see if they have been fertilized and have started to develop into embryos. If they have, several embryos (usually at the two- or four-cell stage) are placed in the woman's uterus through the vagina.

14 to 15 days Immediately before ovulation (which may be induced with drugs), ripe eggs are removed by laparoscopy or by ultrasound-guided needle aspiration through the vagina or abdomen. The eggs are mixed with the man's sperm in a dish, which is then put in an incubator.

DIAGNOSIS AND TREATMENT

A barium enema (see *Barium X-ray examinations*) is usually sufficient to reveal the obstruction. Sometimes the barium enema actually treats the condition; the pressure applied when the enema is introduced can force the prolapsed segment back into position. Otherwise, an operation is carried out. Usually, the intestine is gently squeezed to push out the inner segment, permitting surgery on the cause that led the segment of bowel to telescope. In rare cases, the prolapsed intestine must be cut out.

Invasive

Having the tendency to spread throughout body tissues; the term is usually applied to malignant tumors or harmful microorganisms. An invasive medical procedure is one in which body tissues are penetrated by an instrument. *Angiography* is an example. (See also *Noninvasive*.)

In vitro

The performance of biological processes in the laboratory rather than in the body; in vitro literally means "in glass." Tests successfully carried out in vitro do not always work the same way in the body.

In vitro fertilization

A method of treating *infertility* in which an egg is surgically removed from the ovary and fertilized outside the body. In vitro, which literally means "in glass," refers to the glass Petri dish that is used in the process.

The first successful birth as a result of in vitro fertilization (IVF) occurred in England in 1978.

WHY IT IS DONE
In vitro fertilization may be performed when the woman's *fallopian tubes* are permanently blocked or absent. IVF may also be done if the man's sperm count is very low or if it is thought that antibodies in the woman's cervical mucus are killing the sperm.

HOW IT IS DONE
Stages in the procedure are shown in the illustrated box.

After IVF, the woman's condition is monitored for a few days to determine if the fertilized eggs have become safely implanted in the uterine wall. Once this occurs, the pregnancy usually continues normally, although the early miscarriage rate is high, and multiple births may occur because more than one of the eggs "takes."

OUTLOOK
It is unlikely that in vitro fertilization will become a widespread treatment for infertility, at least in the near future. Currently, this highly specialized procedure is available only at a small number of clinics. It is expensive (costing about $5,000 per implantation attempt) and the success rate is limited.

Research into IVF has shown that half or more of all eggs have abnormal chromosomes and cannot develop into normal embryos; after fertilization, the eggs begin to divide, but the pregnancy miscarries. Only about 10 percent of couples achieve pregnancy on the first attempt, and many tries may be needed before a successful pregnancy is achieved. In addition, the legality of in vitro fertilization is still unclear. In the US, the procedure is prohibited in a number of states because of laws governing the rights of the embryo.

In vivo
Biological processes occurring, or caused to occur, within the body.

Involuntary movements
Uncontrollable movements of the body, usually affecting the face, head, limbs, and trunk. These movements occur spontaneously and may be slow and writhing (see *Athetosis*); rapid, jerky, and random (see *Chorea*); or predictable, stereotyped, and affecting one part of the body, usually the face (see *Tic*). They may be a feature of a disease (*Huntington's chorea*, for example) or a side effect of certain psychotherapeutic drugs.

Iodine
An element essential for the formation of *thyroid hormones* (thyroxine and triiodothyronine). These hormones control the body's *metabolism* (internal chemistry), promote growth and development, burn excessive fat, improve mental processes, and promote the formation of healthy hair, skin, nails, and teeth.

Iodine is found in seafood (the best dietary source), dairy products, bread, and some table salt preparations. Adequate amounts are obtained from a well-balanced diet. Iodine deficiency may cause a *goiter* (enlarged thyroid gland), *hypothyroidism* (underactive thyroid gland), and, in babies, *cretinism*.

MEDICAL USES
Iodine is sometimes given to people to protect against the effects of consuming food or drink contaminated with radioactive iodine (see *Radiation hazards*). Saturation with radiation-free iodine prevents the thyroid gland from absorbing and being damaged by radioactive iodine.

Radioactive iodine is sometimes given to deliberately damage the thyroid gland to treat *thyrotoxicosis* (overactive thyroid gland).

Some iodine compounds are used as *antiseptics*; others are included in *cough remedies*. Iodine is also a constituent of the radiopaque contrast medium used in some X-ray procedures (see *Imaging techniques*).

POSSIBLE ADVERSE EFFECTS
Iodine supplements rarely cause an allergic reaction. Possible symptoms of allergy to iodine include rash, facial swelling, abdominal pain, vomiting, and headache.

Ion
A particle (either an atom or a group of atoms) that carries an electrical charge; positively charged ions are called cations and negatively charged ions are called anions. Important cations in the body include sodium, potassium, hydrogen, and calcium. Important anions include bicarbonate, chloride, and phosphate.

ROLE IN THE BODY
Many vital body processes depend on the movement of ions across cell membranes. For example, the exchange of sodium for potassium across the membranes around nerve and muscle cells is the mechanism by which nerve impulses are transmitted and by which muscle contraction occurs. Calcium also plays an important role in muscle contraction, in addition to being involved in blood clotting and bone growth.

IMPORTANT IONS AND THEIR ROLES

Cations (positively charged ions)	Major roles in body
Ammonium	Acid-base balance; produced by protein metabolism
Calcium	Nerve conduction; muscle contraction; blood clotting; bone and tooth formation; heart action
Hydrogen	Acid-base balance; component of stomach acid
Magnesium	Nerve conduction; muscle contraction; bone and tooth formation; enzyme activation; protein metabolism
Potassium	Nerve conduction; muscle contraction; water balance; acid-base balance
Sodium	Nerve conduction; muscle contraction; water balance; acid-base balance
Anions (negatively charged ions)	
Bicarbonate	Acid-base balance; neutralizes stomach acid
Chloride	Acid-base balance; water balance; component of stomach acid
Phosphate	Acid-base balance; bone and tooth formation; protein metabolism; energy metabolism; structure of cell membranes

Sodium is the principal cation in extracellular fluid (which surrounds all cells in the body), where it affects the flow of water into and out of cells (see *Osmosis*) and thereby influences the concentration of body fluids.

The levels of sodium, potassium, and calcium are regulated by the kidneys, which control the amount lost from the body in the urine. The level of calcium is also affected by hormonal effects on bones.

The acidity of the blood and other body fluids depends on the level of hydrogen cations, which are produced by various metabolic processes. To prevent these fluids from becoming too acidic, hydrogen cations are neutralized by bicarbonate anions in the extracellular fluid and blood, and by phosphate anions inside cells (see *Acid-base balance*).

ION DISTURBANCES

For the body to function normally, the level of each ion must be maintained within narrow limits; any substantial deviation can cause symptoms, such as muscle weakness caused by hypokalemia (too low a level of potassium cations in the blood).

Dehydration caused by insufficient water intake or excessive water loss (from diarrhea, vomiting, or sweating) increases the concentration of all ions. This may cause thirst, muscle cramps, dizziness, and faintness.

Ipecac

A drug used to induce vomiting in the treatment of *poisoning*. Ipecac (also known as ipecacuanha) is derived from a plant native to South and Central America. It is available over-the-counter in syrup form. It should not be used if poisoning has been caused by corrosive or petroleum-based substances, if the victim is not fully conscious, or if the victim is less than 1 year old.

Ipratropium

An *anticholinergic drug* used as a *bronchodilator drug* in the treatment of *asthma* and chronic *bronchitis*. It is also used as a *decongestant drug* in the treatment of *rhinitis*.

IQ

Abbreviation for intelligence quotient, an age related measure of intelligence (see *Intelligence tests*).

Iridectomy

Removal of part of the *iris*, usually to treat narrow-angle *glaucoma*. Iridectomy involves making a small opening near the root of the iris to form a channel through which aqueous humor can drain. Called a "peripheral iridectomy," the opening is made by laser or by operative surgery.

Iridectomy is sometimes performed to remove tumors and to improve the vision of children who have small central cataracts.

Iridencleisis

A surgical procedure that was used in the 1940s and 1950s (to control chronic *glaucoma*) in which an artificial channel was created for the drainage of aqueous humor. Iridencleisis has been replaced by *trabeculectomy*, which is a more reliable procedure.

Iridocyclitis

Inflammation of the *iris* and ciliary body. The term is rarely used today; the condition is now called anterior *uveitis*. (See also *Eye* disorders box.)

Iris

The colored part of the eye that lies behind the cornea. The iris is connected at its outer edge to the ciliary body and has a central perforation called the *pupil* through which light enters the eye and falls on the retina. This loose framework of transparent *collagen* (a fibrous protein) and muscle fibers constantly contracts and dilates to alter the size of the pupil and control the amount of light that passes through the pupil. The color of the iris is mostly due to the amount and distribution of the pigment cells on the back of the iris.

Iritis

An infrequently employed term for inflammation of the *iris*; the condition is now known as *uveitis*.

Iron

A mineral essential for certain *enzymes* (proteins that stimulate chemical reactions) and for the formation of *hemoglobin* (red blood cell pigment) and *myoglobin* (muscle cell pigment).

Iron is contained in a variety of foods, such as liver, eggs, fish, green leafy vegetables, nuts, and beans. Adequate amounts are usually obtained from a well-balanced diet. During pregnancy, iron supplements may be necessary for the healthy development of the baby.

Iron deficiency leading to anemia (see *Anemia, iron-deficiency*) is usually caused by abnormal blood loss, such as that from *menorrhagia* (heavy periods) or a *peptic ulcer*.

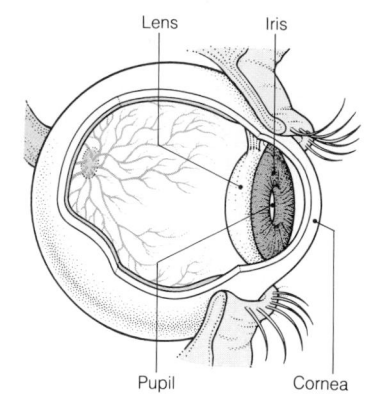

LOCATION OF THE IRIS
The iris lies behind the cornea and in front of the lens. The outer edge of the iris is connected to the ciliary body; at the center is an aperture called the pupil.

Lens   Iris

Pupil   Cornea

Iron supplements may cause nausea, abdominal pain, constipation, or diarrhea. They also color the feces black. Excessive intake of iron may cause *cirrhosis* of the liver.

Iron-deficiency anemia

See *Anemia, iron-deficiency*.

Irradiation

See *Radiation hazards*; *Radiation therapy*.

Irrigation, wound

The cleansing of a deep wound by repeatedly washing it out with a medicated solution or sterile saline.

WHY IT IS DONE

A deep wound is often contaminated with infected foreign material, and, unless it is completely cleansed before repair, it may fail to heal, an abscess may form in it, or, in extreme cases, *gangrene* may result. If the wound contains soil, *tetanus* is a risk.

Irritable bladder

Intermittent, uncontrolled contractions of the muscles in the bladder. Irritable bladder may cause urge incontinence (see *Incontinence, urinary*).

Irritability of the bladder is commonly due to a urinary tract infection (see *Cystitis*), the presence of a catheter within the bladder, a bladder stone (see *Calculus, urinary tract*), or obstruction to the outflow of urine by an enlarged *prostate gland*. In many cases of irritable bladder, however, no underlying cause for the muscular irritability and spasm is found.

Symptoms may be relieved by *antispasmodic drugs*; other treatment is directed at any underlying cause.

Irritable bowel syndrome

A combination of intermittent abdominal pain and irregular bowel habit (i.e., constipation, diarrhea, or both, alternating) that occurs in the absence of demonstrable disease. Alternative names are irritable colon syndrome and spastic colon.

Although symptoms subside and even disappear for periods of time, the condition usually is recurrent throughout life and, without being life-threatening or leading to complications, can cause much distress.

CAUSES AND INCIDENCE
The cause is not fully understood, but the basic abnormality is a disturbance

---

IRRIGATION TECHNIQUES

After removal of contaminated tissue, a wound may be cleansed either by forced syringe (or catheter) irrigation or by using an irrigation chamber.

Forced syringe irrigation
A syringe (sometimes with a catheter attached) is used to flush irrigation fluid repeatedly into and out of the wound until the drained fluid is clear.

Irrigation chamber
A flexible, plastic irrigation chamber is sealed over the wound; irrigation fluid is then run through the chamber until the drained fluid is clear.

---

of involuntary muscle movement in the large intestine. However, there is no abnormality in the intestinal structure and people with irritable bowel syndrome neither lose weight nor become malnourished. It is the most common disorder of the intestine, accounting for more than half the patients seen by gastroenterologists.

The condition is twice as common in women as in men, usually beginning in early or middle adulthood. Sufferers are usually otherwise in good health and have had the condition for some time before seeking medical advice.

A psychological element, particularly anxiety, is believed by some physicians to be the main causative factor; emotional stress tends to exacerbate the condition. However, bowel upset is a normal reaction to stress in many people who do not suffer from the illness.

SYMPTOMS
The symptoms include intermittent cramplike pain in the abdomen, abdominal distention (swelling), often on the left side, transient relief of pain by bowel movement or passing gas, mucus in the feces, sense of incomplete evacuation of the bowels, excessive gas, and symptoms aggravated by food. Various other symptoms may also occur (which are not precisely part of the irritable bowel syndrome), such as heartburn, back pain, weakness, faintness, agitation, tendency to tire easily, reduced appetite, and palpitations.

DIAGNOSIS
Following a careful history and physical examination (which is valuable in both diagnosis and treatment), patients may have their feces tested and may be given a *barium X-ray examination* and a *sigmoidoscopy* (examination of the colon through an endoscope passed via the anus). These tests are intended to exclude conditions, such as cancer and inflammatory bowel disease, that may have similar symptoms.

TREATMENT
Bulk-forming agents, such as bran or methylcellulose, may be prescribed for constipation along with an *antispasmodic drug* to relieve some of the muscular spasm. *Antidiarrheal drugs* (such as loperamide) may be given briefly for prolonged diarrhea. A high-fiber diet is advised for certain types of irritable bowel syndrome. Although these treatments can alleviate the disorder's troublesome symptoms, there is no cure.

Ischemia

Insufficient supply of blood to a specific organ or tissue. Ischemia is usually caused by a blood vessel disease, such as *atherosclerosis*, but may also result from injury to a vessel, constriction of a vessel due to spasm of the muscles in the vessel wall, or inadequate blood flow due to inefficient pumping action of the heart. The symptoms of ischemia depend on the part of the body affected.

Treatment may include *vasodilator drugs* to widen the blood vessels or, in more severe cases, an *angioplasty* or *bypass operation*.

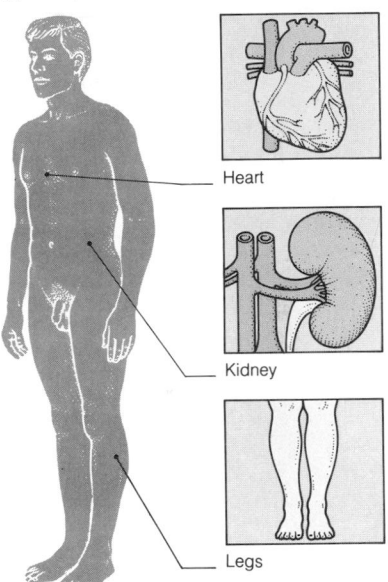

Heart

Kidney

Legs

Symptoms of ischemia
Ischemia (insufficient blood supply) of the heart causes the chest pain of angina pectoris; ischemia of blood vessels in the legs may cause a cramplike pain during exercise. Ischemia may also affect the kidneys (causing renal failure) or the brain (resulting in a stroke).

Isocarboxazid

A monoamine oxidase inhibitor *antidepressant drug*. Like other monoamine oxidase inhibitors, isocarboxazid is not usually prescribed unless other antidepressant drugs are ineffective or the patient is intolerant of other antidepressant drugs.

Possible adverse effects of isocarboxazid include headache, dizziness, blurred vision, tremor, and constipation. If taken with foods containing tyramine (such as cheese and red wine) or certain other drugs, isocarboxazid may cause a dangerous rise in blood pressure.

Isolation

Nursing procedures designed to prevent a patient from infecting others or from being infected by them. In either case, the patient is usually isolated in an individual room.

TYPES

COMPLETE ISOLATION This is used if a patient has a contagious disease, such as *tuberculosis* or *Lassa fever*, that can be transmitted to others both by direct contact and by airborne germs. All nursing staff members wear masks, gowns, caps, and gloves, which afterward are incinerated or sterilized. Bed linen, eating utensils, bedpans, and any other items that come in contact with the patient are also sterilized and, even though they wear gloves, staff members wash their hands thoroughly after each nursing task.

PARTIAL ISOLATION This is carried out if the patient's disease is transmitted in a more limited way—for example, only by respiration (as in *pertussis*) or only by contact with infected skin (as in *impetigo*), blood (as in *AIDS*), or feces (as in *cholera*). In these cases, some of the precautions taken in complete isolation nursing are unnecessary.

Child being nursed in an isolator
The plastic tent and strict sterilization procedures protect the patient from infection.

REVERSE ISOLATION This technique is used to protect a patient whose resistance to infection has been severely lowered. Air entering the room is first filtered. Visiting is drastically limited and all staff members and visitors wear caps, gowns, masks, and gloves. Bed linen and all items used by the patient are sterilized. When these measures do not give enough protection (such as after *bone marrow transplantation*), the patient is placed in an isolator (plastic tent) or in a room ventilated with specially purified air.

Occasionally, long-term reverse isolation is needed for patients with severe combined *immunodeficiency;* these people are born without normal defenses against infection.

Isoniazid

An *antibacterial drug* used to prevent and treat *tuberculosis*. As a preventive measure, isoniazid may be given to close contacts of people suffering from tuberculosis. To treat the disease, isoniazid is given in combination with other antibacterial drugs, usually for at least nine months.

Adverse effects are rare and include nausea, fatigue, numbness, twitching, and insomnia. Because isoniazid may increase the amount of pyridoxine (vitamin B_6) lost from the body, vitamin B_6 supplements are usually given to prevent nerve damage.

Isoproterenol

A *bronchodilator drug* used in the treatment of lung disorders (such as *asthma*, chronic *bronchitis*, and *emphysema*). Isoproterenol widens the airways in the lungs and thus improves air flow and relieves breathing difficulty. Isoproterenol is also given in the emergency treatment of *heart block* (abnormally slow heart beat) before a *pacemaker* is fitted.

Adverse effects are dry mouth, nervousness, dizziness, and palpitations.

Isosorbide dinitrate

A long-acting form of nitroglycerin that acts as a *vasodilator drug*. It is used to reduce the severity and frequency of *angina pectoris* (chest pain due to impaired blood supply to heart muscle). Isosorbide dinitrate is also given to treat severe *heart failure* (reduced pumping efficiency).

Adverse effects include headache, hot flashes, and dizziness.

Isotope scanning

See *Radionuclide scanning*.

Isotretinoin

A drug derived from *vitamin A* used in the treatment of severe *acne* when other treatments have proved ineffective. Isotretinoin is also given to treat *ichthyosis* (a disorder characterized by thickening and scaling of the skin). It works by reducing the formation of sebum (natural skin oils) and keratin (the tough, outer layer of skin).

POSSIBLE ADVERSE EFFECTS

Isotretinoin may cause itching, dryness, and flaking of the skin. Rarely, it may cause liver damage and an increased risk of *coronary heart disease* and *peripheral vascular disease*. Isotretinoin may damage a developing fetus; pregnancy should be avoided during treatment and for at least three months after taking the drug.

Isoxsuprine

A *vasodilator drug* used in the treatment of *peripheral vascular disease*, *transient ischemic attacks* (symptoms of *stroke* lasting less than 24 hours), and *dementia* caused by reduced blood supply to the brain. Its efficacy in the treatment of these disorders is questioned by many physicians.

Isoxsuprine also relaxes muscles in the uterus and is given to suppress contractions in premature labor.

Adverse effects of isoxsuprine include dizziness and palpitations.

Itching

Intense, distracting irritation or tickling sensation in the skin that may be generalized (felt all over the skin's surface) or local (confined to one area). The reason for the sensation is not fully understood.

Itching is the most prominent symptom in skin disease, but does not itself necessarily indicate an underlying skin disorder. People differ in their tolerance to itching, and a person's threshold can be altered by stress, emotions, or other factors. Itching is worse when the skin is warm and when there are few distractions, making it more noticeable at night.

CAUSES

GENERALIZED ITCHING Excessive bathing, which removes the skin's natural oils and may leave the skin excessively dry and scaly, is a common cause of itching. Some people experience itching after taking certain drugs, such as cocaine, codeine, and some antibiotics. Soap, detergents, and roughly textured clothing (e.g., made of wool) also produce itching in some people.

Many elderly people suffer for no apparent reason from dry, itchy skin, especially on their backs. A similar condition affects some younger people in cold weather. Itching commonly occurs during pregnancy.

Many skin conditions produce an itchy rash—for example, *chickenpox*, *urticaria* (hives), *eczema*, and fungal infections (see *Tinea*). Less common causes include *psoriasis* or *dermatitis herpetiformis*.

Generalized skin itchiness can be a result of *diabetes mellitus*, *renal failure*, *jaundice*, and thyroid disorders. Disorders of the blood (such as *leukemia*) and of the lymphatic system (e.g., *Hodgkin's disease*) may occasionally cause itching.

LOCAL ITCHING Pruritus ani (itching around the anal region) occurs in adults, particularly those with such problems as *hemorrhoids*, *anal fissure*, and persistent diarrhea. Pruritus ani often results from irritation caused by overzealous cleansing after defecation. Worm infestation is the most likely cause of itching in children.

Another form of intense skin irritation confined to one area occurs with pruritus vulvae; it affects the external genitalia in women. The condition may be due to *candidiasis*, hormonal changes (at puberty, pregnancy, and the menopause), or to use of spermicides or vaginal suppositories, ointments, and deodorants.

Lice and scabies infestations cause notable itching. Insect bites, too, can produce intense skin irritation.

TREATMENT

Specific treatment depends on the underlying cause, if known. Cooling lotions, such as calamine, relieve irritation; *emollients* reduce dryness.

Soaps often irritate itchy skin, especially if a rash is visible. They should be used only when necessary. Often, extremely mild cleansing lotions or water alone is sufficient to keep most of the skin adequately clean. Itchy skin should be handled very gently. Scratching temporarily relieves itching, but makes the itching worse in the long run. The scratching habit can be suppressed by applying a soothing lotion, salve, or wet compress to the affected areas when the urge to scratch occurs.

-itis

A suffix meaning "inflammation of." Virtually every organ or tissue in the body can suffer inflammation (the most common form of tissue disorder), so "-itis" is by far the most common word ending in medicine. An example of its use is *bronchitis* (inflammation of the bronchi).

The term -itis is applied strictly to cases of inflammation with redness, pain, heat, and swelling. The term should not be used loosely to imply general disorder, for which the ending "-opathy" is appropriate.

IUCD

Abbreviation for intrauterine contraceptive device. (See *IUD*.)

IUD

A mechanical device inserted into the uterus for the purposes of *contraception*. IUDs (intrauterine contraceptive devices) became widely used in the 1960s and 1970s; except for two types, they are no longer being manufactured or sold in the US.

TYPES

Most types of IUD are made of plastic molded into various forms and shapes. They have a plastic string that, once inserted, comes through the cervix into the vagina. The string makes removal easier and indicates the presence of the IUD.

Some IUDs are inert; others contain bioactive substances. Because of their larger size, inert IUDs are more suitable for women who have had at least one child. They must be replaced about every five years.

The bioactive (progesterone-containing) IUDs are much smaller than inert IUDs and may be used by women who have never had children, although most physicians recommend their use only by women who do not plan to have children in the future. Devices containing copper need replacing every two to three years; the progesterone-containing types should be replaced once a year.

HOW THEY WORK

IUDs are about 97 to 98 percent effective, though it is still not certain exactly how they work. It is thought that a foreign body in the uterus prevents pregnancy by creating an inflammation in the uterine lining that destroys sperm as they pass through the uterus. It is also thought that the presence of an IUD may inhibit implantation of the fertilized egg in the uterine wall (see *Implantation, egg*).

Site of an IUD
An IUD is inserted into the uterus; it has a plastic string that hangs down through the cervix and into the vagina.

HOW THEY ARE USED

An IUD is usually inserted by the woman's gynecologist or family practitioner. It can be inserted any time during the menstrual cycle, but the preferred time is during or just after menstruation (because it is unlikely that the woman is pregnant and because the cervix is easier to handle). After a full-term pregnancy, a woman should wait six weeks before having an IUD inserted.

An IUD is inserted through the vagina and cervix into the uterine cavity. Most IUDs are loaded in a small plastic tube that is inserted through the cervical canal; the device is gently pushed out by means of a plunger. Once an IUD is in place, it provides immediate protection. The woman should check once or twice a week that the string is present. If it is not, the string has probably curled up into the uterus, but it is possible that the IUD has been expelled.

WHO SHOULD NOT USE IUDS

Women who have never been pregnant are more likely to have serious complications than women who have had children. Women with no previous pregnancies usually have more pain on insertion, higher expulsion rates, and a heavier menstrual flow. A woman with *fibroids* may be advised not to have an IUD. Any woman with a history of pelvic disease or tubal infection should not use an IUD. Women with multiple partners (or whose partner has other sexual partners) are at increased risk of *pelvic inflammatory disease* (PID) and should probably avoid IUDs. Young women have a higher infection rate than older women. Women with heavy or painful periods may find the IUD makes the symptoms worse.

COMPLICATIONS

Immediately after insertion, there may be heavy bleeding, pain, or vaginal discharge. Menstrual periods after insertion may become irregular, heavier, and more painful.

Women with IUDs also have a higher rate of *ectopic pregnancy*, especially if the pregnancy occurred with the IUD still in place. Pelvic inflammatory disease may be severe and lead to permanent infertility. A rare complication of IUD use is a perforated uterus, in which the device works its way through the wall of the uterus into the abdominal cavity, causing infection.

OUTLOOK

Most pharmaceutical companies have discontinued the manufacture and sale of IUDs in the US because of economic factors. The cost of the large number of lawsuits claiming that IUDs have caused serious complications has been enormous.

IVF

See *In vitro fertilization*.

IVP

The abbreviation for intravenous *pyelography*.

J

Jakob-Creutzfeldt disease

See *Creutzfeldt-Jakob syndrome*.

Jaundice

Yellowing of the skin and the whites of the eyes caused by an accumulation of the yellow-brown bile pigment bilirubin in the blood. Jaundice is the chief sign of many disorders of the liver and biliary system.

TYPES AND CAUSES

Bilirubin is formed from *hemoglobin* (the oxygen-carrying substance in red blood cells) when old red cells are broken down, mainly by the spleen. The pigment is absorbed from the blood by the liver, where it is made soluble in water and is excreted in bile. The process can be upset in any of three ways, causing the main types of jaundice: hemolytic, hepatocellular, and obstructive.

In hemolytic jaundice, the amount of bilirubin produced is too great for the liver to process. This is caused by excessive *hemolysis* (breakdown of red cells), which can have many causes (see *Anemia, hemolytic*). Similar types of jaundice can develop in the newborn as a result of an insufficiently developed capacity of the liver to take up bilirubin. In adults, a type of jaundice similar to hemolytic jaundice can develop as a result of a mild liver disorder called *Gilbert's disease*.

In hepatocellular jaundice, bilirubin builds up in the blood because its transfer from liver cells to bile is prevented, usually as the result of acute *hepatitis* (inflammation of the liver) or *liver failure*.

In obstructive jaundice, bile is prevented from flowing out of the liver because of disorders causing blockage of the bile ducts (see *Bile duct obstruction*) such as *gallstones* or a tumor. Obstructive jaundice can also occur if the bile ducts are not present (as in *biliary atresia*) or have been destroyed within the liver (for example, in primary *biliary cirrhosis*). As a result, bile stagnates in the liver (a condition called *cholestasis*) and bilirubin is forced back into the blood.

SYMPTOMS AND SIGNS

Sometimes (as in acute hepatitis) jaundice is only one of several signs and symptoms. In other cases (such as Gilbert's disease) it may be the sole sign of a disorder.

Obstructive or cholestatic jaundice is usually accompanied by two other characteristic features: pale feces and dark urine. The feces are pale because bilirubin, which normally colors feces brown, does not reach the intestine; the urine is dark due to large amounts of water-soluble bilirubin being filtered into it from the blood. Bilirubin may also be deposited in the skin, causing itching.

In hemolytic jaundice, both urine and feces color are normal. In hepatocellular jaundice, the feces are normal but the urine may be dark.

DIAGNOSIS AND TREATMENT

If excessive hemolysis is suspected, *blood tests* are carried out to determine the amount of water-insoluble bilirubin. A *blood smear* indicates whether large numbers of immature red cells are present; if they are, hemolysis is the suspected cause of the jaundice.

To diagnose hepatocellular jaundice, the blood is tested and a *liver biopsy* (removal of a small sample of tissue for analysis) may be performed.

If the physician suspects obstructive jaundice, *ultrasound scanning*, *liver function tests*, and *cholangiography* may be carried out to determine if the bile ducts are diseased or blocked.

In all cases, treatment is for the underlying cause.

Jaw

The lowest and only mobile bone of the face, also known as the mandible. The term jaw sometimes includes the bone that extends from the inner rims of the eyes to the mouth, more commonly known as the *maxilla*.

The mandible is U-shaped as seen from above and bears the lower teeth on its upper surface. It is connected to the base of the skull at the temporomandibular joints, which can be felt in the cheek just in front of the earlobe. Powerful muscles, arising from the temple on either side, attach to the jaw for movements needed in chewing and biting; other muscles allow side-to-side and downward movement.

Jaw, dislocated

Displacement of the lower jaw from one or both of the temporomandibular joints (the joints between the jaw and the base of the skull). A dislocated jaw is usually caused by a blow or by yawning. The jaw is the most commonly dislocated joint because it is very unstable. Once dislocation has happened, it tends to recur.

SYMPTOMS

There is pain in front of the ear on the affected side or sides and the jaw projects forward. The mouth cannot be fully closed and, as a result, the victim drools and has difficulty speaking.

TREATMENT

A second person can easily correct the dislocation. He or she should stand in front of the victim, place a thumb on the lower back teeth at each side, and press downward. The lower jaw should then click back into position. To avoid causing injury when the teeth snap shut, the thumbs should be wrapped in cloth.

Recurrent dislocation requires an operation to stabilize the joint, such as strengthening the ligaments with stitches. However, surgery is rarely successful in curing the problem.

Jaw, fractured

Fractures of the jaw are most often caused by a direct blow to the face. Because of the shape of the jaw, fracture often occurs not only at the site of the blow, but also on the other side of the jaw.

SYMPTOMS

If the fracture is minor, the only symptoms may be some tenderness, pain on biting, and slight stiffness of

---

ANATOMY OF THE JAW
The U-shaped, mobile bone of the face that meets the skull in front of the ears at the temporomandibular joint. The jaw bears teeth on its upper surface.

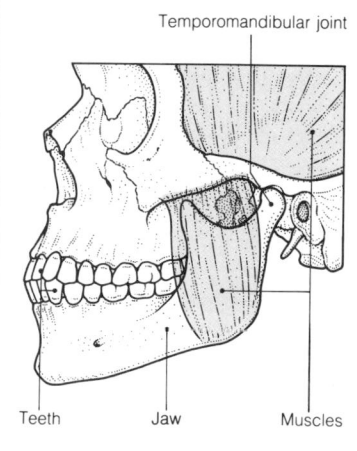

Temporomandibular joint

Teeth   Jaw   Muscles

the jaw. In more severe injuries, teeth may be loosened or damaged, movement of the jaw may be severely limited, and there may be loss of feeling in the lower lip.

DIAGNOSIS AND TREATMENT
If a fracture is suspected, X rays of the area are taken. Minor fractures are normally left to heal on their own.

For severe fractures in which the bones have become displaced, surgical treatment is required. The bone fragments are first manipulated back into the correct position. Teeth too badly damaged to be saved may require extraction. The jaw is immobilized to allow healing to occur, usually by wiring the upper and lower teeth together. If the patient has no teeth, special dentures can be constructed to hold the wires.

Some fractures cannot be adequately immobilized by this method. In such cases, an incision is made in the skin to expose the jaw bone, holes are drilled in each bone fragment, and wires are inserted and twisted together. The skin incision is sewn up with the wires in position.

RECOVERY PERIOD
If the teeth have been wired together, the patient is given a liquid diet. The wires are usually removed after about six weeks.

Jealousy, morbid
Preoccupation with the sexual infidelity of one's partner. The sufferer, usually a man, becomes convinced that his partner is having an affair; he constantly spies on her and often resorts to physical violence.

Morbid jealousy is usually due to *personality disorder*, *depression*, or *paranoia*, but may also occur in those suffering from *alcohol dependence* or organic *brain syndrome*.

Treatment of the underlying disorder may improve the condition, but the outlook is generally poor. Psychiatrists usually recommend separation of the partners, since morbid jealousy is a significant cause of murder within established relationships.

Jejunal biopsy
A diagnostic test in which a small piece of tissue is removed from the lining of the *jejunum* (the middle, coiled section of the small intestine) for laboratory examination under the microscope.

WHY IT IS DONE
The procedure is especially useful in the diagnosis of *Crohn's disease, celiac sprue, lymphoma,* and all other causes

of *malabsorption* because these conditions are associated with recognizable changes in the small intestine.

HOW IT IS DONE
The patient may be sedated slightly before the procedure is started. A small device called a Crosby capsule is attached to a length of fine tubing; both are well lubricated and the patient is asked to swallow the capsule. The tube is guided down the esophagus through the stomach and duodenum until the capsule reaches the jejunum. An X ray is then performed to ensure that the capsule is in the correct position. A syringe is used to withdraw air from the tube, causing a minute piece of tissue to be sucked into the capsule, where it is sheared off. The tube and capsule are then withdrawn and the tissue is taken from the capsule for examination.

Jejunum
The middle, coiled section of the small *intestine*, joining the *duodenum* to the *ileum*. It is wider than the ileum and has a thicker wall, but its function is the same—the digestion of food and the absorption of nutrients from it. Among the few disorders that affect the jejunum are *celiac sprue, Crohn's disease,* and *lymphoma.*

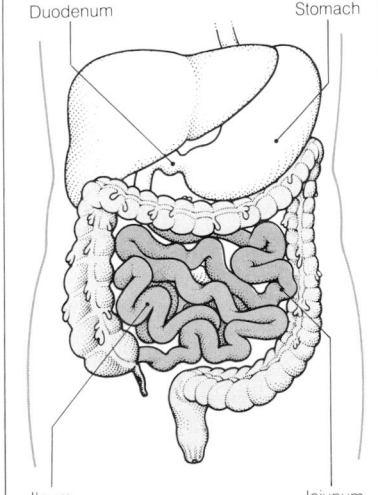

ANATOMY OF THE JEJUNUM
This section of the small intestine joins the duodenum to the ileum. It is wider than the ileum and has a thicker wall.

Duodenum

Stomach

Ileum

Jejunum

Jellyfish stings

Jellyfish, together with corals, sea anemones, and Portuguese men-of-war, belong to a group of marine animals called the coelenterates. These animals have tentacles armed with stinging capsules that discharge when touched. Usually, the result of a sting is no more than an itchy or mildly painful rash, but some jellyfish and Portuguese men-of-war can cause a severe sting. In rare cases, venom entering the bloodstream may cause vomiting, sweating, shock, breathing difficulties, convulsions, and collapse. Dangerous species live mainly in tropical waters.

TREATMENT
If fragments of jellyfish tentacle remain attached to the skin after a sting, vinegar should be applied to inactivate the stinging capsules; the tentacle fragments should then be scraped off. Analgesics (painkillers) may be taken. A severe reaction requires hospitalization and sometimes *cardiopulmonary resuscitation.* Antivenoms effective against the more dangerous species of jellyfish may be available in areas where these species are common.

Jet lag
Interruption of the sleep/wake cycle, fatigue, and other symptoms caused by disturbance of normal body rhythms as a result of flying across different time zones.

CAUSES
Each person has an "internal clock" that determines when the desire to sleep, wake, and eat, the release of various hormones, and many other bodily functions take place in every 24-hour period. The near 24-hour cycle of each activity is called a circadian rhythm. When an air traveler crosses several time zones, his or her day (as timed by an external clock) is longer or shorter than 24 hours, depending on the direction of the flight. Most of the traveler's circadian rhythms are unable to adjust to this shorter or longer day, resulting in jet lag when the flight is over. Jet lag is the desire to sleep during the local day, wakefulness at night, general fatigue, reduced physical and mental activity, and poor memory.

Jet lag tends to be worse after an eastward flight (which shortens the traveler's day) than after a westward one. It is most likely to affect people over 30 who normally follow an established daily routine.

J

TYPES OF JOINTS

Some joints are fixed (e.g., the skull) and some allow a little movement (e.g., the vertebrae). Of the mobile joints, the hinge joint is the simplest. Pivot joints allow rotation only, while ellipsoidal joints allow all types of movement except pivotal. Ball-and-socket joints allow the widest range of movement.

Ball-and-socket joint
A ball-and-socket joint allows the widest range of movement—backward or forward, sideways, and rotation. Examples are the hip and shoulder joints.

Pivot joint
In a pivot joint, movement is limited to rotation, either by means of a bony projection pivoting within a ring, or a ring pivoting around an axis (e.g., the joint between the first and second vertebrae).

Ellipsoidal joint
In an ellipsoidal joint, an oval-shaped part fits into an elliptic cavity, allowing all types of movement except pivotal (an example is the wrist joint).

Hinge joint
This is one of the simplest joints; it allows bending and straightening, as in the fingers. The knee and elbow are modified hinge joints that allow some rotation as well.

STRUCTURE OF A FIXED JOINT

Fixed joints are firmly secured by fibrous tissue. The joints between the bones of the skull are an example.

Sutures
(fixed joints)

STRUCTURE OF A MOBILE JOINT

In mobile joints, the surfaces of the bones are coated with smooth and slippery cartilage to reduce friction during movement. The joint is sealed within a tough fibrous capsule lined with synovial membrane, which produces a clear, sticky fluid that lubricates the joint. Each joint is surrounded by strong ligaments that support it and prevent excessive movement. Movement of the joints is controlled by muscles that are attached to bone by tendons on either side of the joint.

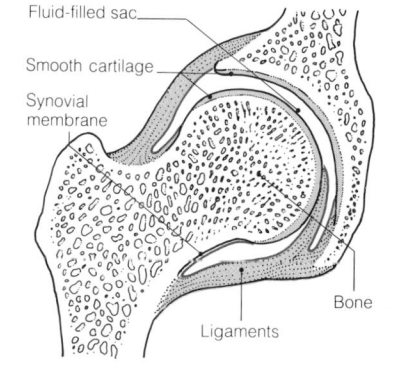

Fluid-filled sac

Smooth cartilage

Synovial membrane

Bone

Ligaments

PREVENTIVE MEASURES

The symptoms of jet lag can be minimized by drinking plenty of nonalcoholic fluids during the flight and avoiding heavy meals. Also, people flying east should go to bed earlier than usual for a few days before the journey; people flying west should do the opposite. If possible, try to arrive in the new time zone in the early evening and go to bed early.

It may take several days to adjust to a new time zone (about half a day to one day for each time zone crossed). The adjustment can be eased by breaking up a long journey with a stopover and by resting after the flight.

Jigger flea

See *Chigoe*.

Jock itch

See *Tinea*.

Joggers' nipple

Soreness of the nipple caused by the rubbing of clothing against it, usually during sports such as jogging or long-distance running. Joggers' nipple, which affects both men and women, can be prevented by applying petroleum jelly to the nipple before prolonged running. Wearing a clean shirt also helps because sweat can aggravate the condition. Treatment involves covering the nipple with a bandage to reduce rubbing.

Joint

The point at which two bones meet. At these junctions, the surfaces of the ends of the bones are covered with cartilage and the joint lined with a synovial membrane. Some joints are fixed (such as those between bones of the skull) and some allow a small amount of movement (those between the bodies—central areas—of the vertebrae, for example). Highly mobile joints are far more common; there are several types capable of different types of movement.

DISORDERS

Common joint injuries include *sprains*, ligament tears, cartilage damage, and tears of the joint capsule.

Dislocation of a joint is usually the result of injury, but is occasionally congenital. A less severe injury may cause *subluxation* (partial dislocation). Rarely, the bone ends are fractured, sometimes leading to *hemarthrosis* (bleeding into the joint) or *effusion* (accumulation of fluid in a joint) due to *synovitis* (inflammation of the lining of the joint).

Joints are commonly affected by forms of *arthritis* (inflammation of a joint). *Bursitis* (inflammation of a bursa) may occur as a result of local irritation or strain.

Permanent joint deformities may be caused by severe injury or arthritis. Temporary deformities may occur in childhood, usually affecting a joint in the legs; they resolve later in life as growth continues. Surgery may be required to relieve certain deformities.

Joint replacement

See *Arthroplasty*.

Joule

The international unit of *energy*, work, and heat. Approximately 4,200 joules (symbol J), or 4.2 kilojoules (kJ), equal one kilocalorie (1,000 calories, or 1 C); 1 kJ equals about 240 C.

Jugular vein

One of three veins on each side of the neck that return deoxygenated blood from the head to the heart. Of the three (internal, external, and superficial) by far the largest is the internal jugular, which arises at the base of the skull, travels down the neck alongside the carotid arteries, and passes behind

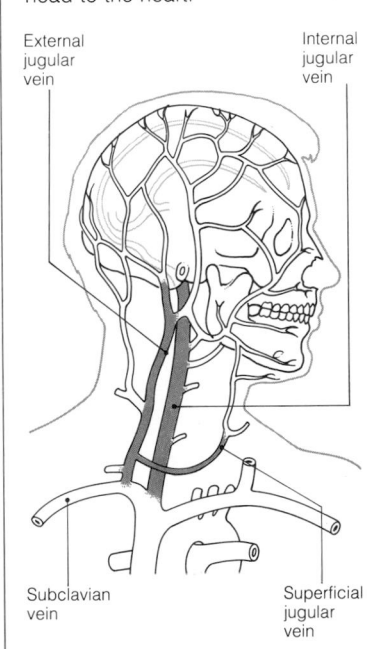

ANATOMY OF THE JUGULAR VEIN
These three veins on each side of the neck return blood from the head to the heart.

External jugular vein

Internal jugular vein

Subclavian vein

Superficial jugular vein

the clavicle (collarbone), where it joins the subclavian vein (the large vein that drains blood from the arms). The jugular is rarely injured because it lies deep in the structures of the neck.

Jumpers' knee

Inflammation of the tendon below the patella (kneecap) usually caused by repetitive exercise such as long-distance running (see *Overuse injury*). Jumpers' knee can also be caused by exercise that strains the kneecap.

Jungian theory

Ideas put forward by the Swiss psychiatrist Carl Gustav Jung (1875-1961). Originally an associate of Sigmund Freud, Jung broke away in 1913 to form his own school of analytical psychology, mainly because he did not believe that sexual drive was the only force behind all human activity. Instead, he theorized that certain ideas (called archetypes) inherited from experiences in our distant past were present in each person's unconscious and controlled the way in which each person viewed the world. Jung called these shared ideas the "collective unconscious."

Although Jung believed that each individual also had a "personal unconscious" containing experiences from his or her life, he regarded the collective unconscious as superior. Therapy was therefore aimed at putting people in touch with this source of profound ideas, particularly through interpretation of dreams.

Jung's therapeutic approach was also based on his theory of personality, which postulated two basic types, the *extrovert* and the *introvert*. He believed that one of these types dominates a person's consciousness and that the other must be brought into consciousness and reconciled with its opposite.

Junk food

 The name commonly applied to refined or processed foods, such as candy, potato chips, and sweetened carbonated beverages. Junk food provides *calories* but few of the other *nutrients* needed for a healthy diet. Small amounts of junk food are not harmful, but people who consume large quantities may not eat enough other foods to provide a well-balanced diet. (See also *Nutrition*.)

Juvenile arthritis

See *Rheumatoid arthritis, juvenile*.

K

Kala-azar

A form of the insect-spread parasitic disease *leishmaniasis*. Kala-azar occurs in many parts of Africa, the Mediterranean area, and India.

Kaolin

An *aluminum* compound used as an ingredient in some *antidiarrheal drugs*. It is thought that kaolin helps treat *diarrhea* by adsorbing *bacteria*, *viruses*, and toxins (poisons) from the intestine and eliminating them from the body when the drug is excreted in the feces.

Kaposi's sarcoma

A condition, characterized by malignant skin tumors, that is a prominent feature of *AIDS*. In the past, Kaposi's sarcoma developed slowly and was seen almost exclusively in elderly Italian and Jewish men. In patients with AIDS, it is highly aggressive and tumors soon become widespread.

The tumors, consisting of blue-red nodules, usually start on the feet and ankles, spread further up the legs, and then appear on the hands and arms. In people with AIDS, tumors also commonly affect the gastrointestinal and respiratory tracts, where they may cause severe internal bleeding.

For mild cases of Kaposi's sarcoma, low-dose *radiation therapy* is usually effective. For more severe cases, *anticancer drugs* may be necessary to slow the spread of the tumors.

Kawasaki disease

An acute childhood illness that affects many systems in the body. It is also called mucocutaneous lymph node syndrome. The condition was first observed in Japan in the 1960s. It is becoming increasingly common in the US in all children, not only those of Japanese ethnic origin. It usually occurs in the first two years of life. The cause is unknown.

SYMPTOMS

Fever is the first symptom; it usually persists for one or two weeks. Other characteristic symptoms are *conjunc-* *tivitis*, dryness and cracking of the lips, and swollen lymph nodes in the neck. Toward the end of the first week of illness, the palms and soles become red, the hands and feet swell, and a rash similar to that of measles appears over the body. By the end of the second week, the skin at the tips of the fingers and toes peels and the other symptoms subside.

TREATMENT AND OUTLOOK

There is no cure, but *aspirin* may help prevent possible heart complications. Most children make a complete recovery. In about 1 to 2 percent of cases, however, sudden death occurs after the acute phase of the illness, usually due to *coronary thrombosis*.

Keloid

A raised, hard, irregularly shaped, itchy scar on the skin. A keloid occurs because of a defective healing process in which an excess of *collagen* forms at the site of a healing scar. Keloids are more common in black people than in white people.

Keloids can occur anywhere on the body, but are most common over the sternum (breastbone) and over the shoulder. They often enlarge after developing and may be unsightly; after some months most flatten and cease to be itchy.

Injections of *corticosteroid drugs* directly into the keloid may reduce itchiness and cause some shrinkage. Surgical removal is of little use since the new scar that forms is almost always a keloid.

Crop of keloids over the breastbone
These overgrowths of scar tissue usually flatten out and become less noticeable over a period of months or years.

Keratin

A fibrous protein that is the main constituent of the outermost layer of the *skin*, *nails*, and *hair*. Keratin is a tough substance that is resistant to damage from a wide range of chemical and physical agents.

Keratitis

Inflammation of the *cornea* (the front part of the eyeball). The term is often used loosely to refer to corneal disorders that do not meet the strict definition of inflammation (since inflammation involves blood vessels and the normal cornea has none). A better general term for disorders of the cornea is *keratopathy*.

True keratitis is rare. One form is interstitial keratitis, which affects about 70 percent of children with congenital *syphilis*. Symptoms include eye pain, excessive watering, and photophobia (sensitivity to bright light); blood vessels grow into the cornea. Treatment with antibiotics usually restores vision.

Keratoacanthoma

A harmless skin nodule that generally occurs singly on the face or arm of elderly people. Initially resembling a small, round wart with a soft center, the keratoacanthoma grows rapidly over a period of about eight weeks. At this point it reaches its maximum size of about 0.8 inch (2 cm) across. The mature nodule has bulging sides and its center may have a whitish appearance. Without treatment, the keratoacanthoma slowly disappears after reaching its mature state.

The cause of the growth is unknown, but it tends to be more common in people who have had years of exposure to strong sunlight and in people taking long-term *immunosuppressant drugs*.

A *biopsy* (removal of a small piece of tissue for analysis) may be necessary to distinguish a keratoacanthoma from a *squamous cell carcinoma*, a form of skin cancer.

Keratoconjunctivitis

A disorder of the cornea associated with *conjunctivitis*. The most common form is epidemic keratoconjunctivitis, caused by a virus that usually causes painful swelling of a small lymph gland in front of the ear. It is highly infectious and is spread mainly by sharing towels or by unsterile instruments and eye drops.

The conjunctivitis is often severe, with notable redness, swelling, or destruction of the surface layer of the conjunctiva, leaving a whitish membrane. Seven to ten days after the onset, tiny opaque spots resembling snowflakes develop in the cornea. The spots may persist for many months and sometimes interfere with vision.

There is no specific treatment for epidemic keratoconjunctivitis. The corneal opacities can sometimes be minimized with *corticosteroid drugs* in eye-drop form. (See also *Keratoconjunctivitis sicca*.)

Keratoconjunctivitis sicca

A condition of persistent corneal and conjunctival dryness caused by deficiency in tear production. Commonly referred to as "dry eye," keratoconjunctivitis sicca occurs in *autoimmune disorders* such as *rheumatoid arthritis*, *Sjögren's syndrome*, and systemic *lupus erythematosus*; all of these conditions can damage the tear-producing glands. Prolonged dryness may cause blurred vision, burning, itching, and grittiness. In severe cases, opacification or ulceration of the cornea may occur. The most effective treatment for dry eyes is artificial tears, which may require frequent use.

Keratoconus

A condition of abnormal corneal growth in which both corneas gradually become thinned and conical.

Keratoconus usually starts around puberty and affects more females than males. It causes increasing *myopia* (nearsightedness) and a progressive distortion of vision that cannot be fully corrected by glasses. Hard contact lenses improve vision in the early stages but are less effective as the condition progresses.

A *corneal graft* is usually performed when vision has seriously deteriorated and contact lenses no longer are helpful. The results of corneal grafting are generally excellent.

Keratolytic drugs

Drugs that loosen and remove keratin (the tough, outer layer of the skin). Keratolytic drugs, which include preparations of *sulfur* and *salicylic acid*, are used in the treatment of skin and scalp disorders, such as *warts*, callosities (see *Callus, skin*), *acne*, *dandruff*, and *psoriasis*.

Keratomalacia

The last stage of corneal damage due to *vitamin A* deficiency. Keratomalacia usually occurs only in severely malnourished children; it is very rare in developed countries.

Prolonged lack of vitamin A causes severe dryness of the eyes with a characteristic foamy patch on the cor-

ners of the conjunctiva. There may also be a gritty feeling in the eyelids and sensitivity to bright light. Until this point, the condition is easily reversible by taking large doses of vitamin A. If the deficiency is not treated, keratomalacia develops and the cornea becomes opaque and ulcerated. Perforation of the cornea is common, usually leading to loss of the eye from infection.

Keratopathy

A general term used to describe a wide variety of disorders of the *cornea* (the front part of the eyeball). The word also forms part of the name of certain specific disorders.

Actinic keratopathy is damage to the outer layer of the cornea by ultraviolet light, either from the sun or from artificial sources, such as sunlamps or arc welding torches. The corneal layer tends to strip off, exposing the nerve endings and causing severe pain. Skiers or mountaineers may suffer a similar effect known as snow blindness.

Exposure keratopathy is damage to the cornea caused by loss of the normal protection afforded by the tear film and the blink reflex. It may occur in a variety of conditions in which the lids cannot cover the cornea, including severe *exophthalmos*, *facial palsy*, and *ectropion*.

Keratoplasty

See *Corneal graft*.

Keratosis

A skin growth caused by an overproduction of *keratin* (the main skin protein). Keratoses occur mainly in the elderly.

TYPES

SEBORRHEIC KERATOSES Often called seborrheic warts, they range from flat, dark brown, rough patches to small, wartlike protrusions and are covered with a greasy, removable crust. Seborrheic keratoses are completely harmless, but can be unsightly.

SOLAR KERATOSES Small, wartlike, red or flesh-colored growths that appear on exposed parts of the body as a result of overexposure to sun over a period of years. Solar keratoses may rarely develop into skin cancer, usually a *squamous cell carcinoma*.

TREATMENT

Unless they are large and unsightly, seborrheic keratoses require no treatment. However, solar keratoses must always be removed because of the risk of skin cancer. Removal is usually

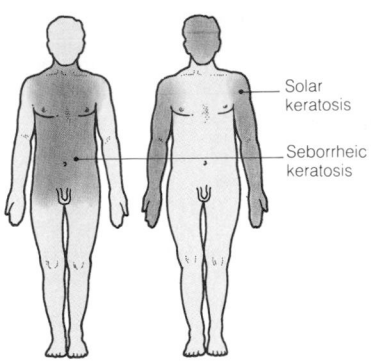

Sites of keratoses
Seborrheic keratoses occur mainly on the trunk; solar keratoses usually affect the face, arms, and hands.

done as an outpatient procedure by *cryosurgery* (the destruction of tissue by extreme cold).

Keratosis pilaris

A very common skin condition in which patches of raised, rough skin appear on the upper arms, thighs, and buttocks. The openings of the hair follicles become distended with hard plugs of *keratin* (the main skin protein) and the hairs that grow in them may be distorted.

The condition occurs most commonly in older children, adolescents, and obese people, and is often worse in winter. It is not serious and usually clears up on its own. In severe cases, symptoms can be improved by rubbing a mixture of salicylic acid and soft paraffin into the affected areas; scrubbing these areas with a loofah may also help.

Keratotomy, radial

A relatively new surgical procedure to reduce *myopia* (nearsightedness).

The results of radial keratotomy vary and the effect is not always per-

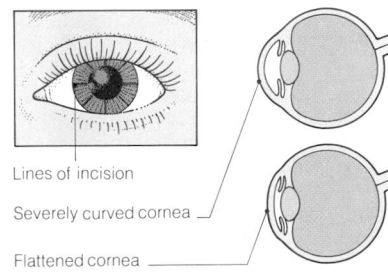

Lines of incision

Severely curved cornea

Flattened cornea

Procedure for keratotomy
Eight or more radial cuts are made in the cornea, avoiding the central zone. During healing, the scars contract, causing the cornea to become flatter and less powerful.

manent. Serious complications may develop. The procedure is not generally recommended for people whose vision can be corrected by glasses or contact lenses.

Kerion

A red, pustular swelling that develops as a reaction to a fungal infection, usually scalp ringworm (see *Tinea*). The inflammation gradually subsides over six to eight weeks but, if severe, may leave a scar and permanent loss of hair from the affected area. It is treated by applying ichthammol paste to the swelling and by taking the antibiotic griseofulvin.

Kernicterus

A rare disorder in which excess bilirubin (a pigment derived from the breakdown of red blood cells) causes brain damage in newborn (especially premature) infants, resulting in a form of mental retardation.

SYMPTOMS AND SIGNS

Excess bilirubin produces signs of *jaundice* in the first few days of life. In addition, the baby becomes more and more listless, sometimes adopting a characteristic posture with arched back and neck. Without treatment, the baby is likely to die at the end of the first week of life. Survivors may be deaf and may suffer from *athetosis* (uncontrollable, writhing movements) and *spasticity* (abnormal muscle stiffness). Mental retardation, bizarre eye movements, difficulty speaking, and a proneness to seizures may follow.

PREVENTION AND TREATMENT

Kernicterus is completely preventable if jaundice is treated promptly; there is no cure for the brain damage if kernicterus has occurred.

Ketoconazole

An *antifungal drug* used in the treatment of severe fungal infections of the lungs, brain, kidney, and lymph glands (see *Fungi*). Ketoconazole is also given to treat *candidiasis* (thrush) of the skin, mouth, or vagina when other antifungal preparations have proved ineffective.

Ketoconazole may cause nausea but it can sometimes be avoided if the drug is taken with food. Other possible adverse effects include rash and, rarely, liver damage.

Ketoprofen

A *nonsteroidal anti-inflammatory drug* (NSAID) prescribed as an *analgesic* (painkiller) in the treatment of injury to soft tissues, such as muscles and ligaments. Ketoprofen is also given to reduce joint pain and stiffness in people with types of arthritis, including *rheumatoid arthritis*, *osteoarthritis*, and *ankylosing spondylitis*.

Ketoprofen may cause abdominal pain, nausea, indigestion, and an increased risk of *peptic ulcer*.

Ketosis

A potentially serious condition in which excessive amounts of ketones accumulate in the body. Ketones are substances chemically related to acetone, which is found in solvents such as nail polish remover. Ketosis results whenever glucose is not available to use as a source of energy, which forces the body to use fats instead. This, in turn, leads to fatty acids being released into the blood; they are then converted to ketones.

The underlying causes of ketosis include fasting or starvation, and untreated or inadequately controlled *diabetes mellitus*, in which the lack of insulin prevents glucose from being used as fuel.

Symptoms and signs may include sweet, "fruity-smelling" breath, loss of appetite, nausea, vomiting, and abdominal pain. If the condition is not treated, confusion, unconsciousness, and death may follow.

Ketosis can be diagnosed by a test to detect ketones in the urine. Treatment is the same as for diabetes unless the cause is fasting or starvation, in which case gradual reintroduction of a nutritious diet is usually effective.

Kidney

The organ responsible for filtering the blood and excreting waste products and excess water in the form of urine. The kidney, ureter, bladder, and urethra make up the *urinary tract*.

STRUCTURE

There are two kidneys, each about 4 to 5 inches long and about 6 ounces in weight. They lie in the abdomen underneath the liver on the right and the spleen on the left. The arteries that supply the kidneys arise directly from the aorta (the main artery of the body leading from the heart). Once within the kidneys, the renal arteries divide into smaller and smaller branches, ending in capillaries in the glomeruli (the kidney's primary filtering units). Each kidney contains about 1 million glomeruli, which pass the filtered blood through long tubules into the medulla (the central collecting

LOCATION OF THE KIDNEYS

The kidneys are situated at the back of the abdominal cavity, just above the waist, on either side of the spinal column. The kidney on the right lies below the liver, while the kidney on the left is situated below the spleen. The arteries that supply the kidneys arise directly from the aorta.

Diaphragm

Rib cage

Left kidney

Adrenal gland

Right kidney

Vena cava

Ureters

Aorta

region of the kidney). The glomeruli and tubules make up the nephrons, the functioning units of the kidney. As people age, the number of functioning nephrons is reduced; this process may be speeded up by disease.

FUNCTION

The main functions of the kidney are to regulate blood and electrolytes and to eliminate waste products. The most important waste products are those generated by the breakdown of proteins. The kidneys also control the body's acid-base balance. When blood and body fluids become too acid or too alkaline, the urine acidity is altered to restore the balance. When excess water is ingested, the kidney excretes it; when water is lost (as a result of diarrhea or sweating), the kidney conserves it (see *ADH*).

The kidney also produces several hormones, including erythropoietin, which regulates the production and release of red blood cells from the bone marrow. *Vitamin D* is converted into active hormonal form by the kidney. Renin, an enzyme released by the kidney when blood pressure falls, acts on a protein in the blood to produce *angiotensin* (a powerful constrictor of small arteries that helps regulate blood pressure). Angiotensin also controls the release of *aldosterone*, an adrenal hormone that acts on the tubules to promote reabsorption of sodium and excretion of potassium.

Kidney cancer

Cancers that have their origins in the kidneys themselves are not rare. Cancer that starts in other organs rarely spreads to the kidneys.

TYPES

There are three main types of cancer arising in the kidneys.

RENAL CELL CARCINOMA This is the most common type of kidney cancer, accounting for about 75 percent of all kidney growths. The tumor usually occurs after the age of 40 and affects twice as many men as women. The most common symptom is *hematuria* (blood in the urine). There may be pain in the loins, a lump in the abdomen, fever, or weight loss. About 25 percent of patients survive five years or more because the tumor often has spread to the lungs, bone, liver, and brain by the time treatment is started.

NEPHROBLASTOMA Also called Wilms' tumor, this cancer accounts for about 20 percent of all cancers in children. It is found mainly in children under the age of 4 years and occurs almost twice as often in males. Nephroblastoma

THE FUNCTION OF THE KIDNEY

The kidney is essential to the regulation of the body's fluid balance and acid-base balance. The kidney contains about 1 million nephrons, each of which consists of a glomerulus and a tubule that drain urine into the renal pelvis. Capillaries feed each glomerulus and surround each tubule.

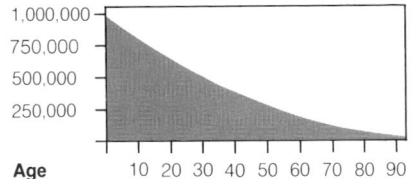

RENAL FUNCTION AND AGE
The efficiency of the kidney diminishes with age as the number of functional nephrons is reduced.

Nephrons per kidney

Fibrous capsule

Cortex

Medulla

Renal artery

Renal vein

Renal pelvis

Calyces

Ureter
The waste fluid (urine) left in the tubules passes into the calyces of the kidney and then into the ureter. The normal daily output of urine is 1 to 2 liters.

Arterioles
Small blood vessels that carry blood to and from each glomerulus and surround each tubule.

Tubule
About 140 liters of fluid pass from the glomeruli into the tubules each day; 99 percent of this salt and water solution is reabsorbed into the surrounding capillaries. The tubules also reclaim other essential substances, such as amino acids, glucose, bicarbonate, calcium, and phosphorus and, when necessary, add potassium and hydrogen to the tubular fluid.

Glomerulus
Each glomerulus acts as a filter, allowing the passage of certain dissolved substances from the bloodstream into the tubule, but preventing cells and large proteins from crossing over.

grows rapidly and is often felt as a lump in the abdomen. This cancer occasionally causes abdominal pain. Nephroblastoma frequently spreads to the lungs, liver, and brain. If treatment is started early, about 50 to 80 percent of children survive.

TRANSITIONAL CELL CARCINOMA This type arises from cells lining the renal pelvis. It develops in tobacco smokers and in people who have consumed very large quantities of analgesics (painkillers) over the course of many years. Hematuria is a common symptom; *hydronephrosis* (distention of the kidney with urine) may occur due to blockage of the ureter. Survival rates vary greatly, depending in part on early detection and treatment of the tumor.

K

DISORDERS OF THE KIDNEY

The kidneys are susceptible to a wide range of disorders. However, only one normal kidney is needed for good health, so disease is rarely life-threatening unless it affects both kidneys and has reached an advanced stage.

Hypertension (high blood pressure) can be both a cause and effect of kidney damage. Other effects of serious disease or damage include the *nephrotic syndrome* (in which large amounts of protein are lost in the urine and fluid collects in body tissues) and acute or chronic *renal failure*.

CONGENITAL AND GENETIC DISORDERS

Congenital abnormalities of the kidneys are fairly common. In *horseshoe kidney*, the two kidneys are joined at their base. Some people are born with one kidney missing, both kidneys on one side, or a kidney that is partially duplicated and gives rise to two ureters (duplex kidney). These conditions seldom cause problems. In rare cases, a baby is born with kidneys that are so underdeveloped that they are barely functional.

Polycystic disease of the kidneys is a serious inherited disorder in which multiple cysts develop on both kidneys (see *Kidney, polycystic*). In *Fanconi's syndrome* and *renal tubular acidosis* (which are rare), there are subtle abnormalities in the functioning of the kidney tubules, so that certain substances are inappropriately lost in the urine.

IMPAIRED BLOOD SUPPLY

Various diseases may cause damage to, or lead to obstruction of, the small blood vessels within the kidneys, impairing blood flow. *Diabetes mellitus* and *hemolytic-uremic syndrome* are examples. In physiological *shock*, blood pressure and flow through the kidneys are seriously reduced; this can cause a type of damage known as acute tubular necrosis. The larger blood vessels in the kidney may be affected by *periarteritis nodosa* and systemic *lupus erythematosus*. In rare cases, there is a defect of the renal artery supplying a kidney, which may lead to hypertension and tissue damage.

AUTOIMMUNE DISORDERS

Glomerulonephritis refers to an important group of autoimmune disorders in which the glomerular filtering units of the kidneys become inflamed. It sometimes develops after infection with streptococcal bacteria.

TUMORS

Benign *kidney tumors* are rare. They may cause *hematuria* (blood in the urine), although most cause no symptoms. Malignant tumors are also rare. Renal cell carcinoma, the most common type, occurs mostly in adults over 40; nephroblastoma (Wilms' tumor) affects mainly children under 4 (see *Kidney cancer*).

METABOLIC DISORDERS

Kidney stones are common in middle age. They are usually caused by excessive concentrations of various substances (such as calcium) or lack of inhibitors of crystallization in the urine. In *hyperuricemia*, there is a tendency for uric acid stones to form (see *Calculi, urinary tract*).

INFECTION

Infection of a kidney is called *pyelonephritis*. An important predisposing factor is obstruction of the flow of urine through the urinary tract, leading to stagnation and subsequent infection spreading up from the bladder. The cause of the obstruction may be a congenital defect of the kidney or ureter, a kidney or ureteral stone, a bladder tumor, or, in a man, enlargement of the prostate gland.

Tuberculosis of the kidney is caused by infection carried by the blood from elsewhere in the body, usually the lungs.

DRUGS

Allergic reactions to certain drugs can cause an acute kidney disease, with most of the damage affecting the kidney tubules. Other drugs may directly damage the kidneys if taken in large amounts for prolonged periods. For example, renal failure can develop after many years of taking excessive amounts of analgesics. Some potent antibiotics can damage the kidney tubules, producing acute tubular necrosis.

OTHER DISORDERS

Hydronephrosis refers to a kidney swollen with urine as a result of obstruction further down the urinary tract. In the *crush syndrome*, kidney function is disrupted by proteins (released into the blood from severely damaged muscles) that block the filtering mechanisms.

INVESTIGATION

Kidney disorders are investigated by *kidney imaging* techniques such as *ultrasound scanning*, intravenous or retrograde *pyelography*, *angiography*, and *CT scanning*; by *renal biopsy* (removal of a small amount of tissue for analysis); by *blood tests*; and by *kidney function tests*, such as *urinalysis*.

DIAGNOSIS AND TREATMENT

Diagnosis is made by intravenous *pyelography* or by renal *angiography*. Treatment consists of *nephrectomy* (removal of the kidney) and sometimes removal of the ureter as well. In the case of a nephroblastoma, nephrectomy is followed by *radiation therapy* and *chemotherapy*.

Kidney cyst

A fluid-filled sac within the kidney. Most are noncancerous.

Simple kidney cysts are found in about half the people over 50; most of them develop for no known reason. The cyst usually produces no symptoms unless it becomes large enough to cause pain in the lower back due to pressure from a buildup of fluid. Multiple cysts sometimes occur in one or both kidneys.

Kidney cysts also occur in polycystic kidney disease (see *Kidney, polycystic*), a hereditary condition that often leads to *renal failure* before the age of 50.

DIAGNOSIS AND TREATMENT

Cysts are frequently discovered only when the person is being examined for some other reason. Treatment is not usually necessary. *Aspiration* of the cyst may be performed to ensure that there is no malignancy or to relieve severe pain. When the cyst is large, fluid often reaccumulates, requiring excision.

Kidney failure

See *Renal failure*.

Kidney function tests

Tests performed to investigate urinary symptoms and kidney disorders. Kidney function tests may also be performed as part of a routine investigation before major surgery, or before prescribing drugs that are eliminated by the kidney. The tests are also performed to determine the function of a transplanted kidney.

TYPES

Urinalysis is a simple kidney function test. Collected urine is examined under the microscope for blood cells, pus cells, and casts (cells and mucuslike material that accumulate within the tubules and pass into the urine). Urine may also be cultured to confirm the presence of infection. It also may be tested for substances that are present only when the kidneys are diseased or damaged.

Kidney function can be assessed by measuring the concentration of substances in the blood (such as *urea* and creatinine) normally eliminated from the body via healthy kidneys. The creatinine clearance test provides an assessment of kidney function by comparing the amount of creatinine in the blood with the amount excreted in the urine over a timed interval, usually 24 hours.

Kidney function may also be assessed by *kidney imaging* techniques, which can help identify whether one or both kidneys are diseased.

Kidney imaging

Techniques for visualizing the kidneys, usually performed for diagnostic purposes.

TYPES

Ultrasound scanning provides remarkably clear pictures of the kidney. It can show an enlarged kidney, indicate the site of any blockage, and show the presence of a cyst or other tumor.

Conventional *X rays* show the outlines of the kidney and most kidney stones. Intravenous *pyelography* (in which a radiopaque contrast material is injected into a vein) gives a good picture of the internal anatomy of the kidney and ureters, as well as the presence of stones. *Angiography* involves injecting a material similar to that used in intravenous pyelograms into the renal arteries or veins to demonstrate the blood supply of the kidneys. When the material is injected into the arteries, it is known as arteriography. Digital subtraction angiography permits imaging of the renal circulation with less contrast material and greater safety.

CT scanning provides a complete cross section of the kidney displayed as computerized X-ray pictures. It is particularly useful for showing abscesses or tumors.

Radionuclide scanning is cheaper than conventional X rays and exposes the patient to less radiation. The two types usually used for the kidney are the DMSA scan and DTPA scan. DMSA is a substance given by intravenous injection that binds to the cells of the kidney tubules and gives a single static picture of the kidneys, indicating their relative size, shape, position, and function. DTPA, also given intravenously, is filtered by the glomeruli and passes out in the urine. Pictures are taken at intervals to record its passage through the renal tract. DTPA provides similar information to that provided by the intravenous pyelogram, although the anatomical details are less clear.

Kidney, polycystic

An inherited disorder in which there are numerous cysts in both kidneys. The cysts gradually increase in size until most of the normal kidney tissue is destroyed; cysts may also occur in the liver and, rarely, in other organs. Polycystic kidney disease is distinguished from multiple simple cysts of the kidneys, which occur commonly with age (see *Kidney cyst*).

TYPES

ADULT POLYCYSTIC DISEASE This disorder shows an autosomal dominant pattern of inheritance (see *Genetic disorders*). Symptoms, which may appear at any time (but usually appear in middle age) include abdominal swelling, pain, *hematuria* (blood in the urine), and frequent *urinary tract infections*. As the disease progresses, *hypertension* and *renal failure* may result.

JUVENILE POLYCYSTIC DISEASE This rare disorder causes *renal failure* in infants and young children. It is usually diagnosed at birth because of massive enlargement of the kidneys.

TREATMENT

There is no effective treatment for preserving kidney function in polycystic kidney disease. Symptoms of renal failure can be treated by *dialysis* (artificial purification of the blood) and *kidney transplant*.

Kidney stone

See *Calculus, urinary tract*.

Kidney transplant

A transplant operation in which the diseased kidney of a person who has chronic *renal failure* is replaced by a transplanted healthy kidney, either from a living donor or a cadaver. One healthy donor kidney is sufficient to maintain the health of the recipient.

Kidney transplantation is more straightforward than the transplantation of any other major organ and is by far the most commonly performed. In addition, the failure of a kidney transplant is far less serious than an unsuccessful heart, liver, or lung transplant because kidney function can be taken over by *dialysis*.

HOW IT IS DONE

For a description of a kidney transplant, see box (next page).

OUTLOOK

Kidney transplants are successful in more than 80 percent of cases. This figure climbs to more than 90 percent if the donor is a close blood relative. The primary danger is rejection of the donated kidney within the first month or two after transplantation. If the kidney is rejected, the patient returns to dialysis (artificial purification of the blood). However, more transplants may be attempted if the patient is in good health otherwise. All kidney transplant patients must take a lifelong course of *immunosuppressant drugs* to prevent rejection.

Kidney tumors

Growths of the kidney. Kidney tumors may be malignant (see *Kidney cancer*) or benign.

Fibromas, *lipomas*, and *leiomyomas* (which are benign) often cause no symptoms and may be discovered only during surgery on the kidney. Occasionally, a *hemangioma* grows very large and is mistaken for a cancer; it may also cause *hematuria* (blood in the urine).

No treatment is necessary for benign tumors unless they are very large or cause pain or bleeding.

Example of a kidney tumor
A malignant tumor of one kidney (sliced in half). Surgical removal of a malignant kidney tumor is always necessary.

K

PROCEDURE FOR A KIDNEY TRANSPLANT

The donated kidney comes from a close (living) blood relative of the patient or from any person who consented to medical use of organs after death (cadaver transplant). To prevent rejection of the kidney by the recipient's *immune system,* the tissue type and blood group of recipient and donor must be a close match (see *Transplant surgery*).

HOW IT IS DONE

Removal
The kidney is removed via an incision under the ribs.

Insertion
The donor kidney is inserted low in the pelvis.

Donor kidney

1 Usually the left kidney is removed from living donors because it has a longer vein than the right and is easier to remove safely. After removal, the kidney is flushed with saline solution.

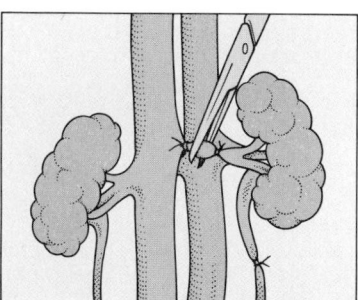

2 The surgeon may remove one or both of the patient's kidneys. Before removing a kidney, it is necessary first to clamp and cut the renal blood vessels that supply the kidney. The ureter must also be clamped and cut.

DIALYSIS AND TRANSPLANTATION IN THE US

About one third to one half of new patients with end-stage kidney failure are suitable for a transplant, but many have to wait some time for a suitable donor kidney to become available; in the meantime they add to the growing number of patients undergoing dialysis.

Year	Transplants	Patients on dialysis
1986	8,976	90,886
1984	6,968	78,483
1982	5,358	65,765
1980	4.697	52,364

Key
Patients on dialysis
Transplants

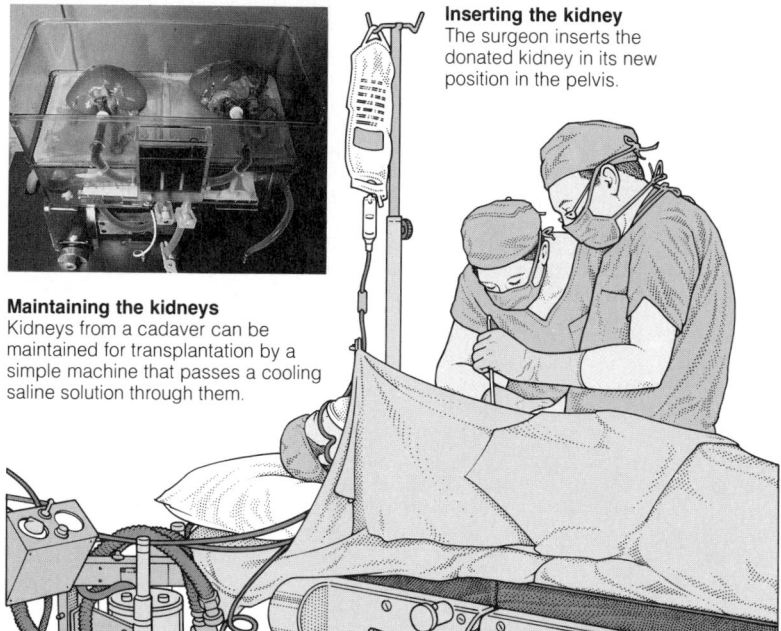

Maintaining the kidneys
Kidneys from a cadaver can be maintained for transplantation by a simple machine that passes a cooling saline solution through them.

Inserting the kidney
The surgeon inserts the donated kidney in its new position in the pelvis.

Donor kidney
Renal artery
Renal vein
Ureter
Bladder

3 The donor kidney is usually placed in the pelvis. The renal artery and vein of the donor kidney are joined to the recipient's artery and vein and the lower end of the donor ureter is connected to the recipient's bladder. The clamps are then removed.

THE DONOR (AFTER THE OPERATION)

The health of the donor is not affected by losing one kidney; the remaining kidney enlarges to take over full function.

Enlarged kidney
Original size

Kilocalorie

The unit of energy equal to 1,000 *calories*. In dietetics, a kilocalorie is often called simply a Calorie.

Kilojoule

The unit of energy equal to 1,000 *joules*, abbreviated kJ.

Kleptomania

A recurring inability to resist the impulse to steal objects that are not necessarily wanted or needed. The condition is rare, although it is often used by shoplifters and other thieves as an excuse.

In true kleptomania, the person experiences an increasing sense of tension before committing the act of theft and a sense of relief or pleasure while carrying it out. The act is not preplanned and little thought is given to the consequences, but later there may be anxiety and depression caused by the fear of being caught.

Kleptomania is usually a sign of an immature personality. It may also be caused by *dementia* and be the result of some forms of brain damage.

Klinefelter's syndrome

A *chromosomal abnormality* in which a male has one or more extra X *chromosomes* in his cells, giving him a chromosome complement of XXY or, more rarely, XXXY, XXXXY, and so on (instead of XY). About one in every 500 male infants born has the syndrome. The chances of a baby having the condition increase with age of the mother.

SYMPTOMS AND SIGNS

The features of Klinefelter's syndrome may pass unnoticed until puberty, when *gynecomastia* (breast enlargement) occurs and the testes remain small. Affected males are infertile due to *azoospermia* (absence of sperm production). They are usually tall and thin, and the body shape looks female rather than male. The incidence of mental retardation is higher in people with Klinefelter's syndrome than in the general population.

DIAGNOSIS AND TREATMENT

Diagnosis is confirmed by *chromosome analysis*. There is no treatment, although mastectomy may be performed if gynecomastia causes psychological distress; hormonal treatment may be used to induce secondary sexual characteristics, such as growth of facial hair. Parents who have had an affected child should receive *genetic counseling*.

Klumpke's paralysis

Paralysis of the lower arm, with wasting of the small muscles in the hand and numbness of the fingers (excluding the thumb) and of the inside of the forearm.

Klumpke's paralysis is caused by injury to the first thoracic nerve (one of the *spinal nerves*) in the brachial plexus (the network of nerves behind the shoulder blade); injury to this nerve is usually the result of dislocation of the shoulder.

In some cases, there may also be drooping of the upper eyelid, constriction of the pupil, and loss of sweating on one side of the face and neck (a collection of symptoms known as *Horner's syndrome*).

The condition is usually permanent. The only treatment consists of exercises to maintain mobility of the joints.

Knee

The joint between the femur (thigh bone) and tibia (shin); the patella (kneecap) lies across the front of the joint. The knee is a modified hinge joint, capable of bending and straightening, and capable of slight rotation in the bent position.

STRUCTURE

Two disks of protective cartilage called menisci (see *Meniscus*) cover the surfaces of the femur and tibia; they reduce friction between the bones during movement. The joint is partly surrounded by a fibrous capsule lined with synovial membrane, which secretes a lubricating fluid that allows the cartilage to move freely.

Strong ligaments on each side of the joint provide support and limit side-to-side movement. *Cruciate ligaments* within the joint, which cross over each other as they run diagonally between the femur and tibia, provide additional support, prevent overbending and overstraightening of the knee, and limit sliding movement between the bones.

Bursas (fluid-filled sacs) are present above and below the patella and behind the knee. The *quadriceps muscles* (which run along the front of the thigh) straighten the knee; the *hamstring muscles* at the back of the thigh bend the knee.

DISORDERS

Sudden twisting of the knee may cause a ligament sprain or tear a meniscus. If a meniscus is torn and a fragment of the cartilage catches between the surfaces of the joint, the knee may become temporarily locked in one position.

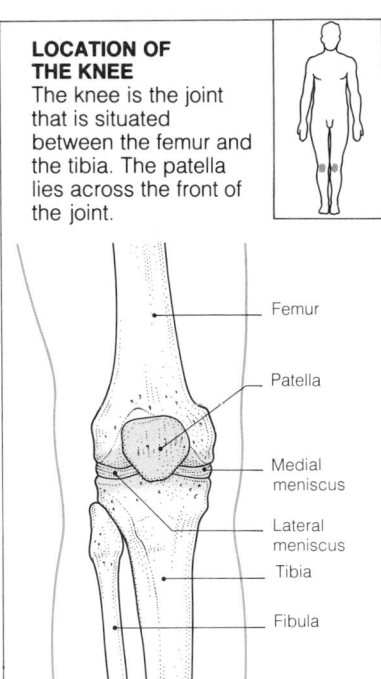

LOCATION OF THE KNEE
The knee is the joint that is situated between the femur and the tibia. The patella lies across the front of the joint.

Femur
Patella
Medial meniscus
Lateral meniscus
Tibia
Fibula

Severe damage to a joint, often as the result of a sports injury, may cause *hemarthrosis* (bleeding into the joint); minor injuries may lead to *synovitis* (inflammation of the joint lining). Repetitive activity, such as running, may cause inflammation of the tendon below the patella. In children, inflammation of the tibial tubercle (the bony prominence beneath the knee) may occur temporarily (see *Osgood-Schlatter disease*).

Bursitis (inflammation of a bursa) usually occurs in response to local pressure on the front of the knee. Fluid escaping from a bursa behind the knee causes a *Baker's cyst*.

Arthritic conditions most likely to affect the knee are *osteoarthritis*, *rheumatoid arthritis*, and retropatellar arthritis (inflammation of the undersurface of the patella). A condition similar to retropatellar arthritis, known as *chondromalacia patellae*, is common in adolescents.

Fractures of the lower femur, upper tibia, or the patella disrupt normal movement of the knee. A sharp blow to the knee may result in dislocation of the patella.

Knock-knee and *bowleg* are common in childhood as temporary deformities that resolve as growth continues; in adults, they may be caused by injury or disease.

K

Knee joint replacement

A surgical procedure to replace a diseased knee joint with an artificial substitute. Early replacement knees were simply large hinges. Today, most artificial knees take the form of metal and plastic implants that cover the worn cartilage. The aim is generally to preserve as much of the original joint as possible.

PROCEDURE FOR A KNEE REPLACEMENT

The surgeon usually makes one long incision, cuts through the joint capsule and synovial membrane, and then pushes aside the patella to reach the joint. Special instruments are used to make precise measurements and to cut away areas of bone so that the artificial components will fit and move correctly.

Femur
Skin incision
Capsular incision
Patella
Tibia
Fibula

1 The lower end of the femur is shaped and holes are drilled into it to accept the femoral component of the prosthesis. Cutting and drilling are done using special instruments.

2 The upper end of the tibia is shaped and holes are drilled into it to accept the tibial component. The cutting and drilling are again carried out using special precision instruments.

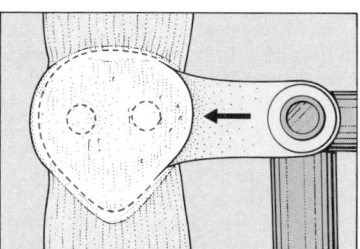

3 The back part of the patella is cut away to leave a flat surface. Small holes are then drilled into this surface to accept the patellar component of the artificial joint.

4 Having achieved a satisfactory fit using trial components, the final prosthesis is cemented in place. Excess cement is then removed and a final check is made of the joint movements.

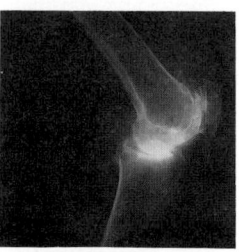

X ray of arthritic knee
Severe wear and tear of the bone and cartilage can easily be seen.

Femoral component
Tibial component

Knee prosthesis
The two main components fit over the femur and tibia.

X ray of artificial knee
The X ray shows the components of the prosthesis in position.

WHY IT IS DONE

Knee joint replacement is most often carried out in older people whose knees are severely affected by pain and impaired motion due to *osteoarthritis* or *rheumatoid arthritis*. An artificial knee is not normally recommended for younger patients because it does not restore the full range of movements and is unlikely to withstand vigorous activity.

RECOVERY PERIOD

The plaster cast fitted after the operation is usually removed after five days and exercises are started to strengthen the quadriceps. The patient can normally put weight on the leg after two or three weeks.

OUTLOOK

Although knee replacements can relieve pain and restore a degree of movement, results are often uncertain and the durability of the artificial parts is limited. However, research continues into the development of stronger materials, better cements (glues), and joint designs that more closely resemble natural joints.

Knock-knee

Inward curving of the legs so that the knees touch, causing the feet to be kept farther apart.

CAUSES

Knock-knee is a part of normal development in some children and is common between the ages of 3 and 5 years. It may also be the result of injury or disease. Among the common causes are diseases that soften the bones (such as *rickets* or *osteomalacia*), *rheumatoid arthritis* or *osteoarthritis* of the knee, or a fracture of the lower femur (thigh bone) or upper tibia

The appearance of knock-knee
This condition is common in toddlers but nearly always disappears by age 7.

K

(shin) that has not healed in a straight, vertical line.

TREATMENT

In children, the condition usually requires no treatment unless it persists after the age of 10, when it may start to strain the joints of the lower leg. Wearing heel wedges in the shoes may help correct the line of the leg, but most people require *osteotomy* (an operation in which the tibia is cut and realigned to straighten the leg).

In adults, treatment consists of osteotomy, or, when the condition has been present for a considerable time, *knee joint replacement*.

Knuckle

The common name for a *finger* joint.

Koilonychia

A condition in which the nails are dry, brittle, and thin, eventually becoming concave (spoon shaped). Koilonychia may be caused by injury to the nail. Other causes include iron-deficiency *anemia* and *lichen planus*; rarely, the condition is inherited.

The appearance of koilonychia
In koilonychia, the nails are flattened and look fragile, bending where they protrude past the finger ends.

Koplik's spots

Tiny, gray-white spots within the mouth (on the inner lining of the cheeks) that appear during the incubation period of *measles*.

Korsakoff's psychosis

See *Wernicke-Korsakoff syndrome*.

Kraurosis vulvae

See *Vulvitis*.

Kuru

A progressive and fatal infection of the brain that affects some natives of the highlands of New Guinea. Kuru is caused by a virus spread by cannibalism. The condition is now rare.

The disease is caused by a "slow" virus (which causes no signs of disease until many months or years after entry into the body) and the incubation period may be as long as 30 years. Symptoms include progressive difficulty in controlling movements and, eventually, *dementia*.

Kuru has aroused special interest recently because of certain similarities between the causative virus and *HIV* (human immunodeficiency virus), which causes *AIDS*. It is known that HIV can cause brain changes similar to those in kuru.

Kwashiorkor

A severe type of malnutrition in young children, occurring mainly in poor rural areas in the tropics. It is chiefly confined to children between 1 and 3 years old. The term kwashiorkor is derived from a Ghanaian word meaning "disease suffered by a child displaced from the breast."

CAUSES

The illness starts when the child is suddenly weaned onto a poor diet low in calories, protein, and certain essential micronutrients such as zinc, selenium, and vitamins A and E. To obtain enough nutrients from the food that is available, the child would need to eat a larger amount than he or she is capable of taking in. The problem is often exacerbated by a poor appetite due to illness. In addition, the lacking micronutrients provide protection against certain chemicals that are produced during infections and which also lead to *edema* (accumulation of fluid in the tissues). Measles and other infections common in the tropics precipitate kwashiorkor in undernourished children.

SYMPTOMS AND SIGNS

Growth is stunted, but edema makes the child look puffy and generally less emaciated than a child with *marasmus*, another form of malnutrition. Affected children are apathetic, weak, irritable, and inactive. Their skin sometimes flakes off, leaving a raw, weeping area beneath, and their hair may lose its curliness, become sparse and brittle, and turn from dark to fair.

The liver often enlarges, dehydration may develop (despite the simultaneous presence of edema), and the child loses resistance against severe infection, which may be fatal. In its severe, advanced stage, the illness is often marked by jaundice, drowsiness, and a fall in body temperature.

DIAGNOSIS AND TREATMENT

Diagnosis is based on a physical examination and the child's medical and dietary history.

The priorities in severe cases are to keep the child warm, replace lost fluids, and treat any infection. Initially, the child is fed milk (in frequent small amounts) and vitamin and mineral tablets, if possible. Zinc is given to prevent more flaking of the skin. When the edema has disappeared and the child's appetite has returned, a high-calorie, protein-rich diet is given.

OUTLOOK

Most children treated for kwashiorkor recover, but those less than 2 years old are likely to suffer permanent stunting of growth. Of the children ill enough to be admitted to a hospital, about 85 percent survive.

Kyphoscoliosis

A combination of *kyphosis* (abnormal backward curvature of the spine) and *scoliosis* (curvature of the spine to one side or the other).

Kyphosis

The medical term for excessive backward curvature of the spine. Kyphosis usually affects the spine at the top of the back, resulting in either a hump or a more gradually rounded back. Less commonly, it affects normally forward-curving parts of the spine at the neck and lower back.

Kyphosis may be caused by any of a variety of spinal disorders, including *osteoporosis* (bone degeneration from softening due to calcium loss), fracture of a vertebra, or a tumor of a vertebra (see *Spine* disorders box). In the past, the main cause of kyphosis was spinal tuberculosis. Treatment, which is rarely successful, is of the underlying disorder.

K

Normal curvature   Kyphosis of the thoracic spine

The appearance of kyphosis
In kyphosis, the thoracic part of the spine is excessively curved, producing a humped (rounded) appearance.

L

Labetalol

A *beta-blocker drug* used to treat *hypertension* (high blood pressure) and *angina pectoris* (chest pain caused by impaired blood supply to the heart).

Possible adverse effects include indigestion, nausea, and, in rare cases, depression and temporary impotence. Labetalol is less likely than some other beta-blocker drugs to cause cramping of the legs or coldness of the hands and feet.

Labia

The lips of the *vulva* (the female external genitalia) that protect the vaginal and urethral openings. There are two pairs of labia. The outer pair, called the labia majora, are fleshy folds that bear hair and contain sweat glands. They cover the smaller, hairless inner folds, the labia minora, which meet to form the hood of the *clitoris*.

LOCATION OF LABIA
The labia majora extend forward from the perineum and fuse at the front at the mons pubis. The labia minora lie within.

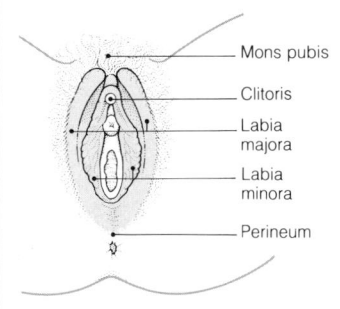

- Mons pubis
- Clitoris
- Labia majora
- Labia minora
- Perineum

Labile

Unstable; likely to undergo change. Vitamins are labile because they are broken down easily by such factors as heat and excess acidity. Blood pressure that has a tendency to fluctuate may be described as labile. In psychiatry, the term is sometimes used to mean emotional instability.

Labor

See *Childbirth*.

Labyrinthitis

Inflammation of the labyrinth (the fluid-filled chambers in the inner ear that sense balance) that results in *vertigo*, a sensation that oneself or one's surroundings are spinning around.

- Labyrinth
- Inner ear
- Middle ear

Mechanism of labyrinthitis
In labyrinthitis, inflammation of the fluid-filled chambers (labyrinth) of the inner ear causes disruption of the individual's sense of balance. The inflammation is usually caused by viral or bacterial infection.

CAUSES
Labyrinthitis is almost always caused by bacterial or viral infection. Viral labyrinthitis may occur during a flulike illness or during illnesses such as measles or mumps. Bacterial labyrinthitis is commonly caused by inadequately treated *otitis media* (infection of the middle ear), particularly if a *cholesteatoma* (an infected collection of debris in the middle ear) has developed and eroded a pathway into the inner ear. Infection may also reach the inner ear (via the bloodstream) from elsewhere in the body. Less commonly, bacterial labyrinthitis results from a head injury.

SYMPTOMS AND TREATMENT
Apart from vertigo, labyrinthitis can cause nausea, vomiting, *nystagmus* (jerky eye movements), *tinnitus* (ringing in the ears), and deafness.

Viral labyrinthitis clears up on its own, but symptoms are relieved by antihistamines such as meclizine. Bacterial labyrinthitis requires immediate treatment with *antibiotic drugs* to eradicate the infection. Otherwise, the infection may lead to permanent deafness or may spread to the tissue covering the brain, causing *meningitis*.

Surgery may be necessary to drain pus from the ear or to remove any cholesteatoma.

Laceration

A torn, irregular wound, as opposed to a straight cut, or *incision*. One example of a laceration is the tearing of the perineum (the area between the vagina and anus) that sometimes occurs during childbirth.

Lacrimal apparatus

The system that produces and drains tears. The lacrimal apparatus includes the main and accessory lacrimal glands and the nasolacrimal drainage ducts. The main glands secrete *tears* during crying and when the eye is irritated; the accessory glands maintain the normal tear film.

STRUCTURE
The main lacrimal glands lie just within the upper and outer margin of the orbit (socket) and drain into the *conjunctiva*. The accessory glands lie within the conjunctiva, secreting directly onto its surface.

Tears drain through the lacrimal puncta, tiny openings toward the inner end of each eyelid. The puncta are connected by narrow tubes to the lacrimal sacs, which lie in shallow hollows in the lacrimal bones. These bones are situated just within the inner margin of the orbit on either side of the nose. Overlying the lacrimal sacs are flat muscles that compress the sacs during blinking. Leading from the sacs are the nasolacrimal ducts, which run down through the bone to open inside the nose.

The action of blinking provides a suction effect to draw away excess fluid by compressing and releasing the lacrimal sacs.

FUNCTION
The principal function of tears is to keep the *cornea* and conjunctiva constantly moist. Moisture is essential to maintain transparency of the cornea and to prevent ulceration. By lubricating the surface of the eye, tears aid movement of the eyelid in blinking. Tears also wash away small foreign bodies and contain a natural antibiotic called lysozyme. Another function is their role in expressing emotion.

Lactase deficiency

A condition in which lactase, an enzyme that breaks down the lactose (milk sugar) present in the cells of the

FUNCTIONS OF THE LACRIMAL APPARATUS

Tear production must be sufficient to compensate for evaporation and maintain the tear film. Accessory lacrimal glands in the conjunctiva perform this function. The main lacrimal glands secrete when excess fluid is required. Surplus tears drain into the nose.

- Upper eyelid
- Accessory lacrimal glands
- Lacrimal gland
- Conjunctiva
- Iris
- Accessory lacrimal glands
- Lower eyelid
- Lacrimal puncta
- Iris
- Lower eyelid
- Lacrimal bone
- Lacrimal sac
- Lacrimal duct (leading to an outlet into the nose)

small intestine, is missing. Lactase deficiency causes lactose intolerance, an inability to digest lactose.

TYPES, INCIDENCE, AND SYMPTOMS

Lactase deficiency may be present at birth, may develop immediately after weaning, or may not become evident until puberty or later.

Congenital lactase deficiency is sometimes permanent, but is more often temporary. This type is caused by delayed enzyme maturation, especially in premature babies.

Permanent lactase deficiency develops in about 80 to 90 percent of blacks and Orientals and in about 5 to 15 percent of whites. Lactase deficiency may also occur as a complication of intestinal diseases (such as *celiac sprue* and *gastroenteritis*). In these cases, the deficiency frequently disappears as the disease improves.

Undigested lactose ferments in the intestine and causes severe abdominal cramps, bloating, flatulence, and diar-rhea; weight loss and malnutrition may also occur.

DIAGNOSIS AND TREATMENT

The diagnosis can be confirmed by tests on blood and feces. Treatment is a lactose-free diet; milk must be avoided but fermented milk products, such as yogurt, can be eaten. Enzyme replacements (which partially or fully break down lactose) may be used.

Lactation

The production and secretion of milk after childbirth. (See *Breast-feeding*.)

Lactic acid

A weak acid produced by cells when they break down glucose to produce energy by anaerobic metabolism (chemical processes that do not require oxygen). This process occurs only when there is too little oxygen for the more usual aerobic metabolism. For example, lactic acid is produced by muscles during vigorous exercise and

is one of the factors that contributes to *cramp*. Lactic acid is also produced in tissues when their blood supply (oxygen) fails due to a *myocardial infarction* (heart attack) or *shock*.

Normally, lactic acid is removed from the blood by the liver; if lactic acid accumulates, a condition called *acidosis* results.

Lactose

One of the sugars present in milk. Chemically, lactose is a disaccharide *carbohydrate*, a sugar made up of two monosaccharide (simple sugar) units.

Lactose is broken down by lactase (an enzyme released by the lining of the small intestine) into the monosaccharides glucose and galactose, which are then absorbed into the bloodstream. *Lactase deficiency* results in a reduced ability to digest lactose. If the diet contains milk, lactose accumulates and ferments in the feces, sometimes causing diarrhea.

Lactose intolerance

The inability to digest lactose, a sugar found in milk. It is usually caused by a deficiency of lactase, an enzyme found in the small intestine (see *Lactase deficiency*). Rarely, it occurs in a person who is not deficient in lactase.

Lactulose

A *laxative drug* used to treat *constipation* and *liver failure*. Lactulose causes water to be absorbed into the feces from the intestinal blood vessels, making the feces softer and easier to pass. It is used to treat liver failure because it helps eliminate ammonia from the bloodstream into the feces.

Lambliasis

Another name for *giardiasis*.

Laminectomy

Surgical removal of part or all of one or more laminae (the bony arches of the vertebrae that surround the spinal cord) to expose the spinal cord. Laminectomy is performed as the first stage of spinal canal decompression, an operation carried out to relieve pressure on the spinal cord or on a nerve root leading from it (see *Decompression, spinal canal*).

HOW IT IS DONE

An incision is made in the patient's back and the laminae are exposed. Enough of one or more adjacent laminae is then chipped away to give the surgeon access to the cord. Rarely, several complete laminae must be removed. In this case, *spinal fusion* (immobilization of the spine with metal rods or bone grafts) is then necessary to prevent subsequent instability of the spine.

Lance
To incise (cut) using a *lancet* or a surgical scalpel.

Lancet
A small, pointed, double-edged knife used to open and drain lesions such as boils and abscesses.

Lanolin
A mixture of a yellow, oily substance obtained from sheep's wool and purified water, used as an *emollient* in the treatment of dry skin. Lanolin is a common ingredient of bath oils and hand creams; it is also used to treat mild *dermatitis*. Occasionally, lanolin may irritate the skin.

Lanugo hair
Fine, soft, downy hair that covers a fetus. Lanugo hair first appears in the fourth or fifth month and usually disappears by the ninth month. It can still be seen in some premature babies.

Lanugo hair sometimes reappears in adults who have cancer, particularly of the breast, bladder, lung, or large intestine. It may also occur with *anorexia nervosa* or be a side effect of drugs (especially *cyclosporine*).

Laparoscopy
A method of examining the abdominal cavity by means of a laparoscope, a type of *endoscope* (viewing tube).

WHY IT IS DONE
Laparoscopy is usually performed to determine the cause of pelvic pain or gynecological symptoms (such as *ectopic pregnancy* or *pelvic inflammatory disease*) that cannot be confirmed by physical examination. It is frequently used to examine the condition of the fallopian tubes when investigating cases of *infertility*. Laparoscopy can also be used to examine the appendix, gallbladder, and liver.

Laparotomy, exploratory
An operation in which the abdomen is opened to look for the cause of an undiagnosed illness. Laparotomy strictly describes any abdominal surgery because, even when the surgeon is operating to treat a known disorder, a thorough examination of the entire abdomen is carried out.

WHY IT IS DONE
The primary reason for a laparotomy is to investigate symptoms and signs whose cause other tests have failed to discover. Common examples include recurrent abdominal pain and *peritonitis* (infection within the abdominal cavity). The operation may also be performed as an emergency procedure if the abdomen has been seriously injured in an accident.

HOW IT IS DONE
A vertical (or, less commonly, a crosswise or oblique) incision is made in the abdomen and the abdominal cavity is opened and explored for signs of disease. Any diseased organ is repaired or removed, after which the incision is sewn up.

The recovery period depends upon the nature and extent of the disease discovered and treated.

Larva migrans

Infections characterized by the presence of the larval (immature) forms of certain worms in the body and by the symptoms caused by movement of the worms.

Visceral larva migrans, better known as *toxocariasis*, is caused by a type of worm that normally parasitizes dogs. Cutaneous larva migrans is caused by hookworm larvae that normally parasitize dogs, cats, or other animals. Also known as creeping eruption, it is contracted by walking barefoot on soil or beaches contaminated with animal feces. The larvae penetrate the skin of the feet and move randomly, leaving intensely itchy red lines sometimes accompanied by blistering.

Both types of larva migrans can be treated with *antihelmintic drugs*, such as thiabendazole.

Laryngeal nerve
One of a pair of nerves that carries instructions from the brain to the larynx (voice box) and sends sensations from the larynx to the brain. Each nerve leaves the brain through a hole in the base of the skull and passes down the neck. The right-hand nerve then hooks around an artery behind the clavicle (collarbone) before returning to the larynx. The other nerve travels farther, hooking around the

---

PROCEDURE FOR LAPAROSCOPY
A hollow needle is inserted into the abdomen just below the navel (using anesthesia), and carbon dioxide gas is pumped through the needle to expand the abdominal cavity. The laparoscope (see below) is then inserted through another incision to view the internal organs. The gas in the abdomen may cause discomfort for a day or two afterward.

Sites of incision

Entry point for surgical instruments

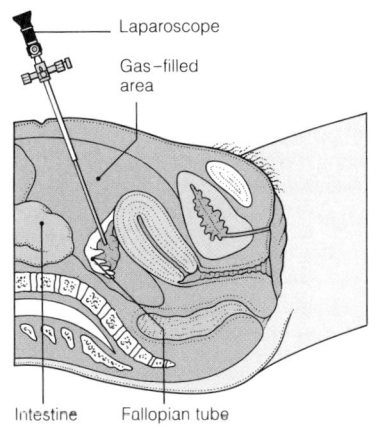

Laparoscope

Gas-filled area

Intestine   Fallopian tube

Gynecological laparoscopy
Laparoscopy is used in diagnosis and for removing ova for in vitro fertilization. Laparoscopic sterilization is a common sterilization procedure for women.

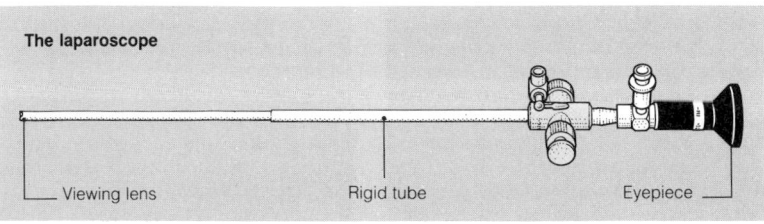

The laparoscope

Viewing lens   Rigid tube   Eyepiece

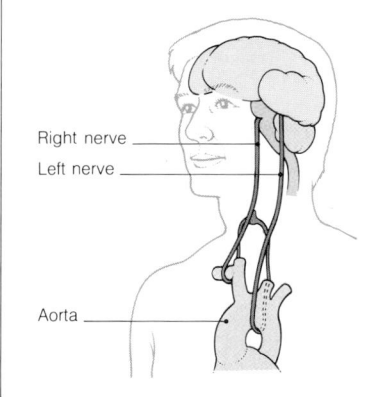

LOCATION OF LARYNGEAL NERVES
Both nerves exit the brain at the base of the skull and pass down the neck. One hooks around an artery behind the right clavicle, the other hooks around the aorta; both return to the larynx.

Right nerve

Left nerve

Aorta

aorta (the major artery leaving the heart) before passing back to the larynx. Damage to one or both nerves causes *vocal cord* paralysis, resulting in loss of voice and sometimes obstruction to breathing.

Laryngectomy

Surgical removal of all or part of the larynx (voice box) to treat advanced cancer of the larynx (see *Larynx, cancer of*). After the operation, the patient is no longer able to speak in the usual fashion.

WHY IT IS DONE

If cancer of the larynx is detected early, the prospects of curing it with *radiation therapy* are good. However, tumors that have grown to a considerable size, and those that are not responding to radiation therapy, require surgical removal.

HOW IT IS DONE

An incision is made in the neck and the larynx is removed, using general anesthesia. The top of the trachea (windpipe) immediately below the larynx is then sewn to the skin around the surgical wound in the neck to form a permanent opening called a stoma, through which the patient will breathe from then on.

RECOVERY PERIOD

Immediately after the operation, a bell or buzzer and pen and paper are given to the patient so that he or she can communicate. A tube is left in the stoma for a few days so that, as the surrounding tissues heal, they do not

close the opening. The air in the patient's room is humidified to reduce the production of mucus in the stoma, and any excess mucus is sucked away.

Initially, all food is passed through a thin tube running from the nose to the stomach. After about 10 days the feeding tube is removed and food (fluid or semisolid at first) can be taken normally again. Speed of recovery depends partly on age and health.

OUTLOOK

With persistence, the patient can learn from a speech therapist a new way of speaking (called esophageal speech). Air is swallowed, then expelled in a controlled way; this noise is modulated by the tongue, palate, and lips to form gruff, though distinguishable, words. The technique requires painstaking practice. Alternatively, patients may use an electronic larynx, a device that emits a buzzing noise and is held against the top of the throat. By mouthing words, the person converts the buzz to speech.

Swimming is not possible, and care must be taken when bathing.

Laryngitis

Inflammation of the larynx (voice box) usually caused by infection and resulting in *hoarseness*. Laryngitis may be acute, lasting only a few days, or chronic, persisting over a long period.

CAUSES

Acute laryngitis is usually caused by a viral infection, such as a cold, but it can also be due to an allergy to a drug, pollen, or some other substance.

Chronic laryngitis may be caused by overuse of the voice, by violent coughing, by irritation due to tobacco smoke, alcohol, or fumes, or by damage during surgery.

SYMPTOMS AND SIGNS

Hoarseness is the most common symptom, and it may progress to loss of voice. There may also be pain or a feeling of discomfort in the throat (especially during swallowing) and a dry, irritating cough. Laryngitis caused by a viral infection is often accompanied by fever and a general sick feeling.

TREATMENT

A person with laryngitis should rest in bed, avoid tobacco and alcohol, keep the throat lining moist with humidifiers, and take *antipyretic drugs* to reduce fever and *analgesic drugs* to relieve pain.

If the symptoms do not subside within four or five days, if sputum (phlegm) is coughed up, or if hoarseness persists for several weeks, a

physician should be consulted. Antibiotic drugs will be prescribed if there is a bacterial infection. If the physician suspects a cause other than infection, diagnostic tests may be required, possibly to check for signs of cancer (see *Larynx, cancer of*), which can be cured if treated at an early stage.

Laryngoscopy

Examination of the larynx (voice box) using a mirror held against the back of the palate (indirect laryngoscopy), or a viewing tube called a laryngoscope (direct laryngoscopy). Either a rigid or a flexible laryngoscope may be required.

WHY IT IS DONE

The larynx is inspected when a person complains of persistent hoarseness or has other change in the voice, when there is persistent stridor (a harsh noise when breathing in), or when someone experiences difficulty inhaling. Laryngoscopy is also useful in examining people who have throat pain or difficulty swallowing.

INDIRECT LARYNGOSCOPY This technique is used to detect *epiglottiditis* (in adults), *laryngitis*, benign or malignant laryngeal tumors, and any reduction of movement in the vocal cords.

DIRECT LARYNGOSCOPY This procedure is used when a biopsy or more careful evaluation is needed (e.g., assessing the extent of a tumor). The laryngoscope also allows more elaborate procedures, such as complete excision of a benign *lesion*, foreign body removal, laser surgery, or injection of polytef into paralyzed vocal cords. Often, a microscope is used with the laryngoscope. Direct laryngoscopy is also done before *intubation*.

HOW IT IS DONE

Indirect and direct laryngoscopy procedures are shown in the illustrated box, next page.

Laryngotracheobronchitis

Inflammation of the larynx, trachea, and bronchi. It is the most common cause of *croup*.

Larynx

The organ in the throat responsible for voice production and for preventing food from entering the airway during swallowing. Its common name is the voice box.

STRUCTURE

The larynx, which lies between the *pharynx* (upper part of the airway) and the *trachea* (windpipe), forms part of the tube in the throat that carries air to and from the lungs. It consists of areas

PROCEDURE FOR LARYNGOSCOPY

There are two techniques. In indirect laryngoscopy, the patient's throat is examined with the use of a mirror. In direct laryngoscopy, the patient's throat is viewed with an instrument called a laryngoscope. If a rigid laryngoscope is used, general anesthesia is required. Only mild sedation is needed if a flexible laryngoscope is used.

INDIRECT LARYNGOSCOPY

Angled mirror

Tongue

Larynx

The patient sticks out his or her tongue and the physician rests an angled mirror on the soft palate. A lamp or mirror on the physician's head illuminates the larynx, which is reflected in the mirror.

DIRECT LARYNGOSCOPY

Laryngo-scope

Larynx

A rigid laryngoscope is passed down the throat via the mouth; a flexible laryngoscope is passed via the nostril.

View of larynx
This view was obtained with a laryngoscope. The vocal cords are at the center and the epiglottis forms the arc at the top.

---

of cartilage (tough but flexible tissue), the largest of which is the thyroid cartilage, which projects at the front to form the Adam's apple. Below it, connecting the thyroid cartilage to the trachea, is the cricoid cartilage, which is shaped like a signet ring with the seal at the back. Situated on top of the seal are the two pyramid-shaped arytenoid cartilages. Between these two cartilages and the interior surface of the Adam's apple stretch two fibrous sheets of tissue, the *vocal cords*, which are responsible for voice production.

Attached to the top of the thyroid cartilage at the entrance to the larynx is the *epiglottis*, a leaf-shaped flap of cartilage that prevents food from entering the larynx during swallowing. The entire larynx is lined with *mucous membrane*, which is of the squamous cell type.

FUNCTION

The most important function of the larynx is to prevent *choking*. When a person is not eating or drinking, the epiglottis stays upright, keeping the

LOCATION OF LARYNX

The larynx, commonly called the voice box, is situated deep in the throat between the pharynx and the trachea (windpipe).

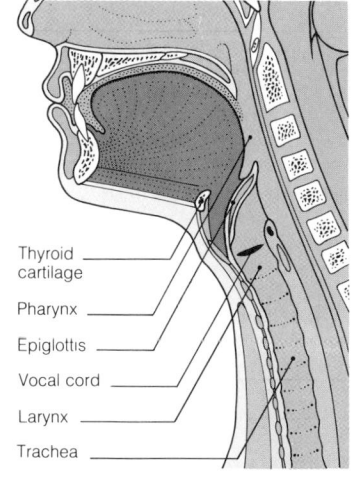

Thyroid cartilage

Pharynx

Epiglottis

Vocal cord

Larynx

Trachea

---

larynx open as part of the airway to the lungs; as soon as swallowing begins, the epiglottis drops like a lid over the larynx, directing food to either side. Closure of the true vocal cords and the false vocal cords just above them also helps protect the airway. The food or drink then passes down the *esophagus* to the stomach.

The secondary function of the larynx is voice production. Air from the lungs passes over the stretched vocal cords. The resultant vibrations are modified by the tongue, palate, and lips to produce *speech*.

Larynx, cancer of

A malignant tumor of the larynx (voice box), often causing persistent hoarseness. Laryngeal cancer represents about 2 percent of all cancers.

CAUSES AND INCIDENCE

The exact causes of this type of cancer are not known, but it occurs most commonly in heavy smokers. Laryngeal cancer is also associated with high alcohol consumption.

In the US, laryngeal cancer primarily affects people over age 60; it is more common in men than in women.

SYMPTOMS

Hoarseness is the main symptom, particularly when the tumor originates on the vocal cords. A tumor that develops elsewhere in the larynx often passes unnoticed until an advanced stage of the disease, when the tumor causes discomfort in the throat, difficulty breathing and swallowing, and coughing up blood.

DIAGNOSIS

Laryngoscopy (examination of the larynx indirectly with a mirror, or directly with an endoscope) reveals any tumor on the larynx. A *biopsy* (removal of a sample of tissue) is carried out in the hospital using local or general anesthesia to determine whether the growth is benign or malignant, and whether the lining of the larynx shows any signs of early cancerous change.

TREATMENT

If the tumor is discovered when it is still small, the outcome is usually favorable. A small cancer of the true vocal cords has about a 95 percent chance of cure, usually by *radiation therapy* alone.

For larger tumors (and for those that do not respond to radiation therapy) partial or total *laryngectomy* (removal of the larynx) is considered for all but frail or elderly patients. The cure rate of surgery varies according to the site and extent of the tumor. In all cases

DISORDERS OF THE LARYNX

Disorders affecting the larynx (voice box) are common. They usually cause *hoarseness* because they interfere with the functioning of the vocal cords. Other symptoms include difficulty breathing, stridor (a harsh noise on breathing in), a painful throat, and coughing. Persistent hoarseness should be reported to a physician.

CONGENITAL DEFECTS

Rarely, a baby is born with a soft, limp larynx, a condition called laryngomalacia. The main signs are stridor and noisy breathing when feeding. The larynx usually attains a normal firmness by age 2.

INFLAMMATION

Laryngitis (inflammation of the larynx) is the most common laryngeal disorder in adults; symptoms are hoarseness, fever,

and discomfort in the throat. In children, *croup* (inflammation and narrowing of the air passages) is very common up to age 4. Much rarer is *epiglottiditis* (inflammation of the epiglottis, the flap of cartilage that closes the larynx during swallowing). This is a life-threatening disorder in young children.

TUMORS

Various kinds of benign growth may develop on the vocal cords. The most common is a polyp, a smooth swelling usually caused by smoking, by an infection such as influenza, or by straining the voice. Warts occasionally develop on a child's vocal cords. Both polyps and warts require removal and microscopic analysis to exclude cancer. *Singers' nodes* are small benign growths that can occur on the vocal cords of people who strain their voices. They give the voice a hoarse tone.

Malignant tumors, which cause

persistent hoarseness, are usually caused by smoking and/or alcohol use (see *Larynx, cancer of*).

OTHER DISORDERS

A tumor, an infection, or, rarely, throat surgery can damage one or both of the nerves supplying the larynx, causing *vocal cord* paralysis, which results in loss of voice and may interfere with breathing.

INVESTIGATION

Disorders of the larynx are investigated by *laryngoscopy*. Sometimes a *biopsy* sample is taken for pathologic analysis; X rays, especially *tomography*, may provide more information.

after losing part or all of the larynx, the patient must master new techniques for producing speech.

If the tumor has spread throughout the larynx, or to other parts of the throat (or, rarely, other parts of the body), the patient is treated with radiation therapy and *anticancer drugs*. This combination relieves symptoms and often temporarily arrests the progress of the disease.

Laser

A device that produces a concentrated beam of light radiation; laser is an acronym for light amplification by stimulated emission of radiation. A laser beam is parallel, of a single specific wavelength (or sometimes of a narrow band of wavelengths), and coherent (that is, all the crests of the individual waves coincide).

Laser treatment

The use of a *laser* beam in a variety of medical procedures.

LOW-INTENSITY TREATMENT

Treatment with low-intensity beams stimulates tissue healing and reduces pain, inflammation, and swelling. It works by improving blood and lymph flow and by reducing the production of *prostaglandins* (hormonelike substances that stimulate inflammation and cause pain). Low-intensity beams are used in the treatment of muscle tears, ligament sprains, and inflamed tendons and joints.

HIGH-INTENSITY TREATMENT

High-intensity treatment destroys cells directly under the beam while leaving adjacent cells undamaged, making it useful in the treatment of some tumors. The beam cuts through tissue and, simultaneously, causes blood clotting, making it a useful surgical tool.

LASERS IN OPHTHALMOLOGY Lasers are used in the treatment of diabetic *retinopathy* (to prevent bleeding from abnormal blood vessels), to prevent and treat retinal detachment (by sealing small tears or areas of degeneration), and to destroy small tumors of the retina. The laser can also be used to make a central hole to restore vision if the lens capsule becomes opaque after *cataract surgery*.

LASERS IN GYNECOLOGY Laser beams are sometimes used to unblock fallopian tubes by removing scar tissue formed after an infection or a *sterilization* procedure. Lasers are used to destroy abnormal cells in the *cervix*.

OTHER USES Lasers are commonly used to remove small birthmarks and tattoos; the results are variable. Early malignant tumors of the larynx can be successfully removed without damaging the vocal cords.

Many new applications are being investigated. Potential uses include the removal of atherosclerotic *plaque* from inside arteries. It may also be possible to use lasers to disintegrate bladder and kidney stones, and to

remove otherwise inaccessible tumors of the brain and spinal cord. (See also illustrated box, overleaf.)

Lassa fever

A dangerous infectious disease, caused by a virus, that was first reported in 1969. The disease occurs in occasional outbreaks in West Africa; a small number of cases have been imported into the US and Europe.

In Africa, where the virus is harbored by a type of rat, infection may be acquired by inhaling droplets of the rat's urine. Medical and nursing staff are at risk of acquiring the virus from the blood of an infected person or from droplets coughed into the air. No one in the US has ever acquired the disease from an infected person.

SYMPTOMS AND TREATMENT

After an incubation period of three to 17 days, the illness starts with fever, headache, muscular aches, and a sore throat. Later, severe diarrhea and vomiting develop. In extreme cases, the patient's condition deteriorates rapidly in the second week. About one quarter to one third of hospitalized patients die from the illness.

Lassa fever can be diagnosed by a blood test. Infected people must be isolated; they are treated by relief of symptoms and injections of the *antiviral drug* ribavirin and of serum containing *antibodies* that are active against the virus.

USE OF A LASER
The concentrated beam of light released by a laser has a variety of medical purposes. When set to low intensity, the laser works to stimulate tissue healing and reduces pain, inflammation, and swelling. At high intensity, the beam destroys cells on which it is focused while leaving adjacent tissue unharmed. It can also cut through tissues without causing bleeding.

Argon laser
Photocoagulation of blood vessels occurs when the blue-green light from this laser is absorbed by hemoglobin.

Protective goggles

Laser

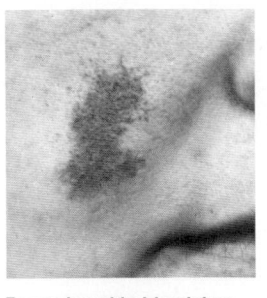

Removing skin blemishes
These photographs, taken before and after laser treatment, show removal of a port-wine stain. In some cases, treatment is less successful, leaving scars.

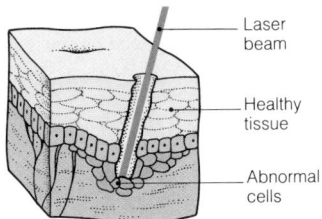

Laser beam

Healthy tissue

Abnormal cells

Focused carbon dioxide laser
This laser is ideal for precision cutting or for destroying abnormal cells because its focused beam leaves surrounding areas of tissue intact.

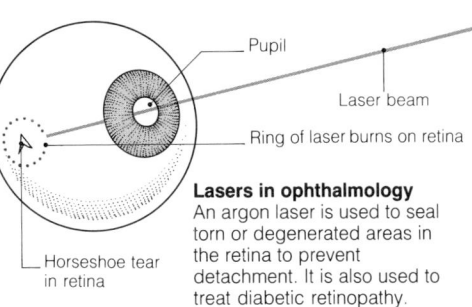

Pupil

Laser beam

Ring of laser burns on retina

Horseshoe tear in retina

Lasers in ophthalmology
An argon laser is used to seal torn or degenerated areas in the retina to prevent detachment. It is also used to treat diabetic retinopathy.

Lassitude
A term describing a feeling of *tiredness*, weakness, or exhaustion.

Lateral
Relating to, or situated on, one side. Bilateral means on both sides.

Laudanum
A solution of *opium* once used as a sedative and painkiller and in the treatment of diarrhea.

Laughing gas
The popular name for *nitrous oxide*, a gas inhaled in combination with oxygen to produce general *anesthesia*. Laughing gas is so called because of the euphoric effects it produces.

Laurence-Moon-Biedl syndrome
A very rare inherited disorder characterized by increasing *obesity*, *retinitis pigmentosa* that may lead to blindness, mild to moderate *mental retardation*, *polydactyly*, and *hypogonadism*.

The condition is probably caused by a disorder of the hypothalamus (part of the brain that controls the hormone balance). There is no treatment; parents should seek *genetic counseling*.

LAV
Lymphadenopathy-associated virus, a name formerly given to the virus responsible for *AIDS*. The virus was renamed *HIV* (human immunodeficiency virus) in 1986.

Lavage, gastric
Washing out the stomach with water, usually to remove poisons.
HOW IT IS DONE
The patient is placed face down with his or her head below the level of the stomach and turned to one side. A lubricated tube is passed down the esophagus into the stomach and a funnel is attached to the top. (If the patient is not fully conscious, a tube is also passed down the throat into the windpipe to prevent regurgitated water and stomach contents from entering the lungs.) Water is poured into the funnel until the stomach is filled. The top of the tube is then lowered, allowing the fluid in the stomach to drain into a bucket. This process is repeated until the water returns clear. An early sample of fluid from the stomach is kept so that the poison can be analyzed. In certain cases, an antidote to the poison (or a substance that neutralizes the poison)

is added to the water or is passed into the stomach after lavage is finished.

Lavage is not used if a corrosive poison has been swallowed because of the risk of the tube perforating tissues. Corrosive acids or alkalis may be diluted by giving large amounts of water or milk (see *Poisoning*).

Laxative drugs

COMMON DRUGS
Bulk-forming *Methylcellulose Psyllium*
Lubricant *Mineral oil*
Saline *Magnesium sulfate Sodium phosphate*
Stimulant *Bisacodyl Senna*
Others *Lactulose*

WARNING
If constipation lasts for more than a week, consult your physician; you may have a serious underlying disorder.

A group of drugs used to treat *constipation*. A high-fiber diet, plenty of liquids, and proper toilet habits may relieve constipation without use of laxative drugs. They may be given to prevent constipation when straining should be avoided (e.g., following childbirth, abdominal surgery, or a *myocardial infarction*). Laxatives are sometimes used to clear feces from the intestine before surgical or investigational procedures.

TYPES

BULK-FORMING LAXATIVES These drugs retain fluid drunk with the laxative, increasing bulk and stimulating propulsion. They increase the volume of feces, making them softer and easier to pass.

STIMULANT LAXATIVES These drugs stimulate the intestinal wall to contract and thus speed up the elimination of feces. Because the feces spend less time in the intestine, less water is reabsorbed into the blood vessels, which helps keep the feces soft.

LUBRICANT LAXATIVES These substances soften and thus facilitate the passage of feces.

SALINE LAXATIVES These drugs increase the concentration of salts within the feces, an action that draws fluids into the intestine from the surrounding blood vessels.

POSSIBLE ADVERSE EFFECTS

Used in excess, laxative drugs may cause diarrhea. Since prolonged treatment may cause dependence on the laxative drug for normal bowel action, laxative use should be stopped as soon as normal habits are reestablished.

Stimulant laxatives and lactulose may cause abdominal cramps and flatulence. Prolonged use of saline laxatives is likely to cause a chemical imbalance in the blood. Lubricant laxatives may coat the intestine and prevent vitamin absorption.

Lazy eye

An ambiguous name for the visual defect that commonly results from *strabismus*. (See *Amblyopia*.)

LD$_{50}$

The abbreviation for median lethal dose, the amount of a drug needed to kill 50 percent of a group of animals. This dose is determined during experiments carried out to assess the toxicity of new drugs.

Lead poisoning

Swallowing or inhaling lead or lead salts can damage the brain, nerves, red blood cells, and digestive system.

Acute poisoning, which is relatively rare but sometimes fatal, occurs when a large amount of lead is taken into the body over a short period. Chronic poisoning results from small amounts of lead being taken in over a longer period. The body excretes lead very slowly, so it accumulates in body tissues (primarily in the bones). There is evidence that lead poisoning may produce no detectable physical effects but can cause mental impairment, particularly in children.

CAUSES AND INCIDENCE

Lead poisoning is most common in children who have licked or eaten old paint that contains high levels of lead. Adults most at risk include workers in industries such as lead mining and smelting, soldering, demolition, and pottery glazing. Drinking liquor from illicit stills with lead piping or inhaling the fumes from burning battery casings containing lead may also cause lead poisoning. So, too, can eating acidic food or drink that is stored or cooked in lead-glazed or lead-soldered containers.

Almost everybody is exposed to lead from exhaust fumes. In recent years, atmospheric lead levels have decreased as a result of legislation requiring vehicles manufactured after 1975 to run on unleaded gasoline. There is also a legal limit to the amount of lead that paint may contain.

SYMPTOMS AND SIGNS

Acute lead poisoning causes severe, colicky, abdominal pain, diarrhea, vomiting, weakness or paralysis of the limbs, seizures, and sometimes death.

In addition to the symptoms of acute poisoning, chronic poisoning may cause mental disturbances ranging from loss of memory, emotional instability, abnormal behavior, incoordination, and headaches to hallucinations, seizures, blindness, and coma. Seizures, behavioral abnormalities, and coma occur chiefly in children. There may also be *anemia*, loss of appetite, and a blue, black, or gray line along the gum margins.

If symptoms progress as far as seizures and coma, the risk of death is high. Even if the person survives, there is a high probability of permanent brain damage.

DIAGNOSIS

Lead poisoning is diagnosed from the patient's condition and history, and from blood tests to measure lead levels, X rays of the bones and abdomen to reveal lead deposits, and urine tests to measure the level of lead breakdown products.

TREATMENT

Treatment consists of avoiding further exposure to lead. The physician will prescribe *chelating agents* to bind to the lead and help the body excrete it at a faster rate. In mild cases, the chelating agent penicillamine may be used alone. In more severe cases, it may be used in combination with other chelating agents, such as edetate calcium disodium (calcium EDTA) and dimercaprol (BAL).

Learning

A change in behavior as a result of experience. Committing facts to memory, often termed "learning by heart," is a separate process. True learning may not be immediately obvious. Whether or not a person has learned a skill or a fact can be judged only on the basis of his or her performance in a real-life situation.

THEORIES OF LEARNING

According to behavioral theories, all learning in humans and animals occurs by *conditioning*. The simplest form (as described by Ivan Pavlov) is classical conditioning, in which a particular stimulus becomes associated with a particular response. In Pavlov's experiments, a bell was rung every time dogs were presented with food; eventually the dogs salivated in response to the bell alone.

A more sophisticated version of learning, termed operant conditioning by B.F. Skinner, relies on a system of rewards, known as reinforcements. Skinner observed that, if a hungry rat wandering about a cage accidentally bumped into a lever that released a food pellet, it learned to press the lever purposefully. The reinforcement need not appear every time for the rat to continue trying. In the same way, an occasional win on a slot machine is often enough to make people continue to play the game.

Rewards can also be used to encourage the development of new forms of behavior. Behavior "shaping" is the basis of animal training, and is used in dealing with behavioral problems in children and the mentally retarded. It can also apply to family and marital difficulties; partners or family members give each other rewards for desirable behavior. (See *Behavior therapy*.)

Another theory of learning proposes that, with experience, an abstract "cognitive" structure is built on which future decisions and behavior is based. Cognitive theorists believe that the simple responses of

L

conditioning are not sufficient to explain the ability to cope with new situations or solve new problems. For these processes, the more abstract mental qualities of *memory*, insight, and understanding are necessary.

The behavioral and cognitive approaches are combined in the "social learning theory," which proposes that learning occurs as a result of observation and imitation of the behavior of others.

No one theory can account for the complexities of learning. It is probable that some things are learned automatically, by conditioning, and others by complex thought processes that take account of many facts. Different factors may be more important at different times in a person's life; trial and error and observational learning are particularly important in young children. The ability to learn is also affected by personal interest in a task or subject, past experiences, and anxiety levels. In general, people learn faster when they are given a little at a time to learn; learning slows down as skill improves.

Learning disabilities

A range of physical and psychological disorders that interferes with learning. Learning disabilities include problems in learning caused by defects in mental activities (such as speech, hearing, and memory), but do not include those due to emotional or environmental deprivation or to poor teaching.

Children of borderline or retarded intelligence have general difficulty learning. So, too, do those with *hyperactivity*, which lowers the attention span. Others have specific problems, such as *dyslexia* (difficulty reading), dyscalculia (inability to perform mathematical problems), or dysgraphia (writing disorders). Some psychologists believe that specific learning difficulties in children of normal intelligence may be caused by forms of *minimal brain dysfunction*, which may be inherited. Attempts to assess and treat such children have so far not been very successful.

Leech

 A type of blood-sucking worm with a flattened body and a sucker at each of its ends. Different types live on land or in water. Land leeches inhabit tropical forests. They can work their way through clothing and attach themselves to the ankles and lower legs. Aquatic, blood-sucking leeches live in warm water and attach themselves to swimmers, sometimes penetrating to the bronchi and the esophagus.

Use of a leech to drain blood
Leeches bite painlessly, introducing saliva into the wound before sucking blood. When they are satiated, they drop off. Here, a leech is being used to drain a hematoma (collection of blood) from a person's outer ear following an injury.

TREATMENT OF BITES
Attached leeches should be startled by applying a lighted match, alcohol, salt, or vinegar. They can then be pulled off gently to prevent the mouth parts from staying attached and becoming infected. A styptic pencil helps stop the bleeding after the leech has been removed. *Endoscopy* (use of an internal viewing tube) may be necessary to remove leeches from inside the body.

MEDICAL USES
Leeches were once attached to a patient's skin to "treat" many illnesses ascribed to excess blood. Today, leeches are sometimes used to drain a *hematoma* (a collection of partially clotted blood) from a wound.

Leg, broken
See *Femur, fracture of*; *Fibula*; *Tibia*.

Legionnaires' disease

 A form of pneumonia (infection of the lungs) named after an outbreak that caused the death of 29 members of the American Legion who were attending a convention in a Philadelphia hotel in 1976. The bacterium responsible was isolated and the genus named *LEGIONELLA*. Tests identified the causative organism as a common contaminant of water systems that had been responsible for earlier epidemics of pneumonia (the cause of which had not been understood at the time).

CAUSES AND INCIDENCE
The bacterium breeds most readily in warm, moist conditions; in most outbreaks the source of infection has been the water or air-conditioning system in a large public building. Infection follows the inhalation of droplets of heavily contaminated water (from air-conditioning outlets and showers, for example). Elderly people, especially heavy smokers or drinkers, are particularly at risk.

The disease occurs both in localized outbreaks and as isolated cases. Over 700 diagnosed cases are reported in the US each year, but the true incidence is probably much higher. One to 2 percent of hospital cases of pneumonia may be caused by legionnaires' disease.

Control of the disease relies on the disinfection of water systems by chlorination or other means.

SYMPTOMS AND SIGNS
The first symptoms develop within a week of infection; they include headache, muscular and abdominal pain, diarrhea, and a dry cough. Over the next few days pneumonia develops, resulting in a high fever, shaking chills, the coughing up of thick sputum (phlegm), drowsiness, and sometimes delirium. Like other types of pneumonia, the illness usually becomes more severe unless treated. This phase lasts about a week, after which either a gradual recovery takes place or progressively serious breathing problems develop.

DIAGNOSIS AND TREATMENT
The patient is admitted to the hospital, where analysis of a sample of sputum (cultured on special media) or a lung biopsy reveals the microorganism responsible for the pneumonia. If it is *LEGIONELLA PNEUMOPHILA*, the patient is given the antibiotic erythromycin, often intravenously, which usually relieves symptoms quickly. Occasionally another antibiotic drug, rifampin, may be required.

OUTLOOK
The outcome of the disease depends on the age and general health of the patient. Younger people generally recover fully, but a substantial proportion of elderly, unfit people die from the illness. Death is usually due to irreversible lung damage.

Leg, shortening of

Shortening of the leg is usually caused by faulty healing of a fractured femur (thigh bone) or tibia (shin). Other causes are an abnormality present from birth, surgery on the leg, or muscle weakness associated with *poliomyelitis* or some other neurological disorder. Also, a deformity of the hip, knee, or spine may make one leg effectively shorter than the other even if the two are in fact of equal length.

If the difference in leg length exceeds 1.5 inches (4 cm), there is usually a noticeable limp; the resultant stress on the lower spine often causes *back pain*. Placing a raised heel on the shoe of the shortened side is a common remedy for a shortened leg.

Leg ulcer

An open sore on the leg that fails to heal, usually resulting from an inadequate arterial blood supply to or insufficient venous drainage from the area. Elderly people are most commonly affected.

Venous ulcer on leg
This type of ulcer, also known as a stasis ulcer, is caused by impaired drainage of blood from the leg by the veins. It is usually accompanied by edema (fluid accumulation) in the lower leg.

TYPES

Varicose ulcers, which occur mainly on the ankles and lower legs, are caused by valve failure in veins ; these ulcers usually appear in conjunction with *varicose veins*.

Bedsores (also called decubitus ulcers) develop on pressure spots on the legs as a result of a combination of poor circulation, pressure, and immobility over a long period.

Leg ulcers may also be due to *peripheral vascular disease*, in which fatty deposits on or thickening of the walls of arteries restricts blood supply to the extremities.

Diabetes mellitus, which increases susceptibility to blood vessel disease and skin infection and impairs sensation, may lead to ulcers.

Ulcers may also develop through neglect of an infected small wound. In the tropics, infection with microorganisms can cause *tropical ulcers*.

PREVENTION AND TREATMENT

Prevention is always easier than cure. In general, anyone susceptible to leg ulcers should attempt to avoid obesity, leg injury, and immobility.

Treatment of leg ulcers, which depends on the cause, should be sought at the earliest sign of trouble. If an ulcer is exuding pus, a wet dressing may be applied under a bandage. This dressing should be changed only every three to seven days to avoid removing new skin from the area.

Leiomyoma

A benign tumor of smooth muscle (a type of muscle not under voluntary control). Leiomyomas usually occur in the smooth muscle of the uterus, where they gradually become replaced with fibrous tissue (hence their popular name, *fibroids*). More rarely, leiomyomas develop from smooth muscle in the wall of blood vessels in the skin, where they form tender lumps.

Leiomyomas are usually multiple and, although they are not malignant (cancerous), they may require surgical removal if they cause symptoms.

Leishmaniasis

 Any of a variety of diseases affecting the skin, mucous membranes, and internal organs, caused by infection with single-celled parasites called leishmania. The parasites are harbored by dogs and rodents in various parts of the world, and are transmitted from infected animals or people to new hosts by the bites of sand flies.

About 12 million people worldwide are thought to be affected. Leishmaniasis is not contracted in the US, but travelers occasionally contract an infection abroad.

TYPES AND INCIDENCE

The most serious form of leishmaniasis, mainly affecting the internal organs, is called kala-azar or visceral leishmaniasis. It is prevalent in some parts of Asia, Africa, and South America, and also occurs in some Mediterranean countries.

In addition, there are at least three varieties of cutaneous leishmaniasis (mainly affecting the skin), one of which is prevalent in the Middle East, North Africa, and in the Mediterranean; the others occur only in parts of Central and South America.

Travelers can minimize the risk of infection by taking common-sense measures to discourage sand-fly bites (see *Insect bites*).

Leishmaniasis ulcer
This skin ulcer, which developed at the site of a sand-fly bite, is typical of the lesions found on the skin of people who are suffering from cutaneous leishmaniasis.

SYMPTOMS

Kala-azar causes a persistent fever, enlargement of the spleen, anemia, and, in the later stages, darkening of the skin. The illness may develop anytime up to two years after the initial infection, and, unless treated, is sometimes fatal.

The cutaneous forms cause the appearance of a persistent ulcer at the site of the sand-fly bite. The ulcer may eventually heal, but can leave an ugly scar. With the South American forms, more extensive tissue damage may occur, often on the face, causing severe disfigurement.

DIAGNOSIS AND TREATMENT

Kala-azar is diagnosed by a *bone marrow biopsy* and a blood test. The cutaneous forms are diagnosed by identifying parasites in scrapings taken from the edge of affected skin patches. All types of leishmaniasis are treated effectively with drugs, such as sodium stibogluconate, which are given by injection into a muscle or into a vein.

Lens

The internal optical component of the eye. Also called the crystalline lens, it is responsible for adjusting focus. This lens is one of two lenses in each eye; the other is the *cornea*, which provides most of the power needed to form an image on the *retina*.

The crystalline lens is situated behind the iris and is suspended on delicate fibers from the ciliary body. It is elastic, transparent, and slightly less

L

LOCATION OF THE LENS

This elastic and transparent organ is situated behind the iris and is suspended on delicate fibers from the ciliary body. Its full name—the crystalline lens—differentiates it from the cornea (another lens).

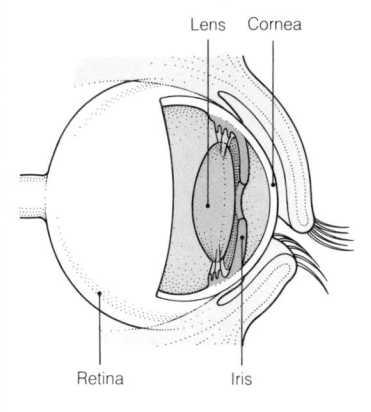

Lens   Cornea

Retina   Iris

L

convex on the front surface than on the back. Changing degrees of curvature alter the focus of the eye so that an image remains sharp whether a near or a distant object is being viewed (see *Accommodation*).

Opacification of the crystalline lens, from any cause, is called *cataract*. (See also *Lens dislocation*.)

Lens dislocation

Displacement of the eye's crystalline *lens* from its normal position. Lens dislocation is almost always caused by an injury that ruptures some or all of the fibers that connect the lens to the ciliary body. In *Marfan's syndrome*, the fibers are particularly weak and lens dislocation is common.

A dislocated lens may slide downward, causing severe visual distortion or double vision in the affected eye, or it may slip backward into the vitreous humor. A lens dislocated forward usually causes a form of *glaucoma* because of closure of the drainage angle of the eye. If the glaucoma is severe, the lens may be removed. (See also *Aphakia*.)

Lens implant

A plastic prosthesis used to replace the removed opaque lens in *cataract surgery*. There are many different designs, which may be positioned in front of the iris, clipped to the pupil, or held in place behind the pupil by delicate plastic loops.

A lens implant usually provides excellent distance vision without glasses. However, most people need reading glasses or bifocal lenses for close vision after the implant.

Lentigo

A flat, discolored area of skin similar to a freckle. Lentigines (the plural of lentigo) are usually light brown and may occur singly or in groups. Unlike freckles they are as common on covered as on exposed parts of the body, and they do not fade in winter. Lentigines are more common in middle-aged and elderly people, especially those who have been exposed to a lot of sun.

Lentigines are harmless and no treatment is necessary. If raised, darker brown areas appear within them, a physician should be consulted; there is a danger that these areas could develop into malignant melanomas (see *Melanoma, malignant*).

Leprechaunism

A very rare congenital disorder in which affected infants have elfin faces, with wide-set eyes, large lips, and large, low-set ears; they also have large hands and feet. Hormonal imbalances cause enlargement of the penis in males and the clitoris and breasts in females, as well as hirsutism (hairiness). Most babies who have leprechaunism die in the first weeks or months of life.

Leprosy

A chronic bacterial infection, also known as Hansen's disease, that damages nerves, mainly in the limbs and facial area, and may also lead to skin damage. Untreated leprosy can have severe complications, which include blindness and disfigurement. Contrary to popular belief, it is not highly contagious.

Performing a lens implant
The photograph shows an operation in which the plastic lens implant is being inserted immediately behind the iris into position over the pupil of the eye.

CAUSES
Leprosy is caused by a bacterium, *MYCOBACTERIUM LEPRAE*, spread in droplets of nasal mucus. A person is infectious to others only during the first stages of the disease. Only people living in prolonged close contact with the infected person are at risk of infection. This, along with the fact that only 3 percent of the population is susceptible to leprosy, means that there is no justification for the practice (still prevalent in some countries) of isolating people with the disease.

INCIDENCE
Worldwide, there are about 20 million sufferers from leprosy, mostly in Asia, Central and South America, and Africa. Probably fewer than 20 percent of these have access to treatment. In the US, there are now more than 4,000 known cases, mainly in California, Florida, Hawaii, Louisiana, New York, and Texas; three quarters of the people affected were born outside the US.

SYMPTOMS AND SIGNS
Leprosy has a very long incubation period—about three to five years. Most of the destructive effects of the bacteria on nervous tissue are caused not by bacterial growth but by a reaction of the body's *immune system* to the organisms as they die. There are two main types of the disease. In lepromatous leprosy, damage is widespread, progressive, and severe. Tuberculoid leprosy is milder.

Initially, damage is confined to the peripheral nerves (those supplying the skin and muscles). There is lightening or darkening of skin areas, with associated reduced sensation and reduced sweating. As the disease progresses, the peripheral nerves swell and become tender. Hands, feet, and facial skin eventually become numb and muscles become paralyzed.

Complications include loss of all sensation in the hands and feet, so that accidental burns or injuries are not noticed, leading to extensive scarring or even to loss of fingers or toes. Muscle paralysis can lead to further deformity. Damage to the facial nerve means that the eyelids cannot be closed; the cornea dries and ulcerates, leading to blindness. Alternatively, direct invasion by bacteria may lead to inflammation of the eyeball, again leading to blindness. The disability caused by the combined effects of blindness and loss of touch sensation is extremely severe.

Cartilage and bone in the nose are often eroded, and bones elsewhere in the body may be destroyed. In addition, the testes may atrophy, leading to sterility.

DIAGNOSIS AND TREATMENT

Early diagnosis of the disease is essential to prevent permanent disfigurement and disability. A provisional diagnosis is made from a physical examination of the patient; the presence of the bacteria is confirmed by a skin *biopsy* (removal of a sample of tissue for analysis).

Treatment is with the drug dapsone, which kills most of the causative bacteria within a few days. Any damage that has already occurred, however, is irreversible. Patients cease to be infectious soon after treatment starts. To prevent a relapse, use of the drug needs to be continued for at least two years after the last signs have disappeared.

Prevention of damage to the feet and other insensitive areas—through the use of proper footwear and health education—is very important. Plastic surgery may be helpful for facial deformities. Nerve and tendon transplants may improve the function of damaged limbs.

In the US, patients are eligible for treatment by the Public Health Service. There are special clinics and hospitals in different areas.

OUTLOOK

Resistance to dapsone is becoming more common worldwide; other curative drugs, such as rifampin and clofazimine, are much more expensive. With no vaccine and so many sufferers in poor countries, the battle against leprosy has only just begun.

Leptospirosis

 A rare disease caused by a spirochete (spiral-shaped) bacterium harbored by rodents and excreted in their urine. It is also known as Weil's disease. About 100 cases of leptospirosis, leading to a few deaths, are reported in the US each year.

SYMPTOMS

After an incubation period of one to three weeks, there is an acute illness with fever, chills, an intense throbbing headache, severe muscle aches, eye inflammation, and a skin rash. In most cases, the kidneys are affected, often severely. Liver damage leading to jaundice is also common.

TREATMENT

Antibiotics are effective against the spirochetes. In about one third of all cases the condition improves promptly. However, many patients suffer a more persistent illness in which kidney and liver function recover only slowly. In these cases, the nervous system may also be affected, often producing signs of *meningitis* (inflammation of the membranes covering the brain and spinal cord).

Lesbianism

Female homosexuality. According to Alfred Kinsey's studies carried out in the 1940s, about 5 percent of women are entirely lesbian in their sexual activity, although some 15 percent have had, by the age of 45, a homosexual experience. Lesbianism is less common than male homosexuality (see *Homosexuality, male*), but relationships tend to be more stable and often are lifelong. Masturbation, oral sex, and mutual rubbing of the clitoris are the usual means of reaching orgasm.

Lesion

An all-encompassing term for any abnormality of structure or function in any part of the body. The term may refer to a wound, infection, tumor, abscess, or chemical abnormality.

Lethargy

A feeling of *tiredness*, drowsiness, or lack of energy.

Leukemia

Any of several types of cancer in which there is usually a disorganized proliferation of white *blood cells* in the bone marrow (from which all blood cells originate). The production of red blood cells, platelets, and normal white blood cells is impaired as they are crowded out from the marrow by the leukemic cells.

Other organs, such as the liver, spleen, lymph nodes, testes, or brain, may cease to function properly as they become infiltrated by the leukemic cells. The number of leukemic cells circulating in the blood may be high.

Leukemias are classified into acute and chronic types; acute leukemia generally develops more rapidly than chronic leukemia. They are also classified according to the type of white cell that is proliferating abnormally. If the abnormal cells are derived from lymphocytes or their immature precursors (lymphoblasts), the leukemia is called lymphocytic or lymphoblastic leukemia. If the abnormal cells are derived from other types of white blood cells or their precursors, it is called myeloid, myeloblastic, or granulocytic leukemia.

There are about 13 new cases of leukemia per 100,000 annually in the US, leading to about six to seven deaths per 100,000. (See also *Leukemia, acute*; *Leukemia, chronic lymphocytic*; *Leukemia, chronic myeloid*.)

Leukemia, acute

A type of leukemia in which the white blood cells produced in excess within the bone marrow are immature cells called blasts. Untreated, acute leukemia can be fatal within a few weeks to months. Treatment today can often prolong life and may even provide a complete cure.

The abnormal cells may be of two types: lymphoblasts (immature *lymphocytes*) in acute lymphoblastic leukemia, and myeloblasts (immature forms of other types of white cell) in acute myeloblastic leukemia. Various subtypes are recognized according to the nature of the abnormal cells.

INCIDENCE AND CAUSES

About six or seven new cases of acute leukemia are diagnosed annually per 100,000 people in the US. The incidences of the two main types (acute lymphoblastic leukemia and acute myeloblastic leukemia) at different ages are shown on the next page.

Both types seem to result from a single white cell mutating (altering in its genetic structure). The cell undergoes an uncontrolled series of divisions until billions of copies of the abnormal cell are present in the bone marrow, blood, and other tissues.

There are a number of possible causes for the original mutation. One type of acute lymphoblastic leukemia is thought to be caused by a virus similar to the one that causes *AIDS*. Exposure to certain chemicals (such as benzene and some anticancer drugs) and to atomic radiation or radioactive leaks from nuclear reactors can be a cause. Inherited factors may play a part; there is an increased incidence in people with certain genetic disorders (such as *Fanconi's anemia*) and chromosomal abnormalities (such as *Down's syndrome*). People with certain other blood disorders, such as chronic myeloid leukemia and primary *polycythemia*, are also at increased risk.

SYMPTOMS AND SIGNS

The symptoms and signs of both types of acute leukemia are caused by overcrowding of the bone marrow by blasts and by infiltration of various organs by the abnormal cells. The overcrowding causes the marrow's failure to produce normal blood cells of all types (see box, next page).

L

LEUKEMIA

In all forms of leukemia, abnormal white cells proliferate in the bone marrow. There are four main types— acute lymphoblastic leukemia (ALL), acute myeloblastic leukemia (AML), chronic lymphocytic leukemia (CLL), and chronic myeloid leukemia (CML). Their incidence varies with age (see right). The acute types have a rapid onset. There is a risk of death from overwhelming infection or blood loss, but modern treatment has greatly improved survival rates (below) and may bring a cure.

The chronic forms of leukemia progress much more gradually but are essentially incurable.

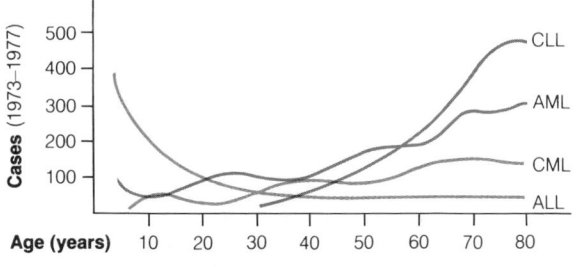

Incidence
The graphs show how the four main types of leukemia vary in incidence with age. Acute lymphoblastic leukemia (ALL) is the common type in children, chronic lymphocytic leukemia (CLL) is the most common after 40.

Survival rates for acute leukemia
The graphs show survival rates for acute lymphoblastic leukemia (ALL) and acute myeloblastic leukemia (AML) for cases diagnosed in the years 1964 to 1973 and 1974 to 1983. The improved survival rates are the result of better treatment.

Symptoms of acute leukemia
Symptoms are caused partly by the abnormal white cells crowding out the bone marrow (so that it fails to produce sufficient normal blood cells of all types) and partly by the invasion of other body organs by abnormal cells.

Gum bleeding
This results from insufficient production of platelet cells by the bone marrow; platelets are needed for the arrest of bleeding.

Bone tenderness
This may be felt as the bone marrow becomes packed with immature white cells.

Frequent bruising
Reduced numbers of platelets may lead to bleeding points in the skin and bruising after mild trauma.

Headache
Headache may be caused by anemia or by abnormal white cells affecting the nervous system.

Enlarged lymph nodes
The lymph nodes in the neck, armpits, and groin may be swollen with huge numbers of immature white cells. The liver, spleen, and testes may also be swollen.

Anemia
Anemia develops if there is insufficient production of red blood cells by the bone marrow. Anemia causes tiredness, breathlessness on exertion, and pallor.

Infections
White blood cells play a major part in the defense against infection. However, in acute leukemia, only immature, nonfunctioning white cells are made, so the patient may suffer from repeated chest or throat infections, herpes zoster, or skin and other infections.

HOW LEUKEMIA ATTACKS THE BODY

Leukemia is a form of cancer, but with the abnormally growing cells—mutated white blood cells— scattered throughout the body in bone marrow, rather than grouped into a single tumor. The abnormal cells may spill into the blood and may infiltrate and interfere with the function of other organs. But worse, the abnormal cells "take over" the marrow and prevent it from making enough normal blood cells—including normal white cells, red cells, and platelets. This leaves the sufferer highly susceptible to serious infections, anemia, and bleeding episodes.

Cell photograph
Shown is blood in acute leukemia. The large cells are abnormal, immature white cells; the smaller, paler cells are red blood cells.

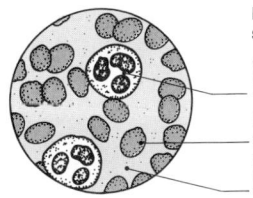

Normal blood smear

White cells fight infection

Red cells transport oxygen

Platelets help blood clot

Blood smear in leukemia

Abnormal white cells—susceptibility to infection

Fewer platelets— bleeding tendency

Fewer red cells— anemia

Appearance of blood in leukemia
In leukemia (above), the blood usually contains many abnormal white cells, and fewer red cells and platelets.

Normal appearance of blood
In a normal blood smear (left), there are large numbers of red cells, many platelets, and a few white cells.

DIAGNOSIS

The diagnosis of acute leukemia is based on a *bone marrow biopsy* that confirms an abnormal number of blast cells. The blast cells are sometimes also seen in the blood. When acute lymphoblastic leukemia is diagnosed, a *lumbar puncture* is usually performed to examine the cerebrospinal fluid for the presence of blast cells.

TREATMENT

Treatment includes giving the patient transfusions of blood and platelets, and the use of *anticancer drugs* to kill the leukemic cells. These drugs tend to make the patient even more susceptible to infection, so powerful antibiotics may also be given.

From the beginning of treatment, it is common for the patient to have inserted into a large vein near the heart a catheter (tube) through which all drugs and transfusions are given. Treatment of leukemic cells in the cerebrospinal fluid is accomplished by the direct injection of drugs into the fluid and by subsequent *radiation therapy* to the head and spinal cord. Radiation therapy is more commonly given in the treatment of acute lymphoblastic leukemia than for acute myeloblastic leukemia.

The course of drug treatment may last for many weeks. When there is no evidence of leukemic cells in the blood or bone marrow, a state of remission is said to have been achieved. However, without repeated courses of treatment, the leukemia often relapses (returns). For this reason, the use of drugs is usually continued for many weeks after remission.

If the leukemia relapses after the first remission, *bone marrow transplantation* may be considered.

OUTLOOK

The outlook for people with acute lymphoblastic leukemia is generally better than it is for acute myeloblastic leukemia, and it is better for children than for adults. Survival rates are shown in the illustrated box.

Leukemia, chronic lymphocytic

A type of leukemia caused by proliferation of mature-looking *lymphocytes* (a type of white *blood cell* important in the body's *immune system*). Although incurable, the disease is not invariably fatal.

INCIDENCE AND CAUSES

There are about four new cases of chronic lymphocytic leukemia annually per 100,000 people in the US. Nearly all patients are over 50. The cause of the disorder is unknown.

SYMPTOMS AND SIGNS

Symptoms develop slowly, often over many years. Many cases are discovered by chance when a blood test is performed. In addition to features common to acute forms of leukemia (see opposite), symptoms and signs may include an enlarged liver and spleen, persistent raised temperature, and night sweats.

DIAGNOSIS AND TREATMENT

Chronic lymphocytic leukemia is diagnosed by finding large numbers of lymphocytes, all of the same type, in the blood and on a *bone marrow biopsy*. The severity of the disease is assessed by the degree of liver and spleen enlargement, anemia, and lack of platelet cells in the blood. Often, no treatment is required if the disease is mild. If more severe, *anticancer drugs* are given by mouth, sometimes combined with *radiation therapy*. Other measures include transfusions of blood and platelets, antibiotics to combat infection, and injections of *immunoglobulins* to boost the patient's immune system.

OUTLOOK

The progression of chronic lymphocytic leukemia is slow. More than half of the patients survive for five years from the time of diagnosis. Eventually, death usually results from overwhelming infection.

Leukemia, chronic myeloid

Also known as chronic granulocytic leukemia, chronic myeloid leukemia results from uncontrolled proliferation of the class of white *blood cell* called granulocytes. Large numbers of these cells, in various stages of maturity, appear in the blood.

INCIDENCE AND CAUSES

There are about two new cases of chronic myeloid leukemia diagnosed per 100,000 people in the US each year. Cases occur mainly among middle-aged to elderly people.

The cause of chronic myeloid leukemia is not known. However, in most cases, the patient's cells contain a specific *chromosomal abnormality* known as the Philadelphia chromosome. Part of one chromosome is attached to another chromosome.

SYMPTOMS

The disease usually has two phases—a chronic phase that may last several years and a more malignant phase in which large numbers of immature granulocytes are produced.

During the chronic phase, symptoms develop slowly; they may include tiredness, fever, night sweats, and weight loss. If the number of white cells in the blood rises very high, the blood may become excessively viscous (sticky), impairing the supply of oxygen to various organs. The effects can include visual disturbances and abdominal pain due to death of tissues within the spleen. *Priapism* (persistent, painful erection of the penis) is sometimes a feature.

The symptoms of the second phase are like those of acute forms of leukemia (see opposite).

DIAGNOSIS AND TREATMENT

The disease is sometimes not apparent until the patient has a blood test for some other reason. The diagnosis is made from the increased numbers of granulocytes in the blood and in the bone marrow (as detected by *bone marrow biopsy*). The presence of the Philadelphia chromosome, found by *chromosome analysis*, may help establish the diagnosis.

Treatment of the chronic phase includes the use of *anticancer drugs*. When the disease transforms into the acute phase, treatment is similar to that given for acute leukemia. If the number of white cells rises very high, the cells may be removed from the patient using a machine known as an apheresis machine.

Treatment of the acute phase is seldom successful; the patient usually dies of bleeding or infection. *Bone marrow transplantation* is now being used in an attempt to cure patients while the condition is still in the chronic phase.

OUTLOOK

The average survival time from first diagnosis is about three years. However, about one fifth of patients survive for 10 years or more. A successful bone marrow transplantation may improve the outlook, but is not without its own risks.

Leukocyte

Any type of white *blood cell*.

Leukodystrophies

A rare group of inherited childhood diseases in which the *myelin* sheaths that form a protective covering around many nerves are destroyed.

Diseases included in this group are metachromatic leukodystrophy (which causes impaired speech, blindness, paralysis, dementia, and death within a few years), Krabbe's disease (which results in blindness, deafness, seizures, paralysis, and death within one year), and Merzbacher-Pelizaeus disease (which causes progressive incoordination, speech difficulties, paralysis, and mental deterioration from infancy until death, which occurs in early childhood).

Leukoplakia

Raised, white patches on the mucous membranes of the mouth or the vulva (the area around the opening to the vagina). Leukoplakia is due to the thickening of tissue and is most common in elderly people.

CAUSES

Leukoplakia in the mouth, which is most common on the tongue, is usually due to tobacco-smoking (particularly pipe-smoking) or to the rubbing of a rough tooth or denture. It is not known what causes the condition to develop on the vulva.

SYMPTOMS AND TREATMENT

The patches, which develop slowly, cause no discomfort and are usually harmless. Occasionally, they result from a malignant change in the affected tissue. For this reason, leukoplakia should always be reported to a physician.

Leukoplakia in the mouth may clear up once the cause has been treated. If the condition persists, the patches are removed using a local anesthetic. Leukoplakia of the vulva is treated in the same way. The removed tissue is examined microscopically for any signs of malignant change. (See also *Mouth cancer*; *Vulva, cancer of.*)

Leukorrhea

See *Vaginal discharge*.

Levodopa

A drug used in the treatment of *Parkinson's disease*, a neurological disorder caused by deficiency of the chemical dopamine in part of the brain.

HOW IT WORKS

Levodopa is absorbed into the brain and converted into dopamine. The drug is usually given with an enzyme (such as carbidopa) that reduces the amount of levodopa broken down by the liver before it can reach the brain. This allows a lower dose of levodopa to be given and thereby reduces the risk of adverse effects.

POSSIBLE ADVERSE EFFECTS

Adverse effects include nausea, vomiting, nervousness, and agitation. Prolonged use often impairs the effectiveness of treatment or increases the severity of adverse effects.

Levonorgestrel

A *progesterone drug* used in some *oral contraceptive* preparations.

Levothyroxine

A synthetic drug preparation related to thyroxine, the most important of the *thyroid hormones*.

LH

The abbreviation for luteinizing hormone—a *gonadotropin hormone* produced by the *pituitary gland*.

LH-RH

The abbreviation for *luteinizing hormone-releasing hormone*. This hormone is released by the *hypothalamus*.

Liability insurance, professional

A protection against lawsuits, traditionally purchased by physicians. As a result of the tremendous growth in the number of suits and size of awards in the 1970s and 1980s, coupled with less stringent interpretation of negligence, insurance companies have dramatically raised premiums, restricted policies to low-risk medical specialties, and, in some cases, stopped providing liability insurance.

Libido

Sexual desire. Libido is a healthy, normal feeling, especially strong in youth and gradually fading with age. Loss of libido is a symptom of numerous physical illnesses, and of *depression*, *drug abuse*, and *alcohol dependence*.

The libido theory of Sigmund Freud describes sexual development in childhood in terms of oral, anal, and genital stages (representing the areas of the body toward which a child's attention is directed at different ages). Freud believed that certain neurotic disorders and abnormal sexual behaviors were due to fixation of libido at one of these stages. By contrast, directing the libido (or "love energy") away from oneself to other people or objects was seen as a sign of maturity. (See also *Narcissism*; *Sexual desire, inhibited*.)

Lice

Small, wingless insects that feed on human blood. There are three species: *PEDICULUS HUMANUS CAPITIS* (the head louse), *PEDICULUS HUMANUS CORPORIS* (the body louse), and *PHTHIRUS PUBIS* (the crab, or pubic, louse). All lice have flattened bodies and measure up to one eighth of an inch (3 mm) across.

HEAD LICE

These lice live on and suck blood from the scalp. They leave red spots that itch intensely, leading to scratching,

dermatitis (skin inflammation), and *impetigo* (a bacterial infection of the skin). The females lay a daily batch of tiny, pale eggs (nits) that are attached to hairs close to the scalp; the nits hatch in about seven days. The adults may live for several weeks.

Head lice affect all social classes. Children are most affected, women occasionally, and men rarely. The lice are spread by direct (although not necessarily head-to-head) contact.

Lotions containing malathion or carbaryl kill lice and nits rapidly. The lotion should be washed off 12 hours after application, and a fine-toothed comb run through the hair to remove dead lice and nits. Shampoos containing malathion or carbaryl are also effective if used repeatedly over several days. Combs and hairbrushes should be treated with very hot water to kill any attached eggs.

BODY LICE

These lice live, and lay eggs, on clothing next to the skin. The lice visit the body only to feed. Body lice transmit epidemic *typhus* and *relapsing fever*, which are rare today, but, in the past, were common in areas affected by war or natural disaster.

Body lice affect only people who rarely change their clothes. These lice can be killed by placing infested clothes in a hot dryer for five minutes, by washing them in very hot water, or by burning them.

CRAB LICE

These lice live in pubic hair or, more rarely, armpits or beards. They are usually passed from one person to another during sexual contact. (See *Pubic lice*.)

Licensure

Physicians must be licensed by the state in which they practice. The qualifications for licensure vary from state to state. In general, however, a physician must graduate from an accredited medical or osteopathic school, complete one year of residency training (internship), and pass a state's licensing examination. Graduates of foreign medical schools may be licensed if they meet the state's requirements for residency training and pass its licensing examination. Only a state licensing board has the legal power to restrict or suspend a physician's license to practice.

Lichenification

Thickening and hardening of the skin caused by repeated scratching. Lichenification is often the result of trying to relieve the intense itching of disorders such as atopic *eczema* or *lichen simplex*.

Lichen planus

A common skin disease of unknown cause that usually affects middle-aged people. Small, shiny, extremely itchy, pink or purple raised spots appear on the skin of the wrists, forearms, or lower legs. There is often a lacy network of white spots covering the inside lining of the cheeks.

Treatment is with *corticosteroid drugs*. Creams, sometimes supplemented by injections in severe cases, are used to treat the skin rash and tablets are used to treat lichen planus in the mouth. Most cases clear up within 18 months.

Lichen simplex

Patches of thickened, itchy, and sometimes discolored skin caused by repeated scratching. Typical sites are the neck, wrist, arm near the elbow,

and ankles. Lichen simplex is most common in women and is psychological in origin; sufferers often rub the patches (without being aware of what they are doing) when agitated or under stressful circumstances.

A cycle is established in which repeated scratching to relieve itching leads to more skin thickening and itching, which in turn requires yet more scratching.

Treatment is with *antihistamine* tablets and *corticosteroid* creams to relieve the itching and thus break the cycle. This permits the disorder to subside and the drug treatment to be effective.

Lid lag

A momentary delay in the normal downward movement of the upper eyelids that occurs when the eye looks down. A characteristic feature of *thyrotoxicosis*, lid lag usually occurs in conjunction with *exophthalmos* (protrusion of the eyeball).

Lidocaine

ANTIARRHYTHMIC LOCAL ANESTHETIC

Liquid Injection Cream Ointment

Ointment available over-the-counter

Available as generic

A local anesthetic (see *Anesthesia, local*). Lidocaine is used to relieve the pain and irritation caused by *sunburn* or *hemorrhoids*. It is given to numb tissues before minor surgical procedures and as a *nerve block* (to numb the area supplied by a particular nerve). Lidocaine is also used topically to relieve discomfort during the insertion of a *catheter* or an *endoscope*.

Lidocaine is given by intravenous injection after *myocardial infarction* to reduce the risk of *ventricular fibrillation* (an irregularity of the heart beat).

POSSIBLE ADVERSE EFFECTS

High doses given by injection occasionally cause nausea and vomiting.

Life expectancy

The number of years a person can expect to live. In most Western countries, life expectancy at birth is about 70 years for men and 75 years for women. This sex difference is thought to be due to the fact that many more men than women smoked in the first half of this century. However, since then, the smoking sex ratio has evened out and there has been an increase in deaths from lung cancer in women. As a result, the sex difference in life expectancy is narrowing.

The expected age of death becomes greater the longer a person lives, so someone aged 70 may have a life expectancy of 15 years; even a 100 year old can expect to live a year or two.

LIFE EXPECTANCY AND LIFE SPAN

Life expectancy should be distinguished from life span. Since records began, some old people have lived well beyond 70 years. Gerontologists agree that, in the absence of disease, the average normal life span is about 85 years (see *Aging*).

The natural life span is determined largely by genetic factors. People whose parents and grandparents lived to be 90 are likely to live to about this age. However, the extent to which individuals fulfill their genetic potential is affected by environmental factors, such as nutrition and accidents, as well as by disease.

The proportion of the population that attains its natural life span

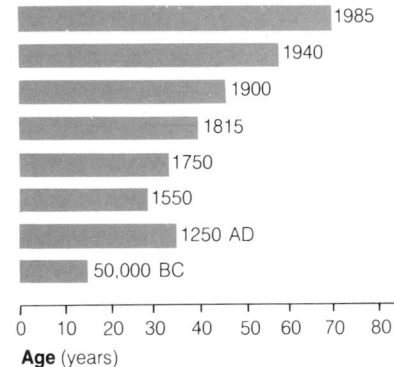

Age (years)

Life expectancy through history
Advances in medicine have dramatically increased life expectancy at birth. Life expectancies in England fluctuated around age 30 to 35 for many centuries, before reaching 40 in the early 19th century and climbing to over 70 in recent decades. Most developed countries follow a similar pattern.

depends on the general health of that population, so life expectancy is a good means of comparing the state of health in different countries or in different parts of the same country.

Life expectancy at birth may be as low as 35 years in some developing countries. However, although statistically accurate, this figure is misleading because it reflects the high mortality during infancy in these countries. Records show that life expectancy at age 40 is not greatly different around the world.

Years 0 10 20 30 40 50 60 70 80

Gender and life expectancy
In rich and poor countries, life expectancy at birth is generally higher for females (gray bars) than males (red). India is an exception.

Nationality and life expectancy
Average life expectancy at birth in most developed countries is now 70 or more; in developing countries it is 40 to 55.

Life support

The process of keeping a person alive by artificially inflating the lungs (see *Ventilation*) and, if necessary, maintaining the heart beat with a *pacemaker*.

Ligament

A tough band of white, fibrous, slightly elastic tissue. Ligaments are important components of joints, binding together the bone ends and preventing excessive movement of the joint. Ligaments also support various organs, including the uterus, bladder, liver, and diaphragm, and help maintain the shape of the breasts.

FUNCTION OF LIGAMENTS
These tough, fibrous bands of tissue bind bone ends together.

Left knee
Femur
Medial ligament
Cruciate ligament
Lateral ligament
Tibia
Fibula

Torn ligament
A common injury of football and soccer players, torn knee ligaments usually result from twisting stress when the knee is turned while weight is on that leg.

Rupture of ligament due to stress

INJURY

Ligaments, especially those in the *ankle joint* and *knee*, are sometimes damaged by injury. Minor sprains are treated with ice, bandaging, and sometimes physical therapy. If the ligament is torn, the joint is either immobilized by a plaster cast to allow healing or repaired surgically.

Ligation

The surgical process of ligating (tying off) a blood vessel to prevent bleeding, or a duct to close it, with a length of thread or other material. The term is used in *tubal ligation*, a form of sterilization in which the fallopian tubes are tied off.

Ligature

A length of thread or other material used for *ligation* (tying off) of a blood vessel or duct.

Lightening

A feeling experienced by many pregnant women when the baby's head drops into the pelvic cavity. Lightening usually occurs in the last three weeks of pregnancy, leaving more space in the upper abdomen and relieving pressure under the ribs, making breathing easier.

Light treatment

See *Phototherapy*.

Limb, artificial

Most artificial legs and arms, known medically as limb prostheses, are fitted to replace all or part of a limb amputated because of disease or severe injury (see *Amputation*). In some cases, however, they are required as a substitute for limbs missing from birth (see *Limb defects*).

To be acceptable, an artificial limb must restore as much as possible the function of the lost limb, be light enough to be worn comfortably, be easy to put on and take off, and look as natural as possible.

CONSTRUCTION AND MATERIALS

Artificial limbs can be obtained ready-made. However, for the best results, they should be constructed by a prosthetist (a specialist in making and fitting artificial limbs) to suit the individual's needs. A mold taken from the stump of the missing limb is used to make a socket for the top of the prosthesis into which the stump can fit closely and comfortably. The socket, made from wood, leather, or plastic, is attached to the stump by suction or by straps.

Each main part of an artificial limb replacing the natural lower leg, thigh, forearm, or upper arm is called an extension. The extension consists of an inner strut made of various materials; it is covered by foam rubber shaped to match the corresponding part of the natural limb. This unit is enclosed by an outer shell of metal, wood, or leather.

Artificial joints are usually made of plastic and metal and today incorporate sophisticated mechanisms that rotate the wrist, stabilize the knee joint, and control the length of stride.

Generally, artificial legs are more useful than artificial arms because the straightforward movements of the natural leg are easier to duplicate than the wide-ranging, often intricate, movements of the arm (especially the hand). Even so, the design of artificial hands is now extremely advanced. Electronic circuitry has been developed to pick up muscle and nerve impulses reaching the stump from the spinal cord. The circuitry transforms the impulses into movements of the prosthesis. People with an artificial arm or hand may have several prostheses (e.g., one with a glove for social use and others with a claw or powered attachments for working).

Limb defects

Incomplete development of one or more limbs at birth. Sometimes an entire limb is missing, sometimes only the hand or foot, or the upper or lower half of a limb, is missing. In other people, hands, feet, or tiny fingers or toe buds are attached to limb stumps or grow directly from the trunk (a condition called phocomelia). Any combination of limbs may be affected.

Limb defects are rare; the incidence in the US is only about one in every 2,000 live births. The sedative drug *thalidomide* is known to have caused phocomelia when taken during pregnancy. (This drug was never sold in the US.) Otherwise, apart from those cases in which limb defects are inherited or part of a syndrome, their cause remains unknown.

MANAGEMENT

A child with a limb defect usually needs to attend a specialized center. Pediatricians, occupational therapists, psychologists, social workers, and other experts will treat the condition and advise on the child's development. A prosthetist will fit an artificial limb (see *Limb, artificial*) and teach the child how to use it.

Limbic system

A ring-shaped area in the center of the brain that consists of a number of connected clusters of nerve cells. The limbic system plays a role in the *autonomic nervous system* (which automatically regulates body functions), in the emotions, and in the sense of smell. The limbic system is extensive, and the different substructures within it

TYPES OF ARTIFICIAL LIMBS

Different types of artificial limbs must restore as much as possible the function of the lost limb, be light enough to be worn comfortably, be easy to put on and take off, and look as normal as possible. Although ready-made prostheses are available and can be quite effective, the best artificial limbs are constructed by specialists and specially adapted to meet an individual's particular needs.

Initiating movement
The nerve impulses that move the prosthesis originate in the brain and pass via the spinal cord to the stump.

Prosthetic movement
Electronic circuitry in the prosthesis picks up nerve impulses in the stump and causes the prosthesis to move in a near-normal way.

Artificial hands
Many devices are available. The prosthesis on the left is servo-mechanism-controlled and battery-operated; it allows finger and wrist movements. The shovel grip is a prosthesis designed to meet a specific need, as are precision tweezers and golf-club grips.

Strap for stump

Thigh extension

Knee mechanism

An artificial leg
Components can be modified for each individual. They are covered with a plastic material to give the limb a natural appearance.

Training with prostheses
Special walking classes enable patients to adjust to their new limbs.

have been named (for example, the hippocampus, the cingulate gyrus, and the amygdala).

Much of our knowledge of the limbic system comes from the observation and investigation of the behavior of animals and people known to have damage to or disease in the limbic area of the brain. The most commonly observed effects are abnormalities of emotional response, such as inappropriate crying or laughing, easily provoked rage, unwarranted fear, anxiety and depression, and excessive sexual interest.

Limp

An abnormal, uneven pattern of *walking* in which the movements of one leg (or of the pelvis on one side of the body) are different from those of the other. A limp may involve dipping of the pelvis to one side, or failure to straighten the leg fully when the foot is placed on the ground.

Lincomycin

An *antibiotic drug* used to treat serious infections of the lungs, skin, bones, joints, and pelvis that are resistant to commonly prescribed antibiotic drugs such as *penicillin*. Lincomycin may rarely cause a type of *colitis* (inflammation of the intestine) called pseudomembranous enterocolitis.

Lindane

A drug used to treat infestation by *scabies* or *lice* and available in the form of a lotion, cream, or shampoo. Lindane sometimes irritates the skin and scalp and causes itching.

Linear accelerator

A device for accelerating subatomic particles, such as electrons, to a speed approaching that of light so that they have extremely high energies. A linear accelerator can also be used to generate high-energy X rays.

In medicine, high-energy electrons or X rays are used in *radiation therapy* to treat certain cancers. This method causes less damage to the healthy tissue around a tumor than does low-energy radiation therapy.

Lip

One of two fleshy folds around the entrance to the mouth. Externally the lips are covered with skin and internally with mucous membrane, the relative transparency of which allows the red-pink of the underlying capillaries to show through.

The main substructure of the lips is a ring of muscle; its functions include keeping food in the mouth, helping to produce speech and other sounds (like whistling), and kissing. Smaller muscles at the corners of the lips are responsible for facial expression.

DISORDERS

These include chapping (see *Chapped skin*), *cheilitis* (inflammation, cracking, and dryness), *cold sores* (blisters on the lips), syphilitic ulcers (see *Chancre, hard*), and *lip cancer*.

L

Lip cancer

A tumor, usually on the lower lip. Lip cancer is largely confined to older people, especially those exposed to a lot of sunlight through working outdoors and those who have smoked cigarettes or a pipe for many years. Lip cancer is the most common form of mouth cancer, but represents only about 1 percent of all cancers.

SYMPTOMS

A white patch develops on the lip and soon becomes scaly and cracked with a yellow crust. The affected area grows, eventually becoming ulcerous; the cancer may spread to the lymph nodes in the jaw and then the neck.

DIAGNOSIS AND TREATMENT

Any lip sore that persists for longer than a month should be seen by a physician. Lip cancer (usually a *squamous cell carcinoma*) is diagnosed by *biopsy* (microscopic examination).

Treatment is surgical removal, *radiation therapy*, or a combination of both. If the tumor has spread to the lymph nodes in the neck, *neck dissection* and more radiation may be necessary.

Lipectomy, suction

A type of *body contour surgery* in which excess fat is suctioned out through a small incision made in the skin.

Lipid disorders

Disorders of metabolism that cause abnormal amounts of *lipids* in the body. The most common of these disorders are the *hyperlipidemias*, which may be inherited or brought on or aggravated by diet or a disorder. In addition, there are also some very rare lipid disorders that are due solely to heredity, such as *Tay-Sachs disease*.

Lipid-lowering drugs

COMMON DRUGS
Drugs that act on the liver
Clofibrate Gemfibrozil Lovastatin
Drugs that act on bile salts
Cholestyramine Colestipol Neomycin

A group of drugs used to treat *hyperlipidemia* (abnormally high levels of one or more types of *lipid*, such as *cholesterol*, in the blood). Lipid-lowering drugs are given to reduce the risk of severe *atherosclerosis* (narrowing of the arteries causing impaired blood flow), usually when dietary measures have not worked.

HOW THEY WORK

Some lipid-lowering drugs alter enzyme activity in the liver to prevent the production of one or more types of lipid from fatty acids. This action reduces the level of lipids in the blood.

Other lipid-lowering drugs interfere with the absorption of bile salts from the intestine into the blood. Bile salts contain large amounts of cholesterol; a decrease in their concentration in the blood stimulates the liver to convert more cholesterol into bile salts, thus reducing the amount of cholesterol in the blood.

POSSIBLE ADVERSE EFFECTS

Lipid-lowering drugs that act on the liver cause increased susceptibility to gallstones. Those that act on bile salts may cause nausea and diarrhea.

Lipids

Often called structural *fats*, lipids are a group of fatty substances that includes triglycerides (the principal forms of fat in body fat), phospholipids (important constituents of cell membranes), and sterols such as *cholesterol*.

Lipoatrophy

Loss of *adipose tissue* (body fat). Patchy lipoatrophy may be caused in diabetics by repeated injections of insulin into one area of skin. Other causes include *malabsorption* of fat from the intestine and lipodystrophies (disorders of fat metabolism).

Lipoma

A common benign tumor of fatty tissue. Lipomas give rise to soft swellings that are slow-growing and often occur in multiples. They may develop anywhere in the body, but occur most commonly on the thigh, trunk, or shoulder. Lipomas are painless and harmless and do not need treatment, although they may be surgically removed for cosmetic reasons.

Liposarcoma

A rare malignant tumor of fatty tissue that usually develops during late middle age. Liposarcomas usually occur in the abdomen or on the thigh, where they produce firm swellings. They can generally be removed by surgery, but have a tendency to recur.

Lipreading

A way of understanding words or conversation through the use of visual clues rather than hearing. Lipreading is invaluable in helping people who are deaf understand more of what is said to them (see *Deafness*).

HOW IT IS DONE

The basis of lipreading is that certain speech sounds are produced by characteristic movements, positions, and relationships of the jaw, lips, and tongue. Because there are more than 40 clearly distinct sounds in the English language, facial expression and context are also important. However, many of the language sounds are produced by similar mouth patterns ("p," "b," and "m" all share the same pattern). There are only about 14 visibly distinguishable mouth patterns; of these, only four or five can be consistently recognized under normal viewing conditions.

EFFECTIVENESS

Tests have shown that the proportion of identified words can rise from 20 to 60 percent after training. Anyone speaking to a deaf person can help improve the effectiveness of lipreading by speaking slightly more slowly than usual, by not covering the mouth when speaking, and by looking directly at the deaf person.

Liquid petrolatum

See *Mineral oil*.

Lisp

The most common form of *speech disorder*. A lisp is due to protrusion of the tongue between the teeth so that the "s" sound is replaced by "th." Most children with a lisp have completely normal structures of the mouth and lips. However, sometimes the speech defect is caused by a cleft palate (see *Cleft lip and palate*).

In most children, lisping disappears without treatment. If it persists after the age of about 4, *speech therapy* may be considered.

Listeriosis

An infection common in animals, including cattle, pigs, and poultry, that also occurs very rarely in humans. It is caused by the bacterium *LISTERIA MONOCYTOGENES*. Possible causes include eating improperly cooked, infected meat or direct spread of the bacteria from an infected live animal.

A fever and generalized aches and pains are the only symptoms that most affected adults develop, but, in the elderly or infirm, the disease can be life-threatening. If an unborn child is infected through its mother's blood, it may be stillborn. *Pneumonia*, *septicemia*, and *meningitis* may develop in a newborn with the disease.

Listeriosis is diagnosed from blood tests and cultures of other fluids obtained from the infected person. Treatment with antibiotics usually clears up the infection.

Lithium

A drug used in the long-term treatment of *mania* and *manic-depressive illness*. Lithium helps prevent mood swings in mania and reduces their frequency and their severity in manic-depressive illness.

HOW IT WORKS

Lithium reduces excessive nerve activity in the brain. It is thought to work by altering the chemical balance within certain nerve cells.

POSSIBLE ADVERSE EFFECTS

High levels of lithium in the blood may cause nausea, vomiting, diarrhea, blurred vision, tremor, drowsiness, rash, and, in rare cases, kidney damage. Regular blood tests are carried out to monitor the level of lithium in the body.

Too much tea and coffee increases the risk of adverse effects. Too much sodium in the diet reduces the effectiveness of treatment.

Lithotomy

Surgical removal of a *calculus* (stone) from the urinary tract, especially from the bladder.

The operation of "cutting for stone" is one of the oldest known surgical procedures. Until the discovery of antiseptic surgical techniques, bladder stones were removed by approaching the organ through incisions between the thighs rather than via the abdomen. The patient would lie back with hips and knees bent and the legs open. Today, this *lithotomy position* is used primarily for gynecological examinations.

The operations of ureterolithotomy and *pyelolithotomy* (removal of ureteral and kidney stones, respectively, by incision) are still occasionally performed. In developed countries, surgical removal of bladder stones is rarely performed, and then only for large stones. Today, bladder stones are usually crushed and dissolved by use of a cystoscope (see *Cystoscopy*) or by *lithotripsy*.

Lithotomy position

Position in which a patient lies on his or her back with knees bent and wide apart. Originally used for *lithotomy* (surgical removal of stones), the position is still used for *pelvic examinations*, childbirth, and many types of pelvic surgery. Stirrups are usually used to support the feet and legs.

Lithotripsy

The process of using shock waves or ultrasonic waves to break up *calculi*

LITHOTRIPSY PROCEDURES

Calculi can sometimes be removed without major surgery. Lithotripsy uses ultrasonic or shock waves to break up the calculi. In percutaneous lithotripsy, the stones are easily removed through a small incision. After extracorporeal shock-wave lithotripsy (ESWL), stone fragments are passed in the urine.

Abdominal calculi
This X ray shows two staghorn calculi in the kidneys. Before lithotripsy, stones such as these could be removed only by major surgery.

PERCUTANEOUS LITHOTRIPSY

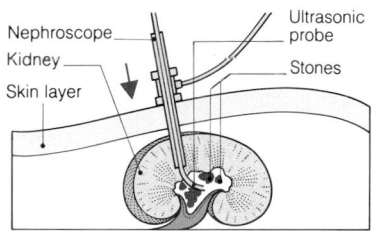

Nephroscope · Ultrasonic probe · Kidney · Stones · Skin layer

1 The surgeon first makes a small incision in the flank and inserts a nephroscope (a type of viewing tube) into the kidney.

Stone fragments removed · Shattered stones

2 A probe is passed through the nephroscope to direct ultrasound waves at the stones, causing them to shatter. Stone fragments are then removed.

EXTRACORPOREAL SHOCK-WAVE LITHOTRIPSY (ESWL)

Arm for positioning shock—wave emitter · Lithotriptor · Control unit · Shock—wave emitter · Movable couch

Ultrasound location transducer · Emitter

Focusing reflector · Skin layer · Kidney stone fragmented

Before · After

Patient receiving ESWL
The patient is given a general or epidural anesthetic. The lithotriptor, placed in contact with the abdomen, produces shock waves that are focused on the stone.

Effects and side effects
Nearly all the shock-wave energy is dissipated in the stone, causing it to shatter. The patient then drinks liberally to clear stone fragments from the urinary system. There may be blood in the urine and abdominal bruising, but serious complications are uncommon.

(stones) for excretion. There are two different procedures—extracorporeal shock wave lithotripsy (ESWL) and percutaneous lithotripsy.

WHY IT IS DONE

Lithotripsy is used to break up kidney and upper ureteral stones (see *Calculus, urinary tract*) into tiny pieces so that they can be excreted in the urine. It is also being investigated as a treatment for gallstones.

ESWL is used to break up smaller stones; percutaneous lithotripsy is used to break up larger stones. Very large stones may be treated with a combination of the two.

HOW IT IS DONE

Both procedures are performed using a general or epidural anesthetic. In some cases, more than one treatment is required.

ESWL This technique uses a machine called a *lithotriptor* to produce external shock waves to break up stones. X-ray imaging systems are used to show the position of the stone and to monitor its destruction into a fine sand, which is passed out of the body in the urine or the bile over the following few weeks. ESWL has radically changed the treatment of kidney stones by eliminating the need for most surgery. The technique may also change the treatment of gallstones.

PERCUTANEOUS LITHOTRIPSY A nephroscope (type of *endoscope*) is inserted into the kidney via a small flank incision. An ultrasonic probe is directed through the nephroscope to break up the stone; fragments are removed through the nephroscope.

RECOVERY PERIOD

There may be hematuria (blood in the urine) for about 12 hours after the treatment. After ESWL there may be some bruising of the skin at the entry and exit points of the shock wave. Most people can return to full activity within a week.

COMPLICATIONS

Renal colic, a sudden, severe pain in the side due to obstruction of the ureter by small fragments of stone, may occur after ESWL. Patients treated for gallstones may need drug treatment to aid the final elimination of stone residue.

Lithotriptor

The machine used in extracorporeal shock wave *lithotripsy* (ESWL) to disintegrate small *calculi* (stones).

Livedo reticularis

A netlike purple or blue mottling of the skin, usually on the lower legs. It is

LOCATION OF THE LIVER

The liver is a roughly cone-shaped, red-brown organ that occupies the upper right-hand portion of the abdominal cavity. It lies immediately beneath the diaphragm, to which its upper side is attached. Its base is in contact with the stomach, right kidney, and intestines. Tucked within a depression on the underside of the liver is the gallbladder.

Diaphragm

Right lobe

Large intestine

Left lobe

Stomach

caused by the enlargement of blood vessels beneath the skin and tends to be worse in cold weather.

Though harmless, the condition is present for life. Livedo reticularis may appear in healthy people, but is more common in those who are abnormally sensitive to cold or in people who have suffered damage to blood vessels just beneath the skin (see *Vasculitis*).

Liver

The largest and one of the most important internal organs, which functions as the body's chemical factory and regulates the levels of most of the main chemicals in blood. Weighing 2.5 to 3.3 pounds (1.1 to 1.5 kg), the liver is a roughly cone-shaped, red-brown organ that occupies the upper right abdominal cavity.

STRUCTURE

The liver lies immediately beneath the diaphragm; it has two main lobes.

The liver receives oxygenated blood from the hepatic artery and nutrient-rich blood via the portal vein (see illustration). The blood drains into the hepatic veins. The liver cells secrete *bile*, a fluid that leaves the liver through a network of ducts, the bile

ducts. Within the liver, the small bile ducts and branches of the hepatic artery and the portal vein form a kind of conduit system known as the portal tracts.

FUNCTION

The liver has many functions vital to the body. One is to produce important proteins for blood plasma. They include albumin (which regulates the exchange of water between blood and tissues), complement (a group of proteins that plays a part in the *immune system's* defenses against infection), coagulation factors (which enable blood to clot when a blood vessel wall is damaged), and globin (a constituent of the oxygen-carrying pigment *hemoglobin*). The liver also produces *cholesterol* and special proteins that help carry fats around the body.

Another function of the liver is to take up glucose that is not required immediately by the body's cells, and store it as glycogen. When the body needs to generate more energy and heat, the liver (under the stimulation of hormones) converts the glycogen back to glucose and releases it into the bloodstream.

The liver also regulates the blood level of amino acids, chemicals that form the building blocks of proteins. When the blood contains too high a level of amino acids (such as after a meal), the liver converts some of them into glucose, some into proteins, some into other amino acids, and some into urea, which is passed to the kidney for excretion in the urine.

Along with the kidneys, the liver acts to clear the blood of drugs and poisonous substances that would otherwise accumulate in the bloodstream. The liver absorbs the substances to be removed from the blood, alters their chemical structure, makes them water soluble, and excretes them in the bile.

Bile carries waste products away from the liver and helps in the breakdown and absorption of fats in the small intestine (see *Biliary system*).

Although extremely complex in its functions, the liver is a remarkably resilient organ. Up to three quarters of its cells can be destroyed or surgically removed before it ceases to function.

Liver abscess

A localized collection of pus in the liver. The most common causes are a spread of bacteria from intestines inflamed by *diverticular disease* or *appendicitis* and invasion of the liver by amebae (single-celled animal parasites) in people infected with *amebiasis*. In some cases, the source of infection cannot be identified.

An affected person is obviously sick, has a high fever and pain in the upper right abdomen, and (especially if elderly) may be confused.

DIAGNOSIS AND TREATMENT
Ultrasound scanning usually shows the abscess. The responsible microorganisms can sometimes be grown in *culture* from a blood sample or direct needle aspiration of the liver.

If possible, the abscess may be drained through a needle inserted through the abdominal wall and guided by ultrasound. Otherwise, abdominal surgery is needed.

Liver biopsy

A diagnostic test in which a small sample of tissue is removed from the liver. The procedure is relatively safe, and complications are rare.

WHY IT IS DONE
The main function of the test is to diagnose liver diseases, such as *cirrhosis* and different types of *hepatitis*. A liver biopsy can also help diagnose diseases such as tumors and *lymphomas*, which spread throughout the body and affect many organs. In addition, the test can

LIVER STRUCTURE AND FUNCTION

The liver is a large organ with numerous functions. It absorbs oxygen and nutrients from the blood, and regulates the blood's glucose and amino-acid levels. It helps break down drugs and various toxins, and manufactures important proteins, such as albumin and blood coagulation factors. The liver also produces bile, which removes waste products and helps process fats in the small intestine.

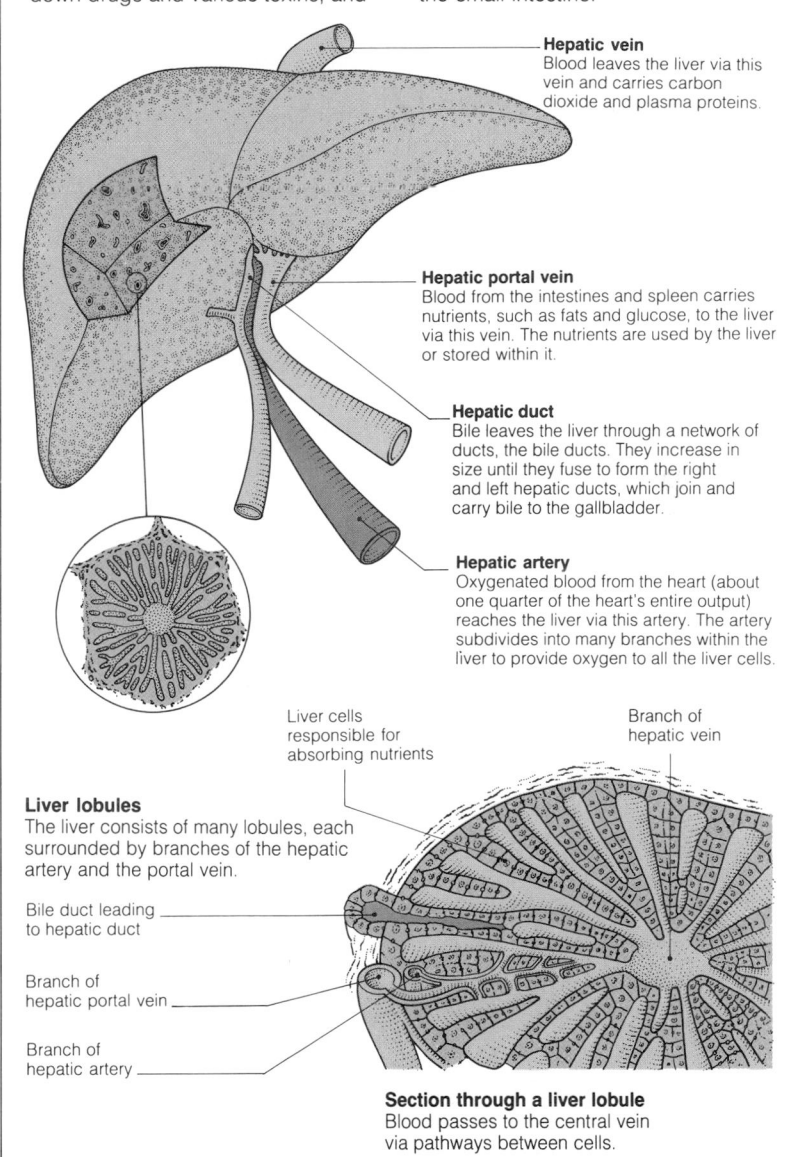

Hepatic vein
Blood leaves the liver via this vein and carries carbon dioxide and plasma proteins.

Hepatic portal vein
Blood from the intestines and spleen carries nutrients, such as fats and glucose, to the liver via this vein. The nutrients are used by the liver or stored within it.

Hepatic duct
Bile leaves the liver through a network of ducts, the bile ducts. They increase in size until they fuse to form the right and left hepatic ducts, which join and carry bile to the gallbladder.

Hepatic artery
Oxygenated blood from the heart (about one quarter of the heart's entire output) reaches the liver via this artery. The artery subdivides into many branches within the liver to provide oxygen to all the liver cells.

Liver cells responsible for absorbing nutrients

Branch of hepatic vein

Liver lobules
The liver consists of many lobules, each surrounded by branches of the hepatic artery and the portal vein.

Bile duct leading to hepatic duct

Branch of hepatic portal vein

Branch of hepatic artery

Section through a liver lobule
Blood passes to the central vein via pathways between cells.

provide an important check on the efficacy of treatment of diseases such as chronic active hepatitis.

HOW IT IS DONE
Most liver biopsies are performed using a local anesthetic. While the patient holds his or her breath, a slim needle is inserted into the liver via a very small incision made over the right lower ribs. The needle is removed with a small sample of liver tissue, the structure and cells of which are examined by a pathologist.

A liver biopsy is sometimes performed during the course of another abdominal operation.

L

DISORDERS OF THE LIVER

By far the most common cause of liver disease in the US and other developed countries is excessive consumption of alcohol (see *Liver disease, alcoholic*). Alcohol-related disorders, which include alcoholic *hepatitis* and *cirrhosis*, outnumber all other types of liver disorder by at least five to one.

Worldwide, the pattern of liver disease is different. In parts of Africa and Asia, up to 20 percent of the population are carriers of the *hepatitis B* virus; in these parts of the world, the most important liver disorders are virus-induced cirrhosis and primary *liver cancer*.

Apart from alcohol- and virus-induced liver disease, the liver may be affected by congenital defects, bacterial and parasitic infection, circulatory disturbance, metabolic disorders, poisoning, and autoimmune processes.

Liver failure (complete loss of liver function) may occur as a result of acute hepatitis, poisoning, or cirrhosis. Enlargement of the liver (hepatomegaly) and *jaundice* are two common signs of liver disease.

CONGENITAL DEFECTS

Defects of liver structure at birth principally affect the bile ducts. A choledochal cyst is a malformation of the hepatic duct (formed from the union of all the small bile ducts in the liver) that may obstruct the flow of bile in infants (causing jaundice); it requires removal. In *biliary atresia*, the bile ducts are absent, again causing jaundice.

INFECTION AND INFLAMMATION

Hepatitis is a general term for inflammation in the liver; it may be caused by viruses such as the hepatitis A, B, and non A, non B viruses (see *Hepatitis, viral*). Bacteria may spread up the biliary system toward the liver to cause *cholangitis* or *liver abscess*. Parasitic diseases that may affect the liver include *schistosomiasis*, *liver fluke*, and *hydatid disease* (caused by various types of worm or fluke) and *amebiasis* (caused by a single-celled parasite).

POISONING AND DRUGS

Apart from alcohol, many drugs and toxins are broken down by the liver, damaging liver cells in the process.

Hepatitis
Inflammation of the liver may be caused by one of the hepatitis viruses, alcohol, or various poisons.

Amebiasis
Infection by amebic parasites can cause painful abscesses in the liver.

Liver cancer
Malignant tumors may arise from the liver itself or may spread from cancer elsewhere in the body.

Choledochal cyst
This congenital malformation blocks the flow of bile through the hepatic duct.

Suicidal overdose with the painkilling drug acetaminophen causes severe liver damage, which may not be obvious until up to two days after the overdose. Some medications, even in normal doses, can cause acute or chronic hepatitis by a direct toxic effect or through drug allergy.

Poisoning by certain types of mushrooms can cause acute liver failure (see *Mushroom poisoning*).

AUTOIMMUNE DISORDERS

Liver cells and bile ducts can be targets for autoimmune reactions (in which the body's immune system attacks its own tissues). A gradual destruction of liver cells is the main problem in autoimmune chronic active hepatitis (see *Hepatitis, chronic active*). The slowly progressive bile duct damage that occurs in primary *biliary cirrhosis* and sclerosing cholangitis possibly also has an autoimmune basis.

METABOLIC DISORDERS

The two main metabolic disorders affecting the liver are *hemochromatosis* (in which there is too much iron in the body) and *Wilson's disease* (in which there is too much copper).

TUMORS

The liver is a common site of malignant tumors that have spread from cancers of the stomach, pancreas, or large intestine. Enlargement of the liver and spleen is a common feature of *leukemias* and *lymphomas*. Primary tumors of the liver are much less common. (See *Liver cancer*.)

OTHER DISORDERS

In *Budd-Chiari syndrome*, the veins draining the liver become blocked by blood clots, causing painful swelling of the liver and severe *ascites* (collection of fluid in the abdomen). Obstruction of the portal vein is one cause of *portal hypertension* (high blood pressure in the portal vein), which can lead to *esophageal varices* (swollen veins in the esophagus) and ascites. Portal hypertension is also one of the usual complications of cirrhosis.

INVESTIGATION

Disorders of the liver may be investigated by physical examination, *liver biopsy, liver function tests, ultrasound scanning,* and *CT scanning.*

Liver cancer

A malignant tumor in the liver. The tumor may be primary (originating within the liver itself) or secondary (spread from elsewhere). There are two main types of primary tumor—a hepatoma, which develops in the liver cells, and a *cholangiocarcinoma*, which arises from cells lining the bile ducts.

CAUSES AND INCIDENCE

Hepatomas are the most common form of cancer worldwide. They are closely linked to hepatitis B (see *Hepatitis, viral*), common throughout Africa, the Middle East, and the Far East. In the US, hepatitis B is a relatively uncommon infection, so hepatomas are rare. There are only about three or four new cases per 100,000 people annually. When a hepatoma does occur, it is usually a complication of *cirrhosis* of the liver.

Secondary liver cancer is relatively common in the US (about 20 times more common than primary cancer); it often originates from cancers in the stomach, pancreas, or large intestine, where the primary tumor may have been small and caused no symptoms.

SYMPTOMS AND SIGNS

The most common symptoms of any liver cancer are weight loss, loss of appetite, and lethargy. In addition, there is often pain in the upper right abdomen. The later stages of the disease are marked by *jaundice* and *ascites* (fluid in the abdomen).

DIAGNOSIS

Liver tumors are usually detected as a result of *ultrasound scanning* that reveals abnormal areas in the liver. The diagnosis is confirmed by *liver biopsy* (removal of a small sample of liver for analysis).

About 80 percent of hepatomas raise the production by the liver of a substance called *alpha-fetoprotein*; measurement of the blood level of this protein is used as a screening test in areas where the cancer is common. *Angiography* is also used to detect hepatomas too small to be seen by other imaging techniques.

TREATMENT

A hepatoma usually remains confined to the liver for a long time. In cases where cirrhosis is not also present (which is rare in the US), complete removal of the tumor, leading to cure, is sometimes possible. In other cases, *anticancer drugs* can help the patient survive longer. A *liver transplant* may occasionally be considered.

There is no cure for secondary liver cancer, but anticancer drugs can help slow the progress of the disease.

Tying off or blocking the hepatic artery or one of its branches to deprive the tumor of its blood supply has been attempted, as has placing a catheter into the artery for continuous administration of anticancer drugs.

Liver, cirrhosis of

See *Cirrhosis*.

Liver disease, alcoholic

Damage to the liver caused by persistent heavy alcohol consumption, with progression to *cirrhosis* (severe structural damage and loss of liver function) and death.

TYPES

Excess fat accumulation in the liver affects almost everyone with a moderate to high alcohol consumption. It is completely reversible through abstinence and, with the reversal, carries a low risk of progression to cirrhosis.

Acute or chronic *hepatitis* can sometimes develop in the persistent drinker. Individual liver cells are destroyed and there is inflammation of the liver with scarring. In people who continue to drink, there is a high risk (about 90 percent) of progression to cirrhosis; in most of those who stop drinking the liver returns to normal. Cirrhosis is irreversible, but abstinence often leads to a notable improvement in liver function.

CAUSES AND INCIDENCE

Until the 1960s, alcoholic liver damage was thought to be caused mainly by the malnutrition associated with alcohol dependence rather than by alcohol itself. It is now accepted that alcohol is directly toxic to the liver.

There is a clear relationship between the total amount of alcohol consumed in a population and the *incidence* of cirrhosis. The *prevalence* of alcoholic liver disease has been rising rapidly in most developed countries since about 1960, and the increase has been particularly steep in women. In the US, the death rate from cirrhosis has risen by about 70 percent since 1960. In New York, alcoholic cirrhosis is now one of the most common causes of death in people 25 to 44.

A person who consumes 7 ounces of alcohol on average per day (contained in about three quarters of a bottle of whisky or two and a half bottles of wine) has a 50 percent chance of cirrhosis within 20 years. A much lower average daily intake of 1.5 ounces (contained in two double shots of whiskey or four glasses of wine) in a man, or half that consumption in a woman, still carries a substantial risk.

SYMPTOMS AND DIAGNOSIS

The first symptoms or signs of liver damage are the same as those of hepatitis or cirrhosis. *Liver function tests* show a characteristic pattern of abnormalities, and *liver biopsy* may be recommended to define the type of damage precisely.

TREATMENT AND OUTLOOK

Abstinence from alcohol is the only method of returning the liver to normal or improving its function and prolonging life expectancy. Treatment methods are as for *alcohol dependence*.

Liver failure

A complication of acute *hepatitis* (inflammation of the liver) in which there is such a severe impairment of liver function that it affects other organs, particularly the brain. Liver failure may also refer to a critical stage in *cirrhosis* of the liver.

SYMPTOMS

The principal symptoms of acute liver failure are those of the underlying hepatitis; later, symptoms of brain dysfunction develop. The brain dysfunction probably occurs because the liver fails to break down certain substances that build up in the blood (such as ammonia), which then poison or alter the transmission of nerve messages in the brain. The symptoms may include agitation and restlessness, followed by drowsiness, confusion, and coma—a condition known as hepatic *encephalopathy*.

When liver failure accompanies cirrhosis, other complications, such as *ascites* (fluid collection in the abdomen) and internal bleeding, may develop in addition to hepatic encephalopathy. The symptoms of brain dysfunction develop more slowly, with recurrent episodes of drowsiness or confusion. These episodes are frequently precipitated by bacterial infections or changes in drug treatment or diet.

DIAGNOSIS AND TREATMENT

A diagnosis is made from the patient's history, physical examination, *liver function tests*, and tests for viruses that can cause acute hepatitis.

Treatment of acute liver failure consists of skilled intensive care. There is no specific cure, although the use of antibiotics and enemas can reduce the number of intestinal bacteria, which are one of the main sources of toxic ammonia entering the bloodstream. A *liver transplant* is occasionally possible and suitable for certain patients. Only about one quarter of patients survive acute liver failure.

L

When brain dysfunction complicates cirrhosis, treatment of precipitating causes (such as infection) often leads to an improvement.

Liver fluke

 Any of various species of flukes (small, flattened, worms) that infest the bile ducts within the liver. The only fluke of any importance in the US is *FASCIOLA HEPATICA*, which causes the disease fascioliasis. The adult flukes normally infest sheep and produce eggs that are passed in the sheep's feces. The eggs are eaten by snails, from which immature forms of the fluke emerge. They then become encysted (enclosed in a sac) on aquatic vegetation, particularly watercress. In the US the disease is confined to some western and southern states.

The disease has two stages. During the first stage, young flukes migrate through the liver, causing liver tenderness and enlargement, fever, night sweats, and sometimes a rash. In the second stage, adult worms are present in the bile ducts. This may lead to *cholangitis* (inflammation of the bile ducts) and *bile duct obstruction*, which can cause *jaundice*. In light infections, there may be no symptoms.

The disease is diagnosed from the presence of fluke eggs in the patient's feces. Treatment with the antihelmintic drug praziquantel may be effective.

A different species, *CLONORCHIS SINENSIS*, is common in the Far East. Infection is acquired from eating raw or uncooked freshwater fish. The symptoms and treatment are broadly similar to those for fascioliasis.

Liver function tests

A series of tests of blood chemistry that can detect changes in the way the liver is making new substances, breaking down and/or excreting old ones, and whether liver cells are healthy or being damaged. The tests are widely used to help in the diagnosis of liver disease, and to assess responses to treatment. They are particularly useful in distinguishing between acute and chronic liver disorders and between *hepatitis* (liver inflammation) and *cholestasis* (failure of bile flow). The most commonly performed tests are shown in the table.

Liver imaging

A technique that produces images of the liver, gallbladder, bile ducts, and blood vessels supplying the liver to detect abnormality or disease.

TABLE OF LIVER FUNCTION TESTS

Test	Significance
Serum bilirubin	Bilirubin is the yellow breakdown product of red blood cells that is passed to the liver and excreted in bile. It is the substance that gives the yellow color to the skin in jaundice. A high bilirubin level in the blood may indicate defective processing of bile by the liver or obstruction to bile flow.
Serum albumin	Albumin is one of the main proteins in blood. Made by the liver, one of its actions is to hold fluid inside the blood vessels. A low level is found in many chronic liver disorders and is often associated with ascites and ankle edema (fluid collection in the abdomen and around the ankles).
Serum alkaline phosphatase	Alkaline phosphatase is an enzyme found in bile. The blood level of this enzyme rises when there is obstruction to the flow of bile (cholestasis).
Serum aminotransferases (transaminases)	The aminotransferases are enzymes released from liver cells into the blood when the liver cells are damaged. The levels will be raised in acute and chronic hepatitis.
Prothrombin time	A normal result in this test of blood clotting depends on the presence in the blood of a protein made by the liver from a fat-soluble vitamin, vitamin K. The test result can be abnormal in two kinds of disorders—when the protein is not made because of liver cell damage, and when there is a blockage to bile flow in the liver, causing a lack of bile in the intestines (which interferes with fat and vitamin K absorption).

TYPES

CONVENTIONAL X-RAY TECHNIQUES *Cholecystography* and *cholangiography* are techniques in which a contrast medium (iodine-containing substance opaque to X rays) is introduced to show up gallstones, tumors, and blockages. *ERCP* (endoscopic retrograde cholangiopancreatography) is an alternative method of examining the biliary system by means of a contrast medium; it is especially useful in detecting blockage or narrowing of a bile duct or a pancreatic duct by a stone or tumor.

Angiography shows up the blood vessels within the liver that supply the liver. It also may be used to confirm the diagnosis of a hemangioma or to plan the treatment of liver tumors and other disorders.

SCANNING TECHNIQUES *Ultrasound scanning* is the most widely used of all liver imaging techniques. It is simple, safe, noninvasive, and produces excellent images, particularly of gallstones. *CT scanning* also provides good images and may be used if ultrasound has proved inconclusive.

Radionuclide scanning can indicate the presence of a cyst or a tumor. It is also useful in recording the progress of radioactive isotopes as they are excreted from the liver in bile.

Liver transplant

Replacement of a diseased liver with a healthy organ removed from a donor who has been declared brain dead. Liver transplantation is a technically difficult procedure, but is now accepted as a feasible and appropriate treatment for some types of advanced liver disease. The chances of surviving for many years with a transplanted liver are improving, but they are not yet as high as the chances of surviving with a kidney transplant.

WHY IT IS DONE

Transplantation is worth considering only for people with life-threatening or severely debilitating liver disease. However, if the disease process is too advanced, the person is unlikely to survive the operation. An assessment must be made of the likely length of survival and the quality of life with and without the operation.

In adults, the best results are obtained in the treatment of advanced liver *cirrhosis* in people with long-standing chronic active *hepatitis* or primary *biliary cirrhosis*. In acute *liver failure*, there can be difficulty in obtaining donor organs at an appropriate time, but people with a slightly less acute illness and those with *Budd-Chiari syndrome* have been successfully treated. People with primary *liver cancer* are rarely considered for transplantation because there is a high risk that the tumor will recur.

In children, congenital *biliary atresia* is the most common reason for transplantation.

HOW IT IS DONE

The donor organ is obtained from someone who has suffered *brain death* but whose liver is still healthy. The organ can be stored in cold salt solutions for a few hours.

A general anesthetic is given and the recipient's abdomen is opened. The diseased liver is removed, the donor organ is inserted in its place, and the major blood vessels and common bile duct are reconnected.

RECOVERY PERIOD

The first few days after the operation are spent in an *intensive-care* unit. *Immunosuppressant drugs* (particularly cyclosporine) are given to reduce the risk of rejection.

OUTLOOK

In some cases rejection occurs and a second transplant operation provides the only hope. There is now a 60 to 80 percent chance of surviving one year, which may mean that more than half of the people now receiving liver transplants will survive for five years. The quality of life is generally excellent, with most people returning to near normal activity within a few weeks of the operation.

Living will
See *Will, living*.

Lobe
One of the clearly defined parts into which certain organs, such as the brain, liver, lungs, and thyroid gland, are divided. The term may also be used to describe any projecting, flat, pendulous part of the body, such as the earlobe.

Lobectomy
An operation to cut out a lobe in the brain (see *Lobotomy, prefrontal*), liver (see *Hepatectomy, partial*), lungs (see *Lobectomy, lung*), or thyroid gland (see *Thyroidectomy*).

Lobectomy, lung
An operation to remove one of the lobes of the lung. Lobectomy is usually performed to remove a malignant tumor, but may also be used to treat localized *bronchiectasis* that has not responded to medical treatment. In the past, lobectomy was carried out to treat tuberculosis, which is treated today by drugs.

After lobectomy, the remaining lobes expand to fill the pleural space.

HOW IT IS DONE

A curved incision is made (using a general anesthetic), starting under the armpit and extending across the back, following the line of the lower edge of the shoulder blade. The muscles are cut through and the ribs are gently spread apart (or one is removed) to expose the lung. The blood vessels and bronchus (air passage) leading to the diseased lobe are then tied off and divided, and the lobe is removed. Before the incision is sewn up, a tube is inserted into the pleural space surrounding the lung to drain off fluid. It is usually removed after 24 hours.

Lobotomy, prefrontal
The cutting of some of the fibers linking the frontal lobes to the rest of the brain. Prefrontal lobotomy was widely used in the 1940s and 1950s to treat serious psychiatric disorders. However, the operation often resulted in harmful personality changes and is now used only as a last resort to treat people with severe, chronic depression. (See also *Psychosurgery*.)

Lochia
The discharge after childbirth of blood and fragments of the lining of the uterus where the placenta was attached. Lochia is bright red for the first three or four days and then becomes paler. The discharge decreases as the placental site heals and usually ceases within six weeks.

Locked knee
See *Knee*.

Lockjaw
A painful spasm of the jaw muscles that makes it difficult or impossible to open the mouth. Lockjaw is the most common symptom of *tetanus*.

Locomotor
Relating to movement of the extremities, as in locomotor *ataxia*, the incoordinated movements and lurching gait that occur in the later stages of untreated syphilis.

Loiasis
 A form of the tropical parasitic disease *filariasis* that is caused by an infestation by the worm *LOA LOA*. The worm travels beneath the skin, producing areas of inflammation known as Calabar swellings.

Loin
The part of the back on each side of the spine between the lowest pair of ribs and the top of the pelvis.

Loose bodies
Fragments of bone, cartilage, or capsule linings that are free to move within a joint. They may occur whenever there is any damage to a joint, as in *osteoarthritis* (degeneration due to wear and tear), fracture, or *osteochondritis dissecans* (inflammation of bone and cartilage due to disrupted blood supply).

SYMPTOMS AND SIGNS

Loose bodies can sometimes be felt. They are troublesome only if they lodge between joint surfaces, where they cause the joint to lock (usually only briefly), resulting in severe pain. The joint usually swells several hours later. Though the swelling subsides, further locking and swelling can recur at any time.

DIAGNOSIS AND TREATMENT

X rays or *arthroscopy* (examination of the interior of the joint through a viewing tube) show whether loose bodies are present.

Occasionally, gentle manipulation of the joint is required to unlock it. If locking occurs frequently, the loose bodies are removed during arthroscopy or by an open operation.

Loperamide
An *antidiarrheal drug* used in the treatment of recurrent and sudden bouts of diarrhea. Loperamide is also given to help regulate bowel action in people who have had an *ileostomy*.

POSSIBLE ADVERSE EFFECTS

Loperamide occasionally produces a rash. Other rare adverse effects, such as fever, abdominal cramps, and bloating, are often difficult to distinguish from symptoms of the disorder causing the diarrhea.

Lorazepam
A *benzodiazepine drug* used to treat *insomnia* and *anxiety*. If use of lorazepam is suddenly stopped after it has been taken regularly for more than three weeks, there may be withdrawal symptoms (see *Drug dependence*).

L

Lordosis

Inward curvature of the spine, which is normally present to a minor degree in the lower back. Lordosis in the lower back can become exaggerated by poor posture (especially in someone who is overweight and has weak abdominal muscles) or by *kyphosis* (backward curvature of the spine) above the lower back.

Normal and abnormal lordosis
The normal inward curvature of the spine (left) is exaggerated in abnormal lordosis (right).

Once pronounced lordosis has developed, it is usually a permanent condition and can lead to *disk prolapse* or *osteoarthritis* of the spine.

Loss of normal lordosis in the lower back or neck can occur when the back or neck muscles are in spasm. The condition corrects itself once the cause is successfully treated.

Lotion

A liquid drug preparation applied to the skin. Lotions have a cooling, soothing effect and are useful for covering large areas. Examples of drugs prepared as a lotion include *calamine* (used to treat skin inflammation) and *lindane* (used in the treatment of scabies and lice infestations).

Lou Gehrig's disease

A name used commonly by the public for amyotrophic lateral sclerosis (see *Motor neuron disease*).

Lovastatin

A lipid-lowering drug approved in 1987 that lowers serum cholesterol levels by inhibiting cholesterol-producing enzymes. Lovastatin should not replace standard diet therapy; it is recommended when dietary measures and other nondrug therapy have been ineffective. Long-term effects are yet to be ascertained.

LSD

A synthetic *hallucinogenic drug* (drug that produces hallucinations) derived from ergot (a type of fungus). LSD is the abbreviation for lysergic acid diethylamide. The drug has no medical role. Its distribution and manufacture are governed by the Controlled Substance Act because of the drug's high potential for abuse.

LSD sometimes produces "bad trips" in which a person experiences panic, fear, and physical symptoms, such as nausea, dizziness, and weakness. In severe cases, sedation in the hospital may be necessary for several days. There may also be "flashbacks" to previous trips months or years afterward. Although there is no evidence that LSD causes *psychosis* (mental illness characterized by a loss of contact with reality), it may act as a trigger in a person predisposed to mental illness. There is evidence that LSD damages chromosomes.

Ludwig's angina

A bacterial infection of the floor of the mouth that becomes life-threatening as it spreads to the throat. The tissues become inflamed, swell, and harden.

The disorder is usually caused by an infected tooth or gum and is most common in people with poor *oral hygiene*. It generally results in fever, pain in the mouth and neck, and difficulty opening the mouth and swallowing. If not treated immediately with antibiotics, the swollen tissues of the throat may cause difficulty breathing. *Tracheostomy* (making a hole in the windpipe and inserting a tube through it) may be necessary to prevent asphyxiation.

Lumbar

Relating to the part of the back between the lowest pair of ribs and the top of the pelvis. The lumbar region of the spine consists of the five lumbar vertebrae between the lowest (12th) thoracic vertebra and the sacrum.

Lumbar puncture

A procedure in which a hollow needle is inserted into the lower part of the spinal canal to withdraw *cerebrospinal fluid* (the watery liquid that surrounds the brain and spinal cord) or to inject drugs or other substances.

WHY IT IS DONE

The main use of the lumbar puncture is to examine cerebrospinal fluid to diagnose and investigate disorders of the brain and spinal cord (such as *meningitis* and *subarachnoid hemor-*

rhage). The procedure is also used to inject drugs into the fluid (such as *anticancer drugs* to treat *leukemia* and other malignant diseases of the central nervous system). Another use of lumbar puncture is to inject a dye that will show up on X ray (see *Myelography*) to produce images of the spinal cord. Finally, lumbar puncture can be used to inject a local anesthetic to achieve extensive anesthesia without causing loss of consciousness.

HOW IT IS DONE

The patient lies on his or her side, chin on chest and knees drawn up, to pull the vertebrae (bones of the spine) apart; the area of skin overlying the lumbar vertebrae at the base of the spine is anesthetized with a local anesthetic. A hollow needle is then inserted between two of the vertebrae and into the spinal canal and is used to withdraw cerebrospinal fluid or to inject drugs, dye, or anesthetic.

After the needle is removed, the puncture site is covered with sterile tape. The procedure takes less than 20 minutes. It usually causes no discomfort; a headache that soon wears off may occur in some people.

Lumbosacral spasm

Prolonged, excessive tightening of the muscles that surround and support the lower part of the spine. Lumbosacral spasm is a cause of *back pain* and may occasionally result in temporary *scoliosis* (curvature of the spine to one side). Treatment may include bed rest, *analgesic drugs* (painkillers), and *muscle-relaxant drugs*.

Lumen

The space within a tubular organ. The term is most commonly used to refer to the cavity of the intestine.

Lumpectomy

An operation to treat breast cancer (see *Mastectomy*).

Lunacy

An outdated term for insanity. It was coined because of the belief that phases of the moon ("luna" in Latin) could bring on mental illnesses, especially illnesses that seemed to come and go. Patients were called lunatics and mental hospitals were known as lunatic asylums.

Lung

The main organ of the *respiratory system*. The two lungs supply the body with oxygen and eliminate carbon dioxide from the blood.

STRUCTURE

The *trachea* (windpipe) branches in the chest into two main *bronchi* (air passages), which supply the left and right lungs. The main bronchi divide again into smaller bronchi and then into bronchioles, which lead to air passages that open out into grapelike air sacs called alveoli. It is through the thin walls of the alveoli that gases diffuse into or out of the blood.

Each lung is enclosed in a double membrane called the *pleura*, which allows the lungs to slide freely as they expand and contract during *breathing*. (See also *Respiration*.)

Lung cancer

One of the most common forms of *cancer* in the US, lung cancer is the leading cause of cancer deaths in men and the second most common cause (after breast cancer) in women. There were about 160,000 deaths from lung cancer in 1986 in the US. The peak age for lung cancer is 65 years for men and 70 years for women. The disease is uncommon before age 40.

CAUSES

Cigarette smoking is the main cause of lung cancer. The more cigarettes smoked per day and the lower the age at which smoking started, the greater the risk of lung cancer. Cigar or pipe smokers have a lower risk of having lung cancer than cigarette smokers, but still have a significantly higher risk than nonsmokers (see *Tobacco smoking*). Passive smoking (the inhalation of tobacco smoke by nonsmokers) has been shown to increase the risk.

Living in an environment with a high level of air pollution or working with radioactive minerals or asbestos may cause some cases of lung cancer.

TYPES

There are several types of lung cancer, the most common being squamous cell carcinoma, small (oat) cell carcinoma, adenocarcinoma, and large cell carcinoma; each has a different natural history (growth pattern) and response to treatment. The squamous cell, small cell, and large cell types are all strongly associated with tobacco abuse; the relation between adenocarcinoma and tobacco use is less clear.

SYMPTOMS AND SIGNS

The first and most common symptom is a cough, occurring in about 80 percent of people with lung cancer. About half of all people with lung cancer have a chronic cough from *bronchitis*. Other symptoms include coughing up blood, shortness of breath, chest pain, and wheezing.

LOCATION AND STRUCTURE OF THE LUNGS

The lungs lie in the chest within the rib cage. Air entering the body via the nose and mouth travels down the trachea to the main bronchi, which divide into smaller bronchi and then into bronchioles. These in turn lead to alveoli, where the oxygen/carbon dioxide exchange takes place. During expiration (breathing out), air leaves the body by the same routes.

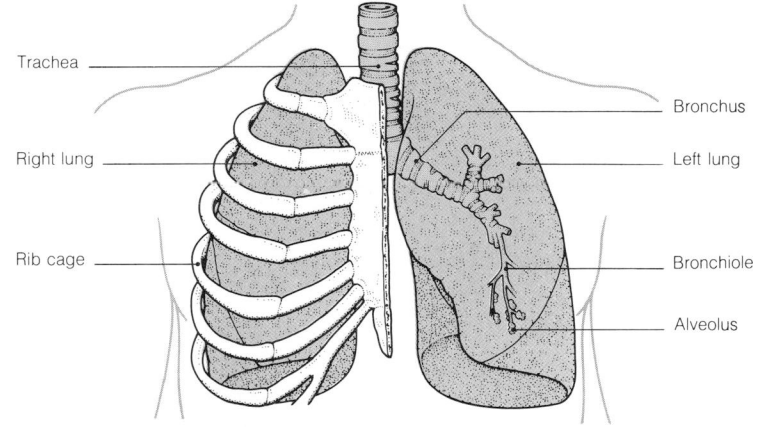

Trachea

Right lung

Rib cage

Bronchus

Left lung

Bronchiole

Alveolus

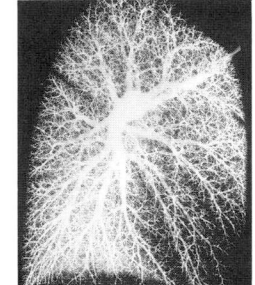

Blood vessels in a lung
The tiniest "twigs" of this extensive blood vessel "tree" form into capillaries that surround the alveoli (air sacs) in the lung. Oxygen and carbon dioxide are exchanged between the alveoli and the capillaries.

Lung cancer can spread locally to affect tissues immediately surrounding the lungs, or can spread to other parts of the body, especially the liver, brain, and bones. Pain may occur in these sites, and weight loss is a frequent symptom. Local spread may cause the collapse of a lung or *pneumonia*, or affect the pleura (membrane covering the lung), causing *pleural effusion* (a collection of fluid between the lung and the chest wall).

DIAGNOSIS

Lung cancer may be suspected during *history-taking* or a physical examination but, most often, it is discovered when a chest X ray shows a characteristic shadow on the lung.

To confirm the diagnosis, tissue must be examined cytologically for the presence of cancerous cells (see *Cytology*). The simplest test is to examine samples of sputum (phlegm), because cancer cells may have been shed into the airways and occur in the sputum.

A *bronchoscopy* may be performed to examine the condition of the lungs or to take a biopsy (small sample of tissue) for analysis or examination. Sometimes biopsy of the suspected tumor is necessary. Cells are obtained through a needle inserted into the chest or by performing an operation to expose the tumor for a direct biopsy (excision of part of the tumor).

TREATMENT

If lung cancer is diagnosed at an early stage, *pneumonectomy* (surgical removal of the lung) or *lobectomy* (removal of part of the lung) may be performed. Surgery is usually possible only when the cancer is still fairly small and confined to one lung, and when the patient's general condition enables a major operation to be performed. *Anticancer drugs* and *radiation therapy* may be used to contain the spread of the tumor or destroy cancerous cells; they are the usual treatment for small cell lung cancer.

L

OUTLOOK

Overall, less than 10 percent of lung cancer patients survive for five years after the disease is diagnosed. After surgery, the five-year survival rate is between 15 and 30 percent; there have been cases of long-term survival in patients treated with chemotherapy for small cell carcinoma.

The highest chance of cure is obtained when the cancer is discovered and treated early. If the cancer has spread beyond the chest, a cure is highly unlikely.

Lung, collapse of
See *Atelectasis; Pneumothorax.*

Lung disease, chronic obstructive
The combination of chronic *bronchitis* and *emphysema*, in which there is persistent disruption of airflow into or out of the lungs.

Lung imaging
A technique that provides images of the lungs to aid in the diagnosis of abnormalities or disease.

TYPES

CONVENTIONAL X-RAY TECHNIQUES A *chest X ray* provides an excellent image of the lungs, from which almost every type of lung disorder can be detected. *Tomography* produces a sharp image of a cross section of an organ at a particular depth and is sometimes used to visualize the interior of a lung that is obscured by an overlying diseased area or to more clearly identify a nodule in the lung.

In pulmonary *angiography*, a contrast medium (a substance opaque to X rays) is injected into the pulmonary artery to detect *pulmonary embolism* (blockage by a blood clot). *Bronchography* (in which the contrast medium is injected into the bronchi) was once widely used to examine bronchi damaged by chronic infections; it has now been largely replaced by *bronchoscopy*. Other imaging techniques are also used.

SCANNING TECHNIQUES *CT scanning* provides a more detailed image of the lungs than is possible with standard X rays and plays an important role in detecting the presence and spread of lung tumors. *Ultrasound scanning* is sometimes used to reveal *pleural effusion* (fluid around a lung).

Other less commonly employed imaging techniques involve the use of *radionuclide scanning* to aid in detecting pulmonary embolism. Digital radiography uses a computer to process a standard X-ray film. The computer removes all unwanted elements (such as the bones of the chest) from the image, leaving a clearer view of the structures to be examined.

Lung tumors
Growths in the lung that may be malignant (see *Lung cancer*) or benign. Benign lung tumors are less common than malignant tumors and, unlike malignant tumors, typically affect younger adults and are unrelated to cigarette smoking.

The most common benign tumor is a bronchial *adenoma*, which arises in the lining of a bronchiole. Adenomas often cause partial bronchial obstruction; hemoptysis (coughing up blood) may also occur. Treatment involves surgical removal of the tumor.

DISORDERS OF THE LUNG
The lungs are continuously exposed to airborne particles, such as bacteria, viruses, and allergens, all of which can cause lung disorders. Most of these disorders do not interfere with oxygen supply; those that do are a major threat to health.

INFECTION

Infective disorders are common, especially *tracheitis* (inflammation of the lining of the windpipe) and *croup* (a virus infection of young children). *Bronchitis* (inflammation of the bronchi), *bronchiectasis* (swelling of the bronchi), and *bronchiolitis* (inflammation of the bronchioles) commonly follow colds or *influenza*. *Pneumonia* (inflammation of the lung) is usually caused by infection by viruses or bacteria. Fungal infections of the lungs, such as *aspergillosis*, *actinomycosis*, *histoplasmosis*, and *candidiasis*, are relatively uncommon.

ALLERGIES

Bronchial *asthma*, in which the muscles of the bronchi contract and obstruct the free passage of air, often occurs in sensitized people exposed to pollens, house mites, fungal spores, animal dander, and many other agents. Allergic *alveolitis* (inflammation of the alveoli) may be caused by many organic dusts, such as moldy hay.

TUMORS

Lung cancer is one of the most common of all malignant tumors; in most cases it is associated with cigarette smoking. Secondary malignant tumors, which have spread from other parts of the body to the lungs, are common. However, benign tumors affecting the lung are uncommon.

INJURY

Lung injury usually results from penetration of the chest wall. *Pneumothorax* (air in the pleural cavity) and *hemothorax* (blood in the pleural cavity) are usually caused by a penetrating injury; either may cause collapse of the lung. Injury can also occur from the inhalation of poisonous dusts, gases, or toxic substances. *Silicosis* and *asbestosis* are caused by inhalation of silica and asbestos, respectively; they may lead to progressive *fibrosis* of the lung.

IMPAIRED BLOOD AND OXYGEN SUPPLY

The most serious disorder is *pulmonary embolism*, in which a blood clot formed in one of the major veins breaks free and is carried to the lungs. The clot may block the pulmonary arteries and cause death. Heart failure may cause pulmonary *edema*, in which the lungs become filled with fluid. *Respiratory distress syndrome*, which may affect newborn babies or adults, has many causes. In this condition, leakage of fluid into the alveoli seriously interferes with oxygen supply. *Emphysema*, in which the walls of the alveoli break down so that the area for oxygen exchange is reduced, is frequently seen in people suffering from chronic bronchitis and asthma.

INVESTIGATION

Lung disorders are investigated by *chest X ray*, *bronchoscopy*, *pulmonary function tests*, *sputum* analysis, *blood tests*, and physical examination. Sometimes a biopsy of lung tissue is taken for analysis.

Other rare benign tumors include *fibromas* (made up of fibrous tissue) and *lipomas* (made up of fatty tissue). No treatment is necessary unless the tumors are causing problems.

Lupus erythematosus

A chronic disease that causes inflammation of *connective tissue*. The more common type, discoid lupus erythematosus (DLE), affects exposed areas of the skin. The more serious and potentially fatal form, systemic lupus erythematosus (SLE), affects many systems of the body, including the joints and the kidneys.

Discoid lupus erythematosus on cheek
The disease causes circular, reddened areas of skin. The patch shown here is healing at its center to form white scar tissue.

CAUSES

Lupus erythematosus is an *autoimmune disorder* in which the body's *immune system*, for unknown reasons, attacks the connective tissue as though it were foreign, causing inflammation. It is probable that the disease can be inherited and that hormonal factors play a part. Sometimes the agent that triggers the immune response (e.g., a viral infection) can be inferred. Certain drugs can induce some of the symptoms of SLE, particularly in elderly people; drugs most frequently responsible are hydralazine, procainamide, and isoniazid.

INCIDENCE

Lupus erythematosus affects nine times as many women as men, usually those of childbearing age. It occurs worldwide, although its incidence is higher in certain ethnic groups, such as blacks in the US, West Indians, and Chinese in the Far East. In high-risk groups the incidence may be as high as one in 250 women.

SYMPTOMS

The symptoms of both varieties of lupus erythematosus periodically subside and recur with varying severity.

In DLE the rash starts as one or more red, circular, thickened areas of skin that later scar. They may occur on the face, behind the ears, and on the scalp, sometimes causing permanent hair loss in affected areas.

SLE causes a characteristic red, blotchy, almost butterfly-shaped rash over the cheeks and bridge of the nose. There is no scarring and the hair grows back between attacks. Most sufferers feel sick, with malaise, fatigue, fever, loss of appetite, nausea, joint pain, and weight loss. There may be iron-deficiency *anemia*, neurological or psychiatric problems, *renal failure*, *pleurisy* (inflammation of the lining of the lungs), *arthritis*, and *pericarditis* (inflammation of the membrane surrounding the heart).

DIAGNOSIS

Blood tests and sometimes a skin *biopsy* (removal of tissue for microscopic examination) are performed to look for specific *antibodies* that occur when the disease is active.

TREATMENT

Treatment aims to reduce inflammation and alleviate symptoms; there is no cure. *Nonsteroidal anti-inflammatory drugs* may be prescribed for joint pain, antimalarial drugs for the skin rash, and *corticosteroid drugs* for fever, pleurisy, and neurological symptoms. Sufferers whose symptoms are made worse by sunlight should avoid sun exposure and use *sunscreens*.

OUTLOOK

The future for patients with SLE has improved dramatically over the past 20 years, although the disease may be life-threatening if the kidneys are affected. Today, many people who have SLE survive for more than 10 years after diagnosis of the disease. This improvement may be due to earlier diagnosis, especially of mild cases, and to more effective treatment of kidney problems.

Lupus pernio

A variant of the disease *sarcoidosis* in which purple swellings appear on the nose, cheeks, or ears. It more commonly affects women than men.

Lupus vulgaris

A form of *tuberculosis* affecting the skin, especially of the head and neck. Painless, clear, red-brown nodules appear and ulcerate; they eventually heal, leaving deep scars.

Luteinizing hormone

A *gonadotropin hormone*, also known as LH, produced by the *pituitary gland*.

Luteinizing hormone-releasing hormone

A naturally occurring hormone released by the hypothalamus in the brain, also prepared synthetically as a drug. Natural luteinizing hormone-releasing hormone (LH-RH) stimulates the release of *gonadotropin hormones* from the *pituitary gland*. Gonadotropin hormones, in turn, control the production of *estrogen hormones* and *androgen hormones*.

WHY IT IS USED

Synthetic LH-RH is given to treat abnormally early onset of puberty. It is also currently under investigation as a male contraceptive and as a treatment for uterine *fibroids*, prostatic cancer (see *Prostate, cancer of*), and certain types of *breast cancer*.

HOW IT WORKS

Synthetic LH-RH reduces the amount of natural gonadotropins released from the pituitary gland and thus the amount of *estrogen hormones* and *androgen hormones* produced by the ovary and testes. This action reduces the level of cell activity in organs stimulated by these sex hormones, such as the uterus, breasts, testes, ovaries, and prostate gland.

POSSIBLE ADVERSE EFFECTS

LH-RH may cause headache, nausea, hot flashes, vaginal dryness, and irregular periods.

Luxated tooth

A tooth displaced in its socket as the result of an accident. The upper front teeth are the most vulnerable. The tooth may be depressed deep into the gum, tilted backward or forward, and loosened. A dentist can usually manipulate a luxated tooth back into position, after which it is usually immobilized with a splint (see *Splinting, dental*). If the tooth's blood vessels are torn and the pulp dies, the tooth requires *root-canal treatment*.

Lyme disease

 A disease characterized by skin changes, flulike symptoms, and joint inflammation. It was first described in the community of Old Lyme, Connecticut, in 1975.

CAUSES AND INCIDENCE

Lyme disease is caused by the bacterium *BORRELIA BURGDORFERI*, which is transmitted by the bite of a tick that usually lives on deer but can infest dogs. Most cases have occurred in the northeastern US, but the disease has also been reported in other parts of the US and in other countries.

L

SYMPTOMS AND COMPLICATIONS

At the site of the tick bite, a red dot may appear and gradually expand into a reddened area several inches across (although in some cases the bite passes unnoticed). Symptoms such as fever, headache, lethargy, and muscle pains usually develop, followed by a characteristic joint inflammation, with redness and swelling typically affecting the knees and other large joints.

The symptoms may vary in severity and occur in cycles lasting a week or so. Unless the disease is diagnosed and treated, symptoms may continue for several years, gradually declining in severity. There is usually no permanent damage to joints.

Complications affecting the heart (such as *myocarditis* and *heart block*) or nervous system (such as *meningitis*) occur in some cases.

DIAGNOSIS AND TREATMENT

Anyone in whom the above symptoms develop, particularly after a tick bite, should consult a physician. The diagnosis of Lyme disease can be confirmed by blood tests.

If diagnosed before joint inflammation occurs, the disease can be quickly cleared up with antibiotics. If the disease is more advanced, *nonsteroidal anti-inflammatory drugs* and sometimes *corticosteroid drugs* are given and a cure may take longer.

Lymph

A milky body fluid that contains lymphocytes (a type of white blood cell), proteins, and fats. Lymph accumulates outside the blood vessels in the intercellular spaces of body tissues and is collected into the *lymphatic system* to flow back into the bloodstream. Lymph plays an important part in the *immune system* and in absorbing fats from the intestine.

Lymphadenitis

A little-used medical term for inflammation of the lymph nodes, a common cause of lymphadenopathy (swollen glands). See *Glands, swollen*.

Lymphadenopathy

The medical term for swollen lymph nodes (see *Glands, swollen*). A condition called persistent generalized lymphadenopathy, which causes generalized swelling of the lymph nodes, develops in some people infected with HIV (the *AIDS* virus).

Lymphangiography

A diagnostic procedure that enables lymph vessels and lymph nodes to be

---

PROCEDURE FOR LYMPHANGIOGRAPHY

To plan and monitor the progress of treatment for certain types of cancer, such as of the testis or cervix, X-ray pictures of the lymph vessels and nodes can be taken to reveal the spread of the cancer throughout the body. A contrast medium is injected into the foot, from where it travels throughout the lymphatic system. The procedure takes about two and a half hours.

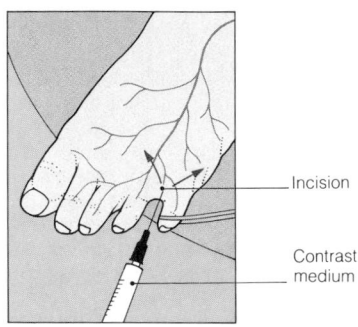

Incision

Contrast medium

1 A blue dye is injected through a needle into the web spaces between the toes of each foot, and into the outside of the little toes. The dye spreads rapidly into the tiny lymphatic vessels along the top of the foot, and makes them visible.

2 After the use of a local anesthetic, an incision is made over a stained lymphatic vessel in each foot. Contrast medium is injected through a needle into the vessels and passes up the legs, into the groin and abdomen. When the limit of diffusion is reached, the needles are removed and the incisions sewn.

Dye spreading through lymphatic system

3 The lymph vessels and nodes containing the dye show up clearly on the X-ray pictures. More lymphangiograms are taken after 24 hours.

---

seen on X-ray film after a contrast medium (a substance opaque to X rays) has been injected into them.

WHY IT IS DONE

Until recently, lymphangiography was frequently used to determine the extent to which a cancer had spread throughout the body (because lymph nodes trap cancer cells). However, the more straightforward techniques of *CT scanning* and *MRI* also clearly reveal abnormal lymph nodes and have largely superseded lymphangiography. Even so, in certain types of cancer (such as cancer of the testis or cervix), the additional information provided by lymphangiography is useful in planning treatment and monitoring progress.

HOW IT IS DONE

A blue dye is injected into the web spaces between all the toes. This dye quickly finds its way into the tiny, usually invisible, lymphatic vessels, allowing the radiologist to see them and select suitable vessels for further examination (see box).

Lymphangiography is sometimes performed on the arms to reveal lymph nodes in the upper body.

Lymphangioma

A rare benign tumor of the skin or tongue consisting of a collection of abnormal lymph vessels. It is usually present from birth.

There are two types of lymphangioma. One consists of a group of clear blisters that may be inconspicuous at birth but are usually obvious by the age of about 2. If the blisters are damaged they fill with blood, giving a red and white appearance to the lymphangioma. The growth often disappears on its own, but some cases require removal.

The other type, known as a cystic hygroma, is a soft swelling that resembles a bunch of small white grapes. It grows just beneath the skin (commonly in the neck), and may become very large and unsightly. It is usually removed at about age 5.

Lymphangitis

Inflammation of the lymphatic vessels as a result of the spread of bacteria (commonly streptococci) from an infected wound. The inflammation is so severe that it causes tender red streaks to appear on the skin overlying the lymphatic vessels. These streaks extend progressively from the site of infection toward the nearest lymph nodes (for example, from an infected finger up the arm toward the lymph nodes in the armpits). The affected nodes become swollen and tender. There is usually fever and a general feeling of illness.

Lymphangitis is a clear indication of a serious infection and requires urgent treatment with *antibiotic drugs*. Upon treatment, the condition usually clears up quickly without complications. (See also *Lymphadenitis*.)

Lymphatic system

A system of vessels (lymphatics) that drains *lymph* from all over the body back into the bloodstream. This system is part of the *immune system*, playing a major part in the body's defenses against infection and cancer.

STRUCTURE AND FUNCTION

All body tissues are bathed in a watery fluid derived from the bloodstream. Much of this fluid returns to the bloodstream through the walls of the capillaries, but the remainder (along with cells and small particles such as bacteria) is transported to the heart through the lymphatic system (see box, next page).

Throughout the course of the lymphatics lie *lymph nodes*, through which the lymph flows. These nodes are, in effect, filters that trap microorganisms and other foreign bodies in the lymph. The nodes contain many lymphocytes (a type of white blood cell), which can neutralize or destroy invading bacteria and viruses. If part of the body is inflamed or otherwise diseased, the nearby lymph nodes become swollen and tender as they limit the spread of the disease (see *Glands, swollen*). If an infection is particularly virulent, the lymphatics may also be inflamed, becoming visible as thin red lines running along a limb (see *Lymphangitis*).

The lymphatic system also plays a part in the absorption of fats from the intestine. While the products of carbohydrate and protein digestion pass directly into the bloodstream, fats pass into the intestinal lymphatics (lacteals); the lymph in them is so rich in fat that it appears milky.

DISORDERS

In some conditions, such as after radical breast surgery (which is rarely performed today), the lymphatics to a limb become obstructed and the limb becomes hard and swollen as a result, a condition known as *lymphedema*.

Cancer commonly spreads via the lymphatic system. A primary tumor invades the lymphatics and fragments (metastases) break off and travel to the local group of lymph nodes, where the metastases continue to grow and produce a secondary tumor. This is particularly evident in *breast cancer*, which tends to spread early to the lymph nodes in the armpit.

Lymphedema

An abnormal accumulation of *lymph* in the tissues, causing swelling of a limb. Lymphedema occurs if lymphatic vessels are blocked, damaged, or removed, resulting in disruption of the normal drainage of lymph (see *Lymphatic system*).

CAUSES

There are various causes. In the tropical disease *filariasis*, for example, the lymphatic vessels may be blocked by parasitic worms. Blockage may also occur if cancer spreads through the lymphatic system and deposits cancer cells in the lymph vessels.

Surgical removal of lymph nodes under the arm or in the groin or radiation therapy for a tumor destroys lymph nodes and vessels, sometimes resulting in lymphedema.

Lymphedema may also occur for no known cause. It may be present from birth or may develop later in life. Lymphedema of unknown cause affects twice as many women as men.

SYMPTOMS AND SIGNS

In about 10 percent of women who have had a radical mastectomy, lymphedema develops in the arm (but not usually in the hand) on the same side as the breast removed. In some such cases, the arm becomes disablingly heavy and cumbersome. The incidence of lymphedema is much lower with newer surgical techniques.

Other than following mastectomy, lymphedema usually causes swelling of one or both legs. Starting with only a slight, intermittent puffiness around one ankle, the swelling gradually extends up the leg. In about half of all cases, the other leg also becomes affected. The swelling is usually painless, but the leg feels heavy.

In some people the legs enlarge to an unsightly and incapacitating degree, but in others the swelling may be only minimal even 40 or more years after the onset of the condition.

TREATMENT

There is no known cure for lymphedema. Treatment consists of taking *diuretic drugs*, massaging the affected limb, wearing an elastic bandage or compression sleeve, and performing exercises with the leg or arm elevated. However, these measures usually produce only a slight improvement. If the leg or arm is so large that it causes disability, the swollen tissue and some of the overlying skin may be removed surgically.

Lymph gland

A popular name for a *lymph node*. (See also *Lymphatic system*.)

Lymph node

Popularly known as a lymph gland, a small organ lying along the course of a lymphatic vessel.

STRUCTURE AND FUNCTION

Lymph nodes vary considerably in size from microscopic to about 1 inch (2.5 cm) in diameter. Each node consists of a thin, fibrous outer capsule and an inner mass of lymphoid tissue. Penetrating the capsule are several small lymphatic vessels (which carry lymph into the gland) and a single, larger vessel (which carries it out).

Lymphoid tissue forms *antibodies* and houses *lymphocytes*, both of which play a very important role in fighting infection. Lymph nodes also contain macrophages, large cells that engulf bacteria and other foreign particles. The nodes act as a barrier to the spread of infection, destroying or filtering out bacteria before they can pass into the bloodstream. (See also *Glands, swollen*; *Lymphatic system*.)

Lymphocyte

Any of a group of white *blood cells* of crucial importance to the adaptive part of the body's *immune system*. The adaptive portion of the immune system mounts a tailor-made defense when dangerous invading organisms penetrate the body's general defenses (such as those provided by other types of white blood cell).

Some lymphocytes retain a memory of invading microorganisms so that the invaders can be dealt with more rapidly when next encountered. It is this memory function that is stimulated by vaccines. Lymphocytes protect against the development of tumors and cause rejection of tissue in organ transplants.

TYPES

There are two principal types of lymphocytes. They are called B- and T-lymphocytes.

B-LYMPHOCYTES This type accounts for about 10 percent of circulating lymphocytes. When a particular *antigen* (foreign protein), such as a

STRUCTURE AND FUNCTION OF THE LYMPHATIC SYSTEM

The lymphatic system is a collection of organs, ducts, and tissues that has the dual role of draining tissue fluid (lymph) back into the bloodstream and of fighting infection. Lymph is drained by a system of channels (the lymphatic vessels). White cells produced by the bone marrow, thymus, and spleen are present in lymph nodes or circulate through the lymphatic system, providing defenses against infection.

The lymphatic network
The lymphatic system consists of a network of lymph nodes connected by lymphatic vessels. The nodes generally occur in clusters, mainly around the neck, armpits, and groin.

Thoracic duct

Liver

Spleen

Cisterna chyli

Lymph nodes

Lymphatic vessels

Right lymphatic duct
Thoracic duct
Right subclavian vein
Left subclavian vein
Lymph
Superior vena cava

Lymphatic drainage
Just below the neck, the thoracic duct and the right lymphatic duct drain into the two subclavian veins. These veins unite to form the inferior vena cava, which passes into the heart; in this way, the lymph fluids rejoin the circulation.

Lymphatic vessels

Collagenous capsule

Primary follicle

Artery

Vein

Lymph

White blood cells

Structure of a lymph node
Any fluid absorbed into the lymphatic system passes across at least one lymph node before it returns to the circulation. The fluid filters through a mesh of tightly packed white blood cells—some of which are grouped into primary follicles consisting of similar cells—which attack and destroy harmful organisms. Every lymph node is supplied by its own tiny artery and vein.

MOVEMENTS OF BODY FLUIDS
Lymph is constantly moving around the body, but the lymphatic system has no central pump equivalent to the heart. Lymph is circulated by the movement of the body's muscles; a system of one-way valves in the lymphatic vessels ensures that it moves in the right direction. Exertion also pushes fluid from body tissues into the bloodstream.

Heart

Arteries

Veins

Lymphatic vessels

Capillaries

Cells   Lymphatic vessel

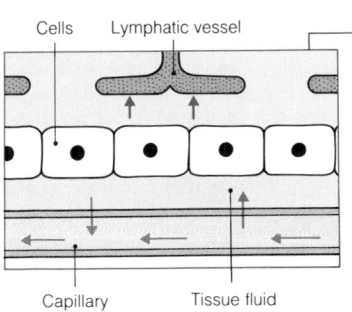

Capillary   Tissue fluid

Fluid exchange
During a 24-hour period, approximately 42 pints of serumlike fluid pass from the bloodstream to the body's tissues. This fluid bathes the cells and provides them with oxygen and nutrients. During the same period of time, approximately 36 pints of fluid pass back from the tissues to the bloodstream, carrying carbon dioxide and other waste products. The remaining 6 pints pass from the tissues to the lymphatic system and return eventually to the circulation from there.

Enlarged lymph nodes
This photograph shows a girl with marked enlargement of the lymph nodes in her neck. In this case, the appearance is due to Hodgkin's disease, a rare cancer that affects the lymph nodes. Enlargement of the lymph nodes may also be due to infection.

substance on the surface of a bacterium, is encountered by the immune system, certain B-lymphocytes are stimulated to enlarge and undergo cell division, transforming into cells called plasma cells. The plasma cells secrete into the blood vast numbers of tailor-made *immunoglobulins* or *antibodies* that attach to the antigen on the surface of the microorganism. This starts a process that leads to the destruction of the microorganism. The protective effect of immunoglobulins is called humoral immunity.

T-LYMPHOCYTES This type accounts for more than 80 percent of circulating lymphocytes. T-lymphocytes are derived from white cells that have at some stage entered the thymus gland, where they were "educated" to fulfill a particular function.

There are two main groups of T-lymphocytes: killer (cytotoxic) and helper cells. The killer T-lymphocytes (like B-lymphocytes) are sensitized and stimulated to multiply by the presence of antigens, in this case by antigens present on abnormal body cells (e.g., cells that have been invaded by viruses, cells in transplanted tissue, and tumor cells). Unlike the B-lymphocytes, the killer cells do not produce antibodies; instead, they travel to and attach to the cells recognized as abnormal. The killer cells then release chemicals known as lymphokines, which help destroy the abnormal cells. This is called cell-mediated immunity.

Helper T cells enhance the activities of the cytotoxic cells and control other aspects of the immune response. In people infected with HIV (the *AIDS* virus) these helper T cells are reduced in number, thus impairing the body's ability to fight certain types of infections and tumors.

MEMORY FUNCTION
Some lymphocytes do not participate directly in immune responses; instead, they serve as a memory bank for the different antigens that have been encountered in the past. These cells may survive for many years.

Lymphogranuloma venereum
A sexually transmitted disease, common in tropical countries. It is caused by a *chlamydial infection* that is common in tropical countries.

The first sign of infection is a small genital blister that appears three to 21 days after infection; this blister heals in a few days without leaving a scar. There may also be fever, headache, muscle and joint pains, and a rash.

The lymph glands, particularly in the groin, become painfully enlarged and inflamed. Abscesses may form and ulcers may develop on the skin over the affected glands; the ulcers take several months to heal.

Treatment of lymphogranuloma venereum is with *antibiotic drugs*.

Lymphoma
Any of a group of cancers in which the cells of lymphoid tissue (found mainly in the lymph nodes and spleen) multiply unchecked.

Lymphomas fall into two categories. If characteristic abnormal cells (Reed-Sternberg cells) are present, the disease is called Hodgkin's lymphoma. All other types are called non-Hodgkin's. (See *Hodgkin's disease*; *Lymphoma, non-Hodgkin's*.)

Lymphoma, non-Hodgkin's
Any cancer of lymphoid tissue (found mainly in the lymph nodes and spleen) other than *Hodgkin's disease*.

Non-Hodgkin's lymphomas vary in their malignancy according to the nature and activity of the abnormal cells. Lymphomas are most malignant when the cells are primitive or are poorly differentiated (unspecialized). These cells tend to take over entire lymph nodes quickly. Low-grade lymphomas consist of cells that are better-differentiated.

CAUSES AND INCIDENCE
In most cases of non-Hodgkin's lymphoma, the cause is unknown. Occasionally, the disease is associated with suppression of the *immune system*, particularly after organ transplantation. One type of non-Hodgkin's lymphoma, called *Burkitt's lymphoma* (common only in the tropics), is thought to be caused by the Epstein-Barr virus. It is suspected that *HIV* (the *AIDS* virus) permits other viruses to cause lymphomas.

About eight new cases of non-Hodgkin's lymphoma are diagnosed annually per 100,000 people in the US. Most sufferers are over 50.

SYMPTOMS AND SIGNS
In most patients, there is painless swelling of one or more groups of lymph nodes in the neck or groin. The liver and spleen may enlarge and lymphoid tissue in the abdomen may be affected, in rare cases causing abdominal pain and bleeding from the intestines, which is revealed as tarry-looking feces or vomiting of blood. Many other organs may also become involved, leading to diverse symptoms ranging from headache to

skin ulceration. Unless it is controlled, spread of the disease (often marked by fever) progressively impairs the immune system, leading to death from infections. The patient may also die of an uncontrolled spread of cancer.

DIAGNOSIS
Diagnosis is based on a *biopsy* (removal of a sample for analysis) of lymphoid tissue, usually from a lymph node. The extent of the disease is assessed by a process called staging. A *chest X ray*, *CT scanning*, *bone marrow biopsy*, and *lymphangiography* (X rays of the lymph glands) of the abdomen may be required.

TREATMENT AND OUTLOOK
If the lymphoma is confined to a single group of lymph nodes, treatment consists of *radiation therapy*. If the disease is more extensive, *anticancer drugs* are given. In some cases both forms of treatment are used. When all else fails, autologous *bone marrow transplantation* and high doses of chemotherapy and/or radiation may be used.

About three quarters of patients with a low-grade localized non-Hodgkin's lymphoma survive at least five years. In more severe types of lymphoma that have spread, 40 to 50 percent of patients survive for two years or more.

Lymphosarcoma
A now uncommonly used name for non-Hodgkin's lymphoma (see *Lymphoma, non-Hodgkin's*).

Lypressin
A synthetic preparation of *ADH* (antidiuretic hormone), a hormone that controls the volume of water excreted in the urine. Lypressin is used as a nasal spray to treat *diabetes insipidus* (a deficiency of ADH causing excessive urination and thirst).

Possible adverse effects are abdominal cramps, an urge to pass bowel movements, and nasal congestion that, if severe, may impair the efficiency of treatment.

Lysis
A medical term for the destruction of a cell by damage to its outer membrane. A common example is *hemolysis*, the breakdown of red blood cells. Lysis may be caused by chemical action, such as that of an *enzyme* (a protein that controls a chemical reaction), or by physical action, such as heat or cold. The term lysis is also occasionally used to refer to a sudden recovery from a fever.

L

M

Macro-
A prefix meaning large, as in macrophage (a large cell that plays an important part in the body's defense system by engulfing bacteria and other foreign particles) or macroglossia (enlargement of the tongue).

Macrobiotics

A diet based on the oriental belief that all foods are either yin or yang (possessed of negative or positive energy), and that a balance of yin and yang must be maintained for health. Foods are classified yin or yang according to many factors, including where they are grown, their color, texture, and taste. There are several levels of macrobiotic diet; the most advanced consists mainly of whole grains. Eating such a diet may lead to severe malnutrition, scurvy, or anemia due to the lack of protein, vitamins, and minerals.

Macroglossia
Abnormal enlargement of the tongue. Macroglossia is a feature of *Down's syndrome*, of *hypothyroidism*, and of *acromegaly*. Tumors of the tongue, such as a *hemangioma* or *lymphangioma*, also cause macroglossia; *amyloidosis* is another possible cause.

In addition to being unsightly, an abnormally large tongue can cause snoring and is sometimes responsible for *sleep apnea*. Treatment is limited and depends on the underlying cause.

Macular degeneration
A progressive disorder that affects the central part of the *retina*, causing gradual loss of vision. Macular degeneration is a painless condition that is common in the elderly. It usually affects both eyes, either simultaneously or one after the other.

The macula is the part of the retina that distinguishes fine detail at the center of the field of vision. Degeneration begins with partial breakdown of an insulating layer between the retina and the *choroid* (layer of blood vessels behind the retina). Fluid leakage occurs, and new blood vessels growing from the choroid destroy the retinal nerve tissue and replace it with scar tissue. The effect is a roughly circular area of blindness, increasing in size until it is large enough to obliterate two or three words at normal reading distance.

With early diagnosis, it is sometimes possible to seal off the leakage with a *laser*. In most cases, however, the disorder is untreatable.

Macule
A spot on the skin (level with the surface) discernible only by difference in color or texture.

Magnesium
A metallic element that plays several vital roles in the body. Magnesium is essential for the formation of bones and teeth, for muscle contraction, for the transmission of nerve impulses, and for the activation of many *enzymes* (substances that promote biochemical reactions in the body). There are about 1.25 ounces (35 g) of magnesium in an average-sized person, much of it in the bones and teeth.

The recommended daily intake of magnesium varies from 50 mg in the newborn to 400 mg in young men. Women require slightly less than men, except during pregnancy and breast-feeding. Dietary sources are green, leafy vegetables, nuts, whole grains, soybeans, milk, and seafood.

MAGNESIUM-CONTAINING DRUGS
Magnesium compounds are used in *antacid drugs* and *laxatives*. Magnesium carbonate and magnesium oxide are common ingredients of antacids; magnesium sulfate is used in laxatives. Magnesium is also a constituent of some mineral supplements.

DEFICIENCY AND EXCESS
A normal diet contains sufficient magnesium. Deficiency (which is rare) usually occurs as a result of an intestinal disorder that impairs absorption of both calcium and of magnesium, a severe kidney disease, alcoholism, or prolonged treatment with *diuretic drugs* or *digitalis drugs*. Symptoms of deficiency include anxiety, restlessness, tremors, palpitations, and depression. There is also thought to be an increased risk of kidney stones or coronary heart disease. Deficiency is treated with supplements.

Magnesium excess is usually caused by taking too much of a magnesium-containing antacid or laxative. Too much magnesium may cause nausea, vomiting, diarrhea, dizziness, and muscle weakness. Very large amounts may lead to heart damage or respiratory failure, especially in people with kidney disease. Mild magnesium excess does not usually require treatment. However, anyone who has taken a substantial overdose may require hospitalization so that breathing and heart activity can be monitored (and supported, if necessary) and drugs can be given to help the body excrete the excess.

Magnetic resonance imaging
See *MRI*.

Malabsorption
Impaired absorption of nutrients, vitamins, or minerals from the diet by the lining of the small intestine.

CAUSES
Malabsorption is caused by many conditions. In *lactose intolerance*, deficiency of the enzyme lactase in the intestine prevents the breakdown and absorption of lactose (sugar found in milk). In *cystic fibrosis* and chronic *pancreatitis*, damage to the pancreas prevents the production of enzymes required for the digestion and absorption of fats and other nutrients.

In *celiac sprue*, many nutrients cannot be absorbed because of damage to the small intestine by sensitivity to the protein gluten. Uncommon diseases in which the intestinal lining is damaged include *Crohn's disease*, *amyloidosis*, *giardiasis*, *Whipple's disease*, and *lymphoma*.

Removal of portions of the small intestine can cause malabsorption, as can stomach operations that cause food to pass through the digestive tract more quickly than normal.

There are also some disorders that interfere with the passage of bile salts to the small intestine or that interfere with their uptake, thus preventing the breakdown and absorption of fats. These disorders include *bile duct obstruction*, primary *biliary cirrhosis*, and Crohn's disease.

SYMPTOMS AND DIAGNOSIS
Common effects are diarrhea and weight loss; in severe cases, there may also be malnutrition (see *Nutritional disorders*), *vitamin* deficiency, *mineral* deficiency, or *anemia*.

The diagnosis is confirmed by examining feces for unabsorbed fat and by blood tests to detect anemia and deficiencies of nutrients, vitamins, and minerals. To determine the cause of malabsorption, tests may be carried out, including *barium X-ray examination* of the small intestine and *jejunal biopsy* (removal of tissue from the jejunum for examination).

TREATMENT AND OUTLOOK
Treatment depends on the underlying cause. In most cases, modifications or supplements to the diet restore the affected person to health. However, if there is severe, irreversible damage to the lining of the intestine, infusion of nutrients into a vein may be necessary (see *Feeding, artificial*).

Maladjustment
Failure to adapt to a change in one's environment, resulting in an inability to cope with work or social activities. Maladjustment is common and can occur at any age as a reaction to stressful situations (such as starting school, changing residence, divorce, physical illness, or retirement). It may be expressed by feelings of *depression* or *anxiety*, or by *behavioral problems in children* and adolescents.

Maladjustment is usually temporary, clearing up when the person is removed from the stressful situation or learns to adapt to it.

Malaise
A vague feeling of being sick or of physical discomfort. It is a general symptom of little value in diagnosis.

Malalignment
Positioning of teeth in the jaw so that they do not form a smooth arch shape when viewed from above or below (see *Malocclusion*). The term is also used to refer to a *fracture* in which the bone ends are not in a straight line. These fractures must be manipulated back into position so that the bone is not deformed when it heals.

Malar flush
A high color over the cheekbones, with a bluish tinge caused by reduced oxygen concentration in the blood. Malar flush is considered to be a sign of *mitral stenosis* (narrowing of one of the heart valves), usually following *rheumatic fever*. However, malar flush is not always present in mitral stenosis, and many people with this coloring do not have heart disease.

Malaria

A serious parasitic disease, spread by the bites of *ANOPHELES* mosquitoes. The disease produces severe fever and, in some cases, complications affecting the kidneys, liver, brain, and blood that can be fatal.

Malaria is prevalent throughout the tropics, affecting up to 300 million people worldwide each year. It is the single most important disease hazard for travelers to warm climates.

CAUSES
The parasites responsible for malaria are single-celled (protozoal) organisms called plasmodia. Four different species can cause disease in humans: *PLASMODIUM FALCIPARUM, PLASMODIUM VIVAX, PLASMODIUM OVALE,* and *PLASMODIUM MALARIAE.* Each of these species spends part of its life cycle in humans and part in *ANOPHELES* mosquitoes (see diagram, overleaf).

Symptoms, including shaking, chills, and fever, appear only when red blood cells, infected with parasites, rupture to release more parasites into the bloodstream.

INCIDENCE
Malaria occurs in much of the tropics, where it is a major health problem (see map). Children in affected countries suffer repeated infections, and many die. Malaria kills about 1 million infants and children every year in Africa alone; those who survive gradually build up immunity. The World Health Organization has undertaken a massive program of malaria control, but little progress has been made in the past 20 years. Mosquitoes have developed resistance to insecticides and, in many areas, the parasites have developed resistance to drugs.

The number of cases diagnosed in the US has increased significantly over the last 15 years, from a few hundred cases annually in the early 1970s to about 1,000 cases in both 1984 and 1985. Part of this rise is attributable to increased travel; about 40 percent of cases occur in people recently returned from the tropics. The risk of contracting the disease in Africa seems particularly high. The remaining 60 percent of cases affect foreign immigrants to the US.

The chance of contracting malaria within the US is very small. Cases have occurred among drug users who have shared needles with an infected person, and in people who have received infected blood transfusions.

SYMPTOMS
The period between the mosquito bite and the appearance of symptoms is usually a week or two, but can be as long as a year if the person has been taking antimalarial drugs (which suppress rather than cure malaria).

The prime symptom of infection is the classic malarial ague (fever). Except for most *P. FALCIPARUM* infec-

tions, this fever has three stages: a cold stage of uncontrollable shivering (rigors), a hot stage in which the temperature may reach 105°F, and finally a sweating stage that drenches the bedding and brings down the temperature. A severe headache, general malaise, and vomiting may accompany the attack. At the end of an attack, the patient is left weak and tired, and sleeps. In many cases, the parasitized red blood cells rupture at the same time in each cycle and the fever develops cyclically, occurring every other day (with *P. VIVAX* and *P. OVALE* infections) or every third day (with *P. MALARIAE*).

P. FALCIPARUM infects all ages of red blood cells, whereas the other varieties attack only young or old cells. Falciparum malaria thus affects a greater proportion of the blood cells and is therefore more severe. It can be fatal within a few hours of the first symptoms. The fever is prolonged and irregular. So many blood cells may be destroyed that they block blood vessels in vital organs, especially the kidneys. The spleen becomes enlarged and the brain may be affected, leading to coma and convulsions. Destruction of blood cells leads to hemolytic *anemia*. Kidney and liver failure are common complications of falciparum malaria.

DIAGNOSIS
Malaria is diagnosed from studying *blood smears* in the laboratory at six- to 12-hour intervals; the parasites are clearly visible under the microscope.

TREATMENT
Malaria, especially falciparum malaria, is a medical emergency that is treated in the hospital.

The antimalarial drug chloroquine, which eradicates the parasites from the blood, is the usual treatment for all types of malaria. However, chloroquine-resistant falciparum malaria is now widespread in many tropical areas. If a chloroquine-resistant form is suspected, or if the number of parasites does not diminish over 24 hours, other drugs, such as quinine or the combination of pyrimethamine and sulfadoxine, may be given.

In serious illness, exchange blood transfusions have been investigated as a lifesaving effort.

For any type other than falciparum malaria, another drug, primaquine, must be taken for another two weeks to eradicate parasites in the liver. Primaquine may cause hemolytic anemia in people who have a disorder called *G6PD deficiency*.

PREVENTION

In countries where malaria is common, most people have acquired some immunity to the disease. However, this does not apply to visitors to the tropics, who should take preventive antimalarial drugs. These drugs should be taken a day or two before entering a malarious area and use should be continued for at least four weeks after leaving it.

The physician will want to know what countries are to be visited before prescribing a drug. For areas where there is no resistance to chloroquine, this drug is recommended; proguanil is recommended for longer term use because it has fewer side effects. For chloroquine-resistant areas there are various possibilities, such as a combination of chloroquine and proguanil, or the combination of pyrimethamine with either sulfadoxine or dapsone. These drugs may then be followed by a course of primaquine, which provides a radical cure of the forms of malaria found in the liver.

Antimalarial drugs should be taken even by pregnant women in highly malarious areas (proguanil or chloroquine are the recommended drugs in this case). Although the drugs present a slight risk to the fetus, it is less than the risk to the fetus if the mother contracts malaria.

In addition, visitors to the tropics should avoid mosquito bites by wearing protective clothing over the arms and legs in the evening; other preventive measures include screens over windows, insecticide sprays, and, if necessary, mosquito nets. People should also avoid entering jungle areas at night.

Even people who take antimalarial drugs and precautions against bites may contract malaria. Anyone in whom a fever and headache develops after returning from the tropics should see a physician as soon as possible and mention the trip abroad so that appropriate blood smears can be arranged to diagnose malaria.

Malformation
A deformity, particularly one resulting from faulty development.

Malignant
A term used to describe a condition that tends to become progressively worse and to result in death. By contrast, a *benign* disorder remains relatively mild and is not usually fatal. The term malignant is primarily used to refer to a *tumor* that spreads from its original location to affect other parts of the body, with potentially life-threatening results.

Malignant melanoma
See *Melanoma, malignant.*

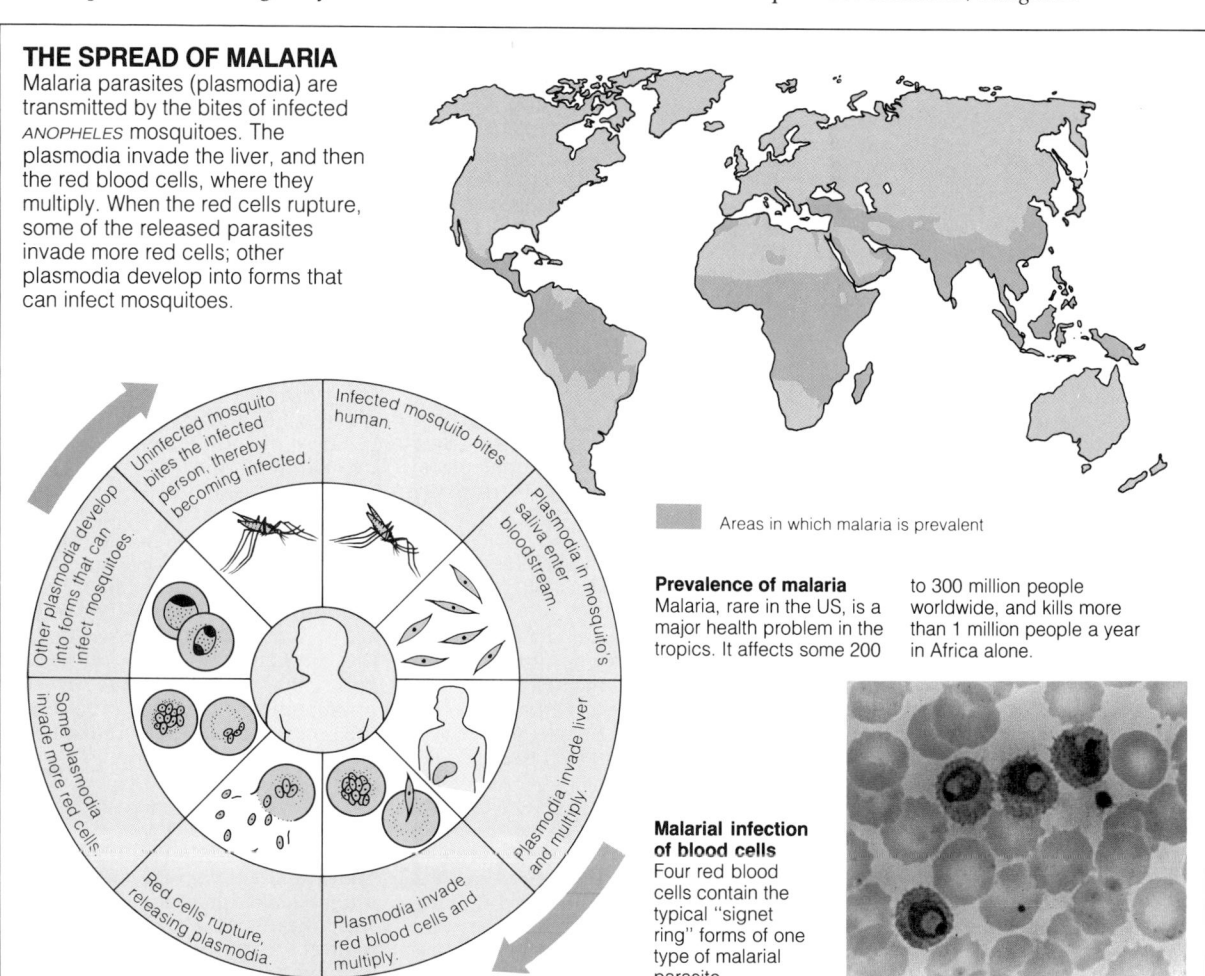

THE SPREAD OF MALARIA
Malaria parasites (plasmodia) are transmitted by the bites of infected ANOPHELES mosquitoes. The plasmodia invade the liver, and then the red blood cells, where they multiply. When the red cells rupture, some of the released parasites invade more red cells; other plasmodia develop into forms that can infect mosquitoes.

Areas in which malaria is prevalent

Prevalence of malaria
Malaria, rare in the US, is a major health problem in the tropics. It affects some 200 to 300 million people worldwide, and kills more than 1 million people a year in Africa alone.

Malarial infection of blood cells
Four red blood cells contain the typical "signet ring" forms of one type of malarial parasite.

Malingering

Deliberate simulation of physical or psychological symptoms for a particular purpose, such as obtaining time off work, avoiding military service, or obtaining compensation. Malingering differs from *factitious disorders*, in which the person feigns illness for no reason other than a wish to gain the attention associated with illness and being a patient. Malingering is also distinguished from a *somatization disorder* (such as *hypochondriasis*), in which symptoms are not under the voluntary control of the person.

Mallet finger

See *Baseball finger*.

Mallet toe

A deformity of one or more toes (excluding the big toe) in one or both feet. The end of the affected toe bends downward so that the toe curls under itself. The cause is unknown. A painful corn may develop on the tip of the toe or over the top of the bent joint. Protective pads can sometimes relieve excessive pressure from footwear; if not, surgical treatment of the toe may be needed. (See also *Clawfoot*.)

Mallory-Weiss syndrome

A condition in which a tear at the lower end of the esophagus causes vomiting of blood. Mallory-Weiss syndrome is particularly common in alcoholics after a bout of excessive drinking accompanied by retching and vomiting. Occasionally, the tear may be produced by violent coughing, a severe asthma attack, or epileptic convulsions. The damage is thought usually to result from violent contractions of the diaphragm during prolonged retching and vomiting.

DIAGNOSIS AND TREATMENT

Diagnosis is made by passing an *endoscope* (a tubelike instrument with a light source and lens attachment) down the esophagus. The tear usually heals within 10 days and no special treatment is required unless the person has lost a considerable amount of blood, in which case blood transfusions may be necessary.

Malnutrition

See *Nutritional disorders*.

Malocclusion

An abnormal relationship between the upper and lower sets of teeth when they are closed. In ideal occlusion the upper incisors and canines (front teeth) slightly overlap the lower ones, the outer ridges of the lower premolars and molars (back teeth) fit into the hollows in the corresponding upper teeth, and, except for the four frontmost incisors, the other upper and lower teeth alternate. This arrangement enables food to be bitten and chewed efficiently.

TYPES OF MALOCCLUSION

Unsatisfactory contact between the upper and lower teeth (malocclusion) is of three main types, shown below.

Type 1 malocclusion
In this (the most common) type, the jaw relationship is normal, but, because the teeth are poorly spaced, tilted, or rotated, the upper and lower set do not meet properly.

Type 2 malocclusion
In this type—called retrognathism—the lower jaw is too far back; the normal small overbite of the upper incisors is greatly increased, and the molar bite is displaced backward.

Type 3 malocclusion
In this (the least common) type (called prognathism), the lower jaw is too far forward; the lower incisors meet, or lie in front of, the upper ones, and the molar bite is displaced forward.

Ideal occlusion is uncommon; most people have some teeth slightly out of position. Only severe malocclusion usually requires treatment.

CAUSES

Malocclusion usually develops in childhood, when the teeth and jaws are growing. Most malocclusion is the result of *heredity*. Other cases may result from *thumb-sucking* beyond a certain age or from a mismatch between the teeth and the jaws (for example, large teeth in a small mouth, leading to *overcrowding*).

TREATMENT

Malocclusion may require treatment to improve appearance, to prevent strain from the abnormal bite (which causes pain, stiffness, and sometimes *arthritis* in the jaw joints), or to facilitate teeth cleaning and thus help prevent *periodontal disease* and decay (see *Caries, dental*).

The dentist may be able to correct uneven contacts between teeth by recontouring opposing tooth surfaces or by fitting an onlay restoration (see *Onlay, dental*) to alter the shape of a tooth. However, most serious abnormalities require orthodontic treatment, which consists mainly of using *orthodontic appliances* (braces) to train teeth to grow into the proper position. In cases of tooth crowding, some teeth may need to be extracted. *Orthognathic surgery* is used to treat recession or protrusion of the lower jaw.

Treatment is best carried out in childhood or adolescence, when the teeth and bones of the jaw are still developing. Problems left until adulthood can be treated successfully, but may take longer to correct than when treated earlier.

Malpractice

See *Liability insurance, professional*.

Malpresentation

A condition in which a baby is not in the usual face downward, head first position during *childbirth*. Only 5 percent of babies enter labor malpresented. Most malpresentations are bottom first (breech position) or head first but face upward (occipital posterior position); some lie transversely across the uterus.

A baby lying bottom first may be delivered by *breech delivery* or *cesarean section*. A baby lying transversely usually is delivered by cesarean section. A baby in the occipital posterior position usually rotates into a normal position during labor; sometimes a cesarean is necessary.

M

Mammary gland

See *Breast*.

Mammography

An X-ray procedure for detecting *breast cancer* at an early stage.

WHY IT IS DONE

Successful treatment of breast cancer depends on early diagnosis (detection of tumors less than about one half inch across). Growths this small may not be discernible on physical examination (see *Breast self-examination*) and can be effectively detected only by mammography. Screening tests using mammography have reduced death rates from breast cancer in women over the age of 50 by 30 percent.

Mammography is also used to aid diagnosis of established breast disease and to help plan treatment.

Mammoplasty

A cosmetic operation to reduce the size of extremely large or pendulous breasts, to enlarge small breasts, or to reconstruct a breast after it has been removed to treat cancer.

BREAST REDUCTION

This operation is performed using a general anesthetic. Incisions are inconspicuous and positioned so that unwanted tissue is easily removed. This procedure reduces the size of the breast and raises its position to correct any drooping.

Most patients are pleased with the results. The nipple scar and the scar beneath the breast are usually well hidden, but the vertical scar is usually evident and may need to be made less obvious at a second, minor operation.

BREAST ENLARGEMENT

This procedure is usually performed using a short-acting general anesthetic. A small opening at the side or below the breast allows a pocket to be made to accommodate the implant.

The immediate results are usually excellent, but internal scar tissue often eventually forms around the implant, altering its shape and making the breast harder. External pressure on the implant to restore its shape or sometimes another minor operation may be necessary.

BREAST RECONSTRUCTION

This operation is carried out either at the same time as a *mastectomy* (breast removal) or at a later date, again using a general anesthetic. Depending on the type of mastectomy, reconstruction takes one of two forms.

Before

After

Reconstruction of a breast
A breast removed at an earlier mastectomy operation can be reconstructed later using a silicone rubber implant.

If the entire breast is removed, a portion of skin and underlying fat and muscle is transplanted from a site near the breast; a silicone rubber implant is incorporated at the same time. In this case, scarring is extensive.

Increasingly often, surgeons remove only the tumor and surrounding tissue, leaving the overlying skin in place; the implant can then be inserted with minimal scarring.

In both operations the size of the other breast may be reduced to make the breasts look balanced.

Mandible

The lower *jaw*.

Mandibular orthopedic repositioning appliance

A device used by some dentists to treat conditions claimed to result from misalignment of the jaw, such as headaches, temporomandibular disorders, scoliosis (curvature of the spine), and loss of balance. A mandibular orthopedic repositioning appliance (MORA) is often mistaken for a mouth protector, but does not perform the same function.

PROCEDURE FOR MAMMOGRAPHY

Mammography is simple, safe, and causes minimal discomfort. Only low-dose X rays are used. The breast may be X-rayed from above, the side, or both; sometimes an oblique (angled) view is taken.

How mammography is done
In the method shown here, the breast is placed on the machine and gently compressed between the X-ray plate below and a plastic cover above. This flattens the breast so that as much tissue as possible can be imaged. Several views may be taken. In another method, the breast hangs freely and is X-rayed from the side.

Mammograms
The normal mammogram (far left) shows a side view of a healthy breast, with the milk ducts appearing as denser areas. In the abnormal mammogram (left), an irregular, dense mass in the upper part of the breast indicates a tumor. A biopsy (removal of a tissue sample for analysis) is necessary to determine whether a tumor is cancerous.

M

PROCEDURE FOR MAMMOPLASTY

One of the most common cosmetic operations, mammoplasty is done to improve the appearance of the breasts by removal of excess fat and skin or by using an implant to increase their size.

BREAST REDUCTION

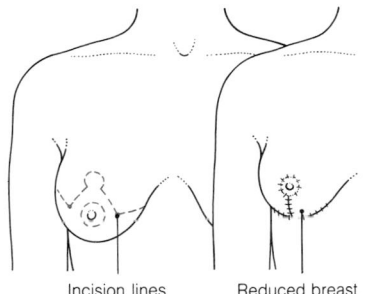

Incision lines   Reduced breast

Incisions are made around the edge of the nipple and in the crease below the breast. These are joined by a third vertical cut. Excess tissue and skin are removed, and the incisions are closed with stitches.

BREAST ENLARGEMENT

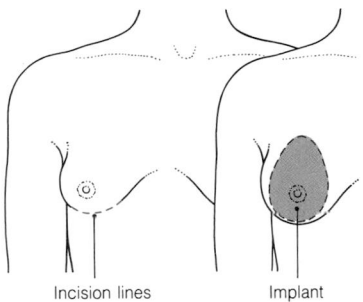

Incision lines   Implant

An incision is made in the armpit or along the crease under the breast, and a pocket is created behind the breast to receive the implant. After the implant has been inserted, the incision is stitched.

Much controversy exists over whether a MORA can improve athletic performance by building strength and endurance. Such claims have not been scientifically proved. In fact, there is evidence that continued use of a MORA may result in severe malocclusion that requires extensive orthodontic or reconstructive treatment.

Mania

A mental disorder characterized by episodes of overactivity, elation, or irritability. Mania usually occurs as part of a *manic-depressive illness.*

SYMPTOMS

The primary symptom of mania is an abnormal increase in activity (for example, the sufferer may make elaborate plans for a constant round of social activity). Other symptoms may include extravagant spending, repeatedly starting new tasks, less need to sleep, increased appetite for food, alcohol, sex, and energetic exercise, outbursts of inappropriate anger, laughter, or sudden socializing, and a grandiose sense of knowing better than others. This may extend to delusions of grandeur (for example, believing oneself to be God). When symptoms are relatively mild, the condition is called hypomania.

Manic attacks usually first appear before the age of 30, and may last for a few days or several months. If attacks begin after age 40, they are frequently more prolonged.

TREATMENT

Severe mania often leads to marked social disruption or even violence; hospital admission is usually required. Treatment is generally by means of *antipsychotic drugs* and relapses are prevented by giving *lithium.* Carbamazepine is sometimes used to augment the effect of lithium.

Manic-depressive illness

A mental disorder in which a disturbance of mood is the major symptom. This disturbance may consist of *depression* or of *mania* (unipolar) or of a swing between the two states (bipolar).

CAUSES

A number of physical illnesses (especially brain disorders), certain drugs, and a clear inherited tendency are all established factors. Research has located at least one of the defective genes responsible on chromosome 11.

Overactivity seems due largely to extra amounts of the neurochemical dopamine in parts of the brain; this may simply represent a manic reaction to an underlying depression caused by loss or grief.

PREVALENCE

Depression is very common, affecting about one in 10 men and one in five women at some time in their lives. About a third of these illnesses are severe. By contrast, mania (unipolar or bipolar) is rare, affecting only about eight per 1,000 people, men and women equally.

TREATMENT

Admission to the hospital is often required for severe manic-depressive illness. *Antidepressant drugs* and/or *ECT* (electroconvulsive therapy) are effective in treating depression. *Antipsychotic drugs* (e.g., chlorpromazine and haloperidol) are used to control manic symptoms. *Lithium* alone or, when inadequate, with carbamazepine may be used during remission to prevent relapse.

Group, family, and individual therapy are useful in treating neurotic disorders and in aiding recovery after a severe episode. *Cognitive-behavioral therapy* may also be helpful.

OUTLOOK

Though often crippling in the acute phase, manic-depressive illnesses have a good prognosis. Abilities are not affected, and more than 80 percent of patients recover.

Repeated, severe illnesses, however, or persistent depression, can seriously disrupt life. A significant number of depressed people commit, or attempt, *suicide.* Others suffer from social isolation, poverty, and problems caused by alcohol dependence. Nevertheless, the widescale use of maintenance treatment with lithium has restored many people who have manic-depressive illness to near normal health.

Manipulation

As a therapy, the skillful use of the hands to move a part of the body or a specific joint or muscle to treat certain disorders. Manipulation at times is carried out by a physician, sometimes using a general anesthetic. The technique of manipulation is widely practiced by physical therapists, osteopaths, and chiropractors.

Manipulation is used to correct deformity by aligning the bones of a displaced *fracture,* putting a joint back into position following *dislocation,* or stretching a *contracture* (shortened muscle or tendon). It may also be used to increase the range of movement of a stiff joint, usually following injury. Occasionally, it is helpful in treating *frozen shoulder,* but does not usually relieve stiffness caused by *arthritis* (inflammation of a joint).

Mannitol

An osmotic *diuretic drug.* Mannitol is used as a short-term treatment for *glaucoma* (raised pressure in the eyeball) before corrective surgery. It is also given to reduce *edema* (fluid retention) in the brain before and after

M

surgical treatment of a *brain tumor* or an intracerebral *hematoma* (blood clot on the brain).

Mannitol is occasionally used to prevent *renal failure* following severe shock. In some cases of drug overdose, mannitol is given to increase urine production and thus the amount of the drug excreted from the body.

Possible adverse effects include headache, nausea, vomiting, dizziness, and confusion.

Manometry

The measuring of pressure (of either liquid or gas) by means of a manometer. The simplest type of manometer is a glass U-shaped tube containing mercury, oil, or water. One limb of the tube is connected by flexible tubing to the pressure source; the other limb is either open to the atmosphere or closed. Increased pressure forces the liquid down in one limb and up in the other; the change in height represents a measure of the pressure. This form of manometer is used to measure blood pressure (see *Sphygmomanometer*) and cerebrospinal fluid pressure.

There are also more sophisticated manometers that measure pressure by a coiled spring, a diaphragm, or an electrical transducer.

Mantoux test

A type of skin test for tuberculosis (see *Tuberculin tests*).

Maprotiline

An *antidepressant drug*. Because maprotiline has a sedative effect, it is useful in the treatment of *depression* accompanied by anxiety or difficulty sleeping. Maprotiline usually takes about six weeks to become fully effective. Possible adverse effects include dizziness, drowsiness, palpitations, and rash.

Marasmus

A severe form of protein and calorie malnutrition (see *Nutritional disorders*) that occurs principally in famine or semistarvation conditions. In developing countries, marasmus is widespread in children under 3 years of age, usually because they have been weaned too early onto an inadequate diet or kept too long on unsupplemented breast milk.

Children with marasmus are stunted and emaciated; they have loose folds of skin on the limbs and buttocks due to loss of muscle and fat. Other signs include sparse, brittle hair, diarrhea, and dehydration.

DIAGNOSIS AND TREATMENT
Marasmus is diagnosed from a physical examination and the child's dietary history. Treatment consists of keeping the child warm and giving a high-calorie, protein-rich diet. Persistent marasmus can cause permanent mental retardation and impairment of growth. (See also *Kwashiorkor*.)

Marble bone disease
See *Osteopetrosis*.

March fracture

A break in one of the *metatarsal bones* (long bones in the foot) caused by repeated jarring. Usually affecting the second or third metatarsal, march fracture is caused by running or walking long distances on a hard surface. The name is derived from the high incidence of this fracture in soldiers after long marches.

Pain, tenderness, and swelling occur around the site of the fracture. However, X rays may not show the fracture until healing has begun, when callus (new bone) appears as a white shadow. Treatment is rest and, occasionally, immobilization in a plaster cast. (See also *Stress fracture*.)

Marfan's syndrome

A rare, inherited disorder of connective tissue that results in abnormalities of the skeleton, heart, and eyes. The incidence of Marfan's syndrome is about two cases per 100,000 people. The precise cause is unknown.

SYMPTOMS AND SIGNS
The features of Marfan's syndrome usually appear after age 10. Affected people grow very tall and thin, the fingers are long and spidery, the chest and spine are often deformed, and the tendons, ligaments, and joint capsules are weak, leaving the sufferer "double-jointed" and prone to joint

Features of Marfan's syndrome
One of the characteristic features of Marfan's syndrome is long, thin, "spider" fingers (arachnodactyly).

dislocation. In 90 percent of cases, the heart or aorta (major blood vessel leading from the heart) is abnormal; in over 60 percent of sufferers, the lens of the eye is dislocated.

DIAGNOSIS
There are no specific diagnostic tests for the syndrome; *echocardiography* may be used to examine the valve deformities in the heart. An eye examination may also be performed.

TREATMENT AND OUTLOOK
Orthopedic braces or surgery may be required to correct spinal deformity. Beta-blockers (such as propranolol) may help control heart problems, but heart surgery is sometimes necessary.

Affected people should receive genetic counseling; there is a 50 percent chance that their offspring will inherit the disease. Women with Marfan's syndrome risk heart complications if they become pregnant.

Sufferers usually do not live beyond 50, with death often caused by heart failure or rupture of the aorta.

Marijuana

The dried leaves and flowering tops of the Indian hemp plant CAN-NABIS SATIVA. Marijuana contains the active ingredient THC (tetrahydrocannabinol), which is also found in cannabis resin (hashish). The chopped leaves are usually smoked alone as a joint, or "reefer," but can be taken as tea or in food.

EFFECTS
When marijuana is smoked, effects occur within minutes and last for an hour or more. When eaten, one half to one hour usually elapses before effects are felt, and they may last for three to five hours.

Physical effects include a dry mouth, mild reddening of the eyes, slight clumsiness, and increased appetite. The main subjective feelings are usually of well-being and calmness, although depression occasionally occurs. Users become dreamy and relaxed, laughing readily and experiencing time as passing very slowly. Sights and sounds become more vivid, imagination increases, and random connections between things seem more relevant.

Large doses may result in panicky states, fear of death, and illusions. Rarely, true psychosis (loss of contact with reality) occurs, producing paranoid delusions, confusion, and other symptoms. These symptoms usually disappear within several days if triggered by the drug, which may

M

merely be acting on an underlying illness. A more permanent state of apathy and loss of concern—the amotivational syndrome—has been attributed to prolonged, regular use.

There is evidence that regular users of marijuana can become physically dependent on its effects. Whether the drug causes brain or other physical damage is much debated. Possession and use of marijuana is subject to legal controls, which vary from state to state.

Marital counseling

Professional therapy for married couples or established partners that is aimed at resolving problems in relationships. Usually the partners attend sessions together on a regular basis. The counselor promotes communication and sorts out differences between the partners.

HOW IT IS DONE

Marital therapy today is largely based on the ideas and methods of *behavior therapy*. It assumes that behavior in a relationship is learned; it also is based on the idea that both people are responsible for problems because they have either failed to reinforce desirable behavior in the partner or have failed to respond themselves with appropriate behavior.

Therapy starts by analyzing the good and bad aspects of the relationship, and then by detailing clearly how each partner would like the other to behave. A contract may be drawn up in which each person agrees to do something that the other wants. Alternatively, each person may be given a supply of tokens, which are used to reward the partner for pleasing or helpful behavior.

EFFECTIVENESS

Although behavioral marital therapy may seem superficial and ineffective, it has radically altered behavior and marital happiness. Research evidence shows that it may be more effective than lengthy personal analysis.

Marrow, bone

See *Bone marrow*.

Marsupialization

A surgical procedure used to drain an abscess of a *Bartholin's gland* (glands on either side of the entrance to the vagina) and to prevent further abscesses from developing. Marsupialization involves cutting out part of the abscess wall and a small piece of vaginal tissue, then stitching the opened abscess wall to the vaginal

wall, forming a pouch. This maneuver is also used to drain certain pancreatic cysts into the bowel.

Masculinization

See *Virilization*.

Masochism

A desire to be physically, mentally, or emotionally abused. The term is derived from the name of the 19th century Austrian novelist Leopold von Sacher-Masoch.

Masochism is often used specifically to refer to the achievement of sexual excitement exclusively or preferably by means of one's own suffering. Activities include bondage, flagellation, and verbal abuse. The condition is usually chronic, and may be life-threatening when people increase the severity of their masochistic acts.

Masochists rarely seek professional treatment; when they do, it is usually at the instigation of a spouse who threatens to leave. (See also *Sadism*; *Sadomasochism*.)

Massage

Rubbing and kneading areas of the body, usually using the hands. Massage is used to relieve painful muscle spasm, treat muscle injury, reduce edema (fluid retention in tissue), and, in the treatment of scars, to prevent tethering of skin and underlying tissue. Massage increases blood flow, reduces pain by counter-irritation (alleviation of deep-seated pain by irritation of nerve endings in the skin), relaxes muscles, and increases the suppleness of the skin.

Mast cell

 A type of cell that plays an important part in the body's allergic response (see *Allergy*). Mast cells are present in most body tissues, but are particularly numerous in connective tissue, such as the dermis (innermost layer) of the skin.

In an allergic response, an allergen stimulates the release of antibodies, which attach themselves to mast cells.

M

SELF-MASSAGE
Although massage is most effective when carried out by another person, self-massage can still be useful; for example, it may help to alleviate pain caused by muscular tension.

Kneading the lower back
For self-massage of the lower back, the hands should be placed with the thumbs pointing forward, and the fingertips close together at the back. Firm finger pressure is required to massage this area.

Finger kneading of the neck and foot
For neck massage, the elbows are rested on a firm surface, such as a table, and the head is supported with one hand while the fingertips of the other hand knead the back and side of the neck. After one side of the neck has been massaged, switch hands and massage the other side. The foot contains few muscles, but many nerve endings, so foot massage is often very soothing.

As a result, the mast cells release substances such as *histamine* (a chemical responsible for allergic symptoms) into the tissue.

Mastectomy

Surgical removal of all or part of the breast. Mastectomy is usually performed to treat *breast cancer* and is often followed by a course of *radiation therapy* or *anticancer drugs*.

The amount of breast and surrounding tissue that is removed depends on the size and location of the tumor, how much the cancer has spread, and the age and health of the patient. The final choice of treatment should be a matter for discussion between the woman and her physician.

TYPES

Until the late 1960s, the standard operation was the radical mastectomy, which involves removal of the affected breast, the chest muscles, all chest and underarm lymph nodes, and additional fat and skin from the chest. When certain chest muscles are left intact, the operation is known as a modified radical mastectomy.

Today, surgeons more often recommend lumpectomy (in which only cancerous tissue is removed) or a quadrantectomy (in which one quadrant of the breast is removed). Another alternative is simple mastectomy, which consists of removing the affected breast and sometimes a portion of the underarm lymph nodes. If possible, surgeons leave the overlying skin intact, or leave plenty of surrounding skin, to allow the breast to be reconstructed.

HOW IT IS DONE

Each of the operations is performed using general anesthesia. For lumpectomy and quadrantectomy, an incision is made over the breast lump, which is cut free and removed (with or without surrounding tissue).

For simple mastectomy, leaving the skin intact, an incision is made along the perimeter of the breast closest to the tumor. For more extensive operations, the incision extends from the armpit to encompass the entire breast. Underlying tissue is then cut free and removed, and a drainage tube is inserted. In all cases, the skin is closed with stitches or clips, which are usually removed after a week. A skin graft is sometimes needed.

RECOVERY PERIOD

Patients can usually go home one to two days after lumpectomy and quadrantectomy, and can resume most activities within two weeks.

TYPES OF MASTECTOMY

The type of operation depends on many factors, including the location of the tumor and the woman's health.

A small tumor may be treated by lumpectomy; other cases may require more extensive surgery.

LUMPECTOMY

Only the area of cancerous tissue is removed. Lumpectomy is the least invasive procedure and leaves the breast looking normal.

QUADRANTECTOMY

The cancerous tissue plus a wedge of surrounding tissue is removed. The lymph nodes in the armpit may also be removed. The breast is slightly smaller after the operation.

SIMPLE MASTECTOMY

An incision is made under the breast and internal breast tissue is removed, leaving most of the skin intact. The nipple is not involved, but the milk ducts leading to it are cut. In some cases, the appearance of the breast is restored by immediate insertion of a silicone rubber implant. More often, however, this is done later.

TOTAL MASTECTOMY

1 A large elliptical incision, encompassing the nipple and sometimes the entire breast, is made. The incision extends into the armpit.

2 All the breast tissue, including the skin and some of the fat, is dissected (cut out) down to the chest muscles. The dissection is continued under the skin into the armpit, to free the upper and outer "tail" of breast tissue with its lymph nodes. All bleeding vessels are tied off before inserting a drainage tube and closing the skin with stitches or clips.

3 The scar after the operation. The woman may wear a prosthesis or may have a silicone implant inserted later.

After other operations, the hospital stay is usually several days, with the drainage tube being removed on the second or third day. Analgesics (painkillers) may be necessary for the first week.

OUTLOOK

Healing is usually very good after lumpectomy and quadrantectomy, with no noticeable scarring. Wound infection is uncommon. Skin scars after more radical procedures may be extensive, but usually fade within a year. Possible long-term complications, particularly of radical mastectomy, include *lymphedema* (accumulation of fluid under the skin) and stiffness of the arm and shoulder.

M

If the entire breast has been removed, the woman may decide to be fitted with a prosthesis (artificial breast). A temporary prosthesis may be worn until the chest scars have healed, when a more permanent prosthesis can be fitted. Alternatively, a plastic silicone implant can be inserted either at the end of the mastectomy operation or at a later operation (see *Mammoplasty*).

Mastication

The process of chewing food. Mastication consists of two stages. In the first, the canines and incisors (front teeth) shear the food. In the second, the tongue pushes the food between the upper and lower premolars and molars (back teeth) to be ground by side-to-side and circular movements of the lower jaws. At the same time, saliva is mixed with the food to help break it down for swallowing.

Any food that spills over between the gums and cheeks is scooped up by rhythmic contractions of the cheeks and lips. The muscles of mastication, which attach the lower jaw to the rest of the skull, are controlled by signals from sensory nerves in the mouth to prevent undue stress on tooth-supporting tissues.

Only gross irregularities in the positional relationship of upper to lower teeth (see *Malocclusion*) prevent normal mastication.

Mastitis

Inflammation of breast tissue often caused by bacterial infection.

CAUSES

Mastitis usually occurs during breast-feeding when bacteria enter the breast through the nipple (especially if it is cracked). Infection with the *mumps* virus is another cause of mastitis.

Changes in levels of sex hormones can cause mastitis in the newborn (due to high levels of hormones from the mother's circulation) and at the start of puberty. Hormonal variations may also be the cause of chronic mastitis in women who are prone to lumpy breasts. This common disorder is known as fibrocystic disease of the breast, fibroadenosis, cystic mastitis, benign mammary dysplasia, or benign breast disease.

SYMPTOMS

Pain, tenderness, and swelling occur in all types of mastitis and may be present in one or both breasts.

In mastitis caused by bacterial infection during breast-feeding, the breasts become red and engorged. The prob-lem tends to occur during the first month of breast-feeding and may result in a breast abscess.

Symptoms of acute mastitis in babies and at puberty usually last for only a few weeks and clear up without specific treatment.

In chronic mastitis, there may be diffuse lumpiness of the breasts or a single breast lump caused by an overgrowth of glandular and fibrous tissue and sometimes resulting in cysts. There may also be a feeling of heaviness in the breast and, occasionally, a discharge from the nipple. The symptoms are worse during the second half of the menstrual cycle and usually affect the upper, outer part of the breast.

DIAGNOSIS AND TREATMENT

If the cause of mastitis is unknown, *mammography* may be performed or a *biopsy* (removal of a small piece of tissue for examination) of a breast lump carried out to exclude the possibility of cancer.

Acute mastitis caused by infection is treated with *antibiotic drugs*, *analgesics* (painkillers), and *expressing milk* to relieve engorgement. Breast-feeding should be continued unless pus begins to drain from the nipple. If a breast abscess develops, it requires surgical drainage.

Breast tenderness caused by chronic mastitis generally requires no specific treatment, although *diuretic drugs* may relieve symptoms. If symptoms are severe, progesterone, danazol, or bromocriptine may be prescribed. Any cysts in the breast may be aspirated (drained by a needle and syringe).

Mastocytosis

An unusual condition, also called urticaria pigmentosa, characterized by numerous itchy, irregular, yellow or orange-brown swellings on the skin. Mastocytosis may affect any part of the body but is most commonly found on the trunk; it is worse after bathing or scratching.

Mastocytosis usually begins in the first year of life and disappears by adolescence. Treatment is difficult, although *antihistamine drugs* sometimes help.

Mastoid bone

The prominent bone behind the ear. Projecting from the temporal bone of the skull, it is honeycombed with air cells, which are connected to a cavity in the upper part of the bone called the mastoid antrum. This bone, in turn, is connected to the middle ear. As a result, infections of the middle ear (see *Otitis media*) occasionally spread through the mastoid bone to cause acute *mastoiditis*.

Mastoiditis

Inflammation of the *mastoid bone*, the prominent bone behind the ear.

CAUSE AND INCIDENCE

The disease is caused by the spread of infection from the middle ear (see *Otitis media*) to the antrum (a cavity in the mastoid bone), and from there to a honeycomb of air cells in the bone.

Mastoiditis has been uncommon since the advent of antibiotic drugs, which control middle-ear infection.

SYMPTOMS AND SIGNS

Mastoiditis causes severe pain, swelling, and tenderness behind the ear, as well as pain within the ear. These symptoms are usually accompanied by fever, a creamy discharge from the ear, progressive hearing loss, and some displacement of the outer ear.

COMPLICATIONS

There is always a risk that the infection may spread to inside the skull, causing *meningitis*, *brain abscess*, or blood clotting in veins within the brain. The infection may also spread outward to damage the facial nerve and cause *facial palsy*.

DIAGNOSIS AND TREATMENT

Prompt diagnosis, based on a physical examination, is essential because of the possible complications.

Treatment is with antibiotics, which usually clear up the infection. If the infection persists, an operation known as a mastoidectomy may be necessary. This procedure involves

M

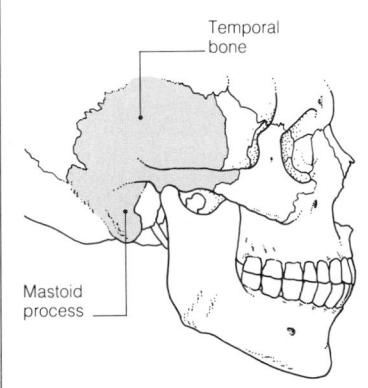

LOCATION OF MASTOID BONE
Forming the prominence behind the ear, the mastoid process (bone) is not a separate bone but is part of the temporal bone.

Temporal bone

Mastoid process

making an incision behind the ear, opening up the mastoid bone, and removing the infected air cells. The wound is stitched up around a drainage tube, which is removed a day or two later.

Masturbation

Sexual self-stimulation, usually to orgasm. It is now accepted as a normal behavior, particularly among teenagers and young adults. Over 90 percent of men and about 65 percent of women masturbate at some time during their lives. Massaging the penis or clitoris with the hand is the usual method.

There is no evidence that masturbation causes any physical or psychological harm, despite the 19th-century belief that it caused insanity, blindness, or other disorders. This notion may have been based on the observation that people who are severely retarded or suffering from *schizophrenia* sometimes masturbate publicly. Such behavior is a sign, not a cause, of mental illness that also occurs in *dementia* and other forms of brain damage.

Maternal mortality

The death of a woman during pregnancy or within 42 days of *childbirth*, *miscarriage*, or elective *abortion* from any cause related to, or made worse by, pregnancy. Maternal mortality is the number of such deaths per year per 100,000 (or sometimes per 1,000 or 10,000) pregnancies.

CAUSES

Maternal deaths may occur as a direct result of complications of pregnancy, or as an indirect result of a medical condition that has been aggravated by pregnancy. The principal direct causes include *pulmonary embolism* (blood clots in the lungs), *hypertension* (high blood pressure), *antepartum hemorrhage* or *postpartum hemorrhage*, *ectopic pregnancy* (development of the fetus outside the uterus), *eclampsia* (a condition characterized by seizures during late pregnancy), abortion, miscarriage, or *cesarean section*, and *puerperal sepsis* (infection of the uterus after childbirth). Important indirect causes are heart disease, *anemia*, *hyperthyroidism* (overactivity of the thyroid gland) or *hypothyroidism* (underactivity of the thyroid gland), *diabetes mellitus*, and some cancers.

RELATED FACTORS

Maternal mortality is highest for the first pregnancy, and for the fifth and subsequent pregnancies. It is also greater in women who are younger than 20 or older than 30. Statistically, it is safest for a woman to have her first baby when she is between 20 and 25 years old; it becomes increasingly less safe after age 30.

Social factors also play a part. Maternal mortality is higher among poor, less well-educated women, and is greater in blacks than in whites. Maternal mortality generally is greater among women who do not receive adequate prenatal care.

TRENDS

Maternal mortality has decreased considerably since about the 1940s. In the US, the death rate has fallen from 74 per 100,000 pregnancies in 1950, to eight per 100,000 in 1983. This dramatic decline is due largely to social improvements, better obstetric care, the development of antibiotics and other drugs to combat infection, and the availability of blood transfusions. In addition, because of the ready availability of contraception, fewer women than formerly have a large number of pregnancies.

Maxilla

One of a pair of bones that forms the upper jaw. At their base the maxillas carry the upper teeth and form the roof of the mouth; at the top they form the floor of the orbits (the sockets that contain the eyes). Each bone contains a large air-filled cavity (called the maxillary sinus) that is connected to the nasal cavity.

LOCATION OF THE MAXILLA
The maxilla is one of a pair of bones that together form the center of the face, the upper jaw, and the roof of the mouth.

Maxilla   Mandible

DISORDERS

The most common disorder affecting the maxilla is *sinusitis* (inflammation of the mucous membrane that lines the maxillary sinuses), usually caused by infection spreading from the nose. Severe sinusitis occasionally leads to *osteomyelitis* (bone infection).

The maxilla is often fractured in motor vehicle accidents, causing a variety of facial deformities, such as backward displacement of the teeth or caving in of the center of the face. Immediate surgery to reposition and secure the bones is necessary to prevent permanent disfigurement.

Various kinds of tumors may develop in the maxillary sinus; 80 percent of them are malignant, and they may eventually alter the shape of the jaw, loosen the teeth, block one of the nasolacrimal ducts (causing the eye to water), push the eyeball upward or outward, or block the nose and cause a bloody, offensive-smelling discharge. Treatment is by *radiation therapy*, followed by surgical removal of the maxilla. About one third of sufferers survive for five years.

McArdle's disease

A rare genetic disorder characterized by muscular stiffness and painful cramps that increase during and after exertion. McArdle's disease is caused by a deficiency of the enzyme in muscle cells that stimulates the breakdown of *glycogen* (a complex carbohydrate) to glucose (a type of sugar). This deficiency results in a build up of glycogen within the muscle tissue and prevents the release of glucose as an essential source of energy during exercise.

Symptoms usually start between the ages of 20 and 30. Myoglobinuria (muscle cell pigment in the urine) occurs because of the damage to muscle cells; rarely, it is severe enough to cause *renal failure*. Affected people are usually healthy apart from the need to restrict their exercise.

There is no treatment, although symptoms may be helped by eating glucose or fructose before exercise.

Measles

A distressing viral illness that causes a characteristic rash and a fever. Measles mainly affects children but can occur at any age. One attack usually confers lifelong immunity.

CAUSES AND INCIDENCE

The measles virus is highly infective and is spread primarily by airborne droplets of nasal secretions. There is

M

an incubation period of nine to 11 days before symptoms appear. Infected children can transmit the virus from shortly after the start of this period up to one week following the development of symptoms. Infants under 8 months old are rarely affected because they have acquired some immunity from their mothers.

Measles was once very common throughout the world, occurring in epidemics. It is now less common in developed countries due to immunization. In the US, where proof of immunization is required before a child can attend school, there are several thousand cases reported annually. Prevention of the illness is important because it can have rare but serious complications. It may also be serious, or fatal, in children with impaired immunity (e.g., those being treated for leukemia).

In developing countries, measles is still common, accounting for more than 1 million deaths a year, especially in malnourished children whose defenses against infection are seriously impaired.

SYMPTOMS AND SIGNS

The illness starts with a fever, runny nose, sore eyes, and cough, and the sufferer is sick. After three to four days a red rash appears, usually starting on the head and neck and spreading downward to cover the whole body. The spots sometimes join to produce large red blotchy areas, and the lymph glands may be enlarged. After three days the rash starts to fade and symptoms subside.

The most common complications are ear and chest infections, which usually occur with a return of fever two to three days after appearance of the rash. Diarrhea, vomiting, and abdominal pain also occur. A more serious complication, occurring in about one in 1,000 cases, is *encephalitis* (inflammation of the brain). It causes headache, drowsiness, and vomiting, starting seven to 10 days after the rash appears. Seizures and coma may follow, sometimes leading to mental retardation or death (however, seizures are common with measles and do not necessarily indicate encephalitis).

Very rarely (in about one in a million cases) a progressive brain disorder (subacute sclerosing panencephalitis) develops years after the acute illness.

Measles during pregnancy results in death of the fetus in about one fifth of cases. There is no evidence that measles causes birth defects.

TREATMENT

Plenty of fluids should be given and acetaminophen taken to treat the fever. Antibiotics are not routinely required but may be needed to treat secondary infections.

IMMUNIZATION

In the US, children are routinely immunized early in the second year of life. The vaccine is given by injection (usually combined with mumps and rubella vaccine), producing immunity in 97 percent of people. Side effects of the vaccine are generally mild. There may be a low fever, slight cold, and rash about one week after vaccination.

The vaccine should not be given to children under age 1 or to those with any of the usual risk factors for vaccination (see *Immunization*). The vaccine may induce a seizure in children who have had one before and if there is a history of epilepsy in the family. In these cases simultaneous injection of measles-specific immunoglobulin (which contains antibodies against the virus) should be given.

A pregnant woman who has never had measles or been immunized against the disease should avoid people with measles. If she does come into contact with an infected person, she should be passively immunized against measles with *immunoglobulin* within five days.

Meatus

A canal or passageway through part of the body. The term usually refers to the external auditory meatus, the canal in the outer *ear* that leads from the outside to the eardrum.

Mebendazole

An *antihelmintic drug* used to treat *worm infestations* of the intestine. Mebendazole is under investigation as a treatment for worms that infest other areas, such as the lungs and liver (as in *hydatid disease*).

Possible adverse effects include abdominal pain and diarrhea.

Meckel's diverticulum

A common congenital anomaly of the digestive tract in which a small, hollow, wide-mouthed sac protrudes from the *ileum* (the final section of the small intestine). Meckel's diverticulum occurs in 2 percent of people.

There are usually no symptoms unless the diverticulum is affected by infection, obstruction, or ulceration. The most common symptom is painless bleeding, which may be sudden and severe, making immediate blood

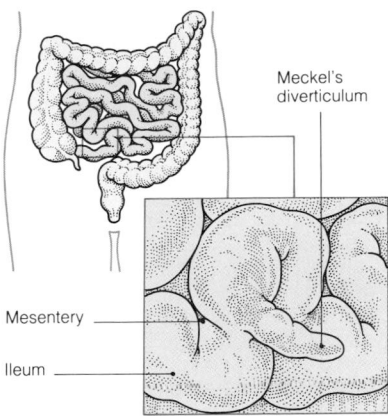

Anatomy of Meckel's diverticulum
In this birth defect, an appendixlike sac protrudes from the ileum (the last part of the small intestine).

transfusion necessary. Sometimes, inflammation causes symptoms so similar to those of acute *appendicitis* that the disorder is diagnosed only when abdominal surgery is carried out. A Meckel's diverticulum occasionally causes *intussusception* (telescoping) or *volvulus* (twisting) of the small intestine.

Disorders are treated by removal of the diverticulum.

Meclizine

An *antihistamine drug* used as an *antiemetic drug*. Meclizine is given to treat nausea, vomiting, and *vertigo* in *motion sickness* and *Meniere's disease* and when these symptoms are due to *anticancer drugs* or *radiation therapy*. Meclizine may cause drowsiness, dry mouth, and blurred vision.

Meclofenamate

A *nonsteroidal anti-inflammatory drug* (NSAID) used to relieve joint pain and stiffness in types of arthritis, such as *osteoarthritis* and *rheumatoid arthritis*. Meclofenamate produces adverse effects, such as diarrhea and nausea, and is normally prescribed only when similar drugs have proved ineffective.

Meconium

The thick, sticky, greenish-black feces passed by infants during the first day or two after birth. Meconium consists of bile, mucus, and sloughed intestinal cells. After the baby starts feeding, the feces gradually change in color and consistency.

Occasionally, the fetus passes meconium into the amniotic fluid in the uterus. This is more common in babies who experience *fetal distress* during labor or who are postmature (that is, over 40 weeks' gestation). Meconium in the amniotic fluid may be inhaled when the baby starts to breathe, sometimes blocking the airways and damaging the lungs.

In some babies with *cystic fibrosis*, the meconium is so thick and sticky that it blocks the intestine and causes intestinal obstruction.

Medial

A medical term meaning situated toward the midline of the body. Less commonly, the word is used to refer to the middle layer of a body structure, particularly of a blood vessel wall.

Median nerve

A branch of the *brachial plexus* (one of the main nerves of the arm) that runs down the arm's full length into the hand. The median nerve controls the muscles of the forearm and hand, which carry out bending movements of the wrist, fingers, and thumb, and which rotate the forearm palm-inward. This nerve also conveys sensations from the thumb, index finger, middle finger, part of the ring finger, and the region of the palm at the base of these digits.

DISORDERS

The nerve may be damaged where it originates from the brachial plexus as a result of injury to the shoulder, just above the wrist by a *Colles' fracture*, or by pressure on the nerve where it passes through the wrist (see *Carpal tunnel syndrome*). The principal symptoms of any damage are numbness and muscle weakness in the areas controlled by the nerve.

Mediastinoscopy

Investigation of the right side of the *mediastinum* (the central compartment of the chest containing the heart, esophagus, and trachea) by means of an *endoscope* (a viewing tube with a light and lens) inserted into the cavity through an incision in the neck. Because more of the heart occupies the left side of the mediastinal cavity, endoscopic investigation of this area is difficult and dangerous; *imaging techniques* are preferred.

Mediastinoscopy is used mainly to perform a *biopsy* (removal of a small sample of tissue for analysis) of a lymph gland to look for disease. Using a general anesthetic, an incision is made in the base of the neck and an endoscope is passed through it into the mediastinum. A tissue sample is

removed by minute blades at the end of the endoscope. After the instrument has been withdrawn, the incision is closed with stitches.

Mediastinum

The space between the lungs and the structures within that space. The mediastinum extends from the sternum (breastbone) in front to the spine behind, and from the inlet of the thoracic duct (one of the main lymphatic vessels) at the top to the diaphragm at the bottom.

It contains the *heart*, *trachea* (windpipe), *esophagus*, *thymus* gland, the major blood vessels entering and leaving the heart, *lymph nodes* and lymphatic vessels, and nerves (including the *vagus nerve* and *phrenic nerve*).

Medicaid

A term applied (in some states) to a federal program that provides funds to support state programs of medical assistance to people receiving or eligible for welfare. Programs vary widely from state to state. (See also *Medicare*.)

Medical examiner

A public official and physician (often a pathologist) who is responsible for determining causes of death not obviously due to natural causes. The medical examiner (a county office in most cases) has largely replaced the office of *coroner*.

Medicare

A federal program that finances medical care for certain dependents. Part A of the program covers many hospital services. Part B helps with physician charges, assuming a retired person elects to pay a monthly insurance premium. (See also *Medicaid*.)

Medication

A term used to describe any substance prescribed to treat illness. (See also *Drug*; *Medicine*.)

Medicine

The study of human diseases, including their causes, frequency, treatment, and prevention. The term is also applied to any substance prescribed to treat illness.

EARLY HISTORY

In many early cultures, medicine was closely associated with religion because disease was regarded as a punishment from the gods. As a result, the victim would turn for help to a priest, who took on the additional function of a medicine man. Medicine

probably became separated from religion with the emergence of people skilled in treating injuries such as broken bones and dislocated joints. These healers attracted patients and, in time, apprentices who wanted to learn the same skills.

By the fifth century BC, the Greek physician Hippocrates had established medicine as a profession with a body of learning and a code of ethics to be passed on to each new generation of physicians (the Hippocratic oath is still used as an ethical guide for the medical profession). The dominant figure after Hippocrates was the second-century, Greek-born Roman physician Galen, who made valuable contributions but whose many false theories about anatomy and physiology were uncritically accepted for more than 13 centuries; these theories effectively held back advances in medical knowledge.

RENAISSANCE DISCOVERIES

With the Renaissance, medicine began to emerge from its long period of stagnation. In 1543 the Flemish anatomist and physician Andreas Vesalius (1514-1564) produced the first truly accurate anatomical text; in 1628 the English physician William Harvey (1578-1657) first demonstrated how blood circulates through the body. Also in the 17th century, the Dutch microscopist Antonj van Leeuwenhoek (1632-1723) became the first to observe and describe microorganisms and the detailed structure of blood, muscles, and sperm.

MODERN MEDICINE

Despite the medical achievements of the Renaissance—and some notable later achievements, such as the English physician Edward Jenner's (1749-1823) discovery of the principle of vaccination in the late 18th century—it was not until the 19th century that the foundations of modern scientific medicine were laid. This was the result of a growing realization that medicine needed to become a true science, systematic in its approach and based on scrupulous observation and experimentation. Significant advances in other disciplines also played an important role. For example, the first practical high-powered microscope was developed during the 19th century; the ophthalmoscope (an instrument for examining the retina of the eye) was invented in 1851; the first practical thermometer was introduced in the 1860s; and X rays were discovered in 1896, an occurrence that revolutionized medical diagnosis. These developments, along with the French scientist Louis Pasteur's (1822-1895) work on the germ theory of disease, brought about an enormous advance in the understanding of a large number of diseases.

Curing and controlling disease was not a reality until the 20th century, however, when vaccines were developed against many serious diseases (including typhoid, cholera, and diphtheria); insecticides and improved sanitation helped control diseases such as malaria, yellow fever, and sleeping sickness.

The early 20th century was also marked by the development of safe anesthesia, effective surgery, and a steady growth in the number of new drugs. In the late 1930s, the first effective antibacterial drugs (the sulfonamides) were produced, followed in the 1940s by penicillin, streptomycin, and the tetracyclines; these drugs saved millions of lives.

Among the important recent developments are the introduction of sophisticated diagnostic techniques, such as MRI, CT scanning, and ultrasound scanning; more effective drugs and other treatments (such as radiation therapy) to treat a wider range of diseases and disorders; and developments in surgical techniques that have made it possible to transplant organs and rejoin severed nerves.

Today, the boundaries between medicine and other sciences are becoming progressively less distinct; medical research is being increasingly undertaken by scientists who have little or no formal medical training. (See also entries for individual medical, surgical, and scientific specialties.)

Medicolegal

Relating to aspects of medicine and law that overlap, particularly to medical matters that come before the courts. Among the matters on which medicolegal experts advise are the laws concerning damages for injuries due to medical negligence or malpractice, medical evidence concerning the extent of injury in a civil action, the use of tests in determining paternity, the mental competence of people who have drawn up wills, and restrictions on the liberty of the mentally ill.

In recent years, new areas of medicolegal study have emerged, notably an individual's right to die (see *Brain death*; *Euthanasia*; *Will, living*); the necessity for informed consent to any surgical procedure; the

legal aspects of *artificial insemination, in vitro fertilization, sterilization*, and *surrogacy*; and a person's right to confidentiality concerning his or her illness, particularly in the context of AIDS. (For medical aspects of criminal law, see *Forensic medicine*.)

Meditation

Concentration on an object, a word, or an idea with the intention of inducing an altered state of consciousness. Meditation of different kinds has traditionally been a feature of many religions, particularly Eastern ones.

At its deepest level, meditation can resemble a trance or be an all-engrossing spiritual experience. More commonly, it is a physically calming therapy for body and mind. Some clinical trials have shown that meditation can be a valuable therapy for reducing stress levels and in helping treat stress-related disorders. The most common form of meditation practiced in the west is transcendental meditation (TM), introduced by the Maharishi Mahesh Yogi in the 1960s.

Medroxyprogesterone

A *progesterone drug* used in the treatment of *endometriosis* and certain types of *breast cancer* and uterine cancer (see *Uterus, cancer of*). Medroxyprogesterone is occasionally given to treat menstrual disorders such as mid-cycle bleeding and *amenorrhea* (absence of menstruation). It is also given with an estrogen drug in *hormone replacement therapy* to reduce the risk of cancer of the uterus.

Injections of medroxyprogesterone are widely used as a contraceptive (see *Contraception, hormonal methods*) in developing countries; this use is not permitted in the US.

Possible adverse effects include weight gain, swollen ankles, and breast tenderness.

Medulla

The innermost part of an organ or body structure; the adrenal medulla is the central region of an adrenal gland, and the medulla of bone is the bone marrow. The term medulla is also sometimes used to refer to the medulla oblongata (part of the *brain stem* joining the spinal cord).

Medulla oblongata

Also known as the medulla, the medulla oblongata is the lowest part of the *brain stem*; it is situated in the skull between the pons (above) and the spinal cord (below).

Medulloblastoma

A type of malignant *brain tumor* that occurs mainly in children (in whom it is the most common type of brain tumor). The tumor usually arises from the cerebellum (the organ at the back of the brain concerned with posture and balance). It grows rapidly and may spread to other parts of the brain and spinal cord.

Several hundred cases of medulloblastoma are diagnosed each year in the US. Typically, a morning headache, repeated vomiting, and a clumsy gait develop, with frequent falls caused by disturbance of the function of the cerebellum. The tumor is diagnosed by *CT scanning* or *MRI* and often responds to *radiation therapy*. This, combined with surgery and the use of *anticancer drugs*, often allows survival for five years or more.

Mefenamic acid

A *nonsteroidal anti-inflammatory drug* (NSAID) used to relieve pain after a minor operation, injury to soft tissues (such as muscles and ligaments), or joint pain and stiffness caused by types of arthritis (including *osteoarthritis* and *rheumatoid arthritis*). It is also used to relieve the pain that can occur with menstruation.

Possible adverse effects include abdominal pain, nausea, vomiting, and, after prolonged use, a *peptic ulcer*.

Mega-

A prefix meaning very large, as in *megacolon*, a condition in which the colon (part of the large intestine) is greatly enlarged. The prefix megalo- is synonymous with mega-.

Megacolon

A grossly distended colon usually accompanied by severe, chronic constipation. Megacolon may be present at birth or may develop later in life; it occurs in all age groups.

CAUSES
In children, the main causes are *Hirschsprung's disease* (congenital absence of nerve cells in part of the colon), *anal fissures*, and psychological factors that may have developed at the time of toilet-training.

In the elderly, megacolon may be caused by long-term use of powerful laxatives, particularly those containing senna, rhubarb, or cascara.

People suffering from chronic depression or schizophrenia, particularly if they live in an institution, often suffer from megacolon. Other rarer causes include *Chagas' disease*,

M

hypothyroidism, neurological disorders (for example, spinal cord injury), and certain drugs (notably the narcotics morphine and codeine).

SYMPTOMS

The symptoms are severe constipation and abdominal bloating; some sufferers lose their appetite, which may result in weight loss. Occasionally there is diarrhea, caused by a leakage of semiliquid feces around the obstructing hard stools.

DIAGNOSIS

The condition is diagnosed by proctoscopic examination of the rectum (see *Proctoscopy*), *barium X-ray examination*, tests of bowel muscle function, and, if Hirschsprung's disease is suspected, *biopsy* (removal of a small sample of tissue for examination) of the large intestine.

TREATMENT

In severe cases, impacted feces are removed manually. Often, however, the large intestine can be emptied by saline enemas.

Megalomania

An exaggerated sense of one's own importance or ability. It may take the form of a *delusion* of grandeur (such as believing oneself to be Napoleon) or of a desire to organize activities that are expensive, large in scale, and involving many people (for example, leasing an ocean liner for a party). Megalomania is not a formal category of psychiatric illness, although such bizarre ideas and behavior often occur in *mania*.

-megaly

A suffix meaning enlargement, as in *acromegaly*, a condition in which there is enlargement of the skull, jaw, hands, and feet during adulthood as a result of excessive production of growth hormone in the fore part of the pituitary gland.

Megestrol

A *progesterone drug* used to treat certain types of *breast cancer* and uterine cancer (see *Uterus, cancer of*). Megestrol is usually prescribed when a tumor cannot be removed by surgery, if a tumor has recurred after surgery, or when other *anticancer drugs* or *radiation therapy* is ineffective.

Possible adverse effects include swollen ankles, loss of appetite, headache, dizziness, rash, and elevation of the blood's calcium level.

Meibomian cyst

See *Chalazion*.

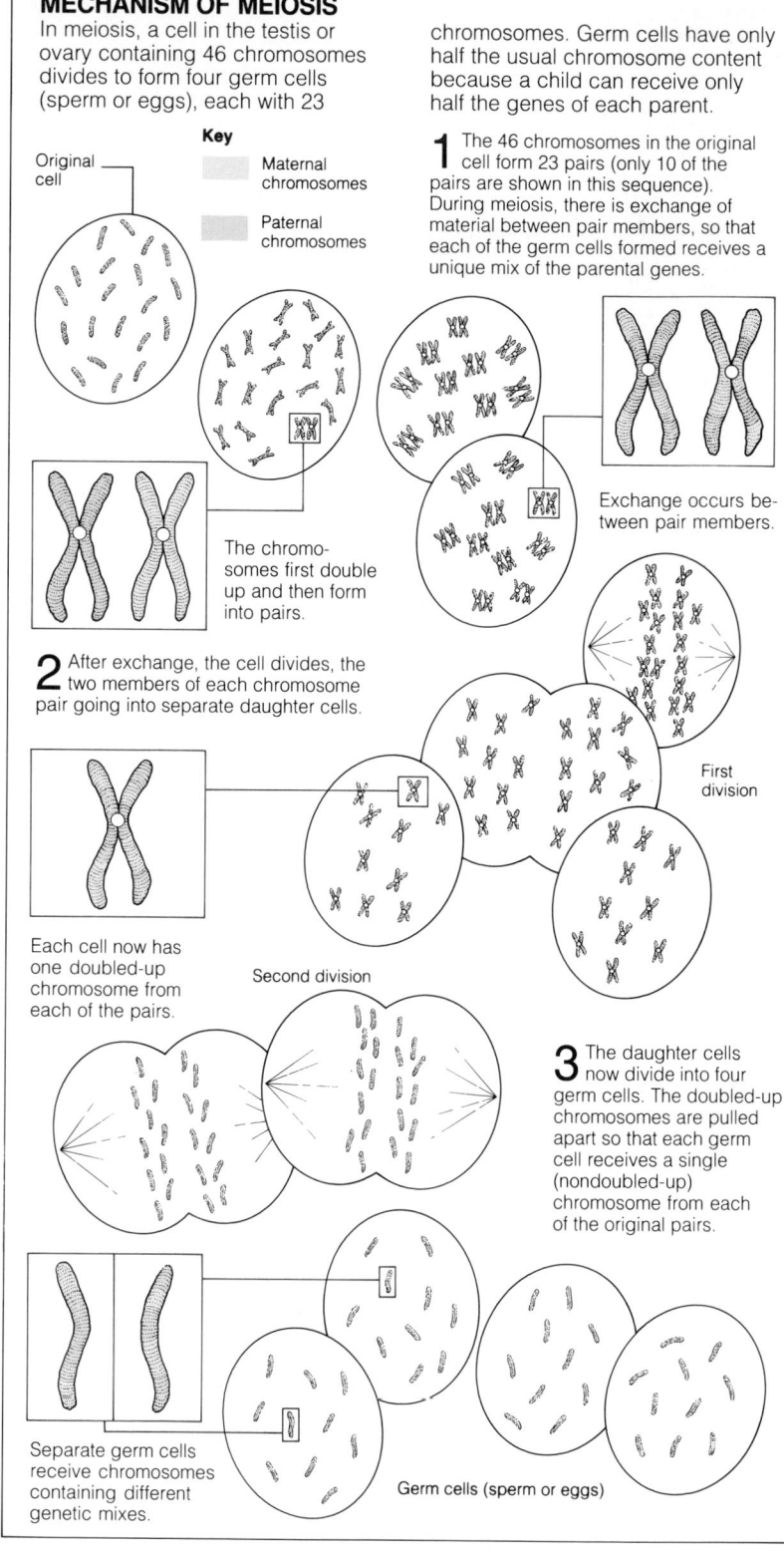

MECHANISM OF MEIOSIS

In meiosis, a cell in the testis or ovary containing 46 chromosomes divides to form four germ cells (sperm or eggs), each with 23 chromosomes. Germ cells have only half the usual chromosome content because a child can receive only half the genes of each parent.

Key
- Maternal chromosomes
- Paternal chromosomes

1 The 46 chromosomes in the original cell form 23 pairs (only 10 of the pairs are shown in this sequence). During meiosis, there is exchange of material between pair members, so that each of the germ cells formed receives a unique mix of the parental genes.

Original cell

Exchange occurs between pair members.

The chromosomes first double up and then form into pairs.

2 After exchange, the cell divides, the two members of each chromosome pair going into separate daughter cells.

First division

Each cell now has one doubled-up chromosome from each of the pairs.

Second division

3 The daughter cells now divide into four germ cells. The doubled-up chromosomes are pulled apart so that each germ cell receives a single (nondoubled-up) chromosome from each of the original pairs.

Separate germ cells receive chromosomes containing different genetic mixes.

Germ cells (sperm or eggs)

Meibomianitis

An inflammation of the glands on the eyelid, which causes the normal, oily secretion to thicken. Meibomianitis usually affects middle-aged people, often those with *blepharitis* (inflammation of the eyelid), and frequently leads to recurrent meibomian cysts (see *Chalazion*).

Meigs' syndrome

A rare condition in which *ascites* (fluid in the abdominal cavity) or a *pleural effusion* (fluid around one of the lungs) accompanies a tumor of the ovary. The fluid usually disappears with removal of the tumor.

Meiosis

A special type of cell division that occurs only within the ovaries and testes. The cells that undergo meiotic division are the forerunners of egg and sperm cells.

In meiosis, the *chromosomes* (inherited genetic material) within the nucleus of a cell are first duplicated. In the course of two successive cell divisions, the chromosomal material is then divided into four parts, each part going into one of four daughter cells. The four daughter cells each acquire only half of the original cell's chromosomal material, and each daughter cell acquires a different "selection" of this material. Consequently, every egg and sperm formed in the ovary or testis is different in its chromosomal content. As a result of meiosis, parents contribute exactly half of their chromosomal material (genes) to each child, and the selection that each child receives is unique.

Meiosis differs fundamentally from *mitosis*, the more common and simpler method of cell division, in which a cell's chromosomes are exactly duplicated in one division into two daughter cells.

Melancholia

An old term for *depression* derived from the Greek word for black bile, an excess of which was believed to be the cause of low spirits. Melancholia is used today to refer to certain symptoms that occur in severe depression. These include loss of pleasure in most activities, lack of reaction to pleasurable stimuli, and inappropriate guilt feelings.

Melanin

The yellow, brown, or black pigment that gives skin, hair, and the iris of the eyes their coloring. The amount of melanin present in a person depends on race and on exposure to sunlight. The pigment is produced by cells called melanocytes, whose activity is controlled by a hormone secreted by the pituitary gland in the brain.

Exposure to sunlight increases the production of melanin, protecting the skin against the harmful effects of ultraviolet rays and darkening skin color in the process.

Localized overproduction of melanin in the skin can result in a pigmented spot called a *nevus*, of which moles and freckles are the most common examples.

Melanoma, juvenile

A raised, reddish-brown skin blemish that sometimes appears on the face or legs in early childhood. A juvenile melanoma is a form of *nevus* that grows rapidly up to almost 1 inch (about 2 cm) across. Most juvenile melanomas are harmless. However, if the growth is unsightly, or if the physician suspects skin cancer, the melanoma can be removed surgically.

Melanoma, malignant

The most serious of the three types of skin cancer (the other two being *basal cell carcinoma* and *squamous cell carcinoma*). Malignant melanoma occurs in the melanocytes, the cells that produce *melanin* (the pigment that colors the skin, hair, and the iris of the eyes).

Development of malignant melanoma
Only one mole in a million becomes malignant, but change of shape, darkening, tenderness, pain, itching, or ulceration are warning signs.

CAUSES AND INCIDENCE
Malignant melanomas account for 2 percent of all cancers that occur and are most common in middle-aged and elderly people with pale skin who have been exposed to strong sunlight for many years.

In the US, the incidence varies with latitude from 22,500 cases per year in the northern states to 65,000 cases in the south. This incidence appears to be rising, probably due to increased recreational exposure to sunlight.

SYMPTOMS AND SIGNS
The growth usually develops on exposed areas of skin, but may occur anywhere on the body, including under the nails and in the eye (see *Eye tumors*). The melanoma usually grows from an existing mole, which may enlarge, become lumpy, bleed, change color, develop a spreading black edge, turn into a scab, or begin to itch. Occasionally, a tumor may develop on normal skin.

DIAGNOSIS AND TREATMENT
Because the tumor is highly malignant and often spreads to other parts of the body, early diagnosis is essential. The diagnosis is made by a skin *biopsy* (removal of a small sample of tissue for microscopic analysis).

Treatment consists of excising (cutting out) the melanoma. To avoid an unsightly scar on exposed areas, a *skin graft* may be carried out at the same time. *Radiation therapy* or *anticancer drugs* may also be necessary.

Melanosis coli

Black or brown discoloration of the lining of the colon, associated with chronic constipation and the use of certain laxatives (e.g., senna, rhubarb, and cascara) in chronic constipation.

Melanosis coli is most common in the elderly and usually produces no symptoms. The discoloration disappears after laxatives are stopped. Rarely, the condition is associated with cancer of the colon.

Melasma

See *Chloasma*.

Melena

Black, tarry feces caused by bleeding, usually in the upper gastrointestinal tract (esophagus, stomach, or duodenum). The blood is blackened by the action of secretions during digestion. Melena is a sign that should never be ignored. It is usually caused by a *peptic ulcer*, but may be an indication of cancer (or other disorders) of the stomach or of the cecum. (An intake of iron, bismuth, or licorice may also color the feces black.)

Melioidosis

An infectious disease, similar to *glanders*, caused by a bacterium that lives in soil and lakes. Melioidosis does not occur in the US and Europe but has been reported in Asia, Africa, and Australia. It may cause a high fever

M

and symptoms of pneumonia. Given early, antibiotics can cure the illness, but in some cases it is rapidly fatal.

Melphalan

An *anticancer drug* used mainly in the treatment of *multiple myeloma* (a cancer of the bone marrow). Melphalan is also prescribed to treat certain types of *breast cancer* and ovarian cancer (see *Ovary, cancer of*).

Possible adverse effects include nausea, vomiting, sore throat, and loss of appetite. Melphalan may also cause aplastic anemia, abnormal bleeding, and increased susceptibility to infection.

Membrane

A layer of tissue, often very thin, that covers a body surface (such as the *meninges*, which cover the surface of the brain); lines a cavity (such as the *peritoneum*, which lines the abdominal cavity); divides a space or organ (such as the tympanic membrane, or eardrum, which separates the *ear* canal from the middle ear); or forms the boundaries of individual *cells*.

Memory

The ability to remember what has happened in the past. It is a complex process, usually thought of as having three stages—registration, long-term memory, and recall (see box).

Many factors determine how well something is remembered, including its familiarity and how much attention has been paid to it. Techniques advertised for improving memory are generally based on teaching people methods of improving their coding systems by consciously associating new material with what is already known. For example, a person might be taught to visualize a well-known street and then think of each building as representing a new fact.

MECHANISM OF MEMORY

It is not known where in the brain the memory process takes place. There seems to be no set memory area; stimulating the brain with electrodes can evoke different memories from the same site. However, disturbances of the temporal lobe and limbic lobe typically cause memory disorders. Stimulation of a particular part of the temporal lobe in patients with temporal lobe *epilepsy* may consistently evoke the same memory.

The mechanisms for storing memory also are unknown. Memory may be held within the chemical structure of some substance within brain

THE STAGES OF MEMORY

Stage 1
In the first stage, known as registration, information is perceived and understood. It is then retained in a short-term memory system that seems to be very limited in the amount of material it can store at one time. Unless refreshed by constant repetition, the contents of short-term memory are lost within minutes, to be replaced by other material.

Stage 2
If information is important enough, it may be transferred into the long-term memory, where the process of storage involves associations with words or meanings, with the visual imagery evoked by it, or with other experiences, such as smell or sound.

Stage 3
The final stage is recall (or retrieval), in which information stored at an unconscious level is brought, at will, into the conscious mind. The reliability of recall depends on how well the material was coded at stage 2.

cells—possibly spare *DNA* that is not being utilized to hold the genetic code. Others stress the role of the brain's electrical circuits in memory storage.

A good memory is usually part of a high *IQ*, although some people have extraordinary "photographic" memories that are unrelated to their other intellectual abilities. Even some severely retarded people have phenomenal memories for specific types of information (the so-called "idiot savant"—learned idiot).

DISORDERS

Disturbances of memory can result from a problem at any of the three stages. Most disturbances involve an inability to recall past events due to failure at the retention or recall stage (see *Amnesia*). In some cases, the problem occurs at the registration stage (for example, in *mania* because the person's attention is continually distracted, or in *depression* as a result of preoccupation with personal thoughts and feelings). Some people with temporal lobe epilepsy have uncontrollable flashbacks of distant past events.

Memory, loss of

See *Amnesia*.

Menarche

The onset of *menstruation*. Menarche usually occurs around age 13, two or three years after the first physical signs of *puberty* start to appear.

Meniere's disease

A disorder of the inner ear characterized by recurrent *vertigo*, *deafness*, and *tinnitus* (ringing or buzzing in the ear). In 80 to 85 percent of cases, only one ear is affected.

CAUSES AND INCIDENCE

The disease is caused by an increase in the amount of fluid in the membranous labyrinth (the canals in the inner ear that control balance). This increase damages the labyrinth and sometimes the adjacent cochlea (a spiral organ that receives sound and transmits it to the brain). The cause of the fluid increase is not known in most cases. Meniere's disease is uncommon before age 50.

SYMPTOMS AND SIGNS

The main symptom is a sudden attack of vertigo, which may be so severe that the person falls to the ground. Vertigo is usually accompanied by nausea, vomiting, nystagmus (jerky eye movement), and, in the affected ear, deafness, tinnitus, and a feeling of pressure or pain. Attacks, which vary considerably in frequency, may last from a few minutes to several hours. However, the deafness and tinnitus tend to persist between the attacks of vertigo.

The cause of Meniere's disease
This condition is caused by excessive fluid in the middle ear, which may become damaged as a result.

DIAGNOSIS AND TREATMENT

Meniere's disease is usually diagnosed from the results of audiometry (see *Hearing tests*), a *caloric test*, and sometimes other tests.

During an attack, the person should rest in bed. An *antiemetic drug* (such as dimenhydrinate or cyclizine) may be given to relieve nausea and tinnitus.

Hearing tends to deteriorate progressively. If deafness becomes total, the other symptoms of the disease usually disappear.

Meninges

The three membranes that cover and protect the brain and the spinal cord. The outermost layer, the dura mater, is tough and fibrous; it lines the inside of the skull and forms a loose sheath around the spinal cord. The middle layer, the arachnoid mater, is elastic and weblike. It is separated from the innermost membrane, the pia mater, by the subarachnoid space, which contains *cerebrospinal fluid*. The pia mater is a thin layer that lies directly next to the brain and follows the folds and furrows of its surface.

Inflammation of the meninges, usually from infection, is called *meningitis*. Tumors of the meninges are called *meningiomas*.

ANATOMY OF THE MENINGES
The pia mater lies on the brain, separated from the arachnoid mater by the subarachnoid space. The dura mater lines the inside of the skull.

Arachnoid   Skull   Subdural space   Dura mater

Subarachnoid space

Pia mater   Brain

Meningioma

A benign *brain tumor* that develops from the meninges (protective coverings of the brain). The tumor arises from cells in the arachnoid (middle layer of the meninges) and usually becomes attached to the dura mater (outer layer).

Meningiomas are rare, with about one new case diagnosed annually per 100,000 population in the US. They may occur at any age. The tumor expands slowly, sometimes becoming large before it causes symptoms.

SYMPTOMS

Symptoms can include headache, vomiting, and impaired mental function from raised pressure within the skull; more specific symptoms include speech loss or visual disturbance due to pressure from the meningioma on underlying brain tissue. The tumor may invade the overlying bone, causing thickening and bulging of a region of the skull.

DIAGNOSIS AND TREATMENT

Meningiomas can be detected by skull *X ray*, *CT scanning*, and *MRI*. Because they are usually well demarcated from underlying brain tissue, meningiomas can often be completely removed by surgery. Tumors that cannot be removed surgically are treated by *radiation therapy*.

Meningitis

Inflammation of the *meninges* (the membranes that cover the brain and spinal cord) that usually results from infection by a variety of microorganisms. Viral meningitis is relatively mild; bacterial meningitis is life-threatening and needs prompt treatment.

CAUSES

The organisms that cause meningitis usually reach the meninges through the bloodstream from an infection elsewhere in the body. Less common means of transmission are through cavities in the skull from an infected ear or sinus, or from the air following a fractured skull.

INCIDENCE

Viral meningitis is far more common than bacterial meningitis, tending to occur in epidemics in the winter months. It affects between 9,000 and 12,000 people, mostly under the age of 30, in the US each year.

Meningococcal meningitis, the most common form of bacterial meningitis, sometimes occurs in small epidemics; more frequently, it occurs in isolated cases. It probably affects between 2,000 and 5,000 young

people—70 percent under the age of 5—in the US each year. Tuberculous meningitis, which is a less common type of bacterial meningitis, occurs particularly in young children in parts of the world where there is a high incidence of tuberculosis.

SYMPTOMS

The main symptoms are fever, severe headache, nausea and vomiting, dislike of light, and a stiff neck. In viral meningitis the symptoms are mild and may resemble influenza.

In meningococcal meningitis the main symptoms develop more rapidly, sometimes over a few hours, and are followed by drowsiness and sometimes loss of consciousness. In about half the cases there is also a red, blotchy skin rash.

In tuberculous meningitis, the sufferer may be sick for several weeks before the typical symptoms of meningitis develop.

DIAGNOSIS AND TREATMENT

Meningitis is diagnosed by *lumbar puncture* and the removal of a small sample of cerebrospinal fluid from the spinal cord for examination.

Viral meningitis requires no treatment. Bacterial meningitis is a medical emergency treated with large doses of intravenous antibiotics.

OUTLOOK

Viral meningitis is usually not serious, clears up within a week or two, and leaves no aftereffects. Patients with bacterial meningitis who receive prompt treatment usually recover; in some cases, however, some brain damage results.

PREVENTION

Vaccination may occasionally be valuable in controlling an epidemic caused by certain strains of bacteria. However, giving antibiotics to people who have come into contact with sufferers is generally more effective than vaccination.

Vaccination against meningitis has achieved only limited success because vaccines exist against only some of the organisms responsible and the protection is of limited duration.

Meningocele

A protrusion of the meninges (protective coverings) of the spinal cord under the skin due to a congenital defect in the spine (see *Spina bifida*). Meningocele is less serious than myelocele, which is protrusion of the spinal cord and of the meninges.

Meningomyelocele

See *Myelocele*.

M

Meniscectomy

A surgical procedure in which the whole or part of a *meniscus* (cartilage disk) is removed from a joint. Meniscectomy is almost always performed on the knee.

WHY IT IS DONE

Meniscectomy is carried out when a meniscus has been badly damaged, usually as a result of injury, causing the knee to lock or give way repeatedly. Removing the damaged part of the meniscus cures these symptoms but may increase the likelihood of premature *osteoarthritis* in the joint. Today, the operation is avoided whenever possible.

HOW IT IS DONE

Arthroscopy (in which a viewing tube is inserted into the joint through a small incision) is performed to confirm that a torn meniscus is the cause of the symptoms and to locate the tear. The torn portion of the meniscus is then removed by means of instruments inserted through the arthroscope. The incision is closed with one stitch, a bandage is applied, and the patient goes home.

Alternatively, the surgeon may need to open up the knee joint through an incision at the side of the patella (kneecap). After the operation, the wound is stitched and an elastic bandage and a plaster splint are applied over the knee.

RECOVERY PERIOD

Patients can usually go home the day of arthroscopic surgery and are able to walk normally within several days. After an open operation, the patient stays in the hospital for a few days. He or she is allowed to put weight on the affected leg after two or three days; the splint is removed after about a week, but normal activities cannot be resumed for four to six weeks.

After either procedure, patients should do exercises to strengthen the thigh muscles, which help to stabilize the knee.

OUTLOOK

The procedures are about equally effective in relieving symptoms and restoring the knee to normal function, although the scar after an open operation is larger. In either case, there may be an increased risk of osteoarthritis in later life, although the risk is less than if the damaged meniscus had been left in place.

Meniscus

A crescent-shaped disk of cartilaginous tissue found in several joints in the body. The *knee* joint has two

MENISCI

The diagram (right) shows the sites of the menisci. The menisci of the knee are shown in detail below.

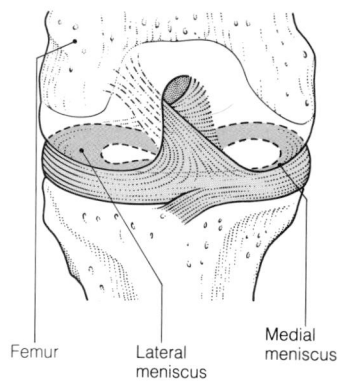

Femur   Lateral meniscus   Medial meniscus

menisci; the *wrist* joint and *temporomandibular joints* (jaw joints) have one each. The main function of the meniscus, which is held in position by ligaments, is to reduce friction during joint movement.

Menopause

The cessation of *menstruation*; the term is commonly used to describe the time in a woman's life when physical and psychological changes occur as a result of reduced production of *estrogen hormones* by the ovaries.

Menopause usually occurs between the ages of 45 and 55. The follicles in the ovaries stop producing ova (eggs) and less estrogen is produced. It is this reduction in estrogen that causes the problems associated with the menopause. Other hormonal changes include increased amounts of *gonadotropin hormones* (produced by the pituitary gland) and higher amounts of androgens (male hormones) present in the blood.

SYMPTOMS AND SIGNS

Hot flashes and night sweats occur in about 70 percent of all menopausal women. These symptoms occur with varying frequency and severity. The flashes are usually present for between two and five years, but may continue longer; in 25 percent of women they are so severe that the woman seeks medical help.

Vaginal dryness is the major symptom of 20 percent of menopausal women. Dryness occurs because the vaginal skin thins and its secretions diminish with the fall in estrogen levels. The vagina itself shrinks, loses elasticity, and becomes prone to minor infections; sexual intercourse is often more difficult and painful due to the dryness (see *Vaginitis*). The neck of the bladder and the urethra undergo similar changes, often resulting in the "urethral syndrome," in which the woman feels the need to empty her bladder frequently.

The skin becomes thinner during the menopause and the sebaceous secretions (the skin's natural oils) diminish, resulting in skin dryness. Body and scalp hair becomes dry and brittle and falls out more easily.

Psychological symptoms are often attributed to the menopause, but it is not clear whether these symptoms are caused by the lack of estrogen or are a reaction to the physical symptoms and the sleep disturbance caused by the night sweats. The most common symptoms are poor memory, poor concentration, tearfulness, anxiety, and loss of interest in sex.

Changes in *metabolism* (internal body chemistry) also occur during the menopause, but may not cause symptoms until later. The bones lose calcium more rapidly, especially in the first two to five years of the menopause; over a period of 10 to 15 years, *osteoporosis* (brittle bones) may develop. Other metabolic effects include a rise in blood pressure and an increase in fats in the blood. These changes result in an increase in *atherosclerosis* (fatty deposits in the arteries) and an increased incidence of *coronary heart disease* and *stroke*.

TREATMENT

If symptoms are severe, *hormone replacement therapy* is recommended to treat the physical and psychological symptoms and also to prevent menopause-related osteoporosis and heart disease. *Beta-blocker drugs* are sometimes given to women for whom hormone replacement therapy is unsuitable (e.g., women who have been treated for breast cancer).

Menorrhagia

Excessive loss of blood during *menstruation*. The average amount of blood lost during a normal menstrual period is about 2 fluid ounces (60 milliliters). A woman with menorrhagia may lose 3 fluid ounces (90 milliliters) or more. Some women regularly have menorrhagia, while others rarely or never do.

Menorrhagia is usually caused by an imbalance of estrogen and progesterone, the hormones that control menstruation. This imbalance causes an excessive buildup of endometrium (lining of the uterus).

Any disorder that affects the uterus can cause menorrhagia, including *fibroids*, polyps of the uterus, the presence of an *IUD*, or a pelvic infection. In some women with menorrhagia no physical cause can be found.

TREATMENT

Treatment depends on the severity of the bleeding, the age of the woman, whether or not she wants children in the future, and on any underlying disorder. A *D and C* (dilatation and curettage) may be performed to investigate the cause of menorrhagia. Hormones may be prescribed to reduce the amount of bleeding, especially if the woman is very young. If the condition is severe, a *hysterectomy* (removal of the uterus) may be considered.

Menotropins

A *gonadotropin hormone* given as a drug to stimulate cell activity in the ovaries and testes. Menotropins is prepared from human menopausal gonadotropin, which is obtained from urine samples of women who have passed the menopause.

WHY IT IS USED

Menotropins is used together with human chorionic gonadotropin (see *Gonadotropin, human chorionic*) in the treatment of certain types of female and male *infertility*. Menotropins prepares the ovary for ovulation and helps stimulate sperm production.

POSSIBLE ADVERSE EFFECTS

In women, menotropins may cause multiple pregnancy, abdominal pain, bloating, and weight gain. In men, breast enlargement may occur.

Menstrual extraction

A procedure in which the endometrium (the lining of the uterus), which is ordinarily sloughed off during *menstruation*, is removed all at one time. The procedure is also known as menstrual regulation. Menstrual extraction is usually performed to terminate a pregnancy.

Menstrual extraction is carried out in the first two weeks after a missed period. The procedure can be performed in a physician's office with or without local anesthetic. A narrow plastic tube is inserted into the uterus and the contents, including any embryo if the woman is pregnant, are suctioned out.

Menstruation

The periodic cyclical shedding of endometrium (lining of the uterus), accompanied by bleeding, that occurs in a woman who has not become pregnant. Menstruation identifies the fertile years of a woman's life. Menstrual periods usually begin at *puberty* and continue until the *menopause*.

MECHANISM

Menstruation is the end result of a complicated series of hormonal interactions. At the beginning of the menstrual cycle, *estrogen hormones* cause the endometrium to thicken to prepare the uterus for the possibility of *fertilization*; this is known as the proliferative or follicular phase of the menstrual cycle. *Ovulation* (egg release) usually occurs around midcycle and is accompanied by the increased production of *progesterone hormone*. This hormone induces marked changes in the endometrium, and the cells become swollen and thick with retained fluid. These changes, which occur during the secretory (or luteal) phase of the menstrual cycle, enable a fertilized egg to implant in the endometrium. If pregnancy fails to occur, the production of estrogens and progesterone from the ovaries diminishes, with the blood-filled lining of the uterus is not required and both the unfertilized egg and the lining are shed about 14 days after the start of ovulation. Uterine contractions force the menstrual discharge to be expelled through the cervix and into the vagina.

Blood loss varies from cycle to cycle and from woman to woman, averaging about 2 fluid ounces (60 milliliters). The menstrual cycle, which is counted from the first day of bleeding to the last day before the next menstrual period, lasts between 24 and 35 days in 95 percent of women, the average being 28 days. The length of bleeding also varies—usually lasting from one to eight days, with the average length being five days. (See also *Menstruation, disorders of*; *Menstruation, irregular*.)

M

THE MENSTRUAL CYCLE

Phase	Menstruation	Proliferative	Secretory		
Egg release and endometrial changes	Endometrium is shed	New egg ripens and endometrium begins to thicken	Egg released	Endometrium thickens further	Unfertilized egg passes through uterus
Day	1 2 3 4 5 6	7 8 9 10 11	12 13 14 15 16 17	18 19 20 21 22 23	24 25 26 27 28

During menstruation, estrogen and progesterone levels are low, and the unfertilized egg and endometrium are shed. Following menstruation, a pituitary hormone stimulates the ovaries to produce egg follicles. The follicles secrete estrogen, and one eventually releases an egg. The empty follicle also produces progesterone, which, with estrogen, prepares the endometrium to receive the egg. If the egg is unfertilized, follicle hormone levels fall and a new menstrual cycle begins.

Menstruation, disorders of

An abnormality in the monthly cycle of menstrual bleeding. Regular *menstruation* depends on development of a healthy endometrium (lining of the uterus) and regular cyclical production of *estrogen hormones* and *progesterone hormone*. This delicate balance is easily upset, making abnormal menstruation one of the most common disorders of women. Any change in a woman's periods can indicate a problem in the pelvic area, such as *fibroids*, *endometriosis*, or *pelvic inflammatory disease*.

Dysmenorrhea (painful periods) is the most common disorder. In most women the cause is unknown.

Amenorrhea (absence of menstruation) is most frequently caused by pregnancy; it may also be caused by a hormonal imbalance, stress, starvation, and *anorexia nervosa*. Polymenorrhea (too frequent menstruation) occurs when the length of the menstrual cycle is reduced to less than 22 days. It is usually due to a hormone imbalance. If the periods occur infrequently or the blood loss is scanty, it is termed oligomenorrhea.

Menorrhagia (excessive bleeding) may be caused by a hormone imbalance, the presence of an IUD, fibroids, or *polyps*.

In metrorrhagia, there are extreme variations in the interval between periods, the duration of bleeding, and the amount of blood lost each month (see *Menstruation, irregular*).

Menstruation, irregular

A variation from the normal pattern of *menstruation*. Menstruation is considered irregular if there are wide variations in the interval between periods, the duration of bleeding, or the amount of blood lost.

CAUSES

Disturbance of a woman's menstrual pattern can be caused by stress, travel, or changing the method of contraception. Because menstruation depends on a balance of estrogen and progesterone hormones, the cause of irregular menstruation is often a hormone disturbance. For the first few years after menstruation starts, and for the few years before the *menopause*, cycles are often irregular and ovulation does not occur.

A common cause of irregularity is unsuspected pregnancy or early miscarriage. Disorders of the uterus, ovaries, or pelvic cavity (e.g., *endometriosis*) can also lead to irregularity. (See also *Vaginal bleeding*.)

Mental hospital

A hospital specializing in the treatment of psychiatric illness. Formerly called asylums (or lunatic asylums), many were built in the 19th and early 20th century and were of enormous size. They became infamous as institutionalized backwaters filled with chronic patients who were commonly neglected and abused. Recently, many mental hospitals have been closed as the trend toward care in the community has increased. Still, the debate continues over how much this has contributed to the number of homeless people and how best to protect and treat old, long-stay patients (many of whom are homeless) and new, long-stay patients (such as those suffering from *schizophrenia* or advanced *dementia*).

Today, most admissions to mental hospitals are for acute psychiatric illness. People are admitted to remove them from a stressful or harmful home environment, to provide treatment possible only in the hospital, or to protect them or others from harm. The majority of these admissions are voluntary, but in some cases legal *commitment* is necessary.

Mental illness

A general term that describes any form of psychiatric disorder. It is common to divide these illnesses into two broad categories, the more severe *psychoses* and the less disturbing *neuroses*. While the former are probably caused by complex biochemical brain disease, the latter seem related to upbringing and personality.

The concept of mental illness is also important, for legal reasons, in determining whether a person can be held responsible for his or her actions. In this respect, there is much uncertainty as to whether *personality disorder*, which is often characterized by antisocial behavior, should be regarded as a form of mental illness.

Mental retardation

Impaired intellectual function that results in an inability to cope with the normal responsibilities of life.

CLASSIFICATION AND PREVALENCE

To be classified as mentally retarded, a person must have an IQ below 70 (see *Intelligence tests*) and impairment must be present before the age of 18. Within this group (which comprises about 1 percent of the population) there are various degrees of severity, resulting in different levels of handicap (see table for classification).

MENTAL RETARDATION

Severity	IQ
Mild	50 to 70
Moderate	35 to 49
Severe	20 to 34
Profound	Under 20

Mild retardation is the most common form, accounting for 80 percent of the retarded population. The other 20 percent have moderate, severe, or profound retardation.

CAUSES

The more severe grades of retardation (IQ below 50) usually have a specific physical cause; their incidence is the same in all social classes. About a quarter are due to *Down's syndrome*, another quarter to other inherited or congenital conditions (such as *phenylketonuria* or brain damage due to *hemolytic disease of the newborn*), and about one third result from trauma or infection around birth or early childhood. In about 15 percent of cases the cause is unknown, but the recently discovered *fragile X syndrome* may account for some of them.

By contrast, mild mental retardation usually has no specific cause, is concentrated in the lowest social classes, and seems to run in families. Poverty and *malnutrition* probably contribute to it along with inheritance.

SYMPTOMS

The mildly retarded usually show no obvious psychological symptoms apart from slowness in carrying out mental tasks, such as arithmetic or problem-solving. Reading is variably impaired and emotions may be expressed in a more childlike manner. However, *hyperactivity*, repetitive involuntary movements, and *autism* are up to four times more common than in the general population.

In more severely retarded people, speech is limited or absent, and epileptic seizures and neurological impairments are common. Fecal and urinary incontinence and self-injury may also occur.

TREATMENT

There is no specific means of eliminating the intellectual deficit. Special training and behavior modification can enhance the skills and quality of life for retarded people, many of whom are cared for in the community rather than in institutions. Family support and counseling can be crucial in preserving a stable home for the retarded person.

MENSTRUATION, IRREGULAR

Any variation in the interval between menstrual periods, the duration of bleeding, or the amount of blood lost, or bleeding that occurs in between normal periods, during pregnancy, or after the menopause. An occasional irregular period is generally no cause for concern if it is normal in other respects.

Absent or reduced bleeding

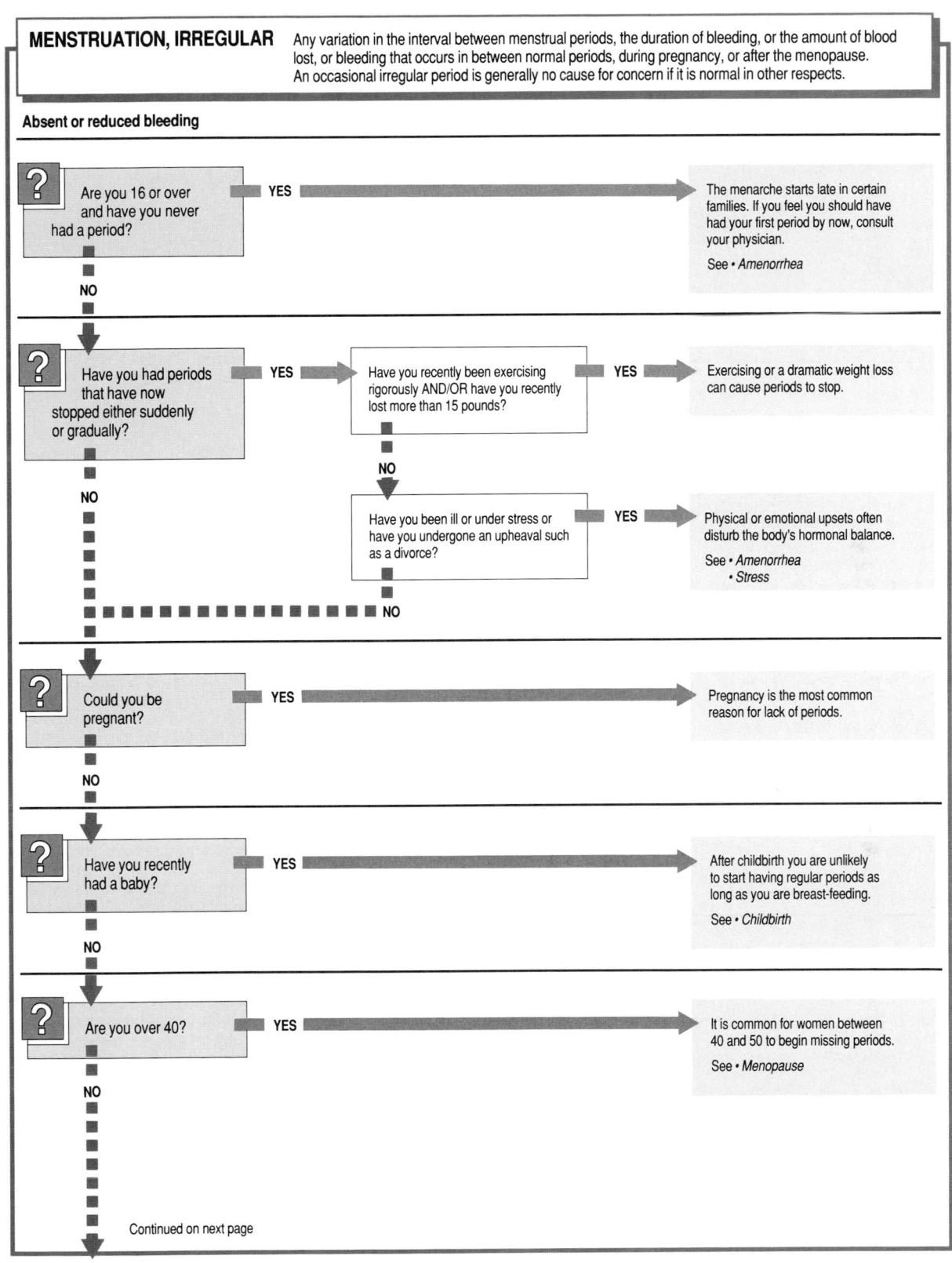

Are you 16 or over and have you never had a period?

YES → The menarche starts late in certain families. If you feel you should have had your first period by now, consult your physician.

See • *Amenorrhea*

NO

Have you had periods that have now stopped either suddenly or gradually?

YES → Have you recently been exercising rigorously AND/OR have you recently lost more than 15 pounds?

YES → Exercising or a dramatic weight loss can cause periods to stop.

NO

Have you been ill or under stress or have you undergone an upheaval such as a divorce?

YES → Physical or emotional upsets often disturb the body's hormonal balance.

See • *Amenorrhea*
 • *Stress*

NO

NO

Could you be pregnant?

YES → Pregnancy is the most common reason for lack of periods.

NO

Have you recently had a baby?

YES → After childbirth you are unlikely to start having regular periods as long as you are breast-feeding.

See • *Childbirth*

NO

Are you over 40?

YES → It is common for women between 40 and 50 to begin missing periods.

See • *Menopause*

NO

Continued on next page

M

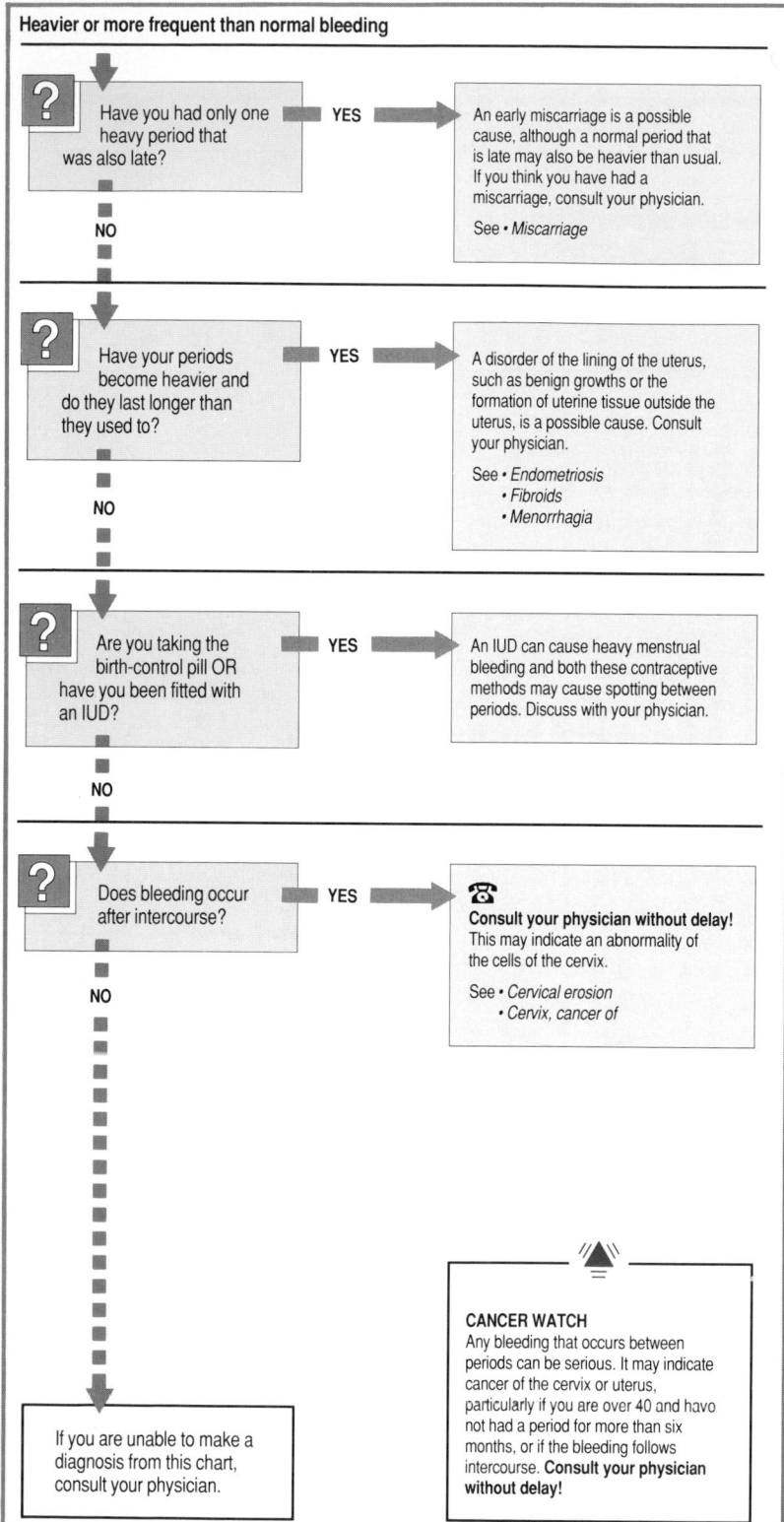

Heavier or more frequent than normal bleeding

? Have you had only one heavy period that was also late? → **YES** → An early miscarriage is a possible cause, although a normal period that is late may also be heavier than usual. If you think you have had a miscarriage, consult your physician.

See • *Miscarriage*

NO

? Have your periods become heavier and do they last longer than they used to? → **YES** → A disorder of the lining of the uterus, such as benign growths or the formation of uterine tissue outside the uterus, is a possible cause. Consult your physician.

See • *Endometriosis*
• *Fibroids*
• *Menorrhagia*

NO

? Are you taking the birth-control pill OR have you been fitted with an IUD? → **YES** → An IUD can cause heavy menstrual bleeding and both these contraceptive methods may cause spotting between periods. Discuss with your physician.

NO

? Does bleeding occur after intercourse? → **YES** → ☎ **Consult your physician without delay!** This may indicate an abnormality of the cells of the cervix.

See • *Cervical erosion*
• *Cervix, cancer of*

NO

If you are unable to make a diagnosis from this chart, consult your physician.

CANCER WATCH
Any bleeding that occurs between periods can be serious. It may indicate cancer of the cervix or uterus, particularly if you are over 40 and have not had a period for more than six months, or if the bleeding follows intercourse. **Consult your physician without delay!**

Anticonvulsant drugs may be needed in the treatment of epilepsy and *antipsychotics* in the treatment of other mental illness that may accompany mental retardation; these drugs help control symptoms ·and thus reduce impairment.

In the future, the incidence of retardation should be reduced by prevention. Preventive measures include *genetic counseling*, the elimination of infections such as *rubella*, reducing the alcohol and drug intake during pregnancy, and the early identification of fetal abnormalities.

OUTLOOK
While caring for a mentally retarded relative is often a demanding and time-consuming task, there is evidence that such people, even if severely impaired, can live rewarding and emotionally stable lives. Handicap is caused not by an absolute limit on achievement, but by delay in acquiring skills; as they grow older, the mentally retarded are able to improve in terms of personal and social function.

Meperidine

A synthetic narcotic *analgesic drug* (painkiller) similar to, but less powerful than, *morphine*. Meperidine, which is used almost exclusively in hospitals, is given as a *premedication* (a drug used to relax and sedate a person before an operation). It is also used to relieve severe pain after a major operation, during childbirth, and, occasionally, in terminal illness.

Since meperidine may cause nausea and vomiting, it is usually given with an *antiemetic drug* to control these symptoms. Used for long periods, meperidine may cause constipation.

ABUSE
Meperidine may cause euphoria and is abused for this effect. Taken regularly, it is likely to cause psychological and physical dependence (see *Drug dependence*).

Meprobamate

An *antianxiety drug* that is used to treat *anxiety* and *stress*. Meprobamate, which also has a muscle-relaxant effect, is combined with aspirin to relieve pain caused by rheumatic disorders (such as *osteoarthritis*) or injury to soft tissues (such as muscles and ligaments).

Since meprobamate has a sedative effect, it may cause drowsiness and dizziness. After long-term use, its discontinuation may be followed by severe withdrawal reactions.

Mercaptopurine

An *anticancer drug* used to treat certain types of *leukemia* (cancer of white blood cells). Mercaptopurine is also used as a treatment for *Crohn's disease* and for *lymphoma* (cancer of lymph nodes) in children.

Possible adverse effects include nausea, vomiting, mouth ulcers, and appetite loss. Rarely, mercaptopurine may cause liver damage, anemia, and abnormal bleeding.

Mercury

The only metallic element that is liquid at room temperature. Mercury is used in *thermometers*, *sphygmomanometers* (instruments for measuring blood pressure), and dental *amalgam*. Various compounds of mercury are used in some paints, pesticides, cosmetics, medicines, and in certain industrial processes.

Mercury poisoning

All forms of mercury are poisonous (except the amalgam in dental fillings), but some forms are absorbed into the body more readily than others and are therefore more dangerous. The liquid metal itself is absorbed very slightly through the intestines, so accidentally swallowing mercury from a broken thermometer is unlikely to lead to poisoning. However, liquid mercury is highly volatile and mercury vapor is readily absorbed into the body via the lungs. Inhalation of mercury vapor—usually as a result of industrial exposure—is the most common cause of poisoning. Mercury compounds (not highly volatile) cause poisoning by absorption through the skin or intestines.

SYMPTOMS AND SIGNS

The initial symptoms of mercury poisoning depend on the part of the body affected. Inhalation of mercury vapor may cause shortness of breath from lung damage; mercury compounds that come into contact with the skin may cause severe inflammation. A swallowed mercury compound can cause nausea, vomiting, diarrhea, and abdominal pain.

After mercury has entered the body, it passes into the bloodstream and later accumulates in various organs, principally the brain and kidneys. Mercury deposits in the brain cause a wide range of symptoms, including tiredness, incoordination, excitability, tremors, numbness in the limbs, and, in severe cases, impairment of vision and sometimes *dementia*. Deposits of mercury in the kidneys

may lead to *renal failure*. Without treatment, severe mercury poisoning may be fatal.

TREATMENT

Mercury poisoning is treated by giving *chelating agents* (such as penicillamine) to detoxify the mercury and help the body excrete it at a faster rate. In some cases, purification of the blood by hemodialysis (see *Dialysis*) may also be performed, especially if the kidneys have been damaged. Inducing vomiting or pumping out the stomach is helpful only if mercury has been swallowed within the previous few hours.

Mescaline

 A drug obtained from the Mexican peyote (or peyotl) cactus and classified as a psychedelic or *hallucinogenic drug*. The dried tops of the cactus, known as peyote buttons, have been used historically by Mexican and North American Indians in religious ceremonies. In modern times, psychologists have used mescaline to study the mechanism of *psychosis*, since the drug induces temporary psychotic symptoms.

The effects, which generally last for four to eight hours, are similar to those of *LSD* and *psilocybin*. Effects include illusions, changes in thought and mood, a sense of being in touch with the unknown, intense self-absorption, and an altered sense of time. Although the "trip" is most often pleasant and seemingly insightful, frightening ideas or experiences leading to panic and injury may occur. True psychosis, persisting after the drug has worn off, and addictive craving may occur.

Mesenteric lymphadenitis

An acute abdominal disorder in which lymph nodes in the mesentery (a membrane anchoring organs to the abdominal wall) become inflamed. Mesenteric lymphadenitis mainly affects children. Its cause is unknown but it may be related to some type of viral infection.

The main symptoms are pain and tenderness in the lower right abdomen, as in appendicitis. There may be mild fever, and sometimes the condition is preceded by a sore throat, chest infection, or swollen neck glands.

The disorder usually clears up rapidly. Analgesics (painkillers) may be given to reduce pain and fever. If the sufferer is no better after six hours or if the symptoms worsen dra-

matically, a *laparotomy* (surgical opening of the abdominal cavity) may be carried out to exclude appendicitis.

Mesentery

A membrane that attaches various organs to the abdominal wall. The term is used particularly to refer to the membranous fold that encloses the small intestine, attaching it to the back of the abdominal wall. The mesentery contains the arteries, veins, nerves, and lymphatic vessels that supply the large and small intestines.

Mesothelioma

A tumor of the pleura (lining of the lung and chest cavity). There are two types of mesothelioma—a solitary growth that remains localized in one area of the pleura and a diffuse malignant form. There is an increased incidence of mesothelioma in people exposed to asbestos dust (see *Asbestosis*), especially smokers.

Mesothelioma may cause no symptoms or it may cause cough, chest pain, and breathing difficulty, especially if a *pleural effusion* (collection of fluid around the lung) develops.

A chest X ray may show abnormal shadowing; the diagnosis can be confirmed by examination of a sample of fluid from any effusion or by pleural *biopsy* (removal of a sample of tissue for examination).

Surgical removal of a solitary tumor may result in complete cure. There is no effective treatment for the malignant form, although *radiation therapy* may help alleviate symptoms.

Mesothelium

A type of *epithelium* (surface cell layer) that lines the body cavities of the *peritoneum* and the *pleura* and makes up the *pericardium* (the saclike covering of the heart).

Mestranol

An *estrogen drug* used in various *oral contraceptive* preparations.

Metabolism

A collective term for all the chemical processes that take place in the body. Metabolism is divided into catabolism and anabolism. A catabolic process is a chemical reaction in which a complex substance is broken down into simpler ones, usually with the release of energy. An example is the "burning" of glucose (sugar) in body cells to produce energy and the by-products carbon dioxide and water. An anabolic process is a chemical reaction in which

M

a complex substance is built up from simpler ones, usually with the consumption of energy (which is provided by catabolism). The synthesis of complex *proteins* from *amino acids* is an anabolic process.

METABOLIC RATE

The basal metabolic rate (BMR) is the energy required to keep the body functioning at rest (that is, to maintain breathing, heart beat, body temperature, and other basic body functions). It is measured in Calories (or joules) per square meter of body surface per hour. The metabolic rate increases in response to factors such as exertion, stress, fear, and illness. It is controlled principally by various endocrine hormones (such as *epinephrine*, *norepinephrine*, *insulin*, *corticosteroid hormones*, and thyroid hormones—see *Thyroid gland*), which influence the rate at which chemical processes are carried out in body cells.

DISORDERS

The primary types of metabolic disorders include inherited abnormalities in which a specific enzyme (a substance that promotes a metabolic reaction) is lacking or malfunctions in some way (see *Metabolism, inborn errors of*). Other metabolic disorders are endocrine disorders in which there is underproduction or overproduction of a hormone that controls metabolic activity. Examples are *Cushing's syndrome*, *diabetes mellitus*, *insulinoma*, *hyperthyroidism* (overproduction by the thyroid gland), and *hypothyroidism* (underproduction by the thyroid).

Metabolism, inborn errors of

Inherited defects of body chemistry. These are *genetic disorders* in which the disturbance of body chemistry is caused by a single gene defect.

TYPES AND INCIDENCE

There are about 180 known inborn errors of metabolism. They vary in severity, from harmless abnormalities to serious diseases that may cause death in a newborn baby or result in severe physical or mental handicap. Examples include *Tay-Sachs disease*, *phenylketonuria*, *galactosemia*, the various *porphyrias*, *Hurler's syndrome* and various other types of *mucopolysaccharidosis*, hereditary fructose intolerance, Lesch-Nyhan syndrome, homocystinuria, glycogen storage diseases, mucolipidoses, and sphingolipidoses.

Individual disorders are rare. Most affect only one child in every 10,000 to 100,000, but the precise incidence is often unknown because sufferers may have only vague symptoms that are never investigated, or because they die before any characteristic features appear. Collectively, these disorders affect about one child in 1,000.

CAUSES

All inborn errors of metabolism are caused by abnormal functioning of a specific *enzyme* (protein that stimulates a chemical reaction) caused by a defect of a *gene*. Most defects show an autosomal recessive pattern of inheritance (see *Genetic disorders*).

Individual disorders vary in their effects. In some cases the abnormal enzyme is nonfunctional; in others there is some residual activity.

SYMPTOMS AND SIGNS

Symptoms are usually present at or soon after birth, although they may not appear until later in childhood. Symptoms may include unexplained illness or failure to thrive in a newborn, developmental delay, floppiness, drowsiness, persistent vomiting, or seizures. Signs may include enlarged body organs, bone deformities, anemia, cataracts, persistent jaundice, unusual body odor, the recurrent development of kidney stones, or a rash brought on by sunlight. The child may be intolerant to specific foods.

Miscarriages, stillbirths, or deaths in early infancy suggest the possibility of an inborn error of metabolism.

DIAGNOSIS

Investigations include tests to measure the levels of various substances in the affected child's blood, including *liver function tests* and *kidney function tests*. Chemical analysis of a *biopsy* specimen (small piece of tissue removed from the body) may be performed to check the level and function of a specific enzyme.

Early diagnosis can be important in preventing serious complications. Routine tests are done in the newborn for some of the more common disorders, such as phenylketonuria. Additional screening may be performed for disorders that are more common in certain countries or racial groups (for example, Tay-Sachs disease in European Jews).

Certain disorders can now be diagnosed prenatally following *chorionic villus sampling* or *amniocentesis*, allowing for an elective abortion.

TREATMENT

Some inborn errors of metabolism do not require treatment. Some respond to avoidance of a specific environmental factor to which an affected person is abnormally sensitive. For example, avoiding exposure to sunlight may help certain types of porphyria, avoiding food containing phenylalanine helps in phenylketonuria.

In some cases, a vitamin supplement can help compensate for defective enzyme function. In others, injections of the defective enzyme are given. Transplanting enzyme-producing cells from a donor has been effective in some cases (such as to treat Hurler's syndrome). Treating inborn errors of metabolism at the gene level is still, however, only theoretical. (See also *Genetic counseling*.)

Metabolite

Any substance that takes part in a metabolic reaction (a biochemical reaction in the body). In the breakdown of glucose (sugar) to produce energy, the metabolites are glucose, carbon dioxide, and water. The term metabolite is sometimes used to refer only to the products of a metabolic reaction. (See also *Metabolism*.)

Metacarpal bone

One of five long, cylindrical bones within the body of the hand. The bones run from the base of each digit to the wrist. On the palm of the hand, they are covered by a thick layer of fascia (fibrous connective tissue); on the back of the hand, they can be seen and felt through the skin. The heads of the metacarpal bones form the knuckles, standing out prominently when the hand is clenched. Fracture of the metacarpal bones is fairly common, usually as the result of a fall on the hand or a blow to the knuckles.

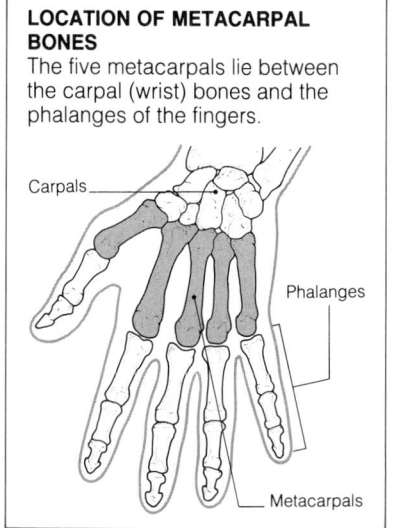

LOCATION OF METACARPAL BONES
The five metacarpals lie between the carpal (wrist) bones and the phalanges of the fingers.

Carpals

Phalanges

Metacarpals

Metaplasia

A change in tissue resulting from the transformation of one type of cell into another. Usually harmless, but occasionally precancerous, metaplasia can affect the lining of various organs, such as the bronchi (airways) and bladder. Metaplasia of the cervix, which occurs in *cervical erosion*, can be detected by a *cervical smear test*.

Metaproterenol

A *bronchodilator drug* used in the treatment of *asthma*, chronic *bronchitis*, and *emphysema*. Possible adverse effects include anxiety, restlessness, tremor, and palpitations.

Metastasis

A secondary malignant tumor (one that has spread from a primary *cancer* to affect other parts of the body). A metastasis in the liver may arise as a result of the spread of a cancer in the colon. The term metastasis also applies to the process by which such spread occurs. The degree of malignancy of a tumor depends largely on its ability to invade surrounding normal tissue and on its ability to send metastases to other parts of the body.

Metastases can spread from one part of the body to another through the lymphatic system, in the bloodstream, or across a body cavity (such as that between the inner and outer layer of the peritoneal membrane in the abdomen).

Metatarsal bone

One of five long, cylindrical bones within the foot. The bones make up the central skeleton of the foot and are held in an arch by surrounding ligaments. Fracture of the metatarsal bones may be caused by a heavy object falling onto the foot, by a twisting

LOCATION OF METATARSAL BONES

The five metatarsals lie between the tarsal bones (which form the ankle and back of the foot) and the phalanges of the toes.

Tarsals

Metatarsals

Phalanges

injury in which the foot turns over on its outside edge, or by prolonged walking or running on a hard surface (see *March fracture*).

Metatarsalgia

Pain in the foot. Causes include a fracture of one of the *metatarsal bones*, *flatfeet*, or a *neuroma* (benign tumor) of one of the nerves in the foot.

Metatarsophalangeal joint

The joint between each *metatarsal bone* and its adjoining toe bone (see *Phalanges*). The metatarsophalangeal joint at the base of the big toe is commonly affected by *gout* and osteoarthritis (see *Hallux rigidus*). Deformity may result in a bunion (see *Hallux valgus*).

Methadone

A synthetic narcotic *analgesic drug* (painkiller) that resembles *morphine*. Methadone causes only mild symptoms when it is withdrawn and is therefore used to relieve withdrawal symptoms in people undergoing a supervised heroin or morphine detoxification program.

Possible adverse effects include nausea, vomiting, constipation, dizziness, and dryness of the mouth.

Methane

A colorless, odorless, highly flammable gas that occurs naturally in the gas from oil wells and in coal mines, where it is an explosion hazard. Methane is also produced by the decomposition of organic matter; it is one of the gases present in intestinal gas (see *Flatus*).

Methanol

A poisonous type of *alcohol* used as a solvent or paint remover, and as an ingredient in some types of antifreeze. Also known as wood alcohol or methyl alcohol, methanol may cause blindness or death if ingested.

POISONING

Methanol is toxic; poisoning usually occurs as a result of drinking it as a substitute for ordinary alcohol (ethanol, or ethyl alcohol), although its inebriating effect is weaker.

Symptoms of poisoning, which develop 12 to 24 hours after drinking the methanol, include headache, dizziness, nausea, vomiting, and unconsciousness. The symptoms are caused by the breakdown in the liver of methanol into formaldehyde and formic acid. These substances may also damage the retina and optic

nerve, causing blurred vision. If methanol is drunk repeatedly, or if a single large dose is taken, permanent blindness may result.

TREATMENT

If somebody has ingested methanol and is conscious, vomiting should be induced and medical help obtained. Treatment may include pumping the stomach (see *Lavage, gastric*) and inducing vomiting, although this is effective only within about two hours of having drunk the methanol (before it has been absorbed into the bloodstream). In addition, ethanol may be given by injection into the bloodstream because it slows the rate at which the liver breaks down the methanol. An intravenous infusion of sodium bicarbonate may be used to neutralize formic acid in the blood. Occasionally, purification of the blood (by *dialysis*) is also necessary.

Methimazole

A drug used in the treatment of *hyperthyroidism* (overactivity of the thyroid gland). Methimazole suppresses the production of thyroid hormones by the thyroid gland.

Possible adverse effects include nausea, rash, dizziness, headache, and aching in the joints. Rarely, methimazole may cause increased susceptibility to infection.

Methocarbamol

A *muscle-relaxant drug* used to relieve stiffness caused by muscle injury and back pain. Methocarbamol is sometimes given to treat symptoms of *tetanus* (lockjaw). During prolonged treatment, methocarbamol may cause drowsiness, dizziness, and, in rare cases, liver damage.

Methotrexate

An *anticancer drug* used in the treatment of *lymphoma* (cancer of the lymph nodes) and certain forms of *leukemia*. Methotrexate is also used to treat some cancers of the uterus, breast, ovary, lung, bladder, and testis. It is given to treat *rheumatoid arthritis* when other treatments have proved ineffective and is sometimes used to treat severe *psoriasis*.

Methotrexate may cause nausea, vomiting, diarrhea, and mouth ulcers. It may also cause anemia, increased susceptibility to infection, and abnormal bleeding.

Methoxsalen

A *psoralen drug* used in the treatment of *psoriasis* and *vitiligo* when other

M

treatments have been ineffective. Potential adverse effects are typical of other psoralen drugs.

Methyclothiazide

A commonly prescribed thiazide *diuretic drug*.

Methyl alcohol

Another name for *methanol*.

Methylcellulose

A bulk-forming *laxative drug* commonly used to treat *constipation*, *diverticular disease*, and *irritable bowel syndrome*. Methylcellulose is also used to increase the firmness of bowel movements in *diarrhea* and to regulate their consistency in people who have had a *colostomy* or *ileostomy*.

In eye-drop form, methylcellulose is given to relieve dryness caused by sun, wind, and other irritants.

POSSIBLE ADVERSE EFFECTS
Methylcellulose may cause bloating, flatulence, and abdominal pain, or even bowel obstruction if sufficient amounts of fluids are not taken.

Methyldopa

An *antihypertensive drug* used in the treatment of *hypertension* (high blood pressure), usually in conjunction with other drugs from this group. Unlike most antihypertensives, methyldopa is safe to use during pregnancy. Adverse effects include drowsiness, depression, and nasal congestion.

Methylprednisolone

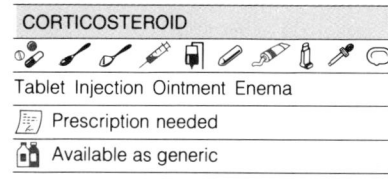

CORTICOSTEROID		
Tablet Injection Ointment Enema		
💊 Prescription needed		
🔲 Available as generic		

A *corticosteroid drug* used to replace hormones in *pituitary* or *adrenal gland* disorders that reduce the body's natural corticosteroid production. Methylprednisolone is also used in the treatment of severe *asthma*, skin inflammation, *inflammatory bowel disease*, and types of arthritis, including *rheumatoid arthritis*.

Possible adverse effects are typical of corticosteroid drugs.

Methysergide

A drug used to prevent *migraine* and cluster *headaches* (recurrent severe headaches). Methysergide is usually given only when other treatments have been ineffective.

Long-term drug treatment with methysergide may cause abnormal tissue growth in the lungs, around the ureters, or around blood vessels (resulting in chest pain, kidney failure, or leg cramps). Other possible adverse effects include dizziness, drowsiness, nausea, and diarrhea.

Metoclopramide

An *antiemetic drug* used to relieve nausea and vomiting caused by *anticancer drugs*, *radiation therapy*, or anesthetic drugs (see *Anesthesia, general*).

Metoclopramide is often given with a *premedication* (drug used to relax and sedate a person before an operation) to empty the stomach's contents and thereby reduce the risk of a person inhaling vomit. Metoclopramide is sometimes used to treat *heartburn*.

HOW IT WORKS
Metoclopramide reduces nerve activity in the part of the brain that stimulates vomiting. It also increases the speed with which fluid and food pass from the stomach.

POSSIBLE ADVERSE EFFECTS
Adverse effects may include rash, dryness of the mouth, agitation, and irritability. Large doses or prolonged use may cause sedation, diarrhea, or uncontrollable movements of the face, mouth, and tongue.

Metolazone

A *diuretic drug* used in the treatment of *hypertension* (high blood pressure). Metolazone is also given to reduce *edema* (fluid retention) in people with *heart failure* (reduced pumping efficiency of the heart), kidney disorders, *cirrhosis* of the liver, or *premenstrual syndrome*.

Metolazone is also a useful treatment for certain types of kidney stones (see *Calculus, urinary tract*) because it reduces the amount of calcium in the urine.

Possible adverse effects include weakness, lethargy, and dizziness caused by an increase in the amount of potassium excreted in the urine.

Metoprolol

A cardioselective *beta-blocker drug* used in the treatment of *angina pectoris* (chest pain due to impaired blood supply to heart muscle) and *hypertension* (high blood pressure). Metoprolol is also prescribed to relieve symptoms of *hyperthyroidism* (overactivity of the thyroid gland). It is occasionally given following a *myocardial infarction* (heart attack) to reduce the risk of further damage to the heart.

Possible adverse effects of metoprolol include lethargy, cold hands and feet, nightmares, and rash.

Metronidazole

An *antibiotic drug* that is particularly effective against infections caused by *anaerobic* bacteria (those that do not depend on oxygen), such as a tooth abscess and *peritonitis*. Metronidazole is also used to treat infections caused by *protozoa*, such as *trichomoniasis*, *amebiasis*, and *giardiasis*.

Adverse effects include nausea and vomiting, loss of appetite, abdominal pain, and dark-colored urine. Drinking alcohol during treatment often produces severe unpleasant effects such as nausea and vomiting, hot flashes, abdominal pain, palpitations, and headache.

Mexiletine

An *antiarrhythmic drug* used in the treatment of certain heart rhythm disorders, usually after a *myocardial infarction* (heart attack).

Adverse effects include nausea, vomiting, dizziness, and tremor.

Miconazole

ANTIFUNGAL		
Injection Vaginal suppository Cream		
💊 Prescription needed		
🔲 Available as generic		

An *antifungal drug* used to treat *tinea* skin infections, such as ringworm and *athlete's foot*, vaginal *candidiasis* (thrush), and rare fungal infections that affect internal organs, such as the lung.

Miconazole in the form of a cream or vaginal suppository causes a burning sensation and rash in rare cases. Injections of miconazole may cause nausea, vomiting, and fever.

Micro-

A prefix meaning small, as in microorganisms, tiny living organisms (such as bacteria, viruses, and protozoa), most of which are too small to be seen by the naked eye.

Microangiopathy

Any disease or disorder of the small blood vessels. Microangiopathy may be a feature of various conditions, including some kidney diseases, such as *glomerulonephritis* (inflammation of the kidneys' filtering units) or *hemolytic-uremic syndrome* (premature destruction of red blood cells accompanied by kidney damage); *eclampsia* (a disorder characterized by seizures in late pregnancy); *septicemia* (blood poisoning); and advanced cancer. When microangiopathy accompanies these conditions, the small blood vessels become distorted, resulting in red blood cells becoming damaged or destroyed. This, in turn, leads to a certain type of anemia called microangiopathic hemolytic anemia (see *Anemia, hemolytic*).

Another cause of microangiopathy is thrombotic thrombocytopenic purpura, a rare, often fatal disease that mainly affects young adults. In this condition, the small blood vessels in many organs throughout the body become blocked and the vessel walls are damaged; hemolytic anemia, fever, and a patchy, purplish rash known as *purpura* develop.

Microbe

A popular term for a *microorganism*, especially one that causes disease.

Microbiology

The study of *microorganisms*, particularly pathogenic (disease-causing) ones. Microbiology began in the 17th century with the discovery by the Dutch microscopist Antonj van Leeuwenhoek (1632-1723) of a wide variety of organisms too small to be seen by the naked eye. However, relatively little progress was made until the 19th century when, largely due to the work of scientists such as Louis Pasteur (1822-1895) and Robert Koch (1843-1910), it was recognized that microorganisms cause many infectious diseases and are also responsible for processes such as fermentation and decay. Microbiology continued to progress with the discovery of viruses, the development of vaccines and antibiotics against many diseases, and studies of the chemical processes fundamental to all living cells. Recently, microbiologists have played an important role in the study of genetics by pioneering techniques of *genetic engineering*.

In hospitals, microbiologists help identify the infectious organisms responsible for a patient's illness; they also advise clinicians on the sensitivity of these organisms to drugs.

Microcephaly

An abnormally small head, usually associated with mental retardation. Microcephaly may occur if the brain is damaged before birth by congenital

rubella (German measles) or if the mother is exposed to X rays during early pregnancy. It may also be the result of brain damage during birth, or of injury or disease in early infancy. Microcephaly may also occur if the skull bones fuse too early (see *Craniosynostosis*). There is also a rare inherited form of microcephaly in which the forehead slopes backward and the top of the head is pointed.

There is no method of treatment for this condition.

Microorganism

 Any tiny, single-celled living organism, usually too small to be seen by the naked eye. In medicine, the most important microorganisms are those that are pathogenic (disease-causing), although this group constitutes a relatively small minority of the vast number of microorganisms known to exist.

The principal pathogenic microorganisms are *bacteria*, which cause certain types of pneumonia, typhoid, diphtheria, and some types of food poisoning; *viruses* (usually classified as microorganisms although they are not true cells), which cause numerous infections, including AIDS, the common cold, influenza, and measles; *protozoa*, which are the causative agents of malaria, giardiasis, and amebic dysentery; *fungi*, which cause disorders such as ringworm and thrush; *rickettsiae*, which cause typhus, Rocky Mountain spotted fever, and Q fever; and chlamydiae, which cause various genital, eye, and respiratory infections (see *Chlamydial infections*).

Microscope

An instrument for producing enlarged images of small objects. There are many types of microscopes, ranging from simple, one-lens instruments (magnifying glasses), to compound microscopes and high-powered electron microscopes.

HISTORY

The single-lens microscope may date from as early as the 15th century, but the first truly powerful lenses were probably made by Antonj van Leeuwenhoek (1632-1723). His single-lens microscopes were capable of magnifying up to about 300 times. With them, he discovered microorganisms, thereby founding the science of *microbiology* and providing the basis for the development of the germ theory of disease. Probably the greatest of the early microscopists was

the Italian Marcello Malpighi (1628-1694), who is generally regarded as the founder of *histology*.

The compound microscope, which has two lens systems, was developed toward the end of the 16th century. However, the single-lens microscope continued to be widely used until the 19th century, when improvements in optical design and glass technology made the compound microscope a practicable instrument.

Light microscopes continued to be refined with the development of the phase-contrast microscope. However, the next major advances were instruments that use electrons in place of light—the transmission electron microscope (TEM), invented in the early 1930s, and the scanning electron microscope (SEM), invented in the middle 1960s.

LIGHT MICROSCOPES

Compound microscopes are the most widely used instruments. They have two lens systems. The objective and eyepiece are mounted at opposite ends of a tube called the body tube. There is also a stage to hold the specimen, a light source, and an optical condenser (see box, overleaf).

For ordinary light microscopes, the maximum magnification is about 1,500 times. By using a beam of electrons, much higher magnifications are possible.

ELECTRON MICROSCOPES

TEMs are similar to light microscopes, except that they use a beam of electrons instead of light, and electromagnetic "lenses" instead of glass ones. Furthermore, because electrons are invisible, the image must be formed on a fluorescent screen or photographic film. Modern TEMs can magnify up to about 5 million times, enabling tiny viruses and large molecules (such as DNA) to be seen.

The SEM works in a different way from the TEM (see box). SEMs have a lower maximum magnification (about 100,000 times) than do TEMs. However, unlike TEMs, SEMs produce three-dimensional images. This makes SEMs particularly valuable for studying the surface structures of cells and tissues.

OTHER MICROSCOPES

Phase-contrast and interference microscopes are types of light microscopes with modified illumination and optical systems that make it possible for unstained transparent specimens to be seen clearly. These microscopes are particularly useful for examining living cells and tissues.

M

TYPES OF MICROSCOPES

Microscopes are indispensable in medicine. For many purposes, the light microscope, with a magnification of up to 1,500 times, is sufficient. Modern research increasingly requires the much higher magnifications (up to about 5 million times) of a transmission electron microscope or a scanning electron microscope.

LIGHT MICROSCOPE

Eyepiece
Objective
Specimen
Optical condenser
Focusing knob
Stage
Illuminator

Shown is a collection of sperm cells.

The compound light microscope

One lens (the objective) forms a magnified image of the specimen; this image is then magnified further by the eyepiece (viewing) lens. The specimen is held on a stage, beneath which is an optical condenser that concentrates light (usually from a built-in illuminator) onto the specimen. Focusing is carried out by altering the distance between the objective and specimen.

TRANSMISSION ELECTRON MICROSCOPE

Electron gun
Electron beam
Condenser
Specimen
Objective "lens"
Projector "lens"
Viewing binoculars
Fluorescent screen

Shown here is the sperm's internal structure.

The transmission electron microscope

An electron beam (generated by a "gun") is concentrated by an electromagnetic condenser, then passes through the specimen. An electromagnetic objective "lens" then produces a magnified "image" of the specimen; this image is further magnified by an electromagnetic projector "lens," which also focuses the image onto a fluorescent screen, where it can be viewed through special binoculars.

SCANNING ELECTRON MICROSCOPE

Electron gun
Electron beam
Condenser
Scanning electromagnets
Fluorescent screen
Detector
Amplifier
Secondary electrons
Specimen

This shows the sperm cells in close detail.

The scanning electron microscope

An electron beam (generated by a "gun") is scanned over the surface of the specimen, causing the emission of a beam of secondary electrons, the intensity of which varies according to the surface features of the specimen. A detector converts the secondary electrons into an electric current, which is then amplified and used to control an electron beam that forms an image on a fluorescent screen.

Another instrument, the fluorescence microscope, is used to study the chemical composition of cells. In fluorescence microscopy, a specimen that has been selectively stained with fluorescent dyes is illuminated with ultraviolet light, which makes the stained parts glow.

Operating microscopes are low-powered compound microscopes with several modifications. They do not have a stage, and the illumination system is arranged to shine light down onto the living tissues rather than up through the specimen.

USES

The microscope is probably the single most important instrument in biological and medical science. Its applications are vast, ranging from the study of molecular structures to *microsurgery*. Microscopes have enabled scientists to examine both the structure and chemical composition of cells (*cytology*) and tissues (histology). They are used to investigate diseased tissues (a specialty called *histopathology*), thereby playing a vital role in diagnosis. In the operating room, microscopes have enabled the development of microsurgery, one application of which is to rejoin individual nerve fibers.

M

TECHNIQUES OF MICROSURGERY

Microsurgery started with ophthalmic surgeons, whose demands for more delicate operating instruments led to the adoption of the operating microscope. The results were so favorable that surgeons working in other specialties began to use the technique for intricate operations.

The operating microscope
This surgeon is performing microsurgery with the aid of an operating microscope. The photograph (below) shows small blood vessels as seen through the microscope.

Replantation microsurgery
A major application of microsurgery is the replantation of severed fingers, toes, hands, feet, or even entire limbs. This is successful only if the severed blood vessels and nerves are accurately rejoined so that regeneration occurs.

MAIN AREAS OF OPERATION
Microsurgery is most commonly employed in ophthalmic, vascular, neurological, gynecological, urological, and otological surgical procedures, in which delicate structures are involved.

Ophthalmology
By using microsurgery, even operations on the delicate retina of the eye are now possible.

Otology
Microsurgery is routinely used for operations on the tiny bones in the middle ear.

Gynecology
With microsurgery, blockages of the fallopian tubes can often be corrected, restoring fertility.

Urology
A vasectomy (male sterilization) can sometimes be reversed by using microsurgery to rejoin the cut ends of the vas deferens.

INSTRUMENTS

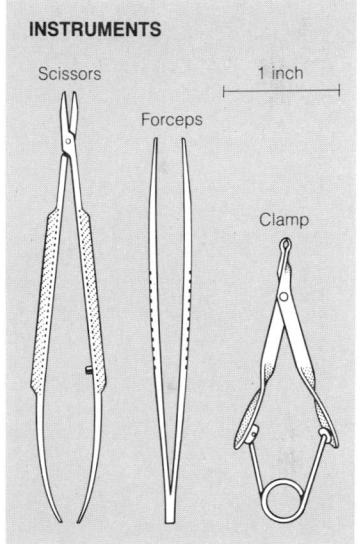

Microsurgery is possible only by using extremely delicate operating instruments, such as the fine scissors, forceps, and clamp shown above (their sizes can be judged from the scale bar).

Microsurgery
Delicate surgery in which the surgeon views the operation site through a special binocular *microscope* with pedal-operated magnification, focusing, and movements.

Microsurgery technique is used for surgery involving minute, delicate, or not easily accessible tissues. It has strikingly improved the success rate of some operations and made others possible that were previously impracticable. These operations include removing a diseased cataract from the eye and implanting a new lens (see *Cataract surgery*); transplanting a new cornea to the eye (see *Corneal graft*); replacing a diseased stirrup bone in the middle ear to treat deafness caused by otosclerosis (see *Stapedectomy*); restoring a severed limb by rejoining disconnected blood vessels and nerves; and unblocking and rejoining obstructed fallopian tubes to restore a woman's fertility.

Micturition
A term for passing *urine*.

Midbrain
Also known as the mesencephalon, the midbrain is the topmost part of the *brain stem*, situated above the pons.

Middle ear

See *Ear*.

Middle-ear effusion, persistent

Fluid accumulation in the middle-ear cavity that causes impaired hearing. Persistent middle-ear effusion is most common in children, often accompanied by enlarged *adenoids*; it frequently occurs with viral upper respiratory tract infections, such as colds. Usually both ears are affected.

CAUSES

The mucus-secreting lining of the middle-ear cavity sometimes becomes overactive, producing large amounts of sticky fluid. If there is blockage of the eustachian tube, which links the middle ear to the back of the nose, the fluid cannot drain away. The fluid subsequently accumulates and inter-

Eardrum

Ossicles

Labyrinth

Cochlea

Excessive fluid in middle ear and eustachian tube

Effects of middle-ear effusion
In this condition, sticky fluid in the middle ear prevents free movement of the eardrum and ossicles, causing deafness.

feres with the movement of the delicate bones in the middle ear.

SIGNS

The first, and often the only, sign is some degree of deafness. The child may be unaware of it and, unless his or her unresponsiveness is noticed by parents or teachers, the condition may pass undetected.

DIAGNOSIS

Middle-ear effusion is sometimes first detected through *hearing tests*, which

should be carried out routinely on all children. Once any hearing loss is detected or suspected in a child, a physician uses an *otoscope* (viewing instrument) to examine each eardrum for the characteristic changes in appearance and color that occur in middle-ear effusion.

TREATMENT

In mild cases the patient is given nose drops containing *decongestant drugs* to unblock the affected eustachian tube, so that the fluid can drain through it.

When the condition is severe, a *myringotomy* (a surgical opening in the eardrum) may be needed to drain the fluid. Removal of the adenoids may also be required (see *Adenoidectomy*).

Middle-ear infection

See *Otitis media*.

Mid-life crisis

A popular phrase that describes the feelings of distress that affect some people in early middle age (35 to 45 years) after realizing that they are no longer young. The term is used most often to describe men who strive to recapture their sense of lost youth by having extramarital affairs, suddenly changing jobs, or adopting youthful fashions. Sometimes anxiety or depression, brought on by fears of declining powers and death, can lead to psychiatric illness. Counseling and support are usually effective in helping people come to terms with the changes of age.

Midwifery

The profession concerned with the assistance of women in pregnancy and childbirth. A midwife provides care and information throughout pregnancy, supervises labor and delivery, and cares for both mother and baby during the period immediately following childbirth.

Certified midwives (called nurse-midwives) have met the graduate training standards of the American College of Nurse-Midwives and are licensed to practice in most states. Unqualified, or lay, midwifery is illegal in most states. The vast majority of qualified midwives practice in hospitals or birthing centers, usually with physician backup in case of complications and emergencies. Others work in private practice, and some midwives deliver in the woman's home.

Migraine

A severe headache, lasting for two hours to two days, accompanied by

disturbances of vision and/or nausea and vomiting. A sufferer may experience only a single attack; more commonly, he or she has recurrent attacks at varying intervals.

CAUSES AND INCIDENCE

Migraine occurs in at least 10 percent of the population and is three times more common in women than in men. It may affect children as young as 3; 60 percent of migraine sufferers have their first attack before the age of 20. It is extremely rare for migraine to appear for the first time after age 50.

There is no single cause of migraine. It tends to run in families, although the exact mechanism of inheritance is not understood. A number of factors, singly or in combination, may bring on an attack in a susceptible person. These factors may be stress-related (such as anxiety, anger, worry, excitement, depression, shock, overexertion, changes of routine, and changes of climate), food-related (particularly chocolate, cheese and other dairy products, red wine, fried food, and citrus fruits), or sensory-related (such as bright light or glare, loud noises, and intense or penetrating smells). Menstruation and the birth-control pill may also trigger migraine.

TYPES

There are two types of migraine: common and classical. In common migraine, the pain of the headache develops slowly, sometimes mounting to a throbbing pain that is made worse by the slightest movement or noise. The pain is often, but not always, on one side of the head only and usually occurs with nausea and sometimes vomiting. Many sufferers, particularly children, recover after they have vomited.

Classical migraine is comparatively rare. The headache is preceded by a slowly expanding area of blindness surrounded by a sparkling edge that increases to involve up to one half of the field of vision of each eye. The blindness clears up after about 20 minutes and is often followed by a severe one-sided headache with nausea, vomiting, and sensitivity to light. Other temporary neurological symptoms, such as weakness in one half of the body, may occur.

DIAGNOSIS

Special tests are rarely necessary. The physician can usually make a diagnosis from the patient's history and a physical examination. However, if there are accompanying persistent symptoms (such as tingling or weakness of a limb) or if the type of headache changes or becomes more severe, a full neurological examination may be carried out to exclude the unlikely possibility of a serious condition, such as a brain tumor.

TREATMENT

If migraine attacks occur less frequently than once a month, treatment of the acute attack is all that is required. If the attacks are more frequent, preventive treatment may be necessary. The simplest form of prevention is to avoid known trigger factors; keeping a careful diary can help the sufferer pinpoint them.

The best treatment for an acute migraine attack is with aspirin or acetaminophen plus an *antiemetic drug* (often provided in suppository form). If this combination is not effective, *ergotamine* may also be prescribed. Certain ergotamine preparations may help prevent an attack if taken in the early phases before the headache begins. Most people find that they recover more quickly if they can then sleep in a darkened room.

If migraine attacks occur more than once a month, prophylactic drugs (for example, *beta-blockers* and *calcium channel blockers*) may be prescribed.

Milia

Tiny, hard, white spots that most commonly occur in clusters on the upper cheeks and around the eyes of young adults. The cause is usually unknown although they may sometimes follow injury or blistering. They are painless and harmless.

Miliaria

Another name for *prickly heat*.

Milk

A *nutrient* fluid produced by the mammary gland of any mammal. Human milk differs considerably from cow's milk in the proportions of its ingredients. It contains about the same amount of fat, but twice as much lactose (sugar) and half as much protein.

Virtually all babies can digest milk, but early in childhood some lose the enzyme that breaks lactose down to simpler sugars (see *Lactase deficiency*). Milk allergy occurs in some infants, caused by a *food allergy* or intolerance to the proteins in cow's milk. (See also *Breast-feeding; Feeding, infant.*)

Milk-alkali syndrome

A rare type of *hypercalcemia* (abnormally high level of calcium in the blood) accompanied by *alkalosis* (reduced acidity of the blood) and *renal failure*. Milk-alkali syndrome is caused by excessive, long-term intake of calcium-containing *antacid drugs* and milk. It is most common in people with the symptoms of a *peptic ulcer* and associated kidney disorders.

The symptoms include weakness, muscle pains, irritability, and apathy. Treatment is to reduce the intake of milk and antacids.

Milk of magnesia

A magnesium preparation used as an *antacid drug* and a *laxative drug*.

Milk teeth

See *Primary teeth*.

Minamata disease

The name given to a severe form of *mercury* poisoning that occurred in the middle 1950s in people who had eaten fish from Minamata Bay, Japan. The fish contained large amounts of mercury as a result of water polluted with industrial mercury waste. By the time the cause of the condition was identified and brought under control, many people had suffered severe nerve damage and some had died.

Mineralization, dental

The deposition of calcium crystals and other mineral salts in developing teeth. (See *Calcification, dental*.)

Mineralocorticoid

The term used to describe a corticosteroid hormone (a hormone produced by the *adrenal gland*) that controls the amount of salts, including potassium and sodium, excreted in the urine. Some corticosteroid hormones (e.g., *aldosterone*) have only a mineralocorticoid action; others (such as *hydrocortisone*) also have a glucocorticoid effect (that is, they help regulate the body's use of carbohydrates).

Mineral oil

A lubricant *laxative drug* obtained from petroleum. Taken orally or given as an enema, mineral oil is used to treat *constipation*. Prolonged use may impair the absorption of vitamins from the intestine into the blood.

Minerals

Defined in *nutrition* as chemical elements that must be present in the diet for the maintenance of health. At least 13 minerals are essential to health. Important among them are potassium, sodium, calcium, magnesium, and phosphorus. Others, such as iron, zinc, and copper, are needed in only tiny amounts (see *Trace elements*). A balanced diet usually contains all the minerals the body requires. (See also chart, next page.)

Mineral supplements

A group of drug preparations containing one or more *minerals*. Mineral supplements, which are available over-the-counter in tablet or liquid form, should be used only when deficiency exists and on the advice of a physician. Most people obtain adequate amounts of minerals from the diet and additional amounts do not have any beneficial effects. Taken in excess, some mineral supplements may have harmful effects.

MEDICAL USES

The most commonly used mineral supplement is iron, which is used to treat iron-deficiency *anemia* and is sometimes needed by a woman who is pregnant or breast-feeding.

Other types of mineral deficiency are rare, with the exception of *magnesium* deficiency, which may occur as a result of alcohol abuse, a kidney disorder, or prolonged treatment with *diuretic drugs*.

Mineral supplements are sometimes needed by people suffering from an intestinal disorder that impairs the absorption of minerals from the diet. (See also individual mineral entries.)

Minilaparotomy

See *Sterilization, female*.

Minimal brain dysfunction

A postulated explanation for a variety of behavioral and other problems occurring in young children for which a physical cause might be expected but for which none is found.

Minimal brain dysfunction may be a cause of attentional difficulties, impulsiveness, *hyperactivity*, and some *learning disabilities*.

Minocycline

A tetracycline *antibiotic drug* used in low doses to treat *acne*. In rare cases, it is used to treat other disorders.

Minoxidil

A *vasodilator drug* used to treat severe *hypertension* (high blood pressure) when other drugs have been ineffective. Prolonged treatment often stimulates hair growth, especially on the face. Minoxidil in lotion form was approved by the FDA in 1988 as a treatment for male pattern *alopecia* (baldness).

M

MINERALS AND MAIN FOOD SOURCES

Mineral	Sources
Calcium	Milk, cheese, butter and margarine, green vegetables, legumes, nuts, soybean products, hard water
Chromium	Red meat, cheese, butter and margarine, whole-grain cereals and breads, green vegetables
Copper	Red meat, poultry, liver, fish, seafood, whole-grain cereals and breads, green vegetables, legumes, nuts, raisins, mushrooms
Fluorine	Fish, fluoridated water, tea
Iodine	Milk, cheese, butter and margarine, fish, whole-grain cereals and breads, iodized table salt
Iron	Red meat, poultry, liver, eggs, fish, whole-grain cereals and breads
Magnesium	Milk, fish, whole-grain cereals and breads, green vegetables, legumes, nuts, hard water
Phosphorus	Red meat, poultry, liver, milk, cheese, butter and margarine, eggs, fish, whole-grain cereals and breads, green vegetables, root vegetables, legumes, nuts, fruit
Potassium	Whole-grain cereals and breads, green vegetables, legumes, fruit
Selenium	Red meat, liver, milk, fish, seafood, whole-grain cereals and breads
Sodium	Red meat, poultry, liver, milk, cheese, butter and margarine, eggs, fish, whole-grain cereals and breads, green vegetables, root vegetables, legumes, nuts, fruit, table salt, processed foods
Zinc	Red meat, fish, seafood, eggs, milk, whole-grain cereals and breads, legumes

Miosis

Constriction (reduction in size) of the pupil of the eye. Miosis may be caused by certain drugs (such as pilocarpine or opium), by a disease affecting the *autonomic nervous system* (such as *Horner's syndrome*), or simply by bright light. A degree of miosis is normal in older people.

Miscarriage

Loss of the fetus before the 22nd week of pregnancy or before viability (the ability to survive outside the uterus without artificial support). The medical term for miscarriage is spontaneous abortion.

INCIDENCE

The incidence of miscarriage is difficult to determine, since not all women who miscarry seek medical attention or even realize they are miscarrying. It is estimated that from 10 to 30 percent of all pregnancies end in miscarriage, with the majority occurring in the first 10 weeks.

CAUSES

A wide range of problems can cause miscarriage. Many miscarriages occur because of abnormalities of the fetus itself, such as *chromosomal abnormalities* or major developmental defects. Severe maternal illness or exposure to toxins may also cause miscarriage. Less common causes of miscarriage include abnormalities such as inadequate progesterone secretion or an *autoimmune disorder* of the pregnant woman.

After the first three months, miscarriage is less common. Of the 3 to 5 percent of pregnancies that miscarry between 12 and 22 weeks, problems include genetic defects, *cervical incompetence* (inability of the cervix to hold the pregnancy), a defect such as a septate (subdivided) uterus, and large uterine fibroid tumors. Severe maternal infection or illness can also trigger a late miscarriage.

SYMPTOMS AND SIGNS

The symptoms of miscarriage are cramping and/or bleeding. Light bleeding during the early months of pregnancy occurs in up to half of all pregnancies and is often caused by low placental implantation or by *cervical erosion*. Many of these pregnancies continue uneventfully to term.

Heavy bleeding with cramping is generally more serious since it may signal impending miscarriage. Spotting and severe pain can be a symptom of either a threatened miscarriage or *ectopic pregnancy*. A gush of clear or pink fluid caused by rupture of the amniotic sac is an ominous sign.

DIAGNOSIS AND TREATMENT

In early pregnancy a woman in whom bleeding and cramping develop is often prescribed bed rest to minimize bleeding (although bed rest probably does not influence the outcome). Ultrasound scanning may be recommended to determine that the pregnancy is intrauterine (i.e., not ectopic) and that it appears to be progressing normally. A pelvic examination may be performed to find out if the size of the uterus feels appropriate and to see if the cervix is open or closed.

If a miscarriage is incomplete or inevitable and bleeding is heavy, a *D and C* (scraping out of the uterus) may be required. If the miscarriage seems complete (i.e., all fetal and placental material has been passed), no further treatment may be needed. Missed abortion may require *induction of labor*. Often, women are given antibiotics and other drugs to minimize bleeding. Rh-negative women are given $Rh_o(D)$ immune globulin to prevent future Rh complications (see *Rh incompatibility*).

After the first trimester, any cramping or spotting merits immediate medical attention; at this stage a significant number of possible miscarriages are caused by treatable problems, such as an incompetent cervix, rather than by severe fetal defects.

If there is evidence of an incompetent cervix, the cervix may be stitched shut. Prolonged bed rest may be recommended and uterine relaxants may be administered to women with uterine or cervical abnormalities.

A woman who miscarries three or more times consecutively is called an habitual aborter. Habitual abortion may be caused by genetic or hormonal

M

TYPES OF MISCARRIAGE

Threatened abortion	The fetus remains alive and has not been expelled from the uterus, despite bleeding from the woman's vagina.
Inevitable abortion	The fetus has died and is being expelled from the uterus. An inevitable abortion may be complete (when all the uterine contents are expelled) or incomplete (when the fetus and/or placenta are not completely expelled).
Missed abortion	The fetus has died but is retained with the placenta in the uterus.

abnormalities, chronic infection, autoimmune disease, or uterine abnormalities. Evaluation includes genetic studies for hormonal and infectious problems as well as *hysterosalpingography* (X-ray imaging of the uterus and fallopian tubes).

OUTLOOK

The majority of women who miscarry can eventually carry a pregnancy to term. Current diagnostic and treatment measures have made the outlook better than ever before. (See also *Abortion*; *Abortion, elective*.)

Mites and disease

 Mites are small, eight-legged animals, less than one twentieth of an inch (1.2 mm) long, similar to tiny spiders. Many have piercing and blood-sucking mouthparts and may parasitize animals and humans.

Mites can cause problems in a variety of ways. One species, the *scabies* mite, lives solely in human skin, where its burrowing activities cause an intense itch. Another, the house-dust mite, is common in bedding; inhaling dust containing dead mite parts can cause *asthma*.

Other types of mites inhabit grassy areas or affect crops. Chiggers (harvest mites) can be picked up when walking through thick grass. Their bites can produce an itchy rash (see *Chigger bites*). Mites in grain or fruit may cause various types of skin irritation, commonly known as grocers' itch or bakers' itch.

In some parts of the world, certain mites transmit disease, particularly scrub *typhus* and rickettsialpox. Both these diseases are caused by *rickettsiae* (organisms intermediate between bacteria and viruses), which normally infect rodents, but which can be transmitted to humans by mites.

The use of insect repellents (such as dimethyl phthalate) is advisable when walking through mite-infested areas.

Mitosis

The way in which most cells divide, so that the *chromosomes* (inherited genetic material) within the nucleus of the original cell are exactly duplicated into two daughter cells.

Each person begins as a single cell (a fertilized egg) and, following successive mitotic divisions of this cell, is born as a multicellular being with trillions of cells, most of which contain exactly the same chromosomal material. Mitotic divisions occur in the body thousands of times every second as dead cells are replaced by new ones formed by the division and multiplication of other cells.

Mitosis can be observed in a cell culture under a microscope. The sequence of events as the original cell divides to form two daughter cells is shown below.

A minority of cells (in the ovaries and testes) undergoes a fundamentally different type of division that results in the daughter cells receiving only half of the original cell's chromosomal material. This process, called *meiosis*, occurs in the formation of egg and sperm cells.

M

THE MECHANISM OF MITOSIS

Mitosis is the simplest type of cell division. It provides new body cells to replace those that have died. The new cells each receive an identical copy of the original cell's chromosomes.

Cell membrane
Nucleus
Chromosomes

1 Chromosomes in a cell nucleus are invisible long threads. Before cell division, the threads replicate, coil up, and shorten, appearing as dark rods. The two copies of each chromosome are joined, so they appear X-shaped.

2 The doubled chromosomes line up in the center of the cell, the cell nucleus breaks down, and threads appear in the cell. The two copies of each chromosome then move apart along the threads.

3 The two identical groups of single chromosomes now gather at opposite ends of the cell, and a nuclear membrane forms around each group. The rest of the cell then divides.

Nuclear membrane

4 When division has finished and new nuclei have fully formed in the two daughter cells, the chromosomes uncoil to resume their invisible, threadlike form. Mitosis is now complete.

Mitral insufficiency

Failure of the mitral valve of the heart to close properly, which allows blood to leak back into the left atrium (upper chamber) when pumped out of the left ventricle (lower chamber). Also known as mitral incompetence or mitral regurgitation, the disorder may occur in conjunction with *mitral stenosis* (narrowing of the valve).

In mitral insufficiency, the left side of the heart must work harder to clear the regurgitated blood. Eventually left-sided (and later, right-sided) *heart failure* may develop; generally, however, this is not a life-threatening condition. A buildup of blood from the left side of the heart can result in pulmonary *edema*.

CAUSES AND INCIDENCE

The most common cause (though much less common than it once was) is damage to the valve as a result of *rheumatic fever*. Other causes include *mitral valve prolapse* (floppy valve syndrome), damage following a *myocardial infarction* (heart attack), and stretching of the valve due to enlargement of the ventricle in left-sided heart failure. Rarely, the disorder may be present from birth or occurs as part of *Marfan's syndrome*.

SYMPTOMS AND SIGNS

The characteristic symptoms are increasing shortness of breath and fatigue, sometimes accompanied by *palpitations*. Later, as right-sided heart failure develops, the ankles swell.

An occasional complication is *endocarditis* (infection of the valve). Another risk is that a thrombus (blood clot) may form in the left atrium and travel to the brain, resulting in a *stroke*.

DIAGNOSIS

The physician makes a diagnosis from the patient's history, from a characteristic heart *murmur* heard through a stethoscope, and from the results of chest *X rays*, *ECG*, *echocardiography*, and cardiac *catheterization*.

TREATMENT AND OUTLOOK

If shortness of breath is troublesome, a *diuretic drug* may be prescribed to reduce fluid in the lungs and other tissues. *Digitalis drugs* may be given to increase the force of the heart's contraction and control rhythm disturbances. *Anticoagulant drugs* may be given to prevent the formation of blood clots. Before undergoing dental or other surgery, a person with mitral valve disease should take *antibiotic drugs* to prevent a blood infection that could cause endocarditis.

Heart valve surgery is considered only if severe heart failure develops or if drug treatment fails to prevent the patient's symptoms from becoming severe and disabling.

The outlook for mitral insufficiency is good whether treated by drugs or by valve surgery. Breathlessness and fatigue cannot be relieved by treatment once there has been permanent heart damage.

Mitral stenosis

Narrowing of the orifice of the mitral valve in the heart. This causes the atrial portion of the left side of the heart to work harder to force blood through the narrowed valve. The consequences are similar to those of *mitral insufficiency* (failure of the valve to close properly), which may accompany stenosis.

CAUSES AND INCIDENCE

Mitral stenosis is almost always due to scarring of the valve from an earlier attack of *rheumatic fever*, although in about half the cases there is no medical record of the illness. Mitral stenosis is four times more common in women than in men.

SYMPTOMS AND SIGNS

Symptoms do not usually develop until adulthood, many years after rheumatic fever. The primary symptom is shortness of breath, which at first occurs only on exertion; as the stenosis worsens, breathing difficulty is felt with less exertion and is eventually present when the person is at rest. Other symptoms and signs include *palpitations*, *atrial fibrillation* (rapid, uncoordinated, irregular heart beat), and deeply flushed cheeks. Congestion of the lungs can lead to recurrent chest infections, coughing up of blood, and fatigue.

Possible complications are as for mitral insufficiency.

DIAGNOSIS

Mitral stenosis is diagnosed from the patient's history, by a physician listening to heart sounds through a stethoscope, and by investigations that may include an *ECG*, chest *X rays*, *echocardiography*, and cardiac *catheterization*.

TREATMENT AND OUTLOOK

Drug treatment (with *diuretic drugs* and *digitalis drugs*) is broadly the same as for mitral insufficiency, as are the precautions to help prevent *endocarditis* (infection of the valve).

If symptoms persist despite drug treatment, *heart valve surgery* may be considered to repair or replace the defective valve. The outlook following surgery is good, although the operation may need to be repeated several years later.

Mitral valve prolapse

A common, slight deformity of the mitral valve, situated in the left side of the heart, that can produce a degree of *mitral insufficiency* (leakage of the valve). Also known as "floppy valve syndrome," the condition affects up to 5 percent of the population and is most common in young to middle-aged women. Mitral valve prolapse causes a characteristic heart *murmur* that may be heard by the physician through a stethoscope during a routine examination.

The cause is not known in most cases, although there is some evidence that the condition is inherited. Occasionally the prolapse results from *rheumatic fever*, *coronary heart disease*, or *cardiomyopathy*.

Usually, there are no symptoms and the condition is of no consequence; treatment is not required. Occasionally, however, it may produce chest pain, *arrhythmia* (disturbance of heart rhythm), or leakage of the valve sufficient to cause *heart failure*. These conditions may require treatment with heart drugs (such as *beta-blockers*, *diuretics*, or *digitalis drugs*) or, rarely, *heart valve surgery*.

Mittelschmerz

Pain in the lower abdomen that occurs in some women at the time of *ovulation* midway through each menstrual cycle. The pain is usually one-sided and lasts only a few hours; slight spotting (vaginal blood loss) may accompany the pain. Mittelschmerz is usually not severe. However, if it is, *oral contraceptives* may be prescribed to suppress ovulation.

Mobilization

The process of making a part of the body capable of movement. Mobilization refers to treatment aimed at increasing mobility in a part of the body recovering from injury or affected by disease. Examples include exercises to treat *frozen shoulder* or joint stiffness caused by *arthritis*, and retraining in walking following a *stroke* or lower limb *fracture*.

Surgeons use the term mobilization to refer to the freeing, during an operation, of an organ or structure from surrounding connective tissue and fibrous adhesions. For example, in a *cholecystectomy*, the gallbladder has to be mobilized from the liver before it can be removed.

Molar

See *Teeth*.

Molar pregnancy

A pregnancy in which a tumor develops from placental tissue and the embryo fails to develop normally. A molar pregnancy may be benign (*hydatidiform mole*) or malignant, when it is called an invasive mole. *Choriocarcinoma* is an invasive mole that has spread outside the uterus.

A different type of molar pregnancy occurs after a missed abortion (a type of *miscarriage* in which the dead embryo and placenta are not expelled from the uterus). The dead tissue is called a carneous mole.

Mold

Any of a large group of *fungi* that exist as many-celled, filamentous colonies. Some molds are the source of antibiotics, such as penicillin. Some can cause disease, such as *aspergillosis*.

Mole

A type of pigmented *nevus*.

Molecule

The smallest complete unit of a substance that can exist independently and still retain the characteristic properties of that substance. Almost all molecules consist of two or more atoms that are linked. A molecule of carbon dioxide comprises one carbon atom linked to two oxygen atoms. Certain unusual molecules, called monatomic molecules, consist of only one atom (e.g., molecules of inert gases such as argon and neon).

Molecules vary enormously in size and complexity. At one extreme are the small, simple ones, such as oxygen, consisting of two linked oxygen atoms. At the other extreme are huge, complicated molecules, such as *DNA* (deoxyribonucleic acid), containing thousands of atoms of carbon, hydrogen, oxygen, nitrogen, and phosphorus that are linked to form a double-helix structure shaped like a spiral staircase.

Molluscum contagiosum

A harmless viral infection characterized by shiny, pearly white papules (tiny lumps) on the skin surface. Each papule is circular, has a tiny central depression, and produces a cheesy fluid if squeezed. A crust forms before healing occurs.

The papules appear in groups, or sometimes alone, on the genitals, the inside of the thighs, the face, or elsewhere. Children or, less commonly, adults may be affected. The infection is easily transmitted by direct skin contact or during intercourse.

Molluscum contagiosum usually clears up in a few months, but may require treatment by a physician.

Mongolian spot

A blue-black pigmented spot found singly or in groups on the lower back and buttocks at birth. The spot may be mistaken for a bruise, although it is a type of *nevus*. Mongolian spots are common in black or Asian children and are caused by a concentration of melanocytes (pigment-producing cells) deep within the skin. They usually disappear by the age of 3 or 4.

Mongolism

The outdated name for the disorder now called *Down's syndrome*.

Moniliasis

See *Candidiasis*.

Monitor

To maintain a constant watch on a patient's condition so that any change can be detected early and appropriate treatment given. The term also refers to any device used to carry out monitoring, such as the cardiac monitor used in intensive-care units. A cardiac monitor displays the patient's *ECG* (a record of the electrical impulses generated by the heart) on a screen and signals the heart rate both visually and audibly.

Monoarthritis

Inflammation of a single joint, causing pain and stiffness. Common causes are *osteoarthritis*, *gout*, and infection.

Monoclonal antibody

See *Antibody, monoclonal*.

Mononucleosis, infectious

An acute viral infection characterized by a high temperature, sore throat, and swollen lymph glands, particularly in the neck (hence its common name, glandular fever).

CAUSES AND INCIDENCE

Infectious mononucleosis is caused either by the Epstein-Barr virus or cytomegalovirus, both members of the herpesvirus family. The disease develops only if the virus is encountered for the first time at an age when the response of the body's *immune system* is most vigorous (that is, during adolescence and early adult life). The peak incidence of the illness occurs around ages 15 to 17. Kissing is thought to be a common method of transmitting the virus.

Once in the body, the virus multiplies in the *lymphocytes* (white blood cells that form part of the immune system). Lymphocytes are also called mononuclear cells. When infected with the virus, the lymphocytes change their appearance and are referred to as "atypical."

Blood smear in mononucleosis
The large cell with one nucleus, surrounded by many red blood cells, is an atypical lymphocyte (it is bigger than normal).

SYMPTOMS AND SIGNS

The illness usually starts with a fever and headache, followed by swelling of the lymph glands in the neck, armpits, and groin and a severe sore throat due to tonsillitis. The enlarged, inflamed tonsils make swallowing difficult and, in rare cases, may obstruct breathing. Occasionally, mild liver damage may occur, leading to jaundice for a few days. A physician may feel an enlarged spleen in the upper left part of the abdomen.

DIAGNOSIS

The diagnosis is often obvious from the symptoms and from examination of a blood smear, which shows many atypical lymphocytes in the blood. A test for the infection—the heterophil antibodies test—may also be carried out. This test looks for antibodies (proteins produced by the immune system to counter the virus) that possess the unique ability to cause clumping of red cells taken from sheep's blood. More specific tests are also available when the diagnosis is in doubt.

TREATMENT AND OUTLOOK

Almost all patients recover after four to six weeks without drugs. If the antibiotic ampicillin is mistakenly given, it may produce a rash and worsening of symptoms. Rest is needed for a month or so to allow the body's immune system to destroy the virus. In rare cases, *corticosteroid drugs* are required to reduce severe inflammation, particularly if breathing is obstructed by swollen tonsils. For two to three months after recovery, patients often feel depressed, lack energy, and feel sleepy during the day. However, the majority of people who have chronic fatigue that they attribute to chronic Epstein-Barr virus disease produce no laboratory results to substantiate this diagnosis.

Monorchism

The presence of only one testis in a male. Unless a testis has been removed surgically (see *Orchiectomy*), the most likely cause of monorchism is *congenital* absence. The term monorchism should not be used to describe an undescended testis (see *Testis, undescended*).

Monosodium glutamate

A *food additive* frequently used as a flavor enhancer and seasoning. Until recently, monosodium glutamate (MSG) was suspected to be the cause of *Chinese restaurant syndrome*, in which a sense of pressure in the face, pain in the chest, and a feeling of burning in the head and upper trunk comes on 20 minutes after a meal and lasts for about 45 minutes. Clinical trials have shown that MSG does not produce exactly this symptom pattern, although it may occasionally cause some of these symptoms in sensitive people.

Monteggia's fracture

Fracture of the ulna (the bone on the inner side of the forearm) just below the elbow, with dislocation of the radius (the bone on the outer side of the forearm) from the elbow joint. Monteggia's fracture can be caused by a fall onto the arm or by a blow to the back of the upper arm.

Treatment usually requires an operation through two incisions on either side of the forearm. First, the radius is replaced in the joint. The fractured bone ends of the ulna are then realigned and fixed with a plate and screws or a long nail. The incisions are sewn up and the limb is immobilized in a plaster cast until healing occurs, which usually takes about 12 weeks.

Montezuma's revenge

A name given to a type of *gastroenteritis* (especially the resulting diarrhea) that is often contracted by tourists visiting Mexico.

Moon face

The rounded facial appearance that is a feature of *Cushing's syndrome*.

MORA

The abbreviation for *mandibular orthopedic repositioning appliance*.

Morbid anatomy

Also known as pathological anatomy, the study of the structural changes that occur in body tissues as a consequence of disease.

The term morbid anatomy refers especially to those changes that are visible to the naked eye during a postmortem examination (in contrast to changes visible only through a microscope).

Morbidity

The state or condition of being diseased. The morbidity ratio is the proportion of diseased to healthy people in a community.

In the US, detailed statistics on morbidity are recorded at the *Centers for Disease Control* in Atlanta, Georgia.

Morbilli

Another name for *measles*.

Morning-after pill

See *Contraception, postcoital*.

Morning sickness

See *Vomiting in pregnancy*.

Moron

An outdated term, derived from the Greek word for dull, for a person with mild *mental retardation* (IQ 50 to 70).

Morphea

A condition in which one or more well-defined, hard, flat, round or oval patches develop on the skin. Morphea is a nonspreading type of *scleroderma* (a disease in which there is progressive hardening of tissues).

The skin patches of morphea are white or reddish, measuring up to several inches in diameter. They usually occur on the trunk, neck, hands, or feet. Loss of hair or ulceration at the affected site may also occur. The condition most often affects middle-aged women. Although harmless, morphea can be disfiguring. There is no treatment.

Morphine

The best known narcotic *analgesic* (painkiller), derived from the unripe seed pods of the opium poppy.

MAJOR CAUSES OF DEATH IN THE US IN A REPRESENTATIVE YEAR

Cause	Total deaths (per 100,000 population)	Male deaths (per 100,000 men)	Female deaths (per 100,000 women)
Circulatory system diseases	421.5	435.3	408.4
Acute myocardial infarction	122.4	145.7	100.3
Other ischemic heart disease	113.8	116.0	111.7
Hypertension	13.6	12.1	15.0
Other forms of heart disease	79.9	81.5	78.4
Stroke	66.5	55.3	77.1
Atherosclerosis	11.3	8.8	13.6
Cancer (all forms)	189.9	209.7	170.1
Colon	19.7	19.7	19.8
Lung, bronchus, trachea	49.2	70.7	28.8
Breast	—	—	31.6
Prostate	—	22.0	—
Accidents	39.5	56.2	23.8
Traffic accidents	18.6	27.1	10.2
Suicide	12.1	19.2	5.4
Homicide	8.5	13.4	3.9
Pneumonia	23.3	24.2	22.4
Bronchitis, emphysema, asthma	8.7	11.3	6.3
Other respiratory diseases	28.1	36.7	19.9
Diabetes mellitus	15.5	12.9	17.9
Other endocrine and metabolic diseases	4.3	4.1	4.4
Chronic liver disease and cirrhosis	11.7	15.4	8.1
Other digestive system disorders	14.3	13.8	14.7
Infections and parasitic diseases	9.3	9.9	8.8
Septicemia	5.7	5.6	5.8

WHY IT IS USED

Morphine is given to relieve severe pain caused by *myocardial infarction* (heart attack), major surgery, serious injury, and cancer. It is occasionally used as a *premedication* (a drug used to prepare a person for surgery).

HOW IT WORKS

Morphine blocks the transmission of pain signals at specific sites (called opiate receptors) in the brain and spinal cord, thereby preventing the perception of pain.

POSSIBLE ADVERSE EFFECTS

Morphine causes drowsiness, dizziness, constipation, nausea, vomiting, and confusion. Short-term use is unlikely to cause *drug dependence*.

ABUSE

The euphoric effects of morphine have led to its abuse. Long-term abuse leads to a craving for the drug and *tolerance* (the need for greater amounts to have the same effect). It also causes physical dependence, with flulike symptoms (such as sweating, shaking, and cramping) when the drug is suddenly withdrawn.

Mortality

The death rate, that is, the number of deaths per 100,000 (or, occasionally, per 1,000 or per 10,000) of the population per year. The total mortality is made up of the individual mortality from different causes (such as accidents, coronary heart disease, and cancer). The study of differences in these proportions between one country and another, or between different periods in the same country, can offer valuable information about the comparative state of health of a population or about disease trends.

Mortality is often calculated for specific groups of the population. For example, *infant mortality* quantifies deaths of live-born infants during the first year of life; perinatal mortality quantifies deaths (including all stillbirths) during the first week (or sometimes month) of life.

Standardized mortality compares the death rate in an occupational or socioeconomic group with the average for the entire population. It is a useful indicator of the relative safety of an occupation, or of whether a specific socioeconomic group is at particular risk. (See also table, left; *Life expectancy*; *Maternal mortality*.)

Mosaicism

The presence of two (or more) groups of cells containing different chromosomal material within one person.

Usually, each of a person's body cells contains 46 chromosomes. They include the two sex chromosomes, termed XX in females and XY in males (see *Chromosomes*). In a mosaic person, some cells may contain 46 and others 45, 47, or other numbers of chromosomes. The probable cause in most cases is a fault in the process of cell division early in embryonic life. The diagnosis is made by *chromosome analysis* of skin or white blood cells.

Mosaicism can give rise to syndromes associated with *chromosomal abnormalities* (such as *Down's syndrome* and *Turner's syndrome*). A girl with Turner's syndrome mosaicism has some cells with a normal chromosome complement and others missing an X sex chromosome. About 3 percent of children with Down's syndrome have mosaicism. These children carry a mixture of normal cells and others containing an extra number 21 chromosome.

Depending on the proportion of abnormal cells and type of abnormality, people with mosaicism range from looking physically normal to having features typical of a chromosomal abnormality syndrome. People with mosaicism are often less severely affected than those with the abnormality in all their cells.

Mosquito bites

Mosquitoes are flying insects found throughout the world. The females require blood from humans or animals to produce eggs; they obtain this blood through their bites. The mosquito eggs are laid and hatched in stagnating water, so mosquitoes are most prevalent close to marshes, ponds, reservoirs, and water tanks, especially after a rainy period. Male mosquitoes do not bite.

Mosquitoes are a nuisance simply because of their bites. However, the main problem with mosquitoes is disease transmission—particularly in the tropics. During a bite, a mosquito may acquire infectious organisms from the blood of an infected person; the organisms multiply within the insect and are transferred to another person during a subsequent bite.

The main disease-transmitting mosquitoes belong to three groups: ANOPHELES, AEDES, and CULEX. They have varying appearances and habits and transmit different diseases (see chart). The only illnesses acquired from mosquito bites in the US are certain types of viral *encephalitis* (inflammation of the brain), such as St. Louis encephalitis, eastern and western equine encephalitis, and California encephalitis. Several thousand cases of these infections occur in the US each year, with features similar to other types of encephalitis. A hundred years ago, malaria was commonly transmitted in parts of the South and middle West.

TREATMENT

Mosquito bites should be washed with soap and water, and a soothing cream applied. A physician should be consulted if mosquito bites cause a severe skin reaction.

PREVENTION

Protective measures against mosquitoes (to limit the chances of infection) should be taken in the tropics and subtropics and in any area where the insects are rampant. The most effective measures are the wearing of long sleeves and socks at dusk to reduce the amount of exposed skin,

DANGEROUS MOSQUITOES

Mosquito	Appearance	Habits	Diseases transmitted
ANOPHELES species	Head and body in straight line and at an angle to surface	Mainly rural; bite at night	Malaria; filariasis
CULEX species	Body parallel to surface; head bent down; whining flight; brown color	Urban or rural; bite in evening or at night	Viral encephalitis; filariasis
AEDES species	Body shape as for CULEX, but tropical species are black and white	Urban or rural; bite during day	Dengue; yellow fever; viral encephalitis

placing mosquito screens over windows, and the use of insect-repellent sprays or slow-burning coils that release a smoke containing insecticide. A mosquito net that surrounds the bed is of value in preventing mosquitoes from biting during sleep.

Attempts to control mosquitoes in the tropics have included direct attack with insecticides, efforts to limit breeding areas, and even the release of vast numbers of sterilized male mosquitoes. However, these efforts have achieved only limited success. (See also *Insect bites; Insects and disease.*)

Motion sickness

A condition produced in some people by road, sea, or air travel. In its mildest form, motion sickness may be only a feeling of uneasiness and a headache; in severe cases, there may be distress, excessive sweating and salivation, pallor, nausea, and vomiting.

Motion sickness is caused by the effect of any constant pronounced movement on the organ of balance in the inner ear. Other factors also play a part, however. Anxiety based on previous attacks, a stuffy or fume-laden atmosphere, a full stomach, or the sight of food can make the condition worse. So, too, can focusing on nearby objects; sufferers should look at a point on the horizon.

PREVENTION
Various *antiemetic drugs* are available to prevent or help control motion sickness. Scopolamine or cyclizine (an *antihistamine drug*) should be taken about an hour before the start of a journey. The longer-acting antihistamines (promethazine or meclizine) need to be taken about a day before the journey.

Motor

A term used to describe anything that brings about movement, such as a muscle or nerve. The word is usually applied to nerves (including those in the part of the brain called the cerebral cortex) that stimulate muscles to contract and thereby produce movement.

Motor neuron disease

A group of rare disorders in which the nerves that control muscular activity degenerate within the brain and spinal cord. The result is weakness and *atrophy* (wasting) of the muscles. The cause is unknown.

INCIDENCE AND TYPES
The most common motor neuron disease is amyotrophic lateral sclerosis (ALS), often referred to as Lou Gehrig's disease. About one or two cases of ALS are diagnosed annually per 100,000 people in the US. ALS usually affects people over 50 and is more common in men than women. About 10 percent of ALS cases are familial (run in the family).

Other motor neuron diseases include progressive muscular atrophy and progressive bulbar palsy. While these diseases start with patterns of muscle weakness different from typical ALS, they usually develop into that disease.

Two motor neuron diseases, usually inherited, affect much younger people. In infantile progressive spinal muscular atrophy (Werdnig-Hoffmann paralysis), children are affected at birth or shortly thereafter. The weakness progresses to death in several months to several years with rare exceptions. A more benign form (chronic spinal muscular dystrophy) begins any time from childhood through adolescence; it causes a progressive weakness that may never result in serious disability.

SYMPTOMS
In ALS, sufferers first note weakness in the hands and arms accompanied by wasting of the muscles. Fasciculations, an involuntary quivering of small areas of the muscle, may also occur. Many sufferers also report cramping or stiffness. Sometimes the weakness starts in the legs but, in every case, all four extremities are soon involved. There is no loss of sensation; bladder function is normal.

The diagnosis is confirmed by *EMG* (measurement of muscle electrical activity) and other tests, such as muscle *biopsy*, blood studies, *myelography*, *CT scanning*, or *MRI*, to rule out other disease.

TREATMENT AND OUTLOOK
The weakness usually progresses to involve the muscles of respiration and swallowing, leading to death in two to four years. Exceptions do occur, however, and some people have lived more than 20 years after diagnosis.

There is no means of slowing the nerve degeneration, although physical therapy can sometimes lessen disability. Wheelchairs, walkers, and other aids are available to help patients maintain independence as long as possible.

The final stages may be especially distressing for the patient and family because, although the victim is unable to speak, swallow, or move, awareness and intellect are maintained. Occasionally, life may be prolonged through the use of feeding tubes and *ventilators*. Care is generally aimed at easing discomfort.

Motor system disease
See *Motor neuron disease.*

Mountain sickness
An illness that can affect mountain climbers, hikers, or skiers who have ascended too rapidly to heights above 8,000 feet (2,400 m) or, more commonly, to above 10,000 feet (3,000 m).

CAUSES
Mountain sickness is caused by the reduced atmospheric pressure—and thus reduced oxygen—at high altitude, but the exact mechanism by which reduced pressure leads to illness is not fully understood. Broadly, reduced oxygen in the blood, along with other changes in blood chemistry, affects the nervous system, muscles, heart, and lungs.

At altitude there is a higher-than-normal blood flow through the lungs and to the brain; this, combined with an apparent increase in the permeability (leakiness) of blood vessels, can lead to *edema* (waterlogging) of these organs.

Mountain sickness is more likely the younger the person, the faster the ascent, and the higher the altitude.

PREVENTION
A person ascending to an altitude above 8,000 feet should do so gradually, stopping for a day or two's rest after each further ascent of 2,000 to 3,000 feet. Ascending higher during the rest day is permissible, provided a return to the lower level is made before night.

SYMPTOMS AND SIGNS
In most cases, mountain sickness is mild and short-lived, with symptoms such as headache, nausea, dizziness, and impaired mental processes. No further ascent should be made until the symptoms disappear. Some cases are more severe. Fluid builds up in the lungs, leading to severe breathlessness, cough, and the production of frothy sputum (phlegm). This is called high-altitude pulmonary edema. If fluid builds up around the brain (cerebral edema) the symptoms may include severe headache, seizures, vomiting, unsteadiness, hallucinations, and sometimes coma.

FIRST AID AND TREATMENT
In serious cases, the victim must be brought down from the mountain and taken to a hospital as quickly as possible. Any delay can result in brain damage and death. Administering

M

pure oxygen, if available, can help. In the hospital, *diuretic drugs* are often given to help reduce edema.

The conditions of patients with high-altitude pulmonary edema often improve rapidly after descending a few thousand feet. Patients with the cerebral form may take days or weeks in the hospital to recover.

Mouth

The mouth, where food is broken down for swallowing, forms the first part of the digestive tract (see *Mastication*); it converts vibrations produced by the larynx (voice box) into *speech*; and it is used in breathing.

STRUCTURE

The roof of the mouth consists of a hard bony *palate* at the front and a soft fleshy palate behind. Most of the floor of the mouth is formed by the *tongue*, which contains specialized cells, sensitive to taste, known as taste buds. Surrounding the palate and tongue are the *teeth*, which are set in the shock-absorbent tissue of the *gums*. Enclosing them all are the cheeks and *lips*, which contain a ring of muscle that helps keep food in the mouth. The inside of the mouth is lined with mucous membrane, which is lubricated with saliva produced by three pairs of *salivary glands*.

DISORDERS

The most common deformities of the mouth, other than alignment of the teeth (see *Malocclusion*), are *cleft lip and palate* (a split in the upper lip and a gap in the roof of the mouth). They may occur alone or together.

Infections of the mouth are common. They include an abscess around the root of a tooth (see *Abscess, dental*) and oral *candidiasis* (thrush), a fungal infection that produces sore, cream-colored patches on the lining of the mouth. Noninfective conditions that also cause discoloration include *leukoplakia* (marked by thickened white or gray patches) and the more rare *lichen planus* (in which a white network of raised tissue develops).

Extremely common are *mouth ulcers*, painful white or yellow open sores that may develop anywhere on the mucous membrane. *Cysts*, fluid- or semisolid-filled swellings, may also occur on the lining of the cheek or the floor of the mouth.

Any lump, sore, or ulcer in the mouth that persists for more than three or four weeks should be seen by a physician. In rare cases, the abnormality is an early sign of a malignant growth (see *Mouth cancer*).

ANATOMY OF THE MOUTH

The mouth has a complicated structure, reflecting its various functions. For example, the tongue, lips, teeth, and palate play an essential role in speech production. Together with the salivary glands, the same mouth parts play a role in eating and drinking.

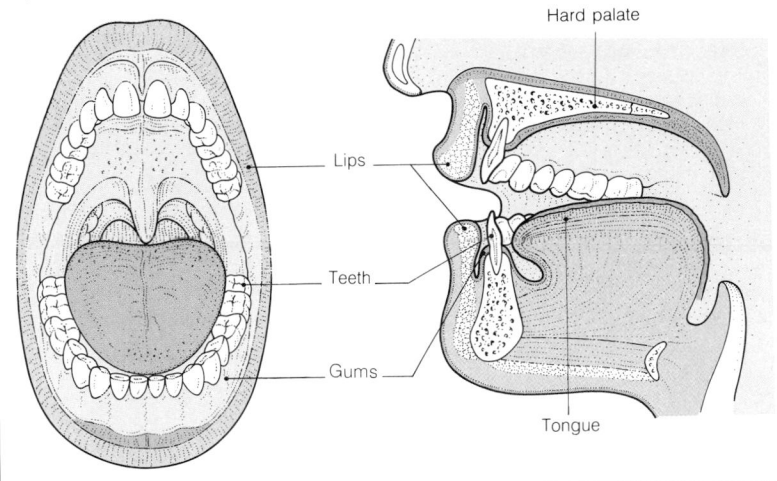

Mouth cancer

Malignant tumors affecting the oral cavity; most common are *lip cancer* and *tongue cancer*. The floor of the mouth, the salivary glands, the inside of the cheeks, the gums, and the palate are less commonly affected. Most are squamous carcinomas.

CAUSES AND INCIDENCE

The main cause of oral cancer is smoking. Tobacco smoke and heat irritate the mucous membrane lining the mouth. The risk to pipe and cigar smokers is as great, or greater, than to cigarette smokers. The other chief causes are chewing tobacco, inhaling snuff, and heavy alcohol consumption. Poor oral hygiene and irritation from ill-fitting dentures or jagged teeth are predisposing factors.

Oral cancers represent about 8 percent of all malignancies. Men are twice as commonly affected as women, and most cases occur in men older than 40.

SYMPTOMS AND SIGNS

Cancer of the lip usually starts with a whitish patch on the lower lip called *leukoplakia*. The lesion is a small ulcer, or a deep, hard-edged fissure, and may be the first sign of a malignant tumor in the mouth. These initial tissue changes may be accompanied by a burning sensation, but are usually painless.

As the tumor grows, it develops into an ulcer that may bleed and that erodes surrounding tissue. If the tongue is affected, it becomes stiff, making chewing, swallowing, and speaking difficult. In its advanced stages, the tumor is usually painful.

DIAGNOSIS

Any lump, discolored patch, or other tissue change on the lip or in the mouth that does not clear up within a month should be reported to a physician. In some cases, a dentist is the first person to detect such a change. The diagnosis is based on a *biopsy* (removal of a small sample of tissue).

TREATMENT AND OUTLOOK

Treatment consists of surgical removal of all cancerous tissue, *radiation therapy*, or a combination of both. Extensive surgery may result in facial disfigurement and problems with eating and speaking, which may require reconstructive surgery. Radiation therapy sometimes damages the salivary glands (see *Mouth, dry*).

The rate of spread of oral cancer varies according to the site. Tongue cancer is the most dangerous, spreading rapidly to nearby lymph nodes. When oral cancer in any form is detected and treated early, the outlook is good, resulting in a cure in three quarters of cases. More than half the people with oral cancer survive for more than five years after treatment.

Mouth, dry

The result of inadequate production of saliva. Dry mouth is usually a temporary condition caused by fear, a salivary gland infection (see *Parotid*

M

MOVEMENT

During life, movement occurs constantly throughout the body. All visible movements are caused by the shortening of muscles, usually for only brief periods at a time. This causes movement of many kinds—of bones, of blood in the vessels, of food in the intestines, of urine from the bladder, of the eye, of facial expression, and of the body as a whole. All movement is either voluntary (willed) or involuntary (automatic).

SKELETAL MOVEMENT

This always involves moving bones relative to one another. Many muscles are involved. Some act to brace certain bones so that different bones can be moved by other muscles.

Combined rotation and displacement

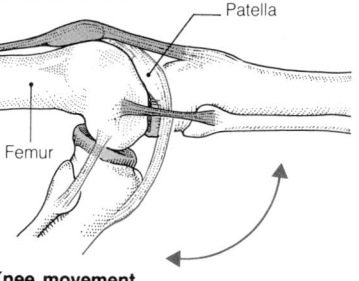

Knee movement
A hinge joint, the knee allows movement in one plane only through an arc of about 130 degrees.

Arm movements
The shoulder—a ball-and-socket joint—allows movement in all directions. Sometimes two or more movements of the arm may be combined.

Yoga and movement
Yoga (right) teaches a wide range of body movements and postures. It helps to increase joint flexibility, to eliminate tension, and to promote relaxation.

EYE MOVEMENT

Six muscles work together on the eyeball to give a range of smooth, precise movements.

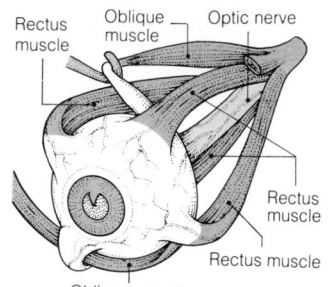

Eye muscles
The four rectus eye muscles run directly back from the eyeball; the oblique muscles are attached to and pull on the eyeball at an angle.

Actions of eye muscles
Two rectus muscles control side-to-side eye movements. The other muscles control up-and-down and rotational movements.

INVOLUNTARY MOVEMENT

Movement of internal organs is not under voluntary control but is regulated by the autonomic nervous system.

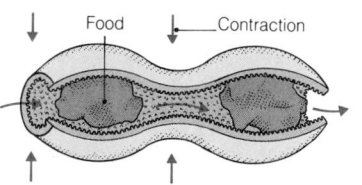

Peristalsis
This is an example of movement caused by involuntary muscle action. Waves of contraction pass along muscles in the intestinal wall, forcing the contents forward and preventing obstruction.

Heart beat
The heart differs from other muscles in that it has an impulse-conducting system that ensures contraction in sequence—the atria (upper chambers) first, then the ventricles (lower chambers).

gland), or the action of *anticholinergic drugs*. Permanent dry mouth is rare. It can occur, for unknown reasons, as part of *Sjögren's syndrome* or may result from *radiation therapy* given to treat a tumor of the mouth. In these cases, dry mouth is usually accompanied by difficulty swallowing and speaking, interference with taste, and tooth decay. Dry mouth may be partially relieved by spraying the inside of the mouth with artificial saliva.

Mouth-to-mouth resuscitation

See *Artificial respiration*.

Mouth ulcer

An open sore caused by a break in the *mucous membrane* lining the mouth. Mouth ulcers take the form of round or oval, shallow, white, gray, or yellow spots with an inflamed red border. They may occur singly or in clusters anywhere in the mouth.

TYPES

The most common type of mouth ulcer is a *canker sore*, which occurs on the inside of the cheek and lip and on the tongue. Also common are ulcers caused by the *herpes simplex* virus, which also causes *cold sores*.

Rare types of mouth ulcer include those occurring in *Behçet's syndrome*, *tuberculosis*, *syphilis*, *Vincent's disease*, *leukemia*, *anemia*, and drug allergy.

A mouth ulcer may be the first stage of *mouth cancer*. Any ulcer that fails to heal within three or four weeks, or that recurs, should be seen by a physician. *Blood tests* and/or a *biopsy* (removal of a small sample of tissue for analysis) may be required to determine the cause.

Mouthwash

A solution for rinsing the mouth. Many mouthwashes make various medicinal claims, but most do no more than leave the mouth feeling fresh and, if used vigorously, remove loose food debris from the teeth (an effect that can be achieved with water). Most antiseptic mouthwashes intended to combat *halitosis* (bad breath) are ineffective because they do not treat the cause of the problem; if used for a prolonged period, they may irritate the mouth.

Some mouthwashes, however, are useful. When the gums are too tender for proper toothbrushing, as in some types of *gingivitis* (inflamed gums), a mouthwash containing hydrogen peroxide can help clean the teeth by its foaming action. Any time routine dental hygiene is not possible (such as

after oral surgery), a mouthwash with chlorhexidine used under the supervision of a dentist acts effectively against the bacteria in dental plaque, the sticky coating on the teeth responsible for decay.

Fluoride mouthwashes are helpful in preventing dental caries, probably by strengthening tooth enamel, and possibly also by acting directly against plaque. A mouthwash of warm salt water can help ease painful inflammation caused by tooth disorders, such as impacted wisdom teeth (see *Impaction, dental*) or *dry socket* (infection at the site of a tooth extraction).

Movement

Bodily movements include skeletal movements and movements of soft tissues and body organs. All movement is brought about by the actions of various types of muscles.

SKELETAL MOVEMENTS

The simplest skeletal movement consists of a change in the relative position of two bones, brought about by shortening of a muscle attached to the two bones and acting across a *joint*. Simultaneously, other muscles and soft tissues, such as skin, tendons, and ligaments, are stretched.

More complex skeletal movements involve many bones, joints, and muscles, which are arranged to allow an enormous range of possible actions, from turning a screwdriver to turning a somersault. Even in a fairly simple movement, several muscles are active, some contracting to initiate and maintain a movement while others that oppose the movement contract to help prevent sudden, uncontrolled movement.

All voluntary (willed) skeletal movements are initiated in the part of the cerebrum (the main mass of the brain) called the motor cortex. Signals are sent down the spinal cord along nerve fibers, and from there along separate nerve fibers to the appropriate muscles. Control relies on information supplied by sensory nerve receptors, in the muscles and elsewhere, that record the position of the different parts of the body and the amount of contraction in each muscle. This information is integrated in specific areas of the brain (including the cerebellum and basal ganglia) that control coordination, initiation, and cessation of movement. Learning complex sequences (such as piano playing) involves the establishment of unconscious patterns of nerve activity in the cerebellum.

Skeletal movements can also occur as simple *reflexes* in response to certain sensory warning signals. In these instances, the movement is automatic and less controlled, involving far fewer nerve connections.

OTHER MOVEMENTS

Not all body movements involve the skeleton. Movements of the eyes and tongue are brought about by contractions of muscles attached to soft tissues. Again, they may be voluntary movements (controlled from the motor cortex) or reflexes. Movements of the internal organs are involuntary; they include the *heart beat* and *peristalsis*. (See also *Muscles*.)

DISORDERS

Disorders of the nervous system, muscles, joints, or bones may impair movement. (See *Nerve injury*; *Neuropathy*; *Brain* disorders box; *Spinal cord*; *Muscles* disorders box.)

Moxibustion

A form of treatment, often used in conjunction with *acupuncture*, in which a cone (moxa) of wormwood leaves or of certain other plant materials is burned just above the skin to relieve internal pain. The burning material is thought to act as a counterirritant (that is, its irritation of nerve endings in the skin alleviates deep-seated pain in the same area). When used in conjunction with acupuncture, the cone of moxa is placed on a needle over an acupuncture point, and the moxa is lit.

MRI

Magnetic resonance imaging. MRI is a diagnostic technique that provides high quality cross-sectional images of organs and structures within the body without X rays or other radiation.

HOW IT WORKS

During the imaging, the patient lies inside a massive, hollow, cylindrical magnet and is exposed to short bursts of a powerful magnetic field. The nuclei (protons) of the body's hydrogen atoms normally point randomly in different directions, but, in a magnetic field, they line up parallel to each other, like rows of tiny magnets. If the hydrogen nuclei are then knocked out of alignment by a strong pulse of radio waves, they produce a detectable radio signal as they fall back into alignment.

Magnetic coils in the machine detect these signals and a computer changes them into an image based on the strength of signal produced by different types of tissue. Tissues that

M

contain a lot of hydrogen (such as fat) produce a bright image; those that contain little or no hydrogen (such as bone) appear black.

WHY IT IS DONE

MRI allows images to be constructed in any plane; it is particularly valuable in studying the brain and spinal cord. This technique reveals tumors vividly, indicating their precise extent, and produces impressive images of the internal structure of the eye and ear.

MRI also produces detailed images of the heart and major blood vessels, provides images of blood flow, and is useful for examining joints and soft tissues, particularly in the knee. The role of MRI in imaging the abdominal organs is becoming established.

Images from MRI are similar in many ways to those produced by *CT scanning*, but MRI generally gives much greater contrast between normal and abnormal tissues.

HOW IT IS DONE

MRI is usually an outpatient procedure. During the examination the patient must lie still; children may be given a general anesthetic. A scan usually takes about half an hour.

RISKS

There are no known risks or side effects to MRI. The technique does not use radiation and can therefore be performed repeatedly with no known adverse effects.

However, any person fitted with a pacemaker, hearing aid, or other electrical device should tell his or her physician before undergoing MRI, since the scanner may interfere with these devices.

OUTLOOK

MRI is a costly test that is not yet widely available; it is still the subject of continuing research. A future application of MRI, known as magnetic resonance spectroscopy, relies on the properties of other chemical elements in the body (such as phosphorus and calcium) and is able to provide information on organ function.

MS

The abbreviation for *multiple sclerosis*.

Mucocele

A swollen sac or cavity within the body that is filled with mucus secreted from cells in its inner lining. An example is a mucocele of the appendix, caused by constriction of the opening of the appendix into the intestine. A mucocele of the gallbladder (*hydrops*) may be caused by a gallstone obstructing its outlet.

MAGNETIC RESONANCE IMAGING (MRI)

A valuable diagnostic technique, MRI has been in use since the early 1980s. The patient lies down surrounded by electromagnets and is exposed to short bursts of powerful magnetic fields and radio waves. The bursts stimulate hydrogen atoms in the patient's tissues to emit signals, which are detected and analyzed by computer to create an image of a "slice" of the patient's body.

MRI computer
A computer linked to the MRI scanner creates an image of the area being scanned and displays it on a monitor.

Mucolytic drugs

Mucolytic drugs (including *acetylcysteine*) make sputum (phlegm) less sticky and easier to cough up.

Mucopolysaccharidosis

Any of a group of inborn errors of *metabolism*. The best known is *Hurler's syndrome*; others include Hunter's, Sanfillippo's, Morquio's, Maroteaux-Lamy, and Scheie's syndromes. They are rare, collectively affecting about one child in 10,000.

All are *genetic disorders* in which there is an abnormality of a specific *enzyme* in body tissues. The enzyme abnormality affects the way carbohydrates are handled within body cells, leading to an accumulation of unwanted substances called mucopolysaccharides in the tissues.

Depending on the disease, features include abnormalities of the skeleton and/or the central nervous system (brain and spinal cord) with mental retardation and, in some cases, a characteristic facial appearance. There may also be corneal clouding, liver enlargement, and joint stiffness. No specific treatment is available; death often occurs during the childhood or teenage years. However, there are also mild varieties that may allow a reasonably normal life. Some children with Hurler's syndrome have been successfully treated by bone marrow transplantation, which provides a continuing source of the enzyme.

Parents with a seriously affected child should receive *genetic counseling* concerning the risk of any future child being affected.

Mucosa

Another term for a *mucous membrane*.

Mucous membrane

The soft, pink, skinlike layer that lines many of the cavities and tubes in the body, including the respiratory tract, alimentary canal, the urinary and genital passages, and eyelids. The mucous membrane secretes a fluid that contains *mucus* to keep such structures moist and well-lubricated. The fluid is produced and released onto the surface of the mucous membrane by millions of specialized cells (goblet cells) within the membrane.

Mucus

The thick, slimy fluid secreted by *mucous membranes*. Mucus moistens, lubricates, and protects those parts of the body lined by mucous membrane, such as the alimentary and digestive tracts. Mucus prevents stomach acid from damaging the stomach wall and

M

prevents enzymes from digesting the intestine, it eases swallowing and lubricates food as it passes through the alimentary tract, it moistens inhaled air and traps smoke and other foreign particles in the airways (to keep them out of the lungs), and it facilitates sexual intercourse.

Mucus method of contraception
See *Contraception*.

Multiple myeloma
A malignant condition of middle to old age, also called myelomatosis. Multiple myeloma is characterized by the uncontrolled proliferation and disordered function of cells called plasma cells in the bone marrow.

Plasma cells are a type of B-*lymphocyte* (class of white blood cell) responsible for making *antibodies*, or *immunoglobulins*, that normally help protect against infection. In multiple myeloma, the proliferating plasma cells produce excessive amounts of a single type of immunoglobulin while the production of other types is impaired, making the patient particularly prone to infection.

Multiple myeloma is rare, with about three new cases annually per 100,000 population.

SYMPTOMS
As the abnormal plasma cells expand within bone, they cause pain and destruction of bone tissue. If the bones in the spine are affected, they may collapse and compress nerves, causing symptoms such as numbness or paralysis. The level of calcium in the blood may increase markedly as bone is destroyed, as may the level of a breakdown product of the immunoglobulin secreted by the plasma cells. These changes in blood chemistry may damage the kidneys, leading to *renal failure*.

In addition to the increased risk of infection, patients may suffer from *anemia* and a bleeding tendency if healthy bone marrow becomes replaced by malignant plasma cells.

DIAGNOSIS, TREATMENT, AND OUTLOOK
The disease is diagnosed from the appearance of a *bone marrow biopsy* specimen, the excess of the single type of immunoglobulin in the blood or urine, and the presence of areas of destroyed bone, as shown by X rays.

Treatment includes the use of *anticancer drugs* to reduce the number of abnormal plasma cells, *radiation therapy* to diseased areas of bone, and supportive measures (including blood transfusions to correct anemia, antibiotics to combat infections, and analgesics to relieve pain).

The severity and prognosis of the illness varies, but only about one fifth of patients survive for four years or longer from the time of diagnosis.

Multiple personality
A rare disorder in which a person has two or more distinct personalities, each of which dominates at different times. The personalities are almost always very different from each other and are often total opposites, as in the story of Dr. Jekyll and Mr. Hyde. They may have no awareness of each other, but are aware of lost periods of time.

Although multiple personality is often called split personality, a phrase also used to describe *schizophrenia*, the two disorders are unrelated. The split in schizophrenia is between thought and feeling.

Multiple pregnancy
See *Pregnancy, multiple*.

Multiple sclerosis
A progressive disease of the central nervous system in which scattered patches of myelin (the protective covering of nerve fibers) in the brain and spinal cord are destroyed. This causes symptoms ranging from numbness and tingling to paralysis and incontinence. The severity of multiple sclerosis (MS) varies markedly among sufferers.

CAUSES
The cause of multiple sclerosis remains unknown. It is thought to be an *autoimmune* disease in which the body's defense system begins to treat the myelin in the central nervous system as foreign, gradually destroying it, with subsequent scarring and damage to some of the underlying nerve fibers.

There seems to be a genetic factor since relatives of affected people are eight times more likely than others to contract the disease. Environment may also play a part—it is five times more common in temperate zones (such as the US and Europe) than in the tropics. Spending the first 15 years of life in a particular area seems to determine future risk. It is thought that a virus picked up by a susceptible person during this early period of life may be responsible for the disease's later development.

INCIDENCE
Multiple sclerosis is the most common acquired (not present at birth) disease of the nervous system in young adults. In relatively high-risk temperate areas the incidence is about one in every 1,000 people. The ratio of women to men sufferers is 3 to 2.

SYMPTOMS AND SIGNS
Multiple sclerosis usually starts in early adult life. It may be active briefly and then resume years later. The symptoms vary with which parts of the brain and spinal cord are affected.

Spinal cord damage can cause tingling, numbness, or a feeling of constriction in any part of the body. The extremities may feel heavy and become weak. *Spasticity* (stiffness) sometimes develops. The nerve fibers to the bladder may be involved, causing incontinence.

Damage to the white matter in the brain may lead to fatigue, vertigo, clumsiness, muscle weakness, slurred speech, unsteady gait, blurred or double vision, and numbness, weakness, or pain in the face.

These symptoms may occur singly or in combination and may last from several weeks to several months. In some sufferers, relapses may be precipitated by injury, infection, or physical or emotional stress.

Attacks vary considerably in their severity from person to person. In some, the disease may consist of mild relapses and long symptom-free periods throughout life, with very few permanent effects. Others have a series of flare-ups, leaving them with some disability, but further deterioration ceases. Some become gradually more disabled from the first attack and are bedridden and incontinent in early middle life. A small group suffers gross disability within the first year.

A person disabled with multiple sclerosis may have problems in addition to the paralysis, such as painful muscle spasms, urinary tract infections, constipation, skin ulceration, and changes of mood between euphoria and depression.

DIAGNOSIS
There is no single diagnostic test for multiple sclerosis; confirmation of the disease is usually by exclusion of all other possible conditions. A neurologist may perform tests to help confirm the diagnosis, including *lumbar puncture* (removal of a sample of fluid from the spinal canal for laboratory analysis), tracing electrical activity in the brain (see *Evoked responses*), CT scanning, and *MRI*.

TREATMENT
The search for a cure is still in progress. Patients are encouraged to

M

adopt as positive an outlook as possible, and to lead as active a life as their disabilities allow. *Corticosteroid drugs* may be prescribed to alleviate the symptoms of an acute episode; other drugs may be given to control specific symptoms, such as incontinence and depression. *Physical therapy* often helps strengthen muscles and various aids can help patients maintain mobility and independence.

Multivitamin

A group of over-the-counter preparations containing a combination of *vitamins* and used to supplement the intake of vitamins in the diet. (See *Vitamin supplements.*)

Mumps

An acute viral illness, mainly of childhood. The chief symptom is inflammation and swelling of the parotid (salivary) glands on one or both sides. Serious complications are uncommon. However, in teenage and adult males, mumps can be a highly uncomfortable illness in which one or both testes become inflamed and swollen. One attack of mumps confers lifelong immunity.

CAUSES AND INCIDENCE

The mumps virus is spread in airborne droplets. There is an incubation

---

FEATURES OF MULTIPLE SCLEROSIS

This disease can affect any area of the white matter of the brain and spinal cord. The plaques of demyelination are areas in which the fatty myelin sheaths of the nerve fibers have been destroyed. Affected fibers cannot conduct nerve impulses, so functions such as movement and sensation may be lost. The patchy distribution of plaques causes very varied effects.

Multiple sclerosis and the spine
Multiple sclerosis often affects nerve fibers in the spinal cord, thus blocking impulses to and from the brain.

Effects of multiple sclerosis
The fiber of the nerve tract is not usually destroyed. But the loss of insulating myelin and its replacement by neuroglia alters normal ion movements, so that the fiber can no longer conduct impulses.

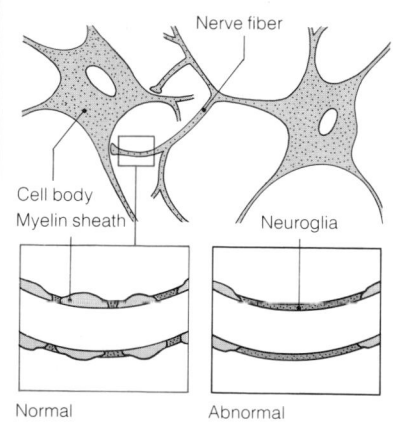

Nerve fiber

Cell body
Myelin sheath

Neuroglia

Normal   Abnormal

RANGE OF OUTLOOKS IN MULTIPLE SCLEROSIS

Dead
Bedridden
Restricted
Mild
No obvious disease

Dead
Bedridden
Restricted
Mild
No obvious disease

Years   0   5   10   15   20   25   30

Progress of multiple sclerosis
Multiple sclerosis is characterized by periods when symptoms are present, alternating with remissions (when symptoms are mild or absent).

5 percent

10 percent

33 percent

Majority

AFFECTED AREAS

Because the brain and spinal cord control all parts of the body, damage to these parts by multiple sclerosis may affect any function or any organ.

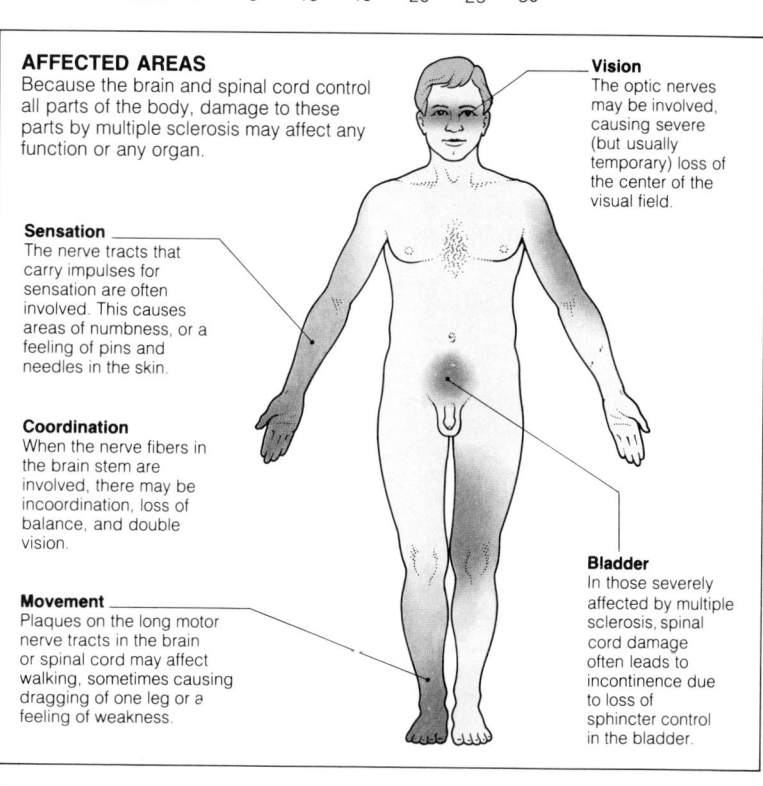

Sensation
The nerve tracts that carry impulses for sensation are often involved. This causes areas of numbness, or a feeling of pins and needles in the skin.

Coordination
When the nerve fibers in the brain stem are involved, there may be incoordination, loss of balance, and double vision.

Movement
Plaques on the long motor nerve tracts in the brain or spinal cord may affect walking, sometimes causing dragging of one leg or a feeling of weakness.

Vision
The optic nerves may be involved, causing severe (but usually temporary) loss of the center of the visual field.

Bladder
In those severely affected by multiple sclerosis, spinal cord damage often leads to incontinence due to loss of sphincter control in the bladder.

period of two to three weeks between infection and the appearance of symptoms. An affected person may spread the virus to others for about a week before and up to two weeks after symptoms appear. Most infections are acquired at school or from infected family members.

In the US, where many states require proof of mumps vaccination for school entry, the incidence has dropped markedly over the last 20 years, from a peak incidence of more than 185,000 cases in 1967 to a few thousand cases per year currently. In countries where immunization is not given routinely in early childhood, the infection remains common, affecting a large proportion of the population at some time between ages 5 and 10.

SYMPTOMS AND COMPLICATIONS

Many infected children have no symptoms or no more than mild sickness and discomfort in the region of the salivary glands (just inside the angle of the jaw). In more serious cases, the child first complains of pain in this region and has difficulty chewing; the glands on one or both sides then become swollen, painful, and tender. Fever, headache, and difficulty swallowing may develop, but the temperature falls after two to three days and the swelling subsides within a week to ten days. When only one side is affected, the second gland often swells as the first is subsiding.

An occasional complication is *meningitis*, which can cause headache, photophobia, drowsiness, fever, and stiff neck. However, these symptoms also resolve without long-term effects in most cases. A less common complication is *pancreatitis*, causing abdominal pain and vomiting.

In males after puberty, *orchitis* (inflammation of the testis) develops in about one quarter of cases. Only one testis is usually affected, becoming swollen, tender, and painful for two to four days. Subsequently, the affected testis shrinks to smaller than normal size. Uncommonly, both testes are affected; extremely rarely this can lead to sterility.

There is no evidence that mumps in pregnancy has any effect on the fetus.

DIAGNOSIS AND TREATMENT

Mumps is usually diagnosed from the patient's symptoms; the diagnosis may be confirmed by culturing the virus from saliva or urine or by measuring antibodies to mumps virus in the blood.

There is no specific treatment, but an affected child may be given

Appearance of mumps
The swelling, especially if present on both sides, may give the affected child a somewhat hamsterlike appearance.

analgesics (painkillers) and plenty to drink. In moderate to severe cases, the child may need to stay in bed during the first few days of the illness and should not go to school until symptoms have subsided.

For males with severe orchitis, a physician may sometimes prescribe a stronger painkiller, and *corticosteroid drugs* to reduce inflammation.

IMMUNIZATION

A safe and effective mumps vaccine is available and routinely given in the US to children in their second year, usually in combination with measles and rubella vaccines. The vaccine should not be given to children under 1, or to anyone with risk factors for vaccination (see *Immunization*).

Males who have already gone through puberty who have never been immunized against mumps or had the infection should avoid contact with any infected person. If symptoms of mumps do develop, passive immunization with antimumps *immunoglobulin* can provide some protection against the development of orchitis.

Münchausen's syndrome

A form of chronic *factitious disorder* in which the sufferer complains of physical symptoms that are pretended or self-induced. Sufferers are not *malingering*, they simply want to play the patient role. Most afflicted people are repeatedly hospitalized for investigations and treatment.

Pain in the abdomen, bleeding, neurological symptoms (such as dizziness and blackouts), skin rashes, and fever are the usual complaints. Sufferers typically invent dramatic, but often plausible, false histories and, once in the hospital, behave in a disruptive manner. Many show evidence of self-injury or of previous treatment (such as numerous scars or detailed medical knowledge).

It is difficult to determine the causes of the disorder; when challenged, the sufferers deny any allegations of deception or immediately discharge themselves from the hospital. Treatment is aimed at protecting these people from unnecessary operations and treatments.

Murmur

A sound caused by turbulent blood flow through the heart, as heard by a physician through a *stethoscope*. Murmurs are a separate phenomenon from other types of normal or abnormal *heart sounds*, which are caused mainly by sudden acceleration or deceleration of blood movement.

Heart murmurs are not necessarily a sign of disease, but an unusual sound is regarded as an indication of possible abnormality in the blood flow. Apart from "innocent" murmurs, the most common cause of extra blood turbulence is a disorder of the heart valves, such as stenosis (narrowing) or insufficiency (leakage) with regurgitation. Murmurs can also be caused by some types of congenital heart disease such as *septal defects* (holes in the heart) or *patent ductus arteriosus*, by *pericarditis* (inflammation of the membrane around the heart), or by other, rarer, conditions, such as a *myxoma* in a heart chamber.

By noting the location on the chest wall at which the murmur is best heard and the timing of the murmur in relation to the basic heart sounds, and by considering these factors in conjunction with other signs and symptoms, the physician can usually arrive at a diagnosis, which may be confirmed by *echocardiography*.

Muscle

A structure composed of bundles of specialized cells capable of contraction and relaxation to create movement, both of the body itself in relation to the environment and of the organs within it. There are three different types of muscle in the body—skeletal, smooth, and cardiac.

SKELETAL MUSCLE

The largest part of the musculature consists of skeletal (voluntary) muscles; the body contains more than 600 such muscles.

Skeletal muscles are classified according to the type of action each muscle performs. An extensor muscle opens out a joint, a flexor closes it; an adductor muscle draws a part of the body inward, an abductor moves it outward; a levator raises it, a

M

THE BODY'S MUSCLES

The most prominent muscles in the body are the skeletal muscles, which account for 40 to 45 percent of body weight. These muscles are called voluntary because they are under conscious control; some important voluntary muscles are indicated on the illustration below. Many internal organs, such as the heart and intestines, also consist partly or entirely of involuntary muscle, which is not under conscious control.

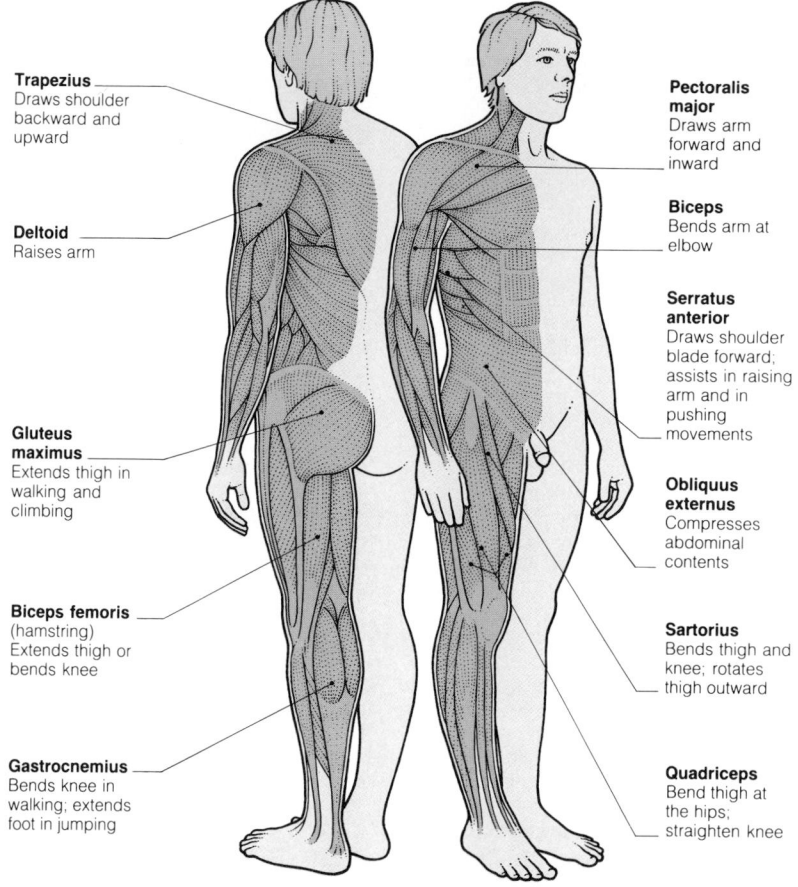

Trapezius
Draws shoulder backward and upward

Deltoid
Raises arm

Gluteus maximus
Extends thigh in walking and climbing

Biceps femoris
(hamstring)
Extends thigh or bends knee

Gastrocnemius
Bends knee in walking; extends foot in jumping

Pectoralis major
Draws arm forward and inward

Biceps
Bends arm at elbow

Serratus anterior
Draws shoulder blade forward; assists in raising arm and in pushing movements

Obliquus externus
Compresses abdominal contents

Sartorius
Bends thigh and knee; rotates thigh outward

Quadriceps
Bend thigh at the hips; straighten knee

M

MUSCLE MOVEMENT

Contraction makes a muscle shorter and draws together the bones to which the muscle is attached.

Two or more muscles may oppose each other's actions (e.g., biceps and triceps).

Biceps muscle
Triceps muscle
Elbow joint

Controlled movement at the elbow relies on coordinated relaxation and contraction of the biceps and triceps.

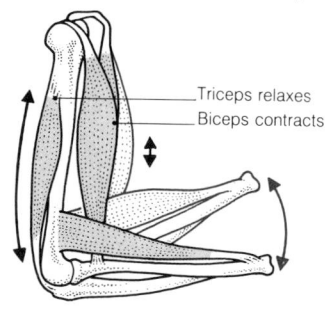

Triceps relaxes
Biceps contracts

MUSCLE TYPES

Skeletal and cardiac muscles appear striped under the microscope, unlike smooth muscles.

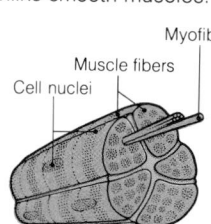

Myofibril
Muscle fibers
Cell nuclei

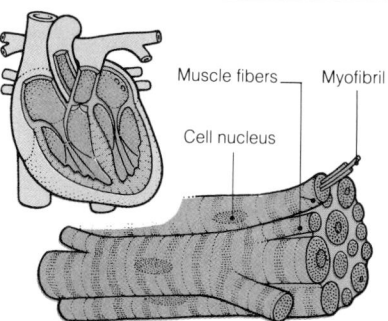

Muscle fibers — Myofibril

Cell nucleus

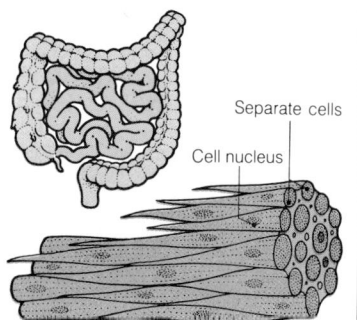

Separate cells

Cell nucleus

Skeletal muscle
Skeletal muscle consists of bundles of fibers (muscle cells), each containing contractile elements (myofibrils).

Cardiac muscle
Cardiac muscle contains short, branching cells that interconnect to help spread the signals that cause contraction.

Smooth muscle
Smooth muscle consists of more loosely woven, tapering cells. Contraction is slower than in other muscle types.

depressor lowers it; and constrictor or sphincter muscles surround and close body orifices.

Skeletal muscles are composed of groups of muscle fibers in an orderly arrangement.

A small muscle may be made up of only a few bundles of fibers, while the major muscles in the body (such as the gluteus maximus that forms the bulk of the buttock) are made up of hundreds of bundles. A muscle fiber is made up of even smaller longitudinal units called myofibrils, the basic working units of which are microscopic filaments called actin and myosin; these are proteins that control contraction.

Movement of the skeletal muscles is under the voluntary control of the brain. Each muscle fiber is supplied with a nerve ending that receives impulses from the brain. The nerve impulse stimulates the muscle by releasing a *neurotransmitter* called acetylcholine. This starts a chain of chemical and electrical events, involving sodium, potassium, and calcium ions, which results in the filaments of myosin sliding over the actin filaments in much the same way as an extendable ladder moves when it is closed. This movement of myosin over actin filaments causes the muscle to shorten in length.

Each muscle contains a set of specialized nerve fibers that registers the force of contraction; another set in the tendon gauges the stretch. The information received by these fibers is transmitted to the brain and is vital in limiting muscle action.

Skeletal muscle is maintained in partial contraction—called muscle tone. *Spasticity* is one form of abnormally increased muscle tone.

Skeletal muscle activity is affected by changes in chemical composition of the fluid surrounding the muscle cells. A fall in potassium ions causes muscle weakness; a decrease of calcium ions causes muscle spasm.

DISORDERS OF MUSCLE

The most common muscle disorder is injury, followed by symptoms caused by a lack of blood supply to a muscle (including the heart). In addition, there are a number of other rarer disorders of muscle.

GENETIC DISORDERS

The *muscular dystrophies* cause progressive weakness and disability. Some types appear at birth, some in infancy, and some develop as late as the fifth or sixth decade.

One type of *cardiomyopathy*, a general term for disease of the heart muscle, is inherited.

INFECTION

The most important infection of muscle is *gangrene*, which may complicate deep wounds (especially those contaminated by soil). *Tetanus* is acquired in a similar way, causing widespread muscle spasm through the release of a powerful toxin.

Viruses (especially influenza B) may also infect muscles (causing *myalgia*), as may the organism causing *toxoplasmosis*. *Trichinosis* is an infestation of muscle with the worm TRICHINELLA SPIRILIS, which is acquired by eating undercooked meat (usually pork).

INJURY

Muscle injuries, such as tears and *sprains*, are very common; they cause bleeding into the muscle tissue. Healing leads to formation of a scar in the muscle, which shortens its natural length. Blunt muscle injury may result in *hematoma* formation from bleeding into the muscle. Rarely, bone may form in the hematoma causing *myositis* ossificans.

TUMORS

Primary muscle tumors may or may not be cancerous. Noncancerous tumors are called *myomas*, those affecting smooth muscle are *leiomyomas*, and those affecting skeletal muscle are rhabdomyomas. Myomas of the uterus (see *Fibroids*) are among the most common of all tumors. Cancerous tumors are called myosarcomas and are very rare; cancers of the skeletal muscle are known as *rhabdomyosarcomas*.

Secondary tumors, which spread from a primary site of cancer elsewhere in the body, very rarely involve muscle.

HORMONAL AND METABOLIC DISORDERS

Muscle contraction depends on the maintenance of proper levels of sodium, potassium, and calcium in and around muscle cells. Any alteration in the concentration of these substances affects muscle function. For example, a severe drop in the level of potassium (hypokalemia) causes profound muscle weakness and may stop the heart. A drop in blood calcium (hypocalcemia) causes increased excitability of muscles and, occasionally, spasms.

Thyroid disease is often associated with muscle disorders, the most common being a swelling of the small muscles that move the eyes, causing a bulging eyeball (see *Exophthalmos*).

Adrenal failure causes general muscle weakness.

IMPAIRED BLOOD SUPPLY

Muscles depend on a good blood supply for normal function. *Cramp* is usually caused by a lack of blood flow, sometimes associated with severe exertion. *Peripheral vascular disease*, which restricts the blood supply,

causes *claudication* (muscle pain on exercise). *Angina pectoris* (chest pain caused by lack of blood supply to heart muscle) occurs in *coronary heart disease*.

The *compartment syndrome* is pain in muscles as a result of swelling that limits the blood supply. It is brought on by injury or exercise, occurring often in athletes with well-developed muscles.

POISONS AND DRUGS

Several toxic substances can damage muscle. They include alcohol, which can cause damage following a prolonged drinking bout. Other substances that may cause muscle damage include aminocaproic acid, chloroquine, clofibrate, emetine, and vincristine.

AUTOIMMUNE DISORDERS

Myasthenia gravis is a disorder of transmission of nerve impulses to muscles; it usually begins by causing drooping of the eyelids and double vision. Other diseases with an autoimmune basis that may affect muscles are *lupus erythematosus*, *rheumatoid arthritis*, *scleroderma*, *sarcoidosis*, and *dermatomyositis*.

INVESTIGATION

Muscle disorders are investigated by *EMG* (electromyography), which measures the response of muscles to electrical impulses, and by muscle biopsy.

M

SMOOTH MUSCLE

This type of muscle is concerned with the movements of internal organs, such as *peristalsis* in the intestine and contractions of the uterus during childbirth. Many other parts of the body, such as the bronchi of the lungs, the bladder, and the walls of the blood vessels, also contain smooth muscle.

Smooth muscle is composed of long, spindle-shaped cells. In most hollow organs, these cells are arranged in bundles organized in an outer longitudinal layer and an inner circular one. However, the mechanism of contraction relies on the same sliding action of actin and myosin as in skeletal muscle.

The nerve supply to smooth muscle comes from the *autonomic nervous system*, which is not under conscious control. Hence, its alternative name—involuntary muscle. Nerves from the autonomic nervous system penetrate into the muscle. There, they divide into many branches from which the neurotransmitter is released to initiate the process that leads to contraction.

In addition to neurotransmitters, smooth muscle responds to a variety of hormones, to the stretch of individual muscle fibers, and to changes in the chemical composition of the fluid surrounding the fibers, such as oxygen levels and acidity.

CARDIAC MUSCLE

This type of muscle, also called myocardium, is found only in the heart; it has unique properties that enable it to contract rhythmically about 100,000 times a day to propel blood through the circulatory system. The structure of cardiac muscle resembles that of skeletal muscle.

Contraction of cardiac muscle is stimulated by the autonomic nervous system, hormones, and stretching of the muscle fibers.

To act as an efficient pump, the muscles of the heart must contract in an orderly, regular manner. Separate muscle fibers are joined end to end by areas of extensive folds that allow contractions to be transmitted rapidly from one fiber to another. The stimulus for cardiac muscle contraction is initiated in an area of the right atrium (called the sinoatrial node), which stimulates a regular rate of contraction. Specialized conducting cells in cardiac muscle form a network capable of transmitting nerve impulses throughout the cardiac muscle fibers, spreading the contraction through both atria and then both ventricles alternately (see *Heart*).

Muscle-relaxant drugs

COMMON DRUGS

Baclofen Carisoprodol
Cyclobenzaprine Dantrolene
Diazepam Methocarbamol Orphenadrine

A group of drugs used to relieve *muscle spasm* and *spasticity*. They are often used in combination with an *analgesic* (painkiller) to relieve muscle stiffness caused by types of *arthritis*, back pain, or a disorder of the nervous system, such as *stroke* or *cerebral palsy*. Muscle-relaxant drugs are occasionally used to relieve muscle rigidity caused by injury.

HOW THEY WORK

With the exception of *dantrolene*, muscle-relaxant drugs partially block nerve signals from the brain and spinal cord that stimulate different muscles to contract.

Dantrolene acts directly on muscles by interfering with the chemical activity in muscle cells necessary for muscle contraction.

POSSIBLE ADVERSE EFFECTS

Because muscle-relaxant drugs reduce the strength of muscle contraction, they may cause weakness that is noticed when performing certain activities. Some muscle relaxants affect the brain and spinal cord, causing drowsiness. In rare cases, dantrolene causes liver damage.

Muscle spasm

Abnormal rigidity of a muscle. Causes include brain damage due to *stroke*, *cerebral palsy*, and severe *head injury*; brain disorders, such as *Parkinson's disease*; and pressure on a nerve from a *disk prolapse*. Other causes include muscle *strain* or injury.

Muscular dystrophy

An inherited muscle disorder of unknown cause in which there is slow but progressive degeneration of muscle fibers. Different forms are classified according to the age at which the symptoms appear, the rate at which the disease progresses, and the way in which it is inherited. (See box at right for main types.)

INCIDENCE

All forms of muscular dystrophy are rare. Duchenne muscular dystrophy is the most common type, affecting about one or two in 10,000 boys. It is inherited through a recessive, sex-linked gene (see *Genetic disorders*) so that only males are affected and only females can pass on the disease.

DIAGNOSIS

Often the diagnosis is suggested to the physician from observing the patient, but tests are needed for confirmation. A blood test may be performed to look for high levels of certain enzymes released from the damaged muscle cells. A test of electrical activity in the

DUCHENNE MUSCULAR DYSTROPHY: A TYPICAL FAMILY TREE

Key

○ Unaffected male

● Affected male

○ Carrier female

? Possible carrier female

○ Unaffected female

Affected males always inherit the gene for the disorder from their mothers, who are carriers of the gene, although unaffected themselves. About half the sons of carriers are affected; the other sons are neither affected nor carriers. The daughters of carriers have a 50 percent chance of being carriers themselves; complex blood tests provide the only means of knowing whether or not a certain daughter (or granddaughter) is a muscular dystrophy carrier.

muscles (see *EMG*) and muscle *biopsy* may be performed.

TREATMENT AND OUTLOOK

There is no effective treatment for muscular dystrophy. Affected children should be active for as long as possible to keep the healthy muscles in good condition. The children should not be allowed to become overweight; surgery to the heel cords may assist walking in some cases. The long-term outlook varies.

PREVENTION

Parents or siblings of an affected child should receive *genetic counseling*. Carriers of sex-linked forms of muscular dystrophy (see box, previous page) can be detected because their blood contains high levels of a particular enzyme.

It is now possible to diagnose some types of muscular dystrophy before birth by *chorionic villus sampling* or *amniocentesis*.

Musculoskeletal

Relating to muscle and/or bone. The musculoskeletal system is the bony skeleton of the body and the hundreds of muscles that are attached to it.

Mushroom poisoning

 There are many species of poisonous mushrooms and toadstools in the US, but only some of them cause poisoning. Many of the others, although poisonous, have an unpleasant taste and thus are unlikely to be eaten in significant amounts.

TYPES, SYMPTOMS, AND TREATMENT

Most fatal cases of mushroom poisoning in the US are caused by *AMANITA PHALLOIDES* (the death cap) and its relatives. This mushroom looks innocuous, bearing a resemblance to the edible field mushroom. However, there are some clear differences. The death cap grows in deciduous woods (mainly beech and oak), has a yellow-olive colored cap, and, most importantly, has white gills on the underside of its cap (not pink-brown as on the edible field mushroom).

The death cap and one or two related species such as *AMANITA VIROSA* (destroying angel) contain highly poisonous peptides called amanitins, which attack cells in the lining of the small intestine, the liver, and, occasionally, the kidneys. Symptoms such as severe abdominal pain, vomiting, and diarrhea usually develop eight to 14 hours after eating the mushroom. Later, there may be liver enlargement and jaundice; about 10 to 15 percent of victims die of liver failure (this stage of the poisoning resembles acute viral hepatitis). There is no effective antidote. Treatment consists of supportive measures in the hospital. For those who survive the poisoning (after about one week), recovery is usually fairly rapid.

Another species, *AMANITA MUSCARIA*, or fly agaric, is very similar in shape to the death cap but has a red cap flecked with white. Symptoms of poisoning, which appear within 20 minutes to two hours, may include drowsiness, visual disturbances, delirium, muscle tremors, and nausea and vomiting. Treatment of this type of mushroom poisoning, and of other types in which symptoms develop rapidly, is by gastric lavage (see *Lavage, gastric*) and the administration of activated charcoal. Full recovery usually occurs within 24 hours. Fatal poisoning by fly agaric has never been reported in the US.

"Magic" mushrooms are a species containing the hallucinogenic substance psilocybin. In addition to hallucinations, they may cause high fever in children, which requires medical attention. The effects usually subside within four to six hours; occasionally they persist longer.

Mutagen

Any physical or chemical agent that, when applied to a group of living cells, increases the rate of *mutation* in those cells. A mutation is a change in the genetic material within a cell, which,

TYPES OF MUSCULAR DYSTROPHY

Duchenne muscular dystrophy	In this type, the child is slow in learning to sit up and walk, and does so much later than normal. The condition is rarely diagnosed before the age of 3, but progresses rapidly. Affected children tend to walk with a waddle and have difficulty climbing stairs. In getting up from the floor, the child "climbs up his legs," pushing his hands against his ankles, knees, and thighs. Sometimes there	is curvature of the spine. Despite their weakness, the muscles (especially those in the calves) appear bulky; this is because wasted muscle is replaced by fat. By about age 12, affected children are no longer able to walk; few survive their teen years, usually dying from a chest infection or heart failure. Affected boys often have below-average intelligence.
Becker's muscular dystrophy	This type produces the same symptoms as the Duchenne type, but starts later in childhood and progresses much more	slowly. Patients often reach the age of 50. Both types of dystrophy have sex-linked inheritance.
Myotonic dystrophy	This form affects muscles of the hands and feet. Infants are floppy and slow to develop. The main feature is that the muscles contract strongly but do not relax easily. Myotonic dystrophy	is associated with cataracts in middle age, baldness, mental retardation, and endocrine problems. The condition has an autosomal dominant pattern of inheritance.
Limb-girdle muscular dystrophy	This type takes different forms. It starts in late childhood or early adult life, and progression is slow. The muscles of the hips and shoulders are mainly	affected. Other nerve and muscle conditions must be eliminated before this form of dystrophy can be diagnosed confidently.
Facioscapulohumeral muscular dystrophy	This form usually appears first between the ages of 10 and 40; it affects only the muscles of the upper arms, shoulder girdle, and face. It is inherited in an autosomal	dominant pattern. In this form of muscular dystrophy, progression of the weakness is slow, and severe disablement is rare.

M

under certain circumstances, can give rise to a cancer or a hereditary disease.

The most important mutagens are ionizing radiation and some chemicals. The former includes X rays and various types of emission from nuclear explosions, radioactive fallout, and leaks from nuclear reactors, including gamma rays and alpha and beta particles (see *Radiation hazards*). Similar types of radiation are also emitted (at a low intensity) from rocks and from the sky (cosmic rays).

Many chemical *carcinogens* are thought to cause cancers by altering the genetic material within cells, thus acting as mutagens. Chief among them are chemicals in tobacco smoke.

Mutation

A change in the genetic material within a living cell—that is, in the *DNA*, the main constituent of a cell's *chromosomes* that provides the coded instructions for the cell's activities.

Many mutations are neutral or harmless; some are harmful, giving rise to cancers, birth defects, and hereditary diseases. Very rarely, a mutation may be beneficial.

CAUSES AND TYPES

A mutation results from a fault in the copying of a cell's DNA to its daughter cells when the cell divides. One of the offspring cells inherits some faulty DNA, and the fault is copied each time the cell divides, creating a population of cells containing the altered DNA.

The change may be a point mutation, affecting only a small part of a section of DNA (called a *gene*). This type may lead to production of defective enzymes or other proteins in the affected cells, thus disrupting their activities. In other cases, entire chromosomes or bits of chromosomes are deleted, added, or rearranged in affected cells, which can produce greater disruptive effects.

The term *mutagen* refers to any physical or chemical agent that makes mutations more likely. The most important mutagens are types of high-energy radiation, and certain chemicals, including some *carcinogens* (cancer-inducing agents).

EFFECTS

The effects of a harmful mutation depend on whether the affected cell is a "germ" cell in an ovary or testis (capable of giving rise to an egg or sperm) or whether it is one of the other cells in the body (somatic cells).

A mutated somatic cell can, at worst, multiply to form a group of abnormal cells within a particular body region. Often these cells die out, are destroyed by the body's immune system, or have only a minor local effect. Sometimes, however, they may form the basis for a tumor.

A mutation in a germ cell can have a dramatically different effect. It may be passed on, via egg or sperm, to a child, who then carries the mutation in all of his or her cells. This may lead to an obvious birth defect or abnormality in body chemistry. Furthermore, the child may pass on the mutation to some of his or her descendants. *Genetic disorders* (such as *hemophilia* and *achondroplasia*) stem originally from point mutations that have occurred to the germ cell of a parent, grandparent, or more distant ancestor. Some of these mutations occur frequently; about one third of all cases of hemophilia are caused by new mutations. *Chromosomal abnormalities* (such as *Down's syndrome*) generally result from mutations in the formation of a parental egg or sperm.

PREVENTION

Some mutations are unavoidable, occurring by chance or as the result of natural background radiation from the sky and from radioactivity in rocks. This background radiation causes random mutations in the population.

Minimizing any further risk of a mutation depends on avoiding known mutagens. It is particularly important for people exposed to radiation in the course of their work to have their exposure closely monitored to ensure that it does not exceed safe limits (see *Radiation hazards*). Younger people and those of reproductive age should have their reproductive organs shielded when undergoing X rays or radiation therapy.

Radioactive leaks or explosions from nuclear reactors can cause a rise in mutation rates that affects large populations. This may lead to an increase in the incidence of various cancers and birth defects in succeeding generations.

The chances of a mutation can also be lessened by avoiding exposure to carcinogens (which are a class of mutagen), the most obvious of which are the chemicals in tobacco smoke.

BENEFICIAL MUTATIONS

Very rarely, a mutation occurs in a germ cell that confers a survival advantage in the face of some environmental stress. People who inherit this mutation tend to survive longer than their peers; some of their children in turn inherit the mutation and pass it on to succeeding generations. Such mutations tend to become more common in a population over many generations as long as the original environmental stress persists.

An example is the mutation that causes sickle cell trait. Carrying this mutation protects against malaria, so it enhances a child's survival chances where malaria is prevalent. The mutation is prevalent in Africa (along with malaria) and affects many people of African origin. A double dose of the mutation (inheriting it from both parents) can lead to *sickle cell anemia*.

Mutism

Refusal or inability to speak. Mutism may occur as a symptom of severe *manic-depressive illness*, catatonic *schizophrenia*, and a rare form of *conversion disorder*. The term may also be applied to those who have taken a vow of silence for religious reasons.

Elective mutism describes a rare childhood disorder usually starting before age 5. The child understands language and speaks properly, but refuses to speak most of the time, preferring to use nods or gestures. A shy, withdrawn personality and anxiety over leaving home for school are important factors, but mild mental retardation or language problems may be the cause. This condition rarely lasts more than a few months.

Akinetic mutism describes a state of inert passivity that is caused by certain deep-seated tumors of the brain or by *hydrocephalus*. Though conscious and able to follow movements with their eyes, these people are incontinent, require feeding, and respond at most with a whispered "yes" or "no."

Treatment of mutism depends on the underlying cause.

Myalgia

The medical term for muscle pain. Myalgia is common in viral illnesses (such as influenza) and also occurs in a number of rheumatic disorders, such as *rheumatoid arthritis*, systemic *lupus erythematosus*, and *polymyalgia rheumatica*. Myalgia is the main symptom of *polymyositis* and *dermatomyositis*, disorders that cause inflammation of muscle tissue.

Myasthenia gravis

A disorder in which the muscles become weak and tire easily. The eyes, face, throat, and limb muscles are most commonly affected. Typically, the sufferer has drooping eyelids, a blank facial expression, and weak, hesitant speech.

CAUSES AND INCIDENCE

Myasthenia gravis is an *autoimmune disorder* in which, for unknown reasons, the body's *immune system* attacks and gradually destroys the receptors in muscles that are responsible for picking up nerve impulses. As a result, affected muscles fail to respond, or respond only weakly, to nerve impulses.

Myasthenia gravis is a rare disease; two to five new cases per 100,000 people are diagnosed annually. It affects more women than men (in a ratio of 3 to 2). Although it can occur at any age, myasthenia gravis usually appears between the ages of 20 and 30 in women and 50 and 70 in men.

SYMPTOMS AND SIGNS

The disease may develop suddenly or gradually. It is extremely variable in the way it affects different people and in how it affects the same person from day to day. The affected muscles become worse with use but may recover completely with rest. Symptom-free periods typically alternate with relapses of the condition.

The eye muscles are the most commonly affected, and most sufferers have drooping eyelids and double vision. Weakness is also common in the muscles of the face, throat, larynx (voice box), and neck. This causes difficulty speaking, so that the voice becomes weak, hoarse, nasal, and slurred toward the end of a conversation. Chewing and swallowing become increasingly difficult as a meal progresses, so that the sufferer may choke or regurgitate food through the nose. Sometimes the jaw must be supported to prevent it from hanging.

In some people, the arm and leg muscles are also affected, producing difficulty combing the hair and climbing stairs. In severe cases of myasthenia gravis, respiratory muscles in the chest may be weakened, causing breathing difficulty.

Infection, stress, menstruation, medications, and other factors can exacerbate the condition.

Abnormalities in the thymus gland are present in about three quarters of affected people and, in about 10 to 15 percent of them, a *thymoma* (tumor of the thymus gland) is found.

DIAGNOSIS

The disease is diagnosed by a physical examination, the patient's history, and various tests. The most commonly used diagnostic test involves the injection of a drug called edrophonium into a vein. Within a minute, power is temporarily restored to the weak muscles. Electromyography (see *EMG*), which detects muscle weakness by measuring the muscle's electrical activity, and blood tests that reveal the presence of certain antibodies may also be carried out.

In some patients, mainly those over 40, *CT scanning* may be performed to look for a thymoma.

TREATMENT

In mild cases of myasthenia gravis, regular medication with drugs to facilitate the transmission of nerve impulses to the muscles is often enough to restore the patient's condition to near normal.

In severe myasthenia gravis, thymectomy (removal of the thymus gland) often considerably improves, and sometimes cures, the condition. Otherwise, regular exchanges of the patient's antibody-containing plasma for antibody-free plasma may be carried out; high doses of *corticosteroid drugs*, which block the immune process, may be given.

OUTLOOK

In mild cases the sufferer is able to live a comparatively normal life. In a minority of patients, progression of the disease cannot be halted and paralysis of the throat and respiratory muscles may lead to death.

Mycetoma

A rare tropical infection affecting skin and bone, caused by fungi or by actinomycetes (bacteria that form long chainlike colonies).

The infection is usually confined to one limb and can be highly disfiguring. It produces a hard swelling covered by the openings of multiple drainage channels, through which pus is discharged. The disease organisms form into visible "grains," which are found in the discharge.

Antibiotic drugs are the main treatment if the disease is caused by actinomycetes. Mycetoma caused by fungal infections may be difficult to treat with drugs; surgical removal of diseased tissue may be necessary.

Mycology

The study of *fungi* and *fungal infections*.

Mycoplasma

Any of a group of microorganisms that are the smallest capable of free existence. Mycoplasmas are about the same size as viruses and, like viruses, have no cell wall. However, unlike viruses, mycoplasmas can reproduce outside living cells.

Most types of mycoplasma are harmless to humans, although many cause respiratory diseases in animals such as cattle, sheep, and poultry. One of the species, MYCOPLASMA PNEUMONIAE, causes a special form of *pneumonia* (primary atypical pneumonia) in humans. The pneumonia is treated effectively with antibiotics such as tetracyclines.

Mycosis

Any disease caused by a fungus. (See *Fungi; Fungal infections*.)

Mycosis fungoides

A type of *lymphoma* (cancerous spread of lymphoid tissue) that primarily affects the skin of the buttocks, back, or shoulders but can also occur in other sites. The cause of this rare disorder is unknown.

The mildest form appears as a red, scaly, nonitching rash; it may spread slowly or remain unaltered for many years. In the more severe forms of the disease, thickened patches of skin and ulcers may develop and lymph glands may enlarge.

DIAGNOSIS, TREATMENT, AND OUTLOOK

A skin *biopsy* (removal of a small sample of tissue for microscopic examination) is carried out. In mild cases, patients are treated with *PUVA* (psoralen drugs plus long-wave ultraviolet light treatment in the A range) or nitrogen mustard applied to the skin. In more severe cases, *anticancer drugs* may be needed.

Mydriasis

Dilation (widening) of the pupil of the eye. Mydriasis, which occurs naturally in the dark, also occurs if a person is emotionally aroused, after the use of eye drops (such as atropine), and after consumption of alcohol. Adie's syndrome is a benign condition in which one pupil constricts slowly in response to light. The condition may last for years.

Myectomy

Surgical removal of part or all of a muscle. Myectomy may be performed to alter the power of an eye muscle to correct *strabismus* (squint), or to remove a fibroid in an operation called a *myomectomy*. Myectomy is also part of the treatment of severely injured and infected muscles.

Myel-

A prefix that denotes a relationship to bone marrow (as in myeloma, a tumor consisting of bone marrow cells) or to the spinal cord (as in myelitis, inflammation of the spinal cord). The prefix myelo- is synonymous with myel-.

Myelin

The fatty material, composed of lipid (a fat) and protein, that forms a protective sheath around some types of nerve fiber. Myelin gives the characteristic appearance to the white matter of the brain, which is composed largely of myelinated nerve fibers.

In addition to having a protective function, myelin acts as an electrical insulator, thereby increasing the efficiency of nerve impulse conduction.

Abnormal breakdown of myelin is called *demyelination*. It occurs in some diseases of the nervous system, notably *multiple sclerosis*.

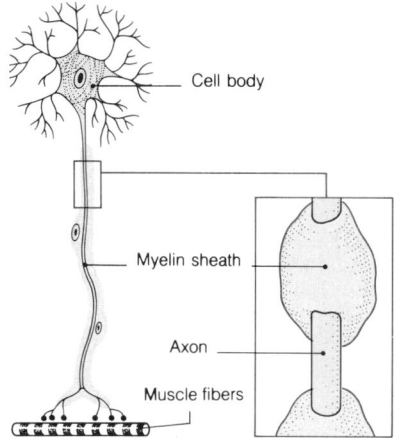

Cell body

Myelin sheath

Axon

Muscle fibers

The myelin nerve sheath
The axon is the long conducting fiber of a nerve. To transmit impulses, each nerve requires an insulating myelin sheath.

Myelitis

Inflammation of the spinal cord. Myelitis may be the result of a viral infection—for example, *poliomyelitis* (commonly called polio), *measles*, or *herpes simplex*. The illness starts suddenly with headache, fever, neck stiffness, and pain in the back and limbs, which are followed in some cases by muscle pain and weakness, and eventually paralysis.

Transverse myelitis is a type of myelitis in which there is inflammation of the spinal cord around the middle of the back. It may follow a viral illness but often occurs without obvious cause. Common symptoms are back pain and gradual paralysis of the legs. Many people recover, but some are left with spastic paralysis of the involved limbs.

Myelocele

A protrusion of the spinal cord and its meninges (protective coverings) under the skin due to a congenital defect in the vertebral column (see *Spina bifida*).

Myelography

X-ray examination of the spinal cord, nerves, and other tissues within the spinal canal after injection of a substance opaque to X rays.

WHY IT IS DONE

In the past, myelography was often performed to examine the lower spinal nerves when a disk prolapse was suspected; it was also important in diagnosing tumors of the spinal cord, and in looking for damaged nerves after certain injuries. The procedure is being replaced today by newer imaging techniques, such as *CT scanning* and *MRI*.

HOW IT IS DONE

The patient lies facedown on the X-ray table. Using local anesthesia, a *lumbar puncture* is performed; X-ray control is used to guide a fine needle into the fluid-filled space that surrounds the spinal cord and spinal nerves. A small sample of fluid is withdrawn for testing, and the radiopaque dye is introduced. By tilting the patient headdown, the dye can be moved up the spinal canal, and X-ray pictures are taken of areas where damage is suspected. The procedure usually takes 15 to 20 minutes. Afterward, the patient must lie down for a few hours with the head slightly raised.

Myeloma, multiple

See *Multiple myeloma*.

Myelomeningocele

See *Myelocele*.

Myelopathy

A term that refers to any disease of the *spinal cord* or of the bone marrow, such as *multiple myeloma* or *leukemia*.

Myelosclerosis

An increase of fibrous tissue within the bone marrow. It is also known as osteosclerosis or myelofibrosis. Myelosclerosis may occur without any obvious cause (primary myelosclerosis) or may result from some other bone marrow disease (such as *polycythemia* or chronic myeloid *leukemia*). The ability of the bone marrow to produce blood components is impaired. However, this function can be partly taken over by the spleen and the liver.

Primary myelosclerosis is a disease of middle age with a gradual onset. The main symptoms are those of *anemia*, which is caused by impaired red blood cell production by the bone marrow. Enlargement of the spleen, night sweats, itching, loss of appetite, and weight loss are other common symptoms of myelosclerosis. In secondary myelosclerosis, there may be other symptoms connected with the underlying disease.

TREATMENT

Treatment of primary myelosclerosis is aimed at the relief of symptoms, mainly through blood transfusions. Anticancer drugs are of little or no use. Only half of patients survive for more than three years, and acute leukemia develops in a small number.

In secondary myelosclerosis, treatment is of the underlying cause.

Myiasis

An infestation of the skin, deeper tissue, or intestines by fly larvae. Myiasis is primarily restricted to the tropical regions of the world.

TYPES AND SYMPTOMS

In Africa, the tumbu fly lays eggs on clothing left outside to dry; the larvae that hatch from these eggs penetrate the skin to cause boillike swellings. Various other flies may lay eggs in open wounds, on the skin, or in the ears or nose. Sometimes the larvae penetrate deeply into the tissues, causing considerable destruction. Intestinal infestation can occur after eating contaminated food.

PREVENTION AND TREATMENT

Myiasis can largely be prevented by keeping flies away from food, by covering open wounds, and, in Africa, by thoroughly ironing clothes dried outdoors.

Cutaneous myiasis is treated by placing drops of oil over the swelling caused by the larva. The oil suffocates the larva, which is forced to come to the surface and can be removed with a needle. Infestation in deeper tissues may require surgical treatment. Intestinal myiasis can be adequately treated with a laxative.

Myo-

A prefix that denotes a relationship to muscle (as in myocarditis, inflammation of the heart muscle).

Myocardial infarction

Popularly known as a heart attack, sudden death of part of the heart muscle characterized, in most cases,

FEATURES OF MYOCARDIAL INFARCTION

Myocardial infarction, in which an area of heart muscle is deprived of blood supply and suffers tissue death as a result, is a major cause of death in developed countries. Atherosclerosis of the coronary arteries is the cause in most cases of myocardial infarction.

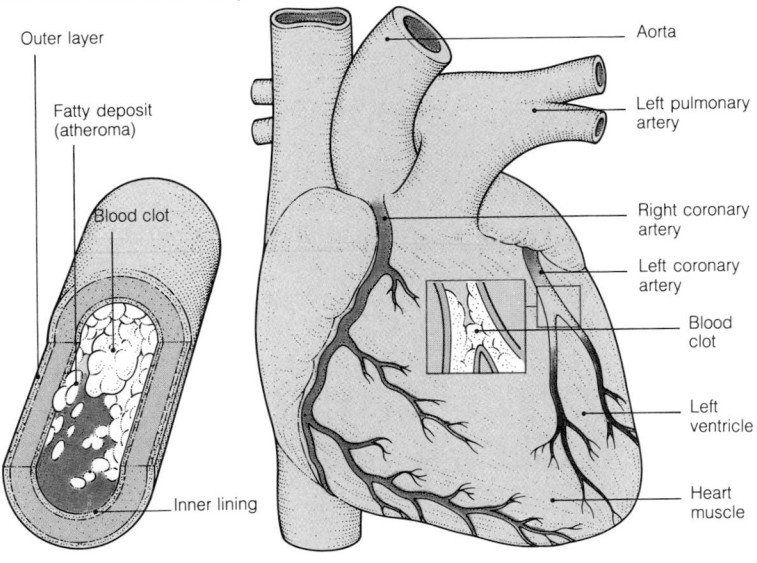

Outer layer

Fatty deposit (atheroma)

Blood clot

Inner lining

Aorta

Left pulmonary artery

Right coronary artery

Left coronary artery

Blood clot

Left ventricle

Heart muscle

Atherosclerosis
Like all other arteries, the coronary arteries may be affected by atherosclerosis. Patchy plaques of atheroma develop on the inner lining of the arteries, restricting the blood flow and encouraging the formation of blood clots. The clotting results in a sudden stoppage of blood flow to the heart.

OUTLOOK AFTER AN ATTACK
Myocardial infarction is fatal within 20 days in about one third of cases, and another 3 to 12 percent of patients die between 20 days and one year of the attack. Some further risk persists for several years, but a significant number of patients (about 30 percent) are still alive 10 years after an attack.

FATALITY RATES

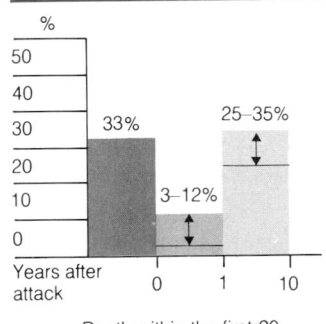

%

50
40
30
20
10
0

33%

3–12%

25–35%

Years after attack

0   1   10

Death within the first 20 days after the attack

Death between 20 days and 1 year after the attack

Death between 1 year and 10 years after the attack

M

PAIN
Many victims of myocardial infarction have a history of angina pectoris, in which the chest pain is relieved by rest. The pain of infarction usually comes on suddenly, and ranges from a tight ache to intense crushing agony. It lasts for 30 minutes or more, and is not relieved by rest.

A central chest pressure, ranging from mild to severe, is common to almost every attack of myocardial infarction from coronary obstruction.

In some cases, pain radiates up into the jaw and through to the back. Sometimes, it occurs only in these places.

In many cases, the pain radiates down the left arm; it may cause a sensation of weakness in the arm muscles.

More rarely, pain may be felt in the upper abdomen. If it occurs only here, it may be mistaken for another disorder.

RISK FACTORS

Uncontrollable factors include a family history of heart disease, old age, and being male.

Habitual cigarette smokers have a substantially increased risk of dying from myocardial infarction.

High blood pressure is a major risk factor, and the risk increases the higher the pressure.

The risk of atherosclerosis and coronary heart disease increases dramatically in those who are more than 30 percent overweight.

A raised blood cholesterol content (for which there may be a genetic tendency) increases the risk. A high-fat diet is also a factor.

Physical inactivity is also a major risk factor.

by severe, unremitting chest pain. Each year in the US about 1 million people have a heart attack; attacks are fatal in about one third of cases and are the single most common cause of death in developed countries.

Men are more likely to suffer heart attacks than women, smokers more than nonsmokers, and the children of someone who has died of a heart attack are more likely to die from this cause. Other risk factors include increased age, unhealthy diet, stress, obesity, and disorders such as *hypertension* (high blood pressure), *diabetes mellitus*, and *hyperlipidemia*.

SYMPTOMS AND COMPLICATIONS

The characteristic symptom is sudden pain in the center of the chest (see box on previous page). The victim may also be short of breath, restless, and apprehensive, have cold clammy skin, feel nauseated or vomit, or lose consciousness.

In mild cases, pain and other symptoms are slight or do not develop at all (in which case the attack is known as a silent infarct). The episode passes unnoticed and may be discovered only by subsequent tests.

Damage to the heart muscle may be so severe that it leads immediately to *heart failure* (reduced pumping efficiency of the heart). *Arrhythmias* (abnormal heart rhythms) are common. Most people who die of a myocardial infarction do so within the first few hours due to a type of arrhythmia called ventricular fibrillation, which seriously interferes with the pumping action. However, if the person can be brought to a hospital, arrhythmias can be controlled with drugs or electrical *defibrillation*.

Possible long-term complications include damage to the mitral valve, leading to *mitral insufficiency*, or the development of a weak area in the wall of the heart or in the muscle dividing the two sides of the heart. Complications may require surgery.

DIAGNOSIS

The diagnosis is made from the patient's history and from special tests. Those performed immediately include *ECG* and the measurement of certain enzymes released into the blood from damaged heart muscle. Emergency coronary artery *angiography* may be performed if surgery is being considered.

TREATMENT

If someone is thought to be having a heart attack, a physician or ambulance should be called immediately. Initial treatment may include strong *analgesics* (painkillers) and *oxygen therapy*. *Diuretic drugs* may be given to treat heart failure, which can lead to accumulation of fluid in the lungs. Intravenous fluids may need to be given for shock, and *antiarrhythmic drugs* may be given to control arrhythmias. *Beta-blocker drugs* are given in some cases to reduce the risk of further muscle damage.

In many hospitals, patients who arrive within three to six hours of a heart attack are now treated with *thrombolytic drugs* to dissolve any blood clot. Other new methods of treatment include angioplasty (widening of narrowed coronary arteries), which may follow the thrombolytic treatment. *Coronary artery bypass* surgery may be considered.

In the past, it was recommended that patients rest in bed for two weeks or more following an attack. Today, patients are encouraged to be out of bed within four or five days.

It is increasingly common for heart attack patients to be supervised in special hospital coronary care units. The nursing and medical staff are trained to recognize and institute early treatment for arrhythmias, and many patients find the environment reassuring. However, some specialists believe coronary care units are actually more stressful and prefer that some patients, particularly the very elderly, be cared for elsewhere in the hospital or at home.

OUTLOOK

Anyone who has suffered a heart attack has an increased risk of suffering another one in the following few years. The chances of surviving for many years can be improved by attention to risk factors (see table on previous page).

It is important for patients to have their conditions assessed by their physicians at regular intervals for life.

Myocarditis

Inflammation of the heart muscle. The diagnosis of myocarditis is sometimes made after death when a young person has died unexpectedly during vigorous exercise. In such cases the pathologist finds evidence of inflammation, which is usually assumed to be due to a virus infection sometimes preceded by a sore throat or a cold. Myocarditis is a feature of *rheumatic fever*, which is rare today. It may also, in rare cases, be caused by drugs or radiation therapy.

People with virus infections affecting the lungs often have mild myocar-

ditis, which may be detected only by an *ECG*. Rarely, the inflammation causes a serious disturbance of the heart beat, breathlessness, chest pain, *heart failure* (reduced pumping efficiency), and cardiac arrest leading to death. Acute *pericarditis* (inflammation of the outer lining of the heart) often accompanies myocarditis.

Most cases clear up without treatment, although occasionally *corticosteroid drugs* are prescribed to reduce inflammation. It is generally believed that exercise is dangerous for people with myocarditis; most physicians recommend that exercise be avoided until a patient's electrocardiogram results have returned to normal. Anyone with symptoms of a viral infection (such as a sore throat) should avoid strenuous exercise to reduce the risk of myocarditis developing.

In Central and South America, the most common cause of myocarditis is the parasitic infection *Chagas' disease*. Many years after the initial infection, the parasitic organisms can cause extensive damage to the heart muscle, leading to progressive and often fatal heart failure.

Myoclonus

Rapid, uncontrollable jerks or spasm of a muscle or muscles that occur at rest or during movement. Myoclonus may be associated with disease of nerves and muscles. It may occur during an epileptic seizure (see *Epilepsy*) or as a symptom of a brain disorder such as *encephalitis* (inflammation of the brain).

Myoclonus also occurs in healthy people, an example being the limb jump that is sometimes experienced just before falling asleep.

Myofacial pain disorder

See *Temporomandibular joint syndrome*.

Myoglobin

The oxygen-carrying pigment in muscles. It consists of a combination of iron and protein, and gives muscles their red color. Like *hemoglobin* (the oxygen-carrying pigment in red blood cells), myoglobin takes up and then stores oxygen, which it releases when the muscle tissues are in need of oxygen to contract.

Myoglobinuria is the presence of myoglobin in the urine. Small amounts of myoglobin in the urine may occur when taking prolonged, vigorous exercise. However, severe myoglobinuria is usually caused by the release of myoglobin from a large area of damaged muscle (which can occur in *crush syndrome*, for instance) and may cause *renal failure*.

Myoma

A noncancerous tumor of muscle. The most common type is a *leiomyoma*, which affects the smooth muscle of the intestine, uterus, and stomach.

Myomectomy

Surgical removal of a *myoma* (a non-cancerous tumor of muscle). The term is commonly applied to the removal of *fibroids* of the uterus.

Myopathy

A disease of muscle, usually degenerative (see *Muscle* disorders box), but sometimes caused by chemical poisoning, by a drug side effect, or by a chronic disorder of the *immune system*. A myopathy is not caused by disease of the nervous system. An example is *muscular dystrophy*.

Myopia

An error of *refraction* in which near objects can be seen clearly while those in the distance appear blurred. Commonly known as nearsightedness, myopia is caused by the eye being too long from front to back. As a result,

---

THE CAUSE OF MYOPIA

Myopia is caused by the combined power of the cornea and lens being too great in relation to the length of the eyeball.

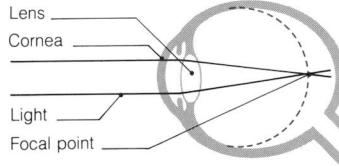

Lens
Cornea

Light
Focal point

Uncorrected myopia
With uncorrected myopia, the images of distant objects are focused in front of the retina and appear blurred.

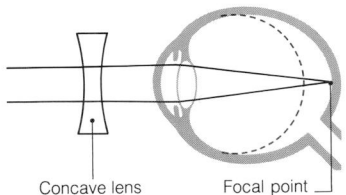

Concave lens   Focal point

Corrected myopia
To see distant objects clearly, the power of the eye must be reduced by a concave (negative) lens.

---

the corneal lens focuses images of distant objects in front of the retina.

Myopia, which tends to be inherited, usually appears around puberty and increases progressively until the early 20s, when it stabilizes. Myopia that starts in early childhood often progresses into adult life, and may become very severe.

If myopia is detected during a *vision test*, *glasses* or *contact lenses* may be prescribed to reduce the focusing power of the cornea.

Myositis

Inflammation of muscle tissues that causes pain, tenderness, and weakness. Types of myositis include *pleurodynia* (a viral infection affecting muscles around the rib cage), myositis ossificans (in which the damaged muscle is replaced by bone), *polymyositis* (inflammation of muscles throughout the body), and *dermatomyositis* (inflammation of muscles and the presence of a rash). Polymyositis and dermatomyositis are rare *autoimmune disorders*.

Myotomy

A procedure that involves cutting into a muscle. An example is pyloromyotomy—cutting into the muscle surrounding the lower end of the stomach to treat *pyloric stenosis* (narrowing of the stomach's exit).

Myotonia

A rare symptom that describes the inability of a muscle to relax after the need for contraction has passed. Myotonia occurs primarily in two neurological diseases. Myotonia congenita is an inherited condition in which muscle stiffness starts during infancy and usually improves as the person grows older. In myotonic dystrophy, myotonia is combined with muscle weakness. Drugs may help reduce myotonia.

Myringitis

Inflammation of the eardrum. Myringitis occurs, to some degree, in every case of *otitis media*.

Myringoplasty

Surgical closure of a perforation (hole) in the eardrum (see *Eardrum, perforated*) by means of a tissue graft. Myringoplasty is done to improve hearing and, sometimes, to stop a recurrent discharge from the ear. The graft material is usually muscle fascia (fibrous lining) taken from the temple or the thigh.

Myringotomy

A surgical opening made through the eardrum to allow drainage of the middle-ear cavity.

WHY IT IS DONE

Myringotomy is usually performed on children to treat persistent *middle-ear effusion*, in which a sticky secretion fills the middle-ear cavity. The fluid causes hearing loss, which may become permanent if the condition is not treated.

Before the advent of antibiotics, myringotomy was performed to treat acute *otitis media* (middle-ear infection) by releasing the pus and thereby relieving pressure on the eardrum.

HOW IT IS DONE

Using a general anesthetic, a small incision is made in the eardrum and most of the fluid is removed by suction. At the same time, a small tube may be inserted in the hole to allow any remaining and subsequently produced fluid to drain into the outer ear. In most cases the child can leave the hospital the following day. The tube usually falls out a few months later as the hole in the eardrum closes. If the condition has not cleared up, a second operation may be required to insert another tube.

Myxedema

A condition in which there is thickening and coarsening of the skin and other body tissues (most noticeable in the face, where the lips become swollen and the nose thickened). Other symptoms usually include weight gain, hair loss, sensitivity to cold, and mental dullness. Myxedema results from *hypothyroidism* and is most common in adults (especially women) over 40. The term myxedema is sometimes used interchangeably with adult hypothyroidism.

Myxoma

A benign, jellylike tumor composed of soft mucous material and loose fibrous strands. Myxomas usually occur singly, and may grow very large. They usually occur under the skin (typically in the limbs or neck), but may also develop in the abdomen, bladder, or bone. Very rarely, a myxoma may grow inside the heart, which can lead to the formation of thrombi (blood clots) and obstruct blood flow through the heart. In most cases, a myxoma can be successfully removed by surgery. Myxomatosis is a highly infectious viral disease of rabbits in which many myxomas develop throughout the rabbit's body; this disease does not affect humans.

N

Nadolol

A *beta-blocker drug* used in the treatment of *hypertension* (high blood pressure), *angina pectoris* (chest pain due to impaired blood supply to heart muscle), certain types of *arrhythmia* (irregularity of the heart beat), and *hyperthyroidism* (overactivity of the thyroid gland).

Possible adverse effects are typical of other beta-blocker drugs.

Nail

A hard, curved plate on the fingers and toes composed of *keratin* (a tough protein that is also the main constituent of skin and hair). A fingernail takes about six months to grow from base to tip, although there are seasonal growth variations. Toenails take twice as long to grow.

DISORDERS
The nails are susceptible to damage through injury, usually as a result of crushing or pressure on the nail. Sometimes the nails become abnormally thick and curved—a condition called *onychogryphosis* that mainly affects the big toes of elderly people.

Nails may be damaged by bacterial or fungal infections, especially *tinea* and *candidiasis*. In *paronychia*, the nail folds are infected. The nails may also be affected by skin disease or by more generalized illnesses.

Examples of the effects of skin disease on the nails include pitting of the nails in *alopecia* areata, pitting and *onycholysis* (separation of the nail from its bed) in *psoriasis*, and scarring and onycholysis in *lichen planus*.

Nail abnormalities may be signs of more generalized disease. Brittle, ridged, concave nails are a sign of iron-deficiency *anemia*, onycholysis is seen in *thyrotoxicosis*, and fibrous growths on the nails are a sign of *tuberous sclerosis*. Splinterlike black marks develop beneath the nails (denoting bleeding into the nail bed) in *endocarditis* and *bleeding disorders*.

Abnormalities of nail color may also signify disease. A greenish discoloration may be caused by bacterial infec-

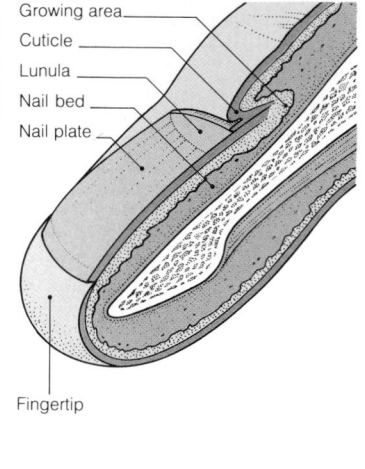

ANATOMY OF A NAIL
The nail bed is the area from which the nail grows. At the base of each nail, a half-moon shape, the lunula, is crossed by a flap of skin, the cuticle. The skin that surrounds the nail is the nail fold. The nail is composed of keratin, a tough protein also found in skin and hair.

Growing area
Cuticle
Lunula
Nail bed
Nail plate
Fingertip

tion under the nail, blue nails may be a sign of heart or respiratory disease, and yellow nails that are hard and curved develop in *bronchiectasis* and *lymphedema*. The nails may also be discolored by the color in nail polish and by nicotine staining.

DIAGNOSIS AND TREATMENT
Nail disorders are usually diagnosed by inspecting the nails and skin, along with a physical examination if necessary. Laboratory examination of nail clippings may be performed.

Treatment of nail disorders is difficult. Creams and lotions seldom penetrate sufficiently; oral medication may take months to be effective.

Nail-biting

A common activity that does not indicate any underlying medical condition. Many children bite their nails during their first years at school, but most grow out of it. Nail-biting sometimes continues as a nervous habit in adolescents and adults. Persistent nail-biting may make the nails unsightly and cause pain and sometimes bleeding.

Various preparations with an unpleasant taste can be painted on the nails, but many people become accustomed to the taste.

Nalidixic acid

An *antibiotic drug* used to treat and, occasionally, to prevent *urinary tract infection*. Nalidixic acid is effective against some types of bacteria that are resistant to other antibiotics.

Adverse effects include nausea, vomiting, increased sensitivity to sunlight, blurred vision, drowsiness, and dizziness.

Naloxone

A drug that blocks the action of *narcotic drugs*. Naloxone reverses breathing difficulty caused by a narcotics overdose. It is also given to newborn babies affected by narcotics used to aid childbirth and to people who have received high doses of a narcotic drug during surgery.

Possible adverse effects include abdominal cramps, diarrhea, nausea, vomiting, and tremors.

Naltrexone

A drug that blocks the euphoric effects of *narcotic drugs*. Naltrexone is given to addicts who have stopped taking narcotics as part of a supervised detoxification program. It helps prevent the recurrence of *drug dependence*.

Possible adverse effects include nausea, loss of energy, depression, and, in rare cases, liver damage.

Nandrolone

An anabolic steroid (see *Steroids, anabolic*) sometimes used with *growth hormone* in the treatment of *short stature*. Nandrolone is also used to treat certain types of *anemia*.

Possible adverse effects include swollen ankles, nausea and vomiting, jaundice, and aggressive behavior. In men, nandrolone may cause difficulty passing urine; in women, irregular menstruation and abnormal hair growth may occur.

Naphazoline

A *decongestant drug* used in the treatment of allergic *rhinitis*, *sinusitis*, or a common *cold*. Naphazoline is also given to clear bloodshot eyes and to relieve minor eye irritation.

Overuse of nasal preparations containing naphazoline may lead to palpitations, headache, drowsiness, restlessness, and "rebound" congestion (worsening of congestion after drug use is stopped).

Naproxen

A *nonsteroidal anti-inflammatory drug* (NSAID) that is used as an *analgesic* (painkiller) in the treatment of headache, menstrual pain, and injury to soft tissues (such as muscles or ligaments). It is also used to reduce joint pain and stiffness in *arthritis*.

Possible adverse effects are nausea, abdominal pain, and *peptic ulcer*.

Narcissism

Intense self-love. The term is derived from the Greek myth of Narcissus, who so loved to stare at his own reflection in the water that he fell in and drowned. In *psychoanalytic theory* there is an early stage in childhood development when the ego (self) feels omnipotent. Failure to deal with the frustrations of discovering that this is not so may result in neurosis later.

A narcissistic personality disorder is characterized by an exaggerated sense of self-importance, constant need for attention or praise, inability to cope with criticism or defeat, and poor relationships with other people.

Narcolepsy

A *sleep* disorder characterized by chronic, excessive daytime sleepiness with recurrent episodes of sleep occurring several times per day. Attacks may last from a few seconds to more than an hour and may be mildly inconvenient or severely disabling, often interfering with work and daily life. *Cataplexy* (sudden loss of muscle tone without loss of consciousness) occurs in about three quarters of cases. Other symptoms may include *sleep paralysis* and vivid hallucinations at the onset of sleep or on awakening.

In narcolepsy, the REM (rapid eye movement) state, which normally occurs only during sleep, intrudes into wakefulness. Narcolepsy is often inherited. Treatment usually involves regular naps, along with *stimulant drugs* to control drowsiness and sleep attacks and *antidepressant drugs* to suppress cataplexy.

Narcosis

A state of stupor usually caused by a drug (see *Narcotic drugs*) or other chemical. Narcosis resembles sleep, being marked by reduced awareness and by diminished ability to respond to external stimulation. However, unlike a sleeper, a person in narcosis cannot be roused completely.

Narcotic drugs

COMMON DRUGS	
Codeine	Meperidine
Morphine	Propoxyphene

A type of *analgesic* (painkiller) used in the treatment of moderate and severe pain. Abuse of narcotic drugs for their euphoric effects often causes *tolerance* (the need for greater amounts to have the same effects) and physical and psychological *drug dependence*.

Nasal congestion

Partial blockage of the nasal passage caused by inflammation of the mucous membrane that lines it. Congestion can be caused by an infection of the nasal passage itself (such as a cold), by an infection that has spread from the sinuses (see *Sinusitis*), or by an allergy (see *Rhinitis, allergic*).

A simple, effective, and time-honored method of alleviating nasal congestion is to inhale the steam from a pot of hot water. This loosens the mucus, which enables the sufferer to blow it out through the nose. *Decongestant drugs* in the form of nasal drops and sprays should be used sparingly since extensive use can make congestion worse. Decongestant tablets and syrups are of doubtful value and may cause drowsiness.

Persistent nasal congestion should be investigated by a physician.

Nasal discharge

The spontaneous emission of fluid from the nose. Nasal discharge is commonly caused by inflammation of the mucous lining and is often accompanied by *nasal congestion*.

In allergic *rhinitis*, the discharge consists of runny, clear mucus. Infection of the nasal passage itself (such as a cold) or infection that has spread from the sinuses (see *Sinusitis*) usually causes a thicker discharge of mucus, often mixed with pus. A newly developed persistent runny discharge may be an early sign of a tumor (see *Nasopharynx, cancer of*).

Bleeding from the nose is usually caused by injury or a foreign body in the nose; it may also be a sign of an underlying bleeding disorder or a tumor (see *Nosebleed*). In rare cases, cerebrospinal fluid may be discharged from the nose as a result of a fracture at the base of the skull.

Nasal obstruction

Blockage of one or both sides of the nasal passage, which interferes with breathing. The most common cause is inflammation of the mucous membrane that lines the passage (see *Nasal congestion*). Other causes include severe deviation of the *nasal septum*, nasal *polyps*, a *hematoma* (a collection

of clotted blood) usually caused by injury, and, rarely, a malignant tumor. In children, enlargement of the adenoids is the most common cause of nasal obstruction.

Nasal septum

The central partition inside the nose that divides it into two cavities. The nasal septum consists of cartilage at the front and bone at the rear, both covered by *mucous membrane*.

DISORDERS

Deviated septum (twisting of the septum to one side) may be present from birth or may be caused by a blow to the nose. It is rarely troublesome, but, if breathing is obstructed, the septum can be straightened by surgery.

Injury can also cause a *hematoma* (a collection of clotted blood) to form between the cartilage of the septum and the wall of one nasal cavity, again sometimes obstructing breathing. The hematoma may become infected, causing an *abscess*, which may require surgical drainage. Occasionally, an abscess develops on a child's septum without prior injury.

Rarely, a hole may be eroded in the septum by *tuberculosis, syphilis, cocaine,* or *Wegner's granulomatosis.*

Destroyed nasal septum
This photograph of the left nostril was taken with a light shined into the right nostril. There is a hole in the septum.

Nasogastric tube

A narrow plastic tube that is passed through the nose, down the esophagus, and into the stomach.

WHY IT IS USED

One of its most common uses is to suck or drain digestive juices from the stomach when the intestine is blocked (as in *pyloric stenosis*) or is not working properly (as may occur after an abdominal operation). The tube is also used to give liquid nourishment to very ill patients who cannot eat (see *Feeding, artificial*), to obtain specimens of stomach secretions for examination, and to wash out the stomach after a drug overdose or after swallowing a poison (see *Lavage, gastric*).

HOW IT IS USED
Inserting the tube is a quick, simple procedure that causes little discomfort and does not require an anesthetic. The tube is lubricated and passed into one nostril; while the patient swallows, it is slid down the throat and into the stomach. To ensure that the tube is in the stomach, a sample of fluid is withdrawn through a syringe and tested on litmus paper for acidity. The stomach contents may then be sucked out through the syringe or through a suction device, or they may be allowed to drain freely into a container. Fluids for lavage or feeding are introduced through a funnel. If the nasogastric tube is to be left in place for some time, the protruding end of the tube is taped to the face.

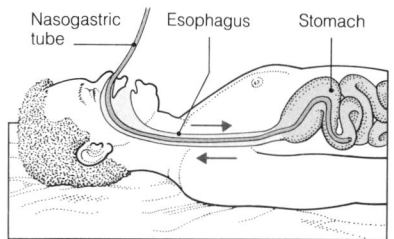

Using a nasogastric tube
The tube is passed via a nostril and the esophagus into the stomach. Substances may be delivered into the stomach via the tube, or the stomach contents may be removed through it.

Nasopharynx
The passage connecting the nasal cavity behind the nose to the top of the throat behind the soft *palate*. Part of the respiratory tract, the nasopharynx forms the upper section of the *pharynx*. During swallowing, the nasopharynx is sealed off (to prevent food from entering it) by the action of the soft palate pressing against the back of the throat.

The nasopharynx contains the openings to the *eustachian tubes* (passages connecting the back of the nose to the middle ear) and, in children, the *adenoids*. The adenoids can enlarge to such an extent that the nasopharynx becomes completely blocked, forcing the child to breathe through his or her mouth.

Nasopharynx, cancer of
A malignant tumor that originates in the *nasopharynx* (uppermost part of the

throat, behind the nose) and usually spreads to the nasal cavity, nasal sinuses, base of the skull, and lymph nodes in the neck. Cancer of the nasopharynx is rare in the West but common in the Far East; it is most common between the ages of 40 and 50 and affects twice as many men as women. One cause is believed to be the *Epstein-Barr virus*.

SYMPTOMS AND SIGNS
Common first signs are recurrent nosebleeds, a persistently runny nose, and voice change. As the tumor spreads, there may be a bloody discharge from the nose, loss of smell, double vision, deafness, paralysis of one side of the face, and severe facial pain.

DIAGNOSIS AND TREATMENT
The diagnosis is made from a *biopsy* (removal of a small sample of tissue for analysis). X rays may be taken to determine to what extent the cancer has spread.

Treatment is with *radiation therapy*. The outlook depends on when treatment began; one third of sufferers survive for more than five years.

Natural childbirth
See *Prepared childbirth*.

Naturopathy
A form of *alternative medicine* based on the principle that disease is due to the accumulation of waste products and toxins in the body, and that symptoms reflect the body's attempt to rid itself of these substances. Practitioners of naturopathy believe that health is maintained by avoiding anything artificial or unnatural in the diet or in the environment.

Nausea
The sensation of needing to vomit. Although nausea may occur independently of vomiting, the causes are the same (see *Vomiting*).

Navel
A popular term for the *umbilicus*, the depression in the abdomen that marks the point at which the umbilical cord was attached to the fetus.

Nearsightedness
See *Myopia*.

Nebulizer
A device used to administer a drug in aerosol form through a face mask. Nebulizers are used to administer *bronchodilator drugs*, especially in the emergency treatment of an attack of

Using a nebulizer
An electric or hand-operated pump sends a stream of air or oxygen across a chamber containing the required drug. This stream of air disperses the drug into a fine mist, which is then conveyed to the face mask and inhaled by the user.

asthma. A nebulizer is much easier to use than a conventional *inhaler* (pressurized aerosol canister).

Neck
In addition to supporting the head, the neck is the passageway between the head and brain and the body. It thus contains a number of vital structures. Decapitation kills because it cuts through the *spinal cord* (which carries nerve impulses to and from the brain) and because it severs the *trachea* (windpipe), the *esophagus*, and major blood vessels leading to and from the head. Strangulation kills by compressing major blood vessels and by cutting off the air supply to the lungs.

DISORDERS
INJURY *Torticollis* (wryneck), in which the head is twisted to one side, may result from birth injury to a neck muscle or from skin *contracture* after burns or other injuries.

Fractures and *dislocations* of any of the vertebrae in the neck can injure the spinal cord, causing paralysis or even death; *whiplash injuries* can also severely damage the spinal cord.

DEGENERATION The joints between vertebrae may be affected by *cervical osteoarthritis*, causing neck pain, stiffness, and sometimes tingling and weakness in the arm and hand. Similar symptoms may be caused by a *disk prolapse*. In *ankylosing spondylitis*, fusion of the vertebrae may result in permanent neck rigidity.

CONGENITAL DEFECT *Cervical rib* (a small extra rib in the neck) often causes no symptoms until middle age, when it may result in pain, numbness, and a pins and needles sensation in the forearm and hand.

N

ANATOMY OF THE NECK

The neck contains many important structures, including the larynx, the thyroid and parathyroid glands, many lymph nodes, and the carotid arteries. The upper seven vertebrae of the spine are in the neck; a complex system of muscles is connected to these vertebrae, the clavicles, the upper ribs, and the lower jaw. Contraction of these muscles allows the head to turn and the jaw to open and close.

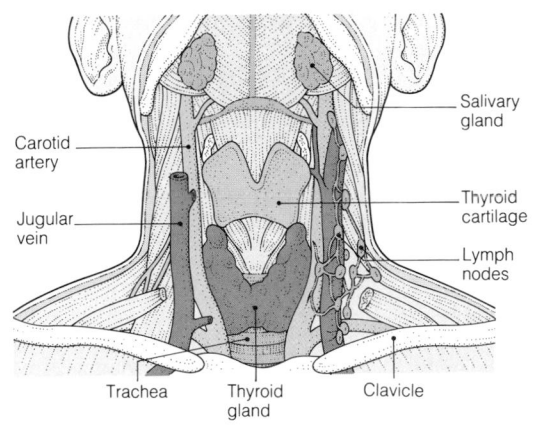

Carotid artery

Jugular vein

Trachea

Thyroid gland

Clavicle

Salivary gland

Thyroid cartilage

Lymph nodes

Muscles of the neck
Muscles on the back and side of the neck support and move the head.

OTHER DISORDERS Because structures in the neck are so closely packed, any condition that causes swelling (such as inflammation, allergy, bleeding, or tumors) may, if large enough, interfere with breathing or swallowing. Enlargement of the lymph nodes usually results from infection, but may be due to other conditions.

Neck pain of unknown origin is very common. As long as neurological symptoms (such as loss of sensation or muscle power) are absent, it is unlikely to be serious. Most sufferers recover within a few weeks.

Neck dissection, radical

A surgical procedure for removing cancerous lymph nodes in the neck. The operation is commonly required as part of the treatment of cancer of the tongue, tonsils, or other structures in the mouth and throat.

A flap of skin on the affected side of the neck is raised (using a general anesthetic) to expose the underlying sternomastoid muscle. The muscle is cut through just above the clavicle (collarbone) and lifted up. The entire lymphatic system in the neck (the vessels as well as the nodes) is then removed, along with the internal jugular vein, lower salivary gland, and other surrounding tissue.

Neck rigidity

Marked stiffness of the neck caused by spasm of the muscles in the neck and spine. Neck rigidity is an important clinical sign of *meningitis* (inflammation of the membranes surrounding the brain and spinal cord). Severe neck rigidity may cause the head to arch backward, especially in babies.

Necrolysis, toxic epidermal

A severe, blistering rash in which the surface layers of the skin peel off, exposing large areas of red raw skin over the body. The effects of toxic epidermal necrolysis are similar to those of a severe third-degree burn, with the same potentially serious risks of widespread infection and loss of body fluid and salts from the exposed body surface.

In newborn babies, the condition is usually caused by staphylococci (a type of bacteria) and is called the scalded skin syndrome. Treatment is with antibiotic drugs and sometimes intravenous fluid replacement.

In adults, the most common cause of toxic epidermal necrolysis is an adverse reaction to a drug, particularly a barbiturate, sulfonamide, or penicillin. The condition usually clears up when use of the drug is discontinued. Intravenous fluid replacement is sometimes necessary.

Necrophilia

A rare sexual perversion in which orgasm is achieved by sexual acts, either heterosexual or homosexual, with dead bodies.

Necropsy

A little-used alternative medical term for an *autopsy* (postmortem examination of a body).

Necrosis

The death of tissue cells. Necrosis can occur as a result of *ischemia* (inadequate blood supply), which may lead to *gangrene*; infection (such as *tuberculosis*); or damage by extreme heat or cold, noxious chemicals (such as acids), or excessive exposure to X rays or other forms of radiation.

The appearance of dead tissue depends on the cause of the necrosis and, usually, on the type of tissue affected. For example, in necrosis due to tuberculosis, the dead tissue is soft, dry, and cheeselike; fatty tissue beneath the skin that has died as a result of damage or infection develops into tough scar tissue that may form a firm nodule.

Nematodes

 The scientific name for a group of cylindrically shaped worms, some of which can be parasites of humans. (See *Roundworms*.)

Neologism

The act of making up new words that have a special meaning for the inventor. The term also refers to the invented words themselves. While inventing words is often considered a creative act in novelists and poets, persistent neologism is a sign of *schizophrenia*, in which it occurs with other disordered thoughts.

Neomycin

An *antibiotic drug* used in the treatment of ear, eye, and skin infections, often in combination with other drugs. Neomycin is given to treat and sometimes prevent some infections of the intestine. It is also used in the treatment of *hyperlipidemia* (high lipid levels in the blood).

Possible adverse effects include rash, itching, diarrhea, nausea and vomiting, hearing loss, dizziness, and ringing in the ears.

Neonate

A newly born infant (see *Newborn*).

Neonatologist

A specialist in the care of newborn babies and their special problems. Problems may be short-term (such as those associated with premature or low-weight babies) or lifelong (such as

N

spina bifida). The neonatologist cares for the baby for the first four weeks of life. After this time, the child's medical care becomes primarily the responsibility of a *pediatrician*.

Neonatology

The branch of *pediatrics* concerned with the care of newborn infants and the treatment of their disorders. (See also *Neonatologist*.)

Neoplasia

A medical term for *tumor* formation, characterized by a progressive, abnormal multiplication of cells. The term neoplasia does not necessarily imply that the new growth is *malignant*; *benign* tumors also develop as a result of neoplasia.

Neoplasm

A medical term for a *tumor* (any new, abnormal growth). Neoplasms may be *malignant* or *benign*.

Neostigmine

A drug used in the treatment of *myasthenia gravis* (a rare autoimmune disorder that causes muscle weakness). Neostigmine is also given to treat abnormal retention of urine (see *Urine retention*) and paralytic *ileus* (temporary paralysis of the intestine).

Neostigmine works by increasing the activity of *acetylcholine*, a *neurotransmitter* (chemical released from nerve endings) that stimulates the contraction of muscles.

Possible adverse effects include nausea and vomiting, increased salivation, blurred vision, diarrhea, abdominal cramps, sweating, muscle cramps, twitching, and rash.

Nephrectomy

Surgical removal of one or both of the *kidneys*.

WHY IT IS DONE

One of the most common reasons for nephrectomy is to remove a malignant tumor (see *Kidney cancer*). A kidney may also be removed if it is not functioning normally due to infection or the presence of stones (see *Calculus, urinary tract*), or is causing severe *hypertension* (high blood pressure). Nephrectomy may also be necessary if a kidney is so badly injured that bleeding cannot be stopped.

HOW IT IS DONE

Nephrectomy is carried out using general anesthesia. The patient lies on his or her side, bent sharply at the waist over an angled operating table. An incision is made along the lower

edge of the ribs, from the spine at the back to the front of the abdomen to expose the kidney. The *ureter* and renal blood vessels are tied off, and the kidney is removed. The incision is stitched up after insertion of a drainage tube, which is left in position for 24 to 48 hours.

OUTLOOK

A person's kidney function becomes virtually normal about six months after removal of a single kidney because the remaining kidney (providing it is healthy) takes over the entire work load. If both kidneys are removed, the patient requires *dialysis* or a *kidney transplant*.

Nephritis

Inflammation of one or both kidneys. Nephritis may be caused by infection (see *Pyelonephritis*), by abnormal responses of the *immune system* (see *Glomerulonephritis*), and by metabolic disorders, such as gout. (See also *Kidney* disorders box.)

Nephroblastoma

See *Kidney cancer*.

Nephrocalcinosis

The deposition of calcium within the substance of one or both kidneys. Nephrocalcinosis is not the same as kidney stones (see *Calculi, urinary tract*), in which calcium particles develop within the drainage channels of the kidney.

Nephrocalcinosis may occur in any condition in which the blood level of calcium is raised. These conditions include *hyperparathyroidism* (overactivity of the parathyroid gland) and *renal tubular acidosis* (in which the kidney produces urine of lower than normal acidity). Nephrocalcinosis may also develop as a result of taking excessive amounts of certain *antacid drugs* or *vitamin D*.

Treatment is of the underlying cause to prevent further calcification.

Nephrolithotomy

The surgical removal of a *calculus* (stone) from the kidney by cutting through the body of the kidney. Nephrolithotomy can be achieved through an abdominal incision, or through a puncture incision made through the skin in the back and directly into the kidney (percutaneous nephrolithotomy). Instruments allow the stone to be grasped or fragmented and withdrawn.

A more straightforward method of stone removal is *pyelolithotomy*, in

which the stone is removed through a cut at the junction between the kidney and ureter.

An alternative approach to dealing with kidney stones is to pulverize them by means of ultrasonic waves (see *Lithotripsy*). Pulverization may also be achieved with an ultrasonic wand passed through the skin (percutaneous *lithotripsy*).

Nephrologist

A specialist in the diagnosis and treatment of kidney disease.

Nephrology

The medical specialty concerned with the normal functioning of the *kidneys*, and with the causes, diagnosis, and treatment of kidney disease.

Methods of investigating the kidneys include kidney *biopsy*, *kidney function tests*, and *kidney imaging* techniques (such as intravenous *pyelography*). Treatment of kidney disorders includes drugs (to control high blood pressure, inflammation, or infection), surgical intervention (for the treatment of stones and tumors), and *dialysis* or, in some cases, a *kidney transplant* (for the treatment of advanced kidney disease).

Nephron

The microscopic unit of the *kidney* that consists of a glomerulus (filtering funnel) and a tubule. There are about 1 million nephrons in each kidney. The nephrons filter waste products from the blood and modify the amount of salts and water excreted in the urine according to the body's needs.

Nephropathy

Any disease or damage to the kidneys (see *Kidney* disorders box).

Obstructive nephropathy refers to kidney damage caused by a urinary tract *calculus* (stone), tumor, scar tissue, or pressure from an organ blocking urine flow and creating back pressure within the kidney.

Reflux nephropathy refers to kidney damage caused by backflow of urine from the bladder toward the kidney. It is caused by failure of the valve mechanism at the lower end of each ureter.

Toxic nephropathy refers to damage caused by various poisons or minerals (such as carbon tetrachloride or lead).

Nephrosclerosis

A process in which normal kidney structures are replaced with scar tissue composed of *collagen*. Nephrosclerosis usually represents the final healing stage of any of the conditions that cause inflammation within the kidney. Such conditions include *diabetes mellitus*, *glomerulonephritis*, and chronic *pyelonephritis*.

Nephrosis

See *Nephrotic syndrome*.

Nephrostomy

The introduction of a small tube into the kidney to drain urine to the abdominal surface, thus bypassing the ureter. Nephrostomy is sometimes performed after an operation (typically, removal of a *calculus*) on the ureter or kidney-ureter junction to allow healing to take place.

Nephrotic syndrome

A collection of symptoms and signs that results from damage to the glomeruli (filtering units of the *kidney*) causing severe *proteinuria* (loss of protein from the bloodstream into the urine). Loss of large amounts of protein in the urine lowers the protein content of the blood and results in edema (fluid retention).

CAUSES

Nephrotic syndrome may be caused by *diabetes mellitus*, *glomerulonephritis* (inflammation of the glomeruli), *amyloidosis* (a condition in which amyloid, an abnormal protein, collects in the tissues and organs), severe *hypertension* (high blood pressure), reactions to poisons (including lead, carbon tetrachloride, and poison ivy), and adverse drug reactions.

SYMPTOMS

Edema causes marked swelling of the legs and face. Fluid may also collect in the chest cavity (producing *pleural effusion*) or within the abdomen (causing *ascites*). Anorexia, lethargy, and diarrhea may also occur.

TREATMENT

Treatment is of the underlying condition. A low-sodium diet may be recommended, and *diuretic drugs* may be given to reduce edema. If the plasma protein concentration is particularly low, protein may need to be given intravenously.

Nerve

A bundle of nerve fibers that travels to a common location. Nerve fibers, also called axons, are the filamentous projections of many individual *neurons* (nerve cells).

The most obvious nerves in the body are the peripheral nerves, which extend from the central nervous system (CNS), consisting of the brain and spinal cord, to other parts of the body. Apart from the *optic nerves*, most nerve fiber bundles within the brain and spinal cord are referred to as nerve tracts or nerve pathways rather than simply "nerves."

STRUCTURE

Including optic nerves, there are 12 pairs of *cranial nerves* (which link directly to the brain) and 31 pairs of *spinal nerves* (which join the spinal cord)—all are peripheral nerves.

In the shoulder and hip regions, the spinal nerves join to form the main nerves to the limbs, such as the median nerve in the arm and the sciatic nerve in the leg. Most nerves divide at numerous points along their length to send branches to all parts of the body, particularly to the sense organs, skin, skeletal muscles, internal organs, and glands.

FUNCTION

Nerve fibers may have a sensory function, carrying information from a receptor or sense organ at the far end of the nerve toward the CNS, or a motor function, carrying instructions from the CNS to a muscle or a gland. Messages are carried by electrical impulses propagated along the fibers. Some nerves carry only sensory or motor fibers, but most carry both.

Nerve functioning is sensitive to cold, pressure, and to a wide variety of injuries (see *Nerve injury*). The peripheral nerves can be damaged by infection, inflammation, poisoning, nutritional deficiencies, and metabolic disorders (see *Neuropathy*).

Nerve block

The injection of a local anesthetic into or around a nerve to produce anesthesia (loss of sensation) in a part of the body supplied by that nerve.

WHY IT IS DONE

A nerve block is performed when it is not possible to inject anesthetic directly into the tissues that are being treated because the area is painfully inflamed or because there is a risk of spreading infection. Nerve block may also be used to anesthetize a large area, or an area not suited for injection because it is deep within the body or is covered with bone.

HOW IT IS DONE

The local anesthetic is injected at an accessible area into or around the nerve at a point remote from the area to be treated (e.g., the palm of the hand may be anesthetized by injecting points up the arm, thus blocking the ulnar and median nerves).

A nerve may be blocked as it leaves the spinal cord, such as in *epidural anesthesia* (used in childbirth) and in *spinal anesthesia* (used mainly for surgery of the lower abdomen and limbs). In a caudal block, anesthetic is injected into nerves leaving the lowest part of the spinal cord; it produces anesthesia in the buttock and genital areas. A caudal block is occasionally used for childbirth, especially a forceps delivery. A pudendal nerve block involves injection of nerves passing under the pelvis into the floor of the vagina; it is used for forceps delivery. (See also *Anesthesia, local*.)

Nerve injury

A cut or crush injury to a nerve that severs some or all of its individual conducting fibers. Surgical repair is the only treatment for a severed nerve, and only the peripheral nerves (those outside the brain and spinal cord) are amenable to such repair. (See *Neuropathy* for nerve damage from causes other than injury.)

CRUSH INJURIES

In a crush injury, individual fibers within a peripheral nerve may be severed while the nerve trunk itself remains intact. The severed fibers degenerate on both sides of the injury, leading to loss of power in the muscles and loss of sensation in the skin area supplied by the fibers. However, if the ends are still aligned, new fibers can regenerate along the channels left by the degenerated fibers. These fibers begin to grow within a few days after an injury and advance at a rate of about 1 inch (2.5 cm) per month.

COMPLETE SEVERANCE

Total severance of a nerve can result from accidental contact with powered devices (such as rotary saws and propellers), from knife and bullet wounds, or from other penetrating injuries (such as from flying glass).

If the ends of the cut nerve are separated, the fibers try to regenerate but, in the absence of directing channels, they simply bunch up to form a lump of tissue; there is no recovery of function. It is therefore essential in the surgical repair of cut nerves to ensure that the ends are meticulously brought together and stitched into place. This is achieved with *microsurgery* and delicate sutures and needles.

Even with the best surgical repair, recovery is rarely complete. While the fibers with a motor function are regenerating, the paralyzed muscles are kept healthy and free from *contractures* by constant *physical therapy*.

N

Regenerating nerve fibers sometimes pass down the wrong channels; as a result, when function is restored, actions may differ from what was intended (for example, an attempt to move the index finger may move the middle finger as well). Movement skills and the interpretation of sensations may need to be relearned.

BRAIN AND SPINAL CORD INJURY

Nerve tracts within the brain and spinal cord are structurally different from the peripheral nerves, and severed fibers there do not regenerate. For example, it is impossible for vision to be restored if the *optic nerves* are cut.

Nerve, trapped

Compression or stretching of a nerve, causing numbness, tingling, weakness, and sometimes pain in the area supplied by the nerve.

Common examples of a trapped nerve include *carpal tunnel syndrome*, in which symptoms appear in the thumb, index, and middle fingers as a result of pressure on the median nerve as it passes through the wrist; a prolapsed disk (see *Disk prolapse*), in which pressure on the nerve root leading from the spinal cord produces symptoms in the back and legs; and *crutch palsy*, in which the radial nerve is pressed against the humerus (upper arm bone), producing symptoms in the wrist and hand.

A damaged nerve may take some time to heal, causing symptoms to persist. Surgical decompression to relieve pressure on the nerve may be necessary in severe cases.

Nervous breakdown

A popular term used to describe unusual behavior that is thought to be part of a crisis of severe anxiety or tension or a psychiatric illness. The term has no technical meaning, but is often applied to people suffering from sudden tearfulness, episodes of shouting and screaming, marked social withdrawal, and concerns about the possibility of illness.

Nervous habit

A nontechnical term for a minor repetitive movement or activity. Sometimes these are involuntary twitches and facial tics, such as in *Gilles de la Tourette's syndrome* and some forms of *dyskinesia*.

Voluntary nervous habits, such as *thumb-sucking* and nose-picking, are common in young children, but usually disappear naturally with time. Also common is *nail-biting*, which often persists into adult life (20 percent of adults bite their nails). Such habits are thought to be a means of releasing inner tension.

All nervous habits increase during tension or anxiety. They may be severe in some forms of *depression*, an *anxiety disorder*, or drug withdrawal.

Nervous system

The body's information-gathering, storage, and control system.

The overall function of the nervous system is to gather information about the external environment and the body's internal state, to analyze this information, and to initiate appropriate responses aimed at satisfying certain drives. The most powerful drive is for survival. Many survival responses, which range from running away from danger to shivering in response to cold, are initiated unconsciously and automatically by the nervous system.

Other drives are more complex, revolving around a need to experience positive emotions (pleasure, excitement) and avoid negative ones (pain, anxiety, frustration).

In carrying out its functions, the nervous system has access to many built-in programs, but it can also improve its performance through *learning*, which relies on *memory*.

STRUCTURE

The nervous system is organized like a computer system that controls a highly complex machine. The central processing unit for the system is the central nervous system (CNS), comprising the brain and spinal cord, which consists of billions of interconnecting *neurons* (nerve cells).

Input of information to the CNS comes from the sense organs. Output (motor) instructions go to the skeletal muscles, muscles controlling speech, internal organs and glands, and the sweat glands in the skin. The cables along which this information is carried are the *nerves* that fan out from the CNS to the entire body. Each nerve is a bundle of the axons (filamentous projections) of many neurons.

In addition to these anatomical divisions of the nervous system, there are various functional divisions. Two of the most important are the *autonomic nervous system*, which is specifically concerned with the automatic (unconscious) regulation of internal body functioning, and the somatic nervous system, which controls the skeletal muscles responsible for voluntary movement.

FUNCTION

The nervous system functions largely through automatic responses to various stimuli (see *Reflex*), although voluntary (willed) actions can also be initiated through the activity of higher, conscious areas of the brain. Certain higher functions (such as visual perception, memory storage, thought, and speech production) are extremely complex and not understood in detail. Overall, however, all nervous activity is based on the transmission of impulses through complex networks of neurons.

DISORDERS

Disorders of the nervous system may result from damage to or dysfunction of its component parts (see *Brain* disorders box; *Spinal cord*; *Neuropathy*; *Nerve injury*). Disorders may also be due to impairment of sensory, analytical, or memory functions (see *Vision, disorders of*; *Deafness*; *Numbness*; *Smell, loss of*; *Agnosia*; *Amnesia*) or of motor functions (see *Aphasia*; *Dysarthria*; *Ataxia*).

Netilmicin

An *antibiotic drug* used in the hospital to treat serious infection, usually when other antibiotic drugs have been ineffective. Netilmicin is often used to enhance the effects of other antibiotics. In rare cases, it causes damage to the inner ear and the kidneys.

Neuralgia

Pain caused by irritation of, or damage to, a nerve. The pain usually occurs in brief bouts, may be very severe, and can often be felt shooting along the affected nerve.

The neuralgia that often occurs in *migraine* consists of attacks of intense, radiating pain around the eye that can last for up to an hour. Postherpetic neuralgia is a burning pain that may recur at the site of an attack of *herpes zoster* (shingles) for months or even years after the illness.

In glossopharyngeal neuralgia, intense pain is felt at the back of the tongue and in the throat and ear. The structures in this area are served by the glossopharyngeal nerve. The pain may occur spontaneously or be brought on by talking, eating, or swallowing; its cause is generally unknown. The same is true of *trigeminal neuralgia*, a severe paroxysm of pain affecting one side of the face supplied by the trigeminal nerve.

TREATMENT

Glossopharyngeal, trigeminal, and postherpetic neuralgia sometimes re-

NERVOUS SYSTEM

The nervous system detects and interprets changes in conditions inside and outside the body and responds to them. The central nervous system analyzes information and initiates responses; the peripheral nervous system gathers information and carries the response signals. Some responses are involuntary; others are dictated by conscious thought. All nervous system activity consists of signals passed through pathways of inter-connected neurons (nerve cells).

Median nerve

Ulnar nerve

Femoral nerve

Posterior tibial nerve

Peripheral nervous system
This system comprises all the nerves connecting the brain and spinal cord to the rest of the body. Of these, 31 pairs (the spinal nerves) connect to the spinal cord and 12 pairs (cranial nerves) connect to the brain. The main nerves of the limbs are labeled.

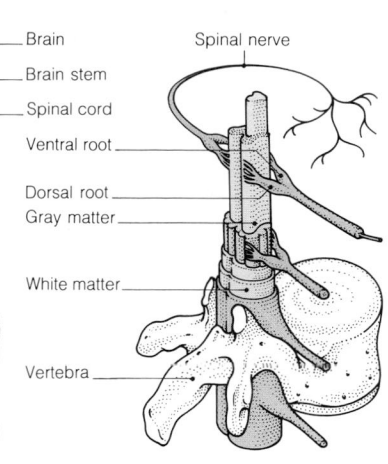

Brain

Brain stem

Spinal cord

Ventral root

Dorsal root

Gray matter

White matter

Vertebra

Spinal nerve

Structure of the spinal cord
The gray matter contains nerve cell bodies; white matter contains their conducting fibers. On joining the cord, spinal nerves split into two. The dorsal root carries sensory fibers; the ventral root carries motor fibers.

Central nervous system
This system consists of the brain and spinal cord, protected by the skull and spine. The CNS receives input from sense organs and receptors and sends signals to muscles and glands, via the peripheral nervous system.

N

HOW IT WORKS

Some possible events in response to a finger touching a hot object are shown. A receptor sends a message, via a sensory fiber, to the spinal cord. This triggers a signal that travels, via a motor fiber, back to a muscle, which contracts to move the finger. This action is called a reflex arc. Other signals pass toward the brain.

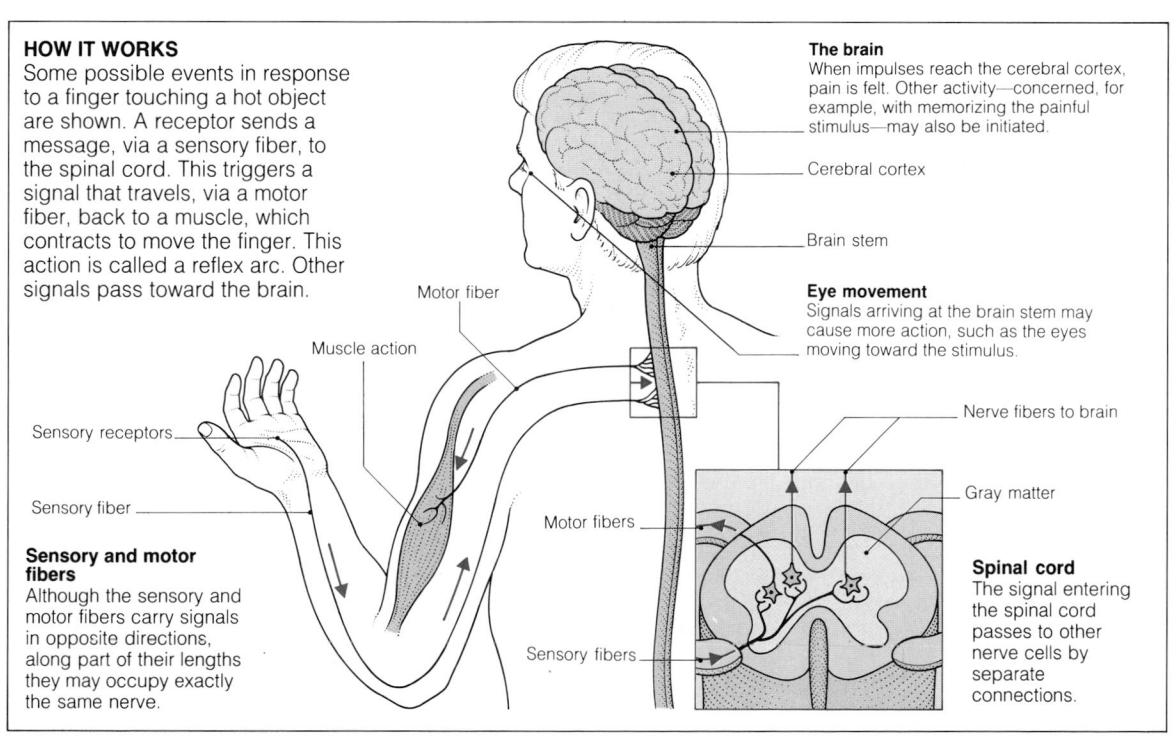

Motor fiber

Muscle action

Sensory receptors

Sensory fiber

Sensory and motor fibers
Although the sensory and motor fibers carry signals in opposite directions, along part of their lengths they may occupy exactly the same nerve.

Motor fibers

Sensory fibers

The brain
When impulses reach the cerebral cortex, pain is felt. Other activity—concerned, for example, with memorizing the painful stimulus—may also be initiated.

Cerebral cortex

Brain stem

Eye movement
Signals arriving at the brain stem may cause more action, such as the eyes moving toward the stimulus.

Nerve fibers to brain

Gray matter

Spinal cord
The signal entering the spinal cord passes to other nerve cells by separate connections.

spond to carbamazepine. They may also be relieved by analgesics (painkillers) such as acetaminophen.

Neural tube defect

A developmental failure affecting the spinal cord or brain in the embryo. Very early in fetal development, there is a ridge of neural-like tissue along the back of the embryo. As the fetus develops, this material differentiates into both the spinal cord and body nerves at the lower end and the brain at the upper end. At the same time, the bones that make up the back gradually surround the spinal cord on all sides. If any part of this sequence goes awry, many defects can appear. The worst is total lack of brain (*anencephaly*). Much more common is *spina bifida*, in which the back bones do not form a complete ring to protect the spinal cord. One to two babies per 1,000 born alive in the US have a neural tube defect; many more fetuses are affected but do not survive birth.

Healthy spine
Skin on back
Spinal cord
Spinal fluid
Vertebra

Spine affected by spina bifida
Skin on back
Spinal fluid
Spinal cord
Vertebra

Neural tube defect
This defect leads to failure of the bony arch to fuse over the back of the spinal cord, thus causing spina bifida.

Neurapraxia

A type of *nerve injury* in which the outward structure of a nerve appears intact, but in which some of the conducting fibers have been damaged or have degenerated and thus do not transmit signals to muscles.

Neurasthenia

An outdated term, meaning literally "nervous exhaustion." It was once used to describe a number of mental and physical symptoms, including loss of energy, insomnia, aches and pains (especially in the chest and abdomen), *depression*, irritability, and reduced concentration.

Neuritis

Literally, inflammation of a nerve. True nerve inflammation may be caused by infection (e.g., by a virus in *herpes zoster* or a bacterium in *leprosy*). The term neuritis is also often applied to nerve damage or disease from causes other than inflammation. Thus, it has become virtually synonymous with *neuropathy*, a term for all disorders of peripheral nerves.

Neuroblastoma

A tumor of the adrenal glands or sympathetic nervous system (the part of the nervous system responsible for certain automatic body functions, notably the *fight or flight response*). Most neuroblastomas develop in the adrenal glands or in the sympathetic nerves along the back wall of the abdomen. Less commonly, they develop in the sympathetic nerves of the chest or neck, or, very rarely, in the brain.

Neuroblastomas are the most common extracranial (outside the skull) solid tumor of childhood. About 80 percent of cases develop during the first 10 years of life, most commonly in the first four years. The incidence is 8.3 cases per 1 million children.

SYMPTOMS AND SIGNS

The symptoms vary according to the site of the tumor and the extent to which it has spread. Common symptoms include weight loss, general aches and pains, paleness, and irritability. There may also be tumors of the abdomen, neck, eyes, or skin. In some cases, the tumor secretes the hormones *epinephrine* and *norepinephrine*, which may cause diarrhea, high blood pressure, and flushing of the skin.

DIAGNOSIS

The condition is diagnosed from the symptoms and signs, and from X rays, blood tests, and urine tests. In some cases, it may be necessary to perform a biopsy (removal of a small sample of tissue for examination) of the bone marrow and any accessible tumors.

TREATMENT AND OUTLOOK

Treatment consists of surgical removal of the tumor, followed by *radiation therapy* and possibly *anticancer drugs*.

The outlook varies greatly because neuroblastomas range from being relatively harmless to highly malignant. Overall, about one third of those affected survive for at least five years after treatment.

Neurocutaneous disorders

A group of conditions characterized by abnormalities of the skin as well as abnormalities of the nerves and/or the central nervous system.

The best known of these disorders is *neurofibromatosis*, in which there are brown patches on the skin and numerous fibrous nodules on the skin and nerves. Another example is *tuberous sclerosis*, characterized by small skin-colored swellings over the cheeks and nose, mental deficiency, and epilepsy.

Neurodermatitis

An itchy, eczemalike skin condition caused by repeated scratching. (See also *Lichen simplex*.)

Neuroendocrinology

The study of the interactions between the *nervous system* and the *endocrine system*. These systems control internal body functions and the way in which the body responds to the external environment. However, the two systems do not act separately. Hormones produced by the endocrine system can affect nervous system functions, including behavior (for example, sex hormones affect mood and sexual motivation). Similarly, special nerve cells, called neurosecretory cells (found mainly in the *hypothalamus*), can release hormones in response to stimulation by the nervous system; these hormones can, in turn, affect various endocrine glands. Stress is initially perceived by the nervous system but ultimately causes the release of hormones by the pituitary and adrenal glands.

Neuroendocrinological investigations range from recording the electrical activity of neurosecretory cells to experiments showing the relationship between hormones and behavior.

Neurofibromatosis

An uncommon inherited disorder, also called von Recklinghausen's disease. Neurofibromatosis is characterized by numerous soft, fibrous swellings (called neurofibromas) that grow from nerves in the skin and sometimes elsewhere in the body. In addition, there are *café au lait spots* (pale, coffee-colored patches) on the skin of the trunk and pelvis.

SYMPTOMS AND SIGNS

In most cases, neurofibromatosis affects only the skin. However, the swellings and spots may be unsightly. If neurofibromas occur in the central nervous system, they can cause *epilepsy* and other complications, sometimes affecting vision and hearing. Rarely, bone deformities occur.

TREATMENT

Surgical removal of neurofibromas is necessary only if they are causing complications. Anyone who has the disorder, and parents of an affected child, should seek *genetic counseling*.

Neurologist

A specialist in the diagnosis and treatment of diseases and disorders of the nervous system. Neurologists conduct examinations of the patient's nerves, reflexes, motor and sensory functions, and muscles to determine the cause and extent of a problem.

Neurology

The study of the nervous system and its disorders, particularly their diagnosis and treatment (the specialty of *neuropathology* is concerned with the causes and effects of neurological conditions). In addition to a detailed knowledge of the structure and function of the brain, spinal cord, and nerves, neurologists must understand the many conditions that can affect them. To aid in the diagnosis of such conditions, extensive use is made of modern imaging techniques (such as *CT scanning* and *MRI*). Because the nervous system is profusely supplied with blood vessels that may be involved in a neurological disorder, *angiography* (an X-ray imaging technique to show blood vessels) is often used in diagnosis.

In the past, relatively few disorders of the nervous system could be treated effectively. Today, however, with better understanding of the biochemical and structural bases of neurological disorders, new treatments are being developed, including the surgical removal of tumors, repair of damaged nerves (see *Neurosurgery*), transplantation of adrenal tissue in *Parkinson's disease*, and drug treatment of some forms of *dementia*.

Neuroma

A benign tumor of nerve tissue that may affect any nerve in the body. In most cases, the cause is unknown; rarely, a neuroma develops as a result of damage to a nerve.

The symptoms vary according to the nerve involved. In general, there is intermittent pain in parts of the body supplied by the nerve. The same areas may also become numb and weak if the neuroma develops in a confined space and presses on the nerve.

If the symptoms are troublesome, the tumor may be surgically removed. (See also *Acoustic neuroma*.)

Neuron

A nerve cell. There are billions of neurons in the nervous system; they act in various combinations to do everything from writing a symphony to scratching a fleabite. The neurons are analogous to the wires in a complex electrical machine.

There are three main types of neuron—interneurons, motoneurons, and sensory neurons (see illustrated box, overleaf).

FUNCTION

The function of a neuron is to signal, or "fire" (that is, to transmit an electrical impulse along its axon), under certain specific conditions. The electrical impulse causes the release of a neurotransmitter from the axon terminals, which in turn may cause a muscle cell to contract, cause an endocrine gland to release a hormone, or affect the next neuron in a circuit.

Different stimuli excite different types of neurons to fire. Sensory neurons may be excited by physical stimuli, such as light of a certain wavelength, pressure, or cold. The activity of most neurons is controlled by the effects of neurotransmitters released from adjacent neurons.

The ability of a neuron to fire depends on a small difference in electric potential between the inside and outside of the cell. Under the direct influence of an excitatory neurotransmitter, a sudden change occurs in this potential at one point on the cell's membrane. The change, called an "action potential," then flows along the membrane (and thus along the axon of the cell) at speeds up to several hundred miles per hour. A neuron may be able to fire in this way several times every second.

There are also neurotransmitters that stabilize neuronal membranes, preventing an action potential. Thus, the firing pattern of a neuron depends on the balance of excitatory and inhibitory influences acting on it.

LIFE SPAN

If the cell body of a neuron is damaged or degenerates, the cell dies and is never replaced. A baby starts life with the maximum number of neurons; their number decreases continuously thereafter. We seem to be born with an excess number of neurons, so problems arise only when disease, injury, or persistent alcohol abuse affects the central nervous system, dramatically increasing the rate of neuron loss.

If a peripheral nerve is damaged, its individual fibers can regenerate (see *Nerve injury*; *Neuropathy*).

Neuropathic joint

A joint damaged by a series of injuries, which pass unnoticed because of neuropathy (loss of sensation) affecting that joint. Neuropathic joints develop in a number of conditions, including *diabetes mellitus* and untreated *syphilis*.

When sensation to pain is lost, abnormal stress and strain on a joint do not stimulate the protective reflex spasm of the surrounding muscles; this allows exaggerated movement that can damage the joint. Severe recurrent damage to a joint may lead to *osteoarthritis*, swelling, and deformity; there is minimal pain because of the lack of sensation.

DIAGNOSIS AND TREATMENT

Severe joint degeneration and deformity are visible on X rays. A brace or caliper splint may be necessary to restrict abnormal joint movement. Occasionally, an arthrodesis (joint fusion) is performed. The nerve damage is irreversible.

Neuropathology

The study of diseases and disorders of the nervous system. Neuropathologists are concerned principally with the causes and effects of neurological conditions rather than with their diagnosis and treatment (usually handled by a *neurologist* or *neurosurgeon*).

Neuropathy

Disease, inflammation, or damage to the peripheral nerves, which connect the central nervous system, or CNS (brain and spinal cord), to the sense organs, muscles, glands, and internal organs. Symptoms caused by neuropathies include numbness, tingling, pain, or muscle weakness, depending on the nerves affected.

TYPES

Most nerve cell axons (the conducting fibers that make up nerves) are insulated within a sheath of a fatty substance called *myelin*, but some are unmyelinated. Most neuropathies arise from damage or irritation either to the axons or to their myelin sheaths. An axon may suffer thinning, complete loss of, or patchy loss of its myelin sheath. This may cause a slowing or a complete block to the passage of electrical signals.

Various types of neuropathy are described according to the site and distribution of damage. For example, a distal neuropathy starts with damage at the far end of a nerve (farthest from the brain or spinal cord). A symmetrical neuropathy

N

STRUCTURE OF A NEURON

A neuron (nerve cell) consists of a cell body and several branching projections called dendrites. Every neuron has a filamentous projection called an axon (nerve fiber). Axons vary in length from a fraction of an inch to several feet. An axon branches at its end to form terminals, via which signals are transmitted to target cells, such as the dendrites of other neurons, muscle cells, or glands. Bundles of the axons of many neurons are known as nerves or, within the brain or spinal cord, as nerve tracts or pathways.

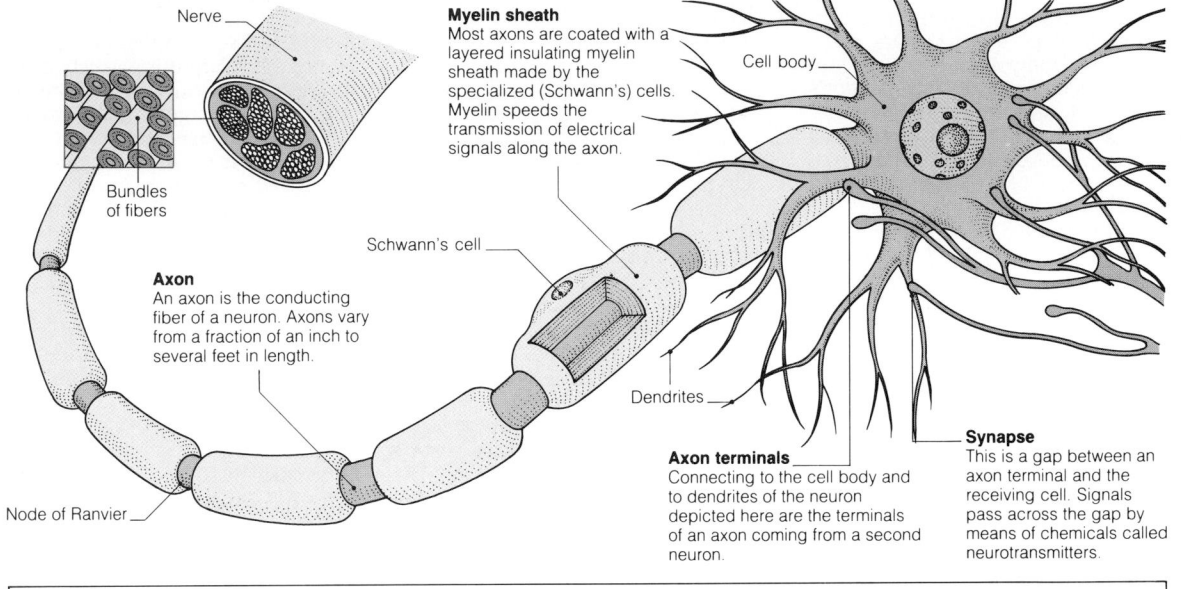

Nerve

Bundles of fibers

Myelin sheath
Most axons are coated with a layered insulating myelin sheath made by the specialized (Schwann's) cells. Myelin speeds the transmission of electrical signals along the axon.

Cell body

Schwann's cell

Axon
An axon is the conducting fiber of a neuron. Axons vary from a fraction of an inch to several feet in length.

Dendrites

Node of Ranvier

Axon terminals
Connecting to the cell body and to dendrites of the neuron depicted here are the terminals of an axon coming from a second neuron.

Synapse
This is a gap between an axon terminal and the receiving cell. Signals pass across the gap by means of chemicals called neurotransmitters.

BASIC TYPES OF NEURON
Sensory neurons carry signals from sense receptors along their axons into the CNS. Motoneurons carry signals from the CNS to muscles or glands; the axon terminals form a motor end-plate. Interneurons form all the complex interconnecting electrical circuitry within the CNS itself. For each sensory neuron in the body, there are about 10 motoneurons and 99 interneurons.

Motoneuron

Muscle fiber

Nucleus

Dendrites

Axon

Motor end-plate

Sensory neuron

Axon terminals

Axon

Nucleus

Interneuron

Sense receptor

Brain neurons
Electron micrograph of interneurons in the brain.

N

affects nerves at the same places on each side of the body. Some neuropathies are described according to their underlying cause (e.g., diabetic neuropathy and alcoholic neuropathy).

The term neuritis is now used virtually interchangeably with neuropathy. Polyneuropathy (or polyneuritis) literally means damage to several nerves; mononeuropathy (or mononeuritis) indicates damage to a single nerve. *Neuralgia* describes pain caused by irritation or inflammation of a particular nerve.

CAUSES
In some cases of neuropathy there is no obvious or detectable cause. Among the many specific causes are *diabetes mellitus*, dietary deficiencies (particularly of B vitamins), persistent excessive alcohol consumption, and metabolic upsets such as *uremia*. Other causes include *leprosy*, *lead poisoning*, or poisoning by drugs.

Nerves may become acutely inflamed. This often occurs after a viral infection (for example, in *Guillain-Barré syndrome*). Neuropathies may result from autoimmune disorders such as *rheumatoid arthritis*, systemic *lupus erythematosus*, or *periarteritis nodosa*. In these disorders, there is often damage to the blood vessels supplying the nerves. Neuropathies may occur secondarily to malignant tumors such as *lung cancer*, or with *lymphomas* and *leukemias*. Finally, there is a group of inherited neuropathies, the most common being *peroneal muscular atrophy*.

SYMPTOMS
The symptoms of neuropathy depend on whether it affects mainly sensory nerve fibers or motor nerve fibers. Damage to sensory nerve fibers may cause numbness and tingling, sensations of cold, or pain, often starting in the hands and feet and spreading toward the body center. Damage to motor fibers may cause muscle weakness and muscle wasting.

Damage to nerves of the autonomic nervous system may lead to blurred vision, impaired or absent sweating, episodes of faintness associated with falls in blood pressure, and disturbance of gastric, intestinal, bladder, and sexual functioning, including incontinence and impotence. Some neuropathies are linked with particular symptoms (for example, very painful neuropathies may arise in diabetes mellitus and in *alcohol dependence*).

DIAGNOSIS
To determine the extent of damage, studies of nerve conduction are performed, along with *EMG* tests, which record the electrical activity in muscles. To determine the cause of neuropathy, *blood tests*, X rays, nerve or muscle *biopsy* (removal of tissue for analysis), and various other tests may be required.

TREATMENT
When possible, treatment is aimed at the underlying cause. For example, in diabetes mellitus, scrupulous attention to the control of the blood sugar level affords the best chances for recovery. Other people may need to stop drinking alcohol, or, if a nutritional deficiency has been diagnosed, may be given injections of vitamins such as thiamine (vitamin B_1).

If treatment is successful and the cell bodies of the damaged nerve cells have not been destroyed, a full recovery from the neuropathy is possible.

Neuropsychiatry
The branch of medicine that deals with the relationship between psychiatric symptoms and distinct neurological disorders. These conditions are usually forms of brain disease, such as *temporal lobe epilepsy*, tumors, or infections. Research and brain imaging are revealing evidence that subtle forms of brain damage underlie certain psychotic illnesses.

Neurosis
A term commonly used to describe a range of relatively mild psychiatric disorders in which the sufferer remains in touch with reality.

Neurotic symptoms are distressing to the afflicted person, who is aware of a change from his or her usual psychological state. By contrast, people suffering from psychotic illnesses do not recognize that they are sick (see *Psychosis*). Neurotic symptoms generally do not lead to distinctly abnormal behavior, although they can severely limit work or social activities. They tend to fluctuate in intensity,

often in response to social or personal stresses. No physical abnormality has been shown to underlie them.

The major neurotic disorders are *depression* (the mild form); *anxiety disorders*, including *phobias* and *obsessive-compulsive behavior*; *somatization disorder*; and *dissociative disorders*. *Psychosexual disorders* have recently been included in this category.

Neurosurgeon
A surgeon who operates on the brain, spinal cord, or other parts of the nervous system (see *Neurosurgery*).

Neurosurgery
The specialty concerned with the surgical treatment of disorders of the nervous system. Many generalized nervous system disorders do not respond to surgical treatment, but neurosurgery can deal with most conditions in which a localized structural change interferes with nerve function.

Conditions treated by neurosurgery include tumors of the brain, spinal cord, or meninges (membranes that surround the brain and spinal cord), certain abnormalities of the blood vessels that supply the brain, such as an *aneurysm* (a bulge in a weak point of an artery), bleeding inside the skull (see *Extradural hemorrhage*; *Intracerebral hemorrhage*; *Subdural hemorrhage*), *brain abscess*, some birth defects (such as *hydrocephalus* and *spina bifida*), certain types of *epilepsy*, and nerve damage caused by illness or accidents. Neurosurgeons are also concerned with the surgical relief of otherwise untreatable pain.

Neurosyphilis
Infection of the brain or spinal cord that occurs in untreated *syphilis* many years after the initial infection.

Damage to the spinal cord due to neurosyphilis may cause tabes dorsalis, characterized by poor coordination of leg movements when walking, urinary incontinence, and intermittent pains in the abdomen and limbs. Damage to the brain may cause *dementia*, muscle weakness, and, in rare cases, extensive neurologic damage (when it is called general paralysis of the insane).

Neurotoxin
A chemical that damages nervous tissue. The principal effects of neurotoxic nerve damage are numbness, weakness, or paralysis of the part of the body supplied by the affected nerve. Neurotoxins are pres-

ent in the venom of certain snakes (see *Snakebites*), and are released by some types of bacteria (such as those that cause *tetanus* and *diphtheria*). Some chemical poisons, such as arsenic and lead, are also neurotoxic.

Neurotransmitter
Although nerve impulses are electrical, the transmission of these impulses from one neuron (nerve cell) to another, or to a muscle cell, is achieved chemically rather than electrically. The chemical that transmits the message is a neurotransmitter. Scores of different chemicals fulfill this function in different parts of the nervous system (see box, overleaf).

Many neurotransmitters are similar to, or identical to, substances used by our bodies as hormones. These neurotransmitters also act as messenger molecules, but are released into the bloodstream to act on their target cells at a distance.

TYPES
One of the most important neurotransmitters is *acetylcholine*. It is released by neurons connected to skeletal muscles (causing them to contract) and by neurons that control the sweat glands and the heart beat. It also transmits messages between neurons in the brain and spinal cord.

Interference with the action of acetylcholine on skeletal muscles is the cause of the disease *myasthenia gravis*; depletion of the nerve cells that release acetylcholine in the brain may be a cause of *Alzheimer's disease*.

Another transmitter, *norepinephrine*, is important in nerve pathways controlling heart beat, blood flow, and response to stress. In addition to being produced in the body by neurons, norepinephrine is made by the *adrenal glands*. Dopamine plays an important role in parts of the brain that control movement, and malfunction of the neurons that respond to dopamine is thought to be important in causing *Parkinson's disease*. *Serotonin* is one of the primary neurotransmitters in parts of the brain concerned with conscious processes.

Over the last 20 years, a whole new family of transmitters, called the neuropeptides, has been discovered. Neuropeptides are small proteins; they are larger molecules than the previously known neurotransmitters, which are all very small molecules. The best studied of these neuropeptides are the *endorphins*, which are used by the brain to control sensitivity to pain.

N

Nevus

A skin blemish that can be flat, raised slightly above the skin's surface, or on a stalk; a nevus can be colored or not colored, and with or without hair growth. Some nevi are present at birth, others develop at any age.

TYPES

There are two main types of nevus: melanocytic (pigmented) nevi, caused by abnormality or overactivity of skin cells producing the pigment *melanin*, and vascular nevi, caused by an abnormal collection of blood vessels.

The most common type of pigmented nevi are *freckles*, which are small, flat, light to dark brown areas found on any part of the body that is exposed to the sun. A *lentigo* is a pale to brown spot very similar to a freckle. *Café au lait spots* are another type of light brown pigmented nevus.

A mole (a brown to dark brown spot that is not usually present at birth) is another common type of nevus. As a child grows, moles may spread, forming an average number of 15 to 20 per person by adulthood. In rare cases these moles become cancerous (see *Melanoma, malignant*).

Unusual types of moles include hairy, pigmented nevi found on the shoulders of some young men, halo nevi (in which the skin surrounding the nevus lightens in color to give a characteristic "halo" appearance), and juvenile melanomas (see *Melanoma, juvenile*), which are red-brown nevi that occur in childhood.

Some nevi have a bluish coloration; these so-called blue nevi are often found on the backs of the hands of young girls. Most black and Asian infants are born with one or more blue-black spots on their lower backs (see *Mongolian spot*).

Another type of nevus is a vascular nevus (*hemangioma*), caused by an abnormal collection of blood vessels; a port-wine mark is an example.

TREATMENT

Most nevi are harmless and do not require treatment. However, if a nevus suddenly appears, grows, bleeds, or changes color, medical advice should be sought without delay to exclude the possibility of cancer. (See also *Spider nevus*.)

Newborn

An infant at birth and during the first few weeks of life.

INITIAL EXAMINATION

Immediately after birth, the newborn baby is briefly checked by the nurse, midwife, or physician in attendance.

HOW NEUROTRANSMITTERS WORK

When an electrical impulse travels down a nerve cell axon, it causes the release of a chemical neurotransmitter at the axon terminals. The chemical is not the same in every case; acetylcholine, norepinephrine, dopamine, and serotonin are all important examples.

Example of neurotransmitter activity
Neurotransmitters enable the pupil to change size in different light conditions.

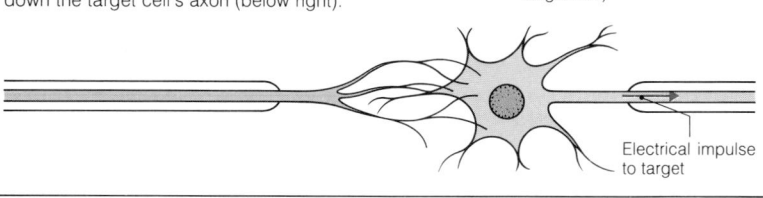

Nerve cell axon

Electrical impulse

Axon terminal

Cell body

Dendrites

1 The impulse travels down the neuronal axon (above), from the cell body toward the axon terminals; neurotransmitter is released from tiny swellings, called synaptic knobs, at the axon terminals.

2 The neurotransmitter crosses the gap, or synapse, to the surface membrane of the target cell (right), where it binds to a protein called a receptor.

3 If sufficient target cell receptors are activated by neurotransmitter binding, an impulse is initiated and passes in turn down the target cell's axon (below right).

Synapse

Receptors

Presynaptic membrane (axon terminal)

Postsynaptic membrane (dendrite of target cell)

Neurotransmitter chemical

Electrical impulse to target

This examination includes checking the heart rate with a *stethoscope* and establishing that breathing is normal. The *Apgar score* and other tests are performed to check the baby's health. The baby's sex is noted and a check made for any obvious *birth defect*.

NURSING PROCEDURE

The baby is labeled with his or her name and date of birth; the birth weight, length, and head circumference are recorded. Usually a handprint or footprint is recorded along with the mother's fingerprint or thumbprint for identification.

At birth, the baby is usually covered with vernix, a greasy, white substance that protects it in the uterus. It is wiped off and the baby is wrapped in a blanket and given to the mother to hold and to feed, or placed in a warm crib. If very small or sick, the baby is kept in an *incubator* and treated in a neonatal intensive-care unit or other intensive-care unit.

The frequency of the baby's urine and *meconium* (the newborn stool) is recorded. During the second week of life, two special blood tests are performed. The *Guthrie test* is performed on all babies to check for *phenylketonuria*. The other test done at this time checks for *hypothyroidism*.

MEDICAL EXAMINATION

Within 24 hours of birth, the baby is usually given a complete medical examination by his or her physician. This examination assesses the baby's general health and identifies any birth defects (such as cleft palate). The skull, eyes, face, abdomen, heart, spine, hips, genitals, and limbs are checked, and the baby's posture, movements, behavior, cry, reflexes, and responsiveness are noted (see *Reflexes, primitive*).

ABNORMALITIES IN THE NEWBORN

The newborn baby may have a swollen or misshapen head due to pressure during labor. Less commonly, there may be more notable evidence of *birth injury*, such as *cephalhematoma* (swelling of the scalp caused by bruising around the skull). Most problems caused by the pressure of delivery resolve themselves within a few days.

Jaundice is extremely common in the newborn, especially if the baby is breast-fed. Usually appearing on the second or third day, the jaundice generally disappears over the next few days. In most cases, jaundice in the newborn is harmless. However, it may be serious if it appears during the first 24 hours or occurs in a very premature infant.

Some newborn girls have slight vaginal bleeding or discharge, and babies of either sex may have enlargement of the breasts. These harmless conditions are caused by maternal sex hormones that reached the fetus through the placenta. Any extra hormones soon leave the baby's body.

The umbilical cord, which may be painted with a dye to prevent infection, usually dries and drops off within a week or so of birth. Serious infections of the cord stump can occur.

Minor, harmless abnormalities of the newborn include *milia* (tiny, white spots on the face), *hemangioma*, *mongolian spot*, and *urticaria* of the newborn (a blotchy, red rash that occurs around the second day). See also *Prematurity*; *Postmaturity*.

Niacin

See *Vitamin B*.

Nickel

A metallic element that is present in the body in minute amounts. Its exact role is poorly understood. Nickel is thought to activate certain *enzymes* (substances that promote biochemical reactions). It also may play a part in stabilizing chromosomal material in the nuclei of cells.

Disease due to a deficiency of nickel is unknown. However, excessive exposure to it—which occurs most commonly in industrial workers— may cause *dermatitis* (inflammation of the skin) or, rarely, *lung cancer*.

Niclosamide

An *antihelmintic drug* used in the treatment of *worm infestation*. Niclosamide acts on tapeworms in the intestine, causing them to loosen their grip and be passed out of the body in the feces.

Adverse effects are uncommon and are typical of those produced by other antihelmintic drugs.

Nicotine

 A drug in tobacco that acts as a stimulant and is responsible for dependence on tobacco. The drug has no medical use, but certain of its derivatives are used as pesticides.

After inhalation, the nicotine in tobacco smoke passes rapidly into the bloodstream. Nicotine in chewing tobacco is absorbed more slowly through the lining of the mouth. Once in the bloodstream, the drug acts on the nervous system until it is eventually broken down by the liver and excreted in the urine.

EFFECTS

Nicotine acts primarily on the *autonomic nervous system*, which controls involuntary body activities such as the heart rate. The effects of the drug vary from one person to another, and also depend on dosage and past usage. In someone unused to smoking, even a small amount of nicotine may slow the heart rate and cause nausea and vomiting. However, in habitual smokers, the drug increases the heart rate, narrows the blood vessels (the combined effect of which is to raise blood pressure), and stimulates the central nervous system, thereby reducing fatigue, increasing alertness, and improving concentration.

Regular tobacco smoking results in tolerance to nicotine, so that a higher intake is needed to bring about the same effect. However, this process is much less notable with tobacco than with other addictive drugs.

NICOTINE AND DISEASE

Although it is the tar in tobacco smoke that damages lung tissue and causes lung cancer, tobacco smoking is also clearly associated with *coronary heart disease*, *peripheral vascular disease*, and other cardiovascular disorders. It is uncertain whether these disorders are caused by the nicotine or by the carbon monoxide content of the smoke.

Excessively large amounts of nicotine can cause poisoning, which may result in vomiting, seizures, and, very occasionally, death.

WITHDRAWAL

Because most smokers are physically dependent on nicotine, stopping smoking often causes withdrawal symptoms, such as drowsiness, headaches, fatigue, and difficulty concentrating. To reduce these symptoms in a person who is trying to stop smoking, a physician may prescribe nicotine chewing gum, which has a less harmful effect on the circulatory system. (See also *Tobacco smoking*.)

Nicotinic acid

See *Vitamin B*.

Nifedipine

A *calcium channel blocker* used mainly to prevent and treat *angina pectoris*. It is also often used to treat *hypertension* (high blood pressure) and disorders affecting the circulation, such as *Raynaud's disease*.

Possible adverse effects are *edema* (fluid retention), flushing, headache, and dizziness.

Night blindness

The inability to see well in dim light. Many people with night blindness show no discernible eye disease. In other people, the condition may be an inherited functional defect of the retina or an early sign of *retinitis pigmentosa*. Night blindness is sometimes caused by vitamin A deficiency.

Nightmare

An unpleasant vivid dream, often accompanied by a sense of suffocation. Nightmares occur during REM (rapid eye movement) *sleep*, in the middle and later parts of the night, and are often clearly remembered if the dreamer awakens completely.

Nightmares are very common, especially in children aged 8 to 10. They are particularly likely to occur when the child's breathing is slightly difficult because of a cold or illness, or when there is anxiety over separation from parents or home. In adults, nightmares may be a side effect of certain drugs, including *beta-blocker drugs* and *benzodiazepine drugs*. Traumatic events (such as accidents, torture, or prolonged imprisonment) seem to be particularly associated with disturbing and repeated nightmares. However, there is no specific relationship to psychiatric illness.

Nightmares should not be confused with hypnagogic *hallucinations*, which occur while falling asleep, or with *night terror*, which occurs in NREM (nonrapid eye movement) sleep and is not remembered the next day.

Night terror

A disorder, occurring mainly in children, consisting of abrupt arousals from sleep in a terrified state. Night terror (also called sleep terror) usually starts between the ages of 4 and 7, and gradually disappears in early adolescence. Episodes occur during NREM (nonrapid eye movement) *sleep*, usually half an hour to three and a half hours after falling asleep.

N

Sufferers awaken screaming in a semiconscious state and remain frightened for some minutes. They do not recognize familiar faces or surroundings, and usually cannot be comforted. Physical signs of agitation, such as sweating or an increased heart rate, are also common. Gradually, the sufferer falls back to sleep and has no memory of the event the next day.

Though distressing to parents, night terror in children has no serious significance. In adults, it is likely to be associated with an *anxiety disorder*.

NIH

The abbreviation for the National Institutes of Health. The institutes are a part of the Department of Health and Human Services and comprise a research hospital, a computerized medical library, and 11 of the largest and best-financed research organizations in the world. One of them concentrates on cancer; the others have broader charters—the National Institute of Allergy and Infectious Diseases, for example, and the National Heart, Lung, and Blood Institute. The major focus of medical and dental research in the US, the NIH finance additional research programs in universities, hospitals, and other nongovernment institutions.

Nipple

The small prominence at the tip of each breast. Each of a woman's nipples contains tiny openings through which milk can pass. The nipple and the surrounding areola are darker than the surrounding skin, darkening more and increasing in size during pregnancy. Muscle in the nipple allows it to become erect.

DISORDERS
Structural defects of the nipple are rare. One or both nipples may be absent, or there may be additional nipples along a line extending from the armpit to the groin.

An inverted nipple is usually an abnormality of development. It can be corrected by drawing out the nipple between finger and thumb daily for several weeks. Inversion of a previously normal nipple in an adult is much more significant and may be due to *breast cancer*.

Cracked nipples are common during the last months of pregnancy and during breast-feeding. Daily washing, drying, and moisturizing of the nipple can help prevent it. In addition to causing discomfort, cracks may lead to infective *mastitis*.

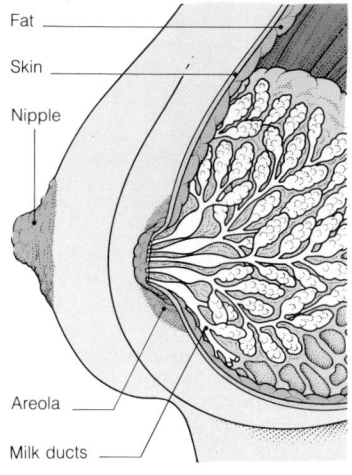

LOCATION OF THE NIPPLE
The protrusion at the tip of the breast, surrounded by the areola. Milk ducts emerge at the nipple.

Fat
Skin
Nipple
Areola
Milk ducts

Papilloma of the nipple is a benign swelling attached to the skin by a stalk. *Paget's disease of the nipple* appears initially as persistent eczema of the nipple. It is caused by a slowly growing cancer arising in a milk duct, and surgical treatment is required.

Discharge from the nipple occurs for a variety of reasons. A clear, straw-colored discharge may develop in early pregnancy. A milky discharge may occur after the period of breast-feeding is over. *Galactorrhea* (discharge of milk in someone who is not pregnant or breast-feeding) may be caused by a hormone imbalance; rarely, it may be due to a galactocele (a cyst under the areola). A discharge containing pus indicates a breast *abscess*. A bloodstained discharge may be due to mammary dysplasia (abnormal tissue), chronic mastitis, or cancer.

Nit

The egg of a louse. Both head lice and pubic lice produce eggs, which they glue to the base of hairs growing from their host's head or pubes. The nits are tiny—about one fiftieth of an inch (0.5 mm) in diameter—and yellow (newly laid) or white (hatched). They hatch within eight days, and the empty eggshells are carried outward as the hair grows.

Louse infestations are often diagnosed from the presence of nits. The distance from the base of hairs to the furthest nits provides a rough approximation of the duration of the infestation. (See *Lice*; *Pubic lice*.)

Nitrate drugs

COMMON DRUGS
Isosorbide dinitrate Nitroglycerin

A group of *vasodilator drugs* used in the treatment of *angina pectoris* (chest pain due to impaired blood supply to heart muscle) and severe *heart failure* (reduced pumping efficiency).

Possible adverse effects of nitrate drugs include headache, flushing, and dizziness. *Tolerance* (the need for greater amounts of the drug to have the same effect) may develop when the drug is used regularly.

Nitrites

Salts of nitrous acid (a nitrogen-containing acid). Some of these chemicals, notably sodium nitrite, are added to certain foods in small quantities (mainly meat products such as sausages) because they act as preservatives and destroy bacteria that cause *food poisoning*. In large amounts, nitrites can cause dizziness, nausea, and vomiting.

Within the intestine, nitrites are converted to substances called nitrosamines. In laboratory tests, nitrosamines have been shown to cause cancer in animals. However, there is no conclusive proof that they have the same effect in humans or that eating food containing nitrites is harmful to health.

Nitrofurantoin

An *antibacterial drug* used in the treatment of *urinary tract infection*.

Nitrofurantoin should be taken with food to reduce the risk of irritating the stomach, which can prompt abdominal pain and nausea. More serious adverse effects, such as breathing difficulty, numbness, and jaundice, are rare.

Nitrogen

A colorless, odorless gas that makes up 78 percent of the Earth's atmosphere. Atmospheric nitrogen has no biological action, although, in scuba diving, bubbles of nitrogen gas may form in body fluids if a diver ascends to the surface too rapidly, causing the condition commonly called the "bends" (see *Decompression sickness*).

Although nitrogen gas cannot be utilized by the body, compounds of nitrogen are essential to life. Probably the most important of such compounds are *amino acids*, the building blocks of *proteins*, which represent the fundamental structural substances of all cells and tissues. Because humans cannot make amino acids, they must be obtained from the diet in the form of animal and plant proteins. The proteins are then broken down into their constituent amino acids so that they can be absorbed and reconstituted into the specific proteins needed by the body. These processes of protein breakdown and reconstitution produce a variety of nitrogen-containing waste products, primarily *urea*, which is excreted from the body in the urine. (See also *Nitrate drugs*; *Nitrites*.)

Nitroglycerin

A *vasodilator drug* used to treat and prevent symptoms of *angina pectoris* (chest pain due to an inadequate blood supply to the heart). Nitroglycerin may cause headache, flushing, and dizziness; adverse effects are usually relieved by a reduction in the dose.

Nitrous oxide

A colorless gas (sometimes called laughing gas) with a sweet taste that is used with oxygen to provide *analgesia* (pain relief) and light anesthesia (see *Anesthesia, general*) during dental procedures, childbirth, and minor surgery. For major surgery requiring deeper anesthesia, nitrous oxide and oxygen need to be combined with other drugs.

The advantages of the combination of nitrous oxide and oxygen over other agents are their rapid action and nonflammability. Possible adverse effects include nausea and vomiting during the recovery period.

NMR

Abbreviation for nuclear magnetic resonance. The preferred term for this technique is magnetic resonance imaging (see *MRI*).

Nocardiosis

An infection caused by a funguslike bacterium. The infection usually starts in the lung and spreads via the bloodstream to the brain and tissues under the skin. The causative organism is present in the soil in all parts of the world and is acquired by inhalation. Nocardiosis is rare except in people with *immunodeficiency disorders* or those already suffering from other serious disease.

The infection causes a pneumonia-like illness, with fever and cough. It fails to settle under normal, short-term, antibiotic treatment, and signs of progressive lung damage occur. Brain abscesses may follow. The condition is diagnosed by microscopic examination of sputum (phlegm). Treatment, which may have to be continued for 12 to 18 months, is with *sulfonamide drugs*, sometimes in conjunction with other antibiotics (such as trimethoprim).

Nocturia

The disturbance of a person's sleep at night by the need to pass urine. In most people, a moderately full bladder does not usually disturb sleep, although light sleepers are more likely to wake to empty their bladders. Drinking alcohol in the evening stimulates urine production and may result in nocturia.

A common cause of nocturia is enlargement of the prostate gland (see *Prostate, enlarged*), which obstructs the normal outflow of urine and causes the bladder to be full at night.

Another common cause is *heart failure* (reduced pumping efficiency of the heart) leading to the retention of excess fluid, which is absorbed into the bloodstream and carried to the kidneys at night to make more urine. Also common is *cystitis* (inflammation of the bladder), in which irritation of the bladder wall increases its sensitivity so that smaller volumes of urine trigger a desire to pass urine.

Rarer causes of nocturia include *diabetes mellitus* (in which greater volumes of urine are produced both day and night) and chronic *renal failure* (in which the kidney loses its ability to produce a reduced quantity of more concentrated urine at night).

Nocturnal emission

Ejaculation that occurs during sleep, commonly called a "wet dream." Nocturnal emission is normal in male adolescents and is a common cause of unnecessary anxiety. Nocturnal emissions may also occur in adult males whose sexual activity is limited.

Node

A small, rounded mass of tissue that may be normal or abnormal. The term most commonly refers to a *lymph node*, which is a normal structure in the lymphatic system. Abnormal nodes are often called *nodules*.

Nodule

A small lump of tissue, usually more than one quarter of an inch (6 mm) in diameter. A nodule may protrude from the skin's surface or it may form deep under the skin. Nodules may be either hard or soft.

Noise

Sound that is disordered, unwanted, or that interferes with hearing.

Hearing may be damaged by exposure to intensely loud noise for a short period (such as an explosion at close range) or by prolonged exposure to lower levels of noise (such as might occur in a machine room or foundry). Any noise above 90 decibels may cause damage; the louder the noise, the shorter the time required for damage to occur (see chart).

HOW NOISE DAMAGES HEARING

Exposure to a sudden very loud noise, usually above 130 decibels, can cause immediate and permanent damage. Normally, muscles in the middle ear respond to loud noise by altering the stiffness of the chain of bones that pass vibrations to the inner ear, thus reducing their efficiency. But when the noise occurs without warning, these protective reflexes have no time to respond. The full force of the vibrations is carried to the inner ear, causing severe damage to delicate hair cells in the cochlea. Occasionally, loud noises can rupture the eardrum.

N

COMPARATIVE NOISE LEVELS

	Safe	Risk of injury	Injury
Jet engine at 30 yards			
Jackhammer at 1 yard			
Loud music			
Normal conversation			
Ticking of a watch			

Decibels: 10 20 30 40 50 60 70 80 90 100 110 120 130

More commonly, damage from loud noise occurs over a period of time, with gradual destruction of the hair cells of the cochlea and permanent hearing loss.

SYMPTOMS OF NOISE DAMAGE

Sound at 90 decibels or above usually causes pain, which is a warning that hearing may be damaged unless the source of the noise is removed. Prolonged *tinnitus* (ringing or buzzing in the ears) that occurs after a noise has ceased is an indication that some damage has probably occurred.

Prolonged exposure to loud noise leads initially to a loss of ability to hear certain high tones. Later, deafness extends to all high frequencies and the perception of speech becomes impaired. Eventually, lower tones are also affected.

PREVENTION OF NOISE DAMAGE

Regulations governing maximum noise levels apply to places of work and to some other potential hazards, such as noise from low-flying aircraft. People who cannot avoid exposure to loud noise (for example, workers using pneumatic drills) should wear earplugs. People who are persistently exposed to loud noise should have their hearing monitored regularly.

Noma

Also known as cancrum oris, death of tissue in the lips and cheeks caused by bacterial infection. Noma is most often seen in (and largely confined to) young, severely malnourished children in developing countries. It may complicate other diseases, especially *measles*, and sometimes occurs during the last stages of *leukemia*.

SYMPTOMS

The first symptom is inflammation of the gums and the inner surface of the cheeks. Without treatment, this leads to severe ulceration (with a foul-smelling discharge) and eventual destruction of the bones around the mouth and loss of teeth. Healing occurs naturally after a time, but scarring may be severe.

TREATMENT

Penicillin drugs and improved nutrition halt the progress of the disease. Plastic surgery may be necessary to reconstruct damaged bones or to improve facial appearance.

Nonaccidental injury

See *Child abuse*.

Noninvasive

A term used to describe any medical procedure that does not involve penetration of the skin or entry into the body through any of the natural openings; examples include *CT scanning* and *echocardiography*. The term noninvasive is sometimes applied to benign tumors that do not spread throughout body tissues.

Nonspecific urethritis

Also called nongonococcal urethritis, inflammation of the urethra due to a cause or causes other than *gonorrhea*. Worldwide, nonspecific urethritis is the most common type of *sexually transmitted disease*.

CAUSES

The name nonspecific urethritis was given to the disorder at a time when few laboratory tests were available for the detection of microorganisms. Today, about 40 percent of cases are known to be caused by CHLAMYDIA TRACHOMATIS (see *Chlamydial infections*); others are caused by HERPESVIRUS HOMINIS (the virus that causes *herpes simplex*) or TRICHOMONAS VAGINALIS infections. In about 50 percent of cases, however, the cause remains unknown.

SYMPTOMS

Nonspecific urethritis has an incubation period of about two to three weeks. In men, the infection usually causes a clear or pus-containing urethral discharge often accompanied by pain or discomfort on passing urine. Sometimes these symptoms are very mild or even absent. Women with nonspecific urethritis may have no symptoms; some have a vaginal discharge, mild discomfort on passing urine, or pain in the pelvic region.

DIAGNOSIS AND TREATMENT

Laboratory tests are performed to find the organism responsible for the infection. Because a woman may have no symptoms, a diagnosis often rests on the fact that she has a male partner with nonspecific urethritis.

Treatment is difficult because in many cases the cause cannot be determined. The cure rate is roughly 85 percent. *Antibiotic drugs*, including oxytetracycline and erythromycin, are given. Because relapses are common, follow-up visits are necessary for three months after treatment to examine the urine and any discharge.

COMPLICATIONS

In men, *cystitis*, *epididymitis*, *prostatitis*, and urethral stricture (narrowing of the urethra) can occur as complications of nonspecific urethritis.

In women, *salpingitis* (inflammation of the fallopian tubes), cysts of the Bartholin's glands, and *cervicitis* may occur. *Ophthalmia* neonatorum, a type of conjunctivitis, sometimes develops in babies born to women with chlamydial cervicitis.

Reiter's syndrome (in which there is arthritis and conjunctivitis as well as urethritis) develops in about 5 percent of people with nonspecific urethritis.

Nonsteroidal anti-inflammatory drugs

COMMON DRUGS

Diflunisal Fenoprofen Ibuprofen Indomethacin Meclofenamate Naproxen Phenylbutazone Piroxicam Sulindac Tolmetin

> **WARNING**
> Report abdominal pain or indigestion to your physician.

A group of drugs that has an *analgesic* (painkilling) action and also reduces inflammation in joints and soft tissues, such as muscles and ligaments. The name nonsteroidal anti-inflammatory drugs is commonly abbreviated NSAIDs.

WHY THEY ARE USED

NSAIDs are widely used to relieve symptoms caused by types of arthritis, such as *rheumatoid arthritis, osteoarthritis,* and *gout.* They do not cure or halt the progress of disease but improve mobility of the affected joint by relieving pain and stiffness.

NSAIDs are also used in the treatment of back pain, menstrual pain, headaches, pain after minor surgery, and soft tissue injuries.

HOW THEY WORK

NSAIDs reduce pain and inflammation by blocking the production of prostaglandins (chemicals that cause inflammation and trigger transmission of pain signals to the brain).

POSSIBLE ADVERSE EFFECTS

Nausea, indigestion, diarrhea, and *peptic ulcer* may occur.

Norepinephrine

A hormone secreted by certain nerve endings (principally those of the *sympathetic nervous system*) and by the medulla (center) of the *adrenal glands*. Norepinephrine's primary function is to help maintain a constant blood pressure by stimulating certain blood vessels to constrict when the blood pressure falls below normal. For this reason, an injection of the hormone may be given in the emergency treatment of *shock* or severe bleeding. (See also *Epinephrine*.)

Norethindrone

A *progesterone drug* that is used with an *estrogen drug* in several *oral contraceptive* preparations and in *hormone replacement therapy*.

On its own, norethindrone is sometimes used to treat women who are suffering from *endometriosis*, *amenorrhea* (absent periods), or irregular menstrual bleeding (see *Menstruation, disorders of*).

Norgestrel

A synthetic *progesterone drug* used in some *oral contraceptive* preparations.

Nortriptyline

An *antidepressant drug* that also has a sedative effect. Nortriptyline is useful in the treatment of *depression* that may follow a *stroke*.

Nose

The uppermost part of the respiratory tract and the organ of *smell*.

STRUCTURE

The nose is an air passage connecting the nostrils at its front to the *nasopharynx* (the upper part of the throat) at the rear. The *nasal septum*, made of cartilage at the front and bone at the rear, divides the passage.

Two small bones, the nasal bones, project from the front of the cranium and form the top of the bridge of the nose; the remainder of the bridge is cartilage. The roof of the nasal passage is formed by bones at the base of the skull, the walls by the maxilla (upper *jaw*), and the floor by the hard *palate*. Projecting from each wall are three conchae (thin, downward-curling plates of bone). The entire nasal passage is lined with *mucous membrane*, which bears tiny hairs that considerably increase the surface area.

The bones surrounding the nose contain air-filled, mucous membrane-lined cavities known as paranasal *sinuses*, which open into the nasal passage. In each wall of the nose is the opening to a nasolacrimal duct, which drains away the tears that bathe the front of the eyeball.

Projecting into the roof of the nasal passage through tiny openings are the hairlike nerve endings of the *olfactory nerves*, which are responsible for the sense of smell.

FUNCTION

One of the main functions of the nose is to filter, warm, and moisten inhaled air before it passes into the rest of the respiratory tract. Just inside the nostrils small hairs trap large dust particles and even larger foreign bodies

ANATOMY OF THE NOSE

The nose is involved in breathing and also in the sense of smell; it is a hollow passage connecting the nostrils and the top of the throat. The upper part of the nose transmits sensations of smell.

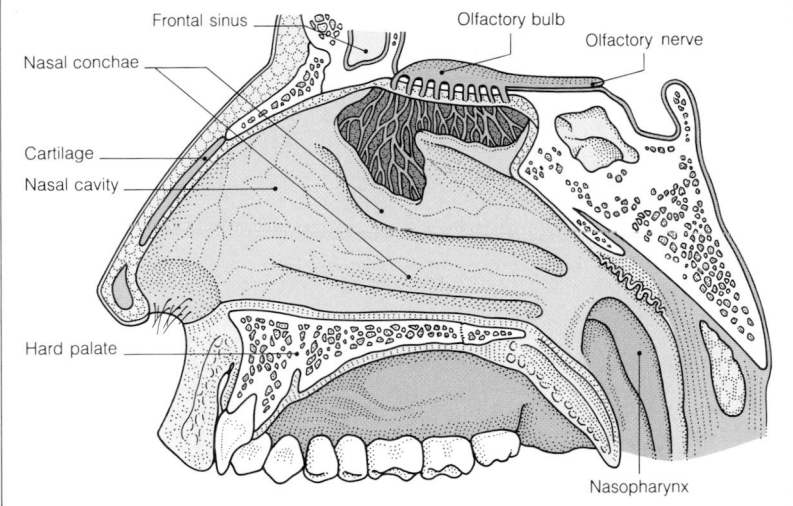

and induce sneezing to remove them. Smaller dust particles are filtered from the air by the hairs of the conchae. All air entering the nose passes over the blood vessels and mucus-secreting cells on the surface of the conchae. The mucus on the conchae flows inward, carrying harmful microorganisms and other foreign bodies back toward the nasopharynx so that they can be swallowed and destroyed by the gastric acid in the stomach.

The nose detects smells by means of the olfactory nerve endings, which, when stimulated by inhaled vapors, transmit this information to the olfactory bulb in the brain.

The nose also is a resonator, giving each voice its characteristic tone. (See also *Nose* disorders box, overleaf.)

Nosebleed

Loss of blood from the mucous membrane that lines the nose, most

FIRST AID: NOSEBLEED

WARNING
If a nosebleed starts after a heavy blow to the head, it could indicate a fractured skull. Take the victim to the hospital immediately.

1 Have the victim sit, ensuring he or she leans forward slightly with the mouth held open so that blood or clots do not obstruct the airway.

2 Pinch the lower part of the nostrils for about 15 minutes. The victim should breathe through the mouth.

3 The nostrils should be released slowly and the victim should avoid touching or blowing the nose. If the bleeding has not stopped after 20 minutes, seek medical attention.

N

N

DISORDERS OF THE NOSE

The nose is susceptible to a wide range of disorders. Infections and allergic conditions, leading to stuffiness or sneezing and sometimes some loss of smell, are common. Because of its prominent position, the nose is also particularly prone to injury.

CONGENITAL DEFECTS

In choanal atresia, one or both nasal cavities fail to develop fully. If both sides are affected, the baby cannot breathe properly. An abnormality affecting one side may not cause any problems until later in life.

Syphilis that is transmitted to a fetus during pregnancy may lead to a failure of full development of the nasal bones, with flattening of the bridge of the nose.

INFECTION

The common *cold*, a virus infection, causes inflammation of the lining of the nasal passages and excessive production of mucus, leading to nasal congestion. Small *boils* (infected hair follicles) are common just within the nostril, where they may cause severe pain. Backward spread of infection from the nose

can rarely cause *cavernous sinus thrombosis*, a serious condition that, without antibiotics, may be fatal.

TUMORS

Hemangiomas (benign tumors of blood vessels) commonly affect the nasal cavity in babies. Many disappear spontaneously before puberty.

Basal cell carcinoma and *squamous cell carcinoma* (skin cancers) may occur in and around the nostril. The nose may also be invaded by cancers originating in the surrounding sinuses.

INJURY

Fracture of the nasal bones (see *Nose, broken*) is a common sports injury that can lead to deformity; it may require corrective surgery. *Nosebleeds* are also common, particularly in children; they may be caused by fragile blood vessels, infection of the lining of the nose, or a blow to the nose.

DRUGS

Repeated sniffing of cocaine interferes with the blood supply to the mucous membrane lining the nose and can cause perforation of the nasal septum. Persistent inhalation of snuff can lead to nasopharyngeal cancer.

ALLERGIES

Allergic rhinitis (hay fever) is one of the most common allergies. Common causative allergens include pollens, animal dander, house mites, and fungal spores. (See *Rhinitis, allergic*.)

OBSTRUCTION

A nasal *polyp* (a projection of swollen mucous membrane) may block a nostril, causing a sensation of congestion.

Young children frequently insert foreign bodies, such as beads, peas, or pebbles, into their nostrils. They often become stuck, causing obstruction and a discharge.

INVESTIGATION

To inspect the inside of the nose, the physician uses a speculum to open up the nostrils. If a fracture is suspected, *X rays* are taken. For suspected cancer, nasal endoscopy and a *biopsy* are done.

often from inside one nostril only. Nosebleeds are most common in childhood, when they are usually insignificant and easily stopped. They are infrequent in healthy young adults, but become more common and more serious in old age.

CAUSES

The most common causes of a nosebleed are a blow to the nose, fragile blood vessels, or dislodging crusts that form in the mucous membrane as a result of a cold or other infection. Rarely, recurrent nosebleeds are a sign of an underlying disorder, such as *hypertension* (high blood pressure), a *bleeding disorder*, or a tumor of the nose or sinuses.

TREATMENT

Most nosebleeds can be controlled by simple first-aid measures (see box on previous page).

If first-aid treatment fails to stop bleeding within 20 minutes, a physician should be consulted. He or she may pack the affected nostril firmly with gauze (to apply constant pressure to the wound) or may cauterize the wound. In rare cases, surgery may be needed to stop the bleeding.

Nose, broken

Fracture of the nasal bones, sometimes with dislocation of the adjacent cartilage. A blow from the side may knock the bones or cartilage out of position or cause displacement of the *nasal septum*. A frontal blow tends to splay the nasal bones out-

X ray showing broken nose
The nasal bones under the bridge of the nose and part of the ethmoid bone, which forms the top part of the nasal septum (partition between the two sides of the nose), have been broken.

ward, depressing the bridge. Usually, the fracture is accompanied by severe swelling of overlying soft tissue, which can mask a minor fracture (revealed only when *X rays* are taken).

A fractured nose is painful and remains tender for about three weeks after the injury.

TREATMENT

Resetting is usually carried out either before the swelling has started or when it has subsided, about 10 days after the injury. Occasionally, the displaced bridge can be manipulated into position using a local anesthetic, but usually a general anesthetic is needed. A plaster splint is sometimes required during healing.

Nose reshaping

See *Rhinoplasty*.

Nuclear energy

Also known as atomic energy, the energy released (principally in the form of heat, light, and "hard" *radiation* such as gamma rays) as a result of changes in the nuclei of atoms. Nuclear energy is released in certain natural processes, such as the spontaneous decay of naturally occurring radioactive substances (uranium ores, for example), and the nuclear reactions that power the sun and other stars. It is also released in man-made devices such as nuclear reactors and nuclear weapons.

Nuclear magnetic resonance
See *MRI*.

Nuclear medicine
Techniques that use radioactive substances to detect or treat disease.

The most important application of nuclear medicine is in diagnosis. Radioactive materials (which are injected or swallowed) are taken up by body tissues or organs in different concentrations, and an instrument called a gamma camera is used to detect and map the distribution of radiation within the body. The technique requires only a small amount of radiation, and produces images that reflect bodily functions—not simply anatomy. (See *Radionuclide scanning*.)

In techniques for treatment, higher doses of radiation are used. Diseased tissues are destroyed by exposing them to an external radioactive source or by inserting a radioactive substance into a body tissue or cavity. (See *Radiation therapy; Interstitial radiation therapy; Intracavitary therapy*.)

Nucleic acids
Substances found in all living matter that have a fundamental role in the propagation of life. Nucleic acids provide the inherited, coded instructions (or "blueprint") for an organism's development; they also provide some of the apparatus by which these instructions are carried out.

There are two types of nucleic acid, called deoxyribonucleic acid (DNA) and ribonucleic acid (RNA). In all plant and animal cells (including humans), it is the DNA that permanently holds the coded instructions; RNA helps transport, translate, and implement the instructions. The DNA is the main constituent of *chromosomes*, which are carried in the nucleus (central unit) of the cell.

STRUCTURE
DNA and RNA are similar in their structure. Both have long, chainlike molecules. The main difference is that DNA usually consists of two intertwined chains, whereas RNA is generally single stranded.

The basic structure of DNA (shown at right) has been likened to a very long rope ladder, the chains of the DNA forming the two sides of the ladder with interlinking structures between the chains forming the rungs. The ladder is not straight, however, but twisted into a helical (spiral) shape, which gives it great stability. This shape is called a double helix.

If the two DNA chains are separated, it is found that each has a "backbone" (the side of the ladder) consisting of a string of sugar and phosphate chemical groups. Attached to each sugar in this string is a chemical called a base. The base can be any of four types, called adenine, thymine, guanine, and cytosine (or A,T,G, and C), and each forms half of one "rung" of the DNA ladder. The four bases can occur in any sequence along the chain (a sequence might be, for example, GTCGTATTTAGTCC). The sequence itself, which may be many millions of individual bases long, provides the code for the activities of the cell, just as the sequence of letters on this page provides a message to the reader (see *Genetic code*).

Because the two bases that form each rung of the ladder conform to certain pairings (A always pairing with T, and G with C), the sequence of bases on one chain always determines exactly the sequence on the second chain. This is of fundamental importance for the copying of DNA molecules when a cell divides.

RNA is like a single strand of DNA, except that the nucleotide base thymine in DNA is replaced by another base, uracil, in RNA, and the sugar and phosphate chain in RNA is slightly different chemically.

FUNCTION
DNA controls a cell's activities by specifying and regulating the synthesis of enzymes and other proteins in the cell, with different *genes* (sections of DNA) regulating the production of different proteins. For a particular protein to be made, an appropriate section of DNA acts as a template for an RNA chain. This "messenger" RNA then passes out of the nucleus into the cell cytoplasm, where it is decoded to form proteins (see *Genetic code; Protein synthesis*).

When a cell divides, identical copies of its DNA must go to each of the two daughter cells. The structure of DNA makes this process possible. Starting at one end of the molecule, the two chains separate, or "unzip." As they do so, two more chains are formed side by side to the original chains (these new chains are formed by the linking of free, unlinked, nucleotides that are present in cells). Because only certain base pairings are possible, the new double chains are identical to the original DNA molecule.

Thus, when a cell divides, it provides an exact copy of its DNA to its daughter cells. Each of a person's cells carries the same DNA replica that was present in the fertilized ovum. The DNA message is thus passed from one generation to another.

N

DNA STRUCTURE
A DNA molecule consists of two intertwined strands, the margins of which are chains of sugar and phosphate groups. The chains are linked by pairs of substances called bases, of which there are four types—adenine, guanine, thymine, and cytosine. An adenine on one chain is always paired with thymine on the second; similarly, cytosine is always paired with guanine. The sequence of bases in one chain thus exactly determines the sequence in the other chain.

Nucleotides
Each base, along with the sugar and phosphate groups to which it is attached, forms a unit called a nucleotide.

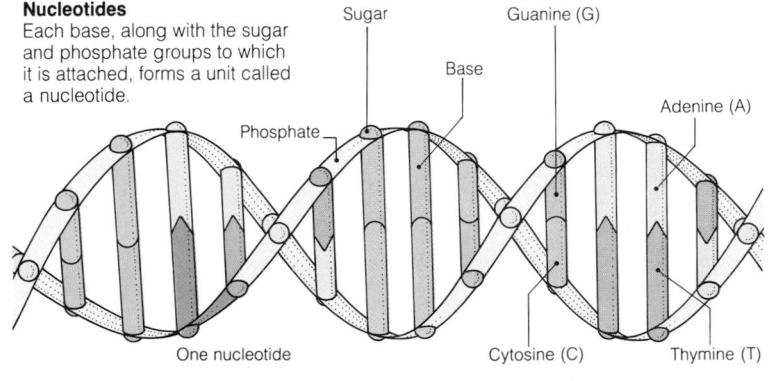

Sugar   Guanine (G)

Base

Phosphate

Adenine (A)

One nucleotide   Cytosine (C)   Thymine (T)

NUMBNESS AND TINGLING
Loss of feeling and/or a pins and needles sensation in any part of the body

? Did you notice the numbness AND/OR tingling after sitting in one position for a long time or after waking from a deep sleep?

YES → Pressure on a nerve, which stretches it, or temporarily cuts off its blood supply, is often the cause of these sensations. Feeling should return to normal in a few minutes.

NO

↓

? Are only your hands affected?

YES → Have you noticed any stiffness in your neck?

YES → These symptoms suggest a disorder of the nerves and bones of the neck, especially if you are over 50.

See • *Cervical osteoarthritis*

NO

NO

↓

Are the symptoms worse at night AND/OR do you have pains that shoot up the hand from your wrist?

YES → This suggests a disorder of the nerves that pass through the wrist.

See • *Carpal tunnel syndrome*

NO

↓

? Does the numbness AND/OR tingling affect only one side of your body?

YES → Have you also noticed one or more of the following symptoms?
• blurred vision
• confusion
• difficulty speaking
• loss of movement in your arms or legs
• dizziness

YES → ☎ **EMERGENCY!**
GET MEDICAL HELP NOW!
Your symptoms may be caused by a disruption of the blood supply to the brain.

See • *Stroke*
• *Transient ischemic attack*

NO

NO

↓

? Do your fingers or toes get numb and turn blue in cold weather, and then become red and painful as feeling returns?

YES → You may have a disorder that affects the small blood vessels in the extremities.

See • *Raynaud's disease*

NO

↓

If you are unable to make a diagnosis from this chart, consult your physician.

N

Nucleus

The central core, structure, or focal point of an object.

The nucleus of a living cell is a roughly spherical unit at the center of the cell. It contains the *chromosomes* (composed mainly of *nucleic acid*) responsible for directing the cell's activities, and is surrounded by a membrane. There are small pores in the membrane through which various substances can pass between the nucleus and the cytoplasm (the rest of the cell).

The nucleus of an atom, composed of protons and neutrons, accounts for nearly all the mass of an atom but only a tiny proportion of its volume. Nuclear energy is produced through changes in the mass and structure of atomic nuclei.

A nerve nucleus is a group of neurons (nerve cells) within the brain and spinal cord that work together to perform a particular function.

Numbness

Loss of sensation in part of the body caused by interference to the passage of impulses along sensory nerves.

CAUSES

Numbness can occur naturally and harmlessly (such as when blood supply to a nerve in the leg is cut off temporarily by sitting cross-legged), it can be induced artificially (e.g., by a dentist anesthetizing a nerve before filling a tooth), or it may be the result of a disorder or damage to the nervous system or its blood supply.

Multiple sclerosis can cause loss of sensation in any part of the body through damage to nerve pathways in the central nervous system (CNS). In *neuropathy*, it is the peripheral nerves (outside the CNS) that are damaged. In a *stroke*, pressure on, or reduced blood supply to, nerve pathways in the brain often causes loss of feeling on one side of the body.

Severe cold, as in frostbite, causes numbness by a direct action on the nerves. Numbness may also be a feature of various psychological disorders, such as *anxiety*, *panic attack*, or a hysterical *conversion disorder*.

DIAGNOSIS AND TREATMENT

Examination by a physician usually reveals an area of sensory loss or impairment that corresponds to the skin distribution of a single peripheral nerve, several nerves, or a sensory area in the CNS. The distribution of the affected area may suggest the site and mechanism of nerve damage. Treatment can then be prescribed.

Nurse

A person trained in *nursing care*. Registered nurses (RNs) are registered and licensed by a state to care for the sick and to promote health. They work in hospitals, nursing homes, physicians' offices, clinics, workplaces, schools, and patients' homes.

Some RNs concentrate on a particular field, engaging in the full-time practice of *anesthesia*, *psychiatry*, *pediatrics*, or *surgery*. Specific types of RN also exist. Nurse-midwives have special training in prenatal and postnatal care, labor, and delivery (see *Midwifery*). Nurse practitioners or nurse clinicians are trained to provide health services (such as preventive care, monitoring of chronic conditions, physical examinations, and health counseling) under the supervision of a physician.

Other types of nurses include licensed practical nurses (LPNs), who are trained to provide basic care for patients under the supervision of physicians and RNs. Nurses' aides assist nurses in hospitals, nursing homes, and clinics.

Nursing

See *Breast-feeding*.

Nursing care

The process by which a patient is helped by a *nurse* to recover from an illness or injury, or to regain as much independence as possible. The nurse is more concerned with the patient's overall reaction to the disorder than with the disorder itself, and is devoted to the control of physical pain, the relief of mental suffering, and, when possible, the avoidance of complications. In terminal cases, the nurse's responsibility is to help the patient meet death with as little distress and as much dignity as possible.

Working closely with physicians and other health care professionals, the nurse exercises continuous surveillance over the patient. This involves the measurement and recording of many bodily functions. The patient's pulse rate, respiratory rate, temperature, weight, and urine output are recorded daily—or more frequently in acute illness. The nurse may also monitor blood pressure and the ECG in an intensive-care unit, and may record the output of fluids and the intake of fluids and food.

In patients recovering from surgery, the nurse monitors the level of consciousness, ensures that there is no obstruction to breathing, maintains the correct rate of flow of any intravenous infusion, and records vital functions, such as pulse rate.

Prevention is another important aspect of nursing care. The nurse moves unconscious or immobile patients every few hours to prevent the development of bedsores; washing out the mouth, cleaning the teeth, and removing urine and feces guards against infection.

The nurse is also responsible for administering drugs.

From the patient's perspective, the most important quality the nurse can offer may be understanding care, which involves listening with patience to anxieties and fears, and providing emotional support and comfort.

Nursing home

A residential facility for the care of elderly people or, in some cases, for people who have serious illnesses or disabilities.

The rapid increase in the number of elderly people in the US (more than 11 percent of the population is now over 65) has resulted in an increased need for provision of long-term care. There are currently some 19,000 nursing homes in the US caring for more than 1.4 million people, including 20 percent of the people over 85.

Nursing homes as they exist today are partly a result of the Social Security Act of 1935, which refused benefits to people who were in public residential institutions. Consequently, many of the people concerned moved to private facilities.

TYPES OF NURSING HOME

There are three basic types of nursing home. Residential care facilities (RCFs) provide accommodation and food; staff members monitor the basic health of the residents. RCFs are appropriate for elderly people who are fairly independent and able, but who want someone to take over responsibility for basic housekeeping chores.

Intermediate care facilities (ICFs) provide food and lodging and regular custodial care for people who are too ill or frail to look after themselves. Recreational activities may be provided, and some ICFs have rehabilitation programs.

Skilled nursing facilities (SNFs) are overseen by physicians and provide 24-hour nursing. These facilities are for people who require intensive medical and rehabilitation care.

Most care in nursing homes is long-term, but short-term homes are available for people who are primarily

N

nursed at home. This allows care-givers (usually family members) some respite from their responsibility.

CARE IN NURSING HOMES

Approximately 50 percent of nursing home residents are demented, and most suffer from a number of medical conditions related to *aging*. In addition, because of changes in the Medicare system, patients tend to be discharged from hospitals to nursing homes at earlier stages in their convalescence. These factors place great demands on the medical care provided by nursing homes.

The ideal nursing home is well equipped with registered nurses as well as nurses' aides, has regular visits from a physician, provides access to advanced medical care facilities, and is closely linked, both organizationally and geographically, to community hospitals. It is also important for a nursing home to have a pleasant atmosphere, to treat its patients in a caring and sensitive manner, and to respect their rights to privacy. (See also *Geriatric medicine*.)

Nutrient

A substance that provides nourishment. Essential nutrients are those necessary for body function that are not synthesized in the body. They include proteins, carbohydrates, fats, vitamins, and minerals.

Nutrition

The science and study of the foodstuffs people eat and drink and the ways they are digested and assimilated. Both physicians and the public have shown growing interest in the relationship between diet and health. Until about 30 years ago the primary concern of nutritionists was dietary deficiencies; their recommendations concentrated on the minimum amounts of nutrients required for health. In Western societies the focus is now on the dangers of too much fat or sugar in the diet, and the effects of food additives, colorings, and preservatives on health.

ELEMENTS OF GOOD NUTRITION

Basic elements of the diet are proteins, carbohydrates, fats, fiber, vitamins, minerals, and water (see also entries on individual nutrients). A balanced diet contains adequate, not excessive, amounts of each (see box).

EATING A BALANCED DIET

People require different amounts of nutrients and energy. A precise assessment of each person's requirements would be ideal, but a general

ESSENTIAL NUTRIENTS

Proteins	The main structural component of tissue and organs. We need proteins for growth and repair of cells. Each protein contains hundreds and sometimes thousands of units called amino acids in specific combinations. In the body there are 20 amino acids; 12 of these are manufactured by the body itself and	the remaining eight are obtained from a balanced diet. A vegetarian diet containing eggs, milk, and cheese provides sufficient amounts of all essential amino acids. A vegan diet, which also excludes dairy products, needs careful planning to prevent protein deficiency (see *Vegetarianism*).
Carbohydrates	The two carbohydrate food groups, sugars and starches, are the main energy sources required for metabolism (chemical processes that take place within cells). Carbohydrates should make up at	least half of our diet. Unrefined (unprocessed) carbohydrates found in cereals and fruit are usually richer in fiber and nutrients than refined carbohydrates, such as sugar and white flour.
Fats	Fats provide energy for metabolism and are a structural component of cells. Most people in developed countries eat too much fat; fats should constitute no more than 30 percent of total calorie intake. There are three kinds of dietary fats—saturated fats (found mostly in meat and dairy products), monosaturated fats (found in olive oil and avocados), and polyunsaturated fats (found in fish and vegetable oils). Saturated fats	tend to increase the amounts of unwanted types of cholesterol in the blood whereas polyunsaturated fats and monosaturated fats have the opposite effect. Studies have indicated that a high level of low-density lipoprotein cholesterol in the blood is associated with coronary heart disease. Our bodies produce enough cholesterol for our needs; any excess is primarily due to eating too much saturated fat.
Fiber	This is the indigestible structural material in plants. Although fiber passes through the intestine unchanged, it is an essential part of a healthy diet. A low fiber diet may lead to constipation, diverticular disease, and other disorders. High fiber diets (including plenty	of fruit, raw vegetables, grains, and cereals) provide bulk without excess calories. Low fiber diets tend to be high in refined carbohydrates and fats, and thus are more likely to encourage obesity, heart disease, and other unwanted effects.
Water	Our bodies are composed of about 60 percent water. Water constitutes a high proportion of many foods and is essential to maintain metabolism	(chemical processes within cells) and normal bowel function. It also determines the volume of blood in our circulation.
Vitamins	Regulators of metabolism. Vitamins ensure the healthy functioning of the brain, nerves, muscles, skin, and bones. Although vitamins do not supply energy, some enable energy to be released from the food. A healthy, balanced diet contains enough vitamins for most people's needs and supplements are not	usually necessary. Indeed, some vitamins, especially A, D, E, and K, are dangerous if taken in excess. Water-soluble vitamins (B and C) are stored in the body less well than fat-soluble vitamins, but even on a very restricted diet vitamin deficiency is rare until several months have elapsed.
Minerals	A balanced diet provides enough minerals for most people. Calcium is necessary for the maintenance of healthy bones and teeth. Other minerals, such as zinc and magnesium, are needed in minute amounts to control cell metabolism.	The only mineral commonly required as a supplement is iron, which is used to prevent anemia in women who experience heavy periods. Sodium chloride (table salt) is needed to maintain fluid balance. Excess may cause *hypertension*.

guide can be useful as well. The figures for the recommended daily allowances (RDAs) are based on average requirements to cover the needs of the majority; the variables are usually body size, age, sex, and lifestyle (active or sedentary).

Nutritional disorders

Nutritional disorders may be caused by a deficiency or an excess of one or more nutrients or by a toxin or poisonous element in the diet.

NUTRIENT DEFICIENCY

A diet deficient in carbohydrate is almost inevitably deficient in protein too (protein-calorie malnutrition). This deficiency is most often seen in people in Africa and Asia as a result of poverty and famine (see *Kwashiorkor; Marasmus*).

Inadequate intake of protein and calories may also occur in people who restrict their diet in an attempt to lose weight (see *Anorexia nervosa*); it can also occur because of mistaken beliefs about diet and health (see *Food fad*) or because of loss of interest in food associated with *alcohol dependence* and *drug dependence*.

In Western societies, deficiency of nutrients is usually associated with a disorder of the digestive system, such as *celiac sprue, Crohn's disease*, or pernicious anemia (see *Anemia, megaloblastic*).

NUTRIENT EXCESS

Obesity and dental *caries* are two of the most common disorders in the US; both are due to excessive intake of nutrients. Obesity is caused by an excess of refined carbohydrates and fat. Dental caries develop mainly in people who eat large amounts of refined carbohydrates.

TOXIC EFFECTS

A nutritional disorder may arise from the presence of toxic substances in the food. These may be naturally occurring substances, such as the *aflatoxin* fungus found on peanuts (which can cause *liver cancer*) or the *ergot* fungus found on rye (which can cause ergotism). Industrial pesticides, fertilizers, pollutants, and other chemicals may also contaminate food.

Nymphomania

A *psychosexual disorder* in which a woman is dominated by an insatiable appetite for sexual activity with numerous different male partners. Nymphomaniacs are often distressed by their own behavior and by their inability to see men as anything other than objects for sexual conquest. Nymphomania is generally thought to be an expression of some deep psychological disorder.

A similar behavior in men is called satyriasis or Don Juanism. It is said to be caused by intense narcissism and the need to control feelings of inferiority through sexual success.

Nystagmus

A condition in which there is involuntary movement of the eyes; the movement is usually horizontal, but can be vertical or rotary. In almost all types, both eyes move together.

CAUSES AND TYPES

In the most common type, called jerky nystagmus, the eyes repeatedly move slowly in one direction and then rapidly in the other, giving a jerking effect. The disorder is almost always congenital and is usually unassociated with any abnormality of the eyes; the cause is unknown. Jerky nystagmus is permanent and, because steady gaze is impossible, there is almost always a moderate to severe defect of visual acuity. Nystagmus also occurs in *albinism* and as a result of any very severe defect of vision, such as congenital *cataract*, retinal disease, or *optic atrophy*, present at birth.

Persistent nystagmus appearing later in life indicates the presence of a disorder of the nervous system (such as *multiple sclerosis* or a brain tumor) or a disorder of the balancing mechanism in the inner ear. Nystagmus may also occur as a normal effect of a person's attempts to follow a sequence of objects rapidly passing the eyes. This phenomenon is known as "opto-kinetic nystagmus."

Electronystagmography, a method of recording eye movements, may be performed to identify different types of nystagmus.

Nystatin

ANTIFUNGAL
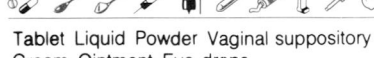
Tablet Liquid Powder Vaginal suppository Cream Ointment Eye drops
Prescription needed
Available as generic

An *antifungal drug* used in the treatment of *candidiasis* (thrush). Nystatin may be safely used during pregnancy. High doses taken by mouth may cause diarrhea, nausea, vomiting, and abdominal pain.

THE FOUR FOOD GROUPS AND RECOMMENDED DAILY SERVINGS

Food group		Typical servings	
Milk group Servings required per day: 2		Milk Yogurt, plain Hard cheese Cheese spread Cottage cheese	8 ounces (1 cup) 1 cup 1¼ ounces 2 ounces 2 cups
'Meat' group Servings required per day: 2		Meat, lean Poultry Fish Eggs Peanut butter	2 to 3 ounces (cooked) 2 to 3 ounces 2 to 3 ounces 2 to 3 4 tablespoons
Fruit and vegetable group Servings required per day: 4		Vegetables Fruits Grapefruit Potato Lettuce	½ cup ½ cup ½ medium 1 medium 1 wedge
Bread and cereal group Servings required per day: 4		Bread Cooked cereal Pasta Rice Dry cereal	1 slice ½ to ¾ cup ½ to ¾ cup ½ to ¾ cup 1 ounce

Essential nutrients are found in differing amounts in foods, so a varied diet is needed to ensure you get all you need. An easy way to plan a balanced diet is to use the above chart to select foods from each of the four basic food groups. Note that the meat group contains other protein-rich foods, such as eggs and peanut butter, as well as meat.

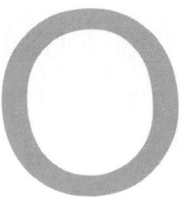

Obesity

A condition in which there is too much body fat. Being obese is not the same as being overweight. A person is usually not considered obese unless he or she weighs 20 percent or more over the maximum desirable weight for his or her height (see *Weight*).

INCIDENCE

It is estimated that about 25 percent of the US population carries too much fat. About 5 to 10 percent of children are overweight or obese. Between 13 and 23 percent of all adolescents (especially girls) are obese; 80 percent of obese teenagers are likely to grow into obese adults.

CAUSES

The reasons why some people become obese are unclear. Although obesity occurs when the net energy intake exceeds the net energy expenditure (that is, when more calories are taken in than are being used by the body), obese people do not always eat considerably more than thin people.

A person's energy requirements are determined partly by his or her basal metabolic rate (the amount of energy needed to maintain vital body functions at rest—see *Metabolism*) and partly by his or her level of physical activity. Obese people may have a very low basal metabolic rate, or they may need fewer calories because they are less physically active.

It is thought that genetic factors play a part in the development of obesity; children of obese parents are 10 times more likely to be obese than children with parents of normal weight. Some hormonal disorders are accompanied by obesity, but the overwhelming majority of obese people do not suffer from such disorders.

COMPLICATIONS

Obesity increases a person's chance of becoming seriously ill. *Hypertension* (high blood pressure) and *stroke* are twice as likely to occur in obese people than in lean people. *Coronary heart disease* is more common, particularly in obese men under the age of 40. Adult-onset *diabetes mellitus* is five times more common among obese people, the risk increasing with the degree and duration of obesity. Increasing degrees of extra weight in men are associated with an increased risk of cancer of the colon, rectum, and prostate. With increasing weight, women show a progressive increase in risk of cancer of the breast, uterus, and cervix. *Osteoarthritis* may be agravated by obesity. Extra weight on the hips, knees, and back places undue strain on these joints. Weight loss does not reverse the disease but does help relieve stress and pain.

TREATMENT

The first line of treatment for obesity is a weight-loss diet (see *Nutrition*; *Weight reduction*). An obese person should follow a diet that provides 500 to 1,000 calories less than his or her energy requirements. The energy deficit is met by using some of the excess stored fat, which is reflected by an average weight loss of 1 to 2 pounds a week. Regular exercise (especially *aerobics*) increases weight loss by burning extra calories and by increasing the metabolic rate.

Fad diets may cause a dramatic weight loss within a short period of time, but, in almost all cases, the weight is quickly regained when normal eating habits are resumed. The use of drugs as appetite suppressants was once popular, but is usually no longer recommended by physicians.

Various radical procedures are available for severely obese people who have failed to lose weight, but because of the possible adverse effects they are attempted only if the person's health is in danger.

Wiring the jaw to prevent the mouth from opening more than about half an inch makes it impossible to chew. Reduced calorie meals in liquid form are taken through a straw. The jaw is usually wired for up to a year and the patient is kept under constant medical supervision. Weight is often regained once the wiring is undone.

An operation in which part of the stomach is stapled together reduces its size and has the effect of making the person feel full after eating a small amount of food.

Intestinal bypass operations were popular in the 1970s but are now uncommon due to the frequency and variety of adverse effects. A large part of the small intestine is bypassed by cutting the jejunum and joining it to the ileum, thus reducing the length of the digestive tract and allowing less food to be absorbed.

OUTLOOK

Some people who have been seriously obese for much of their lives can lose weight without regaining it. As when trying to give up smoking or alcohol, the essential element in weight reduction is psychological motivation.

Obsessive-compulsive behavior

A neurosis in which sufferers are constantly troubled by persistent ideas (obsessions) that make them carry out repetitive, ritualized acts (compulsions). Obsessive-compulsive disorder usually starts in adolescence and runs a fluctuating course.

CAUSES AND INCIDENCE

The condition is partly inherited, but environmental factors also play a part. Personality traits of orderliness and cleanliness are said to be related, as is a tendency for other neurotic symptoms. Certain forms of brain damage (especially *encephalitis*) can result in obsessional symptoms.

Obsessive-compulsive disorder is rare, although minor obsessional symptoms probably occur in about one sixth of the population.

SYMPTOMS

People with this disorder usually suffer from both obsessions and compulsions, often accompanied by *depression* and *anxiety*.

Obsessions are recurrent thoughts or feelings that come into the mind seemingly involuntarily. Sufferers regard these thoughts as senseless and sometimes unpleasant, but are unable to ignore or resist them. Thoughts of violence, fears of being infected by germs or dirt, and constant doubts (e.g., whether or not the front door is shut) are the most common obsessions. One form is obsessional rumination, in which a person broods constantly over a word, phrase, or an unanswerable problem.

Compulsions are repetitive, apparently purposeful acts that are carried out in a ritualized fashion. They are performed for the purpose of warding off fears or relieving anxiety and are thus the physical form of an obsessional state. Sufferers do not usually derive any pleasure from performing the activities, but feel increasingly anxious if they try to resist the compulsion. Handwashing, counting, and checking are the most common compulsions.

Compulsive acts may have to be performed so many times in a particular way that they seriously disrupt work and social life. It may take some sufferers two or three hours just to get up and wash in the morning. In addition, the constant use of soap may irritate the skin.

TREATMENT
Traditionally, obsessive-compulsive symptoms have been treated by *psychoanalysis*. Today, treatment may also consist of *behavior therapy*. It is often combined with *antidepressant drugs* (especially clomipramine) or *antianxiety drugs*.

OUTLOOK
At least two thirds of all people who have obsessive-compulsive disorder respond well to therapy. Symptoms may recur under stress but can usually be controlled. In severe cases, the affected person may become housebound and severely handicapped by indecision. In less than 3 percent of cases, sufferers go on to have psychotic symptoms (see *Psychosis*).

Obstetrician

A physician who specializes in the care of a woman during pregnancy, labor, delivery, and the period immediately afterward. Prenatal care may include periodic examinations of the woman and her developing baby with recommendations for changes in activity or diet. The obstetrician delivers the baby, performing a cesarean section if necessary. In many cases, the obstetrician is also the woman's *gynecologist*.

Obstetrics

The branch of medicine concerned with *pregnancy*, *childbirth*, and *postnatal care*. In conjunction with *gynecology*, obstetrics also involves the study of the structure and function of the female reproductive system (see *Reproductive system, female*).

Obstructive airways disease

See *Lung disease, chronic obstructive*.

Occiput

The lower back part of the head, where it merges with the neck.

Occlusion

Blockage of any passage, canal, opening, or vessel in the body. Occlusion may be the result of disease (as in *pulmonary embolism*) or may be induced for medical reasons (see *Embolism, therapeutic*). The term is also used to refer to the covering of the better-seeing eye during treatment of *amblyopia*. In dentistry, occlusion is the relationship between the upper and lower teeth when the jaw is shut.

Occult

A term meaning hidden or obscure. Occult blood in a sample of feces is invisible to the naked eye but can be detected by chemical tests.

Occult blood, fecal

The presence in the feces of blood that cannot be seen by the naked eye but can be detected by chemical tests. It may be a sign of various disorders of the gastrointestinal tract, including *esophagitis*; *gastritis* (inflammation of the stomach lining); *stomach cancer*; intestinal cancer (see *Intestine, cancer of*); rectal cancer (see *Rectum, cancer of*); *diverticular disease*; *polyps* in the colon; *ulcerative colitis*; or the use of medications that irritate the stomach or intestine, such as aspirin. Bleeding gums or *hemorrhoids* may also cause occult blood in the feces, although in most cases of hemorrhoids the blood is visible.

DETECTION
Screening for colorectal cancer is done by testing the stools of asymptomatic people for occult blood.

A thin film of feces is smeared on a chemically coated paper and a drop or two of oxidizing agent is placed on it. If blood is present, the feces-covered paper turns blue. (See also *Feces, abnormal*; *Rectal bleeding*.)

Occupational disease and injury

Illnesses, disorders, or injuries that occur as a result of work practices or exposure to chemical or physical agents or factors (e.g., dusts, poisons, or radiation) in the workplace. The efforts of specialists in this field mean that serious occupational diseases are much less common than they once were. Overall, however, occupational diseases make up an important and fairly common group of conditions (see table, overleaf).

TYPES
Some of the main types of occupational diseases are described below.

DUST DISEASES *Pneumoconiosis* refers to *fibrosis* of the lung caused by inhaled inorganic and organic dusts. It includes various diseases associated with mining (including coal and quartz mining), china clay processing, metal grinding, and foundry work. *Asbestosis* is a similar hazard for workers in the asbestos, mining, milling, and product manufacturing industries, and in shipbuilders.

Allergic *alveolitis* is a lung condition caused by inhalation of organic dusts (often containing fungal spores). It is

often occupationally related and includes such conditions as *farmers' lung* in agricultural workers.

CHEMICAL POISONING A vast number of industrial chemicals can cause damage to the lungs if inhaled, or to the liver, kidneys, bone marrow, or other organs if they reach the bloodstream via the lungs or skin.

Exposure to the fumes of cadmium (in the welding and electroplating industries) or beryllium (in high-technology industries) can damage the lungs. Lead and arsenic compounds (in metal processing and other industries) and benzene (in various industries where solvents are used) can damage the bone marrow, leading to *anemia* and other blood abnormalities. Carbon tetrachloride and vinyl chloride (in chemicals and plastics manufacture) are causes of liver disease. Many of these compounds can also cause kidney damage.

OCCUPATIONAL SKIN DISEASE Contact *dermatitis* (skin inflammation) can occur as a result of an allergy or of direct irritation by chemicals contacting the skin at work. Many substances may be responsible, from wet cement to processing chemicals used in the rubber goods industry. Other skin problems may also be occupationally related (e.g., severe itching caused by glass fiber or *squamous cell carcinoma* through exposure to tar).

RADIATION HAZARDS People with outdoor occupations in sunny climates are at increased risk of skin disease (such as *basal cell carcinoma*).

Workers in the nuclear energy industry and in some health care professions should use precautions to reduce the risk of developing a disease caused by ionizing radiation (see *Radiation hazards*).

INFECTIOUS DISEASES Rare infectious diseases are more common in certain occupations. They include *brucellosis* and *Q fever* (acquired from livestock) among farmworkers, *psittacosis* (from birds) in pet store owners, and *leptospirosis* (from rats) in sewer workers, miners, ditchdiggers, and fishermen. Viral *hepatitis* and *AIDS* are hazards for people who work with blood and blood products.

MISCELLANEOUS Disorders caused by repetitive actions, or overuse of parts of the body, range from writers' cramp to *carpal tunnel syndrome* and *singers' nodes*. *Raynaud's phenomenon* is associated with the handling of vibrating tools; *deafness* may be caused by exposure to noise and *cataracts* by exposure to intense heat.

O

SAFETY AT WORK

A major method of preventing occupational disease and injury is the use of suitable protective clothing. This may include an air-filter mask in the presence of dust or fumes; earplugs where there is a noise hazard; eye shields to protect against radiation, chemicals, or metal dust; gloves for handling machinery; protective headgear and reinforced footwear where there is a risk of falling objects.

Ear protectors

Tool safety
Before using any power tool, always read the instructions. Never leave the safety guard off.

Eye protectors

Air-filter mask

Chemical safety
Many chemical sprays are toxic. Protection for the eyes and lungs is advisable.

Heavy gloves

Reinforced footwear

OCCUPATIONAL INJURIES OR DISEASES

Injuries or diseases	Approximate no. of cases in US annually	Deaths	Examples
Disabling injuries at work caused by falls	250,000	Many thousands	All types of fractures, wounds, crush and penetrating injuries, sprains, burns, electrical injuries
All other disabling injuries at work	1,650,000		
Skin conditions	40,000	Few	Contact allergic or irritant dermatitis, some squamous cell carcinomas
Disorders associated with repeated trauma or overuse injury	26,000	Very few	Bursitis, tenosynovitis, tennis elbow, singers' nodes
Respiratory diseases caused by inhaled dusts or toxic agents	10,000	Several thousand	Pneumoconiosis, asbestosis, byssinosis, berylliosis, farmers' lung
Disorders caused by effects of physical phenomena	9,000	Few	Cancers, blood disorders (radiation), hearing loss (noise), cataract (heat), Raynaud's phenomenon (vibration)
Other types of poisoning	3,000	Several hundred	Diseases of the liver, kidneys, bone marrow, heart, nervous system, bladder
Other occupational diseases	18,000	Few	Brucellosis (slaughterhouse workers), decompression sickness (divers), viral hepatitis (health-care workers)

O

DIAGNOSIS AND PREVENTION

Sometimes the link between a disease and occupation may be obvious; sometimes it may become apparent only when a patient with mysterious symptoms mentions his or her occupation to the physician. Part of every medical history is a question regarding the patient's occupation. Even when an occupational disease is suspected, it may require extensive investigation at the workplace to determine the exact cause.

In more serious cases, the patient must quit his or her occupation, but then can make a claim for workers' compensation. In all cases, measures to prevent a recurrence are needed.

Occupational medicine

A branch of medicine concerned with the effects of a person's job on his or her health, with preventing *occupational disease and injury*, and with promoting general health in workers.

Occupational medicine has a long history. As early as the middle ages, it was recognized that miners were at risk of lung diseases caused by dust, and attempts were made to improve their working conditions by increasing ventilation. The scope of occupational medicine widened during the industrial revolution as research revealed the hazards of working with metals (such as lead and mercury) and minerals (such as phosphorus).

The occupational physician uses epidemiological (see *Epidemiology*) techniques to analyze patterns of absenteeism, injury, illness, and causes of death in working populations, and investigates and monitors the health of a particular work force. Health risks can be reduced in two ways: by primary prevention—the reduction of exposure to harmful substances and work practices by attention to dust control, safe work stations, and the disposal of wastes—and by secondary prevention, which involves regular screening of workers for early evidence of occupational disorders, such as dust diseases or damage to the liver from chemicals.

Today, the occupational physician is increasingly concerned with psychological stress at work, with the investigation of the hazards (known and unknown) of new technologies, and with promoting healthy personal habits in workers.

Occupational mortality
Death caused by disease contracted at the workplace or by injuries related to a person's work.

The death rate from work-related injuries in the US has been decreasing steadily for 50 years—from about 40 deaths annually per 100,000 working population in the 1930s to about 10 deaths per 100,000 in the middle 1980s. This last figure still represents approximately 10,000 injury-related deaths in the US each year.

In addition, there are several thousand deaths annually in the US attributable to occupational disease—principally to *pneumoconiosis* (dust disease of the lungs)—and to lung disease or cancers caused by exposure to asbestos.

While the precise number is unknown, it is estimated that one person in 200 in the US dies as a direct result of his or her occupation.

Occupational therapy
Treatment aimed at enabling people disabled by physical illness or a serious accident to relearn muscular control and coordination, to cope with everyday tasks (such as dressing), and, when possible, to resume some form of employment. Treatment, carried out by specially trained therapists, usually starts in the hospital and may be continued at an outpatient clinic or in the person's home.

Ocular
Relating to or affecting the eye and its structures. The term is also used to refer to the eyepiece of an optical device, such as a microscope.

Oculogyric crisis
A state of fixed gaze, lasting for minutes or hours, in which the eyes are turned in a particular direction (usually upward). The fixed-eye position is sometimes associated with spasm of the muscles of the tongue, mouth, and neck.

The crisis may occur in people with *parkinsonism* or those who have had *encephalitis*, or it may be induced by drugs (such as *reserpine* or the *phenothiazine* derivatives). It is often precipitated by emotional stress.

Oculomotor nerve
The third *cranial nerve*. The oculomotor nerve stimulates only motor functions. This nerve controls all the muscles that move the eye, except for two—the superior oblique muscle (which rotates the eyeball downward and outward and is controlled by the *trochlear nerve*) and the lateral rectus muscle (which moves the eye outward and is controlled by the *abducent nerve*). The oculomotor nerve also supplies the muscle that constricts the pupil, the ciliary muscle (which focuses the eye), and the muscle that raises the upper eyelid.

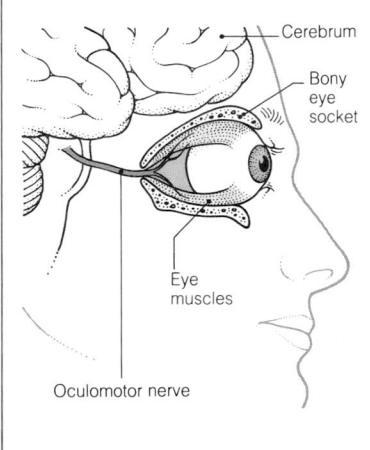

LOCATION OF THE OCULOMOTOR NERVE
The oculomotor nerve originates high in the brain stem and passes forward through a slit in the bony eye socket to reach the muscles that move the eye and eyelids.

Cerebrum

Bony eye socket

Eye muscles

Oculomotor nerve

The oculomotor nerve may be damaged as a result of a basal skull fracture or a disorder that distorts the brain, such as a tumor. Depending on the severity of damage, the following symptoms may occur: *ptosis* (drooping of the upper eyelid), *strabismus* (squint), dilation of the pupil, inability to focus the eye, double vision, and slight protrusion of the eyeball.

Oedipus complex
A term used in *psychoanalytic theory* to describe the unconscious sexual attachment of a child for the parent of the opposite sex and the consequent jealousy of, and desire to eliminate, the same-sexed parent. The name is derived from the Greek myth in which, unknowingly, Oedipus kills his father Laius and marries his mother Jocasta.

Sigmund Freud believed that the Oedipus complex (sometimes called the Electra complex in females) was present in all young children and that normal psychological development depended on the child coming to identify with the parent of the same sex and, later, making sexual attachments with members of the opposite sex outside the family.

Oils
See *Fats and oils*.

Ointment
A greasy, semisolid preparation that is applied to the skin. Ointments are used to apply drugs to an area of skin or to act as a protective agent. Most ointments contain petrolatum or wax and have an *emollient* (soothing, moisturizing) effect.

Olecranon
The bony projection at the upper end of the ulna (the inner bone of the forearm) that forms the point of the *elbow*. The olecranon is commonly known as the "funny bone"; a blow to the nerve that passes across it produces a tingling sensation that passes down the forearm to the fourth and fifth fingertips.

O

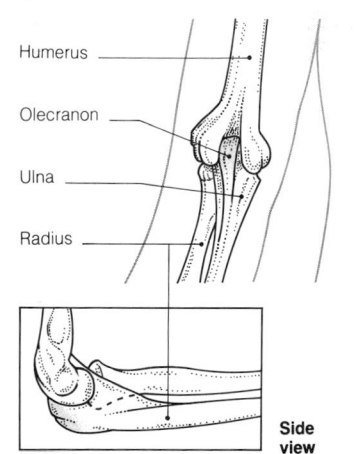

LOCATION OF THE OLECRANON
This is the curved projection at the upper end of the ulna. It acts to prevent elbow overextension.

Humerus

Olecranon

Ulna

Radius

Side view

Olfactory nerve
The first *cranial nerve*, which conveys *smell* sensations (as nerve impulses)

from the *nose* to the brain. Each of the two olfactory nerves detects smells with hairlike receptors (nerve endings specialized in detecting stimuli) in the mucous membrane lining the roof of the nasal cavity. Nerve fibers pass from the receptors through tiny holes in the roof of the nasal cavity and come together to form two structures called the olfactory bulbs. From the bulbs, nerve fibers travel to the olfactory center in the brain.

LOCATION OF OLFACTORY NERVE

Each olfactory bulb lies on top of a thin bony plate in the roof of the nose and connects to the brain via an olfactory nerve. Nerve twigs pass through the bony plate to enter the nasal lining.

Olfactory nerve

Olfactory bulb

Twigs

Damage to the olfactory nerves, which is usually caused by head injury, may result in loss or impairment of the sense of smell.

Oligo-

A prefix meaning few, little, or scanty, as in oligospermia (too few sperm in the semen). The prefix olig- is synonymous with oligo-.

Oligodendroglioma

A rare, slow-growing type of primary *brain tumor* that mainly affects young or middle-aged adults. Several hundred cases of oligodendroglioma occur in the US each year. Symptoms, diagnosis, and treatment are as for other types of brain tumor. Surgical removal of the tumor can, in some cases, lead to a complete cure. About one third of patients survive for five years or more.

Oligohydramnios

A rare condition in which there is an abnormally small amount of *amniotic fluid* surrounding the fetus in the uterus during pregnancy.

CAUSES

Amniotic fluid is normally produced by the placenta, swallowed by the fetus, and excreted as fetal urine. Oligohydramnios may occur if the placenta is not functioning properly, as in severe *preeclampsia* or *eclampsia*. Oligohydramnios may also occur if there is an abnormality of the fetal urinary tract or if a pregnancy continues beyond 41 weeks' gestation.

TREATMENT AND OUTLOOK

In some cases, the underlying disorder can be treated, but sometimes it cannot (particularly if the fetus is abnormal). If oligohydramnios occurs early in pregnancy, it usually results in *miscarriage*. If it occurs later in pregnancy, the pressure of the uterus on the fetus may cause deformity, such as *clubfoot*. If it occurs in an overdue pregnancy, induction of labor or cesarean section may be beneficial.

Oligospermia

A deficiency in the number of sperm per unit volume of seminal fluid; there are normally more than 20 million sperm per milliliter of semen. Oligospermia may be temporary or permanent. It is a major cause of *infertility*, especially when present with certain other disorders of the sperm.

CAUSES

Oligospermia may be caused by a number of different disorders, including *orchitis* (inflammation of a testis), failure of a testis to descend into the scrotum (see *Testis, undescended*), and, infrequently, a *varicocele* (varicose vein of the testis). Stress, cigarette smoking, alcohol abuse, and some drugs may cause temporary oligospermia.

DIAGNOSIS AND TREATMENT

A sperm count is performed as part of *semen analysis*. Treatment is of the underlying cause. *Gonadotropin hormones* may be prescribed for a short period when the cause is unknown. (See also *Azoospermia*.)

Oliguria

The production of a smaller-than-normal quantity of urine in relation to the volume of fluid taken in. Oliguria may be due simply to excessive sweating (without adequate fluid replacement) in a hot climate. In other cases oliguria may be a sign of failure of normal kidney function (see *Renal failure*).

Olive oil

An oil obtained from the fruit of the olive tree OLEA EUROPAEA. Warm olive oil is sometimes used to soften *earwax* before the ears are syringed. Olive oil is also used for its *emollient* (soothing, moisturizing) effect in the treatment of *cradle cap*.

-oma

A suffix that denotes a tumor, as in lipoma, a benign tumor of fatty tissue.

Omentum

An apronlike double fold of fatty membrane that hangs down in front of the intestines. The omentum contains blood vessels, nerves, lymph vessels, and lymph nodes. In addition to acting as a fat store, the omentum may limit the spread of infection within the abdominal cavity by adhering to the affected area.

Omphalocele

An alternative name for *exomphalos*.

Onchocerciasis

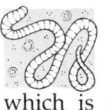

A tropical disease that is caused by infestation with the worm ONCHOCERCA VOLVULUS. The disease, which is a type of *filariasis*, affects more than 20 million people in portions of Central and South America and Africa. Many sufferers are blinded by the condition.

CAUSES AND SYMPTOMS

The disease is transmitted from person to person by small, fiercely biting, black SIMULIUM flies. These flies breed in, and always remain near, fast-running turbulent streams (hence the disease's alternative name, "river blindness").

The transmission of the disease and life cycle of the worm are shown opposite. Blindness may result as an allergic reaction to dead microfilariae (tiny worms) near the eyes.

TREATMENT AND PREVENTION

The microfilariae are quickly killed by the drug diethylcarbamazine. This drug must be used with great care, however, because of the severe reactions caused by the dead worms.

Travelers to areas where the disease is prevalent should take measures to discourage the insects from biting (see *Insect bites*).

Oncogenes

Genes, found in all cells, that are responsible for cells becoming malignant (cancerous). Out of the complete human gene complement of 50,000 genes, fewer than 100 are probably oncogenes; about half of them have been identified.

Cancer cells differ from healthy ones in various ways. Their growth is unrestrained, and they infiltrate and destroy normal tissues (see *Cancer*). These differences are induced by mutations (alterations) in certain key genes—the oncogenes—that cause them to be "switched on." Switching on of a cell's oncogenes may increase its rate of multiplication, alter its responsiveness to hormonal growth factors, or increase its invasiveness.

Oncogenes may be switched on by the various environmental factors that are known to cause cancer, such as ultraviolet light, radioactivity, tobacco smoke, alcohol, asbestos particles, carcinogenic chemicals, and certain viruses. To transform a cell from normal to malignant seems to require the switching on of between two and four oncogenes. Thus, cancer of the cervix may develop in a woman who smokes and whose cervix has been infected with papillomavirus (a potentially cancer-causing virus), whereas either of these factors by itself might not be sufficient to cause cancer.

Oncologist

A specialist in the diagnosis and treatment of *cancer*. Many oncologists specialize in a particular type of cancer, such as leukemia. The oncologist conducts tests to determine the location, type, and extent of the cancer. He or she administers or supervises treatment, which may involve several other specialists and take a number of forms, such as *radiation therapy*, *anticancer drugs*, surgery, or a combination of these.

Oncology

The study of the causes, development, characteristics, and treatment of *tumors*, particularly malignant (cancerous) ones. Because there are many different types of tumors, which can derive from virtually any tissue in the body, oncology encompasses a wide range of experimental techniques and investigative approaches. These include surveying the frequency and distribution of tumors, testing new treatments, investigating the biochemical processes involved in tumor formation, and studying abnormal genes associated with tumors.

Onlay, dental

A tooth restoration of gold made outside the mouth and fixed onto the biting surface and over one or more cusps of a tooth. An onlay may be used to strengthen an extensively restored tooth. It is also sometimes needed to build up teeth in cases of *malocclusion* in which the biting surfaces of certain upper and lower teeth fail to meet when the jaw is closed.

Onychogryphosis

Abnormal thickening, hardening, and curving of the nails, which occurs

Onychogryphosis
This extraordinary thickening and overgrowth, resembling the claws of the mythological griffin, may affect toenails or fingernails.

mainly in elderly people. Its cause is unknown, but onychogryphosis is associated with fungal infection or poor circulation.

Onycholysis

Separation of the nail from its bed, beginning at the tip. It occurs in many skin conditions, including *psoriasis* and fungal infections.

Onychosis

A general term for disease, deformity, or wasting of the *nails*. Onychosis caused by fungal infection is called onychomycosis.

Oophorectomy

Removal of one or both ovaries.

WHY IT IS DONE
Oophorectomy is performed to treat *ovarian cysts* or ovarian cancer (see *Ovary, cancer of*). In women under 40, the surgeon attempts to preserve ovarian function by performing only a partial oophorectomy.

Both ovaries may be removed during a *hysterectomy* if disease has spread from the uterus to the ovaries. Removing both ovaries can also reduce the risk of ovarian cancer in women past the menopause.

HOW IT IS DONE
Oophorectomy is performed using general anesthesia and usually takes less than one hour. The ovaries are removed through an incision in the lower abdominal wall.

RECOVERY PERIOD
There is some pain and tenderness around the operation site. Most activities can be resumed within about a month of surgery, and sexual intercourse after about six weeks.

OUTLOOK
There are usually no adverse effects when one ovary or part of an ovary is

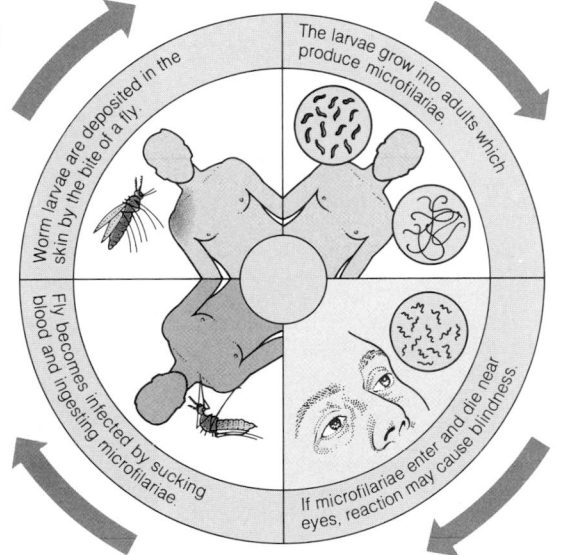

THE CYCLE OF ONCHOCERCIASIS
The infestation is spread by a fly that ingests microfilariae (tiny worms) from an infested person; the worms grow into larvae and are deposited in the skin of a new host when the fly bites.

Worm larvae are deposited in the skin by the bite of a fly.

The larvae grow into adults which produce microfilariae.

Fly becomes infected by sucking blood and ingesting microfilariae.

If microfilariae enter and die near eyes, reaction may cause blindness.

OPERATING ROOM

The operating table can be raised, lowered, and tilted in any direction to allow optimum access to the patient. For some operations it is best for the surgeon to stand but, during delicate procedures, such as microsurgery, the surgeon usually sits. The operating lamp is designed to give brilliant focal illumination but to cast no shadows. The anesthesia machine can maintain breathing in patients who have been given a muscle-relaxant drug.

Operating room technician
Anesthesiologist
Shadowless operating lamp
Intravenous fluid for transfusion
Clocks
X-ray screen
Surgeon
Assistant
Tray of instruments
Antistatic table cushion
Operating table
Padded patient support
Pedal for raising table
Spare gas cylinder
Movable anesthetic apparatus
Anesthetic gas flow rate monitor
Patient pulse and cardiograph monitor
Piped anesthetic gases

O

removed because ovulation and hormone production continue. If both ovaries are removed, *hormone replacement therapy* may be necessary.

-opathy
A suffix that denotes a disease or disorder (often a noninflammatory one), as in neuropathy, any disorder of the peripheral nerves. The suffix -pathy is synonymous with -opathy.

Open heart surgery
Any operation on the heart in which the heart beat is temporarily stopped and its function taken over by a mechanical pump. The early heart surgeons carried out closed operations, inserting their fingers and specially designed knives into the heart (to open the channel of a narrowed valve) while the organ continued to beat. Such operations had only limited scope.

With the development of reliable *heart-lung machines* in the 1950s, the picture changed. Once the pump was connected, the surgeon could open the heart, repair defects, and even reconstruct the main chambers. During the operation, the heart is kept cool through techniques of surgical *hypothermia*, which help prevent damage to the heart muscle from lack of oxygen.

The main applications of open heart surgery have been the correction of congenital heart defects (see *Heart*

disease, congenital), surgery for heart valve insufficiency or narrowed heart valves (see *Heart valve surgery*), and *coronary artery bypass* surgery.

Operable
A term applied to any condition that is suitable for surgical treatment, such as an accessible benign tumor that requires removal because it is causing symptoms. (See also *Inoperable*.)

Operating room
A hospital room in which surgical procedures are performed. The room is designed to reduce the risk of bacteria infecting open surgical wounds. A ventilation system provides a constant supply of clean, filtered air, the walls

and floors are easily washable and are cleaned at least once daily, and there are annexes with foot- or elbow-operated faucets where surgeons, assistants, and nurses use sterile brushes and bactericidal soaps to scrub their hands and forearms before putting on sterile gowns, masks, and gloves. Often built into the walls are light boxes for viewing images obtained by *X ray*, *CT scanning*, or *MRI*.

EQUIPMENT

During an operation using general anesthesia, the anesthesia machine stands at the head of the operating table (see *Anesthesia, general*) connected by tubes to oxygen and various anesthetic gases.

The surgeon's sterile instruments, covered with sterile towels before use, are arranged on stainless steel wheeled tables. There is also a *diathermy* machine, which controls bleeding. If required, other equipment, such as a *heart-lung machine* (which can take over the function of the patient's heart and lungs), is brought into the operating room.

Operation

Any surgical procedure, usually carried out with instruments but sometimes using only the hands (as in the

COMMON SURGICAL OPERATIONS

Operation	No. performed in US per year
Inguinal hernia repair	585,000
Cholecystectomy (gallbladder removal)	490,000
Releasing of peritoneal adhesions	300,000
Appendectomy (removal of appendix)	285,000
Biopsy or local removal of breast abnormality	235,000
Debridement of wound, burn, or infection	220,000
Partial colectomy (excision of large intestine)	170,000
Hemorrhoidectomy	130,000
Free skin graft	120,000
Mastectomy (breast removal)	115,000

manipulation of a simple fracture). Operations range from procedures performed quickly using a local anesthetic (such as draining a skin abscess) to surgery using general anesthesia lasting several hours (such as a heart or liver transplant).

Ophthalmia

A word once used to describe any inflammatory eye disorder; its use is now restricted to the following two specific disorders.

Ophthalmia neonatorum (literally "eye inflammation of the newborn") is a discharge of pus from the eyes of an infant that starts within 21 days of birth. In many cases the cause is an infection (such as *gonorrhea* or a *chlamydial infection*) acquired during birth. It is treated with antibiotics.

Sympathetic ophthalmia is a rare condition that occurs at least 10 days after a penetrating eye injury. If the injured eye is not removed within this time, severe *uveitis* (inflammation of the iris and choroid) that threatens blindness in the uninjured eye may develop. *Corticosteroid drugs* are used to treat the inflammation.

Ophthalmologist

A physician who specializes in care of the *eyes*. Ophthalmologists conduct examinations to determine the quality of *vision* and the need for corrective *glasses* or *contact lenses*. Ophthalmologists also check for the presence of any disorders, such as *glaucoma* or *cataracts*. Ophthalmologists may prescribe glasses and contact lenses, medication, or surgery, as necessary.

Ophthalmology

The study of the *eye*, and the diagnosis and treatment of disorders that affect it. Ophthalmology includes not only the assessment of *vision* and the prescription of *glasses* or *contact lenses* to correct defects, but also the surgery required to treat eye disorders such as *cataracts*, *glaucoma*, *retinal detachment*, and obstruction of tear ducts.

Ophthalmologists frequently work closely with other physicians because many disorders of the retina at the back of the eye are signs of nonoptical disorders, such as *hypertension* (high blood pressure), *atherosclerosis* (narrowing of arteries due to the deposition of fatty material inside them), or *diabetes mellitus*. Careful analysis of a person's field of vision (see *Eye, examination of*) can reveal defects that indicate neurological damage, such as that caused by a brain tumor.

Ophthalmoplegia

Partial or total paralysis of the muscles that move the eyes. Ophthalmoplegia may be caused by disease of the muscles themselves (as in *Graves' disease*) or by one of the conditions affecting the brain or the nerves supplying the eye muscles (including *stroke*, *encephalitis*, *brain tumor*, and *multiple sclerosis*).

Ophthalmoscope

An instrument used to examine the inside of the eye. The ophthalmoscope, by means of a deflecting prism or a perforated angled mirror, allows illumination and viewing of the entire area of the retina, the head of the optic nerve, the retinal arteries and veins, and the vitreous humor.

OPHTHALMOSCOPE

Observer's eyehole

Lens selection ring

Handle containing battery

Opiate

Any drug derived from, or chemically similar to, *opium*. The term opiate is also used to refer to certain *receptors* (specific sites on the surface of cells) with which opiate drugs combine to initiate their effects.

Opium

A milky substance obtained from the unripe seed pods of the poppy *PAPAVER SOMNIFERUM*. Used as a drug for thousands of years, opium has an analgesic (painkilling) effect and may also cause sleepiness and euphoria. Opium and its derivatives, which include *codeine* and *morphine*, are among the drugs collectively known as *narcotic drugs*.

Opportunistic infection

Infection caused by organisms that do not usually produce disease in healthy

O

people; or widespread infection by organisms that normally produce only mild, local, infection.

Many of the causative organisms are normally present on or in the human body and cause disease only when the host's *immune system* is impaired. Impairment of natural defenses may be due to treatment with anticancer and immunosuppressant drugs, to radiation therapy, or to diseases such as leukemia. Opportunistic infections also affect premature or malnourished infants and people with *immunodeficiency disorders*.

Opportunistic infections, especially *pneumocystis pneumonia*, are the cause of death in most *AIDS* patients. Many fungal infections (such as *cryptococcosis* and *candidiasis*) and some viral infections (such as *cytomegalovirus* and the virus that causes *herpes simplex*) are opportunistic infections.

Opportunistic infections are often unavoidable because the underlying defects in the host's defenses cannot easily be rectified. However, treatment with appropriate antimicrobial drugs may be lifesaving.

Optic atrophy

A shrinkage or wasting of the *optic nerve* fibers, which results in some or near total loss of vision. Optic atrophy is caused by disease or injury to the optic nerve and may occur without prior signs of nerve disease, such as inflammation or swelling.

Optic disk edema

Swelling of the head of the *optic nerve*, visible when the eye is examined with an ophthalmoscope. Optic disk edema usually indicates a dangerous rise in the pressure of *cerebrospinal fluid* within the skull, but may also arise from conditions affecting the nerve itself, including damage from restriction of blood supply. Optic disk edema may be followed by *optic atrophy*. (See also *Papilledema*.)

Optician

A person who fits, supplies, and adjusts *glasses* or *contact lenses*. Because their training is limited, opticians may not examine or test eyes or prescribe glasses or drugs.

Optic nerve

The second *cranial nerve*. The nerve of *vision*, the optic nerve consists of a collection of about 1 million nerve fibers that transmit impulses from the *retina* (the layer of light receptors at the back of the eye) to the brain.

THE FUNCTION OF THE OPTIC NERVE

Each optic nerve is a bundle of long fibers originating from nerve cells in the retina and passing to the back of the brain. Because of the arrangement of the nerve fibers, disease or injury at any point causes a unique pattern of visual loss. Charting the pattern of visual loss allows accurate location of damage to the nerve.

Image received by left eye

Image received by right eye

Optic chiasm

Coordinated image

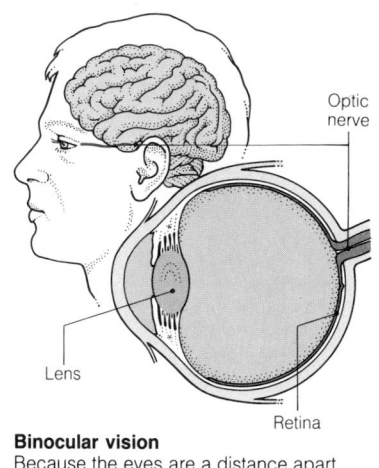

Optic nerve

Lens

Retina

Binocular vision
Because the eyes are a distance apart, they form slightly different images of a nearby object. The fusion of these two images into one provides the illusion of solidity. This is called stereopsis.

The two optic nerves converge at the optic junction behind the eyes, where fibers from the inner halves of the retinas cross over. As a result of this crossing over, nerve fibers from the right halves of both retinas pass to the right side of the occipital lobes at the back of the brain. The nerve fibers from the left halves of the retinas go to the left side of the brain.

Disorders of the optic nerve include *optic neuritis* (inflammation of the optic nerve) and *optic disk edema*, caused by external pressure from disease within the orbit or a brain tumor.

Optic neuritis

Inflammation of the optic nerve that often causes sudden loss of part of the field of vision. Optic neuritis is usually accompanied by pain on moving the eyes and tenderness when the eyes are touched. In some cases, however, there may be little or no pain.

The cause of optic neuritis often remains uncertain, but most cases are thought to be due to *demyelination* (destruction of the myelin sheaths) of the optic nerve fibers, which occurs in *multiple sclerosis*. The condition may also result from inflammation or infection of tissues around the optic nerve.

Optic neuritis causes loss of vision, usually in the central part of the visual field. Vision usually improves substantially within six weeks, but each attack causes damage to a proportion of the optic nerve fibers; recurrent attacks usually lead to permanent loss of visual acuity.

Treatment with *corticosteroid drugs* may aid the return of vision but seems to have little effect on the long-term outcome of the inflammatory process. (See also *Optic atrophy*.)

Optometrist

A specialist trained to examine the *eyes* and to prescribe, supply, and adjust *glasses* or *contact lenses*. Because they are not physicians, optometrists may not prescribe drugs or perform surgery. An optometrist refers patients requiring these types of treatment to an *ophthalmologist*.

Optometry

The practice of assessing *vision* and establishing whether *glasses* or, for certain people, *contact lenses* are needed to correct any visual defect. (See also *Optometrist*.)

Oral

Concerning the mouth.

O

Oral contraceptives

COMMON DRUGS

Estrogens
*Conjugated estrogens Diethylstilbestrol
Ethinyl estradiol*

Progesterones
Norethindrone Norgestrel

> **WARNING**
> If you vomit or have diarrhea while taking an oral contraceptive, follow the advice for missing a pill. If you have missed two consecutive periods, you should have a pregnancy test.

A group of oral drug preparations containing a *progesterone drug*, often combined with an *estrogen drug*, taken by women to prevent pregnancy. All types of oral contraceptives—combined pills, phased pills, and minipills—are commonly known as the pill.

HOW THEY ARE TAKEN

All types of oral contraceptives need to be taken on a monthly cycle for as long as a woman wishes to avoid pregnancy. The first course of pills is started on the first day of a period or on the fifth day after bleeding starts. Additional contraceptive precautions are usually needed for the duration of the first course of combined pills or phased pills or if the minipill is commenced on day 5.

Each course of pills is usually taken as described (right). Some brands of phased pills contain seven additional inactive pills, which may contain an iron supplement, so that the habit of taking a pill each day is not broken. It is possible to take a combined or phased pill continuously and thus avoid bleeding, but most physicians do not recommend this.

In some women, the use of oral contraceptives may cause menstruation to cease.

MISSING A PILL

For maximum contraceptive effect, each type of pill should be taken at approximately the same time each day. This is particularly important with the minipill, which should be taken within three hours of the chosen time each day.

A forgotten combined or phased pill should be taken as soon as remembered even if it means taking two pills the next day. Pills for the rest of the course should be taken at the correct time. A different form of contraception should be used for seven days after missing the pill.

If between three and 12 hours have elapsed from the time a minipill was due to be taken, the pill should be taken and additional contraceptive precautions used for 48 hours. If more than 12 hours have elapsed, the minipill should be taken and additional contraceptive precautions used for as long as your physician advises. (For more information, see the illustration below.)

EFFECTIVENESS

Used correctly, oral contraceptives have a failure rate of less than one

HOW ORAL CONTRACEPTIVES WORK

The combined and phased pills increase the levels of estrogen and progesterone in the body, which interferes with the production by the pituitary gland of two *gonadotropin hormones* called follicle-stimulating hormone (FSH) and luteinizing hormone (LH). This action in turn prevents ovulation.

The minipill works mainly by making the mucus that lines the inside of the cervix (neck of the uterus) so thick that it is impenetrable to sperm.

Pituitary gland

Gonadotropin hormones inhibited

LH

FSH

Hormonal effects
Each month the pituitary produces spurts of FSH and LH, which act on the ovary to cause egg ripening and release. Combined and phased pills interfere with natural hormone production and thus prevent ovulation.

Ripening and release of egg prevented

Ovary

Pill packaging
Most oral contraceptives come in packs that clearly indicate the day on which each pill should be taken.

Effects on eggs
FSH normally brings about egg ripening and LH the egg's release from the ovary; combined and phased pills prevent this.

Combined pill
This pill contains an estrogen and a progesterone drug in fixed doses. A course usually consists of one pill per day

Menstruation

for 21 days, followed by seven tablet-free days, during which bleeding may occur. A new course is then started, whether or not bleeding has occurred.

Change   Change   Menstruation

Phased pill—a typical program
These pills contain both an estrogen and a progesterone drug, but are divided into two or three groups or phases. The dose

of the progesterone drug, and sometimes of estrogen as well, changes from phase to phase. A course lasts for 21 days followed by seven tablet-free days.

Menstruation

Minipill—progesterone only
These pills contain a progesterone drug only in a fixed dose. The pills are taken continuously, one every day with no

tablet-free days. Bleeding usually occurs during the last few days of each cycle. The minipill has a slightly higher failure rate than the combined and phased pills.

O

pregnancy per 100 woman-years (i.e., the number of pregnancies among 100 women using the method for one year). Allowing for incorrect use or other factors, the actual failure rates may be as high as between two and three pregnancies per 100 woman-years for the combined or phased pill, and between two and a half to four pregnancies for the minipill.

Certain other drugs (such as *barbiturate drugs*, *anticonvulsant drugs*, *griseofulvin*, and some *antibiotic drugs*) may impair the effectiveness of oral contraceptives. A woman should always inform her gynecologist if she is taking other medication.

ADVANTAGES AND DISADVANTAGES

In addition to providing excellent protection against pregnancy, the main advantage of oral contraceptives is that they do not interfere with the spontaneity of sex.

Estrogen-containing pills seem to protect against cancer of the uterus and ovaries, *ovarian cysts*, *endometriosis*, and iron-deficiency *anemia*. They also tend to make periods regular, lighter, and relatively free of menstrual pain.

The main disadvantages of oral contraceptives are that they are medically unsuitable for some women and that they may produce adverse effects.

CONTRAINDICATIONS

Estrogen-containing pills increase the risk of certain disorders and are therefore not usually prescribed if a woman suffers from *hypertension* (high blood pressure), *hyperlipidemia* (high levels of fat in the blood), *liver* disease, *migraine*, *otosclerosis* (an ear disorder), or if she has previously had a *thrombosis* (abnormal blood clot).

The chances of a thrombosis occurring are increased in women who smoke or who are over the age of 35. An estrogen-containing pill is usually not given during the first few months after childbirth or in the four weeks before a major operation because of the increased risk of thrombosis. *Obesity* and *diabetes mellitus* also make a woman more susceptible to thrombosis.

Oral contraceptives are not usually prescribed to women with heart or circulatory disorders, a family history of certain disorders, or unexplained vaginal bleeding.

Combined or phased pills interfere with milk production and should not be taken during breast-feeding. The minipill is usually considered unsuitable for a woman who has had an ectopic pregnancy.

POSSIBLE ADVERSE EFFECTS

Estrogen-containing pills may cause nausea and vomiting, weight gain, depression, breast swelling, reduced sex drive, increased appetite, cramps in the legs and abdomen, headaches, and dizziness. A more serious adverse effect of these pills is the risk of a thrombosis causing a *stroke*, *embolism*, or *myocardial infarction* (heart attack). Estrogen-containing pills may also aggravate heart disease or cause hypertension, *gallstones*, *jaundice*, and, very rarely, *liver cancer*.

Medical evidence suggests that cancer of the cervix is more common in women taking estrogen-containing pills. This risk may be outweighed by the reduced risk of other cancers of the reproductive system.

All forms of oral contraception can cause bleeding between periods, but this is especially true of the minipill. Other possible adverse effects of the minipill are irregular periods, ectopic pregnancy, and ovarian cysts.

There is no evidence that use of an oral contraceptive reduces a woman's fertility permanently (although menstruation may be irregular or absent for some months after stopping the pill). Likewise, there is no evidence that a fetus can be harmed if conceived while the woman is taking the pill or has recently stopped doing so.

Adverse effects usually disappear within a few months. If they persist, it may be necessary to change to a different type of pill or to an alternative method of contraception. Because adverse effects are more likely to occur with high doses of estrogen, low-estrogen preparations are prescribed whenever possible. The minipill may be used by women who suffer adverse effects even with low estrogen doses or who should not take estrogen drugs for other medical reasons.

Women taking oral contraceptives should receive checkups, including blood pressure and weight checks and *cervical smear tests*. (See also *Contraception*; *Contraception, hormonal methods*.)

Oral hygiene

Measures that keep the mouth and teeth clean and healthy. Good oral hygiene reduces the incidence of tooth decay (see *Caries, dental*), prevents *gingivitis* and other *gum* disorders, and helps prevent *halitosis* (bad breath). Oral hygiene is broadly divided into personal and professional care.

PERSONAL CARE

The most important aspect of personal oral hygiene is daily removal of dental *plaque* (a sticky, bacteria-containing substance) by thorough *toothbrushing* and use of dental floss (see *Floss, dental*). Use of a fluoride mouth rinse or an oral irrigator (a device that produces a forceful water stream) may also be helpful, but these are aids that cannot remove plaque or replace brushing and flossing. *Disclosing agents* can help make tooth cleaning more efficient by showing the location of plaque. Dentures must always be kept scrupulously clean by brushing every surface and soaking them in a cleansing solution.

PROFESSIONAL CARE

A *dentist* or hygienist (see *Hygienist, dental*) removes stubborn plaque and *calculus* (a hard mineral deposit that forms on the teeth above and below the gums) by *scaling* and polishing. These procedures are usually carried out during a routine checkup; in cases of *periodontal disease*, they may need to be performed more often.

Oral surgeon

A surgeon who specializes in operations on the teeth, jaws, and other parts of the mouth and face (see *Oral surgery*). The qualifications required include a degree in general dentistry and specialization through a four-year training program in oral and maxillofacial (pertaining to the upper jaw and face) surgery. Many oral surgeons also have medical degrees, although it is not required.

Oral surgery

Surgery to treat disease, deformity, or injury of the mouth, face, and jaws.

Among the dental procedures carried out by oral surgeons are the extraction of severely impacted wisdom teeth (see *Impaction, dental*) and *alveolectomy* (removal of part of the jaw that holds the teeth) to improve the fitting of dentures.

More complicated oral surgery includes *orthognathic surgery* to correct deformities of the jaw that result in an abnormal relationship between the upper and lower teeth; repairing a broken jaw; plastic surgery to correct *cleft lip and palate*; and the removal of certain types of benign tumors from tissues within the mouth.

Orbit

The socket in the skull that contains the eyeball, protective pads of fat, and various blood vessels, muscles, and nerves. An opening in the back of the orbit allows the *optic nerve* to pass from the eyeball into the brain.

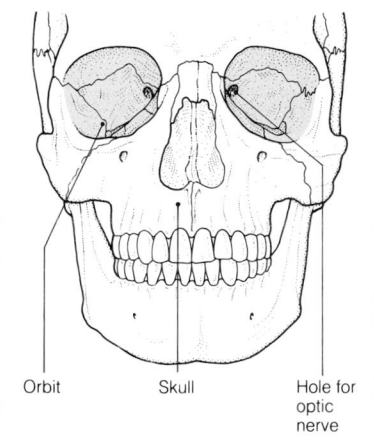

LOCATION OF ORBIT
The orbits are the deep cavities in the skull in which the eyeballs and muscles that move the eyes are protectively enclosed.

Orbit   Skull   Hole for optic nerve

DISORDERS

INJURY A blow of great force, as in a car crash or a sports injury, may fracture the orbit; the eyeball itself often escapes damage because it is squeezed backward by protective muscles during reflex blinking. Many such fractures heal without treatment, but some result in facial deformity that requires corrective surgery. An operation also may be needed to reinforce the floor of the orbit if a fracture causes downward displacement of the eye.

INFECTION Rarely, bacteria infect the fatty tissue lining the orbit, causing orbital *cellulitis*. Usually the infection originates in a nearby sinus, but sometimes it spreads in the blood from a facial infection. The affected eye protrudes, is extremely painful and red, and there is severe swelling of the lids and conjunctiva (the membrane lining the inside of the lids and front of the eye).

Orbital cellulitis is a serious disorder. The pressure on the eye may damage it and there is a slight risk that the infection may spread inward to the meninges (the membranes covering the brain) and the brain itself, causing *meningitis*. Prompt treatment with high doses of antibiotics usually clears up the condition.

Orchiectomy

The surgical removal of a single testis or of both the testes.

WHY IT IS DONE
Orchiectomy may be performed to deal with a testicular cancer (see *Testis,*

cancer of) or *gangrene*, or to reduce production of the hormone testosterone as part of the treatment of cancer of the prostate gland (see *Prostate, cancer of*). Because the prostate gland depends on male sex hormones for its normal growth, orchiectomy is often effective in reducing the growth of a prostatic cancer. It is especially effective in controlling the symptoms of secondary tumors in the bones.

HOW IT IS DONE
The scrotum is cut open (using spinal and local anesthesia), the blood vessels and nerves leading to the scrotum are cut free, the testis is cut away from surrounding tissue and removed, and the skin is stitched.

After the operation, *analgesics* (painkillers) may be needed and an *ice pack* may be applied to the surgical area for the first 24 hours to prevent excessive swelling.

OUTLOOK
Complete healing can be expected without complications. Removal of one testis does not affect sex drive, potency, or the ability to have children. The patient is advised to wear an athletic supporter and to avoid vigorous exercise for a month or so after the operation.

Orchiopexy

An operation in which an undescended testis (see *Testis, undescended*) is brought down into the scrotum. It is usually performed before a boy is 5 to avoid the risk of the condition causing infertility or even cancer of the testis (see *Testis, cancer of*).

An incision is made in the groin (using a general anesthetic) and the testis is gently maneuvered down the inguinal canal leading from the abdomen to the scrotum. The base of the testis is then usually attached to the scrotum with a few stitches to prevent it from retracting.

Pain and swelling are relieved with *analgesics* (painkillers) and an *ice pack*. Healing usually takes place without any complications.

Orchitis

Inflammation of a testis. Orchitis may be caused by infection with the virus that causes *mumps*.

Orchitis develops in about one quarter of males who contract mumps after puberty. It is characterized by swelling and severe pain in the affected testis and a high fever. In *epididymo-orchitis* (which has different causes), the tube that carries sperm from the testis is also inflamed.

Treatment is with *analgesics* (painkillers) and *ice packs* to reduce swelling and pain; antibiotics are usually given. The condition usually begins to subside after three to seven days. Occasionally, orchitis is followed by shrinking of the testis.

Organ

A collection of various *tissues* integrated into a distinct structural unit that performs specific functions. For example, the brain consists of nerve tissue and supporting tissue (called neuroglia) organized to receive, process, and send out information.

Organ donation

The agreement of a person (or his or her relatives) to the surgical removal of one or more organs for use in *transplant surgery*. Most organs used as transplants are removed immediately after death, but a kidney is also commonly taken from living *donors*.

The donation of kidneys by living donors is usually confined to relatives of the transplant patient. This occurs for medical reasons (because a relative is more likely to have the same or a similar tissue type as the patient) and for ethical reasons (because physicians discourage the sale of living organs). The risks of donation are carefully explained and the kidney is removed only after the donor gives clear voluntary consent.

The range of organs removed after death is much greater, including the heart, lungs, liver, pancreas, and kidneys. Most organs can be transplanted successfully only if removed immediately after death; the best results often require surgical removal of organs before the donor's heart has stopped beating. In practice this means that most donations of major organs are made from patients who die in an intensive-care unit and are certified as "brain dead" while still having the heart and lung function maintained by a machine (see *Death*).

People who want to donate some or all of their organs after death should make their intentions clear to their relatives and sign a donor card. In most Western countries the demand for donated organs is far greater than the supply. Some countries have introduced laws that allow physicians to remove organs after death unless the patient has specifically forbidden it. In practice, physicians are reluctant to carry out such legislation and the supply of donor organs continues to depend on voluntary donations. (See

O

also *Corneal graft*; *Heart valve surgery*; *Heart transplant*; *Heart-lung transplant*; *Kidney transplant*; *Liver transplant*.)

Organic

Related to a body organ; having organs or an organized structure; or related to organisms or to substances from them. In chemistry, the term refers to any of the group of compounds that contain carbon, with the exception of carbon oxides (such as carbon dioxide) and sulfides and metal carbonates (such as calcium carbonate). The term also signifies the presence of disease, in contrast to a *functional disorder* or psychosomatic complaint. (See also *Inorganic*.)

Organic brain syndrome

See *Brain syndrome, organic*.

Organism

A general term for any individual animal or plant. Medically, the most important are humans and disease-causing *microorganisms*, such as *bacteria*, *fungi*, *protozoa*, and *viruses*.

Orgasm

Intense sensations resulting from the series of muscular contractions that occur at the peak of sexual excitement. Orgasm is usually followed by physical relaxation and often drowsiness.

In men, contractions of the muscles of the inner pelvis massage seminal fluid from the prostatic area into the urethra, from which it is forcefully propelled from the urethral orifice (see *Ejaculation*). Following orgasm, the penis becomes soft again and there is a refractory period during which there is no physical response to further sexual stimulation.

Orgasm in women is associated with irregular contractions of the voluntary muscles of the walls of the vagina and, in some women, of the uterus, followed by relief of congestion in the pelvic area. Orgasm usually lasts about three to 10 seconds, but can last up to a minute in some women. There is no refractory phase; some women experience multiple orgasms if stimulation is continued.

Both men and women may have problems with orgasm (see *Ejaculation, disorders of*; *Orgasm, lack of*).

Orgasm, lack of

The inability to achieve orgasm. Lack of orgasm is the most common sexual problem in women. Between 30 and 50 percent experience difficulties at some time in their lives. The once-

used term "frigidity" to describe lack of orgasm is outmoded and considered perjorative by many women. Lack of orgasm is rarer in men (see *Ejaculation, disorders of*).

Some women (10 to 15 percent) are not able to achieve orgasm under any circumstances. Others experience orgasm only occasionally or under special circumstances.

CAUSES
Lack of orgasm is usually caused by sexual inhibition, inexperience, lack of knowledge, or psychological factors (such as anxiety or early sexual trauma). In some cases it may be due to alcohol dependence, certain drugs, or pain during intercourse (see *Intercourse, painful*).

Inability to achieve orgasm under any circumstances may stem from poor sex education or lack of familiarity with the body's sexual responses. Psychological attitudes also contribute. Some women are ashamed of their bodies, are inhibited about the sex act, have deep-seated guilt feelings about sexual pleasure, fear pregnancy, feel uncertain about intimacy, or fear "letting go" or losing momentary control during an orgasm. They therefore cannot relax during sex. Additionally, some women have difficulties with physical arousal and never reach or get past the excitement stage (see *Sexual desire, inhibited*) due to not receiving or not allowing sufficient foreplay.

A woman may be able to achieve orgasm through masturbation but fail to achieve orgasm with her partner. This may occur with a new partner who is unfamiliar with the woman's sexual responses. In other cases, a woman may be able to achieve orgasm through stimulation by a partner, but not through intercourse. This is sometimes attributable to the longer time a woman needs to attain coital climax (about 13 minutes for a woman compared to less than three minutes for the average man). Lack of experience or knowledge, impatience, or premature ejaculation of the partner are factors. Problems in a long-term relationship may be due to underlying feelings of hostility, boredom, or distrust. Performance anxiety caused by the pressure to have an orgasm may also be an inhibiting factor, which in time sets up a cycle of failure.

TREATMENT
Any physical problems should be treated. Otherwise, women may be helped to achieve orgasm or to increase the frequency of orgasms

through *sex therapy* or *marital counseling*. *Psychotherapy* may be helpful for women in whom the problem is related to deep-seated feelings of guilt or insecurity.

Ornithosis

A disease of birds that is caused by the microorganism CHLAMYDIA PSITTACI. It can be transmitted to humans, causing *psittacosis*, a feverish illness accompanied by pneumonia.

Orphan drugs

Drugs that have been developed to treat rare conditions but are not manufactured because the potential sales are small while the cost of carrying out the necessary safety tests is high. Reluctance to market an orphan drug may increase if the drug is out of patent (i.e., available for other companies to market) or cannot be patented because it is a known substance. However, changes in the law have made it profitable to provide certain orphan drugs.

An example of an orphan drug is tetrahydroaminoacridine (THA). Although clinical trials suggest THA may improve orientation and memory in people who have *Alzheimer's disease*, it has not been manufactured because the patent has expired.

Orphenadrine

A *muscle-relaxant drug* used to relieve painful muscle spasm caused by injury to soft tissues (such as muscles and ligaments). Orphenadrine is also given to reduce muscle rigidity in *Parkinson's disease*.

Possible adverse effects include dryness of the mouth and blurred vision.

Ortho-

A prefix meaning normal, correct, or straight, as in orthopedics (from the Greek for "straight child"), which originally concerned the correction of skeletal deformities in children. Today it includes all bone or joint problems in any age group.

Orthodontic appliances

Devices, commonly known as braces, worn to correct *malocclusion* (poorly positioned teeth). Braces are most commonly fitted during childhood and adolescence when the teeth and jaws are still developing.

WHY THEY ARE USED
Braces are usually worn to correct overcrowded teeth that splay outward, tilt inward, or rotate (see *Overcrowding, dental*). Braces are fre-

quently used on *buck teeth* (projecting upper front teeth) and may also be used to reposition upper and lower premolars and molars (back teeth) when a faulty relationship between the upper and lower jaws prevents the teeth from meeting properly and interferes with chewing. Sometimes braces are required when permanent teeth fail to develop; in such cases, it may be necessary to move teeth to create room for artificial teeth.

TYPES

FIXED APPLIANCES These braces, which cannot be removed by the wearer, exert a continuous pressure and can move teeth in any direction. They are usually fitted to all the upper and/or lower teeth and are used when many teeth need repositioning.

The tooth-moving part of a fixed appliance is the arch wire, an adjustable, high-tensile steel wire, threaded through a bracket on each tooth.

To allow extra force to be applied to specific teeth, some brackets may be fitted with small hooks to which headgear (straps that fit around the back and over the top of the head) can be attached when the wearer is at rest.

Fixed appliances are kept in the mouth until the teeth have moved into the correct position, which may take a year or more. Thereafter, a fixed or removable retainer plate may need to be worn for anywhere from six months to five years to hold the teeth in their correct place until tooth and jaw growth stop in late adolescence.

Fixed appliances give more precise control over tooth movement than removable braces, but they are more expensive and take longer to fit and adjust. They also trap *plaque* (the sticky coating that forms on teeth and causes decay) and make cleaning of the teeth more difficult.

Lingual braces ("invisible" braces) also can be used by some people in the inner arch (the tongue side) of teeth. These braces pull rather than push teeth into place.

REMOVABLE APPLIANCES These braces are used when only one or several teeth need correcting. They consist of a plastic plate that covers the roof of the mouth (or, much less commonly, the floor of the mouth) with attachments that anchor over the back teeth. Force is applied by means of springs, wire bows, screws, or rubber bands fitted to the plate, sometimes combined with the use of headgear.

Occasionally, removable appliances are used in younger children before facial growth has stopped. They con-

sist of interconnected upper and lower plates that force the jaw into a position of slight tension against the pull of the surrounding muscles, translating this force to move the teeth.

Potential disadvantages of removable appliances are that their bulk may interfere with speech and that wearers may remove them so often that they become ineffective.

HOW ORTHODONTIC APPLIANCES WORK

The tooth sockets are remarkably responsive to sustained pressure against the teeth. Orthodontic appliances, which may be fixed or removable, provide such pressure. Even gentle pressure applied in a particular direction will move teeth. As they move, bone is remodeled so that the new position is stable.

FIXED APPLIANCES

Appearance of brackets and wires
Brackets are fixed appliances cemented to the outer surface of the teeth; they have slots into which arch wires can be fitted.

By careful design of the arrangement of wires and springs, force can be exerted in any direction to move a tooth into the desired position.

Arch wire

Extraction space

Bracket

1 Teeth are removed to create space and an appliance made to correct the alignment of the remaining teeth and to close gaps between them.

Spring for fine adjustment

2 Once the teeth in the upper and lower jaws are aligned, the appliance is adjusted to tip or rotate the teeth to give a good appearance and bite.

Overcrowding
This is frequently associated with malocclusion (poor alignment between upper and lower teeth). Teeth may have to be extracted to make room for those to be straightened.

REMOVABLE APPLIANCES

These are easier to keep clean than fixed appliances and are less obtrusive, but they may interfere with speech; their efficiency relies on patients using them as directed. This type exerts pressure to push the teeth at the sides outward.

Bow device
This simple wire spring acts by exerting force to straighten the tooth. Many bow devices are more complicated.

A removable bow
One of the many forms of orthodontic wire appliance, this bow device exerts pressure on the teeth at the sides, which straightens and moves them outward.

Orthodontics

A branch of dentistry concerned with the prevention and treatment of *malocclusion* (irregularities of the position of teeth or an abnormal relationship between the upper and lower teeth). In most cases, the orthodontist performs orthodontic procedures on children and adolescents while the teeth are still developing and are

O

relatively maneuverable. However, adults are also able to benefit from orthodontic treatment.

Diagnosis of the exact type of malocclusion involved may require making models of the teeth (see *Impression, dental*) to see clearly how they come together when clenched, taking X rays of the head to relate the position of the teeth to that of the facial bones, and taking X rays of the jaws to study their structure and relationship.

Orthodontic treatment consists of moving poorly positioned teeth by means of gentle pressure exerted by *orthodontic appliances* (braces). To achieve this, the orthodontist may first need to extract certain teeth, often the first molars, to provide growing room for the teeth being moved.

Orthodontist

A dentist who specializes in preventing or correcting crooked, crowded, or irregularly spaced teeth and abnormal relationships between the upper and lower teeth (see *Malocclusion*). To achieve this, the orthodontist makes use of various *orthodontic appliances*.

Orthognathic surgery

An operation to correct deformity of the jaw and the severe *malocclusion* (abnormal relationship between the upper and lower teeth) that is invariably associated with it.

HOW IT IS DONE

The operation, which usually requires a stay in the hospital, is carried out using a general anesthetic.

A jaw that projects too far can be shortened by removing a block of bone from each side and maneuvering the front of the jaw backward. A jaw that is too short can be remedied by dividing the bone on each side, sliding the front of the jaw forward, and inserting bone grafts (taken from elsewhere in the body) into the gaps.

After repositioning, the bones often require splinting (see *Splinting, dental*) until healing occurs.

Orthopedics

The branch of surgery concerned with disorders of bones and joints and the muscles, tendons, and ligaments associated with them. Orthopedists perform many tasks, including setting broken bones and putting on casts; treating joint conditions, such as dislocations, slipped disks, arthritis, and back problems; treating bone tumors and birth defects of the skeleton; and surgically repairing or replacing hip, knee, or finger joints.

Orthopedist

A physician who specializes in problems affecting bones, joints, and related structures (see *Orthopedics*).

Orthopnea

Breathing difficulty brought on by lying flat. Orthopnea is a symptom of *heart failure* (reduced pumping efficiency) and is caused by *edema* (fluid collection) in the lungs. It also occurs with *asthma* and chronic obstructive lung disease (chronic *bronchitis* with or without *emphysema*).

Orthoptics

A technique used to measure and evaluate *strabismus* (misalignment of the eyes). Orthoptics sometimes includes eye exercises, which may or may not help the strabismus.

Os

An anatomical term for a bone, as in os coxae, the hip bone. The plural of os is ossa, as in ossa cranii, the skull bones. The term os also refers to an opening in the body, usually the cervical os (entrance to the uterus).

Osgood-Schlatter disease

Painful enlargement of the tibial tuberosity, the bony prominence of the tibia (shin) just below the knee. Osgood-Schlatter disease occurs in children (usually boys) aged 10 to 14.

The condition is caused by excessive, repetitive pulling of the quadriceps muscle (at the front of the thigh) on the patellar tendon, which is attached to the tibial tuberosity. There is usually pain above and below the knee, which is worse during strenuous activity, and the tibial tuberosity is tender when touched.

Osgood-Schlatter disease usually clears up completely without treatment; if pain is severe, the knee may be immobilized in a plaster cast.

Osmosis

The passage of a solvent (such as water) through a semipermeable membrane (one that acts like a sieve) from a less concentrated (weaker) solution to a more concentrated (stronger) one. Osmosis occurs whenever solutions of different strengths are separated by a semipermeable membrane and continues until the two solutions are of equal strength unless the movement of solvent is opposed by applying pressure to the stronger solution. The pressure needed to stop the movement completely is called the osmotic pressure.

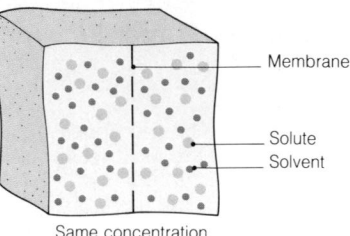

Osmosis

If two solutions, consisting of different concentrations of a solute (e.g., salt) in a solvent (e.g., water), are separated by a semipermeable membrane, solvent moves from the weaker to stronger solution until the two solutions attain equal concentration.

Semipermeable membranes are widespread in the body—they surround all cells. These membranes allow water, salts, simple sugars (such as glucose), and amino acids (but not proteins) to pass through. Consequently, osmosis plays an important part in regulating the distribution of water and other substances.

Ossicle

A small bone, particularly the malleus (hammer), incus (anvil), and stapes (stirrup)—the three tiny bones in the middle *ear* that conduct sound from the eardrum to the inner ear.

Ossification

The process by which *bone* is formed, renewed, and repaired. Ossification begins in the embryo and continues throughout life. There are three main types of ossification: bone growth, during which new bone is formed mainly from *cartilage* at the *epiphyses* (bone ends); bone renewal, which occurs as part of the normal regeneration process; and bone repair, which fuses broken bones after a fracture.

Osteitis

Inflammation of bone. The most common cause is infection (see *Osteomyelitis*). Other causes are *Paget's disease* and *hyperparathyroidism*.

Osteo-

A prefix that denotes a relationship to bone, as in *osteoporosis*, a condition in which the bones become thin and weak. The prefix oste- is synonymous with osteo-.

Osteoarthritis

A joint disease aggravated by mechanical stress. Osteoarthritis is characterized by degeneration of the cartilage that lines joints or by *osteophyte* (bony outgrowth) formation, which leads to pain, stiffness, and occasionally loss of function of the affected joint.

INCIDENCE

Osteoarthritis occurs in almost all people over age 60, although not all have symptoms. Various factors lead to the development of osteoarthritis earlier in life, including an injury to a joint or a congenital joint deformity. Osteoarthritis may occur with *rheumatoid arthritis*. Severe osteoarthritis affects three times as many women as men.

SYMPTOMS

Osteoarthritis causes pain, swelling, creaking, and stiffness of one or more joints. Pain and stiffness may interfere with activities (such as walking and dressing) and may disrupt sleep.

Weakness and shrinkage (*atrophy*) of surrounding muscles may occur if pain prevents the joint from being used regularly. The affected joints become enlarged and distorted by osteophytes, which account for the gnarled appearance of hands affected by osteoarthritis.

DIAGNOSIS AND TREATMENT

A diagnosis is generally made on the basis of a person having a history of joint pain with use and on physical findings of joint tenderness, swelling, and pain on motion. An X ray can confirm cartilage loss and osteophyte formation and assess the extent of the degenerative process. As yet there is no cure for osteoarthritis; symptoms may be relieved by *analgesics* (painkillers) and *nonsteroidal anti-inflammatory drugs*, which reduce joint inflammation. Sometimes a painful joint can be eased by injection of a *corticosteroid drug*.

Physical therapy, including exercises and heat treatment, can often relieve symptoms. If the condition is severe, various aids can make coping at home easier (see *Disability*).

Surgical treatment for severe osteoarthritis includes *arthroplasty* (joint replacement surgery) and *arthrodesis* (immobilization of a joint).

OSTEOARTHRITIS

This differs from rheumatoid arthritis and has a better outlook. It results from excessive wear on joints, sometimes due to obesity or to slight deformity or misalignment of bones in a joint. Inflammation from disease, such as gout, may also proceed to osteoarthritis. Weight-bearing joints, such as those in the neck, the lower back, and the knees and hips, are the most commonly affected by this type of arthritis.

Normal joint surface
The healthy joint is lined with smooth cartilage and lubricated by synovial fluid.

Unaffected cartilage
Lubricating fluid

Osteoarthritic joint
In osteoarthritis (below), the cartilage becomes rough and flaky and small pieces break off to form loose bodies.

Degenerated cartilage

X-ray signs of osteoarthritis
This X ray shows narrowing of the joint space with osteophyte production and an increase in density of the bone ends.

Osteophyte   Characteristic swelling

Osteophytes
These are outgrowths of new bone that tend to occur at the margins of the joint surfaces in osteoarthritis.

TREATMENT AND SELF-HELP MEASURES

An important self-help measure is to shed excess weight to reduce wear and tear on joints. Measures to increase muscle power help to stabilize the affected joint and reduce symptoms.

Swimming
Regular exercise, to strengthen muscles and maintain joint mobility, can be valuable. Swimming in a heated pool increases muscle power without putting undue strain on joints.

Other treatment
Drugs such as aspirin or indomethacin are useful; sometimes corticosteroid injections are advised. There is little evidence that special diets or herbal treatments are effective.

Osteochondritis dissecans

Degeneration of a bone just under a joint surface, causing fragments of bone and cartilage to become separated from surrounding bone.

Osteochondritis dissecans frequently affects the knee and usually starts in adolescence. The exact cause is unknown but the disorder is thought to be caused by damage to a small blood vessel beneath the joint surface, which may be initiated by injury. The separated fragment sometimes reattaches but usually forms a *loose body* within the joint. Symptoms include aching discomfort and inter-

O

mittent swelling of the affected joint. The presence of a loose body may cause locking of a joint in one position.

X rays show damage to the joint and reveal the presence of any loose bodies. If a fragment has not completely separated, the joint may be immobilized in a cast to allow reattachment. Loose bodies of the knee are removed during *arthroscopy*.

The cavity left in the bone by a detached fragment disrupts the smoothness of the joint surface, increasing the likelihood of developing *osteoarthritis* in later life.

Osteochondritis juvenilis

Inflammation of an *epiphysis* (growing area of bone) in children and adolescents. The exact cause is unknown, but the condition is thought to be due to disrupted blood supply to the bone.

There are several distinct types of osteochondritis juvenilis, each involving different bones in the body. *Perthes' disease* affects the epiphysis of the head of the femur (thigh bone), while Scheuermann's disease affects epiphyses of several adjoining vertebrae. Other types affect certain bones in the foot and wrist.

SYMPTOMS AND SIGNS
Osteochondritis juvenilis causes localized pain and tenderness and, if the epiphysis forms part of a joint, restricted movement. Inflammation leads to softening of the bone, which may result in deformity because of surrounding pressure. X rays of the affected area show a patchy appearance and flattening of the bone.

TREATMENT AND OUTLOOK
Immobilization by use of a brace or plaster cast may be used to relieve pain and reduce the risk of deformity. In some cases of Perthes' disease, an operation is required to relieve the pressure on the diseased bone to prevent more deformity.

The bone usually regenerates within three years and rehardens. In many cases, however, deformity is permanent and increases the likelihood of the development of *osteoarthritis* in later life.

Osteochondroma

A benign bone tumor made up of a stalk of bone capped with cartilage. It grows from the side of a bone, usually at the end of a long bone in the region of the knee or shoulder. The osteochondroma develops in late childhood and early adolescence and stops growing when the skeleton is fully developed.

X ray of osteochondroma
The X ray shows a typical osteochondroma protruding from the bone. The tumor has a bony stalk and a cap made of cartilage.

The tumor, which appears as a hard round swelling near a joint, causes problems only if it interferes with the movement of tendons or the surrounding joint. In such cases, surgical removal may be necessary. A large osteochondroma can interfere with skeletal growth, causing deformity.

Osteochondrosis

See *Osteochondritis juvenilis*.

Osteodystrophy

Any generalized defect of the bones caused by a metabolic disorder (an abnormality of the body chemistry). Examples include *rickets*, a childhood condition in which the bones fail to harden properly due to a deficiency of vitamin D; *osteomalacia*, the equivalent condition in adults; *osteoporosis* (wasting away of bone) when it is caused not by aging but by the hormonal disorder *Cushing's syndrome* or by an excessive intake of *corticosteroid drugs*; and bone cysts and reduction of bone mass, which occasionally occur in chronic *renal failure* or *hyperparathyroidism* due to a disturbance in calcium metabolism in the body.

An osteodystrophy is usually reversible if the underlying cause can be treated effectively.

Osteogenesis imperfecta

Abnormally brittle bones from birth caused by a familial (inherited) congenital defective development of the *connective tissue* that forms the basic material of bone.

SYMPTOMS AND SIGNS
Severely affected infants, born with multiple fractures and a soft skull, usually do not survive. Those less severely affected have many fractures, often brought about by minimal force, during infancy and childhood. A physician examining such children

may sometimes find it difficult to determine whether the cause is osteogenesis imperfecta or *child abuse*. Very mild cases may not be detected until adolescence or later.

A common accompanying sign of the disorder is abnormal thinness of the sclera (whites of the eyes), making them appear blue. In addition, sufferers of osteogenesis imperfecta may be deaf due to *otosclerosis*.

Osteogenesis imperfecta
Affected children may suffer recurrent fractures of the limbs that lead to deformity and shortening, and to abnormal growth. At right is an X ray of the leg of a sufferer.

TREATMENT AND OUTLOOK
Fractures are generally treated in the usual way (by immobilization); otherwise, there is no specific treatment for the condition. The fractures usually heal quickly but often cause severe shortening and deformity of limbs, resulting in stunted, abnormal growth. Skull fractures may cause brain damage or death.

Osteogenic sarcoma

See *Osteosarcoma*.

Osteoid osteoma

An abnormal area of bone that causes deep pain, which is usually worse at night. An osteoid osteoma is extremely small—about 0.2 inch (0.5 cm)—and can be definitely diagnosed only by X ray. It most commonly affects a long bone of the arm or leg.

Pain can usually be relieved by *aspirin*. The condition is cured by removing the affected area of bone. (See also *Osteochondroma; Osteoma*.)

Osteoma

A benign bone tumor. It is hard, usually small, and may occur on any bone. An osteoma is usually harmless, but surgical removal may be necessary if the tumor causes symptoms by pressing on surrounding structures.

Osteomalacia

Softening, weakening, and demineralization of the bones in adults due to *vitamin D* deficiency (in children, the condition is called *rickets*).

The development of healthy bone requires an adequate intake of calcium and phosphorus from the diet, but these minerals cannot be absorbed by the body without a sufficient amount of vitamin D. A deficiency of this vitamin, which is obtained from certain foods and from the action of sunlight on the skin, results in softening and weakening of the bones, which then become vulnerable to distortion and fractures.

CAUSES

Osteomalacia is usually caused by any of the following, alone or in combination: an insufficient amount of vitamin D in the diet (due to a lack of milk, butter, eggs, or fish liver oils), insufficient exposure to sunlight, or inadequate absorption of vitamin D from the intestine (see *Malabsorption*), which may be caused by a disorder such as *celiac sprue* or by intestinal surgery. Rare causes include *renal failure*, *acidosis* (increased acidity of body fluids), and certain metabolic disorders that are inherited.

Osteomalacia is rare in developed countries. Most commonly affected are people with an inadequate diet, people who rarely or never go outdoors, and dark-skinned immigrants living in a country that has much less sunlight than their countries of origin.

SYMPTOMS AND SIGNS

Osteomalacia causes pain in the bones (particularly those in the neck, legs, hips, and ribs), muscle weakness, and, if the blood level of calcium is very low, *tetany* (muscle spasms) in the hands, feet, and throat. If the bones become greatly weakened, they may break after a minor injury.

DIAGNOSIS AND TREATMENT

Osteomalacia is diagnosed from the symptoms and signs, along with blood tests, urine tests, and bone X rays. In some cases, a bone *biopsy* (removal of a small sample of bone for examination) is performed.

Treatment consists of a diet that is rich in vitamin D and regular supplements of the vitamin. Supplements are usually taken as tablets; if tablets cannot be absorbed by the intestine, injections may be necessary. In some

cases of osteomalacia due to malabsorption, calcium supplements may also be taken.

Osteomyelitis

Infection of bone and bone marrow, usually by bacteria. It can affect any bone in the body, is more common in children, and most often affects the long bones of the arms and legs and the vertebrae. In adults, it usually affects the pelvis and the vertebrae. In developed countries, adequate nutrition and a generally high resistance to infection have made the disease, which may be acute or chronic, much rarer than it once was.

ACUTE OSTEOMYELITIS

The infecting microorganism (generally the bacterium *STAPHYLOCOCCUS AUREUS*) enters the bloodstream via a skin wound or an infection (usually in the nose or throat) and is carried to the bone in the blood. The infected bone and marrow become inflamed and pus forms, causing fever, severe pain and tenderness in the infected bone, and inflammation and swelling of the skin over the affected area.

The diagnosis may be confirmed by blood *culture*, bone scanning, and bone *X rays*. Treatment is with high doses of *antibiotic drugs* over several weeks or months. With prompt antibiotic treatment, acute osteomyelitis usually clears up completely. If the condition fails to respond to antibiotics, an operation is performed to expose the bone, to clean out the areas of infected and dead bone, and to drain the pus.

CHRONIC OSTEOMYELITIS

This form may develop when an attack of acute osteomyelitis is neglected or fails to respond to treatment. It may also occur after a compound *fracture* or, occasionally, as a result of *tuberculosis* spreading from another part of the body.

Chronic osteomyelitis causes constant pain in the affected bone. Complications include persistent deformity and, in children, arrest of growth in the affected bone. In the later stages of the disease (which may have been recurring for many years) *amyloidosis* (harmful deposits of a starchy substance in vital organs) may develop.

Chronic osteomyelitis requires surgical removal of all affected bone, sometimes followed by a *bone graft* to replace the removed bone; antibiotics are also prescribed. If the cause is tuberculosis, antituberculous drugs are prescribed for at least one year after surgery.

Osteopathic medicine

A system of diagnosis and treatment that recognizes the role of the musculoskeletal system (bones, muscles, tendons, tissues, nerves, and spinal column) in the healthy functioning of the human body.

Osteopathic medicine was founded on the Missouri frontier in 1874 by Andrew Taylor Still, MD. It is based on the concept of the human body as a unified organism, with the musculoskeletal system as central to the patient's well-being.

The Doctor of Osteopathy (DO) is a fully licensed physician with additional training in osteopathic palpatory diagnosis and manipulative therapy. The DO prescribes drugs and is qualified to practice all branches of medicine and surgery.

Osteopathic physicians emphasize that all body systems operate in unison, and that disturbances in one system can alter the functions of other systems in the body.

The osteopathic physician uses manipulation techniques, as well as traditional diagnostic and therapeutic procedures, to diagnose and treat dysfunction. Manipulation includes thrusting techniques and rhythmic stretching and pressure to restore motion to the joints.

Osteopetrosis

A rare, inherited disorder in which bones harden and become more dense. The growth of healthy bone is a balance between the activity of its two constituent cells, bone-forming osteoblasts and bone-reabsorbing osteoclasts. In osteopetrosis, there is a deficiency of osteoclasts, which results in the disruption of normal bone structure.

The mildest form of osteopetrosis may not cause any symptoms. More severe forms can result in greater susceptibility to fractures, stunted growth, deformity, and anemia. Pressure on nerves may cause blindness, deafness, and facial paralysis.

Bone marrow transplants have been attempted on an investigational basis. The transplant supplies the recipient with cells from which healthy osteoclasts might develop.

Osteophyte

A localized outgrowth of bone that forms at the boundary of a joint. Osteophytes are a characteristic of *osteoarthritis* and are partly responsible for the deformity and restricted movement of affected joints.

O

OSTEOPOROSIS

In osteoporosis, the density of bones decreases, and their brittleness increases, although there is no change in size or composition. Women past the menopause are the most commonly affected because their ovaries no longer produce estrogen, which helps to maintain bone mass. The risk of the condition is greater in a woman who undergoes the menopause early, or whose mother had osteoporosis.

Normal bone cross section
Bone consists of fibers of collagen (a protein), which give elasticity, and calcium, which gives hardness.

Osteoporotic bone
Thinning is mainly due to loss of collagen, which takes calcium with it. Both hard and spongy bone tissue are affected.

Bone loss with age
The graph at right shows how the percentage of bone lost increases in both sexes from age 30 onward, with the losses particularly marked in women after the menopause. By age 75, about half of all women have sustained at least one fracture due to osteoporosis, a much higher proportion than in men.

Graph: Decrease % versus Age, showing curves for Women and Men, with Age axis marked 10, 20, 30, 40, 50, 60, 70, 80, 90, 100 and Decrease % axis marked 10, 20, 30.

Spine affected by osteoporosis
The X rays show progressive thinning of the vertebrae, giving a characteristic "codfish" appearance to the spine.

Osteoporosis

Loss of protein matrix tissue from bone, causing it to become brittle and easily fractured.

Many physicians do not discriminate between osteoporosis and *osteomalacia*, diagnosing any decreased density of bone (thinning) as osteoporosis. In fact, decreased density may be caused by osteomalacia or by osteomalacia with osteoporosis.

Osteoporosis is a natural part of aging. By age 70, the density of the skeleton has diminished by about one third. However, for hormonal reasons, the condition is much more common in women than in men. Also, for reasons that are unknown, osteoporosis is more common in whites than in blacks.

CAUSES
Bone naturally becomes thinner as a person ages, but women are especially vulnerable to osteoporosis after the *menopause* because their ovaries no longer produce *estrogen hormone*, which helps maintain bone mass.

Other causes of the disorder include removal of the ovaries; a diet deficient in calcium, which is essential for bone health; certain hormonal disorders, such as *Cushing's syndrome*, or prolonged treatment with *corticosteroid drugs*; and prolonged immobility.

Osteoporosis is more common in smokers and drinkers and, for unknown reasons, is associated with chronic obstructive lung disorders, such as *bronchitis* and *emphysema*.

SYMPTOMS AND SIGNS
In many cases, osteoporosis produces no obvious symptoms; the first sign is often a fracture after a fall that would not cause a fracture in a young adult. Typical sites for such fractures are just above the wrist and the top of the femur (thigh bone). Another type of fracture that occurs in osteoporosis is a spontaneous fracture of one or several vertebrae, which causes the bones to be compressed, leading to a progressive loss of height or to pain due to compression of a spinal nerve.

DIAGNOSIS
The condition is diagnosed from the symptoms and from bone X rays. In some cases, blood tests and a bone *biopsy* (removal of a sample of bone for examination) may also be necessary to exclude osteomalacia.

TREATMENT AND PREVENTION
Lost bone tissue cannot easily be replaced, but more bone loss can be minimized by preventive measures. For example, both men and women should ensure that their *calcium* intake is adequate. The richest dietary sources of this mineral are milk and milk products, green leafy vegetables, citrus fruits, sardines, and shellfish. Calcium tablets may be needed.

Exercise also helps to build bones, but anything less than three brisk three-mile walks a week (or the equivalent) is unlikely to be of much benefit in preventing osteoporosis.

Hormone replacement therapy to compensate for reduced estrogen production after the menopause has been shown to prevent osteoporosis in women; in the US, it has halved the rate of fractures caused by osteoporosis in menopausal women.

Osteosarcoma

A malignant bone tumor that occurs primarily in adolescent and elderly people. It spreads rapidly to the lungs and, less commonly, to other areas.

In young people, osteosarcoma develops for no known reason; in elderly people, it is a late, rare complication of *Paget's disease*.

SYMPTOMS AND DIAGNOSIS
The most common site of the tumor in young people is in a long bone of the leg or arm, or around the knee, hip, or shoulder. The first symptom is usually a painful visible swelling of the affected bone (if it is near the surface) or a deep-seated pain (if the affected bone cannot be felt through the skin).

As a complication of Paget's disease, an osteosarcoma may develop in several bones; its pain may be indistinguishable from that caused by the original disease.

Diagnosis is usually based on *X rays* of the bone. Other imaging techniques (e.g., *MRI*) may also be used.

TREATMENT AND OUTLOOK

Although *radiation therapy* is sometimes used to treat the tumor, the bone is usually surgically removed. In most cases, this means *amputation* of a limb; in some cases, a prosthesis can be fitted immediately after the amputation (see *Limb, artificial*). The tumor can also be treated by removal and bone graft or bone transplant.

Treatment with *anticancer drugs* is usually given for several months after the operation to destroy any cancer cells that may have spread to other parts of the body. With this additional treatment, the outlook is good; about half of all patients whose disease is discovered early are cured.

Osteosclerosis

Increased bone density, usually detected on *X-ray* film as an area of extreme whiteness.

Localized osteosclerosis may be caused by a severe injury that compresses the bone; by *osteoarthritis*, in which bone around affected joints thickens; by chronic *osteomyelitis*, in which healthy bone next to the infected area thickens and becomes more dense; or by an *osteoma* (benign bone tumor), which consists of a hard, dense, usually harmless outgrowth of normal bone tissue.

Osteosclerosis occurs throughout the body in *osteopetrosis*, an inherited bone disorder.

Osteotomy

An operation in which a bone is cut to change its alignment or to shorten or lengthen it.

WHY IT IS DONE

Osteotomy is performed on a deformity of the big toe that has caused a bunion (see *Hallux valgus*). It is also performed to straighten a long bone that has healed crookedly after a *fracture* or to shorten the uninjured leg after a fractured leg has shortened during healing (see *Leg, shortening of*).

Osteotomy may be used to correct the deformity caused by congenital dislocation of the hip (see *Hip, congenital dislocation of*) that has not been detected until after about age 10. It is also used to correct *coxa vara* (hip deformity usually caused by injury).

Bone cut here

Example of an osteotomy
This procedure is performed to correct a hallux valgus (outward protrusion of the joint at the base of the toe), usually because it has caused a bunion. Part of the top of the first metatarsal bone is removed.

HOW IT IS DONE

Using general anesthesia, bones are straightened by cutting through them and repositioning the ends; sometimes a wedge of bone is inserted or removed to achieve the correct alignment. Bones can be lengthened by making an oblique cut and displacing the two parts slightly before rejoining them. Bones can be shortened by cutting out a section of bone and rejoining the two parts.

After the operation, bones that were corrected during surgery are held in position by a metal plate or nail or by a plaster cast or splint.

Ostomy

The term used to describe a surgical opening or junction of two hollow organs (e.g., *colostomy* and *ileostomy*).

Ot-

A prefix that denotes a relationship to the ear, as in otitis, inflammation of the ear. The prefix oto- is also used to denote the ear.

Otalgia

The medical term for *earache*.

OTC

The abbreviation for over-the-counter. OTC refers to drug preparations that may be purchased from a drugstore without a prescription from a physician.

Otitis externa

Also called swimmers' ear, inflammation of the outer-ear canal that is caused by infection.

CAUSES

Generalized infection, affecting the whole canal and sometimes also the pinna (the external ear), may be caused by bacteria or by fungi, which produce a persistent inflammation known as otomycosis. Bacterial infection may also cause a localized infection in the form of a *boil*. In some cases, the outer-ear canal becomes inflamed as part of a generalized skin disorder, such as atopic *eczema* or seborrheic *dermatitis*.

Malignant otitis externa is an uncommon and occasionally fatal form of the disorder caused by the bacterium *PSEUDOMONAS AERUGINOSA*. It usually affects elderly diabetics, whose resistance to infection is reduced, and spreads rapidly into surrounding bones and soft tissue.

SYMPTOMS AND SIGNS

Otitis externa usually causes redness and swelling of the skin of the ear canal, a discharge from the ear, and sometimes an area of eczema around the opening of the ear. The ear may itch only in the early stages, but can become painful. Occasionally, pus blocks the ear, causing deafness.

DIAGNOSIS AND TREATMENT

The physician examines the ear with an *otoscope* (a viewing instrument) and may take a sample of any pus for laboratory analysis.

Often the only treatment required is a thorough cleaning and drying of the ear by the physician, sometimes using a suction apparatus. Antibiotic, antifungal, or anti-inflammatory drugs are often necessary. Oral antibiotics are used for the treatment of severe bacterial infections. If the ear canal is very swollen, a wick should be placed in the canal to allow drops to enter. The sufferer should avoid getting the ear canal wet until the infection has cleared up.

Otitis media

Inflammation of the middle ear (the cavity between the eardrum and the inner ear).

CAUSES

The inflammation occurs as the result of an upper respiratory tract infection (such as a cold) extending up the eustachian tube, the passage that connects the back of the nose to the middle ear. The tube may become blocked by the inflammation or sometimes by enlarged *adenoids*, which are often associated with infections of the nose and throat. As a result, fluid produced by the inflammation—along with pus in bacterial infections—is not drained off through the tube but accumulates in the middle ear.

The chronic phase of otitis media (otitis media with effusion) follows an upper respiratory infection that has produced acute otitis media.

O

INCIDENCE

Children are particularly susceptible to otitis media, probably because of the shortness of their eustachian tubes. About one in six children suffers from the acute form in the first year of life and about one in 10 in each of the next six years. Some children have recurrent attacks. Chronic otitis media is much less common because, in most cases, attacks of acute middle-ear infection clear with treatment.

SYMPTOMS AND SIGNS

Acute otitis media is marked by sudden, severe earache, a feeling of fullness in the ear, deafness, tinnitus (ringing or buzzing in the ear), and fever. Sometimes the eardrum bursts, relieving the pain and resulting in a discharge of pus. In this case, healing usually occurs in several days.

In chronic otitis media, pus constantly exudes from a perforation in the eardrum and there is some degree of deafness. Complications of the condition include *otitis externa* (inflammation of the outer ear); damage to the bones in the middle ear, causing more deafness (sometimes total) in the affected ear; or a *cholesteatoma* (a matted ball of sometimes infected skin debris). In rare cases, infection spreads inward from an infected ear, causing *mastoiditis* or a *brain abscess*.

DIAGNOSIS

The diagnosis is usually made from examining the ears with an *otoscope* (a viewing instrument). A swab may be taken of any discharge so that the organism responsible for the infection can be cultured and identified.

TREATMENT

Acute otitis media is treated by giving antibiotic drugs and analgesics (painkillers). Usually, the condition clears up completely with treatment, but in some cases there is continual production of sticky fluid in the middle ear, a condition known as persistent *middle-ear effusion*.

Chronic otitis media is treated by sucking out pus and infected debris from the ear as necessary. Antibiotic ear drops may be given if this does not adequately control the condition.

Otolaryngologist, head and neck surgeon

A specialist in the medical and surgical treatment of disorders of the head and neck, excluding the brain, eyes, spinal cord, and spinal column. The term "head and neck surgery" refers to surgical procedures on certain tumors of the sinuses, throat, and neck, and to facial plastic surgery.

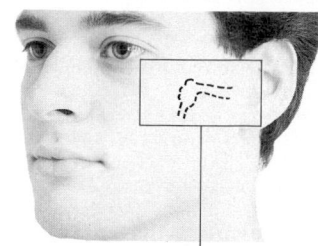

EAR INFECTIONS

Inflammation of the middle ear (otitis media) or ear canal (otitis externa) usually results from infection and may cause an earache. Otitis media is more common in children and may be acute (with sudden onset of pain) or chronic (continuing painlessly over a long period).

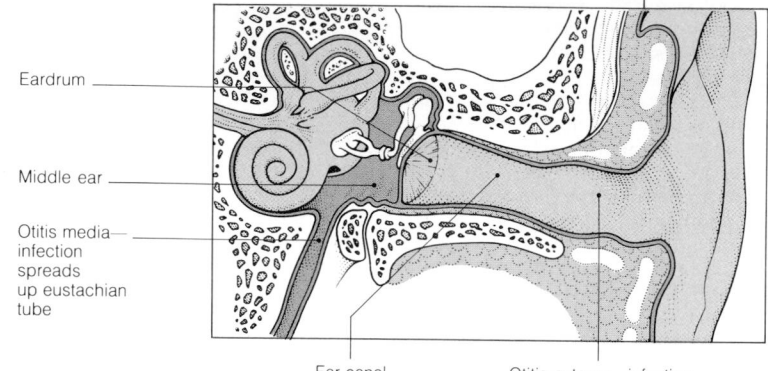

Eardrum

Middle ear

Otitis media— infection spreads up eustachian tube

Ear canal

Otitis externa—infection spreads from outside

Otitis media
This usually occurs through spread of infection from the back of the nose to the middle ear via the eustachian tube.

Otitis externa
The ear canal is susceptible to infection if it is moist (after swimming) or damaged by attempts to remove earwax.

Much of an otolaryngologist's time is spent treating common conditions, such as *sinus* infections, acute *otitis media* (middle-ear infection), persistent *middle-ear effusion*, *tonsillitis*, and minor hearing loss. The otolaryngologist is often faced with complex and difficult problems, such as *otosclerosis*, *Meniere's disease*, airway problems in children, uncontrollable bleeding from the nose, and cancer of the larynx and sinuses.

Otoplasty

Cosmetic or reconstructive surgery on the outer ear. Otoplasty is usually performed to flatten protruding ears. It may also be done to construct or repair a missing or badly damaged ear.

PROTRUDING EARS

The operation, as described at right, is usually done as an outpatient procedure using local anesthesia. After the operation, the ear is dressed until the wound has healed 10 to 14 days later, when the stitches are removed. The scar is hidden in the crease between the ear and scalp.

LACK OF AN OUTER EAR

Some children are born with part or all of the outer ear missing. These chil-

dren may also lack an external ear passage; in some cases there is also underdevelopment of the same side of the face.

Treatment involves transferring a piece of rib cartilage, which is sculpted to resemble the normal ear, to a pocket of skin in the position that the ear will be placed. The procedure usually involves three operations. Hearing in the reconstructed ear may be abnormal but, if the child has a normal range of hearing in the other ear, no attempt is made to improve hearing in the reconstructed ear.

Otoplasty for protruding ears
A strip of skin is removed from behind each ear. The underlying cartilage is remolded and the two edges of the wound stitched together, thus pulling the ear closer to the head. The appearances before and after are shown.

O

Otorhinolaryngology

The full title for the surgical specialty concerned with diseases of the ear, nose, and throat (see *Otolaryngologist, head and neck surgeon*).

Otorrhea

The medical name for a discharge from the ear (see *Ear, discharge from*).

Otosclerosis

A disorder of the middle ear that causes progressive deafness. Otosclerosis is often inherited.

CAUSES AND INCIDENCE

Otosclerosis occurs when, for unknown reasons, an overgrowth of bone immobilizes the stapes (the innermost bone of the middle ear). This prevents sound vibrations from being passed to the inner ear, resulting in conductive *deafness*. In most cases of otosclerosis, both ears are ultimately affected.

About one person in 200 is affected by the disease, which usually starts in early adulthood. It is more common in women than in men and often develops during pregnancy.

SYMPTOMS AND SIGNS

Sound is heard as muffled but is more distinguishable when there is background noise. Affected people tend to talk quietly. Hearing loss progresses slowly over a period of 10 to 15 years and is often accompanied by *tinnitus* (noises in the ear) and sometimes by *vertigo* (dizziness). Some sensorineural deafness (caused by damage spreading to the inner ear) may eventually occur, making high tones difficult to hear and resulting in the sufferer speaking loudly.

DIAGNOSIS AND TREATMENT

The diagnosis is based on abnormal results of *hearing tests*. A *hearing aid* is an excellent treatment for otosclerosis; the deafness can be cured only by *stapedectomy*, an operation in which the stapes is replaced with an artificial substitute. Stapedectomy is usually performed on only one ear at a time because there is a risk that total deafness may result in the operated ear.

Otoscope

An instrument for examining the ear. An otoscope includes magnifying lenses, a light, and a speculum (a funnel-shaped tip that is inserted into the ear canal). The instrument allows easy inspection of the outer-ear canal and the eardrum. With an otoscope it is also possible to detect certain diseases of the middle ear through the semitransparent eardrum.

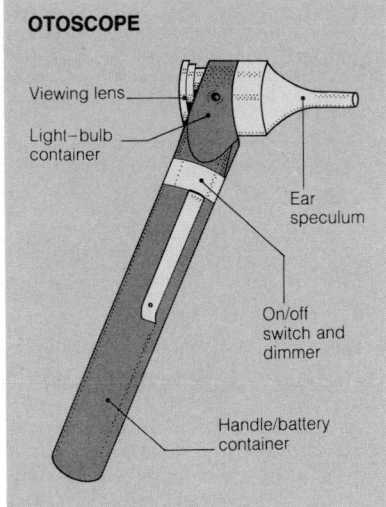

OTOSCOPE

Viewing lens

Light–bulb container

Ear speculum

On/off switch and dimmer

Handle/battery container

Ototoxicity

Having a poisonous effect on the ear. High doses of certain drugs (especially aminoglycoside *antibiotic drugs*) can damage the cochlea and the semicircular canals in the inner ear, impairing hearing and balance.

Outpatient treatment

Medical care given to a person on a day basis in a clinic or other facility.

Ovarian cyst

An abnormal, fluid-filled swelling in an ovary. Ovarian cysts are common and are benign in about 95 percent of cases. Many ovarian cysts disappear without treatment.

TYPES

The most common type of ovarian cyst is a follicular cyst, in which the egg-producing follicle of the *ovary* enlarges and fills with fluid. Cysts may also occur in the corpus luteum, a yellow mass of tissue that forms from the follicle after *ovulation*.

Other types of ovarian cysts include *dermoid cysts* and malignant cysts (see *Ovary, cancer of*).

SYMPTOMS AND SIGNS

Ovarian cysts often cause no symptoms, but some cause abdominal discomfort, pain during intercourse, or menstrual irregularities including *amenorrhea* (lack of menstruation), *menorrhagia* (heavy periods), or *dysmenorrhea* (painful periods). Severe abdominal pain, nausea, and fever, which necessitate surgery, may develop if twisting of a cyst occurs.

DIAGNOSIS AND TREATMENT

A cyst may be discovered during a routine *pelvic examination*. *Ultrasound*

scanning or a *laparoscopy* (examination of the abdominal cavity through a viewing tube) may be necessary to confirm the diagnosis and to determine the size and position of the cyst.

Simple cysts (thin-walled and filled with fluid) often go away on their own, but complex cysts (such as dermoid cysts) do not. They often require surgical removal. In many cases, only the cyst needs to be removed, but if a cyst is large it is sometimes necessary for the surgeon to remove the entire ovary (see *Oophorectomy*).

Ovary

One of a pair of almond-shaped glands situated on either side of the *uterus* immediately below the opening of the *fallopian tube*. Each ovary is about 1.25 inch (30 mm) long and 0.75 inch (20 mm) wide and contains numerous cavities called follicles in which egg cells (see *Ovum*) develop. In addition to producing ova, the ovaries also produce the female sex hormones estrogen and progesterone.

DISORDERS

Absence or failure of normal development of the ovaries is a rare disorder usually caused by a chromosomal abnormality (see *Turner's syndrome*).

Oophoritis (inflammation of the ovary) may be caused by the *mumps* virus or by other infections such as *gonorrhea* or *pelvic inflammatory disease*.

Ovarian cysts may develop at any age; about 95 percent of them are benign. *Polycystic ovary* syndrome, in

O

ANATOMY OF THE OVARY

Each ovary consists of glandular cells and egg-producing follicles. After ovulation, each follicle forms a corpus luteum.

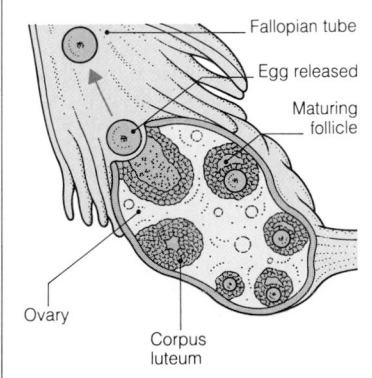

Fallopian tube

Egg released

Maturing follicle

Ovary

Corpus luteum

which multiple ovarian cysts form, is an uncommon disorder thought to be due to the body's inappropriate hormonal stimulation of the ovaries. The cysts may produce male sex hormones, leading to *amenorrhea*, *infertility*, and *hirsutism*.

Cancer of the ovary (see *Ovary, cancer of*) occurs mainly in women over 50 and usually causes few symptoms (if any) in the early stages, although it can cause symptoms similar to those of an ovarian cyst.

Ovarian failure, in which the ovaries cease to function, causes premature *menopause* in about 5 percent of all women.

Ovary, cancer of

Malignant growth of the *ovary*. Ovarian cancer is the fourth leading cause of cancer death in women. Cancer of the ovary can occur at any age but is most common after 50. It is three times more common in women who have never had children and less common in women who have taken oral birth-control pills.

The growth may be primary (arising in the ovary) or may be a secondary growth that has spread to the ovary from some other part of the body, often the breast.

SYMPTOMS AND SIGNS

In most cases ovarian cancer causes no symptoms until it is widespread. The first symptom is usually vague abdominal discomfort and swelling. There may be digestive disturbances, such as nausea and vomiting, abnormal vaginal bleeding, and *ascites* (excess fluid in the abdominal cavity). A physical examination may reveal a swelling in the pelvis.

DIAGNOSIS AND TREATMENT

A *laparoscopy* (examination of the abdominal cavity through a viewing tube) or *laparotomy* (opening of the abdomen wall) may be necessary to confirm the diagnosis. Treatment is surgery to remove the cancer or as much of the malignant tissue as possible. This usually involves *salpingo-oophorectomy* (removal of the ovaries and fallopian tubes) and *hysterectomy* (removal of the uterus). Surgery is usually followed by *radiation therapy* and *anticancer drugs*.

OUTLOOK

If the growth is confined to one or both ovaries, 60 to 70 percent of patients survive at least five years. If the growth is more widespread, only about 10 to 20 percent of patients survive five years. New drug combinations may improve this survival rate.

Overbite

Overlapping of the lower front teeth by the upper front teeth. A slight degree of overbite is normal because the upper jaw is larger than the lower one. In *malocclusion*, overbite may be greater than normal or may be reversed (with the lower teeth projecting in front of the upper ones).

Overcrowding, dental

Excessive crowding of the teeth so that they are unable to assume their normal positions in the jaw.

Severe case of overcrowding
The front teeth are crowded together because the two molars, just behind them, have grown too far forward.

CAUSES

Overcrowding frequently occurs through heredity when the teeth are relatively too large or there are too many for a person's jaw. The condition also can occur or worsen with the premature loss of primary molar teeth. This can cause the permanent teeth growing beneath them to move out of position and leave insufficient space for the developing permanent teeth further forward in the mouth.

PROBLEMS

Overcrowded teeth may lead to *malocclusion* (incorrect relationship between the upper and lower teeth) and may prevent certain teeth from erupting through the gum (see *Impaction, dental*). There is an increased risk of dental decay in crowded teeth because they are more difficult to clean. Overcrowding can also increase the risk of *periodontal disease* because of more difficult cleaning and more unusual stress being placed on supporting tissues.

TREATMENT

An orthodontist decides whether one or more teeth should be extracted to allow room for others to grow. Often the remaining teeth require fitting with an *orthodontic appliance* to move them into their correct positions.

Overuse injury

A term for any injury that has been caused by repetitive movement of part of the body. A common example is *epicondylitis*, painful inflammation of one of the epicondyles (bony prominences) at the elbow, caused by the pull of the attached forearm muscles during gardening, painting, or playing certain sports (see *Golfers' elbow*; *Tennis elbow*).

Overuse injuries of the finger and wrist joints may affect assembly line workers and typists. Musicians are also prone to a variety of problems; the thumb may be affected in players of woodwind instruments and the neck may be affected in violinists.

Symptoms, which usually disappear with rest, include pain and stiffness in the affected joints and muscles. It is sometimes possible to avoid a recurrence by altering technique during the activity.

Overweight

See *Obesity*.

Ovulation

The development and release of an *ovum* (egg) from a follicle within the *ovary*. Ovulation occurs midway through the menstrual cycle and is regulated by hormones. During the first half of the cycle, the follicle-stimulating hormone (FSH) causes several ova to mature in the ovary. At mid-cycle, the luteinizing hormone causes one ripe ovum to be released. The follicle then forms a small mass of yellow tissue called the corpus luteum, which secretes the hormone *progesterone* during the second half of the menstrual cycle.

After its release, the ovum travels along the fallopian tube and, unless *fertilization* occurs, is shed during *menstruation*. Regular menstruation usually means that a woman ovulates, but this is not always the case, especially around *puberty* and approaching the *menopause*.

Some forms of contraception (see *Contraception, periodic abstinence*) are based on predicting when ovulation occurs each month and avoiding sexual intercourse at that time. Signs of ovulation include a rise in body temperature and changes in the amount and consistency of cervical mucus; there may also be mild abdominal pain (see *Mittelschmerz*).

If a woman does not ovulate, she cannot conceive. Investigation of female *infertility* includes tests to determine whether ovulation occurs.

Ovum

 The egg cell (female cell) of reproduction. Each ovum measures about 0.04 inch (0.1 mm) in diameter. There are about 1 million immature ova present in each ovary at birth; only about 200 per ovary ever mature to be released at *ovulation* during a woman's fertile years. If *fertilization* occurs, the ovum develops into an *embryo*.

Oxacillin

A *penicillin*-type *antibiotic drug*. Oxacillin is especially useful in the treatment of *staphylococcal infections* resistant to other antibiotic drugs.

Oxandrolone

An anabolic steroid (see *Steroids, anabolic*) used after a major illness or injury to help increase weight. It is also sometimes used in the treatment of *hyperlipidemia*.

Oxandrolone may cause swollen ankles and, in women, irregular periods. Rare adverse effects include nausea, vomiting, jaundice, and, in men, difficulty passing urine.

Oxazepam

A *benzodiazepine drug* used in the treatment of *anxiety* and *insomnia*. Like other benzodiazepines, oxazepam may cause dependence if taken regularly for more than two weeks (see *Drug dependence*).

Oxtriphylline

A *bronchodilator drug* related to *theophylline*, used in the treatment of *asthma* and *bronchitis*. Oxtriphylline may cause adverse effects, such as nausea, vomiting, and headache.

Oxycodone

A narcotic *analgesic* (painkiller) derived from *morphine*. It is used in the treatment of severe pain.

Oxygen

A colorless, odorless gas that makes up 21 percent of Earth's atmosphere. Oxygen is essential for almost all forms of life, including humans, because it is necessary for the metabolic "burning" of foods to produce energy—a process known as *aerobic* metabolism.

To reach the body cells, where aerobic metabolism takes place, oxygen in the air is absorbed through the lungs and into the blood, where it binds to the *hemoglobin* in red blood cells. In this form, the oxygen is distributed throughout the body, being released from the hemoglobin and taken up by cells in areas where the oxygen level is low.

Oxygen is used therapeutically to treat conditions such as severe *bronchitis* or *hypoxia* (an inadequate supply of oxygen to body tissues). In some cases, high pressure oxygen (see *Hyperbaric oxygen treatment*) is used to treat the bends (*decompression sickness*) or poisoning from *carbon monoxide*. (See also *Ozone*.)

Oxygen therapy

Supplying a person with oxygen-enriched air to relieve severe *hypoxia* (inadequate oxygen in the tissues).

In hospitals, oxygen is usually piped to a terminal at the patient's bedside and is administered as necessary through a face mask or nasal cannulas (tubes inserted into the nostrils). The concentration of oxygen is varied according to the patient's needs.

People at home can be supplied with oxygen in cylinders for use during acute attacks of hypoxia (which occur in severe *asthma*). People with persistent hypoxia due to severe, chronic *bronchitis* or *emphysema* may benefit from long-term oxygen therapy. These patients may be supplied with a machine called an oxygen concentrator, which separates oxygen from the air and remixes it in a higher-than-normal concentration. Oxygen-rich air is then piped to different rooms for prolonged inhalation.

People receiving oxygen therapy should not smoke, since smoking not only presents a fire risk but also reduces the oxygen-carrying capacity of the blood and aggravates the underlying condition for which the oxygen is being given. (See also *Hyperbaric oxygen treatment*.)

Oxymetazoline

A *decongestant drug* used in the treatment of allergic *rhinitis* (hay fever), *sinusitis*, and the common *cold*. Oxymetazoline has a longer-lasting effect than other decongestants; it needs to be taken only twice a day.

Oxymetazoline may irritate the nose. Prolonged use causes rebound congestion (increased congestion when the drug is withdrawn).

Oxytetracycline

A type of *antibiotic drug* known as a *tetracycline drug*. Oxytetracycline is used to treat *chlamydial infections* such as *nonspecific urethritis*, *psittacosis*, and *trachoma*. It is also used to treat a variety of other infections, including *bronchitis*, pneumonia caused by *mycoplasma*, *syphilis*, *brucellosis*, *Rocky Mountain spotted fever*, and *cholera*. Oxytetracycline may be used to treat severe *acne*.

POSSIBLE ADVERSE EFFECTS
Oxytetracycline occasionally causes nausea, vomiting, diarrhea, rash, or increased sensitivity of the skin to sunlight. It may also discolor developing teeth and is therefore not prescribed for children under 12 or during pregnancy.

Oxytocin

A hormone produced by the *pituitary gland* that causes contractions of the uterus during labor and stimulates the flow of milk in nursing women.

USE AS A DRUG
Synthetic oxytocin is commonly used to induce childbirth (see *Induction of labor*). It is sometimes used to help expel the placenta (afterbirth) after delivery or to empty the uterus after an incomplete *miscarriage* or a fetal death. Oxytocin is sometimes given as a nasal spray to stimulate milk flow.

POSSIBLE ADVERSE EFFECTS
Contractions may be stronger and more painful than usual, increasing the need for stronger *analgesic drugs* (painkillers). Rare adverse effects include nausea, vomiting, palpitations, seizures, and coma.

Ozena

A severe and rare form of *rhinitis* (inflammation of the mucous membrane in the nose) in which the membrane atrophies (wastes away) and a thick nasal discharge dries to form crusts. It often causes severe *halitosis* (bad breath).

Ozone

A rare form of oxygen, ozone is a poisonous, faintly blue gas that is produced by the action of electrical discharges (such as lightning) on oxygen molecules.

Ozone occurs naturally in the upper atmosphere (about 15 to 20 miles above the Earth's surface), where it screens the Earth from most of the sun's harmful ultraviolet radiation.

However, there are claims that the ozone layer is being depleted by various environmental chemicals (notably the chlorofluorocarbons in aerosols). The result is that stronger and more potent forms of ultraviolet radiation are reaching the Earth's surface. Increased ultraviolet levels could lead to an increase in the incidence of skin cancer and cataracts.

O

PABA
The abbreviation for *para-aminobenzoic acid*, a sunscreen ingredient.

Pacemaker
A device that supplies electrical impulses to the heart to maintain the heart beat at a regular rate. A pacemaker consists of a small electronic device and power source connected to the heart via an electrical wire.

In a healthy heart, the beat is maintained by a nucleus of specialized muscle called the sinoatrial node; it sends out regular electrical impulses that pass through the heart muscle and trigger heart contractions. An artificial pacemaker is implanted when a person's sinoatrial node is not functioning properly, or when there is some impairment to the passage of the normal electrical impulses (see *Heart block; Sick sinus syndrome*). Each year, tens of thousands of Americans have a pacemaker implanted.

Two main types of pacemaker—fixed rate and demand—are shown in the box below. More advanced types can increase the heart rate during exercise. Dual-chamber devices utilize one electrode in the atrium and another in the ventricular wall.

IMPLANTATION
Implantation is carried out using local anesthetic. Patients can expect complete healing without complications and should return to normal work and activity as soon as possible. Vigorous exercise should be avoided for two weeks after the operation.

Modern microelectronic circuits require little power and lithium batteries have a long life. Unless the demand on the battery is excessive, a pacemaker usually runs satisfactorily for several years. Battery replacement requires a minor operation.

PRECAUTIONS
Modern pacemakers are relatively insensitive to interference but may be affected by powerful electromagnetic pulses. Anyone with a pacemaker should avoid powerful radio or radar transmitters and should not pass through security screens at airports. Precautions may also be required with some physical therapy or surgical *diathermy* machines.

Paget's disease
A common disorder of middle-aged and elderly people in which the normal process of bone formation is disrupted, causing the affected bones to weaken, thicken, and become deformed. Also known as osteitis deformans, Paget's disease usually involves only limited areas of the skeleton. The bones usually affected are the pelvis, skull, collarbone, vertebrae, and long bones of the leg.

CAUSE AND INCIDENCE
The normal maintenance of healthy bones by the body involves a balance between the actions of cells that break down bone tissue and those that rebuild it. In Paget's disease, this balance is disturbed. The disease varies in frequency from one part of the country to another, suggesting an infective cause, which is thought to be

---

PACEMAKERS
A pacemaker may be external (worn on a belt) or internal (implanted in the chest), like those shown below.

External pacing is used only as a temporary measure. There are two main methods of implantation.

TYPES OF PACEMAKERS
The two main types are shown. In some cases, an external programmer can adjust the rate.

Transvenous implantation
An insulated wire is inserted into a major vein in the neck and guided down into the heart until the electrode at its far end is secured within the part of the heart muscle to be stimulated. The free end is connected to the pacemaker, which is fitted into a pocket created under the skin of the abdomen or below the collarbone.

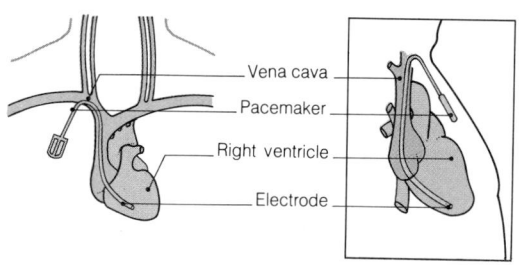

Vena cava
Pacemaker
Right ventricle
Electrode

Side view
The pacemaker is usually well hidden by overlying tissue

Epicardial implantation
The electrode is attached to the outer surface of the part of the heart muscle to be stimulated and the pacemaker is fitted into a pocket constructed underneath the skin of the abdomen.

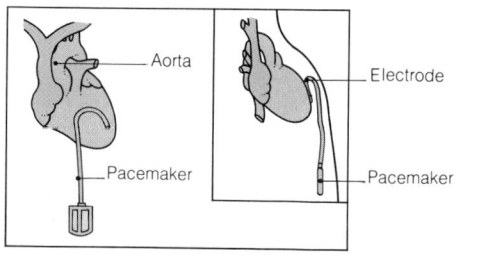

Aorta
Pacemaker
Electrode
Pacemaker

FIXED RATE

Impulse

No response to heart beat

Fixed-rate pacemaker
This type discharges impulses at a steady rate, irrespective of the heart's activity.

DEMAND

Impulse when beat is missed

Pacemaker suppressed by heart beat

Demand pacemaker
This type discharges impulses only when the heart rate slows or a beat is missed. A normal heart rate and beat suppresses the pacemaker.

viral. Overall, Paget's disease affects about 3 percent of the population over the age of 40, the incidence increasing with age. The disorder has a tendency to run in families and affects more men than women.

SYMPTOMS AND SIGNS

Paget's disease often causes no symptoms and is usually discovered from an X ray taken for some other reason. The most common symptoms are bone pain and deformity, especially bowing of the legs. Affected bones are prone to fracture.

Changes in the skull may lead to leontiasis (distortion of the facial bones that produces a lionlike appearance) and to inner-ear damage, sometimes resulting in deafness, tinnitus (ringing in the ear), vertigo, or headaches. Enlarged vertebrae may press on the spinal cord, causing pain and sometimes paralysis of the legs. If the pelvis is affected, it can result in severe arthritis of the hips. Occasionally, *bone cancer* may develop, and, in rare cases, when many bones are involved, increased blood flow through the affected bones may cause *heart failure*.

DIAGNOSIS

X rays reveal areas of porous, thickened bone. *Blood tests* that show an elevated level of the enzyme alkaline phosphatase (which is associated with bone cell formation) give an indication of the extent and activity of the disease.

TREATMENT AND OUTLOOK

Most people with the disorder do not require treatment, and many others simply need to take *analgesic drugs* (painkillers). In severe cases, the hormone *calcitonin* may be prescribed. It relieves pain, reduces alkaline phosphatase levels, and promotes normal bone formation. Other drugs that have the same effect (including disodium etidronate and plicamycin) may also be used. Surgery may be required to correct deformities or treat secondary arthritis.

Paget's disease of the nipple

A rare *breast cancer* in which the tumor starts in the milk ducts of the nipple. Paget's disease of the nipple looks similar to *eczema*, causes the nipple to itch and burn, and may feature a sore on the nipple that will not heal. Usually only one nipple is affected. If left untreated, the tumor may gradually spread into the breast. Eczema of the nipple should be reported to a physician and a *biopsy* of the underlying breast taken.

Pain

A localized sensation that can range from mild discomfort to an unbearable and excruciating experience. Pain is the result of stimulation of special sensory nerve endings following injury or caused by disease.

THE MECHANISM OF PAIN

The basic mechanism of pain is shown in the illustrated box on the next page. The skin contains many specialized nerve endings (nociceptors). Stimulation of these receptors leads to transmission of pain messages to the brain. Nociceptors have different sensitivities, some responding only to severe stimulation, such as cutting, pricking, or heating the skin to a high temperature; others respond to warning stimuli, such as firm pressure, stretching, or temperatures not high enough to burn. Pain receptors are present in structures other than the skin, including blood vessels and tendons. Most internal organs have few, if any, nociceptors. The large intestine, for example, can be cut without causing any pain. It does, however, have nociceptors that respond to stretching, which, in severe cases, may cause pain.

PSYCHOLOGICAL ASPECTS OF PAIN

Pain is usually associated with distress and anxiety, and sometimes with fear. People vary tremendously in their pain thresholds (the level at which the pain is felt and the person feels compelled to act). The cause and circumstances of the pain may also affect the way it is perceived by the sufferer. The pain of cancer, because of fear of the disease, may seem much greater and cause more suffering than similar pain resulting from persistent indigestion. Unexplained pain is often worse because of the anxiety it can cause; once a diagnosis is made and reassurance given, the pain may be perceived as less severe.

The experience of pain may be reduced by arousal (e.g., an injury sustained during competitive sport or on the battlefield may go unnoticed in the heat of the moment); strong emotion can also block pain. Some people believe that mental preparation for pain (e.g., in childbirth or in experiments to test pain) can greatly reduce the response.

A person's response to pain is greatly modified by past experience; the outcome of previous episodes of pain may affect the way the individual copes with subsequent pain. Factors such as insomnia, anxiety, and depression, which often accompany

incapacitating illness, lower pain tolerance. Treatment for these symptoms is given along with treatment for the pain to allow the minimum dose for pain relief.

Cultural differences exist in the expression of pain. In some parts of the world self-inflicted torture and the ability to withstand great pain are a mark of a person's strength and character. However, the pain of even mild torture inflicted by captors may be perceived as much worse than a similar degree of pain that occurs under different circumstances.

TYPES OF PAIN

Many adjectives are used to describe different types of pain. Common descriptive terms include throbbing, penetrating, gnawing, aching, burning, and gripping. The extent to which a patient is accurately able to describe his or her pain to the physician is highly variable, even though it can be a vital clue to the diagnosis.

Attempts have been made to categorize pain according to intensity, ranging from a minor cut or sore throat at the lower end to childbirth and renal or biliary colic at the upper.

If the pain comes from an internal organ it is often difficult for the sufferer to pinpoint its origin with any precision. For example, in the early stages of appendicitis, pain may be felt in the region above the navel. In the later stages, when infection has caused inflammation of the peritoneum (lining of the abdominal cavity), the pain becomes localized above the right groin.

Pain may be felt at a point some distance from the disorder. This is called *referred pain* (see illustrated box overleaf). A person who has lost a limb may experience pain that seems to come from the amputated limb (see *Phantom limb*). Sometimes the person can localize the pain (e.g., to a toe, despite having had a mid-thigh amputation). See also *Endorphins; Enkephalins*.

Painful arc syndrome

A condition in which pain occurs when the arm is lifted between 45 degrees and 160 degrees away from the side of the body. Movement either side of this range is pain-free. Painful arc syndrome is usually caused by inflammation of tendons or bursae (see *Bursa*) around the shoulder joint. The pain is caused by the inflamed tendon or bursa being squeezed between the upper parts of the shoulder blade and the *humerus*.

PAIN

Pain mechanisms exist to provide a useful warning of possible injury or to caution against repeating an action that has led to injury. Certain diseases, such as arthritis and extensive cancer, may set off these same mechanisms, causing chronic pain that has no apparent function.

Reflex action

The nerve pathways that warn of noxious stimuli (through the sensation of pain) may also initiate automatic, reflex actions that help prevent harm.

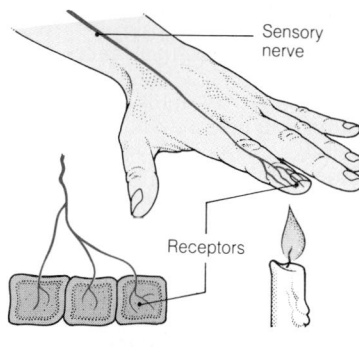

Sensory nerve

Receptors

Spinal cord

1 Receptors in the fingertip detect heat. Signals are sent along a sensory nerve to the spinal cord.

Motor nerve

Sensory nerve

Spinal cord

Ganglion

Sensory nerve

Motor nerve

Muscle

Finger

2 The signals arriving in the spinal cord pass instantaneously to a motor nerve that connects to a muscle in the arm. The signals received via the motor nerve cause the muscle in the arm to contract, moving the arm away from the source of danger (the flame).

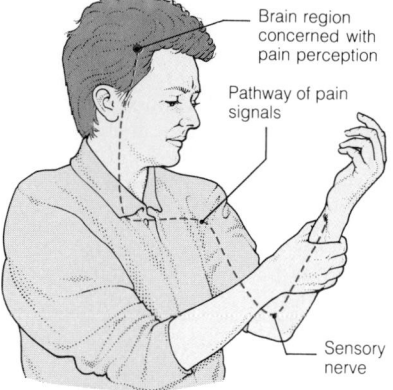

Brain region concerned with pain perception

Pathway of pain signals

Sensory nerve

Perception of pain

When an injury occurs, signals pass along nerve pathways concerned with pain, first to the spinal cord and then to the thalamus in the brain; there the pain is perceived.

REFERRED PAIN

A referred pain is one felt in a site other than an injured or diseased part. Sensory nerves from certain body areas converge before they enter the brain, causing confusion about the source of pain signals.

Tooth to ear region
A toothache may be felt in the ear, because the same sensory nerve supplies both parts.

Diaphragm to right shoulder
Inflammation of the diaphragm, often due to pneumonia, may be felt as a pain in the right shoulder.

Heart to left arm
Angina, a pain caused by reduced blood supply to the heart muscle, is often felt in the left shoulder or arm.

Knee to hip
Disorders affecting the knee, such as arthritis, may be felt as pain in the hip.

Pain message
Nerve ending
Prostaglandin
Damaged cell

Initiation of pain signals

The signals are set off by stimulation of special nerve endings—by pressure, heat, or release of chemicals, including prostaglandins, by damaged cells.

Nerve cells
Chemical transmitter
Pain signal

Signal transmission to brain

Within the brain and spinal cord, pain signals pass between nerve cells by means of chemicals that cross the gaps between the cells.

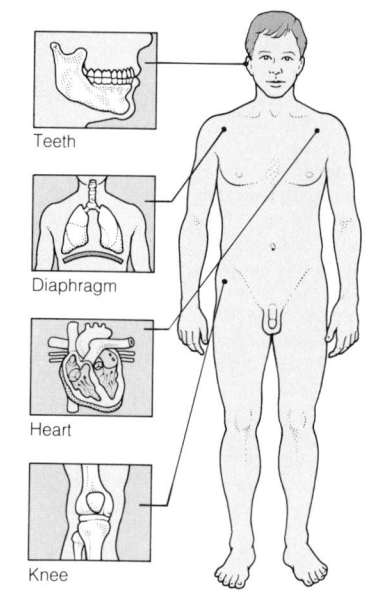

Teeth

Diaphragm

Heart

Knee

Painkillers

See *Analgesic drugs*.

Pain relief

The treatment of *pain*, usually with *analgesic drugs*. Methods of treatment depend on the severity, duration, location, and cause of the pain.

DRUG TREATMENT

Mild analgesics, available over-the-counter, are usually effective in the treatment of mild pain, such as headache, toothache, or dysmenorrhea (menstrual pain). *Acetaminophen* and *aspirin* are the most widely used drugs in this group.

Mild or moderate pain, such as that caused by arthritis or sports injuries, is often treated with a *nonsteroidal anti-inflammatory drug* (NSAID).

Severe pain, such as that caused by serious injury or kidney stones, may require treatment with a *narcotic* analgesic. Narcotic analgesics are also

P

used to prevent pain after surgery. Long-term use of narcotic analgesics may be necessary to prevent or relieve pain in cancer.

NONDRUG TREATMENT

Massage, ice packs, or *poultices* may be used for the relief of localized pain caused by muscle spasm, inflammation, or injury.

Chronic or recurrent pain that has not responded to drug treatment may be relieved by *acupuncture* or *hypnosis.*

Surgical procedures to relieve pain may be performed if all other treatments have failed. These procedures may involve destruction of nerves that transmit pain (as is done in a *cordotomy*). Alternatively, nerve fibers in the thalamus (the part of the brain that responds to pain) may be cut to prevent perception of pain.

Palate

The roof of the mouth. The palate separates the mouth from the nasal cavity. Covered with *mucous membrane*, it consists, in the front, of the hard palate, whose substructure is a plate of bone forming part of the *maxilla* (upper jaw). At the rear is the soft palate, a flap of muscle and fibrous tissue that projects into the *pharynx* (throat). During swallowing, the soft palate presses against the rear wall of the pharynx, preventing food from being regurgitated into the nose.

About one in 500 babies is born with a gap along the midline of the palate (see *Cleft lip and palate*).

Palliative treatment

Therapy that relieves the symptoms of a disorder but does not cure it. Treatment for the symptoms of widespread cancer is considered palliative.

Pallor

Abnormally pale skin, particularly of the face. Pallor may be a symptom of disease, but more often has an innocent explanation. Possible causes include a deficiency of the skin pigment *melanin*, constriction of the small blood vessels in the skin, or *anemia.*

Melanin deficiency may result from lack of exposure to the sun, occurring in people (such as nightworkers or miners) who spend very little time in daylight. A deficiency of melanin can also be hereditary when it is associated with *albinism.*

Constriction of small blood vessels in the skin may occur in response to shock, severe pain, injury, heavy blood loss, fainting, or extreme cold. Cutting off the blood flow to the skin

LOCATION OF THE PALATE
The palate forms the floor of the nasal cavity and roof of the mouth, providing a surface against which the tongue can push during chewing and swallowing.

Tongue
Nasal cavity   Hard palate   Soft palate

ensures that the brain and other vital organs are adequately supplied and that body heat is conserved. In anemia, pallor results from lack of *hemoglobin* pigment in blood vessels in the skin.

Certain kidney disorders, such as *pyelonephritis* and *renal failure,* produce a sallow appearance akin to pallor, as does *hypothyroidism.* Rare conditions that give rise to pallor include *scurvy* and lead poisoning.

Palpitation

Awareness of the heart beat.

CAUSES

A palpitation is usually felt after strenuous exercise, in tense situations, or after a severe scare, when the heart is beating harder and/or faster than normal. When experienced at rest or in a calm mood, palpitation is usually due to *ectopic heart beats* (premature beats followed by a prolonged pause) and is felt as a fluttering or thumping in the chest, sometimes with a brief but alarming sense that the heart has stopped beating. Ectopic beats do not normally indicate heart disease; they are often caused by heavy smoking, alcohol, or a large intake of caffeine.

An *arrhythmia* (irregularity of the heart beat) may cause palpitation. An example of an arrhythmia is atrial *tachycardia,* a condition in which the heart suddenly starts to beat very rapidly; the affected person may feel

faint and breathless. The pulse may be as high as 200 beats per minute but remains regular. In *atrial fibrillation,* the atria (upper chambers of the heart) beat in a disorganized manner and the impulses passed to the ventricles (lower pumping chambers) are very irregular. *Hyperthyroidism* (overactive thyroid gland) may cause palpitation by speeding up the heart beat.

DIAGNOSIS AND TREATMENT

If palpitation lasts for several hours or recurs over several days, or if it causes chest pain, breathlessness, or dizziness, a physician should be consulted as soon as possible, as there may be a serious underlying disorder. Recurrent palpitations can be investigated by means of a *Holter monitor* and *thyroid function tests.* Treatment depends on the underlying cause.

Palsy

A term applied to certain forms of *paralysis.* Examples are *cerebral palsy,* Bell's palsy (paralysis of one side of the face), and Erb's palsy (paralysis of the upper arm and shoulder on one side of the body).

Panacea

A remedy for all diseases; a cure-all. No such remedy is known, despite claims to the contrary made by numerous quacks through the ages.

Pancreas

An elongated, tapered gland that lies across the back of the abdomen, behind the stomach. Its right-hand end (called the head) is the broadest part and lies in the loop of the duodenum. Tapering from the head, the main part of the gland (the body) extends left and slightly upward; the left-hand, narrower end (the tail) terminates near the spleen.

STRUCTURE

Most of the pancreas consists of exocrine tissue, embedded in which are "nests" of endocrine cells (the islets of Langerhans). The exocrine cells secrete digestive enzymes into a network of ducts that meet to form the main pancreatic duct. This duct joins the common bile duct (which carries bile from the gallbladder) to form a small chamber, called the ampulla of Vater, that opens into the duodenum. The islets of Langerhans are surrounded by many blood vessels into which they secrete hormones.

FUNCTION

The pancreas has two functions: digestive and hormonal. The exocrine tissue secretes various digestive

P

LOCATION OF THE PANCREAS

This organ lies under the stomach, except for its head, which lies within the curve of the duodenum.

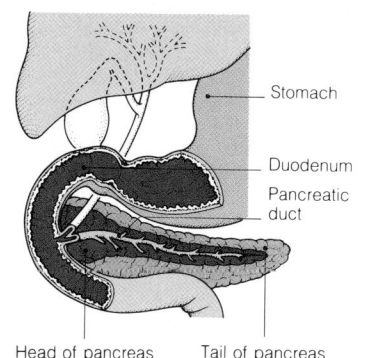

Stomach

Duodenum

Pancreatic duct

Head of pancreas   Tail of pancreas

enzymes that break down carbohydrates, fats, proteins, and nucleic acids (see *Digestive system*). Most of these enzymes are secreted in inactive form and are activated in the duodenum by other enzymes. Also secreted by the exocrine tissue is bicarbonate, which neutralizes stomach acid entering the duodenum. The endocrine cells in the islets of Langerhans secrete the hormones *insulin* and *glucagon*, which regulate the level of glucose in the blood. (See also *Pancreas* disorders box.)

Pancreas, cancer of

A malignant tumor of the exocrine tissue of the *pancreas* (the main tissue in the gland). The cause of the condition is unknown, although it has been linked to heavy smoking and to certain dietary factors, such as a high intake of fats or alcohol.

The incidence of pancreatic cancer in the US has increased threefold during the past 50 years, to about 11 per 100,000 people. Today, it is the fourth most common cancer in men, and the sixth most common in women. Approximately 80 percent of cases occur in people older than 50.

SYMPTOMS AND DIAGNOSIS

The most common symptom is pain in the upper abdomen, which often spreads to the back. Other common symptoms are appetite and weight loss, and jaundice. There may also be indigestion, nausea, vomiting, diarrhea, and tiredness. In most cases, the symptoms do not appear until the cancer is well advanced, often not until it has spread to other parts of the body (typically to the liver or lungs).

Diagnosis of pancreatic cancer usually requires *ultrasound scanning* or *CT scanning* of the upper abdomen, or endoscopic examination of the ducts of the pancreas (see *ERCP*). In some cases, the condition is detected during exploratory surgery on the abdomen (see *Laparotomy, exploratory*).

TREATMENT AND OUTLOOK

If the condition is detected in its early stages, surgical removal of the malig-

DISORDERS OF THE PANCREAS

Serious disruption of pancreatic function occurs only when the secretory tissue of the gland has been damaged or destroyed in advanced disease. The most common pancreatic disorder is *diabetes mellitus*, in which the insulin-producing cells in the gland are destroyed.

CONGENITAL AND GENETIC DISORDERS

About 85 percent of people with the genetic disorder *cystic fibrosis* produce totally inadequate quantities of pancreatic digestive enzymes, which results in *malabsorption* of fats and proteins. This, in turn, may produce steatorrhea (excess fat in the feces) and muscle wasting.

Genetic factors are thought to play some part in diabetes mellitus, although they are not the primary cause of the disease.

Chronic *pancreatitis* (inflammation of the pancreas) may, in rare cases, be hereditary; chronic pancreatitis often causes diabetes.

INFECTION

Acute pancreatitis may result from certain viral infections, especially infection with the *mumps* virus. Other viruses, such as coxsackievirus and echoviruses, may

also cause pancreatitis. In some cases, coxsackievirus infection may contribute to the development of diabetes.

TUMOR

Pancreatic cancer is one of the most common cancers in the US (see *Pancreas, cancer of*). It is difficult to diagnose and often has spread extensively by the time it is detected.

TRAUMA

Injury to the pancreas—which may result from a powerful blow to the abdomen, for example—may cause acute pancreatitis. The mechanism by which this happens is not fully established, but it is believed that pancreatic enzymes (most of which are inactive until they reach the intestine) are released within the tissue of the gland and then activated, with the result that they digest the pancreas.

POISONS AND DRUGS

Excessive alcohol intake is a common cause of pancreatitis. It can also be caused by various drugs, such as sulfa drugs, estrogens (including estrogen-containing contraceptive pills), and thiazide *diuretic drugs; corticosteroid drugs* may also cause pancreatitis.

AUTOIMMUNE DISORDERS

The cause of the damage to the pancreas in diabetes mellitus remains controversial. However, there is increasing evidence that, possibly in response to a viral infection, the body's immune system produces *antibodies* (proteins with a role in the defense against infection) that inappropriately attack and destroy the pancreatic cells.

OTHER DISORDERS

Other than alcohol overuse, the condition most commonly associated with pancreatitis is *gallstones*. They occasionally block the exit of the pancreatic duct into the duodenum, which leads to inflammation of the pancreas.

INVESTIGATION

Diagnosis of pancreatic disorders may involve *ultrasound scanning* of the abdomen, tests to measure levels of pancreatic enzymes in the blood or duodenum, and endoscopic examination of the gland (see *ERCP*).

nant tissue (see *Pancreatectomy*) along with *radiation therapy* and *anticancer drugs* may cure it. However, in most cases the cancer is not diagnosed until it is well advanced, and little can be done apart from relieving the pain with *analgesics* (painkillers), alleviating any other symptoms, and bypassing the growth if it is causing obstruction of the bile duct or bowel. In such cases, the outlook is poor; death occurs in about 90 percent of the cases within a year of diagnosis.

Pancreatectomy

Removal of all or part of the pancreas. Pancreatectomy may be performed to treat *pancreatitis* (inflammation of the pancreas), localized pancreatic cancer (see *Pancreas, cancer of*), or carcinoma of the ampulla of Vater (the small chamber formed by the union of the common bile duct and pancreatic duct that opens into the duodenum). Rarely, it is done to treat some endocrine tumors, such as *insulinomas* (*insulin*-producing tumors).

Removal of all or part of the gland depends on the disorder involved and/or on how much of the pancreas is affected. Obstruction of the pancreatic duct may require removal of only the tail of the gland (the narrower end, nearest the spleen) and the linking of the duct with a small piece of small intestine. Disease of the head of the pancreas (the broader end, situated in the loop of the duodenum) may necessitate removal of both the pancreatic head and duodenal loop (Whipple's operation).

COMPLICATIONS

Because the pancreas produces insulin and a variety of digestive enzymes, removal of the entire gland results in *diabetes mellitus* (which requires insulin therapy) and *malabsorption* (which requires oral supplements of pancreatic enzymes). Such treatment may also be necessary after a partial pancreatectomy, depending on how much function remains.

Pancreatin

A drug obtained from the pancreas of pigs and used to supplement a deficiency of pancreatic *enzymes* (proteins that stimulate digestion of nutrients).

Pancreatitis

Inflammation of the pancreas. In acute pancreatitis, the gland usually returns to normal after a single attack (although sometimes attacks recur). In chronic pancreatitis, there is permanent damage to the structure and to the function of the pancreas due to persistent inflammation, which causes fibrosis (the formation of fibrous scar tissue) in the gland.

CAUSES

The principal causes of acute pancreatitis are *gallstones* and alcohol abuse. Less commonly, pancreatitis results from a viral infection (such as *mumps*), injury (such as through surgery on the biliary tract or a blow to the abdomen), or certain drugs (such as *tetracycline*).

The most common cause of chronic pancreatitis is alcohol abuse. It may also result from *hemochromatosis* (excess iron in the body) or, rarely, it may be hereditary. In some cases, severe acute pancreatitis causes it.

SYMPTOMS AND DIAGNOSIS

Acute pancreatitis produces a sudden attack of severe upper abdominal pain, often accompanied by nausea and vomiting. The pain may spread to the back and is made worse by movement; sitting up may relieve it. An attack, which usually lasts for about 48 hours, is accompanied by the release of pancreatic enzymes into the blood; measurement of these enzymes is an important diagnostic test. *Ultrasound scanning* or *CT scanning* of the abdomen may also be performed.

Chronic pancreatitis usually produces the same symptoms as the acute form, although the pain may last from hours to several days, and attacks become more frequent as the condition progresses. However, in some cases there may be no pain and the principal signs may be *malabsorption* (due to a deficiency of pancreatic enzymes) or *diabetes mellitus* (due to insufficient *insulin* production by the pancreas). Measuring pancreatic enzyme levels in the blood is of little value in diagnosing chronic pancreatitis, although measuring the output of such enzymes into the duodenum may be useful. Abdominal X rays or scans are the principal diagnostic methods, along with endoscopic examination of the ducts of the gland (see *ERCP*) to visualize the extent of tissue damage.

COMPLICATIONS

If acute pancreatitis causes severe damage to the gland, hypotension (low blood pressure), failure of the heart, kidneys, and respiratory system, and *ascites* (accumulation of fluid in the abdomen) may occur. In some cases, cysts or abscesses may develop in the damaged gland.

Ascites and cysts may also develop as a result of chronic pancreatitis.

Other possible complications include obstruction of the common bile duct (which drains the gallbladder and joins the pancreatic duct), permanent diabetes mellitus, and blood clots in the splenic vein (which drains the spleen and pancreatic veins).

TREATMENT

There is no specific remedy for acute pancreatitis. Treatment consists of giving fluids and salts by intravenous infusion to replace those lost through vomiting; pain is relieved by giving narcotic analgesics. Nothing is given by mouth, because anything in the digestive tract stimulates pancreatic activity and makes the symptoms worse. A recurrence of the condition may be prevented by treating the underlying cause, when possible. Occasionally, surgery is necessary to remove the pancreas (see *Pancreatectomy*) or any gallstones that are blocking the drainage of pancreatic juice.

Chronic pancreatitis is treated by providing pain relief, controlling blood sugar levels by giving insulin, and giving preparations of pancreatic enzymes to correct the underproduction that the condition causes. In some cases, a pancreatectomy may be necessary to relieve pain.

Pancreatography

Imaging of the pancreas or its ducts. The methods usually used include *CT scanning*, *ultrasound scanning*, *X rays* (with a radiopaque dye) during exploratory surgery of the pancreas, and endoscopic retrograde cholangiopancreatography (see *ERCP*), an X-ray procedure in which a radiopaque dye is introduced into the ducts of the pancreas through an *endoscope* (flexible viewing tube).

Pancrelipase

A preparation of *enzymes* (proteins that stimulate chemical reactions) obtained from the pancreas of pigs.

Pancrelipase is given by mouth to supplement a deficiency of pancreatic enzymes and thus prevent *malabsorption* of fats, carbohydrates, and proteins. Deficiency may be caused by *pancreatectomy* or by disorders that affect the pancreas, such as chronic *pancreatitis*, cancer of the pancreas, and *cystic fibrosis*.

Pandemic

A medical term applied to a disease that occurs over a large geographical area (sometimes the whole world) and affects a high proportion of the population; a widespread *epidemic*.

P

Panic attack

A brief period of acute *anxiety*, often dominated by an intense fear of dying or losing one's reason. Panic attacks occur unpredictably at first, but tend to become associated with certain places, such as a crowded supermarket or a cramped elevator.

The symptoms begin suddenly and usually include a sense of breathing difficulty, chest pains, palpitations, feeling light-headed and dizzy, sweating, trembling, and faintness. *Hyperventilation* (fast, shallow breathing) often accompanies and worsens the symptoms, leading to a *pins and needles sensation*, and to feelings of *depersonalization* and *derealization*.

Most often, these symptoms are the result of underlying emotional conflicts (such as a fear of being trapped or fear of loss of dependency). Psychoanalytically, the person is often unconsciously feeling threatened by the loss of his or her relationship with the mother. Anxiety about heights may represent the fear of losing emotional support. Fear of being closed in may symbolize fear of being trapped or overwhelmed.

Although unpleasant and frightening, panic attacks last for only a few minutes, cause no physical harm, and are rarely associated with serious physical illness. The symptoms of hyperventilation may be relieved by covering the mouth and nose with a small paper bag and breathing into the bag for a few minutes.

In general, panic attacks are a symptom of *panic disorder*, *agoraphobia* (if they lead to avoidance of certain situations), or other *phobias*. Less often they are part of a *somatization disorder* or *schizophrenia*.

Panic disorder

A common form of *anxiety disorder* dominated by repeated *panic attacks* that are not caused by other illnesses or brought on by intense exercise or truly dangerous situations. A panic disorder runs a fluctuating course, tending to become worse during periods of stress. Underlying emotional anxieties cause panic reactions.

Psychotherapy is an effective treatment. Medication is often effective in treating the symptoms.

Papaverine

A *vasodilator drug* sometimes used in the treatment of patients with *peripheral vascular disease* (reduced blood supply to the legs and sometimes the arms) and in those with *transient ischemic attacks* and *impotence* of unknown cause.

Possible adverse effects of papaverine include flushing, nausea, loss of appetite, and drowsiness.

Papilla

Any small, nipple-shaped projection from the surface of a tissue, such as the mammary papilla (the nipple of the breast) and the lingual papillae (the numerous projections from the surface of the tongue, some of which contain taste buds).

Papilledema

Optic disk edema (swelling of the head of the optic nerve) caused by a rise in pressure within the brain. Papilledema, which is visible through an *ophthalmoscope*, may be a sign of a *brain tumor*.

Papilloma

A usually nonmalignant tumor, often resembling a wart, that arises from *epithelium* (the cell layer that forms the skin and mucous membranes, and that lines most of the hollow organs of the body). Although papillomas may develop from epithelium anywhere in the body, they are most common on the skin, tongue, or larynx (voice box), and in the urinary tract, digestive tract, or breasts.

Skin papilloma
This harmless type of growth is common in elderly people. It can easily be snipped off at skin level and the base cauterized.

Pap smear

See *Cervical smear test*.

Papule

A small, solid, slightly raised area of skin. Papules are usually less than half an inch (1 cm) in diameter and may be rounded or flat, with a smooth or warty texture. Papules may be the color of surrounding skin or pigmented. Many skin conditions, including *acne* and *lichen planus*, start as papules.

Par-/para-

Prefixes with several meanings: beside or beyond, as in the parathyroid glands (which are situated behind the thyroid at its sides); closely related to or closely resembling, as in paratyphoid fever (a disease that is similar to typhoid); faulty or abnormal, as in paresthesia (abnormal sensation); or associated with an accessory capacity, as in paramedical workers (personnel who supplement the work of physicians).

Para-aminobenzoic acid

The active ingredient in many *sunscreen* preparations, commonly abbreviated to PABA.

Paracentesis

A procedure in which a body cavity is punctured with a needle from the outside. Paracentesis is most often performed to remove fluid for analysis to aid diagnosis of conditions causing *ascites*, in which fluid collects in the abdominal cavity. It may also be performed to relieve pressure due to excess fluid or to instill drugs. Abdominal or thoracic paracentesis is most common, but other sites include the pericardium and the scrotum.

The procedure is usually carried out using local anesthesia; it is quick and relatively painless.

Paraffinoma

A tumorlike swelling under the skin caused by prolonged exposure to paraffin. Paraffinomas may occur in the lungs due to inhalation of paraffin, usually in someone who uses liquid paraffin as a laxative. They were once an uncommon side effect of augmentation *mammoplasty* (enlargement of the breast) when paraffin wax was used in this operation.

Paraldehyde

An unpleasant-smelling hypnotic sedative that has been used in the treatment of alcohol withdrawal. Paraldehyde is administered as an enema or by injection. This drug dissolves plastic, so a glass syringe must be used to inject it.

Paralysis

Complete or partial loss of controlled movement caused by the inability to contract one or more muscles. Weakness, rather than complete loss of movement, is often referred to as *paresis*. Paralysis may be temporary or permanent, and can affect a range of muscles—from a small facial muscle to

P

many of the major muscles in the body. Loss of feeling in the affected parts may accompany the inability to move them.

TYPES
Paralysis of one half of the body is called *hemiplegia*; paralysis of all four limbs and the trunk is called *quadriplegia*. *Paraplegia* is paralysis of both legs and sometimes part of the trunk. *Palsy* is an outdated general term for paralysis; it is still used in the names of certain disorders (such as *cerebral palsy*).

Paralysis may be flaccid, which gives the limbs a floppy appearance, or spastic, in which case the affected parts of the body are rigid.

CAUSES
Muscles that control movement of the body are stimulated to contract by impulses originating in the motor cortex of the brain; they travel via the spinal cord and peripheral nerves to reach the muscle. Paralysis may be caused by any form of injury or disorder anywhere along this nerve pathway, or by a muscle disorder.

BRAIN DISORDERS A very common cause of paralysis is a *stroke*, in which damage to part of the brain is caused by bleeding from or blood clotting in a blood vessel that supplies that area of the brain. Because motor fibers cross in the brain stem, paralysis occurs on the side opposite to the site of the brain damage.

Hemiplegia can be caused by any brain disorder in which the portion of the brain that controls movement is damaged—by a *brain tumor*, *brain abscess*, *brain hemorrhage*, *cerebral palsy*, or *encephalitis* (brain infection).

Some forms of paralysis are caused by damage to those parts of the nervous system concerned with the fine control of movement (such as the *cerebellum* and *basal ganglia*). *Parkinson's disease* is caused by lack of dopamine in the basal ganglia.

SPINAL CORD DISORDERS Paralysis can be caused by damage to the spinal cord from a fractured spine caused by a motor vehicle accident. Pressure on the spinal cord may cause paralysis in *disk prolapse* or *cervical osteoarthritis*. Muscles supplied by nerves below the damaged area are affected.

Diseases affecting nerves in the spinal cord (e.g., *multiple sclerosis*, *poliomyelitis*, *myelitis*, *Friedreich's ataxia*, *meningitis*, and *motor neuron disease*) may also cause paralysis.

PERIPHERAL NERVE DISORDERS A range of disorders (known as *neuropathies*) affects the peripheral nerves and causes paralysis of varying degrees. A neuropathy may be caused by a variety of conditions, including *diabetes mellitus*, vitamin deficiency, liver disease, cancer, and the toxic effects of some drugs or metals (such as lead); it may also occur as an inherited disorder.

A type of neuropathy that often causes paralysis of the shoulder, arm, or hand is injury to the *brachial plexus* (a collection of nerves that serves the arm and hand).

MUSCLE DISORDERS *Muscular dystrophy* causes progressive muscular weakness and may lead to paralysis. Temporary paralysis sometimes occurs in *myasthenia gravis*.

TREATMENT
The underlying cause is treated if possible. *Physical therapy* is used to prevent joints from becoming locked into useless positions, which is important in both temporary and permanent paralysis. When the paralysis is temporary (such as in a mild stroke), physical therapy is used to retrain and strengthen the muscles and joints so that some degree of mobility is possible after recovery.

For paralyzed people confined to bed or a wheelchair, nursing care is essential to avoid complications (such as bedsores, deep vein thrombosis, urinary tract infections, constipation, and limb deformities) of prolonged *immobility*. In addition, various aids are available to help the totally or partially paralyzed person.

Paralysis, periodic

A rare, inherited condition that affects young people. Periodic paralysis is characterized by episodes of weakness and paralysis of limb muscles that may last from a few minutes to two days, occurring every six weeks or so. The attacks often begin during the night and wake the sufferer.

The exact cause of periodic paralysis is unknown, although, in many cases, there is a drop in the level of potassium (which is essential for normal muscle function) in the blood. A meal that is rich in carbohydrates often triggers an attack.

The frequency of attacks can be lessened by reducing the intake of carbohydrates and by taking *acetazolamide* or other potassium-sparing, weak *diuretic drugs*. An episode can sometimes be curtailed by taking potassium or by gentle exercise at the first sign of muscle weakness. The condition often disappears without treatment by the age of 30.

Paramedic

A person trained to provide emergency resuscitation after an accident or when someone has collapsed from a myocardial infarction (heart attack) or other medical condition. Paramedics work from ambulances and in the emergency room.

The term is also used as an abbreviation for paramedical, to describe any health care worker other than a physician, nurse, dentist, or podiatrist. Examples of paramedical staff include physical therapists, X-ray technologists, and laboratory technicians.

Paranoia

A condition whose central feature is the *delusion* (a false idea not amenable to reasoned argument) that people or events are in some way specially related to oneself. The term is also used popularly to describe a person's feelings of persecution.

A person suffering from paranoia gradually builds up an elaborate set of beliefs based on the interpretation of chance remarks or events. Typical themes include persecution, jealousy (see *Jealousy, morbid*), love, and grandeur (belief in one's own superior position and powers).

TYPES AND CAUSES
Psychoanalytically, paranoia stems from deep, underlying insecurity. Chronic paranoia may result from brain damage, amphetamine or alcohol abuse, *schizophrenia*, or *manic-depressive illness*. The condition is especially likely to develop in people with paranoid *personality disorder*—suspicious, oversensitive people who seem emotionally cold and take offense easily.

Acute paranoia, lasting for less than six months, may occur in people who have experienced radical changes in their environment, such as immigrants, refugees, people entering military service, or people leaving home for the first time.

In shared paranoia (folie à deux), delusion develops as a result of a close relationship with someone who already has a delusion.

SYMPTOMS
Feelings and activities often seem relatively normal in that they are appropriate for the beliefs held. There are usually no other symptoms of mental illness apart from occasional *hallucinations*. However, anger, suspiciousness, and social isolation mark an increasing change in the person toward difficult and eccentric behavior. Paranoid individuals rarely

P

see themselves as ill and usually receive treatment only when brought by friends or relatives.

TREATMENT AND OUTCOME

When acute illness is treated early with *antipsychotic drugs*, the outlook is good. In chronic disorders, delusions are usually firmly entrenched, although antipsychotic drugs may make them less prominent. However, long-term control through medication is difficult in someone with poor insight into his or her illness.

Paraparesis

Partial *paralysis* or weakness of both legs and sometimes part of the trunk.

Paraphilia

See *Deviation, sexual.*

Paraphimosis

Constriction of the penis behind the glans (head) by an extremely tight foreskin that has been retracted (pulled back), causing swelling and pain. Paraphimosis often occurs as a complication of *phimosis* (an abnormally tight foreskin).

Often the foreskin can be returned to its normal position manually. The swelling in the glans may be reduced by first applying an ice pack and then squeezing the glans. If manual return proves impossible, an operation to cut the foreskin (using a general anesthetic) or an injection may be necessary. *Circumcision* (surgical removal of the foreskin) is usually required to prevent recurrence.

Paraplegia

Weakness or *paralysis* of both legs, and sometimes part of the trunk; it is often accompanied by loss of sensation and by loss of urinary control.

Paraplegia is a result of nerve damage in the brain or spinal cord. It is usually caused by a motor vehicle or sports accident, a fall, or gunshot wounds. Twice as many men as women are victims, and the incidence is highest between the ages of 19 and 35 years.

Parapsychology

The branch of psychology dealing with experiences and events that cannot be accounted for by scientific understanding. Such paranormal phenomena include telepathy (communicating thoughts from one person's mind to another), telekinesis (the movement of objects simply by thinking), clairvoyance (the ability to "see" events at a distance without

using one's eyes), and precognition (being able to see into the future). These are all forms of extrasensory perception (ESP).

The basis of most paranormal experiences can probably be explained by various brain disorders (see *Brain disorders box*) and mental disturbances. Thought broadcasting (in which individuals have the impression that their thoughts can be heard by others) is a common symptom of *schizophrenia.*

Other apparently paranormal experiences are a result of coincidence or self-deception, while some, such as psychic surgery (removal of objects from the body apparently without an incision), are no more than sleight-of-hand trickery.

Paraquat

A poisonous defoliant weedkiller that, if swallowed, causes respiratory failure, acute or progressive lung damage, and kidney failure, which

may be fatal. The main symptom of paraquat poisoning is difficulty breathing. It may be severe, depending on the amount swallowed.

If paraquat poisoning is known or suspected, medical help should be obtained immediately. First-aid treatment consists of having the victim eat charcoal or fuller's earth (a clay-containing earthy substance), which inactivate paraquat.

In some cases, medical treatment may include hemodialysis (removal of toxic substances from the blood, see *Dialysis*) and other measures to remove the chemical from the body.

If paraquat has been splashed into the eyes or onto the skin, it should be washed away immediately with plenty of water.

Marijuana is sometimes contaminated with paraquat. Smoking it can cause any or all of the following: stinging eyes, a burning sensation in the mouth and throat, vomiting, and mouth ulcers.

PARASITES

Head louse	Bedbug	Cat flea	Tapeworm	Hookworm

ECTOPARASITES (present in skin or on body surface)

Common examples	Activities	How acquired
Head lice Ticks Bedbugs Cat fleas Aquatic leeches	Suck host's blood.	Through contact with other people (lice, scabies mites, warts), animals (ringworm fungi, ticks), vegetation (ticks, mites), water (aquatic leeches), or locker-room floors (some fungi). Bedbugs live in bedroom walls or mattresses and visit their host at night. Cat and dog fleas may visit humans when the pet is absent.
Scabies mites	Burrow in skin.	
Ringworm fungi	Multiply in skin.	
Wart viruses		

ENDOPARASITES (live within body)

Tapeworms Flukes Roundworms Pinworms Hookworms	Adults live in human gut, blood vessels, bile ducts, or elsewhere and produce eggs that are passed out of body.	By eating infected meat, swallowing eggs on food, contaminating fingers with fecal material, or contact with infected water.
Various disease-causing protozoa, fungi, bacteria, and viruses	Organisms multiply locally or spread throughout the body, causing disease.	By inhalation, water- or food-borne transmission, sexual transmission, or blood-borne infection, among other mechanisms.

P

Parasite

Any organism living in or on any other living creature and deriving advantage from doing so, while causing disadvantage to the host. The parasite satisfies its nutritional requirements from the host's blood or tissues or from the host's diet, which allows the parasite to reproduce and multiply.

Parasites may remain permanently with their host or may spend only part of their life cycles in association. Some cause few symptoms, others cause disease and even death of the host.

Animal parasites of humans include various *protozoa* (single-celled animals), *worms*, *flukes*, *leeches*, *lice*, *ticks*, and *mites*. *Viruses* and disease-causing *fungi* and *bacteria* are also essentially parasites. Some types of bacteria actually benefit their hosts (by helping to control the populations of more harmful organisms), so they are not strictly parasites.

Parasitology

The scientific study of organisms that treat others as their living environment (see *Parasite*), especially the study of their life cycles and reproductive behavior, the ways in which they cause disease, and their susceptibility to drug treatment and other methods used to halt their multiplication. Although viruses and many types of bacteria and fungi are parasites, their study is conducted under the general title of *microbiology*.

Medical parasitology is concerned primarily with animal parasites of humans, especially the protozoa, worms, flukes, and arthropod parasites (insects and related animals) such as lice and the scabies mite.

Parasuicide

See *Suicide, attempted*.

Parasympathetic nervous system

One of the two divisions of the *autonomic nervous system*. In conjunction with the other division (the sympathetic nervous system), the parasympathetic system controls the involuntary activities of the organs, glands, blood vessels, and other tissues in the body.

Parathion

An agricultural organophosphate insecticide that is highly poisonous to both humans and animals. Poisoning may occur by absorption through the skin, inhalation, or swallowing and is most common in agricultural workers.

Symptoms of poisoning include nausea, vomiting, abdominal cramps, involuntary defecation and urination, excessive salivation and sweating, blurred vision, headache, confusion, and muscle twitching. If poisoning is severe, there may also be difficulty breathing, palpitations, seizures, and unconsciousness. Without treatment, parathion poisoning may be fatal.

If parathion has been swallowed, treatment consists of inducing vomiting or washing out the stomach (see *Lavage, gastric*). If poisoning occurred through skin absorption, clothing is removed and contaminated areas of skin are thoroughly washed. To counteract the effects of the poison, injections of atropine and pralidoxime may be given. It may also be necessary to support breathing by giving oxygen and/or artificial ventilation. With rapid treatment, many people survive doses of parathion much greater than the usual fatal dose.

Parathyroidectomy

The surgical removal of abnormal parathyroid tissue. Parathyroidectomy may be performed to treat *hyperparathyroidism* (excess secretion of parathyroid hormone) when it is caused by an *adenoma* (a small, benign tumor) of a parathyroid gland or, less commonly, by overgrowth of all of the glands or by parathyroid cancer.

In the case of an adenoma, usually only one of the glands is involved and requires removal. If all glands are enlarged and overactive, all but a whole gland or a half of a gland may require excision (cutting out). Removal of all parathyroid tissue leads to a dangerously low level of calcium in the blood and the condition of *tetany* (painful, cramplike spasms).

The operation is performed using general anesthesia. An incision is made in the neck, just beneath the Adam's apple. A section of suspected abnormal tissue is taken and examined to decide how much should be removed. It is then cut out, and the incision sewn up.

The average hospital stay for the operation is less than a week. Patients can expect complete healing without complications, although some people need treatment for *hypoparathyroidism*.

Parathyroid glands

Two pairs of oval, pea-sized glands, located adjacent to the two lobes of the thyroid gland in the neck. Occasionally, only one or (rarely) an extra gland is present in the neck or chest.

LOCATION OF THE PARATHYROID GLANDS These glands, situated near the thyroid, keep blood calcium levels within close limits.

Thyroid cartilage
Thyroid gland
Superior parathyroid glands
Inferior parathyroid gland
Trachea

FUNCTION

The glands produce parathyroid hormone, which helps control the level of calcium in the blood. This requires constant regulation, since even small variations from normal can impair muscle and nerve function.

If the blood's calcium level drops, the parathyroid glands respond by increasing their output of hormone. This causes the bones to release more calcium into the blood, the intestines to absorb more from food, and the kidneys to conserve calcium. These actions quickly restore the blood calcium level. If the blood level of calcium rises too high, the glands reduce their output of hormone, reversing the above processes.

In rare cases, the glands may become overactive (see *Hyperparathyroidism*), causing thinning of the bones (*osteoporosis*) and *calculi* in the urinary tract. In other cases, the glands become underactive (see *Hypoparathyroidism*), resulting in painful spasms or seizures.

Parathyroid tumor

A growth within one of the parathyroid glands. A parathyroid tumor may result in excess secretion of parathyroid hormone into the bloodstream, leading to the symptoms of *hyperparathyroidism*.

Most parathyroid tumors are benign *adenomas*. Cancers of the parathyroid are very rare (with an incidence of less than one per 100,000 population per year) and are not highly malignant, although occasionally they may spread to other organs in the body.

When a tumor is causing hyperparathyroidism, it is surgically removed (see *Parathyroidectomy*). If the tumor is an adenoma, surgery usually gives a complete cure. Occasionally the tumor may recur or, after surgery, the patient may need treatment for *hypoparathyroidism*.

In people who have parathyroid cancer, surgery allows long-term survival without recurrence, provided the entire tumor can be completely removed before it has spread.

Paratyphoid fever

An illness identical in most respects to *typhoid fever*, except that it is caused by a slightly different bacterium, SALMONELLA PARATYPHI, and is usually less severe. The causative organism is spread in a similar way to the typhoid bacterium, but long-term carriers of infection are less common.

Parenchyma

The functional tissue of an organ, as distinct from accessory structures such as the framework (*stroma*) and the fibrous outer layer (capsule) that holds the organ together.

Parenteral

A term applied to the administration of drugs or other substances by any route other than via the gastrointestinal tract (e.g., by injection into a blood vessel or muscle or by suppository into the vagina).

Parenteral nutrition

See *Feeding, artificial*.

Paresis

Partial *paralysis* or weakness of one or several muscles.

Paresthesia

Altered sensation in the skin that causes *numbness* or tingling (see *Pins and needles sensation*).

Parietal

A medical term that refers to the wall of a body cavity or organ, as in the parietal peritoneum (the membrane that lines the walls of the abdomen and pelvis and the underside of the diaphragm), or to the parietal bones

(the two joined bones that form much of the top, sides, and upper back part of the skull), as in the parietal lobes of the brain (the parts of the cerebral hemispheres that are covered by the parietal bones).

Parkinsonism

A neurologic disorder characterized by a masklike face, rigidity, and slowness of movements. The most common type, which is of unknown cause, is *Parkinson's disease*.

Known causes of parkinsonism include *antipsychotic drugs*, the rare *encephalitis lethargica* infection, *carbon monoxide* poisoning, *cerebrovascular disease*, and the use of certain *designer drugs* of abuse.

Parkinson's disease

A brain disorder that causes muscle tremor, stiffness, and weakness. The characteristic signs are trembling, a rigid posture, slow movements, and a shuffling, unbalanced walk.

CAUSE OF PARKINSON'S DISEASE

This disorder results from damage, of unknown origin, to the basal ganglia (nerve cell clusters in the brain). The difference between the healthy state and Parkinson's disease is shown below.

Healthy state
During movement, signals pass from the brain's cortex, via reticular formation and spinal cord (pathway A), to muscles, which contract. Other signals pass, by pathway B, to the basal ganglia; these damp the signals in pathway A, reducing muscle tone so that movement is not jerky. Dopamine, a nerve transmitter made in the basal ganglia, is needed for this damping effect. Another transmitter, acetylcholine, inhibits the damping effect.

Parkinson's disease
In Parkinson's disease, degeneration of parts of the basal ganglia causes a lack of dopamine within this part of the brain. The basal ganglia are thus prevented from modifying the nerve pathways that control muscle contraction. As a result, the muscles are overly tense, causing tremor, joint rigidity, and slow movement. Most drug treatments increase the level of dopamine in the brain or oppose the action of acetylcholine.

P

CAUSES AND INCIDENCE

Parkinson's disease is caused by degeneration of or damage to nerve cells within the *basal ganglia* in the brain. The way this affects muscle tension and movement is shown in the illustrated box at left.

About one person in 200 (mostly elderly) is affected by the disease, with 50,000 new cases a year in the US. Men are more likely to be affected than women. The incidence of Parkinson's disease is lower among smokers.

SYMPTOMS AND SIGNS

The disease usually begins as a slight tremor of one hand, arm, or leg. In the early stages, the tremor is worse when the hand or limb is at rest; when it is used, the shaking virtually stops.

Later, the disease affects both sides of the body and causes stiffness and weakness, as well as trembling, of the muscles. Symptoms include a stiff, shuffling, overbalancing walk that may break into uncontrollable, tiny, running steps; a constant trembling of the hands, more marked at rest and sometimes accompanied by shaking of the head; a permanent rigid stoop; and an unblinking, fixed expression. Eating, washing, dressing, and other everyday activities gradually become very difficult to manage.

The intellect is unaffected until late in the disease, although speech may become slow and hesitant; handwriting usually becomes very small. Depression is common.

TREATMENT

Although there is no cure for Parkinson's disease, much can be done for sufferers to improve their morale and mobility through exercise, special aids in the home, and encouragement. Organizations exist to provide help and advice for sufferers and their families. This is often all that is needed in the early stages of the disease.

Later, treatment is with drugs, which minimize symptoms but cannot halt the degeneration of brain cells. Such treatment is often complex because several different types of drugs may need to be administered in various combinations.

Levodopa, which the body converts into dopamine, is usually the most effective drug and is often the first drug tried. The beneficial effects of levodopa often suddenly wear off, when another drug usually can be given; levodopa usually can be successfully reintroduced some weeks later.

Drugs used in conjunction with or as substitutes for levodopa include bromocriptine and amantadine. Other drugs that provide effective relief for specific symptoms, such as tremor, include *anticholinergic drugs*.

Occasionally, an operation on the brain may be performed to reduce the tremor and rigidity. This operation is reserved for relatively young, active sufferers who are otherwise in good health and who are in the early stages of the illness.

OUTLOOK

Untreated, the disease progresses over 10 to 15 years to severe weakness and incapacity. However, with modern drug treatment, a person suffering from Parkinson's disease can obtain considerable relief from the illness and a much improved quality of life. About one third of patients do eventually show signs of *dementia*.

Experimentation with transplantation of dopamine-secreting adrenal tissue is now taking place.

Paronychia

An infection of the skin fold at the base of the nail. Paronychia is usually caused by *CANDIDA ALBICANS* (a yeast), although in some cases bacteria are responsible.

The condition is most common in women—particularly those who have poor circulation and whose work involves frequent hand washing. Paronychia is also likely to develop in people with skin disease that affects the nail fold.

Treatment is with *antifungal drugs* or *antibiotic drugs*. It is important to keep the hands as dry as possible (by wearing rubber gloves for wet work and by drying the hands thoroughly each time they are washed). If an abscess forms, it may be drained surgically.

Parotid glands

The largest of the three pairs of *salivary glands* (the other two are the sublingual glands and submandibular glands). The parotid glands lie, one on each side, above the angle of the jaw, below and in front of the ear. The parotid glands continuously secrete saliva, which passes along the duct of the gland and into the mouth through an opening in the inner cheek, level with the second upper molar tooth. The output of saliva is increased substantially by thinking about or seeing food.

DISORDERS

Certain conditions, including *dehydration* and *Sjögren's syndrome*, may cause reduced secretion of saliva by the gland, resulting in a dry mouth (see *Mouth, dry*).

LOCATION OF THE PAROTID GLANDS

The glands are situated deep in the angle of the jaw and secrete saliva into the mouth. Mumps is a viral infection of the glands.

Parotid duct
Parotid gland

Parotitis, inflammation of the gland, is usually due to infection with the mumps virus but may also be caused by a bacterial infection due to poor oral hygiene, by dehydration, or by severe illness. In some cases, an *abscess* forms in the inflamed gland.

Calculi (stones) may block the duct of the parotid gland, causing a painful swelling of the gland. Painless enlargement may be caused by *sarcoidosis*, *tuberculosis*, a *lymphoma*, or a benign tumor. Rarely, carcinoma (a type of malignant tumor) of the gland causes a hard, painful growth.

Paroxysm

A sudden attack, worsening, or recurrence of symptoms or of a disease; a *spasm* or *seizure*.

Parturition

The process of giving birth (see *Childbirth*).

Passive-aggressive personality disorder

Failure to keep up with tasks at home or at work as a result of passive resistance to demands for improved performance rather than of active refusal to cooperate. People with the disorder may delay or "forget" to perform tasks, or be deliberately inefficient. Their resulting ineffectiveness and unreliability prevents promotion at work and interferes with social func-

P

tioning. Depression often compounds the problem. Hidden aggression is thought to be the cause of passive-aggressive personality disorder.

Pasteurization

The process of heating foods, usually milk and milk products, to destroy or retard the development of pathogenic (disease-causing) microorganisms and thus protect against putrefaction and fermentation.

The process is named for its inventor, the French scientist Louis Pasteur (1822-1895).

Pasteurization consists of heating food to a moderate temperature for a specific period, then cooling it rapidly. For example, milk is heated to between 145°F and 150°F (63°C and 66°C) for 30 minutes, then its temperature is raised to 161°F (72°C) for 15 seconds, and finally it is quickly cooled. This process does not sterilize the milk, but it does destroy most types of pathogenic microorganisms. Pasteurization has been an important factor in dramatically decreasing the incidence of milk-borne diseases, such as tuberculosis.

Patella

The medical name for the kneecap, the triangular bone at the front of the knee joint. The patella is held in position by the *quadriceps muscle* (at the front of the thigh), the lower end of which surrounds the patella and is attached to the upper part of the tibia (shin) by the patellar tendon. The patella protects the knee.

DISORDERS

Dislocation of the patella is usually due to a congenital abnormality, such as underdevelopment of the lower end of the femur (thigh bone) or excessive laxity of ligaments that support the knee. Fracture is usually caused by a direct blow.

Inflammation and roughening of the undersurface of the patella, resulting in knee pain that worsens when bending the knee or climbing stairs, is caused by *chondromalacia patellae* in adolescents and by retropatellar inflammation in adults.

Patent

In medicine, a term meaning open or unobstructed, as in *patent ductus arteriosus*, a condition in which the ductus arteriosus (a blood vessel that enables blood to bypass the lungs in the fetus) remains open after birth. The term patent is also applied to nonprescription medications.

Patent ductus arteriosus

A type of heart defect present at birth.

CAUSES AND INCIDENCE

The ductus arteriosus is a channel between the pulmonary artery and the aorta (two large vessels emerging from the heart) through which, in the fetus, blood pumped by the right side of the heart is able to bypass the lungs (see *Fetal circulation*).

The duct usually closes at or shortly after birth so blood will go to the lungs. However, in some babies born prematurely or with breathing difficulties, this closure fails to happen. Some of the blood pumped by the left side of the heart and intended for the body is misdirected via the duct to the lungs. As a result, the heart must work harder to pump sufficient blood to the body.

Patent ductus arteriosus accounts for about 8 percent of all heart defects present from birth (see *Heart disease, congenital*), affecting about 60 babies per 100,000.

SYMPTOMS AND SIGNS

Usually, the defect is not severe enough to cause symptoms. Occasionally, however, when a large amount of blood is misdirected, strain is placed on the heart; as a result, the baby fails to gain weight, becomes short of breath on exertion, and has frequent chest infections. Eventually, *heart failure* (reduced pumping efficiency) may develop. Bacterial *endocarditis* (inflammation of the lining of the heart) is a common complication of patent ductus arteriosus.

DIAGNOSIS AND TREATMENT

The diagnosis is made by a physician listening to the heart with a stethoscope (the defect produces a characteristic *murmur*), from *chest X rays*, and from an *ECG* (electrocardiogram) and *echocardiography*.

The drug indomethacin often causes the duct to close in premature babies. If this treatment fails, the channel is closed surgically. The operation is straightforward, carries little risk, and enables the child to thrive normally.

Paternity testing

The use of blood tests to help decide whether a particular man is or is not the father of a particular child. Tests are carried out on blood samples taken from the child, from the man who is suspected to be the father, and, if available, from the child's mother.

WHY IT IS DONE

The investigation may be requested, or ordered by a court, in any of various legal situations in which the paternity of a child is disputed.

HOW IT IS DONE

The blood tests are performed by a special investigator, who examines the samples for the presence of various genetically determined substances. These substances may include proteins found on the surface of red blood cells that determine *blood groups*, other proteins in the blood plasma, *histocompatibility antigens*, and short lengths of *DNA*, the genetic material itself. Comparison of these genetic markers in the different blood samples can provide useful information. For example, if a particular marker is present in the child but not in the mother, it must be determined by a gene present in the real father. If the man claimed to be the father does not display this marker in his blood, he can be excluded from paternity.

Techniques have advanced to the stage where it is now possible, through extensive tests, to exclude a wrongly named father in nearly 100 percent of cases. Until recently, it was never possible to prove beyond reasonable doubt that a man was the father of a particular child; the new technique of DNA fingerprinting (see illustrated box opposite) changes this situation almost beyond doubt. Using this technique, an investigator may be able to state that the similarities between a man's and a child's DNA could have occurred by chance with a probability of just one in 30 billion—which would amount to positive proof of paternity.

Patho-

A prefix denoting a relationship to disease, as in pathogen, a disease-causing agent.

Pathogen

Any agent, particularly a *microorganism*, that causes disease.

Pathogenesis

The processes by which a disease (or disorder) originates and develops. Pathogenesis applies particularly to the cellular and physiological events involved in these processes.

Pathognomonic

A medical term applied to a symptom or sign that is itself characteristic of a specific disease or disorder, and is therefore sufficient to establish a diagnosis. Koplik's spots (small red spots with white centers) on the lining of the mouth are pathognomonic of measles.

PATERNITY TESTING USING DNA FINGERPRINTS

A new method of paternity testing, DNA fingerprinting, is replacing older techniques because it gives a decisive result in more cases.

Blood samples are taken from the mother, child, and suspected father, and some DNA (hereditary material) from each is specially processed.

PATERNITY ESTABLISHED

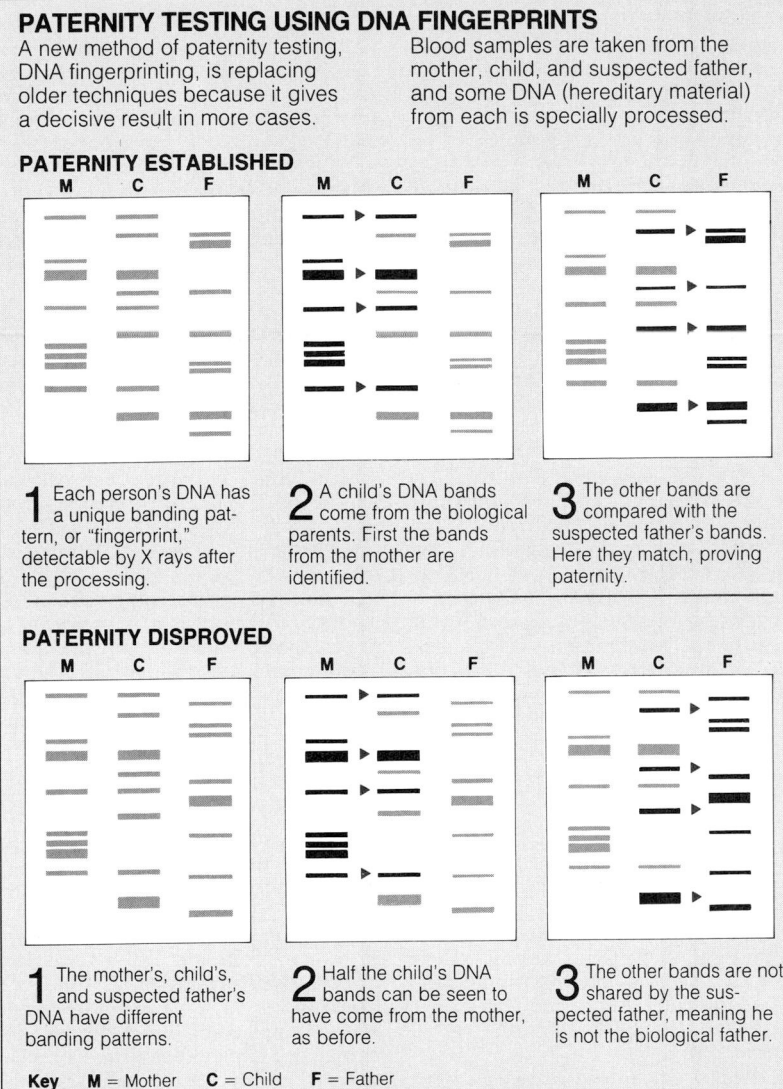

1 Each person's DNA has a unique banding pattern, or "fingerprint," detectable by X rays after the processing.

2 A child's DNA bands come from the biological parents. First the bands from the mother are identified.

3 The other bands are compared with the suspected father's bands. Here they match, proving paternity.

PATERNITY DISPROVED

1 The mother's, child's, and suspected father's DNA have different banding patterns.

2 Half the child's DNA bands can be seen to have come from the mother, as before.

3 The other bands are not shared by the suspected father, meaning he is not the biological father.

Key **M** = Mother **C** = Child **F** = Father

Pathological

Relating to disease or to *pathology* (the study of disease).

Pathologist

A physician who conducts the laboratory studies of tissues and cells that help other physicians reach accurate diagnoses and who supervises other laboratory personnel in the testing and microscopic examination of blood and other body fluids. Pathologists also conduct *autopsies*. (See also *Pathology*.)

Pathology

The study of disease, its causes, mechanisms, and effects on the body.

Various factors can cause pathological changes in tissues and cells. These factors include pathogens (disease-causing microorganisms), poisonous chemicals, radiation, *inflammation*, degeneration (see *Degenerative disorders*), the accumulation of abnormal substances (see *Infiltrate*), metabolic defects (see *Metabolism, inborn errors of*), *nutritional disorders*, and *carcinogens* (agents that cause *cancer*).

The study of the pathological changes that occur in cells is known as cytopathology (a branch of *cytology*); histopathology (a branch of *histology*) is concerned with changes in tissues. Both rely on examining cell or tissue samples under the *microscope*.

It was the growth of postmortem pathology in the 18th and 19th centuries that formed the basis of modern scientific medicine. Study of the body after death enabled a patient's symptoms to be linked with observable changes in the internal organs. It also made it possible for physicians to assess the accuracy of their diagnoses and the effects of their treatment.

Pathology, cellular

Also called cytopathology, the branch of *cytology* concerned with the effects of disease on cells.

Pathophysiology

The study of the effects of disease on body functions (e.g., how bronchitis impairs lung function).

-pathy

A suffix that denotes a disease or disorder, as in myopathy, any disorder of the muscles. The suffix -opathy is synonymous with -pathy.

Peak flow meter

A piece of equipment that measures the maximum speed at which air can flow out of the lungs. Because narrowed airways slow the rate at which air can be forced from the lungs, a peak flow meter is useful in assessing the severity of *bronchospasm* (narrowing of the airways in the lungs).

The most common use of a peak flow meter is to monitor patients with *asthma* and to assess their response to treatment with *bronchodilator drugs*. It is also useful to confirm whether people who suffer from intermittent coughing or breathing difficulty without wheezing have asthma.

People with asthma are encouraged to measure their peak flow every day as a means of monitoring their health, just as diabetics measure their blood sugar level. A diary of readings is kept to record the difference in airflow when symptoms are present and during other times in the day.

The peak flow is measured by taking a deep breath in and then breathing out with maximum effort through the mouthpiece of the meter.

Peau d'orange

A condition in which the skin resembles orange peel. The skin remains a normal color but develops a dimpled appearance due to retention of fluid in the nearby lymph vessels. Causes of blockage of the lymph vessels include *breast cancer* in the region of the nipple and *elephantiasis*.

P

Pectoral

A medical term that means relating to the chest, as in the major and minor pectoral muscles.

The pectoralis major is a large, fan-shaped muscle that covers much of the upper part of the front of the chest; it arises from the sternum (breastbone) and cartilages of the second to sixth ribs, and converges on the humerus (upper arm bone) just below the shoulder. Its main function is to move the arm across the body.

The pectoralis minor is a smaller, triangular muscle that underlies the pectoralis major; it arises from the third to fifth ribs, and converges on the scapula (shoulder blade), which it moves down and forward.

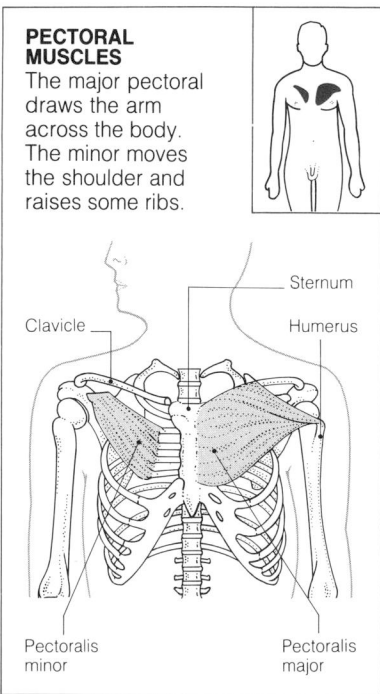

PECTORAL MUSCLES
The major pectoral draws the arm across the body. The minor moves the shoulder and raises some ribs.

Sternum
Clavicle
Humerus
Pectoralis minor
Pectoralis major

Pediatrician

A specialist in the care of children from infancy through adolescence (usually to age 18, occasionally into the early 20s). Pediatricians advise on the care of the child and conduct periodic "well baby" examinations to assess general health and detect any problems. They also give vaccinations and treat childhood disorders. (See also *Neonatologist*.)

Pediatrics

The branch of medicine concerned with the growth and development of children, and the diagnosis, treatment, and prevention of childhood diseases. Special aspects of pediatrics include the care of newborn infants and disabled children.

Pedicle

A stemlike structure by which some tumors are attached to tissue and through which they receive their blood supply. Also called pedicles are the two bars of bone that extend backward from the body of each vertebra and form the sides of the bony arch that surrounds the spinal cord.

Pediculosis

Any type of louse infestation. (See *Lice; Pubic lice*.)

Pedophilia

An illegal sexual perversion in which sexual activity with a prepubertal child is the preferred recurrent means of reaching orgasm. Pedophiles are almost exclusively male (heterosexual, bisexual, or homosexual) and are rarely diagnosed as suffering from psychosis. However, they often show personality problems and little concern for the effect of their behavior on the minor.

Pedophiles fantasize about sex with a child, and fondle the child more commonly than they have intercourse. Actual research is rudimentary. However, the prevalence of child prostitution and of child sexual abuse within families seems much higher than previously thought. Nearly 10 percent of women in some studies report some form of sexual interference in childhood or early adolescence. (See also *Child abuse; Incest*.)

Peduncle

A stalklike connecting structure. The term usually refers to bands of nerve fibers that connect different parts of the brain, or to the ropelike connection of a polyp to the surface of the organ to which it is attached.

Peer review

Various processes by which physicians review the work, including clinical decisions and scientific writings, of other physicians.

Pellagra

A nutritional disorder caused by a deficiency of niacin (see *vitamin B complex*), resulting in dermatitis, diarrhea, and dementia. Pellagra occurs primarily in poor rural communities in parts of India and southern Africa where people subsist on corn.

CAUSES

Although the niacin content of corn is no lower than that of some other cereals, much of the vitamin occurs in an unabsorbable form unless it is first treated with an alkali such as lime water. (People living in communities in Mexico who prepare the cereal in this way before making tortillas do not suffer from the disease.)

Corn is also low in tryptophan, an amino acid that is converted into niacin in the body. Certain disorders, such as *carcinoid syndrome* (which increases the breakdown of tryptophan) and *inflammatory bowel disease* (which reduces its absorption from the intestine) may also cause pellagra.

SYMPTOMS

The first symptoms are weakness, weight loss, lethargy, depression, irritability, and itching and inflammation of skin exposed to sunlight. In acute attacks, weeping (leaking) blisters may develop on the affected skin; the tongue becomes bright red, swollen, and painful. In chronic cases, the exposed skin darkens, thickens, and becomes rough and dry. Diarrhea is a common symptom, and severe mental disturbance, including confusion and memory loss, may develop.

DIAGNOSIS AND TREATMENT

Pellagra is diagnosed from the patient's physical condition and dietary history. Daily intake of a regulated amount of niacin and a varied diet rich in protein and calories usually are enough to bring about a complete cure.

Pelvic examination

Examination of a woman's external and internal genitalia, performed as part of a complete physical examination or to investigate the cause of abdominal pain or symptoms. A pelvic examination is sometimes performed by the primary care physician, who may refer the woman to a *gynecologist* for more tests.

A pelvic examination should be a part of a physical examination; it may also be performed as part of contraceptive counseling. Women with symptoms such as abdominal pain, vaginal bleeding or discharge, urinary incontinence, or infertility require a pelvic examination to establish the cause of the symptoms. During childbirth, a pelvic examination is performed to help assess the position and descent of the baby.

The main aspects of a pelvic examination are shown in the illustrated box opposite.

P

PROCEDURE FOR PELVIC EXAMINATION

The examination is usually performed with the woman lying on her back with knees bent. If it is carried out because of uterine prolapse or incontinence, she may be asked to lie on her side. The physician usually begins by inspecting the external genitals for ulceration or swelling and then does an internal examination.

Use of speculum
A speculum is inserted into the vagina to hold apart the vaginal walls; this gives the physician a clear view of both the vagina and cervix. A *cervical smear test* may also be performed at this time.

Manual examination
The physician inserts two fingers into the vagina and palpates (feels) the abdomen to evaluate the size and position of the uterus and ovaries, and to detect any abnormal pelvic swelling or tenderness.

Pelvic floor exercises

A program of exercises to strengthen the muscles and tighten the ligaments at the base of the abdomen. These muscles and ligaments, which form the pelvic floor, support the uterus, vagina, bladder, urethra, and rectum. Stretching or slackening of the pelvic floor is common during childbirth and is also a part of the aging process.

Performing pelvic floor exercises, especially during pregnancy and following childbirth, tones these structures and may help to prevent prolapse of the uterus (see *Uterus, prolapse of*) and urinary stress incontinence (see *Incontinence, urinary*).

Pelvic floor exercises also can sometimes help women who are having difficulty achieving orgasm.

One exercise, carried out during urination, involves stopping and starting the flow of urine several times by contracting and then relaxing the muscles around the vagina, each time for a count of six. Another exercise involves placing two fingers inside the vagina and contracting the muscles around the fingers. The exercises should be done two or three times a day for at least a month.

Pelvic infection

An infection in the female reproductive system. Severe or recurrent pelvic infection is referred to as *pelvic inflammatory disease* (PID). The infection can result in damage to the fallopian tubes and can cause female infertility.

Occasionally, nongynecologic conditions affecting surrounding organs, such as *appendicitis* and *inflammatory bowel disease*, can cause damage to the female genital tract.

Pelvic inflammatory disease

Infection of the internal female reproductive organs. Pelvic inflammatory disease (PID) is one of the most common causes of pelvic pain in women. The infection may not have any obvious cause, but often occurs after a sexually transmitted disease, such as *gonorrhea* or a *chlamydial infection*. PID may also occur after miscarriage, abortion, or childbirth. *IUD* users have a higher incidence of PID, as do young, sexually active women.

SYMPTOMS AND SIGNS

Abdominal pain and tenderness, fever, and an unpleasant-smelling vaginal discharge are the most common symptoms of PID. The pain often occurs immediately after menstruation and may be worse during intercourse. There may also be malaise, vomiting, or backache.

DIAGNOSIS AND TREATMENT

The physician performs a *pelvic examination* and takes samples of any discharge for analysis. A *laparoscopy* may be done to detect any abscess or abnormal growth.

Antibiotic drugs are prescribed to clear up the infection, and *analgesics* may be given. If the woman has an IUD, it may need to be removed.

OUTLOOK

Some women have repeated attacks of PID with or without reinfection. PID may cause *infertility* or an increased risk of *ectopic pregnancy*, primarily due to scarring in the fallopian tubes that prevents the egg from traveling down the tube into the uterus.

Pelvic pain

See *Abdominal pain*.

Pelvimetry

Assessment of the shape and dimensions of a woman's pelvis. Pelvimetry is usually carried out about the 37th week of pregnancy to determine whether the woman is likely to have difficulty delivering her baby.

A rough indication of the size of the pelvic outlet can be obtained during an internal examination by the gynecologist checking the distance between the ischial tuberosities (the prominent bones in the lower pelvis). Radiological pelvimetry (assessing the dimensions by X ray) allows more precise measurement and may be carried out in unusual circumstances. However, the risk of subsequent development of leukemia or solid tumors in children exposed to this procedure mandates great care in balancing the benefit with the risk of the procedure.

P

Pelvis

The ring of bones in the lower trunk, bounded by the coccyx and the hip bones. The pelvis protects abdominal organs such as the bladder, rectum, and, in women, the uterus.

STRUCTURE

The pelvis consists of two innominate bones (hipbones), which are joined by rigid sacroiliac joints to the sacrum (the triangular spinal bone below the lumbar vertebrae) at the back; the hipbones curve forward to join at the pubic symphysis at the front. Attached to the pelvis are the muscles of the abdominal wall, the buttocks, the lower back, and the insides and backs of the thighs.

Each innominate bone consists of three fused bones: the ilium, ischium, and pubis. The ilium, the largest and uppermost, consists of a wide, flattened plate with a long curved ridge (called the iliac crest) along its upper border. The ischium is the bone that bears much of the body weight when sitting. The pubis is the smallest pelvic bone; from the ischium it extends forward and round to the pubic symphysis, where it is joined to the other pubis bone by tough fibrous tissue. All three bones meet in the acetabulum, the cup-shaped cavity that forms the socket of the hip joint.

The pelvis varies considerably between men and women. In women, the pelvis is generally shallow and broad, and the pubic symphysis joint is less rigid than a man's. These differences facilitate childbirth. In men, the pelvis is usually larger and built more heavily to bear a greater body weight.

DISORDERS

Fractures of the pelvis may be caused by a direct blow, or by a force transmitted through the femur (thigh bone). Considerable force is required to cause such a fracture, and it is usually the result of a motor vehicle accident; motorcycle riders are particularly at risk. The fracture itself often heals without problems, but it is frequently accompanied by damage to internal organs within the pelvis, especially the bladder, which may require immediate surgical treatment.

Osteitis pubis (inflammation of the pubic symphysis) is usually caused by repeated stress on the pelvis. It is most common in soccer players as a result of continually kicking a ball. The symptoms include pain in the groin and tenderness over the front of the pelvis. In most cases, the condition clears up with rest.

STRUCTURE OF THE PELVIS

The pelvis is a basin-shaped bony structure at the base of the trunk. It consists of the sacrum and coccyx at the back and, at the sides, the two hipbones, which curve around to meet at the front. The pelvis supports the upper half of the body and protects the lower abdominal organs. The female pelvis is shallower and wider.

Male pelvis

Sacroiliac joint
Iliac crest
Ilium
Sacrum
Coccyx
Pubis
Ischium
Femur
Pubic symphysis

Female pelvis

Pemoline

A central nervous system *stimulant drug* used in the treatment of *narcolepsy* (a rare condition characterized by paroxysms of sleep) and *hyperactivity* in children. Pemoline may cause insomnia, loss of appetite, and, in rare cases, drowsiness, depression, and hallucinations.

Pemphigoid

An uncommon, chronic skin disease in which large, soft blisters form on the skin. The blisters in pemphigoid are intensely itchy, unlike those in *pemphigus*, a similar, but more serious, disorder. Pemphigoid, which is considered to be an *autoimmune disorder* (one in which the body reacts against its own tissues), primarily affects elderly people.

The diagnosis is confirmed by a skin *biopsy* (removal of a small sample of tissue for analysis). Treatment is usually a long-term course of *corticosteroid drugs* or, in some cases, *immunosuppressant drugs*.

Pemphigus

An uncommon, serious skin disease in which blisters appear on the skin and on mucous membranes in the mouth and sometimes elsewhere. Pemphigus primarily affects people between the ages of 40 and 60.

SYMPTOMS AND SIGNS

The blisters usually begin in the mouth (and sometimes the nose), then appear on the skin. They rupture easily, forming raw, often painful areas that may become infected and that later crust over. Apparently unaffected skin may also blister after gentle pressure. When the blisters occur over a great area of the body, the resultant severe skin loss can lead to secondary bacterial infection and, sometimes, death.

Pemphigus on back
The typical appearance is of numerous large, raw areas of skin where the fragile blisters have broken down.

DIAGNOSIS AND TREATMENT

A diagnosis of pemphigus is confirmed by a skin *biopsy* (removal of a small sample of tissue for analysis).

The usual treatment is with *corticosteroid drugs* given over long periods to keep the disease under control. In addition, other *immunosuppressant drugs* may help. *Antibiotic drugs* may need to be taken for skin and secondary infections.

Penicillamine

An *antirheumatic drug* sometimes used to treat *rheumatoid arthritis* when symptoms are severe and not relieved by *nonsteroidal anti-inflammatory drugs* (NSAIDs).

Penicillamine is also a *chelating agent* used in the treatment of copper, mercury, lead, or arsenic poisoning. It is used to treat *Wilson's disease* (a rare brain and liver disorder caused by copper deposits in these tissues) and primary *biliary cirrhosis* (a liver disorder). Penicillamine has also been given to people with cystinuria (excessive excretion of cystine in the urine) to prevent stones from forming in the urinary tract.

POSSIBLE ADVERSE EFFECTS
Penicillamine frequently causes allergic rashes, itching, nausea, vomiting, abdominal pain, and loss of taste. Infrequently, it causes blood disorders or impaired kidney function.

Penicillin drugs

COMMON DRUGS

Amoxicillin Ampicillin Penicillin G Penicillin

The first group of *antibiotic drugs* to be discovered, natural penicillins are derived from the mold PENICILLIUM. Also made synthetically, penicillins are used in the treatment of many infections, including *tonsillitis, pharyngitis, bronchitis,* and *pneumonia*.

Penicillins are also given to prevent the recurrence of *rheumatic fever* and to treat bacterial *endocarditis, syphilis, gonorrhea,* and *Vincent's disease*.

POSSIBLE ADVERSE EFFECTS
The most common adverse effect is an allergic reaction that causes a rash. Any person who has an allergic reaction to one type of penicillin should not be given any other type of penicillin or its derivatives without great caution. Other adverse effects include vomiting and diarrhea.

Penile implant

A prosthesis inserted into the penis to help a man suffering from *impotence* to achieve intercourse. Penile implants are usually used for men who are permanently impotent.

INFLATABLE PENILE IMPLANT
There are various types of penile implants for the treatment of impotence. The type below gives full control over erection. It is implanted surgically, entirely within the body.

Inflatable cylinders in the penis

Reservoir implanted under abdominal muscles

Pump positioned in scrotum

Liquid is pumped from the reservoir

Cylinders fill

Pump squeezed with fingers

Operation
The device is operated by squeezing the pump in the scrotum. Fluid flows from the reservoir and inflates the cylinders.
A small release valve on the pump is pressed to allow the penis to return to a flaccid state.

One treatment involves inserting a silicone splint between the loose skin of the upper surface of the penis and the underlying tissue. The penis can be inserted into the vagina, but does not become erect or increase in size.

Alternatively, an inflatable prosthesis may be implanted in the penis. This type makes the penis larger and firmer for intercourse and is operated by squeezing a small bulb placed in the scrotum.

Penile warts

See *Warts, genital*.

Penis

The male sex organ through which urine and semen pass. The penis consists mainly of three cylindrical bodies of erectile tissue (spongy tissue full of tiny blood vessels) that run the length of the organ. Two of these bodies, the corpora cavernosa, lie side by side in the upper part of the penis. The third, the corpus spongiosum, lies centrally beneath them, expanding at its end to form the tip of the penis, the glans.

Through the center of the corpus spongiosum runs the *urethra*, a narrow tube that carries urine and semen out of the body through an opening at the tip of the glans. Surrounding the erectile tissue is a sheath of fibrous connective tissue enclosed by skin. Over the glans, the skin forms a loose fold known as the *foreskin*, which is sometimes removed soon after birth (see *Circumcision*).

DISORDERS
The most common congenital abnormality is *hypospadias*, in which the urethra opens on the undersurface of the penis anywhere from the base of the glans to the root. *Pseudohermaphroditism*, which is also congenital,

ANATOMY OF THE PENIS
The corpora cavernosa and spongiosum are the erectile tissues of the penis. A network of nerves controls the blood flow into them.

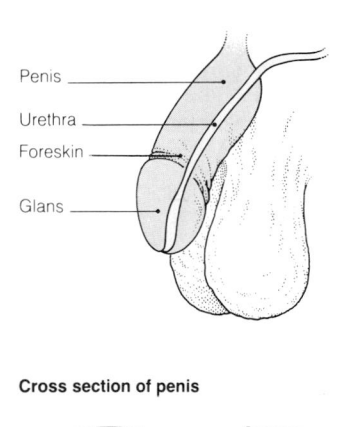

Penis

Urethra

Foreskin

Glans

Cross section of penis

Corpora cavernosa

Corpus spongiosum

Urethra

P

causes the penis to be very small; it is usually complicated by hypospadias.

Balanitis (inflammation of the glans and foreskin) is usually caused by *candidiasis*, although other organisms, including those that cause *gonorrhea* and *syphilis*, may cause inflammation. Balanitis may lead to *phimosis* (abnormally tight foreskin) or *paraphimosis*, in which the foreskin retracts at erection but is too tight to move over the glans.

Penile warts (see *Warts, genital*) are caused by a sexually transmitted virus. Cancer of the penis is rare and is more common in uncircumcised men (see *Penis, cancer of*).

Impotence (failure to attain or maintain an erection) is usually psychological in origin. However, it may be caused by nerve damage associated with *diabetes mellitus*, *alcohol dependence*, *atherosclerosis*, or spinal cord injury. The causes of *priapism*, in which an erection is painful and prolonged, and of *Peyronie's disease*, in which the erect penis bends to one side, are unknown.

Penis, cancer of

A rare form of malignant tumor that is more common in uncircumcised men whose personal hygiene is poor. Both virus infection and smoking have been shown to be additional factors.

The tumor usually starts on the glans (head) of the penis or on the foreskin as a dry, painless, wartlike lump or a painful ulcer, and develops into a cauliflowerlike mass. The growth usually spreads slowly, but a highly malignant tumor can spread to the lymphatic glands in the groin within a few months; the glands swell and the skin over them may ulcerate.

Any growth or sore area on the penis that persists for more than two or three weeks should be reported to a physician. A *biopsy* (removal of a sample of tissue for analysis) will show whether the condition is due to cancer or to some other cause, such as warts (see *Warts, genital*) or *syphilis*.

Because it spreads slowly, cancer of the penis can usually be treated successfully by *radiation therapy* if it is reported early. Otherwise, surgical removal of part or all of the penis may be necessary.

Pentazocine

A narcotic *analgesic drug* (painkiller) used as a *premedication* (drug used to prepare a person for an operation). Pentazocine is also given to relieve pain caused by *cancer*, during *childbirth*, and, occasionally, after a *myocardial infarction* (heart attack).

Possible adverse effects are typical of other narcotic analgesics. Such effects include depression of respiration and the cough reflex and an ability to induce addiction.

Pentobarbital

A *barbiturate drug* sometimes used to treat *insomnia*. Pentobarbital is also used as a *premedication* (drug used to prepare a person for an operation). Possible adverse effects are typical of other barbiturate drugs.

Pentoxifylline

A drug related to *caffeine* that is promoted for the relief of *claudication* (leg pain during exercise) in *peripheral vascular disease*.

Possible adverse effects include dizziness, headache, nausea, flushing, and, in rare cases, chest pain and palpitations.

Peppermint oil

An oil obtained from the peppermint plant MENTHA PIPERITA. It is used as a flavoring in some drug preparations. Peppermint oil may cause *heartburn*.

Peptic ulcer

A raw area that occurs in the gastrointestinal tract, where it is bathed by acid gastric juice. A peptic ulcer may occur in the esophagus, stomach, or duodenum. Rarely, it occurs in the jejunum (as it does in *Zollinger-Ellison syndrome*) or ileum (as in *Meckel's diverticulum*). Usually about 0.33 inch to 1 inch (10 to 25 mm) across, and about 0.01 inch deep, an ulcer may occur singly or in several places. The typical symptom is a gnawing pain in the abdomen when the stomach is empty.

CAUSES AND INCIDENCE

The lining of the stomach and duodenum is constantly at risk of erosion from acid produced by the stomach wall. The lower esophagus is at risk only when reflux of acid juice from the stomach occurs. Ulcers in the jejunum occur only with massive outpouring of gastric acid, while ulcers in a Meckel's diverticulum occur when misplaced gastric lining grows there. Some of the main factors that may be involved in causing peptic ulcer are shown in the illustrated box opposite. In some people, there is a strong family history of peptic ulceration. Psychological stress may play a part in making an existing ulcer worse.

In the US, a duodenal ulcer develops in about one in 10 people at some time in their lives; a gastric ulcer develops in about one in 30. The incidence of gastric ulcers is about equal in men and women, but more males than females suffer from duodenal ulcers. Middle age is the most likely time for either type of ulcer to develop, although the peak age for duodenal ulcers to develop is somewhat earlier than the peak age for gastric ulcers.

SYMPTOMS

Many people found to have a peptic ulcer have no symptoms, but a greater number complain of a burning or gnawing pain in the abdomen, which sometimes wakes them at night. The pain of a duodenal ulcer is often relieved by eating, but usually recurs a few hours later.

Other symptoms accompanying both types of ulcer include loss of appetite (though sometimes a duodenal ulcer increases appetite), belching, feeling bloated, weight loss, nausea, and vomiting (which usually relieves the pain).

COMPLICATIONS

In some cases, complications develop, usually bleeding from the ulcer, which, if considerable, results in vomiting blood and passing black feces; this is a medical emergency. Chronic blood loss may cause iron-deficiency *anemia*.

Rarely, an ulcer may penetrate (make a hole in) the back wall of the digestive tract and extend to the pancreas, usually causing pain that spreads through to the sufferer's back. If the affected area is on the front wall of the duodenum, the leaking digestive juices may cause *peritonitis* (inflammation of the abdominal lining), producing sudden, severe pain and requiring emergency hospital admission.

Chronic ulcers can cause extensive scarring of the stomach or duodenum, narrowing the outlet of the stomach into the duodenum (a condition called *pyloric stenosis*) and obstructing the passage of food. This may cause vomiting and rapid weight loss.

A small number of gastric ulcers are malignant and should be removed as soon as they are diagnosed.

DIAGNOSIS

The condition can be diagnosed with certainty only after a *barium X-ray examination* or *endoscopy* (inspection through a viewing tube) of the stomach and duodenum.

SITES AND CAUSES OF PEPTIC ULCER

A peptic ulcer develops in about one in eight Americans at some time in their lives. Some of the mechanisms involved in causing ulcers are shown below. Most ulcers respond to self-help measures or to drug treatment, but occasionally surgery is necessary.

Gastric ulcer
This photograph of an ulcer in the wall of the stomach was taken via a viewing tube passed down the esophagus.

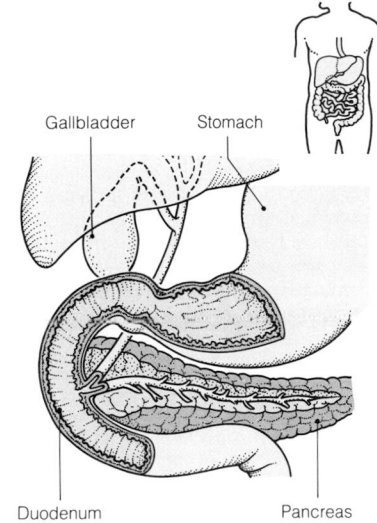

Gallbladder   Stomach

Duodenum   Pancreas

Site of ulcers
Peptic ulcers are most common in the first part of the duodenum or lower half of the stomach, but esophageal ulcers also occur.

ULCER CARE

Self-help methods

Avoid smoking, the most important step in self-help.

Avoid drinking alcohol, coffee, and tea.

Avoid using aspirin and nonsteroidal anti-inflammatory drugs.

Eat several small meals a day, at regular intervals, rather than two or three large ones.

Drug treatment

Antacids neutralize acid in the stomach.

H_2-blockers, such as ranitidine, cimetidine, and famotidine, reduce acid secretion by blocking nerve receptors on acid-producing cells.

Drugs such as sucralfate work by forming a protective coat over the ulcer crater.

HOW AN ULCER IS FORMED

1 Gastric glands in the lining of the stomach secrete acid and the enzyme pepsin, which help break down food. The acid and pepsin would quickly eat away the stomach and duodenum if other cells in the lining did not secrete a protective mucus.

2 Peptic ulcers may be caused by one or more of the following: increased acid secretion; reduced mucus production; or factors that irritate the lining, such as alcohol. Drugs of the aspirin group act as irritants and reduce mucus production.

3 If damaging influences overcome the protective factors in the stomach or duodenal lining, the mucous layer and mucus-secreting cells are eroded and an ulcer forms. Stress is probably not a prime cause of ulcers but may aggravate an existing ulcer.

TREATMENT AND OUTLOOK

Antacid drugs neutralize excess acidity and assist in the healing of ulcers. They ultimately relieve pain if taken regularly, and, along with the other self-help measures listed below, may be enough to heal the ulcer. If not, and if symptoms persist, professional treatment is necessary. It usually consists of *ulcer-healing drugs* (such as cimetidine, ranitidine, or famotidine), which reduce acid production, or sucralfate, which may form a protective covering on the ulcer.

In more than two thirds of cases, the drugs promote healing within six to eight weeks of the start of treatment. In the remaining one third, long-term drug treatment is usually required; very rarely, if the ulcer fails to respond to medication, surgery is necessary. Usually the surgery is a *vagotomy* (cutting the fibers of the vagus nerve that control digestive acid production).

Occasionally, a partial *gastrectomy* (surgical removal of a portion of the stomach) is performed to treat the ulcer and reduce acid production.

Substantial bleeding from an ulcer sometimes requires a *blood transfusion* to be performed.

Perforation, obstruction, or penetration into the pancreas usually necessitate surgery to correct the problem. In some cases of perforation, however, passing a suction tube into the stomach via the nose to drain off digestive juices may be treatment enough. This procedure sometimes allows the perforation to heal of its own accord in the absence of irritation from acidic juices.

Peptide

A fragment of protein consisting of two or more *amino acids*. Peptides are formed by the linking of amino acids by chemical bonds (peptide bonds) between the amino and carboxyl groups of adjacent acids. Larger peptides, consisting of many linked amino acids, are known as polypeptides; still longer chains of amino acids, made up of linked polypeptides, are called *proteins*.

Peptides are widely distributed in the body's endocrine and nervous systems. Many hormones are peptides, including some *gastrointestinal hormones* and several pituitary hormones, such as *oxytocin*, *ADH* (antidiuretic hormone), and *ACTH* (adrenocorticotropic hormone). In the nervous system, peptides are found in nerve cells throughout the brain and the spinal cord; examples include *endorphins* and substances involved in the control of the pituitary gland.

Perception

The interpretation of a sensation. People receive information about the environment through the five senses—*taste*, *smell*, *hearing*, *vision*, and *touch*—but the way in which this information is interpreted depends on other factors.

First, the information must be organized into a pattern. Objects must be distinguished from their background and recognized as moving or stationary. The object then requires identification (e.g., as a chair or a friend), a process that relies on memory. The final interpretation depends on an individual's attitudes, expectations, and current mood. Valued objects often appear larger, and hungry people are more likely to notice food sooner than those who have just eaten.

False perceptions, which occur in the absence of sensory stimuli, are *hallucinations*. They are a symptom of psychotic illness (see *Psychosis*).

Percussion

A diagnostic technique for examining the chest or abdomen by tapping it with the fingers and listening to the resonance of the sound produced. In this way, the condition of internal organs can be deduced. For example, a fluid-filled lung produces a dull note when tapped, as opposed to the hollow sound yielded by air filling one side of the chest in *pneumothorax*. (See also *Examination, physical*.)

Percutaneous

A medical term meaning performed through the skin. Percutaneous procedures include the injection of drugs into veins, muscles, or other body tissues, and biopsies in which tissue or fluid is removed with a needle.

Perforation

A hole made in an organ or tissue by a disease or injury. Among the more common types of perforation due to a disorder are a hole in the wall of the stomach or duodenum (the first part of the small intestine) caused by a *peptic ulcer*, and a rupture of the eardrum, usually caused by middle-ear infection (see *Eardrum, perforated*).

Perforating *wounds* (which penetrate through outer layers of tissue to an internal organ or cavity) usually require exploratory surgery to check for and remove any foreign material; they are then repaired.

Peri-

A prefix meaning around, as in pericardium, the membranous sac that surrounds the heart.

Periarteritis nodosa

An uncommon disease of small and medium-sized arteries, also called polyarteritis nodosa. Areas of arterial wall become inflamed, weakened, and liable to the formation of *aneurysms* (ballooned out segments). Many different groups of blood vessels may be involved, including the coronary arteries that supply blood to the heart muscle, or the arteries of the kidneys, intestine, skeletal muscles, and nervous system. The seriousness of the condition depends on which organs are affected and how severely they are affected.

CAUSES AND INCIDENCE

The disease seems to be the result of a disturbance of the *immune system* (body's defenses against infection), triggered in some cases by exposure to the *hepatitis B* virus. It may develop at any age but is most common in adults. More men than women are affected.

SYMPTOMS AND COMPLICATIONS

In the early stages the patient has a fever and aching muscles and joints. There is general malaise, loss of appetite and weight, and, if blood vessels supplying nerves are affected, nerve pain. Damage to blood vessels leads to obstruction of the blood supply, causing *hypertension* (raised blood pressure), muscle weakness, ulceration of the skin, and *gangrene* (tissue death). If the coronary arteries are affected, *myocardial infarction* (heart attack) may occur. Because blood vessels supplying the intestines are frequently affected, a high proportion of patients suffer abdominal pain, nausea, vomiting, and diarrhea, and pass blood in the feces.

DIAGNOSIS

The condition is diagnosed by examination of the blood vessels in a *biopsy* specimen taken from an affected organ. Inflammation is seen under the microscope. *Angiography* (X rays of blood vessels injected with radiopaque dye) may show areas of narrowing, irregularity of the walls, and/or aneurysms.

TREATMENT AND OUTLOOK

Corticosteroid drugs in large doses, supplemented, if necessary, by *immunosuppressant drugs*, are effective in improving an otherwise unfavorable outlook. Without treatment, few victims of the condition survive for five years; death often occurs from a heart attack, *renal failure*, severe bleeding into the intestine, or from complications of hypertension. With modern drug treatment, however, about 50 percent of patients survive for five years or more.

Pericarditis

Inflammation of the *pericardium* (the membrane that encloses the heart), leading, in many cases, to chest pain and fever. In addition to inflammation, there may be an effusion (increased amount of fluid) in the pericardial space, which separates the two smooth layers of the pericardium. This excess fluid may compress the heart, restricting its action.

Long-standing inflammation can cause constrictive pericarditis, in which the pericardium becomes scarred, thickens, and contracts, interfering with the heart's action.

CAUSES

There are many causes of pericarditis. They include certain bacterial, viral, and fungal infections; *myocardial infarction* (heart attack); cancer spreading from a nearby tumor in the lung or breast or by way of the blood from a remote site; and injury to the pericardium from a penetrating wound or after open heart surgery. Pericarditis sometimes accompanies *rheumatoid arthritis*, systemic *lupus erythematosus*, and *renal failure*. It can also occur for no known reason.

SYMPTOMS AND SIGNS

The characteristic symptom of pericarditis is pain behind the breastbone, sometimes spreading to the neck and shoulders. The pain often becomes more severe if the person takes a deep breath, changes posture, or even swallows; sitting up and leaning forward sometimes relieves it. Fever is another common symptom.

When pericarditis is due to infection, pus may accumulate in the pericardial space. When, rarely, the cause is a tumor, blood may collect there. If heart action is impeded, heart output and blood pressure fall—a condition known as cardiac tamponade. This results in breathing difficulty and in swollen neck veins. The main symptom of constrictive pericarditis is *edema* (an accumulation of fluid in the tissues) of the legs and abdomen, causing them to swell.

DIAGNOSIS

The condition is diagnosed by the findings of the physician during a physical examination, including listening to the heart with a stethoscope, and from the result of an *ECG* (electrocardiogram) and chest *X rays*. *Echocardiography* may be used to confirm that enlargement of the heart shown on X rays is due to effusion.

TREATMENT

Treatment is aimed at the underlying cause whenever possible. *Analgesics* (painkillers) or *anti-inflammatory drugs* may be given to relieve pain. If effusion is seriously affecting heart action, the excess fluid is drawn off through a needle inserted through the chest wall into the pericardial space.

Severe constrictive pericarditis may require surgical removal of the thickened pericardium.

Pericardium

The membranous bag that completely envelops the heart and the roots of the major blood vessels that emerge from the heart. The pericardium has two layers. The outer layer is tough, inelastic, and fibrous and is attached to the diaphragm below. It is attached to the sternum (breastbone) in front by fibrous bands. The inner layer is separated into two sheets. Of these, the innermost is firmly attached to the heart and the outer is attached to the fibrous layer. The space between the smooth, inner surfaces of these sheets is called the pericardial space; it contains a small quantity of fluid that lubricates the movements of the heart.

Perimetry

A visual field test to determine the extent of peripheral vision. Perimetry, which is not usually done as a routine procedure, may be performed to pro-

vide vital information in certain neurological disorders, such as a brain tumor. (See *Eye, examination of.*)

Perinatal

Relating to the period just before or just after birth. Perinatal is often defined more precisely as the period from the 28th week of pregnancy to the end of the first week after birth. Perinatal mortality is a statistical expression of the number of stillbirths and infant deaths occurring during the first week after birth.

Perinatologist

An obstetrician who specializes in caring for mother and baby during late pregnancy and after birth.

Perinatology

A branch of *obstetrics* and *pediatrics* concerned with the study and care of mother and baby during the late stages of pregnancy and early days after birth.

Perineum

There are two definitions. Internally, the perineum is bounded by the pelvic floor (the muscles that form the supportive base of the pelvis) and the surrounding bony structures. The perineum is pierced by the genitourinary and digestive organs. Externally, the perineum is represented by the area between the thighs that lies behind the genital organs and in front of the anus.

Periodic fever

An inherited condition causing recurrent bouts of fever. (See *Familial Mediterranean fever.*)

Period, menstrual

See *Menstruation.*

Periodontal disease

Any disorder of the periodontium (the tissues surrounding and supporting the teeth). The most common type is chronic *gingivitis* (inflammation of the *gums*), which, if untreated, leads to *periodontitis* (inflammation of the periodontal membranes around the base of the teeth and erosion of the bone holding the teeth).

Periodontics

The branch of dentistry concerned with the study and treatment of diseases that affect the periodontium (the structures that surround and support the teeth). Of particular concern are *gingivitis* (inflammation of the

gums) and *periodontitis* (inflammation of the periodontium).

A periodontist makes considerable use of X rays in diagnosis (to detect erosion of the bones in which the teeth are embedded) and is concerned with *preventive dentistry*. Treatment includes *scaling*, curettage (see *Curettage, dental*), *gingivectomy*, and root planing (removal of the *calculus* from the root surface).

Periodontitis

Inflammation of the periodontium (the tissues that support the teeth). There are two types. Periapical periodontitis is a complication of neglected dental *caries* and affects the area around a root tip. Chronic periodontitis is a complication of untreated *gingivitis* (inflammation of the gums). It affects the whole of the periodontium and is the major cause of tooth loss in adults.

Periodontal disease
The gums are inflamed and have receded. Many of the teeth are eroded at their bases; the tooth sockets may also be in decay.

CAUSES

If dental caries is untreated, enamel and the dentin beneath eventually are destroyed, allowing bacteria to enter the tooth pulp. From there, bacteria spread to the root tip and into the surrounding tissues, sometimes leading to the formation of a dental *abscess*, *granuloma*, or dental *cyst*.

If gingivitis, which is usually the result of poor *oral hygiene*, is neglected, inflamed gum tissue at the base of the teeth becomes damaged and pockets form between the gums and the teeth. Dental *plaque* (a sticky deposit of mucus, food particles, and bacteria) and calculus (a hard, mineralized coating that forms from plaque and saliva) then collect in these pockets. The bacteria in the plaque and calculus attack the periodontal tissues, causing them to become inflamed and detached from the teeth. The bacteria also eventually erode the bones surrounding

P

the teeth. In time, the teeth become loose in their sockets and fall out.

SYMPTOMS AND SIGNS

In periapical periodontitis, there may be localized toothache, especially when biting. An abscess may cause some bone and ligament destruction, thus causing the tooth to become loose; a large dental cyst may cause visible swelling of the jaw.

In chronic periodontitis, the signs of gingivitis are present (red, soft, shiny, tender gums that bleed easily) along with an unpleasant taste and bad breath. The deepening pockets in the gums gradually expose the sensitive dentin of the roots of the teeth, causing aching when hot, cold, or sweet food or liquids are consumed.

Occasionally, there is a discharge of pus from the gums or a gumboil (an abscess in the gum); in late stages of chronic periodontitis, there may be bone loss and loosening of teeth.

DIAGNOSIS AND TREATMENT

In periapical periodontitis, the dentist usually finds a deep cavity beneath a filling, and X rays may show bone destruction around the root tip.

The condition is treated either by draining pus through the root canal and then cleaning and filling the tooth or, if the tooth cannot be salvaged, by dental *extraction*. A minor operation may be required to remove dental cysts or large granulomas. Root canal treatment may also be necessary.

The dentist assesses the extent of chronic periodontal disease by measuring the depth of the gum pockets and by taking X rays to determine the extent of bone loss. If the disease has not reached an advanced stage, regular, scrupulous cleaning of the teeth can, by preventing further plaque and calculus formation, halt destruction of the tissues surrounding the teeth. The dentist removes the plaque and calculus by *scaling* and, in some cases, root planing.

Gingivectomy (surgical trimming of the gums using a local anesthetic) may be required to reduce the size of the gum pockets; curettage (see *Curettage, dental*) may be carried out to remove the diseased lining from the pocket so that healthy underlying tissue will reattach itself to the tooth.

Loose teeth can sometimes be anchored to firmer ones by splinting (see *Splinting, dental*); if they are very loose, they may require extraction and replacement with dentures.

Period pain

See *Dysmenorrhea*.

Periosteum

The tissue that coats all the bones in the body except the surfaces inside joints. Periosteum contains small blood vessels that supply nutrients to the underlying bone, and nerves that respond to pain caused by injury or disease. New bone is produced by the periosteum in the initial stages of healing after a *fracture*.

Periostitis

Inflammation of the *periosteum* (connective tissue covering bone). The usual cause is a blow that presses directly onto bone. Rarely, periostitis is caused by infection, such as syphilis. Symptoms include pain, tenderness, and swelling over the affected area of bone.

Peripheral nervous system

All the nerves that fan out from the central nervous system (brain and spinal cord) to the muscles, skin, internal organs, and glands (see *Nerve; Cranial nerves; Spinal nerves*).

Diseases and disorders affecting the peripheral nerves are grouped under the heading *Neuropathy*.

Peripheral vascular disease

Narrowing of blood vessels in the legs, and sometimes in the arms, restricting blood flow and causing pain in the affected area. In severe cases, *gangrene* (death of tissue supplied by the vessels) may develop, requiring amputation of the limb.

TYPES AND CAUSES

In most cases, peripheral vascular disease is caused by *atherosclerosis*, in which fatty plaques form on the inner walls of arteries. Factors that contribute to the risk of atherosclerosis, such as *hypertension* and inadequately controlled *diabetes mellitus*, are associated with peripheral vascular disease. However, the greatest risk factor is cigarette smoking; more than 90 percent of patients are, or were, moderate to heavy smokers.

Diseases affecting the peripheral arteries that are not caused by atherosclerosis include *Buerger's disease* (which mainly affects smokers) and *Raynaud's disease*; deep vein *thrombosis* and *varicose veins* are diseases of the peripheral veins.

SYMPTOMS AND COMPLICATIONS

When narrowing of the arteries develops gradually because of atherosclerosis, the first symptom is usually an aching, tired feeling in the leg muscles when walking. It occurs most often in the calf, but may be felt anywhere in the leg. Typically, the pain is relieved by resting the leg for a few minutes, but recurs after roughly the same amount of walking as before. This symptom is called intermittent *claudication*. Prolonged use of the arms may produce a similar symptom.

As the disease worsens, the amount of activity possible before symptoms develop decreases, until eventually pain is present at rest. This pain may be severe and continuous, disturbing sleep; to relieve it, the sufferer may dangle the limb over the edge of the bed. At this stage, an affected leg is dangerously short of blood supply; the foot and lower leg are cold and often numb, the skin is dry and scaly, and *leg ulcers* tend to develop after minor injury. In the final stage there is gangrene, which usually starts in the toes and then spreads upward.

Sometimes, sudden arterial blockage occurs. It may be caused by a clot developing rapidly on top of a plaque of atherosclerosis, by a dissecting *aneurysm* (splitting of an arterial wall), or by an *embolism* arising from a clot formed in the heart and carried to obstruct a peripheral artery. Blockage causes sudden severe pain in the affected limb, which becomes cold and either pale or blue. There is no pulse in the limb, and movement and sensation in it are lost.

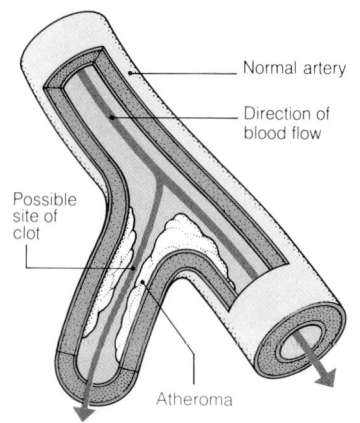

HOW PERIPHERAL VASCULAR DISEASE DEVELOPS

The disease usually starts with the formation of fatty plaque on artery walls. Smokers are among those at highest risk.

Normal artery

Direction of blood flow

Possible site of clot

Atheroma

Clot formation

Clots may form on top of the plaque, restricting blood flow to tissues. This may cause pain and tissue death.

DIAGNOSIS

The diagnosis is based on comparing blood pressure readings taken at the ankle, calf, upper thigh, and arm and use of *Doppler* ultrasound blood velocity detection or *plethysmography*, which traces the pulse pattern.

TREATMENT

By far the most important part of treatment is for the sufferer to stop smoking. Exercise is also extremely important; an affected person should walk for up to an hour each day, stopping whenever claudication occurs and resuming when it stops.

Regular inspection of the feet and scrupulous care of them (ideally by a *podiatrist*) are essential to prevent infection, which can lead to gangrene. Feet should be washed and stockings changed daily. Shoes should fit well to avoid pressure on the feet, and toenails should be cut straight across.

Surgery on the diseased blood vessels is sometimes required (*arterial reconstructive surgery* to bypass them, *endarterectomy* to remove the obstructing fatty deposits on their linings, and balloon *angioplasty* to widen them).

In severe cases in which gangrene has developed, *amputation* is necessary, usually to just below the knee to leave a suitable stump for fitting an artificial limb.

Peristalsis

Wavelike movement as a result of contraction and relaxation of the muscles in the walls of the digestive tract and of the ureters. Peristalsis is responsible for the movement of food and waste products through the digestive system and for transporting urine from the kidneys to the bladder.

Peristalsis occurs in the esophagus during swallowing so that food can be moved toward the stomach even when the body is upside down. Stomach peristalsis helps to mix food with gastric juices and moves the partially digested food into the duodenum. In the small intestine, peristalsis changes to a slow back-and-forth churning motion that allows more time for absorption of nutrients.

In the large intestine, peristaltic contractions occur only once every 30 minutes. Two or three times a day, usually following a meal, a strong, sustained wave of peristalsis passes over the colon. This forces the contents into the rectum and prompts the urge to defecate.

Peritoneal dialysis

See *Dialysis*.

Peritoneum

The two-layered membrane that lines the wall of the abdominal cavity and covers the abdominal organs; it contains blood vessels, lymph vessels, and nerves. The peritoneum has a large surface area equal to that of the entire skin surface.

The most important functions of the peritoneum are to support the abdominal organs, to produce a lubricating fluid that allows the organs to glide smoothly over each other and the abdominal wall, and to protect against infection. In addition, the peritoneum is able to absorb fluid; it is a natural filtering system made use of in peritoneal *dialysis*.

The peritoneum may become inflamed as a complication of an abdominal disorder (see *Peritonitis*).

Peritonitis

Inflammation of the peritoneum (the membrane that lines the wall of the abdomen and covers the abdominal organs). It is a serious, usually *acute*, and painful condition, almost always due to bacterial infection caused by another abdominal disorder.

CAUSES

The most common cause of peritonitis is *perforation* of the stomach or intestine, which allows bacteria and digestive juices to escape from the digestive tract into the abdominal cavity. The perforation is usually the result of a *peptic ulcer*, *appendicitis*, or *diverticular disease*. Less commonly, intestinal contents may leak into the abdominal cavity after surgery on the intestine. Peritonitis may also be associated with acute *salpingitis*, *cholecystitis*, or *septicemia*.

SYMPTOMS AND SIGNS

Peritonitis is usually marked by severe abdominal pain, either localized (in one place) or generalized (covering a larger area). Occasionally, however, pain may be mild or absent. After a few hours, the muscles in the abdominal wall go into spasm, making the abdomen feel hard, and *peristalsis* (wavelike contractions of the intestinal muscles) stops (see *Ileus, paralytic*). Other symptoms include fever, bloating, nausea, and vomiting. Dehydration and shock may occur.

DIAGNOSIS AND TREATMENT

The condition, diagnosed from a physical examination, requires immediate admission to the hospital.

Prompt surgery may be needed to deal with any underlying cause—for example, removal of a perforated appendix (see *Appendectomy*) or repair of a perforated peptic ulcer. When the cause is unknown, an exploratory operation called a *laparotomy* may be performed. *Antibiotic drugs* are often given, sometimes requiring a delay in surgery. Dehydration is treated by an *intravenous infusion* of fluid.

OUTLOOK

In most cases, the patient makes a full recovery following treatment.

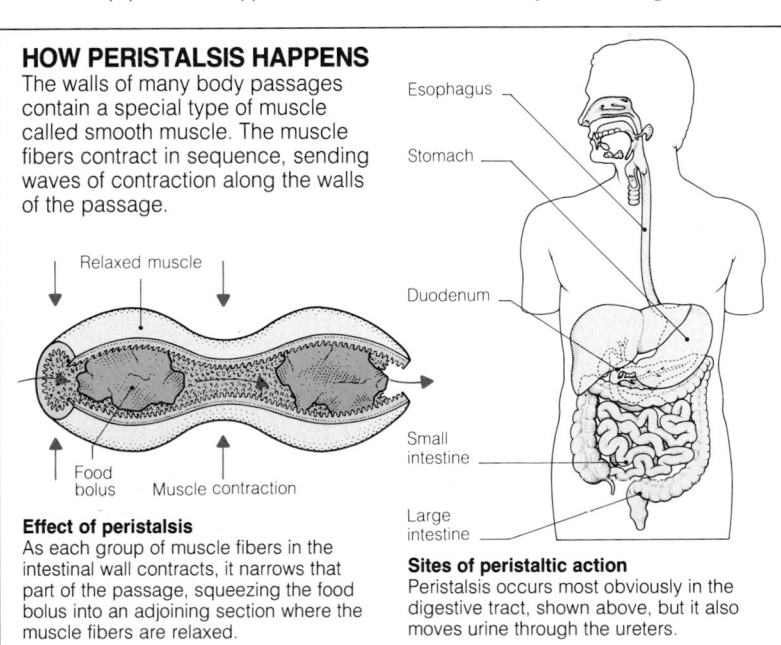

HOW PERISTALSIS HAPPENS

The walls of many body passages contain a special type of muscle called smooth muscle. The muscle fibers contract in sequence, sending waves of contraction along the walls of the passage.

Relaxed muscle

Food bolus   Muscle contraction

Effect of peristalsis
As each group of muscle fibers in the intestinal wall contracts, it narrows that part of the passage, squeezing the food bolus into an adjoining section where the muscle fibers are relaxed.

Esophagus

Stomach

Duodenum

Small intestine

Large intestine

Sites of peristaltic action
Peristalsis occurs most obviously in the digestive tract, shown above, but it also moves urine through the ureters.

P

Occasionally, however, an abscess develops within the abdomen, requiring more surgery. Intestinal obstruction, resulting from the formation of *adhesions* (fibrous bands of scar tissue between loops of the intestine), may occur later.

Peritonsillar abscess

See *Quinsy*.

Permanent teeth

The second *teeth*, which usually start to replace the primary teeth at about age 6. There are 32 permanent teeth, 16 in each jaw. Each set of 16 consists of four incisors (biting teeth) at the front, flanked by two canines (tearing teeth), with four premolars and six molars (grinding teeth) at the back of the mouth. (See also *Eruption of teeth*.)

Pernicious anemia

A type of anemia caused by failure to absorb vitamin B_{12}, which is essential for normal red blood cell production in the bone marrow. A deficiency leads to the production of abnormal, large, red cells. The vitamin is also essential for normal nerve cell metabolism. (See *Anemia, megaloblastic*.)

Pernio

An itchy, purple-red swelling, usually on a toe or finger, caused by excessive constriction of small blood vessels below the surface of the skin in cold weather conditions.

Pernios are most common in the young and the elderly, and women are more susceptible than men. Pernios generally heal without treatment; talcum powder may partially relieve itching. Those susceptible to pernios can help prevent them by keeping feet and hands warm in cold weather.

Peroneal muscular atrophy

A rare, inherited disorder characterized by wasting of the muscles, first in the feet and calves and then in the hands and forearms. The condition, also known as Charcot-Marie-Tooth disease, is a result of degeneration of some of the peripheral nerves. It can affect both sexes, but is more common in boys, and usually appears in late childhood or adolescence.

SYMPTOMS AND SIGNS
Wasting of the muscles stops abruptly halfway up the arms and legs, giving them the appearance of inverted bottles; sensation may be lost in the affected areas. Muscle weakness in the legs causes a characteristic high-stepping walk and clawing of the toes.

TREATMENT AND OUTLOOK
No treatment is available but the condition tends to progress so slowly that the sufferer rarely becomes completely incapacitated; sometimes the deterioration stops for no apparent reason. Life expectancy for an affected person is normal.

Perphenazine

A *phenothiazine*-type *antipsychotic drug* used to relieve symptoms in certain psychiatric disorders, especially in *schizophrenia* and *mania*. Perphenazine is also often used as an *antiemetic drug* to relieve nausea and vomiting caused by anesthesia, *radiation therapy*, chemotherapy, and certain drugs.

Possible adverse effects include abnormal movements of the face and limbs, drowsiness, blurred vision, stuffy nose, and headache. Long-term use may cause *parkinsonism*.

Personality

The sum of a person's traits, habits, and experiences. There is much disagreement as to precisely what personality is, what defines it, and how it can be assessed. However, three different aspects are usually considered to be important in any definition: temperament, intelligence, and emotion and motivation.

The notion of temperament originates from the four ancient humors, which divided people into choleric, melancholic, sanguine, and phlegmatic types. It reflects differences in the nature and speed of an individual's responses. For example, some people are easily angered, while others are placid and react slowly. Intelligence defines a person's capabilities in comparison with a theoretical norm, while emotion and motivation describe feelings, attachments to others, moral standards, and aspirations.

The development of personality seems to depend on the interaction of two basic factors: heredity (the qualities a person is born with) and environment (a person's life experiences that affect his or her ways of thinking and behaving).

Personality disorders

A group of conditions characterized by a general failure to learn from experience or adapt appropriately to changes, resulting in personal distress and impairment of social functioning.

Personality disorders are not forms of illness, but ways of behaving that may become especially obvious during periods of stress. They are usually first recognizable in adolescence and continue throughout life, often leading to *depression* or *anxiety*. Some people realize that they have personality problems; others fail to see their personalities as in any way unusual or difficult, blaming circumstances, bad luck, or other people for their constant failures in life.

TYPES
Specific types of personality disorders are divided into three groups; there is often overlap among types, particularly within each group. The first group is characterized primarily by eccentric behavior. Paranoid people show unwarranted suspiciousness and mistrust of others, schizoid people are cold emotionally and have difficulty forming social relationships, and schizotypal personalities show oddities of behavior similar to those of *schizophrenia*, but less severe.

In the second group, behavior tends to be dramatic and emotions intensely expressed. Histrionic individuals are very excitable and constantly crave stimulation, narcissists have an exaggerated sense of their own importance (see *Narcissism*), and those with *antisocial personality disorder* consistently fail to conform to social standards.

General anxiety and fear characterize people in the third group. Included are people with *avoidant personality disorder*, who are extremely sensitive to criticism; dependent personalities, who lack self-confidence and cannot function independently (see *Dependence*); compulsive people, who are perfectionists, rigid in their habits, and emotionally cold (see *Obsessive-compulsive behavior*); and passive-aggressive types, who resist demands from others to improve their performances at work and at home (see *Passive-aggressive personality disorder*).

TREATMENT AND OUTLOOK
The usual forms of treatment are counseling and individual *psychotherapy*. Because such people are often uncooperative, it may be difficult to attain even simple goals, such as avoiding the complications of drug abuse or hospitalization, or maintaining personal relationships and jobs. Drug therapy is used only for treating additional illnesses.

In *psychoanalysis*, a therapeutic, helping relationship may be established between sufferer and therapist. Ideally, this forms a foundation for gradual changes in personality as the sufferer begins to understand the causes that motivate his or her maladaptive behavior.

Personality tests

Questionnaires designed to define various *personality* traits or types. Personality tests are used to assist in psychiatric diagnosis, in research, and to assess the suitability of candidates or employees for positions in colleges or industry. The validity and reliability of the tests are uncertain.

The Minnesota Multiphasic Personality Inventory (MMPI) has more than 500 questions, some relating to psychiatric symptoms (such as *depression* or *paranoia*) and others relating to underlying personality traits (such as *intelligence*). Another personality test is said to measure "extroversion-introversion" (how outgoing or reserved a person is) and "neuroticism" (predisposition to developing neurotic illness). Closely related to this test is a third questionnaire, in which a person is rated on pairs of factors, such as tense versus relaxed, or timid versus adventurous.

Perspiration

The production and excretion of sweat from the *sweat glands*. Perspiration is another name for sweat.

Perthes' disease

Inflammation of an epiphysis (growing area) of the head of the *femur*. A type of *osteochondritis juvenilis*, Perthes' disease is thought to be due to disrupted blood supply to the bone.

The condition most commonly occurs in children aged 5 to 10, and usually affects one hip. Symptoms include pain in the thigh and groin and a limp on the affected side. Movement of the hip is restricted and painful. X rays may show fragmentation and, at a later stage, shrinking of the head of the femur.

Treatment may consist of rest for a few weeks until the pain subsides, followed by splinting of the hip to reduce pressure on the femur, or an *osteotomy* operation to change the angle of the head of the femur so that it fits more securely into the pelvis.

Perthes' disease usually clears up by itself within three years, but may leave the hip permanently deformed. Severe deformity may increase the likelihood of *osteoarthritis* later in life.

Pertussis

A distressing infectious disease, also called whooping cough, that mainly affects infants and young children. Paroxysms of coughing, often ending in a characteristic "whoop" as breath is drawn in, are the main symptoms of the illness, which may last for weeks and can have some serious complications. Before the introduction of a vaccine against pertussis in the 1950s, this disease killed more children every year in the US than all other infectious diseases combined.

DEATH RATE FROM PERTUSSIS IN US

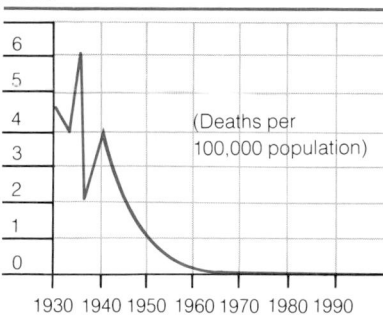

(Deaths per 100,000 population)

1930 1940 1950 1960 1970 1980 1990

The decline of pertussis
Pertussis caused thousands of deaths annually in the 1930s and 1940s. Now there are just a handful of deaths each year.

CAUSES AND INCIDENCE
Pertussis is caused by a bacterium, *BORDETELLA PERTUSSIS*, that is spread from an infected person to others in coughed-out airborne droplets. The disease leads to inflammation of the entire respiratory tract. The illness occurs worldwide. Infants are susceptible from birth, and the illness is most dangerous in infants. Adults are occasionally affected.

In developed countries such as the US, most infants are vaccinated in the first year of life. However, the vaccine is not completely effective in preventing the illness, and not all children are suitable for vaccination, so epidemics of the illness still occur. Probably about 20,000 to 30,000 cases occur annually in the US, although not all of them are reported.

Experience has shown that, if the percentage of children vaccinated drops significantly (as occurred in the UK in the 1970s), the number affected in epidemics climbs severalfold. Because the illness is potentially serious, it is important that as many infants as possible who are suitable for vaccination be vaccinated. The risks of vaccination are far less than the dangers of having pertussis.

PREVENTION
Pertussis vaccine is usually given in combination with diphtheria and tetanus vaccines to children at 2, 4, and 6 months of age in the US; a "booster" dose is given at age 5.

An infant often becomes mildly feverish or fretful for a day or two after an injection, but this is no cause for concern. Giving the child a dose of acetaminophen before the vaccination helps reduce the side effects.

Very rarely (in about one in 100,000 cases), a baby may have a severe reaction, with high-pitched screaming or seizures and, in about one in 300,000 cases, may suffer permanent brain damage. To lessen these already very small risks, the vaccine is not given to an infant who has a history of seizures, who has a feverish illness, or who has suffered a previous reaction to the pertussis vaccine.

Infants should be kept away from anyone with pertussis.

SYMPTOMS AND COMPLICATIONS
After an incubation period of one to three weeks, the illness starts with a mild cough, sneezing, nasal discharge, fever, and sore eyes; this is the period when the child is most infectious. After a few days, the cough becomes more persistent and severe. Whooping occurs in most but not all cases. Sometimes the cough induces vomiting. In infants, there is a risk of temporary *apnea* (cessation of breathing) after a coughing spasm.

The illness continues for up to 10 weeks and can be exhausting for the whole family, especially if the child's coughing continues at night. Complications include the development of *pneumonia*; the mechanical effects of the coughing may cause nosebleeds and bleeding from blood vessels on the surface of the eyes. Recurrent vomiting can cause dehydration and malnourishment.

DIAGNOSIS AND TREATMENT
Pertussis is diagnosed by identifying the causative bacterium in a culture grown from a nasal swab in the early stages of the illness.

Antibiotics are not particularly helpful once the severe coughing stage of the illness has begun. However, if the illness is recognized early, erythromycin is often given; it reduces the child's infectivity to others and may shorten the length of the illness.

A child with pertussis should be kept warm, given small, frequent meals and plenty to drink, and protected from stimuli that can cause coughing (such as drafts or smoke). An infant or child who becomes blue or keeps vomiting after coughing needs to be admitted to the hospital.

Perversion

See *Deviation, sexual*.

P

Pes cavus
See *Clawfoot*.

Pessary
One of a variety of devices placed in the vagina. Some types of pessaries are used to correct the position of the uterus (see *Uterus, prolapse of*).

Pesticides
Poisonous chemicals used to eradicate pests of any kind. The most frequently used types are insecticides, herbicides (weedkillers), and fungicides. Most cases of pesticide poisoning occur in children who have swallowed a garden herbicide or insecticide, such as *paraquat* or a chlorate pesticide (see *Chlorate poisoning*). However, poisoning also occurs in agricultural workers, usually by inhalation or absorption through the skin—as in *parathion* poisoning.

In addition, indirect exposure to pesticides can occur through eating food in which the chemicals have accumulated as a result of repeated crop spraying. Some authorities believe the result of eating such foods may be insidious long-term damage to health. For this reason, and because of environmental dangers, pesticide manufacturers in the US must reveal the results of their toxicity studies before the Environment Protection Agency will approve a new product. (See also *DDT*; *Defoliant poisoning*.)

Petechiae
Red or purple, flat, pinhead spots that occur in the skin or mucous membrane. Petechiae are caused by a localized hemorrhage from small blood vessels. They occur in *purpura* (a group of bleeding disorders) and sometimes in bacterial *endocarditis*.

Petit mal
A type of seizure that occurs in *epilepsy*. Petit mal attacks occur in children and adolescents but rarely persist into adult life. They are characterized by a momentary loss of awareness; an observer may think that the sufferer is daydreaming. Petit mal attacks may occur hundreds of times a day and sometimes last as long as half a minute each.

Petroleum jelly
A greasy substance obtained from petroleum, also known as petrolatum and yellow soft paraffin. Petroleum jelly is commonly used as an *ointment* base, as a protective dressing, and as an *emollient* to soothe the skin.

PET scanning
Positron emission tomography, a diagnostic technique based on the detection of positrons (positively charged particles) that are emitted by labeled substances introduced into the body. PET scanning produces three-dimensional images that reflect the metabolic and chemical activity of tissues being studied.

HOW IT WORKS
Substances that take part in biochemical processes in the body are labeled with radioisotopes (radioactive forms of elements, such as carbon 11, nitrogen 13, or oxygen 15). These substances are injected into the blood and are taken up in greater concentrations by areas of tissue that are more metabolically active. In the tissue, the substances emit positrons, which, in turn, release photons. It is the detection of these photons that actually forms the basis of PET scanning.

By surrounding the patient with an array of detectors linked to a computer, the origin of the photons can be computed and a picture built of the distribution of the radioisotope within body tissues.

PET scan images of brain sections
Features within the brain appear as light or dark areas according to their uptake of radioactively labeled glucose.

WHY IT IS DONE
PET scanning is particularly valuable for investigating the brain. It is used for detecting tumors (which are more or less metabolically active than surrounding brain tissue), for locating the origin of epileptic activity within the brain, and for examining brain function in various mental illnesses.

OUTLOOK
PET scanning equipment is expensive to buy and operate; it is available in only a few centers where there is also a cyclotron, which makes the necessary isotopes. However, because PET scanning can provide valuable information not obtainable by other techniques, it seems likely that its use will become more widespread in the future.

Peutz-Jeghers syndrome
An inherited condition in which numerous polyps occur in the small intestine and small, flat, brown spots appear on the lips and in the mouth. The syndrome usually produces no symptoms but occasionally the polyps cause abdominal pain, bleed, or lead to *intussusception* (in which the intestine telescopes in on itself and causes obstruction).

Tests may include *barium X-ray examination* of the small and large intestines and *colonoscopy* (inspection through a viewing tube). Bleeding polyps may be removed.

Peyote
A cactus plant found in northern Mexico and the southwestern US, the dried blossoms of which are prepared as an *hallucinogenic drug*. The active ingredient is *mescaline*, which produces visual hallucinations and altered consciousness lasting for several hours.

Peyronie's disease
A disorder of the *penis* in which part of the sheath of fibrous connective tissue within the penis thickens. Peyronie's disease causes the penis to bend at an angle during erection, usually to one side, often making intercourse difficult and painful. The disorder usually affects men over 40 and the cause is unknown.

The thickened area can usually be felt as a firm nodule when the penis is flaccid. Eventually, some of the erectile tissue (spongy tissue in the penis responsible for erection) may also thicken, interfering with erection.

In some cases, Peyronie's disease improves without treatment. Local injections of *corticosteroid drugs* sometimes improve the condition. If it persists, the thickened area may be removed surgically and replaced with a graft of normal tissue. The drawback to this operation is that it sometimes results in more scarring, making the problem worse.

pH
A measure of the acidity or alkalinity of a solution. The pH scale ranges from 0 to 14, with 7 denoting neutrality; the smaller the pH value below 7, the more strongly acidic a solution is; the larger the value above 7, the more strongly alkaline it is.

The pH of body fluids must be maintained very near 7.4 (close to neutrality) for the body's metabolic reactions to proceed properly (see

Acid-base balance). If the pH falls below about 7.3, a condition called *acidosis* results; if it rises above about 7.5, *alkalosis* results.

Phagocyte

 A cell capable of surrounding, engulfing, and digesting microorganisms (such as bacteria and viruses), foreign particles that have entered the body (such as dust inhaled into the lungs), and cellular debris.

Phagocytes form part of the body's *immune system* (natural defenses against infection) and are found in the blood, spleen, and lymph nodes, in the alveoli (small air sacs) within the lungs, and elsewhere.

Some types of white *blood cells*, especially granulocytes and some monocytes, are phagocytes. They are "free" phagocytes, able to wander through the tissues and engulf organisms and debris.

Phalanges

The small bones that make up the skeleton of the fingers, thumb, and toes. Each finger has three phalanges, the thumb and big toe have two, and the other toes have three.

Phallus

Any object that is considered to symbolize the penis.

Phantom limb

The perception that a limb is present after *amputation*. Impulses from the nerves in the remaining stump are interpreted by the brain as if they were coming from the original limb.

Pharmaceutical

Any medicinal drug. The term is also used to describe the manufacture and sale of drugs.

Pharmacist

A person who is professionally concerned with the preparation and dispensing of drugs.

Pharmacokinetics

The term used to describe how the body deals with a drug, including how the drug is absorbed into the bloodstream, distributed to different tissues, broken down, and excreted from the body.

Pharmacologist

A specialist in the composition of drugs and their effects on the body. A pharmacologist also undertakes

research to help develop new drugs and find new ways to use existing drugs. Although most drugs come in prepackaged forms and dosages, the clinical *pharmacist* is often called upon in a hospital to develop special preparations for special needs, and to advise on dosage, methods of administration, and side effects.

Pharmacology

The branch of science concerned with the discovery and development of drugs; with their chemical structure and the ways in which they act in the body; with their uses in the prevention or treatment of disease; and with their side effects and toxicity. Pharmacological chemists are also concerned with devising methods of synthesizing naturally occurring drugs, producing completely new synthetic drugs, finding new combinations of drugs, and modifying existing drugs to extend or improve their effectiveness.

Pharmacopeia

Any book that lists and describes almost all drugs used in medicine, especially an official national publication, such as the United States Pharmacopeia (USP).

Used as a standard book of reference by physicians and pharmacists, a pharmacopeia describes sources, preparations, doses, and tests that can be used to identify individual drugs and to determine their purity. Pharmacopeias may also contain additional information, such as how a drug works, and possible adverse effects.

Pharmacy

The practice of preparing drugs and making up prescriptions, or a place where this activity is carried out.

Pharyngitis

Acute inflammation of the pharynx (the part of the throat between the tonsils and the larynx), the chief symptom of which is a *sore throat*.

CAUSES

Pharyngitis is most often caused by a viral infection; sometimes it is due to infection by bacteria, such as streptococci, mycoplasma, or chlamydial infection. A common symptom of a cold (see *Cold, common*) or *influenza*, pharyngitis may also be an early feature of mononucleosis (see *Mononucleosis, infectious*) or *scarlet fever*. *Diphtheria* is a rare, but serious, cause of pharyngitis.

Pharyngitis may also be caused by swallowing substances that scald, corrode, or scratch the lining of the throat. The condition can be aggravated by smoking or excess consumption of alcohol.

SYMPTOMS AND SIGNS

In addition to a sore throat, there may be discomfort when swallowing, slight fever, earache, and tender, swollen lymph nodes in the neck. In severe cases, the fever may be high and the soft palate and throat may swell so much that breathing and swallowing become difficult. One potential complication is edema (an accumulation of fluid in the tissues) of the larynx (voice box), which is a life-threatening condition.

TREATMENT

Other than gargling with warm salt water, avoiding lying flat, and taking *analgesics* (painkillers), no treatment is usually required; pharyngitis most often clears up on its own. Antiseptic lozenges and sprays may aggravate the condition and should therefore not be used.

Particularly severe and/or prolonged sore throats should be reported to a physician, who may take a throat culture and prescribe *antibiotic drugs*. Severe edema of the larynx may require *intubation* (establishment of an air passage by placing a tube through the larynx into the trachea) or *tracheostomy* (creating an opening in the trachea to insert a breathing tube).

Pharyngoesophageal diverticulum

An abnormal blind-ending sac that bulges back and down from the back of the throat or top of the esophagus. (See *Esophageal diverticulum*.)

Pharynx

The passage that connects the back of the mouth and the nose to the esophagus. This muscular tube, lined with *mucous membrane*, forms part of the respiratory and the digestive tract. The uppermost part, the *nasopharynx* (an air passage), connects the nasal cavity to the region behind the soft *palate* of the mouth. The middle section, the oropharynx (a passage for both air and food), runs from the nasopharynx to below the tongue. The lowest portion, the laryngopharynx (a passage for food only), lies behind and to each side of the larynx and merges with the esophagus.

DISORDERS

Acute *pharyngitis* (inflammation of the pharynx), which causes sore throat, is

P

the most common disorder affecting the pharynx. A foreign body, such as a fish bone, may become lodged in the pharynx, causing pain and *choking*.

Pharyngoesophageal diverticulum (also called Zenker's diverticulum) is a rare disorder in which a small sac develops in the rear wall of the laryngopharynx.

Malignant tumors of the nasopharynx (see *Nasopharynx, cancer of*), though common in the Far East, are rare in the West, as are cancer of the oropharynx and laryngopharynx (see *Pharynx, cancer of*). The latter two are found in association with smoking and heavy drinking.

LOCATION OF THE PHARYNX
The pharynx, or throat, plays an essential part in breathing and eating and can change shape to help form vowel sounds in speech. It has a mucous membrane lining.

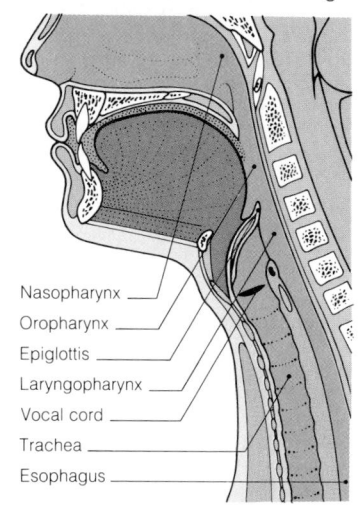

Nasopharynx

Oropharynx

Epiglottis

Laryngopharynx

Vocal cord

Trachea

Esophagus

Pharynx, cancer of
A malignant tumor of the *pharynx* (the passage that connects the back of the nose with the esophagus). It usually develops in the squamous (flattened, scalelike) cells of the *mucous membrane* that lines the passage. Tumors of the nasopharynx, the uppermost part of the passage, have different causes and symptoms than those occurring elsewhere in the pharynx (see *Nasopharynx, cancer of*).

CAUSES AND INCIDENCE
In the West, almost all pharyngeal cancer is related to smoking (of pipes and cigars as well as cigarettes) and drinking alcohol, with the highest incidence in those who both smoke and drink.

In the US, the incidence of the disease is about six cases per 100,000 population per year. The incidence rises with age, and the disorder is more common in men.

SYMPTOMS AND SIGNS
Malignant tumors of the oropharynx (the middle section of the pharynx, running from behind the soft palate to below the tongue) usually cause difficulty swallowing, often with a sore throat and earache. In addition, blood-stained sputum (phlegm) may be coughed up. Sometimes the disease causes no more than the feeling of a lump in the throat or a visible enlarged lymph node in the neck.

Cancer of the laryngopharynx (the lowest part of the pharynx), which lies behind the larynx and merges with the esophagus, initially causes an uncomfortable sensation of incomplete swallowing. As the tumor spreads, symptoms include a muffled voice, hoarseness, and increased difficulty swallowing. A sensation of incomplete swallowing may have a different, harmless cause, but it should always be reported to a physician.

DIAGNOSIS
Biopsy (removal of a small sample of tissue for analysis) of suspicious pharyngeal lesions is mandatory and is often done in the operating room in conjunction with *laryngoscopy*, *bronchoscopy*, and *esophagoscopy* (inspection through a viewing tube of the larynx, lungs, and esophagus).

TREATMENT AND OUTLOOK
The growth may be removed surgically or treated with *radiation therapy*; *anticancer drugs* may be given. The outlook varies considerably according to the site and type of tumor, its degree of malignancy, the stage of the disease at the time of treatment, and the age of the patient.

Phenazopyridine
An *analgesic drug* (painkiller) used to relieve pain in the urinary tract (caused, for example, by *cystitis* or the insertion of a *catheter*). When pain is due to an infection, phenazopyridine is given with an *antibiotic drug*.

Phenazopyridine may cause abdominal discomfort, orange or red discoloration of the urine, and, rarely, headache and dizziness. Diabetics may find that the drug causes false readings of urine sugar test results.

Phenelzine
A monoamine oxidase inhibitor *antidepressant drug*. Like other drugs of this type, phenelzine may cause a dangerous increase in blood pressure if taken with certain drugs, foods, or drinks. For this reason, it is usually given only when other antidepressant drugs are ineffective.

Phenelzine may cause dizziness, and, rarely, jaundice and rash. Headache, unexplained sweating, nausea, and vomiting may indicate a dangerous rise in blood pressure.

Phenobarbital
A *barbiturate drug* used mainly as an *anticonvulsant drug*. Although phenobarbital has to some extent been replaced by newer anticonvulsant drugs, it is widely used with *phenytoin* to treat *epilepsy* in children.

Phenobarbital is occasionally used as a daytime sedative and is combined with *antispasmodic drugs* for the treatment of *irritable bowel syndrome*.

Possible adverse effects include drowsiness, clumsiness, dizziness, excitement, and confusion.

Phenothiazine drugs

COMMON DRUGS

Chlorpromazine Fluphenazine Perphenazine Thioridazine Trifluoperazine

A group of drugs derived from the chemical phenothiazine. These drugs are widely used to treat psychotic illness (see *Antipsychotic drugs*) and are also commonly used as *antiemetic drugs* and *antihistamine drugs*.

Phentermine
An *appetite suppressant* promoted for the treatment of *obesity*. Phentermine may cause dryness of the mouth, palpitations, and *insomnia*.

Phenylbutazone
A *nonsteroidal anti-inflammatory drug* (NSAID) used to relieve the symptoms of certain types of arthritis, such as *ankylosing spondylitis* and *rheumatoid arthritis*. Because of the risk of adverse effects, phenylbutazone is not commonly given; it is usually prescribed only when other similar drugs have proved ineffective.

Phenylbutazone is sometimes given illegally to lame horses to improve their performance.

POSSIBLE ADVERSE EFFECTS
Phenylbutazone may cause nausea, fluid retention, rash, and *peptic ulcer*. It may also increase the risk of *blood disorders*, such as agranulocytosis (lack of white blood cells). Regular blood tests are therefore carried out if treatment lasts for longer than two weeks.

P

Phenylephrine

DECONGESTANT

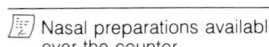

Eye drops Nose drops Nasal spray
Nasal jelly

Nasal preparations available over-the-counter

Available as generic

A *decongestant drug* commonly used in the treatment of seasonal allergic *rhinitis* (hay fever) and the common *cold*. Phenylephrine is also used to relieve pain in *conjunctivitis* and to dilate the pupils during examination of or surgery on the eyes.

Combined with a local anesthetic (see *Anesthesia, local*), phenylephrine slows down the anesthetic's spread into surrounding tissues (by narrowing blood vessels) and thereby prolongs its effect.

POSSIBLE ADVERSE EFFECTS
Eye drops may irritate the eyes. High doses or prolonged use of nasal preparations may lead to worse congestion and may cause headache, blurred vision, and raised blood pressure.

Phenylketonuria

An inherited disorder in which the enzyme that converts phenylalanine (an amino acid) into tyrosine (another amino acid) is defective. Unless phenylalanine is excluded from the diet, it builds up in the body and causes severe mental retardation.

INCIDENCE AND DIAGNOSIS
About one baby in 16,000 has phenylketonuria (PKU). All newborn babies are routinely given the *Guthrie test* (sometimes called a PKU test), in which a sample of blood is taken from the baby's heel so that the level of phenylalanine can be checked. If the level of phenylalanine is high, more sensitive tests are carried out during the first few weeks of life.

SYMPTOMS AND SIGNS
Newborn babies show few signs of abnormality, but, early in infancy, neurologic disturbances, including *epilepsy*, become evident. Affected children have an unpleasant, musty, mousy smell due to the excretion in the sweat and urine of a breakdown product of phenylalanine. Ninety percent of those affected have blond hair and blue eyes. Some skeletal changes are associated with phenylketonuria, such as a small head, short stature, and flat feet. About one third to half the patients have eczema.

TREATMENT
The only treatment is to restrict the intake of phenylalanine, which is a natural constituent of most protein-containing foods. Babies must be given special milk substitutes. After weaning, they are given a very low-protein, mainly vegetarian, diet. Some physicians believe that a strict low-protein diet should be followed throughout life. Other physicians maintain that a normal diet can be introduced at the age of 10 to 12 years; the special diet must be followed during pregnancy.

Phenylpropanolamine

DECONGESTANT

Tablet Capsule Liquid Lozenge

Available over-the-counter

Available as generic

A *decongestant drug* commonly used in the treatment of seasonal allergic *rhinitis* (hay fever), *sinusitis*, and the common *cold*. Phenylpropanolamine is also given to relieve stress incontinence (see *Incontinence, urinary*) and is sometimes promoted as an *appetite suppressant* in the treatment of *obesity*.

Prolonged use of phenylpropanolamine as a decongestant may cause a worsening of the condition. High doses may cause anxiety, nausea, and a rise in blood pressure.

Phenytoin

An *anticonvulsant drug* commonly used in the long-term treatment of *epilepsy*. Phenytoin is used occasionally to treat *migraine* and infrequently to control certain types of *arrhythmia* (irregular heart beat). Prolonged use may cause slurred speech, dizziness, confusion, and overgrowth of the gums.

Pheochromocytoma

A rare, nonmalignant tumor of cells secreting the hormones epinephrine and norepinephrine, which regulate heart rate and blood pressure. The tumor increases production of these hormones, causing intermittent or sustained hypertension (high blood pressure). Pheochromocytomas may be single or multiple, and usually develop in the medulla (core) of one or both adrenal glands. Sometimes they occur in similar tissue in the brain and elsewhere. The tumors may develop at any age but are most common in young to middle-aged adults.

SYMPTOMS AND SIGNS
Most patients have hypertension, but, for much of the time, there are usually no other signs or symptoms. However, pressure on the area of the tumor, emotional upset, a change in posture, or taking *beta-blocker drugs* can cause a surge of hormones from the tumor, bringing on a sudden rise in blood pressure, rapid pulse, palpitations, headache, nausea, vomiting, clammy skin, and sometimes a feeling of impending death.

DIAGNOSIS AND TREATMENT
Diagnosis involves blood and urine tests to check for excessive epinephrine and norepinephrine and their metabolites. *CT scanning* and investigational *radioisotope scanning* may be used to locate tumors.

Treatment consists of surgical removal of the tumors. Before surgery, drugs are usually given to control the patient's blood pressure. The outlook after treatment is very good in almost all cases. In some patients, hypertension recurs and requires treatment with drugs.

Pheromone

An odorous chemical, released by an animal, that affects the behavior or development of other individuals of the same species. Many animals secrete pheromones to attract mates or mark their territory. However, although humans also give off distinctive body odors, whether or not these are true pheromones, able to alter the behavior of other humans, remains open to debate.

Phimosis

Tightness of the foreskin, preventing it from being drawn back over the underlying glans (head) of the penis.

In uncircumcised males, some degree of phimosis is normal until the age of 6 months. In some boys it persists for several years after, sometimes making urination difficult and causing the foreskin to balloon out. Phimosis prevents proper cleaning of the glans, leading to *balanitis* (infection of the glans and foreskin). There may also be an increased risk of cancer (see *Penis, cancer of*). Phimosis makes erection painful and *paraphimosis* may occur as a complication. The condition is treated by *circumcision*.

Phlebitis

Inflammation of a vein, often accompanied by clot formation. The preferred medical name for this condition is *thrombophlebitis*.

P

Phlebography

The obtaining and interpretation of X-ray images of veins after they have been injected with a radiopaque substance. (See *Venography*.)

Phlebotomy

Puncture of a vein for the purpose of letting blood. (See *Venesection*.)

Phlegm

See *Sputum*.

Phobia

A persistent, irrational fear of, and desire to avoid, a particular object or situation. Many people have minor phobias, experiencing some anxiety when unable to avoid contact with spiders, for example. However, these phobias do not impair the ability to cope with day-to-day life. It is only when a fear causes significant distress and interferes with normal social functioning that it is considered a psychiatric disorder.

TYPES

Simple phobias, also known as specific phobias, are the most common. They may involve fear of particular animals (most often dogs, snakes, spiders, or mice) or of particular situations, such as enclosed spaces (*claustrophobia*), heights, or air travel. Animal phobias usually start in childhood, but other forms may develop at any time. Treatment is not usually required, unless the feared object is so common that it is not easily avoided (e.g., fear of elevators in a person who lives in a large city).

Agoraphobia (fear of open spaces or entering public places) is a more serious type of phobia, often causing severe impairment and disruption of family life. It is the most common phobia for which treatment is sought. The disorder usually starts in the late teens or early 20s.

Social phobia, which is relatively rare, is fear of being exposed to the scrutiny of others. Examples include fear of eating, speaking, or performing in public, using public toilets, or writing in the presence of others. The disorder usually begins in late childhood or early adolescence.

CAUSES

According to some theories, simple phobias are a form of learned response (see *Conditioning*). People with such phobias often have been brought up by someone with a similar fear or have had an early frightening experience that has become associated with the feared object or situation. According to other theories, the phobia has a symbolic meaning (e.g., a fear of snakes may result from repressed sexual feelings).

Separation anxiety in childhood, an introverted or dependent personality, and an unstable or conflict-ridden background may predispose a person to the development of agoraphobia.

SYMPTOMS

Exposure to the feared object or situation causes intense *anxiety* and sometimes a *panic attack*. Phobic individuals may also suffer from *depression* and generalized anxiety and may indulge in minor obsessional rituals (see *Obsessive-compulsive behavior*). People with agoraphobia or social phobia may attempt to relieve their anxiety with alcohol, barbiturates, or antianxiety drugs, and may become psychologically dependent on them, thus compounding the problems.

TREATMENT

The most effective treatment is *psychotherapy*, sometimes combined with *antidepressant drugs*. People with social phobia may benefit from training in social skills.

Phocomelia

A type of *limb defect* in which the feet and/or the hands are joined to the trunk by short, stubby stumps resembling seal fins. The condition is rare and was seen in people whose mothers took the drug *thalidomide* early in pregnancy.

Phosphates

Salts containing a combination of phosphorus, oxygen, and another element such as *sodium* or *calcium*. Phosphates are an essential part of the diet and are present in cereals, dairy products, eggs, and meat.

FUNCTION

About 85 percent of the body's phosphate is combined with calcium to form the structure of bone and teeth. The remainder is deposited in small amounts in most of the body's tissues and plays a part in maintaining the acid-alkaline balance of the blood, urine, saliva, and other body fluids. Adenosine triphosphate (see *ATP*) is a phosphate compound that provides energy for chemical reactions in cells.

DISORDERS

In most people, the kidneys maintain a constant level of phosphates in the body by regulating the amount excreted in the urine. A slight deficiency of phosphates in the diet is compensated for by a reduction in the amount lost in the urine.

Hypophosphatemia (an abnormally low level of phosphates in the blood) may occur in some forms of kidney disease, *hyperparathyroidism*, long-term treatment with *diuretic drugs*, *malabsorption* (inadequate absorption of incompletely digested foods from the intestine), or prolonged starvation. Hypophosphatemia causes bone pain, weakness, seizures, and, in severe cases, coma and death.

Accidental poisoning with a phosphate-containing fertilizer may cause hyperphosphatemia (excessive levels of phosphates in the blood). Although this condition does not usually cause symptoms, it sometimes leads to the formation of calcium deposits in tissues.

DRUG THERAPY

Phosphates may be taken by mouth as tablet preparations or milk to treat hypophosphatemia. Phosphates are also used to treat *hypercalcemia*. Diarrhea is a possible side effect of phosphate drugs.

Phosphorus poisoning

There are two forms of phosphorus—yellow and red. Yellow phosphorus is readily absorbed by the body and is highly poisonous. Red phosphorus cannot be absorbed and is nontoxic.

Yellow phosphorus is used in matches, fireworks, some insecticides, and certain rodent poisons. Most cases of poisoning occur in industrial workers who accidentally ingest the chemical or inhale its vapor. Acute poisoning, due to absorption of comparatively large amounts of phosphorus over a short period, causes damage to the liver, kidneys, central nervous system, and other organs. Symptoms of acute poisoning include burning abdominal pain, an odor of garlic on the breath, nausea, vomiting, bloody diarrhea, jaundice, and symptoms of kidney failure (see *Renal failure*) and *liver failure*. In severe cases, or untreated milder ones, delirium, seizures, unconsciousness, and death may occur within about 48 hours of poisoning.

Chronic poisoning, caused by taking in small amounts of phosphorus over a relatively long period, may cause gradual destruction of the jaw bones (phossy jaw), *cirrhosis* of the liver, and kidney damage.

Treatment of acute poisoning consists of washing out the stomach (see *Lavage, gastric*) with copper sulfate, along with injections of calcium and treatment for any resultant liver or kidney failure.

P

Photocoagulation

The destructive heating of tissue by intense light focused to a fine point, as with *laser treatment*. Photocoagulation is used to treat disorders of the retina, especially diabetic retinopathy.

Photophobia

An abnormal sensitivity or intolerance to light. Photophobia causes pain and occurs with some eye disorders, such as corneal abrasion and ulceration, acute *keratitis* (inflammation of the cornea), acute *uveitis* (inflammation of the iris and the ciliary body), and congenital *glaucoma*.

Photophobia is commonly, and inaccurately, used to describe any discomfort caused by bright light.

Photosensitivity

Abnormal reaction to sunlight. Photosensitivity usually takes the form of a skin rash that occurs as a reaction to the effects of light on the skin. It often occurs because a substance has been ingested or topically applied to the skin. Examples of such substances, called photosensitizers, are certain drugs, dyes, chemicals used in perfumes and soaps, and plants such as buttercups, parsnips, and mustard.

Photosensitivity is also a feature of certain disorders that affect internal organs as well as the skin, such as systemic *lupus erythematosus* and *porphyria*; exposure to light may worsen the disease.

TREATMENT

Known photosensitizers should be avoided when possible. If the reaction occurs independently of photosensitizers, a susceptible person should avoid exposure to sunlight, especially between 10 AM and 4 PM (when the light is at its most intense), and should use a *sunscreen*.

Phototherapy

Treatment with light. Phototherapy may involve the use of sunlight, nonvisible ultraviolet light, visible blue light, or *lasers*.

Moderate exposure to sunlight is the most basic form of phototherapy. It is helpful in treating about 75 percent of people with *psoriasis* and probably accounts for its lower incidence in sunny climates.

A newer form of phototherapy is *PUVA*, which combines the use of long-wave ultraviolet light with a *psoralen drug* (such as methoxsalen), which sensitizes the skin to light. PUVA is particularly effective in treat-ing psoriasis and is also used in treating some other skin diseases, such as *vitiligo* and *mycosis fungoides*. Short-wave ultraviolet light, sometimes combined with application of coal tar, may also be used to treat psoriasis. Several treatments are given; the exposure time is gradually increased according to the reaction of the patient's skin to the therapy.

Visible blue light is used in treating *jaundice* in the newborn (caused by accumulation of the bile pigment bilirubin as a result of an insufficiently developed liver). The light is thought to cause the chemical breakdown of bilirubin, allowing it to be excreted in urine. With eyes shielded, the infant is completely exposed to the light for 12 hours or more; he or she may need additional fluids to compensate for water loss.

Phrenic nerve

The principal nerve supplying the *diaphragm*. It carries all the motor impulses to, and some of the sensory impulses from, the diaphragm, and plays an important part in controlling breathing. Each of the two phrenic nerves arises from the third, fourth, and fifth cervical nerves in the neck, and passes down through the chest to one side of the diaphragm. Injury to, or surgical cutting of, one of the

LOCATION OF PHRENIC NERVES
There are two phrenic nerves, one on each side of the body. Each follows a tortuous course from its origin in the neck, through the chest, to the diaphragm.

Cervical nerves

Cervical vertebrae

Heart

Diaphragm

Phrenic nerve

nerves results in paralysis of the corresponding half of the diaphragm.

The phrenic nerve may be deliberately crushed by a surgeon to produce temporary paralysis of the diaphragm after an operation to repair a *hiatal hernia*, or, very rarely, as a treatment for intractable *hiccup*. Crushing the nerve was once commonly performed as a part of the treatment for lung disorders such as *tuberculosis* and *bronchiectasis*.

Physical examination

See *Examination, physical*.

Physical medicine and rehabilitation

A medical specialty that concentrates on patients recovering from or overcoming disabilities or impairments caused by injury (especially of the joints and muscles), illness, or neurological conditions such as paralytic strokes. The physician specializing in rehabilitation examines and tests the patient, establishes a rehabilitation program, and supervises a team of therapists who help the patient carry out the program.

Physical therapy

Treatment of disorders or injuries with physical methods or agents, such as exercise, *massage*, *heat treatment* (including *ultrasound treatment* and short-wave *diathermy*), cold (see *Ice packs*), water (see *Hydrotherapy*), light (see *Phototherapy*), and electrical currents (see illustrated box overleaf).

Exercises may be passive, in which the physical therapist moves parts of the patient's body, or active, in which the patient is taught to contract and to relax certain muscle groups or to perform specific movements.

Physical therapy is used to prevent or reduce joint stiffness and to restore muscle strength in the treatment of arthritis or after a fracture has healed. It is also used to reduce pain, inflammation, and muscle spasm, and to retrain joints and muscles after stroke or nerve injury.

Physician

A person licensed to practice medicine and surgery in all branches of medicine. The term commonly refers to a doctor of medicine (MD) or a doctor of osteopathy (DO). However, the term is popularly used by other practitioners of the healing arts whose licenses to practice may be more limited (e.g., doctors of podiatric medicine). See also *Licensure*.

TECHNIQUES OF PHYSICAL THERAPY

Physical therapy may be given after a stroke, nerve damage, or a fracture, or for muscle pain or arthritis. In addition to the techniques shown, heat and electrical treatments are often used.

Passive exercise
The therapist moves the affected part. This preserves joint mobility and is valuable after nerve injuries and in the treatment of patients with polio.

Active exercise
This may help restore function to weak muscles. Stroke patients may benefit, for example, by exercises in which the stronger arm supports the weaker.

THERAPEUTIC MASSAGE

Massage
Massage is given mainly to relieve muscle pain and spasm. Long, sweeping strokes can be alternated with "circling" techniques.

Physiology

The study of the functioning of the body, that is, the physical and chemical processes of its cells, tissues, organs, and systems, including their various interactions. Along with *anatomy* (the study of body structure), physiology constitutes the foundation of all medical science.

Strictly, physiology is concerned with normal functioning, but the boundary between normality and abnormality is not always distinct. Thus a specialty has developed called pathophysiology, which is concerned with the functional changes associated with diseases and disorders. There are also other physiological specialties, such as renal physiology (the study of kidney function), neurophysiology (the study of the functioning of the nervous system), and endocrine physiology (the study of the functions of endocrine glands and their hormone secretions).

Physiotherapy

See *Physical therapy*.

Physostigmine

A drug used as eye drops in the treatment of *glaucoma* (raised pressure in the eyeball), often with *pilocarpine*.

Phytonadione

A *hemostatic drug* used to treat certain *bleeding disorders*. A synthetic preparation of *vitamin K*, phytonadione is used to treat bleeding caused by certain *anticoagulant drugs*, malnutrition, or the inadequate absorption or production of vitamin K in the intestine.

Phytonadione is also used to prevent bleeding in newborns because it carries less risk of anemia and jaundice than other hemostatic drugs.

Possible adverse effects include dizziness, flushing, and, rarely, an unpleasant taste in the mouth.

Pica

A craving to eat substances (such as dirt, coal, chalk, or wood) that are not food. Pica sometimes occurs during pregnancy and may be a feature of various nutritional or iron deficiency disorders. It may also occur in severe psychiatric disorders.

Pickwickian syndrome

An unusual disorder characterized by extreme *obesity*, abnormally shallow breathing, excessive sleepiness, and *sleep apnea*. It is named for the fat boy Joe in Charles Dickens' "Pickwick Papers." The cause of the disorder is unclear; symptoms usually improve with weight loss.

PID

See *Pelvic inflammatory disease*.

Pigeon toes

A minor abnormality in which the leg or foot is rotated, forcing the foot and toes to point inward.

Pigmentation

Coloration of the skin, hair, and iris of the eyes by the *melanin* (a yellow, brown, or black pigment) produced by special cells called melanocytes. The greater the amount of melanin, the darker the coloration. The amount of melanin produced is determined by heredity and by exposure to sunlight. Blood pigments can also color skin (such as in a bruise).

ABNORMALITIES OF PIGMENTATION

LIGHTENED SKIN Patches of pale skin occur in various skin disorders. In *psoriasis*, *pityriasis alba*, and *tinea versicolor*, skin scales flake off, resulting in loss of melanin. In *vitiligo*, areas of skin stop producing melanin.

The rare, inherited disorder *albinism* is caused by generalized melanin deficiency, resulting in pale skin and white hair. In *phenylketonuria*, another

Appearance of pigeon toes
This is a common condition in toddlers. In almost all cases it corrects itself by age 7. Severe cases may require surgery.

genetic condition, sufferers have a reduced melanin level, making them paler-skinned and fairer-haired than other members of the family.

DARKENED SKIN Patches of dark skin mingled with lighter areas may follow an episode of *eczema* or psoriasis, or may occur in tinea versicolor. In *chloasma*, hormonal changes cause dark areas to develop on the face; this may occur in women taking oral contraceptives, or during pregnancy or the menopause. Dark facial patches may also be caused by some perfumes and cosmetics, particularly when they contain chemicals that cause *photosensitivity*. All such patches of discoloration usually fade with time.

Permanent areas of pronounced deep pigmentation are usually due to an abnormality in the melanocytes, as is the case with moles and freckles (see *Nevus*). *Acanthosis nigricans*, which may be inherited or acquired, is characterized by dark patches of velvetlike, thickened skin, primarily in body creases.

Darkening of the skin, unrelated to sun exposure, may occur in certain hormonal disorders, such as *Addison's disease* and *Cushing's syndrome*.

OTHER SKIN DISCOLORATION Some abnormal skin pigmentation is caused by an excessive blood level of other pigments. An excess of the bile pigment bilirubin in *jaundice* turns the skin yellow and too much iron in *hemochromatosis* turns the skin bronze. Discoloration may also be caused by an abnormal collection of blood vessels, such as the one that produces a port-wine stain (see *Hemangioma*).

Piles
A common name for *hemorrhoids*.

Pill, birth-control
See *Oral contraceptives*.

Pilocarpine
A drug obtained from the plant *PILOCARPUS*, used for *glaucoma* (raised pressure in the eyeball). Because pilocarpine causes the pupils to constrict, it is also used to reverse dilation (widening) of the pupils (which may be caused by drugs given during surgery or examination of the eyes).

Pilocarpine often causes blurred vision. Other possible effects include headache and irritation of the eyes.

Pilonidal sinus
A pit in the skin, often containing hairs, in the upper part of the cleft between the buttocks. It is usually harmless, but it can become infected, resulting in recurrent painful abscesses that discharge pus. The condition is probably due to hair fragments burrowing inward. Pilonidal sinus is most common in young, hairy, white males, but is frequently found in others.

Treatment of an infected sinus is by surgically removing a wide area around the infection; the wound is usually left open to allow slow healing from below. Recurrence of infection is common, and plastic surgery is occasionally required.

Pimozide
A drug used in the treatment of *Gilles de la Tourette's syndrome* (a rare neurological disorder). Pimozide may cause sedation, dry mouth, constipation, and blurred vision.

Pimple
The common name for a small *pustule* or *papule*. Pimples are usually found on the face, neck, or back, particularly in adolescents suffering from *acne*.

Pindolol
A *beta-blocker drug* used in the treatment of *angina pectoris* (chest pain due to inadequate blood supply to heart muscle), *arrhythmias* (irregularities of the heart beat), and *hypertension* (high blood pressure). Pindolol is currently under investigation as a treatment for control of *glaucoma* (raised pressure in the eyeball).

Pindolol is less likely than some beta-blockers to cause *bradycardia* (abnormally slow heart beat). Otherwise, possible adverse effects are typical of other beta-blockers.

Pineal gland
A tiny, cone-shaped body within the brain, whose sole function appears to be the secretion of the hormone melatonin. The amount of hormone secreted varies over a 24-hour cycle, being greatest at night. Control over this secretion is possibly exerted through nerve pathways from the retina in the eye; a high light level seems to inhibit secretion. The exact function of melatonin is not understood, but it may help to synchronize circadian (24-hour) or other *biorhythms*.

The pineal gland is situated deep within the brain, just below the back part of the corpus callosum (the band of nerve fibers that connects the two halves of the cerebrum). In rare cases, it is the site of a tumor.

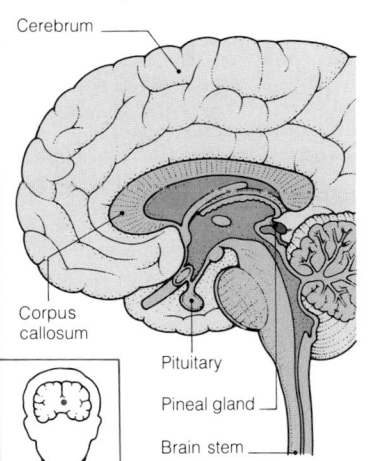

LOCATION OF THE PINEAL GLAND
Long considered a mystery, this gland is now thought to act as a sort of body clock.

Cerebrum

Corpus callosum

Pituitary

Pineal gland

Brain stem

Pinguecula
A small, benign, yellowish spot on the *conjunctiva* over the exposed areas of the white of the eye. Pingueculas are common in the elderly and are caused by ultraviolet radiation in sunlight. Occasionally, a pinguecula enlarges and may threaten to extend onto the cornea to cause a *pterygium*. In such cases the pinguecula may be removed.

Pinkeye
A common name for *conjunctivitis*.

Pink puffer
A term sometimes used by physicians to describe one of the two main categories of patients with the lung disease *emphysema*. The other category is the *blue bloater*.

Pink puffers are able to maintain adequate oxygen in their bloodstream—and thus remain "pink" despite serious lung damage—through an increase in their breathing rate. However, this causes almost constant shortness of breath. (Treatment is described under *Emphysema*.)

Pinna
The fleshy part of the outer *ear*, formed of a flap of cartilage and skin. It is also known as the auricle. The pinna appears to have little practical value; its loss barely affects hearing.

Cosmetic problems affecting the pinna, such as *cauliflower ear*, can usually be corrected by plastic surgery (see *Otoplasty*).

P

Pins and needles sensation

Medically called paresthesia, a tingling or prickly feeling in an area of skin. It is usually associated with *numbness* (loss of sensation) and occasionally with a burning sensation. Temporary pins and needles sensation is caused by a disturbance in the conduction of impulses through nerves that carry sensation from the skin to the brain (e.g., after sleeping with an arm bent awkwardly under the body). Persistent pins and needles sensation may be caused by *neuropathy* (a group of nerve disorders).

Pinta

A skin infection occurring in some remote villages in tropical America. The organism responsible, *TREPONEMA CARATEUM*, is closely related to the bacterium that causes syphilis. It is uncertain how the disease is transmitted. A large spot, surrounded by smaller ones, appears on the face, neck, buttocks, hands, or feet, and, one to 12 months later, is followed by red skin patches that turn blue, then brown, and finally white. A course of penicillin or tetracycline clears up the infection, but the skin may be left permanently disfigured.

Pinworm infestation

A common infestation with a small parasitic worm, *ENTEROBIUS VERMICULARIS*, that lives in the intestines. This species is also sometimes called threadworm.

CAUSES, INCIDENCE, AND SYMPTOMS

The pinworm primarily affects children; it is the most common worm parasite of children in temperate areas. Possibly one fifth of all children in the US are affected at any time.

The female adult pinworms are white and about a third of an inch (10 mm) long. They lay eggs in the skin around the anus, and their movements cause tickling or itching in the anal region, often at night, which may cause the child to scratch. Eggs are transferred directly via the fingers to the mouth to cause reinfestation, or are carried on toys or blankets to other children. Swallowed eggs hatch in the intestine and the worms reach maturity after two to six weeks.

DIAGNOSIS AND TREATMENT

Pinworm infestation is easily diagnosed by a physician seeing the worm eggs under a microscope (after the worm eggs have been picked up from the patient's anal area with some sticky tape).

Ointments may be used to relieve the anal itching and the physician may prescribe an *antihelmintic drug*. Treatment of all members of the family is advisable.

Preventive and self-help measures include the wearing of pajamas to discourage scratching, keeping fingernails short, and washing the hands scrupulously before meals. Sheets and nightwear should be changed frequently, washed at high temperature, and ironed.

Piperazine

An *antihelmintic drug* used in the treatment of intestinal *worm infestations*. Rare adverse effects include nausea, vomiting, and diarrhea.

Piroxicam

A *nonsteroidal anti-inflammatory drug* (NSAID) used to relieve the symptoms of types of arthritis, such as *osteoarthritis, rheumatoid arthritis*, and *gout*. Piroxicam is also used to relieve pain in *bursitis, tendinitis*, and after minor surgery. Piroxicam may cause nausea, indigestion, abdominal pain, *peptic ulcer*, and swollen ankles.

Pituitary gland

Sometimes referred to as the master gland, the pituitary is the most important of the endocrine glands (glands that release hormones directly into the bloodstream). The pituitary regulates and controls the activities of other endocrine glands and many body processes (see *Endocrine system*).

LOCATION OF PITUITARY GLAND
This master gland is itself controlled by the hypothalamus, located immediately above it.

Cerebrum

Hypothalamus

Pituitary

Brain stem

STRUCTURE
The pituitary is a pea-sized structure that hangs from the base of the brain, just below the optic nerves, and lies in a cavity in the skull. It is attached by a short stalk of nerve fibers to the *hypothalamus*, a region of the brain that controls the function of the pituitary by nervous stimulation and by hormone-releasing factors. The pituitary consists of three parts—the anterior lobe, the intermediate lobe, and the posterior lobe.

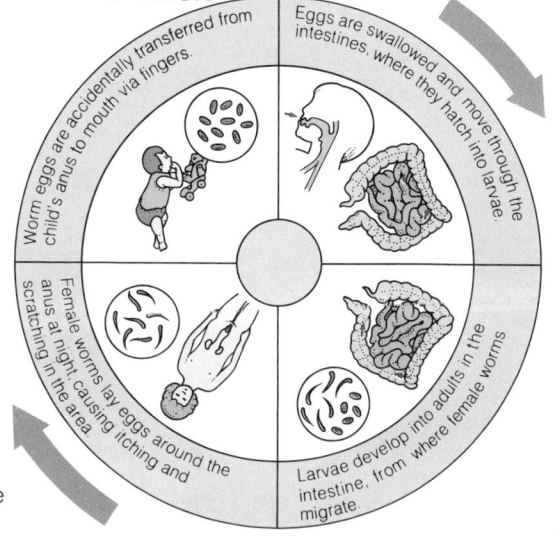

CYCLE OF PINWORM INFESTATION
This is probably the most common worm infestation of humans. The adult worms live in the large intestine, from where the females migrate to lay eggs around the anal region. Eggs may be transferred to the mouth (via fingers, sheets, or toys), are swallowed, and hatch to start a new infestation. Occasionally, in a girl, an adult worm migrates into the vagina or bladder, leading to a discharge or to cystitis.

Worm eggs are accidentally transferred from child's anus to mouth via fingers.

Eggs are swallowed and move through the intestines, where they hatch into larvae.

Female worms lay eggs around the anus at night, causing itching and scratching in the area

Larvae develop into adults in the intestine, from where female worms migrate.

HORMONES SECRETED BY THE PITUITARY GLAND

Growth hormone
stimulates cell division and protein synthesis in tissues such as bone and cartilage, leading to growth.

Thyroid-stimulating hormone (TSH)
stimulates the thyroid gland to secrete various hormones vital to body metabolism.

Adrenocorticotropic hormone (ACTH)
stimulates the adrenal glands to secrete hormones, with multiple effects on metabolism.

Prolactin
stimulates female breast development, and, in response to sucking of the infant, milk production.

Luteinizing and follicle-stimulating hormones (LH and FSH)
help control the function of male and female sex organs.

Melanocyte-stimulating hormone (MSH)
controls skin darkening by stimulating pigment cells.

Antidiuretic hormone (ADH)
acts on the kidneys to decrease water loss in the urine and thus reduces urine volume.

Oxytocin
stimulates contraction of the uterus during childbirth and milk release from the breasts.

FUNCTION
The different lobes of the pituitary produce a range of hormones.

The anterior pituitary produces six hormones: *growth hormone*, which stimulates growth; prolactin, which stimulates the production of milk after giving birth (see *Breast-feeding*); *ACTH* (adrenocorticotropic hormone), which stimulates hormone production by the adrenal glands; TSH (thyroid-stimulating hormone), which stimulates hormone production by the *thyroid gland*; and the *gonadotropins* FSH (follicle-stimulating hormone) and LH (luteinizing hormone), which stimulate the *gonads*.

The intermediate part of the pituitary secretes one hormone, melanocyte-stimulating hormone (MSH), which controls darkening of the skin.

The posterior pituitary produces two hormones—*ADH* (antidiuretic hormone), which increases reabsorption of water into the blood by the kidneys and therefore decreases urine production; and *oxytocin*, which stimulates contractions of the uterus during labor and the ejection of milk during breast-feeding.

Pituitary tumors
Growths that arise in the pituitary gland. Pituitary tumors are rare, comprising about 10 percent of primary *brain tumors*. Most are benign (noncancerous). However, because the pituitary is situated in a bony hollow at the base of the skull, enlargement of the tumor is upward, where it tends to press on the optic nerves, causing visual field defects.

CAUSES AND TYPES
The causes of pituitary tumors are unknown. The most common type is called an endocrine inactive tumor. As it grows, it leads to destruction of some of the hormone-secreting cells in the gland, which causes hypopituita-

---

DISORDERS OF THE PITUITARY GLAND

Any abnormality of the pituitary gland usually means that it produces either too much or too little of one or more hormones, and this causes changes elsewhere in the body. Locally, serious effects may be caused by enlargement of the gland; for example, it may press on the nearby optic nerves and cause visual defects.

CONGENITAL AND GENETIC DISORDERS
Deficiency of *growth hormone* may be a genetic disorder, or it may be due to congenital absence or undergrowth of the pituitary, or to damage to the gland sustained during birth. Whatever the cause, deficiency of growth hormone leads to *short stature*.

Congenital growth hormone deficiency may also be associated with deficiency of other pituitary hormones, notably *ACTH* (adrenocorticotropic hormone), *gonadotropin hormones*, and thyroid-stimulating hormone (TSH).

TUMORS
Pituitary tumors are usually benign but may cause either excess production of pituitary hormones (hyperpituitarism) or reduced production (hypopituitarism), depending on the type of cell involved.

INJURY
Birth injury or a later head injury may cause loss of pituitary function.

IMPAIRED BLOOD SUPPLY
Rarely, the pituitary may suffer deprivation of its blood supply as a result of pressure on its blood vessels from a growing tumor. This may cause a sudden loss of pituitary function, which may be fatal, or a more gradual loss, which produces signs of general underactivity of the gland. A similar deprivation of blood supply may occur as a complication of massive blood loss associated with childbirth (Sheehan's syndrome). This may lead to failure of milk production, and a range of secondary effects due to the resultant underactivity of other endocrine glands.

Impaired blood supply may also occur from *vasculitis*, or from pressure on the gland from an *aneurysm* of a nearby artery.

RADIATION
Radiation therapy for a pituitary tumor may cause general underactivity of the gland.

INVESTIGATION
Techniques used to investigate pituitary disorders include analysis of the levels of pituitary hormones in the blood or urine, and of hormones from other endocrine glands under pituitary control; *X rays, CT scanning*, or *MRI* of the pituitary; and *angiography*, to show displacement of blood vessels by a pituitary tumor. A visual field test (see *Vision tests*) may be done.

P

rism (reduced hormone production). This often leads to a failure of sexual function, with cessation of menstrual periods in women and reduced sperm production in men.

Other types of tumors cause the gland to produce too much of a certain hormone. For example, a tumor of the anterior pituitary can cause excess growth hormone production, leading to *gigantism* or *acromegaly*. Too much thyroid-stimulating hormone (TSH) can lead to *hyperthyroidism* and excess adrenocorticotropic hormone (ACTH) can cause *Cushing's syndrome*. Finally, an increased production of prolactin can cause *galactorrhea* (abnormal milk production), absence of menstrual periods, and infertility in women. In men, increased production can cause impotence, infertility, feminization, and galactorrhea.

Tumors that affect the posterior pituitary may disrupt production of antidiuretic hormone (ADH) and lead to *diabetes insipidus*.

DIAGNOSIS AND TREATMENT
The diagnosis is made from measurements of the levels of different hormones in the blood and urine, from *CT scanning* or *MRI* of the brain, and from visual field testing (see *Vision tests*).

Treatment may be by surgical excision of the tumor, *radiation therapy*, or replacement of missing hormones, or a combination of these techniques. The drug bromocriptine is sometimes used for hormone-secreting tumors because it suppresses production of some of the hormones.

Pityriasis alba

A common skin condition of children and adolescents in which irregular, fine, scaly, pale patches appear on the face, usually the cheeks. The condition is caused by mild *eczema* and is often more pronounced after exposure to sun because the patches tan poorly. The condition usually clears up with emollients.

Pityriasis rosea

A common mild skin disorder in which flat, scaly-edged, round or oval, dark pink or copper colored spots appear over the trunk and upper arms, usually in a "T-shirt" distribution. The rash is preceded about a week beforehand by a single, larger, round spot (called a herald patch) of the same type on the trunk. The condition, which is not contagious, mainly affects children and young adults. Its cause is unknown.

The rash, which lasts for about six to eight weeks, can occasionally cause itching but is otherwise symptomless. Although the rash usually clears up without treatment, a physician should be consulted to rule out other conditions that cause similar rashes.

Calamine lotion alleviates mild itching; more severe itching can be relieved by *antihistamine drugs*.

PKU test
See *Guthrie test*.

Placebo

A chemically inert substance given in the place of a *drug*. Some physicians may prescribe a placebo if a person's symptoms, such as fatigue, are not caused by an illness that requires drug treatment. The benefit gained from taking a placebo occurs because the person taking it believes it will have a positive effect.

Since the effectiveness of any drug may be due in part to this "placebo effect," which is based on a person's expectations of the drug, many new drugs are tested against a placebo preparation. The placebo is made to look and taste identical to the active preparation; volunteers are not told which preparation they are taking.

A comparison of the results enables a more accurate assessment of the drug's efficacy.

Placenta

The organ that develops in the uterus during pregnancy and links the blood supplies of the mother and baby.
STRUCTURE
The placenta develops from the chorion (the outermost layer of cells that develops from the fertilized egg). It is firmly attached to the lining of the woman's uterus and is connected to the baby by the umbilical cord. By the end of pregnancy it is about 8 inches (20 cm) wide and 1 inch (2.5 cm) thick. Shortly after the baby is born, the placenta is expelled (thus its common name, "afterbirth").
FUNCTION
The placenta acts as an organ of respiration and excretion for the fetus. It transfers oxygen from the mother's circulation into the fetus's circulation, and removes waste products from the fetus's blood into the mother's blood for excretion by her lungs and kidneys. The placenta also conveys nutrients from mother to baby.

The placenta produces three hormones—*estrogen*, *progesterone*, and human chorionic gonadotropin

---

FUNCTION OF THE PLACENTA

The mother's and baby's blood do not completely mix in the placenta, but are brought sufficiently close so that exchange of nutrients and oxygen (from mother to baby) and waste products (from baby to mother) can occur between the two blood circulations.

Pool of mother's blood

Maternal blood vessels

Umbilical cord

Chorionic villi

Placenta

How the mother's and baby's blood are brought together
The baby's blood flows via the umbilical cord to the placenta, where it enters numerous tiny blood vessels arranged in "fingers" (chorionic villi). These are surrounded by a pool of maternal blood brought to the placenta by a major artery.

P

(HCG; see *Gonadotropin, human chorionic*). High levels of HCG appear in the woman's urine during pregnancy and detection of them in the urine forms the basis of *pregnancy tests*. The hormones enter the mother's blood to help her body adapt to the conditions of pregnancy; they also prepare the breasts for lactation (see *Breastfeeding*).

Placenta previa

Implantation of the placenta in the lower part of the uterus, near or over the cervix. Placenta previa occurs in approximately one in 200 pregnancies; it is less common in first pregnancies.

The condition varies in severity, depending on how much of the placenta is situated close to the cervix. In some cases, mild placenta previa is detected by *ultrasound scanning* but has no adverse effect on the pregnancy. More severe placenta previa often causes sudden painless vaginal bleeding in late pregnancy, when placental tissue separates from the uterus.

If the bleeding is minor and the pregnancy still has several weeks to run, bed rest may be all that is necessary. If the bleeding stops, the woman may be allowed to get up but she will probably be advised to remain resting in bed until the baby is born because of the risk of sudden severe hemorrhage. The baby is usually delivered by cesarean section at the 38th week.

If the bleeding is heavy or if the pregnancy is near term, an immediate delivery is carried out.

Plague

A serious infectious disease that mainly affects rodents but is transmissible to humans by the bites of rodent fleas. Plague has been a scourge to people since early history. One of the largest pandemics (worldwide epidemics) was the "black death" of the 14th century, which killed 25 million people in Europe alone. Today, human plague occurs sporadically in various parts of the world (including the US), but can be treated with antibiotics.

CAUSES, TYPES, AND INCIDENCE

The bacterium responsible for the disease, YERSINIA PESTIS, circulates among rodents and their fleas in many parts of the world. The great pandemics of the past were caused by spread of plague from wild rodents to rats in cities and then to humans (via rat fleas) when the rats died. Today, human disease is usually the result of

SPREAD OF PLAGUE

1 Plague bacteria circulate mainly among wild rodents, such as prairie dogs, ground squirrels, and chipmunks, in the US. They are spread from rodent to rodent by rodent fleas.

2 Sometimes so many wild rodents die that the fleas transfer to and infest new wild hosts, such as rats, or even humans who enter plague-affected areas.

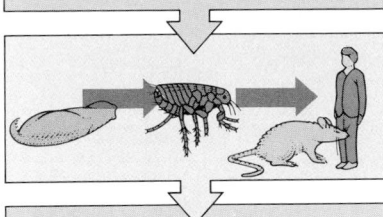

3 The real danger is of plague spreading to, and killing, large numbers of urban rats; rat fleas might then transfer from dead rats to humans en masse, causing an epidemic.

being bitten by fleas of wild rodents. A bite from an infected flea leads to bubonic plague, a form of the disease characterized by swollen lymph glands (called "buboes"). Pneumonic plague, which affects the lungs, can occur as a complication of bubonic plague; it is also spread from person to person in infected droplets expelled during coughing.

In recent years, outbreaks of plague have been confined mainly to parts of Africa, South America, and Southeast Asia. In the US, plague is present in rodents such as ground squirrels, prairie dogs, and marmots in parts of Arizona, New Mexico, California, Colorado, and Nevada. Some 10 to 50 cases of human plague occur in these areas of the US each year, mainly in the spring or summer.

PREVENTION

There is a constant risk of plague spreading to urban rat populations, and the main measures to prevent this are rat control and surveillance of the disease in wild rodents. Hikers in areas where plague is present should not touch rodents or any carcass.

A vaccine against plague is available for people in high-risk occupations, such as agricultural workers within plague areas and workers conducting research on the plague organism.

SYMPTOMS AND SIGNS

Bubonic plague usually starts two to five days after infection with fever, shivering, and severe headache. Soon the buboes appear. They are smooth, oval, reddened, intensely painful swellings usually in the groin, less commonly in the armpits, neck, or elsewhere. There may be bleeding into the skin around the buboes, resulting in dark patches. The victim may have seizures and, in about half the cases, will die if not treated. Occasionally, *septicemia* (blood poisoning) is an early complication and may cause death before buboes appear.

In pneumonic plague, there is severe coughing that produces a bloody, frothy sputum (phlegm) and labored breathing. Death is almost inevitable unless the disease is diagnosed and treated early.

DIAGNOSIS AND TREATMENT

A sample of fluid taken from a bubo, or of sputum in the case of suspected pneumonic plague, is cultured to confirm the presence of plague bacteria and establish the diagnosis.

Prompt treatment with the antibiotics streptomycin, chloramphenicol, or tetracycline reduces the risk of death to less than 5 percent.

All contacts of anyone with pneumonic plague are watched closely and their temperatures checked regularly for a week. Antibiotics are given as a preventive measure and at the first suspicion of illness.

Plantar wart

A hard, horny, rough-surfaced area on the sole of the foot caused by a virus called a papillomavirus. Plantar warts (verrucae plantaris) may occur singly or in mosaiclike clusters.

Infection is usually acquired from contaminated floors in swimming pools and communal showers. Because of pressure from the weight of the body, the wart is flattened and forced into the skin of the sole, sometimes causing discomfort or pain when standing or walking.

P

TREATMENT

Many plantar warts disappear without treatment, but some persist for years or may recur. To relieve discomfort, a foam pad may be worn in the shoe. Plantar warts can be removed by *cryosurgery, electrodesiccation, curettage, laser treatment,* or applying salicylic acid plasters.

Plants, poisonous

Several species of plants are poisonous to eat or can cause a severe allergic reaction if their leaves brush against the skin.

SKIN CONTACT

In the US, poison ivy, poison oak, and poison sumac can cause severe skin reactions. They grow as vines or bushes, and the leaves have three leaflets (poison ivy, poison oak) or a row of paired leaflets (poison sumac). Itching, burning, and blistering develop at the site of skin contact. In some people, these skin reactions can be extremely severe.

First-aid treatment includes thorough washing of the affected area, sponging with alcohol, and application of calamine lotion. Washing any clothing that may have come in contact with the plant is also advised. In the case of a severe reaction, it is wise to consult a physician, who may prescribe *corticosteroid drugs* to be taken by mouth or injection.

INTERNAL POISONING

Plants that are poisonous to eat include foxglove, aconite, hemlock, laburnum seeds, and many types of berry, including the berries of deadly nightshade (which are black) and holly (red). Young children are the most commonly affected as a result of eating colorful berries. Symptoms of poisoning vary according to the plant but may include abdominal pain, vomiting, excitement, flushing, breathing difficulties, delirium, and coma. Medical help should be sought at once. The usual treatment is gastric *lavage* and measures to relieve symptoms as they arise.

Fatal poisoning is rare. Children should be taught not to sample berries or any type of wild plant.

Paradoxically, many poisonous plants are a source of useful drugs (e.g., *atropine* from deadly nightshade and *digitalis drugs* from foxglove). See also *Mushroom poisoning.*

Plaque

The term given to an area of *atherosclerosis* (a disease that affects the inner lining of arteries). The

---

POISONOUS PLANTS

There are hundreds of different poisonous plants—including many common houseplants and flowers—in addition to those shown. Therefore, it is best to eat only plants known to be harmless.

Poison ivy
Poison ivy occurs throughout the US, growing as a bush or vine; each leaf consists of three shiny leaflets. On skin contact, an oily substance on the surface of the plant causes irritation, which can be severe.

Nightshade
Sometimes called belladonna, the nightshade is about 3 feet high, with shiny black berries. Eating any part can lead to symptoms such as rash, blurred vision, swallowing difficulty, confusion, and coma.

Foxglove
This plant has purplish pink flowers; it is a source of the heart drug digitalis. Eating the plant irritates the mouth and causes abdominal pain, diarrhea, and disturbance to the heart beat.

---

atheromatous plaques give no indication of their presence until they become so large that they reduce blood flow in a vessel or until some disturbance of the plaque surface develops, causing *thrombosis* (clotting of blood) at the site. When this occurs in a small or medium-sized vessel, blockage is likely (see *Peripheral vascular disease*). Plaques in the coronary arteries (which supply blood to the heart muscle) are the cause of *coronary heart disease.*

Plaque, dental

A rough sticky coating on the teeth that consists of saliva, bacteria, and food debris. It is the chief cause of tooth decay (see *Caries, dental*) and *gingivitis*; if allowed to accumulate, plaque forms the basis of a hard deposit (see *Calculus, dental*).

Plaque begins to form on teeth within a few hours of cleaning and is responsible for the furry feeling of unbrushed teeth. Salivary mucus, consisting mainly of proteins, forms on the teeth. Bacteria that live in the mouth then multiply within this mucus, building up a layer of plaque. Some of these microorganisms, notably *STREPTOCOCCUS MUTANS,* break down the sugar in the remains of carbohydrate food that stick to the mucus, adding to the plaque and creating an acid that erodes enamel.

Plaque should be thoroughly removed at least once a day by *toothbrushing* and use of dental floss (see *Floss, dental*). It can be made more visible by the use of harmless dyes known as *disclosing agents.*

Plasma

The fluid part of blood that remains if the blood cells are removed. It is a solution containing many important nutrients, salts, proteins, and other chemicals (see *Blood*).

Plasmapheresis

A procedure, also called plasma exchange, for removing or reducing the concentration of unwanted substances in the blood. Blood is withdrawn from the patient in the same way as for *blood donation,* and the plasma portion of the blood is removed by special machines called cell separators. The blood cells are then mixed with a plasma substitute and returned to the circulation in the same way as for *blood transfusion.* The procedure usually takes approximately two hours.

The main use of plasmapheresis is to remove damaging antibodies or antibody-antigen particles (immune complexes) from the circulation in some *autoimmune disorders,* such as *myasthenia gravis, Goodpasture's syndrome,* kidney disease associated with systemic *lupus erythematosus*, and thrombotic *thrombocytopenia*.

Plasma proteins

All the proteins present in blood plasma (see *Blood*). They include *albumin*, fibrinogen, and other substances important to *blood clotting* and *immunoglobulins* (proteins with a role in the *immune system*).

Apart from their specific roles, the plasma proteins help maintain blood volume by preventing loss of water from the blood into the tissues. The proteins keep the water in the blood by a phenomenon called osmotic pressure (see *Osmosis*).

Plasminogen activator

See *Tissue plasminogen activator*.

Plaster of Paris

A white powder composed of a calcium compound that reacts chemically with water, giving off heat and producing a paste that can be molded and shaped before it sets. Plaster of Paris is used for constructing *casts* to immobilize parts of the body and for making dental models (see *Impression, dental*).

Plastic surgeon

A surgeon who uses special techniques to repair visible defects of skin and underlying tissue present from birth or caused by burns, injuries, certain types of operation, aging, or disease (see *Plastic surgery*). Plastic surgeons also perform operations to improve the appearance of healthy people (see *Cosmetic surgery*).

Plastic surgery

Any operation carried out to repair or reconstruct skin and underlying tissue that has been damaged or lost by injury or disease, has been malformed since birth, or has changed with aging. Every attempt is made to maintain function of the affected part of the body and to create as natural an appearance as possible.

Operations performed mainly to improve appearance in a healthy person are known as *cosmetic surgery*.

WHY IT IS DONE

Plastic surgery is usually performed to treat damage caused by severe burns or injuries, cancer, certain types of operation, such as *mastectomy* (breast removal), or the effects of aging. Among the more common congenital conditions that may require correction by plastic surgery are *cleft lip and palate*, *hypospadias*, and imperforate anus (see *Anus, imperforate*).

HOW IT IS DONE

A variety of techniques is used to provide skin cover for damaged areas, including *skin grafts*, *skin and muscle flaps*, *Z-plasty*, and tissue expansion (in which skin is stretched by inserting a silicone balloon beneath the surface and gradually increasing its size). These techniques may be combined with a *bone graft* or *implants* to provide underlying support.

The scope of plastic surgery has been much broadened over the past 10 years by the use of microsurgical techniques (see *Microsurgery*) to join blood vessels, thus allowing the transfer of blocks of skin and muscle from one part of the body to another.

-plasty

A suffix meaning shaping by surgery; performing plastic surgery on. *Rhinoplasty* is plastic surgery on the nose; *mammoplasty* is reshaping or reconstruction of the breasts.

Platelet

The smallest type of blood particle, also called a thrombocyte (see *Blood cells*). Platelets play a major role in *blood clotting*. A deficiency of platelets (*thrombocytopenia*) can cause *bleeding disorders* or *purpura*.

Electron micrograph of platelets
Normal and activated (spiky) platelets can be seen. Activated platelets clump to seal defects in blood vessel walls after injury.

Platyhelminth

 A flat, or ribbon-shaped, parasitic worm. Flukes, *tapeworms*, and schistosomes are types that cause disease in humans. (See *Liver fluke*; *Schistosomiasis*.)

Play therapy

A method used in the *psychoanalysis* of young children. Play therapy is based on the principle that all play in children has some symbolic significance.

The child is allowed to choose from the toys, drawing materials, and games in the therapist's room. Watching the child at play helps the therapist diagnose the source of the child's problems; the child can then be helped to "act out" particular thoughts and feelings that are causing anxiety. An improvement in the child's state may be indicated by changes in play, such as drawing smiling faces.

Plethora

A florid, bright-red, flushed complexion. It may be caused by dilation of blood vessels near the skin surface, or, more rarely, by *polycythemia* (excessive numbers of red blood cells).

Plethysmography

A method of estimating the blood flow in vessels by measuring changes in the size of a body part. Plethysmography

P

DEVELOPMENT OF PLAQUE

Plaque starts with a deposit of salivary mucus on the teeth. The mucus is colonized by various types of bacteria. Initially, the predominant bacteria are spherical cocci. After a day or two, long filamentous colonies of bacteria spread over the surface of the teeth.

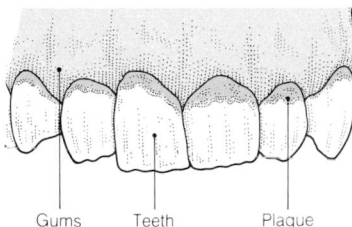

Areas of plaque buildup
Plaque develops predominantly at the margin of teeth and gums. If the gums are inflamed or otherwise unhealthy, the plaque tends to develop more rapidly.

Mature plaque
This picture, taken with a scanning electron microscope, shows a mass of filamentous bacterial colonies in plaque, magnified about 2,000 times.

is used on the penis to establish whether a patient with *impotence* gets an erection during sleep. It is occasionally used in the investigation of deep vein *thrombosis* to detect an obstruction of the blood flow back toward the heart.

Pleura

A thin membrane with two layers, one lining the outside of the lungs and the other the inside of the chest cavity. Fluid between the two layers provides lubrication and thus allows smooth, uniform expansion and contraction of the lungs during breathing.

DISORDERS

Pleurisy (inflammation of the pleura) is usually caused by a lung infection, such as *pneumonia* or *tuberculosis*, and may lead to *pleural effusion* (excessive fluid between the layers of the pleura). *Pneumothorax* (air in the pleural cavity) may occur spontaneously or be caused by a penetrating injury.

Pleural effusion

An accumulation of fluid between the layers of the *pleura* (the membrane lining the lungs and chest cavity). Pleural effusion may be caused by *pneumonia*, *heart failure*, *cancer*, *pulmonary embolism*, or *mesothelioma* (pleural tumor). The effusion may affect one or both sides of the chest.

Pleural effusion causes compression of the underlying lung, leading to breathing difficulty. Diagnosis is confirmed by *chest X ray*. To determine the cause of the effusion, some of the fluid may be aspirated (removed with a needle and syringe) and examined. A *biopsy* (removal of a tissue sample for microscopic analysis) of the pleura may also be necessary.

Treatment is of the underlying cause. The fluid may require draining with a needle or tube to help breathing. In some cases, depending on the cause, *tetracycline* or *anticancer drugs* are injected into the pleural space to prevent a recurrence.

Pleurisy

Inflammation of the *pleura* (the membrane lining the lungs and chest cavity). Pleurisy is usually caused by a lung infection, such as *pneumonia* or *pleurodynia* (a viral infection). Rarer causes include *pulmonary embolism*, *lung cancer*, and *rheumatoid arthritis*.

Pleurisy causes a sharp chest pain that sometimes travels to the tip of the shoulder on the involved side. The pain, which is worse when breathing in, arises because the two inflamed membranes rub across each other. Treatment is of the underlying cause, along with *analgesics* (painkillers).

Pleurodynia

Pain in the chest due to an infectious disease. Sometimes called Bornholm disease, pleurodynia is caused by coxsackievirus B and often occurs in epidemics; it usually affects children but can occur at any age.

Symptoms include sudden severe pain in the lower chest or upper abdomen, with fever, sore throat, headache, and malaise. The disease usually settles in three or four days without treatment, but sometimes recurs several times over a period of weeks. Occasionally, pleurodynia is complicated by *orchitis* (inflammation of the testis), *pericarditis* (inflammation of the lining of the heart), or *meningitis* (inflammation of the lining of the brain and spinal cord).

Plexus

A network of interwoven nerves or blood vessels, such as the *brachial plexus* (a network of nerves in the neck and upper arm) and the choroid plexus (in the brain).

Plication

A surgical procedure in which tucks are taken in the walls of a hollow organ and then stitched to decrease the organ's size. One type of plication is fundoplication, used to treat *hiatal hernia*. In this operation, the fundus (upper part) of the stomach is folded up around the lower end of the esophagus to create an inkwell-like valve to prevent reflux of gastric acid from the stomach into the esophagus.

Plummer-Vinson syndrome

Difficulty swallowing caused by the formation of webs of tissue across the upper esophagus, and usually occurring with severe iron-deficiency *anemia*. The condition primarily affects middle-aged women.

The diagnosis is made by a barium swallow (see *Barium X-ray examinations*) and by inspection of the esophagus with an *endoscope* (flexible viewing instrument). Treatment of the anemia usually relieves symptoms; swallowing is relieved when the web is broken, which often occurs at the time of endoscopy.

Plutonium

A radioactive metallic element that occurs naturally only in infinitesimal amounts in uranium ores; it is produced artificially in breeder reactors by the bombardment of uranium with neutrons. Plutonium is used as a fuel in nuclear reactors and as an explosive in nuclear weapons, such as the atomic bomb that was dropped on Nagasaki in 1945. The element is highly toxic if it enters the body because of its high rate of *radiation* emission (in the form of alpha particles) and its specific absorption in bone marrow.

PMS

See *Premenstrual syndrome*.

Pneumaturia

The presence of gas in the urine. Pneumaturia usually indicates that a *fistula* (an abnormal connection) has developed between the bladder and the intestine. It is an unusual complication of a number of disorders, including *Crohn's disease*, *cancer*, or *diverticular disease*.

Pneumo-

A prefix meaning related to the lungs, to air, or to the breath. Pneumonia is a disease in which there is inflammation and the accumulation of cells and fluid in the lungs; pneumothorax is air in the pleural space in the chest.

Pneumoconiosis

Any of a group of lung diseases caused by the inhalation of certain mineral dusts. These dusts originate from nonfibrous materials, so they do not include asbestos (see *Asbestosis*).

Only dust particles smaller than about one five thousandth of an inch across—small enough to reach the smallest air passages and alveoli (air sacs) in the lungs—are likely to cause harm. The dust particles cannot be destroyed within or removed from the lungs, so they accumulate and eventually cause thickening and scarring. The lungs become less efficient in supplying oxygen to the blood.

TYPES, CAUSES, AND INCIDENCE

The main types of pneumoconiosis are coal workers' pneumoconiosis (caused by coal dust) and silicosis, caused by dust containing silica (a constituent of sand and many types of rock, and the sole constituent of quartz). Silicosis is a hazard for workers in occupations such as quartz mining, stone cutting, blasting, and tunnel construction.

The risk of having either disease develop is directly related to the amount of dust inhaled over the years. Both diseases primarily affect workers over 50, although acute cases of silicosis can occur with 10 months' exposure to a high level of dust.

Other, far less common, types of pneumoconiosis are caused by dusts containing beryllium (used in various high-technology industries), kaolin (from china-clay processing), shale, or hematite (from mining iron ore).

Overall, about 1,700 new cases of pneumoconiosis, causing about 1,000 premature deaths, are diagnosed each year in the US. The incidence is falling due to better preventive measures (e.g., by enforcing maximum permitted dust levels in industry and by use of protective clothing).

SYMPTOMS AND COMPLICATIONS

Pneumoconiosis is often detected by a *chest X ray* before it causes any symptoms; if exposure to the dust is stopped at this point, further progression of the disease is sometimes prevented. In other cases, the main symptom is shortness of breath, which gradually gets worse.

In severe cases, *cor pulmonale* (a type of failure of the right side of the heart caused by the lung damage) may develop. There is also a variant of the disease called progressive massive fibrosis, in which damage continues relentlessly (mainly affecting the upper parts of the lungs) even though exposure to dust has stopped.

Complications include the development of *emphysema* and an increased risk of *tuberculosis* in people who have silicosis. One type of pneumoconiosis—caused by hematite—is associated with an increased risk of lung cancer.

DIAGNOSIS, TREATMENT, AND OUTLOOK

The diagnosis depends on *pulmonary function tests*, a chest X ray, and a history of exposure to dusts.

There is no treatment for pneumoconiosis aside from treating complications such as lung infections and cor pulmonale. Further exposure to dust must be avoided.

Anyone in whom pneumoconiosis develops at an early age or in whom progressive massive fibrosis develops at any age is at increased risk of a premature death. In the US, compensation can be claimed by anyone in whom pneumoconiosis develops.

Pneumocystis pneumonia

An infection of the lungs that is caused by the microorganism *PNEUMOCYSTIS CARINII*, a type of protozoan (single-celled) parasite. Pneumocystis pneumonia is an *oppor-*tunistic infection that is dangerous only to people with impaired immunity (resistance) to infection—such as people who are suffering from *AIDS* or *leukemia*. Pneumocystis pneumonia is a major cause of death in people who have AIDS.

Symptoms include fever, dry cough, and shortness of breath. They may last from a few weeks to a few months. Diagnosis is by examination of the sputum (phlegm) or a lung *biopsy*. High doses of antibiotics may help eradicate the infection, although it can recur.

Pneumonectomy

An operation to remove an entire lung. Pneumonectomy is sometimes performed to treat *lung cancer*. It once was used to treat *tuberculosis*, *bronchiectasis*, and lung infection, but these conditions are usually treated today by drugs or removal of only part of the lung (see *Lobectomy, lung*).

Before a pneumonectomy is performed, *pulmonary function tests* are carried out to make sure that the remaining lung is healthy enough to cope with the increased demands that will be placed on it.

HOW IT IS DONE

Using general anesthesia, a curved incision is made (starting under the armpit and extending across the back) following the line of the lower edge of the shoulder blade. The muscles are cut through and the ribs gently spread apart to expose the lung. Sometimes a rib is removed for better exposure. The arteries, veins, and bronchi (air passages) leading to the lung are tied off and divided, and the lung is removed. A drain is usually inserted into the pleural space (see *Pleura*) and the incision is then stitched.

RECOVERY PERIOD

The drain is usually removed the day after the operation, and the stitches are taken out after about 10 days, when the patient can usually leave the hospital. Many patients require *ventilator* support for hours to days after the operation. At home, normal activities should be resumed slowly; most people are able to return to work after about two months.

Pneumonia

Inflammation of the lungs due to infection. Pneumonia is the sixth most common cause of death in the US, primarily because it is a common complication of any serious illness. It is more common in males, during infancy and old age, and in those who have reduced immunity to infection (such as alcoholics).

There are two main types of pneumonia: lobar pneumonia and bronchopneumonia. In lobar pneumonia one lobe of one lung initially is affected. In bronchopneumonia, inflammation starts in the bronchi and bronchioles (airways) and then spreads to affect patches of tissue in one or both lungs.

CAUSES

Most cases of pneumonia are caused by viruses or bacteria. Causes of viral pneumonia include adenovirus, respiratory syncytial virus, or a coxsackievirus. The most common bacterial pneumonia is caused by *STREPTOCOCCUS PNEUMONIAE*. Other causes of bacterial pneumonia include *HEMOPHILUS INFLUENZAE*, *LEGIONELLA PNEUMOPHILIA* (see *Legionnaires' disease*), and *STAPHYLOCOCCUS AUREUS*. Pneumonia may also be caused by a *mycoplasma* (an organism that is intermediate between a bacterium and a virus) or by a *chlamydial infection*; *Q fever* is a type of pneumonia caused by a *rickettsia*.

Rarely, pneumonia may be due to a different type of organism, such as fungi, yeasts, or protozoa. These types usually occur only in people with *immunodeficiency disorders* (e.g., pneumocystis pneumonia, caused by a protozoon, commonly occurs in people with *AIDS*).

SYMPTOMS AND SIGNS

Symptoms and signs typically include fever, chills, shortness of breath, and a cough that produces yellow-green sputum and occasionally blood. Chest pain that is worse when breathing in may occur because of *pleurisy* (inflammation of the membrane lining the lungs and chest cavity).

Potential complications include *pleural effusion* (fluid around the lung), *empyema* (pus in the pleural cavity), and, rarely, an *abscess* in the lung.

DIAGNOSIS

The physician gives the patient a physical examination, listening to chest sounds through a stethoscope. The diagnosis may be confirmed by a *chest X ray* and by examination of sputum and, occasionally, of blood for microorganisms.

TREATMENT

Patients with mild pneumonia can usually be treated at home, but hospitalization is necessary in severe cases. The drugs prescribed depend on the causative microorganism; they may include *antibiotic drugs* or *antifungal drugs*. Aspirin or acetaminophen may be given to reduce fever. In severe cases, *oxygen therapy* and artificial *ventilation* may be required.

OUTLOOK
The majority of sufferers recover completely within two weeks. However, some elderly or debilitated people fail to respond to treatment; progressively more lung tissue is affected and death occurs as a result of respiratory failure.

Pneumonitis
Inflammation of the lungs that causes coughing, breathing difficulty, and sometimes wheezing. Pneumonitis may be due to a wide range of causes, including infection, allergic reaction caused by inhalation of dust containing animal or plant material (see *Alveolitis*), exposure to radiation (see *Radiation hazards*), and inhalation of vomit. It may also occur as a rare side effect of some drugs, such as acebutolol and azathioprine.

Pneumothorax
A condition in which air enters the pleural cavity (the space between the two layers of pleura lining the lungs and the chest wall) from the lungs or from the outside.

PNEUMONIA
Pneumonia is not a single disease, but the name for several types of lung inflammation caused by infectious organisms. In some cases, accidental inhalation of vomit or a liquid starts the infection. The symptoms, treatment, and outcome vary greatly, depending on the cause and on the general health of the patient.

Lobar pneumonia
In this type, which is rare in most developed countries today, the inflammation is usually confined to just one lobe of one lung—often a lower lobe.

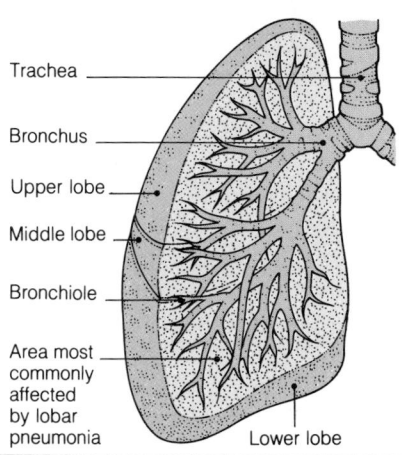

Trachea
Bronchus
Upper lobe
Middle lobe
Bronchiole
Area most commonly affected by lobar pneumonia
Lower lobe

Chest X ray in bronchopneumonia
The X ray clearly shows bronchopneumonia. The blotchy, white areas within the darker areas correspond to patches of inflamed lung.

TYPES, CAUSES, AND TREATMENT OF PNEUMONIA

Types	Causes	Symptoms	Drug treatments	Other treatments
Pneumonias always or usually caused by bacteria				
Lobar pneumonia	*Streptococcus pneumoniae*	Cough, painful breathing, high temperature, rust-colored sputum	Penicillin	Machine ventilation of the lungs to help breathing may be required in some cases. Respiratory therapy to clear sputum out of the lungs may also be needed.
Bronchopneumonia	*Hemophilus influenzae* or other organisms	Cough, often a fever, green or yellow sputum	Antibiotics	
Aspiration pneumonia	Various organisms. Occurs following inhalation of sputum, vomit, liquids, and so on.	Fever, cough	Antibiotics	
Legionnaires' disease	*Legionella pneumophila*	Fever, cough, chest pain, headache, aches and pains	Erythromycin	
Pneumonias not caused by bacteria				
Viral pneumonia	Chickenpox virus, influenza virus, and adenovirus	Cough, fever, not much sputum	Antibiotics (if lungs become infected by bacteria)	Machine ventilation of the lungs to help breathing may be required in severe cases.
Psittacosis	*Chlamydia psittaci*, a bacterialike organism caught from birds	Cough, raised temperature, not much sputum	Tetracycline or erythromycin	
Q fever	*Coxiella burnetti*, a rickettsia	Cough, raised temperature, not much sputum	Tetracycline or erythromycin	
Mycoplasmal pneumonia	*Mycoplasma pneumoniae*, a bacterialike organism	Cough, raised temperature, not much sputum	Tetracycline or erythromycin	

P

CAUSES

Spontaneous pneumothorax, which usually occurs for no apparent reason, is six times more common in men than women. Most often, it occurs in thin young adults who have no underlying lung disease; in many cases, it is thought to be due to rupture of a congenital blister (*bleb*) at the top of the lung. There is a 30 percent chance of a recurrence of spontaneous pneumothorax, usually on the same side. Pneumothorax may also be a complication of lung disease (particularly *asthma* or *emphysema*) or it may follow a penetrating injury (e.g., rib fracture).

A pneumothorax may be caused accidentally when a catheter is inserted into a vein in the neck for artificial *feeding*.

SYMPTOMS

A pneumothorax may cause chest pain or shortness of breath. The degree of breathlessness is proportional to the size of the pneumothorax and any underlying lung disease may be severe. If there is continual leakage of air, the pneumothorax may become progressively bigger and produce a tension pneumothorax, which may occasionally be life-threatening because of compression of the heart.

DIAGNOSIS AND TREATMENT

A chest X ray confirms the diagnosis and may also show any underlying lung disease.

A small pneumothorax in a healthy adult usually disappears within a few days without treatment. A larger pneumothorax, or a small one in the presence of underlying lung disease, requires treatment. Treatment usually involves removing the air from the pleural cavity through a suction tube inserted through the chest wall; the tube often needs to stay in place for several days. A small pneumothorax can be treated by drawing out the air through a needle and syringe. If the lung fails to expand, or if the pneumothorax recurs, surgery may be required to seal the pleural cavity.

Pocket, gingival

See *Periodontitis*.

Podiatrist

A specialist in diagnosing, treating, and preventing diseases and malfunctions of the foot (see *Podiatry*). A podiatrist earns a Doctor of Podiatric Medicine (DPM) degree after completion of college and four years of podiatric medical education (some podiatrists take additional years of residency training).

Podiatrists are licensed to prescribe medications and perform surgery. While most surgery can be performed in the podiatrist's office or in an ambulatory care facility, podiatrists may also use hospital facilities. Podiatrists often work closely with physicians to assure that comprehensive care is provided to the patient.

Podiatry

The branch of medicine that deals with the examination, diagnosis, treatment, and prevention of diseases and malfunctions of the foot and its related structures. Podiatric medicine is concerned with many different types of foot problems, including walking disorders in children, ankle injuries among adolescents, fractures among athletes and joggers, *bunions* and *hammer toes* among men and women of all ages, and care of foot ulcers, toenails, and infections among people who have diabetes.

Podophyllin

A drug used in the treatment of genital warts (see *Warts, genital*). It may damage normal skin if not applied carefully. Overuse may in rare cases cause serious adverse effects, such as kidney damage and reduced production of white blood cells.

Poison

A substance that, in relatively small amounts, disrupts the structure and/or function of cells. Although *toxin* is often used interchangeably with poison, toxin refers strictly and specifically to poisonous proteins produced by pathogenic (disease-causing) bacteria, some animals, and certain plants. (See also *Drug poisoning; Poisoning*.)

Poisoning

Poisons enter the body by various routes. They may be swallowed, inhaled, absorbed through the skin, or injected under the skin (as with an *insect sting* or *snakebite*). They may also originate within the body itself.

For example, bacteria can produce poisonous *endotoxins*, *enterotoxins*, or *exotoxins*. Various disorders, such as *renal failure*, *liver failure*, and certain metabolic disorders (see *Metabolism*), may cause poisonous substances to be produced or to accumulate within the body.

Poisoning may be acute or chronic. In acute poisoning, a large amount of poison enters, or is produced in, the body over a short time (as may occur in *food poisoning*). Chronic poisoning results from the gradual accumulation of a poison.

FIRST AID: POISONING

DO NOT
- make the victim vomit if he or she has swallowed corrosives

1 If the victim is conscious, quickly ask what he or she has swallowed.

2 Call an ambulance and say what the victim has taken.

3 If the victim is unconscious but breathing, place him or her in the *recovery position*.

4 If the victim is not breathing, *artificial respiration* is necessary. Use the mouth-to-nose method to avoid contact with the poison.

5 If you are certain the victim has swallowed only tablets or berries, it may help to induce vomiting by placing your fingers at the back of the throat.

P

Accidental poisoning is one of the most common types of accident in the home. It occurs primarily in young children, although adults sometimes accidentally poison themselves, often by mistaking the dosage of a prescribed drug (see *Drug poisoning*) or, less commonly, by unthinkingly taking very high doses of certain vitamin or mineral supplements. Exposure to poisonous substances in industry is another important cause of unintentional poisoning in adults, as is *drug abuse*.

Poisoning may be a deliberate attempt to commit *suicide*. However, most such attempts are unsuccessful or are not intended to prove fatal. Taking a drug overdose (often in combination with alcohol, which increases the toxicity of many drugs) is a common method of suicidal poisoning. (See also *Poisoning* first-aid box and articles on individual poisons.)

Poison ivy

See *Plants, poisonous*.

Polio

An abbreviation of *poliomyelitis*.

Poliomyelitis

An infectious disease once known as infantile paralysis but now usually called polio. Poliomyelitis is caused by a virus, which usually provokes no more than a mild illness. However, in more serious cases it attacks the central nervous system (brain and spinal cord). This may lead to extensive paralysis (including paralysis of the muscles involved in breathing) or may be fatal.

Since the development of effective vaccines in the 1950s, polio has virtually been eliminated from the US and Europe; cases still occur in people who have not been fully vaccinated. Polio also remains a serious risk for anyone not vaccinated and traveling in southern Europe, Africa, or Asia.

INCIDENCE OF PARALYTIC POLIO (US)

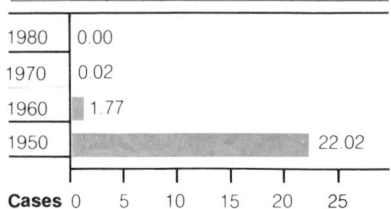

Year	Cases
1980	0.00
1970	0.02
1960	1.77
1950	22.02

Cases 0 5 10 15 20 25

New cases per 100,000 population
The incidence has dropped dramatically since the 1950s. In 1986, there were just three reported cases in the entire US.

CAUSES AND INCIDENCE

There are three closely related polioviruses. Infected people pass large numbers of virus particles in their feces, from where they may be spread indirectly, or directly via fingers, to food to infect others. Airborne transmission also occurs.

In countries where standards of hygiene and sanitation are low, most children become infected and immunity to polio develops early in life, when the infection rarely causes serious illness. In countries with better standards of hygiene, children do not become immune in this manner; if they are not vaccinated, disastrous epidemics occur. Immunization is thus of vital importance.

Wasted limb of polio patient
Muscle bulk is severely reduced in the paralyzed (right) leg. Muscle function can sometimes be helped by physical therapy.

PREVENTION

Vaccination is given during infancy, usually in doses at 2, 4, and 18 months of age in the US, with an optional extra dose at 6 months and a booster dose at 5 years (see *Immunization*). The vaccine contains all three types of poliovirus, and immunity develops against each in turn. There are two alternative types of vaccine: IPV (inactivated polio vaccine), which contains dead viruses and is given by injection, and OPV (oral poliovirus vaccine), which contains live but harmless strains of virus and is given by mouth. OPV is the vaccine of choice in the US, except for children who have an *immunodeficiency disorder*, which lowers resistance to infection.

There is an extremely small risk (about one in 5 million doses) of the live vaccine causing polio in the vaccinated person or in a close contact.

SYMPTOMS AND SIGNS

Minor forms of polio are by far the most common. About 85 percent of children infected with the virus have no symptoms at all. In the rest, after an incubation period of three to five days, there is a short illness with slight fever, sore throat, headache, and vomiting. This lasts for a few days, after which the majority of children recover completely.

In some children, however, after a short period of apparent health there is a major illness with symptoms of *meningitis* (inflammation of the coverings of the brain and spinal cord). The symptoms are fever, severe headache, stiffness of the neck and back, and aching in the muscles, sometimes with widespread twitching. In some cases the condition progresses, often in the course of a few hours, to extensive paralysis of muscles. The legs and lower trunk are the most frequently paralyzed. If infection spreads to the brain stem (lowest part of the brain), the result may be difficulty (or inability) swallowing and breathing.

DIAGNOSIS

To make a firm diagnosis, the causative virus must be isolated from a sample of cerebrospinal fluid, taken by *lumbar puncture*, or from a throat swab or sample of feces. Muscle paralysis combined with an acute feverish illness is so characteristic of severe polio that it usually enables an immediate diagnosis to be made.

TREATMENT

There is no effective drug treatment for polio. Nonparalytic patients do not usually need treatment except for bed rest and *analgesics*. When muscles are paralyzed, *physical therapy* is essential to prevent muscle damage while the virus is active. Later, during convalescence, it is needed to help retain muscle function.

When the lower part of the body is paralyzed, the bladder does not function properly and may need catheterization (see *Catheterization, urinary*). Respiratory paralysis requires *tracheostomy* (making an opening in the windpipe to insert a breathing tube) and artificial *ventilation*.

OUTLOOK

Recovery from nonparalytic polio is complete. Of those who become paralyzed, more than half eventually make a full recovery, more than a quarter suffer only minor permanent muscle weakness, less than a quarter are left with severe disability, and less than one in 10 dies (mainly adults and those in whom the brain stem has been severely affected). Years after extensive paralysis with some recovery, there is a "postpolio" deterioration with new weakness and pain of some of the recovered muscles.

Pollution

Contamination of the environment by poisons, microorganisms, or radioactive substances.

Serious public concern about pollution developed in the 1950s with the growing realization that *pesticides* were destroying wildlife and poisoning the food chain, and that atmospheric nuclear tests were disseminating radioactive fallout over a wide area (see *Radiation*). This concern was strengthened by incidents of industrial pollution, such as the release of mercury waste into Minamata Bay, Japan (see *Minamata disease*); the release into the atmosphere of the poisonous chemical dioxin by a factory explosion in Italy (see *Defoliant poisoning*); damage to seabirds and beaches from oil tanker spillages; and, more recently, acid rain and radioactive fallout from the nuclear reactor explosion at Chernobyl in the Soviet Union.

Probably the most serious pollutant in its long-term effects is *carbon dioxide*, vast amounts of which are discharged into the atmosphere by the burning of fossil fuels. The continual increase in the atmospheric carbon dioxide level is producing what is called the "greenhouse effect," which is increasing the average global temperature. If the level continues to increase, many experts believe it could cause catastrophic climatic changes within the next 50 years.

Perhaps as serious is the gradual destruction of the *ozone* layer (which blocks harmful ultraviolet radiation from the sun) as a result of the extensive use of aerosols. Other important pollutants include lead (see *Lead poisoning*), cadmium (see *Cadmium poisoning*), *DDT*, and agricultural pesticides, such as *parathion*.

Poly-

A prefix that means many, much, or excessive, as in polymyositis (inflammation of many muscles) and polyuria (excessive urination).

Polyarteritis nodosa

Another name for *periarteritis nodosa*.

Polycystic disease of the kidney

See *Kidney, polycystic*.

Polycystic ovary

A condition, also known as Stein-Leventhal syndrome, characterized by oligomenorrhea (scanty menstruation) or *amenorrhea* (absence of menstruation), *infertility*, *hirsutism* (excessive hairiness), and *obesity*. Often, but not always, the ovaries contain multiple cysts.

In most women with polycystic ovaries, menarche (the onset of menstruation) occurs at the normal age. After a year or two of regular menstruation, the periods become highly irregular, and then cease. Hirsutism, which often becomes evident around menarche, occurs in about 50 percent of cases, as does obesity.

CAUSE
The condition is due to an imbalance between the pituitary *gonadotropin hormones* luteinizing hormone (LH) and follicle-stimulating hormone (FSH); there is excessive stimulation of the ovaries by LH and a relative deficiency of FSH. This results in lack of *ovulation* and in increased *testosterone* production by the ovaries.

DIAGNOSIS
Tests to determine the level of hormones in the blood are needed to confirm the diagnosis. *Ultrasound scanning* of the ovaries and/or *laparoscopy* may be helpful.

TREATMENT
Methods include drug treatment with clomiphene, progestins, luteinizing hormone-releasing hormone, or oral contraceptives. In rare cases, surgical removal of a wedge of ovarian tissue is performed. The method of treatment used depends on the severity of the symptoms and on whether the woman wishes to become pregnant. Spontaneous ovulation is not unusual in women with polycystic ovary.

OUTLOOK
Since women with polycystic ovary often have high estrogen levels and irregular menstrual periods, they are at increased risk of heavy periods at menopause and, subsequently, are at increased risk of endometrial (uterine) cancer. Treatment with progesterone may be recommended to restore hormonal balance and decrease the risk of this cancer.

Polycythemia

A condition characterized by an unusually large number of red cells in the blood due to increased production of red cells by the bone marrow. This condition usually results from some other disorder or is a natural response to *hypoxia* (reduced oxygen in the blood and tissues). In such cases, it is called secondary polycythemia. Rarely, it occurs for no apparent reason and is called polycythemia vera or primary polycythemia.

SECONDARY POLYCYTHEMIA
Polycythemia occurs naturally in people living at (or visiting) high altitudes due to the reduced air pressure and level of oxygen. It can also result from any disorder that impairs the supply of oxygen to the blood (e.g., chronic *bronchitis*). In these cases, the low blood oxygen stimulates production of the hormone erythropoietin by the kidneys, which in turn stimulates the bone marrow to produce more red cells. The result is an increase in the oxygen-carrying efficiency of the blood, which compensates for the reduced oxygen supply. Descending to sea level, or effective treatment of an underlying disorder, soon returns the blood to normal.

Polycythemia can also be secondary to *liver cancer* or certain kidney disorders that cause excess production of erythropoietin. Treatment of the underlying disorder quickly returns the blood to normal.

POLYCYTHEMIA VERA
This rare disorder of the bone marrow develops primarily in people over 40. The estimated incidence is about five new cases per million people annually in the US.

The large number of red cells results in an increased volume and thickening of the blood, which may cause headaches, blurred vision, and *hypertension* (high blood pressure). There may also be a flushed skin, dizziness, night sweats, and widespread itching, particularly after a hot bath. Often, the sufferer's spleen is enlarged. In addition, there may be abnormalities in the platelets in blood, causing a tendency to bleed or to form blood clots. Other complications include *stroke* and, at a late stage, other types of bone marrow disease, such as *myelosclerosis* or myelogenous leukemia (see *Leukemia, chronic myeloid*).

The diagnosis is made from a physical examination and *blood tests* and by ruling out any other causes of polycythemia. Treatment of polycythemia vera consists of regular *venesection* (removal of blood through a vein), sometimes in combination with *anticancer drugs* or with radioactive phosphorus taken by

P

mouth to control the overproduction of red cells in the marrow.

Treatment enables most patients to survive for 10 to 15 years. Death usually occurs from a stroke or other complications of the disease.

Polydactyly

A *birth defect* in which there is an excessive number of fingers or toes. The extra digits may be fully formed and look like the other fingers or toes or they may be fleshy stumps.

Polydactyly affects about 50 babies in every 100,000. It often runs in otherwise normal families, but may also occur as part of the *Laurence-Moon-Biedl syndrome*.

Polydactyly affecting the feet
The extra toes can cause problems with footwear and are usually removed surgically during childhood.

Polydipsia

A medical term for persistent excessive thirst. Polydipsia is an important symptom in people with *diabetes mellitus* and *diabetes insipidus* (see *Thirst, excessive*).

Polyhydramnios

See *Hydramnios*.

Polymyalgia rheumatica

An uncommon disease of elderly people that is marked by pain and stiffness in the muscles of the hips, thighs, shoulders, and neck.

CAUSES AND INCIDENCE

The cause of polymyalgia rheumatica is unknown, but it may be associated with *temporal arteritis*, *rheumatoid arthritis*, systemic *lupus erythematosus*, and, sometimes, cancer.

The disorder affects twice as many women as men and is unusual before the age of 50.

SYMPTOMS

The pain and stiffness, which may develop gradually or suddenly, make movement difficult. Morning stiffness is notable and often makes getting out of bed a problem. Weight loss and depression may also occur.

DIAGNOSIS AND TREATMENT

The diagnosis, which is often difficult to confirm, is based on a physical examination, the patient's history, and blood tests (including an *ESR*). If temporal arteritis is suspected, a *biopsy* (removal of a small sample of tissue for analysis) may be performed on an artery in the temple.

Small doses of *corticosteroid drugs* (higher doses when temporal arteritis is present) usually bring about a notable improvement in the disorder within a few days. The dosage is gradually reduced and use of the drug may be discontinued within two years.

Polymyositis

A rare disease in which the muscles become inflamed and weak. Polymyositis shares the features of *dermatomyositis*, but there is no rash.

Polymyxins

A group of *antibiotic drugs* derived from the bacterium *BACILLUS POLYMYXA*. Polymyxins, which include *colistin* and polymyxin B, are commonly given in drop or ointment form to treat eye, ear, and skin infections. Polymyxins are very infrequently given by injection to treat severe infections but in this form may cause nerve or kidney damage. Taken orally, colistin is associated with pseudomembranous enterocolitis (a severe, sometimes life-threatening diarrhea caused by some antibiotics).

Polyp

A growth that projects, usually on a stalk, from the lining of the nose, the cervix, the intestine, the larynx, or any other *mucous membrane*.

Polyps may need to be removed surgically if they are responsible for symptoms. Some polyps are liable to develop into cancer.

Polypeptide

A compound that consists of many *amino acids* linked by *peptide* bonds.

Polypharmacy

The practice of prescribing several different drugs to one person at the same time. Polypharmacy increases the risk of drug interactions (effects that differ from those occurring when a drug is taken alone) and, thus, the risk of adverse effects.

Polyposis, familial

A rare, inherited disorder, also known as polyposis coli, in which numerous (often a thousand or more) polyps are present in the colon and rectum. The probability of one or more polyps becoming cancerous is extremely high. Without preventive treatment, the development of cancer of the colon (see *Intestine, cancer of*) by age 40 is almost a certainty.

SYMPTOMS AND DIAGNOSIS

The polyps are not present at birth but usually appear by the age of 10 and may cause bleeding and diarrhea. However, there are often no symptoms until cancer has developed; it is therefore extremely important that a diagnosis be made as early as possible. The polyps are detected by air contrast *barium X-ray examination* and *colonoscopy* (investigation of the colon with a viewing tube).

PREVENTION AND TREATMENT

Since there is a 50 percent chance that the children of an affected parent will inherit the disease, close medical surveillance is necessary from the age of about 10. This screening, by the diagnostic methods mentioned, is performed every two years until the age of about 40, after which time it is unlikely that polyps will appear.

Because there is such a high risk of cancer, preventive treatment is usually carried out. This often takes the form of total *colectomy* (removal of the entire colon) and the creation of an artificial opening of the ileum (the lower part of the small intestine) through the abdominal wall (see *Ileostomy*). Alternatively, the end of the ileum is joined to the rectum so that a normal passage for bowel movements exists. However, the rectum must be examined regularly to detect polyps, which must be treated immediately before there is a chance for cancerous changes to occur.

Polyuria

See *Urination, excessive*.

Pompholyx

An acute form of *eczema* in which itchy blisters form over the palms and/or soles. The condition, often called dyshydrotic eczema, often develops for no apparent reason but is sometimes due to an allergic response to a substance in contact with the skin. It rarely is associated with *ringworm*.

Treatment is with an astringent, which causes the skin to shrink and dry, or with a *corticosteroid drug*.

Pons

The middle part of the *brain stem*, situated between the midbrain (above) and the medulla oblongata (below).

Pore

A tiny opening. The term usually describes an opening in the skin that releases sweat or sebum (an oily substance secreted by sebaceous glands). Most of the pores from which sebum arises are also hair follicles.

Porphyria

Any of a group of uncommon inherited disorders caused by the accumulation in the body of substances called porphyrins. Victims often have a rash or skin blistering brought on by sunlight and may have abdominal pain and nervous system disturbances from certain drugs.

CAUSES, TYPES, AND INCIDENCE

The porphyrins are chemicals with a complex structure and are precursor substances formed in the body during the manufacture of heme—a component of *hemoglobin* (the oxygen-carrying pigment in blood) and of various other important body substances.

The porphyrias result from blocks in the chemical processes by which heme is formed, resulting in accumulation of porphyrins. The blocks are the results of deficiencies of various enzymes in the body; these deficiencies are inherited, usually in an autosomal dominant pattern (see *Genetic disorders*).

Six types of porphyria are recognized—acute intermittent porphyria, variegate porphyria, and porphyria cutanea tarda (the more common types); and hereditary coproporphyria, protoporphyria, and congenital erythropoietic porphyria (all very rare). The prevalence of each varies throughout the world. The combined prevalence in the US is unknown, but is probably about one affected person per 10,000 to 50,000 population.

SYMPTOMS

Features are as follows.

ACUTE INTERMITTENT PORPHYRIA This type usually first appears in early adulthood with attacks of abdominal pain, which may mimic appendicitis. Limb cramps, muscle weakness, and psychiatric disturbances are common. There are no skin symptoms, but the patient's urine turns red when left to stand. A large number of drugs are known to precipitate attacks, including barbiturates, phenytoin, birth-control pills, and tetracyclines.

VARIEGATE PORPHYRIA This type is similar in many respects to acute intermittent porphyria, but with blistering of sun-exposed skin. Attacks may be brought on by the same drugs that precipitate acute intermittent porphyria.

HEREDITARY COPROPORPHYRIA This type of porphyria is similar to acute intermittent porphyria, with additional skin symptoms in some sufferers.

PORPHYRIA CUTANEA TARDA This type also causes blistering on sun-exposed skin, but no abdominal or nervous system disturbance. Wounds are characteristically slow to heal. The urine is sometimes pink or brown. Many cases are precipitated by liver disease, including alcoholic liver disease.

PROTOPORPHYRIA This type usually causes mild skin symptoms after exposure to sunlight.

CONGENITAL ERYTHROPOIETIC PORPHYRIA This type is extremely rare; it is characterized by red discoloration of urine and teeth, excessive hair growth, severe skin blistering and ulceration, and hemolytic *anemia*. Death may occur in childhood.

DIAGNOSIS AND TREATMENT

The porphyrias are diagnosed by finding abnormal levels of porphyrins in the urine. More specific tests are available for some types.

Treatment is difficult. Avoiding exposure to sunlight and/or to precipitating drugs is the most important measure. Attacks of acute intermittent porphyria, variegate porphyria, and hereditary coproporphyria can sometimes be helped by administration of glucose or a drug called panhematin,

which is chemically related to heme. Porphyria cutanea tarda can be helped by *venesection* (removal of blood through a vein).

Portal hypertension

Increased blood pressure in the portal vein, a large blood vessel that carries blood from the stomach, intestine, and spleen to the liver. The pressure in the veins of the upper stomach and lower esophagus is raised, causing them to widen (a condition known as *esophageal varices*) and sometimes to rupture. In addition, fluid is forced from the overloaded portal vein, resulting in *ascites*, an accumulation of fluid in the abdomen.

CAUSES

The most common cause of portal hypertension is the liver disease *cirrhosis*; the scarring and regenerative tissue that form in the organ obstruct the portal vein. Another cause is *thrombosis* (blood clotting) in the vein. This may occur shortly after birth or later in life, when it is usually the result of narrowing of the vein by cirrhosis, compression by enlarged lymph nodes, or inflammation resulting from an infection. Portal hypertension may also be caused by narrowing of the vein from birth.

Rarely, the disorder is due to an abnormal connection between the

P

PORTAL HYPERTENSION

The most common cause of this condition is liver cirrhosis or some other obstruction to blood flow through the liver. The portal vein becomes congested with blood, and back pressure develops through the system of veins that join the portal vein.

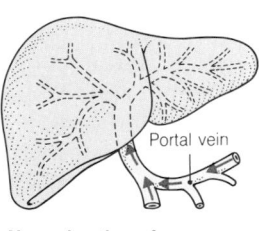

Normal action of portal vein
The vein carries nutrient-rich blood from the abdominal organs to the liver for processing.

Features of portal hypertension
The portal vein becomes congested, the pressure in it rises, fluid is forced out into the abdomen, and veins that supply the portal vein are widened and may rupture.

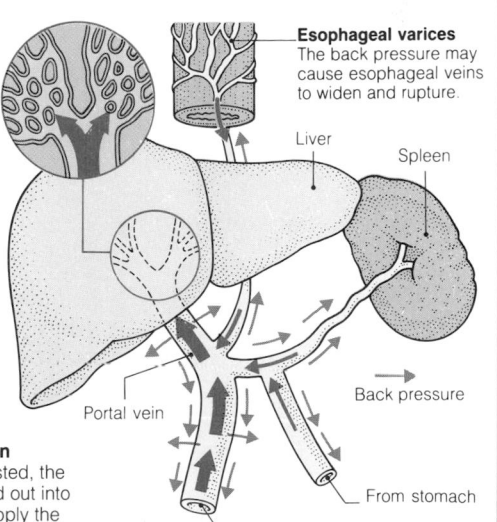

Portal vein

Esophageal varices
The back pressure may cause esophageal veins to widen and rupture.

Liver

Spleen

Back pressure

Portal vein

From stomach

From intestines

portal vein and an artery (*arteriovenous fistula*), usually as the result of injury. It can also be caused by increased blood flow from the spleen if disease has caused this organ to enlarge.

SYMPTOMS AND SIGNS
If the veins in the esophagus and stomach rupture, it causes massive recurrent vomiting of blood and the passing of black feces. Ascites results in abdominal swelling and discomfort and sometimes difficulty breathing.

DIAGNOSIS
Portal hypertension is usually diagnosed from the patient's symptoms and signs. The cause can be determined by examining the liver and surrounding blood vessels by means of *ultrasound scanning* and arteriography (see *Angiography*).

TREATMENT
Bleeding from ruptured blood vessels is stopped by sclerotherapy, which consists of injection of a solution into or around the veins. This induces inflammation, subsequent scarring, and consequent thickening of the vessels' walls so that the veins are blocked off. Ascites is controlled by dietary sodium chloride (salt) restriction and *diuretic drugs*, which increase urine production.

In some cases, an operation known as a *shunt* may be carried out to divert blood from the portal vein to some other blood vessel, thus relieving the high pressure.

However, studies fail to show any substantial improvement in survival time using sclerotherapy or a shunt for esophageal varices.

The outlook depends on how successfully the underlying cause of the condition can be treated.

Port-wine stain
A large, purple-red birthmark that is level with the skin's surface. A port-wine stain is a permanent and often unsightly type of *hemangioma*.

Positron emission tomography
See *PET scanning*.

Postcoital contraception
See *Contraception, postcoital*.

Posterior
Relating to the back of the body. In human anatomy, the term is synonymous with *dorsal*.

Postmaturity
A condition in which a pregnancy persists for longer than 42 weeks; the average length of a normal pregnancy is 40 weeks from the first day of the last menstrual period (see *Gestation*). Postmaturity may be due to a family tendency to prolonged pregnancy, or it may be an indication that the head is bigger than the mother's pelvis and that the baby is unable to descend properly (see *Engagement*). Many obstetricians attempt to avoid postmaturity by *induction of labor* as the pregnancy nears 42 weeks' gestation.

COMPLICATIONS
Because the postmature baby is larger than average and the bones of the baby's skull harder and able to mold less readily, postmaturity is associated with a prolonged labor and an increased risk of a traumatic delivery. The major risk of postmaturity is fetal death and consequent stillbirth; the risk of this occurring doubles by the 43rd week of pregnancy and triples by the 44th week when compared to the normal 40 week pregnancy. This increase in fetal death is in part a consequence of diminished placental efficiency, resulting in the fetus being starved of nutrients and oxygen.

Postmortem examination
Another term for an *autopsy*.

Postmyocardial infarction syndrome
Another name for *Dressler's syndrome*.

Postnasal drip
A watery or sticky discharge from the back of the nose into the *nasopharynx* (the uppermost part of the throat, behind the nose). As the fluid trickles down the throat, it may cause a cough, hoarseness, or a foreign body sensation. The condition is usually caused by *rhinitis* (inflammation of the mucous membrane in the nose); treatment is of the underlying cause.

Postnatal care
Care of the mother after *childbirth* until about six weeks after delivery.

After delivery the mother's temperature, pulse, and blood pressure are monitored, especially after a *cesarean section* or if there have been any complications, such as *pre-eclampsia* or kidney disease.

The length of stay in the hospital depends on whether or not there have been any complications; typically, in the US, women stay one to three days after delivery. During the hospital stay, a daily check is made for any signs of *puerperal sepsis* (infection of the genital tract after childbirth), including inspection of the *lochia* (vaginal discharge after childbirth). If the woman had an *episiotomy* or tears around the vagina, the wounds are checked daily.

The woman is encouraged to walk as soon as possible after delivery to reduce the risk of *thrombosis* (abnormal blood clots). If necessary, help is given with infant feeding techniques (see *Bottle-feeding*; *Breast-feeding*). There may also be instruction on various abdominal and *pelvic floor exercises*, which can help restore muscle tone.

A final postnatal checkup usually takes place about six weeks after delivery. The obstetrician checks the woman's blood pressure and weight, examines the uterus and bladder to make sure they are in the correct position, and ensures that any wounds are healing properly. Advice on contraception may also be given.

Postnatal depression
See *Postpartum depression*.

Postpartum depression
Depression in a woman after childbirth. It is probably caused by a combination of sudden hormonal changes and a variety of psychological and environmental factors. Psychological stress is the major component. Postpartum depression ranges from an extremely common and short-lived attack of mild depression ("baby blues") to a depressive psychosis in which the woman is severely depressed and requires admission to the hospital to prevent harm to herself or her baby.

MILD DEPRESSION
Probably more than two thirds of mothers have the "blues," usually starting about four to five days after childbirth. The woman feels miserable, discouraged, irritable, sometimes mentally confused, and may cry easily. Apart from hormonal changes, psychological factors may play a role, including a sense of anticlimax after the birth or an overwhelming sense of responsibility for the baby's care. With reassurance and support from family and friends, the depression usually passes in two or three days.

MORE SEVERE DEPRESSION
In about 10 to 15 percent of women the depression is more marked and persists for weeks. There may be a constant feeling of tiredness, difficulty sleeping, loss of appetite, and restlessness. This type of postpartum depression seems more likely to develop if the woman has a strained relationship with her partner, no support from her

P

family, financial or other worries, or a *personality disorder*. At particular risk are women who suffered from depression or anxiety during the pregnancy, first-time mothers, and single-parent mothers. The condition usually clears up of its own accord or responds to treatment with *antidepressant drugs*.

DEPRESSIVE PSYCHOSIS

This severe form of postpartum depression occurs in about one in 1,000 pregnancies and usually starts two to three weeks after childbirth. Since psychosis tends to run in families, its appearance after childbirth probably results from the triggering of latent emotional conflicts by the stress of the birth. Depressive psychosis is marked by severe mental confusion, feelings of worthlessness, threats of suicide or of harm to the baby, and sometimes *delusions*. The woman's moods may change rapidly.

Treatment requires sensitive counseling and *family therapy. Antidepressant drug* therapy may be necessary.

Postpartum hemorrhage

Excessive blood loss after *childbirth*. Postpartum hemorrhage occurs in about 2 percent of all births. It is more common after a long labor, after a multiple birth, or if the woman required general anesthesia. Before the development of *blood transfusion*, postpartum hemorrhage was a common cause of maternal death.

CAUSES

Most cases of postpartum hemorrhage occur immediately after delivery and are due to excessive bleeding from the site where the placenta was attached to the uterus. Such bleeding may be caused by failure of the uterus to contract efficiently after delivery or by the retention of placental tissue within the uterus.

Postpartum hemorrhage immediately after delivery may also be caused by tears anywhere along the birth canal. Tearing is more likely to occur during a *forceps delivery* or breech delivery. In some cases, postpartum hemorrhage occurs because the mother has a *bleeding disorder*.

Occasionally, postpartum hemorrhage occurs with pain and fever between five and 10 days after delivery. In these cases, the cause of the hemorrhage is usually infection of a retained fragment of placenta.

TREATMENT

A blood transfusion may be given to replace lost blood and emergency treatment may be needed for shock. Other treatment depends on the cause of the hemorrhage. Any retained placental tissue may need to be removed using a general anesthetic, an injection of *ergonovine* may be given to stimulate uterine contractions, and any lacerations in the vagina or on the cervix are sutured. *Antibiotic drugs* are used to treat infection.

Post-traumatic stress disorder

A specific form of *anxiety* that comes on after a stressful or frightening event. Common causes include natural disasters (such as earthquakes), violence, rape, torture, and serious physical injury. The condition may also result from military combat, when it is sometimes known as battle fatigue or shell shock.

The symptoms include recurring memories or dreams of the event, a sense of personal isolation, and disturbed sleep and concentration. There may be a deadening of feelings, or irritability and painful feelings of guilt, sometimes building to form a true depressive illness (see *Depression*). Symptoms may begin immediately after the trauma or may develop many months later. The symptoms are made worse by any reminder of the traumatic experience.

Most people recover given time, emotional support, and counseling. However, prolonged physical deprivation (such as that experienced in a concentration camp) may scar people psychologically for life.

Postural drainage

A technique that assists a person whose lungs are clogged with sputum (phlegm) or other secretions to drain them. The person lies in such a way that the secretions drain by gravity into the trachea (windpipe), from

P

TECHNIQUES OF POSTURAL DRAINAGE

The patient lies in one or a series of positions on a bed, to drain different areas of the lung. "Huffing" and chest clapping by an assistant may be performed from time to time to loosen secretions in the lung.

Huffing
This technique—breathing out forcibly while "flapping" one or both elbows—is performed in the drainage position and repeated in an upright position (left) after treatment.

Typical drainage posture
The posture shown is used to drain secretions from part of the lower lobe of the right lung. The patient lies with a pillow under the hips. The foot of the bed is raised 18 inches. The shoulders should not rest on the pillow at the head of the bed.

Chest clapping
The helper claps with a cupped hand on the chest wall. This helps loosen sticky secretions in the lungs.

where they are coughed up. Postural drainage is used to treat disorders in which stagnant secretions have become infected (as in acute chest infections in those suffering from chronic *bronchitis*) or are at risk of becoming infected (as in *bronchiectasis* or *cystic fibrosis*).

Postural drainage is sometimes done in association with chest clapping (in which another person gently strikes the chest), theoretically to loosen sticky secretions.

HOW IT IS DONE

The affected person lies on a bed and each lobe of the lung is drained in turn by the adoption of a different position (see illustration). The different postures are achieved by the person lying supine, prone, or on his or her side; by raising the foot of the bed by varying amounts; and by the use of pillows to elevate different parts of the body. At the same time, the secretions are loosened by the person "huffing" (breathing out forcibly) and raising and lowering the elbows, and by the helper clapping with a cupped hand on the chest wall. A mechanical *vibrator* may be used.

Postural hypotension

See *Hypotension*.

Posture

The relative position of different parts of the body at rest or during movement. Good posture consists of efficiently balancing the body weight around the body's center of gravity in the lower spine and pelvis. It is dependent on the shape of the *spine* and on balanced contraction of *muscles* around the spine and in each limb. Maintaining good posture helps prevent neck pain and *back pain*.

Many people have bad posture as the result of habit, such as sitting slumped in a chair or standing with the shoulders and back hunched. Obesity increases the likelihood of bad posture because it increases the strain on muscles. Poor posture may also be caused by neurological disorders (such as *Parkinson's disease*), by muscle disorders (such as *muscular dystrophy*), or by disorders of the joints or bones (such as *ankylosing spondylitis*).

Potassium

A mineral that, in combination with *sodium* and calcium, maintains normal heart rhythm, regulates the body's water balance, and is responsible for the conduction of nerve impulses and the contraction of muscles.

The body of an average-sized person contains about 5 ounces (140 g) of potassium. Blood levels of the mineral are controlled by the kidneys, which eliminate any excess in the urine. Almost all foods contain potassium, so dietary deficiency is rare. Particularly rich sources include lean meat, whole grains, green leafy vegetables, beans, and many fruits (especially bananas and oranges).

POTASSIUM DEFICIENCY

A low level of potassium in the blood (called hypokalemia) usually occurs as a result of *gastroenteritis* or some other digestive tract disorder that causes loss of potassium-rich gastrointestinal fluids through diarrhea and/or vomiting. Children are especially vulnerable to this type of potassium loss.

Other potential causes of hypokalemia include prolonged treatment with *diuretic drugs* or *corticosteroid drugs*; overuse of *laxative drugs*; *diabetes mellitus*; *Cushing's syndrome* (overproduction of steroid hormones by the adrenal cortex); *aldosteronism* (overproduction of the hormone aldosterone by the adrenal cortex); certain kidney diseases; excessive intake of sugar, coffee, or alcohol; and extremely profuse sweating.

The effects of mild hypokalemia include fatigue, drowsiness, dizziness, and muscle weakness. In more severe cases, there may be abnormalities of heart rhythm and paralysis of the muscles.

POTASSIUM EXCESS

Much less common than hypokalemia is an excess of potassium in the blood, a condition called hyperkalemia. It may be caused by taking more than the daily potassium requirement, usually in the form of supplements to correct hypokalemia; by severe *renal failure*; or by *Addison's disease*.

The effects of hyperkalemia include numbness and tingling, muscle paralysis, heart rhythm disturbances, and, in severe cases, *heart failure*.

Potassium permanganate

A drug that has an *antiseptic* and *astringent* effect, useful in the treatment of *dermatitis* (skin inflammation). Potassium permanganate is sometimes applied to a dressing, may be placed in water as a soak, or may be applied directly to the skin.

Potency

The ability of a man to perform sexual intercourse; the strength of a drug assessed from its ability to cause certain desired effects.

Pott's fracture

A combined fracture and dislocation of the *ankle* caused by excessive or violent twisting. In a Pott's fracture, the fibula (the outer of the two bones of the lower leg) is broken just above the ankle, and the tibia (shin) also breaks or the ligaments tear, resulting in dislocation.

Treatment consists of manipulating the bones back into position using a general anesthetic, followed by immobilization of the foot, ankle, and lower leg in a cast for eight to 10 weeks. Screws may be inserted to hold the bone fragments in place.

Severe fracture-dislocations may result in stiffness of the ankle; they increase the likelihood of *osteoarthritis* in later life.

Poultice

A warm pack consisting of a soft, moist substance (such as *kaolin*) spread between layers of soft fabric. Poultices were once widely used for reducing local pain or inflammation and improving local circulation.

Pox

Any of various infectious diseases characterized by blistery skin eruptions (e.g., chickenpox). Pox is an outdated term for *syphilis* and still survives as slang.

Praziquantel

An *antihelmintic drug* used to treat *tapeworm* and *fluke* infestations. Adverse effects include dizziness, drowsiness, and abdominal pain.

Prazosin

A *vasodilator drug* used as an *antihypertensive drug* in the treatment of *hypertension* (high blood pressure). Prazosin is usually given with a *diuretic drug* and sometimes with other antihypertensive drugs.

Prazosin is also used to treat *heart failure* (reduced pumping efficiency) and *Raynaud's phenomenon* (a circulatory disorder characterized by cold, painful hands and feet).

Prazosin may cause dizziness and fainting by lowering the blood pressure too much. Other possible adverse effects are nausea, headache, and dry mouth.

Precancerous

A term applied to any condition in which cancer has a tendency to develop. There are three types of such conditions. In the first, there are no tumors present but the condition is

P

known to carry an increased risk of cancer. Examples include *ulcerative colitis* (which carries an increased risk of malignant tumors of the colon or rectum) and *Down's syndrome* (which carries an increased risk of leukemia).

In the second type, there are benign tumors that tend to become malignant themselves or are associated with the development of malignant tumors elsewhere in the body. Examples of this type include *neurofibromatosis* (von Recklinghausen's disease), in which there are large numbers of tumors on the nerves, any of which may become malignant; and *tuberous sclerosis*, in which cancer may develop in the brain, the back of the eye, and various endocrine glands.

The third type comprises disorders that have chronic, sometimes inflammatory or irregular features from the beginning, but which do not always become fully malignant. Disorders within this group include cervical dysplasia (see *Cervix, cancer of*); *leukoplakia* of the mouth (see *Mouth cancer*); and papillomas of the bladder (see *Bladder tumors*).

Predisposing factors

Factors that lead to increased susceptibility to a disease. Predisposing factors that make a person more likely to have coronary heart disease are a family history of the disease, tobacco smoking, high blood pressure, high *lipid* levels in the blood, being overweight, lack of regular exercise, and mental stress.

Prednisolone

A *corticosteroid drug* used to reduce inflammation and improve symptoms in a variety of disorders, including *eczema, psoriasis, conjunctivitis, iritis, ulcerative colitis, rheumatoid arthritis,* and *asthma*.

Prednisolone is also used in the treatment of blood disorders, such as *thrombocytopenia* and *leukemia*.

High doses or prolonged treatment may cause adverse effects typical of other corticosteroids, including facial rounding, *acne, hypertension, osteoporosis, peptic ulcer,* and *diabetes mellitus*.

Prednisone

CORTICOSTEROID
Tablet Liquid
Prescription needed
Available as generic

A *corticosteroid drug* used to reduce inflammation and improve symptoms in a variety of disorders, including *rheumatoid arthritis* and *ulcerative colitis*. Prednisone is also used in the treatment of severe *asthma*.

Other disorders that are occasionally treated with prednisone include *Addison's disease* and blood disorders, such as *leukemia*. Prednisone is also used to prevent organ rejection after *transplant surgery*.

Large doses taken over a prolonged period may cause adverse effects typical of other corticosteroid drugs.

Preeclampsia

A serious condition in which *hypertension* (high blood pressure), *edema* (fluid retention), and *proteinuria* (protein in the urine) develop in a woman in the second half of pregnancy. Additional symptoms include headache, nausea and vomiting, abdominal pain, and visual disturbances.

Preeclampsia affects about 7 percent of pregnancies. It is more common in first pregnancies and in women under 25 or over 35; it is also more common if *diabetes mellitus*, hypertension, or kidney disease already exists. Untreated preeclampsia may lead to *eclampsia*, which is characterized by seizures; eclampsia may cause maternal or fetal death.

TREATMENT

For mild cases of preeclampsia, the woman is confined to bed, and *antihypertensive drugs* may be used to reduce blood pressure. If the woman is close to term or if eclampsia is imminent, emergency *induction of labor* and delivery may be necessary.

Pregnancy

The period from conception to birth. Pregnancy begins with conception, the *fertilization* of an ovum (egg) by a sperm and the subsequent implantation of the egg. The fertilized egg develops into the *placenta* and *embryo*, and later into the *fetus*. Most fertilized eggs implant into the uterus. However, occasionally, an egg implants into an abnormal site, such as a fallopian tube, resulting in an *ectopic pregnancy*. (See boxes overleaf on the stages and features of pregnancy and on the effects of hormones during pregnancy.)

WEIGHT GAIN DURING PREGNANCY

The average increase in pregnancy is 28 pounds (12.7 kg)—70 percent of it occurring during the last 20 weeks. At term, the typical fetus weighs 7.5 pounds (3.4 kg) and the placenta and

fluid together weigh another 3 pounds (1.4 kg). The remaining weight is largely due to water retention and increased fat stores. Within six weeks of delivery, most women return to their pre-pregnancy weight.

STAYING WELL

Provided the pregnancy is desired and the woman takes care of herself and has adequate *prenatal care*, there is no reason why she should not overcome some of the early symptoms and feel healthy during pregnancy.

A balanced and nutritious diet is important. Appetite will increase, but pregnant women should avoid filling up on high-calorie snacks, such as potato chips, that are low in nutritional value. It is better to eat frequent, smaller meals. Many physicians prescribe *folic acid* and *iron* supplements during pregnancy.

Tobacco smoking and *alcohol* should be avoided throughout pregnancy, and no other drug should be taken except under medical supervision (see *Pregnancy, drugs in*).

Exercise can be continued during pregnancy but overexertion and potentially dangerous sports are generally best avoided.

Sex can continue throughout pregnancy (unless there is bleeding or if the waters break). Adopting different positions may make intercourse more comfortable. Libido may decrease during early and late pregnancy, but many women enjoy sex throughout pregnancy.

PROBLEMS DURING PREGNANCY

In addition to the expected features of pregnancy, such as nausea and tiredness, some women experience other minor problems. The symptoms may be troublesome but generally disappear after delivery.

During pregnancy, food passes through the intestine more slowly, which enables more nutrients to be absorbed for the fetus, but which also tends to cause *constipation*. *Hemorrhoids* are fairly common during late pregnancy, as is *heartburn* due to *acid reflux*. The gums may become spongy and bleed easily. *Pica* (a craving to eat substances other than foods, such as clay or coal) is fairly common.

Swollen ankles are common during the second half of pregnancy, especially during the evening. *Varicose veins* may appear in the later months in susceptible women. Leg cramps, backache, and breathlessness are also common during late pregnancy. Pigmentation tends to increase and may cause *chloasma* (mask of pregnancy).

P

STAGES AND FEATURES OF PREGNANCY

Pregnancy typically lasts 40 weeks, counted from the first day of the pregnant woman's last menstrual period, and is conventionally divided into three trimesters, each lasting three months. For the first eight weeks following conception, the developing baby is called an embryo; thereafter, it is known as a fetus. It is during the early part of pregnancy (first trimester) that the growing baby is most vulnerable to damage.

During this first stage, all the major organ structures are developing.

The fetus, now with features that are recognizably human, grows rapidly in size.

The fetal organs mature in preparation for birth and life outside the uterus.

First trimester (0 to 12 weeks)
The first sign of pregnancy is usually the absence of a menstrual period, though some women have breakthrough bleeding. The breasts start to swell and may become tender as the mammary glands develop to prepare for *breast-feeding*. The nipples start to enlarge and the veins over the surface of the breasts, become more prominent. A supportive bra should be worn.

Nausea and vomiting are common, are often worse in the morning, and usually persist for six to eight weeks (see *Vomiting in pregnancy*). Urine is passed more frequently and there is often a creamy white discharge from the vagina. Many women feel unusually tired during the early weeks. Some notice a metallic taste in the mouth or a craving for certain foods. Weight begins to increase.

Second trimester (13 to 28 weeks)
From 16 weeks, the enlarging uterus is easily felt and the woman begins to look noticeably pregnant. The nipples enlarge and darken, and skin pigmentation may deepen. Some women may feel warm and flushed. Appetite tends to increase and weight rises rapidly. Facial features tend to become heavier. By 22 weeks (usually between the 18th and 20th weeks), most pregnant women have felt the baby moving around (sometimes called "quickening").

During the second trimester, nausea and frequency of urination diminish, and the woman may feel generally better and more energetic than during the early weeks. The heart rate increases, as does the volume of blood pumped by the heart, to allow the fetus to develop properly. These changes put an extra strain on the heart of women who have preexisting heart disease.

Third trimester (29 to 40 weeks)
In some women, stretch marks develop on the abdomen, breasts, and thighs. A dark line may appear running from the umbilicus to the pubic hair. *Colostrum* can be expressed from the nipples.

Minor problems are common. Many women become hot and sweat easily, as body temperature rises slightly. More rest may be needed at this stage, though many women find it difficult to find a comfortable position. *Braxton Hicks' contractions* may get stronger.

The baby's head engages (drops down low into the pelvis) around the 36th week in a first pregnancy, but not until a few weeks later in subsequent pregnancies. This "lightening" may relieve pressure on the upper abdomen and on breathing, but increases pressure on the bladder and may result in more vaginal discharge.

Urinary tract infections are more common during pregnancy, and stress incontinence (see *Incontinence, urinary*) may occur, especially during the later weeks. Vaginal *candidiasis* (thrush) is also more common when a woman is pregnant.

Women may find that their moods are more changeable, which may be the result of hormonal effects on the brain. In addition, women often feel more lethargic than usual, and may experience bouts of depression, may be easily annoyed or angered, and may be prone to bouts of crying.

For complications of pregnancy, see *Antepartum hemorrhage*; *Diabetic pregnancy*; *Hydramnios*; *Miscarriage*; *Preeclampsia*; *Prematurity*; *Rh incompatibility*; *Vomiting in pregnancy*. (See also *Childbirth*; *Fetal heart monitoring*; *Pregnancy, multiple*.)

Pregnancy, drugs in

Drugs taken during pregnancy may pass from the mother through the placenta to the developing baby. Although only several drugs have been proved to cause harm to a developing baby, no drug should be considered completely safe, especially during early pregnancy. For this reason, a pregnant woman should not take any drug (including over-the-counter drugs) without first consulting her physician.

Drug treatment during pregnancy is usually prescribed only if the potential benefits of treatment outweigh any risk to the baby. Treatment for long-term conditions, such as *epilepsy* or *diabetes mellitus*, is continued during pregnancy but drug therapy may require modification (sometimes even before the woman conceives if pregnancy is planned).

Problems in a developing baby may also be caused if a pregnant woman drinks alcohol (see *Alcohol* in pregnancy box) or smokes tobacco (see *Tobacco smoking*).

EFFECTS OF HORMONES DURING PREGNANCY

A pregnant woman undergoes many changes that enable her to maintain the pregnancy, nourish the baby, and prepare for breast-feeding.

These adaptations are brought about by increased levels of the female sex hormones *estrogen* and *progesterone*, and by the action of two other

hormones, human chorionic gonadotropin (HCG) and human placental lactogen (HPL), produced only by the placenta.

EFFECTS OF HORMONES DURING PREGNANCY

Progesterone	Decreases excitability of smooth muscle, so helps prevent uterine contractions and premature labor. Induces constipation and esophageal acid reflux as a result of its effects on smooth muscle. Increases body temperature. Affects mood. Increases breathing rate.	**Estrogens**	Are important for the development of the reproductive system and breasts. Stimulate growth of the uterine muscle to enable the powerful contractions of labor. Increase vaginal secretions. Increase size of nipples and help the development of milk glands in breasts. Increase protein production, which is essential for healthy growth of woman and fetus. Alter collagen and other substances to allow body tissues to soften and stretch in preparation for labor. Relax ligaments and joints. May cause sciatica and backache, and contribute to formation of varicose veins as a result of effects on body tissue.
Human placental lactogen (HPL)	Increases energy production necessary for fetal development. Causes enlargement of breasts and development of milk glands. Induces temporary diabetes mellitus (gestational diabetes) in susceptible women as a result of its effects on metabolism.		
Human chorionic gonadotropin (HCG)	Increases energy production necessary for fetal development. Induces gestational diabetes in susceptible women.	**Melanocyte-stimulating hormone (MSH)**	Stimulates pigmentation (in combination with estrogens), particularly of the nipples. May also produce chloasma (darkening of facial skin).

Drug abuse during pregnancy can cause serious problems. The babies of women who use *heroin* during pregnancy tend to have a low birth weight and have a higher death rate than normal during the first few weeks after birth. They may suffer withdrawal symptoms, such as feeding and sleeping difficulties, trembling, and seizures. Babies born to women who are intravenous drug abusers have a high risk of being infected with HIV, the *AIDS* virus.

RISKS

Drugs taken during the first three months of pregnancy may interfere with the normal formation of the baby's organs, causing *birth defects*.

Drugs taken later in pregnancy may slow the rate at which the baby grows, causing a low birth weight. Or they may damage specific fetal tissue, such as developing teeth, which may be damaged by *tetracycline drugs*.

Drugs taken toward the end of pregnancy or during labor and delivery may cause problems for the newborn baby. Narcotic analgesics, for example, may cause breathing difficulty. (See also *Childbirth* pain relief box.)

Pregnancy, false

An uncommon psychological disorder, medically known as pseudocyesis, in which a woman has the physical signs of pregnancy, including morning sickness, amenorrhea (lack of periods), breast enlargement, and abdominal swelling. Although the results of *pregnancy tests* prove negative and the fetal heart cannot be heard during examination, the woman believes she is pregnant.

Many women with pseudocyesis are childless or approaching the menopause and have an intense desire to have children.

Treatment of pseudocyesis may involve counseling or *psychotherapy*. (See also *Conversion disorder*.)

Pregnancy, multiple

The presence of more than one fetus in the uterus. Multiple pregnancy can occur if two or more ova (eggs) are released from the ovary and fertilized at the same time. It can also result if a single fertilized ovum divides at an early stage of development. Today, most pregnancies in which there are three or more babies result from the use of *fertility drugs*.

INCIDENCE

Twins occur in about one in 90 pregnancies, triplets in about one in 8,000 pregnancies, and quadruplets in about one in 73,000 pregnancies.

Multiple pregnancies are more common than average in women who are successfully treated with fertility drugs or if multiple fertilized ova are implanted during *in vitro fertilization*.

DIAGNOSIS AND TREATMENT

During the woman's prenatal examination, the physician may be able to feel more than one fetus, and may find that the abdomen is larger than expected for the duration of gestation. The physician may also be able to hear more than one fetal heart beat when listening through a stethoscope. *Ultrasound scanning* may confirm the diagnosis.

P

The woman is advised to rest during pregnancy and to increase her protein intake. Iron and folic acid tablets are usually recommended.

COMPLICATIONS

Hypertension (high blood pressure), *hydramnios*, *postpartum hemorrhage*, and *malpresentation* occur more frequently in a multiple pregnancy. *Prematurity* is a common complication, and the weight of each baby is usually less than that of a single baby. Cesarean section is necessary more often than in single pregnancies.

Pregnancy tests

Tests on urine or blood performed to determine whether or not a woman is pregnant; some can be performed at home. Pregnancy tests check for the presence of human chorionic gonadotropin (HCG; see *Gonadotropin, human chorionic*), which is produced by the placenta.

HOW IT IS DONE

Urine tests are used most often. Most can detect pregnancy about two weeks after a missed period, although some of the newer tests can detect pregnancy within five days. The test is usually done on an early morning midstream urine specimen (because HCG is most concentrated at this

MULTIPLE PREGNANCY

About one pregnancy in 89 is multiple (e.g., twins or triplets). The rate is highest among women in their 30s. Problems arise more often in multiple pregnancies than in single pregnancies. For example, twins are much more likely than single babies to be born prematurely.

— Placenta

— Amniotic fluid

— Fetal limb

— Fetal heads

— Division between amniotic sacs

— Wall of uterus

Ultrasound scan revealing twins
Ultrasound scanning of the woman's uterus can reveal twins within the first several weeks of pregnancy. Here, two fetal heads, a limb belonging to the fetus on the right, and the membrane dividing the two amniotic sacs are visible.

time). Urine tests are about 97 percent accurate if the result is positive and about 80 percent accurate if the result is negative. If the result is negative and there is no menstrual period within about a week, the pregnancy test should be repeated.

Blood tests are normally used only when a very early diagnosis of pregnancy is needed. Blood tests measure

PREGNANCY TEST KIT

Just one of the many types of pregnancy test kit is shown. No kit is 100 percent accurate. Whether a test indicates pregnancy or gives a negative result despite a missed period, it is wise to consult a physician for confirmation.

Components of test kit
The kit has three main parts—a dropper tube containing a test solution, a test tube with stopper, and an indicator stick.

Indicator stick

Dropper with test solution

Stopper

Test tube

1 The end of the dropper tube is squeezed gently to introduce the test solution into the test tube, which is held upright in a stand provided.

3 Five drops of urine are added to the solution in the test tube. The stopper is put in the test tube, the contents shaken, and the stopper removed.

2 The lid of the test kit is used to collect a urine sample early in the morning. Some urine is drawn up into the dropper tube by squeezing and releasing.

Negative

Positive

4 The indicator stick is placed in the test tube. The result can be read after 30 minutes. If the end of the stick changes color, it signifies a pregnancy.

P

the level of HCG in the blood by a laboratory technique called *immunoassay*. It produces a result within nine to 12 days of conception but is more expensive to perform.

Premature ejaculation
See *Ejaculation, disorders of.*

Prematurity
Birth of a baby before 37 weeks' *gestation*. A premature labor carries little risk for the mother, but the premature infant may be insufficiently developed to cope with independent life and needs special care.

Prematurity was once a major cause of infant mortality, but improved medical techniques have dramatically increased survival rates of premature infants in developed countries. Approximately 10 percent of babies in the US are born prematurely.

CAUSES
Some 40 percent of all premature deliveries occur for no known reason. The remainder are due to conditions affecting the mother or fetus.

Preeclampsia is the most common maternal cause of premature labor. Other maternal causes include *hypertension* (high blood pressure), long-standing kidney disease, *diabetes mellitus*, and heart disease. Women who have any of these conditions carry an increased tendency to go into labor prematurely. However, more commonly, the pregnancy is curtailed early by *cesarean section* or *induction of labor* by the obstetrician to avoid further risk to mother and baby.

Similarly, *antepartum hemorrhage*, which may result if the *placenta* separates from the uterus before the baby is born, may result in premature labor due to the irritant effect of blood within the uterus. It sometimes makes induction of labor necessary. Other common causes of premature labor are intrauterine infection or premature rupture of membranes.

The most common fetal cause of prematurity is multiple pregnancy (see *Pregnancy, multiple*), which accounts for approximately 15 percent of all premature births. Multiple pregnancy may cause problems in the mother that make cesarean section or induction of labor necessary, or it may cause excessive stretching of the uterus, which stimulates contractions and leads to premature labor. A similar mechanism may occur with *hydramnios* (excessive amniotic fluid) or if the woman's uterine cavity is smaller than normal.

PREVENTION
If labor begins prematurely and there is no underlying cause, the obstetrician may attempt to stop labor by administering a drug (such as ritodrine) that inhibits contractions of the uterus.

THE PREMATURE INFANT
The premature infant is not only smaller than a full-term baby but has a characteristic physical appearance— the infant lacks subcutaneous fat, is covered with downy hair called lanugo, and has a very thin, gelatinous skin.

The baby's internal organs are also immature and incompletely developed, making it necessary for the baby to be monitored in a special hospital environment until he or she has developed sufficiently to sustain independent life.

The major complication for a premature infant is *respiratory distress syndrome*, which results from lung immaturity. Other organs, particularly the liver, may also be immature, leading to increased risk of brain hemorrhage, *jaundice*, and *hypoglycemia* (low blood sugar). A premature baby has a limited ability to suck and to maintain body temperature. Additionally, the immune system is poorly developed and the baby is more prone to infection.

TREATMENT
Premature infants are usually nursed in a special baby unit that provides intensive care. The baby is placed in an *incubator*, which provides warmth and allows easy observation. Other special care may include artificial *ventilation* to assist breathing, artificial feeding through a stomach tube or into a

---

PREMATURITY
A premature baby may need to be nursed in an incubator where the temperature and humidity are carefully controlled and the baby can be closely observed. If breathing difficulties develop, they may be treated by artificial ventilation. Very small babies cannot suck so they must be fed intravenously or via a tube passed into the stomach. If jaundice develops, it may be treated by *phototherapy* (light therapy), which breaks up the bilirubin that causes the yellow discoloration of the skin.

Premature infant
This baby girl was born several weeks prematurely. She is being fed via a flexible tube that passes via the nose and esophagus into the stomach.

FEATURES AND COMPLICATIONS OF PREMATURITY

Physical features	Complications
Low birth weight (often less than 5.5 pounds)	Increased risk of birth injury
Small size	Respiratory distress syndrome
Relatively large head and hands	Recurrent bouts of breathing arrest
Thin, smooth, shiny skin	Jaundice
Veins visible under the skin	Infection
Little fat under the skin	Poor temperature control
Wizened, wrinkled features	Anemia
Soft, flexible ear cartilage	Hypoglycemia (low blood sugar level) and other disturbances of body chemicals
Short toenails	Rickets
Downy (lanugo) hair	Increased bleeding tendency
Reduced vernix (greasy substance that covers newborn)	Brain hemorrhage
Protuberant abdomen	Necrotizing enterocolitis (severe intestinal inflammation)
Enlarged clitoris (girls)	
Small scrotum (boys)	
Feeble, whining cry	
Irregular breathing	
Poor sucking and swallowing ability	
Tendency to regurgitate	

P

vein, and treatment with *antibiotic drugs* and iron and vitamin supplements. The baby is usually kept in the hospital until he or she reaches a weight of at least 5 pounds (2.25 kg).

OUTLOOK

The survival chances of a premature baby increase with the length of the pregnancy. With modern techniques, some infants now survive even if they are born as early as 23 weeks' gestation and while weighing less than 2 pounds (1 kg), but this remains exceptional. Of babies born at 28 weeks' gestation, approximately 80 percent survive. Most premature babies catch up with full-term babies before the end of their first year.

Premedication

The term applied to drugs given one to two hours before an operation to prepare a person for surgery. Premedication usually contains a narcotic *analgesic* (painkiller) to help relieve pain and anxiety and to reduce the dose of anesthesia needed to produce unconsciousness (see *Anesthesia, general*). An *anticholinergic drug* is also sometimes included because it reduces secretions in the airways.

Premenstrual syndrome

The combination of various physical and emotional symptoms that occurs in women the week or two before *menstruation*. Premenstrual syndrome (PMS) begins at or after *ovulation* and continues until the onset of menstruation. PMS affects more than 90 percent of fertile women at some time in their lives and in some women is so severe that work and social relationships are seriously disrupted.

CAUSES

Many theories exist for the cause of PMS. Hormonal changes that occur throughout the menstrual cycle clearly influence PMS, but an imbalance between estrogen and progesterone levels has not been consistently found. Similarly, deficiencies of vitamins E and B_6 (pyridoxine), magnesium, or prostaglandins have been suggested but not confirmed.

SYMPTOMS AND SIGNS

The most frequent emotional symptoms of PMS are irritability, tension, depression, and fatigue. Physical symptoms include breast tenderness, fluid retention, headache, backache, and lower abdominal pain.

TREATMENT

No single method of treatment has proved completely successful. Treatments that may relieve specific symptoms include relaxation techniques to relieve anxiety and tension; *diuretic drugs* to relieve fluid retention; and dietary changes during the latter half of the menstrual cycle (such as avoidance of salt, caffeine, and chocolate). Taking vitamin B_6 or evening primrose oil may help some women with breast symptoms, irritability, and depression. *Oral contraceptives*, by eliminating the normal menstrual cycle, can be effective. Progesterone supplements are widely used but do not help all women.

Premolar

One of eight permanent grinding *teeth*, two on either side in each jaw, located between the canines and molars. (See also *Permanent teeth*; *Eruption of teeth*.)

Prenatal care

Care of a pregnant woman and her unborn baby throughout pregnancy with the aim of making sure both are healthy at delivery. Such care involves regular tests on the woman and the fetus to detect disease, defects, or potential hazards, and advising the woman on general aspects of pregnancy, such as diet and exercise.

FIRST VISIT

A woman should see her obstetrician as soon as she believes she is pregnant. At this time, he or she will take down the medical history of the woman and her family. The physician then examines the woman to confirm that she is actually pregnant and to check her general health. A vaginal examination is carried out to check that the reproductive organs and pelvis are normal and will not present any problems at delivery and to confirm the estimated date of the pregnancy, calculated from the first day of the woman's last period.

The first of a series of screening tests to detect any abnormalities in the woman or baby may be carried out at this visit—see the prenatal screening procedures chart. Some of these tests, such as *ultrasound scanning*, to detect any gross abnormality, usually need to be carried out only once; others, such as *blood tests* to detect *anemia* or *diabetes mellitus* in the woman, may be performed periodically throughout the pregnancy.

At this first visit, too, the woman is given advice about diet and the need not to drink any alcohol and not to smoke, since smoking can stunt the baby's growth and alcohol can result in *fetal alcohol syndrome*.

SUBSEQUENT VISITS

If there are no problems, the woman visits the physician every month until the 28th week, then every two weeks until the 36th week, and then weekly until the delivery date, which on average is the 40th week from the mother's last menses (menstrual period). If the pregnancy is a high-risk one—for example, if the woman is over 35 years old or is suffering from *hypertension* or diabetes—or if problems develop, visits will be more frequent and, in some cases, the woman may need to be admitted to the hospital for closer observation.

At each visit, as well as undergoing the tests detailed in the chart, the woman is weighed, her blood pressure is taken, and the size of the uterus is estimated to confirm that the baby is growing well.

After the 32nd week, the position of the baby in the uterus (whether it is head-down as it should be) is determined, and the degree of engagement (how far the baby's head has descended into the woman's pelvis) is regularly recorded. The woman is also asked about the baby's movements; frequent pronounced movements indicate an active, healthy baby.

PREPARATION FOR CHILDBIRTH CLASSES

Childbirth preparation classes (see *Prepared childbirth*) are given in hospitals, physicians' offices, community meeting places, or private homes. Such classes aim to provide information on all aspects of pregnancy, labor, and delivery, including advice on exercise, diet, and sexual activity. The woman learns what happens during labor and the different types of pain relief available during it, and may learn breathing exercises to help her cope with labor and delivery.

Prepared childbirth

A program of classes for pregnant women and their partners that encourages active involvement in the process of childbirth. Prepared childbirth, also known as natural childbirth or psychoprophylaxis, involves learning relaxation techniques to cope with labor pains so that the use of anesthesia or analgesia (medications for *pain* relief) can be minimized. An important feature of the prepared childbirth method is the involvement of a partner, usually the baby's father, who learns relaxation techniques and breathing exercises along with the expectant mother. The partner provides encouragement, support, and comfort during labor.

PRENATAL SCREENING PROCEDURES

When performed	Procedure	Reason for procedure
First visit	Blood tests	To check the woman's *blood group* and, sometimes, to check for presence of *hepatitis B* virus which might be transmitted to the baby.
	Cervical smear test (Pap smear)	To test for an early cancer of the cervix (if a test has not been performed recently).
First visit and throughout the pregnancy	Blood tests	To check for *anemia* in the woman and, in women with Rh-negative blood groups, to look for the presence of Rhesus antibodies.
	Urine test	To check for *proteinuria*, which could indicate a *urinary tract infection* or *preeclampsia*.
	Blood and urine test	To check for *diabetes mellitus*.
	Blood pressure check	To screen for *hypertension*, which interferes with blood supply to the placenta and is a sign of preeclampsia.
First visit and after any infection	Blood tests	To screen for *rubella*, which can cause defects in the baby, and for *syphilis* and HIV (the *AIDS* virus), which can also be passed on.
First 12 weeks	Chorionic villus sampling	May be performed if there is a risk of certain genetic (inherited) disorders being passed on.
16 to 18 weeks	Ultrasound scanning	Is carried out to date the pregnancy accurately and to detect any abnormalities present in the fetus.
	Amniocentesis	Carried out on older women and those who have children with *spina bifida* or *Down's syndrome* to detect possible abnormalities in the fetus.
	Blood test	In some cases, the amount of *alpha-fetoprotein* in the blood is tested to determine whether the baby has spina bifida.
	Fetoscopy and fetal blood sampling	In some cases, these are carried out if there is doubt about the normality of the baby.
High-risk or overdue pregnancies	Blood and urine tests	May be administered to assess placental function and well-being of the fetus.
	Electronic fetal monitoring	To check on the fetal heart beat.
	Ultrasound scanning	Extra scans may be recommended to assess fetal growth and development, the location of the placenta, and the amount of amniotic fluid.

There are a number of prepared childbirth organizations. In the US, prepared childbirth is often associated with the Lamaze method, which began in the 1940s.

METHODS

Prepared childbirth classes are taught by midwives or other qualified childbirth educators. The weekly classes usually begin during the last three months of pregnancy. Most classes are small, containing from six to 10 couples. Information is provided about female anatomy, the physiology of pregnancy, fetal development, labor, delivery, and the postnatal period. Other topics (such as nutrition, breast-feeding, and parenting skills) are also covered.

The primary purpose of the classes is to teach relaxation techniques, often using breathing exercises to help expectant women cope with the pain of uterine contractions and labor. For example, a woman may be taught to concentrate on her breathing pattern, inhaling slowly and deeply initially, then increasing the rate and reducing the depth as the pain of contractions increases. At the end of each contraction, the woman breathes out slowly and relaxes completely. Relaxation techniques help the mother to be aware of muscle tension and to relax during labor.

OUTCOME

Of women who use psychoprophylactic preparation for childbirth, about 45 percent require no analgesia during labor; another 45 percent request some analgesia. The remaining 10 percent of women who have attended classes require epidural anesthesia or some other method of pain relief.

Prepuce
See *Foreskin*.

Presbycusis

The progressive loss of hearing that occurs with age. Presbycusis is a form of sensorineural *deafness* (degeneration of the hair cells and nerve fibers in the inner ear), which makes sounds less clear and tones, especially higher tones, less audible.

SYMPTOMS AND CAUSES

People with presbycusis often have difficulty understanding speech and are usually unable to hear well in the presence of background noise. The severity and progression of the condition vary considerably from person to person (some people who are 80 have far better hearing than others who are only 60).

The natural process of presbycusis may be exacerbated by exposure to high *noise* levels, diminished blood supply to the inner ear due to an arterial disease such as *atherosclerosis*, and toxic damage to the inner ear by certain drugs (such as aminoglycoside; see *Antibiotic drugs*).

TREATMENT

Hearing aids can help most people, except for those with a poor ability to discriminate among speech sounds (and who thus have difficulty understanding what is being said). A person speaking to someone with presbycusis should remember to speak loudly, slowly, and clearly. (If the person with presbycusis is wearing a hearing aid, there is no need to speak in a loud voice.)

Presbyopia

The progressive loss of the power of *accommodation* for near vision. The focusing power of the eyes weakens with age until, around 65, little or no focusing power remains. Presbyopia is usually noticed around the age of 45 when the eyes cannot accommodate within normal reading distance. Large print can still be seen, but small print may be impossible to focus on; newspapers may need to be read at arm's length.

Simple, convex lens reading *glasses* are used to correct presbyopia. They may need to be changed four to five times over the course of about 20 years, until eventually all the focusing is being done by the glasses.

Prescription

An instruction written by a physician that directs the *pharmacist* to dispense a particular drug in a specific dose. A prescription also details how often the drug must be taken, how much is to be dispensed, and any other relevant facts. Drugs that require a prescription (prescription medicines) are available only on the authorization of a physician because they are dangerous, powerful, habit-forming, or used to treat a disease that needs to be monitored by a physician.

All prescriptions must bear the name and address of the patient and the physician's signature. The pharmacist keeps a record of all prescriptions dispensed.

Preservative

A substance that prevents foods and drugs from spoiling. Preservatives include sulfur dioxide and nitrates. (See also *Food additives*.)

Pressure points

Places on the body where arteries lie near the surface and where pressure can be applied to limit severe arterial *bleeding*. Applying pressure at these points will not stop venous bleeding.

Arterial bleeding can be identified because blood from arteries is bright red and is pumped in regular spurts as the heart beats. To stop bleeding, pressure is applied by hand to compress the appropriate artery against the underlying bone. (See illustrated box, below.)

Pressure sores

Another common name for *bedsores* (decubitus ulcers).

Prevalence

The total number of cases of a disease in existence at any one time in a defined population. Prevalence is usually expressed as the number of cases per 100,000 people. Prevalence is one of the two chief measures of how common a disease is; the other is *incidence*. (See also box on next page.)

Preventive dentistry

An aspect of dentistry concerned with the prevention of tooth decay and gum disease rather than their treatment. Preventive dentistry consists of encouraging the practice of good *oral hygiene* and a reduced intake of sugary foods, *fluoride* treatment to strengthen tooth enamel, and *scaling* to remove any accumulated dental *plaque* and *calculus* from the teeth. (See also *Public health dentistry*.)

Preventive medicine

The branch of medicine that deals with the prevention of disease by public health measures, such as the provision of pure water supplies; by health education aimed at discouraging smoking and the overuse of alcohol, promoting exercise, and giving advice about a prudent diet; by specific preventive treatments, such as immunization against infectious diseases; and by screening programs to detect diseases such as glaucoma, tuberculosis, and cancer of the cervix before they cause symptoms.

FIRST AID: PRESSURE POINTS

Mechanism of indirect pressure
If direct pressure on a wound fails to control bleeding, apply indirect pressure by compressing a major artery at a point between the wound and the heart where the artery can be pressed against a bone. In the example at right, the brachial pressure point is used, pressing the artery against the bone of the upper arm, between the armpit and the elbow.

THE MAJOR PRESSURE POINTS

Temporal
At the side of the head in front of the ear (for control of scalp bleeding)

Brachial
Middle part of upper arm (for control of arm bleeding)

Radial
Lower part of arm (for control of bleeding in hand and forearm)

Femoral
Center of the fold in the groin (for control of upper leg bleeding)

Carotid
At the side of the neck, below the jaw (for control of head and neck bleeding)

Subclavian
Between the collarbone and first rib (for control of bleeding in armpit, shoulder, and upper chest)

Popliteal
The back of the knee joint (for control of lower leg bleeding)

Most of the increase in the world's population during the 19th century was due to improvements in public health, particularly improvements in the overall standard of nutrition, and the provision of pure water supplies and proper sanitation. Today, these measures remain the priorities of preventive medicine in developing countries, and, along with a program of immunization in childhood, have been targeted as major objectives by the World Health Organization.

However, in developed countries, the primary objective is to persuade the adult population to adopt a healthier life-style. In the US, most premature deaths in adults (that is, deaths before the age of 65) are preventable, being due to accidents and/or linked to such factors as an unhealthy diet, smoking, and excessive drinking. Adoption of a healthier life-style, the wider use of screening for cancers, and measures to reduce accidents could lead to substantial improvements in the nation's health.

Priapism

Persistent, painful erection of the penis without sexual arousal. Priapism is a dangerous condition that requires emergency treatment.

CAUSES

Priapism occurs because blood fails to drain from the spongy tissue of the penis, keeping the penis erect. Possible causes include damage to nerves that control the supply of blood to the penis; a blood disease (such as *leukemia* or *sickle cell anemia*) that causes partial clotting of blood in the penis; and, rarely, blockage of the normal outflow of blood from the penis as a result of an infection (such as *prostatitis* or *urethritis*).

TREATMENT

Urgent treatment is needed because of the risk of permanent damage to the penis. Treatment may involve *spinal anesthesia* (injection of local anesthetic into the spinal cord) or withdrawal of blood from the penis through a wide-bore needle.

Prickly heat

An irritating skin rash that is associated with profuse sweating. The medical name for prickly heat, miliaria rubra, literally means "red millet seeds." This term describes the numerous tiny, red, itchy spots that cover the mildly inflamed, affected areas of skin. Prickly heat is accompanied by aggravating, prickling sensations. The irritation tends to affect

sites on the body where sweat collects, particularly the waist, upper trunk, armpits, and insides of the elbows.

A milder type (miliaria crystallina) sometimes precedes true prickly heat and produces clear, shiny, fluid-filled blisters that tend to dry up quickly without treatment.

CAUSES

The mechanism by which prickly heat is caused is not fully understood, but unevaporated sweat is known to be an important factor. The skin becomes unhealthy and waterlogged. Sweat ducts become blocked with debris and eventually leak sweat into the skin. Sleep is often possible only in cool surroundings, and lack of sleep combined with the intense irritation of the rash can make the sufferer irritable.

TREATMENT AND PREVENTION

Frequent cool showers and sponging the affected areas relieve the itching, although ordinary soap should not be used on affected areas. Application of calamine lotion and dusting powder can further relieve the discomfort.

Clothing should be clean, starch-free, and loose fitting to help sweat evaporation. The chances of developing prickly heat are much reduced by slow acclimation to hot weather. If the sweating has occurred because of fever, *antipyretic drugs* (such as aspirin or acetaminophen) may be helpful.

Primaquine

A drug used in the treatment of *malaria*. Primaquine is often given after prophylactic treatment with *chloroquine*. It is not effective in the prevention of a malaria attack but kills the parasites in the liver. Primaquine is also used to treat *Chagas' disease*.

Adverse effects include nausea, vomiting, and abdominal pain. In people with *G6PD deficiency*, primaquine may cause hemolytic *anemia*.

Primary

A term applied to a disease that has originated within the organ or tissue affected, and is not derived from any other cause or source. Primary liver

PREVALENCE OF VARIOUS CHRONIC CONDITIONS IN THE US

(Number of people with the condition per 100,000 population)

Prevalence	Categorization	Examples
More than 25,000	Extremely common	Myopia (nearsightedness)
5,000 to 25,000	Very common	Male-pattern baldness, partial or total deafness, hypertension (high blood pressure), osteoarthritis
1,000 to 5,000	Common	Alcohol dependence, asthma, chronic bronchitis, coronary heart disease, all types of diabetes mellitus, psoriasis, schizophrenia
200 to 1,000	Fairly common	Blindness, epilepsy, rheumatoid arthritis, symptomatic gallstones
50 to 200	Uncommon	Ankylosing spondylitis, celiac sprue, Down's syndrome, megaloblastic anemia, multiple sclerosis, Parkinson's disease, ulcerative colitis
5 to 50	Rare	Autism, cystic fibrosis, Crohn's disease, gout, myasthenia gravis, sarcoidosis, sickle cell anemia, systemic lupus erythematosus
0.5 to 5	Very rare	Achondroplasia, albinism, galactosemia, polycythemia vera, periarteritis nodosa
Less than 0.5	Extremely rare	Alkaptonuria, congenital erythropoietic porphyria

P

cancer, for example, is the result of some cancer-producing change in liver cells. Secondary liver cancer results from the spread of cancer cells from another part of the body to the liver.

The term primary is also applied to the first of several diseases to affect a tissue or organ in turn. For example, when a viral infection of the lungs is succeeded by a bacterial infection, the viral infection is called primary and the bacterial infection is termed secondary. Primary also occasionally is used to mean "of unknown cause."

Primary teeth

The first teeth (also known as deciduous, or milk, teeth), which usually start to appear at the age of 6 months and are gradually replaced by the permanent teeth from about the age of 6 years.

There are 20 primary teeth, 10 in each jaw. Each set of 10 consists of four incisors (biting teeth) at the front, flanked by two canines (tearing teeth), with four molars (grinding teeth) at the back. (See also *Teeth*; *Eruption of teeth*; *Teething*.)

Primidone

An *anticonvulsant drug* used in the treatment of *epilepsy* and, occasionally, *tremor*. Primidone is usually prescribed with another anticonvulsant. Adverse effects include drowsiness, clumsiness, and dizziness.

Probenecid

A drug used in the long-term treatment of *gout* that reduces the level of uric acid in the body by increasing the amount excreted in the urine.

Probenecid also slows the excretion of *antibiotic drugs* (such as *penicillin drugs* and *cephalosporin drugs*) from the kidneys and is therefore occasionally prescribed with these drugs to boost their levels and thus their effects.

Probenecid may cause nausea and vomiting. It also increases the risk of kidney stones in some people.

Probucol

A *lipid-lowering drug*. Probucol is often prescribed with other lipid-lowering drugs to boost their effect. Treatment is usually monitored by blood tests.

Possible adverse effects include diarrhea, flatulence, abdominal pain, and, rarely, dizziness.

Procainamide

An *antiarrhythmic drug* used in the treatment of certain types of *tachycar-*

dia (abnormally rapid heart beat) or certain ventricular *arrhythmias*.

Procainamide may cause nausea, vomiting, loss of appetite, and, rarely, confusion. Prolonged treatment may induce *lupus erythematosus*, causing fever, joint pain, swelling, and rash.

Procaine

A local anesthetic (see *Anesthesia, local*) used before surgical or dental treatment and, sometimes, during childbirth. Procaine has largely been replaced by drugs that are quicker to take effect or are longer-acting.

Occasionally, procaine causes an allergic reaction, with a rash or swelling of the face, lips, mouth, or throat. Rare adverse effects include anxiety, drowsiness, or ringing in the ears.

Procarbazine

An *anticancer drug* particularly useful in the treatment of *lymphomas*. Procarbazine is also used to treat brain tumors and certain cancers of the skin, lungs, and bone marrow.

In addition to typical anticancer drug adverse effects, procarbazine may cause a sudden rise in blood pressure if taken with certain foods or drinks (e.g., cheese and red wine).

Prochlorperazine

A *phenothiazine*-type *antipsychotic drug*. Prochlorperazine is used to relieve the symptoms of certain psychiatric disorders, including *schizophrenia* and *mania*. In smaller doses, it is also used as an *antiemetic drug* to relieve nausea and vomiting.

Prochlorperazine may cause involuntary movements of the face and limbs, lethargy, dry mouth, blurred vision, and dizziness.

Procidentia

A medical term for severe prolapse (displacement of an organ from its normal position in the body), usually of the uterus.

Proctalgia fugax

A severe cramping pain in the rectum unconnected with any disease. It may be due to muscle spasm, sometimes associated with stress or anxiety. The pain, which may occur at any time, is of short duration and subsides of its own accord.

Proctitis

Inflammation of the rectum, causing soreness, bleeding, and sometimes a discharge of mucus and pus. Proctitis commonly occurs with inflammation

of the colon as a feature of *ulcerative colitis*, *Crohn's disease*, or *dysentery*. In cases where inflammation is confined to the rectum, the cause is often unknown. However, especially in male homosexuals, it is sometimes due to *gonorrhea* or another sexually transmitted disease. Rare causes include *tuberculosis*, *amebiasis*, *bilharziasis*, injury, certain drugs, allergy, or radiation injury.

DIAGNOSIS AND TREATMENT

The diagnosis is made by *proctoscopy* (inspection of the rectum with a viewing tube). A *biopsy* (removal of a small sample of tissue for laboratory analysis) is sometimes required to determine the precise cause of the rectal inflammation.

Successful treatment of any underlying cause usually clears the problem. *Corticosteroid drugs*, in the form of suppositories or enemas, may relieve symptoms, especially in cases of ulcerative colitis or Crohn's disease.

Proctoscopy

Examination of the anal canal and rectum by means of a proctoscope (a rigid viewing tube) inserted through the anus. A short, flexible sigmoidoscope (see *Sigmoidoscopy*) is sometimes used and is more comfortable for the person being examined.

Procyclidine

An *anticholinergic drug* used in the treatment of *Parkinson's disease*. Procyclidine reduces excessive salivation and muscle rigidity and may also improve tremor. Possible adverse effects include dry mouth, blurred vision, and urinary symptoms.

Prodrome

An early warning symptom of illness. A *migraine* headache attack may be preceded by paresthesia (pins and needles sensation) of an extremity or by an aura composed of visual symptoms—both are prodromes. Awareness of this prodromal period enables a migraine headache sufferer to use certain preventive medications that are far less effective once the headache is established.

Progeria

Premature old age. There are two distinct forms of the condition, both of which are extremely rare.

In Hutchinson-Gilford syndrome, aging starts around the age of 4, and by 10 or 12 the affected child has all the external features of old age, including gray hair, baldness, and loss of fat, resulting in thin limbs and sagging skin on the trunk and face. There are also internal degenerative changes, such as widespread *atherosclerosis* (fatty deposits lining the artery walls). Death usually occurs at puberty.

Werner's syndrome, or adult progeria, starts in early adult life and follows the same rapid progression as the juvenile form.

The cause of progeria is unknown, although cells taken from affected people show only a few generations of cell division before they stop reproducing, instead of the 50 or so generations that occur in cells taken from healthy young people.

Progesterone drugs

COMMON DRUGS

Hydroxyprogesterone Medroxyprogesterone Megestrol Norethindrone Norethisterone Norgestrel

A group of drugs similar to *progesterone hormone*, including natural progesterone and synthetic progesterone derivatives.

WHY THEY ARE USED
Progesterone drugs are used in birth-control pills, either on their own (in the mini pill) or with *estrogen drugs* (in combined and phased pills). They work by making the cervical mucus impenetrable to sperm, altering the lining of the uterus so that it prevents the implantation of a fertilized egg, and reducing the production of *gonadotropin hormones*, which may prevent eggs from ripening in the ovary (see *Oral contraceptives*).

Progesterone drugs are also prescribed, sometimes with estrogens, to treat menstrual problems (see *Menstruation, disorders of*).

In *hormone replacement therapy*, a progesterone drug is used in combination with an estrogen drug to reduce the risk of cancer of the uterus (see *Uterus, cancer of*) that occurs if estrogens alone are taken over a long period. The progesterone induces the monthly shedding of the uterine lining.

Progesterone drugs are used also to treat *premenstrual syndrome*, *endometriosis* (a disorder in which fragments of the lining of the uterus occur elsewhere in the pelvic cavity), and *hypogonadism* (underdevelopment of the ovaries). Progesterone drugs are sometimes effective as *anticancer drugs* in the treatment of certain types of cancers (such as uterine endometrial cancer) that are sensitive to progesterone hormones.

POSSIBLE ADVERSE EFFECTS
Adverse effects include weight gain, *edema*, appetite loss, headache, dizziness, rash, irregular periods, breast tenderness, and *ovarian cysts*.

Progesterone hormone
A female sex hormone essential for the healthy functioning of the female reproductive system. Progesterone is produced in the ovaries during the second half of the menstrual cycle (see *Menstruation*) and by the placenta during *pregnancy*. Small amounts of progesterone are also produced in the adrenal glands and testes.

Following *ovulation*, increased production of progesterone causes the endometrium (lining of the uterus) to thicken in preparation for the implantation of a fertilized egg. If fertilization does not take place, the production of progesterone and also of *estrogen hormones* falls, resulting in shedding of the uterine lining and unfertilized egg in the monthly period.

During pregnancy, progesterone is essential for normal functioning of the placenta and thus for the healthy development of the baby. Progesterone also passes into the developing baby's circulation, where it is converted in the adrenal glands to corticosteroid hormones. At the end of pregnancy, a fall in the level of progesterone helps initiate labor.

Other effects of progesterone produce changes in the cervix and vagina during the menstrual cycle, increased deposition of fat, and increased *sebum* production by glands in the skin.

Progestin
Another name for a *progesterone hormone* or a synthetic *progesterone drug*.

Prognathism
Abnormal protrusion of the lower jaw or both jaws. If the condition interferes with biting and chewing (see *Malocclusion*) or is disfiguring, *orthognathic surgery* may be performed.

Prognosis
A medical assessment of the probable course and outcome of a disease. It is based on the recorded history of the disease (e.g., 90 percent of people with small cell carcinoma of the lung die within five years of the condition developing), the physician's own experience of treating the disease, and the patient's general condition and age. However, every prognosis is no more than an informed guess, and any patient may prove it wrong.

Progressive muscular atrophy
A type of *motor neuron disease* in which the muscles of the hands, arms, and legs become weak and wasted and twitch involuntarily. This is a progressively debilitating condition that eventually spreads to other muscles in the body.

Prolactinoma
A benign tumor of the pituitary gland that causes overproduction of the hormone prolactin. In a woman, prolactinoma may result in *galactorrhea* (breast secretion at any time other than a few days before childbirth or during breast-feeding), *amenorrhea* (absence of periods), or *infertility*. In a man, a prolactinoma may cause *impotence* and *gynecomastia* (breast enlargement). In either sex, it may cause headaches, *diabetes insipidus*, and, if it presses on the optic nerves, gradual loss of the outer field of vision.

The condition is diagnosed from blood tests to measure prolactin levels, and from *CT scanning* or *MRI* of the brain. Treatment may consist of removal of the tumor, *radiation therapy*, or the drug bromocriptine, which inhibits prolactin secretion.

Prolapse
Displacement of part or all of an organ or tissue from its normal position. Common structures that prolapse include the uterus (see *Uterus, prolapse of*) and the disk between two vertebrae (see *Disk prolapse*).

Promazine
A *phenothiazine*-type *antipsychotic drug* sometimes used as a sedative. Promazine also acts as an *antiemetic drug* and is used to relieve nausea and vomiting after anesthesia.

Possible adverse effects include abnormal movements of the face and limbs, drowsiness, lethargy, dry mouth, constipation, and blurred vision. Long-term treatment may be associated with *parkinsonism*.

Promethazine
An *antihistamine drug* used to relieve itching in a variety of skin conditions, including *urticaria* (hives) and *eczema*. Promethazine is also used as an *antiemetic drug* to relieve nausea and vomiting caused by *motion sickness* and *Meniere's disease*.

Promethazine has a sedative effect and is therefore sometimes used as a *premedication* (drug used to prepare a person for surgery) and as a short-term sleeping drug for children. Occa-

P

sionally, promethazine is given to produce sedation during *childbirth*.

Adverse effects of promethazine may include dry mouth, blurred vision, and drowsiness.

Pronation
The act of turning the body to a prone (facedown) position, or the hand to a palm backward position. The opposite movements are called *supination*.

Propantheline
An *antispasmodic drug* used in the treatment of *irritable bowel syndrome* and certain types of urinary *incontinence*. Propantheline is rarely used today in the treatment of certain forms of *peptic ulcer*.

Possible adverse effects include dry mouth, blurred vision, and abnormal retention of urine.

Prophylactic
A drug, procedure, or piece of equipment used to prevent disease; the term prophylactic is popularly used to refer to a *condom*.

Propoxyphene
A weak narcotic *analgesic* (painkiller) sometimes combined with other analgesics, such as *aspirin* or *acetaminophen*, to boost their effects.

Propoxyphene may cause drowsiness, dizziness, nausea, and vomiting. Used long-term, it may produce dependence (see *Drug dependence*).

Propranolol
A *beta-blocker drug* used to treat *hypertension* (high blood pressure), *angina pectoris* (chest pain due to inadequate blood supply to the heart muscle), and cardiac *arrhythmias* (irregularities of the heart beat). It is also used to reduce the risk of further damage to the heart after *myocardial infarction*.

Propranolol is used to relieve symptoms of *hyperthyroidism* (overactivity of the thyroid gland) or of *anxiety* (e.g., stage fright), and to prevent attacks of *migraine*.

Possible adverse effects are typical of other beta-blocker drugs.

Proprietary
A drug patented for production by one company. The patent protects the drug's name, ingredients, and process of manufacture.

Proprioception
The body's internal system for collecting information about its position relative to the outside world and the state of contraction of its muscles. This is achieved by means of sensory nerve endings within the muscles, tendons, joints, and sensory hair cells in the balance organ of the inner ear. These structures are called proprioceptors (literally "position sensors").

Information from the proprioceptors passes to the spinal cord and brain and is used to make adjustments in the state of contraction of muscles so that posture and balance are maintained. During movement, there is a continuous feedback of information to the brain from the proprioceptors and from the eyes. This helps ensure that actions are smooth and coordinated.

Proptosis
A term for protrusion of the eyeball (see *Exophthalmos*).

Propylthiouracil
A drug used to treat *hyperthyroidism* (overactivity of the thyroid gland) or to control symptoms before *thyroidectomy* (removal of the thyroid gland).

Possible adverse effects include itching, headache, rash, and joint pain. Propylthiouracil may reduce the production of white blood cells by the bone marrow and thus increase the risk of infection.

Prostaglandin
One of a group of *fatty acids* that is made naturally in the body and that acts in a similar way to *hormones*. Prostaglandins are divided into broad groups according to their chemical structure. They were first discovered in semen but are now known to occur in many different body tissues, including the uterus, brain, and kidneys. Some prostaglandins are prepared synthetically for use as drugs (see *Prostaglandin drugs*).

EFFECTS
Prostaglandins produce a wide range of effects on the body, including causing pain and inflammation in damaged tissue, protecting the lining of the stomach and duodenum against ulceration, and stimulating contractions during labor (see box).

Certain drugs counteract the effects of prostaglandins on the body. *Nonsteroidal anti-inflammatory drugs* (NSAIDs), *aspirin*, and *corticosteroid drugs* relieve pain and inflammation by reducing prostaglandin production in tissues. Taken long-term, however, NSAIDs and aspirin may increase the risk of a *peptic ulcer*, in part by reducing production of prostaglandins that protect the stomach lining.

Prostaglandin drugs
Synthetically produced *prostaglandins* that have a variety of therapeutic uses.

Dinoprostone is an E_2 prostaglandin used to stimulate contractions of the uterus for *induction of labor* at full term, after a fetal death, or to induce a late abortion (see *Abortion, elective*).

Carboprost and dinoprost are F_2 prostaglandins that resemble dinoprostone by inducing contractions of the uterus.

Alprostadil is an E_1 prostaglandin used (temporarily) to treat newborn infants awaiting surgery for certain types of congenital heart disease. Alprostadil is also being investigated for use in the treatment of people with *Raynaud's disease*.

Other prostaglandin drugs are under investigation for use in a variety of disorders, including *peptic ulcer*.

Prostate, cancer of
A malignant growth arising in the outer zone of the *prostate gland*. Cancer of the prostate is the second most common cancer in men. It sometimes develops in middle age but most often occurs in the elderly. While its precise cause is unknown, the hormone *testosterone* appears to be involved.

EFFECTS OF SOME PROSTAGLANDINS

Type	Effect
PGA_1	Lowers blood pressure Protects against peptic ulcer
PGD_2	Causes inflammation
PGE_1	Stimulates contractions of the uterus Lowers blood pressure Protects against peptic ulcer Reduces stickiness of platelets in blood
PGE_2	Causes inflammation Widens airways Increases stickiness of platelets in blood Stimulates contractions of the uterus
PGF_2	Stimulates contractions of the uterus Narrows airways
PGG_2	Causes inflammation
PGI_2	Reduces stickiness of platelets in blood

P

SYMPTOMS AND SIGNS

Symptoms are caused by enlargement of the prostate (see *Prostate, enlarged*) and include difficulty starting urination, poor flow of urine, and increased frequency of urination. Eventually the flow of urine may cease completely either because the urethra is completely blocked or because the cancer has spread to the bladder and ureters. In advanced cases, pain may be caused by involvement of nerves within the pelvis or by spread of cancer to bones anywhere in the body.

DIAGNOSIS

Cancer of the prostate is usually diagnosed at a physical examination in which the physician feels the prostate through the rectum; a diseased gland feels hard and knobby. The diagnosis may be confirmed by *ultrasound scanning*, *pyelography*, and prostatic biopsy (removal of a sample for analysis). Blood tests and a bone scan may be performed to assess the extent to which a cancer has spread.

TREATMENT

Treatment may be by *prostatectomy* (surgical removal of the prostate) or *radiation therapy*; if the disease has spread to other parts of the body, patients may be helped by reducing the level of testosterone. This may be done by *orchiectomy* (surgical removal of the testes), by giving *estrogen drugs*, or by giving drugs that resemble *luteinizing hormone-releasing hormone*.

OUTLOOK

When the growth is discovered at an early stage, the outlook is very good. However, if the cancer has spread outside the prostate gland and does not respond to hormone treatment, the prognosis is poor. The cancer is so advanced in a majority of people discovered to have cancer of the prostate that radical surgery offers little hope for cure.

Prostatectomy

An operation to remove part or all of the *prostate gland*. Prostatectomy is usually performed when enlargement of the gland is causing obstruction to the flow of urine (see *Prostate, enlarged*). The operation may also be performed to treat cancer of the prostate (see *Prostate, cancer of*) and, in some cases, *prostatitis*.

HOW IT IS DONE

The most common method is transurethral prostatectomy, which is performed by means of *cystoscopy*. If the prostate gland is very enlarged, retropubic prostatectomy may be performed (see box, overleaf).

RECOVERY PERIOD

After removal of the catheter and drainage tube, the patient can begin to pass urine as the bladder fills in the normal way. Initially, urination may be frequent and sometimes painful; occasionally, there is mild incontinence for a few weeks. Patients are encouraged to drink large amounts of fluid to help wash out remaining blood in the urine.

Rarely, bleeding after the operation is severe, and blood transfusions are required. Blood clots that may form within the bladder can be washed out through the catheter.

The hospital stay is about three to five days for transurethral prostatectomy and about eight to 10 days for the retropubic operation. After several weeks, patients may resume all activities, including intercourse.

OUTLOOK

The operation may affect potency or sexual sensation in a small percentage of men. The majority of men are sterile after prostatectomy because semen is expelled backward into the bladder instead of being ejaculated. Seminal fluid in the bladder is not harmful and is excreted in the urine.

Prostate, enlarged

Often called benign prostatic hypertrophy, an increase in size of the inner zone of the *prostate gland*, usually affecting men over 50. The cause is unknown.

SYMPTOMS AND SIGNS

Symptoms usually develop gradually as the enlarging prostate compresses and distorts the urethra. The flow of urine is obstructed, and there is difficulty starting urination and a weak stream.

Initially the bladder muscle becomes overdeveloped to force urine through the obstructed urethra. Eventually the bladder is unable to expel all the urine (see *Urine retention*) and becomes distended, causing abdominal swelling.

There may be *incontinence* due to overflow of small quantities of urine, and the bladder may become overactive, resulting in frequency of urination (see *Urination, frequent*). This is a sign of bladder muscle failure and usually means surgery is required.

Severe abdominal pain and the ability to pass only a few drops of urine indicates acute urinary retention and requires immediate treatment.

DIAGNOSIS

Enlargement of the prostate can be detected during a *rectal examination* (in which the physician inserts a gloved finger into the rectum). The physician also feels the abdomen for signs of bladder distention.

A sample of urine may be tested for infection and a blood test performed to provide a measurement of kidney function. *Ultrasound scanning*, *pyelography*, and a recording of the strength of urine flow may be performed to give additional information about the severity of the obstruction and any effects elsewhere in the urinary system, especially the kidneys.

TREATMENT

Mild symptoms of prostatic enlargement do not require treatment. If symptoms are more severe, the usual treatment is *prostatectomy* (removal of the prostate). Retention of urine is treated initially by urinary *catheterization* and then by prostatectomy. If surgery is considered too dangerous because of age or ill health, a catheter is sometimes kept in place permanently to drain urine.

Prostate gland

A solid, chestnut-shaped organ surrounding the first part of the urethra in the male. The prostate gland is situated immediately under the bladder and in front of the rectum.

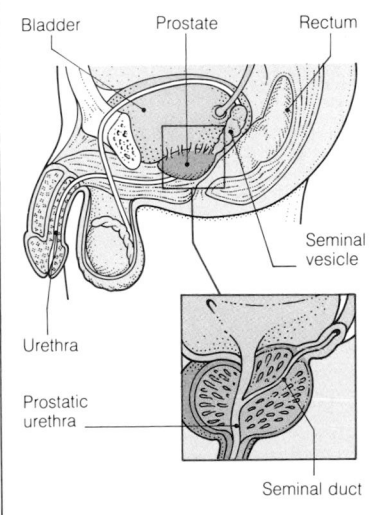

LOCATION OF PROSTATE GLAND
Located under the bladder and in front of the rectum, the prostate gland secretes substances into the semen as the fluid passes through ducts leading from the seminal vesicles into the urethra.

Bladder   Prostate   Rectum

Seminal vesicle

Urethra

Prostatic urethra

Seminal duct

P

The prostate gland produces secretions that form part of the seminal fluid during ejaculation. The ejaculatory ducts from the seminal vesicles pass through the prostate gland to enter the urethra.

The prostate gland weighs only a few grams at birth. Enlargement starts at puberty from the effect of *androgen hormones* and stops at around the age of 20, when it reaches its adult weight of about 20 grams. In most men, the prostate begins to enlarge further after the age of 50.

The prostate gland consists of two main zones: an inner zone (which produces secretions responsible for keeping the lining of the urethra moist) and an outer zone (which produces seminal secretions).

DISORDERS

Prostatic problems very rarely occur before the age of 30. *Prostatitis* (inflammation of the prostate) is usually caused by bacterial infection and may be sexually transmitted. It usually affects men in their 30s and 40s, but can occur later in life.

Enlargement of the prostate (see *Prostate, enlarged*) usually affects men over 50 and may interfere with urination by compressing the urethra.

Cancer of the prostate (see *Prostate, cancer of*) is common in old age and may cause symptoms similar to those that occur with enlargement of the prostate gland.

Prostatism

Symptoms resulting from enlargement of the prostate gland (see *Prostate, enlarged*).

PROSTATECTOMY—REMOVAL OF THE PROSTATE GLAND

Of the two possible methods of removal shown, the transurethral method is the most commonly used.

It avoids the disadvantages of an abdominal incision and usually permits a shorter stay in the hospital.

The retropubic method may be necessary if the prostate is very enlarged or if a cancer is suspected.

TRANSURETHRAL PROSTATECTOMY

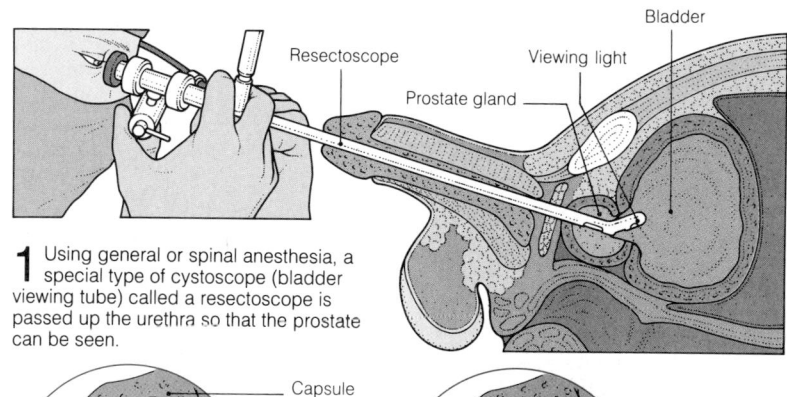

Resectoscope · Viewing light · Bladder · Prostate gland

1 Using general or spinal anesthesia, a special type of cystoscope (bladder viewing tube) called a resectoscope is passed up the urethra so that the prostate can be seen.

Capsule · Prostate gland · Bladder · Cutting edge

Tissue washed out · Electrode cauterizes bleeding vessels

2 A heated wire loop, or sometimes a cutting edge, is inserted through the resectoscope and used to cut away as much of the prostatic tissue as possible.

3 The pieces of tissue are washed out through the resectoscope and any bleeding vessels are cauterized by means of an electrode passed up the tube.

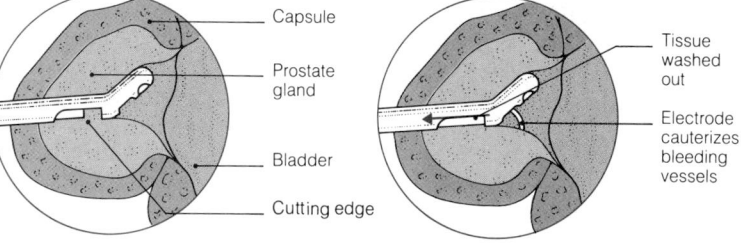

4 The resectoscope is then withdrawn and a catheter passed via the urethra into the bladder. The catheter is left in place for several days to drain urine from the bladder and allow blood to be washed out.

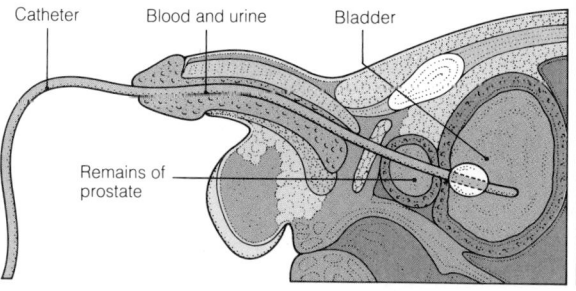

Catheter · Blood and urine · Bladder · Remains of prostate

RETROPUBIC PROSTATECTOMY

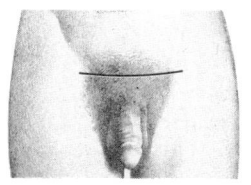

Site of incision

1 Using general anesthesia, an incision is made in the abdomen to expose the bladder and prostate. The surgeon cuts open the capsule containing the gland.

Capsule · Enlarged prostate gland

2 The surgeon then removes the prostatic tissue by hand. Bleeding vessels are cauterized and a catheter passed up the urethra to drain urine from the bladder.

Drainage tube · Stitching

3 A tube is inserted into the empty capsule to drain fluid and blood; the abdomen is sewn up. The tube and catheter are left in for about a week.

Prostatitis

Inflammation of the *prostate gland*, usually affecting men between the ages of 30 and 50. Prostatitis is often caused by a bacterial infection that has spread from the urethra. The infection may or may not be sexually transmitted. Presence of a urinary catheter increases the risk of prostatitis.

SYMPTOMS AND SIGNS

Prostatitis causes pain when passing urine and increased frequency of urination; it sometimes causes fever and a discharge from the penis. There may be pain in the lower abdomen, around the rectum, and in the lower back, and blood in the urine.

DIAGNOSIS AND TREATMENT

The physician examines the prostate by inserting a gloved finger into the rectum; the gland will be tender and enlarged. To investigate the cause of infection, tests are carried out on a urine sample and on urethral secretions obtained after massaging the prostate gland.

Treatment is with *antibiotic drugs*, although the condition may be slow to clear up and tends to recur. If an abscess develops, surgical drainage may be necessary.

Prosthesis

An artificial replacement for a missing or diseased part of the body. Examples of a prosthesis used to restore normal function include a false leg or arm fitted after amputation (see *Limb, artificial*) or an artificial heart valve used to replace a valve damaged by disease (see *Heart valve surgery*).

Prostheses are also used for cosmetic reasons. Examples include a breast prosthesis fitted after *mastectomy* (removal of a breast) and a glass eye inserted following removal of a diseased eye (see *Eye, artificial*).

Prosthodontics

The branch of dentistry concerned with the replacement of missing teeth and their supporting structures. Prosthodontics includes three basic kinds of replacement—partial or complete *dentures* (which are easily removed for cleaning), semipermanent appliances such as overdentures (fittings that are attached over existing teeth), and permanent restorations such as crowns and bridges (see *Crown, dental; Bridge, dental*).

Proteins

Large molecules that consist of hundreds or thousands of *amino acids* linked (by peptide bonds) to form long chains, which are often folded in various ways. In addition to amino acids, proteins may contain constituents such as sugars and lipids.

There are two main types of proteins: fibrous and globular. Fibrous proteins are insoluble and form the structural basis of many body tissues, such as hair, skin, muscles, tendons, and cartilage. Globular proteins are soluble and include all *enzymes* (substances that promote biochemical reactions in the body); many *hormones*, such as growth hormone and prolactin; and various proteins in the blood, including *hemoglobin* and *antibodies*. In addition, the *chromosomes* in cell nuclei are formed of proteins linked with *nucleic acids*; proteins linked with lipids constitute a major part of cell membranes (see *Cell*).

PROTEINS AND DIET

Proteins are needed in the diet primarily to supply the body with amino acids. Ingested proteins are broken down in the *digestive system* to amino acids, which are then absorbed and rebuilt into new body proteins (see *Protein synthesis*). In general, animal proteins have a higher nutritional value than do plant proteins, because they have more essential amino acids. (See also *Nutrition*.)

Protein synthesis

The formation of *protein* molecules inside cells through the linking of much smaller substances called amino acids. Because proteins provide many of the structural components and the *enzymes* that promote biochemical reactions in the body, their manufacture—in the correct numbers and order—is essential to all aspects of development and growth.

Different cells manufacture a different range of proteins. The instructions for their manufacture are held by the hereditary material—the *genes*, which consist of *DNA* (deoxyribonucleic acid)—within the nucleus of the cell. Protein synthesis starts with a gene (a particular length of DNA) acting as a template for the manufacture of a strand of a substance called messenger RNA. Like DNA, RNA is a *nucleic acid* and consists of a string of building blocks called nucleotide bases. There are four different types of nucleotide bases; their sequence in the strand of messenger RNA provides the coded instructions (the *genetic code*) for making a certain protein.

The strand of messenger RNA passes out of the cell nucleus, where it is then decoded (see diagram, next page) to cause a polypeptide chain (string of amino acids) to be produced. Several polypeptide chains may be manufactured and combine to form one protein molecule.

The rate of protein synthesis is regulated through adjustments in the amount of the relevant messenger RNA formed within the cell nucleus. Highly complex mechanisms exist for "blocking" or "unblocking" messenger RNA copying from DNA; this ensures that the cell makes the right type of proteins, in the right quantities, and at the right time.

Proteinuria

The passage of increased amounts of protein in the urine. Proteinuria may result from damage to the glomeruli (filtering units in the *kidney*), allowing proteins to leak from the blood into the urine (see *Glomerulonephritis*). The condition may also result from damage to the kidney tubules, preventing the normal reabsorption of protein from the urine. Increased protein in the urine may also occur because of a generalized disorder (such as *myeloma*) that causes an increase in the blood protein level.

Proteinuria rarely causes any symptoms, although the urine may appear frothy. The condition is usually discovered during a routine *urine test* or during investigation of an underlying disorder.

Protoplasm

An obsolescent term for the entire contents of a cell, including the cytoplasm and organelles such as the nucleus. Today, the word protoplasm has largely been replaced by specific terms for the individual cell components (see *Cell*).

Protozoa

The simplest, most primitive type of animal; each protozoon consists of a single cell. All types of protozoa are of microscopic size, but bigger than bacteria. The more advanced types are capable of excretion, respiration, and engulfing food particles; they move around through jellylike movements or the use of whiplike or hairlike attachments called flagella. Some protozoa are parasites of larger animals during various stages of the life cycle.

About 30 different types of protozoa are troublesome parasites of humans. Included among them are the organisms that cause *amebiasis* and

STEPS IN PROTEIN SYNTHESIS

Proteins consist of one or more subunits called polypeptides. These are formed, within cells, from building blocks called amino acids, which are provided to each cell as raw materials. The instructions for making polypeptides are encoded in the DNA within the cell nucleus.

1 To make a specific protein or polypeptide, the relevant section of DNA (or *gene*) in a cell nucleus is used as a template to make a strand of a substance called messenger RNA. Like DNA, this consists of a string of substances called nucleotide bases.

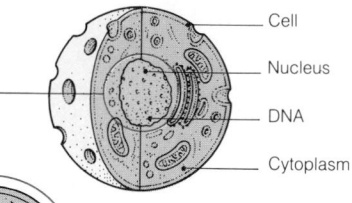

Cell

Nucleus

DNA

Cytoplasm

DNA

Nucleus

Messenger RNA

2 The messenger RNA passes out of the cell nucleus into the cytoplasm, where it is latched onto by several decoding particles called ribosomes. Starting at one end, the ribosomes travel along the RNA strand.

Ribosome

Nucleotide bases

Amino acids

3 As it moves along the RNA, each ribosome connects a chain of amino acids, using special chemical "keys" (called transfer RNAs) within the cell. The correct order of the amino acids is coded by the sequence of bases in the messenger RNA.

Finished polypeptide

4 At the end of the RNA strand, the ribosome parts from the amino acid chain, which folds up to form the finished polypeptide or protein.

---

giardiasis (intestinal infections that cause diarrhea); the sexually transmitted infection *trichomoniasis*; and the insect-borne tropical diseases *malaria, sleeping sickness,* and *leishmaniasis. Toxoplasmosis* (a disease acquired from cats) is also caused by a protozoon.

Protriptyline

An *antidepressant drug*. Protriptyline is especially useful in treating narcolepsy and when *depression* is accompanied by lethargy and tiredness, because it is less likely than other antidepressants to cause drowsiness.

Proximal

Describing a part of the body that is nearer to a central point of reference, such as the trunk of the body. The hip joint is proximal to the knee; the knuckle is proximal to the fingernail. The opposite of proximal is *distal*.

Prurigo

A nonspecific term for an itchy rash.

Pruritus

The medical term for *itching*. Types include pruritus ani (itching of the skin around the anus) and pruritus vulvae (itching of the external genital area in women).

Pseud-/pseudo-

Prefixes that mean false, as in pseudocyesis (a false pregnancy).

Pseudarthrosis

A false joint. The term is used to describe an operation in which the ends of two opposing bones in a joint are removed and a piece of tissue (usually muscle) is fixed between the resulting gap to act as a cushion.

The procedure is used to restore mobility and reduce pain when a hip *arthroplasty* (joint replacement operation) has failed. It results in shortening of the affected leg and instability of the joint. A walking aid is usually required after the operation.

Pseudarthrosis also describes a rare condition in children in which congenital abnormality of the bone of the lower half of the tibia (shin) leads to spontaneous fracture without injury. Treatment of this condition consists of inserting a nail through the bone ends and applying a *bone graft*. If the bone ends fail to unite, amputation of the leg, followed by fitting of an artificial limb, may be necessary.

Pseudocyesis

See *Pregnancy, false*.

P

Pseudodementia

A form of severe *depression* in elderly people that mimics *dementia*. Features of both illnesses include intellectual impairment and loss of memory. Nearly one in 10 of those initially thought to be suffering from dementia may turn out to have a depressive illness. Unlike dementia, depression is treatable; many people respond well to *antidepressant drugs*.

Pseudoephedrine

A *decongestant drug* used to relieve *nasal congestion*. Pseudoephedrine is an ingredient of a variety of cough and cold remedies.

High doses may cause anxiety, nausea, dizziness, and, occasionally, hypertension (high blood pressure), headache, and palpitations.

Pseudoepidemic

An outbreak of an illness in a community or in an institution (such as a school) that has no detectable physical cause but is thought to be due to a form of *hysteria*. Typically, the symptoms are vague and mild—headache and a general feeling of sickness—and are induced by group suggestibility combined with anxiety provoked by contact with somebody who has the symptoms. *Sick building syndrome* is an example of a condition that may be a pseudoepidemic.

Pseudogout

A form of *arthritis* that results from the deposition of calcium pyrophosphate crystals in a joint. The underlying cause of pseudogout is unknown; in rare cases, it is a complication of *diabetes mellitus, hyperparathyroidism,* and *hemochromatosis.*

Symptoms include intermittent attacks of arthritis similar to *gout.* Pseudogout can be distinguished from gout only by examining a sample of the joint fluid under a microscope to identify the crystals, which are different from the urate crystals found in gout.

Treatment is with *nonsteroidal anti-inflammatory drugs.*

Pseudohermaphroditism

A congenital abnormality in which the external genitalia resemble those of the opposite sex. Thus, a female pseudohermaphrodite may have an enlarged clitoris resembling a penis and enlarged labia resembling a scrotum. Conversely, a male may have a very small penis and a divided scrotum resembling labia.

Pseudohermaphroditism is usually caused by an endocrine disorder, such as *adrenal hyperplasia.*

The condition differs from true *hermaphroditism;* in pseudohermaphroditism, the person has only ovarian or testicular tissue and not both.

Psilocybin

A *hallucinogenic drug* similar to *LSD.*

Psittacosis

 A rare illness resembling *influenza* that is caused by a microorganism, CHLAMYDIA PSITTACI, and is spread to humans from birds such as parrots, pigeons, or poultry.

The infection is contracted by inhaling dust contaminated by the droppings of infected birds. Most cases occur among poultry farmers, pigeon owners, and pet store owners, although anyone who acquires a pet parrot is at slight risk. A hundred or so cases are reported in the US each year, though there are probably many more undiagnosed cases.

SYMPTOMS, DIAGNOSIS, AND TREATMENT
The illness in birds is occasionally serious or even fatal, but often causes no more than lethargy.

Human illness is extremely variable in its features, the most common symptoms being fever, severe headache, and cough. They develop a week or more after exposure to infected birds. Other symptoms include muscle pains, sore throat, nosebleed, lethargy, and depression. In some severe cases, there is also breathing difficulty.

The cause of the condition is often suspected from the patient's occupation; it is diagnosed by the finding of *antibodies* (proteins with a defense role) specific to the causative organism in the patient's blood. Treatment with tetracycline antibiotics is usually effective. Without treatment, the illness may continue for several weeks or months before subsiding; it may occasionally be fatal if unrecognized and not treated.

Psoas muscle

A muscle that bends the hip upward toward the chest. The psoas muscle is composed of two parts (psoas major and psoas minor) that originate from the lower spine.

The lower end of psoas minor is attached to the margin of the pelvis; the lower end of psoas major is joined to the prominence just below the neck of the femur (thigh bone).

LOCATION OF PSOAS MUSCLE

The muscle has two parts—major and minor. The psoas major acts to flex the hip (bend it upward toward the trunk) and rotates the thigh inward. The psoas minor acts to bend the spine down toward the pelvis.

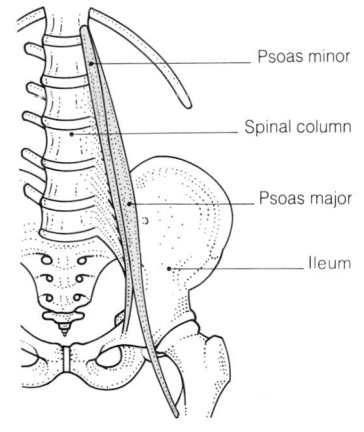

Psoas minor

Spinal column

Psoas major

Ileum

A rare disorder of the psoas muscle is an *abscess* (collection of pus), which develops as a complication of *osteomyelitis* (bone infection) of the spine, usually caused by *tuberculosis.*

Psoralen drugs

COMMON DRUGS
Methoxsalen Trioxsalen

WARNING
During psoralen treatment, always protect eyes and lips from the sun and avoid overexposure to ultraviolet light.

Drugs containing chemicals called psoralens, which occur in certain plants (such as buttercups) and are present in some perfumes. When absorbed into the skin, psoralens react with *ultraviolet light* to cause darkening or inflammation of the skin. Psoralen drugs may be taken by mouth or applied to the skin.

WHY THEY ARE USED
Psoralen drugs may be used to treat *psoriasis* and *vitiligo* (a disorder in which patches of skin lose color).

HOW THEY WORK
Used in *phototherapy* in conjunction with ultraviolet light, psoralen drugs stimulate the production of skin pigment and, in psoriasis, slow the rate at which skin cells grow and multiply.

P

POSSIBLE ADVERSE EFFECTS

Overexposure to ultraviolet light during psoralen treatment or too high a dose of a psoralen drug may cause redness and blistering of the skin. Psoralens in perfumes may cause a rash when the skin is exposed to ultraviolet light (see *Photosensitivity*). The use of psoralens in suntanning preparations is prohibited in the US because these chemicals can cause *sunburn*.

Psoriasis

A common skin disease characterized by thickened patches of inflamed, red skin, often covered by silvery scales. Although psoriasis does not usually cause itching, the affected area may be so extensive that great physical discomfort and social embarrassment may result.

Distribution and appearance of psoriasis
The knees, elbows, scalp, trunk, and back are common sites for psoriasis. The usual appearance is of patches of thickened skin covered by dry, silvery, adherent scales.

CAUSES AND INCIDENCE

The exact cause of psoriasis is not known but it tends to run in families. Psoriasis occurs in about 2 percent of people in the US and Europe and is probably less common in blacks and Asians. It affects men and women equally. Psoriasis usually appears between ages 10 and 30, but infants occasionally suffer from the condition and it may also sometimes develop in old age.

The underlying abnormality in psoriasis is that new skin cells are produced about 10 times faster than normal, but the rate at which old cells are shed remains unchanged. As a result, the live cells accumulate and form the characteristic thickened patches covered with dead, flaking skin.

Psoriasis tends to recur in attacks of varying severity; attacks may be triggered by a number of factors, such as emotional stress, skin damage, and physical illness.

The skin eruption is sometimes accompanied by a painful swelling and stiffness of the joints that can be highly disabling (see *Arthritis*).

TYPES

The disease has different forms that may need different treatment.

DISCOID OR "PLAQUE" PSORIASIS In this type, the most common form, patches appear on the trunk and limbs, particularly the elbows and knees, and on the scalp. In addition, the nails may become pitted, thickened, or separated from their beds.

GUTTATE PSORIASIS This form occurs most frequently in children. It consists of numerous small patches that develop rapidly over a wide area of skin, often after a sore throat.

PUSTULAR PSORIASIS This form is characterized by small pustules, all over the body or confined to the palms, soles, and other isolated locations.

TREATMENT

Mild psoriasis may be helped by moderate exposure to sunlight or an ultraviolet lamp (see *Phototherapy*) and use of an emollient (soothing cream). Moderate attacks are usually treated with an ointment containing coal tar or anthralin. Other methods of treating psoriasis include *corticosteroid drugs*, *PUVA* (a type of phototherapy), and some types of *anticancer drugs*, such as methotrexate.

The arthritis is treated with *nonsteroidal anti-inflammatory drugs*, *antirheumatic drugs*, or methotrexate.

OUTLOOK

For most people, psoriasis is a long-term condition with no permanent cure, although individual attacks can be completely relieved with appropriate treatment.

Psych-

A prefix meaning mental processes or activities, as in psychiatry.

Psyche

A term meaning mind (as opposed to body) that was derived from the ancient Greek for soul or spirit. The most influential description is provided by Freud's *psychoanalytic theory*, which treats the psyche as an organ of the body that is divided into the conscious and unconscious. Each has its own set of functions.

Psychedelic drugs

Drugs (many illicit) that may produce hallucinations, also known as *hallucinogenic drugs*.

Psychiatrist

A physician who specializes in the treatment of mental, emotional, or behavioral problems. A psychiatrist conducts physical examinations, performs laboratory tests, and traces the patient's personal and family history to seek the cause of the problem. Treatment may include medication with counseling or *psychotherapy* (individually or in groups), *psychoanalysis*, or *behavior therapy*.

Psychiatry

The branch of medicine concerned with the study, prevention, and treatment of mental illness and emotional and behavioral problems. Psychiatry is differentiated from *psychology*, which is principally concerned with the normal mental processes and behavior of people.

Psychiatry is broad in scope; it approaches the understanding and treatment of mental problems from psychological, social, and physical aspects. Some psychiatrists assert that major mental illness is due to genetic and biochemical factors, while psychoanalytically oriented psychiatrists believe that environmental experiences are still the major cause of mental illness. Laboratory investigations and drug treatments have played an increasingly important role in modern psychiatry.

Within psychiatry there are a number of subspecialties, including child and adolescent psychiatry, social psychiatry (focusing on social factors as a cause of mental illness), community psychiatry (addressing care of the mentally ill outside psychiatric hospitals), forensic psychiatry (dealing with legal issues, such as rape), and neuropsychiatry (relating to brain disorders with mental symptoms).

Psychoanalysis

A treatment for mental illness based on *psychoanalytic theory*. The system was developed by Sigmund Freud at the beginning of the 20th century as a result of treating, under hypnosis, patients who were supposedly suffering from hysteria. He believed that mental disorders were a result of the failure of normal emotional development during childhood. By encouraging the patient to reenact these years and verbalize any problems (past or present), Freud believed that the cause of any internal strife would be uncovered and resolved, and the illness would be cured.

WHY IT IS DONE

Psychoanalysis can help *neurosis* and *personality disorders*. A modified psychoanalytic approach has also been used to treat *psychosis* (when medication is often an important adjunct). Psychoanalysis aims to help the patient understand his or her emotional development and to help the person make appropriate adjustments in particular situations.

HOW IT IS DONE

The treatment involves interviews between a trained analyst and the patient, each lasting perhaps an hour, repeated up to six times a week and continuing for an indefinite period, usually for several years. Traditionally, the patient lies on a couch with the analyst behind and out of sight, although some therapists prefer to face the patient, who sits in a chair. In dealing with psychotic patients, the psychoanalyst refrains from having the patient lie down on a couch because, in some cases, the structure and reality of face-to-face contact with the psychiatrist is an extremely important element.

The patient is encouraged to talk as freely as possible about his or her life history and any problems that may have occurred in the past or are currently causing concern. This stream of talk is one of free association, with one word or idea leading to another without conscious control so that any repressed material has the opportunity to surface. The analyst interprets these associations in the light of psychoanalytic theory, paying particular attention to areas of resistance that may contain clues to the person's problem. This leads to different trains of thought, more experiences relived, and sometimes exposure of reasons for symptoms.

Psychoanalysis relies on a number of other key processes. A very close relationship develops with the analyst, who eventually comes to be associated in the patient's mind with important people in his or her history (e.g., mother, father, or sister). This experience is called *transference*.

Interpretation of the patient's dreams is another important aspect of the treatment. It is believed that material normally repressed comes to the surface while the patient dreams, usually in the form of symbolic representations (see *Dream analysis*).

The patient is often reluctant to accept the analyst's interpretations and may introduce *defense mechanisms* (such as denial) to cope with the unfolding explanation of his or her behavior. This reaction is a defense against the anxiety that is stimulated as these repressed conflicts break through into consciousness. Understanding the self-destructive patterns of living is an essential aspect of psychoanalytic treatment.

Psychoanalyst

A person who treats people with certain mental illnesses using the methods of *psychoanalysis*.

The psychoanalyst is usually a doctor of medicine. Following a residency in psychiatry, the psychiatrist is accepted to an accredited institute for psychoanalysis. Finally, the psychiatrist undergoes his or her own psychoanalysis at the institute to resolve as much as possible his or her own emotional problems.

Psychoanalytic theory

A system of ideas developed by Sigmund Freud early in this century that explains the development of personality and behavior in terms of unconscious wishes and conflicts.

Psychoanalytic theory has undergone considerable distillation by psychoanalysts over the years. However, its basic concepts and the use of *psychoanalysis* (therapy based on the concepts of psychoanalytic theory) have dominated psychiatry in the US for half a century.

KEY FEATURES OF FREUDIAN THEORY

Freud placed great emphasis on the importance of sexuality (in its broadest sense) in psychological development. His theory postulates that, during the first 18 months, an infant passes through three phases—oral, anal, and genital—each representing the area of the body that the child devotes attention to at a particular age. After these phases, the child is able to direct attention to people outside himself or herself. Sexual attraction to the parent of the opposite sex develops with consequent desire to eliminate the other parent, who prevents fulfilment of the desire—the *Oedipus complex*.

By the age of 5 or 6, sexual feelings become latent, but reemerge at puberty. At this time, psychological and emotional problems may occur if the individual has not developed normally through the successive stages and has become fixed at a primitive level (see *Fixation*). Problems may also occur if the Oedipus complex has not been successfully dealt with.

Less specifically sexual aspects of psychological development are seen as depending on the interaction among the three parts that make up the personality—the id, ego, and superego. The id is the basic component that guides the individual unconsciously and instinctively toward pleasure; the ego mediates, by conscious reasoning, between internal desires and the reality of the outside world; the superego is also a controlling force but is unconscious, being derived from moral and social standards indoctrinated by parents and other authorities.

It is thought that mental illness results if conflict between the three aspects of personality cannot be satisfactorily resolved. Freud believed that under normal circumstances tension is dealt with by (among other *defense mechanisms*) repression (in which painful ideas or unacceptable thoughts are kept out of consciousness) and sublimation (in which emotional drives that cannot openly be expressed are channeled into an acceptable activity, such as sports). These normally healthy unconscious processes can become harmful if they occur inappropriately or in excess.

Psychoanalysis has, however, progressed since Freud. In general, modern psychoanalysis is based on the observation that emotional problems for the most part are the result of troubled childhood experiences in the family. The pre-Oedipal problems that are caused by difficulties in the early mother-child relationship are probably even more important than later Oedipal conflicts. Such conflicts can form the basis of later neurotic or psychotic disturbances.

It is necessary for the child to separate from the mother to become an individual and comprehend reality. A healthy mother and father help the child to become an individual. Conflict-ridden parents distort reality and program patterns of disturbed self-destructive behavior. Psychoanalysis in practice attempts to bring to light these unconscious conflicts with the parent (which have led to distortions

P

of reality). The aim is to free the individual from the past and help him or her become a real person in the present. The relationship and interaction between physician and patient is an essential part of this process.

Psychodrama

An adjunct to *psychotherapy* in which the patient acts out certain roles or incidents. They may relate to people closely involved with the patient or may concern situations that he or she finds particularly stressful. The aims of psychodrama are to bring out hidden concerns and to allow a person's disturbing feelings to be expressed. Psychodrama is often carried out with a partner or in a group of patients; music, dance, and pantomime may also be used.

Psychogenic

A symptom or disorder that originates from psychological or emotional problems and is not produced or caused by any physical illness.

Psychologist

A nonmedical specialist in the diagnosis and treatment of mental and emotional problems. Because psychologists are not physicians, they cannot prescribe drugs. Their role with patients generally involves testing, *counseling*, or *psychotherapy*.

Psychology

The scientific study of mental processes. Psychology deals with all internal aspects of the mind, such as *memory*, feelings, *thought*, and *perception*, as well as external manifestations, such as *speech* and behavior. It also addresses *intelligence*, *learning*, and the development of *personality*. Methods employed in psychology include direct experiments, observations, surveys, study of personal histories, and special tests (such as *intelligence tests* and *personality tests*).

Within psychology, a number of different approaches are used. Neuropsychology attempts to relate human behavior to brain and body functions. Behavioral psychology studies the way people react to events and learn to adapt accordingly. Cognitive psychology concentrates on thought processes; it is based on the theory that what a person thinks about his or her behavior is of equal importance to the behavior itself. Psychoanalytic psychology stresses the role of the unconscious and childhood experiences (see *Psychoanalytic theory*).

There are many specialized areas within the science. Educational psychologists study learning and intelligence, clinical psychologists work with emotional and behavioral problems, social and industrial psychologists consider the effects of work and the environment on behavior, and experimental psychologists concentrate on research into new ways of understanding mental events. The emergence of developmental psychology as a specialist area is due to the work of the Swiss psychologist Jean Piaget, who noted that there are certain stages in a child's intellectual development—from simple motor skills to logical and abstract thought.

Psychometry

The measurement of psychological functions. Psychometry includes statistical assessment of intelligence and personality (see *Intelligence tests*; *Personality tests*) as well as numerous methods of testing specific aptitudes, such as memory, logic, concentration, and speed of response. The design of such measurements has become increasingly sophisticated, but the validity of many tests (that is, whether they measure what they are supposed to measure) is less certain.

Psychoneurosis

A term now used interchangeably with *neurosis*. Neurosis originally referred to any disorder of the nerves; psychoneurosis specifically described nervous disorders associated with psychological symptoms.

Psychopathology

The study of abnormal mental processes. There are two main approaches in psychopathology—the descriptive and the psychoanalytic.

Descriptive psychopathology aims to record, as objectively as possible, the symptoms that make up a diagnosis of psychiatric illness. It is particularly concerned with *thought disorders* (such as *delusion*), with mood disturbances, and with the various forms of *hallucination*. The ability to recognize such symptoms when interviewing patients is an important part of the psychiatrist's job.

The psychoanalytic approach is concerned with the unconscious feelings and motives of the individual; they are studied by *psychoanalysis*.

Psychopathy

An outdated term for *antisocial personality disorder*.

Psychopharmacology

The study of drugs that affect mental states. Since the early 1950s, more effective medications for a wide range of mental illness have been developed. Particular advances have occurred in the treatment of psychotic illnesses, with the development of *antipsychotic drugs* and *antidepressant drugs*. *Antianxiety drugs* have proved to be extremely effective in relieving symptoms in neurotic illness, but the dangers of dependence have been recognized recently.

Psychosexual disorders

A range of conditions related to sexual function. Psychosexual disorders are assumed to stem from psychological problems, although some (e.g., *impotence*) may also be caused by physical injury or illness. Psychosexual disorders include *transsexualism* (a sense that one's anatomical sex is inappropriate), *psychosexual dysfunction* (interference with the normal process of sexual response), and sexual deviations (sexual behavior in which intercourse between adults is not the final aim; see *Deviation, sexual*).

Psychosexual dysfunction

A disorder in which there is interference with the normal process of sexual response in the absence of any known organic cause. Psychosexual dysfunctions are very common in both men and women. They usually start in early adult life, often disappearing spontaneously with experience and increased confidence.

The main dysfunctions affecting men are lack of sexual desire (see *Sexual desire, inhibited*), *impotence*, and premature ejaculation (see *Ejaculation, disorders of*); those affecting women are lack of sexual desire, painful intercourse (see *Intercourse, painful*), *vaginismus*, and lack of orgasm (see *Orgasm, lack of*).

Most psychosexual problems start in early adult life. Some are associated with certain personality traits, including anxiety and obsessiveness. Unpleasant early experiences, such as sexual interference in childhood or problems with the first sexual encounters, are especially likely to inhibit later sexual performance. Unrealistic ideas about normal sexual behavior or a strict upbringing may also increase the likelihood of sexual problems. Many different kinds of feelings and conflicts (basically nonsexual) can be expressed sexually or interfere with normal sexual expression.

P

Psychosexual dysfunctions are common and not usually evidence of serious illness. About 80 percent of people respond well to *sex therapy*, which is usually brief behavioral therapy with the couple. Sex therapy is also done with an individual or a group of solo men and solo women. Instructors offer sex education and instructions for home practice of helpful techniques in relaxation and sensual pleasuring.

Psychosis

A severe mental disorder in which the individual loses contact with reality. It contrasts with *neurosis*, which describes the milder group of mental illnesses. Neurotic individuals generally know they are ill, but psychotic illness so disturbs the ability to think, perceive, and judge clearly that sufferers often do not realize they are sick. Psychosis is what people commonly think of as "madness."

TYPES

Three main forms of psychosis are generally recognized, although the symptoms overlap and there is considerable debate as to whether each is truly a separate category. They are *schizophrenia*, *manic-depressive illness*, and organic brain syndrome (see *Brain syndrome, organic*).

Paranoid illness (see *Paranoia*) is sometimes regarded as a fourth form of psychosis, but many psychiatrists see it as a distinctive disorder.

SYMPTOMS

The main feature of psychotic symptoms is that they may lead the person to view life in a distorted way. Symptoms include *delusions*, *hallucinations*, *thought disorders*, loss of *affect* (emotion), *mania*, and *depression*.

CAUSES

Some physicians believe that psychotic symptoms are due to disordered brain function. Psychoanalytically oriented physicians tend to believe that psychotic behavior is a result of deep disturbances in the mother-child relationship and overwhelming emotional trauma.

Research is centered on the role of *neurotransmitters* (chemicals released by nerve endings), such as dopamine, and on the importance of the limbic system and frontal lobes of the brain. As yet no specific physical abnormality that might be isolated by a blood test or X ray has been clearly related to psychosis. However, a new form of brain imaging, *PET scanning*, may begin to reveal hints as to the causes of these disorders.

TREATMENT AND OUTLOOK

Antipsychotic drugs are usually very effective in controlling symptoms, usually as an adjunct to *psychotherapy*. Treatment may need to be long-term, but many sufferers are able to lead normal working lives. The relationship of patient to therapist (see *Transference*) is extremely important because in many cases it is through this relationship that the patient reestablishes contact with reality.

Psychosomatic

A term used to describe physical disorders that seem to have been caused, or worsened, by psychological factors. Just as a physical reaction (such as crying) may be due to emotion, so it is presumed that worries or unpleasant events can cause physical illness.

For a disorder to be labeled psychosomatic, the psychological factor and physical effect must be closely connected in time and repeatedly related. This is because many chronic illnesses constantly vary in severity, regardless of a person's psychological state, and because there is a tendency to assume that an event was stressful just because a person has become ill.

Common examples of conditions that may fit the psychosomatic label are headache, breathlessness, nausea, *asthma*, *irritable bowel syndrome*, *peptic ulcer*, and certain types of *eczema*. (See also *Somatization disorder*.)

Psychosurgery

Any operation on the brain carried out as a treatment for mental symptoms. Psychosurgery is performed only as a last resort to treat severe mental illnesses that have not responded to other forms of treatment.

TYPES

Prefrontal *lobotomy* was once the most widely used form of psychosurgery, but it often resulted in harmful side effects and has now largely been replaced by other, safer operations.

The most commonly performed operations today are forms of *stereotaxic surgery*. In these operations, a small hole is drilled in the skull above one temple. A scalpel or diathermy probe is inserted and, under X-ray control, guided to specific areas of the brain, where small cuts are made in nerve fibers. Stereotaxic procedures are most often carried out to provide relief of severe *depression* or *anxiety* or to treat disabling *obsessive-compulsive behavior*.

Performed less often are the more complex, "open" operations, in which a complete portion of the skull is cut through and lifted up to expose the brain so that specific areas can be removed. Parts of the temporal lobe are cut out to treat *temporal lobe epilepsy*. In rare cases, complete lobes are removed in an attempt to treat violent or aggressive behavior.

OUTLOOK

Psychosurgery has produced good results in some people, enabling those who would otherwise be chronically disabled to lead more useful lives. However, the operations often have inconsistent and unpredictable results, and can produce adverse changes in personality and intellect. They remain a controversial form of treatment for psychiatric illness.

Psychotherapist

Any person who uses *psychotherapy* as a formal method of treatment. Treatment varies according to the approach used (e.g., if it is based on *Freudian theory* or *Jungian theory*). Many psychotherapists have no medical background, but certain personal characteristics are deemed especially important, notably empathy (the ability to understand what a patient is feeling), genuineness (the therapist appears to mean what he or she says), and warmth. The psychotherapist also requires sufficient maturity and experience to be able to cope with the demanding task of dealing with the mental and emotional problems of his or her patients.

Psychotherapy

The treatment of mental and emotional problems by psychological methods. In psychotherapy, the patient talks to a therapist about symptoms and problems and establishes a therapeutic relationship with the therapist.

WHY IT IS DONE

Psychotherapy is used to help people suffering from *neurosis* or *personality disorders*, as well as individuals with specific personal problems. The aim is to help patients learn about themselves, develop new insights into past and present relationships, and change fixed patterns of behavior.

HOW IT IS DONE

Counseling is the simplest form of psychotherapy, consisting of advice and psychological support. At the opposite end of the spectrum is *psychoanalysis*, which attempts to explore the deep unconscious feelings and early childhood experiences of the individual.

P

Dynamic psychotherapy is based on psychoanalytic principles. The therapist tries to understand and interpret the patient's unconscious messages (without the benefit of formal psychoanalysis) so that the individual can develop a better understanding of his or her underlying feelings and cope with them more effectively.

A course of treatment may be brief, consisting of two or three sessions, or it may extend over many years, depending on the problems involved. It may vary in intensity from a simple, supportive approach during a difficult period to an in-depth analysis aimed at reconstructing the personality.

Psychotherapy may involve one person, a couple (see *Marital counseling*), a family (see *Family therapy*), or a group (see *Group therapy*).

Psychotropic drugs

Drugs that have an effect on the mind. They include *hallucinogenic drugs, sedative drugs, sleeping drugs, tranquilizer drugs,* and *antipsychotic drugs.*

Psyllium

A bulk-forming *laxative drug* used in the treatment of *constipation, diverticular disease,* and *irritable bowel syndrome.* Psyllium is also given to increase the firmness of bowel movements in a person with an *ileostomy.*

Adverse effects include bloating, excess gas, and abdominal pain.

Pterygium

A wing-shaped thickening of the *conjunctiva* that extends across the margin of the cornea toward the center. Pterygium is caused by prolonged exposure to bright sunlight and is common in tropical areas. Unless vision is notably affected, no treatment is usually necessary. If the pterygium is surgically removed, it may be followed by a recurrence that is larger than the original.

Appearance of pterygium
The conjunctiva (outer lining of the eyeball) has extended onto the cornea (transparent front part of the eye).

Ptomaine poisoning

An obsolescent general term for any form of *food poisoning* caused by bacteria or bacterial poisons.

Ptosis

A drooping of the upper eyelid. Ptosis may be congenital or may occur as a result of disease (e.g., *myasthenia gravis*) or injury. It is usually due to a weakness of the levator muscle of the lid or to interference with the nerve supply to the muscle.

Ptosis in a child
This condition, present from birth, should be corrected surgically to prevent any disturbance of visual development.

Severe congenital ptosis, in which the drooping lid covers the pupil, should be surgically corrected to avoid the development of *amblyopia* (failure of visual development).

Acquired ptosis without obvious cause may be a sign of neurologic disease, such as a brain tumor or an aneurysm, and should be investigated by a physician.

Ptyalism

Excessive salivation caused by irritation of the inside of the mouth by ill-fitting dentures, digestive tract disorders (such as *esophagitis* or a *peptic ulcer*), or, rarely, damage to the nervous system (e.g., by *mercury poisoning* or infection with *rabies*).

Puberty

The period when secondary sexual characteristics develop and the sexual organs mature, allowing reproduction to become possible. Puberty is the term used for the physical changes that underlie the emotional changes of *adolescence.* It usually occurs between the ages of 10 and 15 in both sexes; it is initiated by the *pituitary gland* producing hormones (known as *gonadotropins*) that stimulate the *ovaries* to increase secretion of *estrogen hormones* and the *testes* to increase secretion of *testosterone.* It is not known what triggers this action by the pituitary gland.

Puberty is accompanied by a significant growth spurt and increase in weight. Body weight may double during this period, due primarily to muscle growth in boys and increased fat in girls.

PUBERTY IN GIRLS

The first sign of puberty in girls is usually breast budding, which occurs around the age of 11; in about one third of girls, pubic hair appears first. The rate of growth of the breasts may be unequal but any difference usually disappears by the time full maturity is reached. The first menstrual period usually does not occur for a year or more, by which time pubic and underarm hair are in the fully developed adult pattern.

Other secondary sexual characteristics, such as the wider pelvis and the female distribution of fat, develop progressively during this period. Puberty is considered to be complete when menstrual periods occur at regular, predictable intervals.

The age at which menstruation starts has been decreasing for the past century, probably because of a general improvement in nutrition and living standards, but has now become stable. Girls who are overweight tend to start menstruating earlier than the average; those who are malnourished start later. Strenuous sports or other hard physical activity (such as ballet) and debilitating disease can also delay the onset of periods.

PUBERTY IN BOYS

In boys, puberty is heralded by a sudden increase in the rate of growth of the testes and scrotum, followed by the appearance of pubic and facial hair. The penis begins to grow around the age of 13 and reaches its adult size about two years later. However, there is a wide range of variation so that, at the age of 14, some boys may be sexually mature while others still have immature genitals.

The body's increased secretion of testosterone stimulates sperm production and causes the prostate gland and seminal vesicles to mature. It leads to the development of the typical male distribution of hair on the face, chest, and abdomen. The larynx enlarges and the vocal cords become longer and thicker, causing the pitch of the voice to drop.

ABNORMAL PUBERTY

Extremely rarely there are instances in which the normal events of puberty occur at a very young age, sometimes within the first five years of life; the youngest mother on record gave birth to a healthy baby at the age of 5 years 8 months. This precocious puberty can occur in either sex. In boys it is often caused by a brain tumor; in girls the cause is usually not known.

Pubes
The pubic hair or the area of the body covered by this hair.

Pubic lice
 Small, wingless insects that live in the pubic hair and feed on blood. Also called crabs (because of their crablike claws, which they use to grasp hair), they are usually spread by sexual contact. Their scientific name is *PHTHIRUS PUBIS*.

Each louse has a flattened body, up to one twelfth of an inch (2 mm) across, and can be seen with the naked eye. The females lay minute, pale eggs (called nits) on the hair, where they hatch about eight days later. Pubic lice do not transmit infection.

SYMPTOMS AND SIGNS
Both lice and eggs can be seen on close inspection. On hairy men the lice may also be found in hair around the anus, on the legs, and on the trunk, and occasionally even in facial hair. The bites sometimes cause itching. Pubic lice can infest children, usually by transmission from parents. In children, the lice may attach to the eyelids.

TREATMENT
An insecticide lotion containing malathion or carbaryl kills the lice and eggs soon after application. An infested person's sexual partner should also be treated; clothes and bedding should be washed in water hotter than 140°F (60°C) before use.

Public health
A branch of medicine that developed in the 19th century as physicians became aware of the importance to health of the provision of pure water supplies and safe systems for the disposal of sewage. The medical pioneers in this field instigated the construction of reservoirs and of water and sewage systems. Later, they turned their attention to working conditions in factories and mines, and to improvements in the care of women during pregnancy and of infants in the first few years of life, with programs to improve nutrition and provide immunization against infectious diseases.

Today, the functions of the public health physician are so extensive that they are divided among many different agencies, ranging from the Centers for Disease Control and its reporting laboratories to the Food and Drug Administration.

Public health dentistry
The aspect of dentistry, sometimes also known as community dentistry, that deals with the dental health of the population at large rather than of the individual. It includes studying the distribution and prevalence of dental disorders, particularly tooth decay (see *Caries, dental*); making sure that enough dentists are trained to cope with demand for treatment; providing information on the need for *oral hygiene*; monitoring *fluoridation* of water supplies to reduce the incidence of tooth decay; and providing special dental facilities for people who have disabilities.

Pudenda
See *Genitalia*.

Pudendal block
A type of *nerve block* used during childbirth to provide pain relief for a *forceps delivery*. A local anesthetic (see *Anesthesia, local*) is injected into either side of the floor of the vagina near the pudendal nerve, which passes under the bony prominences on each side of the lower pelvis. The lower part of the vagina becomes insensitive to pain within about five minutes.

Puerperal sepsis
Infection that originates in the genital tract within 10 days after childbirth, miscarriage, or abortion. Puerperal sepsis is rare, occurring in between 1 and 3 percent of pregnancies. Infection usually starts in the vagina and spreads to the uterus.

CHANGES OF PUBERTY
There is considerable variation in the age of onset of puberty, but girls, on average, undergo puberty earlier than boys. The entire process takes about three to four years to complete. In addition to the sex-specific changes, height and weight both increase rapidly.

10 to 12   15 to 16   12 to 14   15 to 18

Girls
Puberty most often starts between the ages of 10 and 12 in girls. Major changes include growth of breasts and pubic hair, widening of the hips, enlargement of the uterus, and the onset of menstruation.

Boys
The main changes are enlargement of the sex organs, widening of the shoulders, deepening of the voice, and the growth of facial and pubic hair. The onset is usually between the ages of 12 and 14.

P

CAUSES

Infection may be caused by bacteria that normally inhabit the vagina but usually cause harm only if the woman's resistance is low or if placental tissue has been retained in the genital tract. Puerperal sepsis may also be caused by bacteria entering the genital tract from other parts of the body or from outside.

SYMPTOMS AND TREATMENT

The main symptoms are fever, offensive-smelling *lochia* (vaginal discharge after childbirth), headache, chills, and pain in the lower abdomen. If infection spreads to the fallopian tubes (see *Salpingitis*), the tubes may become blocked and cause *infertility*. Further spread of infection may lead to *peritonitis* and *septicemia*, which may be fatal.

Treatment includes *antibiotic drugs* and removal of any remaining placental remnants.

Puerperium

The period of time following *childbirth* during which the woman's uterus and genitals return to their state before the pregnancy.

Pulmonary

Pertaining to the lungs. For example, the pulmonary artery is the blood vessel that carries blood from the heart to the lungs.

Pulmonary embolism

Obstruction of the pulmonary artery or one of its branches in the lung by an *embolus*, usually a blood clot that originated in a vein in the leg or pelvis as a complication of deep vein thrombosis (see *Thrombosis, deep vein*). If the embolus is large enough to block the main pulmonary artery leading from the heart to the lungs, or if there are many clots, the condition is life-threatening. Pulmonary embolism affects about twice as many women as men; recent surgery, pregnancy, and immobility increase the risk. Pulmonary embolism is responsible for 50,000 deaths in the US each year.

SYMPTOMS

Symptoms depend partly on the size of the embolus. A massive embolus that blocks the main pulmonary artery can cause sudden death. Smaller emboli may cause severe shortness of breath, a rapid pulse, dizziness due to low blood pressure, sharp chest pain that is worse when breathing, and coughing up blood. Small pulmonary emboli may produce no symptoms, but, if recurrent, may eventually lead

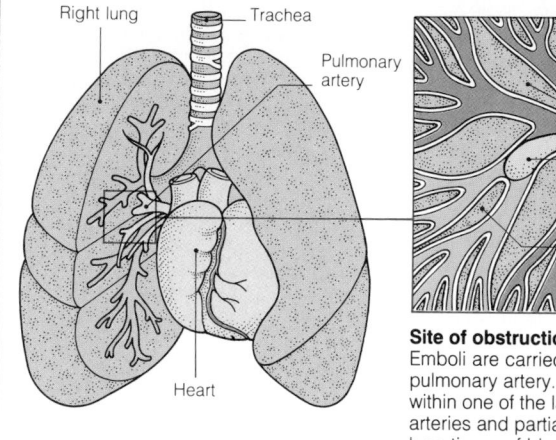

PULMONARY EMBOLISM

This condition results when one or more emboli (fragments of material) break off from a blood clot in a vein and are carried, via the heart, to the lungs. The effects depend on the size and numbers of emboli and on the general health of the person's lungs and heart.

Right lung — Trachea

Pulmonary artery

Heart

Unaffected artery

Unaffected lung tissue

Embolus

Lung tissue deprived of blood

Site of obstruction
Emboli are carried into the lungs by the pulmonary artery. Most of them lodge within one of the larger or medium-sized arteries and partially deprive a section of lung tissue of blood.

to *pulmonary hypertension* (increased pressure of blood flow in the lungs).

DIAGNOSIS

Investigation of the lung may include a *chest X ray*, *radionuclide scanning*, and pulmonary *angiography*. An *ECG* may show changes in the electrical activity of the heart, and *venography* helps determine the source of the embolus.

TREATMENT

Treatment depends on the size and severity of the embolus. A small embolus gradually dissolves but there is a risk of more emboli developing. *Anticoagulant drugs* (such as heparin and warfarin) are usually given to reduce the clotting ability of the blood and to reduce the chance of more clots occurring. *Thrombolytic drugs* may hasten the process of clot dissolution. If the embolus is very large, an emergency operation may be necessary to remove it.

Pulmonary fibrosis

Scarring and thickening of lung tissue, usually as a result of previous lung inflammation, such as *pneumonia* or *tuberculosis*. Pulmonary fibrosis may occur throughout both lungs (see *Interstitial pulmonary fibrosis*) or may affect only part of one lung.

Shortness of breath is a common symptom. Diagnosis is confirmed by chest X ray. Treatment depends on the underlying cause, but the fibrosis may be irreversible.

Pulmonary function tests

A group of procedures used to evaluate the function of the lungs and confirm the presence of some lung disorders. Pulmonary function tests are also performed before any major operation on the lungs, such as *lobectomy* (removal of a lobe of the lung), to ensure that the person will not be disabled by the reduction in his or her lung capacity.

Spirometry and measurement of lung volume are performed to detect any restriction of normal lung expansion or to detect obstruction of air flow. A *peak flow meter* is used to assess the degree of *bronchospasm* (narrowing of the airways), while a test of *blood gases* (measurement of the concentration of oxygen and carbon dioxide in the blood) demonstrates the efficiency of gas exchange in the lungs.

Another test of lung function (diffusing capacity) shows the efficiency of the lungs in absorbing gas into the blood. This is done by measuring the volume of carbon monoxide breathed out after a known volume of the gas has been inhaled.

Pulmonary hypertension

A disorder in which the blood pressure in the arteries supplying the lungs is abnormally high. Pulmonary hypertension develops in response to an increased resistance to blood flow through the lungs. To maintain an

P

adequate blood flow, the right side of the heart, which pumps blood to the lungs, must contract more vigorously than was necessary before. This causes an enlargement of the heart's muscle wall. Eventually, right-sided *heart failure* may develop.

CAUSES

Several conditions can lead to increased resistance to blood flow through the lungs. The most important is an inadequate supply of oxygen to the lungs' small air sacs (e.g., due to chronic *bronchitis* or *emphysema*). The oxygen lack causes the small branches of the arteries in the lungs to constrict and to thicken their muscular walls, thus causing a permanent increase in resistance. Other causes are *pulmonary embolism* (in which a blood clot blocks off one or several arteries in the lungs) and *interstitial pulmonary fibrosis* (thickening and scarring of lung tissue, which can have many causes).

Primary pulmonary hypertension is the term used to describe cases in which the cause of the increased lung resistance is not known.

SYMPTOMS AND SIGNS

As long as the enlargement and strengthening of the right side of the heart is sufficient to maintain a normal blood circulation, there is little indication of trouble. But, with the onset of *heart failure* as the right side of the heart falters in its work load, symptoms develop. Symptoms include enlargement of veins in the neck, enlargement of the liver, and generalized *edema* (swelling due to fluid collection in tissues).

TREATMENT

Treatment is directed at the underlying disorder (if known) and to the relief of the effects of right-sided heart failure. *Diuretic drugs* may be valuable in relieving edema and *oxygen therapy* is sometimes useful.

Pulmonary insufficiency

A defect of the pulmonary valve at the exit of the ventricle (lower, pumping chamber) on the right side of the heart. The valve fails to close properly after each contraction of the ventricle, allowing blood pumped out of the chamber to leak back again.

Pulmonary insufficiency is a rare type of heart valve defect. When it does occur, it is usually the result of *rheumatic fever*, *endocarditis*, or severe *pulmonary hypertension* (raised pressure in the pulmonary artery). It may cause a heart *murmur* that is audible through a stethoscope.

Usually the condition is of little significance. When accompanied by pulmonary hypertension, the eventual result may be right-sided *heart failure*. In such cases, the condition is usually approached by treating the pulmonary hypertension rather than by attempting to repair or replace the defective valve.

Pulmonary stenosis

A heart condition in which the outflow of blood from the ventricle (lower, pumping chamber) on the right side of the heart is obstructed. With pulmonary stenosis, the heart muscle must work much harder to pump blood to the lungs.

The obstruction may be caused by narrowing of the pulmonary valve at the exit of the chamber, by narrowing of the pulmonary artery (large blood vessel beyond the valve) that carries blood to the lungs, or by narrowing within the upper part of the ventricle itself.

CAUSES AND INCIDENCE

Pulmonary stenosis is nearly always congenital (present from birth). About one baby in 8,000 is born with the defect alone or as part of a more complex set of heart defects, called the *tetralogy of Fallot*. Very rarely, pulmonary stenosis develops later in life, usually in a person who has had *rheumatic fever*.

SYMPTOMS

In severe cases, a newborn baby's heart begins to enlarge as soon as breathing is established. If the blood supply to the lungs is inadequate, the baby becomes breathless, and damming of blood behind the valve may lead to liver and abdominal swellings. The baby may also not nurse. This is an emergency that can often be helped by surgery.

In less severe cases (which are more common), symptoms may not appear until the child gets older and becomes more active. The main symptom is breathlessness. Marks resembling *pernios* may appear on the cheeks, hands, and feet as a result of the slower blood circulation. In mild cases there are no symptoms, and the condition is detected only when a physician hears a heart *murmur* through a stethoscope.

When pulmonary stenosis exists with other heart defects, such as a *septal defect* (hole in the heart), some deoxygenated blood bypasses the lungs and goes back into the general circulation, leading to *cyanosis* (blue-purple skin coloration).

Pulmonary stenosis that occurs in later life may lead to the symptoms of *heart failure*.

DIAGNOSIS

A *chest X ray* may show enlargement of the heart. *ECG* (measurement of the electrical activity of the heart), *echocardiography*, and Doppler *ultrasound* techniques (imaging of the heart using sound waves) can help diagnose the severity of the narrowing.

P

PULMONARY HYPERTENSION

In this condition, there is increased resistance to blood flow through the lungs (red arrows), usually due to lung disease. The result is a rise in pressure in the pulmonary artery, the right side of the heart (gray lines and arrows), and in the veins that bring blood to the heart.

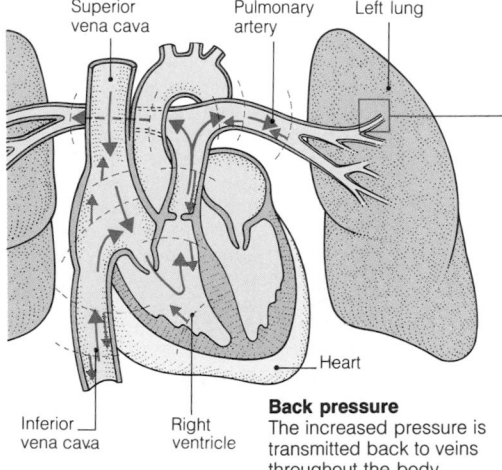

Superior vena cava
Pulmonary artery
Left lung
Heart
Inferior vena cava
Right ventricle

Back pressure
The increased pressure is transmitted back to veins throughout the body.

Causes
The most common cause of increased resistance to blood flow through the lungs is constriction of the small arteries in the lungs and thickening of their muscular walls. This thickening usually results from a lung disease such as chronic bronchitis or emphysema.

TREATMENT

In some cases a *balloon catheter* is used to relieve the narrowing without the need to open the chest. Alternatively, *heart valve surgery* or other types of *open heart surgery* are often successful in correcting or improving it.

Pulp, dental

The soft tissue in the middle of each tooth. It receives a rich supply of blood vessels and contains nerves that respond to heat, cold, pressure, and pain. (See also *Teeth*.)

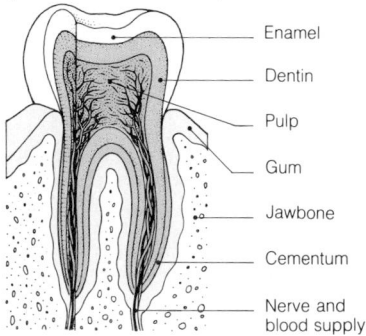

Enamel
Dentin
Pulp
Gum
Jawbone
Cementum
Nerve and blood supply

Location of the dental pulp
The pulp forms the soft core at the center of a tooth. If tooth decay reaches as far as the pulp, the latter degenerates rapidly and must be removed to save the tooth.

Pulpectomy

The complete removal of the pulp of a tooth (the soft tissue inside the tooth that contains blood vessels and nerves). The procedure is part of *root-canal treatment*.

Pulpotomy

Removal of part of the pulp of a tooth (the soft tissue inside the tooth that contains blood vessels and nerves) when it has become inflamed, usually as a result of bacterial infection. The infection is most commonly the result of extensive dental *caries* (tooth decay) or a dental *fracture* that exposes the pulp. Successful pulpotomy prevents further degeneration of the pulp.

Using a local anesthetic, the dentist removes the damaged pulp and covers the wound with a dressing that encourages it to heal. The gap in the overlying dentin and enamel is then sealed with a restoration such as amalgam (see *Filling, dental*). If the treatment is unsuccessful, *root-canal treatment* may be required.

Pulse

The rhythmic expansion and contraction of an artery as blood is forced through it, pumped by the heart.

The pulse is usually checked during the course of a *physical examination* because it can give clues to the patient's state of health or illness. It is detected by pressing one or more fingers or thumb against the skin over an artery, usually at the wrist, although it can also easily be felt in the neck or the groin. The pulse may be visible at the temple or in the neck.

The pulse can be described in terms of its rate (number of expansions per minute), rhythm, strength, and whether the blood vessel is hard or soft. The rate is easily determined by counting the beats in a set period (minimum 15 to 20 seconds) and multiplying to give the beats per minute. The pulse rate usually corresponds to the *heart rate*, which varies according to the person's state of relaxation or physical activity.

Abnormally high or low rates, or abnormal rhythms, may be a sign of a heart disorder (see *Arrhythmia*). When the heart is beating very fast, some of its beats may be too weak to be detectable in the pulse, making the pulse rate slower than the heart rate.

Taking the pulse
Two fingertips are pressed against the wrist just below the base of the thumb to feel the pulse in the radial artery.

If the pulse feels weak, it may be a sign of *heart failure*, *shock*, or an obstruction to the blood circulation. A weak or absent pulse in one or both legs is a sign of *peripheral vascular disease*. The vessel wall should feel soft when the pulse is felt. If the vessel wall feels hard, it may be a sign of *arteriosclerosis*.

Pump, infusion

A machine for the administration of a continuous, controlled amount of a drug or other fluid through a needle that may be inserted into a vein or under the skin.

An infusion pump consists of a small battery-powered pump that controls the flow of fluid from a syringe into the needle. The pump, which is strapped to the patient, is preprogrammed to deliver fluid at a constant rate.

Infusion pumps are frequently used in administering morphine and other drugs to patients suffering from cancer. They are also used to give insulin to patients who have diabetes mellitus (see *Pump, insulin*; see also *Intravenous infusion*).

Pump, insulin

A type of infusion pump (see *Pump, infusion*) used to administer a continuous dose of insulin in some patients with *diabetes mellitus*.

The needle of the insulin pump is inserted under the skin, usually in the upper arm or the abdominal wall. The rate of flow is adjusted so that the level of blood glucose (sugar) is constantly controlled.

Punchdrunk

A condition characterized by slurred speech, impaired concentration, and slowed thought processes. It develops as a result of brain damage caused by several episodes of brief loss of consciousness as a result of a head injury. The name punchdrunk comes from the high incidence of the condition in boxers.

Pupil

The circular opening in the center of the *iris*. In bright conditions, the pupil constricts (narrows) to reduce the amount of light admitted to the *eye*; in dim light, it dilates (widens) to allow more light to reach the retina. Constriction and dilation are controlled by muscles in the iris.

Several drugs affect the size of the pupil. For example, *atropine* eye drops dilate the pupil and *pilocarpine* eye drops constrict it.

DISORDERS

The pupil may be congenitally small, irregular in shape, or displaced to one side; there may also be a coloboma (a missing segment or fissure in the iris). Adie's pupil is a condition in which the affected pupil is larger than the other, with poor constriction in response to light and slow dilation in

P

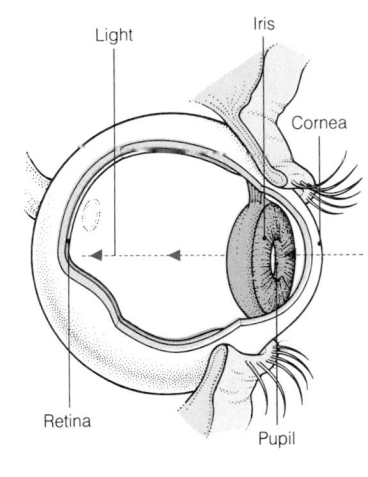

LOCATION OF THE PUPIL
The pupil can be widened or narrowed by muscles in the iris to adjust the amount of light entering the eye.

Light

Iris

Cornea

Retina

Pupil

the dark. The Argyll Robertson pupil, usually caused by *syphilis*, is small and irregular; it does not constrict in response to light but does so when an effort at *accommodation* is made.

Injury to the iris frequently affects the pupil, producing either permanent dilation of the pupil or distortion of its shape.

Purpura
Any of a group of disorders characterized by purplish or reddish-brown areas or spots of discoloration, visible through the skin, and caused by bleeding within underlying tissues. Purpura also refers to the discolored areas themselves, which can range from the size of a pinhead to an inch or so in diameter. The smaller bleeding points are sometimes called *petechiae*; larger, darker areas of discoloration are called bruises or ecchymoses.

TYPES AND CAUSES
There are many different types and causes of purpura.

Common purpura, also called senile purpura, is the most frequent of all bleeding disorders, affecting primarily middle-aged or elderly women. Large discolored areas appear on the thighs or the back of the hands and forearms. They are caused by thinning of the tissues supporting blood vessels beneath the skin, which as a result rupture easily. Bleeding may also be visible under the membrane that lines the mouth.

Schönlein-Henoch purpura (also called anaphylactoid purpura) is caused by inflammation of blood vessels beneath the skin, sometimes as a result of an allergic reaction. Similar changes may occur in patches within the gastrointestinal tract.

Purpura can also occur as a result of a lack of platelets in the blood—a condition called *thrombocytopenia*. Platelets are the small blood cells that play a crucial role in clotting. A lack of platelets may occur as a result of a disease of the bone marrow (such as *leukemia* or aplastic *anemia*), as a side effect of certain drugs or excessive radiation, or for no apparent reason.

Other types of purpura include that seen in *scurvy* due to vitamin C deficiency and forms of the condition caused by damage to blood vessels by certain infections, *autoimmune disorders*, *septicemia* (blood poisoning), or blood chemical disturbances such as uremia (see *Renal failure*).

DIAGNOSIS AND TREATMENT
Purpura is investigated by a physician studying the signs and symptoms and by a full examination and testing of the blood, including *blood-clotting tests*. The state of the blood platelets is of primary interest. It is essential for the physician to determine exactly the type and cause of the purpura, because treatment depends on the exact type.

Common purpura may be helped by estrogen replacement therapy or by *corticosteroid drugs*, but these often do little to help in Schönlein-Henoch purpura. In this form, *immunosuppressant drugs* can help; in severe cases, *plasmapheresis* (removal of blood, replacement of plasma, and retransfusion) has been effective. Platelet deficiency is treated according to the cause. In some cases, transfusions of platelets must be given. Autoimmune thrombocytopenia (sometimes called

Appearance of senile purpura
This common condition of middle to old age is caused by thinning of the tissues that support blood vessels beneath the skin.

idiopathic thrombocytopenic purpura) is usually treated with corticosteroid drugs or *splenectomy*.

Purulent
A term that means containing, producing, or consisting of *pus*.

Pus
A pale yellow or green, creamy fluid found at the site of bacterial infection. Pus is composed of millions of dead white blood cells, partly digested tissue, dead and living bacteria, as well as minute quantities of other substances. A collection of pus in a solid tissue is called an *abscess*.

The main pus-forming organisms include streptococci, pneumococci, and *ESCHERICHIA COLI*. Many bacteria produce a distinctive type of pus (*PSEUDOMONAS AERUGINOSA* produces pus with a bluish tinge).

Pustule
A small skin blister containing pus. Pustules may occur in a hair follicle or on ordinary skin, and may or may not be the result of infection; the pustules in *acne* are noninfective. A *stye* is a type of pustule that develops at the root of an eyelash.

PUVA
A type of *phototherapy* used to treat certain skin conditions, especially *psoriasis*. PUVA combines the use of a *psoralen drug*, which sensitizes the skin to sunlight, and a controlled dose of long wavelength ultraviolet light. The abbreviation stands for psoralens and ultraviolet A.

Pyelitis
See *Pyelonephritis*.

Pyelography
A procedure for obtaining X-ray pictures of the urinary system. Also known as urography, the technique involves the introduction of a radiopaque, iodine-based dye into the kidneys, ureters, and bladder so that they show up well on X rays.

WHY IT IS DONE
Pyelography is performed to help diagnose disorders of the urinary system. It is sometimes recommended for people who have recurrent urinary tract or kidney infections, *hematuria* (blood in the urine), or suspected urinary tract *calculi* (stones). The investigation may also be performed in young people who have *hypertension* (high blood pressure) to discover whether kidney disease is the cause.

P

Retrograde pyelogram
The bright, rodlike object at bottom in this X ray is a cystoscope (viewing tube) that has been passed into the bladder. Via a catheter passed through the cystoscope, a radiopaque dye was introduced into the left ureter. As the dye filled the dilated ureter (bright area at right), X rays were taken. Part of the ureter did not fill with dye, indicating a tumor.

HOW IT IS DONE

INTRAVENOUS PYELOGRAPHY (IVP) Radiopaque dye is injected into the bloodstream via a vein in the arm; it travels from there to the kidneys and urinary tract. Before an IVP, the patient does not drink fluids for eight to 12 hours and is given a laxative to empty the bowel (to improve the quality of the X-ray films).

With the patient lying down, X rays of the complete abdomen are taken before the injection, immediately after it, and then five, 10, and 30 minutes later. Between the five- and 10-minute films, pressure may be applied to the abdomen to improve the definition of the central cavities of the kidneys. After the bladder has filled with dye, the patient is asked to urinate while another X ray is taken.

RETROGRADE PYELOGRAPHY Using an anesthetic, a cystoscope (viewing tube) is passed into the bladder (see *Cystoscopy*); a fine tube is threaded through the cystoscope and up the ureter to the kidney. A small quantity of dye is injected and X rays are taken.

RESULTS

The X rays obtained by IVP allow the radiologist to see the size, shape, and position of the kidneys, the course of the ureters, the size and position of the bladder, and whether there are any obvious obstructions in the ureters. The X ray taken after urination shows whether the bladder has emptied completely.

Retrograde pyelography shows up obstructions of the upper urinary outflow tract particularly clearly.

COMPLICATIONS

Pyelography is generally very safe, but must not be used in people who are sensitive to iodine. With retrograde pyelography, there is a risk of aggravating any infection that may be present in the urinary system.

Pyelolithotomy

An operation performed to remove a *calculus* (stone) from the kidney. The surgeon approaches the kidney via a longitudinal incision to the right or left of the spine, the junction between the kidney and ureter is cut open, and the calculus is removed with a forceps.

Pyelolithotomy is being replaced by ultrasonic wave therapy as a means of dealing with kidney stones (see *Lithotripsy*; *Lithotriptor*).

Pyelonephritis

Inflammation of the kidney, usually caused by a bacterial infection. Pyelonephritis may be acute, taking the form of a sudden attack, or chronic, in which repeated or inadequately treated attacks may cause permanent scarring of the kidney.

ACUTE PYELONEPHRITIS

Acute pyelonephritis is more common in women and more likely to occur in pregnancy. It usually results from *cystitis* (infection of the bladder) spreading up to the kidney.

Symptoms include a high fever, chills, and back pain. Treatment consists of *antibiotic drugs*, which may need to be given by intravenous infusion in severe cases. *Septicemia* (blood poisoning) is a possible complication.

CHRONIC PYELONEPHRITIS

Chronic pyelonephritis often starts in childhood. It is usually caused by *reflux* of urine from the bladder back into one of the ureters, often because the child has a congenital abnormality of the valve where the ureter enters the bladder.

Persistent reflux of urine causes repeated kidney infection, leading to inflammation and scarring, which, over a period of years, causes permanent kidney damage. Children in whom recurrent urinary tract infections develop require testing by a physician. A voiding *cystourethrogram* may help identify the presence of reflux so that the underlying abnormality can be corrected surgically.

Possible complications of chronic pyelonephritis include *hypertension* (high blood pressure) and *renal failure*.

Pyloric stenosis

Narrowing of the pylorus (the lower outlet from the stomach) that obstructs the passage of food into the duodenum (the first part of the small intestine). Pyloric stenosis occurs in babies and in adults.

CAUSES AND INCIDENCE

In infants, the condition is caused by a thickening of the pyloric muscle that occurs, for unknown reasons, soon after birth; one in 4,000 are affected.

PYLORIC STENOSIS IN INFANTS

In infantile pyloric stenosis, the muscle surrounding the outlet from the stomach is abnormally thickened, as shown in the enlarged drawing (below). The condition occurs more often in male than female babies and tends to run in families—infants of a woman who was affected with pyloric stenosis as a baby are liable to develop it.

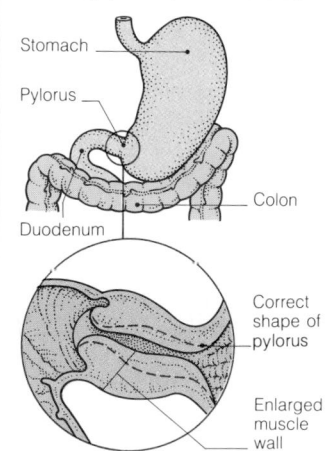

Stomach
Pylorus
Colon
Duodenum
Correct shape of pylorus
Enlarged muscle wall

Barium X ray of pylorus
The X ray shows the blockage to the flow of the barium meal at the lower end of the stomach. Surgery is performed to cut through the thickened muscle around the outlet and relieve the blockage.

P

In adults, the narrowing is usually the result of scarring caused by a *peptic ulcer* or of a malignant tumor of the lower stomach (see *Stomach cancer*).

SYMPTOMS AND DIAGNOSIS
Three to four weeks after birth, an affected infant starts projectile vomiting (profuse, forceful vomiting in which the stomach contents may be ejected a distance of several feet) after feeding. Adults with the disorder vomit undigested food several hours after a meal.

In an infant, a physician can feel the thickened muscle through the abdominal wall, but a barium meal (see *Barium X-ray examinations*) may be required to confirm the diagnosis.

In adults, pyloric stenosis is diagnosed by a barium meal, which shows the narrowing, and by *gastroscopy* (examination of the stomach with a flexible viewing tube).

TREATMENT
Infant pyloric stenosis is sometimes treated with drugs. However, in most cases the only satisfactory treatment is an operation known as pyloromyotomy. While the patient is under a general anesthetic, the abdomen is opened and the obstruction relieved simply by making an incision along the length of the thickened muscle.

In adults, surgery is necessary to correct the underlying cause.

Pyloroplasty

An operation in which the pylorus (the outlet from the stomach) is widened to ensure the free passage of food into the intestine. Pyloroplasty may be performed as part of the surgical treatment for a *peptic ulcer*; it prevents tightening of the pyloric muscles following *vagotomy* (cutting of the vagus nerve to reduce stomach acid production).

While the patient is under general anesthesia, a lengthwise incision is made across the pylorus. The beginning and end of the incision are pushed inward till they meet, and the opening, which is now at right angles to the original incision, is sewn up. This creates an extra wide passage for the movement of food.

Pyo-

A prefix (py- is also used) that denotes a relationship to pus, as in pyuria, pus in the urine.

Pyoderma gangrenosum

A rare condition characterized by ulcers, usually on the legs, that turn into hard, painful areas surrounded by discolored skin. It occurs as a complication in about 5 percent of people with *ulcerative colitis*.

Pyrantel

An *antihelmintic drug* used to treat intestinal *worm infestations*. Possible adverse effects include nausea, loss of appetite, and abdominal pain.

Pyrazinamide

A drug used in the treatment of *tuberculosis* when other drugs have not been effective. Pyrazinamide is prescribed in combination with other antituberculous drugs.

Possible adverse effects are nausea and an increased risk of gout. There may also be liver damage, resulting in loss of appetite and jaundice. Regular blood tests are performed during treatment with pyrazinamide to check liver function.

Pyrexia

A medical term for *fever*.

Pyrexia of uncertain origin

Persistent fever for which no cause is readily apparent despite extensive medical investigations. The cause is usually an illness that is difficult to diagnose or a common disease that presents itself in an unusual way.

Common causes include various viral infections; *tuberculosis*; cancer, particularly *lymphoma* (cancer of the lymphoid tissue); and *collagen diseases* such as systemic *lupus erythematosus*, *temporal arteritis*, and, in children, Still's disease (see *Rheumatoid arthritis, juvenile*).

Occasionally, fever of uncertain origin occurs as a reaction to a drug.

Pyridostigmine

A drug used in the treatment of *myasthenia gravis* (an *autoimmune disorder* causing muscle weakness). Pyridostigmine significantly improves muscle strength in sufferers of myasthenia gravis but does not cure the condition.

Possible adverse effects of pyridostigmine include abdominal pain, nausea, diarrhea, and, rarely, an allergic skin rash.

Pyridoxine

One of the B_6 group of vitamins (see *Vitamin B complex*). Pyridoxine is used to treat people with dietary deficiency, in cases of *neuritis* (nerve inflammation) caused by certain drugs, and to relieve the symptoms that occur in *premenstrual syndrome*.

Pyrilamine

An *antihistamine drug* used to treat seasonal allergic *rhinitis* (hay fever) and *urticaria* (hives). Unlike some other types of antihistamines, pyrilamine rarely causes drowsiness.

Pyrimethamine

A drug used to prevent and treat attacks caused by certain strains of *malaria* parasite and also to treat *toxoplasmosis*. It is usually given in combination with a *sulfonamide drug*.

Possible adverse effects include loss of appetite, vomiting, and, rarely, rash. Long-term use may reduce blood cell production by the bone marrow, causing *anemia*, abnormal bleeding, or susceptibility to infection.

Pyrogen

A fever-producing substance. The term is usually applied to proteins that are released by white blood cells in response to bacterial or viral infections. These proteins act on the temperature-controlling center within the brain, causing the body temperature to increase.

The word pyrogen is also sometimes used to refer to chemicals released by the microorganisms themselves—such as bacterial *endotoxins*, which also have a temperature-raising effect on the body.

Pyromania

A persistent impulse to set fires. The typical pyromaniac becomes fascinated with fires as a child, obtains relief of tension (or even pleasure) from setting fire to something and watching it burn, and has no other motive (such as money) for doing so. The disorder is more often diagnosed in males, and is associated with a low IQ, alcohol abuse, and *psychosexual disorder* (some people seem to be sexually aroused by fires). Pyromaniacs are often dangerous and difficult to treat; imprisonment is not unusual.

Pyuria

The presence of white blood cells (pus cells) in the urine. Pyuria is usually an indication of infection and inflammation in the kidney or urinary tract.

Microscopic examination and *culture* of the urine are performed to look for a causative microorganism so that appropriate *antibiotic drugs* may be given. In some cases, pyuria occurs when no microorganisms are present and may indicate inflammation of the kidney due to another cause (e.g., interstitial *nephritis*).

P

Q fever

An uncommon illness with symptoms similar to *influenza*. Q fever occurs throughout the world; an effective vaccine is available.

The causative organism, COXIELLA BURNETTI, is a type of *rickettsia* harbored by farm animals. It occurs in the urine, feces, milk, flesh, and, particularly, placentas of infected animals. In dry areas, Q fever may be contracted by inhaling dust contaminated with feces, urine, or birth products. The disease may also, in rare cases, be spread by tick bites.

About 20 days after infection, the illness begins suddenly with a high fever (which may persist for up to two weeks), severe headache, muscle and chest pain, and cough. During the second week, a form of pneumonia develops. The patient then usually recovers. In some cases, however, the disease is prolonged; *hepatitis* develops in one third of these people and some suffer *endocarditis*. In less than 1 percent of cases, the illness is fatal unless treated.

A diagnosis of Q fever may be confirmed by a *blood test*. Treatment is with *antibiotic drugs*.

Quackery

A false claim by someone to have both the ability and experience to diagnose and treat disease.

Quadriceps muscle

A muscle with four distinct parts that is situated at the front of the thigh. The quadriceps muscle straightens the knee.

The most common disorder of the quadriceps is a *hematoma* (a collection of blood) caused by a direct blow. Bruising may follow a few days later; in rare cases, bone forms within the hematoma, restricting movement of the affected leg.

Sudden stretching of the leg may tear the muscle, especially in middle-aged or elderly people. Any knee disorder that brings on pain or swelling, limiting full extension of the leg,

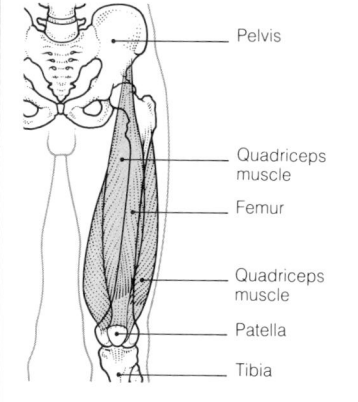

Pelvis

Quadriceps muscle

Femur

Quadriceps muscle

Patella

Tibia

causes the quadriceps muscle to begin wasting away within 48 hours, making the knee feel as though it is giving way when weight is placed on the affected leg.

Quadriparesis

Muscle weakness in all four limbs and the trunk.

Quadriplegia

Paralysis of all four limbs and the trunk. Quadriplegia is caused by damage to the spinal cord in the neck region. The condition results in loss of feeling and power in the affected parts. (See also *Paraplegia*.)

Quarantine

Isolation of a person or persons recently exposed to a serious infectious disease. The aim is to prevent the spread of a disease by an infected, but symptomless, person.

Today, the reduced incidence of most serious infectious diseases and the widespread availability of *immunization* against many of them makes quarantine procedures rarely necessary. In some cases (principally to prevent the spread of *yellow* fever), quarantine has been replaced by compulsory vaccination for travel between certain countries. The contacts of people with highly infectious diseases (such as pneumonic *plague*) may have restrictions placed on their travel in addition to being given preventive immunization against the disease.

The principal remaining quarantine regulations apply to animals imported into countries that are free from *rabies*.

Quickening

The stage of pregnancy when the movements of the fetus are first felt by the pregnant woman. Quickening usually occurs between 16 and 20 weeks of gestation.

Quinacrine

A drug used during World War II to suppress malaria and now to treat *giardiasis*, an intestinal infection. Possible adverse effects include nausea, vomiting, and yellow discoloration of the skin and urine. Prolonged use can cause blood disorders or psychological disturbance.

Quinestrol

A synthetic *estrogen drug* used to treat symptoms of the *menopause* (see *Hormone replacement therapy*).

Quinidine

An *antiarrhythmic drug* used to treat irregular or abnormally fast heart beat. Quinidine may cause nausea, vomiting, diarrhea, and, occasionally, a dangerous drop in blood pressure or a worsening of the *arrhythmia*.

Quinine

The oldest drug treatment for *malaria*. Quinine is now used mainly to treat strains of the disease that are resistant to other antimalarial drugs. Large doses are needed and there is a high risk of adverse effects, including headache, nausea, hearing loss, ringing in the ears, and blurred vision.

Quinine is frequently prescribed to help prevent painful leg cramps at night; low doses are used and adverse effects are rare.

Quinsy

An abscess around the tonsil, usually occurring as a complication of *tonsillitis*. The infection causes a painful throat, high temperature, headache, impaired speech, drooling, and swollen, tender lymph glands in the neck. The uvula (the protuberance that hangs down from the soft palate at the back of the mouth) is displaced to the unaffected side of the throat.

Antibiotic drugs taken at an early stage sometimes clear up the infection. Otherwise, the abscess requires surgical incision and drainage. Once healing is complete, the tonsils are usually removed to prevent the infection from recurring.

R

Rabies

An acute viral infection of the nervous system, also known as hydrophobia. Rabies primarily affects animals, but it can be transmitted from a rabid animal to a human by a bite or by a lick over a break in the skin. The causative virus, present in the animal's saliva, travels from the wound along nerve pathways to the brain, where it causes inflammation that results in delirium, painful muscle spasms in the throat, and other severe symptoms. Once symptoms develop, human rabies is usually fatal.

CAUSES AND INCIDENCE
The geographical distribution of rabies, and some important animal species affected, are shown on the map below.

Most human cases are the result of a bite from a rabid dog. However, the possibility of rabies must be considered whenever any mammal—domestic or wild—bites a human in a country where the rabies virus is present.

Worldwide, there are an estimated 15,000 cases of human rabies each year. Annually in the US, the number of human cases is generally less than five as a result of an intensive dog vaccination program and of prompt medical attention to animal bites.

SYMPTOMS AND SIGNS
The incubation period between bite and appearance of symptoms ranges from nine days to many months (the average is four to eight weeks), depending largely on the site of the animal bite.

The initial symptoms are low-grade fever, headache, and loss of appetite leading to restlessness, hyperactivity, disorientation, and, in some cases, seizures. Often the victim has an intense thirst, but attempts to drink induce violent, painful spasms in the throat (hence the term hydrophobia). Eye and facial muscles may become paralyzed. Coma and death follow three to 20 days after the onset of symptoms.

TREATMENT
Once symptoms have appeared, the features of the disease are treated with sedative drugs and analgesics (painkillers). A very small number of people with established rabies are reported as having survived as a result of intensive care aimed at maintaining breathing and the action of the heart. However, the main emphasis must be on preventing the disease.

PREVENTION
In areas of the US where rabies exists in wild animals, domestic dogs are vaccinated annually and stray dogs are killed. All people with high-risk occupations (e.g., veterinarians and animal trappers) require regular vaccinations. Countries that are free from rabies impose strict quarantine regulations on the importing of dogs and other mammals.

Following any bite, the wound should be thoroughly cleansed (see *Bites, animal*). The wound should not be sutured (stitched). If the bite occurs in a country where rabies is present, medical opinion should be sought immediately on whether postexposure *immunization* is necessary. If there is any risk of rabies, passive immunization is given with human rabies immune globulin (ready-made antibodies against the rabies virus), and rabies vaccine is given by a course of injections lasting several weeks. (Because the vaccine has changed, these shots are no longer administered through the stomach.)

Passive immunization is omitted for persons who have been vaccinated before exposure. The vaccines used today have only mild side effects when compared with the ones used before the 1970s.

Every attempt is made to capture and confine the biting animal. If it appears rabid, it is killed and its brain examined for the presence of rabies inclusion bodies (microscopic findings in the nuclei of affected cells). If no evidence of antibodies can be found or if a healthy animal remains symptom-free after five days, treatment of the bitten person is stopped.

If immunization is given within two days of the bite, rabies is almost always prevented. The chances of prevention decrease with delay, but immunization can still be effective when given weeks or months after a bite.

Rachitic
A term used to describe bony or other abnormalities associated with, or

---

GEOGRAPHICAL DISTRIBUTION OF RABIES
In most rabies-affected areas, the disease circulates mainly among wild animals. Some of the principal animal "reservoirs" of rabies are shown at right, but other mammals may also be affected—e.g., raccoons and bats in North America. Most human cases result from the bite of a rabid dog. The dog may have acquired the virus through contact with a wild animal, but, in some areas, such as the Far East, stray dogs are themselves principal carriers. Vaccination of dogs can largely prevent human rabies.

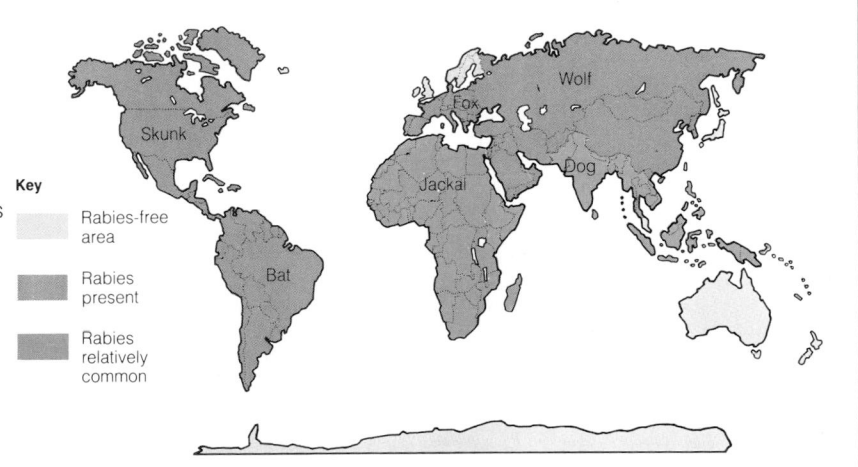

Key

Rabies-free area

Rabies present

Rabies relatively common

suggestive of, *rickets* (the disease produced by a deficiency of vitamin D). Rachitic is also used to refer to people or populations that are particularly afflicted by rickets.

Rad

A unit of absorbed dose of ionizing radiation (see the *Radiation* units box, opposite). Rad is an acronym for radiation absorbed dose.

Radial nerve

A branch of the *brachial plexus*, the radial nerve is one of the main nerves of the arm, running down its full length into the hand. The radial nerve controls muscles that straighten the wrist so that the back of the hand is in line with the forearm. It also conveys sensation from the back of the forearm; from the thumb, second, and third fingers; and from an area at the base of the thumb.

DISORDERS
The radial nerve winds around the shaft of the humerus (upper arm bone) and so may be damaged by a fracture of this bone. The nerve may also be damaged by persistent pressure on the armpit (e.g., from a crutch). Such damage may result in *wristdrop* (inability to straighten the wrist) and numbness in the areas of skin supplied by the radial nerve.

Radiation

There are two main types of radiation—ionizing and nonionizing. Ionizing radiation is capable of forcibly ejecting one or more of the electrons that orbit the nucleus of an atom, thereby creating an entity called an *ion* that has an electrical charge and is capable of chemical combination with other ions. When ionization occurs in the atoms of molecules that play an important role in the body, it can lead to biological damage.

Nonionizing radiation has a different effect on molecules. It tends to cause excitation of the molecules' constituent atoms (somewhat like shaking them) but it does not impart enough energy to the atoms to displace electrons and form ions.

IONIZING RADIATION
There are three types of ionizing radiation—X rays, gamma rays, and particle radiation. X rays are electromagnetic waves (i.e., they are part of the same continuous spectrum—the electromagnetic spectrum—that includes radio waves, infrared radiation, visible light, ultraviolet light, and gamma rays) of very short wavelength and very high frequency. X rays are produced by special electrical machines (X-ray generators). X rays have no mass and no electrical charge; their penetrating power depends on their energy, which, in turn, depends on the voltage used to generate them. X rays generated at a few tens of thousands of volts can penetrate only a few millimeters of tissue, whereas those generated at about 100,000 volts are just energetic enough to pass completely through the body and produce X-ray images. X rays used in *radiation therapy* are generated at several million volts and are sufficiently energetic to destroy deep-seated tumors.

Gamma rays have almost identical properties to X rays. The principal difference between the two is that gamma rays are produced by the spontaneous decay of radioactive materials rather than by a machine. They also tend to have shorter wavelengths and higher frequencies than X rays, although there is some overlap between the two.

Particle radiation—unlike X rays and gamma rays—has mass and may also have electrical charge. It represents parts of atoms, such as electrons (beta particles, which have a negative electrical charge and a very small mass), protons (positively charged particles, each with a mass about 1,800 times that of an electron), or neutrons (particles with the same mass as protons but no electrical charge). The nuclei of small atoms such as helium (helium nuclei are also known as alpha particles) and even larger atomic nuclei may be the source of particle radiation. Particle radiation may be produced during the decay of radioactive atoms or by machines.

SOURCES OF IONIZING RADIATION
Ionizing radiation may originate from natural or man-made sources. One natural source is cosmic rays, which come from remote parts of the universe as well as from the sun. These rays consist largely of very high energy protons, along with a few atomic nuclei (principally helium nuclei). Cosmic rays are highly energetic and not only can irradiate people on the Earth's surface, but can also pass through many feet of soil and rock. The amount of cosmic rays an individual receives depends on the altitude at which he or she lives. A person who is living in Denver, Colorado, at an altitude of about 6,000 feet, receives more than twice the annual radiation dose of cosmic rays than a person living at sea level.

Secondary radiation is another natural source. It is generated in the upper atmosphere from cosmic rays and consists mainly of gamma rays and high-energy electrons. The annual dose from such secondary radiation varies with the latitude, being greatest at the Earth's poles and least at the equator.

The other principal natural source of radiation is radioactivity. Many minerals contain unstable atomic nuclei that spontaneously disintegrate (a process known as radioactive decay), thereby emitting alpha or beta particles and/or gamma rays. The naturally occurring radioactive isotope potassium 40 (isotopes are varieties of an element that are chemically identical but differ in some physical properties) is the principal source of radiation from within the body. Many other natural materials are radioactive and, in some areas, *radon* from soil, rocks, and/or building materials is a major contributor to the annual radiation dose.

Medical X rays—used to diagnose and/or treat numerous diseases and disorders—are the greatest artificial source of radiation to which the general public is exposed. In the US, the average yearly radiation dose from medical X rays is almost equal to that from all natural sources. Radioactive isotopes, also used in diagnosis and treatment, are another medical source of radiation (see *Radionuclide scanning*). Radioisotopes that emit gamma rays are most commonly used (although particle-emitting radioisotopes are also employed); the types selected are usually short-lived to reduce the dose to the patient.

Nuclear reactors are not only sources of direct radiation (such as gamma rays and neutrons, which are normally absorbed by thick reactor shielding to prevent them from escaping into the environment), but are also prolific producers of radioactive isotopes. *Uranium* is the most commonly used fuel, often enriched so that it contains more of the fissionable isotope uranium 235 than is present in natural uranium ores. In the reactor it undergoes fission (splitting), thereby producing heat and leaving behind a wide variety of radioactive isotopes. Radioisotopes of iodine, ruthenium, tellurium, and cesium are among those produced in the greatest amounts, although others of greater biological importance, such as *strontium* isotopes, are also produced. In fast-breeder reactors, *plutonium* is used as the main fuel; uranium 238 is the source from which additional plutonium fuel is made.

Nuclear weapons, including atomic bombs of the types used at Hiroshima and Nagasaki (in which either uranium or plutonium undergoes rapid fission) and hydrogen bombs (which combine nuclear fission and fusion) are intense sources of man-made radiation. However, except for the relatively small battlefield weapons and the "radiation-enhanced" weapon (the so-called neutron bomb), the lethal effects from direct irradiation occur only comparatively near the point of explosion, whereas the lethal effects of blast and heat extend over a considerably larger area.

NONIONIZING RADIATION

The most widespread type of nonionizing radiation is ultraviolet light, a component of sunlight (although much is absorbed by the atmosphere); it is also produced by sunlamps. This type of radiation can penetrate only superficial layers of body tissue but it damages the RNA (ribonucleic acid) and DNA (deoxyribonucleic acid) molecules in cells, which may lead to skin cancer.

Microwave ovens cook food by means of radio-frequency electromagnetic radiation, which can also heat body tissues and thereby damage them. This type of injury is unlikely to occur because modern appliances are shielded to prevent microwaves from escaping; they also have safety cutoffs that stop radiation emission when the door is opened. Radio and television transmissions are harmless forms of electromagnetic radiation.

The other types of nonionizing radiation to which people are subjected are magnetic fields and *ultrasound*. Weak magnetic fields are generated around all wires carrying electricity, and strong fields are used in medicine for magnetic resonance imaging (*MRI*). The effects of such fields are currently being studied, but they are not thought to be harmful; some authorities believe that they may even be beneficial. Ultrasound (inaudible high-frequency sound waves) is used in medicine for diagnosis and, on occasion, treatment. Its effects depend on the power used and the duration of exposure. The low power levels and relatively short durations used in medicine are harmless, but exposure to ultrasound at high power levels and/or for a long time may cause tissue damage. (See also *Radiation hazards; Radiation sickness*.)

RADIATION UNITS

Becquerel	The SI unit of radioactivity. One becquerel (symbol Bq) is defined as one disintegration (or other nuclear transformation) per second. Although the number of becquerels is a measure of how strongly	radioactive a particular source is, it takes no account of the different effects of different types of radiation on tissue; for medical purposes, the sievert is generally more useful.
Gray	The SI unit of absorbed dose of ionizing radiation, the gray (symbol Gy) has superseded the rad. One gray is defined as an energy	absorption of 1 joule per kilogram of irradiated material. One gray is equivalent to 100 rads.
Rad	An acronym for radiation absorbed dose, the rad is a unit of absorbed dose of ionizing radiation. One rad is equal to an energy absorption of 100 ergs (an erg is a unit of work or	energy) per gram of irradiated material. The rad has been superseded by the gray (the corresponding SI unit); 1 rad is equivalent to 0.01 grays.
Rem	An acronym for roentgen equivalent man, the rem is the absorbed dose of ionizing radiation that produces the same biological effect as 1 rad of X rays or gamma rays. The rem was introduced as a result of the observation that some types of ionizing radiation, such as neutrons, produce a greater biological effect for an equivalent amount of absorbed energy than X rays or gamma rays. In short, the rem is a measure of the biological effectiveness of irradiation. For X rays and gamma rays, the rem is	equal to the rad. For other types of radiation, the number of rems equals the number of rads multiplied by a special factor (called the quality factor or relative biological effectiveness) that depends on the type of radiation involved. The rem has been superseded by the sievert in the SI system of units; 1 rem is equivalent to 0.01 sieverts.
Sievert	The SI unit of equivalent absorbed dose of ionizing radiation, the sievert (symbol Sv) has superseded the rem. One sievert is the absorbed dose of radiation that	produces the same biological effect as 1 gray of X rays or gamma rays. One sievert is equivalent to 100 rems.

Measurement of radiation levels

In the SI system (the internationally agreed system of units), three main units are used to measure radiation levels—the becquerel, the gray, and the sievert. These three units are defined above, along with two other radiation units (the rad and rem) that have now been largely superseded but are still occasionally used for some purposes.

Radiation hazards

Hazards from radiation may arise from exposure to external sources of radiation (such as X rays or gamma rays) and from internal irradiation from radioactive materials taken into the body (see *Radiation*). Two topics of particular public concern are whether there are any radiation hazards associated with visual display terminals (VDTs) or with the irradiation of food. In fact, there is no evidence that either of them poses such a hazard. VDTs do not emit significant amounts of penetrating radiation and food that has been irradiated does not itself become radioactive.

TYPES OF HAZARDS AND THEIR EFFECTS

The effects of radiation depend critically on the dose received and the duration of exposure.

Some forms of radiation damage occur when the total radiation dose exceeds a certain threshold, usually 1 sievert or more (see *Radiation* units box above). Above the threshold, damage increases, including *radiation sickness* (an early reaction to radiation) and radiation *dermatitis*, *cataracts*, or failure of various organs, which may occur only many years after exposure. These hazards can be avoided by keeping the cumulative radiation exposure below the threshold dose.

R

For other radiation hazards, the severity of damage does not depend upon the specific radiation dose, but the risk that damage will occur increases with increasing doses. *Cancer* is the major example of this type of radiation damage. It usually occurs many years after exposure, typically five to 15 years for leukemia, and 40 years or longer for skin, lung, breast, and other cancers. Heritable genetic damage is another form of radiation damage.

The International Commission on Radiological Protection has concluded that the total risk factor for death from radiation-induced cancers is about one in 100 per sievert of radiation absorbed. The risk of a hereditary disorder occurring within the first two generations following irradiation of either parent is also thought to be about one in 100 per sievert, and the additional risk to subsequent generations is thought to be the same.

Radiation sickness

The term applied to the acute effects of ionizing *radiation* on the whole, or a major part, of the body when the dose is greater than about 1 gray (1 Gy) of X rays or gamma rays, or 1 sievert (1 Sv) of other types of radiation (see previous page).

SYMPTOMS

The effect of exposure to radiation depends critically on the dose and the time course over which it is received. Above acute exposures of 30 to 100 Gy, there is a rapid onset of nausea, vomiting (which may be repeated and severe), anxiety, and disorientation. Within a few hours, the victim usually loses consciousness and dies as a consequence of direct damage to the nervous system from the radiation, and to edema (accumulation of fluid) of the brain; these effects are known as the central nervous system syndrome.

People who have received radiation doses of 10 to 30 Gy also experience an early onset of nausea and vomiting, which tend to start within about two hours of exposure but disappear a few hours later. However, such individuals invariably die within four to 14 days of exposure as a result of radiation damage to the gastrointestinal tract—which causes severe and frequently bloody diarrhea (known as the gastrointestinal syndrome)—and overwhelming infection due to radiation damage to the *immune system*.

At doses of 1 to 10 Gy, transient nausea and occasional vomiting may occur, but these early symptoms usually disappear rapidly and are often followed by a two- to three-week period of relative well-being. However, by the end of this period, the effects of radiation damage to the bone marrow and immune system begin to appear, with repeated infections (which may be fatal unless treated with antibiotic drugs), and petechiae (pinpoint spots of bleeding under the skin). Some victims may be treated successfully by *bone marrow transplantation* or by isolation in a sterile environment until their own bone marrow recovers.

Radiation damage to other tissues, such as the skin and lining of the respiratory tract, may cause complications, but total-body doses of less than 2 Gy are unlikely to be fatal to an otherwise healthy adult. However, despite the most intensive medical care, few people survive doses of more than 6 Gy.

Radiation therapy

Treatment of *cancer* (and occasionally other diseases) by X rays or other sources of radioactivity, both of which produce ionizing *radiation*. The radiation, as it passes through the diseased tissue, destroys or slows the development of abnormal cells. Provided the correct dosage of radiation is given, normal cells suffer little or no damage.

WHY IT IS DONE

Radiation therapy has various applications in the treatment of cancer. In cancer of the larynx (see *Larynx, cancer of*), in certain kinds of *mouth cancer*, *basal cell carcinoma*, and *squamous cell carcinoma* (a type of skin cancer), in cancer of the cervix (see *Cervix, cancer of*), in cancer of the uterus (see *Uterus, cancer of*), in *Hodgkin's disease* (a cancer of lymphoid tissue), and in *leukemia* it may be used by itself in an attempt to destroy all the abnormal cells.

Radiation therapy is often used after surgical excision of a malignant tumor (such as in the treatment of *breast cancer*) to destroy any remaining tumor cells. It is also used to reduce the size of a tumor to relieve the symptoms of a cancer that is too far advanced to be curable. Examples of palliative treatment include relieving pressure from a tumor on the esophagus that prevents swallowing (see *Esophagus, cancer of*), relieving pain caused by bone cancer, and relieving headaches or paralysis caused by a *brain tumor*.

If the benefits of destroying diseased tissue far outweigh the risk of damage to healthy tissue, radiation therapy may be used to treat non-malignant diseases. A common example is the destruction of part of an overactive thyroid gland with radioactive iodine when it is producing severe symptoms (see *Thyrotoxicosis*).

HOW IT IS DONE

Some of the main techniques of radiation therapy are shown opposite. Radiation is usually passed through diseased tissues by means of X rays (or sometimes electrons) produced by a machine called a linear accelerator. This device has largely supplanted apparatus containing radioactive cobalt, which has the drawback of producing ionizing radiation that is both less intense than that of X rays and incapable of being shut off.

Some malignant tumors are treated not by radiation from an external source, but by inserting radioactive material directly into the growth or surrounding tissue (see *Interstitial radiation therapy*) or into a body cavity (see *Intracavitary therapy*). Both procedures require an anesthetic.

Radiation used to treat thyrotoxicosis is given as a liquid form of radioactive iodine, which the patient drinks through a straw and which concentrates in the thyroid gland.

COMPLICATIONS

Radiation therapy may produce unpleasant side effects, including fatigue, nausea and vomiting (for which *antiemetic drugs* may be prescribed beforehand), and loss of hair from irradiated areas. Rarely, there may be reddening and blistering of the skin, which can be alleviated by *corticosteroid drugs*.

RESULTS

Radiation therapy cures most skin cancers and cancer of the larynx. The cure rate for other types of cancer varies depending on how early the treatment is begun, but the cure rate can be 80 percent or higher.

Radical surgery

Extensive surgery aimed at eliminating a major disease by removing all affected tissue and any surrounding tissue that might be diseased.

In the past, radical surgery was commonly done in an attempt to cure cancer. Radical *mastectomy* for *breast cancer* involved removing the entire affected breast, along with chest muscles, underarm lymph nodes, and other tissue. Such operations are rarely performed today.

Amputation, usually to prevent the spread of *gangrene* (tissue death), is another form of radical surgery.

RADIATION THERAPY

Before treatment, calculations are made of the doses of radiation needed and of the directions from which the rays should be aimed. The areas of the patient's body to be targeted are marked directly on the patient or on a plastic coat that he or she wears. The treatment is usually performed on an outpatient basis, with the patient receiving treatment several times a week.

Radiation therapy machine in use

The patient lies on a table under the machine in a room designed to prevent radiation leakage. A radiation technologist operates the machine, which sends X rays, in the predetermined directions and amounts, through the diseased area of the patient's body. The procedure causes no discomfort and usually lasts just a few minutes.

Machine can be tilted to allow radiation of the tumor from various directions

Radiation generator

Table with adjustable height/tilt

EXAMPLES OF RADIATION THERAPY

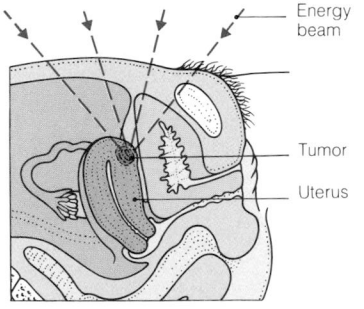

Energy beam

Tumor

Uterus

Rays from different directions
By targeting relatively low-energy rays coming from many directions at a tumor, a large enough dose is achieved in the locality of the tumor to destroy it. Tissues through which the rays pass are unharmed.

Hollow needle

Radioactive pellets

Pituitary gland

Use of radioactive pellets
Another technique is to insert a source of radiation, in the form of tiny radioactive pellets, directly into the tumor via a hollow needle. Pituitary tumors are sometimes treated in this way.

Before treatment
The patient has a keratoacanthoma, a benign skin tumor.

After treatment
The tumor is healing well after radiation therapy.

R

Radiculopathy

Damage to the nerve roots that enter or leave the spinal cord. Radiculopathy may be caused by *disk prolapse*, spinal *arthritis*, thickening of the meninges (the membranes that cover the brain and spinal cord), and sometimes *diabetes mellitus* or ingestion of heavy metals, such as lead.

Symptoms are severe pain and, occasionally, loss of feeling in the area supplied by the affected nerves, and weakness, paralysis, and wasting of muscles supplied by the nerves.

Treatment is of the underlying cause if possible; otherwise, symptoms may be relieved by analgesics (painkillers), *physical therapy*, or, in some cases, surgery.

Radioactivity

The emission of alpha particles or beta particles and/or gamma rays that occurs when the nuclei of certain unstable substances spontaneously disintegrate. Natural radioactivity is due to the disintegration of naturally occurring radioactive substances, such as uranium ores. However, most elements can be induced to become radioactive by bombarding them with high-energy particles (such as neutrons)—so-called artificial radioactivity. (See also *Radiation*.)

Radioimmunoassay

A very sensitive laboratory technique that employs radioactive isotopes to measure the concentration of specific proteins in a person's blood. Proteins that can be detected by radioimmunoassay include hormones, parts of microorganisms, and antibodies formed against microorganisms or allergens. (See *Immunoassay*.)

Radioisotope scanning
See *Radionuclide scanning*.

Radiologic technician
See *X-ray technician*.

Radiologist
A physician (also known as a roentgenologist) who is specially trained and certified in the use of X rays, nuclear imaging devices, radioactive substances, ultrasound, and magnetic resonance to see into the body and diagnose and treat problems. In general, a radiologist (either at an outpatient clinic or in a hospital) is seen only on referral by another physician. Other specialists licensed by the nuclear regulatory agency may also use radioisotopes (radionuclides) for diagnosis and treatment.

Radiology
The medical specialty that uses *X rays*, *ultrasound*, *MRI*, and *radionuclide scanning* for investigation, diagnosis, and treatment. Other specialists may also employ radionuclide scanning.

Radiologic tests can provide images of almost any organ, system, or part of the body in a *noninvasive* way so that diagnoses can be made and treatment planned or monitored frequently without the need for the patient to undergo exploratory surgery.

Radiologic techniques also enable instruments (such as needles and catheters) to be accurately guided into different parts of the body both for diagnosis and, increasingly, for treatment. This subspecialty is known as interventional radiology.

Radiolucent
Almost transparent to radiation, especially to X rays and gamma rays (objects that are entirely transparent to radiation are radiotransparent). See also *Radiopaque*.

Radionuclide scanning
A diagnostic technique based on the detection of radiation emitted by radioactive substances introduced into the body. Different radioactive substances, known as radionuclides, are taken up in greater concentrations by different types of tissue, so that specific organs can be studied. For example, the thyroid gland takes up more radioactive iodine than other parts of the body. The images pro-

vided by radionuclide scanning reflect the function of an organ better than other techniques, although they provide less anatomical detail.

HOW IT WORKS
Radionuclide is swallowed or injected into the bloodstream and accumulates in the target organ. Radiation in the form of gamma rays (similar to X rays but of shorter wavelength) is emitted from the organ and detected by a "gamma camera." The camera contains a scintillation crystal that reacts to gamma rays by emitting minute quantities of light (photons). These are used to produce an image that can be displayed on a screen or in digital (numerical) form.

Using a principle similar to *CT scanning*, cross-sectional images (slices) can be constructed by a computer from radiation detected by a gamma camera that rotates around the patient. This specialized form of radionuclide scanning is known as SPECT (single photon emission computerized tomography).

It is also possible to create moving images with the aid of a computer by recording a series of images immediately following the administration of the radionuclide.

WHY IT IS DONE
Radionuclide scanning can detect certain disorders earlier than other imaging techniques because changes in the functioning of an organ often occur before the structure is affected. For example, infection of bone results in increased activity of bone cells, resulting in radionuclide being taken up in greater amounts by diseased bone before structural changes show on conventional X rays. The technique is also useful for detecting disorders that affect only function (e.g., some *thyroid* disorders).

Moving images can provide information on functions such as blood flow, the movements of the heart walls, urine flow through the kidneys, and bile flow through the liver.

RISKS
Radionuclide scanning is a safe procedure. It requires only minute doses of radiation and, since the radionuclide is ingested or administered by intravenous injection, it also avoids the risks associated with some X-ray procedures in which a radiopaque dye is administered by inserting a catheter into the organ (as in cardiac *catheterization* and coronary *angiography*). In addition, unlike radiopaque dyes, radionuclides carry virtually no risk of toxicity or allergy.

OUTLOOK
Advances in radionuclide scanning depend on the continuing development of radionuclides specific to certain tissues. The fact that monoclonal antibodies (see *Antibody, monoclonal*) can now be produced for use against almost any antigen means that it should be possible to target almost any tissue. Experiments are being carried out using labeled antitumor monoclonal antibodies to assess tumor spread and recurrence.

Radiopaque
Blocking the passage of radiation, especially X rays and gamma rays. Many body tissues are *radiolucent* to X rays (bones being a notable exception). Thus, in diagnostic X-ray imaging, it is sometimes necessary to introduce special radiopaque dyes into the body to make organs stand out more clearly. In intravenous *pyelography*, for example, radiopaque iodine compounds are excreted by the kidney into the lower urinary tract to make the structures clearly visible on X-ray photographs.

Radiotherapy
See *Radiation therapy*.

Radium
A rare radioactive metallic element that does not occur naturally in its pure form but is present as various compounds in *uranium* ores, such as pitchblende and carnotite. Radium has four naturally occurring isotopes (varieties of the element that are chemically identical but differ in some physical properties). In order of decreasing abundance they are radium 226, radium 228, radium 224, and radium 223. Artificial radium isotopes have also been produced.

The most important isotope is radium 226, which is produced by the decay of naturally radioactive elements of the uranium series. It is relatively long-lived (with a *half-life* of about 1,600 years), and itself decays to form the gas *radon*, which then decays further to form other, solid, radioactive decay products. During these decay stages, *radiation* is emitted in the form of alpha and beta particles and gamma rays. Radium 226 was once used to treat tumors but has now been superseded by other radioisotopes, such as cobalt 60 and cesium 137. It was also once used in some luminous paints until it was discovered that the radium caused leukemia and bone tumors in those using the paint.

Radius

The shorter of the two long bones of the forearm; the other is the *ulna*. The radius is the bone on the thumb side of the arm.

The shaft of the radius has a broad base that articulates with the lower end of the ulna and with the upper bones of the wrist. The disk-shaped head of the radius, which is smaller than the base, articulates with the lower end of the *humerus* (the bone of the upper arm) to form part of the elbow joint.

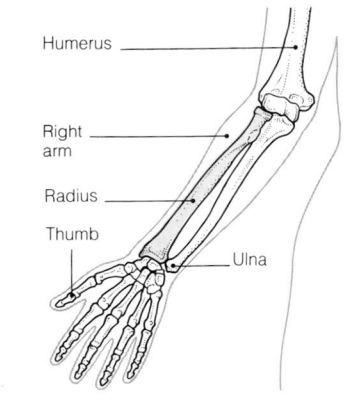

LOCATION OF THE RADIUS
The radius is the bone on the inside of the forearm with the palm facing down, or on the outside with the palm facing up.

Humerus

Right arm

Radius

Thumb

Ulna

The radius takes most of the strain when weight is placed on the wrist and is a common site of fractures (see *Radius, fracture of*; *Colles' fracture*). A fall or blow sometimes causes dislocation of the radius from the elbow joint along with fracture of the ulna, a condition known as *Monteggia's fracture*.

Radius, fracture of

Fractures of the *radius* are among the most common of fractures and are usually caused by a fall on an outstretched hand.

Fracture of the radius just above the wrist is the most common of all fractures in people over 40. It is usually caused by falling on the palm, resulting in backward displacement of the wrist and hand (see *Colles' fracture*).

Fracture of the disk-shaped head of the bone just below the elbow joint is one of the most common fractures in young adults. Treatment consists of immobilizing the forearm (bent at a right angle to the upper arm) and the

elbow in plaster to allow the fracture to heal. If the head of the bone is crushed or splintered, it may require removal by surgery before it is immobilized in a cast.

Fracture of the shaft of the radius often results in displacement of the bone ends. An operation is usually required to reposition the bone ends and fix them together with wires or plates and screws, but sometimes the bones can be externally manipulated back into position. In both cases, the limb is finally immobilized using a plaster cast.

Radon

A colorless, odorless, tasteless, radioactive gaseous element produced by the radioactive decay of *radium*. Radon has three naturally occurring isotopes (varieties of the element that are chemically identical but differ in some physical properties)—radon 219, radon 220, and radon 222. Each of these is short-lived (radon 219 has a *half-life* of roughly 4 seconds, radon 220 of about 51 seconds, and radon 222 of about 3.8 days). They disintegrate—with the emission of *radiation* (in the form of alpha particles)—to form solid radioactive materials known as radon daughters, which themselves emit alpha and beta particles and gamma rays. In addition to radon's naturally occurring radioisotopes, more than a dozen artificial ones have been produced.

The parent sources of radon occur naturally in many materials, such as soil, rocks, and building materials, and the gas is released continually into the atmosphere. As a result, radon makes the largest single contribution to radiation doses received by humans from naturally radioactive materials. This fact has led some researchers to suggest that radon may be a significant causative factor in some cases of cancer (particularly lung cancer). However, this claim has yet to be tested scientifically.

Ranitidine

An *ulcer-healing drug*, similar to *cimetidine* and *famotidine*, belonging to the *histamine-2 receptor antagonist* group of drugs. Ranitidine is used to prevent and treat *peptic ulcers* and to treat peptic *esophagitis*.

Ranitidine and famotidine are less likely to interact with other drugs or to produce any major side effects. Possible minor side effects include headache, skin rash, nausea, constipation, and lethargy.

Rape

Forcible sexual intercourse with an unwilling partner.

Rape is a felony in every state. While the statutory definition may be expressed somewhat differently by the legislature of each state, the elements of the offense are essentially the same. Rape is defined as sexual intercourse by the use or threat of force or violence and against the victim's will or without the victim's consent.

In some states, the term aggravated sexual assault (including penetration of any body orifice without consent) is used instead of rape. In certain states, the law recognizes some forms of rape in marriage.

While rape has traditionally been considered to be an offense committed by a man against a woman, many states have amended their laws to remove the gender identification and to expand the scope of the law to include homosexual rape and other sexual offenses, such as incest.

Society, police, and the courts are attempting to do more for rape victims and there is generally a greater understanding of the traumatic effects the crime can have on the victim. Studies have clarified the nature of the crime, revealing that, contrary to popular belief, rape most often occurs between people who know each other, is not always accompanied by physical violence, and is not provoked by a girl or woman.

INCIDENCE
In recent years, there has been a considerable increase in reported rape cases (see graph on next page). It is difficult to know whether these figures reflect a genuine increase in incidence or a greater willingness on the part of victims to report the crime. Nevertheless, rape is still one of the least reported of all crimes. It is estimated that 70 percent of rapes in the US are unreported due to the victim's shame, fear of family rejection, fear of reprisal by the rapist, or fear of the publicity and trauma associated with going through a trial.

MOTIVES
Rape is a violent crime motivated by a need to dominate the victim. The rapist may use forcible sex as one of many forms of abusive, dehumanizing behavior, being motivated by a profound hostility toward women.

Rarely is rape sexually motivated; rape is a crime of dominance and anger, not of passion. There is also evidence of a significant link between alcohol abuse and rape.

R

INCIDENCE OF REPORTED RAPE

Number of cases reported

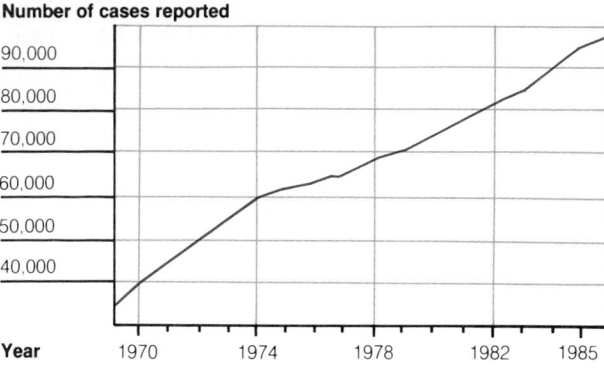

The graph shows the marked and alarming increase in rapes reported annually in the US since 1970. It is difficult to know whether the figures reflect a genuine increase in the incidence of rape or a greater willingness on the part of the victims to report the crime.

About 20 percent of rapists are reconvicted of sexual offenses; up to 80 percent subsequently commit other crimes and often have a long history of violent crime.

EFFECTS

The rape victim may suffer a variety of physical injuries, usually as a result of beating or choking. Severe injury to the genitals is rare, but there may be swelling of the labia, bruising of the vaginal walls or cervix, and, occasionally, tearing of the anus or perineum (area between the genitals and the anus).

Even in the absence of physical injury, the psychological effects of rape are often severe, including significant *anxiety, depression*, or *post-traumatic stress disorder*. Nightmares or daytime flashbacks of the event may also occur.

FORENSIC TESTS

The physician examining a rape victim performs a physical examination, noting signs of bruising or injury, particularly to the genital area. The examination includes inspection of the vaginal canal with a *speculum*. A woman is usually present to support the victim.

For laboratory analysis, the physician collects swabs from any suspected bite marks, from soiled areas of the body, and from the vagina, anus, or throat; fingernail scrapings or clippings; and any torn-out strands of head or pubic hair. These may be matched with samples of blood or saliva taken from suspects.

Clothing worn by the victim at the time of the assault is also retained for forensic examination.

TREATMENT

Physical injuries are treated as required. If conception results from the rape, elective *abortion* may be considered. Treatment for sexually transmitted disease may be required in some cases.

For psychological trauma, rape crisis counseling is highly beneficial. Psychiatric support may also be needed. Help is readily available today, often from rape support groups in most community hospitals through the social work department.

PREVENTION

There are a number of important ways to reduce the incidence of rape. First, rape cases should be moved quickly and effectively through the reporting, arrest, and trial process so that violent criminals are quickly removed from society. It must be clear to victims that they will be dealt with fairly and sympathetically by police and the court system. Rape victim advocacy groups have been established in many areas of the country to provide counseling and support to victims. Women's shelters can provide a temporary place to live, since many women need shelter from a current or previous partner who has become abusive.

Children should be told that there are people who may harm or hurt them due to their mixed-up sexual feelings. They should be instructed never to go into cars, alleys, or secluded places without permission.

True prevention may require more basic and complex changes. While society's emphasis on male machismo is no excuse for committing violent crimes, eliminating the concept of women as sexual objects (rather than as sexual partners) would help. There has also been a "blame the victim" mentality toward rape victims that must be eliminated; the onus must be placed solely on the perpetrator.

There is a place for assertiveness training and self-defense training for women. Although it is in no way the victim's fault that she is molested, learning assertive behavior patterns and even self-defense techniques can head off an attacker. Some of the best approaches teach women common-sense tips, such as how to recognize whether someone is testing you to see if you would make a good victim.

Rash

A group of spots or an area of red, inflamed skin. A rash is usually temporary and only rarely is a sign of a serious underlying problem. It may be accompanied by itching or fever.

TYPES

A rash may be localized (affecting only a small area of the skin) or generalized (covering the entire body). Physicians also describe rashes as blistering (either bullous or vesicular), macular,

AGE WHEN VICTIMIZED BY RAPE

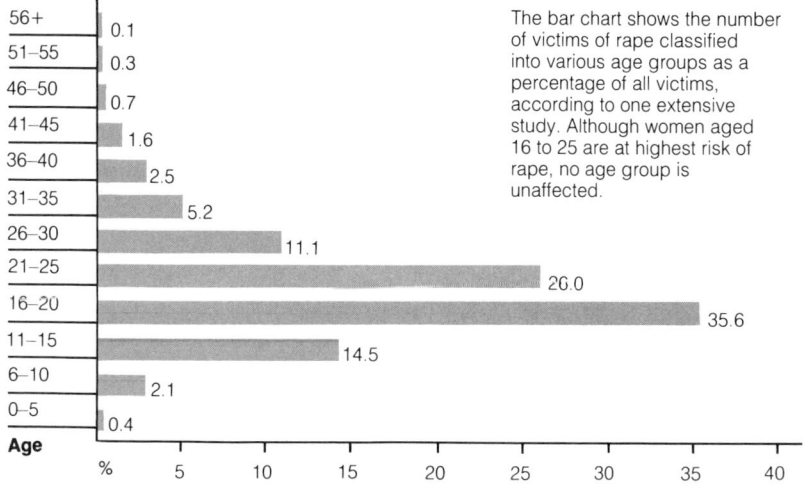

The bar chart shows the number of victims of rape classified into various age groups as a percentage of all victims, according to one extensive study. Although women aged 16 to 25 are at highest risk of rape, no age group is unaffected.

RASH WITH FEVER
Spots, discolored areas, or blisters on the skin combined with a temperature of 100°F (38°C) or above. The most likely cause is one of the childhood infectious diseases.

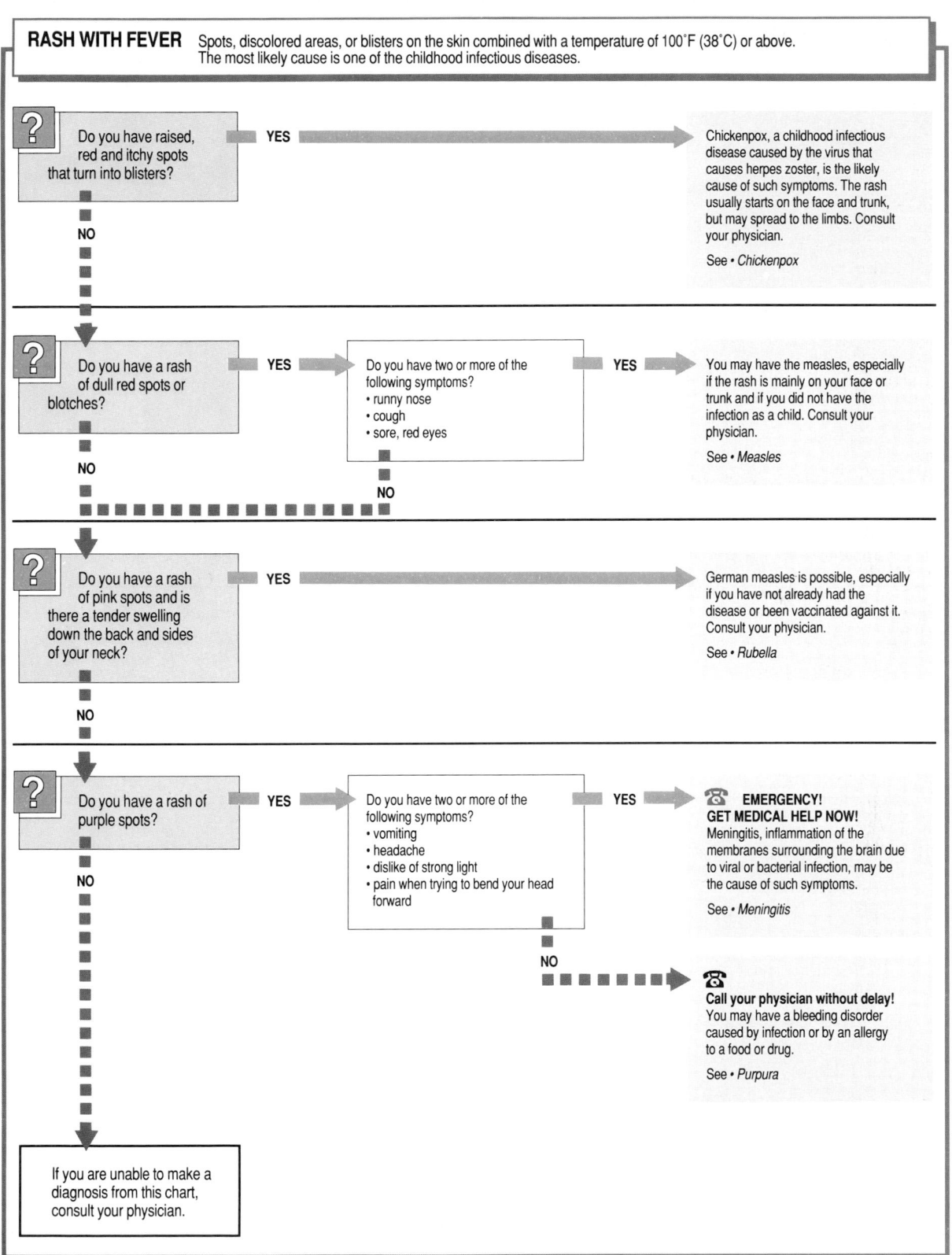

? Do you have raised, red and itchy spots that turn into blisters?

YES → Chickenpox, a childhood infectious disease caused by the virus that causes herpes zoster, is the likely cause of such symptoms. The rash usually starts on the face and trunk, but may spread to the limbs. Consult your physician.

See • *Chickenpox*

NO

? Do you have a rash of dull red spots or blotches?

YES → Do you have two or more of the following symptoms?
• runny nose
• cough
• sore, red eyes

YES → You may have the measles, especially if the rash is mainly on your face or trunk and if you did not have the infection as a child. Consult your physician.

See • *Measles*

NO

NO

? Do you have a rash of pink spots and is there a tender swelling down the back and sides of your neck?

YES → German measles is possible, especially if you have not already had the disease or been vaccinated against it. Consult your physician.

See • *Rubella*

NO

? Do you have a rash of purple spots?

YES → Do you have two or more of the following symptoms?
• vomiting
• headache
• dislike of strong light
• pain when trying to bend your head forward

YES → ☎ **EMERGENCY!**
GET MEDICAL HELP NOW!
Meningitis, inflammation of the membranes surrounding the brain due to viral or bacterial infection, may be the cause of such symptoms.

See • *Meningitis*

NO

NO → ☎
Call your physician without delay!
You may have a bleeding disorder caused by infection or by an allergy to a food or drug.

See • *Purpura*

If you are unable to make a diagnosis from this chart, consult your physician.

R

RASH WITH ITCHING Itchy spots or discolored and/or raised areas of itchy skin.

Do you have a red, flaky, or moist rash that fades away into the surrounding skin?

YES → Is the rash in a place where you have been wearing a new cosmetic or a new item of clothing or jewelry?

YES →

NO ↓

Could you have come into contact with a plant to which you may be sensitive, such as a primrose, or poison ivy, poison oak, or poison sumac?

YES →

This may be an allergic reaction to a substance with which the skin has come into contact. Consult your physician.

See • *Dermatitis*
 • *Eczema*

NO ↓

Is the rash only on your hands AND have you spent a lot of time working with detergents or other substances that might irritate the skin?

YES →

NO →

NO ↓

Do you have a raised, light red rash with clearly defined edges?

YES →

This may be an allergic reaction to something that has been ingested, such as shellfish, strawberries, or drugs. Such a rash may also occur when the skin is exposed to extremes of heat or cold. Consult your physician.

See • *Urticaria*

NO ↓

Do you have a widespread red rash that is particularly itchy at night?

YES →

Have you noticed tiny gray lines or red infected-looking spots between your fingers or on your wrists?

YES →

This may be due to a parasitic infection, particularly if you have been in close physical contact with someone who has the same problem. Consult your physician.

See • *Scabies*

NO ↓

NO ↓

Continued on next page

R

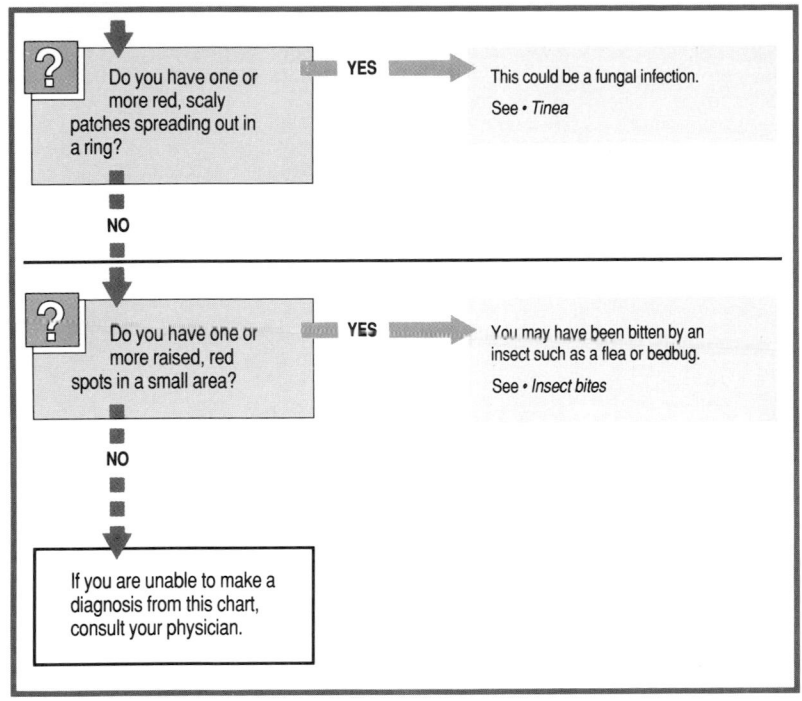

Do you have one or more red, scaly patches spreading out in a ring? **YES** → This could be a fungal infection. See • *Tinea*

NO

Do you have one or more raised, red spots in a small area? **YES** → You may have been bitten by an insect such as a flea or bedbug. See • *Insect bites*

NO

If you are unable to make a diagnosis from this chart, consult your physician.

nodular, papular, or pustular—according to the type of spots present.

CAUSES

A rash is the main sign of many childhood infectious diseases (such as *chickenpox* and *scarlet fever*) and of many other infections, ranging from ringworm (see *Tinea*) to *Rocky Mountain spotted fever*.

Rashes are a feature of many *skin disorders*, such as *eczema* and *psoriasis*. A rash may also indicate an underlying medical problem. Examples include the purple-red spots characteristic of *purpura* (a bleeding disorder); the rash of *scurvy* or *pellagra*, caused by vitamin deficiency; and the rashes appearing in *lupus erythematosus* and other *autoimmune disorders*.

The rashes of *urticaria* (hives) or of contact *dermatitis* may be caused by an allergic reaction to something that has been eaten or with which the skin has come in contact. Drug reactions, particularly to barbiturates and antibiotics, are also a common cause of rash.

DIAGNOSIS AND TREATMENT

The physician makes a diagnosis based on the appearance and distribution of the rash, the presence of any accompanying symptoms, and the possibility of allergy (e.g., to drugs).

Any underlying cause is treated if possible. An itching rash may be relieved by a soothing lotion or an *antihistamine drug*.

RAST

An abbreviation for radioallergosorbent test. RAST is a type of radioimmunoassay and is used to detect antibodies to specific allergens. (See *Immunoassay*.)

Rats, diseases from

 Rats are shy but potentially aggressive rodents that live close to human habitation; in many cities they outnumber humans. Rats damage and contaminate crops and food stores and can spread disease.

Various microorganisms harbored by rats can cause illness if spread to people. The organisms responsible for *plague* and one type of *typhus* are transmitted to humans by the bites of rat fleas. *Leptospirosis* (Weil's disease) is caused by contact with anything (usually water) contaminated with rat's urine. Rat-bite fever is a rare infection, transmitted directly by a rat bite. Either of two types of bacterium may be responsible. Symptoms may include inflammation at the site of the bite and of nearby lymph nodes and vessels, bouts of fever, a rash, and, in one type, painful joint inflammation. Antibiotics are effective in treating either type of infection.

Effective control of urban rat populations is important in the prevention of rat-borne epidemic diseases.

Raynaud's disease

A disorder of the blood vessels in which exposure to cold causes the small arteries that supply the fingers and toes to contract suddenly. This action cuts off blood flow to the digits, which become pale. The fingers, usually on both hands, are more often affected than the toes. Young women are the most commonly affected.

When the symptoms develop with no known cause, the disorder is called Raynaud's disease. When symptoms are secondary to some other condition, the disorder is termed *Raynaud's phenomenon*; it may have more serious long-term consequences.

SYMPTOMS AND SIGNS

On exposure to cold, the digits turn white because of lack of blood. As sluggish blood flow returns, the digits become blue; when they are warmed and normal blood flow is re-established, they turn red. During an attack, there is often a feeling of tingling, numbness, or burning in the affected fingers or toes.

In rare cases, the walls of the arteries gradually thicken, permanently reducing blood flow and eventually leading to painful ulceration or even to *gangrene* (tissue death) at the tips of the affected digits.

DIAGNOSIS AND TREATMENT

The condition is diagnosed from the patient's history. A person with Raynaud's disease should keep the hands and feet as warm as possible. Cigarette smokers should stop because smoking further constricts the arteries. *Vasodilator drugs* may be prescribed to relax the walls of the blood vessels. *Sympathectomy* (an operation in which the nerves that control the caliber of the arteries are cut) has been tried in severe cases.

Raynaud's phenomenon

A circulatory disorder affecting the fingers and toes marked by the same mechanism, symptoms, and signs as those of *Raynaud's disease* but resulting from a known underlying disorder.

Possible causes of the condition include arterial diseases (such as *Buerger's disease, atherosclerosis, embolism,* and *thrombosis*); connective tissue diseases (e.g., *rheumatoid arthritis, scleroderma,* and systemic *lupus erythematosus*); and various drugs (such as *ergotamine, methysergide,* and *beta-blocker drugs*). Raynaud's phenomenon is a recognized occupational disorder of people who use pneumatic drills, chain saws, or other vibrating machinery; it is sometimes seen in

R

TYPES OF RECEPTOR

Sensory receptors (below) are the free endings of sensory nerve cells—or special structures forming the endings of these cells. They respond to specific stimuli (such as light of a certain wavelength) and send a signal indicating the presence of the stimulus to the spinal cord and/or the brain.

Cell surface or chemical receptors (right) are tiny structures on the outer surface of a cell. They allow certain chemicals to bind to the cell and trigger some change within it.

Skin receptors
The skin contains many types of receptor that respond to stimuli such as pressure, cold, heat, and hair movement, allowing the sensations of touch, temperature, and pain. They include such structures as pacinian corpuscles and Merkel's disks and are all special types of nerve cell ending.

- Hair shaft
- Merkel's disk
- Meissner's corpuscle
- Pacinian corpuscle
- Organ of Ruffini
- Subcutaneous fat

HOW CELL SURFACE OR CHEMICAL RECEPTORS WORK
Most cells have many surface receptors (only one is shown below). Their existence allows the activity of the cell to be influenced from outside.

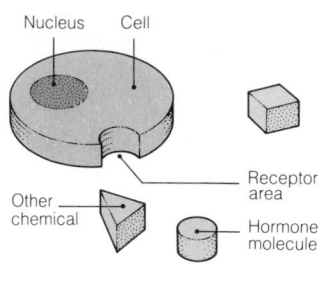

- Nucleus
- Cell
- Receptor area
- Other chemical
- Hormone molecule

1 A receptor allows only one specific chemical—which may be a hormone, or a neurotransmitter substance—to bind to it. The chemical must have a configuration that "fits" the receptor.

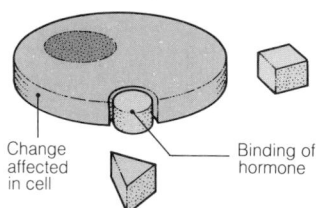

- Change affected in cell
- Binding of hormone

2 The binding of chemical to receptor alters the outer cell membrane and triggers a change—such as contraction of a muscle cell or increased activity of an enzyme-producing cell.

Receptors in tongue

Each taste bud (below) consists of many receptor cells. Each has surface receptors that respond to chemicals in food.

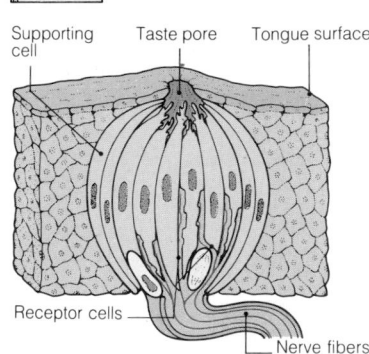

- Supporting cell
- Taste pore
- Tongue surface
- Receptor cells
- Nerve fibers

Receptors in eye
The retina, located at the back of the eye, contains receptor cells, called rods and cones, which are responsive to light.

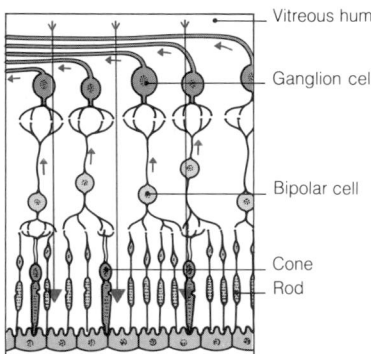

- Vitreous humor
- Ganglion cell
- Bipolar cell
- Cone
- Rod

typists, pianists, and others whose fingers suffer repeated trauma.

Treatment is the same as for Raynaud's disease, along with treatment of the underlying disorder.

Reagent
A general term for any chemical substance that takes part in a chemical reaction. The term usually refers to a chemical (or mixture of chemicals) used in chemical analysis or employed to detect a biological substance.

Receding chin
Underdevelopment of the lower jaw. The condition can be corrected by *cosmetic surgery* in one of three ways—lengthening each side of the jaw by inserting a wedge of bone into it, increasing the bulk of the bone at the front of the chin by a bone graft, or implanting a plastic bone substitute at the front of the chin.

Receptor
A general term for any sensory nerve cell—that is, one that converts stimuli into nerve impulses (see box).

The term receptor is also used to refer to a specific area on the surface of a cell with a characteristic chemical and physical structure. Many natural body chemicals must bind to receptors on cells to exert their effects. For example, epinephrine binds to three different types of receptors (called alpha-, beta$_1$-, and beta$_2$-receptors) that are found on the cells of organs such as the heart and lungs.

Recombinant DNA
A section of genetic material (*DNA*) from one organism that has been artificially spliced into the existing DNA of another organism, often a viral or bacterial cell. The new section may be the genetic code for a hormone such as insulin. If the recipient cell can be encouraged to multiply, large amounts of the hormone can be obtained. See also *Genetic engineering*.

Reconstructive surgery
See *Arterial reconstructive surgery*; *Plastic surgery*.

Recovery position
The correct position in which to place a casualty who is breathing, while waiting for help to arrive (see box).

FIRST AID: THE RECOVERY POSITION

DO NOT:
- Leave an unconscious victim alone.
- Put the victim into the recovery position if you suspect fractures to the neck or spine.

1 Turn the victim's head toward you, tilting it back, to open the airway.

2 Put the arm nearest you by the victim's side and slide it under his or her buttock.

3 Lay the other arm across the chest and cross the leg farthest from you over the near one at the ankle.

4 Grasp clothing at the hip farthest from you with one hand and support the head with the other. Pull the victim toward you to rest against your knees.

5 Bend the uppermost arm and leg to support the body and stop the victim from rolling onto his or her face. The other arm should now be free. Readjust the head to make sure it is tilted well back and check to see if the airway is clear.

Rectal bleeding

Bleeding from the rectum or anal canal. The blood may range from bright red to dark brown or black. It may be mixed with (or on the surface of) feces or passed separately and it may or may not be accompanied by pain. Rectal bleeding requires investigation by a physician.

CAUSES

The type of bleeding often gives a clue to its origin. *Hemorrhoids* are the most common cause of rectal bleeding in the form of small amounts of bright red blood found on the surface of the feces or on toilet paper. *Anal fissure, anal fistula, proctitis,* or *rectal prolapse* may also cause this type of bleeding.

Some disorders of the colon, such as *diverticular disease,* may cause dark red feces. Cancer of the intestine (see *Intestine, cancer of*), cancer of the rectum (see *Rectum, cancer of*), or polyps can also cause bleeding. Bloody diarrhea may be due to *ulcerative colitis, amebiasis,* or *shigellosis.*

Bleeding high in the digestive tract, usually from a *peptic ulcer,* may cause *melena* (black, tarry feces).

DIAGNOSIS

The physician may be able to make a diagnosis by *rectal examination. Proctoscopy, sigmoidoscopy, colonoscopy,* and air-contrast *barium X-ray examination* may also be performed.

Rectal examination

Examination of the anus and rectum, performed to assess symptoms and to check for the presence of tumors of the rectum or prostate.

A rectal examination is performed as a part of a physical examination or when a person reports abdominal or pelvic pain, or a change in bowel habits. It may also be performed if a man complains of urological symptoms and, sometimes (along with a pelvic examination), if a woman has gynecological problems.

The patient usually lies on his or her left side, with the knees bent toward the chest. (The prostate may be examined while the patient stands bending at the waist.) The physician inserts a gloved, lubricated finger into the rectum to feel for any tenderness or abnormalities, such as ulcers or growths, and to examine the prostate or cervix, which can be felt through the rectum.

Rectal prolapse

Protrusion outside the anus of the lining of the rectum, usually brought on by straining to defecate. The condition

R

causes discomfort, a discharge of mucus, and rectal bleeding.

In infants and young children, prolapse is usually temporary. In elderly people it tends to be permanent because of weakening of the tissues that support the *perineum*. Rectal prolapse may occur along with prolapsing *hemorrhoids*. If the rectal prolapse is large, leakage of feces may be a problem.

In younger people, a fiber-rich diet may be all that is necessary. Older people may undergo surgery, which is not uniformly successful.

Rectocele

A protrusion into the back of the vaginal wall caused by the rectum pushing against weakened tissues in the vaginal wall. It is usually associated with a *cystocele* (protrusion of the bladder into the front wall of the vagina) or with a prolapsed uterus (see *Uterus, prolapse of*).

Depending on its size, a rectocele may cause no symptoms or may lead to constipation by interfering with muscle contraction in the rectum.

Exercises to strengthen the muscles of the pelvic floor may help relieve symptoms (see *Pelvic floor exercises*). If they do not, surgery may be attempted to tighten the tissues at the back of the vagina to improve support to the rectum.

Rectum

A short, muscular tube that forms the lowest part of the large intestine and connects it to the *anus*. Feces collect in the rectum before defecation.

STRUCTURE

Like the rest of the colon, the very first part of the rectum consists of four layers—the outermost serous layer; the muscular layer; the submucous layer; and the innermost mucous layer, which lubricates the rectum. There is no serous layer in the last 3 to 4 inches (8 to 10 cm) of the rectum.

FUNCTION

The urge to defecate occurs when feces distend the rectum. Pressure on the rectal wall causes nerve impulses to pass to the brain, which, under voluntary control, sends messages to the muscles in the anus to relax, permitting defecation.

DISORDERS

In rare cases, a baby is born with no rectum or anus (see *Anus, imperforate*).

Disorders of the colon may also affect the rectum. They include inflammation (see *Proctitis*), *polyps* (noncancerous, grapelike growths),

STRUCTURE OF THE RECTUM

The rectum is 6 to 8 inches long. Its wall consists mainly of longitudinal and circular muscle; an inner, mucous layer provides lubrication.

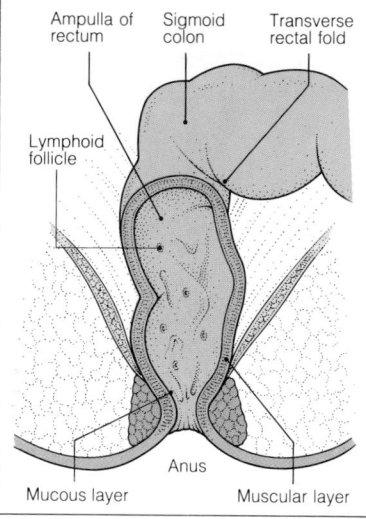

Ampulla of rectum · Sigmoid colon · Transverse rectal fold · Lymphoid follicle · Anus · Mucous layer · Muscular layer

familial *polyposis* (a condition characterized by numerous polyps that usually become cancerous), and cancer (see *Rectum, cancer of*).

The rectum can become obstructed as a result of narrowing caused by *radiation therapy*, *granuloma inguinale* (a sexually transmitted disease), or pelvic infection. Rarely, an ulcer develops in the rectum, causing bleeding and discharge. Similar symptoms may result from injury to the rectum due to anal intercourse or the insertion of foreign objects.

Rectal prolapse occurs when the lining of the rectum protrudes outside the anus. In a *rectocele*, the rectum and rear wall of the vagina are displaced downward into the vagina.

Rectal disorders are usually diagnosed by physical examination (see *Rectal examination*) and by *proctoscopy* or *sigmoidoscopy* (examination with a viewing tube).

Rectum, cancer of

A malignant tumor in the muscular tube that forms the lower part of the colon (large intestine).

CAUSES AND INCIDENCE

The cause of this cancer is unknown, but dietary and genetic factors are thought to play a part in its development (see *Intestine, cancer of*). Certain

diseases of the colon (e.g., familial *polyposis* and *ulcerative colitis*) increase the risk of colorectal cancer.

Colorectal cancer is responsible for about 20 percent of all cancer deaths in the US. Rectal cancer accounts for one fourth to one third of tumors of the large intestine; it is more common between the ages of 50 and 70.

SYMPTOMS

The earliest symptom may be rectal bleeding during defecation; blood may appear in the feces. There may also be a change in bowel habits—diarrhea or constipation—and a sensation of incomplete emptying of the bowel. Later, pain may occur. Untreated, the cancer eventually may cause severe bleeding and pain and block the intestine, preventing the passage of feces. It may also spread to other organs in the pelvis and to other sites, such as the liver.

DIAGNOSIS

A physician can often detect rectal cancer by an examination with a gloved finger. The diagnosis is confirmed by *proctoscopy* or *sigmoidoscopy* (examination of the rectum with a rigid or flexible viewing tube) and *biopsy* (removal of a sample of tissue for analysis).

TREATMENT

In most cases surgery is performed. If the tumor is in the uppermost part of the rectum, the abdomen is opened, the upper rectum and descending colon are removed, and the two ends are sewn together. To promote healing of the joined bowel, a temporary *colostomy* (which diverts feces through a surgical opening in the abdomen) may be performed.

If the growth is in the lower rectum, the colon is cut through above the rectum, an incision is made around the anus, and the entire rectum and anus are removed. The wound is closed and, because there is no longer any outlet for the feces, a permanent colostomy is created.

Both operations take two to three hours to perform. Patients who have undergone surgery are examined at regular intervals to ensure that the tumor has not reappeared or spread to other parts of the body.

In elderly or generally sick people unable to undergo major surgery, *diathermy* (the application of high-frequency electric current) may be used to destroy the surface of the tumor and control local symptoms. Other forms of treatment when surgery is not possible are *radiation therapy* and, less commonly, *anticancer drugs*.

OUTLOOK

The long-term outlook depends on how far the tumor has spread before treatment takes place. About 50 percent of all people operated on for rectal cancer are alive three years later and almost 40 percent ten years later. Survival rates are considerably higher when the disease is diagnosed and treated early.

Red eye

Another name for *conjunctivitis*.

Reducing

See *Weight reduction*.

Reduction

The process of manipulating a displaced part of the body back to its original position. Reduction may be carried out to realign fractured bone ends (see *Fracture*), to replace a dislocated joint in its socket (see *Dislocation, joint*), or to treat a *hernia* by pushing the protruding intestine back through the abdominal wall.

Referred pain

Pain felt in a part of the body at some distance from its cause. Referred pain occurs because some apparently remote parts of the body are served by the same nerve or the same nerve root (group of nerves that joins the spinal cord at one point). Nerve impulses reaching the brain from one of these areas may be misinterpreted as coming from the other (see *Pain*).

Common examples of referred pain are the pain down the inside of the left arm caused by *angina pectoris* or *coronary thrombosis*; the pain felt in the tip of the shoulder from irritation of the diaphragm; the pain felt in a testis when the ureter is stretched by a urinary tract *calculus*; and the pain felt in the leg or foot from compression in the spine by a *disk prolapse*.

Reflex

An action that occurs automatically and predictably in response to a particular stimulus, independent of the will of the individual. Both the sensing of the stimulus and initiation of the action are carried out by components of the nervous system.

In the simplest reflex, a sensory nerve cell, perhaps at the skin surface, reacts to a stimulus such as heat or pressure. It sends a signal along its nerve fiber to the central nervous system (brain or spinal cord). There, the end of the fiber connects to another nerve cell, which becomes

stimulated in turn. Activity in this second cell then causes a muscle to contract or a gland to increase its secretory activity. The passage of the nerve signal from original sensation to final action is called a reflex arc.

Sometimes the reflex is more complicated. Sensory signals may be sent from thousands of sensory receptors to groups of nerve cells within the central nervous system. Complex analysis of these signals may be carried out before responses are initiated.

INBORN REFLEXES

Many reflexes are inborn, including those that control basic body functions. Examples include shivering automatically in response to cold, increased breathing in response to a rise in carbon dioxide in the blood, and contraction of the bladder to expel urine once it has filled beyond a certain point.

The part of the nervous system that is concerned with these processes is called the *autonomic nervous system*. Parts of the *brain stem* and the *hypothalamus* in the forebrain are processing centers for the system. Some autonomic system reflexes are under partial voluntary (willed) control—emptying of the bladder can be voluntarily delayed. Ultimately, however, reflex is stronger than will.

Simple knee-jerk reflex
A tap with a rubber hammer just below the kneecap stretches a tendon of one of the thigh muscles. A signal passes via a sensory neuron (nerve cell) to the spinal cord, activating a motor neuron, which contracts the muscle, jerking the lower leg upward.

Some inborn reflexes occur only in babies (see *Reflex, primitive*). An example is the grasp reflex when a finger is placed in the palm.

Any physical examination usually includes testing some simple, inborn reflexes, such as the knee jerk, plantar reflex (irritation of the sole of the foot causes the toes to curl), and pupil constriction in response to light. Changes in these reflexes may indicate damage to the nervous system. Part of a complete neurological examination may also include the testing of several other reflexes.

The examination of vital reflexes controlled by the brain stem is the basis for diagnosing *brain death*.

CONDITIONED REFLEXES

Reflexes acquired (rather than inborn) as a result of experience are called conditioned reflexes. They result from the formation of new pathways and connections within the nervous system during life. The process by which these reflexes are acquired is called *conditioning*. One type, operant conditioning, is a particularly important process in *learning*. Once a satisfactory response to a new situation has been discovered (often by a process of trial and error) and repeated several times, it is eventually automatically elicited by that situation or stimulus and thus becomes a sort of reflex. For example, a person walking home from work may follow a familiar route without needing to make any conscious effort to do so.

Reflex, primitive

An automatic movement in response to a stimulus; it is present in newborn infants but disappears during the first few months. Primitive reflexes are thought to represent actions that may have been important for survival in earlier stages of our evolution.

Because some of these reflexes can give an indication of the condition of an infant's nervous system, they are tested by the pediatrician at the first examinations after birth. Any abnormality of the primitive reflexes may indicate a nervous system disorder.

The main primitive reflexes are the grasp reflex, Moro's reflex, the tonic neck reflex, the walking or stepping reflex, and the rooting reflex (see chart on next page).

Reflux

An abnormal backflow of fluid in a body passage due to failure of the passage's muscle to close fully. The most common types of reflux are

R

TYPES OF PRIMITIVE REFLEX

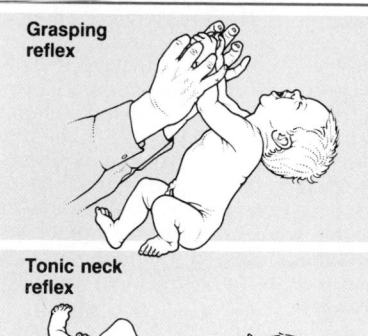

Grasping reflex

Certain automatic reflexes are present early in life before the baby becomes capable of voluntary movement. These reflexes disappear as the nervous system matures. For about the first four months, any object placed in the infant's palm will be firmly grasped.

Tonic neck reflex

When the very young baby turns the head to one side, the arm and leg on that side are stretched out and the arm and leg on the opposite side bend. This reflex normally disappears after the first week, except in premature babies. A strong reflex suggests brain damage.

Walking reflex

When the baby is held upright with the feet touching the ground, a forward stepping movement is made by each leg as the weight is placed on the other foot. This occurs during the first two months of life, and then is lost. It returns at about the age of 6 months.

Moro's reflex

If the baby's head is momentarily left unsupported, the arms will be swung outward and then brought together in an embracing movement. At the same time the legs are extended and the baby cries. This symmetrical reflex should persist for three or four months.

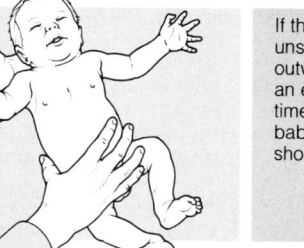

Rooting reflex

This reflex enables the baby to find the nipple; it is evoked by touching the baby's cheek with the fingertip near the corner of the mouth. The head turns so that the finger can enter the mouth. The reflex is best shown if tried near the normal feeding time.

regurgitation of acid fluid from the stomach into the esophagus (see *Acid reflux*) and the backflow of urine from the bladder into one or both ureters. Persistent urinary reflux may lead to kidney damage (see *Nephropathy*).

Refraction

The bending of light rays as they pass from one substance to another. In the eye, refraction provides the mechanism by which an image is focused on the retina, thereby permitting vision.

The term is also used to describe the testing of the eye to determine whether there is any refractive error, such as *myopia*, *hyperopia*, or *astigmatism* (see *Vision tests*).

Regenerative cell therapy

A treatment that claims to revitalize the skin. One such technique—developed in the 1930s and still popular—involves the injection of preparations made from a mixture of animal endocrine glands. Similar claims have been made for skin creams containing sex hormones or animal placentas. There is no evidence that any of these treatments works.

Regression

A term used in *psychoanalytic theory* to describe the process of returning to a childhood level of behavior. Sigmund Freud suggested that humans progress psychologically through various stages of development from infancy to adulthood. Disturbed people, though superficially mature, may be unconsciously fixated at an earlier level. When frustrated or under stress, they undergo regression to immature forms of behavior, such as thumb-sucking or exposing the genitals. (See also *Fixation*.)

Regurgitation

A backflow of fluid. The term is used in medicine to describe the return of swallowed food or drink from the stomach back into the mouth. Regurgitation is very common in babies immediately after feeding, when some of the milk is brought up with gas. Acid juices may also be regurgitated from the stomach into the mouth (see *Acid reflux*).

Regurgitation also describes the backflow of blood through a heart valve that has not closed fully because of a disorder such as *mitral insufficiency* or *aortic insufficiency*. (See also *Reflux*.)

Rehabilitation

Treatment aimed at enabling a person to live an independent life following injury, illness, or drug or alcohol dependence (see *Alcohol dependence*; *Drug dependence*). Treatment may include *physical therapy*, *occupational therapy*, and *psychotherapy*.

Rehabilitation is often carried out in centers, some of which are residential, where people from different specialties work together to assess the severity of an individual's *disability* or dependence and develop a tailor-made treatment program. Industrial rehabilitation centers provide job retraining for people who are unable to return to their previous employment. Drug and alcohol rehabilitation centers help people through the period of withdrawal and provide psychological support to reduce the risk of relapse.

Rehydration therapy

The treatment of *dehydration* by the administration of fluids and salts by mouth (oral rehydration) or by

R

intravenous infusion. The amount of fluid necessary depends on the person's age, weight, and on the degree of dehydration (amount of fluids lost).

In mild dehydration (common in young children who have *diarrhea*), rehydration can usually be carried out with solutions given by mouth. Oral rehydration preparations are available commercially in liquid form, or in powder or tablet form to be added to water. The simplest products contain only sodium chloride and glucose; others also include salts containing potassium and bicarbonate. Any unused solution should be discarded 24 hours after preparation.

If commercial preparations are not available, a homemade oral rehydration solution may be prepared by adding one half teaspoon of salt, 2 teaspoons of sugar, and one quarter of a teaspoon of sodium bicarbonate (baking soda) to 1 pint (0.47 liter) of boiled water.

In severe dehydration, or if the patient is unable to take fluids by mouth because of nausea or vomiting, an intravenous infusion of saline (sodium chloride) solution, glucose solution, or a combination of both, sometimes supplemented with potassium chloride, may be given in the hospital. Additional treatment may be necessary depending on the underlying condition.

Reimplantation, dental

Replacement of a tooth in its socket after an accident so that it can become reattached to supporting tissues. Front teeth are the most commonly involved. The alternative is to fill the gap with a false tooth or, if the jaws are still growing, to maintain the gap with an *orthodontic appliance*.

HOW IT IS DONE

The dentist rinses the tooth in a sterile solution, replaces it in the socket, and maintains it with a splint (see *Splinting, dental*), often for several weeks.

OUTLOOK

Successful reimplantation relies on replacing the tooth soon after the accident (ideally within 30 minutes). Keeping the tooth moist and sterile (for example, with saliva) also increases the chances of success.

Reiter's syndrome

A condition in which there is a combination of *arthritis* and *urethritis*; there may also be *conjunctivitis*. Reiter's syndrome is more common in men and is the most common cause of arthritis in young men.

CAUSES AND INCIDENCE

Reiter's syndrome usually develops after *nonspecific urethritis*; it affects about 2 percent of men with this disorder and may also occur after an attack of bacillary *dysentery*. Although Reiter's syndrome is induced by infection, it develops only in people with a genetic predisposition. About 80 percent of those with the syndrome have a certain tissue type (HLA-B27 positive; see *Histocompatibility antigens*).

SYMPTOMS AND SIGNS

Reiter's syndrome usually starts with a urethral discharge followed by conjunctivitis and then arthritis. The arthritis seldom affects more than one or two joints and is often associated with fever and malaise. The affected joints, commonly the knee or ankle, are warm, painful, and stiff, and the inflammation persists for periods varying from a few days to several months. Tendons and ligaments (especially the Achilles tendon) may also become inflamed, as may fibrous tissue in the soles of the feet. Skin rashes are common.

DIAGNOSIS AND TREATMENT

Diagnosis and treatment are based on the symptoms. *Analgesic drugs* and *nonsteroidal anti-inflammatory drugs* relieve pain and inflammation but may have to be taken for a long period. Antibiotics are of no value in treating the arthritis.

OUTLOOK

Relapses occur in about one third of cases, especially after more episodes of nonspecific urethritis.

Relapse

The recurrence of a disease after apparent recovery or the return of symptoms after a *remission*.

Relapsing fever

An illness caused by infection with spirochetes (spiral-shaped bacteria) transmitted to humans by ticks or lice and characterized by high fever.

CAUSES AND INCIDENCE

Ticks acquire the spirochetes by feeding on infected rodents. The spirochetes can survive in a population of ticks for years; they are transmitted to humans when the ticks bite. In the US, occasional cases of tick-borne relapsing fever occur in the southwestern and mountain states from Texas to Idaho. Louse-borne infection, transmitted from person to person, is rare in the US.

SYMPTOMS AND SIGNS

Relapsing fever starts with a sudden high fever—up to 104°F (40°C)—accompanied by shivering, headache, muscle pains, nausea and vomiting. The symptoms persist for three to six days, culminating in a crisis, with a risk of collapse and death. The affected person then returns to normal but, seven to 10 days later, suffers another attack. In tick-borne fever, several of these relapses, each progressively milder, are common.

DIAGNOSIS AND TREATMENT

A blood smear reveals the presence of the spirochetes. Relapsing fever can be effectively treated with an *antibiotic drug* (such as penicillin).

Relaxation techniques

Methods of consciously releasing muscular tension and achieving a state of mental calm.

WHY THEY ARE DONE

Relaxation techniques can benefit people who suffer from *anxiety* symptoms, can help to reduce *hypertension* (high blood pressure), and are a useful means of relieving the stress caused by a busy job or personal problems. They are taught in *prepared childbirth* classes to help pregnant women cope with the pain of labor.

TYPES

Active relaxation consists of (in turn) tensing and then relaxing all the muscles in the body, usually starting with the head and moving down to the feet. Passive relaxation may also be used. It involves clearing the mind of everything to concentrate on a single phrase or sound. In both techniques, control of the breathing rate is emphasized (see *Breathing exercises*), since *hyperventilation* (rapid, shallow breathing) often brings on or worsens anxiety. Taped instructions or *biofeedback training* may help to reinforce learning. Once mastered, the techniques can be put into practice in potentially stressful situations.

Traditional methods of concentration, such as *yoga* and *meditation*, employ similar techniques.

EFFECTIVENESS

Relaxation is a safe treatment; it may be useful in conjunction with other forms of therapy.

Rem

A unit of equivalent absorbed dose of ionizing radiation (see *Radiation* units box). Rem is an acronym for roentgen equivalent man.

Remission

A temporary diminution or disappearance of the symptoms of a disease, or the period during which this occurs.

R

Remissions occur in many long-term diseases; the most notable example is *multiple sclerosis*, which typically follows a pattern of alternating remissions and *relapses*. Initially, remissions may last months or years; however, they usually become shorter and may eventually disappear.

Renal

The medical term for anything related to the *kidney*.

Renal biopsy

A procedure in which a small portion of *kidney* tissue is removed and examined under a microscope. Renal *biopsy* is usually performed as part of the investigation and diagnosis of various kidney disorders, such as *glomerulonephritis, proteinuria, nephrotic syndrome*, or acute *renal failure*. It may also be used to assess the status of a *kidney transplant*. Percutaneous (through the skin) needle biopsy of the kidney may not be performed if the person has a bleeding disorder, only one functioning kidney, or chronic renal failure with small, contracted kidneys.

HOW IT IS DONE

The procedure for performing a percutaneous needle biopsy of the kidney is shown at right.

If a percutaneous needle biopsy is not advisable, an open end renal biopsy may be performed. Using general anesthesia, the surgeon makes a small incision in the flank to visualize the kidney and then cuts a small wedge of renal cortex (the biopsy specimen).

In both cases, the renal tissue is sent to a pathologist for examination under a light microscope, electron microscope, or immunofluorescent microscope (see *Microscope*).

RECOVERY PERIOD

The patient may have slight pain in the back for some hours after the biopsy and a small amount of blood may be passed in the urine. Provided there are no complications (such as severe bleeding), the patient can return home the following day.

Renal cell carcinoma

The most common type of kidney cancer (see *Kidney cancer*).

Renal colic

Intermittent spasms of severe pain on one side of the back, usually caused by a kidney stone (see *Calculus, urinary tract*). Each spasm usually lasts for several minutes.

Renal disorders

See *Kidney* disorders box.

Renal failure

The reduction in the ability of the *kidneys* to filter waste products from the blood and excrete them in the urine, to control the body's water and salt balance, and to regulate the blood pressure. The resultant buildup of waste products (and other chemical disturbances in the blood and tissues) leads to symptoms that vary in severity. This combination of symptoms is sometimes called uremia.

PERCUTANEOUS RENAL BIOPSY

This procedure is performed with a local anesthetic injected into the skin and tissues over the kidney; it is virtually painless. There is a risk of bleeding from the kidney into the abdominal cavity.

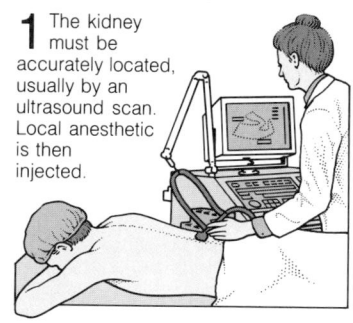

1 The kidney must be accurately located, usually by an ultrasound scan. Local anesthetic is then injected.

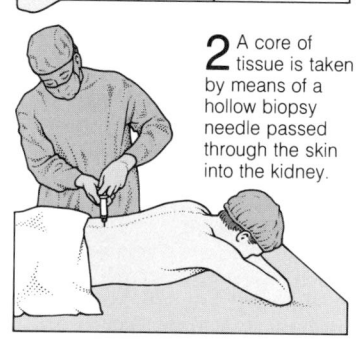

2 A core of tissue is taken by means of a hollow biopsy needle passed through the skin into the kidney.

Kidney glomerulus (filtering unit) as seen under microscope

3 The core of kidney tissue is embedded in wax and cut into thin slices, which are mounted on slides for staining and microscopic examination.

TYPES AND CAUSES

Renal failure can be acute (of sudden onset) or chronic (developing more gradually). In acute renal failure, kidney function usually returns to normal once the underlying cause has been discovered and treated; in chronic failure, function is usually irreversibly lost.

Acute renal failure most often occurs in people who have suffered a severe injury or are seriously ill with some other underlying condition and are suffering from physiological *shock*. Severe bleeding or burns can reduce blood volume and pressure to the extent that the supply of blood to the kidneys is dramatically reduced. A *myocardial infarction* (heart attack) or acute *pancreatitis* can have a similar effect. The kidneys are particularly susceptible to reduced blood flow, which can cause damage to their filtering units.

Obstruction to urine flow as a result of a stone (see *Calculus, urinary tract*), *bladder tumor*, or enlargement of the prostate gland can also cause acute renal failure, as can certain rapidly developing types of kidney disease, such as *glomerulonephritis* and *hemolytic-uremic syndrome*.

Chronic renal failure can result from any disease that causes progressive damage to the kidneys, such as *hypertension* (high blood pressure), *diabetes mellitus*, polycystic kidney disease (see *Kidney, polycystic*), or *amyloidosis* (see also *Kidney* disorders box). It can also result from excessive use of *analgesics* (painkillers) over several years.

Chronic renal failure may progress over months or years to an advanced, life-threatening condition called end-stage renal failure.

SYMPTOMS AND SIGNS

In acute renal failure, the most noticeable symptom may be a much reduced volume of urine. Production of less than a pint of urine per day is called *oliguria* and usually means that waste products are not being cleared effectively from the blood. Production of less than 50 ml (one ninth of a pint) in 24 hours is called *anuria* and results in a serious buildup of waste products. In some cases, however, the person passes normal amounts of urine despite the loss of the filtering and cleansing function; this is called nonoliguric acute renal failure. Within a short time of the development of acute renal failure, more symptoms (such as drowsiness, nausea, vomiting, and breathlessness) appear. In many cases, symptoms of the

R

underlying cause of failure (e.g., symptoms of shock such as pale skin and weak pulse) precede those of the renal failure itself.

Symptoms of chronic failure develop more gradually and may include nausea, loss of appetite, and weakness. Unless the progress of the kidney damage is slowed or arrested, symptoms of end-stage failure may appear (including severe lethargy, headache, vomiting, a furred tongue, unpleasant breath, intense, rashless skin itching, and, eventually, collapse, coma, and death).

COMPLICATIONS

Complications of acute renal failure may include infections such as pneumonia, bleeding into the stomach, and deep vein *thrombosis*. In chronic failure, complications may include high blood pressure (which is both a cause and result of kidney failure), *anemia*, *osteomalacia*, *hyperparathyroidism*, *neuropathy*, or *myopathy*. All result from various disturbances in blood chemistry.

DIAGNOSIS

A person with suspected renal failure should undergo *kidney function tests*, which include measuring the urea and creatinine (two waste products) in the blood; raised levels indicate renal failure. *Urinalysis* and blood pressure measurements are also performed. Unless there is an obvious cause of renal failure (such as severe bleeding), immediate testing is carried out to determine a cause. Techniques include examination of the urine sediment and the blood, intravenous *pyelography*, *renal biopsy*, *ultrasound scanning*, and *radionuclide scanning*.

TREATMENT

In acute renal failure, emergency treatment is given for any cause of shock, such as severe bleeding. Blood volume and pressure must be brought back to normal through saline *intravenous infusion* or *blood transfusions*. Surgery may be required for obstruction caused by stones or enlargement of the prostate gland. Treatment of other causes may be complex and sometimes controversial, but may include the use of *corticosteroid drugs* and other drugs (as is done for certain forms of *glomerulonephritis*). *Diuretic drugs* may also be given to improve urine flow and rid the body of excess fluid. In many cases of acute failure, temporary *dialysis* (artificial methods of removing waste products from the blood) may be required until the kidneys recover their function.

Dietary treatment is an important part of the treatment of all types of renal failure. The diet must be high in carbohydrates and low in protein (the main source of waste products) to reduce the work load on the kidneys; the salt content must also be controlled. Fluid intake is carefully balanced against urine output. If the patient has been taking certain drugs (whose breakdown products are removed from the blood by the kidneys), use of these drugs may be stopped or their dosages reduced.

If hypertension develops, drugs are prescribed to keep the blood pressure under control. In end-stage renal failure, long-term dialysis or, ideally, a *kidney transplant* is the only satisfactory form of treatment.

OUTLOOK

The outlook varies according to the cause of the failure and the patient's response to treatment. Most people with acute renal failure eventually make a full recovery, but some require a transplant or lifelong dialysis. In chronic failure, it may be several years before such measures are required. Well over half the people with end-stage renal failure that is treated by dialysis are able to lead comparatively normal lives for more than five years; a successful kidney transplant improves the outlook.

Renal transplant

See *Kidney transplant*.

Renal tubular acidosis

A condition in which the kidneys are unable to excrete normal amounts of acid generated by the body's *metabolism* (internal chemistry). In renal tubular acidosis, the blood is more acid than normal and the urine is less acid than normal.

The cause of the renal metabolism disorder is often unknown. Possible causes include kidney damage due to disease, drugs, or a genetic disorder. Renal tubular acidosis may lead to *osteomalacia* (softening of the bones), kidney stones (see *Calculus, urinary tract*), *nephrocalcinosis* (calcification of the kidney), and hypokalemia (an abnormally low level of potassium in the blood).

Sodium bicarbonate (to counteract the blood acidity) and potassium supplements may be prescribed.

Renin

An enzyme involved in the regulation of blood pressure. When blood pressure falls, the kidneys release renin, which converts an inactive substance called angiotensinogen to the protein *angiotensin* I (also inactive). This protein is then rapidly converted to an active form, angiotensin II, which constricts blood vessels and so increases blood pressure. In addition, angiotensin II stimulates the release of the hormone *aldosterone*, which also increases blood pressure.

Blood pressure can be lowered by drugs that affect the renin-angiotensin system (e.g., *beta-blocker drugs*, which inhibit the production of renin, and *ACE inhibitor drugs*, which interfere with its actions).

Renography

A type of *radionuclide scanning* used for investigation of the kidney. A radionuclide—either hippuran or pentetic acid—is injected into the bloodstream and passes through the kidney into the urine. Radiation counts are taken continuously during the procedure. The information is recorded graphically as a renogram (a curve of counts per second against time). Both kidneys are examined simultaneously so that a comparison can be made of their functions.

Renography is used when obstruction to the passage of urine is suspected. Normally, the radiation count rate increases rapidly for about 30 seconds after injection, rises more slowly for about five minutes, and then decreases as the radionuclide passes into the bladder. If obstruction is present, the radionuclide accumulates in the kidney and the count rate continues to rise, producing a differently shaped renogram.

Renography is performed quickly and painlessly; it utilizes only a small dose of radiation.

Reportable diseases

Medical conditions that must be reported by the physician responsible for the affected person to the local health authorities who, in turn, report some of them to the national *Centers for Disease Control*.

The notification of certain potentially harmful infectious diseases is important because it enables public health officers to take the necessary steps to control the spread of infection (e.g., by isolation or by offering *immunization* to contacts). Reporting also provides valuable statistics on the *incidence* and *prevalence* of a disease; they may be used in formulating health policies such as immunization programs or improvements in sanita-

R

INCIDENCE OF SOME REPORTABLE DISEASES IN US (per 100,000 population)

Disease	1950	1960	1970	1980	1985
Diphtheria	3.8	0.5	0.2	0.0	0.0
Poliomyelitis	22.0	1.8	0.0	0.0	0.0
Measles	211.0	245.4	23.2	6.0	1.2
Rubella	...	...	27.7	1.7	0.3
Tuberculosis	80.5	30.8	18.2	12.2	9.3
Pertussis	79.8	8.2	2.1	0.8	1.5
Syphilis	16.7	9.1	10.9	12.1	11.5
Gonorrhea	192.4	145.3	297.2	445.0	384.6
Viral hepatitis, types A and B*	...	23.1	31.9	21.2	20.9
Salmonellosis (excluding typhoid)	...	3.8	10.8	14.9	27.4

*Excluding New York City

Note the dramatic decline in the incidence of diphtheria, poliomyelitis, and measles since the 1950s, and the gentler decline of tuberculosis. The incidence of gonorrhea peaked in the late 1970s but may now be in decline. The incidence of pertussis has fluctuated in recent years around a low level. Meanwhile, other reportable diseases such as salmonellosis and AIDS have become more common.

tion. Examples of reportable infectious diseases are chickenpox, AIDS, hepatitis, tetanus, malaria, syphilis, and gonorrhea.

Some categories of disease other than infections must also be reported. These include some *birth defects* and certain types of *occupational disease*.

Reproduction, sexual
The process of producing a new generation to continue the existence of the species by the fusion of two cells from different individuals; this is achieved in humans by the fusion of one *sperm* and one *ovum*. This fusion, called *fertilization*, is achieved by *sexual intercourse* or *artificial insemination*.

Reproductive system, female
The organs that enable a woman to produce ova (eggs), to have *sexual intercourse*, to nourish a fertilized *ovum* until it has developed into a full grown *fetus*, and to give birth. Apart from the *vulva* (external genitalia), the female reproductive organs lie within the pelvic cavity.

Ova are released each month from the *ovaries*, two small egg-shaped glands. The glands also secrete sex hormones (see *Estrogen hormones; Progesterone hormones*), which control the reproductive cycle. Adjacent to each ovary is a *fallopian tube*, which carries ova to the *uterus*, a hollow, pear-shaped organ that is situated between the bladder and the rectum. If, on its journey along the fallopian tube, an ovum unites with a sperm, *fertilization* takes place.

Sperm travel upward through the *cervix* and uterus on their journey to the fallopian tubes. The cervix projects into the top of the *vagina*, a muscular passage that forms the lower part of the birth canal and that receives ejaculated sperm during sexual intercourse. Surrounding and protecting the opening of the vagina are the fleshy folds of the *vulva*.

Fertility, the normal functioning of the reproductive system, begins at *puberty* (when it is signaled by the onset of *menstruation*) and ceases at the time of the *menopause*.

Reproductive system, male
The organs that enable a man to have *sexual intercourse* and to fertilize ova (eggs) with *sperm*. Sperm and male sex hormones (see *Androgen hormones*) are produced in the *testes*, a pair of ovoid glands suspended in a pouch known as the *scrotum*. From each testis, sperm pass into an *epididymis*, a long coiled tube behind the testis, where they slowly mature and are stored.

Shortly before *ejaculation*, sperm are propelled from the epididymis into a long duct called the *vas deferens*, which carries the sperm to the seminal vesicles, a pair of sacs that lies behind the bladder. These sacs produce seminal fluid, which is added to the sperm to produce *semen*.

Semen travels from the vesicles along two ducts to the urethra, a tube that acts as a passage for urine and semen. The ducts pass through the *prostate gland*, a chestnut-shaped organ lying beneath the bladder and surrounding the upper urethra. The prostate produces secretions that are added to the semen.

TOP 20 REPORTABLE DISEASES IN US IN 1986

	No. of cases reported
Gonorrhea	900,868
Chickenpox	183,243
Salmonellosis (excluding typhoid fever)	49,984
Syphilis	27,883
Viral hepatitis, type B*	26,107
Viral hepatitis, type A*	23,430
Tuberculosis	22,768
Shigellosis	17,138
AIDS	12,932
Viral meningitis	11,374
Mumps	7,790
Measles	6,282
Pertussis	4,195
Viral hepatitis, non-A non-B	3,634
Amebiasis	3,532
Meningococcus infections	2,594
Encephalitis, primary	1,302
Malaria	1,123
Legionnaires' disease	948
Rocky Mountain spotted fever	760

*Excluding New York City.

R

FEMALE REPRODUCTIVE SYSTEM

Each month an ovum from one ovary is carried along the fallopian tube. If fertilized, it begins to divide and implants into the lining of the uterus to develop into an embryo. At birth, the baby is forced out via the cervix, the usually narrow passage that forms the neck of the uterus.

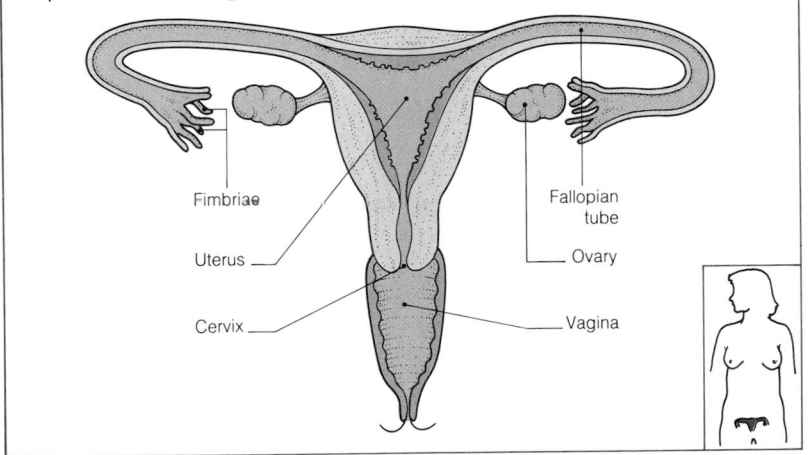

At *orgasm*, semen is ejaculated from the urethra through the erect *penis*, which is placed in the woman's vagina during sexual intercourse.

Resection

Surgical removal of all or part of a diseased or injured organ or structure. An anterior resection is an operation that removes part of the colon as a treatment for cancer.

Reserpine

An *antihypertensive drug*, derived from an Indian plant, used alone or with a *diuretic drug* in the treatment of *hypertension* (high blood pressure). Reserpine is also used in the long-term treatment of *Raynaud's disease* (a circulatory disorder).

Possible adverse effects include nasal congestion, dry mouth, *bradycardia* (slow heart beat), depression, lethargy, and nightmares.

Resident

A medical school graduate undergoing postgraduate training as a hospital staff member. A first-year resident used to be called an intern.

Resistance

A term that has several different medical usages. Blood vessels exert a dynamic resistance to the flow of blood. The resistance increases as the diameter of blood vessels decreases, whether due to normal physiological processes or narrowing as a result of disease. An increase in resistance leads to a rise in blood pressure backward from the narrowed vessels.

In *psychoanalysis*, resistance refers to the blocking off from consciousness of repressed material (e.g., memories or emotions). One task of the psychoanalyst is to help the patient break down this resistance.

Resistance may also refer to an ability to withstand attack from noxious agents (such as poisons, irritants, or microorganisms). A person's resistance to infection is called *immunity*; it varies according to age, nutritional and general health, the integrity of the person's *immune system*, and previous exposure to infective organisms.

Drug resistance refers to the ability of some microorganisms to withstand attack from previously effective drugs. Certain bacteria have acquired *genes* (units of hereditary material) that confer protection against specific antibiotics. Overuse of these antibiotics encourages the multiplication and spread of the resistant strains, which include some varieties of the organisms responsible for *gonorrhea*, *typhoid fever*, *salmonella* poisoning, *shigellosis* (bacterial dysentery), and other serious infections. In addition, some malarial parasites have become resistant to chloroquine, an important antimalarial drug.

When any dangerous infectious disease can no longer be treated with the established remedies, the situation is potentially serious. The development of new drugs has, to date, largely kept pace with the threat. Strategies to prevent the emergence of new resistant strains have included the cyclical use of different antibiotics to treat particular types of infection in hospitals (i.e., if a strain of bacteria resistant to one drug emerges, it is usually knocked out by the next drug in the cycle). Physicians are also learning to avoid indiscriminate use of antibiotic drugs, which encourages the emergence of resistance.

Resorption, dental

Loss of substance from a tooth. Resorption may be external (affecting the surface of the root) or internal (affecting the wall of the pulp cavity).

CAUSES AND INCIDENCE

External resorption of tooth roots, which causes the teeth to become

MALE REPRODUCTIVE SYSTEM

Sperm made in the testis pass via the vas deferens to the seminal vesicle. Secretions from the prostate increase the volume of the semen, which is ejaculated from the penis via the urethra during orgasm.

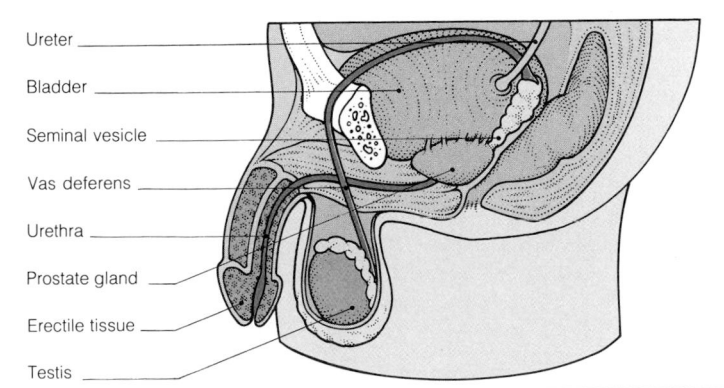

R

RESPIRATION

The function of respiration is to provide the energy needed by body cells. Cells obtain this energy mainly by metabolizing glucose with oxygen, so they require a constant supply of oxygen. In addition, the waste products of the metabolic process—mainly carbon dioxide—must be carried away from the cells.

Respiration includes the breathing of air into the lungs, the transfer of oxygen from the air to the blood, the transport of oxygen in the blood to the body cells, the metabolism of glucose with oxygen in the cells, and the transport of carbon dioxide to the lungs to be breathed out.

During exercise, respiration increases to compensate for higher energy demands by muscle cells.

Artery
Vein
Alveolus
Network of capillaries

1 Air, containing oxygen, is breathed into the lungs and enters the alveoli (tiny air sacs). Oxygen diffuses from the air into the blood vessels surrounding the alveoli.

Glucose $C_6H_{12}O_6$

Oxygen O_2

Carbon dioxide CO_2

Water H_2O

Energy

2 The oxygen-saturated blood passes from the lungs via the pulmonary veins to the left side of the heart.

CO_2 Carbon dioxide

O_2 Oxygen

Trachea

Lung

Alveoli

Pulmonary vein

Bronchiole

Aorta

Bronchus

Pulmonary artery

Left side of heart

Right side of heart

3 From the left side of the heart, the oxygenated blood is pumped via the aorta to the body tissues. The oxygen is carried within the blood by red cells.

O_2

CO_2

6 Carbon dioxide is carried back in the blood to the heart, then to the lungs, where it diffuses into the alveoli and is breathed out of the body.

5 Within body cells, glucose and oxygen take part in a complex series of reactions, which provides energy to power the cells. During this cellular respiration (left), glucose is converted to carbon dioxide and water.

Oxygen

Glucose

Blood

Carbon dioxide

Water

Tissues

4 As the blood passes through tissue capillaries, it gives up oxygen (and nutrients such as glucose) to the body tissues and cells and picks up the waste products of cellular respiration—carbon dioxide and water.

BREATHING VOLUMES

One way the body copes with varied demands for oxygen is through changes in breathing volume. The tidal volume—the amount breathed into and out of the lungs at each breath—may vary from 0.5 liter at rest, up to 4.5 liters (near the maximum or vital capacity) during heavy exercise.

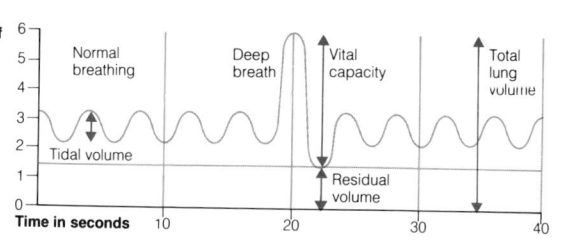

Volume of air in lungs (liters)

Normal breathing

Deep breath

Vital capacity

Total lung volume

Tidal volume

Residual volume

Time in seconds   10   20   30   40

loose, is part of the process by which *primary teeth* are shed. It is thought to be activated by pressure from the underlying *permanent teeth* as they erupt (see *Eruption of teeth*).

Some degree of external resorption, affecting the roots, occurs in most adults as part of the aging process. External resorption may also be caused by injury to a tooth, periapical *periodontitis* (inflammation of tissues around the root tip), or pressure from an *orthodontic appliance*, a tumor, or an impacted tooth. Completely impacted teeth occasionally undergo resorption of both the crown and the root.

The cause of internal resorption, which is a rare form of tooth resorption, occurring in about 1 percent of adults, is unknown. The condition sometimes spreads outward from the pulp cavity, producing a pink spot that shows through the crown.

DIAGNOSIS AND TREATMENT
Resorption is usually detected by taking *dental X rays*. Treatment of external resorption is of the underlying cause (such as removing an impacted tooth). Internal resorption can usually be successfully halted by *root-canal treatment*.

Respiration

A term for the processes by which oxygen reaches body cells and is utilized by them in metabolism and by which carbon dioxide is eliminated.

The various stages in respiration are illustrated in the box opposite. (See also *Metabolism*; *Respiratory system*.)

Respirator

See *Ventilator*.

Respiratory arrest

Sudden cessation of breathing. Respiratory arrest results from any process that severely depresses the function of the respiratory center in the brain. Causes include prolonged *seizures*, an overdose of *narcotic drugs*, *cardiac arrest*, *electrical injury*, serious *head injury*, *stroke*, or *respiratory failure*.

Respiratory arrest leads to *anoxia* (lack of oxygen to tissues) and, if untreated, to cardiac arrest, brain damage, coma, and death. These effects may occur within a few minutes. The victim should be given *artificial respiration* or placed on a *ventilator* without delay. The underlying cause is treated if possible.

Respiratory distress syndrome

A lung disorder that causes increasing difficulty in breathing; this results in a life-threatening deficiency of oxygen in the blood. The condition affects premature babies and adults whose lungs have been damaged by illness or injury. It is the most common cause of death in premature babies.

CAUSES AND INCIDENCE
Respiratory distress syndrome occurs in premature babies who are deficient in surfactant, a chemical that keeps open the *alveoli* in the lungs.

In adults, the disorder is caused by a stiffening of lung tissue associated with an increase of fluid in the interstitial (between the alveoli) part of the lungs. The many possible causes include severe *pneumonia*; inhaling vomit, an irritant gas (such as smoke or chlorine), or a high concentration of oxygen; partial drowning; an overdose of a narcotic drug, such as heroin or morphine; certain other drugs, among them nitrofurantoin; and certain *autoimmune disorders*.

SYMPTOMS AND SIGNS
The condition starts with an increase in breathing rate. Breathing then becomes labored and more rapid. Babies with respiratory distress syndrome make grunting noises and draw in the chest wall when they breathe. If the condition worsens, progressive deoxygenation of the blood makes the sufferer turn blue and eventually, if no treatment is given, death may result.

DIAGNOSIS AND TREATMENT
Respiratory distress syndrome is confirmed by listening to the lung with a stethoscope, by a *chest X ray*, and by analysis of *blood gases*. In adults, more tests may be needed to ensure that the heart is not malfunctioning.

Patients are treated in an *intensive-care* unit. In the early stages, oxygen is given by mask. If the condition does not worsen, this may be the only treatment required and is continued until the patient recovers. If respiratory distress increases, an *endotracheal tube* is inserted through the nose or mouth or a *tracheostomy* (insertion of a breathing tube into a hole made in the windpipe) performed; breathing is then maintained by a *ventilator*. Any underlying cause is treated if possible.

OUTLOOK
About 3 percent of premature babies die of respiratory distress syndrome. With modern intensive care, the survival rate for newborn babies with respiratory distress syndrome approaches 90 percent; for adults it is between 25 and 50 percent. However, some survivors are left with permanent lung damage.

Respiratory failure

A condition in which there is a buildup of carbon dioxide and a fall in the level of oxygen in the blood (see *Hypoxia*). Respiratory failure may be caused by any disorder that disrupts the normal transfer of gases in the blood, including lung disorders (such as *emphysema*, severe *asthma*, or chronic *bronchitis*). Failure may also be due to damage to the respiratory center in the brain from an overdose of *narcotic drugs*.

Symptoms include breathlessness, cough, cyanosis (blue discoloration of the skin), shallow breathing, an increased respiratory rate, and, less commonly, a reduced respiratory rate.

Respiratory failure usually requires *oxygen therapy*, in which a carefully controlled dose of oxygen is given. In severe cases, the patient must be placed on a *ventilator*. The underlying cause is also treated.

Respiratory function tests

See *Pulmonary function tests*.

Respiratory system

The organs responsible for carrying oxygen from the air to the bloodstream and for expelling the waste product carbon dioxide.

Air passes from the nose or mouth, via various respiratory passages, to millions of balloonlike sacs, the alveoli, in the lungs. Oxygen in the warmed and moistened inhaled air

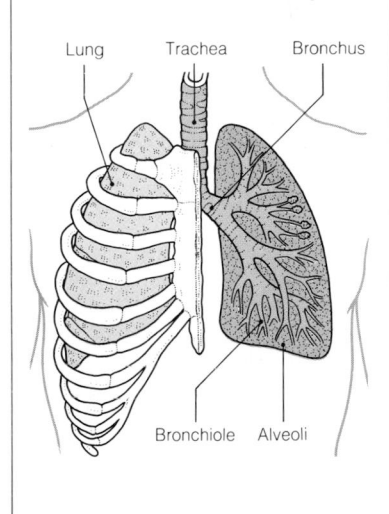

LOCATION OF THE RESPIRATORY SYSTEM
The system includes the upper air passages, lungs, and the muscles that control breathing.

Lung   Trachea   Bronchus

Bronchiole   Alveoli

R

passes through the thin walls of the alveoli into the bloodstream, and carbon dioxide passes from the blood into the alveoli to be breathed out (see *Respiration*).

Air is inhaled and exhaled by the actions of the chest muscles and diaphragm (see *Breathing*).

DISORDERS

Disorders of the respiratory system can affect the air passages (obstructing the passage of air into or out of the lungs) or the lung tissues (resulting in a poor exchange of oxygen and carbon dioxide). The functioning of the respiratory system can also be impaired by disorders, such as poliomyelitis, that affect the chest muscles and diaphragm and make it difficult to inflate the lungs. (See also articles on individual organs of the respiratory system; *Respiratory tract infection*.)

Respiratory therapy

A paramedical discipline concerned with the maintenance of breathing capacity in people with impaired lung function or the prevention and treatment of pulmonary complications following surgery.

Working under the supervision of a physician, respiratory therapists treat severe respiratory diseases (such as chronic *bronchitis*) and care for the respiratory needs of patients who are on *ventilators* or recovering from major operations. Techniques include the administration of oxygen, drugs, or moisture to the lungs through a *nebulizer*; *postural drainage*; *percussion*; and *breathing exercises*.

Respiratory therapists must successfully complete the examination of the National Board for Respiratory Care (NBRC).

Respiratory tract infection

Infection of the breathing passages, which extend from the nose to the alveoli. Most of these illnesses, which are classified as upper or lower respiratory tract infections, are caused by viruses or bacteria.

Upper respiratory tract infections affect the nose, throat, sinuses, and larynx. They are among the most common of all illnesses, especially in early childhood. The most familiar upper respiratory tract infections are the common *cold*, *pharyngitis*, *tonsillitis*, *sinusitis*, *laryngitis*, and *croup*.

Lower respiratory tract infections, which affect the trachea, bronchi, and lungs, include acute *bronchitis*, acute *bronchiolitis*, and *pneumonia*.

Restless legs

A syndrome that features unpleasant tickling, burning, pricking, or aching sensations in the muscles of the legs. Symptoms tend to come on at night in bed, although prolonged sitting sometimes triggers the discomfort; relief may be obtained only by movement, such as walking.

Restless legs affects as many as 15 percent of the population, although many cases are very mild. It tends to run in families and is most common in middle-aged women, in people who consume a lot of caffeine, in smokers, and during pregnancy. The disorder often develops in people with rheumatoid arthritis.

The exact cause is unknown; there is no apparent nerve, muscle, or circulatory problem. Symptoms may be relieved by cold compresses or by keeping the legs warm.

Restoration, dental

The process of reconstructing part of a tooth that has been damaged by disease or injury. Restoration also refers to the material or substitute part used to rebuild the tooth.

Small areas are usually repaired by first removing the decayed or diseased area and then *filling* the tooth with an inactive material. For more extensive repairs, it may be necessary to fit a dental *onlay*, *inlay*, or *crown*. They are constructed outside the mouth and then cemented into place. For repairing chipped front teeth the dentist may use a *bonding* technique, in which the surface of the tooth is etched with an acid solution and then plastic or porcelain material is attached to the roughened surface.

Restricted growth

See *Short stature*.

Resuscitation

See *Artificial respiration*; *Cardiopulmonary resuscitation*.

Retainer

A type of *orthodontic appliance*.

Retardation

See *Mental retardation*.

Reticular formation

A network of nerve cells scattered throughout the *brain stem*.

Reticulosarcoma

An obsolescent term for non-Hodgkin's lymphoma (see *Lymphoma, non-Hodgkin's*).

Retina

The light-sensitive membrane that lines the inside of the back of the *eye* on which images are cast by the cornea and lens. The retina contains specialized nerve cells (the rods and cones) that convert light energy into nerve impulses. The retina also contains a network of connecting and integrating cells, some with very long fibers, that convey these impulses back along the *optic nerve* to the brain.

The rods are exceptionally sensitive, responding to very dim light. The cones are less sensitive but are responsible for color vision; different cones produce impulses that vary in strength with the color of the light striking them (see *Color vision*).

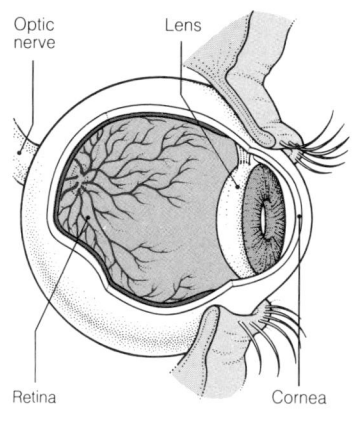

LOCATION OF THE RETINA
The retina is like the light-sensitive film in a camera. It forms a concave membrane over the back inner surface of the eye.

Optic nerve — Lens — Retina — Cornea

Near the center of the retina is the fovea. Here, retinal blood vessels are absent; the light-sensitive cells (almost all cones) are packed so that vision has the highest resolution.

Retinal artery occlusion

Blockage of the main artery feeding blood to the *retina* or of one of its branches. Retinal artery occlusion is most commonly caused by a *thrombosis* (abnormal blood clot formation) or by an embolus (a clot or fatty deposit carried by the blood from another area).

If the main artery is blocked long enough, permanent blindness results in the affected eye. If a small branch is blocked, there is loss of part of the field of vision.

DISORDERS OF THE RETINA

Despite its small size, the retina is subject to a wide variety of disorders, many of which seriously affect the vision or, in some cases, produce blindness.

CONGENITAL AND GENETIC DISORDERS

Color blindness (see *Color vision deficiency*), an abnormality of retinal cones (color receptors in the retina), usually has a genetic basis. *Macular degeneration* (genetic predispositions leading to degeneration of the macula) may appear at any age. Other degenerative disorders of the retina with a genetic basis include *Tay-Sachs disease* and *retinitis pigmentosa*.

Retinopathy may result from exposure of a premature baby to excessive oxygen concentration. Abnormalities occur in the retinal vessels and *retrolental fibroplasia* may occur.

INFECTION

Toxoplasmosis is a common infection of the retina. The infection is often acquired before birth and recurs later in life, with progressive damage to the retina. The parasite that causes toxoplasmosis is found in cat feces and raw beef.

TOXOCARA CANIS worm larvae may lodge in the retina and cause severe retinal destruction, producing a white mass resembling a tumor. *Onchocerciasis*, a worm infestation, may cause severe retinal damage. Bacterial and fungal infections elsewhere in the body can be carried by the blood to the retina. People whose immune systems are impaired are more susceptible to viral infections of the retina.

TUMORS

Retinoblastoma is a malignant tumor that usually appears in the first three years of life. The affected eye may have visual loss and a visible whiteness in the pupil; *strabismus* often develops. The tendency to this cancer can be inherited. Secondary malignant tumors, spreading to the eye from primary tumors elsewhere in the body, can occur. A variety of benign tumors occurs in the retina. Malignant melanoma can arise from the *choroid* (layer beneath the retina) and spread throughout the body.

INJURY

The retina may be torn (see *Retinal tear*) due to severe penetrating or nonpenetrating injury. Permanent damage may be caused by a retinal burn, sometimes caused by looking at an eclipse of the sun.

METABOLIC DISORDERS

Diabetes mellitus may cause retinopathy with fluid leakage, tiny aneurysms of the capillaries, and hemorrhage into the retina. The growth of new, fragile blood vessels on the surface of the retina can be a feature of this type of retinopathy, and these vessels bleed readily. Hemorrhage into the vitreous gel may occur from blood vessels, and fibrous tissue can grow forward onto the gel in cases of proliferative retinopathy. This is a major cause of permanent loss of vision.

IMPAIRED BLOOD SUPPLY

Retinal vein occlusion (or artery occlusion), a common cause of blindness, results from blockage of the central vein or artery of the retina. Hypertensive retinopathy is damage to the retina caused by high blood pressure, which leads to narrowing of the blood vessels of the retina. *Atherosclerosis* of the retinal arteries is common and frequently leads to retinal damage.

POISONS

Methanol causes widespread and permanent destruction of certain retinal tissues, leading to blindness.

A combination of heavy tobacco smoking, heavy alcohol intake, and poor nutrition may lead to visual loss. Both vitamin and lead poisoning may cause visual damage and loss.

DRUGS

Many drugs can damage the retina. *Chloroquine*, used in large doses over a long period for the treatment of conditions such as rheumatoid arthritis, may damage the retina. *Phenothiazine drugs*, used to treat psychiatric disorders, may, in rare cases, damage vision.

OTHER DISORDERS

Age-related macular degeneration, causing progressive loss of vision, is common in older people. *Retinal detachment* often occurs in the absence of injury and may be more common in people with severe *myopia* (nearsightedness).

INVESTIGATION

Retinal disorders are investigated by checking the visual acuity and the visual fields (see *Vision tests*). After dilating the pupils with drops, the retinas are inspected by means of an *ophthalmoscope* and a camera. *Fluorescein* can be injected into a vein, where it is carried by the blood to the retina for investigation. Electrophysiologic tests may be performed to study certain retinal diseases. *Ultrasound scanning* can be used to study tumors in or under the retina.

R

Retinal detachment

Separation of the light-sensitive inner surface of the back of the eye from the outer layers.

CAUSES AND INCIDENCE

Retinal detachment is usually preceded by a break or tear in the retina (see *Retinal tear*), which may be due to natural degeneration or to pulling on the retina by contracting strands in the vitreous gel. Vitreous fluid collects between the delicate nerve membrane and the underlying pigment layer, thus separating them. Retinal detachment may occur after major injury to the eye, but in most cases the condition occurs spontaneously.

Detachment is more common in highly myopic (nearsighted) people who have thinned retinas with areas of degeneration and in those who have had cataract surgery.

SYMPTOMS AND SIGNS

Retinal detachment is painless and the symptoms are exclusively visual. The first indication is the appearance of bright flashes of light, seen at the edge of the field of vision and accompanied by *floaters*. The flashes are caused by strong stimulation of the light-sensitive cells as the tear occurs, and the floaters by the release of blood or pigment into the vitreous gel.

These symptoms do not always occur; the affected person may be unaware of the detachment until a black "drape" obscures vision. This drape descends in a lower detachment, ascends in an upper detachment, enters from the right in a left detachment, and so on.

TREATMENT

Retinal detachment is an emergency. An ophthalmologist must be consulted before the macula (the site of central vision) becomes detached. Once detachment has occurred, normal central vision may not be restored. With a lower detachment (descending drape), the affected person may safely stand in an upright position. If there is upper detachment, there is a risk that the accumulating fluid will strip off the macula and it is safer to lie flat on the back.

Treatment usually involves surgery, in which a soft silicone rubber sponge may be sewn in place on the outside of the sclera overlying the detachment. This indents the sclera and leads to absorption of the subretinal fluid, causing the retina to settle back into place. Cryopexy (involving the application of extreme cold) or a heating *diathermy* may be used to fix the retina in place by causing an inflammatory adhesiveness of the underlying tissues. If the macula has not been detached, the results can be excellent. If a retinal hole is found prior to retinal detachment, the hole may be sealed by laser or cryopexy.

Retinal hemorrhage

Bleeding into the *retina* from one or more blood vessels. Retinal hemorrhage may be caused by *diabetes mellitus*, which leads to the formation of abnormal, small blood vessels that are fragile and bleed easily. Retinal hemorrhages also occur in *hypertension* and *retinal vein occlusion* (blockage of a vein that drains blood from the retina).

When the macula (site of central vision) is involved, vision is severely disturbed. Peripheral hemorrhages may pass unnoticed and may be detected only when the eye is examined with an ophthalmoscope.

Retinal tear

The development of a split in the *retina*, usually caused by degeneration. Retinal tear is more common in people with severe *myopia* (nearsightedness). A retinal tear may also be caused by severe injury to the eye, especially a penetrating injury. *Retinal detachment* often follows a retinal tear.

Retinal vein occlusion

Blockage of the main vein that carries blood away from the *retina* or of one of its branches, usually as a result of *thrombosis* (abnormal blood clot) formation in the vein. Retinal vein occlusion is more common in people who have *glaucoma* and usually causes disturbance of vision in the affected eye. Retinal vein occlusion may also cause glaucoma and can result in complete blindness.

Retinitis

Inflammation affecting the *retina*. (See also *Retinopathy*.)

Retinitis pigmentosa

A degeneration of the rods and cones of the *retina* in both eyes. The condition usually has a genetic basis, but seldom appears before a person reaches adolescence and may not appear until middle age.

The first symptom of retinitis pigmentosa is usually an awareness that vision in dim light is very poor (night blindness). Testing of the fields of vision shows a ring-shaped area of blindness that, over the course of years, gradually extends to destroy an increasing area of the field. The cones in the macula seem more resistant than the peripherally placed rods, so central vision is retained, often for many years. Progression and severity are variable.

Examination of the retinas by ophthalmoscopy shows numerous masses of branching black pigment distributed in areas corresponding to the areas of visual loss.

Retinoblastoma

A malignant tumor (cancer) of the retina that affects babies and infants; the tendency to the disease is usually inherited. It occurs in approximately one baby in 20,000.

Retinoblastoma often first shows itself as a visible whiteness in the pupil. An affected eye may be blind and *strabismus* frequently develops. Retinoblastoma can spread from the eye to the orbit and along the optic nerve to the brain. Treatment is removal or *radiation therapy* of the affected eye. If both eyes are affected, the eye with the larger tumor may be removed and the other eye given radiation therapy.

In many instances retinoblastoma is inherited. If retinoblastoma runs in your family, genetic counseling and prompt and regular eye examinations of newborns are important.

Retinoids

See *Vitamin A*.

Retinol

The principal form of *vitamin A* found in the body.

Retinopathy

Disease or disorder of the retina. The term is usually used to describe damage to the retina caused by persistent *hypertension* (high blood pressure) or *diabetes mellitus*. (See also *Retina* disorders box.)

Retractor

A surgical instrument used to hold an incision open or hold back surrounding tissue so that the surgeon has free access to the underlying area being operated on. Some retractors are held by the nurse or an assisting physician; self-retaining retractors have a locking device that keeps them in position without support.

Retrobulbar neuritis

Sudden total or partial loss of the central field of vision, usually in one eye, accompanied by pain during eye movement and a feeling of pressure in the eyeball.

The symptoms are caused by inflammation of the optic nerve, although the exact reason for the inflammation is often unknown. Sometimes, the condition is thought to be caused by a demyelination process in the nerve fibers similar to that which occurs in *multiple sclerosis*.

The visual loss usually lasts for about six weeks and, although recovery usually seems nearly complete, repeated attacks are likely to lead to permanent loss of some central vision. However, after recovering from one episode, a person may be free of further symptoms.

Although no treatment can affect the long-term outcome, *corticosteroid drugs* may sometimes be prescribed.

Retrolental fibroplasia

Also called the retinopathy of prematurity, a condition that primarily affects the eyes of premature infants. Retrolental fibroplasia can occur when premature infants with a very low birth weight need to be given high concentrations of oxygen to treat *respiratory distress syndrome* and other effects of prematurity.

The tissues at the margin of the retina (as well as other immature tissues) respond to excess oxygen by shutting down their blood vessels.

R

When normal oxygen concentrations are resumed, these tissues can sometimes send out strands of new vessels and fibrous (scar) tissues into the vitreous gel behind the lens, which may seriously interfere with vision and lead to *retinal detachment*.

Retroperitoneal fibrosis

Inflammation and scarring of tissues at the back of the abdominal cavity that occasionally leads to obstruction of both ureters. The resultant blockage of urine flow from the kidneys, if severe, causes *renal failure*.

Most cases of retroperitoneal fibrosis occur in middle-aged men and are of unknown cause. The condition may also be caused by long-term treatment with the drug *methysergide*.

Retrosternal pain

Pain in the central region of the chest in the area of the sternum (breastbone). The most serious cause of such pain is a *myocardial infarction* (heart attack); it is more likely to be due to irritation of the esophagus or *angina pectoris*. (See also *Chest pain*.)

Rett's syndrome

A recently discovered brain disorder that affects girls only. This rare condition was first described in the 1960s by an Austrian, Andreas Rett, but became medically recognized only during the 1980s. Rett's syndrome affects about one in every 15,000 female babies born and is thought to be caused by a *genetic disorder*.

The health and development of an affected baby appear normal until symptoms occur, usually when the child is 12 to 18 months old. Skills that had been acquired, such as walking and talking, gradually disappear and the girl becomes progressively handicapped and may appear autistic (see *Autism*). Odd, repetitive writhing movements of the hands and limbs are characteristic of the condition, and there are often inappropriate outbursts of crying or laughter.

There is no cure for Rett's syndrome; sufferers need constant care and attention because of the level of handicap. Parents of an affected child should receive *genetic counseling*.

Reye's syndrome

A rare disorder characterized by brain and liver damage following an upper respiratory tract infection, chickenpox, or influenza. Reye's syndrome is almost entirely confined to children under age 15.

CAUSES

Evidence suggests that Reye's syndrome is often (but not invariably) related to taking aspirin for a viral infection. Physicians recommend that children be given acetaminophen instead of aspirin for viral infections or fever of unknown origin.

SYMPTOMS AND SIGNS

Reye's syndrome develops as the child is recovering from the infection, starting with uncontrollable vomiting, often with lethargy, memory loss, disorientation, or delirium. Swelling of the brain may cause seizures, deepening coma, disturbances in heart rhythm, and cessation of breathing. Jaundice indicates severe liver involvement.

TREATMENT

Swelling of the brain is controlled by *corticosteroid drugs* and infusions of *mannitol. Dialysis* or *blood transfusions* may be carried out to correct the changes in blood chemistry caused by damage to the liver. If breathing stops, the patient is placed on a *ventilator*.

OUTLOOK

With increasing knowledge of the condition, the death rate has dropped dramatically from about 60 percent to around 10 percent. The outlook is worse for those who have seizures, deep coma, and who stop breathing. Those who survive a serious attack may suffer brain damage.

Rhabdomyolysis

Destruction of muscle tissue accompanied by the release of the oxygen-carrying red muscle pigment *myoglobin* into the blood. The most common cause is a severe, crushing muscle injury (see *Crush syndrome*). Other causes include *polymyositis* (a viral infection of muscles) and, rarely, excessive physical exercise.

Rhabdomyolysis usually causes temporary paralysis or weakness of the affected muscle. Unless the muscle is severely injured, it usually regenerates and the condition clears up without treatment.

Rhabdomyosarcoma

A very rare, malignant tumor of muscle. Rhabdomyosarcoma may develop during infancy, usually affecting the throat, bladder, prostate gland, or vagina, or it may occur in old age, when it commonly affects a large muscle in the arm or leg. The tumor grows rapidly and spreads to other tissues. Treatment includes surgical removal, combined with *radiation therapy* and *anticancer drugs*.

Rheumatic fever

A disease that causes inflammation in various tissues throughout the body. Rheumatic fever is very rare in most developed countries but has been reported to be on the increase again in parts of the US.

Joint inflammation occurs, but without crippling effect. Of importance is the frequency with which the disease permanently damages the heart. The nervous system may also be affected, causing *Sydenham's chorea*.

CAUSES AND INCIDENCE

Rheumatic fever always follows a throat infection with certain strains of streptococcal bacteria. It is not caused by the presence of the bacteria in the affected tissues and is generally believed to be some form of *autoimmune disorder* (one in which the body's immune system attacks its own tissues) induced by streptococci. It can usually be prevented by prompt treatment of streptococcal throat infections with antibiotic drugs.

Children between 5 and 15 are the most commonly affected. In developed countries, the incidence of rheumatic fever has been dropping for many years. In the US, there are a few cases each year. However, in the poorer countries of Asia and Africa, rheumatic fever remains a common and significant cause of heart disease.

SYMPTOMS AND SIGNS

There is fever with pain, inflammation, and swelling of one or more of the larger joints. As one joint improves, symptoms tend to develop in another, although sometimes several joints are affected simultaneously. If damage to the heart is to occur (it does not always occur), it develops insidiously; there may be no symptoms until years later. The heart may be affected in various ways, the most common and most serious being a thickening and scarring of the *heart valves*, leading to narrowing and/or leaking of valves (see *Mitral stenosis; Mitral insufficiency*). These effects are permanent and progressive. *Heart valve surgery* may be needed.

Sydenham's chorea in children occurs when rheumatic fever affects the nervous system. There are irregular, uncontrollable, aimless, jerky movements, and usually some emotional upset.

Pea-sized nodules situated beneath the skin (often over bony prominences) and a rash are other signs.

DIAGNOSIS AND TREATMENT

There are no specific tests for rheumatic fever, but tests may be performed

R

to look for antibodies (proteins made by the *immune system*) directed against streptococci. The diagnosis may be suspected when arthritis moves from joint to joint, but the condition may be discovered only when late heart damage, with symptoms of *heart failure* or a heart *murmur*, is noted.

As soon as the diagnosis of acute rheumatic fever is made, penicillin is used to eradicate streptococci. Sodium salicylate (aspirin) is used to control the joint pain and inflammation and to try to minimize heart damage, but *corticosteroid drugs* may be needed. Sedative and tranquilizer drugs are helpful in treating Sydenham's chorea.

OUTLOOK

The outlook depends on the degree to which the heart has been affected and on whether recurrences can be avoided. The use of penicillin, taken daily for many months or years, may be necessary to prevent further infection with streptococci.

Rheumatism

A popular term for any disorder that causes pain and stiffness in muscles and joints, including minor aches and twinges as well as disorders such as *rheumatoid arthritis*, *osteoarthritis*, and *polymyalgia rheumatica*.

Rheumatoid arthritis

A type of *arthritis* (joint inflammation) in which the joints of the fingers, wrists, toes, or other joints in the body become painful, swollen, stiff, and, in severe cases, deformed.

The frequency of attacks, the number of affected joints, and the severity of symptoms are variable. The disease usually takes the form of recurring moderate attacks.

CAUSES AND INCIDENCE

Rheumatoid arthritis is an *autoimmune disorder* (in which the *immune system* attacks the body's own tissues). The disorder usually starts in early adulthood or middle age but can develop at any age (see *Rheumatoid arthritis, juvenile*). It affects two to three times more women than men.

SYMPTOMS AND SIGNS

The disease's onset is usually gradual, with mild fever and generalized aches and pains preceding specific joint symptoms. In some cases, joint inflammation develops suddenly.

Affected joints become swollen, red, warm, painful, and stiff. Structures around the joint may also become inflamed, resulting in weakness of the ligaments, tendons, and surrounding muscles.

RHEUMATOID ARTHRITIS

One of the most serious forms of joint disease, rheumatoid arthritis may occur as a single episode or a succession of progressively severe attacks. It results from a disturbance in the body's defenses against infection, causing these defenses to attack various body tissues. In the worst cases, joints are completely destroyed, but modern treatment has reduced the incidence of severe disability.

X ray of the hand in rheumatoid arthritis
Note the destructive changes in the joints and the way the finger bones curve away from the thumb side of the hand.

Affected joints
Rheumatoid arthritis can affect virtually any joint, but especially the fingers, wrists, shoulders, knees, hips, and spinal joints in the neck.

Disease progression
The synovium (membrane lining the capsule of an affected joint) becomes inflamed and thickened (right). Later, inflammation may spread to the cartilage and bone.

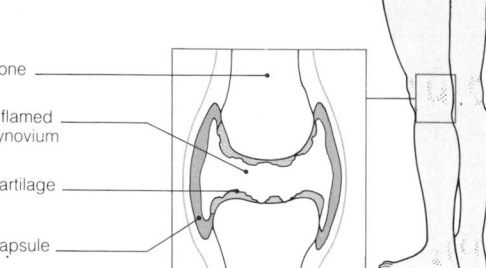

Bone

Inflamed synovium

Cartilage

Capsule

TREATMENT OF RHEUMATOID ARTHRITIS

Drug treatment
may include antirheumatic drugs to slow the progress of the disease, nonsteroidal anti-inflammatory drugs to relieve joint pain, and immunosuppressants to dampen the activity of the immune system.

Occupational therapy
can help people who are disabled by rheumatoid arthritis. Sufferers are shown how to cope with everyday tasks, provided with aids for use in the home, and taught principles of joint protection.

Prostheses
Many joints, such as the hip, can now be replaced with substitutes made from hard-wearing metal and plastic materials. Prostheses may be the only satisfactory solution if a joint becomes seriously damaged.

Physical therapy
aids in the relief of pain and stiffness and helps sufferers to regain use of affected joints and muscles. The physician may recommend removable splints to relieve pain in the hands and wrists.

The finger joints are the most commonly affected, resulting in a weak grip. Swelling of the wrist and *carpal tunnel syndrome* (tingling and pain in the fingers caused by pressure on the median nerve) are also common. *Tenosynovitis* (inflamed painful tendon sheaths) may develop in the wrist and the fingers may turn white on exposure to cold, a condition known as *Raynaud's phenomenon*. Involvement of the feet causes pain in the ankles, arches, and toes. Some of the other joints affected are shown above.

In some cases, soft nodules develop beneath the skin over bony surfaces; in others, *bursitis* occurs, in which the fluid-filled sac around a joint becomes

R

inflamed. When the knee is affected, a fluid-filled swelling known as a *Baker's cyst* may develop behind it.

Many sufferers feel fatigued as a result of the *anemia* that usually accompanies the disease. Early morning stiffness is common, and sufferers may require help getting out of bed and dressing.

DIAGNOSIS

The diagnosis is based on the patient's condition and history, the continuance of symptoms for at least six weeks, X rays of affected joints, and *blood tests* (including a check for specific antibodies known as rheumatoid factor). If rheumatoid factor is absent from a person who otherwise appears to have rheumatoid arthritis, the condition is known as seronegative rheumatoid arthritis.

TREATMENT

Some of the main treatment options are outlined in the box opposite. *Nonsteroidal anti-inflammatory drugs* (NSAIDs) may be used to relieve joint pain and stiffness. *Antirheumatic drugs*, such as gold or penicillamine, may be used to arrest or slow the progress of the disease.

Immunosuppressant drugs, such as *corticosteroid drugs* or azathioprine, are given to suppress the body's immune system if antirheumatic drugs fail to control the disorder or if they produce severe side effects. Corticosteroid drugs may be injected into the joint to provide local pain relief.

Physical therapy and *occupational therapy* are often important.

Destroyed joints can sometimes be replaced with artificial substitutes (see *Arthroplasty*). Hip and knee replacements are the most common.

COMPLICATIONS

In severe cases of rheumatoid arthritis, inflammation may also affect the covering of the heart (causing *pericarditis*), the small blood vessels (resulting in poor circulation and ulcers on the hands and feet), the lungs (leading to *pleural effusion* or *pulmonary fibrosis*), the eyes or mouth (making them dry; see *Sjögren's syndrome*), the lymph glands (producing tender swellings in the neck, armpit, and groin), and the spleen (causing *hypersplenism*).

OUTLOOK

Most sufferers must take drugs for the rest of their lives, but effective control of symptoms usually allows a near-normal level of activity. Modern methods of treatment have reduced the incidence and severity of deformity and disability.

Rheumatoid arthritis, juvenile

A rare form of *arthritis* (joint inflammation) that affects children and lasts more than three months. Juvenile arthritis occurs more often in girls than in boys, and most commonly starts between the ages of 2 and 4 or around puberty.

TYPES AND SYMPTOMS

There are three main types of juvenile arthritis. Still's disease (systemic onset juvenile arthritis) starts with an illness characterized by fever, rash, enlarged lymph glands, abdominal pain, and weight loss. These symptoms last several weeks; joint pain, swelling, and stiffness may not begin for several months. A second type, called polyarticular juvenile arthritis, starts with pain, swelling, and stiffness in a number of joints. In the third type, pauciarticular juvenile arthritis, four or fewer joints are involved.

DIAGNOSIS

Diagnosis is based on the symptoms and signs and the exclusion of other disorders that can cause joint symptoms in children, such as viral or bacterial infections, rheumatic fever, Crohn's disease, ulcerative colitis, hemophilia, sickle cell anemia, and leukemia. Blood tests may help identify the cause of the arthritis.

COMPLICATIONS

Possible complications include short stature, anemia, pleurisy, pericarditis (inflammation of the outer lining of the heart), and enlargement of the liver and spleen.

Uveitis (inflammation of the iris and the surrounding muscles in the eye) may develop and, if untreated, may damage vision. Rarely, *amyloidosis* (deposition of a starchy substance in body organs) may occur; if the kidney is involved, *renal failure* may develop.

TREATMENT

Joint pain and stiffness may be relieved by aspirin, *nonsteroidal anti-inflammatory drugs*, and, in very severe cases, *antirheumatic drugs* (such as gold, penicillamine, chloroquine, or azathioprine) or *corticosteroid drugs*.

Splints may be worn during the day to rest acutely inflamed joints and at night to reduce the risk of deformities. *Physical therapy* reduces the risk of muscle wasting and contractures. Excessive physical exercise should be avoided and special shoes worn to reduce the risk of foot deformity.

OUTLOOK

In most children the arthritis disappears after several years. However, some are left with permanent stiffness and joint deformity.

Rheumatoid spondylitis

See *Ankylosing spondylitis*.

Rheumatologist

A physician who diagnoses and treats arthritis, rheumatism, and other afflictions of the joints, muscles, or connective tissues (see *Rheumatology*).

Rheumatology

The branch of medicine concerned with the causes, development, diagnosis, and treatment of joint, muscle, and *connective tissue diseases*. Rheumatologists use a wide variety of investigative techniques, ranging from X rays of joints to tests of muscle function and blood analysis. Treatment is similarly varied; it includes courses of anti-inflammatory drugs or analgesics and rest.

Rh incompatibility

A mismatch between the blood of a pregnant woman and that of her baby with respect to the Rh (Rhesus) *blood group*. In certain circumstances, this mismatch can lead to *hemolytic disease of the newborn*.

CAUSE

Blood groups are determined by substances called factors on the surface of red blood cells, which differ among individuals. The best known grouping is the A,B,O system. The Rh system (first identified in Rhesus monkeys) was discovered early in this century. It consists of several factors, one of which (D factor) is the most important cause of Rh incompatibility. People can have blood that is Rh positive (carry the D factor in their blood) or Rh negative (do not carry it). Having a positive or negative blood type is determined by *genes* (i.e., it is an inherited trait).

Rh incompatibility can arise only when a woman's blood is Rh negative and her baby's blood is Rh positive. This can happen only if the baby's father's blood is also Rh positive. There are usually no problems during a woman's first pregnancy with a baby whose blood is Rh positive. However, as shown in the diagram (overleaf), the baby may sensitize the woman to Rh-positive blood; if she has a subsequent pregnancy with an Rh-positive baby, there is a risk of hemolytic disease of the newborn. A woman whose blood is Rh negative can also be sensitized if she is mistakenly given a transfusion of Rh-positive blood.

INCIDENCE

Among white people in the US, about one person in six has Rh-negative

R

blood; in about one pregnancy in 11 the mother's blood is Rh negative and the baby's blood is Rh positive. In the past, hemolytic disease of the newborn was a common cause of stillbirth and of a severe fetal condition called erythroblastosis fetalis, in which destruction of fetal blood cells led to severe fetal disease or death. Hemolytic disease of the newborn due to Rh sensitization is becoming rare, primarily due to the development of $Rh_o(D)$ immune globulin. When given by injection to a woman within 72 hours of delivery, it prevents 99 percent of Rh sensitization.

In addition, $Rh_o(D)$ immune globulin is given to women after a miscarriage, elective abortion, amniocentesis, or any other procedure that might result in exposure of the mother to the fetal blood cells. $Rh_o(D)$ immune globulin is also generally given to women with Rh-negative blood who are seven months pregnant.

The injection contains antibodies to Rh factor, which destroy any of the baby's blood cells that may have entered the woman before they have a chance to sensitize her.

Rh incompatibility is less common in black and Oriental families than in white families due to comparative rarity of the Rh-negative blood group in nonwhites.

DIAGNOSIS AND TREATMENT
A pregnant woman's blood groups are checked at the first prenatal visit. Women who have Rh-negative blood are tested for the presence of Rh antibodies at this and subsequent visits. The management of the pregnancy and childbirth, if antibodies are present and there is a risk to the baby, is as described under *hemolytic disease of the newborn*.

Rhinitis
Inflammation of the mucous membrane that lines the nose, usually manifested by some combination of nasal obstruction, nasal discharge, sneezing, and facial pressure or pain.

TYPES
VIRAL RHINITIS A feature of the common cold (see *Cold, common*), rhinitis due to viral infection may lead to *sinusitis*.

ALLERGIC RHINITIS Also known as hay fever, this type may be seasonal, due to pollens, or year-round, due to house dust, molds, or pets (see *Rhinitis, allergic*). It most commonly occurs with vasomotor rhinitis.

VASOMOTOR RHINITIS This type of rhinitis is an intermittent or continual condition. The nose becomes overresponsive to stimuli, including pollutants such as tobacco smoke, temperature and humidity changes or extremes, certain foods, certain medicines, and/or certain emotions. The condition is common in pregnancy and in those taking the estrogen-progestogen contraceptive pill or other estrogen medication.

HYPERTROPHIC RHINITIS Repeated nasal infections can cause hypertrophic rhinitis, in which tissue in the nasal mucosa thickens and veins become chronically congested. This results in constant stuffiness, and sometimes impairment of the sense of smell. In extreme cases, part of the swollen tissue may be removed.

ATROPHIC RHINITIS This wasting of the mucous membrane can result from aging, chronic bacterial infections, or extensive nasal surgery. Other features of the disorder can include persistent nasal infection, a discharge that dries to a crust, loss of smell, and an unpleasant odor. Treatment is with *antibiotic* and *estrogen drugs*.

Rhinitis, allergic
Inflammation of the mucous membrane that lines the nose due to an allergy to pollen, dust, or other airborne substances. Also known as hay fever, the disorder causes sneezing, a runny nose, and nasal congestion.

CAUSES
In some people, inhaling particles of certain harmless substances provokes an exaggerated response by the *immune system*, which forms antibodies against them (see *Allergy*). The otherwise harmless substances, known as allergens, trigger the release of histamine and other chemicals that cause inflammation and fluid production in the lining of the nose and sinuses (air cavities around the nose). The most common of the allergens that cause allergic rhinitis are tree, grass, and weed pollens; molds; animal skin scales, hair, or feathers; house dust; and house-dust mites.

Pollen-induced allergic rhinitis is seasonal. Tree pollens are most prevalent in spring, grass pollens in summer, and weed pollens in summer and early fall. Sufferers are worst affected on days when the pollen count is high—that is, during hot and windy weather, especially in heavily vegetated, low-lying areas.

People affected by household allergens, such as dust, tend to have less severe symptoms but are affected throughout the year.

INCIDENCE
Allergic rhinitis is a common complaint, affecting as many as 5 to 10 percent of the population. It is more common in people who have other allergies, such as asthma or eczema; like these disorders, it has a tendency to run in families. The condition usually develops before the age of 30 and affects more women than men.

SYMPTOMS AND SIGNS
Exposure to the allergen produces an itching sensation in the nose, palate, throat, and eyes. This is followed by sneezing, stuffiness, a runny nose, and, usually, watering eyes. The eyes may also be affected by *conjunctivitis*, which makes them red and sore.

PREVENTION AND TREATMENT
Skin tests help identify the allergen responsible for the disorder. Once the

---

HOW Rh INCOMPATIBILITY OCCURS
Without preventive treatment, an Rh-negative woman who is exposed to D factor (a substance present only in Rh-positive blood) may develop antibodies that will attack the red blood cells of any future Rh-positive babies.

First pregnancy

Rh-negative mother

Rh-positive baby

At birth, baby's blood enters mother's circulation

Subsequent pregnancies

Antibodies against Rh-positive blood formed in mother

Antibodies cross placenta and destroy red blood cells of subsequent Rh-positive babies allergen is known, exposure should be avoided or kept to a minimum, although this is difficult when the cause is pollens.

For mild attacks of allergic rhinitis, occasional use of a *decongestant* spray or drops may clear up symptoms, but use for more than three or four days can make the condition worse. For many sufferers, treatment is with *antihistamine drugs*. Antihistamines reduce the symptoms of itching and some degree of nasal congestion and runny nose, but many have the disadvantage of causing drowsiness. Treatment of allergic rhinitis may also include *corticosteroid drugs*, which can be used in the nose.

The drug cromolyn sodium, inhaled regularly throughout the pollen season, may help to prevent attacks by blocking the allergic response.

Desensitization to a particular pollen allergen by injecting gradually increasing amounts of it into the skin over a period of years can result in long-term relief of symptoms (see *Immunotherapy*).

Rhinophyma

Bulbous deformity and redness of the nose occurring almost exclusively in elderly men. Rhinophyma is a complication of severe *rosacea* (a skin disorder of the nose and cheeks). The tissue of the nose thickens, small blood vessels enlarge, and the sebaceous glands become overactive, making the nose excessively oily.

Rhinophyma can be remedied by an operation. With the use of a general anesthetic, the swollen tissue is cut away until the nose is restored to a satisfactory shape. Skin grafting is not necessary, since the remaining tissue rapidly regenerates.

Example of rhinophyma
This disfiguring condition is remedied by paring away the excess tissue. The skin soon regenerates after treatment.

Rhinoplasty

An operation that alters the structure of the nose to improve its appearance or to correct a deformity caused by injury or disease.

Incisions are made within the nose (to avoid visible scars) using either a local or a general anesthetic. The septum (the vertical wall of cartilage and bone that divides the nose) may be altered if breathing passages are blocked. Then the cartilage and bone of the nasal structure are reshaped. Occasionally, a bone or cartilage graft is used. The nose is splinted in position for about 10 days.

Rhinoplasty usually causes considerable bruising and swelling, and the results may not be clearly visible for weeks or months. Rare complications include recurrent nosebleeds due to persistent crusting at the incision sites and breathing difficulty due to narrowing of the nasal passages.

Rhinorrhea

The discharge of watery mucus from the nose, usually due to *rhinitis* or to the flow of cerebrospinal fluid from the nose following a head injury. (See *Nasal discharge*.)

Rh isoimmunization

The development of antibodies formed against Rh-positive blood in a person who has Rh-negative blood. (See *Rh incompatibility*; *Hemolytic disease of the newborn*.)

Rh₀(D) immune globulin

An *antiserum* that contains antibodies against Rh (Rhesus) D factor (a substance present on the red blood cells of people who have Rh-positive blood). It is given to a woman who has Rh-negative blood after she has given birth to a baby whose blood is Rh positive or if she has had a miscarriage or elective abortion.

Rh₀(D) immune globulin is also given to a pregnant woman with Rh-negative blood after she has had amniocentesis or bleeding episodes or in other instances in which she might be exposed to fetal blood cells, as well as in the seventh month of pregnancy. The injected antibodies destroy any red cells from the fetus that have entered the woman's blood. This is important to prevent or reduce the risk of the woman forming her own antibodies against Rh-positive blood, which might adversely affect any subsequent pregnancies. (See *Rh incompatibility*; *Hemolytic disease of the newborn*.)

Rhythm method

See *Contraception, periodic abstinence*.

Rib

Any of the flat, curved bones that form a framework for the chest and a protective cage around the heart, lungs, and other organs.

There are 12 pairs of ribs, each joined at the back of the rib cage to a vertebra in the spine. Their arrangement is shown in the illustration on the next page. Between the ribs, and attached to them, are thin sheets of muscle that help to expand and relax the chest during breathing. The spaces between the ribs also contain nerves and blood vessels.

DISORDERS

The ribs can easily be fractured by a fall or blow (see *Rib, fractured*).

A rib is one of the more common sites for a benign *bone tumor* or for a *metastasis* (a secondary malignant tumor that has spread from cancer elsewhere in the body).

In rare cases a person is born with one or more extra ribs lying above the uppermost normal rib. Known as *cervical ribs*, the additional ribs may press on nerves supplying the arm or cause other problems.

Rib, fractured

Fracture of a rib is usually caused by a fall or blow, but occasionally it is caused by minor stress on the rib cage, such as that produced by prolonged coughing or even laughing.

The fracture causes severe pain that is made worse by deep breathing, and tenderness and swelling of the overlying tissue. The diagnosis is confirmed by X rays. Pain is relieved by *analgesics* (painkillers) or, occasionally, by an injection of a long-acting, local anesthetic drug.

Most rib fractures are undisplaced (i.e., the bone ends remain in alignment) and, in these cases, healing is usually spontaneous and straightforward. A displaced or splintered fracture may cause complications if the sharp ends or fragments rupture the *spleen* or pierce a lung, causing lung collapse (see *Pneumothorax*). Multiple rib fractures can result in *flail chest*.

Strapping is rarely used to aid healing because it hinders chest expansion and thus increases the risk of *pneumonia*. Instead, the patient is encouraged to take deep breaths while holding the injured side. If several ribs are fractured and displaced, an operation may be performed to wire them back in position.

R

ANATOMY OF THE RIBS

There are seven true ribs attached to the sternum, three false ribs, each attached to a rib above, and two floating ribs on each side. They are joined to the spine and sternum so that, when pulled up by the intercostal muscles (between the ribs), they expand the chest, drawing air into the lungs. The front ends of the ribs are linked to the sternum by cartilages.

Right lung — Sternum — Fixed ribs — Floating ribs

Riboflavin

The chemical name of vitamin B_2 (see *Vitamin B complex*).

Rickets

A nutritional deficiency disease of childhood that affects the skeleton. Because inadequate amounts of calcium and phosphate are incorporated into an affected child's bones as they grow, the bones become deformed. In adults, a similar process leads to *osteomalacia*.

CAUSES AND INCIDENCE

The most common cause of rickets is deficiency of vitamin D, which is vital for the absorption of calcium from the intestines into the blood and for its incorporation into normal bone. Vitamin D is found in fat-containing animal substances, such as oily fish, butter, egg yolk, liver, and fish liver oils. There are also small amounts in human and animal milk. The vitamin is also made in the body through the action of sunlight on the skin.

Rickets occurs primarily in poor countries and in communities where babies receive inadequate vitamin D in the diet and simultaneously do not get enough sunlight. Breast milk alone cannot provide all a baby's needs for vitamin D, so a breast-fed baby who gets little sun should be given vitamin D supplements.

Rickets is now rare in the US and in other developed countries where vitamin D supplements are given to infants, where the vitamin is added to foods such as cow's milk, margarine, and breakfast cereals, and where most children and babies eat a varied diet and get adequate exposure to the sun. The disorder is seen only in vulnerable groups, such as premature babies, strict vegetarians, and some food faddists who avoid the foods rich in vitamin D listed above.

Rickets occasionally develops as a complication of an intestinal disorder that causes *malabsorption* (failure to absorb nutrients from the intestines). It also occurs in certain rare forms of kidney and liver disease and in children undergoing long-term therapy with *anticonvulsant drugs* (which interfere with the action of vitamin D).

SYMPTOMS AND DIAGNOSIS

The most striking feature of advanced rickets is deformity of the bones, especially of the legs and spine. Typically, there is bowing of the legs and, in infants, flattening of the head as a result of the softness of the skull. Infants with rickets often sleep poorly and show delay in crawling and walking. Other features include *kyphoscoliosis* (spinal curvature), enlargement of the wrists, ankles, and ends of the ribs, pelvic pain, a tendency to fractures, and muscle weakness.

TREATMENT

A child with rickets is treated with vitamin D supplements; he or she should also be given plenty of milk to provide calcium. Treatment continues until X rays show healing. The child should not be given excessive vitamin D supplements, however, as they can lead to *hypercalcemia*.

Treatment of other causes of rickets depends on the underlying disorder.

Rickettsia

A type of parasitic microorganism. Rickettsiae resemble small bacteria, but they are able to multiply only by invading the cells of another life form; in this respect they are more like viruses.

Rickettsiae are primarily parasites of the arthropods (insects and insectlike animals), such as lice, fleas, ticks, and mites. However, these arthropods can transmit rickettsiae to larger animals (such as rodents, dogs, or humans) via the saliva of biting ticks or through their feces being deposited on the skin, with the rickettsiae passing to the blood via a small skin break.

Human diseases caused by different types of rickettsiae include *Rocky Mountain spotted fever*, *Q fever*, and the various forms of *typhus*.

Rifampin

An *antibacterial drug* used in the treatment of *tuberculosis*. Rifampin is also used to treat *leprosy*, *endocarditis*, and *osteomyelitis*. It is also used to treat certain asymptomatic people who are *meningitis* bacteria carriers.

The drug is usually prescribed with other antibacterial drugs because some strains of bacteria quickly develop *resistance* to rifampin alone.

Rifampin causes harmless, orange-red discoloration of the urine, saliva, and other body secretions. Other side effects include muscle pain, nausea, vomiting, diarrhea, jaundice, flulike symptoms, rash, and itching.

Rigidity

Increased tone in one or more muscles, causing them to feel tight; the affected part of the body becomes

R

stiff and inflexible. Causes of rigidity include injury to a muscle, arthritis affecting a nearby joint, a neurological disorder, such as Parkinson's disease or stroke, or the tightening of an abdominal muscle overlying an area of inflamed peritoneum (see *Peritonitis*). See also *Spasticity*.

Rigor
Popularly called a chill, a violent attack of shivering, often associated with a fever. Rigor may also refer to stiffness or rigidity of body tissues, as in *rigor mortis*.

Rigor mortis
The stiffening of muscles that occurs after death. It starts some three to four hours after death and is usually complete after about 12 hours; however, stiffness gradually disappears over the next 48 to 60 hours. The greater the amount of physical exertion before death, the sooner rigor mortis begins. Similarly, the sooner rigor mortis begins, the sooner it passes. These facts have important medicolegal implications and, along with other factors, are used to assess the time of death.

Ringing in the ears
See *Tinnitus*.

Ringworm
A popular name for fungal skin infections (commonly of the feet, groin, scalp, nails, or trunk). Ringworm is marked by ring-shaped, reddened, scaly, or blistery patches. (See *Tinea*.)

Patch of ringworm
The name arises from the tendency for certain skin fungus infections to spread uniformly outward, leaving normal skin inside the ring.

Ritodrine
A drug used to prevent or delay premature labor (see *Prematurity*) by relaxing the muscles of the uterus.

Ritodrine causes an increased heart rate if given intravenously. Other side effects include tremor, palpitations, nausea, vomiting, chest pain, breathlessness, and nightmares.

River blindness
See *Onchocerciasis*.

RNA
 Ribonucleic acid, one of the two types of chemicals that carry the inherited, coded instructions within a cell for the cell's activities, or that assist in the decoding of these instructions; the other type is deoxyribonucleic acid (*DNA*). In all animal and plant cells, it is DNA that holds a permanent record of the instructions; RNA helps decode the instructions. In some viruses, the instructions for viral multiplication are held by RNA. (See also *Nucleic acids*; *Protein synthesis*.)

Rocky Mountain spotted fever
 A rare, infectious disease caused by a rickettsia (a microorganism similar to a bacterium) and transmitted from rabbits and other small mammals by the bites of ticks. The disease occurs most commonly on the Atlantic seaboard (it was initially recognized in the Rocky Mountain states). Its incidence has risen steadily since 1980, and there are now more than 1,000 cases of Rocky Mountain spotted fever reported annually.

SYMPTOMS AND SIGNS
About a week after the tick bite, mild fever, loss of appetite, and slight headache may develop gradually. However, sometimes symptoms (e.g., high fever, prostration, aching, tender muscles, severe headache, nausea, and vomiting) come on suddenly and are severe. Two to six days after the onset of symptoms, small pink spots appear on the wrists and ankles. The spots then spread over the body and darken, enlarge, and bleed.

The illness usually subsides after about two weeks; in untreated cases marked by extremely high fever, death may occur from pneumonia or heart failure.

DIAGNOSIS AND TREATMENT
Diagnosis may be difficult because, initially, Rocky Mountain spotted fever resembles several other infections. Laboratory tests on blood and tissue samples can confirm the diagnosis. Treatment with the antibiotic drugs chloramphenicol or tetracycline usually cures the disease.

PREVENTION
People living in tick-infested areas should use an insect repellent, examine the body daily for the presence of ticks, and gently pull away with forceps any ticks that are found.

Roentgenography
See *X rays*; *Radiology*.

Role-playing
The acting out of a role (the pattern of behavior expected of an individual in a given social situation). The conscious adoption of different roles is a useful technique for learning about oneself, other people, or particular situations.

The phrase "sick role" describes the type of passive behavior expected and allowed of a patient; people who have social or emotional problems may unconsciously adopt this role as a means of escaping from social obligations and of gaining the sympathy and understanding of others.

Root-canal treatment
A dental procedure performed to save a tooth in which the pulp (the living tissue within a tooth) has died or become untreatably diseased, usually as the result of extensive *caries*.

HOW IT IS DONE
The main steps in root-canal treatment are shown in the diagrams on the overleaf. X rays are taken to establish the length of the pulp cavity. A local anesthetic may be given. The tooth is isolated from the saliva with a *rubber dam* (a small sheet of rubber) to prevent infection. A hole is drilled in the crown of the tooth, the pulp is removed, and the crown is then sealed with a temporary filling.

About one week later the dentist removes the filling to ensure that the cavity is free of infection; if it is not, an antibiotic paste is applied and the tooth is resealed. When no infection can be detected, the cavity is filled and the chamber is sealed.

COMPLICATIONS
If the pulp cavity has not been filled completely, bacteria may enter, leading to apical *periodontitis* (inflammation of the tissues around the root tips). It may then be necessary to make an opening in the gum and bone overlying the affected root to allow pus to drain. In some cases, a small portion of the root tip may be removed and the area filled with amalgam.

RESULTS
Teeth whose pulp cavities have been filled may function well for as long as normal teeth. However, the teeth

R

ROOT-CANAL TREATMENT

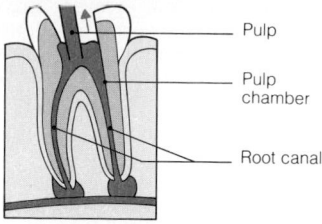

Pulp

Pulp chamber

Root canal

1 A hole is drilled into the crown so that all infected material can be removed from the pulp chamber. The root canals are then slightly enlarged and shaped with long, fine-tipped instruments.

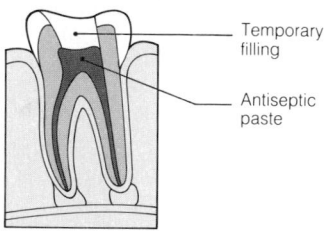

Temporary filling

Antiseptic paste

2 Antibiotic paste is packed into the cavity and a temporary filling fitted. After a week or so, the filling is removed and the canals are checked for sterility.

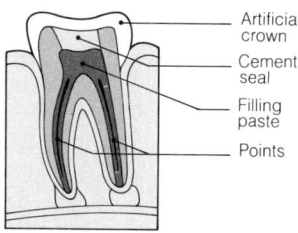

Artificial crown

Cement seal

Filling paste

Points

3 The canals are filled with filling paste and/or tapering solid "points" made of gutta-percha resin mixed with zinc and bismuth oxides. The roots are then sealed with a cement and an artificial crown is fitted.

sometimes turn slightly gray; if this is unsightly, bleaching, a crown, or a facing can restore the appearance.

Rorschach test

A test in which the subject reveals his or her attitude, conflicts, and emotions by responding to a set of inkblot pictures. The inkblot pictures are standardized, but of such a nature that the individual tends to project his or her unconscious attitude. The inkblot test was devised by the Swiss psychiatrist Hermann Rorschach early this century. (See also *Personality tests*.)

Rosacea

A chronic skin disorder in which the nose and cheeks are abnormally red.

The exact cause of rosacea is unknown, but sometimes it is caused by overuse of *corticosteroid* creams in the treatment of other skin disorders. The condition affects about one in 500 people and is most common among middle-aged women.

Rosacea usually begins with temporary flushing, often after drinking a hot beverage or alcohol, eating spicy food, or entering a hot environment. It may then develop into permanent redness of the skin, sometimes accompanied by pustules resembling those of *acne*. In some elderly men, the condition leads to *rhinophyma* (bulbous swelling of the nose).

TREATMENT

A lengthy course of the *antibiotic drug* tetracycline usually suppresses rosacea but it does not cure it. Rosacea may recur over a period of five to 10 years, after which the condition usually disappears on its own.

Roseola infantum

A common infectious disease that primarily affects children aged 6 months to 2 years. Roseola infantum is probably caused by a virus and is characterized by the abrupt onset of irritability and a fever. The temperature may rise as high as 105°F (40.5°C). However, on the fourth or fifth day, it drops suddenly back to normal. At about the same time, a rash appears on the trunk, often spreading quickly to the neck, face, and limbs. The rash rarely lasts longer than a day or two. Other symptoms may include a sore throat and enlargement of lymph nodes in the head and neck.

Occasionally, a child may have a febrile *seizure* during the course of the fever, but the illness has no serious results or complications. There is no specific treatment other than to keep the child cool and give acetaminophen to reduce the fever.

Rotator cuff

A reinforcing structure around the shoulder joint composed of four muscle tendons that merge with the fibrous capsule enclosing the joint.

The rotator cuff may be torn as the result of a fall. A partial tear may cause *painful arc syndrome* (pain when the arm is lifted in a certain arc away from the body). A complete tear seriously limits the ability to raise the arm and, in cases of severe disability, may require surgical repair.

Roughage

See *Fiber, dietary.*

Roundworms

Also known as nematodes, a class of elongated, cylindrically shaped worms. A dozen or so types are the main parasites of humans (the accompanying table summarizes the main ones). In many cases, the adult worms inhabit the human intestines, usually without causing symptoms unless there is a large number of worms. Sometimes, passage of worm larvae through various parts of the body is the main cause of symptoms. Most infestations are treated relatively easily with *antihelmintic drugs*.

In temperate areas, such as the US, the only common type of roundworm disease is *pinworm infestation* (which mainly affects children). *Ascariasis*, *whipworm infestation*, and *trichinosis* are also fairly common, although they often cause no symptoms. *Toxocariasis* occasionally occurs. In tropical countries, roundworm diseases are much more common; they include those mentioned above and *hookworm infestation*, *strongyloidiasis*, *guinea worm disease*, and different types of *filariasis*.

Rubber dam

A rubber sheet used to isolate one or more teeth during certain dental procedures. The dam acts as a barrier against saliva and prevents the inhalation of debris or small instruments. To fit a dam, the dentist punches small holes in the sheet for the teeth to protrude, and secures the sheet with clamps and a frame.

Rubella

A viral infection, also known as German measles (although the similarities to measles are few). Rubella causes a trivial illness in children and a slightly more troublesome one in adults. It is serious only when it affects a woman in the early months of pregnancy, when there is a chance that the virus will infect the fetus, which can lead to any of a range of severe birth defects, known as rubella syndrome.

CAUSES AND INCIDENCE

Apart from mother-to-baby transmission, the rubella virus is spread from person to person in airborne droplets. Symptoms develop after an incubation period of two to three weeks.

Once common worldwide, rubella is now much less prevalent in most developed countries as a result of vaccination programs. The aim in the US has been to eradicate the virus by compulsory vaccination of all children before school entry; the results are encouraging. By 1986 the incidence

R

in the US had been reduced to 551 reported cases of rubella and only 14 cases of rubella syndrome.

SYMPTOMS AND COMPLICATIONS

The infection usually occurs between the ages of 6 and 12 and is almost invariably mild. A rash appears on the face, spreads to the trunk and limbs, persists for a few days, and then disappears. There may be a slight fever and enlargement of lymph nodes at the back of the neck. In some cases, the entire infection passes unnoticed. In adolescents and adults, there may be more marked symptoms, such as headache before the rash appears and a more pronounced fever. The virus may be transmitted to others from a few days before the symptoms appear until a day after they disappear. Polyarthritis (inflammation affecting several joints) is an occasional short-lived complication, starting shortly after the rash has faded.

CONGENITAL INFECTION

Rubella is a risk to the unborn baby only if the mother is infected during the first four months of pregnancy. The earlier in pregnancy infection occurs, the more likely the infant is to be affected, and the more serious the abnormalities tend to be. In very early pregnancy, miscarriage may occur. An affected infant may have one or many defects. The most common abnormalities, in order of frequency, are *deafness*, congenital *heart disease*, *mental retardation*, *cataract* and other eye disorders, *purpura*, *cerebral palsy*, and bone abnormalities. About 20 percent of affected babies die in early infancy. An affected infant continues to harbor the virus and may infect others via his or her urine, stools, and saliva for a year or more after birth.

DIAGNOSIS AND TREATMENT

Rubella is easily confused with other conditions such as rashes caused by other viruses, drugs, and *scarlet fever*. It can be positively diagnosed only by laboratory isolation of the virus from a throat swab or by tests to look for antibodies to the virus in the blood. There is no specific treatment for rubella. Acetaminophen can be given to reduce fever. Treatment of rubella syndrome is of the defects exhibited.

PREVENTION

Rubella vaccine is highly effective in providing long-lasting immunity to the disease; it is given to all babies (usually combined with measles and mumps vaccine) at about 15 months of age. Reactions to the vaccine are usually negligible. Rubella infection itself also provides immunity.

DISEASES CAUSED BY ROUNDWORMS (NEMATODES)

Disease	Adult length	Distribution	How acquired
Ascariasis (common roundworm)	6–15 inches	Worldwide	By swallowing worm eggs that have contaminated food or fingers
Enterobiasis (pinworm)	0.1–0.5 inches	Worldwide	By swallowing worm eggs that have contaminated fingers
Trichuriasis (whipworm)	1–2 inches	Worldwide	By swallowing worm eggs that have contaminated food or fingers
Ancylostomiasis (hookworm)	0.5 inches	Tropics	By penetration of skin of feet by worm larvae in soil
Strongyloidiasis	0.1 inches	Tropics	By penetration of skin of feet by worm larvae in soil
Toxocariasis	A few inches	Worldwide	By swallowing worm eggs from dirt or dog feces
Trichinosis (pork worm)	0.05 inches	Worldwide	By eating undercooked pork containing encysted worm larvae
Filariasis	1–20 inches	Tropics	By mosquito and other insect bites

Any female of childbearing age (or approaching it) who is unsure whether she has been immunized or has had rubella, should have her immune status checked. If she is not immune, vaccination is performed only if there is no chance that she is pregnant because of the risk of the vaccine causing rubella in the fetus.

A nonimmune pregnant woman must avoid contact with anyone who has rubella; if such contact occurs, she should immediately seek a physician's advice. Passive immunization with immune globulin may help prevent infection of the fetus.

Rubeola

Another name for *measles*.

Running injuries

Many of the millions of people who jog or run to keep fit sustain a variety of injuries as a result. Most running injuries can be prevented by taking simple precautions.

TYPES

Common injuries include *tendinitis* (inflammation of a tendon); *stress fracture* of the tibia (shin), the fibula (the other long bone in the lower leg), or a bone in the foot; plantar *fasciitis* (inflammation of tissue in the sole of the foot); and other *overuse injuries*.

Tearing of the hamstring muscles at the back of the thigh is common in sprinting. Long-distance runners are more likely to suffer back pain due to jarring of the spine, tibial *compartment syndrome* (painful cramp in the lower leg caused by muscle compression), or *shin splints* (pain along the inner edge of the tibia).

PREVENTION

Shoes should fit snugly to provide stability but should not cramp the foot; they require insoles to cushion the jarring force on legs and spine. Shoes should not be allowed to become worn, since this can cause abnormal positioning of the foot during running, leading to foot strain.

Before running, warm-up exercises should be performed to reduce the risk of injury. Beginners should run short distances at first, and experienced runners should keep their running within sensible bounds.

Running should be done in an upright posture, with the trunk, neck, and arms relaxed. Long periods of running uphill, downhill, or along the side of a slope should be avoided because they increase stress on the ankle and knee.

Rupture

See *Hernia*.

R

Sac
A pouch, or baglike organ or body structure. The amniotic sac is the thin, membranous, fluid-filled bag that surrounds the fetus.

Saccharin
An *artificial sweetener*.

Sacralgia
Pain in the *sacrum* (the triangular spinal bone below the lumbar vertebrae) caused by pressure on a spinal nerve in this area. Sacralgia is usually the result of a *disk prolapse*. In rare cases, however, it may be due to *bone cancer*. (See also *Back pain*.)

Sacralization
Fusion of the fifth (lowest) lumbar vertebra with the upper part of the *sacrum* (the triangular spinal bone below the lumbar vertebrae). Sacralization may occur as a birth anomaly, in which case it usually produces no symptoms and is discovered only when an X ray of the back is taken for some other reason. Sacralization may also be performed as a surgical procedure to treat a *disk prolapse* or *spondylolisthesis*, in which a vertebra is displaced over the one below it. (See also *Spinal fusion*.)

Sacroiliac joint
One of a pair of rigid joints between each side of the *sacrum* (the triangular spinal bone below the lumbar vertebrae) and each ilium (the largest of the bones that form the outer walls of the *pelvis*). The bony surfaces within the joint are lined with cartilage and have a small amount of synovial fluid (see *Synovium*) between them. Strong ligaments between the sacrum and ilium permit only minimal movement at the joint.

DISORDERS
The sacroiliac joint may be strained (usually as a result of childbirth or overstriding when running), producing pain in the lower back and buttocks. It may also become inflamed, a condition called *sacroiliitis*.

Sacroiliitis
Inflammation of the *sacroiliac joint* (one of a pair of joints between each side of the sacrum and each ilium). Sacroiliitis can be caused by *ankylosing spondylitis*, *rheumatoid arthritis*, or, in rare cases, by an infection that has spread through the bloodstream from elsewhere in the body.

The principal symptom is pain in the lower back, buttocks, groin, and back of the thigh. The pain may be accompanied by fever and malaise if the underlying cause is an infection. If the cause is ankylosing spondylitis, pain may be accompanied by stiffness in the back and hips that is worse after rest and alleviated by exercise.

Sacroiliitis is diagnosed by X rays and blood tests. If infection is suspected, fluid may be removed from the joint and checked for microorganisms. Treatment is with *nonsteroidal anti-inflammatory drugs* or, if the joint is infected, *antibiotic drugs*.

Sacrum
The large triangular bone in the lower spine. Its broad upper part articulates with the fifth (lowest) lumbar vertebra, and its narrow lower part with the *coccyx* (tailbone). The sides of the sacrum are connected by *sacroiliac joints* to the iliums (the largest of the bones that form the *pelvis*). Thus, the sacrum sits like a wedge in the center of the back of the pelvis.

STRUCTURE OF THE SACROILIAC JOINT
The joint forms an interface between the sacrum at the back of the pelvis and the ilium (hip bone) on each side of the body.

Ilium

Lumbar vertebrae

Sacroiliac ligaments

Sacroiliac joint

Sacrum

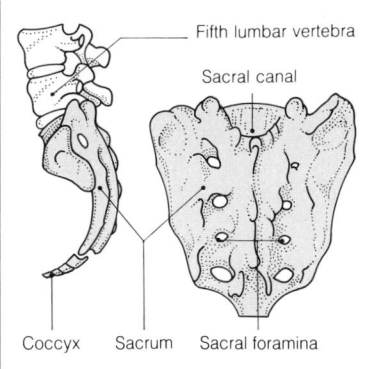

STRUCTURE OF THE SACRUM
The sacrum consists of five vertebrae (spinal bones) that are fused together to form a single solid structure.

Fifth lumbar vertebra

Sacral canal

Coccyx   Sacrum   Sacral foramina

The sacrum is a strong bone and is rarely fractured. If a fracture does occur, it is usually a result of a fall or of a powerful direct blow to the bone. Other disorders include *sacralgia* (pain in the sacrum, sometimes due to a *disk prolapse*); *spondylolisthesis*, in which the fifth lumbar vertebra slips over the sacrum; and a birth anomaly in which the sacrum is fused to the fifth lumbar vertebra (see *Sacralization*). See also *Bone* disorders box; *Spine* disorders box.

Sadism
A love of cruelty and inflicting pain on other people. The term is derived from the name of the French novelist the Marquis de Sade.

Sadism often refers specifically to the achievement of orgasm through hurting, humiliating, or torturing one's partner or other victim. It is more common in men and often accompanied by *masochism* (a desire to be abused). Sadistic activities include beating, whipping, and bondage, usually accompanied by verbal abuse. Sadists rarely inflict serious physical damage (the genuinely sadistic murderer is rare) but *rape* often has a sadistic basis. Only in rare cases do sadists seek help from a psychiatrist. (See also *Sadomasochism*.)

Sadomasochism
Sexual arousal caused by inflicting pain or punishment (*sadism*) or by receiving abuse (*masochism*). Sadism

and masochism may be combined in a person, although one trait usually predominates. The sadomasochist is generally male and may practice other sexual *deviations*, such as *fetishism*.

Researchers have found sadomasochistic literature to be a common form of pornography. The practice may be more widespread than is generally known; biting is a common sex practice. In a broad sense, any relationship in which there is one very dominant and one submissive partner can be said to have sadomasochistic elements.

SADS
Seasonal affective disorder syndrome, an incompletely studied and proved phenomenon in which mood changes are alleged to occur with the seasons.

Safe period
See *Contraception, periodic abstinence*.

"Safe" sex
A term used to describe preventive measures taken to reduce the risk of acquiring a sexually transmitted disease. "Safe" sex has been publicized recently because of the spread of *AIDS*, but the same principles apply to prevention of other sexually transmitted diseases, such as *hepatitis B*, *herpes*, and *gonorrhea*.

Sexual intercourse is completely safe only if you and your partner are monogamous (have not had sex with anyone else) and did not receive a blood product infusion before 1985, when blood products began to be tested for the AIDS virus. To reduce the risk of acquiring AIDS, casual sex and sex with multiple partners should be avoided. People with a higher risk of carrying AIDS include intravenous drug abusers, bisexual and homosexual men, prostitutes, promiscuous men or women, hemophiliacs and their partners, and people from areas where there is a very high incidence of AIDS (e.g., Central Africa and Haiti).

Antibody testing to show whether a person has been exposed to the AIDS virus is being used by dating organizations. Members are issued a "safe sex card" if their test results are negative; they are retested every six months. This procedure provides no guarantee against contracting AIDS. It can take six months to produce antibodies after exposure to the virus.

Known methods of transmitting the AIDS virus include vaginal intercourse, anal intercourse, oral sex, sharing sex aids such as vibrators, and any sexual activity that causes bleeding in the vagina or anus. Any sexual practice that involves contact with urine or feces also poses a risk. Sex during menstruation is particularly dangerous if the woman is a carrier. "Dry kissing," cuddling, caressing, massage, or mutual masturbation (providing there is no broken skin or ejaculation of semen near the vagina) are not believed to transmit the virus.

To reduce the risk of acquiring AIDS or any other sexually transmitted disease, a condom should be worn. If a condom fails to prevent transmission, the cause is most likely to be incorrect use or a torn condom (especially during anal intercourse).

Salicylic acid
A *keratolytic drug* used in the treatment of skin disorders, including *dermatitis*, *eczema*, *psoriasis*, *ichthyosis*, *acne*, *warts*, and callosities (see *Callus*, *skin*). Salicylic acid is sometimes used to treat fungal infections.

Salicyclic acid may cause inflammation and skin *ulcers* if used over a long period or applied to a large area.

Saline
Salty, or consisting of or containing salt (sodium chloride). The term is also used to refer to a solution of salt, particularly one that has the same concentration as body fluids (known as physiological, or normal, saline). This solution, found in tears, is a component of contact lens solution.

Physiological saline may be given in large amounts (by injection or infusion into a vein) to replace body fluids in cases of dehydration. It is sometimes used in small quantities to dissolve drugs for injection.

Saliva
The watery, slightly alkaline fluid secreted into the mouth by the *salivary glands* and the mucous membranes that line the mouth. Saliva contains the digestive enzyme amylase, which helps break down carbohydrates (see *Digestive system*). It also keeps the mouth moist, lubricates food to aid swallowing, and makes it possible to taste food (taste buds are stimulated only by dissolved substances). In addition to amylase, saliva contains chemicals, such as sodium, potassium, calcium, and chloride; pro-

S

HOW TO USE A CONDOM
Using a condom is not a guarantee against transmission of HIV (the AIDS virus) or other sexually transmitted disease, but it does reduce the risks. Whether a condom is used to prevent disease transmission or to prevent conception, it should be used in conjunction with a spermicide preparation.

1 The penis should be fully erect before the condom is put on. The condom should be in place before any vaginal or anal penetration by the penis and before oral sex.

2 Use a brand of condom that has been approved by a regulatory authority. Do not use a condom that has no teat, is time-expired, or appears defective.

3 The teat-end should be squeezed free of air and the condom unrolled fully over the penis. Do not stretch the condom tightly; a tight condom is more likely to burst.

4 The penis should be withdrawn soon after ejaculation. During withdrawal, the base of the condom should be held to prevent spilling the semen.

teins; mucin (the principal constituent of mucus); urea; white blood cells; and debris from the lining of the mouth.

Salivary glands

Three pairs of glands that secrete *saliva*, via ducts, into the mouth. The largest pair, the *parotid glands*, lies over the angle of the jaw, just below and in front of the ears; the ducts of these glands run forward and inward to open inside the cheeks.

The sublingual glands are situated in the floor of the front of the mouth, where they form a low ridge on each side of the frenulum (the central band of tissue that attaches the underside of the tongue to the floor of the mouth). This ridge has a row of small openings through which saliva is secreted.

The submandibular glands lie toward the back of the mouth close to the sides of the jaw. Their ducts run forward to open under the tongue on two small swellings, one on either side of the frenulum.

DISORDERS

Among the most common salivary gland disorders is infection of the parotid glands with the *mumps* virus. Another principal disorder is the formation of *calculi* (stones) in a duct or within the substance of a gland. A stone in a duct causes a swelling that enlarges during eating because of damming of the saliva flow; it may

ANATOMY OF THE SALIVARY GLANDS

Each gland consists of thousands of saliva-secreting sacs. Tiny ducts carry the saliva into the main ducts leading to the mouth.

Parotid gland

Parotid duct

Tongue

Submandibular gland

Sublingual gland

also be painful. Surgical removal of a stone in a duct is straightforward, but a stone in a gland itself may necessitate removal of the entire gland.

Occasionally, the parotid glands are affected by *sarcoidosis*, which may cause considerable swelling. In rare cases, sarcoidosis also affects the facial nerve, which may result in *facial palsy*.

If oral hygiene is poor, the salivary glands may become infected by bacteria spreading from the mouth, which can lead to the development of an abscess in the affected glands.

Tumors of the salivary glands are rare, except for a type of parotid tumor that is usually slow-growing, painless, and benign (but which occasionally becomes malignant).

Insufficient secretion of saliva, causing a dry mouth (see *Mouth, dry*), may result from *dehydration* or *Sjögren's syndrome*. Certain drugs also decrease salivation as a side effect. (See also *Salivation, excessive*.)

Salivation, excessive

The production of too much saliva occurs in numerous disorders, including mouth irritation caused by jagged teeth or dental *caries*, *toothache*, *gingivitis* (inflammation of the gums), *mouth ulcers*, any painful mouth injury, and *esophagitis* (inflammation of the esophagus).

A variety of conditions that affect the nervous system can also cause excessive salivation, among them *Parkinson's disease*, *rabies*, *mercury poisoning*, and overactivity of the parasympathetic division of the *autonomic nervous system* (which controls the salivary glands), usually due to disease or drugs.

Salmonella

An important group of bacteria. One type of salmonella causes *typhoid fever*; others are a common cause of bacterial *food poisoning*.

Salpingectomy

Surgical removal of one or both *fallopian tubes*. Salpingectomy may be performed if the tube has become infected (see *Salpingitis*), as a method of contraception (see *Sterilization, female*), or to treat an *ectopic pregnancy*. (See also *Salpingo-oophorectomy*.)

Salpingitis

Inflammation of a *fallopian tube* (the tube that runs from the ovary to the top of the uterus), commonly caused by infection spreading upward from the vagina, cervix, or uterus.

CAUSES AND INCIDENCE

Salpingitis may be a result of a *chlamydial infection* or a bacterial infection, especially *gonorrhea*. Although salpingitis usually results from a sexually transmitted disease, it may also follow childbirth, miscarriage, or elective abortion. Other causes include *peritonitis* (inflammation of the abdominal lining), or, rarely, a blood-borne infection, such as tuberculosis.

SYMPTOMS AND SIGNS

Symptoms and signs include severe abdominal pain, fever, and frequent urination. The abdomen is very tender and the sufferer is usually most comfortable lying on her back with her legs bent at the knee. Vaginal examination is painful.

DIAGNOSIS

The presence of infection may be confirmed by a blood test showing a high number of white blood cells. A culture of a swab sample of the vaginal discharge allows identification of the causative microorganism. *Laparoscopy* (examination of the inside of the abdominal cavity with a viewing tube) may be performed to confirm the diagnosis and to exclude the possibility of ectopic pregnancy or appendicitis, which can cause similar symptoms.

COMPLICATIONS

Pus may collect within the fallopian tube itself (pyosalpinx), sometimes followed by fluid collection within the tube (hydrosalpinx). Pus collection within the abdominal cavity causes a pelvic abscess. Occasionally, the infection persists despite treatment and causes a variety of symptoms, such as persistent back pain that is worse before menstruation, frequent heavy periods, and pain during intercourse. If the infection damages the inside of the tubes, eggs may be unable to pass the blockage, resulting in *infertility* or an increased risk of *ectopic pregnancy*.

TREATMENT

Treatment includes bed rest, fluids, *analgesics* (painkillers), and *antibiotic drugs*. Surgery is performed to drain a pyosalpinx, hydrosalpinx, or pelvic abscess. If infection persists despite antibiotics, the damaged tubes may be removed, sometimes with the uterus and most of the ovary. (See also *Salpingectomy*; *Salpingo-oophorectomy*.)

Salpingography

See *Hysterosalpingography*.

Salpingo-oophorectomy

Removal of one or both *fallopian tubes* and *ovaries*. Salpingo-oophorectomy may be performed to treat persistent

S

salpingitis (inflammation of the fallopian tubes), cancer of the ovary (see *Ovary, cancer of*), cancer of the uterus (see *Uterus, cancer of*), or *choriocarcinoma* (a malignant tumor derived from placental tissue). The operation is often carried out with a *hysterectomy* (removal of the uterus and cervix).

Salpingo-oophorectomy is carried out using a general anesthetic. Removal of the fallopian tube or tubes is a brief, straightforward procedure and the short recovery period is usually problem-free.

Salt
Any compound of an acid and a base. In general usage, the term usually refers specifically to one such compound—common table salt, known chemically as sodium chloride (see *Sodium*). The term salt may also be applied to a particular chemical salt or mixture of salts used medicinally (often as a purgative), as in magnesium sulfate and sodium sulfate. (See also *Saline*.)

Salve
A term for a healing, soothing, often medicated, ointment.

Sand-fly bites

Sand flies are tiny, delicate, long-legged flies that inhabit most warm parts of the world and, in some areas, transmit disease to humans via their bites. Sand flies are about one eighth of an inch (3 mm) long and can breed in a variety of habitats, including forests, sand, and city rubble.

In the US, sand flies are common in many areas, although they do not transmit disease. Elsewhere, diseases spread by these flies include various forms of *leishmaniasis* in tropical and subtropical regions and *bartonellosis* in the western Andes. Sand-fly fever is an influenzalike illness of short duration that is caused by a virus spread by the flies in parts of the Mediterranean and Asia.

Sand flies primarily bite after dusk. In areas where they are numerous, the best protection is to wear insect repellents and clothing that covers the arms and legs and is snug at the wrists and ankles (see *Insect bites*).

Sanitary protection
Articles used to protect clothing from blood stains during *menstruation*. Disposable sanitary napkins or tampons are available in different absorbencies to meet individual needs.

Sarcoidosis
A rare disease of unknown cause in which inflammation occurs in lymph nodes and other tissues throughout the body, usually the lungs, liver, skin, and eyes. The disorder occurs primarily in young adults.
SYMPTOMS AND SIGNS
Acute sarcoidosis is associated with fever and generalized aches. It may also cause enlargement of lymph nodes in the neck and elsewhere, breathlessness, arthritis, or *erythema nodosum* (red-purple swellings on the legs). Chronic sarcoidosis can cause a variety of symptoms, including fever, a purple rash on the face, painful joints, a painful, bloodshot eye, and areas of numbness. Sometimes, the disease produces no symptoms.

Complications include scarring and thickening of the lung tissues (*fibrosis*) and *hypercalcemia* (an abnormally high calcium level in the blood), which may damage the kidneys.
DIAGNOSIS AND TREATMENT
A diagnosis may be suggested from a chest X ray (which shows enlarged lymph nodes) and from the rash. A biopsy of the lung, skin, lymph gland, or liver confirms the diagnosis.

Many people with sarcoidosis are not seriously ill; the disease may resolve without treatment. About 90 percent of patients recover completely within two years, with or without treatment, but persistent, chronic disease develops in 10 percent.

Corticosteroid drugs are prescribed to treat persistent fever or persistent erythema nodosum, to prevent blindness in an affected eye, and to reduce the risk of permanent lung damage. *Chloroquine* is sometimes used to treat skin abnormalities.

Sarcoma
A cancer of connective tissue (such as cartilage), blood vessels, or the fibrous tissue that surrounds and supports organs. Types of sarcoma include *osteosarcoma* and *chondrosarcoma* (both arising in bones), *Kaposi's sarcoma* (which mainly affects the skin and is common in people who have *AIDS*), and *fibrosarcoma*.

Saturated fats
See *Fats and oils*.

Scab
A crust that forms on the skin or on a mucous membrane at the site of a healing wound or infected area. A scab is composed of fibrin and serum that has leaked from the wound and dried, along with skin scales, pus, and other debris. A similar term is eschar, used in connection with burns.

Scabies
A skin infestation caused by the mite *SARCOPTES SCABIEI*, which burrows into the skin, where it lays eggs. Scabies is highly contagious. Hatched mites can pass from an infested individual to a person standing close beside him or her, although infestation is more likely through physical contact (such as sexual intercourse). The disorder is most common in infants, children, young adults, or in people who are institutionalized.
SYMPTOMS
The openings of the mite's burrows can be seen on the skin as tiny, gray, scaly swellings, usually between the fingers, on the wrists and genitals, and in the armpits. Later, reddish lumps may appear on the limbs and the trunk. The infestation causes intense itching, particularly at night, and scratching results in the formation of scabs and sores.
TREATMENT
The condition is treated by applying an insecticide lotion (such as *lindane*) to all skin below the sufferer's head. The lotion usually kills the mites, but itching may persist for up to two weeks. All members of the affected person's household (even if they show no signs of infestation) should be treated simultaneously.

Scald
To burn with hot liquid or steam (see *Burns*).

Scaling, dental
Removal of *calculus* (a hard, chalky deposit) from the teeth, performed to prevent or treat *periodontal disease* (disorders of the gums and other tissues supporting the teeth).

Scaling is carried out with an instrument called a scaler. It may have a sharp, scraping edge or be an ultrasonic model with a tip that vibrates at high speed to chip away the deposit. After scaling, the teeth are usually polished with a mild abrasive paste and motorized buffers.

Scalp
The region of the skin and underlying tissue layers of the head that is normally covered with hair. Scalp skin differs from other areas of skin because it is tougher and it is attached to an underlying sheet of muscle

S

(called the epicranius) that extends from the eyebrows, over the top of the head, and to the nape of the neck. This muscle is only loosely attached (by connective tissue) to the skull, making it comparatively easy for areas of scalp to be torn off (e.g., as a result of catching the hair in machinery). Because the scalp is richly supplied with blood vessels, wounds bleed profusely.

The scalp may be affected by a variety of hair or skin disorders. The most common are *dandruff*; hair loss, particularly in men (see *Alopecia*); *sebaceous cysts*; *psoriasis*; fungal infections, such as ringworm (see *Tinea*); and parasitic infestations such as *lice*. *Cradle cap*, a harmless form of seborrheic *dermatitis* in which greasy, crusty patches appear on the scalp, is common in infants.

Scalpel
A surgical knife for cutting tissue. Scalpels with steel blades are used for most operations, but in some cases (e.g., eye surgery) sharper diamond or ruby blades are used.

Scanning techniques
Images of the body organs can be produced by a variety of scanning techniques that record, process, and (depending on the technique) analyze the sound waves, radio waves, or X rays that pass through or are generated by body tissues.

The scanning technique used most widely in medicine is *ultrasound*, in which inaudible, ultrahigh frequency sound waves are passed into the region being examined. These sound waves are reflected more strongly by some structures than others, and the pattern of reflections is detected by one or more transducers and displayed on a screen. Ultrasound was originally developed by the military for the detection of submarines beneath the sea. However, in the past 20 years, it has been refined and developed for the examination of a fetus and also the heart, liver, kidney, and other organs.

CT scanning uses X rays to measure variations in the density of the organ being examined; it compiles an image or picture by computer analysis.

Radionuclide scanning involves the injection into the body of radioactive substances that are taken up in different amounts by different organs. Radioactive iodine, for example, becomes concentrated in the thyroid gland. A radioactivity detector, such as a gamma camera, is positioned near the organ under study, and the pattern of radiation being emitted is recorded and displayed on a screen.

MRI (magnetic resonance imaging) uses a powerful electromagnet to align the nuclei of atoms of hydrogen, phosphorus, or other elements in the body. The nuclei are then knocked out of position by radio waves; in realigning themselves with the magnetic field, they produce a radio signal that can be detected and transformed into a computer-generated image. (See also *PET scanning*.)

Scaphoid
One of the wrist bones. The scaphoid is the outermost bone on the thumb side of the hand in the proximal row of carpals (the row of wrist bones nearest the elbow).

A fracture of the scaphoid is one of the most common wrist injuries, usually occurring as a result of a fall on an outstretched hand. A characteristic symptom of this injury is tenderness in the space between the two prominent tendons at the base of the thumb on the back of the hand. This symptom may be a more positive indication of a scaphoid fracture than an X ray. Treatment consists of immobilizing the wrist in a cast.

An undiagnosed, untreated scaphoid fracture may not heal, which can lead to *osteoarthritis* or, in some cases, necrosis (death) of part of the bone. These complications may result in persistent pain in the wrist and restriction of its movement.

Scapula
The anatomical name for the shoulder blade. The scapula is a flat, triangular bone situated over the back of the upper ribs. On its rear surface is a prominent spine (which can be felt under the skin) that runs diagonally upward and outward to a bony prominence (called the acromion) at the shoulder tip. The acromion articulates with the end of the *clavicle* (collarbone) to form the *acromioclavicular joint*. Just below the acromion is a socket (called the glenoid cavity) into which the head of the humerus (upper arm bone) fits to form the shoulder joint.

The scapula serves as an attachment for certain muscles and tendons of the arm, neck, chest, and back, and is involved with movements of the arm and shoulder.

Because the scapula is well padded with muscle, great force is required to fracture it. Treatment of a fracture consists of putting the shoulder in a *sling* until the fracture has healed. *Physical therapy* may be needed to restore movement to the joint.

Scar
Any mark left on damaged tissue after it has healed. Scar tissue forms not only on the skin but on all internal wounds (e.g., after a muscle tear or where surgery has been performed).

The body repairs a wound, ulcer, or other lesion by increasing production of the tough, fibrous protein *collagen* at the site of the damage. The collagen helps form new connective tissue, which covers the area of the lesion. If the edges of an incision are brought together when healing takes place, the resultant scar is narrow and pale; if the edges are left apart, the scar is more extensive (see *Healing*).

ABNORMAL SCAR FORMATION
A hypertrophic scar is a large, unsightly scar that may develop at the site of a wound that has become infected. Some people have a family tendency toward hypertrophic scars for no apparent reason.

A *keloid* is a large, irregularly shaped scar that continues to grow in size as the body continues to produce extra collagen after a wound has healed; this type of scar is more common in black than in white people.

Adhesions are areas of scar tissue that form between unconnected parts of internal organs; they are a potential complication of intestinal surgery.

Scarlatina
Another name for *scarlet fever*.

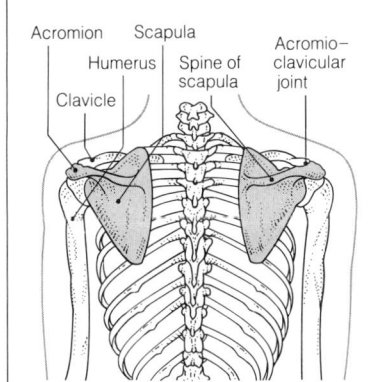

LOCATION OF THE SCAPULAE
The two scapulae are the prominent wing-shaped bones in the upper back. They facilitate many arm and shoulder actions.

Acromion   Scapula
Humerus   Spine of   Acromio-
scapula   clavicular
Clavicle   joint

S

Scarlet fever

An infectious disease of childhood that is caused by a strain of streptococcal bacteria. Characterized by a sore throat, fever, and rash, scarlet fever is far less common and dangerous than it once was.

CAUSES AND SYMPTOMS

The bacteria are spread in droplets coughed or breathed into the air. After an incubation period of two to four days, a sore throat, headache, and fever develop in an infected child. A rash soon appears, caused by a toxin released by the bacteria. The rash begins as a mass of tiny red spots on the neck and upper trunk and spreads rapidly. The face is flushed (except for an area around the mouth) and a white coating with red spots may develop on the tongue. After a few days the coating peels to reveal a bright red appearance. Soon afterward, the fever subsides, the rash fades, and there is frequently some skin peeling, especially on the hands and feet.

As with other types of sore throat caused by streptococci (see *Strep throat*), there is a risk of *rheumatic fever* or *glomerulonephritis* (inflammation in the kidneys) if the infection is not treated promptly.

DIAGNOSIS AND TREATMENT

The physician diagnoses scarlet fever from the symptoms and signs and, if necessary, by *culture* of the bacteria from a throat swab.

Treatment is with *antibiotic drugs*, usually penicillin (or erythromycin if the person has a penicillin allergy). Treatment usually leads to a rapid recovery. During the illness, the child should rest, drink plenty of fluids, and be given acetaminophen to relieve discomfort and reduce fever.

Schistosome

A type of fluke (flattened worm). Three types of schistosomes are parasites of humans, causing the disease *schistosomiasis* in tropical regions of the world.

Schistosomiasis

A parasitic disease, also known as bilharziasis, that occurs in most tropical countries and afflicts over 200 million people worldwide.

CAUSES AND INCIDENCE

The disease is caused by any of three species of flukes called schistosomes and is acquired from bathing in infested lakes and rivers in the tropics. Forms of schistosome (cercariae) penetrate the bather's skin and develop within the body into adult flukes (see life-cycle diagram at right). Eggs produced by the adult females provoke inflammatory reactions, which in turn may cause symptoms.

The infestation causes bleeding, ulceration, and *fibrosis* (scar tissue formation) in the bladder or intestinal walls; infestation may also cause inflammation and fibrosis in other organs, such as the liver.

SYMPTOMS

Symptoms vary considerably. Some infested people have no symptoms, others become severely ill and suffer serious complications.

The first symptom is usually tingling and an itchy rash where the cercariae have penetrated the skin. Many weeks later, when the adults start producing eggs, an influenzalike illness may develop. Sometimes severe, the illness is marked by high fever, chills, aching, and pains. Subsequent symptoms may include blood in the urine or feces, abdominal or low back pain, and enlargement of the liver and/or spleen. Complications of long-term infestation may include liver *cirrhosis*, *bladder tumors*, and *renal failure*.

DIAGNOSIS AND TREATMENT

The diagnosis is made from a special blood test for antibodies to the parasites (see *Immunoassay*) and from microscopic examination of a sample of urine or feces to detect eggs.

Since the early 1980s, treatment has been revolutionized by a new drug (praziquantel), a single dose of which kills the flukes and thus prevents, or limits, damage to internal organs.

PREVENTION

Since no vaccine is available against the disease, visitors to areas where schistosomiasis is present (i.e., much of the tropics) should regard all lakes and rivers as unsafe for swimming.

Control of the disease rests on the provision of latrines and their regular use by the population. The Chinese claim to have achieved some success through measures directed against snails and through imposing strict sanitary regulations.

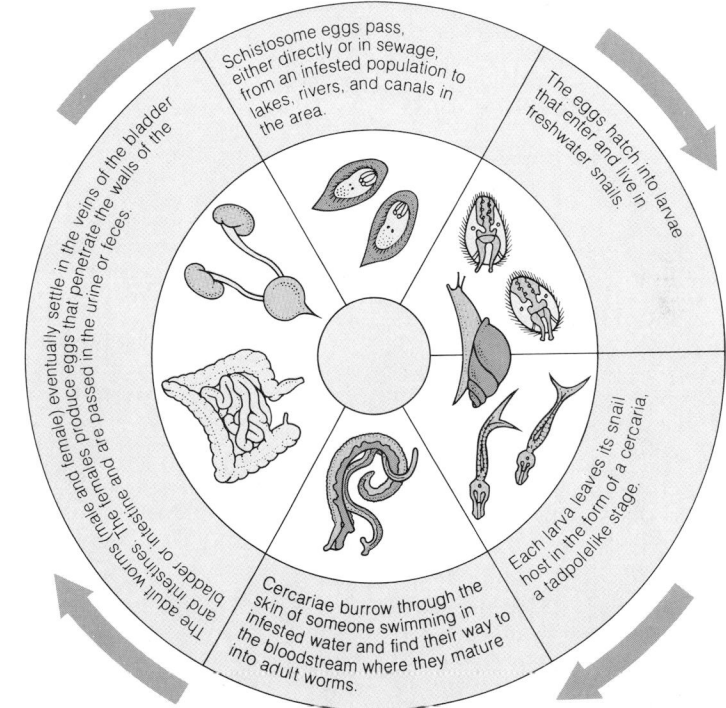

Cycle of schistosomiasis
The disease affects a large proportion of the population in some parts of the world, such as the Nile valley in Egypt. Many methods have been tried to break the cycle of the disease in affected areas, with varying success. Methods used have included strict sanitary regulations and measures to eradicate freshwater snails.

S

Schizoid personality disorder

Inability to relate socially to other people. People with this trait, which is apparent from childhood, are often described as "loners" and have few, if any, friends. They are markedly eccentric, seem to lack warmth or concern for others, and may be vague and detached from day-to-day activities. Psychoanalysts believe the condition results from an impoverished mother-child relationship.

Schizophrenia develops in about 10 percent of people diagnosed as having a schizoid personality. However, not all schizophrenics initially have schizoid personalities.

Although the marital and employment prospects for schizoid people are severely impaired, some succeed in socially isolated occupations. (See also *Avoidant personality disorder*.)

Schizophrenia

A general term for a group of psychotic illnesses characterized by disturbances in thinking, emotional reaction, and behavior. Schizophrenia is sometimes referred to as "split personality" because the sufferer's thoughts and feelings do not relate to each other in a logical fashion. However, the disorder should not be confused with *multiple personality*. Schizophrenia is a disabling illness with a prolonged course that almost always results in chronic ill health and some degree of personality change.

PREVALENCE

Schizophrenia is the most common form of psychotic illness. It has an average lifetime prevalence throughout the world of just under 1 percent. Approximately 1.5 million US citizens are currently affected. For reasons that are not understood, the disorder is more common in certain geographic areas (e.g., Western Ireland and inner-city populations).

Onset is usually between the ages of 15 and 25, being, on average, five years later in women than in men; otherwise, males and females are equally affected.

CAUSES

Inheritance has been shown to play a role in the development of schizophrenia. First-degree relatives (parents, children, or siblings) of schizophrenics have a 10 percent chance of the illness; more distant relatives have a lower risk. If both parents are schizophrenic, one in three of their children becomes ill, and, if schizophrenia develops in one identical twin, the other twin has approximately a one in two chance of being affected. However, factors other than genetics must also play a part or the illness would inevitably develop in both twins.

Biological studies have shown that certain forms of brain damage (such as temporal lobe epilepsy, tumors, and encephalitis) tend to be related to schizophrenic symptoms. Brain imaging techniques, especially *CT scanning* and *PET scanning*, have revealed abnormalities of structure and function in the brains of schizophrenics. It has also been demonstrated that certain drugs, such as amphetamines, can cause a schizophrenic illness and that drugs blocking the action of the brain chemical dopamine often relieve schizophrenic symptoms.

It seems likely that schizophrenia is possibly worsened by stress in the individual's personal life.

SYMPTOMS

Schizophrenia may begin insidiously, with the individual becoming slowly more withdrawn and introverted, and losing his or her drive and motivation. The change may not be noticed for months or years, until it becomes apparent that the individual is suffering from *delusions* (false ideas that do not respond to reasoned argument) or *hallucinations* (a sensory experience in the absence of an external stimulus). In other cases, the illness comes on more suddenly, usually in response to some external stress.

Delusions may take a variety of forms, ranging from single ideas, such as the belief that one is Jesus Christ or Napoleon, to elaborate delusional systems in which special significance is attached to everyday objects or events. In paranoid schizophrenia, the illness is dominated by delusions of grandeur, persecution, or jealousy.

Hallucinations frequently are experienced as voices that comment on behavior or thoughts, occasionally in the form of conversations in which the sufferer is referred to as he or she. This type of auditory third person hallucination occurs exclusively in schizophrenia. True visual hallucinations are rare in Western cultures, but distortions of visual perception do occur; faces or objects may look sharper or change shape. Bodily sensations, such as tingling, are common.

Most schizophrenics also suffer from a variety of thought disorders, which impair concentration or clear thinking. Sufferers describe their thoughts as being blocked, or inserted into or withdrawn, from their minds by some outside force. They may also feel that their thoughts are being broadcast to others; in rare cases, the thoughts are experienced as echoes inside the head.

Disordered thinking is reflected in muddled and disjointed speech. Disturbance of association results in the schizophrenic jumping between subjects that are seemingly unrelated. Inability to think in abstractions often leads to bizarre responses to questions. For example, when a girl was asked why she was turning in a circle, she said she felt she was in a knot and was trying to unravel herself. In some cases, speech disintegrates, becoming a "word salad" of odd phrases, *neologisms* (made-up words), and detached syllables.

In a rare form of schizophrenia, catatonia may occur, in which sufferers adopt prolonged rigid postures or engage in outbursts of repeated movement.

Symptoms of *manic-depressive illness* may accompany schizophrenia, especially in the early stages. However, as the illness progresses, emotions usually become severely blunted, there is increasing detachment from other people, and there is a loss of interest in hobbies or occupations. Behavior becomes more eccentric and self-neglect is common.

DIAGNOSIS

For a diagnosis of schizophrenia to be made by current US standards, the individual must have continuous signs of a profound break with reality and evidence of fragmentation (disorganization) of the personality for at least six months during some time in his or her life. This six-month period must include at least one phase when there are symptoms of hallucinations, delusions, or marked thought disorders.

TREATMENT

The main form of treatment consists of *antipsychotic drugs* (such as chlorpromazine), some of which can be given as long-acting *depot injections*, which reduces the symptoms and makes the person more amenable to *psychotherapy*. Drug treatment is effective in suppressing the more obvious symptoms, such as hallucinations, but may result in side effects, particularly *dyskinesia* (abnormal muscular movements) and tremor.

Schizophrenics may be treated initially in the hospital; once the major symptoms are controlled, most return to the community. Adequate provision of day centers, decent housing, and vocational opportunities can do much to further control symptoms, improve the sufferer's self-reliance, prevent relapse, and reduce the stigma attached to mental illness. If the patient is to live at home, the family needs to be provided with support and guidance, since some schizophrenics may be difficult to live with. A certain number relapse, especially if they do not take their medication regularly.

OUTLOOK

While some 10 percent of those in whom schizophrenia develops remain severely impaired for life, the majority can return to varying degrees of independence. About 30 percent return to normal lives and occupations.

The particular form of the illness is important in determining the outlook. Individuals who have schizophrenia combined with manic-depressive symptoms often recover fully, as do many with catatonia. Paranoid schizophrenics, because of the preservation of their personalities, are often able to function well, albeit as somewhat eccentric members of the community. Schizophrenia that comes on slowly, starting around puberty, often causes significant impairment.

Although drugs have improved the outlook for most schizophrenics, inadequate community care frequently results in relapse, neglect, vagrancy, or imprisonment.

Schönlein-Henoch purpura

Inflammation of the blood vessels, causing leakage of blood into the skin, joints, kidneys, and intestine. The disease is most common among young children, especially boys, and often occurs after an infection such as a sore throat. The precise cause of Schönlein-Henoch purpura is unknown, although some experts believe it is due to an abnormal allergic reaction in response to an infection.

SYMPTOMS

The main symptom is a slightly raised, purplish rash on the buttocks and backs of the legs and arms. The joints are often painful, the hands and feet may be swollen, and the child may complain of colicky abdominal pain. Infrequently, bleeding from the intestine occurs, which gives rise to blood in the feces. The kidneys may become inflamed, resulting in *hematuria* (blood in the urine).

DIAGNOSIS AND TREATMENT

The condition must be distinguished from blood-clotting disorders by performing *blood-clotting tests*.

No specific treatment is required other than bed rest and mild *analgesics* (painkillers). Most children recover within a month, although complications may arise if *nephritis* (inflammation of the kidneys) persists. In severe cases, the physician may prescribe *corticosteroid drugs*.

Sciatica

Pain that radiates along the *sciatic nerve*. The pain sometimes extends from the buttock down the leg to the foot, although usually only part of this area is affected (usually the buttock and thigh). In severe cases, the pain may be accompanied by numbness and/or weakness in the affected area.

CAUSES

The most common cause of sciatica is a prolapsed intervertebral disk pressing on a spinal root of the nerve (see *Disk prolapse*). Less commonly, it may be caused by pressure on the nerve from a tumor, abscess, or blood clot, or simply from sitting in an awkward position. Any disorder that involves nerves (such as certain infections, *diabetes mellitus*, or *alcohol dependence*) may affect the sciatic nerve and produce sciatica.

TREATMENT

Treatment is directed toward the underlying cause, but in many cases the cause is not identified. Thus, treatment consists of measures to relieve the pain, including taking *analgesics* (painkillers) and resting in bed. With such treatment, the pain usually disappears within a few days. In severe cases, the pain may persist for several weeks. Sciatica tends to recur.

Sciatic nerve

The primary nerve of the leg and the largest nerve in the body. The sciatic nerve is a branch of the sacral plexus (nerve network) in the pelvis, and is formed from several lumbar and sacral *spinal nerves*. From the sacral plexus, the sciatic nerve passes below the sacroiliac joint (at the back of the pelvis, near the sacrum) and backward to the buttock, from where it passes behind the hip joint and runs down the back of the thigh. Above the back of the knee, the sciatic nerve divides into two main branches, called the tibial nerve and the common peroneal nerve.

The upper part of the sciatic nerve, above the point of division, supplies the hip joint, many of the thigh muscles, and the skin on the back of the thigh. The lower part—the tibial and peroneal nerves—supplies the

LOCATION OF THE SCIATIC NERVE
The diagram below shows the nerve in a cutaway of the right thigh and knee, as seen from behind.

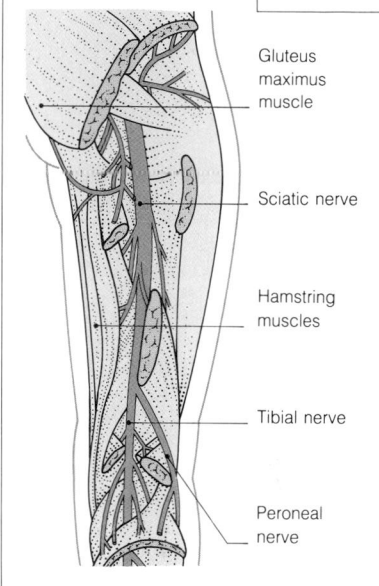

Gluteus maximus muscle

Sciatic nerve

Hamstring muscles

Tibial nerve

Peroneal nerve

knee and ankle joints, all the muscles of the lower leg and foot, and most of the skin below the knee.

DISORDERS

Probably the most common disorder of the sciatic nerve is *sciatica*, which is often due to a prolapsed intervertebral disk pressing on a spinal root of the nerve (see *Disk prolapse*). The upper part of the nerve may also be damaged by dislocation of the hip joint, which, in severe cases, may result in paralysis of muscles below the knee and widespread numbness of the skin in that part of the body.

Damage to the peroneal nerve, often due to a fracture of the upper *fibula* (the outer bone of the lower leg), may produce *footdrop* and numbness of the skin at the side of the lower leg and back of the foot.

The tibial nerve is deeply buried in body tissues and thus is rarely injured. However, it is sometimes damaged by dislocation of the knee, which may cause paralysis of the lower leg and foot, and numbness in the sole of the foot.

Scintigraphy

A less common, alternative name for *radionuclide scanning*.

S

Scirrhous

A medical term meaning hard and fibrous. The word is usually applied to malignant tumors that have dense, fibrous tissue within them.

Sclera

The white outer coat of the *eye*, visible through the transparent *conjunctiva*. The sclera is composed of dense, fibrous tissue formed from *collagen*, which is strong and protects the inner structures of the eye from injury. It may, however, be penetrated by sharp objects.

Disease of the sclera is uncommon, but *scleritis* (inflammation of the sclera) may occur, usually with a *collagen disease* such as *rheumatoid arthritis*. The healthy sclera sometimes shows a blue tinge from the underlying choroid. If the sclera is exceptionally thin, which occurs in *osteogenesis imperfecta*, this blue appearance is striking.

LOCATION OF THE SCLERA
The sclera is about one seventieth of an inch thick and continuous with the cornea at the front of the eye. It is extremely tough.

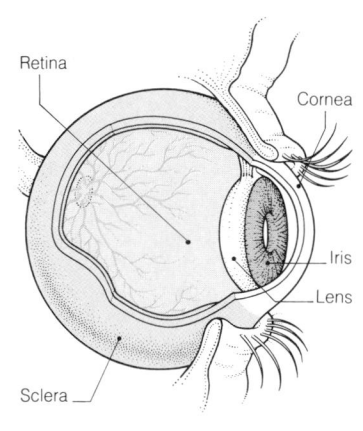

Retina

Cornea

Iris

Lens

Sclera

Scleritis

Inflammation of the *sclera* (white of the eye). Scleritis usually accompanies a *collagen disease*, such as rheumatoid arthritis. It also occurs in *herpes zoster ophthalmicus*, and in *Wegener's granulomatosis*, when it may lead to areas of local thinning and possible perforation of the sclera.

Scleritis is persistent, but often responds well to *corticosteroid* eye drops. In severe cases, these drugs may increase the risk of perforation.

Scleroderma

A rare condition, also known as systemic sclerosis, that can affect many organs and tissues in the body, particularly the skin, arteries, kidneys, lungs, heart, gastrointestinal tract, and joints. Scleroderma is an *autoimmune disorder* (in which the body's immune system attacks its own tissues). Scleroderma is twice as common in women and is most likely to appear between the ages of 40 and 60.

SYMPTOMS AND SIGNS

The number and the severity of symptoms varies dramatically. The most common symptom is *Raynaud's phenomenon*, a painful, three-color (white, red, blue) response of the hands and/or feet to cold exposure; it may be present for many years without any other symptoms.

Also common are changes in the skin (especially of the face and fingers), which becomes shiny (as if it had been waxed), tight, and thickened. There is often puckering around the mouth, giving the sufferer a characteristic masklike appearance. The pulled skin often leads to difficulty performing certain maneuvers, such as bending the fingers or opening the mouth.

In some people, other parts of the body are affected, leading to problems such as difficulty swallowing, shortness of breath, palpitations, high blood pressure, joint pain, stiffness, and muscle weakness. There are wide variations from person to person in the degree to which different parts of the body are involved and the rate at which the disease progresses. Progression is often rapid in the first few years and then slows down or even stops. In a small number of people, degeneration is rapid, usually leading to death from *heart failure*, *respiratory failure*, or *renal failure*.

DIAGNOSIS AND TREATMENT

A physical examination is usually sufficient to confirm the diagnosis, but a blood test and a skin *biopsy* (removal of tissue for microscopic examination) may be performed.

There is no cure for scleroderma, but treatment can relieve symptoms and associated problems. *Vasodilator drugs* and avoiding exposure to cold can relieve Raynaud's phenomenon. *Physical therapy* may be recommended for joint problems. *Antihypertensive drugs* may be given to treat high blood pressure and *dialysis* may be undertaken for renal failure. *Corticosteroid drugs* are sometimes prescribed if the muscle is involved.

Scleromalacia

Softening of the *sclera* (the white portion of the eye). Scleromalacia is frequently a complication of *scleritis* (inflammation of the sclera), especially when the scleritis is caused by rheumatoid arthritis.

Scleromalacia perforans is a rare, severe form of the condition in which the entire thickness of sclera is involved; the underlying choroid bulges through and sometimes perforates the sclera.

Sclerosis

A medical term for hardening of a body tissue. It is usually used to refer to hardening of blood vessels, as in *atherosclerosis* (hardening of arteries), or to hardening of nerve tissue due to deposition of abnormal connective tissue, which occurs in the later stages of *multiple sclerosis*.

Sclerotherapy

A method of treating *varicose veins* (distended, tortuous veins), especially in the legs. *Hemorrhoids* (varicose veins in the anus) and *esophageal varices* (swollen veins at the bottom of the esophagus that may bleed) are sometimes treated this way.

The vein is injected with a strongly irritating solution (called a sclerosant). This causes inflammation in the lining of the vein, blocking it, and eventual fibrosis (scar tissue formation), which leads to the vein's obliteration. For a varicose vein in the leg, the process is assisted by first emptying the vein of blood. After injection, firm pressure is applied so that the walls of the vein are pressed together. Compression is maintained by tight bandaging.

Scoliosis

A deformity in which the spine is bent to one side. The thoracic (chest) or lumbar (lower back) regions are the most commonly affected.

TYPES AND CAUSES

Scoliosis usually starts in childhood or adolescence and progressively becomes more marked until the age at which growth stops. In many such cases, another part of the spine curves toward the opposite side of the body to compensate for the scoliotic curvature, resulting in the spine becoming S-shaped. The cause of juvenile scoliosis is unknown; if the condition is not corrected, it may lead to severe deformity.

More rarely, scoliosis develops as a result of a congenital abnormality of the vertebrae, *poliomyelitis* that has

S

weakened the spinal muscles on one side of the body, or tilting of the pelvis due to one leg being shorter than the other. Occasionally, a spinal injury (such as a *disk prolapse* or ligament sprain) causes temporary scoliosis. In such cases, the spinal curvature appears suddenly and is accompanied by back pain and *sciatica*.

DIAGNOSIS AND TREATMENT

Scoliosis is diagnosed by a physical examination of the spine, hips, and legs, along with X rays of the spine.

If the cause of the condition is known, treatment is directed toward that cause (e.g., bed rest for a disk prolapse or wearing an orthopedic shoe with a raised heel to correct a pelvic tilt due to unequal leg lengths).

Scoliosis of unknown cause may not require treatment if the curvature is slight. However, regular measurement of the spine is necessary to assess the progress of the condition. If it seems to be worsening—or if the curvature is already marked—it may be treated by immobilization of the spine in a hinged plaster jacket or adjustable metal brace, followed by surgery and bone grafting to fuse the affected spinal vertebrae in a straight line (see *Spinal fusion*). A steel rod with hooks or some other metal device may be used to keep the spine straight until the bones become fused.

Scopolamine

An *antispasmodic drug* used to treat *irritable bowel syndrome*, nausea, and *motion sickness*. Scopolamine is also a *premedication* (drug given to prepare a person for surgery). Adverse effects may include drowsiness, dry mouth, and blurred vision.

Scorpion stings

 Scorpions are eight-legged creatures with flexible tails ending in a poison reservoir and a sharp stinger. They are present in most warm regions of the world and are nocturnal, spending the day in dark crevices under rocks and in the loose bark of trees. Sometimes scorpions enter human habitation and crawl into shoes or clothing. If accidentally disturbed, a scorpion is likely to sting, which is achieved by arching its tail over its back.

Some highly venomous species are found in Mexico, North Africa, South America, parts of the Caribbean, and India. About 40 species exist in the US, but only one, found in southern states, is dangerous to humans.

SYMPTOMS

The effects of many types of scorpion stings are little worse than a bee sting, with mild to moderate pain and tingling or burning at the site of the puncture wound. With more dangerous species, there may be sweating, restlessness, diarrhea, and vomiting (caused by stimulation of the *autonomic nervous system*) in addition to severe pain. The venom may also affect the rhythm and strength of the heart's contractions. Fatalities are uncommon in adults; young children and the elderly are at greater risk.

TREATMENT

Any person stung by a scorpion should seek immediate medical attention. For children, or if there are symptoms other than pain, admission to the hospital is advisable.

If pain is the only symptom, mild *analgesics* (painkillers) and cold compresses may be all that is needed. In severe cases, local anesthetics and powerful painkillers may be required, and an *antivenin* to deactivate the venom may be given by intravenous infusion. Antivenins active against the venoms of local, dangerous types of scorpions are available in most parts of the world where such species exist.

PREVENTION

In areas where scorpions are common, clothes and footwear should be shaken out before being put on. Scorpions can be discouraged from entering a house by barriers, such as a porch elevated at least 8 inches above the ground.

Scotoma

An area of abnormal vision within the *visual field*.

Screening

The testing of apparently healthy people with the aim of detecting disease at an early, treatable stage. The ideal screening test is reliable, with a low rate of false-positive results (the results of the test are positive even though the people tested do not in fact have the disease) and a low rate of false-negative results (the results of the test are negative even though the people tested have the disease). An ideal test is also inexpensive, simple, and acceptable to people, causing neither discomfort nor danger. For a screening test to be of practical use, people found to have the disease must benefit from early diagnosis.

Screening for unsuspected diabetes is of no use since there is no evidence that the late complications of the disease are lessened by diagnosis before symptoms develop. (See also *Cancer screening*.)

Scrofula

Tuberculosis of the lymph nodes in the neck, often those just beneath the angle of the jaw. Scrofula was once a common disorder, usually caused by the drinking of contaminated milk. Abscesses would form in the lymph nodes and, after bursting through the skin, leave scars on the neck.

Today scrofula is rare in developed countries. It occasionally develops in Asian or African immigrants in whom the infection has spread from tuberculosis elsewhere in the body. *Antibiotic drugs* clear up the condition in most cases.

Scrotum

The pouch that hangs below the penis and contains the *testes*. The scrotum consists of an outer layer of thin, wrinkled skin over a layer of muscle-containing tissue.

Swelling of the scrotum may be caused by an inguinal *hernia*, a swelling of one of the testes, a *hydrocele* (a fluid-filled sac around one of the testes), or, in severe heart failure, *edema* (fluid retention).

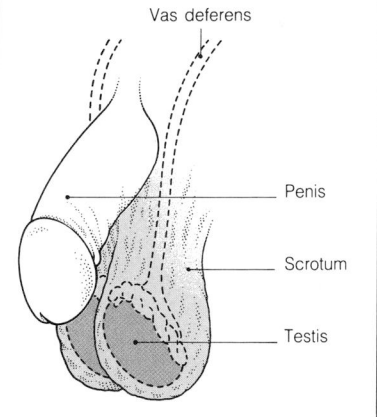

LOCATION OF THE SCROTUM
The scrotum has oil-secreting glands and thinly scattered hairs on its surface. Internally it is divided by a membrane into two halves, each containing a testis.

Vas deferens

Penis

Scrotum

Testis

Scuba-diving medicine

A minor medical specialty concerned with the physiological hazards of underwater diving with self-contained underwater breathing apparatus (S.C.U.B.A.).

S

THE MAIN HAZARDS

Most diving hazards stem from the increase in pressure with depth. At a depth of 33 feet (10 m), the total pressure is twice the surface pressure. At 99 feet (30 m), it is four times the surface pressure.

MECHANICAL EFFECTS OF PRESSURE CHANGE

During descent, divers must introduce gas into their middle-ear cavities and facial sinuses to prevent damage as the pressure mounts. This mounting pressure is what airline passengers experience during descent and repressurization (see *Barotrauma*).

Whatever depth they attain, divers must be supplied with breathing mixtures at a pressure equal to the external water pressure. Thus, at 99 feet (30 m), a diver breathes gas at four times the surface pressure. During ascent, gas in the lungs expands and can rupture the lung tissues if the diver panics and inadvertently holds his or her breath—a serious condition known as pulmonary barotrauma (burst lung). Symptoms may include coughing up blood, inability to urinate, breathing difficulties, and unconsciousness.

TOXIC EFFECTS OF GASES

Amateur divers breathe compressed air, which consists mainly of nitrogen and oxygen. These gases are harmless at surface pressures (oxygen is essential to life), but they become toxic at high pressure. Nitrogen impairs the nervous system when air is breathed at depths from about 80 feet (24 m) downward, causing slowed mental functioning and other symptoms that mimic alcohol intoxication (nitrogen narcosis). Oxygen becomes toxic when air is breathed at about 260 feet (80 m), when it can cause convulsions or lung damage.

To attain greater depths without risking nitrogen and oxygen poisoning, professional divers use gas mixtures other than air. A typical mixture consists of helium, with only small amounts of oxygen and nitrogen; the helium is relatively nontoxic.

THE BENDS

At depth, divers accumulate in their tissues excess quantities of any inert gas they are breathing (nitrogen, if air is being breathed). If pressure is released too quickly (i.e., the diver ascends too fast) and if a large amount of gas has accumulated because the diver remained at depth for too long, this gas can no longer be held in the tissues and may form bubbles, causing *decompression sickness*.

OTHER HAZARDS

Additional hazards include *hypothermia* (dangerous chilling) due to immersion in cold water, bites or stings from marine animals (see *Bites, animal*; *Venomous bites and stings*), and risk of *drowning*.

ACCIDENT PREVENTION AND TREATMENT

Any person taking up scuba diving should first receive a medical checkup and undergo thorough training at a recognized diving school.

Pressure-related accidents, such as burst lung and decompression sickness, are treated by recompression of the diver in a special pressure chamber so that any bubbles or pockets of gas in the blood or tissues are reabsorbed. This is followed by slow release of the pressure.

Treatment of other accidents (such as hypothermia and near drowning) is as for nondivers.

Scurvy

A disease caused by inadequate intake of *vitamin C*. Scurvy is rare today in developed countries as a result of increased consumption of fresh fruit and vegetables. Body stores of vitamin C give protection against scurvy for about three months.

CAUSES AND SYMPTOMS

Inadequate supplies of vitamin C disturb the body's normal production of *collagen* (connective tissue). Collagen continues to be produced but it is unstable, causing weakness of small blood vessels and poor healing in wounds. Hemorrhages may occur anywhere in the body. They are most obvious in the skin, where they result in widespread bruising. Bleeding from the gums and loosening of the teeth are common; bleeding into muscles and joints also occurs in scurvy, causing pain.

Scurvy is especially serious in children because bleeding into the membranes surrounding the long bones may cause separation of the growing ends of the bones and interference with growth. Major, and sometimes fatal, hemorrhages into and around the brain can occur.

Scurvy is often associated with other vitamin deficiencies and *anemia* is common.

PREVENTION AND TREATMENT

A modest intake of fruit (particularly citrus fruit) and vegetables provides the body with sufficient vitamin C to

RECOMPRESSION CHAMBER FOR DIVING ACCIDENTS

Divers suffering from the bends or other pressure-related accidents are often treated in a recompression chamber. The patient is usually accompanied in the recompression chamber by a physician.

Relief valves

Patient

Sealed entrance hatch

Physician

Supply of air or other gas mixture under pressure

How it works
A gas mixture (usually air) is pumped into the chamber. As pressure increases, bubbles (pockets of gas) in the diver's tissues are reabsorbed, and symptoms disappear. Once all symptoms have gone, the pressure is slowly released.

S

prevent scurvy. Other sources are milk, liver, kidneys, and fish.

Scurvy is treated with large doses of vitamin C. Bleeding stops in 24 hours, healing resumes, and muscle and bone pain quickly dissipate.

Sealants, dental

Plastic materials applied to the chewing surfaces of the molars and premolars to help prevent decay. Back teeth have minute surface grooves in which food debris and bacteria can collect and cause decay (see *Caries, dental*). Sealing the teeth stops harmful material from getting into the grooves. Sealants are of the most benefit to children and should be applied as soon as possible after the permanent teeth have erupted.

Teeth to be sealed often require no drilling or anesthesia. The tooth surface may be acid-etched to roughen it so that the sealant will adhere better (see *Bonding, dental*). The semiliquid sealant is then applied and is usually hardened by directing a narrow beam of intense light at the treated tooth for a few seconds. Some sealants are premixed with a chemical activator that causes them to set.

Seasickness

A type of *motion sickness*.

Seasonal affective disorder syndrome

See *SADS*.

Sebaceous cyst

A nonspecific term for a large, smooth nodule under the skin (also called a wen when it is on the scalp). The most common sites of sebaceous cysts are the scalp, face, ear, and genitals.

Although harmless, sebaceous cysts may grow very large and sometimes become infected by bacteria, in

Massive sebaceous cyst
Cysts rarely grow as large as this one, located on the back of the neck. Cysts are harmless and easily removed surgically.

which case they are very painful. Large cysts or cysts that have been infected should be removed using local anesthetic. The physician makes a small incision in the skin and removes the cyst. If the entire cyst wall is removed, recurrence is rare.

Sebaceous glands

Minute glands in the skin that secrete a lubricating substance called *sebum*. Sebaceous glands either open into hair follicles or discharge directly onto the surface of the skin. They are most numerous on the scalp, face, and anus; they do not occur on the palms of the hands or soles of the feet. The production of sebum by the sebaceous glands is partly controlled by *androgen hormones* (male sex hormones).

Disorders of the sebaceous glands may lead to *seborrhea*, seborrheic *dermatitis*, or *acne* vulgaris.

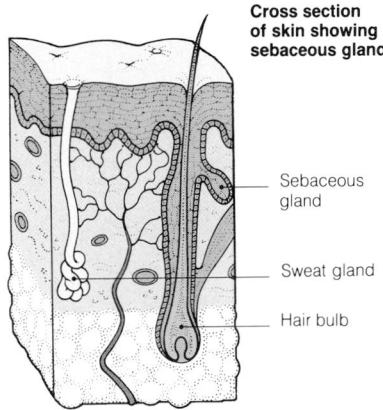

Cross section of skin showing sebaceous gland

Sebaceous gland

Sweat gland

Hair bulb

Seborrhea

Excessive secretion of *sebum*, causing increased oiliness of the face and a greasy scalp. The exact cause is uncertain, although *androgen hormones* (male sex hormones) are known to play a part. The condition is most common in adolescent boys.

Seborrhea usually disappears by adulthood without treatment. However, people with seborrhea are more likely than the average to have other skin conditions, particularly seborrheic *dermatitis* and *acne* vulgaris.

Seborrheic dermatitis

See *Dermatitis*.

Sebum

The oily secretion produced by the *sebaceous glands* of the skin. Sebum is composed of fats and waxes; it lubricates the skin, keeps it supple, and protects it from becoming sodden

when immersed in water or cracked when exposed to a dry atmosphere. Sebum also protects the skin from invasion by bacteria and fungi.

Oversecretion causes a greasy skin, called *seborrhea*. It may lead to seborrheic *dermatitis* or *acne* vulgaris.

Secobarbital

A *barbiturate drug* sometimes used as a *premedication* (drug given to prepare a person for surgery) because of its sedative effect. Secobarbital is seldom used today as a sleeping drug because of its short-lived action and the risk of *drug dependence*. Other possible adverse effects include daytime drowsiness, clumsiness, dizziness, confusion, and rash.

Secondary

A term applied to a disease or disorder that results from or follows another disease (which is called the *primary* disease). For example, secondary *hypertension* (high blood pressure) occurs as a result of some underlying primary disorder, such as a hormonal or kidney disease. The term secondary is also used to refer to a *metastasis* (a malignant tumor that has spread from a primary cancer to affect another part of the body).

Secretion

The manufacture and release by a cell, gland, or organ of chemical substances (such as *enzymes* or *hormones*) that are needed for metabolic processes elsewhere in the body. In contrast, *excretion* is the production and release of waste products. The term secretion is also used to refer to the secreted substances themselves.

The secretions of *exocrine glands* (e.g., the salivary glands) are carried away in ducts; the secretions of *endocrine glands* (e.g., the thyroid) are released directly into the bloodstream.

Security object

A significant item, such as a special blanket, an old garment, or a favorite soft toy, that provides comfort and reassurance to a young child. In many cases, a child settles down to sleep more easily if his or her security object is near. Some children are unable to sleep without their security objects.

Sometimes referred to as transitional objects, these items represent to the child something partway between a person and a thing. The child may become deeply attached to the object and may become highly distressed if an attempt is made to remove it.

S

Security objects are often important during the toddler stage and may be used for several years. Most children grow out of the need for such an item by the time they are 7 or 8 years old, but close attachments to special toys may persist. There is no evidence that security objects are in any way harmful. (See also *Thumb-sucking*.)

Sedation

The use of a drug to calm a person. Sedation is used to reduce excessive *anxiety* and occasionally to control dangerously aggressive behavior. It may also be used as part of *premedication* to produce relaxation before an operation or before an uncomfortable procedure such as *gastroscopy*. (See also *Sleeping drugs*.)

Sedative drugs

A group of drugs used to produce *sedation* (calmness). Sedative drugs include *sleeping drugs*, *antianxiety drugs*, *antipsychotic drugs*, and some *antidepressant drugs*. A sedative drug is often included in a *premedication* (drug given to prepare a person for surgery).

Seizure

A sudden episode of uncontrolled electrical activity in the brain. If the abnormal activity remains confined to one area, the person may experience tingling or twitching of only a small area of the body, such as the face or an extremity.

Other possible symptoms include hallucinations or intense feelings of fear or familiarity (*déjà vu*). If the abnormal electrical activity spreads

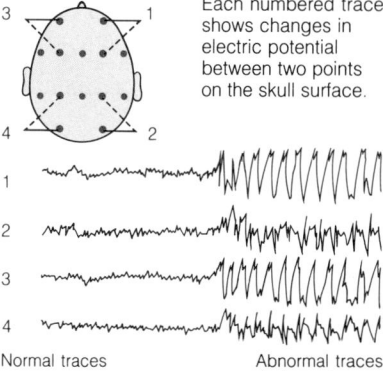

Each numbered trace shows changes in electric potential between two points on the skull surface.

1

2

3

4

Normal traces   Abnormal traces
                     during seizure

EEG changes during a seizure
The traces are recordings of electrical activity in a patient's brain, obtained from electrodes placed at various locations on the scalp and linked to an EEG machine. They show the change in activity at the onset of a seizure.

throughout the brain, consciousness is lost and a *grand mal* seizure results. Recurrent seizures are called *epilepsy*.

Seizures may be caused by many different neurological or medical problems, including *head injury*, infection, cerebrovascular accident (*stroke*), brain tumor, metabolic disturbances, or *alcohol* (withdrawal or hereditary intolerance of alcohol).

Seizure, febrile

Twitching or jerking of the limbs with loss of consciousness occurring in a child after a rapid rise in temperature. Febrile seizures are common; about one child in 20 experiences one or more attacks. The seizures tend to run in families, are usually not serious, and occur mainly in children between 6 months and 5 years.

CAUSES AND SYMPTOMS
Febrile seizures are caused by a disturbance in the normal electrical activity in the brain, but in most cases there is no underlying brain disorder. The fever that triggers the seizure usually develops with an acute infectious illness, such as *tonsillitis* or *otitis media* (inflammation of the middle ear).

The child loses consciousness and his or her arms and legs twitch uncontrollably for a few minutes. After regaining consciousness, the child may be drowsy.

TREATMENT
During a seizure, objects that could be harmful should be moved out of the child's way. Biting the tongue is rare and absolutely no attempt should be made to prevent it by wedging the mouth open. This can cause cuts and broken teeth. Once the seizure is over, the child should be placed in the *recovery position*.

If the child has not had a seizure before, a physician should be consulted; if the seizure lasts for more than five minutes, an ambulance should be called.

If something other than a fever is suspected of causing the seizure, the physician may perform investigative tests, such as a *lumbar puncture* to determine whether *meningitis* is the cause. No treatment is needed for the seizure, but treatment may be given for the underlying infection.

PREVENTION AND OUTLOOK
If an infectious illness develops in a susceptible child, parents can prevent further seizures by reducing the child's temperature. Acetaminophen should be given immediately at the first signs of fever at the full dose for the child's weight given on the

package. The dose can be repeated every four hours. Bedclothes should be removed and a fan directed toward the child. Sponging the child's face and body with lukewarm water may be comforting but is of dubious value in lowering temperature.

Most children who have one or more febrile seizures are completely normal and suffer no ill effects from the attacks. A second febrile seizure occurs in about 30 to 40 percent of cases, usually within the following six months. Recurrences are more likely if the child is abnormally mentally developed, if there was a complex or prolonged (longer than 15 minutes) first febrile seizure, and if there are family members with *epilepsy*. Children with all of these handicaps have about a one in 10 chance of having epilepsy develop. In healthy children, the risk of epilepsy is small.

Selenium

A *trace element* that helps preserve the elasticity of body tissues, thereby slowing the aging process. Selenium also improves the oxygen supply to the heart and helps form prostaglandins (substances that help prevent abnormal blood clotting and high blood pressure).

A balanced diet supplies the minute amount of selenium required by the body. The richest dietary sources are meat, fish, whole grains, and dairy products. The selenium content of vegetables depends on the amount of the mineral in the soil in which they were grown.

DEFICIENCY AND EXCESS
Neither deficiency nor excess of selenium usually has any effect on health. However, prolonged selenium deficiency—as a result of a poor diet or subsistence on vegetables grown in selenium-poor soil—may possibly cause premature aging, muscle pain, and, eventually, heart disease.

Excessive intake as a result of taking supplements or, rarely, from eating vegetables grown in soil with an abnormally high selenium content (as is found in some intensively irrigated areas) may cause baldness, loss of nails and teeth, fatigue, vomiting, and, with massive doses, death.

MEDICAL USES
Selenium is a constituent of some *multivitamin* and *mineral* preparations. Selenium sulfide is used in some anti-dandruff shampoos.

Self-help organizations

See special section at back of book.

S

Self-image
An individual's view of his or her personality. Some psychologists believe that neurosis stems from incongruity between self-image and how others see one (as occurs in an *inferiority complex*). *Psychotherapy* treats neurosis by bringing about a change in the person's perception of the self.

Self-mutilation
The act of deliberately injuring oneself. Self-mutilation usually takes the form of cutting the wrists or burning the forearms with cigarettes. It most often occurs in young adults with *personality disorders*, many of whom are also drug or alcohol abusers, and is three times more common in women. Self-mutilators often have had a violent upbringing and may also suffer from *mental retardation*. The reasons self-mutilators give for their behavior include aggressive impulses, relief of tension, and sadomasochistic fantasies.

More unusual forms of self-harm, such as gouging out the eyes or mutilating the genitals, are almost always due to *psychosis*.

Self-destructive biting is a feature of Lesch-Nyhan syndrome, a rare metabolic disorder that causes gout and mental retardation.

Semen
Fluid produced by the male on *ejaculation*. Semen is composed of fluid from the seminal vesicles (which produce the greatest part of the semen volume), fluid from the *prostate gland*, and *sperm*.

An important constituent of the fluid from the seminal vesicles is fructose (a sugar), which stimulates the sperm to become mobile. The concentration of fructose, the production of sperm, and the volume of the semen is dependent on the presence of the male sex hormone *testosterone*.

Semen analysis is performed as part of the investigation of male *infertility*.

Semen analysis
A method of determining the concentration, shape, and motility (ability to move) of sperm. Semen analysis is important in the investigation of male *infertility*. It is also performed some weeks after *vasectomy* (male sterilization) to ensure that the semen no longer contains sperm.

The semen specimen is produced by masturbation and should be as fresh as possible for successful analysis in the laboratory. The volume of semen is measured and the specimen examined under the microscope.

Normal semen contains from 20 million to 200 million sperm per milliliter. Semen analysis may show a deficiency in the number of sperm (*oligospermia*), a complete absence of sperm (*azoospermia*), altered shape, or diminished motility.

Semen, blood in the
A harmless condition, also called hemospermia, in which a small amount of blood is present in the semen. The blood, which is usually seen as a darkish stain in the semen at *ejaculation*, usually comes from small blood vessels in the region of the prostate gland or seminal vesicles. In the majority of cases, no cause is found.

Seminoma
See *Testis, cancer of.*

Senile dementia
See *Dementia.*

Senility
Changes in mental ability caused by old age. Most people over age 70 suffer from some degree of impaired memory and reduced ability to concentrate. With age, there is an increasing risk of *dementia*, which affects about one in five of those over 80. Depressive illness (see *Depression*) and *confusion* due to physical disease are also common, but there is a reduced prevalence of neurotic illness.

Senna

A *laxative drug* obtained from the leaves and pods of the Arabian shrubs CASSIA *ACUTIFOLIA* and CASSIA *ANGUSTIFOLIA*. Senna stimulates bowel contraction and is used to treat severe *constipation*; it may color the urine yellow-brown or red.

Sensate focus technique
A method taught to couples who are experiencing sexual difficulties caused by psychological rather than organic factors. The aim of the technique is to make each partner more aware of his or her pleasurable bodily sensations as well as those of the partner, and to reduce anxiety about performance.

Sensate focus technique is particularly useful in treating loss of sexual desire, failure to become sexually

STEPS IN THE SENSATE FOCUS TECHNIQUE

The technique is useful in treating a variety of sexual problems, including impotence and difficulties in reaching orgasm.

1 In the first stage (left), each partner gives the other as much pleasure as possible by caressing any part of the body other than the breasts or genitals.

2 The second stage (above) progresses to stimulation of the genitals and breasts but stops short of orgasm. Intercourse is still not permitted at this stage.

3 The final stage consists of sexual intercourse. Both partners concentrate on enjoyment rather than on orgasm, which is not the main goal.

S

PRINCIPAL SENSORY PATHWAYS INTO THE BRAIN

Destinations of sensory information
Some of the information entering the brain passes via the brain stem and/or thalamus to the cerebral cortex (outer surface of the brain), where sensations are perceived. Other information does not lead to conscious sensation. This includes certain data about body posture, processed in the cerebellum, and about internal body functioning, processed in the brain stem.

aroused (see *Sexual desire, inhibited*), or inability to achieve orgasm (see *Orgasm, lack of*), and in helping overcome *impotence* or premature ejaculation (see *Ejaculation, disorders of*).

HOW IT IS DONE
The technique, which should ideally be practiced in a relaxed, romantic or erotic setting, has three stages (see illustrated box on previous page). If premature ejaculation is a problem, one of the techniques to prevent it can be used (see *Sex therapy*).

EFFECTIVENESS
The sensate focus technique has an extremely high success rate—between 80 and 98 percent, depending on the sexual problem.

Sensation
A feeling or impression (such as a sound, an odor, touch, or hunger) that has entered consciousness. The senses are the faculties by which information about the external environment and about the body's internal state is collected and brought to the central nervous system (brain and spinal cord).

SENSORY RECEPTORS
Information is collected by millions of microscopic structures (called *receptors*) throughout the body. Receptors are found in the skin, muscles, and joints, in the internal organs, in the walls of blood vessels, and in special sense organs, such as the eye and inner ear. Receptors are attuned to a particular stimulus, such as light of a particular wavelength, chemical molecules of a certain shape, vibration, or temperature. They fire (send an electrical signal) when excited.

Some receptors are the terminals (free nerve endings) of long nerve cell fibers, others are specialized cells that connect to such fibers. When a receptor fires, a signal passes along the appropriate nerve fiber to the spinal cord, to the brain, or to both.

The principal pathways and destinations of sensory information entering the brain are shown in the diagram above. Only a proportion of this information reaches sensory areas of the cerebral cortex (outer surface of the brain) and is consciously perceived (see *Sensory cortex; Brain*).

THE SPECIAL SENSES
The special senses include *vision, hearing, taste,* and *smell*. The receptor cells for these senses are collected into special organs—the retina in the eyes, the auditory apparatus in the ears, the taste buds in the tongue, and the apparatus for smell in the nose. Information from these organs passes directly to the brain via *cranial nerves*. Much of the information passes to the cerebral cortex, although some goes to other areas of the brain (e.g., from the eyes to the cerebellum, where it is used to help maintain balance).

INTERNAL AND TOUCH SENSES
These senses include the pain, proprioception (position), pressure, and temperature sensations. Proprioception relies on receptors in the muscles and joints to provide information on the position in space of parts of the body. Pain is one of the most primitive senses; it warns of noxious stimuli through receptors at the skin surface and inside.

Many types of receptors are found in the skin. Some are sensitive to pressure, others to the movement of hairs, others to temperature change. Skin receptors are made up of the terminals of nerve fibers, which are wrapped around the roots of hairs, formed into disks, or surrounded by a series of membranes to form onionlike structures (called pacinian corpuscles). Different patterns of stimulation of these receptors give rise to such sensations as pain, tickling, firm or light pressure, heat or cold. Certain skin areas (the lips, palms of the hands, and genitals) have a particularly high concentration of receptors.

Most of the signals from these receptors pass, via the cranial or spinal nerves and tracts in the brain or spinal cord, to the thalamus and then to two regions of the sensory cortex called the somatosensory cortices. Sensations perceived at certain points within these regions correspond to the parts of the body from which the signals originated. Much larger areas of cortex are devoted to sensations originating from the hands and lips than from less sensitive parts.

Sensation, abnormal

Unpleasant, dulled, or otherwise altered sensations without obvious stimulus (e.g., a burning sensation when there is no heat). Abnormal sensations result from damage to, or pressure on, sensory nerve pathways.

TYPES AND CAUSES

The most common types are *tinnitus* or *numbness* and/or a *pins and needles sensation*, sometimes combined with *pain* and, in some cases, with coldness or burning sensations. *Neuralgia* is characterized by pain with a stabbing, brief, repetitive quality.

More unusual disturbances include the feeling that fluid is trickling down the skin, that part of the body is being constricted by a tight band, or that insects are crawling over the skin (formication). The special senses can also be impaired or altered by damage to the relevant sensory apparatus or nerve tracts (see *Vision, disorders of*; *Smell*; *Deafness*; *Tinnitus*).

Neuropathy (damage to peripheral nerves) from thiamine deficiency in alcoholics, from *diabetes mellitus*, or from heavy metal (such as lead) poisoning is a common cause of abnormal sensation. The sufferer may complain of tingling or a feeling of walking on cotton. The peripheral nerves may also be damaged or irritated by infections such as *herpes zoster* (shingles) or by a tumor pressing on a nerve, often causing severe pain. *Spinal injury*, *head injury*, *stroke*, and *multiple sclerosis* are other causes of damage or degeneration of nerve pathways in the brain or spinal cord.

Damage to the thalamus (a relay station for sensory pathways in the center of the brain) can produce particularly unpleasant results, such as a spreading sensation resembling an electric shock that occurs after a simple pinprick. Damage to the parietal lobe in the brain can lead to loss of the ability to locate or recognize objects by touch.

DIAGNOSIS AND TREATMENT

Many tests (including tests of sensation, testing of *reflexes*, *blood tests*, *urinalysis*, and *CT scanning* or *angiography*) may be required to discover the cause of abnormal sensation.

Pressure on or damage to nerves can sometimes be relieved by surgery or by dietary or other treatments to remove or treat the underlying cause. In other instances, severe intractable pain or other abnormal sensation can be relieved only by cutting the relevant sensory nerve fibers or by giving injections to chemically block the transmission of signals along them.

Senses

See *Sensation*.

Sensitization

The initial exposure of a person to an allergen or other substance recognized as foreign by the body's *immune system*, which leads to an immune response. On second and subsequent exposures to the same substance, there is a much stronger and faster immune reaction. This action forms the basis of *allergy* and other types of *hypersensitivity* reaction.

Sensory cortex

A region of the outer part of the *cerebrum* (the main mass of the brain) in which sensory information comes to consciousness. The sensory cortex contains several layers of interconnected neurons (nerve cells) with complex interconnections.

Pressure, pain, and temperature sensations from the skin, muscles, joints, and internal organs are perceived in regions of the parietal lobe (upper side part of the cerebrum) on both sides of the brain. These regions are called the somatosensory cortices. Taste sensations are also perceived in the parietal lobes. Light, color, shape, and other visual sensations are perceived in the occipital lobes at the back of the cerebrum; sounds are perceived in the temporal lobes at the sides.

Sensory deprivation

Removing the normal sights, sounds, and physical feelings from a person. Sensory deprivation can produce a variety of mental changes, demonstrated by studies in which volunteers lie immobile in bed (or in a tub of warm water) wearing masks and gloves in a sound-deadened room. After long periods, reported effects generally include feelings of unreality, difficulty thinking, and hallucinations; EEG recordings show a slowing of brain activity.

Prisoners kept in solitary confinement experience similar symptoms, and infants deprived of the companionship and presence of others tend to be disturbed in later life. (See also *Bonding*; *Emotional deprivation*.)

Separation anxiety

The feelings of distress that a young child experiences when parted from his or her parents or home. Separation anxiety is a normal aspect of infant behavior that increases in intensity until about 2 years of age, but is often minimal by 3 to 4 years. When threatened with separation, the child usually reacts by crying, clinging to the parent, and demanding to be cuddled. Such signs are indicative of *bonding*, which is considered essential to a child's emotional development.

Separation anxiety disorder is a childhood illness in which the reaction to separation is greater than that expected for the child's level of development. The anxiety may manifest itself in the form of headaches, nausea, toothaches, dizziness, or difficulty sleeping. When separated, the child may worry that he

S

NEUROLOGIC SENSORY TESTING

Light touch
With the patient's eyes closed, a piece of cotton is brushed lightly across the face.

Pinprick
The prick tests pain sensation and may be repeated at different locations on the patient's body.

Pain pinch
Pain sense may be further tested by pinching the Achilles tendon at the back of the heel.

Vibration
A vibrating tuning fork is held against a prominent bone, such as the ankle bone or mastoid bone.

Position sense
The patient, with eyes closed, tells in which direction his or her finger is moved.

Two-point discrimination
Measures ability to distinguish two pinpricks from a single prick.

Standard tests
When examining a patient's nervous system, a physician usually includes several standard tests of touch, position, pain, and vibration senses, such as those above.

or she will never be reunited with the parents or that they will be killed. Some children refuse to visit friends or attend school. Separation anxiety disorder may be a feature of *depression*.

Sepsis

Infection of a wound or body tissues with bacteria that leads to the formation of pus (see *Suppuration*) or to multiplication of the bacteria in the blood. If the blood becomes infected with bacteria that the *immune system* can eradicate entirely or prevent from multiplying excessively, the condition is known as *bacteremia*. However, if bacteria that form toxins are present in the blood in large numbers and are multiplying rapidly, the condition (as a result of the toxemia and bacteremia) is called *septicemia* (blood poisoning). See also *Septic shock*.

Septal defect

A heart abnormality, developed before birth, in which there is a hole in the septum (partition) between the left and right sides of the heart. Commonly known as a hole in the heart, septal defect varies in its effects according to the size and position of the defect.

TYPES

When the hole is in the septum separating the two ventricles (lower chambers of the heart), the abnormality is known as a ventricular septal defect; when it is in the septum between the two atria (upper chambers), it is called an atrial septal defect. In both types, the hole allows some of the freshly oxygenated blood in the left half of the heart (which supplies tissues throughout the body) to flow into the right half, mix with deoxygenated blood, and recirculate through the lungs. If the hole is large, the misdirection of blood results in a greatly reduced oxygen supply to the tissues and excessive blood flow through the lungs.

Some children are born with both atrial and ventricular septal defects; either type may be accompanied by one or more other heart abnormalities and/or other birth defects.

CAUSES AND INCIDENCE

The precise cause of this defect is unknown in most cases. (For information on factors influencing the development of congenital heart abnormalities, see *Heart disease, congenital* and *Birth defects*.)

Ventricular septal defects are the most common type of congenital heart abnormality, occurring in about 30 percent of all cases of congenital heart disease and affecting about 200 babies in every 100,000. Atrial septal defects occur in about 8 percent of cases (50 babies per 100,000).

SYMPTOMS AND SIGNS

A small defect of either kind produces little or no effect. With a large ventricular hole, *heart failure* may develop six to eight weeks after birth, causing breathlessness, feeding difficulties, pallor, and sweating. With large atrial defects, however, heart failure may not develop for many years or may not develop at all.

With both types of defect, *pulmonary hypertension* (high blood pressure in the arteries supplying the lungs) may develop. This is more likely, and occurs at an earlier age, in large ventricular defects.

With ventricular defect there is also a slight risk of *endocarditis* (inflammation of the lining of the heart); in atrial septal defect, *atrial fibrillation* (rapid, irregular beating of the atria) may occur after age 30.

DIAGNOSIS

The diagnosis is made by a physician who hears, through a stethoscope, a heart *murmur* (a type of abnormal heart sound made by turbulent blood

Ventricular septal defect

Aorta
Pulmonary artery
Pulmonary veins
Deoxygenated blood
Oxygenated blood
Hole in ventricular septum

Atrial septal defect

Aorta
Pulmonary artery
Hole in atrial septum
Oxygenated blood
Deoxygenated blood

Two types of septal defect
In both cases, oxygenated blood is forced from the left to the right side of the heart through the hole in the septum. Too much blood passes to the lungs (via the pulmonary artery) and too little to the body tissues (via the aorta).

flow through the hole). Diagnosis also includes chest X rays and an ECG. The diagnosis can be confirmed by Doppler *echocardiography*.

TREATMENT

Atrial septal defects are repaired only if they cause symptoms or if examination and tests suggest that complications may develop.

As the child grows, small ventricular holes often become smaller, or even close, on their own. If a large ventricular defect is causing heart failure, it is treated with *diuretic drugs* and with *digitalis drugs* in babies. If the hole does not close spontaneously, it is repaired by *open heart surgery*, usually before the child reaches school age. The operation has an extremely high safety and success rate.

OUTLOOK

Modern surgery is so effective in dealing with large septal defects that it enables most affected people to lead normal lives.

Septicemia

Rapid multiplication of bacteria and the presence of their toxins in the blood, a condition commonly known as blood poisoning. As distinct from *bacteremia* (in which bacteria are present in the blood but do not always multiply), septicemia is always a serious, life-threatening condition.

CAUSES

Septicemia usually arises through escape of bacteria from a focus of infection somewhere in the body (such as from an abscess or from a urinary tract or intestinal infection, or because of pneumonia or meningitis). Septicemia is more likely in people whose natural resistance to infection has been lowered by an *immunodeficiency disorder* or by *immunosuppressant drugs*, allowing the bacteria to multiply unchecked.

SYMPTOMS AND SIGNS

A person in whom septicemia develops suddenly becomes seriously ill, with a high fever, chills, rapid breathing, headache, and often clouding of consciousness. Skin rashes or jaundice may occur and sometimes the hands are unusually warm. In many cases, especially when large amounts of toxins are produced by the circulating bacteria, the person passes into a state of *septic shock*, a life-threatening condition.

DIAGNOSIS AND TREATMENT

A diagnosis of septicemia can be confirmed, and the infective bacteria identified, by growing a *culture* of the organisms from a blood sample.

S

Treatment is started as soon as septicemia is suspected by giving an *intravenous infusion* (slow introduction into a vein) of *antibiotic drugs* and of glucose and/or saline solution.

The focal site of infection is sought immediately and may be surgically removed. Provided the infection is recognized and treated promptly, there is usually a full recovery.

Septic shock

A highly dangerous condition in which there is tissue damage and a dramatic drop in blood pressure as a result of *septicemia* and *toxemia* (the multiplication of bacteria and the presence of their toxins in the blood).

In many cases, the toxins are the main cause of trouble because they can cause damage to cells and tissues throughout the body, promote clotting of blood in the smallest blood vessels, and seriously interfere with the normal blood circulation. Damage occurs especially to tissues in the kidneys, heart, and lungs. The toxins may cause leakage of fluid from blood vessels and a reduction of the ability of the vessels to constrict, leading to a drop in blood pressure.

CAUSES AND INCIDENCE
Septic shock is most common in people hospitalized with such major disorders as *diabetes mellitus*, *cancer*, or liver *cirrhosis* and who have a focus of infection somewhere in the body (often the intestines or urinary tract) that has led to septicemia. Progression to septic shock is especially likely in people who have an *immunodeficiency disorder*, in people taking *immunosuppressant drugs* for cancer, or in people given prolonged and inappropriate antibiotic treatment. Newborn infants are also particularly susceptible if septicemia develops.

SYMPTOMS AND SIGNS
The symptoms vary with the extent and site of major tissue damage. Broadly, they are the same as in septicemia, with additional symptoms including cold hands and feet, often with *cyanosis* (blue-purple coloration) due to slowed blood flow, a weak, rapid pulse, and markedly reduced blood pressure. There may be vomiting and diarrhea. A poor output of urine may indicate that damage to the kidneys is occurring and that there is a risk of *renal failure*. *Heart failure* and abnormal bleeding may also develop.

TREATMENT
Septic shock requires immediate treatment, including the use of *antibiotic drugs* and sometimes surgery to remove the focus of infection. Rapid fluid replacement by infusion and the maintenance of urine flow to prevent the effects of renal failure are other essential procedures. Measures are also taken to raise the blood pressure and to promote better blood supply to tissues. These measures include *intravenous infusions* and *oxygen therapy*.

Despite treatment, septic shock remains a grave condition; survival rates are no better than 50 percent.

Septum

A thin dividing wall within or between parts of the body. The nasal septum is the sheet of cartilage and bone that separates the nostrils.

Sequela

A condition that results from or follows a disease, disorder, or injury. The term is usually used in the plural (sequelae) to refer to the complications of a disease. The sequelae of a common cold may include *bronchitis*, *sinusitis*, and *otitis media* (inflammation of the middle ear).

Sequestration

A term used in medicine to refer to a portion of diseased or necrotic (dead) tissue being separated from, or joined abnormally to, surrounding healthy tissue. The term usually refers to a complication of *osteomyelitis* (bone infection) in which part of a bone dies and becomes separated from healthy bone. Sequestration may also refer to a rare congenital abnormality of the lungs in which part of a lobe is not directly connected to a bronchus (airway) but may be connected to surrounding alveoli (air sacs).

Serology

A branch of laboratory medicine concerned with analysis of the contents of blood *serum* (the clear fluid that separates from clotted blood).

Various serological techniques are extremely useful in the diagnosis of infectious diseases. If a person has been exposed to a particular infectious organism, *antibodies* (proteins with a role in immunity) directed specifically against the organism appear in that person's serum some days after exposure. Their presence or absence in the blood can be detected by such laboratory techniques as *immunoassay*, including the ELISA test and radioimmunoassay. The absence of specific antibodies detected by serology may allow a physician to exclude a particular infection as the cause of the illness; a rising level of antibody may give good evidence that a particular infection is present.

In other cases, serological techniques are used to identify parts of infectious organisms (*antigens*) by studying the reaction between the antigens (obtained by *culture* of a specimen taken from a patient) and serum samples known to contain certain antibodies. A series of tests may be carried out in which the unknown antigen is added to various *antiserums* (preparations containing specific antibodies) in test tubes; a positive reaction is sometimes revealed by a color change.

In addition to devising and carrying out such diagnostic tests, serologists may be involved in developing antiserums for passive *immunization*.

Serologists may also test blood samples for various genetically determined protein markers, including substances that determine blood groups. Such tests can help resolve paternity suits (see *Paternity testing*) or cases in which blood left at the scene of the crime can be compared with blood taken from suspects.

Serotonin

A substance found in many tissues, particularly blood platelets, the lining of the digestive tract, and the brain. Serotonin has a variety of effects in the body. It is released from platelets at the site of bleeding, where it constricts small blood vessels, thus reducing blood loss. In the digestive tract, it inhibits gastric secretion and stimulates smooth (involuntary) muscles in the intestinal wall. In the brain, it acts as a *neurotransmitter* (a chemical involved in the transmission of nerve impulses between nerve cells). Serotonin is thought to be involved in controlling states of consciousness and mood; its action in the brain is disrupted by certain hallucinogenic drugs, notably *LSD*.

Serum

The clear fluid that separates from blood when it clots. Serum does not contain blood cells or the protein (fibrinogen) in blood that helps form clots. Serum does contain salts, glucose, and other proteins (including various *antibodies* formed by the body's *immune system* to protect against infection).

Serum prepared from the blood of a person (or animal) who has been infected with a microorganism usually

S

contains antibodies that can protect against that organism if the serum is injected into someone else. This is called an *antiserum*, and its use forms the basis of passive *immunization*.

Serum sickness

A short-lived illness that may develop about 10 days after injection with an *antiserum* of animal origin (e.g., antirabies serum equine, obtained from horses). Serum sickness is a type of *hypersensitivity* reaction similar to an allergy. A similar illness can occur after taking certain drugs.

CAUSES

Antiserums are preparations obtained from human or animal blood containing specific *antibodies* (substances with a role in immunity). Antiserums are sometimes given to protect against dangerous infections. When an antiserum is prepared from animal blood, a protein in the serum may be misidentified by the body's *immune system* as a potentially harmful foreign substance (*antigen*). In serum sickness, the immune system produces antibodies that combine with the antigen to form particles called immune complexes. They are deposited in various tissues, stimulate more immune reactions, and lead to inflammation and symptoms.

Certain drugs can cause a similar response, though the drug molecules probably combine with a protein in the blood or tissues before they are misidentified as antigens. Penicillin is the most important drug capable of causing serum sickness.

Serum sickness is different from *anaphylactic shock*, another type of hypersensitivity reaction that can also develop in response to antiserums, drugs, and other substances. Anaphylactic shock is a more severe, immediate reaction.

SYMPTOMS AND TREATMENT

A week or two after exposure to the antiserum or drug, symptoms appear. There may be an itchy rash, pain in the joints, fever, and enlargement of lymph nodes. In severe cases, a state similar to *shock*, with low blood pressure, develops. All symptoms usually clear up within a few days provided (in the case of a drug) that its use is stopped.

Soothing lotions can help relieve itching. The physician may prescribe a *nonsteroidal anti-inflammatory drug* to relieve joint pain and an *antihistamine drug* to shorten the duration of the illness. In severe cases, a *corticosteroid drug* may be prescribed.

People who have had serum sickness or anaphylactic shock should note the name of the injection or drug to which they are sensitive. Mention should also be made in the medical records to warn health care personnel against future use of the drug.

Sex

Another term for gender and a commonly used term for *sexual intercourse*.

Sex change

Radical surgical procedures, usually combined with sex hormone therapy, that alter a person's anatomical gender. Sex change operations are performed on transsexuals (see *Transsexualism*) or on people with ambiguous genitalia (see *Pseudohermaphroditism*; *Hermaphroditism*).

WHY IT IS DONE

Sex change operations on transsexuals are performed to give the person a physical appearance that he or she believes coincides with his or her psychological *gender identity*.

Sex change operations on people with ambiguous genitalia (i.e., with external sex organs resembling those of the opposite sex) are performed to modify or improve the anatomical gender and thus provide a more defined sexual identity.

HOW IT IS DONE

TRANSSEXUALS Sex change involves a series of major operations on the genitourinary tract carried out after hormone therapy and counseling.

The male-to-female sex change is the more common procedure. Prosthetic breasts may be implanted to augment the breast growth that has resulted from hormone therapy. An operation removes the erectile tissue of the penis and repositions the urethra. The skin of the penis is used to make the lining of a vagina, which is created in the *perineum*. The testes are removed and the skin of the scrotum is used to make the labia.

In the female-to-male sex change, a mastectomy is performed to remove the breasts. Afterward, removal of the uterus and ovaries is carried out. This may be followed by a penile graft, which involves constructing a new urethra by grafting an abdominal skin flap over a catheter; the graft and the surrounding skin are then separated to make a penis. The upper end is inserted into the perineum and the lower end is detached.

AMBIGUOUS GENITALIA Operations are usually carried out in infancy. Babies with ambiguous genitalia are assigned

a sex as soon as possible after birth, given appropriate surgical and hormonal treatment, and reared as a member of the assigned sex.

Operations on adults who have ambiguous genitalia are uncommon today. In general, they are similar to those performed on transsexuals, with variations depending on specific anatomical problems.

OUTLOOK

The degree to which transsexuals adjust to their new gender varies. Some make a complete adjustment but others are left with serious psychological problems. Hormone therapy may need to be continued for life to maintain secondary sexual characteristics such as body shape, hair distribution, and voice change. Female transsexuals can have intercourse but cannot conceive. Males cannot impregnate or ejaculate; they achieve an erection only with mechanical aids (e.g., *penile implants*).

Sex chromosomes

A pair of chromosomes that determines gender. Sex chromosomes are found in each of a person's cells along with 44 other chromosomes (autosomes). In women, the sex chromosomes are of similar appearance and are called X chromosomes. In men, one sex chromosome is an X and the other, a smaller chromosome, is a Y. Thus, the normal sex chromosome complement for women is XX, and for men, XY.

FUNCTION

Like all chromosomes, the X and Y chromosomes exert their effects in the body through the activities of their constituent *genes*. These genes contain the coded instructions for chemical processes within cells and aspects of growth and development within the body as a whole.

The X and Y chromosomes differ in one fundamental way. Genes on the Y chromosome are concerned solely with gender. Their presence ensures a male, their absence a female. The X chromosome, which is common to both sexes, contains many genes vital to general body development and functioning. Absence of the X chromosome is incompatible with life.

The presence of a single X chromosome and 44 autosomes appears to provide the blueprint for general body functioning and development, which seems to have an underlying female pattern. This is demonstrated in people with *Turner's syndrome*, who

S

have only one sex chromosome, an X. Although full female sex characteristics never develop, these people are nevertheless unmistakably female in appearance and identity. Full female sex characteristics develop only in the presence of a second X chromosome. Addition of a Y chromosome converts the female to the male pattern.

Sex determination

The factors that determine biological sex. The underlying determinants are the *sex chromosomes* in a person's cells—two X chromosomes in females, and one X and one Y chromosome in males. During early life in the embryo, these chromosomes cause the development of different gonads (primary sex organs)—the testes in males and the ovaries in females. In males, the testes then produce hormones that cause the development of a male reproductive tract, including a penis. In females, absence of these male hormones leads to a different pattern of development, with the formation of fallopian tubes, uterus, and vagina. Many years after birth, another surge of hormones from the gonads leads to the development of secondary *sexual characteristics*, such as facial hair in males and breasts in females.

Defects can arise in this process, leading, in some cases, to ambiguous sex. Some people acquire an abnormal complement of sex chromosomes (see *Chromosomal abnormalities*) and all the characteristics of one sex do not develop. In some female fetuses, a metabolic defect causes the production of large amounts of male hormones (see *Adrenal hyperplasia, congenital*), causing masculinization of the female genitals (such as enlargement of the clitoris to form an appendage resembling a penis). Conversely, in some male fetuses, male hormones are not produced or they are produced but fail to cause masculinization; the child's genitals are feminized to some degree (the extreme case of this is called *testicular feminization syndrome*). Finally, there are very rare cases of true *hermaphroditism*, in which a child is born with both testicular and ovarian tissue and may have both a vagina and a penis.

These ambiguities are different from *transsexualism*, in which a person's biological sex is not in doubt, although it conflicts with his or her psychological disposition.

When an infant is born with ambiguous genitals, the cause of the ambiguity is investigated and the child is assigned the sex believed to offer the best chance for a healthy life. The decision depends on the possibilities for establishing one sex or another through hormonal and/or surgical treatment. In most cases, a satisfactory male or female appearance and sexual capacity can be achieved. Full reproductive potential (ability to have children) can be achieved in some cases.

Sex hormones

Hormones that control the development of primary and secondary sexual characteristics and regulate various sex-related functions in the body, such as the menstrual cycle and the production of eggs or sperm. There are three main types of sex hormones—*androgen hormones* (male sex hormones), *estrogen hormones* (female sex hormones), and *progesterone hormones* (which have the specialized function of preparing for and maintaining *pregnancy*).

Sex-linked

Pertaining to a trait or a disorder determined by the *sex chromosomes* in a person's cells or by the *genes* carried on those chromosomes.

Most people carry two sex chromosomes in their cells. Disorders caused by an abnormal number of sex chromosomes include *Turner's syndrome* (which affects females only and is caused by a missing X chromosome) and *Klinefelter's syndrome* (which affects males only and is caused by one or more extra X chromosomes).

Most other sex-linked traits or disorders are caused by recessive genes on the X chromosome (see *Genetic disorders*). These traits or disorders, which almost exclusively affect males, include such conditions as *hemophilia*, Duchenne *muscular dystrophy*, and *color vision deficiency*.

Sex therapy

Counseling for and treatment of *psychosexual dysfunction* (sexual difficulties not due to a physical cause). Sex therapy is usually undertaken in conjunction with *marital* (or relationship) *counseling*.

It is estimated that at least 50 percent of couples experience some form of sexual problem at some stage in their relationships; in most cases, the problem is psychological in origin. Sex therapy can help by changing the general attitude of one or both partners toward sex, by increasing each person's understanding of his or her sexual needs and those of the partner, and by teaching techniques to deal with specific problems at home. Both partners attend the therapy sessions, but individual sex therapy may also be useful.

TECHNIQUES

In the *sensate focus technique*, the couple explores pleasurable, relaxed, sensual rather than sexual, bodily sensations. The goal of this technique is to reduce anxiety about sexual performance and increase individual awareness of how to give and receive pleasure for at least 15 minutes.

To prevent premature ejaculation (see *Ejaculation, disorders of*), the most common sexual difficulty in men, two techniques are taught. One is the squeeze technique (see illustration below). The other technique requires both partners to stop thrusting a moment before ejaculation is imminent. In both cases, once the man has achieved control of this reflex, sexual activity is resumed. The techniques can be repeated as many times as required. They can be learned and are highly successful.

THE SQUEEZE TECHNIQUE
This technique is used for treating and preventing premature ejaculation in men.

Pressure

Method
Either partner squeezes the penis when the man is about to ejaculate, pressing just beneath the glans (head of the penis) using the thumb and two fingers.

Women who rarely or never experience orgasm (see *Orgasm, lack of*) or who have *vaginismus* (spasm of the vaginal muscles, preventing intercourse) may be treated individually, conjointly, or at group therapy sessions. The woman is encouraged to come to terms with her sexuality. She is taught exercises for relaxing and tightening the pelvic muscles and

S

to stimulate the clitoris to achieve orgasm (through masturbation) as a preliminary to intercourse.

RESULTS

Sex therapy has proved successful for many sexual problems, with particularly effective results in treating vaginismus, premature ejaculation, lack of orgasm, impotence, and failure to consummate marriage.

Sexual abuse

The subjection of a person to sexual activity that is likely to cause physical or psychological harm. There is a federal law mandating that child-adult sexual contact be reported to a child protection agency. (See also *Child abuse*; *Rape*.)

Sexual characteristics, secondary

Physical features appearing at *puberty* that indicate the onset of adult reproductive life.

In girls, the earliest secondary sexual characteristic is enlargement of the nipples and breasts. Soon thereafter, pubic and underarm hair appears, and body fat increases around the hips, stomach, and tops of the thighs to produce the female body shape.

In boys, enlargement of the testes is the first change, followed by thinning of the skin of the scrotum and enlargement of the penis. Pubic, facial, and other body hair appears, the voice deepens, and muscle bulk and bone size increase.

Sexual desire, inhibited

Lack of sexual desire or of the ability to become physically aroused during sexual activity (see *Sexual intercourse*). Either form of the condition may be physical or psychological.

CAUSES

LACK OF DESIRE A high proportion of women and some men experience loss of sexual desire at some point in their lives. Common physical causes include fatigue, ill health, and vaginal tenderness after childbirth. Certain drugs can also reduce sexual desire, including sleeping pills, antidepressants, antihypertensives, oral contraceptives, and alcohol. Psychological factors include *depression*, anxiety, severe stress, a conflictual relationship with or grief at the death of a sexual partner, or an unwanted pregnancy, an abortion, or a traumatic sexual experience such as *rape* or *incest*.

LACK OF PHYSICAL AROUSAL It is rare for a woman or a man to be incapable of physical sexual arousal. The most

common reason for failure is the partner's poor or insensitive sexual overtures or technique, although hostility, anxiety, guilt about the sex act, or fear of sexual inadequacy may contribute to the problem. In rare cases, an individual is simply unable to respond to a particular partner but can respond to another, making the sexual problem selective.

TREATMENT

Problems that have a psychological basis or that are caused by the partner's sexual technique can often be successfully treated by *sex therapy* or *marital* (relationship) *counseling*. Sexual problems with a physical or chemical cause often improve once the underlying condition is resolved.

Sexual deviation

See *Deviation, sexual*.

Sexual dysfunction

See *Psychosexual dysfunction*.

Sexual intercourse

The act in which a man's penis is inserted into a woman's vagina with her consent and cooperation. Sexual intercourse provides pleasurable sensations that may result in *orgasm* for one or both partners. The ejaculation of the man's *sperm* into the woman's reproductive tract is the usual means by which reproduction is achieved.

Couples bring many variations to the sexual act in terms of emotions, positions, and techniques used. However, for most, kissing, tenderness, and foreplay precede penetration. During sexual intercourse, a series of physiological responses occurs.

PHASES OF INTERCOURSE

Physiologically, intercourse can be divided into four phases—arousal, plateau, orgasm, and resolution.

DISORDERS

Problems with intercourse may have physical or psychological origins. (See also *Intercourse, painful*; *Psychosexual dysfunction*; *Sexual problems*.)

Sexuality

A general term for the capacity, behavior patterns, impulses, emotions, and sensations connected with reproduction and the use of the sex organs. In biology, sex refers specifically to the anatomical differences between male and female. Sexual attraction, distraction, control, and expression make sexuality a powerful factor in the workplace, as a marketing tool, and in the pursuit of personal or mutual gratification.

Heterosexuality is sexuality directed toward the anatomically opposite sex; in *homosexuality* the attraction is toward the same sex. The term *bisexuality* refers to people who experience sexual attraction to members of either sex. (See also *Gender identity*.)

Sexually transmitted diseases

Infections transmitted primarily, but not exclusively, by sexual intercourse.

HISTORY AND INCIDENCE

Also known as venereal diseases, sexually transmitted diseases (STDs) are acquired more often by people who have many new sex partners each year. Some of the major STDs are also transmitted by blood and thus occur in drug addicts who share needles.

Until about 25 years ago, STDs were thought to be limited to *syphilis*, *gonorrhea*, *chancroid*, and *lymphogranuloma venereum*. Today, however, these four diseases account for only 10 to 15 percent of all STDs seen in STD clinics. The most common conditions are *chlamydial infections*, *trichomoniasis*, genital herpes (see *Herpes, genital*), *pubic lice*, genital warts (see *Warts, genital*), and *AIDS*. Some other diseases, including viral *hepatitis*, *scabies*, *candidiasis*, and *molluscum contagiosum*, can also be transmitted by sexual intercourse, but they are not usually classified as STDs.

During the second world war, STDs became more prevalent in the US and Europe; they declined when the introduction of penicillin provided a cure for syphilis and gonorrhea. In the 1960s and 1970s, however, STDs increased again with the introduction of oral contraception. The birth-control pill led not only to women having more sex partners, but also to fewer couples using barrier contraceptives, which provide some protection against infection in addition to preventing pregnancy.

Also in the 1970s, genitourinary physicians recognized that so-called *nonspecific urethritis* was usually due to chlamydia. By the early 1980s a diagnosis of nonspecific urethritis was being made in about 25 percent of all people who visited STD clinics; in most of these people, careful laboratory testing showed evidence of chlamydial infection.

Throughout the 1970s and the early 1980s, most patients with an STD could expect a rapid cure with an antibiotic. In the late 1970s, however, it became apparent that certain STDs (notably herpes and hepatitis B) could not be cured by drugs and that herpes

S

SEXUAL INTERCOURSE

The term sexual intercourse usually refers to the act during which the male penis is inserted into the female vagina. However, some people use the term more broadly to refer to a much wider range of sexual activity. Physiologically, intercourse falls into four main stages—arousal (which generally includes a period of foreplay), a plateau phase (during which penetration usually occurs), orgasm, and resolution. The duration of each stage of intercourse varies.

Arousal in men
Sexual thoughts, the sight and feel of his partner's body, and foreplay may sexually arouse a man. Blood enters the penis so that it becomes firm and erect.

Plateau phase in men
Vaginal penetration usually takes place during this phase and thrusting movements begin. The penis reaches maximum size and the testes elevate.

Orgasm in men
Muscular contractions in the ducts connecting the testes, prostate, and penis force semen out of the penis, accompanied by intensely pleasurable sensations.

Resolution in men
The penis returns to half its fully erect size and the testes descend.

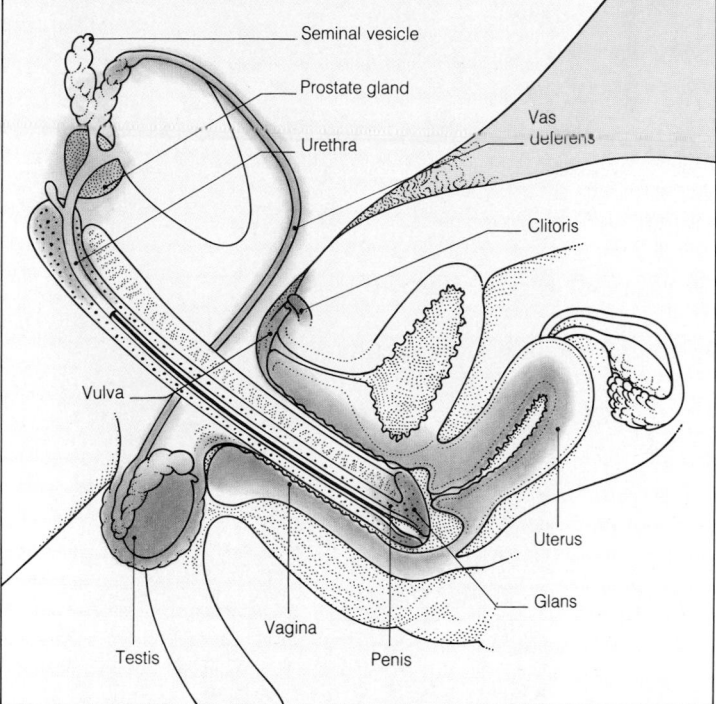

Seminal vesicle
Prostate gland
Vas deferens
Urethra
Clitoris
Vulva
Uterus
Glans
Vagina
Testis
Penis

Arousal in women
Similar factors lead to arousal in women as in men, though foreplay may be more important. The clitoris lengthens, the vagina enlarges, and its walls secrete a lubricating fluid.

Plateau phase in women
Muscular contractions in the walls of the vagina help grip the penis. The uterus rises, and the clitoris pulls back beneath its hood of skin.

Orgasm in women
The walls of the outer part of the vagina contract rhythmically and strongly several times and an intense sensual feeling spreads from the clitoris and throughout the body.

Resolution in women
The clitoris subsides and, more gradually, the vagina relaxes and the uterus falls.

BREATHING RATE
Breaths per minute

50
40
30
20
10

A   P   O   R

HEART RATE
Beats per minute

250
200
150
100
50

A   P   O   R

BLOOD PRESSURE
Millimeters of mercury (mm Hg)

300
250
200
150
100

A   P   O   R

Key ••• Men   ••• Women   **A** = arousal   **P** = plateau   **O** = orgasm   **R** = resolution

Breathing rate
Both men and women breathe faster and louder as sexual excitement builds. The rate rises gradually, peaking at about twice the normal rate at orgasm.

Heart rate
Intercourse provides vigorous exercise for the heart. The heart rate increases rapidly during arousal, peaks as high as 200 beats per minute at orgasm, then drops.

Blood pressure
Systolic blood pressure rises in a similar pattern to heart rate, peaking at orgasm. The rise may be more marked in men than in women.

S

INCIDENCE OF GONORRHEA IN THE US

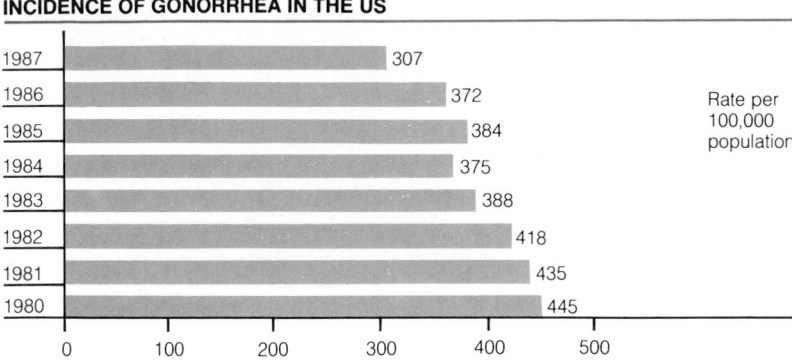

Rate per 100,000 population

Year	Rate
1987	307
1986	372
1985	384
1984	375
1983	388
1982	418
1981	435
1980	445

Gonorrhea
The incidence of gonorrhea peaked in the 1970s but has shown an almost uninterrupted decline in the 1980s. It remains, however, the most common of all reportable diseases.

INCIDENCE OF PRIMARY AND SECONDARY SYPHILIS IN THE US

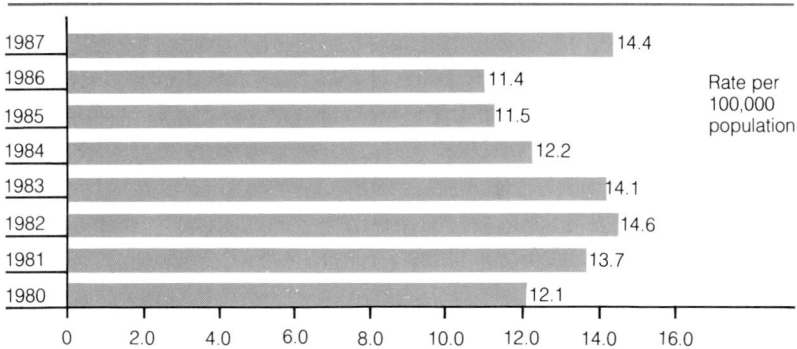

Rate per 100,000 population

Year	Rate
1987	14.4
1986	11.4
1985	11.5
1984	12.2
1983	14.1
1982	14.6
1981	13.7
1980	12.1

Syphilis
Syphilis is uncommon in the US today. Its incidence increased in the late 1970s and early 1980s, then declined in the middle 1980s—possibly helped by a move toward "safe" sex after the appearance of AIDS. There was an unexpected increase in 1987.

INCIDENCE OF NEW CASES OF AIDS IN THE US

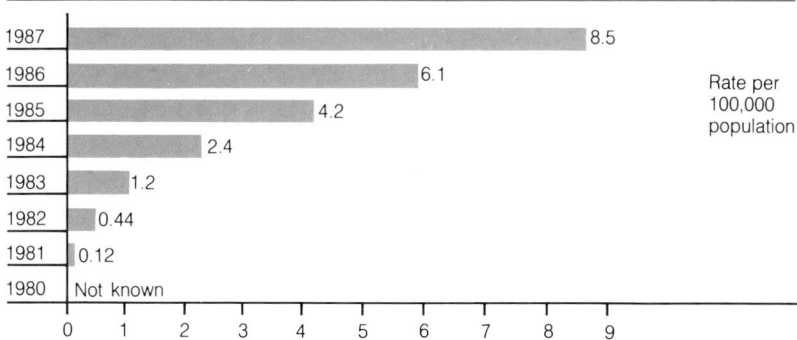

Rate per 100,000 population

Year	Rate
1987	8.5
1986	6.1
1985	4.2
1984	2.4
1983	1.2
1982	0.44
1981	0.12
1980	Not known

AIDS
New cases of AIDS roughly doubled each year from 1982 to 1985, but it was two years before cases doubled again. This may reflect a reduction in the rate of spread of the virus from about 1982 onward, due to greater awareness of the disease.

could become chronic and hepatitis could be fatal. With the recognition of AIDS in 1982, STDs became a threat to life. Promiscuous sex is now a high-risk activity.

DIAGNOSIS AND TREATMENT
Diagnosis and treatment are given at special STD clinics or from specialists in genitourinary medicine and infectious disease. The physician determines which STDs are present (there may be more than one) and then assesses the sensitivity of the infection to various antibiotics. Once drugs have relieved the symptoms, tests are performed to ensure that the patient is no longer infectious.

PREVENTION AND OUTLOOK
To prevent transmitting infection, treatment is made available to all recent sexual partners. The confidential tracing and treatment of contacts is an essential part of the management of STDs (see *Contact tracing*).

The incidence of most STDs (with the exception of AIDS) fell in the middle 1980s. There were 372 new cases of gonorrhea per 100,000 in 1986 compared with 470 cases in 1976. However, a resurgence of penicillin-resistant gonorrhea in 1988 suggested that efforts to educate people on *"safe"* sex measures had yet to take effect.

Sexual problems
Sexual problems are a common reason for consultation with physicians, psychiatrists, marital guidance counselors, and sex therapists. A sexual problem may be perceived by both partners in a relationship, by one partner who is affected by a disorder that lies primarily with the other, or by a person worried about his or her sexual identity or behavior.

CAUSES
Many problems affecting a person's sexual performance or behavior are partly or wholly psychological in origin because of inhibitions, lack of knowledge, anxieties, or a couple's conflicts (see *Psychosexual dysfunction; Deviation, sexual; Transvestism*).

Sometimes, sexual problems are due to organic disease, such as blood flow or hormonal problems. Disorders of the sexual organs may cause pain during intercourse (see *Intercourse, painful*). Some types of chemicals can affect sexual performance; examples include alcohol, *antihypertensive drugs*, and *oral contraceptives*.

People with disabilities may have sexual problems that often go unrecognized. Normal sexual desire may be present but gratification may be difficult to achieve because of physical difficulty with mobility for intercourse or because the disabled person may be avoided sexually by other people.

The mentally handicapped and cognitively impaired may not show normal personal control of their sexual behavior. Sexual molestation and pregnancy may occur.

S

TREATMENT

Many sexual problems disappear when the underlying cause is treated. In other cases, people may benefit from sex education and counseling.

Sézary syndrome

A rare condition in which there is an abnormal overgrowth of lymphoid cells (*lymphocytes*) in the skin, liver, spleen, and lymph nodes. Sézary syndrome primarily affects middle-aged and elderly people.

The first symptom is the appearance of red, scaly patches on the skin that spread to form a severe, flaky, itchy rash. There may also be an accumulation of fluid beneath the skin, baldness, and distorted nail growth; *leukemia* may also be associated with Sézary syndrome. Treatment includes *anticancer drugs* and *radiation therapy*.

Shellfish poisoning

See *Food poisoning*.

Shigellosis

An acute infection of the intestine by bacteria belonging to a group called shigella. Also known as bacillary dysentery, shigellosis causes diarrhea and abdominal pain.

CAUSES AND INCIDENCE

The source of infection is the feces of infected people. The causative bacteria may be spread by an infected person failing to wash his or her hands after defecation and then handling food, or by flies in areas of inadequate sanitation. Endemic in some countries, shigellosis occurs in isolated outbreaks in the US, where about 15,000 cases are reported annually. It is particularly prevalent in children's day-care centers, institutions for the elderly, and mental hospitals.

SYMPTOMS AND SIGNS

The disease usually starts suddenly, with watery diarrhea, abdominal pain, nausea, vomiting, generalized aches, and fever. After a few days, the need to defecate becomes frequent and urgent, and small, watery feces containing pus and blood are passed. Persistent diarrhea may cause *dehydration*, especially in babies and older people. Occasionally, toxemia (the presence of bacterial poisons in the blood) develops, resulting in a high fever and sometimes delirium.

The illness usually subsides after a week or so, but in severe cases may last several weeks. Death is rare, usually occurring only in dehydrated babies and older people.

DIAGNOSIS AND TREATMENT

The diagnosis is confirmed by growing a *culture* of the causative bacteria from a sample of feces.

Dehydration is treated by *rehydration therapy*. Solid food should not be eaten for 24 to 48 hours after the onset of symptoms. In certain cases, *antibiotic drugs* may be prescribed. Infected people should be cared for in isolation until their feces are found to be free of the causative bacteria.

Shingles

See *Herpes zoster*.

Shin splints

A condition characterized by pain in the front and sides of the lower leg that develops or worsens during exercise. There may also be tenderness over the shin and edema (accumulation of fluid) of the surrounding tissues. Shin splints are a common problem in runners.

CAUSES

Shin splints may be caused by various disorders, including *compartment syndrome* (buildup of pressure in a muscle as a result of exercise), *tendinitis* (inflammation of a tendon), *myositis* (inflammation of a muscle), a muscle tear, or *periostitis* (inflammation of the outer layer of a bone).

DIAGNOSIS AND TREATMENT

Diagnosis is based on the symptoms, along with an X ray or radionuclide bone scan (see *Bone imaging*) to exclude the possibility of a stress fracture of the tibia (shin bone), which produces similar symptoms.

In most cases, shin splints clear up after a week or two of rest. However, if the pain is severe or recurrent, other treatment may be necessary, such as a course of *nonsteroidal anti-inflammatory drugs* or *corticosteroid drugs*; infrequently, a surgical operation is performed to alleviate excessive pressure in a muscle. Some people benefit from *physical therapy* instruction that includes stretching and strengthening exercises for the legs.

Shivering

Involuntary trembling of the entire body caused by the rapid contraction and relaxation of muscles. Shivering is the body's normal automatic response to cold; it also occurs in association with *rigors* and fever.

When the body becomes cold, temperature-sensitive nerve cells in the *hypothalamus* (part of the brain) act as a thermostat, initiating the shivering reflex. This causes muscles to con-

tract, generating heat. Shivering caused by cold usually disappears as soon as the body is warmed.

Shivering during rigors and fever is caused by the release of certain substances by the white blood cells. The substances effectively "reset" the thermostat at a higher point, causing the body to shiver when it needs to lose, rather than retain, heat. The trigger for this release is usually an infection, but fever also occurs in some metabolic, autoimmune, and malignant diseases, and as a side effect of certain types of drugs.

Shock

A dangerous reduction of blood flow throughout the body tissues that, if untreated, may lead to collapse, coma, and death. Shock in this sense is physiological shock—different from the mental distress (*posttraumatic stress disorder*) that may follow a physically or emotionally traumatic experience. Reduced blood pressure is, in most cases, a major factor in causing physiological shock and is one of its main features.

CAUSES

Shock is a common accompaniment to severe injury or illness. It may develop in any situation in which blood volume is reduced (through blood or fluid loss), in which blood vessels are abnormally widened, in which the heart's action is weak, in which blood flow is obstructed, or through a combination of these factors. Causes include severe *bleeding* or *burns*, persistent *vomiting* or *diarrhea*, *myocardial infarction* (heart attack), *pulmonary embolism* (blockage of blood flow to the lungs), *peritonitis* (inflammation of the abdominal cavity, often due to perforation of an organ), *spinal injury*, and some types of *poisoning*. *Septic shock* results from bacteria multiplying in the blood and releasing toxins. *Anaphylactic shock* is a type of severe *hypersensitivity* or allergic reaction to an injected substance, such as insect venom or sometimes a drug. Shock is made worse by pain and anxiety.

SYMPTOMS AND TREATMENT

Symptoms of all types of shock include rapid, shallow breathing; cold, clammy skin; rapid, weak pulse; dizziness; weakness; and fainting.

First aid for shock after an injury includes measures to arrest bleeding (see *Bleeding, treatment of*), maintenance of an open airway, keeping the victim flat, reducing heat loss with blankets, and reassurance. A physician or ambulance should be called

S

FIRST AID: SHOCK

> **DO NOT**
> ■ let the victim eat or drink—
>   vomiting may result.
> ■ use a hot-water bottle to
>   warm the victim.

1 Lay the victim down and raise the legs about 12 inches so that blood flows from the legs to the upper body.

2 Loosen tight clothing and wrap the victim in a coat or blanket to prevent heat loss. Seek medical help immediately.

immediately; in the interim, no alcohol or food should be given. Emergency treatment in the hospital involves an *intravenous infusion* of fluid or a blood transfusion, *oxygen therapy*, and, if necessary, morphine or similar powerful painkillers. Further treatment depends on the underlying cause. (See also *Toxic shock syndrome*; *Shock, electric.*)

Shock, electric

The sensation caused by an electric current passing through the body and its effects and aftereffects. A mild shock may produce a sense of having been slightly shaken. A current of an appreciable size and duration can cause loss of consciousness, cardiac arrest (cessation of the heart beat), respiratory arrest, burns, and tissue damage. (See *Electrical injury*.)

Shock therapy

The use of electricity or other agents to produce a sudden and severe disturbance in the nervous system as a means of treating mental illness, particularly severe *depression*. The mechanism of action is unknown.

Only *ECT* (electroconvulsive therapy) is regularly used today. Insulin coma therapy (in which coma was induced by repeated injections of insulin) was a form of shock therapy used in the 1940s and 1950s; it was abandoned because of the risk of permanent, severe brain damage. Another earlier method, involving the use of drugs to stimulate the nervous system, was abandoned because patients often suffered injuries due to violent seizures.

Short stature

A height markedly below the average for a person's age.

CAUSES

In developed countries, restricted growth in children is usually due to heredity factors or to slow bone growth that eventually speeds up, resulting in normal development. Much less commonly, short stature has an abnormal cause, such as a specific growth disorder. The most common types are *growth hormone* deficiency; thyroid hormone deficiency (see *Hypothyroidism*), which also affects brain development; and *achondroplasia*, a hereditary disorder in which primarily the ends of the long bones fail to grow, resulting in disproportionately short limbs.

In certain other disorders, restricted growth occurs as one of several features. Such disorders include those that impair absorption of nutrients, vitamins, or minerals, such as *cystic fibrosis* and *celiac sprue*; chronic infections, such as *tuberculosis*; chronic *asthma*; chromosomal disorders, such as *Down's syndrome* and *Turner's syndrome*; and metabolic disorders, such as *phenylketonuria*.

Other causes of restricted growth in children include certain drugs, particularly *corticosteroid drugs* and *anti-*

cancer drugs. Undernourishment and emotional deprivation, both common in abused or neglected children, can also cause short stature.

INVESTIGATION

The physician takes into account the parents' height and looks for signs of any possible underlying disease.

Most importantly, the child's growth rate is determined by means of regular measurements of height plotted on a chart. If the growth rate is normal, it indicates that the child's short stature is probably due to heredity or to temporary slow skeletal development. Slow growth rate suggests that short stature has an abnormal cause. A sudden drop in growth rate can indicate the onset of disease such as a glandular disorder (e.g., of the thyroid gland).

Other tests may include *X rays* to determine bone age (see *Age*) and *blood tests* to measure hormone levels. More testing is done to ascertain whether the cause is *failure to thrive*.

TREATMENT

Any underlying disorder is treated. Growth hormone is given not only for growth hormone deficiency but also to treat short stature due to Down's syndrome or Turner's syndrome; it is sometimes given in combination with the anabolic steroid *oxandrolone*. (See also *Growth, childhood*.)

Shoulder

The area of the body where the arm attaches to the trunk. The rounded bony surface at the front of the shoulder is the upper part of the *humerus* (upper arm bone); the bony surfaces that form the top and back of the shoulder are parts of the *scapula* (shoulder blade). The *clavicle* (collarbone) articulates with the acromion (the bony prominence at the outer top part of the scapula) at the *acromioclavicular joint* and extends across the top of the chest to the *sternum* (breastbone), to which it is attached at the sternoclavicular joint.

Just below the acromion, on the outer wall of the scapula, is a socket (called the glenoid cavity) into which the head of the humerus fits to form the shoulder joint. A *bursa* (fluid-filled sac) under the acromion reduces friction at the joint. The shoulder joint is a ball-and-socket joint with a wide range of movement produced by part of the *biceps muscle*, several small muscles that make up the *rotator cuff*, various muscles in the chest wall, and the *deltoid* muscle (the muscle at the top of the upper arm and shoulder).

S

STRUCTURE OF THE SHOULDER

Three bones meet at the shoulder—the scapula (shoulder blade), clavicle (collar bone), and humerus (upper arm bone). The shoulder is an example of a ball-and-socket joint.

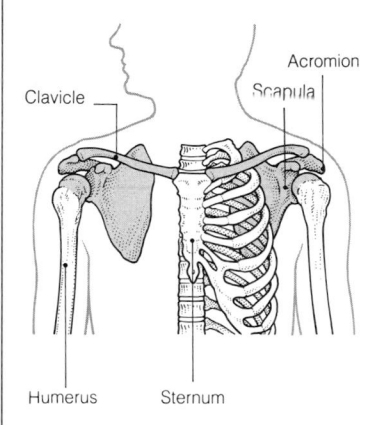

DISORDERS

Shoulder injuries are relatively common, including dislocation of the shoulder joint (see *Shoulder, dislocation of*) or acromioclavicular joint, and *fractures* of the clavicle or the upper part of the humerus. Fractures of the scapula are less common.

The shoulder joint may be affected by any joint disorder, including *arthritis* and *bursitis* (inflammation of a bursa). In severe cases, a joint disorder may lead to *frozen shoulder* (in which movements at the joint are extremely restricted). Movement of the shoulder may also be painful and/or restricted as a result of *tendinitis* (inflammation of a tendon) that affects the tendons of the shoulder muscles. (See also *Bone* disorders box; *Joints; Painful arc syndrome.*)

Shoulder blade

The common name for the *scapula*.

Shoulder, dislocation of

Displacement of the head of the humerus (upper arm bone) out of the shoulder joint. The most common type of dislocation is a forward and downward displacement, caused by a fall onto an outstretched hand or onto the shoulder itself. A backward dislocation may occur as a result of a powerful direct blow to the front of the shoulder or as a result of violent twisting of the upper arm (such as that caused by an electric shock or seizure).

Either type of dislocation may be accompanied by a fracture, usually of the humerus (see *Humerus, fracture of*).

SYMPTOMS AND DIAGNOSIS

The main symptom is pain in the shoulder and upper arm that is made worse by movement. A forward dislocation often produces obvious deformity of the shoulder; a backward dislocation usually does not.

A dislocation is diagnosed by X rays, which also reveal whether there is an accompanying fracture.

TREATMENT

Treatment consists of reduction (maneuvering the head of the humerus back into the joint socket), which is usually performed using an anesthetic. After reduction, X rays are taken to ensure the head of the humerus has been correctly repositioned; the shoulder is then immobilized in a sling for about three weeks. When the humerus has been fractured, treatment is usually the same, although the arm may require a longer period of immobilization.

COMPLICATIONS

A dislocation may damage nerves, which may cause weakness and numbness in the shoulder. Such nerve damage is usually temporary, with full recovery occurring within two to three months. Occasionally, a dislocation damages one of the arteries in the upper arm, causing pain and discoloration of the arm and hand. In severe cases, *arterial reconstructive surgery* may be necessary.

A violent dislocation may damage the muscles that support the shoulder, resulting in the joint being susceptible to recurrent dislocation after only minor injuries. These cases can often be successfully treated by a surgical operation to tighten one of the supporting muscles.

Shoulder-hand syndrome

Pain and stiffness in the shoulder and hand of one side of the body; the affected hand may also become hot, sweaty, and swollen. Because of the pain and stiffness, the arm cannot be used properly and the arm muscles may wither as a result of lack of use.

The precise cause is unknown, but it may occur as a complication of *myocardial infarction* (heart attack), *stroke*, *herpes zoster* (shingles), or a burn or other injury to the shoulder.

In most cases spontaneous recovery occurs within about two years. This period may be shortened by *physical therapy* and treatment with *corticosteroid drugs*. In rare cases, a cervical

DISLOCATION OF SHOULDER

In this injury, the rounded head of the humerus (upper arm bone) has been forced out of its socket just beneath the acromion (tip of the shoulder blade).

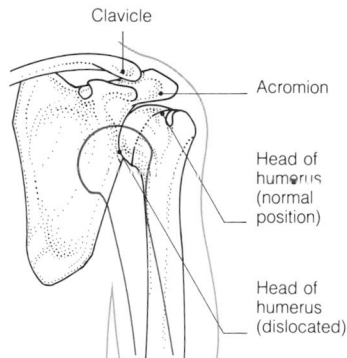

Forward dislocation of left shoulder
A forward and downward dislocation, as shown above, is the most common type.

Backward dislocation
A pit can be seen in this woman's right shoulder where the head of the humerus is normally situated.

sympathectomy (severing of nerves of the sympathetic nervous system on one side of the neck) is performed.

Shunt

An operation performed to relieve abnormal fluid pressure from excess fluid around the brain in *hydrocephalus* or in the portal veins in *portal hypertension*. A shunt between an artery and a vein is installed to provide easy access to the bloodstream for hemodialysis (see also *Arteriovenous fistula*).

SHUNT FOR HYDROCEPHALUS

The shunt for hydrocephalus consists of two catheters and a valve to prevent backflow. The first catheter is inserted through the skull to drain fluid from the ventricles of the brain. The second is passed into another body cavity, usually the abdominal cavity or the right atrium of the heart, where the excess fluid is absorbed.

S

Problems with this procedure include the need to replace the catheter as a child grows and the need to revise the operation two or three times in the first 10 years. The shunt also may become blocked or infected.

SHUNT FOR PORTAL HYPERTENSION

A variety of surgical procedures is used to reduce pressure in the portal system (the veins that carry blood from the digestive organs and spleen to the liver) and thus reduce the risk of bleeding from *esophageal varices*. Shunts are made by creating a direct link between the portal system and the vena cava. Shunt operations prevent bleeding but do not improve liver function and, in fact, may worsen it. The operation itself carries a fairly high mortality that is related to the severity of the disease. Although bleeding is controlled, it is questionable whether survival is prolonged.

Shy-Drager syndrome

A rare degenerative condition that causes progressive damage to the *autonomic nervous system*. The cause of Shy-Drager syndrome is unknown. It begins gradually, affecting people between the ages of 60 and 70, and occurs in more men than women.

The main symptoms are postural *hypotension* (dizziness and fainting when arising or after standing still for a long time), urinary incontinence, reduced ability to sweat, impotence, and *parkinsonism* (muscle tremor, rigidity, and slow movements). The condition worsens over several years, leading to disability and sometimes premature death.

Although there is no cure and no means of slowing the inevitable degeneration, many of the symptoms, particularly the parkinsonism and low blood pressure, can be relieved by drug treatment.

SIADH

An abbreviation for syndrome of inappropriate antidiuretic hormone (secretion). SIADH is a rare condition in which there is excessive production of *ADH*, resulting in retention of water and a low level of sodium in the body.

CAUSES

SIADH may be associated with various underlying disorders, including cancers such as small cell carcinoma of the lung (see *Lung cancer*), cancer of the pancreas or duodenum, or *Hodgkin's disease*; certain lung diseases, such as *pneumonia* or chronic obstructive lung disease (see *Lung disease, chronic obstructive*); or brain disorders, such as *encephalitis*, a brain hemorrhage, or brain damage that results in the pituitary gland overproducing ADH. In addition, certain drugs (such as *chlorpropamide* or *oxytocin*) may increase ADH production and lead to SIADH.

SYMPTOMS AND DIAGNOSIS

The symptoms of SIADH include weakness, tiredness, confusion, and weight gain due to excessive *edema*. The condition is diagnosed from the symptoms and from the results of tests that measure the level of ADH in the blood and compare the concentration of sodium in the blood and the urine.

TREATMENT

Treatment includes restriction of water intake, *diuretic drugs* to increase water loss, and saline infusions to increase the concentration of sodium in the body. However, these measures treat only the symptoms; the underlying cause must be treated successfully to bring about a cure.

Siamese twins

Two babies that are born physically joined. Also called conjoined *twins*, they are named for the first recorded pair, Chang and Eng, who were born in Thailand (formerly Siam) in 1811 and lived for 63 years joined at the hip. Siamese twins are essentially identical twins that fail to develop normally from a single fertilized egg. The cause is unknown.

Siamese twins range from two well-developed individuals, connected only by skin and superficial tissue, to a person with only one extra body part (such as one leg) as evidence of the second twin. Between these extremes are Siamese twins with two heads and two trunks joined at the waist but with only two legs. In some cases one of the twins is very small and poorly developed. The internal organs and brains may be separate, or some or all may be shared.

TREATMENT

If the twins survive birth, and if each one is sufficiently developed to function independently, complete separation by surgery may be possible.

Sibling rivalry

A term that describes the intense competition that is normal between siblings (brothers and/or sisters). An obvious example occurs after the birth of a new baby, when an older sibling constantly seeks to command the parents' attention. Feelings of rivalry may persist through life.

Sick building syndrome

A collection of symptoms sometimes reported by people who work in modern office buildings; the symptoms include loss of energy, headaches, and dry, itching eyes, nose, and throat.

The cause of the syndrome is unknown, although it has been attributed to air conditioning, fluorescent lighting, loss of natural ventilation and light, and psychological factors, especially frustration at being unable to control physical conditions (such as temperature and ventilation) in the working environment. Some authorities believe that many outbreaks of sick building syndrome may be *pseudoepidemics* (conditions without physical causes that are thought to be a form of *hysteria*).

Treatment using environmental agents, such as ionizers, has been unsuccessful. Modification to the building may be the only solution if a large proportion of the work force is affected and the syndrome is thought not to be a pseudoepidemic.

Sickle cell anemia

 An inherited blood disease that occurs primarily in blacks and, less commonly, in individuals of Mediterranean origin. In sickle cell anemia, the red cells are abnormal, resulting in a chronic, very severe form of *anemia* (reduced oxygen-carrying capacity of the blood).

CAUSE

The red cells of affected people contain an abnormal type of *hemoglobin* (oxygen-carrying pigment) called hemoglobin S. In the blood capillaries, where blood is less oxygenated, the deficiency of oxygen causes hemoglobin S to crystallize, distorting the red cells into a sickle shape. This makes the cells fragile; they are easily destroyed, leading to hemolytic anemia. Also, the abnormal cells are unable to pass easily through tiny blood vessels, so they may intermittently block blood flow to various organs, causing sickle cell crises.

Sickle cell anemia occurs in a person who has inherited hemoglobin S from both parents. If hemoglobin S is inherited from one parent, the person has sickle cell trait and is usually free of symptoms. If two such carriers have a child, there is a 1 in 4 chance that the child will have sickle cell anemia, a 2 in 4 chance that the child will have sickle cell trait, and a 1 in 4 chance that the child will have neither.

S

INCIDENCE

In the US, about 150 black children in every 100,000 suffer from sickle cell anemia. About one in 12 blacks has sickle cell trait.

SYMPTOMS AND SIGNS

The symptoms of sickle cell anemia usually first appear after 6 months of age. Chronic hemolytic anemia causes fatigue, headaches, shortness of breath on exertion, pallor, and *jaundice*. Sickle cell crises are sometimes brought on by an infection, cold weather, or dehydration caused, for example, by prolonged vomiting and diarrhea. However, the crises may also occur for no apparent reason. They start suddenly and attack or damage various parts of the body. The sufferer may experience pains (especially in bones), blood in the urine (from kidney damage), or damage to the lungs or intestines. The brain may also be affected, leading to *seizures*, a *stroke*, or unconsciousness.

In some children, the spleen enlarges and traps red cells at a particularly high rate, causing a severe, life-threatening form of anemia. From adolescence onward, the spleen usually shrivels and ceases to function; as a result, the person is at risk of *septicemia* (blood poisoning) if infected by certain types of bacteria.

Children with sickle cell anemia have an increased risk of pneumococcal *pneumonia*, for which prophylactic penicillin has been beneficial. There is also an increased risk of *gallstones*.

DIAGNOSIS

The diagnosis is made from examination of a specially treated *blood smear* for the presence of sickle-shaped red cells and from *electrophoresis* to check for the presence of hemoglobin S.

TREATMENT

There is no cure for the disease. Chronic hemolytic anemia is treated with a lifelong course of folic acid supplements. Affected children should be immunized with pneumococcal vaccine and adolescents and adults may be advised to take penicillin to guard against septicemia.

Because sickle cell crises can be life-threatening, they require prompt treatment. *Intravenous infusions* of fluids are given for dehydration, *antibiotic drugs* are given to treat and prevent infections, *oxygen therapy* is carried out to increase blood oxygenation, and *analgesic drugs* are given to relieve severe pain.

If a severe crisis does not respond to the above measures, an exchange *blood transfusion* may be performed to effect a temporary replacement of hemoglobin S. This may be done regularly for people who suffer frequent severe crises. Exchange transfusions may be carried out during pregnancy to reduce the risk of a crisis (with possibly fatal consequences for mother and child) and before surgery, since anesthesia presents a hazard to patients who have sickle cell anemia (and, to a lesser degree, to those with sickle cell trait).

OUTLOOK

Until about 30 years ago, sickle cell anemia usually proved fatal in childhood. Today, although the mortality is still high in those under 5, improving methods of treatment have enabled more sufferers to survive into adulthood; some are having children.

Blacks and relatives of anyone with sickle cell anemia are advised to have a blood test to determine whether or not they carry the sickle cell gene. A couple, both of whom have sickle cell anemia and/or trait, should obtain *genetic counseling* before starting a family. Tests can be performed in early pregnancy to determine whether a fetus has inherited a double dose of the sickle cell gene.

Sick sinus syndrome

Abnormal function of the sinoatrial node (the heart's pacemaker) that leads to episodes of *bradycardia* (slow heart rate), alternating bradycardia and *tachycardia* (fast heart rate), or very short episodes of cardiac arrest (complete stoppage of the heart beat). The most common cause of sick sinus syndrome is *coronary heart disease*, but the condition can also be caused by a *cardiomyopathy*.

Symptoms include light-headedness, dizziness, fainting, and, occasionally, palpitations (awareness of the heart beat). The diagnosis is confirmed by a 24-hour *ECG* (*Holter monitor*) recording.

Side effect

A reaction or consequence of medication or therapy that is additional to the desired effect. The term usually (although not always) refers to an unwanted or adverse effect. It is not usually applied to the toxic effects produced by a drug overdose, but to a secondary effect of a normal dose.

A side effect may occur as a result of the primary object of therapy continuing beyond its desired limits (e.g., when bleeding results from treatment with *anticoagulant drugs*). Alternatively, the side effect may be com-pletely unrelated, such as when drowsiness results from *antihistamine drugs* prescribed to alleviate allergic *rhinitis* (hay fever). However, an unwanted side effect in one circumstance may be a desired effect in another (drowsiness is the desired effect when antihistamines are used as sedatives).

The aforementioned unwanted side effects are examples of predictable effects; that is, they are expected from the known actions of a particular drug and occur in most patients taking that drug. These side effects are known as type I effects. Type II side effects occur in a minority of patients and are usually unpredictable—until the physician discovers the connection between a particular drug and a patient's idiosyncratic response to it. Type II effects may be caused by factors in the patient, such as a genetic disorder (e.g., the lack of a specific enzyme that usually inactivates the drug) or an allergic reaction. Common type II side effects include a rash, swelling of the face, or jaundice. The occurrence of a type II side effect usually necessitates withdrawal of the drug. (See also *Drug*.)

Siderosis

Any of a variety of conditions in which there is too much iron in the body. Excess iron in the blood or tissues without associated damage is usually called *hemosiderosis*.

SIDS

An abbreviation for *sudden infant death syndrome*.

Sievert

The SI unit of equivalent absorbed dose of ionizing radiation (see *Radiation* units box).

Sight

See *Vision*.

Sight, partial

Loss of vision short of total *blindness*. Partial sight may involve a loss of *visual acuity*, of *visual field*, or of both.

Sigmoid colon

Also known as the pelvic colon, the S-shaped part of the *colon* in the lower abdomen that extends from the brim of the pelvis, usually down to the third segment of the *sacrum* (the triangular bone immediately below the lumbar vertebrae). The sigmoid colon is connected to the descending colon above and the rectum below.

S

Sigmoidoscopy

Examination of the rectum and the sigmoid colon (last part of the large intestine) with a viewing instrument called a sigmoidoscope or proctosigmoidoscope (see *Endoscopy*).

WHY IT IS DONE

Sigmoidoscopy is performed to investigate symptoms such as bleeding from the rectum or lower colon and to inspect the passage for evidence of disorders such as polyps (small benign growths), *ulcerative colitis*, or cancer (see *Intestine, cancer of*). Attachments on the end of the instrument allow the physician to perform a *biopsy* (removal of a small sample of tissue for analysis) if necessary.

Sigmoidoscopy is usually performed as a followup to a rectal examination, in which the physician examines the rectum by inserting a gloved finger. Sigmoidoscopy may also be preceded by *proctoscopy* (examination of the anal canal and rectum with a viewing instrument).

HOW IT IS DONE

The procedure for sigmoidoscopy, along with a typical view through a sigmoidoscope, is shown in the illustrated box at right.

Sign

An objective indication of a disease or disorder (e.g., *jaundice*) that is observed or detected by a physician, as opposed to a *symptom* (e.g., pain), which is noticed by the patient.

Silicone

Any of a specific group of silicon compounds. Silicones are defined as polymeric (long-chain), organic (carbon-containing) compounds of silicon and oxygen. They exist and are used medically in the form of oils, greases, plastics, or rubbers.

Synthetic silicones are widely used as implants in *cosmetic surgery* because they are resistant to body fluids, permeable to oxygen, and are not rejected by the body. Silicone oil in a silicone rubber bag is used in breast reconstruction or breast enlargement (see *Mammoplasty*).

Silicosis

A lung disease caused by the inhalation of dusts containing silica—a common mineral found in sand, quartz, and various types of rock. (See *Pneumoconiosis*.)

Silver nitrate

An *astringent* used to prevent a serious form of *conjunctivitis* in the newborn

---

PROCEDURE FOR SIGMOIDOSCOPY

This is an office procedure taking less than half an hour and needing no anesthetic. Either a rigid or a flexible endoscope (viewing tube) may be used. An *enema* may be used beforehand. The patient lies on the left side with knees drawn up. The entry of the lubricated instrument causes little discomfort.

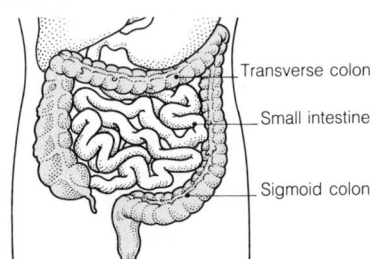

Transverse colon
Small intestine
Sigmoid colon

View through sigmoidoscope

Wall of colon

Sigmoidoscope

Value of sigmoidoscopy

If the bowel is properly cleared of feces beforehand and distended by air pumped in through the instrument, a good view of the lining of the rectum and lower colon may be obtained. This area is often affected by benign growths, ulcers, or cancer. Direct observation of disorders allows early diagnosis and treatment.

(ophthalmia neonatorum). Silver nitrate may also be used on dressings for burns and wounds.

Silver nitrate may cause irritation or pain and, if used over long periods, may result in a permanent blue-black discoloration of the skin.

Silver sulfadiazine

An *antibacterial drug* applied in a cream to prevent infection in burns or after *skin graft*. Possible adverse effects are an allergic reaction, causing a burning sensation, rash, or itching. In rare cases, long-term use may produce serious blood disorders (symptoms of which may include sore throat, fever, or jaundice) or kidney damage.

Simethicone

A drug used on its own or combined with *antacid drugs* to relieve *flatulence*. Simethicone is also used to disperse gas bubbles in the stomach before

gastroscopy (examination of the stomach with a viewing tube) is performed by a physician. There are no known adverse effects.

Sinew

A common nonmedical term for a *tendon*, a tough fibrous cord that joins a muscle to a bone.

Singers' nodes

Small, grayish-white lumps that develop on the vocal cords as the result of constant voice strain. They occur in singers, schoolteachers, politicians, and other people who use their voices excessively, causing hoarseness or loss of voice.

A *biopsy* (removal of a small sample of tissue for microscopic examination) may be performed to rule out a malignant tumor (see *Larynx, cancer of*). Treatment consists of removal of the nodules and voice training.

Sinoatrial node

The heart's natural pacemaker. The sinoatrial node consists of a cluster of specialized muscle cells within the wall of the right atrium (upper chamber) of the heart. Without any external influence, these cells emit electrical impulses at a rate of 100 per minute, which initiate the contractions (beats) of the heart. Various hormones and nervous system activity can affect the node, causing it to emit impulses at a different rate, thus slowing down or speeding up the heart. (See also *Heart rate*.)

Sinus

A cavity within a bone, in particular one of the mucous membrane-lined, air-filled spaces in the bones surrounding the nose (see *Sinus, facial*).

The term sinus also refers to any wide channel that contains blood, such as the venous sinuses in the outermost covering of the brain.

Sinus is also a term for an abnormal, often infected, tract.

Sinus bradycardia

A slow, but regular, heart rate (less than 60 beats per minute). Sinus bradycardia is caused by reduced electrical activity in the sinoatrial node (the heart's pacemaker). Unlike *heart block*, there is no impairment to the transmission of electrical impulses through the heart.

Sinus bradycardia is normal in athletes and in people who exercise regularly; it can be achieved by relaxation techniques.

Sinus bradycardia may also be caused by *hypothyroidism*, a *myocardial infarction* (heart attack), or drugs such as beta-blockers or digoxin.

Sinus, facial

Any of the mucous membrane-lined, air-filled cavities in the bones surrounding the nose. The facial sinuses comprise the two frontal sinuses in the frontal bone of the forehead just above the eyebrows; the two maxillary sinuses in the cheekbones; the two ethmoidal sinuses, honeycomblike cavities in bones that lie between the nasal cavity and the eye sockets; and the sphenoidal sinuses, a collection of air spaces in the large, winged bone behind the nose that forms the central part of the base of the skull. Mucus drains from each sinus along a narrow channel that opens into the nose.

Infection, usually spreading from the nose, may cause *sinusitis* (inflammation of the lining of the sinuses).

LOCATION AND FUNCTION OF THE SINOATRIAL NODE

The sinoatrial (SA) node is a small mass of muscle cells in the right atrium of the heart. It sends out impulses at an inherent rate of over 100 impulses per minute. External control, mainly by the vagus nerve, reduces the rate to about 70 per minute at rest.

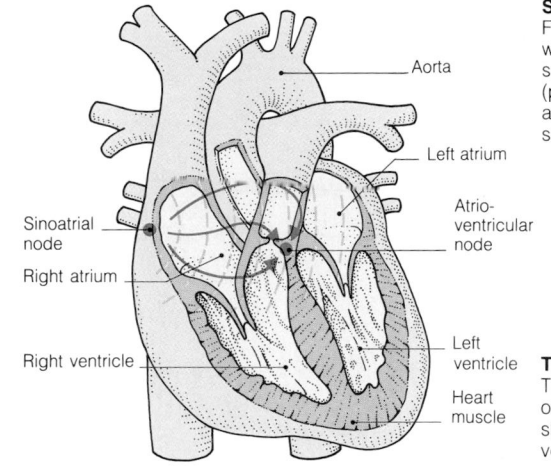

Spread of the impulse
From the SA node, the waves of contraction spread over both atria (pink area) and then to the atrioventricular node serving the ventricles.

Wave of excitation spreading over atria | Excitation spreading over ventricles

The electrocardiogram
The spread of excitation over the two atria is fairly slow; the spread over the ventricles is rapid.

Sinusitis

Inflammation of the membrane lining the facial *sinuses* (the air-filled cavities in the bones surrounding the nose) caused by infection. The ethmoidal sinuses, between the eyes, and the maxillary sinuses, in the cheekbones, are commonly affected.

CAUSES AND INCIDENCE
Most sinusitis is caused by infection spreading to the sinuses from the nose along the narrow passages that drain mucus from the sinuses into the nose. The disorder is usually the result of a bacterial infection that develops as a complication of a viral infection, such

LOCATION OF SINUSES

The air spaces, or sinuses, in the skull bones lighten the skull and improve the resonance of the voice. The sinuses surround and drain into the nose, although the position of the outlets is not always ideal for free drainage.

Cross section through skull

Frontal sinus · Ethmoidal sinus · Frontal sinus · Sphenoidal sinus · Maxillary sinus · Ethmoidal sinus · Maxillary sinus

S

as the common *cold*. Less commonly, infection may arise from an abscess in an upper tooth (see *Abscess, dental*), from infected water being forced into the sinuses when a person jumps feet first into water without covering the nose, or from a severe facial injury.

Sinusitis is extremely common; many people suffer an attack after every common cold. It seems that once the tendency to sinus infection is established, recurrence is more likely with each cold.

SYMPTOMS AND SIGNS

Sinusitis usually causes a feeling of tension or fullness in the affected area and sometimes a throbbing ache. It may also result in fever, a stuffy nose, and loss of the sense of smell.

A common complication is the formation of pus in the affected sinuses, causing pain and a nasal discharge. Other rare complications include orbital cellulitis (see *Orbit*), *osteomyelitis*, and *meningitis*.

DIAGNOSIS AND TREATMENT

X rays are sometimes taken to determine the location and extent of the disorder; a *culture* may be grown from a lavage (washing) of the maxillary sinus to identify the infective bacteria. *Antibiotic drugs* are given immediately to combat the infection, but the antibiotic chosen may be changed after the result of the culture is known. *Decongestant* drops or a spray, by reducing inflammation of the mucous membranes, restores drainage of the sinuses. Steam inhalations moisten the secretions and are helpful in removing them. If sinusitis persists, surgical drainage of the affected sinuses (by creating a new opening in them) may be performed.

Sinus tachycardia

A fast, but regular, heart rate (more than 100 beats per minute). Sinus tachycardia is caused by increased electrical activity in the sinoatrial node (the heart's pacemaker). It is normal during sudden stressful or anxious moments and during (and for a short time after) exercise. Persistent sinus tachycardia at rest may be caused by fever, *hyperthyroidism*, and other disorders. (See *Tachycardia*.)

Situs inversus

An unusual condition in which the internal organs are situated in the mirror image of their normal positions. No treatment is required unless there is an associated abnormality of any of the organs, in which case surgery may be necessary. (See also *Dextrocardia*.)

BONES OF THE SKELETON

There are two main parts to the skeleton—the axial and appendicular skeletons (shown below). Some parts, such as the skull and pelvis, consist of several fused or associated bones. The function of the skeleton is not merely mechanical; bones are active living structures that are constantly producing blood cells and interchanging minerals with the blood.

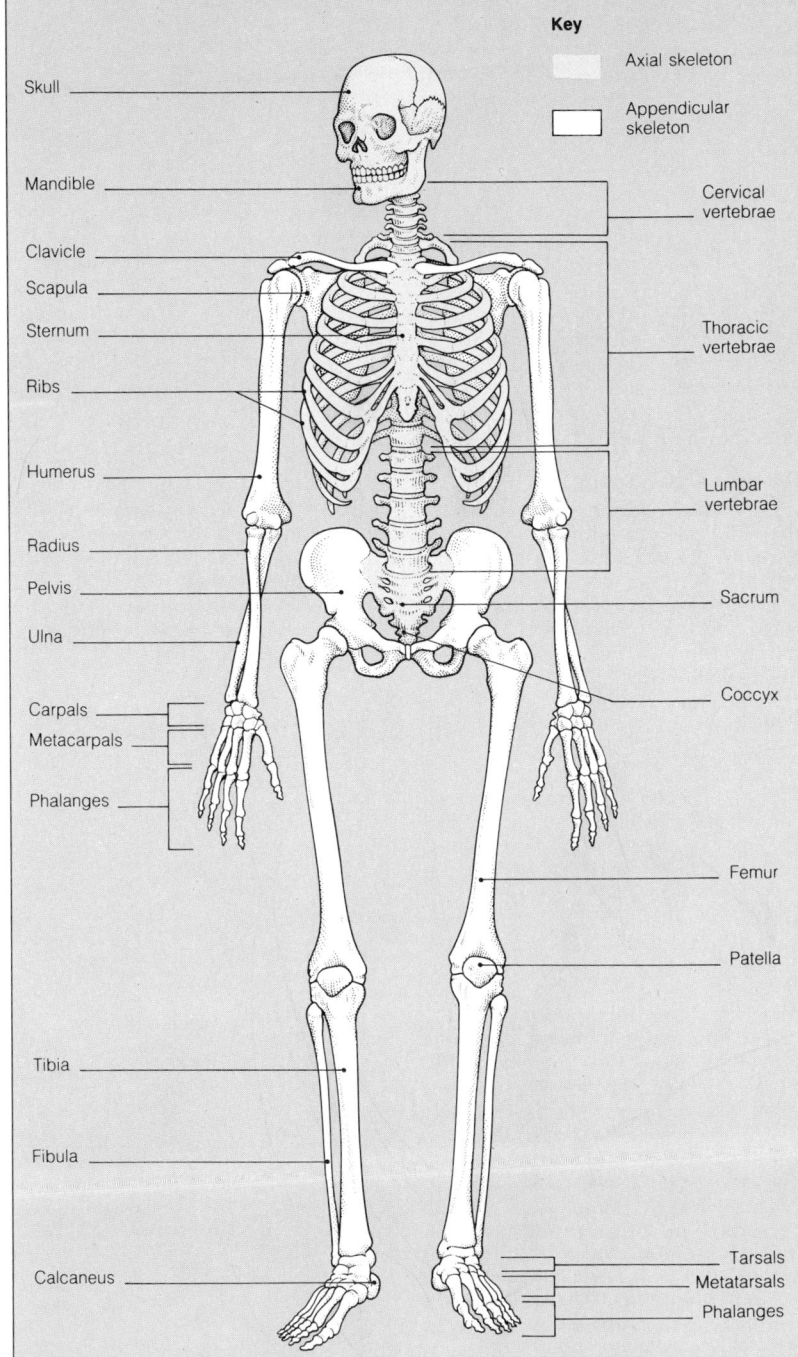

Key

☐ Axial skeleton

☐ Appendicular skeleton

Skull

Mandible

Clavicle

Scapula

Sternum

Ribs

Humerus

Radius

Pelvis

Ulna

Carpals

Metacarpals

Phalanges

Tibia

Fibula

Calcaneus

Cervical vertebrae

Thoracic vertebrae

Lumbar vertebrae

Sacrum

Coccyx

Femur

Patella

Tarsals

Metatarsals

Phalanges

S

Sjögren's syndrome

A condition in which the eyes, mouth, and vagina become excessively dry. Sjögren's syndrome tends to occur with certain *autoimmune disorders*, such as *rheumatoid arthritis* or systemic *lupus erythematosus*. The exact cause is unknown. However, because the body's defense system is upset with the autoimmune disorder, it begins to destroy the glands that produce lubricating secretions.

Ninety percent of sufferers are women—mostly middle-aged and often postmenopausal.

The most characteristic and troublesome feature of the condition is *keratoconjunctivitis sicca* (dry eye), which causes itching and burning of the eyes and creates the sensation of a foreign body under the eyelid. Artificial tears can be used to moisten the eye. Lack of saliva leads to an increased risk of dental caries; good oral hygiene and dental care are therefore essential. A water-soluble lubricating jelly may be used to facilitate sexual intercourse.

Skeleton

The average human adult skeleton has 206 *bones* joined with *ligaments* and tendons to form a protective and supportive framework for the attached muscles and underlying soft tissues of the body. In some people, however, there may be a variation in the number of vertebrae or there may be additional small bones (called sesamoids) in tendons around the joints.

STRUCTURE

The skeleton consists of two main parts, known as the axial and appendicular skeletons. The axial skeleton comprises the *skull, spine, ribs,* and *sternum* (breastbone). Together, they represent a total of 80 bones—29 in the skull (including the *hyoid* bone and three pairs of auditory *ossicles*), 26 in the spine (seven cervical, 12 thoracic, and five lumbar *vertebrae,* the *sacrum,* and the *coccyx*), and 25 in the chest (12 pairs of ribs and the sternum).

The appendicular skeleton consists of the two limb girdles (the *shoulder* and *pelvis*) and their attached limb bones. The appendicular skeleton includes 126 bones, 64 in the shoulders and upper limbs and 62 in the pelvis and lower limbs. There are two bones in each shoulder—the *clavicle* (collarbone) and *scapula* (shoulder blade); three in each arm—the *humerus* (upper arm bone) and the *radius* and *ulna* (forearm bones); eight carpals in each *wrist;* five *metacarpals* in each palm; and 14 *phalanges* in the digits of each hand (two in each thumb and three in each finger).

The pelvic girdle consists of two innominate (hip) bones, and each of the lower limbs has 30 bones—a *femur* (thigh bone), *patella* (kneecap), and *tibia* and *fibula* (lower leg bones) in each leg; seven tarsals in the *ankle,* heel (see *Calcaneus*), and back part of the foot; five *metatarsals* in the middle of each foot; and 14 phalanges in the toes (two in each big toe and three in each other toe).

There are only minor differences between the skeletons of men and women. In general, men's bones tend to be slightly larger and heavier than the corresponding bones in women; the female pelvic cavity is wider to facilitate childbirth.

The individual bones of the skeleton are connected by three types of *joints,* which differ in the amount of mobility they permit through the various planes and ranges of movement.

FUNCTION

The skeleton plays an indispensable role in movement by providing a strong, stable, yet mobile, framework on which the muscles can act. In effect, it consists of a series of independently movable internal levers on which the muscles can pull to move different parts of the body.

The skeleton also supports and protects body organs, notably the brain and spinal cord (which are encased in the skull and spine) and the heart and lungs (which are protected by the ribs). The ribs also make breathing possible by supporting the chest cavity so that the lungs are not compressed, and by helping in the breathing movements themselves.

The skeleton is not an inert frame, however. It is an active organ that produces blood cells (formed in bone marrow) and acts as a reservoir for minerals such as calcium, which can be drawn on, if required, by other parts of the body.

Skin

The outermost covering of body tissue, which protects the internal organs from the environment. The skin is the largest organ in the body. Its cells are continually being replaced as they are lost by wear and tear.

STRUCTURE

The skin consists of a thin outer layer (the epidermis) and a thicker inner layer (the dermis). Beneath the dermis is the subcutaneous tissue, which contains fat. The *hair* and *nails* are extensions of the skin and are composed mainly of *keratin,* which is the main constituent of the outermost part of the epidermis.

S

STRUCTURE OF SKIN

The skin consists essentially of two layers—dermis (true skin), which contains most of the living elements, and epidermis, which is a protective and disposable covering with a dead outer layer.

Pore · Hair · Horny (dead) layer · Epidermis · Melanocyte · Basal cell (living) layer · Nerve · Dermis · Blood vessels · Subcutaneous layer · Sweat gland · Hair follicle · Hair erector muscle

DISORDERS OF THE SKIN

The skin is the largest and most vulnerable organ of the body. Although skin conditions are seldom life-threatening, many can be severely debilitating and cause psychological problems.

CONGENITAL DISORDERS

A *birthmark* is a type of *nevus* (pigmented skin blemish) present from birth. Nevi include moles, freckles, *Mongolian spots*, and *hemangiomas*, such as port-wine stains and strawberry marks.

INFECTION AND INFLAMMATION

Viral infections of the skin include *cold sores, warts, chickenpox, molluscum contagiosum*, and *herpes zoster* (shingles). Bacterial infections include *boils, cellulitis, erysipelas*, and *impetigo*. Fungal infections, such as *tinea*, cause *athlete's foot* and ringworm.

Inflammation of the skin occurs in *dermatitis* and *eczema*; it may be caused by an allergic reaction to a substance (such as nickel), a detergent, a plant, or a drug. *Psoriasis* is a common and persistent skin disease of unknown cause that consists of large, red patches with silvery, scaly surfaces. *Prickly heat* is an irritating rash that is caused by blockage of the sweat glands.

TUMORS

Benign (noncancerous) tumors of the skin are extremely common; these include seborrheic *keratoses* and most types of nevi. *Bowen's disease* is a skin disorder that may slowly become cancerous. Three common forms of skin cancer are *basal cell carcinoma, squamous cell carcinoma*, and malignant melanoma (see *Melanoma, malignant*). Less common skin cancers include *Paget's disease of the nipple, mycosis fungoides*, and *Kaposi's sarcoma*.

INJURY

The skin is vulnerable to many minor injuries, including cuts and bites (see *Bites, animal*; *Insect bites*) as well as more serious *wounds*. *Burns* can be among the most serious of all skin injuries and may cause extensive scarring or death.

HORMONAL DISORDERS

Acne is partially related to the action of *androgens* on the sebaceous glands; it is common among adolescents.

NUTRITIONAL DISORDERS

Deficiency of vitamins B and C can cause *rashes*.

IMPAIRED BLOOD SUPPLY

Leg ulcers, which are particularly common in the elderly, may be caused by poor blood flow to the skin as a result of *atherosclerosis*, by poor drainage of blood through *varicose veins*, or by the leg swelling associated with heart failure.

DRUGS

Many drugs, including antibiotics, barbiturates, and sulfonamides, may cause a rash. Some cause *urticaria* (hives), others cause *eczema* or a rash similar to the measles rash, and some cause *photosensitivity*.

RADIATION

All forms of radiation are potentially damaging to the skin. Overexposure to sunlight (ultraviolet radiation) causes premature aging of the skin and increases the risk of skin cancer (see *Sunlight, adverse effects of*). High doses of other forms of radiation, such as X rays, may cause severe injury to the skin and may lead to cancer.

AUTOIMMUNE DISORDERS

These disorders include *lupus erythematosus*, a disorder that may affect the skin alone or the skin and other organs; *vitiligo*, characterized by pure white patches and caused by destruction of the skin's pigment cells; *dermatomyositis*, which is characterized by a specific skin rash and muscle weakness; *morphea* and *scleroderma*, in which there is progressive hardening of the skin and other tissues; and *pemphigoid* and *pemphigus*, in which large blisters develop on the skin.

OTHER DISORDERS

A *keloid* is an abnormally large and protruding *scar* caused by the continuing production of scar tissue long after healing would usually be complete. *Striae* (stretch marks) often develop during pregnancy and may also develop as a side effect of treatment with *corticosteroid drugs*.

Erythema simply means redness and has many possible causes. *Petechiae* are pinpoints of blood in the skin; in certain conditions, petechiae give rise to *purpura* or larger bruises.

Xanthelasma are yellowish patches that tend to occur on the eyelids; they are a result of the deposition of cholesterol.

INVESTIGATION

Most skin disorders can be diagnosed from their physical characteristics. A skin *biopsy* (removal of a tissue sample for microscopic analysis) may also be performed, usually to aid in the diagnosis of a skin problem or to exclude skin cancer.

EPIDERMIS The epidermis is made up of flat cells that resemble paving stones when viewed under the microscope. Its thickness varies depending on the part of the body, being thickest on the soles and palms and very thin on the eyelids. It is generally thicker in men than in women and normally becomes thinner with age.

The outermost part of the epidermis is composed of dead cells, which form a tough, horny, protective coating. As these dead cells are worn away, they are replaced. The new cells are produced by rapidly dividing living cells in the innermost part of the epidermis. Between the outer and inner parts is a transitional region that consists of both living and dead cells.

Most of the cells in the epidermis are specialized to produce keratin, a hard protein substance that is the main constituent of the tough, outermost part of the epidermis. Some of the cells produce the protective pigment *melanin*, which determines skin color.

DERMIS The dermis is composed of connective tissue interspersed with various specialized structures, such as hair follicles, *sweat glands*, and *sebaceous glands*, that produce an oily substance called *sebum*. The dermis also contains blood vessels, lymph vessels, and nerves.

FUNCTION

The skin's most important function is to protect. It acts as the main barrier between the environment and the internal organs of the body, shielding them from injury, the harmful rays of sunlight, and invasion from infective agents, such as bacteria.

The skin is a sensory organ containing many cells that are sensitive to touch, temperature, pain, pressure, and itching. It also plays a role in keeping body temperature constant. When the body is hot, the sweat glands produce perspiration (which cools the body) and the blood vessels in the dermis dilate to dissipate the heat; if the body gets cold, the blood vessels in the skin constrict, which conserves the body's heat.

The epidermis contains a unique fatty substance that makes the skin waterproof—thus making it possible to sit in a bath without soaking up the water like a sponge. The outer epidermis also has an effective water-holding capacity, which contributes to its elasticity and serves to maintain the body balance of fluid and electrolytes. If the water content drops below a certain level, the skin becomes cracked, reducing its efficiency as a barrier.

Skin allergy

A large number of substances can provoke an allergic reaction through direct contact with the skin of a susceptible person. However, the substance first must have sensitized the person's *immune system* during a previous contact or contacts. If the skin reaction is truly an allergic one, the causative substance produces symptoms only in susceptible people. Many substances that cause skin reactions (fiberglass spicules, for example) are irritant by nature, rather than allergenic, and can affect anyone, not just a sensitive few.

There are two main types of allergic skin reactions. Contact allergic *dermatitis* consists of red, itchy patches, which may blister or form crusts. The patches correspond to the area of contact with the causative substance and develop between a few hours and two days of contact. Substances that can produce such a reaction are adhesives, poison ivy, elastic, nickel in jewelry, some cosmetics, and chromium salts used in hat and shoe manufacture.

Contact *urticaria* (red, itchy, raised areas on the skin) may develop within a few minutes to half an hour of skin contact with some medications, chemicals, plants, insect saliva (from an insect bite), and foods such as shellfish. Urticaria can also be a symptom of an allergic reaction to something eaten, but the majority of cases of urticaria are probably not allergic in origin. Many drugs can cause skin eruptions, some of which resemble urticaria. However, not all of them are allergic in nature (see *Rash*).

Atopic *eczema* is an itchy skin condition that is most common in babies and children, particularly those with a family history of allergic-type illnesses such as asthma. It does not seem to be caused by skin contact with an allergen, but in some cases may be the result of a food allergy.

In many skin allergies, the causative substance is obvious and contact with it should be minimized. In other cases, it may be difficult to know which ingredient (e.g., of a cosmetic) is the cause of allergy. The causative agent may be discovered only through exhaustive tests in which the skin is challenged by exposure to various suspected substances (see *Skin tests*).

Skin and muscle flap

A surgical technique in which a section of skin and underlying tissue, sometimes including muscle, is moved to cover an area from which skin and deeper tissue have been lost or damaged.

WHY IT IS DONE

Unlike a *skin graft*, a flap retains its blood supply—either by remaining attached at one end to the donor site or through reattachment of its blood vessels to vessels at the new site. This makes a flap particularly useful for covering an area (such as exposed bone or tendon) that has lost its blood supply and on which a graft would not "take." Flaps are also used for regions that require thick covering to protect them (e.g., bony prominences such as the hip). In addition, because flaps are less likely to contract than skin grafts, they are useful for releasing tension from scarred areas. Skin flaps may be preferable to skin grafts because healing is more reliable and cosmetic results are better.

HOW IT IS DONE

When the area to be covered is relatively small and there is sufficient skin nearby, the flap may be left

---

TECHNIQUE FOR MOVING A SKIN AND MUSCLE FLAP

A flap of skin and muscle can be moved to a new site to replace tissue loss; if its blood supply is maintained, the flap will adhere well. Microsurgery to rejoin blood vessels facilitates the technique.

1 The donor area needs a good blood supply if muscle is to be taken.

2 The ends of the donor area need to be tapered to allow satisfactory closure.

3 The skin may have to be undercut and freed before the wound is closed.

An artery and a vein of suitable size must be available at the recipient site to be joined to blood vessels in the flap.

Skin and muscle flaps are useful when there has been much loss of deep tissue. The results are usually excellent.

S

attached at one end and moved by stretching, rotating, or transposing it. Otherwise, the flap is removed from another area of the body and its vessels are attached to new arteries and veins at the site of the graft using microsurgical techniques (see illustrated box on previous page). The area left bare by cutting the flap is closed with stitches or, if necessary, by a skin graft. (See also *Microsurgery*.)

Skin biopsy

Removal of a portion of diseased skin for laboratory analysis. Skin *biopsy* may be performed when *skin cancer* is suspected or to confirm the diagnosis of certain skin disorders (such as *pemphigus* or *dermatomyositis*).

Using a local anesthetic, the skin is removed with a *scalpel* or a *curet*. When a highly malignant condition (such as *melanoma*) is suspected, all of the affected area is cut away with skin around and beneath it. Otherwise, only a small portion of tissue is removed. The wound usually requires minimal stitching and leaves little or no scar.

Skin cancer

A malignant tumor in the skin. Skin cancer is one of the most common forms of cancer.

Basal cell carcinoma, squamous cell carcinoma, and malignant *melanoma* are common forms of skin cancer related to long-term exposure to sunlight. *Bowen's disease*, a rare skin disorder that can become cancerous, also may be related to sunlight exposure.

Less common types of skin cancer include *Paget's disease of the nipple* and *mycosis fungoides*; both produce inflammation similar to that of eczema. *Kaposi's sarcoma* is a type of skin cancer commonly found in patients with *AIDS* (although elderly patients may have Kaposi's sarcoma and not have AIDS).

Basal cell carcinoma
This is the most common form of skin cancer. Also called rodent ulcer, it develops most often on the face.

Even though most skin cancers can be easily cured if treated early, many people die because they delay seeking treatment, especially from squamous cell carcinoma and malignant melanoma. Changed or new growths should be reported to a physician.

Skin graft

A technique used in plastic surgery to repair areas of lost or damaged skin. A piece of healthy skin is detached from one part of the body and transferred to the affected area. New cells grow from the graft and cover the damaged area with fresh skin.

Skin taken from an identical twin can be used for a graft, but skin from another person or an animal is soon rejected by the recipient's body (although it may provide useful temporary cover).

WHY IT IS DONE
A skin graft is performed because the area is too large to be repaired by stitching or because natural healing would result in scarring that might be unsightly or restrict movement.

TYPES
There are two basic types of skin graft—split-thickness and full-thickness (see illustrated box below).

TYPES OF SKIN GRAFT

The two main types of skin graft are split-thickness (in which less than the full thickness of skin is removed from the donor site) and full-thickness. There are advantages to each of these types.

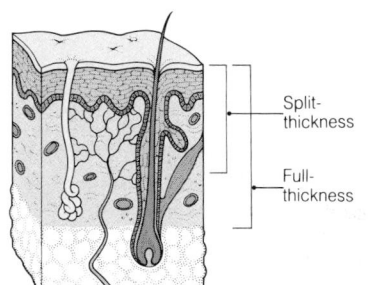

Split-thickness graft
When large areas need to be covered, such as after burns, split-thickness grafts are used and the donor sites are left to regenerate, which they do in a few days. Such sites can be repeatedly harvested.

Full-thickness graft
Full-thickness skin grafts are usually preferred for the face because they more closely approximate the appearance of normal skin. However, donor sites are limited and must be sutured (stitched).

HOW A FULL-THICKNESS GRAFT IS DONE

Most skin grafts are performed using general anesthesia. Full-thickness grafts are easily cut with a scalpel. Subcutaneous fat is avoided and any bleeding at the recipient site prevented.

1 Skin for a full-thickness graft is often taken from behind the ear.

2 The graft must be larger than the area to be covered, to allow for shrinkage.

3 Precise fitting and firm pressure are needed to ensure there is a satisfactory "take."

Instruments
Split-skin grafts are cut, usually from the abdomen or thigh, with an instrument called a dermatome. If necessary, the skin can be expanded into a trellislike mesh on the donor site.

S

In some cases, underlying muscle is removed with the full thickness of skin (see *Skin and muscle flap*).

HOW IT IS DONE
Most grafts are done by removing skin from the donor site and transferring it to the recipient site (see box).

RESULTS
All grafts leave scars. Full-thickness grafts yield more natural color and texture and contrast less than split-thickness grafts. However, full-thickness grafts are less likely to take.

Skin infections
See *Skin* disorders box.

Skin peeling, chemical
A cosmetic operation to remove freckles, acne scars, delicate wrinkles, or other surface skin blemishes. A paste containing phenol (carbolic acid) or some other caustic agent is applied to the skin, left for a half hour, and then scraped off. The outer layers of the skin peel away with the paste, thus removing the blemishes.

Because of *photosensitivity*, the raw area must not be exposed to sunlight until new skin layers have fully grown. Permanent discoloration of the skin is common; it may be improved by wearing makeup.

Skin tag
A small, brown or flesh-colored, protruding flap of skin caused by unsatisfactory healing of a wound or occurring spontaneously. Anal tags often occur as a complication of *anal fissures* or hemorrhoids. Skin tags usually can be removed.

Skin tests
Procedures for determining the body's reaction to various substances by injecting a small quantity of the substance underneath the skin or by applying it to the skin.

Patch tests are widely used in the diagnosis of contact allergic *dermatitis* (a type of skin allergy). Various suspected substances are applied by means of adhesive patches to the skin. After a specific period of time, the patches are removed and the reactions observed. If one substance has caused reddening or blistering, the person is probably allergic to the substance and should avoid it in the future.

Substances injected under the skin may help identify allergens responsible for *asthma*, allergic *rhinitis* (hay fever), or other allergic-type illnesses, even though skin symptoms are not one of the primary features of these conditions. The tests may also be used to test immunity to certain infectious diseases (such as in the *tuberculin test*).

Skin tumors
A growth on or in the skin that may or may not be cancerous (see *Skin cancer*).

Very common types of benign (noncancerous) skin tumors include *keratoses* (wartlike growths caused by overproduction of keratin) and squamous *papillomas* (small, raised, flesh-colored growths).

Other benign skin tumors include *sebaceous cysts*, cutaneous *horns* (hard protrusions from the skin), *kerato-acanthomas* (rapidly growing, flesh-colored nodules), and *hemangiomas* (birthmarks formed by a collection of blood vessels in the skin).

Skull
The bony skeleton of the head. The skull has several functions. It encases and protects the brain, houses organs of the special senses, provides points of attachment for muscles of the head and neck, and helps form the first parts of the respiratory and digestive tracts. Many of the bones are hollow, reducing the weight of the skull and adding to the resonance of the voice.

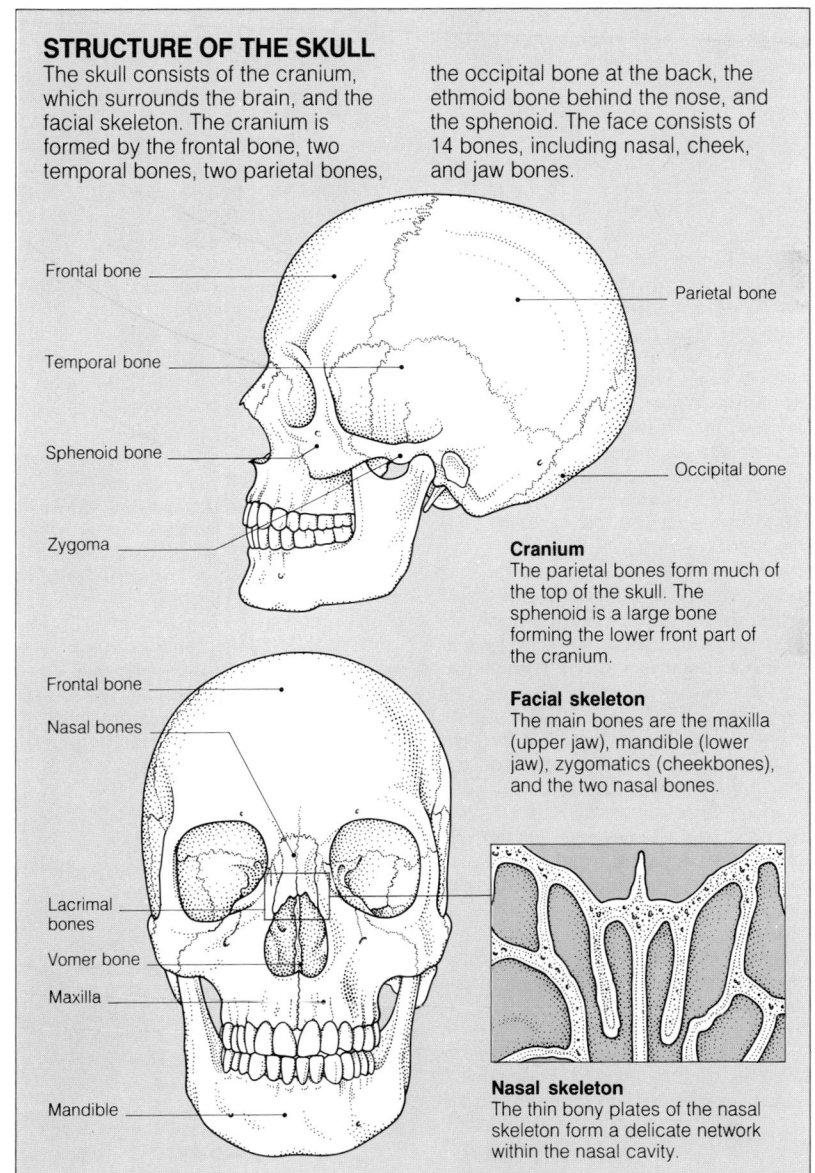

STRUCTURE OF THE SKULL
The skull consists of the cranium, which surrounds the brain, and the facial skeleton. The cranium is formed by the frontal bone, two temporal bones, two parietal bones, the occipital bone at the back, the ethmoid bone behind the nose, and the sphenoid. The face consists of 14 bones, including nasal, cheek, and jaw bones.

Frontal bone
Temporal bone
Sphenoid bone
Zygoma
Parietal bone
Occipital bone

Frontal bone
Nasal bones
Lacrimal bones
Vomer bone
Maxilla
Mandible

Cranium
The parietal bones form much of the top of the skull. The sphenoid is a large bone forming the lower front part of the cranium.

Facial skeleton
The main bones are the maxilla (upper jaw), mandible (lower jaw), zygomatics (cheekbones), and the two nasal bones.

Nasal skeleton
The thin bony plates of the nasal skeleton form a delicate network within the nasal cavity.

S

STRUCTURE

The arrangement of the bones in the skull is shown in the illustrated box on the previous page. All the skull bones, except the mandible, are fixed to each other by immovable joints called sutures. The mandible articulates with the temporal bones at the freely movable temporomandibular joints.

Closely associated with, but not strictly part of, the skull are the hyoid (a small bone in the back of the tongue) and the auditory ossicles (the three tiny bones in each middle ear).

The skull contains several cavities, including the cranial cavity (which houses the brain), the nasal cavity (which is involved in smell and breathing), and the orbits (which house the eyeballs and their associated muscles). Part of the mouth is also formed by the skull.

Several of the skull bones, notably the maxillas, sphenoid bone, frontal bone, and ethmoid bone, contain *sinuses* (air-filled spaces); these sinuses are called the paranasal sinuses. In addition, there are spaces in the temporal bones that house the structures of the middle and inner ear.

In the cranium are many holes (called foramens) for the passage of nerves and blood vessels. Passing through are the *cranial nerves* (which supply most of the sensory structures and muscles of the head and neck) and blood vessels such as the *carotid arteries* and *jugular veins* (which carry blood to and from the brain). The largest of the holes, the foramen magnum, is situated in the occipital bone (which forms part of the base and back of the cranium); this hole allows the brain stem to enter the spinal canal, where it continues as the spinal cord.

The skull rests on the first cervical vertebra (called the atlas), a ring-shaped bone that articulates with the occipital bone and permits nodding movements of the head. Turning the head is a function of the joint between the atlas and the second cervical vertebra (axis). The occipital bone, atlas, and axis are connected by numerous small muscles.

DISORDERS

The skull may be affected by any bone disorder (see *Bone* disorders box) that involves the skeleton, such as *Paget's disease*, but the most common disorder is injury. A blow to the head may cause a fracture (see *Skull, fractured*), which may result in damage to the brain, and, if a foramen is involved, in damage to a blood vessel or cranial nerve. (See also *Head injury*.)

Skull, fractured

A break in one or more of the skull bones caused by a head injury. Because the skull is extremely strong, most fractures are closed and cause no complications. Closed fractures are also called simple fractures—that is, the bone is cracked without any displacement of the broken pieces. However, severe injury to the head may result in an open (also called depressed) fracture in which the bone fragments are displaced, usually inward. In this case, the blood vessels in the *meninges* (the membranes that cover the brain) may be ruptured, resulting in an epidural hemorrhage (bleeding into the space between the skull and the outer membrane) or a *subdural hemorrhage* (bleeding into the space between the outer and middle membranes). The resultant blood clot may press on and displace brain tissue. Less commonly, all the meninges may be torn, and the brain itself may be damaged.

SYMPTOMS AND SIGNS

The degree of brain injury does not always correlate with damage to the skull. Severe brain injury can occur with no skull fracture and, in some cases of closed fracture, little or no brain injury may occur. The symptoms and signs of skull fractures (see *Head injury*) depend mainly on the degree of brain damage sustained. Leakage of cerebrospinal fluid (the liquid that bathes the brain and spinal cord) through the nose or ears indicates rupture of the meninges by an open fracture of the base of the skull.

DIAGNOSIS AND TREATMENT

Any person who has suffered a significant blow to the head—particularly one that has caused unconsciousness—should consult a physician even if there are no symptoms. If the physician suspects a hemorrhage, *CT scanning* may be performed.

Multiple skull fracture
This side-view X ray shows the cranium smashed into several pieces. Some pieces have been surgically removed.

A person with a closed fracture is hospitalized and observed closely for 12 to 24 hours for signs of complications. If no signs develop, treatment is generally not necessary because the fracture usually heals by itself.

An open fracture often requires treatment by a neurosurgeon. A hemorrhage may necessitate a *craniotomy* to drain the blood and repair damaged vessels. When deeply depressed fractures have penetrated the meninges and brain tissue, an operation is performed to raise or remove the pieces of fractured bone and repair the damaged tissue. After such an operation, there can be some degree of skull distortion.

Antibiotic drugs are given for all open fractures because of the risk of infection of the meninges (see *Meningitis*) or of the brain itself (see *Encephalitis*).

Skull X ray

A technique for providing images of the skull.

WHY IT IS DONE

A skull X ray is usually taken after a *head injury* to look for a fracture (see *Skull, fractured*) or locate any foreign bodies in the soft tissues.

A normal skull X ray does not rule out significant brain injury. If such an injury is suspected, or if a skull fracture is found, *CT scanning* of the brain is also performed.

Skull X rays are also useful in evaluating a variety of conditions that affect the bones of the skull, such as *pituitary tumors* or metabolic disorders (such as *hyperparathyroidism*), and in evaluating tumors that have spread to the bones of the skull.

HOW IT IS DONE

A skull X-ray examination is a procedure performed by an *X-ray technician*. It is not uncomfortable and, depending on the number of views taken, takes about 20 minutes. The films are interpreted by a *radiologist*.

SLE

The abbreviation for the disorder systemic *lupus erythematosus*.

Sleep

The natural state of lowered consciousness and reduced *metabolism*. Sleep consumes about one third of an average person's life.

PHYSIOLOGY

EEG recordings of the electrical impulses produced by the brain during sleep show that there are two distinct types of sleep, known as REM (rapid eye movement) and NREM

S

(nonrapid eye movement) sleep. They alternate in cycles lasting roughly 90 minutes throughout the sleep period. NREM sleep, which accounts for the major part of sleep, starts with drowsiness; brain waves become increasingly deeper and slower until brain activity and metabolism fall to their lowest level. Dreams are infrequent.

In REM sleep, the brain suddenly becomes more electrically active (with a wave pattern resembling that of an awake person) and its temperature and blood flow increase. The eyes move rapidly and *dreaming*, often with elaborate story lines, occurs. REM sleep, also known as paradoxical sleep, periodically interrupts NREM sleep. The first REM period usually takes place 90 to 100 minutes after the onset of sleep and lasts about five to 10 minutes. REM sleep periods grow progressively longer as sleep continues; the last of a night's four or five REM sleep periods may last about an hour. REM sleep occupies about one half of sleep time in babies and about one fifth of sleep time in adults.

FUNCTIONS OF SLEEP

Sleep is a fundamental human need, as is shown by the detrimental effects of *sleep deprivation*. However, it is not understood exactly in what way sleep is beneficial, or why a few, extremely rare individuals sleep very little yet suffer no ill effects. Apart from the obvious theory that the brain and metabolic processes require periodic rest to function efficiently, it has been suggested that dreaming is necessary to enable the brain to sort out information gathered during waking hours.

SLEEP REQUIREMENTS

The need for sleep decreases with age. A 1-year-old baby requires about 14 hours of sleep a day, a child of 5 about 12 hours, and adults about seven to eight hours. These amounts can vary from person to person. Some adults need to sleep 10 hours or more a day, others function efficiently on half that amount or less. As people age, their ability to sustain sleep generally declines; the elderly get less sleep at night but doze more during the day than younger adults.

SLEEP DISORDERS

More than 100 disorders of sleeping and waking have been identified. They are divided into four main categories—problems with falling or staying asleep (the *insomnias*), problems with staying awake, problems with adhering to a consistent sleep/wake schedule, and problems with sleep-disruptive behaviors.

Problems with falling or staying asleep trouble one in three adults in the US. Insomnias are classified as transient—lasting up to several nights, usually resulting from excitement or minor stress; short-term—lasting up to two or three weeks, related to major stress or illness; and chronic—frequent or continued poor sleep, a complex disorder with many causes, including physical illnesses, psychological factors, a poor sleeping environment, and life-style. Insomnia is not a disease; it is a symptom warranting medical attention.

Problems with staying awake are the prime reason people seek help at sleep disorders centers, of which more than 200 now exist in the US. The primary causes of this symptom are *sleep apnea*, a potentially life-threatening disorder in which breathing intermittently stops during sleep, and *narcolepsy*, a disorder in which REM sleep intrudes into wakefulness, causing sudden daytime sleep "attacks."

Problems with a consistent sleep/wake schedule involve difficulty sleeping and difficulty staying awake as a result of disruptions of the internal clocks that regulate sleeping and waking. A common example is *jet lag*, in which body clocks are desynchronized by rapid travel across several time zones. Shift workers on rotating schedules, who frequently change their hours for work and sleep, commonly suffer "occupational jet lag." Shift workers, particularly those working at night, complain more about poor sleep and daytime drowsiness than do day workers.

Behaviors that interfere with sleep include *sleepwalking*, *night terrors* (partial awakening from sleep in a terrified state), and *enuresis* (bed-wetting).

SLEEP PATTERNS

The brain does not rest when a person is sleeping, but there is some reorganization of activity within it.

EEGs (electroencephalograms) and other recordings reveal cyclical patterns to this activity.

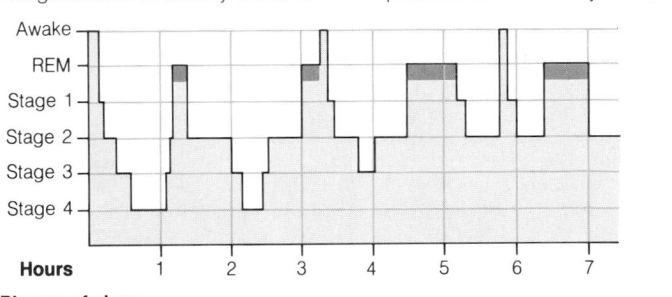

Key

■ REM sleep

□ NREM sleep

Phases of sleep

There are two types of sleep, REM (rapid eye movement) and NREM (nonrapid eye movement). They can be distinguished by the presence or absence of REMs and by EEGs or other recordings. The chart shows how a sleeper passes in cycles between the four stages of NREM sleep during the night, with bursts of REM sleep.

Awake

Stage 1

Stage 3

Stage 4

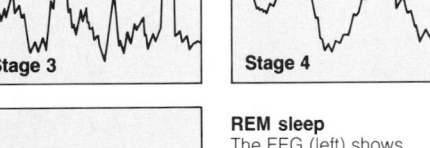

REM sleep

REM sleep

The EEG (left) shows high-frequency, low-voltage waves. People awakened during REM sleep often report dreams.

NREM sleep

This is sometimes called orthodox sleep; in adults it makes up about 80 percent of the sleeping pattern. It has four stages of progressively greater "depth" of sleep, characterized by EEG waves (left) of increasingly larger voltage (amplitude) and slower frequency (number of waves per second). People awakened during NREM sleep often report they were "thinking" about everyday matters but rarely report dreams.

S

Sleep apnea

Episodes of cessation of breathing, lasting 10 seconds or longer, during sleep. Failure to breathe triggers the brain to reinitiate breathing. The wakeful arousals are so brief that they generally go unremembered in the morning. Rather than complaining of restless nights, people with severe sleep apnea typically complain of excessive sleepiness during the day. The sleepiness may be so profound that it disrupts work and social life, causing sleep at inappropriate times and contributing to motor vehicle accidents. Difficulty with concentration and memory also may occur.

Severe sleep apnea may induce high blood pressure, heart failure, heart attack, and stroke.

INCIDENCE AND CAUSES

The most common and severe form of sleep apnea, obstructive sleep apnea, affects an estimated one in 100 men aged 30 to 50, most often overweight, heavy snorers. However, sleep apnea occurs in both sexes and all ages. It has been implicated in some cases of *sudden infant death syndrome* and becomes increasingly common with age.

In obstructive sleep apnea, the most frequent reason for difficulty is excessive relaxation during sleep of muscles of the soft palate at the base of the throat and the uvula (the small, conical, fleshy tissue hanging from the center of the soft palate). These sagging muscles obstruct the airway, making breathing labored and causing extremely loud snoring. If a complete blockage occurs, breathing stops and the sleeper falls silent. Pressure to breathe makes muscles of the diaphragm and chest work harder; opening of the blockage is signaled by a gasp and a brief arousal as breathing restarts. Obstructive sleep apnea may also be caused by enlarged tonsils and adenoids or individual anatomic differences such as a large tongue or small airway opening.

In another form of sleep apnea, central sleep apnea, the airway remains open but the diaphragm and chest muscles fail to work. Snoring may not occur. The fault is believed to lie in a disturbance in the brain's regulation of breathing during sleep.

People with sleep apnea commonly experience mixed apnea, in which a brief period of central apnea precedes a longer period of obstructive apnea. In mixed apnea, snoring is common.

TREATMENT

Weight reduction helps those who are overweight, as is the case in the majority of people with severe sleep apnea. Alcohol should not be consumed within two hours of bedtime and *sleeping drugs* generally should not be used; both drugs slow the activity of breathing muscles and may contribute to a worsening of the disorder.

An effective treatment developed in recent years, continuous positive airway pressure, involves wearing a mask over the nose and mouth during sleep. Air from an air compressor is forced through the mask into nasal passages and into the airway to keep it open. Supplemental oxygen and the drug protriptyline benefit some people. Surgical procedures helpful in some cases include removal of excess tissue at the back of the throat, removal of enlarged tonsils or adenoids, and creation of an opening in the windpipe (*tracheostomy*), which permits air to flow directly to the lungs during sleep, bypassing the obstructed upper airway.

Sleep deprivation

An insufficient amount of *sleep*. Studies of sleep-deprived volunteers have shown that irritability and a shortened attention span may occur after a night in which there was less than three hours' sleep.

After longer periods without sleep, individuals become increasingly unable to concentrate and their performance of tasks deteriorates as they continually slip into short periods of "microsleep." People with epilepsy are more prone to *seizures* after sleep deprivation. Three days or more without sleep may lead to visual and auditory *hallucinations* and, in some cases, *paranoia*.

Sleep deprivation has been employed in torture, to extract confessions, and as a brainwashing technique.

Sleeping drugs

COMMON DRUGS
Barbiturates
Secobarbital
Benzodiazepines
Flurazepam Temazepam Triazolam
Others
Chloral hydrate
Diphenhydramine
Glutethimide

A group of drugs used in the treatment of *insomnia*. Prescription sleeping drugs include *benzodiazepine drugs, barbiturate drugs, antihistamine drugs, antidepressant drugs,* and *chloral hydrate.* Certain antihistamines are sold as nonprescription sleep aids.

WHY THEY ARE USED

Sleeping drugs are given to reestablish the habit of sleeping after self-help measures (e.g., a warm bath or drinking hot milk at bedtime) have not worked and after causes of insomnia, such as breathing disorders or abnormal leg muscle activity, have been ruled out. These drugs promote sleep by reducing nerve cell activity within the brain.

HOW THEY ARE USED

Sleeping drugs always should be taken in the smallest effective dose for the shortest period of time. Generally, this means taking the drugs for no longer than three weeks and, preferably, not every night.

POSSIBLE ADVERSE EFFECTS

The morning after a sleeping drug has been taken, a hangover effect (drowsiness and unsteadiness) may occur. It may impair concentration and the ability to operate machinery.

A sleeping drug may be dangerous if the person awakens during the night and gets out of bed. This poses a special danger to elderly people, who are more prone to falls than others. Use of sleeping drugs may induce *tolerance* and *dependence*.

Sleeping drugs may interact dangerously with alcohol and adversely with other drugs, including those used in the treatment of duodenal ulcers, heart disease, and depression. No sleeping drugs have been determined as safe for use in pregnancy.

Sleeping sickness

A serious infectious disease of tropical Africa caused by the protozoan (single-celled) parasite *TRYPANOSOMA BRUCEI.* Sleeping sickness is spread by the bites of tsetse flies, which transmit the protozoa to people and animals. Within humans, the parasites multiply and spread to the bloodstream, lymph nodes, heart, and, eventually, the brain.

There are two forms of sleeping sickness. One, occurring in West and Central Africa, is spread primarily from person to person. The other occurs in East Africa and mainly affects wild animals, but is occasionally transmitted to humans.

Sleeping sickness is controlled by eradication measures directed against the tsetse fly. Nevertheless, tens of thousands of Africans—and some visitors to safari parks—still contract the disease each year.

S

SYMPTOMS AND SIGNS

With both forms of sleeping sickness, a painful nodule develops at the site of the tsetse fly bite. In the West African form, the disease then takes a slow course, with bouts of fever and lymph gland enlargement. After months or years, spread to the brain occurs, causing headaches, confusion, and, eventually, severe lassitude. The victim may become completely inactive, have drooping eyelids, and a vacant expression (hence, sleeping sickness). Without treatment, coma and death follow. The East African form runs a faster course. A severe fever develops within a few weeks of infection; effects on the heart may be fatal before the disease has spread to the brain.

DIAGNOSIS, TREATMENT, AND PREVENTION

Microscopic examination of the blood, lymph fluid withdrawn from a lymph gland, or cerebrospinal fluid obtained by a *lumbar puncture* reveals the presence of the parasites.

Drugs are effective against the parasites but may cause severe side effects. In most cases, a complete cure can be achieved, although there may be residual brain damage if the infection has already spread to the brain.

To avoid sleeping sickness, visitors to rural parts of Africa should take measures to protect themselves against tsetse fly bites (see *Insect bites*).

Sleep paralysis

The sensation of being unable to move at the moment of going to sleep or when waking up. The experience may be accompanied by *hallucinations*, which often are frightening. Sleep paralysis most often occurs in people with *narcolepsy*, but occasionally it affects otherwise healthy people. Although alarming, the sensation rarely lasts for more than a few seconds. (See also *Cataplexy*.)

Sleep terror

See *Night terror*.

Sleepwalking

Walking while sleeping. Sleepwalking, also known as somnambulism, occurs during NREM (nonrapid eye movement) *sleep* and does not represent the acting out of dreams. It affects perhaps 5 percent of adults; probably 75 percent of children, especially boys, walk in their sleep at least once. Some people show a regular tendency to sleepwalk.

Usually the child calmly gets out of bed, wanders around aimlessly for a few minutes, and then goes back to

CYCLE OF SLEEPING SICKNESS

The life cycle of the trypanosomes that cause sleeping sickness is shown. They multiply in a person's blood and lymph vessels and may spread to the brain or heart with serious effects.

Trypanosomes
The parasites are shown here in blood.

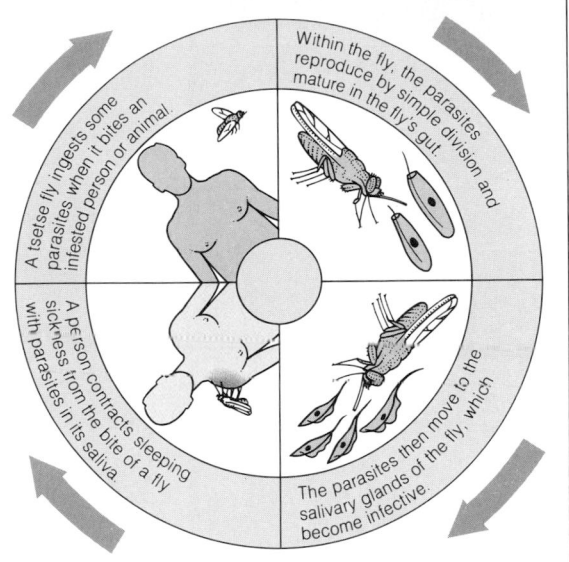

A tsetse fly ingests some parasites when it bites an infested person or animal.

Within the fly, the parasites reproduce by simple division and mature in the fly's gut.

The parasites then move to the salivary glands of the fly, which become infective.

A person contracts sleeping sickness from the bite of a fly with parasites in its saliva

bed. Sometimes sleepwalking arises from a *night terror*, in which case the child's behavior is more frantic and may involve shrieking or thrashing. The child sometimes talks (usually simple words or phrases) during the sleepwalk or urinates in an inappropriate place and may get into the wrong bed. Waking the child is difficult and unnecessary; steer him or her gently back to bed. Take precautions, such as blocking off the stairs, to avoid injury.

Sleepwalking in children is seldom associated with psychological problems; although it may be aggravated by anxiety, it tends to disappear naturally with age. Sleepwalking in adults may be related to anxiety. It may be associated with sleeping pill use, especially in the elderly.

Sling

A device used to immobilize, support, or elevate an upper limb. A sling is usually made from a triangular *bandage*, although an emergency sling can be created from a belt, tie, or scarf.

An arm sling may be used as a first-aid measure to support the arm following a fracture, sprain, or other injury (see illustrated box overleaf). It may also be used to provide relief during infection or after an operation on the hand or arm.

An elevation sling is used in first aid to hold the hand in a well-raised position to control bleeding or to prevent movement of the arm and shoulder if the clavicle (collarbone) is broken.

This type of sling is applied in a similar fashion to an arm sling, except the victim's arm is placed across the chest with the fingers nearly touching the opposite shoulder.

Slipped disk

See *Disk prolapse*.

Slipped femoral epiphysis

See *Femoral epiphysis, slipped*.

Slit lamp

An illuminated microscope used to examine the internal structures of the front part of the eye. When special contact lenses are applied, the slit lamp may be used to examine the retina. (See also *Eye, examination of*.)

Slough

Dead tissue that has been shed from its original site. Examples of sloughing include the loss of dead skin cells from the skin's surface and the shedding of the lining of the uterus during menstruation. Sloughing also occurs as part of the healing process of wounds and ulcers.

Slow virus diseases

A group of diseases of the central nervous system (brain and spinal cord) that occurs many months or years after infection with a virus. The diseases take a slow course in which there is gradual widespread destruction of nerve tissue. This causes progressive loss of brain function and, at present, a fatal outcome.

FIRST AID: ARM SLING

1 If there is no triangular bandage available, improvise with a folded scarf or use a strong piece of fabric such as linen.

2 Ease the bandage into position, leaving the point protruding beyond the elbow. Take the top end around the neck and let the other end hang.

3 Bring the other end up to the neck and tie the ends using a square knot on the injured side. The knot should sit in the hollow above the collarbone.

4 Tuck the surplus bandage behind the elbow and bring the point forward, securing it with a pin.

The group of slow virus diseases includes *Creutzfeldt-Jakob syndrome*, *kuru*, possibly one form of *Alzheimer's disease*, subacute sclerosing panencephalitis (a very rare complication of measles), and possibly the brain disease that occurs in some people infected with the *AIDS* virus.

Small-cell carcinoma

The most dangerous and rapidly spreading form of lung cancer. Also called oat-cell carcinoma, this type of tumor accounts for about 25 percent of lung cancers. Most small-cell carcinomas reach an inoperable stage by the time a diagnosis is made. Life extension from surgery is achieved in about 10 percent of cases, but, even in these cases, the outlook is poor. Spread to other parts of the body is almost inevitable.

Treatment is usually with *anticancer drugs* with or without *radiation therapy*.

Because this treatment must be given in very high doses, bone marrow transplants are being tried.

Smallpox

A highly infectious viral disease, common in the nineteenth century and before, with the distinction of having been totally eradicated by a successful worldwide vaccination campaign. The World Health Organization declared smallpox extinct in 1980.

Smallpox was transmitted from person to person; it was characterized by an illness resembling influenza and a rash that spread over the body and eventually developed into pus-filled blisters. The blisters became crusted and would sometimes leave deeply pitted scars. Complications included blindness, pneumonia, and kidney damage. There was no effective treatment for the disease, which killed up to 40 percent of its victims.

Eradication was achieved through the cooperative international use of a highly effective vaccine. Eradication was possible because smallpox affected only humans, cases of infection were easily recognized, and victims of the disease were infectious to others only for a short time. These characteristics are shared by some other diseases (e.g., measles, another possible candidate for eradication).

Smallpox vaccination certificates are no longer required for travel abroad, and most countries have discontinued vaccination because the risk of the disease is zero and because there is a risk of encephalitis from the vaccine. The virus responsible for smallpox is still maintained at laboratories at the Centers for Disease Control in Atlanta and at a research institute in Moscow.

Smear

A specimen for microscopic examination prepared by spreading a thin film of the cells to be examined onto a glass slide. Common examples are a *blood smear* and a *cervical smear test*.

Smegma

An accumulation of sebaceous gland secretions beneath the foreskin in an uncircumcised male, usually as a result of poor hygiene.

Fungal or bacterial infection of smegma may cause *balanitis* (inflammation of the glans). In a child with *phimosis* (tight foreskin), smegma occasionally hardens into a small stone, known as a smegma pearl. The higher incidence of cancer of the penis in uncircumcised men who smoke may be due to the buildup of cancer-inducing substances in the smegma.

An uncircumcised man should regularly wash his penis with the foreskin retracted to prevent a buildup of smegma.

Smell

One of the five senses. The mechanisms by which smell is perceived are shown in the illustrated box opposite.
DISORDERS
Disturbance of the sense of smell may consist of anosmia (loss of the sense of smell, which may be complete or partial, temporary or permanent) or dysosmia (abnormal smell perception). Because the senses of smell and taste are so closely connected, disturbances of smell usually result in disturbances of taste.

Temporary partial anosmia frequently results from conditions in which the nasal mucous membrane becomes inflamed, such as the common *cold*, *influenza*, and several forms of *rhinitis*, notably allergic rhinitis (hay fever). Cigarette smoking also commonly causes anosmia. In hypertrophic rhinitis, the mucous membrane thickens, burying and sometimes distorting the olfactory nerve endings, which may cause permanent anosmia unless the condition is treated. In atrophic rhinitis, the nerve endings waste away, causing some degree of permanent anosmia; there is also a foul-smelling discharge that may overpower other odors.

The olfactory nerves can be torn in a head injury. If both nerves are torn, complete, permanent anosmia results; during recovery from less severe damage, dysosmia, in the form of illusory bad smells, may occur.

Rarely, anosmia is caused by a *meningioma* (tumor of the meninges, the membranes that surround the brain) or a tumor behind the nose (see *Nasopharynx, cancer of*).

Dysosmia, in the form of illusory, unpleasant odors, may occur as a feature of various psychological disorders, such as *depression* or *schizophrenia*. It may also occur in some forms of *epilepsy* and during "drying out" periods in severe *alcohol dependence*. A person with dysosmia may believe the source of the smell is his or her body and, despite reassurance to the contrary, may wash excessively and tend to avoid others.

Smelling salts

A preparation of *ammonia* that causes a person to withdraw from the pungent substance. Smelling salts were once used to prevent fainting or to revive a person who had fainted.

THE SENSE OF SMELL

The smell receptors are specialized nerve cell endings situated in a small patch of mucous membrane lining the roof of the nose. The axons (fibers) of these sensory cells pass up through tiny perforations in the overlying bone to enter the two elongated olfactory bulbs lying on top of the bone. These bulbs are swellings at the ends of the olfactory nerves; the nerves contain millions of nerve fibers and enter the brain on its lower surface. The olfactory nerves carry sensory information to smell centers situated within the brain.

Smell centers
The centers in the brain concerned with smell include parts of the limbic system and frontal lobes.

Olfactory bulbs
Here, the receptor cell fibers are linked to the nerves that run into the brain.

Nasal cavity
In the nose, hairlike projections from the smell receptor cells lie in the mucous membrane layer.

Olfactory nerve

Olfactory bulb

Limbic system

Nerve pathway

Frontal lobe

Olfactory bulb

Nasal hairs

Olfactory bulb

Axon

Lamina cribrosa

Receptor cell

Supporting cell

Cilia

Cilia

Receptor sites

Layer of mucus

Odor molecules

Ether

Garlic

Bleach

Physiological basis of smell
The receptor cell bodies are swollen at their lower ends; each one gives off several cilia that extend down to the surface of the mucous membrane. The cilia contain the receptor sites at which stimulation by the molecules of odorous substances gives rise to nerve impulses passing up to the brain. We know that we are able to distinguish several thousand different odors, but the exact basis of this high degree of specificity is uncertain. No microscopic difference can be detected among different receptors.

Probable mechanism
The smell process probably is based on a physical "fit" between the odor molecules and the receptor sites. For example, the receptors on some cells may fit only with ether molecules, others with molecules of bleach.

The molecules must dissolve in the mucus before they can stimulate the receptors. The sensitivity of the system is remarkable; as few as four molecules can give a recognizable smell.

S

VENOMOUS SNAKES IN THE US

The distribution of eight of the more dangerous or commonly biting poisonous snakes in the US is shown below. Apart from the eastern coral snake, all are pit vipers. These snakes have stout bodies, broad heads, retractable front fangs, slitlike eyes, and are 2 to 8 feet in length. Heat-sensitive pits between the eyes and nostrils help them locate warmblooded prey in the dark.

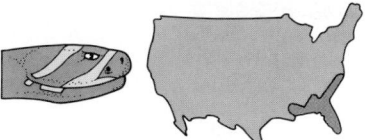

Eastern diamondback rattlesnake
A brown snake, up to 8 feet long, with a diamond pattern on its body. Like all rattlesnakes, it has a rattle on its tail.

Prairie rattlesnake
This rattler, found in the Great Plains, is greenish-gray to brown in color, and 3 to 4 feet long.

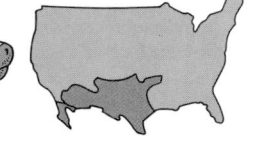

Western diamondback rattlesnake
Similar to the eastern species, but often reddish in color with less distinct diamonds. Widespread in dry habitats.

Water moccasin (cottonmouth)
This snake lives in or near water. When alarmed, its mouth opens to show a white interior. It has no tail rattle.

Timber rattlesnake
This snake lives in forests, swamps, and rocky hillsides. It has a pale brown body with black bands and a black tail.

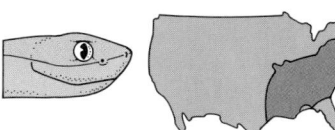

Copperhead
This species has a russet-colored body with dark bands and a yellowish top to its head. It vibrates its tail when angry.

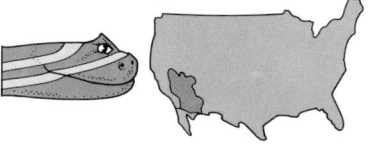

Sidewinder rattlesnake
This smaller, desert-living snake has a pale brown body and distinctive hornlike "eyelash" scales above the eyes.

Eastern coral snake
This snake is up to 4 feet long and slender, with a yellow-black-yellow-red recurring ring pattern.

AVOIDING SNAKEBITES
Anyone working, camping, or walking in areas known to be inhabited by venomous snakes should take these precautions:

- Wear long pants and boots
- Keep to cleared tracks when hiking through the brush
- If moving large rocks or logs, use a stick
- Never sleep on the ground
- Never disturb a snake or try to kill one. Move quietly away
- Burn garbage, which attracts rodents, which in turn attract snakes

Smoking
See *Tobacco smoking*.

Snails and disease

Snails act as host to various types of parasitic flukes (flattened, wormlike animals), which, at different stages in their life cycles, infest people. The flukes include *liver flukes* and the parasites responsible for *schistosomiasis* and various other tropical diseases. Control of snail populations can be important in combating these diseases. There is no risk to eating thoroughly cooked snails anywhere in the world.

Snakebites

Every year, hundreds of thousands of people worldwide are bitten by snakes. However, the chance of death or even serious injury occurring from a bite is relatively small. The majority of bites are by non-poisonous species; in only a proportion of bites by poisonous snakes is venom actually injected. Furthermore, modern medical treatment is effective in treating most serious cases, provided the victim is transported to the hospital quickly. It takes hours or days, not minutes or seconds, for even the most powerful snake venom to kill.

Venomous snakes are found throughout North America, except in Maine, Alaska, and northern Canada. In the US each year, about 45,000 people are bitten by snakes, including 1,500 by poisonous species. The number of deaths annually is less than 20.

VENOMOUS AND NONVENOMOUS SPECIES
Three quarters of the 3,000 types of snakes worldwide belong to the colubrid family. They have slender, tapered bodies and are mostly non-venomous. Most North American snakes are harmless colubrids.

In the US, most venomous bites are caused by pit vipers, which are widespread. The pit vipers, which belong to the crotalid family, include the copperhead, water moccasin (cottonmouth), and about 30 different species of rattlesnake. Rattlesnakes carry a horny rattle on the tail that they vibrate when disturbed. If disturbed, any pit viper is likely to bite, striking quickly and withdrawing at once.

The only other venomous snake in the US is the coral snake. It belongs to a group of snakes called the elapids, which have slender, tapering bodies, narrow heads, round eyes, and small

S

nonretractable fangs. Other members of the group are the cobras, kraits, and mambas of Africa and Asia. Coral snakes are about 4 feet (1.2 m) long, and decorated with black and brightly colored bands. Their colors are mimicked by other, nonvenomous, species, but the coral snakes have red bands bordered by yellow or white; the mimic snakes have red bands bordered by black.

Other venomous snakes include the true vipers, which are not found in North America, and sea snakes, which rarely bite humans.

EFFECTS OF A BITE

The effects of a venomous bite vary considerably and depend on the species of snake, its size, the amount of venom injected, and the age and health of the victim.

Rattlesnakes and other pit vipers make two distinct puncture wounds in the skin. There is an immediate burning pain at the site of the wound and swelling of the bitten limb. Over the next 20 minutes the pain increases in severity and the victim becomes dizzy, nauseated, pale, and sweaty. Blood pressure falls and there is an increase in heart rate. Thirst, headache, and a pins and needles sensation are other common symptoms.

The venom may prevent the blood from clotting, causing bleeding from the fang wounds and bruises beneath the skin. There may also be bleeding into the urine or from the mouth, rectum, or vagina. Internal bleeding further lowers the blood pressure. There is also widespread tissue destruction around the wound.

Coral snakes and other elapids typically make two small puncture wounds with their fangs; they may also chew the skin, producing several wounds. A bite from a coral snake usually causes little pain or swelling. The venom primarily affects the nervous system. Serious symptoms develop from 10 minutes to eight hours after the bite and may include drooping eyelids, slurred speech, and double vision. The victim becomes drowsy or delirious and may have convulsions. Eventually, if treatment is not given, respiratory paralysis causes death.

TREATMENT

Any person accompanying a victim of a snakebite should administer first aid (see box) and then obtain medical help. Antibiotics and injections of tetanus antitoxin are given for all bites, whether venomous or not, to prevent bacterial infection or tetanus.

FIRST AID: SNAKEBITE

DO NOT
- let the victim move
- raise the injured limb; this allows the venom to spread
- cut into the bite or attempt to cauterize it

1 Let the victim rest in a comfortable position and offer reassurance.

2 Apply a pad or sterile dressing to the wound and immobilize the limb.

3 Bandage the wound firmly. Summon medical help, but do not leave the victim alone.

For a severe venomous bite, the victim is given a highly effective injection of *antivenin* (a serum containing antibodies against the poison). In the US, one antivenin is available to treat a bite by any pit viper and another is available for coral snakebites.

In the most severe cases, kidney *dialysis* to treat *renal failure* or artificial *ventilation* to overcome respiratory paralysis may be required.

Modern treatment of venomous snakebites is so advanced that almost all victims who receive prompt medical care survive and do so with minimal aftereffects.

Sneezing

The involuntary, convulsive expulsion of air through the nose and mouth as a result of irritation of the upper respiratory tract. The irritation may be caused by inflammation of the tract, which occurs in the common *cold*, *influenza*, and allergic *rhinitis* (hay fever); by mucus; or by inhaling an irritant (e.g., dust or pepper).

Snellen's chart

A standard method of measuring *visual acuity* used during *vision tests*. Snellen's chart, bearing rows of letters of standard, decreasing size, is set at a distance of 20 feet (6 m) from the patient. One eye is covered and the patient is asked to read as far down the chart as possible. The procedure is repeated with the other eye.

Normal vision (20/20 vision) requires that all the letters in a line near the bottom of the chart be read correctly. If the person being tested can read only the letters twice as large as those on the 20/20 line (which a normal eye would be able to read at 40 feet), the acuity is said to be 20/40.

S

Snoring

Noisy breathing through the open mouth during sleep, produced by vibrations of the soft palate. Snoring is usually caused by any condition that hinders breathing through the nose, such as a common *cold*, allergic *rhinitis*, or enlarged *adenoids*. It is more common while sleeping on the back, when the lower jaw tends to drop open. In some people who snore because of upper airway obstruction, snoring alternates with *sleep apnea* (temporary cessation of breathing).

A sometimes effective way to prevent snoring is to sew an object into the pajama top near the small of the back, thus making it uncomfortable to sleep on the back.

Snuff

A preparation of powdered tobacco (often with other substances) for inhalation into the nose; it is also made into a wad for chewing. Snuff is irritating to the nasal lining, which may waste as a result of prolonged snuff inhalation. Also, because it contains *nicotine*, snuff is addictive.

The increased use in North America and northern Europe of "smokeless" tobacco has provoked interest in its carcinogenic (cancer-causing) effects. Chewing tobacco and snuff are carcinogens. There is a direct proportion between the amount used, the period over which it is used, and the likelihood of cancer. Carcinogens are also present in betel nut and in pan (which is a combination of betel nut, lime, and tobacco).

Among practicing Mormons (who use neither tobacco nor alcohol), *squamous cell carcinomas* of the head and neck are uncommon. In contrast, the majority of people with head and neck cancers have a history of heavy alcohol and tobacco use.

Cultural differences in the way tobacco is used have led to great variation in the location of cancers, in accordance with the principle that increased exposure to heavy concentrates of tobacco carcinogens results in an increased risk of tumor development in the tissue exposed.

A striking example of this has been observed among the women of a certain area of India, where carcinoma of the hard palate (roof of the mouth), which is rare in the rest of the world, has a high incidence. It is correlated with the local custom of reverse chutta smoking, in which the lit end of a slow-burning cigarette is held in the mouth and seldom removed.

Similarly, about one half of all cancer in Bombay, India, is cancer of the buccal mucosa (cheek pouch), which is associated with the custom of chewing pan. Pan is held in the user's cheek throughout the day and sometimes kept in place during sleep. The majority of tumors develop in the place in the mouth where the pan is stored. The practice of dipping snuff among the women of North Carolina has been shown to increase the risk of cancers of the cheek and gum 50 times more than the population at large.

Sociopathy

An outdated term for *antisocial personality disorder*.

Sodium

A mineral that, along with potassium and other substances, regulates the body's water balance, maintains normal heart rhythm, and is responsible for the conduction of nerve impulses and the contraction of muscles.

The body of an average-sized person contains about 2 ounces (55 grams) of sodium. The level of sodium in the blood is controlled by the kidneys, which eliminate any excess of the mineral in the urine.

Almost all foods contain sodium naturally or as an ingredient added during processing or cooking. The principal forms of sodium in food are sodium chloride (table salt) and sodium bicarbonate (baking soda). Apart from table salt, the main dietary sources of sodium are processed foods, cheese, breads and cereals, and smoked, pickled, or cured meats and fish. Pickles and snack foods contain large amounts; sodium is also present in water treated with water softeners.

DEFICIENCY AND EXCESS

Because most foods contain sodium, deficiency is very rare. In fact, most Western diets contain too much sodium. While many nutritionists suggest a daily intake of only 0.04 to 0.1 ounces (1 to 3 grams), the average consumption is 0.1 to 0.25 ounces (3 to 7 grams) per day. There is no official recommended daily allowance.

Sodium deficiency is usually the result of excessive loss of the mineral through prolonged or excessive treatment with *diuretic drugs*. It may also be caused by persistent diarrhea or vomiting or by profuse sweating. Rarely, deficiency is due to *cystic fibrosis*, underactivity of the adrenal glands, or certain kidney disorders. Symptoms of deficiency include tiredness, weakness, muscle cramps, and

dizziness. In severe cases, there may be a drop in blood pressure, leading to confusion, fainting, and palpitations. Treatment consists of taking sodium supplements. In very hot conditions, supplements may also help prevent exhaustion that occurs as a result of sodium loss from excessive sweating.

Excessive sodium intake is thought to be a contributory factor in the high incidence of *hypertension* (high blood pressure) in Western countries. In people whose blood pressure is already raised, excessive sodium may increase the risk of heart disease, *stroke*, and kidney damage. Another adverse effect is fluid retention, which, in severe cases, may cause dizziness and swelling of the legs.

Sodium bicarbonate

An over-the-counter *antacid drug* used to relieve *indigestion*, *heartburn*, and pain caused by a *peptic ulcer*.

Sodium bicarbonate often causes belching and abdominal discomfort. Long-term use may cause swollen ankles, muscle cramps, tiredness, weakness, nausea, and vomiting. Sodium bicarbonate should not be taken by people with *heart failure* or a history of kidney disease.

Sodium salicylate

An *analgesic drug* used to relieve minor musculoskeletal pain and reduce inflammation.

Soft-tissue injury

Damage to one or more of the tissues that surround bones and joints (e.g., to a *ligament*, *tendon*, or *muscle*). Soft-tissue injuries include ligament *sprain*, *tendinitis* (inflammation of a tendon), and muscle tears (see *Strain*). See also *Sports injuries*.

Soiling

The accidental passing of soft, unformed feces into the clothes after the age at which bowel control is usually achieved (about age 3 or 4). More than half the children with this problem also wet the bed (see *Enuresis*). Soiling is distinct from *encopresis* (the deliberate passing of normal feces in inappropriate places).

Causes of soiling include slowness in developing bowel control, longstanding *constipation* (in which fecal liquid leaks around hard feces blocking the large intestine), poor *toilet-training*, and psychological stress (such as starting school). Soiling is usually distressing to the child, who may hide the messy clothes.

S

Soiling due to constipation usually responds to treatment. If there is no physical cause, it may pass after a discussion involving the child, the parents, and the physician; if not, *psychotherapy* may be used.

Solar plexus

The largest autonomic *plexus* (nerve network) in the body (see *Autonomic nervous system*). Also known as the celiac plexus, the solar plexus is situated behind the stomach, where it surrounds the celiac artery and lies between the adrenal glands. The solar plexus incorporates the greater and lesser splanchnic nerves (part of the sympathetic nervous system) and branches of the *vagus nerve*, the most important component of the parasympathetic nervous system. The solar plexus sends out branches to the stomach, intestines, and most other abdominal organs.

Solvent abuse

The practice of inhaling the intoxicating fumes given off by certain volatile liquids. Glue sniffing is the most common form of solvent abuse, but many other substances are used, especially those containing toluene or acetone. The usual method of inhalation is from a plastic bag containing the solvent, but sometimes aerosols are sprayed into the nose or mouth.

INCIDENCE

Solvent abuse is common among boys in poor urban areas. It is usually a group activity that is indulged in for no more than a few months. Solitary abuse over a longer period is frequently associated with a disturbed family background and delinquency.

EFFECTS

Inhaling solvent fumes produces an effect similar to that of becoming drunk or getting high on drugs, sometimes including hallucinations. If carried on for any length of time, it can bring about headache, vomiting, stupor, confusion, and coma. Occasionally, death occurs as the result of a direct toxic effect on the heart, a fall, choking on vomit, or asphyxiation due to a clinging plastic bag.

Long-term harmful effects include erosion of the membrane lining the nose and throat and damage to the kidneys, liver, and nervous system.

DIAGNOSIS AND TREATMENT

The signs of solvent abuse include intoxicated behavior, a flushed face, ulcers around the mouth, a smell of solvent, and personality changes, such as moodiness and nervousness.

Solvent abusers should be warned of the serious risks to health. Professional counseling may be needed. Acute symptoms resulting from solvent abuse, such as vomiting or coma, require urgent medical attention.

Somatic

A term that means related to the body (soma), as opposed to the mind (psyche), or related to body cells, as opposed to germ cells (eggs and sperm). The term somatic also refers to the body wall, in contrast to the viscera (internal organs).

Somatization disorder

A condition in which the individual complains over several years of various physical problems for which no physical cause can be found. The disorder, previously classified as *hysteria*, usually begins before age 30 and leads to numerous tests by many physicians. Unnecessary surgery and other treatments often result.

This disorder may be slightly more prevalent in women, many of whom have a family history of *antisocial personality disorder* in male relatives. Symptoms most commonly complained of are neurological (e.g., double vision, seizures, weakness), gynecological (painful menstruation, pain on intercourse), and gastrointestinal (abdominal pain, nausea). Associated features may include *anxiety* and *depression*, threats of *suicide*, and various forms of substance abuse.

These physical symptoms are caused by underlying emotional conflicts, anxiety, and depression that the person is unable to confront and which are unconsciously displaced onto the body. It is thought that it is easier for the person to view the problem as physical than face the emotional conflicts from which he or she is trying to escape. (See also *Conversion disorder*; *Hypochondriasis*.)

Somatoform disorders

A group of conditions in which there are physical symptoms for which no physical cause can be found, and for which there is definite or strong evidence that the underlying cause is psychological. Somatoform disorders include *conversion disorder*, *hypochondriasis*, and *somatization disorder*.

Somatotype

The physical build of an individual. A variety of attempts have been made to classify people according to body type and to identify corresponding personality traits.

In the 1920s, the German psychiatrist Ernst Kretschmer divided people into three types, each of which he

---

BODY TYPES AND PERSONALITY

The idea that the features of the psyche (mind) are related to those of the soma (body) is not always borne out in practice. Even so, there is a very general relationship between the two.

Endomorph
Tends to be sociable, easygoing, pleasure-loving, relaxed, and convivial.

Mesomorph
Is often physically active, strong, athletic, ready for action, and aggressive.

Ectomorph
Is more sensitive, self-conscious, restrained, introspective, and quiet.

S

thought was more prone to certain types of mental illness—asthenic (thin) types seemed more likely to have a schizoid personality or schizophrenia; pyknic (stocky) types were more prone to manic-depressive illness; athletic (muscular) types were not associated with any single disorder, but there was more delinquency within this group.

An American psychologist, working in the 1940s, believed that people did not fit into rigid categories of body type. Instead he identified three structural tendencies (each associated with certain personality traits), which everyone had in different proportions. They were ectomorphic—a tall, thin physique, with light bones and muscles, linked with a restrained, self-conscious personality; endomorphic—a heavy physique, with poorly developed bones and muscles, associated with a sociable, loving personality; and mesomorphic—strong, well-developed bones and muscles, paired with a physical, adventurous personality.

Somatrem

A preparation of human *growth hormone*. Somatrem is given to children to treat *short stature* caused by growth hormone deficiency. A year's treatment with somatrem costs between $10,000 and $20,000.

Somnambulism

See *Sleepwalking*.

Sore

A term used to describe an ulcer, septic wound, or any disrupted area of the skin or mucous membranes. The word is also used to describe an area that is tender or painful.

Sore throat

A rough or raw feeling in the back of the throat that causes discomfort, especially when swallowing.

Sore throat is an extremely common symptom that is usually caused by *pharyngitis*, and occasionally by *tonsillitis*. It may also be the first symptom of the common *cold*, *influenza*, *laryngitis*, infectious *mononucleosis*, and many common childhood viral illnesses, including *chickenpox*, *measles*, and *mumps*.

A *streptococcal infection* produced by the beta-hemolytic streptococcus produces a sore throat that must be diagnosed. Left untreated, this type of sore throat may result in acute *glomerulonephritis* or *rheumatic fever*.

Treatment consists of gargling with salt water or, for adults, taking aspirin. If a sore throat persists for more than 48 hours or a *rash* develops, a physician should be consulted. (See also *Strep throat*.)

Space medicine

A minor medical specialty concerned with the physiological and pathological effects of spaceflight.

During lift-off, there is a large upward acceleration that makes the astronaut feel many times heavier. There is also a tendency for blood to pool downward. To prevent loss of consciousness as a result of blood draining from the brain, the astronaut must lie in a reclining seat and wear a special suit that exerts pressure on certain parts of the body (such as the limbs) and helps redistribute the flow of blood toward the head.

Once in orbit, the effects of gravity (which pulls spacecraft and astronaut toward Earth) and velocity (which is vertically opposed to this pull) combine to make the astronaut feel weightless. One effect of weightlessness is on the body's balance mechanisms. The brain may be unable to make sense of the lack of signals from the balance organ in the inner ear; one manifestation is *motion sickness*.

Changes also occur in the cardiovascular system (heart and blood vessels) because, in the absence of weight, body fluids are redistributed toward the head. Other effects may include loss of bone and muscle tissue. Such effects could ultimately limit space travel, unless a means can be found to recreate weight within spacecraft. (See also *Aviation medicine*.)

Spasm

An involuntary, often powerful, muscle contraction. A spasm may affect one or more muscles and may occur once or more; pain is not necessarily an accompanying feature.

Examples include *hiccups* (in which the diaphragm goes into spasm), muscle cramps (which often affect the muscles in the calves), and *tics* (which frequently affect facial muscles).

Less commonly, a spasm may be the result of an abnormality in the central nervous system or a symptom of a muscle disorder. Spasms caused by disease of the nervous system include *myoclonus* and *chorea*. Conditions characterized by spasm include *trigeminal neuralgia* (which affects the muscles of the face and head), *tetany* (spasm caused by a drop of the

calcium level in the blood), and *tetanus* (an infectious disease). Rare causes of widespread spasm are *rabies*, *strychnine poisoning*, and the bite of the black widow spider.

Other types of muscle spasm include *bronchospasm* (contraction of muscles in the small airways of the lungs), which occurs in asthma, and vasospasm (tightening of the muscles in the blood vessels).

Spasticity

Increased rigidity in a group of muscles, causing stiffness and restriction of movement. Spasticity can occur with or without *paralysis* or muscle weakness. *Cerebral palsy* causes spasticity and paralysis; *Parkinson's disease* and *multiple sclerosis* may cause spasticity without paralysis. *Tetanus* causes spasticity, initially of the muscles in the face and neck (lockjaw) and then of other body muscles.

Spastic paralysis

The inability to move a part of the body accompanied by rigidity of the muscles; the immobilized parts are frozen in one position. Causes of spastic paralysis include *stroke*, *cerebral palsy*, and *multiple sclerosis*. (See also *Paralysis*.)

Spatulate

Shaped like a spatula (i.e., with a broad, blunt, flattened, spoonlike end). Spatulate fingers are normal and do not indicate disease.

Specialist

A physician with advanced training and knowledge in a particular branch of medicine or surgery. A nephrologist is a specialist in the function and disorders of the kidneys. (See also individual entries, e.g., *Cardiologist*; *Gastroenterologist*; *Pediatrician*.)

Specific gravity

Also called relative density, the ratio of the *density* of a substance to that of water. Materials with a relative density of less than 1 are less dense ("lighter") than water; those with a relative density of more than 1 are denser ("heavier") than water. The specific gravity of urine shows if it has a large amount of material dissolved in it (near 1.030) or if it is almost water (near 1.010).

Specimen

A sample of tissue, body fluids (such as blood), waste products (such as urine), or an infective organism taken

S

for the purpose of examination, identification, analysis, and/or diagnosis. The term is also applied to a sample of a tissue or organism specially prepared for examination under a *microscope*. (See also *Blood tests*; *Urinalysis*.)

SPECT

The abbreviation for single photon emission computerized tomography, a type of *radionuclide scanning*.

Spectacles

See *Glasses*.

Speculum

A device designed to hold open a body orifice (opening), enabling a physician to perform an examination. A speculum is made of plastic or metal.

TYPES

There are many types of speculum designed for use on different parts of the body. The speculum used to examine the eardrum is funnel-shaped, with a narrow end inserted into the ear canal and a wide end attached to an *otoscope*. The speculum used to hold open the walls of the vagina during a pelvic examination may be shaped either like a duck's bill, with wide, smooth, curved edges and a self-retaining lock to hold them in position, or like a shoehorn bent at both ends at an angle of 90 degrees.

Speech

The most frequently used method of human communication.

LANGUAGE AND SPEECH

The terms "speech" and "language" are often used interchangeably, but have different meanings. Language is the representation of objects and ideas by strings of symbols, which form words. These symbols may be speech sounds, written characters, or hand signals. There are two main facets of language ability—understanding the meaning of words (comprehension) and generating words, in grammatical order, to express something meaningful (expression).

Speech is just one method by which language can be communicated to others. Writing and hand signals are others. Each method relies on sequences of muscle movements. Speech involves the muscles used in breathing, the larynx, tongue, palate, lips, jaw, and face.

LANGUAGE CENTERS

Language comprehension and expression take place in two areas of the cerebral cortex (the outer layer of the cerebrum and main mass of the brain)

LANGUAGE AND SPEECH DEVELOPMENT IN CHILDHOOD

3 months	Period of babbling begins. The child produces strings of sounds for pleasure. Babbling is important in building movement sequences, which will be used	later to produce meaningful speech sounds.
9 months	Child echoes the speech of others, but words are not yet used with meaning. By listening to and copying adults, the child learns that clusters of sounds	refer to specific objects, people, or situations.
12 to 18 months	The child begins to utter simple words with meaning, often accompanied by gestures. Examples are "bye-bye," "dog," "hot," and "daddy." Only single	words are used, with vocabulary gradually increasing from two or three words initially.
18 to 24 months	The child begins to combine concepts to form two-word sentences (e.g., "Hello John" or "That hot!"). By age 2, the child	may be using 100 or more different words.
2 to 3 years	The child's sentences expand in length (e.g., "I like cake" or "Peter hit Mary"). He or she begins to incorporate adjectives and adverbs into sentences (e.g., "That's daddy's old coat" or "I want lunch now"). By 3	years, average sentence length is four words. Most sounds have developed, with "th," "r," "j," "ch," and "sh" possible exceptions.
3 years and up	More elaborate sentences with several nouns, verbs in past and future tenses, and linked phrases begin to be used—for example "We went to Amy's and we had milk and cookies" or "I think mommy went downstairs."	However, mistakes are often made, such as "What did you played?", reflecting the child's linguistic immaturity. Language skills continue to develop throughout childhood.

called Wernicke's and Broca's areas. Both are in the dominant cerebral hemisphere (the left hemisphere in most people). In Wernicke's area, incoming messages (heard or read) are scanned and compared with information held in the memory to extract meaning. In Broca's area, words and sentences are composed from vocabulary and from grammatical rules stored in the memory.

SPEECH PRODUCTION

The movement sequences for speech sounds originate from two regions of the cerebral cortex on either side of the brain. These regions are linked to the center for language expression (Broca's area). The signals for movement pass down nerve pathways to the muscles controlling the larynx, tongue, and other parts involved in speech. The cerebellum (a region at the back of the brain) plays a part in coordinating these movements.

Air from the lungs is vibrated by opening and closing the vocal cords in the larynx. This produces a noise, which is amplified in the hollow cavities of the throat, nose, and sinuses. The sound of vibrated or non-vibrated air is modified by movements of the tongue, mouth, jaw, and lips to produce speech sounds. Vibrated air blown through top teeth resting on lower lips gives "v" or, if the air is not vibrated, "f." Consonants are produced mainly by contact among the tongue, roof of the mouth, teeth, and lips; vowels are produced by changing the shape of the mouth cavity.

LANGUAGE AND SPEECH DEVELOPMENT

Normal development of language and speech in a child depends on maturation of the nervous system and muscles, on the child's exploration of his or her environment (which should be stimulating), and on interaction with adults. Through play, the child

S

acquires many concepts (sets of ideas) about different aspects of the world. From adults, the child acquires the verbal labels for objects and concepts that are vital to language development. Normal hearing is, therefore, essential. Language and speech are learned through listening to the speech of others and monitoring one's own speech.

Stages in the development of language and speech in a child, with the significance of each, are shown in the table (see previous page).

Speech disorders

Defects or disturbances can arise in various parts of the nervous system, muscles, and other apparatus involved in *speech*, leading to an inability to communicate effectively. Some of these disorders are, strictly, disturbances of language rather than of speech, since they result from an impaired ability to understand or to form words in the language centers of the brain, rather than from any fault of the apparatus of speech production.

DISORDERS OF LANGUAGE
Damage to the language centers of the brain (usually as a result of a *stroke*, *head injury*, or *brain tumor*) leads to a disorder known as *aphasia*. Both children and adults can be affected. The ability to speak and write and/or to comprehend written or spoken words is impaired, depending on the site and extent of the damage.

Delayed development of language in a child is characterized by slowness to understand speech and/or slow growth in vocabulary and sentence structure. Delayed development has many causes, including hearing loss, lack of stimulation, or emotional disturbance (see *Developmental delay*).

DISORDERS OF ARTICULATION
Articulation is the ability to produce speech sounds; a defect of articulation is sometimes referred to as *dysarthria*. Damage to nerves passing from the brain to muscles in the larynx (voice box), mouth, or lips can cause speech to be slurred, indistinct, slow, or nasal. The sources of such damage are similar to those that cause aphasia (e.g., stroke, head injury, tumors, *multiple sclerosis*, *Parkinson's disease*) but the affected regions of the brain are different. Damage to the cerebellum, for example, produces a characteristic form of slurred speech. Structural abnormalities of the mouth, such as cleft palate (see *Cleft lip and palate*) and malaligned teeth, can also cause poor articulation.

Delayed development of articulation, characterized by an inability to make sounds at appropriate ages, may cause incomprehensible speech. Causes are hearing problems or slow maturation of the nervous system.

DISORDERS OF VOICE PRODUCTION
These disorders include hoarseness, harshness, inappropriate pitch or loudness of the voice, and abnormal nasal resonance. In many cases, the cause is a disorder affecting closure of the vocal cords (see *Larynx* disorders box). A voice pitched too high or low or that is too loud or soft may be caused by a hormonal or psychiatric disturbance or by severe hearing loss.

Abnormal nasal resonance is caused by too much air (hypernasality) or too little air (hyponasality) flowing through the nose during speech. Hypernasality may result from damage to the nerves supplying the palate (roof of the mouth) or be a result of cleft palate. It causes a deterioration in the intelligibility of speech. Hyponasality is caused by blockage to the nasal airways by excess mucus and has the sound of someone speaking with a cold.

DISORDERS OF FLUENCY
Nonfluent speech is marked by repetitions of single sounds or whole words and by blocking of speech; the underlying cause is not understood (see *Stuttering*).

Speech therapy

A form of therapy that attempts to help people with a variety of communication problems.

WHY IT IS DONE
Any person with a disturbance of language or a disorder of articulation, voice production, or fluency of speech (see *Speech disorders*) may be helped by speech therapy. These problems may occur as part of a broader problem, such as a physical handicap, learning difficulty, or hearing loss. Speech therapists work with all age groups.

HOW IT IS DONE
The therapist—a person trained in the causes, assessment, and treatment of speech and language problems—usually begins by taking a history from the client or from a relative or friend, asking how and when the difficulties developed. Relevant medical details are also sought from the client's physician, if necessary.

The client may be asked to provide a sample of speech (which may be recorded) or of writing for detailed analysis. An examination of the physical structures of speech and a hearing test may be performed. The therapist may also assess language comprehension by observing the client's reaction to written or spoken requests.

After making an assessment, the therapist decides on the form of treatment, which is carried out in two parts. A program of exercises is started to improve a specific aspect of language ability or speech performance (e.g., a technique to improve speech fluency). Also, the therapist works with the people most involved with the client (e.g., family, teachers, or friends), explaining to them the nature of the difficulties and how they can help. The aim of therapy is to create a climate that will provide the client with opportunities for effective communication.

Sperm

The male sex cell, also known as spermatozoon (singular) or spermatozoa (plural), responsible for *fertilization* of the female ovum. Sperm are microscopically tiny, measuring 0.002 inch (0.05 mm) in length.

Sperm are produced within the seminiferous tubules of the *testes* by a process known as spermatogenesis. The production and development of sperm is dependent on the male sex hormone *testosterone* and on *gonadotropin hormones* produced by the *pituitary gland*. Sperm production commences at *puberty*.

The original cell from which a sperm develops contains 46 chromosomes, including the XY pair of male sex *chromosomes*. By a process of *cell division*, the number of chromosomes in the sperm is halved to 23, including either the X or the Y from the original pair of sex chromosomes. This X or Y is responsible for determining the sex of an embryo that develops after fertilization of the ovum by the sperm (see *Sex determination*).

Human sperm magnified 350 times
Each sperm consists of a head that contains the hereditary material and a long, whiplike tail that propels it along.

The final stage of spermatogenesis takes place in the *epididymis*, where the sperm grow tails that will propel them through the woman's reproductive tract after *ejaculation* during sexual intercourse.

Spermatocele

A harmless cyst of the *epididymis* (the tube that transmits sperm from the testis) that contains fluid and sperm. If the spermatocele grows to a large size or becomes uncomfortable, it is usually removed surgically. Although the operation is straightforward, it may result in an interruption of the passage of sperm, which may render the testis on the affected side infertile.

Spermatozoa

See *Sperm*.

Spermicides

Contraceptive preparations that kill sperm. Spermicides are usually recommended for use with a barrier device, such as a condom or diaphragm, to increase the final contraceptive effect (see *Contraception, barrier methods*).

Some spermicides, such as nonoxynol, may protect against the organisms that cause various *sexually transmitted diseases*, including *gonorrhea* and *AIDS*.

A possible adverse effect is irritation of the genitals of either partner.

Sphenoid bone

The bat-shaped bone in the center of the base of the cranium (the part of the *skull* that encases the brain). The central body of the bone contains the sphenoidal sinus (air space) and, in the upper surface, a depression in which the *pituitary gland* is situated. The wings support part of the temporal lobe of the brain (see *Cerebrum*) and form part of the back and side walls of the orbits (eye sockets). There are various canals and foramens (holes) in the wings to enable the optic and other cranial nerves to pass through.

Spherocytosis, hereditary

An inherited disorder so named because of the large number of unusually small, round, red blood cells (spherocytes) in the circulation. These cells have an abnormal membrane (outer envelope), which makes them fragile, and a much reduced life span because they are readily trapped, broken up, and consumed when blood passes through

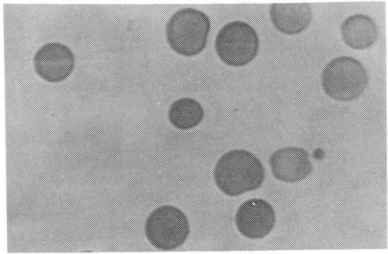

Spherocytes in blood
A person with hereditary spherocytosis has a large number of these unusually small, round, fragile, red cells in the blood.

the *spleen*. At times, the rate of hemolysis (red cell destruction) exceeds the rate at which new cells can be made in the bone marrow, leading to *anemia* (reduced level of the oxygen-carrying pigment *hemoglobin* in the blood due to lack of red cells).

INCIDENCE
Hereditary spherocytosis is the most common form of inherited hemolytic anemia in people of northern European extraction. About one person in 4,500 in the US has the condition. The disorder is inherited in autosomal dominant fashion (see *Genetic disorders*). Each of an affected person's children has a 50 percent chance of inheriting the defective gene responsible for the abnormality.

SYMPTOMS, DIAGNOSIS, AND TREATMENT
Symptoms of anemia, such as tiredness, shortness of breath on exertion, and pallor, may develop at any age. Other symptoms include *jaundice* (caused by the high rate of blood cell destruction) and enlargement of the spleen. Occasionally, there are crises (triggered by infections) when all the symptoms worsen. *Gallstones*, also caused by the high rate of bilirubin release, are a frequent complication.

The diagnosis is made from the presence of spherocytes in the blood of someone with anemia and from tests to ascertain the structure of the red cell membrane.

The treatment is *splenectomy* (removal of the spleen). The red cells remain abnormally shaped, but the rate at which they are destroyed drops markedly, leading to a striking, and usually permanent, improvement in the patient's health.

Sphincter

A ring of muscle around a natural opening or passage that acts like a valve, regulating inflow or outflow. For example, the outlet of the stomach into the duodenum is called the pyloric sphincter. It controls the stomach's outflow. The anal sphincter at the rectal outlet is partly under voluntary control, permitting us to decide when to empty the bowel.

Sphincter, artificial

A surgically created valve or other device used to treat or prevent urinary or fecal *incontinence*.

An artificial urinary sphincter consists of an inflatable cuff that is inserted around the base of the bladder or upper part of the urethra. When inflated, the cuff prevents urine from leaking from the bladder. The patient deflates the cuff by using a pump, which is usually situated in the scrotum in males or adjacent to the labia in females.

An artificial sphincter to prevent fecal incontinence may be created after removal of the colon and rectum. This operation, an alternative to a conventional *ileostomy*, involves using a loop of ileum to create a pouch in which bowel contents collect. Evacuation of feces is controlled by an artificial sphincter, surgically fashioned from a section of ileum.

A similar "continent ileostomy" may be provided for a person whose bladder has been removed to treat cancer and whose ureters are then joined to a segment of ileum that is formed into a pouch. This procedure is still under development and considered experimental, as are other methods of continent *urinary diversion*.

Sphincterotomy

A surgical procedure that involves cutting the muscle that closes a body opening or that constricts the opening between body passages. In rare cases, sphincterotomy is performed on the anal sphincter to treat an *anal fissure*. It is also performed on the ampulla of Vater (the opening of the common bile duct into the duodenum) to release an impacted *gallstone*.

Sphygmomanometer

An instrument for measuring blood pressure. It consists of a cuff with an inflatable bladder that is wrapped around the upper arm, a rubber bulb to inflate the bladder, and a device that indicates the pressure of blood. This pressure device may consist of a calibrated glass column filled with mercury, a spring gauge and dial, or, in more modern instruments, a digital readout display. (For an explanation of how a sphygmomanometer is used, see *Blood pressure*.)

S

Spider bites

Nearly all spiders produce venom, which they inject, via a pair of fangs, to paralyze and kill their prey. However, only a few species are harmful to humans. In the US, the two most dangerous types are the black widow spider (*LATRODECTUS MAC-TANS*) and the brown recluse spider (*LOXOSCELES RECLUSA*).

The black widow is a small, shiny black spider, less than half an inch (1 cm) long but with a leg span of up to 2 inches (5 cm). It has a red hourglass-shaped marking on its underside. This spider can be found in most parts of the US in woodpiles, sheds, and the bowls of outside toilets, from which it may deliver a bite to a person's buttocks or genitals.

A bite from a black widow can cause severe pain and muscle spasms (starting near the site of the bite and spreading), heavy sweating, stomach cramps, nausea, vomiting, tightness in the chest, breathing difficulty, and a sharp rise in blood pressure. These symptoms may continue for several days. Deaths from *cardiac arrest* or *respiratory failure* occur occasionally in children or the elderly, but are uncommon in adults. Treatment consists of *analgesics* (painkillers) and an intravenous injection of a solution of calcium gluconate, which relieves the muscle cramps. If symptoms are very severe, or if the patient is a young child, an *antivenin* active against the spider venom may also be given.

Recluse spiders are brown or brown-yellow. They occur in southern and southwestern states, where they inhabit crevices in or around houses. Their bite causes severe pain, reddening, blistering, and death of tissue at the site of the wound, followed by a deep ulcer. Treatment consists of analgesics, care of the wound to prevent infection, and measures to deal with complications, which can include hemolytic *anemia* and *renal failure*. Fatalities have occurred in children.

Other dangerous spiders include relatives of the black widow spider, and the "funnel web" spider of Australia. The hairy tarantula of southern Europe is relatively harmless, although its bite is painful.

Spider nevus

A discolored patch of skin that takes the form of a red, raised dot the size of a pinhead with small blood vessels radiating from this dot. Also called telangiectasia, spider nevi represent

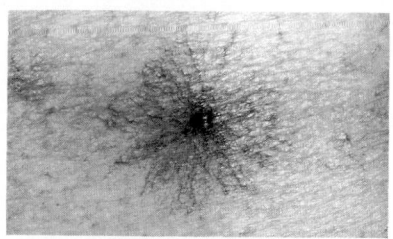

Typical spider nevus
The nevus consists of a tiny, red, raised dot from which widened blood capillaries radiate outward in all directions.

the outward appearance of a dilated arteriole (small artery) and its connecting capillaries.

Small numbers of spider nevi are common in children and pregnant women. However, in larger quantities, spider nevi may be a sign of an underlying disorder, such as advanced *cirrhosis* of the liver. Lesions resembling multiple spider nevi (but without the "spider legs") may be a sign of hereditary hemorrhagic telangiectasia, a disorder of the blood vessels that causes bleeding and iron-deficiency anemia.

Spina bifida

A congenital defect in which part of one (or more) *vertebrae* fails to develop completely, leaving a portion of the *spinal cord* exposed. Spina bifida can occur anywhere on the spine but is most common in the lower back. The severity of the condition depends on how much nerve tissue is exposed.

CAUSES AND INCIDENCE
The cause of spina bifida remains unknown; it is thought that many factors are involved.

The incidence is about one case per 1,000 babies born. The incidence increases with either very young or old maternal age. A woman who has had one affected child is ten times more likely than the average of having another affected child.

TYPES
There are four known distinct forms of spina bifida.

SPINA BIFIDA OCCULTA This is the most common and the least serious form. There is little external evidence of the defect apart from a dimple or a tuft of hair over the area of the underlying abnormality. Spina bifida occulta often goes completely unnoticed in otherwise healthy children, although occasionally there are accompanying abnormalities of the lower part of the spinal cord. Symptoms, which include leg weakness, cold and blue

feet, and urinary incontinence, may be present from birth or may develop later in life.
MYELOCELE Also known as meningomyelocele, this is the most severe form of spina bifida. The nature of the defect is shown in the illustrated box on the opposite page.

A child with myelocele is usually severely handicapped. The legs are partially or completely paralyzed, with loss of sensation in all areas below the level of the defect; hip dislocation and other leg deformities are common. *Hydrocephalus* (excess cerebrospinal fluid within the skull) is common and may result in brain damage. Associated abnormalities include *cerebral palsy, epilepsy, mental retardation,* and visual problems. Paralysis of the bladder leads to urinary incontinence or urinary retention, repeated urinary tract infections, and eventual kidney damage. The anus may be paralyzed, causing chronic constipation and leakage of feces.
MENINGOCELE This form is less severe than myelocele. The nature of the defect is shown in the box opposite.
ENCEPHALOCELE This is a rare type of spina bifida in which the protrusion occurs through the skull. There is usually severe brain damage.
DIAGNOSIS
Closure of the vertebral canal usually occurs within four weeks of conception, meaning that meningomyelocele can often be diagnosed at an early stage in the pregnancy by *ultrasound scanning*. High levels of *alpha-fetoprotein* in the amniotic fluid or maternal blood may indicate spina bifida.

After birth, spina bifida is easy to recognize if there is a protruding sac. Spina bifida occulta can be diagnosed only by spinal X ray.
TREATMENT
In cases that are not severe, surgery may be performed to close the defect and thus prevent further damage to the spinal cord. Ideally, the operation should be performed in the first few days of life. If the abnormality is serious, surgery may allow the child to survive, although he or she may have gross physical and mental handicap.

If hydrocephalus develops, a *shunt* (tube) is inserted into the brain to relieve the buildup of fluid. Retention or incontinence of urine is relieved by an indwelling catheter (which is changed every four to six weeks); in older children, self-catheterization can be taught (see *Catheterization, urinary*). Laxatives or enemas may be needed for constipation.

S

TYPES OF SPINA BIFIDA

There are different forms of spina bifida. In one type (spina bifida occulta), the only defect is a failure of the fusion of the bony arches behind the spinal cord. When the bone defect is more extensive, there may be a meningocele, with protrusion of the meninges (the membranes surrounding the cord) or, more seriously, a myelocele, with change in the spinal cord itself.

MENINGOCELE

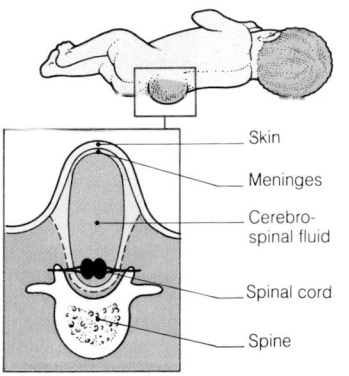

Skin

Meninges

Cerebro-
spinal fluid

Spinal cord

Spine

Meningocele
In this type, the nerve tissue of the spinal cord is usually intact; there is skin over the bulging sac and there are therefore usually no functional problems. However, repairs are necessary early in life.

MYELOCELE

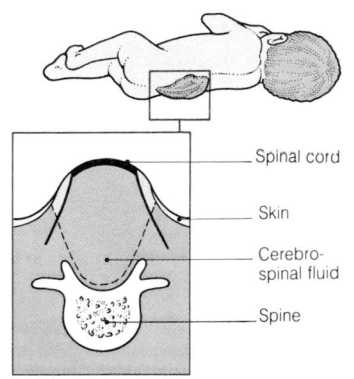

Spinal cord

Skin

Cerebro-
spinal fluid

Spine

Myelocele
In this type, the baby is born with a raw swelling over the spine. It consists of malformed spinal cord, which may or may not be contained in a membranous sac. The child is likely to be very handicapped.

Physical therapy encourages mobility and independence; for the more severely affected, wheelchairs and other walking aids may be required. Depending on the degree of disability, special schooling and training for employment may be needed.

PREVENTION
Parents who have had one child with spina bifida should undergo *genetic counseling* if they are considering another pregnancy.

Spinal accessory nerve
The eleventh *cranial nerve*. The spinal accessory nerve differs from the other cranial nerves in that only a small part of it originates from the brain; most of the nerve comes from the spinal cord.

The part of the nerve originating from the brain supplies many muscles of the palate, pharynx (throat), and larynx (voice box). Damage to this part of the nerve may give rise to dysphonia (difficulty speaking) and dysphagia (difficulty swallowing).

The spinal part of the nerve supplies some large muscles of the neck and back, notably the sternomastoid (which runs from the breastbone to the side of the skull) and the trapezius (a large, triangular muscle of the upper back, shoulder, and neck). Damage to the spinal fibers of the nerve paralyzes these muscles. Such damage usually occurs as a result of surgery for cancer in which lymph nodes in the neck are removed.

Spinal anesthesia
A method of blocking pain sensations before they reach the central nervous system by injecting an anesthetic into the cerebrospinal fluid in the spinal canal. The technique is primarily used to accompany surgery on the lower abdomen and legs. Operations on the hip and prostate gland are commonly performed using spinal or *epidural anesthesia*. The decision as to which anesthesia to use is made after discussion among the patient, anesthesiologist, and surgeon.

The procedure is performed by inserting a delicate needle between two vertebrae in the lower part of the spine (see *Lumbar puncture*) and introducing anesthetic into the cerebrospinal fluid surrounding the spinal cord and its terminal nerve roots. Because the nerves emerging from the spinal cord are bathed in cerebrospinal fluid, they absorb the anesthetic. The position of the injec-

tion and subsequent controlled spread of the local anesthetic solution determines the area that is anesthetized.

After spinal anesthesia, a headache may develop in between 1 and 5 percent of patients.

Spinal cord
A cylinder of nerve tissue, about 18 inches long and roughly the thickness of a finger, that runs down the central canal in the *spine*. It is a downward extension of the brain. The spinal cord and brain can be considered parts of a single unit—the central nervous system (CNS).

STRUCTURE
At the core of the spinal cord is a region with a butterfly-shaped cross section, called the gray matter. It contains the cell bodies of neurons (nerve cells) along with glial (supporting) cells. Some of the nerve cells are motor neurons, whose axons (long, projecting fibers) pass out of the spinal cord in bundles within the *spinal nerves* and extend to glands or muscles in the trunk and limbs. Others are interneurons (nerve cells contained entirely within the central nervous system), which act to convey messages between other neurons. Also entering the gray matter are the axons of sensory neurons (which have their cell bodies outside the spinal cord). These axons connect with the motor neurons or interneurons.

Surrounding the gray matter are areas of white matter, which consist of bundles of nerve cell axons running lengthwise through the cord.

Sprouting from the spinal cord on each side at regular intervals are two nerve bundles—the spinal nerve roots, which contain the fibers of motor and sensory nerve cells. They combine to form the spinal nerves, which emerge from the spine and are the communication cables between the spinal cord and all regions of the trunk and limbs.

The whole of the spinal cord is bathed in *cerebrospinal fluid* and surrounded by a protective sheath, a continuation of the *meninges* that protect the brain.

FUNCTION
The nerve tracts that make up the white matter of the spinal cord act mainly as highways for sensory information passing upward toward the brain (ascending tracts) or motor signals passing downward (descending tracts). However, the cord is also capable of handling some of the sensory information itself and of provid-

S

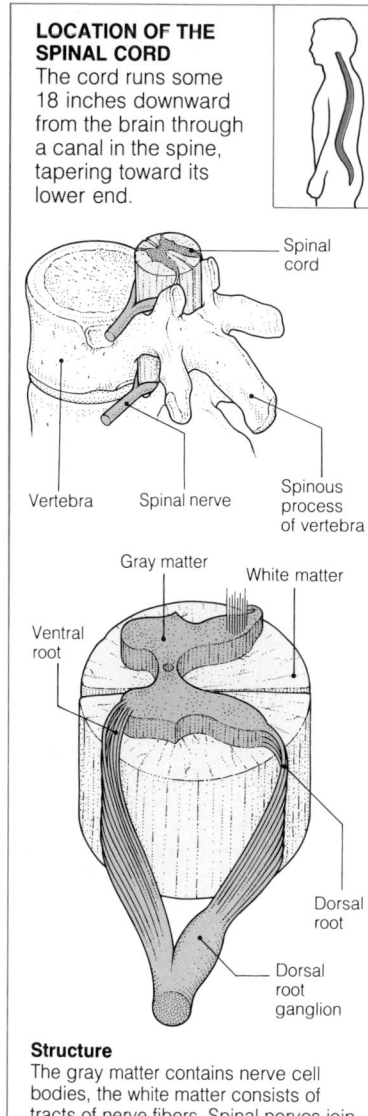

LOCATION OF THE SPINAL CORD
The cord runs some 18 inches downward from the brain through a canal in the spine, tapering toward its lower end.

Spinal cord

Vertebra — Spinal nerve — Spinous process of vertebra

Gray matter — White matter

Ventral root

Dorsal root

Dorsal root ganglion

Structure
The gray matter contains nerve cell bodies, the white matter consists of tracts of nerve fibers. Spinal nerves join the cord at regular intervals.

ing appropriate motor responses without recourse to the brain. Many *reflex* actions (such as the knee jerk reflex) are controlled in this way by the spinal cord.

DISORDERS
The spinal cord may be injured as a result of trauma to the spine (see *Spinal injury*). If an ascending or descending tract is severed, it interrupts communication between the brain and parts of the body served from parts of the cord below the injury. This can lead to a variety of patterns of paralysis and/or loss of sensation, which are usually permanent because

nerve cells and fibers within the cord do not regenerate. However, reflexes controlled by the spinal cord are usually maintained.

Pressure on the cord (e.g., by a blood clot, an abscess, or tumor) can similarly affect movement and sensation. However, the effects of pressure can often be relieved by surgery.

Infections of the spinal cord (including *poliomyelitis*) are relatively rare but can cause serious damage. In *multiple sclerosis*, a degenerative disease, there is patchy loss of the insulating sheaths around nerve fibers.

Spinal fusion
A major surgical procedure to join two or more adjacent vertebrae, the bones that make up the spine.

WHY IT IS DONE
Spinal fusion is performed if abnormal movement between adjacent vertebrae (as revealed by X rays) causes severe back pain or may damage the spinal cord. Such abnormal movement may be due to various spinal disorders, including *spondylolisthesis*, dislocated facet joints (the movable joints that connect vertebrae), *scoliosis*, *osteomyelitis*, a tumor or injury destroying one or more vertebrae, or *osteoarthritis* that causes degeneration of spinal joints.

HOW IT IS DONE
Using a general anesthetic, the affected vertebrae are exposed. *Arthrodesis* (joint fusion) is then carried out, sometimes with a *bone graft*, using bone chips taken from the pelvis. A temporary fixation is made with a plate or screws.

The recovery period includes bed rest for up to six weeks. When mobility is resumed, the patient may initially need to wear a plaster jacket. Full fusion of the vertebrae takes up to six months.

Results are usually good, but fusing the vertebrae may place greater strain on the rest of the spine and cause more back pain. The potential gain must be weighed against the risks.

Spinal injury
Damage to the *spine* and sometimes to the *spinal cord*, in which case the injury may cause loss of sensation and muscle weakness or paralysis.

CAUSES
Spinal injury is usually caused by one of three types of severe force—longitudinal compression, hinging, and shearing. Longitudinal compression, usually due to a fall from a height, crushes the vertebrae (seg-

ments of spine) lengthwise against each other. Hinging, which can occur in a whiplash injury suffered in an automobile accident, subjects the spinal column to sudden, extreme bending movements. Shearing, which may occur when a person is knocked over by a motor vehicle, for example, combines both hinging and rotational (twisting) forces.

Any of these forces can dislocate the vertebrae, fracture them, or rupture the ligaments that bind them together. In severe dislocations and fractures, the vertebrae, accumulated fluid, or a blood clot may press on the spinal cord, or the cord may be torn or even severed. In all of these cases the function of the spinal cord is impaired or destroyed. An unstable injury is one in which there is the possibility that vertebrae will shift and cause damage, possibly severing the spinal cord. Other injuries are called stable.

SYMPTOMS AND SIGNS
Damage to the vertebrae and ligaments usually causes severe pain and swelling of the affected area. Damage to the spinal cord results in loss of sensation and/or motor function below the site of injury. Injuries below the neck may cause *paraplegia* (weakness or paralysis of the legs and sometimes part of the trunk); damage to the cord in the neck may result in *quadriplegia* (weakness or paralysis of all four limbs and the trunk) or may be fatal. Weakness or paralysis is often accompanied by loss of bladder or bowel control, resulting in urinary or fecal incontinence or retention.

Pressure on the spinal cord may cause motor abnormalities, such as muscle weakness or paralysis. It may also cause abnormalities of sensation, such as pain, tingling, or burning sensations.

DIAGNOSIS AND TREATMENT
After an accident in which a spinal injury may have occurred, the victim should be moved only by someone trained in all aspects of first aid. X rays of the spine are carried out to determine whether the spine has been injured and the extent of any damage.

In a stable injury, the patient must rest in bed until comfortable movement is possible; he or she may then need to wear an orthopedic *collar* or *corset* for support or to relieve pain in the injured area.

The priority in an unstable injury is to stabilize the affected bones. If they are dislocated, the surgeon usually manipulates them back into position using a general anesthetic. Some

S

unstable fractures are treated by skeletal *traction* to align the bone ends and hold them in position until healing occurs (which may take up to three months). Other unstable fractures require an operation to fasten the bone ends together permanently with a metal plate or wires.

Surgical repair of damaged nerve tracts in the spinal cord is not possible. Treatment is directed toward preventing the development of problems secondary to the main symptoms. For example, the patient is turned regularly in bed to prevent *bedsores* from forming as the result of immobility and lack of sensation in the skin. *Physical therapy* is carried out to stop joints from locking and muscles from contracting as the result of paralysis. Retention of urine or feces may require catheterization (see *Catheterization, urinary*) or *enemas*.

OUTLOOK
Recovery is usually complete when the spinal cord has not been damaged, although there may be some residual pain and stiffness. When there has been pressure on the spinal cord, surgery to remove the source of the pressure can bring variable improvement in symptoms. Even when there is damage to the cord, some improvement may occur for up to 12 months. In such cases, the patient's recovery can be aided by a program of *rehabilitation*. This may include forms of physical and occupational therapy, which can help morale and independence.

Spinal nerves
A set of 31 pairs of nerves that connects to the spinal cord.

STRUCTURE
The spinal nerves emerge in two rows from either side of the spinal cord and leave the spine through gaps between adjacent vertebrae (segments of spine). Because the spinal cord runs only two thirds of the way down the canal in the center of the spine, the lowest nine pairs of nerves must travel some distance down the canal before finally leaving the backbone. They form a spray of nerves in this area known as the cauda equina.

The distribution and branching of the spinal nerves ensures that all parts of the trunk, arms, and legs are supplied with a network of sensory and motor nerve twigs.

FUNCTION
Like all nerves, the spinal nerves consist of bundles of the axons (long fibers) of individual neurons (nerve cells). Some of these fibers carry information from sensory receptors in the skin, muscles, and elsewhere toward the spinal cord; other motor fibers carry signals from the spinal cord to muscles and glands. Just before it connects to the spinal cord, each spinal nerve splits into two bundles, one of which carries only sensory fibers and the other of which carries only motor fibers. These bundles are sometimes called spinal nerve roots.

DISORDERS
Damage to the shock-absorbing disk of cartilage between two vertebrae sometimes leads to pressure on a spinal nerve root, causing pain (see *Disk prolapse*). Injury to a spinal nerve may lead to loss of sensation and movement in a part of the body. Damage or degeneration from such causes or from infection, diabetes, vitamin deficiency, and poisoning can lead to neurological symptoms such as pain, numbness, or twitching (see *Nerve injury; Neuropathy*).

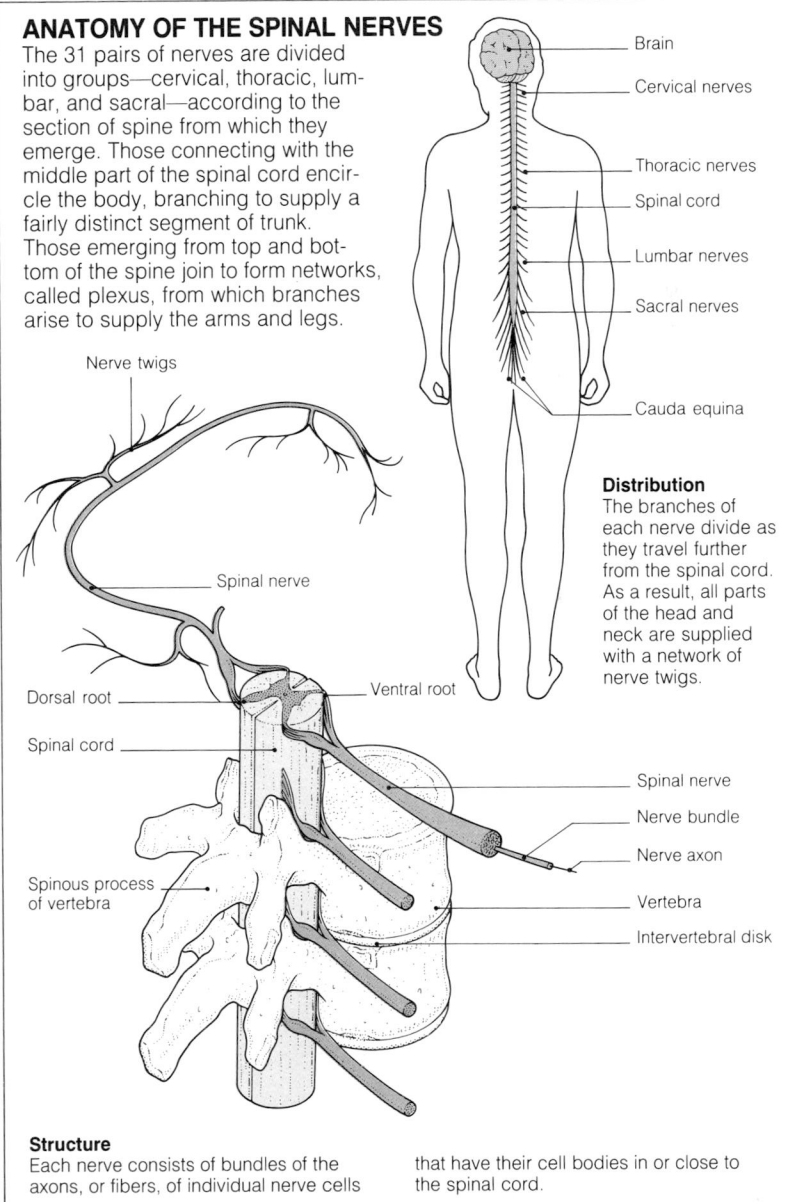

ANATOMY OF THE SPINAL NERVES
The 31 pairs of nerves are divided into groups—cervical, thoracic, lumbar, and sacral—according to the section of spine from which they emerge. Those connecting with the middle part of the spinal cord encircle the body, branching to supply a fairly distinct segment of trunk. Those emerging from top and bottom of the spine join to form networks, called plexus, from which branches arise to supply the arms and legs.

Brain

Cervical nerves

Thoracic nerves

Spinal cord

Lumbar nerves

Sacral nerves

Cauda equina

Nerve twigs

Spinal nerve

Dorsal root

Ventral root

Spinal cord

Spinous process of vertebra

Spinal nerve

Nerve bundle

Nerve axon

Vertebra

Intervertebral disk

Distribution
The branches of each nerve divide as they travel further from the spinal cord. As a result, all parts of the head and neck are supplied with a network of nerve twigs.

Structure
Each nerve consists of bundles of the axons, or fibers, of individual nerve cells that have their cell bodies in or close to the spinal cord.

S

Spinal tap

See *Lumbar puncture*.

Spine

The column of bones and cartilage that extends from the base of the skull to the pelvis, enclosing and protecting the *spinal cord* and supporting the trunk and head.

STRUCTURE AND FUNCTION

The spine is made up of 33 roughly cylindrical bones called *vertebrae*. Each pair of adjacent vertebrae is connected by a joint, called a facet joint, which both stabilizes the vertebral column and allows movement in it. Between each pair of vertebrae lies a disk-shaped pad of tough fibrous cartilage with a jellylike core (nucleus pulposus) called an intervertebral disk (see *Disk, intervertebral*). These disks act to cushion the vertebrae during movements such as running or jumping.

The whole of the spine encloses the spinal cord, a column of nerve tracts running from the brain. Peripheral nerves (see *Peripheral nervous system*) branch off from the spinal cord to every part of the body, their roots passing between the vertebrae.

The vertebrae are bound together by two long, thick ligaments running the length of the spine and by smaller ligaments between each vertebra.

Several groups of muscles are attached to the vertebrae. These muscles control movements of the spine and also help to support it.

In a normal spine the cervical section curves forward, the thoracic section backward, the lumbar section forward (particularly in women), and the pelvic section backward.

Spirochete

 A spiral-shaped bacterium. Spirochetes cause *syphilis*, *pinta* and *yaws* (both related to syphilis), and *leptospirosis*, *relapsing fever*, and *Lyme disease*.

Spirometry

A *pulmonary function test* used to help diagnose or assess a lung disorder or to monitor treatment.

The procedure is shown in the illustrated box below. The spirometer records the total volume of air breathed out, known as the forced vital capacity (FVC). It also records the volume of air breathed out in 1 second, known as the forced expiratory volume in 1 second (FEV_1).

In obstructive lung disease (such as *asthma*, *emphysema*, and chronic bronchitis), the FEV_1/FVC ratio is reduced because the airways are narrowed, thus slowing expiration. In a restrictive lung disease (such as *interstitial pulmonary fibrosis*), the FVC and FEV_1 are reduced almost equally with little change in the ratio. This is because lung expansion is limited but the airways are not narrowed.

Spironolactone

A potassium-sparing *diuretic drug*. Combined with thiazide or loop diuretics, spironolactone is given to treat

---

STRUCTURE OF THE SPINE

The spine is made up of a column of 33 roughly cylindrical bones called vertebrae. Running through the center of this bony structure is the spinal cord.

Cervical spine
Seven vertebrae, the topmost of which supports the skull.

Thoracic spine
Twelve vertebrae that run down the rear wall of the chest. A pair of ribs is attached to each vertebra.

Lumbar spine
Five vertebrae. This section is the one under the most pressure during lifting.

Sacrum
Five fused vertebrae.

Coccyx
Four fused vertebrae.

SPIROMETRY

This technique is used to assess certain lung conditions and the patient's response to treatment. It records the rate at which a patient exhales air from the lungs and the total volume exhaled.

Spirometer

How it is done
The patient exhales forcibly through a mouthpiece into the spirometer. This causes the spirometer to produce a graph like that shown at right.

Volume (expired liters)

Time (seconds)

Normal
FEV_1 (forced expiratory volume of the first second) is the volume of air exhaled in the first second and is normally 60 to 80 percent of FVC (forced vital capacity), the total volume exhaled.

Volume (expired liters)

Time (seconds)

Asthma
A patient with asthma cannot exhale air as fast as normal, due to narrowing of the airways, so FEV_1 is reduced in comparison with FVC.

DISORDERS OF THE SPINE

Many disorders of the spine, despite their different causes, result in just one symptom—*back pain*.

CONGENITAL DISORDERS

Some children are born with a gap in the vertebrae that leaves part of the spinal cord exposed. This condition (*spina bifida*) results in leg paralysis and incontinence.

INFECTION

Osteomyelitis (infection of bone and bone marrow) may in rare cases affect a vertebra, destroying both bone and disk. The most common cause is the spread of an infection, such as tuberculosis, from elsewhere in the body.

INFLAMMATION

In *ankylosing spondylitis*, and in some cases of *rheumatoid arthritis*, the joints in the spine become inflamed and later fuse, causing permanent stiffness. *Osteochondritis juvenilis* (inflammation of the growing area of bone in children and adolescents) can affect the vertebrae, when the disease may cause deformity of the spine.

INJURIES

Lifting heavy objects, twisting suddenly, or adopting bad posture can cause any of the following spinal injuries—a sprained ligament, torn muscle, *spondylolisthesis* (dislocated vertebrae), dislocated facet joint, or *disk prolapse* (rupture of the tough outer layer of the disk).

A direct blow, a fall from a height, or sudden twisting can result in fracture of one or more vertebrae. Overexercising the spine can have the same effect (see *Stress fracture*).

TUMORS

Tumors of the spine are usually malignant; in most cases, they have spread from cancer elsewhere in the body (see *Bone cancer*).

DEGENERATION

Osteoarthritis (degeneration of joint cartilage due to wear and tear) affects the joints in the spines of virtually everyone over 60, particularly people who do heavy manual work or people whose spines have already been affected by disease or injury.

Osteoporosis (thinning and softening of bone), which is most common in older women, can weaken the vertebrae. Under the weight of the trunk, the vertebrae may then fracture.

OTHER DISORDERS

In some people the spine becomes abnormally curved. The excessive curvature may be inward in the lower back (see *Lordosis*), outward in the upper back (see *Kyphosis*), or to one side (see *Scoliosis*). Causes include infection, osteoporosis, congenital spine disorder, and muscle disorders.

INVESTIGATION

Spinal disorders are investigated by *X rays*, *CT scanning*, and *myelography*. Other *bone imaging* techniques, including *MRI*, may sometimes be performed, as may other tests.

---

hypertension (high blood pressure) and *edema* (fluid retention).

Spironolactone may cause numbness, weakness, nausea, and vomiting. Less common adverse effects include diarrhea, lethargy, impotence, rash, and irregular menstruation in women. High doses of spironolactone may cause abnormal breast enlargement in men.

Spleen

An organ that removes and destroys worn-out red blood cells and helps fight infection. Weighing about 7 ounces (200 grams), the spleen is a fist-sized, spongy, dark purple organ lying in the upper left abdomen behind the lower ribs.

STRUCTURE

The spleen is covered with a capsule from which many fibrous bands run inward to give the organ a spongelike structure. The spaces between the bands are filled with lymph tissue, composed of *lymphocytes* and *phagocytes* (cells that ingest other cells or foreign particles), and red blood cells. Blood is supplied to the spleen by a large artery that branches extensively within the organ.

FUNCTION

One of the two main functions of the spleen is to control the quality of circulating red blood cells. It accomplishes this by removing and breaking down all worn-out red cells approximately 120 days after they have been produced in the bone marrow and by destroying other red cells that are misshapen or defective.

The other role of the spleen is to help fight infection by producing some of the *antibodies*, phagocytes, and lymphocytes that destroy invading microorganisms.

In the fetus, the spleen produces red blood cells. After birth, this function is taken over by the bone marrow. However, in certain diseases that affect cell production in the bone marrow (such as *thalassemia*), the spleen may resume production.

Despite its functions, the spleen is not an essential organ. If it is removed, its activities are largely taken over by other parts of the lymphatic system, although the individual is more susceptible to infection.

DISORDERS

The spleen enlarges in many diseases, including infections such as *malaria*, *infectious mononucleosis* (glandular fever), *schistosomiasis*, *tuberculosis*, and *typhoid fever*; in *leukemia* and thalassemia; in some diseases that cause hemolytic *anemia* (such as *sickle cell anemia*); and in tumors of the spleen. The enlargement, which can often be felt as a swelling in the upper left abdomen, is sometimes accompanied by *hypersplenism*.

Lymphomas (tumors of lymphoid tissue) may develop in the spleen and elsewhere in the lymphatic system.

The spleen is sometimes ruptured by a severe blow to the abdomen, usually in an automobile crash or by a fall from a height. A rupture is much more likely if the spleen is enlarged or if overlying ribs are fractured. Rupture can cause severe bleeding, which may be fatal. For this reason, the injury requires an emergency operation to remove the spleen and tie off the artery supplying it (see *Splenectomy*).

Splenectomy

Surgical removal of the *spleen*.

WHY IT IS DONE

Splenectomy is usually performed after the spleen has been seriously injured, causing severe hemorrhage.

S

The organ is removed because it is difficult to repair and because, in an adult, its absence has virtually no known ill effects. Its function is largely taken over by other parts of the lymphatic system and by the liver.

The spleen is also removed to treat primary *hypersplenism* and certain types of anemia, such as hereditary *spherocytosis*. Splenectomy may be performed during *laparotomy* (surgical exploration of the abdomen) as part of a process (called staging) to assess the extent of *Hodgkin's disease*.

HOW IT IS DONE
Using a general anesthetic, a vertical or horizontal incision is made in the upper left abdomen, exposing the spleen. After attachments to other tissues have been cut and blood vessels leading into and out of the spleen have been clamped and severed, the organ is removed. The operation takes about an hour.

RECOVERY PERIOD AND OUTLOOK
Patients usually leave the hospital six to 10 days after the operation. Complications, such as infection of the operation site, are rare.

In an adult, absence of the spleen slightly increases the risk of contracting infections; children become markedly more susceptible, particularly to pneumococcal pneumonia. A child who has undergone a splenectomy should be immunized with pneumococcal vaccine and given long-term *antibiotic drugs*. Healthy fragments of a removed spleen are occasionally reimplanted in a child immediately after splenectomy; in some cases, these fragments regenerate to form an efficient new spleen.

Splint
A device used to immobilize part of the body. Splints may be made of acrylic, polyethylene foam, plaster of Paris, or aluminum. Ambulances may carry inflatable splints. In an emergency, a splint can be constructed from a piece of wood or a rolled magazine or newspaper that is secured to the extremity.

Splinting
The application of a *splint*. Splinting is used as a first-aid measure (see illustrated box) to prevent movement of a fractured limb or to immobilize a suspected fracture of the spine; this is especially important when the victim is being moved.

Splinting is sometimes required for leg fractures that are being treated by *traction*. Other uses of splint-

ing include treatment of finger injuries, such as fracture or *baseball finger*, and of rheumatic disorders affecting the fingers, such as *tenosynovitis* (inflammation of tendon linings) and *rheumatoid arthritis*.

Splinting, dental
The mechanical joining of several teeth to hold them firmly in place while an injury heals or *periodontal disease* is treated.

Splints may be used to secure teeth that have been fractured (see *Fracture, dental*) or loosened (see *Luxated tooth*). They may also be used after a tooth has been reimplanted (see *Reimplantation, dental*). Occasionally, teeth loosened by periodontal disease may be splinted to adjacent, firmer teeth. Splints may also be required after *orthognathic surgery*.

Splints are fashioned directly in the mouth with a variety of materials,

such as wire, quick-setting plastic, and plastic crowns that can be bonded together. (See also *Wiring of the jaws*.)

Split personality
A term used to describe two distinct disorders—*multiple personality*, in which an individual has two or more personalities, each of which dominates at different times, and *schizophrenia*, in which the sufferer's feelings and thoughts are not logically related to each other.

Spondylitis
Inflammation of the joints between the vertebrae in the spine. Spondylitis is usually caused by a rheumatic disorder, such as *ankylosing spondylitis* or *rheumatoid arthritis*. In rare cases, spondylitis is due to a bacterial infection that has spread from elsewhere in the body.

FIRST AID: SPLINTS

1 If help is coming, do not move the victim but support the limb by placing one hand above the fracture and the other below it.

2 If the ambulance is delayed or if the victim must be moved out of danger, first immobilize the leg. Place soft padding, such as a roll of cotton rolled around a splint, between the victim's knees and ankles and gently bring the uninjured leg to the injured one.

3 Tie the victim's ankles and feet together with a figure-of-eight bandage. Secure the bandage on the victim's uninjured side.

4 Tie bandages around the knees, thighs, and legs, being careful to avoid the fracture site. Tie all knots on the uninjured side.

S

Spondylolisthesis

The slipping forward (or occasionally backward) of a vertebra over the one below it. A forward slippage of the fifth (lowest) lumbar vertebra over the top of the sacrum is the most common form of the condition, but it may also occur between the fourth and fifth lumbar vertebrae or between two cervical (neck) vertebrae.

CAUSES AND SYMPTOMS

Lumbar spondylolisthesis, which involves two lumbar vertebrae or the fifth lumbar vertebra and the sacrum, is usually due to *spondylolysis* (in which the bony arch of a lumbar vertebra is abnormally soft and thus liable to slip under stress) or to *osteoarthritis* of the spine (in which the joints between the vertebrae become worn and unstable).

The principal symptoms of lumbar spondylolisthesis include pain in the back that is worse when standing and *sciatica*.

Cervical spondylolisthesis may be caused by a neck injury, congenital abnormality of the cervical spine, or *rheumatoid arthritis* (in which the supporting ligaments of the cervical spine are weakened or the joints between the vertebrae become worn). The main symptoms are pain and stiffness in the neck and, in severe cases, pain, numbness, or weakness in the sufferer's hands and arms.

DIAGNOSIS AND TREATMENT

Spondylolisthesis is diagnosed by X rays of the spine. Treatment may include *traction*, immobilization of the affected area in a plaster jacket or cervical collar, and *physical therapy*. In severe and rare cases (in which there is nerve compression damage or severe back pain), an operation to fuse the affected vertebrae may be necessary (see *Spinal fusion*).

| Normal spine | Spondylolisthesis |

Lumbar vertebra slips forward — Defect

Spinal nerves becomes distorted

Sacrum

Lumbar spondylolisthesis
If the lowest lumbar vertebra slips forward on the sacrum, it may distort or press on a spinal nerve, causing symptoms such as backache or sciatica.

Spondylolysis

A spinal disorder in which the arch of the fifth (or, rarely, the fourth) lumbar vertebra consists of relatively soft fibrous tissue instead of normal bone. As a result, the arch is weaker than normal and is more likely to be deformed or damaged under stress, which may produce *spondylolisthesis* (forward slippage of a vertebra over the one below it). Otherwise, spondylolysis is usually symptomless.

Sponge, contraceptive

A disposable, circular piece of polyurethane foam impregnated with *spermicide* that is inserted into the vagina as a method of birth control. (See *Contraception, barrier methods*.)

Sporotrichosis

A chronic infection caused by the fungus *SPOROTHRIX SCHENCKII*, which grows on moss and other plants. The infection is most often contracted through a skin wound; gardeners and florists are particularly vulnerable. An ulcer develops at the site of the wound and is followed by the formation of nodules (which can be seen as a chain of protuberances beneath the skin) in lymph channels around the site. Potassium iodide solution taken by mouth usually clears up the infection.

Rarely, in people whose resistance to disease has been lowered, sporotrichosis spreads to the lungs, joints, and other parts of the body. This condition may require prolonged treatment with the *antifungal drug* amphotericin B.

Sports, drugs and

The use of drugs to improve athletic performance has been universally condemned by authorities because it endangers the health of athletes and gives users of drugs an unfair advantage. Random urine tests to detect drug abuse are performed in most sports, both during competition and at other times during the season.

Certain drugs may be taken legitimately by athletes for medical disorders such as asthma or epilepsy. Care should be used, however, when taking a drug to treat diarrhea, nasal congestion, or cough because some common medications contain prohibited substances.

TYPES OF DRUGS ABUSED

Four types of drugs are abused to enhance physical or mental condition.

STIMULANTS Drugs of this group are taken to prevent fatigue and to increase self-confidence. However, they also impair judgment and may cause excessive aggression, which increases the risk of injury to the user or an opponent.

Stimulants, such as *amphetamine drugs*, carry the risk of causing *arrhythmias*; prolonged use may cause *heart failure* (reduced pumping efficiency) and increase the risk of a *brain hemorrhage*. Some cold and cough remedies contain low doses of prohibited drugs and should be avoided before competition.

Caffeine contained in coffee, tea, and cola drinks, and available in tablets, is another popular stimulant. Most authorities only prohibit the use of caffeine in high doses.

HORMONES Two types of hormone drugs may be abused—anabolic steroids (see *Steroids, anabolic*) and growth hormone.

Anabolic steroids are substances similar to the male sex hormone testosterone. They are used because they speed the recovery of muscles after strenuous exercise. This permits a more demanding training schedule and causes an increase in muscle bulk and strength. Anabolic steroids are used primarily by weight lifters, field event athletes, and bodybuilders.

Risks of anabolic steroids include liver damage, liver tumors, and adrenal gland damage. In men they may cause infertility and impotence; in women they may cause *virilization*. If taken during childhood, anabolic steroids may cause short stature by affecting the growing areas of bones.

Growth hormone is abused to stimulate growth of muscle; it is likely to cause *acromegaly* (excessive bone growth leading to deformity of the face, hands, and feet) and may cause *diabetes mellitus*.

PAINKILLERS Only narcotic *analgesics* are prohibited but the use of any painkiller (even a weak analgesic such as acetaminophen) may aggravate an injury or lead to permanent damage by allowing the individual to participate with his or her pain masked.

BETA-BLOCKER DRUGS *Beta-blocker drugs* are taken to reduce tremor in sports in which a steady hand is vital. Many authorities now prohibit these drugs in the absence of a specific medical disorder that requires them.

Sports injuries

Any injury that arises during participation in sports. Most sports injuries are not actually specific to sports; they can also occur as the result of other activities.

S

The wide range of sports injuries includes all types of *fracture*, *head injury* (including *concussion*), muscle tear (see *Strain*), ligament *sprain* or tears, *tendinitis* (inflammation of a tendon) or tendon rupture, joint *dislocation* or *subluxation* (partial dislocation), or injury to a specific organ (such as an *eye injury*).

Injuries specific to sports activities are mostly comparatively trivial. Examples include *joggers' nipple* (nipple soreness caused by friction) and *baseball finger* (tendon rupture in a finger caused by the ball striking the end of the finger).

Many injuries are given a sports prefix to their names, but can also be caused by injury unrelated to sports. *Tennis elbow* (painful inflammation of the bony prominence on the outside of the elbow) is a type of *overuse injury* that may occur from playing tennis, but more commonly results from an activity such as sawing wood.

Treatment of a sports injury depends on the body part involved and the severity of the damage. Recovery is not complete until the damaged area is free of pain during exercise. Exercises under the guidance of a sports physician or physical therapist may be required to ensure full recovery of movement, balance, and coordination of the injured part and to restore general fitness to reduce the likelihood of further injury.

Sports medicine
The branch of medicine concerned with assessment and improvement of *fitness* and the treatment and prevention of medical disorders related to sports. Sports medicine physicians give advice about exercises that improve endurance, strength, and flexibility; perform fitness tests; offer nutritional advice to improve performance; regulate the abuse of drugs by athletes (see *Sports, drugs and*); and provide on-site medical care at sporting events.

Preventive work in sports medicine includes advising the individual on footwear, clothing, and protective equipment to reduce the likelihood of injury, and on fluid requirements to prevent dehydration. In addition, the sports physician advises professional athletes on immunization requirements before competition abroad, on coping with *jet lag*, and on changes in altitude and climate. In conjunction with the physical therapist (see *Physical therapy*), a sports physician diagnoses and treats *sports injuries*.

Spouse abuse
Repeated deliberate physical injury inflicted by one spouse on the other, most often by a man on a woman.

PREVALENCE
About one third of all reported assaults are by males on their female partners, and about one third of women filing for divorce describe physical abuse. There is little doubt that in addition to reported cases of spouse abuse many cases go unreported. In about 20 percent of reported cases the abuse continues for more than 10 years.

CAUSES
Men who abuse their spouses have usually learned domestic violence from their parents' behavior, have an immature personality and low self-esteem, and acquire macho attitudes from their peer groups. Aggravating factors including *alcohol dependence*, *drug abuse*, *stress*, and obsession with the partner's sexual fidelity (see *Jealousy, morbid*).

Abused women in many cases stay with their partners for a combination of reasons, the most common of which are feelings of personal inadequacy, a sense of guilt leading to the belief that the violence is justified, fear of the social stigma involved in telling others about the abuse, underlying love for the partner, financial dependence, unwillingness to break up the family, social isolation, and depression (producing apathy).

MANAGEMENT OF THE PROBLEM
Shelters have been opened in some areas to provide a temporary refuge for abused women and their children. More effective means of enforcing alimony payments by the courts would provide women with the financial resources needed to leave their partners. *Marital counseling* also has a role, provided the couple wishes to address the problem openly.

The best long-term approach to reducing the scale of the problem probably lies through education and a downgrading of the traditional macho view of acceptable male behavior.

Sprain
Tearing or stretching of the ligaments that hold together the bone ends in a joint, caused by a sudden pull. The fibrous capsule that encloses the joint may also be damaged. The most commonly sprained joint is the ankle; it is usually sprained as a result of "going over" the outside of the foot so that the complete weight of the body is placed on the ankle.

A sprain causes painful swelling of the joint, which cannot be moved without increasing the pain. There may also be spasm (involuntary contraction) of surrounding muscles.

TREATMENT
An X ray of the joint is usually performed to exclude the possibility of fracture. Treatment consists of applying an ice pack to reduce swelling, wrapping the joint with a compression bandage, resting it in a raised position until the pain and swelling begin to subside, and taking *analgesics* (painkillers) to relieve pain. Once the joint is no longer painful, it should be gently exercised.

If ligaments are badly torn, *nonsteroidal anti-inflammatory drugs* may be prescribed to speed healing. In extremely severe cases, surgical repair may be necessary.

Sprue
A disorder of the intestines that causes failure to absorb nutrients from food. There are two forms of sprue. One occurs mainly in tropical regions (see *Sprue, tropical*); the other, *celiac sprue*, occurs more widely and is due to sensitivity to the wheat protein gluten.

Sprue, tropical
A disease characterized by chronic *malabsorption* (impaired absorption of nutrients from the diet by the small intestine) and, as a result, *malnutrition*. As in *celiac sprue*, villi (frondlike projections) on the lining of the intestine become flattened, decreasing their surface for absorption.

CAUSE AND INCIDENCE
The cause of tropical sprue is unknown, but it may result from an infection of the intestine. The disease occurs in tropical regions (e.g., the Caribbean, Far East, and India).

SYMPTOMS AND TREATMENT
Symptoms include loss of appetite, weight loss, megaloblastic *anemia* (caused by a deficiency of folic acid and vitamin B_{12}), an inflamed mouth, sore tongue, and greasy diarrhea.

The diagnosis is confirmed by a jejunal *biopsy* (removal of a small sample of tissue from the upper small intestine for analysis). The disease responds well to treatment with *antibiotic drugs* and dietary supplements of folic acid, vitamin B_{12}, and other vitamins and minerals if necessary.

Sputum
Mucous material produced by the cells lining the respiratory tract. Also known as phlegm, sputum is released

S

FIRST AID: SPRAINS

> **WARNING**
> A severe sprain may be indistin-
> guishable from a broken bone. If
> in doubt, treat as a *fracture*.

1 The victim may not be able to move the affected joint or stand up if the knee or ankle is injured. Help the victim into a comfortable position and raise the injured body part.

2 If the sprain is recent, apply a cold compress to the affected area and leave for about 30 minutes. This will reduce blood flow and swelling.

3 Cover the area with a roll of cotton and secure with a bandage. Make two turns around the foot, bring it across the top, and around the ankle.

4 Continue figure-of-eight turns, with each turn of the bandage overlapping the last turn by three fourths of its width.

5 Bandage until the foot (not toes), ankle, and lower leg are covered. Secure the loose end. Seek medical aid—an X ray may be necessary.

from glands in the walls of the bronchi (airways) and from cells lining the nose and sinuses.

Sputum production may be increased by infection (see *Respiratory tract infection*), by an allergic reaction (see *Asthma*; *Rhinitis, allergic*), or by inhalation of irritants, such as tobacco smoke (see *Cough, smokers'*). The presence of sputum in the bronchi triggers a reflex *cough*.

The character of sputum varies. A bacterial infection usually causes yellow or green sputum, an allergic reaction normally produces colorless sputum, and pulmonary *edema* (fluid retention in the lungs) may result in frothy, pink sputum. *Hemoptysis* (blood in the sputum) may be caused by infection or *lung cancer*.

Sputum may be examined under a microscope or prepared to *culture* any bacteria that might be present.

Squamous cell carcinoma

One of the three most common types of skin cancer; the others are *basal cell carcinoma* and malignant *melanoma*.

CAUSES AND INCIDENCE
Squamous cell carcinoma arises from flattened, scalelike cells in the skin, usually areas that have been exposed to strong sunlight for many years and that may already have developed actinic or solar *keratoses*. This cancer is most common in pale-skinned, fair-haired people older than 60. The incidence is also higher in people whose work has exposed them to compounds such as arsenic, tar, coal, paraffin, or heavy oils.

A squamous cell carcinoma
This tumor has spread slowly to cover much of the area in front of the patient's ear. It can be treated by radiation therapy.

SYMPTOMS AND SIGNS
The tumor starts as a small, firm, painless lump or patch (usually on the lip, ear, or back of the hand) and slowly enlarges, often resembling a wart or ulcer. If untreated, it may spread to other parts of the body and prove fatal. All suspicious skin lesions should be reported to a physician.

DIAGNOSIS AND TREATMENT
The diagnosis is based on a skin *biopsy* (removal of a small sample of tissue for analysis). The tumor is either removed surgically or destroyed by *radiation therapy* or *cryosurgery* (application of extreme cold). Treatment with *anticancer drugs* may also be necessary.

Any person who has had a squamous cell carcinoma should limit his or her exposure to sunlight. A follow-up examination is required to check for recurrence.

S

Squint

See *Strabismus*.

Stable

Unmoving, fixed, resistant to change, or in a state of equilibrium. A patient's condition is described as stable when it is neither deteriorating nor improving; a stable personality is one that is not susceptible to abnormal behavioral excesses or mental illness. In chemistry, a stable substance is one that is resistant to changes in its chemical composition or physical state, or is not radioactive.

Stage

A term used in medicine to refer to a period or phase in the course of a disease, particularly in the progression of *cancer*. In assessing most types of cancer, a method (staging) is used to determine how far the cancer has progressed. The cancer is described in terms of how large the main tumor is, the degree to which it has invaded surrounding tissue, and the extent to which it has spread to lymph glands or other areas of the body. In *Hodgkin's disease*, staging also takes into account whether the lymph nodes on both sides of the diaphragm are affected, and whether the spleen is involved.

Staging not only helps to assess outlook (in general, the more advanced the stage, the worse the outlook) but also the most appropriate treatment. For example, a cancer at a particular stage may respond better to radiation therapy than to surgery.

Staining

The process of dyeing specimens of cells, tissues, or microorganisms so that they are clearly visible or easily identifiable under a *microscope*. Staining is also sometimes carried out to detect or identify certain chemical substances in cells.

Before a specimen can be examined under a microscope, it must be preserved and then sliced (or smeared) extremely thinly. After these procedures, most specimens are almost transparent, so staining is necessary to make them easily visible. In *cytology* (the study of cells), cells are most commonly stained by the Papanicolaou (Pap) method; in *histology* (the study of tissues), the most commonly used stain is hematoxylin-eosin, a double stain that colors nuclei blue and cytoplasm pink.

Many other stains can be used to identify particular structures or products within cells. These stains may be used in addition to hematoxylin-eosin to clarify a diagnosis or to identify a particular microorganism in tissues.

In bacteriology, *Gram's stain* is widely used to identify and differentiate between groups of bacteria. A more recent development is the use of special fluorescent dyes that stain specific chemical constituents of cells or tissues; when illuminated with ultraviolet light, the stained constituents glow.

Another widely used technique called immunoperoxidase staining involves labeling (washing) the cells with antibodies to various cell components or cell chemicals. The antibodies are tagged with a dye that can be seen under the microscope as red-brown, enabling the observer to identify certain components if they are present within the cell.

Stammering

See *Stuttering*.

Stanford-Binet test

A type of *intelligence test*.

Stanozolol

A steroid drug (see *Steroids, anabolic*).

Stapedectomy

An operation to treat hearing loss caused by *otosclerosis*. In this disorder, the base of the *stapes* (the innermost of the three sound-conducting bones in the middle ear) becomes fixed to the entrance of the inner ear by an overgrowth of spongy bone. As a result, the stapes can no longer move freely to transmit sound to the inner ear. This form of deafness, often familial, is helped by a hearing aid but is curable only by surgery.

HOW IT IS DONE

Using a local or general anesthetic, an incision is made in the ear canal and the eardrum is folded forward. All or most of the stapes is removed and a plastic or metal prosthesis is inserted into the entrance to the inner ear; the other end is attached to the incus (the middle auditory ossicle). In this way, sound can once again be successfully transmitted to the inner ear. The eardrum is then repaired.

OUTLOOK

The operation improves hearing considerably in more than 90 percent of cases. However, in about 1 percent of patients, hearing deteriorates or is lost altogether. Because of this risk, a stapedectomy is usually carried out on only one ear at a time, although otosclerosis usually affects both ears.

Stapes

Also known as the stirrup because of its shape, the stapes is the innermost of the three tiny, sound-conducting bones in the middle ear called auditory ossicles (see *Ear*); it is the smallest bone in the body. The head of the stapes articulates with the incus (the middle auditory ossicle) and its base fits into the oval window in the wall of the inner ear.

Overgrowth of bone that causes the stapes to become fixed in position (*otosclerosis*) can cause deafness.

Staphylococcal infections

 A group of infections caused by bacteria of the staphylococcus family. Staphylococci, which grow in grapelike clusters, are a common cause of skin infections but can also cause serious internal disorders.

Staphylococcal bacteria are present harmlessly on the skin of most people. If the bacteria become trapped within the skin by a blocked sweat or sebaceous gland, they may cause superficial skin infections, such as *pustules, boils, abscesses, styes*, or *carbuncles*. Infection of deeper tissues may result if the skin is broken (see *Wound infection*). In newborn babies, toxins released by bacteria on the skin can cause a severe, blistering rash called the scalded skin syndrome (see *Necrolysis, toxic epidermal*).

Staphylococcal bacteria are also harmlessly present in the membranes that line the nose and throat. When mucus is not cleared from the lungs, such as after a viral infection, organisms may accumulate in the lungs and cause *pneumonia*.

In menstruating women (particularly those using highly absorbent tampons), toxin-producing staphylococci may colonize the mucous membranes lining the vagina, causing *toxic shock syndrome*. A different type of staphylococcus can cause *urinary tract infection*.

Sometimes staphylococci enter the bloodstream as a result of spread from a skin infection or as a result of introduction from a needle, leading to *septic shock*, infectious *arthritis, osteomyelitis*, or bacterial *endocarditis*.

Staphylococcal *food poisoning* is caused by ingestion of toxins produced by the bacteria. A common source of contamination is a pustule on the skin of a food handler.

Starch

See *Carbohydrates*.

S

Starvation

A condition caused by lack of food over a long period, resulting in weight loss, changes in *metabolism* (body chemistry), and extreme hunger. (See also *Anorexia nervosa; Fasting; Nutritional disorders*.)

Stasis

A reduction or cessation of flow. For example, in venous stasis there is diminution or complete stoppage of blood flow through one or more veins.

Statistics, medical

The science of medical statistics has grown rapidly in recent years as physicians feel increasing pressure from insurance companies and the public to evaluate and choose among the numerous medical treatments available. As a result, all medical research institutions today employ statisticians to advise on the design and interpretation of medical trials, and on the interpretation of data obtained from such trials.

For example, when two treatments are to be compared (or the results of surgical treatment are to be compared with not operating), the statistician advises on how many patients are required in the trial to establish a valid conclusion. He or she also advises on other aspects of methodology, including how to allocate patients to various treatment groups, how frequently to take measurements of the outcomes of the treatments, and how to analyze the mathematical results.

In addition to assessing treatments, statisticians are involved in the analysis of other medical data, which may be as diverse as the *incidence* and *prevalence* of various disorders and diseases, infection rates after surgery, waiting times in outpatient clinics, and the frequency of side effects from drugs. (See also *Statistics, vital*.)

Statistics, vital

Assessment of the health of a country's population, which relies on the collection of data on birth and death rates and the causes of death (see *Mortality*). In most Western countries today, all deaths are certified (usually by a medical practitioner) and recorded in a national register. They are then classified by cause and analyzed according to factors such as age, sex, occupation, social class, and ethnic group. Particular attention is paid to deaths associated with childbirth (see *Maternal mortality; Infant mortality*) or with factors that cause public concern, such as alcohol or drug abuse, accidents, violence, or diseases such as AIDS, coronary heart disease, and cancer.

Comparison of the vital statistics of different countries (or regions within a country) gives a measure of the relative health of their populations as a whole. A detailed comparison may also show variations between social classes or ethnic groups. (See also *Life expectancy; Statistics, medical; Centers for Disease Control*.)

Status asthmaticus

A severe and prolonged attack of *asthma*. Status asthmaticus is a serious and potentially life-threatening condition that requires urgent treatment.

Status epilepticus

Prolonged or repeated epileptic seizures without any recovery of consciousness between attacks. Status epilepticus is a medical emergency that may be fatal if not treated promptly. It is more likely to occur if *anticonvulsant drugs* are taken erratically or if they are withdrawn suddenly. (See *Epilepsy*.)

STDs

See *Sexually transmitted diseases*.

Steatorrhea

The presence of excessive fat in the feces. Steatorrhea causes diarrhea characterized by offensive-smelling, bulky, loose, greasy, pale-colored feces, which tend to float in the toilet and are difficult to flush away. Steatorrhea is a symptom of diseases that interfere with the breakdown and absorption of fat in the diet (notably *pancreatitis* and *celiac sprue*) and of the removal of large segments of small intestine. It is also a side effect of some lipid-lowering drugs.

Stein-Leventhal syndrome

See *Polycystic ovary*.

Stenosis

Narrowing of a duct, canal, passage, or tubular organ, such as a blood vessel or the intestine. *Aortic stenosis* is narrowing of the aortic valve opening from the left ventricle (lower chamber of the heart); *pyloric stenosis* is narrowing of the pylorus (the lower outlet from the stomach).

Stereotaxic surgery

Brain operations carried out by inserting delicate instruments through a surgically created hole in the skull and guiding them, using *X rays* or *CT scanning*, to a specific area.

WHY IT IS DONE

Stereotaxic procedures are used in the treatment of pituitary gland tumors, in which the gland is cut out or a radioactive implant is inserted into the gland to destroy it.

Other uses include a brain *biopsy* (taking a small sample of tissue for analysis), insertion of permanent stimulating wires to control otherwise intractable pain, and destruction of areas of the brain to treat disabling neurological disorders, such as severe *depression* (see *Psychosurgery*) or, in rare cases, *temporal lobe epilepsy*. Stereotaxic surgery is also occasionally used to treat people with *Parkinson's disease* in whom severe tremor has not responded to drugs.

HOW IT IS DONE

With the use of a general or local anesthetic, an adjustable metal frame is attached to the skull with screws. The area to be treated is located by X rays or CT scanning and the best position for inserting the instrument is calculated mathematically. The skull is then entered by means of a *burr hole* or *craniotomy*, and the angle of the frame is adjusted to hold and guide a hollow tube into the brain at the correct angle. The required instrument (a needle for biopsies, a scalpel or diathermy probe for cutting or destroying areas) is then inserted through the tube and the operation is performed; more X rays or scans may be taken during the procedure.

Sterility

The state of being germ-free, or a term for permanent *infertility*.

Sterilization

A term that refers to the complete destruction or removal of living organisms or to any procedure that renders a person unable to reproduce (see *Sterilization, female; Vasectomy*).

The elimination of microorganisms is vitally important in preventing the spread of infection. It may be achieved by various physical or chemical means, such as by boiling, steaming, or autoclaving (steaming under high pressure); irradiation with ultraviolet light or X rays; or applying *antiseptics* or *disinfectants*. Sometimes, more than one method is used (e.g., bed linen may be disinfected and then autoclaved). Liquids can also be sterilized by passing them through extremely fine filters that trap microorganisms as tiny as viruses.

S

Sterilization, female

A usually permanent method of *contraception* in which the fallopian tubes are sealed or cut to prevent the male sperm from reaching the ova.

Sterilization is a common method of contraception; nearly 10 percent of women over the age of 30 and one fourth of women with five or more children have been sterilized.

WHY IT IS DONE

Women who have completed their families or do not plan to have children may choose to be sterilized to avoid the inconvenience or side effects of other methods of contraception. Sterilization may also be chosen by a woman in whom a pregnancy would be a serious threat to health, or in whom there is an unacceptably high risk of children being affected by a serious hereditary disease.

HOW IT IS DONE

The illustrated box shows common procedures for female sterilization, performed using *laparoscopy*.

Alternatively, the surgeon may work directly through a small incision just below the navel. Known as a minilaparotomy, this procedure is carried out in the first few weeks after a woman has delivered a baby, when the uterus is high in the abdomen and the fallopian tubes can be reached easily. In other cases, the surgeon may approach the fallopian tubes via the vagina. The tubes are cut and tied off.

Surgical removal of the uterus, fallopian tubes, or ovaries to treat specific disorders also results in sterilization. These operations are performed through a larger abdominal incision and today are considered too drastic to be performed only for sterilization.

In an investigational method, a hysteroscope (a type of endoscope) is passed through the vagina into the uterus; the exits to the fallopian tubes are plugged from the inside.

Most sterilization techniques are performed on an outpatient basis. Surgical removal of the uterus (see *Hysterectomy*) or fallopian tubes and ovaries (see *Salpingo-oophorectomy; Oophorectomy*) requires a hospital stay.

OUTLOOK

Sterilization has a small failure rate; if pregnancy does occur after sterilization, the chance of an *ectopic pregnancy* is 10 times greater than the normal rate. Although sterilization should be considered permanent, microsurgical techniques may be successful in restoring fertility; 70 to 75 percent of women who undergo such surgery later achieve pregnancy.

Sterilization, male

See *Vasectomy*.

Sternum

The anatomical name for the breastbone, the long, narrow, flat plate of bone that forms the central part of the front of the chest. The sternum consists of three main parts—an upper, triangular portion, called the manubrium; a long, narrow middle part, the body; and, at the lower end, a small, slightly flexible, leaf-shaped projection, the xiphoid process. The upper part of the manubrium articulates with the inner ends of the two *clavicles* (collarbones); attached to the sides of the manubrium and body are the seven pairs of costal cartilages that join the sternum to the *ribs*. Between the manubrium and body is a type of joint known as a *symphysis*. It allows slight movement between these two parts of the sternum when the ribs rise and fall during breathing.

The sternum is very strong and requires great force to fracture it. The principal danger of such an injury is not the fracture itself, but the possibility that the broken bone may be driven inward and damage the heart (which lies behind the sternum).

Steroid drugs

COMMON DRUGS

Nandrolone Oxandrolone Stanozolol

A group of drugs that includes the *corticosteroid drugs*, which are similar to hormones produced by the cortex of the *adrenal glands*, and the anabolic steroid drugs (see *Steroids, anabolic*), which have an effect similar to that of the hormones produced by the male sex organs.

Steroids, anabolic

Drugs that have an anabolic (protein-building) effect similar to *testosterone* and other male sex hormones.

FEMALE STERILIZATION

Laparoscopic sterilization (below) is the most common method. Both fallopian tubes must be cut, sealed, or otherwise obstructed so that eggs and sperm cannot meet for fertilization to occur.

Laparoscopic sterilization
An endoscope (viewing tube) and an operating instrument are passed through separate small incisions in the abdomen.

Instruments
The trocar is a sharp-pointed inner stylus surrounded by a close-fitting tube, the cannula. The instrument can be passed through the abdominal wall. After insertion, the trocar is removed, leaving the hollow cannula in place. Other instruments are passed through the hollow cannula.

Cutting
A small loop of the fallopian tube may be drawn up, secured by a tight ligature, and then cut off.

Constriction
The loop is constricted by a tight band. Reversal is possible with this sterilization technique.

Clipping
A plastic or metal clip may be applied to obstruct egg passage. In theory, this method is also reversible.

Cautery
Electrocoagulation (diathermy) can be used to burn through and thus seal the fallopian tube.

Cannula

Trocar

Laparoscopic operating instruments

S

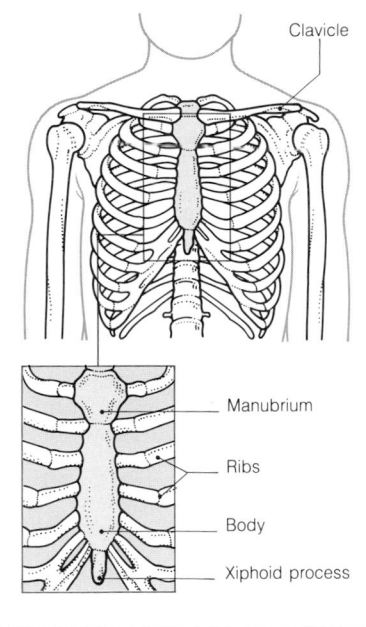

Clavicle

Manubrium

Ribs

Body

Xiphoid process

WHY THEY ARE USED

Anabolic steroids, by mimicking the anabolic effects of testosterone, build tissue, promote muscle recovery following injury, and help strengthen bones. They are given to treat some types of *anemia* and, infrequently, to treat postmenopausal women who have *osteoporosis*.

ABUSE

Anabolic steroid drugs have been widely abused by athletes despite the serious risks to health (see *Sports, drugs and*).

POSSIBLE ADVERSE EFFECTS

Adverse effects include acne, *edema*, liver and adrenal gland damage, infertility, impotence in men, and *virilization* in women.

Stethoscope

An instrument for listening to sounds in the body, particularly those made by the heart or lungs.

The standard stethoscope consists of a Y-shaped flexible plastic tube with an earpiece at the end of each arm of the Y, and a sound-detecting device at the base. One side of this device consists of a thin plastic diaphragm; the other side has a concave bell that has a hole in its center. A physician presses the diaphragm against a patient's chest or back to hear high-pitched sounds. The concave bell side is placed in gentle contact with the skin to hear low-pitched sounds.

Stevens-Johnson syndrome

A rare skin condition characterized by severe blisters and bleeding in the mucous membranes of the lips, eyes, mouth, nasal passage, and genitals. Stevens-Johnson syndrome is a severe form of *erythema multiforme*.

Sticky eye

A common description of one of the symptoms of *conjunctivitis* (inflammation of the conjunctival membrane) in which the eyelids become stuck together with discharge.

Stiff neck

A very common symptom, usually due to spasm (involuntary contraction) in muscles at the side or back of the neck. In most cases, the spasm occurs suddenly and for no apparent reason. It is usually first noticed as a stiff neck upon waking and is called *torticollis*, or wryneck. Torticollis is thought to occur as a result of a minor neck injury—such as a ligament *sprain* or *subluxation* (partial dislocation) of a cervical (neck) joint—that has passed unnoticed but has caused irritation of the cervical spinal nerves; this, in turn, leads to spasm of the neck muscles. A stiff neck due to muscle spasm may also be caused by a *disk prolapse* or by a *whiplash injury* in the cervical spine.

A relatively rare, but potentially serious, cause of a stiff neck is *meningitis* (infection of the meninges, the membranes that surround the brain and spinal cord). In such cases, the stiffness is usually accompanied

STETHOSCOPE

Earpieces

Tubing

Diaphragm

Bell

by headache, vomiting, fever, photophobia (abnormal sensitivity to light), and intense pain when bending the neck.

Stiffness

A term used to refer to difficulty in moving a joint, to restriction of movement in a joint, or to difficulty stretching a muscle.

Causes of joint stiffness include *arthritis* (inflammation of joint surfaces) and *capsulitis* (inflammation of the joint lining). In *rheumatoid arthritis*, severe joint stiffness may last up to two hours after waking. Causes of muscle stiffness include *cramp* and *spasticity* (increased rigidity).

Stillbirth

A baby born dead after the 28th week of *pregnancy*. Stillbirth is also called late fetal death. Stillbirths must be reported and the cause of death recorded on the death certificate.

INCIDENCE

The incidence of stillbirth has decreased dramatically in developed countries over the last 50 years. In the US the incidence fell from 19.2 stillbirths per 1,000 total births (i.e., live births plus stillbirths) in 1950 to 9.2 stillbirths per 1,000 total births in 1980. In general, stillbirths are more common in poor communities, among older women, and when good prenatal and obstetric care are lacking.

CAUSES

The precise cause of stillbirth is unknown in at least one third of cases. Severely malformed babies, particularly those with *anencephaly*, *spina bifida*, or *hydrocephalus*, account for at least one fifth of stillbirths.

A maternal disorder, such as *antepartum hemorrhage*, *hypertension* (high blood pressure), or any other condition affecting the function of the *placenta*, may result in stillbirth, often because the fetus is deprived of oxygen. Another cause is *Rh incompatibility* between mother and baby.

Some infectious diseases (including measles, chickenpox, influenza, toxoplasmosis, rubella, cytomegalovirus, herpes simplex, syphilis, and malaria) may harm the fetus if contracted during pregnancy. In general, the more severe the infection, the greater the risk of stillbirth. A pregnant woman who is exposed to an infectious disease to which she is not immune should consult her physician.

PSYCHOLOGICAL EFFECTS

The loss of a baby is deeply distressing. The bereaved parents usually

S

experience a sense of loss that is just as intense as if any other loved person had died, and often they experience feelings of depression, guilt, anger, and inadequacy. Emotional support from friends, relatives, and self-help groups is useful, as is counseling by a medical professional.

Still's disease

See *Rheumatoid arthritis, juvenile.*

Stimulant drugs

COMMON DRUGS

Nerve stimulants
Caffeine Dextroamphetamine
Methylphenidate

Respiratory stimulants
Doxapram Nikethamide

Drugs that increase nerve activity in the brain by initiating the release of *norepinephrine* from nerve endings (see *Neurotransmitter*).

TYPES

There are two main groups of stimulant drugs—nerve stimulants (including *amphetamine drugs*), which reduce drowsiness and increase alertness by their action on the reticular activating system in the *brain stem,* and respiratory stimulants (see *Analeptic drugs*), which act on the respiratory center in the brain stem.

WHY THEY ARE USED

Nerve stimulants are given to treat *narcolepsy* (characterized by excessive sleepiness). Paradoxically, they have also been found useful in the treatment of *hyperactivity* in children. Nerve stimulants also suppress the appetite but their use in the treatment of *obesity* has decreased because of their adverse effects.

Despite the risk of adverse effects, nerve stimulants are sometimes abused because they prevent fatigue, increase alertness, and may improve self-confidence. The use of nerve stimulants by athletes is widely condemned by physicians and sports organizations (see *Sports, drugs and*).

POSSIBLE ADVERSE EFFECTS

Effects include shaking, sweating, palpitations, nervousness, sleeping problems, hallucinations, paranoid delusions, and seizures. Long-term use may lead to *tolerance* (the need for greater amounts to have the same effects) and *drug dependence.*

Stimulus

Anything that evokes a response (i.e., an agent or event that directly results in a change in the activities of the body as a whole or of any individual part). For example, the sight and smell of food stimulate salivation. Certain nerve cells (known collectively as *receptors*) are specialized to respond to specific stimuli. One example of such nerve cell specialization is the rods and cones in the retina of the eye that respond to light.

Stings

Stinging animals include scorpions and some insects (such as bees and wasps), jellyfish and related marine animals (such as anemones and corals), and some fish (such as stingrays). There are marked differences among these groups in the way the sting is delivered and its effects. (See *Insect stings; Scorpion stings; Jellyfish stings; Venomous bites and stings*.)

Nettles and some other plants carry minute stinging hairs that hold an irritant liquid. The hairs penetrate and break off in the skin; the liquid enters the wound and has an immediate irritant effect, which rarely lasts more than an hour or two. Washing the affected area and applying calamine lotion can provide relief. Contact with poison ivy and related plants may result in a more severe allergic reaction, sometimes requiring medical attention (see *Plants, poisonous*).

Stitch

A temporary, sudden, sharp pain in the abdomen or side that occurs during severe or unaccustomed exercise, usually running. The cause of a stitch is unknown.

Stitch is also commonly used to refer to a suture used to close a wound (see *Suturing*).

Stokes-Adams syndrome

Recurrent episodes of temporary loss of consciousness caused by insufficient blood flow from the heart to the brain. This deficient blood supply is due to very rapid or very slow arrhythmia (see *Arrhythmia, cardiac*), which markedly reduces the pumping efficiency of the heart, or to complete *heart block* (abnormally slow conduction of electrical impulses through the heart muscle), resulting in temporary cessation of the heart beat.

SYMPTOMS AND TREATMENT

In a typical attack, the person faints suddenly and turns blue if the period of unconsciousness is prolonged. The breathing rate increases and a very slow pulse can be felt. Occasionally, lack of oxygen supply to the brain may cause a *seizure* (convulsion).

In most cases, the heart soon starts beating again, the skin flushes, and consciousness is regained. If this fails to happen, *cardiopulmonary resuscitation* should be carried out promptly to prevent brain damage.

Most sufferers are fitted with a *pacemaker* to maintain normal heart beat and prevent future attacks.

Stoma

A term meaning mouth or orifice. A stoma in the abdomen acts as an artificial anus; it may be temporary (diverting feces from a healing wound in the intestine) or permanent (because part of the intestine has been removed). See also *Colostomy; Ileostomy.*

Stomach

A hollow, saclike organ of the *digestive system* that is connected to the esophagus and the duodenum (the first part of the small intestine). The stomach lies in the left side of the abdomen under the diaphragm.

STRUCTURE

The stomach is flexible, allowing it to expand when food is eaten; in an adult, the average capacity is about 3

LOCATION OF THE STOMACH
Food enters the stomach from the esophagus and exits into the duodenum. The stomach lining secretes gastric juice and protective mucus.

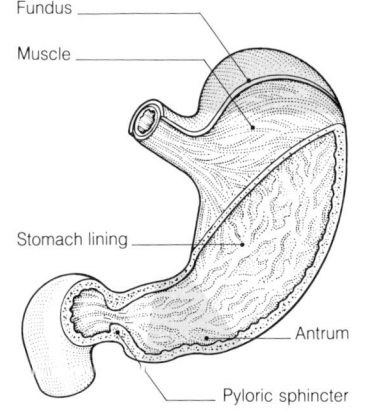

Fundus

Muscle

Stomach lining

Antrum

Pyloric sphincter

Parts of the stomach
The fundus and antrum are two of the main stomach parts; the lower esophageal segment and pyloric sphincters control entry and exit of food.

DISORDERS OF THE STOMACH

Disorders of the stomach have a variety of causes. Because the stomach is a reservoir, disorders in the process of emptying the stomach contents occur. Other problems relate to the stomach's role in the preparation of ingested food for digestion.

INFECTION

The large amount of hydrochloric acid secreted by the stomach protects the stomach from some infections by destroying many of the bacteria, viruses, and fungi that are taken in with food and drink. When the protective power is insufficient, a variety of gastrointestinal infections may occur.

TUMORS

Stomach cancer causes about 15,000 deaths annually in the US. Early symptoms are often mistaken for *indigestion* and diagnosis is often delayed until it is too late for a cure. Any change in the customary functioning of the digestive system is important, especially after fifty. A persistent feeling of fullness, or pain before or after meals, should never be ignored. Unexplained loss of appetite or frequent nausea should always be reported. A tumor in the upper part of the stomach, near the opening of the esophagus, can cause obstruction and difficulty in swallowing. Sometimes a stomach tumor remains "silent" and the first signs are due to the appearance of secondary growths elsewhere in the body.

Benign (noncancerous) *polyps* can also develop in the stomach.

ULCERATION

The acid and other digestive juices secreted by the stomach sometimes attack the stomach lining. The healthy stomach is prevented from digesting itself mainly by the protective layer of mucus secreted by the lining and by the speed with which damaged surface cells are replaced by the deeper layers. Many influences can upset this delicate balance. One of the most important is excessive acid secretion. The resulting *peptic ulcers* are probably the most common serious stomach disorder. Peptic ulcers are sometimes caused by stress, or by severe injury, such as major burns, accidents, and after surgery and severe infections; often they occur for no apparent reason. The stomach lining can be damaged by large amounts of aspirin or alcohol, sometimes causing *gastritis* (inflammation of the stomach lining). This may lead to ulceration of the stomach lining.

AUTOIMMUNE DISORDERS

Pernicious anemia is caused by the failure of the stomach lining to produce intrinsic factor, a substance whose role is to facilitate the absorption of vitamin B_{12}. Failure to produce the intrinsic factor occurs if there is atrophy of the stomach lining, which also causes failure of acid production. Tests that determine a person's ability to absorb vitamin B_{12} are important in the investigation of this condition. Pernicious anemia is usually due to an *autoimmune disorder*.

OTHER DISORDERS

Enlargement of the stomach may be caused when scarring from a chronic peptic ulcer occurs at the stomach outlet. It may also be a complication of *pyloric stenosis*, a rare but serious condition caused by narrowing of the stomach outlet. Rarely, the stomach may become twisted and obstructed, a condition called *volvulus*.

INVESTIGATION

Stomach disorders are investigated primarily by *barium X-ray examinations* and/or *gastroscopy*. Occasionally, a *biopsy* (removal of a tissue sample for microscopic analysis) is performed.

---

pints (1.5 liters). The stomach wall consists of layers of longitudinal and circular muscle, lined by special glandular cells that secrete gastric juice, and supplied by blood vessels and nerves. A strong muscle at the lower end of the stomach forms a ring called the pyloric sphincter that can close the outlet leading to the duodenum.

FUNCTION

Although the main function of the stomach is to continue the breakdown of food that is started in the mouth and completed in the small intestine, it also acts as a storage organ, enabling food to be eaten only two or three times a day. Food would have to be eaten every 20 minutes or so if storage were not possible.

The sight and smell of food and the arrival of food in the stomach stimulate gastric secretion. The gastric juice secreted from the stomach lining contains pepsin (an enzyme that breaks down protein), hydrochloric acid (which kills bacteria taken in with the food and which creates the most suitable environment for the pepsin to work in), and intrinsic factor (which is essential for the absorption of vitamin B_{12} in the small intestine). The stomach lining also contains glands that secrete mucus, which helps provide a barrier to prevent the stomach from digesting itself.

The layers of muscle produce rhythmic contractions about every 20 seconds that churn the food and gastric juice; the combined effect of this movement and the action of the digestive juice convert the semisolid food into a creamy fluid. This process takes varying lengths of time, depending on the nature of the food. Generally, however, the richer the meal, the longer it takes to be emptied from the stomach. The partially digested food is squirted into the duodenum at regular intervals by the contractions of the stomach and relaxation of the pyloric sphincter.

Stomach cancer

A malignant tumor that arises from the lining of the stomach, also called gastric cancer.

CAUSES AND INCIDENCE

The cause of stomach cancer remains uncertain but evidence suggests that an environmental factor, probably diet, plays a part. Recent speculation has centered on an association between stomach cancer and eating quantities of salted, pickled, or smoked foods. Certain other factors, such as megaloblastic *anemia*, partial *gastrectomy*, and belonging to blood group A, seem to increase the risk of this cancer developing.

S

Stomach cancer rarely affects people under the age of 40 and is twice as common in men as in women. There is marked geographic variation—with a very high rate of 80 to 90 cases per 100,000 people in Japan compared with fewer than 10 per 100,000 in the US, where it causes around 15,000 deaths per year. There has been a dramatic decrease in the worldwide incidence of stomach cancer over the past 50 years.

SYMPTOMS AND SIGNS
The symptoms of stomach cancer (if any) are often indistinguishable from those of *peptic ulcer*. In the advanced stages, there is usually loss of appetite, the sensation that the stomach is filling up quickly, nausea and vomiting, and weight loss.

DIAGNOSIS AND TREATMENT
The condition is suggested by *barium X-ray examination* and confirmed by *gastroscopy* (examination of the stomach by a flexible viewing tube). A *biopsy* of the stomach lining (removal of a tissue sample for microscopic examination) may also be performed using a gastroscope.

The only effective treatment is gastrectomy. However, only about 20 percent of patients are able to undergo such surgery; in the rest, the tumor has spread too widely at the time of diagnosis. In inoperable, advanced cases, *radiation therapy* and *anticancer drugs* may be used.

OUTLOOK
If the cancer is detected at a very early stage (before it has spread beyond the stomach lining), a high cure rate is possible. In Japan, where mass screening by gastroscopy is performed, 85 percent of people are still alive five years after treatment by surgery. In advanced disease, however, the outlook is not good, with less than 10 percent of patients surviving longer than five years.

Stomach imaging
See *Barium X-ray examinations.*

Stomach pump
See *Lavage, gastric.*

Stomach ulcer
A raw area in the stomach lining, also called a gastric ulcer. If nonmalignant, it is a *peptic ulcer.*

Stomatitis
Any form of inflammation or ulceration of the mouth. Examples include *mouth ulcers, cold sores, candidiasis* (thrush), and *Vincent's disease.*

Stones
Small, hard aggregates of solid material within the body. Also called calculi, they are formed from substances that are present to excess in fluids such as urine or bile. (See *Calculus, urinary tract; Gallstones.*)

Stool
Another word for *feces.*

Stork bite
A small, flat, harmless, pinkish-red skin blemish found in 30 to 50 percent of newborn babies. Such marks, which are also called salmon patches, are a type of *hemangioma* usually found around the eyes and at the nape of the neck. Stork bites around the eyes usually disappear within the first year; those at the base of the neck may persist indefinitely.

Strabismus
A condition in which there is abnormal deviation of one eye in relation to the other. Strabismus, also known as squint, may be convergent (cross-eye), in which one eye is directed too far inward, or divergent (walleye), in which one eye is directed outward. Occasionally, one eye is directed upward or downward relative to the other (vertical strabismus).

CAUSES
Strabismus usually starts in early childhood because of a failure in the

Convergent strabismus
This boy is using his right eye (note the light reflection in the center of the pupil). Left visual development has stopped.

Divergent strabismus
Simultaneous perception with both eyes would cause double vision, so the brain suppresses the image from the deviating eye.

proper development of the mechanisms that align the two eyes. A common contributory factor is *hyperopia* (farsightedness), which forces the child to *accommodate* (focus to see clearly) excessively and causes the eyes to turn inward.

In children who are acquiring the capacity to see simultaneously with two eyes, strabismus causes double vision and noncorresponding, different images from the malaligned eyes. Because of the double vision, the brain rapidly suppresses the image from the deviating eye. Strabismic *amblyopia* (visual loss) may occur.

In adults, strabismus may occur as a result of various disorders of the brain, of the nerves controlling the eye muscles, or of the eye muscles themselves. It may be a symptom of *stroke, diabetes mellitus, multiple sclerosis,* tumor, or thyroid eye disease. Strabismus that develops in adults causes double vision; although untreated strabismus may disappear, treatment is usually needed.

TREATMENT
Treatment in young children may include covering the normal eye with a patch to force the child to use the weak (amblyopic) eye. This treatment attempts to allow development of normal vision in the affected eye by establishing the functional connections between the eye and the brain. Glasses and/or surgery can be used to try to correct the deviation of the eyes. Patching to try to improve the poor vision in the weak eye may be tried until age 10; surgery can be performed later to improve appearance.

Strabismus acquired later in life always causes double vision and requires medical investigation of the underlying cause. If the strabismus does not clear up, then special glasses or surgery may be tried.

Strain
Tearing or stretching of muscle fibers as a result of suddenly pulling them too far. There is bleeding into the damaged area of muscle, causing pain, swelling, and muscle spasm; a bruise usually appears a few days after the injury. Muscle strain of the back is a common cause of nonspecific *back pain.* Strains are most common in athletes.

Treatment consists of applying an ice pack to the affected area to reduce swelling, wrapping it with a compression bandage, and resting the limb in a raised position for 48 hours. Analgesics (painkillers) may also be

S

taken to relieve pain. After resting the muscle, *physical therapy* involving stretching exercises should be started to prevent possible shortening of the muscle as a result of scar tissue forming in it. In some cases, *nonsteroidal anti-inflammatory drugs* may be prescribed to speed healing.

The risk of muscle strain can be reduced by performing warm-up exercises before any sports activity.

Strangulation

The constriction, usually by twisting or compression, of a tube or conduit in the body, blocking blood flow and interfering with the function of the affected organ. This may occur with a *hernia* or after twisting of the testis (see *Testis, torsion of*).

Strangulation of the neck with the hands or with a ligature, such as a cord or scarf, may be deliberate or accidental. The primary lethal effect arises from compression of the jugular veins in the neck. This prevents blood from flowing out of the brain and head, where it stagnates and its oxygen content is quickly used up. In addition, compression of the windpipe restricts breathing and impairs oxygenation of the blood. The victim's face becomes congested with blood and takes on a livid purple-blue coloration. He or she loses consciousness and, some minutes later, brain damage and death occur from lack of oxygen.

Any constricting ligature must be removed as quickly as possible and medical help summoned. If the victim is not breathing, *artificial respiration* should be performed until an ambulance or physician arrives.

FIRST AID: STRAIN

1 Make the victim as comfortable as possible, then steady and support the injured part.

2 Apply a cold compress to reduce pain and swelling. Seek medical aid.

To prevent accidental strangulation, a child's environment should be kept free of potential ligatures—such as cords on toys or clothing or dangerous restraining apparatus. Children should be discouraged from playing with lassos.

Strangury

A symptom characterized by a painful and frequent desire to empty the bladder, although only a few drops of urine can be passed. Causes of strangury include *prostatitis* (inflammation of the prostate gland), *cystitis*, and bladder cancer (see *Bladder tumors*).

Strapping

The application of adhesive tape to part of the body to exert pressure and hold a structure in place. Strapping is used to reduce pain and swelling caused by soft tissue injuries, such as sprains and muscle tears. It may also be applied to joints to prevent injury due to excessive movement, or to strengthen a joint that has been injured to help prevent recurrence.

Strawberry nevus

A bright red, raised birthmark that is a type of *hemangioma*.

Strep throat

An infection of the throat caused by certain bacteria of the streptococcus group. Strep throat is most common in children and is spread by droplets (containing the bacteria) that are coughed or breathed into the air.

In some people, the bacteria cause few or no symptoms, but a proportion suffer a sore throat, fever, general malaise, and enlarged lymph nodes in the neck. In some cases, toxins released by the bacteria lead to a rash, a condition known as *scarlet fever*.

The diagnosis is usually made by identifying the bacteria in a culture grown from a throat swab. The infection is treated with penicillin or with another antibiotic drug if the person is allergic to penicillin.

An untreated strep throat infection may lead to the serious complications of *glomerulonephritis* (inflammation in the kidneys) or *rheumatic fever*.

Streptococcal infections

A group of infections caused by bacteria of the streptococcus family. Streptococci are spherical bacteria that grow like strung beads; they are among the most common disease-causing bacteria in humans.

Certain types of streptococci are present harmlessly in most people's mouths and throats. If the bacteria gain access to the bloodstream (sometimes after dental treatment), they are usually destroyed. However, in some people with heart valve defects there is a risk of the bacteria settling in the heart to cause bacterial *endocarditis*. Another type of streptococcus is present harmlessly in the intestines but can spread, via the urethra, to cause a *urinary tract infection*.

Other types of streptococci cause *tonsillitis*, *strep throat*, *otitis media* (middle-ear infection), *pneumonia*, *erysipelas*, or wound infections.

Beta-hemolytic streptococcal infection may be the cause of any of the aforementioned, or may result in *scarlet fever* (characterized by a rash).

Infections from these same streptococci may also give rise to the serious complications of *rheumatic fever* and *glomerulonephritis*. These infections are prevented through prompt treatment with *antibiotic drugs* (most often penicillin).

People in whom rheumatic fever has developed are advised to take an antibiotic drug before, during, and after dental treatment and certain diagnostic and surgical procedures.

Streptokinase

A *thrombolytic drug* used to dissolve blood clots in *myocardial infarction* (heart attack) and *pulmonary embolism*. Streptokinase is most effective in dissolving newly formed clots. Given by injection in the early stages of a heart attack, streptokinase may limit the amount of damage that is caused to the heart muscle.

Treatment with streptokinase is strictly supervised because of the risk of allergic reaction or excessive bleeding. Other adverse effects include rash, fever, wheezing, and *arrhythmias* (irregularities of the heart beat).

Streptomycin

An *antibiotic drug* used to treat a number of uncommon infections, including *tularemia*, *plague*, *brucellosis*, and *glanders*. Streptomycin is sometimes given with a *penicillin drug* to treat *endocarditis* (inflammation of the lining of the heart and heart valves).

Once used to treat a wide range of other infections, streptomycin has now been largely superseded by newer, more effective drugs with less serious side effects. Discovered in the 1940s, streptomycin was the first effective drug treatment for *tuber-*

S

culosis; it is still sometimes used to treat resistant strains.

POSSIBLE ADVERSE EFFECTS

Most seriously, streptomycin may damage nerves in the inner ear, disturbing balance and causing dizziness, ringing in the ears, and deafness. Other possible adverse effects include numbness of the face, tingling in the hands, headache, malaise, nausea, and vomiting.

Stress

Any interference that disturbs a person's healthy mental and physical well-being. A person may experience stress in response to a wide range of physical and emotional stimuli, including physical violence, internal conflicts, and significant life events (e.g., death of a loved one, the birth of a baby, or divorce). Some people are more susceptible than others to stress-related medical problems.

EFFECTS

When faced with a stressful situation, the body responds by increasing production of certain hormones, such as *cortisol* and *epinephrine*. These hormones lead to changes in heart rate, blood pressure, metabolism, and physical activity designed to improve overall performance. However, at a certain level, they disrupt an individual's ability to cope. Less than 20 percent of people are effective in crises such as fires or floods.

Continued exposure to stress often leads to mental and physical symptoms, such as *anxiety* and *depression*, *dyspepsia*, palpitations, and muscular aches and pains. *Posttraumatic stress disorder* is a direct response to a specific stressful event. (See also *Relaxation techniques*.)

Stress fracture

A *fracture* that occurs as a result of repetitive jarring of a bone. Common sites include the metatarsal bones in the foot (see *March fracture*), the tibia or fibula (lower leg bones), the neck of the femur (thigh bone), and the lumbar region of the spine. Stress fractures are most common among runners, particularly those who run on hard surfaces with inadequate footwear (see *Sports injuries*).

The main symptoms include pain and tenderness at the fracture site. Diagnosis is by X rays, although sometimes a stress fracture does not show up on an X ray until it has started to heal. Occasionally, a radionuclide bone scan (see *Bone imaging*) may be performed to confirm the diagnosis.

Treatment consists of resting the affected area for four to six weeks. In some cases, it is also necessary to immobilize the fracture in a plaster cast. After recovery, modification of exercise routines and the use of suitably cushioned footwear may help to prevent a recurrence.

Stress ulcer

An acute *peptic ulcer* that sometimes develops after shock, serious burns, severe injuries, or during a major illness. Stress ulcers are usually multiple and are most common in the stomach; they differ from chronic peptic ulcers in that the raw area does not spread deep into the stomach lining.

The exact cause is unknown. Treatment is primarily preventive; patients in intensive-care units are commonly given *antacid drugs* and/or *histamine-2 receptor antagonists*.

Stretcher

A frame covered with fabric that is used in first aid for carrying the sick, injured, or deceased.

Many stretchers are available, including the standard stretcher, which consists of canvas stretched between two long poles on each side, and the trolley bed, a more sophisticated, adjustable stretcher on wheels that is carried in ambulances.

Stretchers can be improvised by passing two poles through holes made in the corners of canvas bags, or by rolling up poles in parallel sides of a strong rug or blanket. An overcoat may also be used. Ideally, stretchers should be fairly rigid. The ends of a loaded stretcher should be lifted simultaneously.

Stretch mark

The common name for *stria*.

Stria

Commonly called a stretch mark, a line on the skin caused by thinning and loss of elasticity in the dermis (underlying skin layer). Striae first appear as red, raised lines. Later they become purple, eventually flattening and fading to form shiny streaks, usually between a quarter of an inch and a half inch wide.

S

STRESS AND HEART RATE

The graph shows how a person's heart rate varies over a typical day. Exercise and stress both activate the body's "fight or flight" system and increase heart rate, but repeated alerting of the system without accompanying physical activity is probably harmful.

Stress levels through the day
Although the home and workplace both present stress, for many city dwellers the most taxing parts of the day are those spent commuting.

Appearance of striae
Commonly known as stretch marks, striae often develop on the abdomen, thighs, and breasts of pregnant women.

USING A STRETCHER

Stretchers are used to carry injured or seriously ill people to avoid the risk of further injury. Any type of stretcher should be fairly rigid and should always be tested for strength before use.

Keeping the victim warm
Place a blanket diagonally on the stretcher. Lift the victim carefully onto the blanket and tuck in the corners.

Improvising a stretcher
Turn the sleeves of two coats inside out. Pass two strong poles through the sleeves and button the coats.

Striae often develop on the hips and thighs during the adolescent growth spurt, especially in athletic girls. They are a common feature of pregnancy, developing in about 75 percent of pregnant women, and tend to occur on the breasts, thighs, and lower abdomen. Purple striae characteristically develop in people with *Cushing's syndrome*.

Striae are possibly caused by an excess of *corticosteroid hormones*, which are known to suppress fiber formation in the skin and to cause collagen in the skin to waste away. There is no effective means of prevention or treatment.

Stricture

Narrowing of a duct, canal, or other passage in the body. A stricture may result from infection and inflammation; damage to and subsequent formation of scar tissue in or around a passage; the development of a tumor; spasm of muscles in a passage wall; or excessive growth of tissue around a passage, which occurs in *prostatism* when the enlarged prostate gland constricts the urethra (the passage between the bladder and outside). In some cases, a stricture is *congenital*.

Stridor

A noisy, high-pitched breathing sound caused by abnormal narrowing of the *larynx* or *trachea*.

Stridor is most common in young children. It usually occurs in *croup*, which is caused by a viral infection of the upper airways. A less common, but more serious, cause is the bacterial infection *epiglottiditis*. Other causes of stridor include an inhaled *foreign body* and certain disorders of the *larynx*, such as tumors, vocal cord paralysis, and laryngomalacia (softening of the cartilage of the larynx).

Stroke

Damage to part of the brain caused by interruption to its blood supply or leakage of blood outside of vessel walls. Sensation, movement, or function controlled by the damaged area is impaired. Strokes are fatal in about one third of cases and are a leading cause of death in developed countries.

CAUSES
The main types and causes of stroke are shown in the box overleaf.

Certain factors increase the risk of having a stroke. The two most important are *hypertension* (high blood pressure), which weakens the walls of arteries, and *atherosclerosis* (thickening of the lining of arterial walls), which narrows arteries.

Other factors that increase the risk of a stroke include *atrial fibrillation* (a type of irregular heart beat), a damaged *heart valve*, and a recent *myocardial infarction* (heart attack). All of these conditions can cause blood clots in the heart that may break off and migrate to the brain. *Polycythemia* (a raised level of red cells in the blood), *hyperlipidemia* (a high level of fatty substances in the blood), *diabetes mellitus*, and smoking also increase the risk of stroke by increasing the risk of hypertension and/or atherosclerosis. Oral contraceptives increase the risk of stroke in women under 50.

INCIDENCE
In the US, the overall incidence of stroke is about 200 people per 100,000 population annually. The incidence rises steeply with age and is higher in men than in women.

SYMPTOMS AND SIGNS
Damage to a specific area of the brain impairs bodily sensation, movement, or function controlled by that part of the brain. Some of the possible symptoms and signs are shown in the illustrated box overleaf. A stroke that affects the dominant of the two cerebral hemispheres in the brain (usually the left hemisphere) may cause disturbance of language and speech (see *Aphasia*).

Movement on one side of the body is controlled by the cerebral hemisphere on the opposite side. Thus, damage to areas controlling movement in the right cerebral hemisphere results in weakness or paralysis on the left side of the body. Such one-sided weakness or paralysis, known as *hemiplegia*, is one of the most common effects of a serious stroke.

When symptoms last for less than 24 hours and are followed by full recovery, the episode is known as a *transient ischemic attack*. Such an attack, which usually lasts for only a few minutes, is a warning signal that a sufficient supply of blood is not reaching part of the brain.

About a third of major strokes are fatal, a third result in a permanent handicap, and a third result in no lasting ill effects.

COMPLICATIONS
Possible complications of a major stroke include *pneumonia* and the formation of blood clots in the veins of the leg (see *Thrombosis, deep vein*), which may travel to the artery supplying the lung to cause a potentially fatal *pulmonary embolism*.

DIAGNOSIS
If someone is thought to have had a stroke, a physician or ambulance should be summoned immediately. In about two thirds of cases, symptoms are serious enough to require admission to the hospital.

CT scanning of the brain is performed to determine whether the symptoms are caused by a stroke or by some other disorder, such as a *brain tumor*, *brain abscess*, *subdural hemor-*

S

TYPES AND CAUSES OF STROKE

Stroke may be caused by any of three mechanisms (below). Thrombosis and embolism both lead to cessation of the blood supply to part of the brain and thus to infarction (tissue death). Rupture of a blood vessel in or near the brain may cause an *intracerebral hemorrhage* or a *subarachnoid hemorrhage*. Any part of the brain may be affected by a stroke; accordingly, the symptoms vary considerably.

CEREBRAL THROMBOSIS

Area deprived of blood

Thrombus blocks artery

Thrombosis
Blockage by a thrombus (clot) that has built up on the wall of a brain artery accounts for 40 to 50 percent of strokes.

CEREBRAL EMBOLISM

Area deprived of blood

Embolus blocks artery

Embolism
Blockage by an embolus (usually a clot) swept into an artery in the brain accounts for 30 to 35 percent of cases.

Tissue death within brain
The photograph at left shows a vertical slice through the brain of someone who died of a stroke. A large region of tissue death (dark area), caused by bleeding and oxygen deprivation, can be seen on one side.

HEMORRHAGE

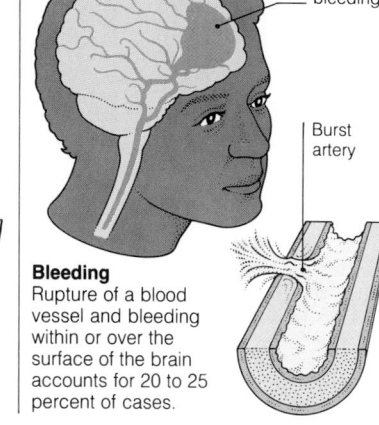

Area of bleeding

Burst artery

Bleeding
Rupture of a blood vessel and bleeding within or over the surface of the brain accounts for 20 to 25 percent of cases.

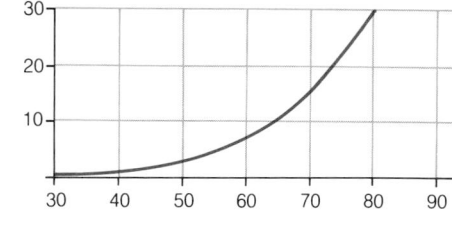

Estimated incidence per 1,000 population

Age

Incidence with age
Strokes are rare to uncommon under the age of 60, but thereafter the chances of one occurring increase rapidly.

SYMPTOMS

The symptoms of a stroke usually develop over minutes or hours, but occasionally over several days. Depending on the site, cause, and extent of damage, any or all of the symptoms at right may be present, in any degree of severity. The more serious cases lead to rapid loss of consciousness, coma, and death or to severe physical or mental handicap, but some strokes cause barely noticeable symptoms.

Hemiplegia
Weakness or paralysis on one side of the body is one of the more common effects of a serious stroke.

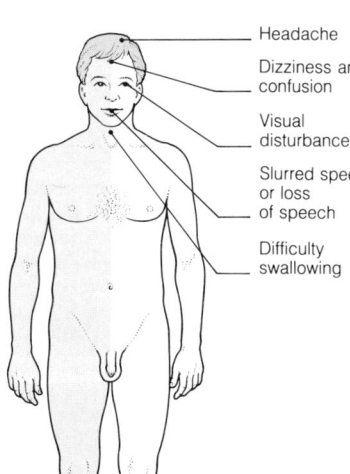

Headache

Dizziness and confusion

Visual disturbance

Slurred speech or loss of speech

Difficulty swallowing

RISK FACTORS

Age
High blood pressure
Atherosclerosis (narrowed artery channels)
Heart disease
Diabetes mellitus
Smoking
Polycythemia
Hyperlipidemia
Use of estrogens

S

rhage (bleeding into the space between the outermost and middle membranes covering the brain), or *encephalitis* (inflammation of the brain). A *lumbar puncture* may be necessary to exclude the possibility of *meningitis* (inflammation of the membranes covering the brain and spinal cord).

To further examine the cause and extent of brain damage, investigations may include an *ECG, chest X rays, blood tests, angiography,* and *MRI.*

TREATMENT
In the hospital, patients who are unconscious or semiconscious require a clear airway, feeding by means of *intravenous infusion* or a *nasogastric tube,* and regular changing of position to avoid bedsores or pneumonia. Any *edema* (accumulation of fluid) within the brain caused by the stroke may be treated with *corticosteroid drugs* or *diuretic drugs.*

When a stroke has been caused by an embolism, *anticoagulant drugs* may be prescribed (in many cases for the rest of the patient's life) to help prevent recurrences. In other instances, aspirin is prescribed or vascular surgery performed to reduce the risk of subsequent stroke.

Every effort is made to restore any lost movement or sensation by *physical therapy* and to remedy any speech disturbance by *speech therapy.*

OUTLOOK
About half of patients recover more or less completely from their first stroke. Many people paralyzed by a stroke learn to walk again. Any intellectual impairment, however, is often permanent. Survivors left with some form of permanent handicap may require *occupational therapy* and aids in the home. About 5 percent require long-term institutional care.

Stroma
The tissue that forms the framework of an organ, as distinct from the functional tissue (called the *parenchyma*) and the fibrous outer layer that holds the organ together. The stroma of the ovaries is the supporting tissue in which the ovarian follicles (the parenchyma) are embedded. The ovarian stroma consists of fibrous tissue, smooth muscle cells, spindle-shaped cells, and a rich supply of blood vessels.

Strongyloidiasis
An infestation of the intestines by a tiny parasitic worm, *STRONGYLOIDES STERCORALIS.* The disease is widespread in the tropics, especially the

Far East. In the US, it is occasionally found in Vietnam War veterans and refugees, but is otherwise rare.

Strongyloidiasis is contracted in affected areas by walking barefoot on soil contaminated with feces. Worm larvae penetrate the skin of the feet and, via the lungs and throat, migrate to the small intestine. There they develop into adults, which burrow into the intestinal wall to produce larvae. Most larvae are passed in the feces, but some enter the bloodstream to begin a new cycle. Thus, an infestation may persist in one person for many years.

SYMPTOMS AND TREATMENT
The larvae cause itching and raised red patches where they enter the skin. In the lungs they may cause bleeding (resulting in the coughing up of blood) or pneumonia. Intestinal infestation may produce no symptoms but, if heavy, causes discomfort, a swollen abdomen, and diarrhea. Occasionally, an infested person dies of complications, such as *septicemia* or *meningitis,* many years after contracting the infection. Pneumonia may occur more readily in a person whose immune system has been compromised.

The disease is diagnosed from microscopic examination of a sample of feces. Strongyloidiasis is treated with an *antihelmintic drug,* which eradicates the worms.

Strontium
A metallic element that does not occur naturally in its pure form but is present as various compounds in certain minerals (notably strontianite and celestite), seawater, and marine plants. It is also found in food and, although not essential to the body, is metabolized in a manner similar to calcium and incorporated into bone.

In addition to the compounds, there are several radioisotopes (radioactive varieties) of the element, of which strontium 90 is medically the most important. It does not occur naturally, but is produced in relatively large amounts during nuclear fission reactions and is also present in the fallout from some nuclear bomb explosions. Strontium 90 emits *radiation* (in the form of beta particles) for a comparatively long time (the *half-life* of this radioisotope is about 28 years), and accumulates in bone, where the radiation may cause *leukemia* and/or *bone tumors.*

Other radioisotopes of strontium have also been used in medicine to diagnose and treat bone tumors.

Strychnine poisoning
 Strychnine is an extremely poisonous chemical found in the seeds of species of *STRYCHNOS,* a group of tropical plants. Although once used as a tonic and general stimulant, strychnine is no longer used therapeutically. Its principal use today is as an ingredient in some rodent poisons; most cases of strychnine poisoning occur in children who accidentally eat such poisons. However, the extremely bitter taste of strychnine and its lack of easy availability makes this form of poisoning rare.

SYMPTOMS AND TREATMENT
The symptoms of poisoning begin soon after strychnine has been eaten. If untreated, death may occur. Initial symptoms include restlessness, stiffness of the face and neck, and increased sensitivity of sight, hearing, taste, and smell. These symptoms are followed by alternating episodes of seizures and floppiness. Eventually, death occurs from respiratory arrest.

The primary objectives of treatment are to prevent seizures and maintain breathing. The victim is given intravenous injections of a tranquilizer or barbiturate, which counteract the effects of strychnine and thus help prevent seizures. To maintain breathing, the victim may be placed on a ventilator. With prompt medical treatment, recovery usually occurs within about 24 hours.

Stuffy nose
See *Nasal congestion.*

Stump
The end portion of a limb that remains after *amputation.*

Stupor
A state of almost complete *unconsciousness* from which a person can be aroused only briefly and only by vigorous external stimulation. (See also *Coma.*)

Sturge-Weber syndrome
A rare, congenital condition that affects the skin and the brain. Characteristically, a large purple *hemangioma* (a birthmark caused by abnormal distribution of blood vessels) extends over one side of the face, including the eye. A similar malformation of blood vessels in the brain may cause some degree of weakness on the opposite side of the body, progressive *mental retardation,* and *epilepsy. Glaucoma* (increased pressure within the eyeball)

S

949

Appearance of Sturge-Weber syndrome
The characteristic birthmark, shown here on the lower part of the face, extends over the left eye and temple.

may develop in the affected eye, leading to a partial or complete loss of vision.

The birthmark can be disguised with masking creams; seizures can usually be controlled with *anticonvulsant drugs*. In severe cases, surgery on the affected part of the brain may need to be performed.

Stuttering

A speech disorder in which there is repeated hesitation and delay in uttering words or in which sounds are unusually prolonged. Stuttering, also known as stammering, usually starts in childhood, beginning before age 8 in 90 percent of sufferers.

INCIDENCE

Stuttering occurs in about 1 percent of the adult population. It is also fairly common temporarily in children aged 2 to 4. About half the children whose stutter persists until age 5 continue to stutter in adult life. The problem is more common in boys, twins, and left-handed people.

SYMPTOMS

People who stutter have problems with different words and sounds. The severity of the stutter is also related to circumstances. Some people find that the stuttering is worse when they are anxious (such as during public speaking or when using the telephone), while others experience more difficulty when relaxed. Problems rarely occur during singing or reading in unison (possibly because less communication is involved). Some stutterers also have *tics* and *tremors*.

CAUSES

The cause of stuttering is uncertain, although it tends to run in families. Some researchers believe that stuttering is due to a subtle form of brain damage; others regard it as a primarily psychological problem.

TREATMENT

Stuttering can often be improved by *speech therapy*, which may include teaching the person to give equal weight to each syllable. Electronic aids to mask the speaker's voice or to relay speech back to the speaker via headphones are also employed.

St. Vitus' dance

An outdated term for the disorder now called *Sydenham's chorea*.

Stye

Also called a hordeolum, a small, pus-filled *abscess* near the eyelashes caused by infection. If the stye is painful, warm compresses may help the pus to discharge. Antibiotic eye ointment can help prevent recurrence.

Stye on upper eyelid
A stye most often forms near the inner corner of an eye but may develop at the base of any of the eyelashes.

Subacute

A medical term applied to a disease that runs a course in time between *acute* and *chronic*. In subacute *meningitis*, the symptoms persist over a period of several weeks; in the acute form, the entire illness may last several days or a couple of weeks.

Subarachnoid hemorrhage

A type of brain hemorrhage in which blood from a ruptured blood vessel spreads over the surface of the brain.

CAUSES AND INCIDENCE

The most common cause of subarachnoid hemorrhage is a burst *aneurysm* (bulge in a weakened wall of an artery), frequently on the circular arrangement of blood vessels at the base of the brain, less commonly a ruptured *angioma* (abnormal proliferation of blood vessels within the brain). Bleeding takes place in the space between the arachnoid and the pia mater (the middle and the innermost of the three *meninges* that cover the brain). This space also contains *cerebrospinal fluid*, which becomes mixed with blood.

Subarachnoid hemorrhage usually occurs spontaneously, without any head injury, although it may follow unaccustomed physical exercise. In the US each year, about five to 10 people per 100,000 suffer a subarachnoid hemorrhage. It is somewhat less common than *intracerebral hemorrhage* (another form of *stroke*), in which bleeding occurs within the brain itself. Subarachnoid hemorrhage is particularly common between the ages of 35 and 60.

SYMPTOMS

An attack may cause immediate loss of consciousness or a sudden violent headache, often followed by loss of consciousness. If the person remains conscious, other symptoms such as *photophobia* (dislike of bright light), nausea, vomiting, drowsiness, and stiffness of the neck may develop. Unconscious patients may recover, but attacks during the ensuing day or weeks are common and often fatal.

DIAGNOSIS

The diagnosis is confirmed by *CT scanning* and by the presence of large amounts of blood in the cerebrospinal fluid following *lumbar puncture*. The site of the burst blood vessel is investigated by *angiography* (injection of a radiopaque substance into the bloodstream followed by X rays), which may not be performed until the patient's condition has stabilized.

TREATMENT

Treatment consists of general life-support procedures, bed rest, and measures aimed at reducing the risk of recurrence—principally, control of high blood pressure. In some cases, a burst aneurysm is surgically accessible. Angiomas can also sometimes be surgically removed, blocked off, or obliterated. Surgery is usually delayed some weeks after the acute attack.

About one third of patients make a full recovery; another one sixth recover but have some residual disability, such as paralysis, mental deterioration, or epilepsy. The remaining patients (about half) die due to the initial or a recurrent attack.

Subclavian steal syndrome

Recurrent attacks of blurred or double vision, loss of coordination, or dizziness caused by reduced blood flow to the base of the brain when one arm (usually the left) is moved. The underlying cause is narrowing of the major arteries that carry blood to the arms (usually due to *atherosclerosis*). The left subclavian artery is particularly affected. Blood supply to the affected arm is weak, but it is sufficient providing the arm is kept at rest. When the arm is moved, its muscles require an increased amount of blood, which must be diverted from the base of the brain.

A physician confirms the diagnosis by finding a weak pulse and low blood pressure in the affected arm. *Angiography* (injection of radiopaque dye into the blood vessels followed by X rays) establishes the site of the narrowed artery. Treatment is by *arterial reconstructive surgery*.

Subclinical

A medical term applied to a disorder that produces no symptoms or signs because it is so mild or because it is in the early stages of development. A subclinical infection may not produce any symptoms, but may cause damage to organs such as the liver.

Subconjunctival hemorrhage

Bleeding under the *conjunctiva* (transparent membrane covering the white of the eye). The small blood vessels of the conjunctiva are fragile, poorly supported, and frequently leak. Subconjunctival hemorrhage may occur spontaneously or after coughing or vomiting, which increases pressure in the veins. Subconjunctival hemorrhage is usually harmless and only rarely signals a serious disorder.

Subconjunctival hemorrhage
The bleeding causes a bright red area to appear in the white of the eye. This may look alarming but is usually harmless.

Subconjunctival blood disappears without treatment, usually within 10 to 14 days. Recurrences sometimes occur as a result of local weakness in a conjunctival blood vessel.

Subconscious

A term describing mental events (e.g., thoughts, ideas, or feelings) that one is temporarily unaware of but that can be recalled under the right circumstances. In *psychoanalytic theory*, the subconscious refers to that part of the mind through which information passes on its way from the *unconscious* to the conscious mind.

Subcutaneous

A medical term meaning beneath the skin, as in a subcutaneous injection, one in which a drug is injected into the tissue under the skin.

Subdural hemorrhage

Bleeding into the space between the dura mater, the tough outer layer of the *meninges* (coverings of the brain) and the arachnoid (middle meningeal layer). The trapped blood slowly forms a large hematoma (enlarging blood clot) within the skull. The most common cause is torn veins on the inside of the dura mater following a blow to the head. Subdural hemorrhage most often affects elderly or alcoholic people who have fallen.

SYMPTOMS
The bleeding occurs slowly; it may be weeks or months before the hematoma enlarges sufficiently to cause symptoms by raising pressure within the skull and displacing and pressing on brain tissue. The symptoms, which tend to fluctuate, consist of headache, episodes of confusion and drowsiness, and the development of one-sided weakness or paralysis.

Any person in whom such symptoms develop should consult a physician immediately. Because the symptoms are similar to those of a *stroke*, it is important that mention be made of any head injury that occurred within the previous few months.

DIAGNOSIS AND TREATMENT
The diagnosis is confirmed, and the location of the hematoma investigated, by means of *angiography* (injection of a radiopaque dye into the bloodstream followed by X rays) and *CT scanning*.

Surgical treatment is by drilling burr holes into the skull (see *Craniotomy*), drainage of the blood clot, and repair of damaged blood vessels, which usually allows a full recovery if carried out soon enough. (See also *Head injury*; *Extradural hemorrhage*.)

Sublimation

The unconscious process by which primitive, unacceptable impulses are redirected into socially acceptable forms of behavior. Aggression, for example, may be channeled into sports. *Psychoanalytic theory* regards sublimation as a healthy process, characteristic of mature personalities.

Subluxation

Incomplete *dislocation* of a joint—that is, displacement of the bony surfaces in a joint so that they no longer face each other exactly but remain in partial contact. In a dislocation, the joint surfaces are displaced so that there is total loss of contact between them. In general, subluxation causes less damage to the joint and surrounding tissues than a dislocation.

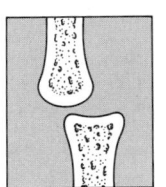

Normal
The diagram at left shows the normal position of the bony surfaces in a simple joint, such as the joint in the middle of a finger.

Subluxation
In a subluxation, the surfaces of the bones are slightly displaced from their normal positions relative to each other but are still in contact.

Dislocation
Here, there is almost complete loss of contact between the bone surfaces and usually considerable damage to surrounding tissues.

Submucous resection

An operation to correct a deviated *nasal septum* (the central partition inside the nose) when it is causing breathing difficulty. With the use of a local anesthetic, an incision is made in the mucous membrane covering the septum; displaced cartilage and bone are then cut away. The membrane is closed with absorbable stitches, which do not require removal. Because some deviation is normal, a second opinion is often recommended.

Subphrenic abscess

An *abscess* under the diaphragm.

Substrate

A substance on which an *enzyme* acts. The digestive enzyme amylase acts on the substrate starch (a polysaccharide) and breaks it down into smaller saccharide (sugar) units.

Sucking wound

An open wound in the chest wall through which air passes, causing the lung on that side to collapse (see *Lung, collapse of*). The mediastinum (central

S

partition of the chest) may also shift to the other side, causing partial collapse of the other lung.

A sucking wound causes severe breathlessness and a life-threatening lack of oxygen. Emergency first-aid treatment is vital. Cover the wound with your hand (or first cover it with a piece of impermeable material, such as a plastic bag). The wound must be kept tightly sealed until medical attention is obtained.

Sucralfate

An *ulcer-healing drug* used to treat *peptic ulcer*. Sucralfate forms a protective barrier over the ulcerated stomach or duodenal lining and thus protects it from further attack by the digestive juices and allows an ulcer to heal.

Antacid drugs should not be taken within an hour of taking sucralfate as they may reduce its effectiveness. Constipation is an adverse effect. Sucralfate may interfere with the absorption of drugs, such as tetracycline and digoxin. Prolonged treatment may impair the absorption of certain vitamins.

Suction

The removal of unwanted fluid or semifluid material from the body with a syringe and hollow needle or with an intestinal tube and a mechanical pump. Among the many uses of suction is cleaning secretions from the throats of newborn babies and from surgical patients after an operation using general anesthesia. Suction is also used to drain blood and other fluids from the abdominal cavity during or after surgery.

Suction lipectomy

See *Body contour surgery*.

Sudden death

Death that occurs unexpectedly in a person who previously seemed healthy and who had not complained of any symptoms of illness (deaths due to *accidents* are excluded).

The most common cause of sudden death is *cardiac arrest*. People older than about 35 who die from cardiac arrest are frequently found at autopsy to have had *coronary heart disease*; younger victims are often found to have had a congenital heart abnormality. Sudden death may also occur in people suffering from unsuspected *myocarditis* or as a result of a *stroke*.

To reduce the risk of sudden death from heart disease, any person about to begin an exercise program after a period of inactivity should consult a physician for a checkup, especially if exertion causes chest pain, breathlessness, extreme fatigue, or palpitations, or if he or she is overweight, smokes, or has a family history of coronary heart disease. (See also *Sudden infant death syndrome*.)

Sudden infant death syndrome

The sudden, unexpected death of an infant, which often cannot be explained even after an autopsy. Such deaths, also known as crib deaths, typically occur in apparently healthy babies who seem well when put to sleep but later are found dead.

CAUSES AND INCIDENCE
In developed countries, sudden infant death syndrome (SIDS) is the most common form of death between the ages of 1 month and 1 year; three quarters of these occur in babies under 6 months old. SIDS is slightly more common among boys, among second children, and in winter. More deaths seem to occur between midnight and 9 AM and on weekends.

Much of the research has been focused on possible risk factors. They include *prematurity* and low birth weight; bottle-feeding; cold weather; young, single mothers; smoking, drug addiction, or anemia in the mother; poor socioeconomic background; the death of a sibling as a result of SIDS; and so-called "near miss" infants who have been found near death and have been resuscitated just in time.

Most experts believe there is no single cause of SIDS. It seems probable that some babies die of a sudden overwhelming respiratory infection and others of undetected inborn errors of metabolism (see *Metabolism, inborn errors of*). Most deaths are thought to be caused by some abnormality in the breathing and heart rate. Abnormal breathing rhythms may be due to a fault in the brain stem, the lungs may have abnormally sensitive airway reflexes, or there may be an abnormality of surfactant (a substance that prevents the air sacs of the lungs from collapsing).

Even though most deaths seem to occur without warning, it is becoming clear that some babies may have been suffering from minor symptoms (such as a cold with a stuffy nose) for several days before death or have shown an inexplicable weight loss.

PREVENTION
Possible preventive measures include good *prenatal care*, avoidance of smoking and unnecessary taking of drugs during pregnancy, good obstetric care, breast-feeding, and close observation of the baby for several days after a minor illness.

Parents of a child who has died from SIDS and parents of "near miss" infants may be reassured by use of an alarm that sounds if the baby stops breathing. However, there is no evidence that the use of such alarms lowers the risk of death, and the number of false alarms that occurs may increase, rather than allay, the parents' anxiety.

EFFECTS
The death of an infant from SIDS is a highly distressing experience.

Grief may manifest itself in a variety of ways, ranging from withdrawal and anger to physical symptoms. There may be feelings of intense guilt; family relationships may be badly strained by misplaced blame and by severe and persistent grief. The family should be prepared for a visit from the coroner's office and the local police.

Parents may lose confidence in their ability to properly care for any other children. They should be reassured that they did not cause the death of their babies.

Siblings are also affected by the death; their grief may be expressed through misbehavior, nightmares, bedwetting, or regression to habits long outgrown. Sometimes siblings fear they will die in the same way.

Professionals, such as the pediatrician, family physician, social worker, and minister, can provide support. Group therapy with other parents who have been through the experience can provide great comfort.

Sudeck's atrophy

Swelling and loss of use of a hand or foot after a fracture or other injury.

Pain, swelling, and stiffness (especially in the joints) develop in the affected hand or foot about two months after the original injury, usually after the plaster cast has been removed. The nails may stop growing normally and hair on the affected limb may fall out. Despite physical therapy and attempts to start using the hand or foot again, the pain, swelling, and stiffness persist.

The condition is diagnosed by X rays, which usually show thinning of the bones (see *Osteoporosis*).

Treatment of Sudeck's atrophy includes elevation of the affected hand or foot, gentle exercise, and different forms of heat. A full recovery is usually made within about

S

four months. However, if pain persists, a *nerve block* may be tried and, if this procedure proves temporarily successful, *sympathectomy* may be attempted.

Suffocation

A condition in which there is a lack of oxygen due to an obstruction to the passage of air into the lungs. Suffocation may be caused by blockage of the nose and mouth, by blockage of the pharynx or larynx, or by blockage of the trachea. (See also *Asphyxia*; *Choking*; *Strangulation*.)

Sugar

See *Carbohydrates*.

Suicide

The act of intentionally killing oneself. In the US, suicide accounts for about 35,000 deaths (about 1 percent of all deaths) each year.

FIRST AID: SUFFOCATION

1 Immediately remove any obstruction and move the victim into fresh air.

2 If the victim is conscious, offer reassurance. If unconscious but breathing normally, place in the *recovery position*.

3 If breathing is difficult or has stopped, begin *artificial respiration* immediately.

CAUSES

More than 90 percent of suicides occur as the result of a psychiatric illness. Among people who take their own lives are about 15 percent of people suffering from severe *depression*, about 10 percent of those with *schizophrenia* (particularly young males in the early stages of the illness), about 7 percent of those suffering from *alcohol dependence*, about 5 percent of those with an *antisocial personality disorder*, and a smaller percentage of people suffering from some form of *neurosis*. An underlying depression is also associated with these disorders.

Suicide results from a person's reaction to a perceived overwhelming problem, such as social isolation, death of a loved one (especially a spouse), a broken home in childhood, serious physical illness, growing old, unemployment, financial problems, and drug abuse.

INCIDENCE

The incidence of suicide shows wide variation from one country to another (see table). Published figures may not reflect the true number of suicides in some countries, especially where there are poor systems of reporting deaths or where suicide is considered to be sinful or shameful.

In the US the average age of suicide is 49.3 years, with the highest rate among the elderly. However, in recent years there has been a steady increase in the suicide rate among young people. Over the last 30 years, suicide has tripled in those aged 15 to 19; suicide is now the third most common cause of death in students, after accidents and homicide.

More men than women commit suicide, although women attempt the act more often (see *Suicide, attempted*). Marital status is also a factor. Suicide is most common in divorced people, less so in the single and widowed, and least common in those who are married. For unknown reasons, the peak months for suicide are May and June.

METHODS

The most common method of committing suicide is poisoning, usually by taking an overdose of analgesics (painkillers) or sleeping tablets or by inhaling car exhaust fumes. Violent methods of committing suicide, such as shooting, are far more common in men than in women.

PREVENTION

One myth about suicide is that only people who are not serious about suicide talk about it beforehand. In fact, many people who commit suicide

SUICIDE RATES (per 100,000 population, age standardized to world population)

Country	Year	Rate
Hungary	1986	35.2
Finland	1986	22.6
Austria	1986	22.3
Denmark	1985	22.0
Belgium	1984	18.4
Switzerland	1986	18.1
France	1985	17.5
Japan	1986	16.4
Czechoslovakia	1985	15.7
Sweden	1985	14.5
West Germany	1986	14.0
Norway	1985	12.5
Bulgaria	1985	12.1
Poland	1986	11.8
Canada	1985	11.3
US	1984	10.7
Australia	1985	10.4
The Netherlands	1985	9.3
New Zealand	1985	9.3
Portugal	1986	7.4
England and Wales	1985	7.1
Italy	1983	5.7
Greece	1985	3.2

Suicide rates compared
This table is a comparison of suicide rates in selected countries. The suicide rate in the US is less than one third that in Hungary, which has by far the highest national suicide rate in the world.

repeatedly threaten to take their own lives; relatives and friends should always take such threats seriously. Suicidal people usually feel desperately lonely, and the opportunity to talk to a sympathetic, understanding listener is sometimes enough to prevent the despairing act. It was for this reason that suicide prevention centers were established to provide 24-hour telephone counseling service for suicidal people.

A psychiatrist should be consulted immediately so that the person's depression can be treated. Hospitalization (or frequent sessions with the psychiatrist) may be necessary to provide enough support to help the sick person through the risky period.

Following a suicide threat, family or friends should remove any obvious tools for committing the act and should watch the person closely.

Suicide, attempted

Any deliberate act of self-harm that is or is believed to be life-threatening but that in effect proves nonfatal. Most attempted suicides, or parasuicides, are carried out in a setting that makes rescue possible. They must therefore be viewed as cries for help by people in extreme distress.

S

CAUSES AND INCIDENCE

People who attempt suicide constitute a sociologically different group from those who actually kill themselves (see *Suicide*), although there is some overlap between the two. Parasuicide is three times more common in women than in men and is most common in the 15-to-30 age group and in single and divorced people. The rate is highest among people who have personality disorders, those who live in deprived urban areas, and those who have problems with alcohol or drugs. Common precipitating factors include an argument with a relative or sexual partner, recent death of a loved one, financial worries, or severe loss of any kind that results in depression.

Suicide attempts far outnumber actual suicides and, since the 1950s, have become one of the primary reasons for hospital admission. The most common method used is to take an overdose of drugs, most often analgesics (painkillers) or sleeping tablets, often with alcohol.

TREATMENT AND PREVENTION

If someone is discovered to have taken a drug overdose, emergency help should be summoned; if the person is unconscious or not breathing, first-aid measures should be carried out (see *Drug poisoning*). In other cases, appropriate measures depend on the victim's condition.

All suicide attempts should be treated seriously. Twenty to 30 percent of people who attempt suicide repeat their attempt within a year, and 10 percent eventually kill themselves, especially socially isolated men in whom a physical or mental illness has developed.

The most important aspect of treatment is for the person to see a psychiatrist as soon as possible to help resolve the underlying depression.

Sulfacetamide

A *sulfonamide*-type *antibacterial drug* used in the treatment of *conjunctivitis*. Sulfacetamide is also sometimes given to treat chronic *blepharitis* (inflammation of the eyelids) and to prevent infection after an eye injury or the removal of a foreign body.

Sulfacetamide may cause stinging of the eye. Itching, redness, and swelling of the eyelids are occasionally caused by an allergic reaction.

Sulfamethoxazole

A *sulfonamide*-type *antibacterial drug* used to treat *conjunctivitis* and ear infections. Sulfamethoxazole com-

bined with *trimethoprim* (another antibacterial drug) is also given to treat a variety of respiratory tract infections (including *pneumocystis pneumonia*), urinary tract infections, *gastroenteritis*, and *gonorrhea*.

Possible adverse effects include rash, nausea, vomiting, diarrhea, and, rarely, headache, dizziness, muscle pain, and joint pain.

Sulfasalazine

A drug used to relieve inflammation in the intestinal disorders *ulcerative colitis* and *Crohn's disease*.

Sulfasalazine may cause nausea, vomiting, headache, abdominal pain, and loss of appetite. An allergic reaction, causing fever and rash, occasionally occurs. Prolonged treatment may cause *folic acid* deficiency, resulting in *anemia*.

Sulfinpyrazone

A drug used to treat *gout* (a metabolic condition associated with an excessive level of uric acid in the blood, sometimes causing painful arthritis and kidney stones). Sulfinpyrazone does not relieve the symptoms of gout but does reduce the frequency of attacks.

Sulfinpyrazone is also given to reduce *hyperuricemia* (raised levels of uric acid in the blood) caused by certain drugs, such as thiazide *diuretic drugs* and some *anticancer drugs*. Sulfinpyrazone reduces the amount of uric acid in the blood by increasing the amount excreted in the urine.

POSSIBLE ADVERSE EFFECTS

Adverse effects include nausea, vomiting, headache, flushing, cloudy or bloodstained urine, rash, itching, wheezing, and breathlessness.

Sulfisoxazole

A *sulfonamide*-type *antibacterial drug* used in the treatment of urinary tract and eye infections. Given with a *penicillin drug*, sulfisoxazole is used to treat ear and chest infections resistant to penicillin alone.

Sulfisoxazole may cause nausea, vomiting, loss of appetite, diarrhea, headache, dizziness, or rash.

Sulfonamide drugs

COMMON DRUGS
Sulfacetamide Sulfamethoxazole Sulfisoxazole

A group of *antibacterial drugs*. Before the advent of *penicillin drugs*, sulfonamide drugs were widely used to treat infectious diseases. Today,

they are used mainly to treat urinary tract infections. Often prescribed in combination with *trimethoprim*, sulfonamide drugs are sometimes used to treat *bronchitis*, certain types of *pneumonia*, skin infections, and infections of the middle ear.

Sulfur

A mineral that plays several important roles in the body. Sulfur is a constituent of vitamin B_1 and of several essential amino acids (building blocks of proteins). In particular, sulfur is necessary for the manufacture of *collagen* (which helps to form bones, tendons, and connective tissue) and is a constituent of *keratin* (the chief component of hair, skin, and nails).

Sulfur-rich foods
The main sources of sulfur in the diet are protein-rich foods such as eggs, fish, lean meat, nuts, and dried beans.

DEFICIENCY AND EXCESS

A balanced diet contains enough sulfur for the body's needs; only people who eat little protein (such as those on extremely restricted vegetarian diets) are likely to suffer from sulfur deficiency. People deficient in sulfur have the symptoms of general protein deficiency, such as weakness and tiredness.

MEDICAL USES

Sulfur is used in some ointments, creams, and skin preparations for the treatment of various skin disorders, including acne, dandruff, psoriasis, scabies, diaper rash, and certain fungal infections.

Sulindac

A *nonsteroidal anti-inflammatory drug* (NSAID) used to relieve joint pain and stiffness caused by various types of *arthritis*.

Adverse effects are typical of other NSAIDs, including indigestion, *peptic ulcer*, rash and itching, and wheezing and breathlessness.

Sunburn

Inflammation of the skin caused by overexposure to the sun. The ultraviolet rays in sunlight destroy cells in the outer layer of the skin and damage tiny blood vessels beneath.

Sunburn is most common in fair-skinned people, whose skin produces only small amounts of the protective pigment *melanin*, and in people attempting to acquire a tan in strong sunlight too quickly. The affected skin turns red and tender and may become blistered. In severe cases, the sunburn may be accompanied by symptoms of sunstroke—such as vomiting, fever, and collapse. Several days later the dead skin cells are shed by peeling.

Repeated overexposure to sunlight can age the skin prematurely, producing yellowish, wrinkled skin through which capillary vessels may be seen. Overexposure can also increase the risk of skin cancer (see *Sunlight, adverse effects of*).

PREVENTION
Exposure to strong sunlight should be limited to 15 minutes on the first day, particularly if the person has fair skin, and should be increased very gradually. This applies even if conditions are hazy. Until a tan is acquired, the skin should be protected with a high protection factor *sunscreen*.

TREATMENT
Calamine lotion or a sunburn cream should be applied to soothe the burned skin, which should be protected from further sun exposure until healing takes place. *Analgesic drugs* (painkillers) may be required to relieve tenderness. A person with severe sunburn should consult a physician, who may prescribe a cream containing *corticosteroid drugs* to speed healing.

Sunlight, adverse effects of

Some exposure to ultraviolet radiation from the sun is necessary for the body to produce vitamin D. Overexposure can have various harmful effects, particularly in fair-skinned people, who produce only small amounts of the protective skin pigment *melanin*.

Short-term overexposure causes *sunburn* and, in intense heat, can result in *heat exhaustion* or *heat stroke*. Repeated overexposure over a long period can cause premature aging of the skin and the production of wartlike growths called solar *keratoses*. Most seriously, it considerably increases the risk of *skin cancer*.

Photosensitivity (skin rash resulting from abnormal sensitivity to sunlight) may be triggered by taking certain drugs. The condition may also occur in people who have systemic *lupus erythematosus* or *porphyria*.

Sunscreens

> **WARNING**
> Some suntanning preparations do not contain a sunscreen and therefore provide no protection against sunburn.

Preparations that protect the skin from the harmful effects of sunlight (see *Sunlight, adverse effects of*). Sunscreens are used mainly to prevent *sunburn*. They are also used to treat rash caused by *photosensitivity*.

Most sunscreens, including the very common *para-aminobenzoic acid* (PABA), work by absorbing ultraviolet rays. Some, such as titanium dioxide, reflect the sun's rays.

Sunscreen products are labeled with a sun protection factor (SPF), with the highest factor affording the greatest protection. Choice of product should depend on skin type (see box). A sunscreen with a lower SPF may be used once the skin tans. During prolonged sunbathing, sunscreens should be reapplied at regular intervals and also after swimming.

Some people are allergic to sunscreen chemicals and a skin rash develops. This is more common with preparations containing PABA.

Sunstroke

The most common type of *heat stroke*, usually brought on by overexposure to direct sun in a person who is unaccustomed to a hot climate.

Suntan

Darkening of the skin after exposure to sunlight. Specialized cells in the outer layer of the skin respond to the ultraviolet rays in the sunlight by producing more of the protective pigment *melanin*. People who spend a lot of time in the sun are likely to experience premature aging and wrinkling of the skin and run a greatly increased risk of skin cancer. (See also *Sunlight, adverse effects of*; *Sunburn*.)

Superego

The part of the personality, described in *psychoanalytic theory*, that is responsible for maintaining an individual's standards of behavior. Popularly termed a person's "conscience," the superego arises as a result of the child incorporating the ideals and moral views of those in authority (usually parents). The superego can create feelings of guilt and anxiety by criticizing the *ego* (the conscious "I") when the ego gives way to the primitive impulses of the *id* (the pleasure-seeking part of the personality).

An excessively strong superego is said to be the cause of severe, puritanical personality types and of *obsessive-compulsive behavior*. By contrast, failure to develop an appropriate superego leads to impulsive and immoral behavior.

In psychoanalytic theory, a harsh, self-punishing superego is said to result from childhood experience with a harsh parent.

Superficial

Situated near the surface, as in the superficial blood vessels (the capillaries that lie near the surface of the skin and play an important role in the regulation of body temperature and blushing).

Superinfection

A second infection that occurs during the course of an existing infection. The term usually refers to an infection by a microorganism that is resistant to drugs being used against the original infection. The second microorganism may be a resistant strain of the first infection, a different pathogen (disease-causing microorganism), or a member of the body's normal flora (microorganisms that are normally present in the body without producing ill effects) that has proliferated excessively because other microorganisms that normally keep it in check have been killed by drug

S

SAFE EXPOSURE TIMES USING SUNSCREENS OF DIFFERENT STRENGTHS

Protection factor	4	8	15
Skin type	Safe exposure time		
Fair	10 minutes	40 to 80 minutes	1.5 to 2 hours
Medium	50 to 80 minutes	2 to 2.5 hours	5 to 5.5 hours
Dark	1.5 to 2 hours	3.5 to 4 hours	all day
Black	4 hours	all day	all day

therapy. For example, tetracycline therapy may result in superinfection of the mouth, vagina, and/or anus with the fungus that causes candidiasis (thrush).

Superiority complex

An exaggerated and unrealistic belief that one is better than other people. *Adlerian theory* suggests that a superiority complex develops in some people in response to the natural feelings of inferiority that everyone is born with. In more modern psychoanalytic terms, a superiority complex is a compensation for unconscious feelings of inadequacy or low self-esteem.

Supernumerary

More than the normal number, as in supernumerary nipples, additional nipples that are not usually associated with underlying glandular tissue; they develop along a line that extends from the armpit to the groin. (See also *Supernumerary teeth*.)

Supernumerary teeth

One or more teeth in excess of the usual number (20 deciduous and 32 permanent). An extra tooth may be a duplicate of an existing tooth or it may have an abnormal shape and position (usually appearing as a small conical protrusion from the gum above the existing teeth in the upper front jaw).

Supernumerary (extra) tooth
This X ray of the upper jaw shows a supernumerary incisor tooth on the roof of the mouth behind the normal incisors.

Supernumerary teeth may interfere with the proper *eruption of teeth* and are usually extracted.

Supination

The act of turning the body to a supine (lying on the back with the face upward) position or the hand to a palm forward position. Movements in the opposite direction to supination are called *pronation*.

Suppository

A solid, cone- or bullet-shaped object containing a drug and an inert (chemically inactive) substance, usually derived from cocoa butter or another type of vegetable oil. The suppository is placed in the vagina or rectum and melts at body temperature, releasing the active ingredient.

Vaginal suppositories are used to treat vaginal disorders, such as *candidiasis* (thrush) or *trichomoniasis*, or to introduce contraceptive *spermicides* into the vagina.

Rectal suppositories are used to treat rectal disorders, such as *hemorrhoids* or *proctitis*. They may also be used to soften feces and stimulate a bowel movement. A rectal suppository is also used to administer a drug into the general circulation via blood vessels in the rectum if vomiting is likely to prevent absorption or if the drug would cause irritation of the stomach lining.

Drugs given by suppository include antifungal drugs, local anesthetics, corticosteroid drugs, nonsteroidal anti-inflammatory drugs, antibiotic drugs, and antiemetic drugs.

Suppuration

The formation or exudation of *pus*. Suppuration occurs at the site of bacterial infection, where the pus may accumulate, forming an *abscess* in solid tissue or a *boil* or *pustule* on the skin. Open sores often suppurate, particularly when they are slow to heal, because the exposed underlying tissue tends to become repeatedly infected with bacteria.

Suprarenal glands

Another name for the *adrenal glands*.

Supraspinatus syndrome

See *Painful arc syndrome*.

Supraventricular tachycardia

An abnormally fast but regular heart rate of between 140 and 180 beats per minute (or, rarely, of up to 300 beats per minute in certain arrhythmias) that occurs in intermittent episodes lasting for several hours or days. Supraventricular tachycardia is caused by abnormal electrical impulses arising within the atria (upper chambers) of the heart taking over control of the heart beat from the *sinoatrial node* (the heart's pacemaker).

Symptoms may include palpitations, breathlessness, chest pain, or fainting (see *Stokes-Adams syndrome*). Diagnosis of the condition is made by

an *ECG* (electrocardiogram). An attack can sometimes be terminated by *Valsalva's maneuver* or by drinking cold water. Recurrent attacks are treated with *antiarrhythmic drugs*. Rarely, the condition may require treatment by electrical conversion of the heart rhythm (by applying an electric shock to the heart).

Surfactant

A wetting agent (i.e., a substance that reduces surface tension). Soaps, detergents, and emulsifiers are surfactants. Pulmonary surfactant is a substance secreted by the alveoli (air sacs) in the lungs that prevents them from collapsing during exhalation.

Surfers' nodules

Multiple *exostoses* (bony outgrowths) occurring on bones in the foot and on the tibial tubercle (the bony prominence below the knee at the top of the shin). Surfers' nodules are caused by the repeated banging of the surfboard against the knees and tops of the feet as the surfer kneels to paddle the board. They can be avoided by paddling in a lying position.

Surgeon

A physician who performs operations that involve cutting body tissue. Surgery may be done to diagnose illness, remove diseased tissue and organs, repair injuries, or correct malfunctioning parts. General surgeons perform a variety of operations on almost all parts of the body. Other surgeons operate only on particular parts of the body. (See also *Surgery*.)

Surgery

The treatment of disease, injury, or other disorders by direct physical intervention, usually with instruments. The term is also used to denote those aspects of medical practice that deal with the study, diagnosis, and management of all disorders treated by operative surgery (as distinct from those treated by drugs, diet, or modification of life-style).

Operative surgery involves incision (cutting) into the skin or other organ, inspection, removal of diseased tissues or organs, relief of obstruction, replacement of structures to their normal position, redirection of body channels, transplantation of tissues or whole organs, and implantation of mechanical or electronic devices.

Surgery may be minor or major. Minor operations are usually, but not always, performed using local

S

anesthesia. Major operations are usually performed using general anesthesia, although local anesthesia is sometimes used. Neurosurgeons and ophthalmologists, for instance, often operate using local anesthesia.

Surgery has for many years been divided into specialties, such as orthopedic surgery, neurosurgery, obstetrics and gynecology, ophthalmology, gastrointestinal surgery, and plastic surgery. In recent years there has been an increasing trend toward further subspecialization; some surgeons now confine their practices to such narrow limits as surgery of the hand, the cornea, the small blood vessels, or the skin.

Surrogacy

The agreement by a woman to become pregnant and give birth to a child with the understanding that she will surrender the child after birth to the contractual parents. Surrogacy became publicized with the advent of *in vitro fertilization*, in which the egg and sperm are brought together in the laboratory. The fertilized egg can be transferred to the uterus of any woman who is at the appropriate stage of the menstrual cycle.

Another means of accomplishing surrogacy is through the *artificial insemination* of the surrogate mother with the contracting father's sperm.

The ethical and legal aspects of surrogacy have yet to be resolved. In most countries a woman who wishes to act as a surrogate for her infertile sister can be helped to do so. Surrogacy for financial reward has been forbidden by law in some countries but not in others. In the US (in 1988), the issue was still before the courts. If surrogacy-for-money agreements were deemed illegal, it would not be possible for either party to go to the courts to enforce a contract.

Susceptibility

A total or partial vulnerability to an infection, disease, or disorder. In *AIDS*, the immune system is impaired and the sufferer is vulnerable to a wide range of infections and diseases.

Suture

A type of *joint* (found only between the bones of the *skull*) in which the adjacent bones are so closely and firmly joined by a thin layer of fibrous connective tissue that movement between them is impossible. The term suture is also used to refer to a surgical stitch (see *Suturing*).

METHODS OF SUTURING

Suturing is carried out using a general or local anesthetic. The type of stitch used depends on the nature of the wound or incision (two types are shown below). In all cases the surgeon sews the wound edges together to produce minimal distortion of tissue.

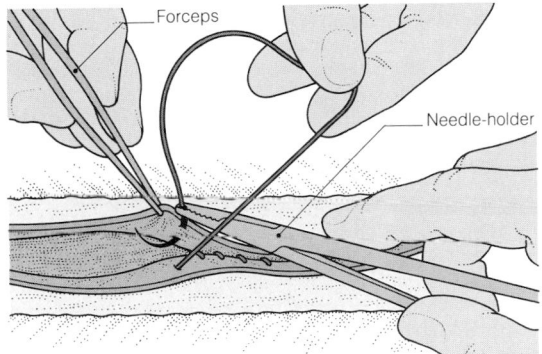

Technique
The surgeon grasps the edge of the wound with forceps held in one hand and, with the other hand, inserts the needle through the skin. In this illustration, the surgeon is shown using a needle-holder, which gives greater control for very fine stitches. In other cases, the needle may be held in the hand.

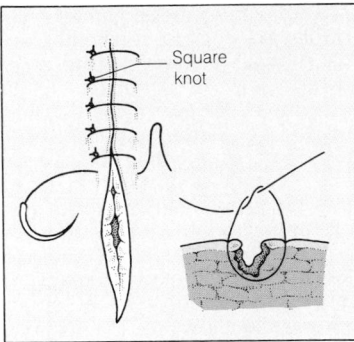

Standard interrupted sutures
The needle is passed into one skin edge, through the full depth of the wound, and out the other skin edge. Each stitch is tied at the side using a square knot.

Mattress sutures
For deeper wounds, the needle is passed through the wound twice: first shallowly, close to the skin edges, and then more deeply, farther from the edges.

OTHER METHODS OF CLOSURE

Alternatives to suturing include removable staples and clips (staples are also used internally) and adhesive tape.

Adhesive tape
When the wound is shallow, tape may be applied directly. For deeper wounds, absorbable stitches are first inserted just below the skin.

Inserting staples
The wound edges are held up with forceps and equally spaced staples are inserted using an automatic stapling device.

S

Suturing

The closing of a surgical incision or a wound by sutures (stitches) to promote healing.

MATERIALS USED

A variety of sterile materials is used as sutures, including catgut (obtained from sheep intestines); linen, silk, or synthetic fiber thread; and stainless steel wire. These materials vary considerably in the length of time they retain their strength, the reaction they provoke in tissues, and the likelihood of their allowing minute pockets of infection to form. In addition, certain materials, such as catgut, are absorbable (i.e., they eventually dissolve in the body). The choice of which material to use for an operation is made by the surgeon. The thickness of sutures varies from almost 0.04 inch (1 mm), used for the repair of major injuries, to a barely visible 0.004 inch (0.01 mm), used for delicate eye and blood vessel surgery.

Most surgical needles are curved and often have a point with a cutting edge. The needle is held in a tweezerlike instrument; larger needles may be held with the fingers.

HOW IT IS DONE

The method of suturing a typical incision, and some alternative methods of skin closure, are shown in the illustrated box on the preceding page. Deep incisions or wounds may need to be sutured at several levels to achieve full closure throughout the depth of tissue, thus preventing collection of blood below the surface.

Internal sutures, made of absorbable material, are left in place permanently. Skin sutures are removed painlessly after one to two weeks.

Swab

A wad of absorbent material used in surgery or to obtain a sample of bacteria from an infected patient.

One type of swab, a surgical sponge, is commonly a folded piece of cotton gauze held in the hand or in a clamp. It is used to apply cleansing and antiseptic solutions to the skin before an incision is made and to soak up blood and other fluids during an operation. The swab often contains material opaque to X rays to enable it to be detected if it is accidentally left in the body, an occurrence that is usually prevented by a "sponge count" made before the operation begins and again before the patient is stitched up.

A bacteriological swab consists of a twist of cotton at the end of a thin stick that is sealed in a container and sterilized. It is applied to an infected area of the body to absorb pus or mucus, from which a *culture* can be grown to identify bacteria.

Swallowing

The process by which food or liquid is conveyed from the mouth to the stomach via the esophagus. The first stage is voluntary (under conscious control), but is so familiar that little thought is given to it. Once food has been well chewed and mixed with saliva (which greatly facilitates swallowing), the tongue pushes it to the back of the mouth and the voluntary muscles in the palate push the food into the pharynx (throat).

The rest of the swallowing act is involuntary (automatic), brought about by a series of *reflexes*; once started, it is rapid, powerful, and difficult to stop. Entry of food into the pharynx causes the epiglottis (a flap of cartilage) to close over the larynx (voice box) leading to the trachea (windpipe). A sphincter (circular muscle) at the top of the esophagus relaxes, and the muscles of the pharynx seize the food and squeeze it in the form of a bolus (rounded lump) into the esophagus. Powerful waves of contraction then pass down the esophagus, propelling the food toward the stomach. Finally, the muscle at the entry to the stomach relaxes and allows the bolus to pass.

Swallowing difficulty

A fairly common symptom with a wide variety of causes, known medically as dysphagia.

CAUSES

Temporary swallowing difficulty may be caused by a foreign object (such as a fish bone) lodging at the back of the throat or in the esophagus. Most foreign objects are able to pass on to the stomach, but a scratch in the lining of the throat or esophagus may cause discomfort. Swallowing difficulty may also result from insufficient production of saliva (see *Mouth, dry*).

Disorders of the esophagus that may disrupt normal swallowing include *esophageal spasm* (uncoordinated contractions of the esophagus), *esophageal stricture* (narrowing) caused by scar or tumor (see *Esophagus, cancer of*), *esophagitis* (inflammation), *achalasia* (abnormal contraction of the muscles at the lower end of the esophagus), or a *pharyngoesophageal diverticulum* (hernia of part of the esophagus through a weak area in the surrounding muscle).

Esophageal atresia (closure or failure of the esophagus to open) can cause feeding problems in the newborn.

Difficulty swallowing may also be caused by a nervous system disorder (e.g., *myasthenia gravis*, *stroke*, or, rarely, *poliomyelitis*).

Pressure on the outside of the esophagus may obstruct the passage of food. In rare instances, pressure is exerted by a *goiter*, an aortic *aneurysm*, or cancer of the bronchus.

DIAGNOSIS AND TREATMENT

Any person who experiences persistent swallowing difficulty should be examined without delay. Investigations may include *esophagoscopy* (examination of the esophagus with a viewing tube) or barium swallow (see *Barium X-ray examinations*). Treatment depends on the cause.

Sweat glands

Minute structures deep within the skin that produce sweat. Each gland is made up of a coiled tube, in which the sweat is secreted, and a narrow passageway, which carries the sweat to the skin surface. The average person has about 3 million sweat glands.

TYPES

There are two types of sweat glands—eccrine and apocrine. Eccrine glands are the most common, especially on the palms and soles; these glands open directly to the skin surface. Apocrine glands, which develop at puberty, occur only in hairy areas, particularly the armpits, pubic region, and around the anus. These glands produce cellular material as well as sweat; they open into a hair follicle before reaching the skin surface.

FUNCTION

Sweat is composed mainly of water (99 percent) and minute quantities of dissolved substances, including sodium chloride (salt).

The activity of the sweat glands is controlled by the *autonomic nervous system*. Usually the glands are stimulated to produce sweat to keep the body cool, in which case sweating is heaviest on the forehead, upper lip, neck, and chest. Sweating can also be caused by anxiety or fear, in which case sweat appears mainly on the palms and soles and in the armpits. Sweating also occurs in many illnesses in which fever is a feature.

Sweat is odorless until bacteria act upon it, producing body odor.

DISORDERS

The most common problem affecting the sweat glands is *prickly heat*, an intensely irritating skin rash caused by

S

blockage of the glands with debris and sweat. Less common disorders of the sweat glands include *hyperhidrosis* (excessive sweating), *hypohidrosis* (reduced sweating), and abnormal or excessive skin odor.

Sweating
The process by which the body cools itself. Sweating also occurs as a response to psychological stress or fear. (See *Sweat glands; Heat disorders*.)

Sweeteners, artificial
See *Artificial sweeteners*.

Swimmers' ear
A common name for *otitis externa*.

Sycosis vulgaris
Inflammation of the beard area, also called barbers' itch. The condition is caused by infection of hair follicles, usually with STAPHYLOCOCCUS AUREUS bacteria contracted from infected razors and towels. Pus-filled blisters or boils develop around the follicles, sometimes resulting in severe scarring unless treated.

Treatment is usually with *antibiotic drugs*; growing a beard may help prevent a recurrence.

Sydenham's chorea
A childhood disorder of the central nervous system, once called St. Vitus' dance. The condition is characterized by involuntary, irregular, jerky movements and usually follows an attack of *rheumatic fever*.

Sydenham's chorea is rare in the US today but remains a common disorder in developing countries.

Restlessness and irritability usually precede the chorea, which affects the head, face, limbs, and fingers. The involuntary fidgets are random and unrepetitive. Voluntary movements are clumsy and the limbs are often floppy. Early signs are slurred speech and deteriorating handwriting.

Treatment is bed rest and antibiotics. Sedation is sometimes necessary if the fidgeting is extreme. The condition usually clears up after two to three months and has no long-term adverse effects. Thereafter, the person may be given antibiotics before surgical or dental treatment to prevent heart disease.

Sympathectomy
An operation in which the ganglia (nerve terminals) of sympathetic nerves are destroyed to interrupt the nerve pathway and thus improve blood supply to a limb or relieve chronic pain.

WHY IT IS DONE
The sympathetic nerves form part of the *autonomic nervous system* and control involuntary activities in the body, including the caliber of blood vessels. In *peripheral vascular disease* (narrowing of blood vessels in the legs and sometimes the arms), stimulation from the sympathetic nerves produces spasms in the blood vessels that worsen constriction. Sympathectomy prevents spasms from occurring and thus may improve blood supply to the affected area. Sometimes this response is limited only to the vessels of the skin when it is the blood flow to the muscles that needs to be improved.

The sympathetic nerves also play an important part in producing the sensation of pain. In some cases of *causalgia* (a persistent severe pain usually caused by nerve injury), sympathectomy offers the only prospect of relieving the pain.

HOW IT IS DONE
The surgeon may first perform a trial procedure, injecting local anesthetic into the nerves that supply the affected area. If this provides considerable temporary relief of the symptoms, a sympathectomy is usually performed.

Destruction of the nerve ganglia, which lie near the spinal cord, can be accomplished by injecting a sclerosing solution, which causes inflammation and subsequent degeneration of the nerves. Symptoms in the upper part of the body are controlled by an injection into the cervicodorsal sympathetic nerves at the base of the neck. To treat disorders of the lower part of the body, sclerosing solution is injected into the lumbar sympathetic nerves in the middle of the back.

Alternatively, nerve ganglia may be destroyed surgically while using a general anesthetic. In a cervicodorsal sympathectomy, this is done through an incision made in the armpit; in a lumbar sympathectomy, the incision runs horizontally from the spine in the lower back almost to the navel.

RESULTS
Sympathectomy performed to widen blood vessels is variable in its results. Results generally depend on the disease for which it is being performed. In controlling severe pain, however, the operation usually proves successful. Lumbar sympathectomy in men occasionally results in inability to ejaculate.

Sympathetic nervous system
One of the two divisions of the *autonomic nervous system*. In conjunction with the other division (the parasympathetic nervous system), this system controls many of the involuntary activities of the glands, organs, and other parts of the body.

Sympatholytic drugs
A group of drugs that blocks the action of the *sympathetic nervous system*. Sympatholytic drugs include *beta-blocker drugs, guanethidine, hydralazine*, and *prazosin*. They work either by reducing the release of the stimulatory *neurotransmitter* norepinephrine from nerve endings, or by occupying the receptors that the neurotransmitters epinephrine and norepinephrine normally bind to, thereby preventing their normal actions.

Symphysis
An anatomical term for a type of joint in which two bones are firmly joined by tough, fibrous cartilage. Such joints occur between the bodies of the vertebrae (the parts of the bones that are separated by the intervertebral disks), between the two pubic bones at the front of the *pelvis*, and between the manubrium (upper part) and body (middle part) of the *sternum*.

Symptom
An indication of a disease or disorder (such as pain) that is noticed by the sufferer. Presenting symptoms are those that prompt a person to obtain medical advice, but they are not necessarily the first to appear. The indications that a physician notes are called signs. The overall clinical picture (syndrome), including the symptoms and signs, helps the physician to identify a disease.

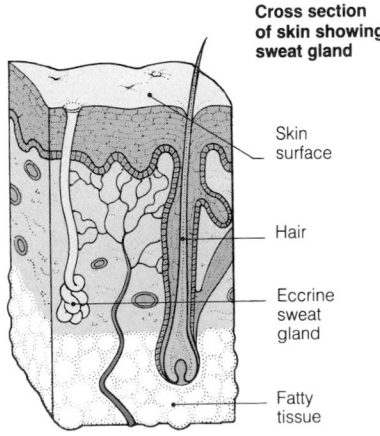

Cross section of skin showing sweat gland

Skin surface

Hair

Eccrine sweat gland

Fatty tissue

S

The distinction between symptoms and signs is not always clear. For example, fever is felt by the patient and observed by the physician. Similarly, in *appendicitis*, pain is a cardinal symptom; tenderness, which is pain felt only when pressure is applied, is a sign generally elicited by the physician, but it may also be elicited by the patient pressing on his or her own abdomen.

In some conditions, an accurate recollection and description of symptoms is extremely important. For example, because physical signs are often absent in *angina pectoris*, diagnosis of this condition may depend almost entirely on the patient's description of the chest pain.

Symptothermal method

See *Contraception, periodic abstinence*.

Synapse

A junctional connection between two neurons (nerve cells) across which a signal can pass. A single neuron may form thousands of these connections with adjacent nerve cells.

A typical neuron has one long fiber (axon) that projects from its cell body; it splits into several smaller branches and twigs, each ending in a terminal that forms a synapse, usually close to the cell body of an adjacent neuron. At a synapse, the two neurons do not come directly into contact; their surface membranes are separated by a gap called the synaptic cleft. When an electrical signal passes along a neuronal axon and reaches a synapse, it cannot bridge the cleft directly; instead, it causes the release of a chemical, called a *neurotransmitter*. The chemical travels across the cleft and is received at the surface membrane of the next neuron, where it changes the electrical potential of the membrane.

The axonal membrane from which the neurotransmitter is released is called the presynaptic membrane; the neuronal membrane at which it is received is called the postsynaptic membrane. Signals can be transmitted across a synapse in one direction only—from presynaptic to postsynaptic membrane.

A synapse may be excitatory or inhibitory. When a neurotransmitter passes across an excitatory synapse, the effect is to excite the postsynaptic membrane, making it more likely that the receptor neuron will "fire" and propagate an electrical impulse in turn. Inhibitory synapses decrease the excitation of the next neuron.

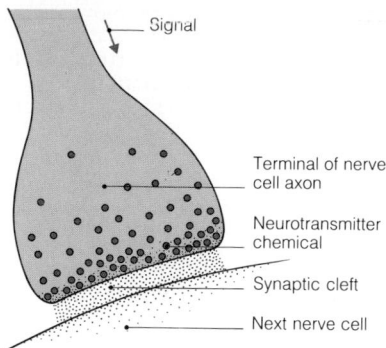

Structure of a synapse
When a signal arrives at the terminal of a nerve cell axon, it causes release of a neurotransmitter, which crosses the synaptic cleft and affects the next cell.

Labels: Signal; Terminal of nerve cell axon; Neurotransmitter chemical; Synaptic cleft; Next nerve cell

Most drugs affecting the nervous system work through their effects on synapses. They may modify neurotransmitter release or may modify the effects of neurotransmitters on postsynaptic membranes.

Syncope

The medical term for *fainting*.

Syndactyly

A congenital (present at birth) defect in which two or more fingers or toes are joined. The toes of one or both feet are more frequently affected. Often inherited and more common in boys, syndactyly is caused by incomplete development of the digits at the embryo stage, or by constriction of the digits by tissue within the uterus later in fetal development.

In mild cases, only the skin between the affected fingers or toes is joined. More seriously, the bones of adjacent digits are fused, as is the overlying skin, and there may be only one nail.

Treatment is usually by one or more operations during early childhood to separate the affected digits.

Syndactyly
In this case, the middle and ring fingers in both hands are partly joined. Sometimes, syndactyly occurs in association with other birth defects.

Syndrome

A group of symptoms and/or signs that, occurring together, constitutes a particular disorder. For example, *irritable bowel syndrome* is characterized by a combination of any or all of the following—intermittent pain in the lower abdomen (usually relieved by bowel movement or passing gas), abdominal swelling, irregular bowel movements (often with a sense of incomplete evacuation of the bowel afterward), mucus in the feces, excessive gas, and worsening of symptoms after eating.

Synovectomy

Surgical removal of the *synovium* (thin membrane lining a joint capsule) to treat recurrent or persistent *synovitis* (inflammation of the synovium), usually in sufferers from severe *rheumatoid arthritis*. The operation is usually performed only if the condition is severely disabling and has not responded to injections of *corticosteroid drugs* or to the taking of *nonsteroidal anti-inflammatory drugs* or *antirheumatic drugs*.

The joint may be opened while using a general anesthetic and the synovium cut away, or the operation may be performed by means of *arthroscopy*. After the operation, the joint is kept mobile to inhibit scarring. Synovectomy is a temporary expedient that usually improves symptoms for no more than about two years; further surgery may then be required.

Synovitis

Inflammation of the *synovium* (thin membrane lining a joint capsule). The condition may be acute (of sudden onset and short duration), in which case it is usually caused by infection, injury, or overuse of the joint, or chronic (recurrent or persistent), as in a disorder such as *rheumatoid arthritis*.

The inflammation causes the synovium to secrete an abnormal amount of lubricating fluid, which makes the joint swollen, painful, and often warm and red. To determine the cause of the condition, an arthrocentesis (removal of fluid from a joint) or a biopsy (removal of a sample of the synovium) may be required.

Symptoms are relieved by rest, supporting the joint with a splint or cast, *analgesics* (painkillers), *nonsteroidal anti-inflammatory drugs*, and, occasionally, an injection of *corticosteroid drugs*. Any causative infection is treated with *antibiotic drugs*. Chronic

S

synovitis that does not respond to drug treatment or injection may be treated by *synovectomy* (surgical removal of the synovium).

Synovium

A thin membrane that lines the fibrous capsule surrounding a movable joint. The synovium also forms a sheath for certain tendons of the hands and feet, lining the fibrous or bony tunnels through which they glide. The membrane secretes synovial fluid, a clear, sticky liquid resembling egg white that lubricates the joint or the tendon. The synovium can become inflamed; in a joint lining this is known as *synovitis*, in a tendon sheath it is known as *tenosynovitis*.

LOCATION OF SYNOVIUM

Every movable joint is enclosed within a fibrous capsule. The inner lining of the capsule is known as the synovium.

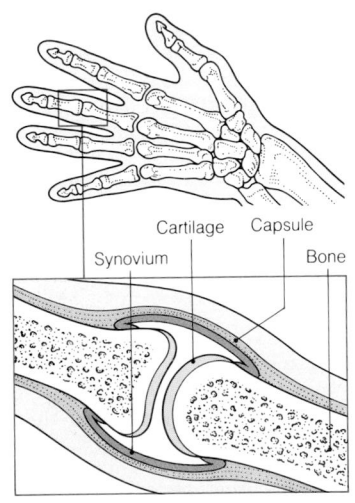

Cartilage Capsule
Synovium Bone

Function
The membrane secretes a thick fluid that lubricates the joint; it may accumulate and cause pain if the joint is injured.

Syphilis

A sexually transmitted or *congenital* (existing at birth) infection of worldwide distribution, first recorded as a major epidemic in Europe in the last decade of the 15th century following the return of Columbus from America. Today, infection is transmitted almost exclusively by sexual contact. Congenital syphilis, once very common, is now rare.

CAUSES
Syphilis is caused by *TREPONEMA PALLIDUM*, a spirochete (spiral-shaped bacterium) that penetrates broken skin or *mucous membranes* in the genitalia, rectum, or mouth during sexual intercourse. Infection may be acquired by kissing or by intimate bodily contact with an infected person. The risk of infection during a single contact with an infected person is about 30 percent. After gaining access, the organism passes quickly by way of the bloodstream and lymphatic system to all parts of the body; within hours, the organism has spread beyond hope of local treatment.

INCIDENCE
The incidence of syphilis in the US increased during the late 1970s and early 1980s, especially in homosexual men, but has demonstrated a marked decrease since 1982. This decrease may be attributed to changes in sexual practices since *AIDS* was first publicized. However, a resurgence of penicillin-resistant *gonorrhea* in 1988 suggested that efforts to educate people on the avoidance of sexually transmitted diseases had yet to take effect.

SYMPTOMS AND SIGNS
Untreated syphilis usually passes through the following stages.

PRIMARY The first symptom is a primary sore (chancre) that usually appears three to four weeks after contact. The chancre is a painless ulcer with a hard, wet base that is covered with serum teeming with spirochetes. The usual site is the genitals but may be the anus, mouth, rectum, or fingers. Often, the chancre is inconspicuous and may be missed. The lymph nodes connected with the area containing the chancre become painlessly enlarged and rubbery but are not tender. The chancre heals in four to eight weeks.

SECONDARY Six to 12 weeks after infection, the secondary stage begins. The most obvious feature is a skin rash, which may be transient, recurrent, or may last for months. In whites, the rash is conspicuous, with crops of pinkish or pale red, round spots; in blacks, the rash is pigmented and appears darker than the normal skin color. The rash is associated with extensive lymph node enlargement; there is often headache, aches and pains in the bones, loss of appetite, fever, and fatigue. Meningitis may occur. The hair may fall out in clumps and, in moist skin areas, thickened, gray or pink patches called con-

dylomata lata may develop. They are highly infectious. The secondary stage may persist for about a year.

LATENT During this stage, which may last for a few years or for the rest of the person's life, the infected person appears normal. However, about 30 percent of untreated cases proceed, eventually, to tertiary syphilis.

TERTIARY This stage usually starts within ten years of infection, but may appear as early as three years or as late as 25 years. The effects are varied. Tissue destruction, by a process called gumma formation, may involve the bones, palate, nasal septum, tongue, skin, or almost any organ of the body. Among the more serious effects are cardiovascular syphilis, which affects the aorta (the main artery of the body) and leads to aneurysm formation and heart valve disease; neurosyphilis, with progressive brain damage and general paralysis (once called "general paralysis of the insane"); and tabes dorsalis, which affects part of the spinal cord.

DIAGNOSIS
Primary syphilis can be readily diagnosed by microscopic demonstration of the active spirochetes in the chancre serum. Confirmation is given by tests such as the Venereal Disease Research Laboratory (VDRL) test or the fluorescent treponemal antibody absorption test. Secondary, latent, and tertiary syphilis give strongly positive results with these and similar tests. In

Congenital syphilis
This baby's mother had syphilis during pregnancy. A rash and other signs of infection developed in the baby early in life. Congenital syphilis is very rare today.

neurosyphilis, it may be necessary to perform these tests on a sample of cerebrospinal fluid.

TREATMENT

The significance of the disease has been altered since the introduction of penicillin. It remains the drug of choice for all forms of the disease. Early syphilis can often be cured by a single large *depot injection*; later forms of syphilis require a longer course of treatment. Although penicillin is, in general, a very safe drug, the treatment of syphilis is not without danger. More than half of those treated suffer a severe reaction within six to 12 hours, caused by the body's response to the sudden killing of large numbers of spirochetes. Organ damage already caused by the disease cannot be reversed.

PREVENTION

Promiscuous and frequent heterosexual or homosexual intercourse inevitably involves a risk of infection with syphilis. Infection can be avoided by maintaining monogamous relationships. Condoms offer some measure of protection but do not offer absolute protection (see *"Safe" sex*). People with syphilis are infectious in the primary and secondary stages but not in the late latent and tertiary stages.

Syringe

An instrument for injecting fluid into, or withdrawing fluid from, a body cavity, blood vessel, or tissue. Most syringes consist of a barrel with a plunger at one end and, at the other, a nozzle to which a hollow needle can be attached. The barrel is calibrated to enable the correct dosage of medication to be given. Most modern syringes are disposable plastic instruments that are presterilized and packed in sealed bags.

A hypodermic syringe is, strictly, one used for giving injections just beneath the skin. However, identical instruments are used for intramuscular (into a muscle) and intravenous (into a vein) injections. Thus, the term hypodermic syringe (or sometimes simply syringe) is used for all types.

Syringing of ears

A procedure for removing excessive *earwax* or, less commonly, a foreign body from the outer-ear canal (see *Ear, foreign body in*).

The physician first examines the ear to see if there is a condition (e.g., perforated eardrum) that indicates syringing should not be done. If there is no such indication, any hard wax

may first require softening by putting drops of oil in the ear. The earwax is then washed out using the procedure shown in the illustrated box below. Afterward, the canal is dried, sometimes with the help of alcohol drops. As an alternative to flushing out, wax and other debris may be removed by suction or by small instruments.

Ear syringing may be an uncomfortable procedure. Sudden acute pain or dizziness may indicate a perforation of the eardrum and the need to stop the procedure.

Syringomyelia

A very rare, usually congenital condition in which a cavity forms in the brain stem or at neck level in the spinal

EAR SYRINGING

This procedure should be carried out only by a physician or nurse; amateur attempts can damage the eardrum.

1 The nozzle of a large syringe is placed just inside the ear canal, which is straightened out by pulling the external ear upward and backward.

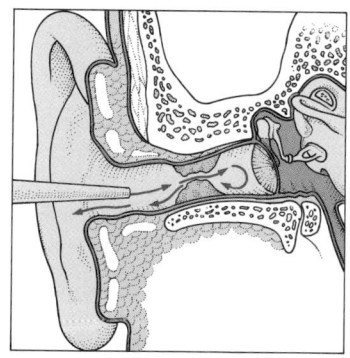

2 A jet of warm water or sodium bicarbonate solution is directed along the upper wall of the patient's ear canal in order to dislodge the blockage.

cord. The cavity gradually expands, filling with cerebrospinal fluid, eventually causing damage to nerve fibers.

The first symptoms usually appear in early adulthood. Affected persons are unable to feel pain or temperature changes in the neck, shoulders, arms, and hands, causing them to suffer burns and injure themselves without realizing it. The muscles in the same region gradually become weak, wasted, and cold, and there is some loss of the sensation of touch.

In people with advanced syringomyelia, there is spasticity (abnormal stiffness and rigidity) in the legs, nasal speech, and sometimes difficulty swallowing. Many severely affected people are confined to wheelchairs.

No drug treatment is available. In some cases, surgical treatment to relieve pressure in the affected region (see *Decompression, spinal canal*) may arrest what is otherwise an inevitably progressive disease.

System

A group of interconnected or interdependent organs that acts to perform a common function. For example, the different parts of the *digestive system* (the mouth, salivary glands, esophagus, stomach, intestines, gallbladder, pancreas, and liver) act together to ingest, break down, absorb, and excrete food.

The term system may also be applied to a method of classification, as in the ABO system for classifying *blood groups*.

Systemic

A term applied to something that affects the whole body rather than a specific part of it. For example, fever is a systemic symptom, whereas swelling is a localized symptom. The term systemic is also applied to the part of the blood circulation that supplies all parts of the body except the lungs.

Systemic lupus erythematosus

See *Lupus erythematosus*.

Systole

A period of muscular contraction of a chamber of the heart that alternates with a resting period, called *diastole*. With each heart beat, the atria (upper chambers) contract first (atrial systole), squeezing blood into the ventricles (lower chambers). The ventricles then contract (ventricular systole), pumping blood out of the heart into the arteries.

S

T

Tabes dorsalis
A complication of *syphilis*, once common but now rare, that affects the spinal cord, causing abnormalities of sensation, sharp pains, incoordination, and incontinence. Symptoms appear several years after infection.

Tachycardia
A heart rate of over 100 beats per minute in an adult. Most people have a rate of between 60 and 100 beats per minute, with an average of 72 to 78 beats. Tachycardia occurs in healthy people during exercise, when the heart is stimulated to work faster and thus increase blood flow to muscles. Tachycardia at rest may be caused by *fever, hyperthyroidism, coronary heart disease* or any other cause of heart disease or heart failure, a high intake of caffeine, or treatment with an *anticholinergic drug* or some *decongestant drugs*. Types of tachycardia include *atrial fibrillation, sinus tachycardia, supraventricular tachycardia*, and *ventricular tachycardia*.

Symptoms of tachycardia may include *palpitations, breathlessness*, and lightheadedness, depending on how fast the heart is beating and on how effectively it is pumping blood.

Tachypnea
An abnormally fast rate of breathing. Tachypnea may be caused by exercise, anxiety, a lung disorder (such as emphysema), or a cardiac disorder (such as heart failure).

T'ai chi
A Chinese exercise based on a series of more than 100 postures between which many slow, continuous, deliberate movements occur. T'ai chi is characterized by outer movement and inner stillness; its purpose is to exercise the muscles and achieve integration of mind and body. Devotees believe that continuous flow of movement is important in performing the exercises because it prevents "blockage" of the internal flow of chi—the essential life energy.

Talipes
A congenital deformity in which the foot is twisted out of shape or position. There are many different varieties of talipes, all of which are commonly labeled clubfoot. The causes are not fully understood, but there is a genetic factor (relatives of affected people have a higher incidence of the disorder).

The most common, and serious, form of talipes is an equinovarus deformity in which the heel is turned inward and the rest of the foot is bent downward and inward. The arch of the foot is higher than normal and there may be underdevelopment of the muscles in the lower leg above the affected foot.

Talipes equinovarus
This birth defect affects about one baby in 1,500. Treatment is by gentle manipulation, repeated several times a day.

TREATMENT
Treatment of talipes equinovarus, which should begin soon after birth, consists of repeated manipulations of the foot and ankle over several weeks. Between manipulations, the foot is held in the corrected position by a plaster cast, metal splint, or adhesive strapping. If this procedure is not effective, an operation to cut the tight ligaments and tendons is performed and the foot is then immobilized in a plaster cast for at least three months. Treatment undertaken after age 2 cannot restore the foot to normal, but function can be improved by transferring a tendon from one bone to another (see *Tendon transfer*) or by lengthening a tendon.

Other types of talipes can usually be corrected by repeated stretching of the foot into a normal position. Occasionally, immobilization in a plaster cast is required.

Tamoxifen
An *anticancer drug* used in the treatment of certain types of *breast cancer*. Tamoxifen is also sometimes effective in the treatment of other cancers, such as those of the prostate.

In women of childbearing age, tamoxifen stimulates *ovulation* (egg release) and is therefore under investigation as a treatment for certain types of *infertility*.

Tamoxifen works by blocking *estrogen hormone* receptors. It has fewer adverse effects than most anticancer drugs, but may cause hot flashes, nausea, vomiting, swollen ankles, and irregular vaginal bleeding.

Tampon
A plug of absorbent material, such as cotton, that is inserted into a wound or body opening to soak up blood or other secretions. The term usually refers to a sanitary tampon that is inserted into the vagina to absorb menstrual blood.

Tamponade
Compression of the heart. Tamponade may occur in *pericarditis* (inflammation of the outer lining of the heart) due to fluid collecting under the lining; it may also result from blood and blood clots surrounding the heart after heart surgery or a penetrating injury of the chest.

Symptoms include breathlessness and, sometimes, collapse because the heart is unable to pump blood efficiently to the lungs and brain. The diagnosis may be best made by using *echocardiography*.

Treatment involves immediate removal of any fluid that is pressing on the heart via a hollow needle guided through the chest wall. If blood clots are present, a *thoracotomy* is usually performed to open the chest wall and remove them.

Tan
See *Suntan*.

Tannin
Also known as tannic acid, an organic chemical that occurs in many plants, particularly in oak gallnuts, the barks of oak, sumac, and mangrove trees, and tea.

Tannin has been used in medicine to stop bleeding, to control diarrhea, and as an antidote to plant poisons. It is no longer used therapeutically because more effective agents are available and because it can cause liver damage. Although tea contains significant amounts of tannin, drinking moderate amounts is unlikely to lead to liver damage. However, it may cause constipation.

Tantrum

An outburst of bad temper, common in toddlers, usually indicating frustration and anger. Tantrums occur in many children between 15 months and 4 years, but are especially likely in 2 year olds.

During a tantrum, the child may scream, cry, yell, kick, bang feet and fists, roll on the floor, go red in the face, spit, and bite. In some cases, the toddler develops the habit of holding his or her breath during tantrums, and may even turn blue and, in rare cases, lose consciousness momentarily (see *Breath-holding attacks*).

CAUSES

Tantrums occur at the age when a child starts to gain independence and becomes frustrated by restraints imposed by others, but is not yet able to express these feelings verbally. The outbursts are more likely when the child is tired, and are often brought on by a disagreement between child and parents. Tantrums may start with the birth of another baby, when the child may believe the baby is getting all the parents' attention.

Most children have occasional tantrums; frequent outbursts may indicate a *behavioral problem*, sometimes due to emotional strain or to a communication problem.

TREATMENT

Try to ignore tantrums as much as possible; becoming angry only excites the child further. Firm and consistent treatment is essential. Do not punish the child and then give in to his or her demands. With calm, quick thinking you can often divert your child's attention to a game or project. This often works better than trying to argue with a 2 year old. Most children grow out of tantrums as they develop the ability to express their feelings through speech, which should be encouraged.

If parents are unable to cope with the tantrums, or the child does not seem to be growing out of them, a physician should be consulted. *Child guidance* may be necessary.

Tapeworm infestation

 Tapeworms, also called cestodes, are ribbon-shaped parasitic worms that live in human or animal intestines. They are typically acquired from eating undercooked meat or fish. Each adult tapeworm bears suckers or hooks on its head, by which it attaches itself to the intestinal wall. The rest of the worm consists of a chain of flat segments.

CAUSES, TYPES, AND INCIDENCE

Human tapeworms have life cycles that usually also involve another animal host. A typical life cycle is shown in the illustration below.

Three large types of tapeworm, acquired by eating undercooked, infected beef, pork, and fish, all have life cycles of this type. The adults may grow to 20 or even 30 feet (6 to 9 meters) long. All occur worldwide, but, in developed countries, infestations are largely prevented by measures such as adequate meat inspection and sanitary disposal of sewage. In the US, the pork tapeworm is extremely rare and the beef and fish tapeworms are uncommon.

The much smaller dwarf tapeworm, which is only 1 inch (2.5 cm) long, has a different life cycle. An infested person may directly cause an infestation of someone else through accidental transfer of worm eggs from feces to fingers to mouth. The dwarf tapeworm is found worldwide, but especially in the tropics; it primarily affects children.

Humans may act as intermediate host to the larvae of a tapeworm for which dogs are the main host. The larvae grow and develop into cysts in the liver and lungs, a condition called *hydatid disease*.

SYMPTOMS, DIAGNOSIS, AND TREATMENT

Despite their size, beef, pork, and fish tapeworms rarely cause symptoms, except mild abdominal discomfort or diarrhea. However, segments of the worm may detach and emerge through the anus or may appear in the feces. In rare cases, fish tapeworms cause *anemia*. Dwarf tapeworms can cause diarrhea and abdominal discomfort.

Tapeworm infestation is diagnosed by a physician finding worm segments and/or eggs excreted in the feces; infestation is treated by drugs (such as niclosamide) which effectively kill the worms.

Treatment of pork tapeworm must be carried out carefully because there is a risk of worm eggs being released and regurgitated into the stomach. The patient may then accidentally become the host to the worm larvae, which burrow into the tissues and form cysts. This leads to a condition called cysticercosis, the symptoms of which may include muscle pains and convulsions. Cysticercosis is treated with drugs such as praziquantel.

Tarsalgia

Pain in the foot at the point where it forms the ankle joint, usually associated with *flatfoot*.

Tarsorrhaphy

An operation in which the upper and lower eyelids are sewn together.

WHY IT IS DONE

Tarsorrhaphy may be performed as part of the treatment of *corneal ulcer*. The eyelids act as a bandage to promote healing of the cornea. Frequently, tarsorrhaphy is used to protect the corneas in people who cannot close their eyelids because of

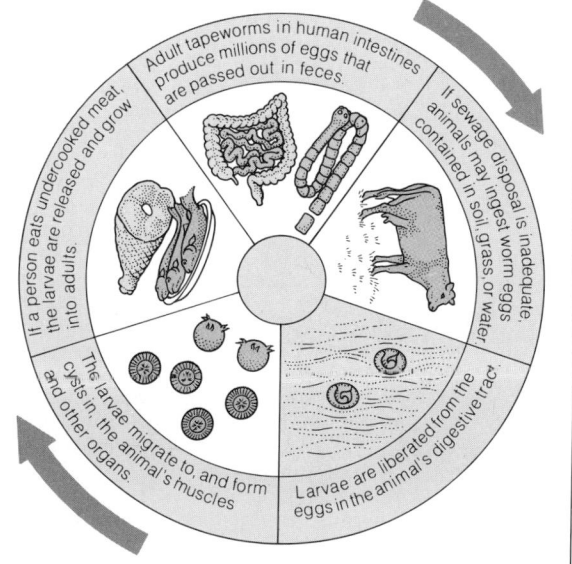

LIFE CYCLE OF TAPEWORM
Many tapeworms have life cycles in which the adult and larval worms infest different hosts. In the cycle at right, the adult worms infest humans and the larvae infest cattle (called the intermediate hosts). Pigs and fish may also act as intermediate hosts to human tapeworms, and humans may act as intermediate hosts to dog and pig tapeworms.

Adult tapeworms in human intestines produce millions of eggs that are passed out in feces.

If sewage disposal is inadequate, animals may ingest worm eggs contained in soil, grass, or water.

Larvae are liberated from the eggs in the animal's digestive tract.

The larvae migrate to, and form cysts in, the animal's muscles and other organs.

If a person eats undercooked meat, the larvae are released and grow into adults.

nerve or muscular disorders or scarring. Tarsorrhaphy is also occasionally performed to protect the cornea in people with *exophthalmos*.

HOW IT IS DONE
A strip of tissue is removed from the upper and lower lid edges. The raw surfaces of the lids are then stitched together. By about two or three weeks after the operation, the eyelids have grown together and the stitches can be removed. The eyelids are cut apart and allowed to open when the original abnormality subsides.

Tartar
See *Calculus, dental.*

Taste
One of the five special senses. Alone, taste is a relatively crude sense, able to distinguish only between sweet, salty, sour, and bitter. In practice, however, many different flavors can be distinguished because of the combination of the sense of taste and the much more discriminating sense of *smell*. This combination explains why loss of the sense of smell (caused by a common cold, for example) also apparently causes loss of taste (see *Taste, loss of*). The full sensory appreciation of food also involves other factors, such as the appearance of food (which helps stimulate saliva-

tion) and the consistency and temperature of the food. The mechanisms and structures on the tongue involved in taste are illustrated below.

Taste, loss of
Loss of *taste* usually occurs as a result of loss of the sense of *smell* (usually due to a common cold or influenza), which contributes greatly to taste.

Loss of taste without loss of smell is relatively rare. A possible cause is any condition that results in a dry mouth (see *Mouth, dry*), because taste buds can detect the substances responsible for flavors only when those substances are dissolved in saliva.

THE SENSE OF TASTE
Tastes are detected by special structures called taste buds, of which everyone has some 10,000, mainly on the tongue, with a few at the back of the throat and on the palate. These taste buds surround pores within papillae (protuberances) on the tongue surface and elsewhere. Four types of taste buds exist—sensitive to sweet, salty, sour, and bitter chemicals. All tastes are formed from a mixture of these four basic elements.

Olfactory bulb

Tongue

Glosso-pharyngeal nerve

Vallate papillae

Taste pore

Taste bud

Vallate papillae

Filiform papillae

Fungiform papillae

Fungiform papillae
These mushroom-shaped papillae occur in small numbers at random over the tongue surface, mainly in the middle.

Filiform papillae
These smaller peak-shaped protuberances occur in large numbers over all except the back of the tongue's upper surface, and on the palate.

How a substance is tasted
Chemicals in food or drink dissolve in saliva and enter pores in the papillae on the tongue. Around these pores are groups of taste receptor cells—the taste buds. The chemicals stimulate hairs projecting from the receptor cells, causing signals to be sent from the cells along nerves to taste centers in the brain.

Magnified photograph of tongue surface
The photograph shows large (fungiform) and small (filiform) papillae. Taste buds are arranged around pores in the surface of the papillae.

Taste centers on the tongue
Taste buds sensitive to sweet, salty, sour, and bitter chemicals tend to be grouped into particular areas on the surface of the tongue.

Bitter

Salt

Salt

Sour

Sweet

T

Complete or partial loss of taste may result from damage to the taste buds themselves as a result of *stomatitis* (inflammation of the mouth), *mouth cancer* or *radiation therapy* (which also eliminates salivation by damaging the salivary glands) to treat mouth cancer, the side effects of certain drugs, or, most commonly, the natural degeneration of the taste buds with age.

Loss of taste may also be caused by damage to the cranial nerves that convey taste sensations to the brain. Nerve damage may occur as a result of a head injury, a tumor of the brain or of the cranial nerves associated with taste, or surgery on the head or neck. In these cases, loss of taste is usually accompanied by facial paralysis.

Disturbances of taste occur in some psychiatric disorders, usually taking the form of taste hallucinations rather than true loss of taste.

Tattooing

The introduction of permanent colors under the surface of the skin, usually to create a picture. Practiced for thousands of years, tattooing was originally used as a means of identification. Today it is almost always carried out for decorative purposes.

Tattooing, even by professionals, is potentially dangerous; if the tattooist does not follow strict sterile procedures, *hepatitis* and *AIDS* may be transmitted through the needles used to introduce the dyes.

Removal of a tattoo is usually difficult and unsatisfactory; a scar almost always results. Small tattoos are best treated by complete removal of the colored area of skin and the stitching together of the edges of the wound. Larger tattoed areas can sometimes be removed by *dermabrasion* or *laser treatment*.

Tay-Sachs disease

A serious inherited brain disorder that results in very early death. Tay-Sachs disease was formerly known as amaurotic familial idiocy.

CAUSES AND INCIDENCE

Tay-Sachs disease is caused by a deficiency of hexosaminidase, a certain *enzyme* (a protein essential for regulating chemical reactions in the body). Deficiency results in a buildup of a harmful substance in the brain.

The disease is most common among Ashkenazi Jews. The incidence in this group is around one in 2,500, which is 100 times higher than in any other ethnic group. The gene for Tay-Sachs disease is recessive and an Ashkenazi

Jew has a one in 25 chance of carrying it. If two carriers marry, there is a one in four chance that they will have an affected child.

SYMPTOMS AND SIGNS

Signs of the illness, which appear during the first six months of life, are blindness, dementia, deafness, seizures, and paralysis. An exaggerated startle response to sound is an early sign. Symptoms progress rapidly and the affected child usually dies before age 3.

DIAGNOSIS

The diagnosis is based on family history and physical examination; it is confirmed by enzyme analysis of any tissue sample—tears, serum, blood cells, or hair roots.

TREATMENT AND PREVENTION

There is no treatment for Tay-Sachs disease. Programs for detecting carriers of the gene have been introduced in some countries. Carriers and those with an affected child or relative should receive *genetic counseling* before starting a family or planning another pregnancy. If *prenatal screening* shows that a fetus may be affected, the parents may choose to have an abortion.

TB

An abbreviation for *tuberculosis*.

T cell

One of the two main classes of *lymphocytes* (a type of white blood cell). T cells play an important role in the body's *immune system* (defenses against infection and against cancer cells).

Tears

The salty, watery secretion produced by the lacrimal glands, part of the *lacrimal apparatus* of the *eye*. The tear film over the *cornea* and the *conjunctiva* consists of three layers—an inner, mucous layer secreted by glands in the conjunctiva; an intermediate layer of salt water; and an outer, oily layer secreted by the meibomian glands.

A deficiency in tear production causes *keratoconjunctivitis sicca* (dry eye). Excessive tear production may cause *watering eye*.

Tears, artificial

Preparations used to supplement inadequate production of tears in *keratoconjunctivitis sicca* and other conditions causing dryness of the eyes. To be effective, artificial tears must be applied at frequent intervals. Artificial tears may also be used to relieve

discomfort caused by irritants, such as smoke or dust, but provide only temporary relief.

Many preparations contain a preservative that can irritate the eyes. Contaminated preparations may cause serious eye infections.

Technetium

A radioactive metallic element that does not occur naturally either in its pure form or as compounds; technetium is produced during nuclear fission reactions. It was the first element to be made artificially (in 1937). Several isotopes (varieties of the element that are chemically identical but differ in some physical properties) have been synthesized, of which the most important medically is a form known as technetium 99m. This radioisotope, incorporated in various chemical substances, is used in *radionuclide scanning* of numerous organs, including the brain, heart, lungs, liver, kidneys, and bones.

Teeth

Hard structures set in the jaw that are used for *mastication* (chewing) of food. The teeth also give shape to the face and help people to speak clearly. In humans, there are two sets of teeth—the *primary teeth* (of which there are 20) and the *permanent teeth* (of which there are 32). The primary teeth usually erupt between the ages of 6 months and 3 years and start to be replaced by the permanent teeth at about age 6 (see *Eruption of teeth*). In some people, the teeth fail to grow in the correct relationship to each other, resulting in *malocclusion* (incorrect bite). The arrangement of the teeth is shown in the box opposite.

Although the enamel that covers the crown of each tooth is the hardest substance in the body, it can be eroded by acid created when bacteria in the mouth break down the carbohydrates in food, resulting in *caries* (decay). To help prevent decay, good *oral hygiene* is essential, consisting of daily *toothbrushing* and flossing (see *Floss, dental*). See also *Gum*.

Teeth, care of

See *Oral hygiene*.

Teething

The period when a baby cuts his or her first set of teeth. The primary teeth usually begin to erupt at about 6 or 7 months (see *Eruption of teeth*). On average, the first set of teeth is complete soon after the second birthday.

T

STRUCTURE AND ARRANGEMENT OF TEETH

At the heart of each tooth is the living pulp, which contains blood vessels and nerves. A hard substance called dentin surrounds the pulp. The part of the tooth above the gum, the crown, is covered by enamel. The roots of the tooth, which fit into sockets in the jawbone, are covered by a sensitive, bonelike material, the cementum. The periodontal ligament connects the cementum to the gums and to the jaw. It acts as a shock absorber and prevents jarring of the teeth and skull when food is being chewed.

Cross section

- Enamel
- Dentin
- Pulp
- Neck of tooth
- Gum
- Jawbone
- Root
- Cementum
- Blood vessels
- Periodontal ligament
- Nerve

- Central and lateral incisors (7 to 9 years)
- First and second premolars (10 to 12 years)
- Second molars (11 to 13 years)
- Third molars (17+ years)
- First molars (6 to 7 years)
- Canines (12 to 14 years)

The permanent teeth

The illustration above shows the arrangement in the jaw of the permanent teeth—eight incisors, four canines, eight premolars, and 12 molars. The ages when these teeth erupt are indicated.

X ray of teeth

The panoramic X ray at left shows all the teeth of the upper and lower jaw (there are no wisdom teeth) and their surrounding structures. The tooth roots, buried in the jaw bones, can be clearly seen; several teeth have been filled.

Molars | Premolars | Canines | Incisors | Canines | Premolars | Molars

Third | Second | First

Molars

The molars are large, strong teeth, efficient at grinding food. The third molars, or wisdom teeth, are the last to erupt; in some people, the wisdom teeth never appear.

Premolars

Also known as bicuspids, because of their two distinct edges, the premolars are concerned with grinding food. There are no premolars among the baby teeth.

Incisors

These teeth have a chisel-shaped, sharp cutting edge ideal for biting. The upper incisors overlap the lower incisors slightly when the jaws are closed.

Canines

The canines are sharp, pointed teeth, ideal for tearing food. They are larger and stronger than the incisors, with very long roots. The upper canines are often known as eye teeth.

SYMPTOMS AND SIGNS

While teeth are erupting, a baby may be irritable, fretful, clinging, have difficulty sleeping, and may cry more than usual. Extra saliva may be produced, resulting in dribbling, and the baby tends to chew on anything that he or she can hold.

Before a tooth comes through, the overlying gum may become red and swollen and the erupting tooth can be felt through the gum as a hard lump.

When molars erupt, the cheek may feel warm and red on the affected side.

Teething should never be considered the cause of a very high temperature, vomiting, diarrhea, prolonged loss of appetite, earache, convulsions, cough, or diaper rash. These are symptoms of illness and a physician should be consulted.

TREATMENT

Give the baby something firm to chew on, such as a piece of apple, or rub the swollen gum with a finger to ease the irritation. A small dose of a simple analgesic, such as acetaminophen, may be necessary if the child is very uncomfortable. Painkilling dental creams or gels are also available to rub on the gums.

Telangiectasia

An increase in the size and number of the small blood vessels in an area of skin, causing redness. Telangiectasia is most common on the nose and cheeks. It is often a result of overexposure to sunlight or long-term high alcohol consumption.

Appearance of telangiectasia
Although sometimes referred to as broken veins, the blood vessels are in fact simply more numerous and larger than usual.

Telangiectasia is a feature of *rosacea* and also of *lupus erythematosus, dermatomyositis,* and *psoriasis*. A common, localized form of telangiectasia is the *spider nevus*. Hereditary hemorrhagic telangiectasia is a rare condition in which frequent bleeding occurs from small, rounded patches of widened blood vessels around the mouth and nose or elsewhere in the skin or gastrointestinal tract.

Temazepam

A *benzodiazepine drug* used in the short-term treatment of *insomnia*.

Temperature

For the body to function optimally, its temperature must be maintained within narrow limits. The generally accepted figure for the average normal body temperature (measured in the mouth) is 98.6°F (37°C). However, in practice, body temperature varies not only among individuals, but also in the same person, being affected by factors such as exercise, sleep, eating and drinking, time of day (lowest at about 3 AM and highest at about 6 PM), and, in women, the stage of the menstrual cycle (lowest at menstruation and highest at ovulation). In most people, body temperature varies between 97.8°F (36.5°C) and 99°F (37.2°C). The temperature is higher in the rectum, by about 0.5 to 0.7°F (0.3 to 0.4°C), and lower in the armpit, by about 0.3 to 0.5°F (0.2 to 0.3°C).

TEMPERATURE REGULATION

Body temperature is maintained within optimal limits by the *hypothalamus*, an area of the brain that acts like a thermostat, constantly monitoring blood temperature and automatically activating mechanisms to compensate for changes.

When body temperature falls, the hypothalamus sends nerve impulses to stimulate *shivering* (which generates heat by muscle activity) and to constrict blood vessels in the skin, which reduces heat loss. Conversely, when body temperature rises, the hypothalamus stimulates *sweating* and dilates blood vessels in the skin to increase heat loss.

A variety of factors—such as infections, certain disorders (notably those of the thyroid gland), unusual symptoms of a tumor, and overexposure to cold or extreme heat—may disrupt the body's heat-regulating system, resulting in *fever, heat stroke,* or *hypothermia*.

Temperature method

See *Contraception, periodic abstinence*.

Temporal arteritis

An uncommon disease of elderly people in which the walls of the arteries that pass over the temples in the scalp become inflamed. Other arteries in the head and neck may also be affected, as may the aorta (the large artery that carries oxygenated blood from the heart) and its main branches. The inflamed blood vessels become narrowed, and blood flow through them is reduced. The disease is also known as giant cell arteritis.

CAUSES AND INCIDENCE

The cause of temporal arteritis is unknown, but it is often associated with *polymyalgia rheumatica* (pain and stiffness in the muscles of the hips, thighs, shoulders, and neck).

In the US, about 10 cases of temporal arteritis are diagnosed per 100,000 population each year. Nearly all patients are over 50, and more women than men are affected.

SYMPTOMS AND SIGNS

The most common symptom is a headache, usually severe, on one or both sides of the head. The temporal artery (located at the side of the head above the earlobe) may be prominent and the scalp may be tender. In nearly one half of sufferers, the ophthalmic arteries supplying the eyes may become affected, resulting in partial loss of vision or even sudden blindness.

Other symptoms and signs of temporal arteritis include low fever, poor appetite, and lethargy.

Involvement of the aorta or its main branches results in circulatory disorders, such as intermittent *claudica-*

TEMPORAL ARTERITIS
In this disorder, the temporal artery and other arteries in the head are inflamed. Early reporting of symptoms is vital, since, in untreated cases, there is a risk of sudden blindness.

Site of pain

Temporal artery

Telltale symptoms
If the temporal artery is inflamed, it is usually prominent and there is a persistent severe headache and scalp tenderness in the area shown.

Normal blood flow

Normal artery
A normal artery has a smooth lining, and blood flow is sufficient to meet the needs of the tissues it supplies.

Reduced blood flow

Inflamed artery
In arteritis, the walls of the artery become disrupted and thickened, and blood flow is markedly reduced.

tion (pain in the legs on walking) or *Raynaud's phenomenon* (pallor in the fingers on exposure to cold).

DIAGNOSIS AND TREATMENT

Early reporting of symptoms to a physician is essential because of the risk of blindness. The diagnosis is made by a *biopsy* (removal of a small sample of tissue for analysis) of the temporal artery and *blood tests* to detect the presence of a raised *ESR* (erythrocyte sedimentation rate).

The disease responds rapidly to a *corticosteroid drug*, which is initially given in high doses to prevent blindness. Most people need to take the drug, at a reduced dosage, for one or two years. If the disease fails to respond to the corticosteroid, or if the drug causes serious side effects, *immunosuppressant drugs* (such as azathioprine) may be given.

OUTLOOK

With treatment, the disease usually clears up within two years. Most people are not left with any lasting disability. However, if one or both eyes become blind before treatment has become effective, the blindness may be permanent.

Temporal lobe epilepsy

A form of *epilepsy* in which abnormal electrical discharges in the brain are confined to a localized region on one side, the temporal lobe. The seizures therefore differ from the generalized disturbances that occur in a grand mal seizure or in an absence seizure (petit mal).

LOCATION OF THE TEMPORAL LOBE
The temporal lobe forms much of the lower side of each half of the cerebrum (main mass of the brain).

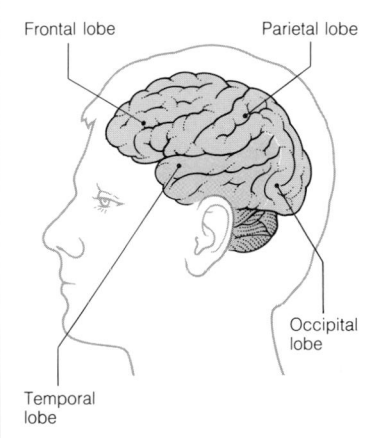

Frontal lobe

Parietal lobe

Occipital lobe

Temporal lobe

CAUSE

There is usually an area of damage within one of the temporal lobes that acts as a focus for the abnormal development of electrical discharges in attacks. Damage may be caused by a *birth injury, head injury, brain tumor, brain abscess,* or *stroke*. The temporal lobes are concerned with such functions as smell, taste, hearing, visual associations, and some aspects of memory. Abnormal electrical activity in a lobe may thus cause peculiarities in any of these functions.

SYMPTOMS AND SIGNS

People affected by temporal lobe epilepsy suffer dreamlike states that range from partial loss of awareness to total disregard. The person may have unpleasant hallucinations of smell or taste. Also common during attacks is the perception of an illusory scene or the phenomenon of *déjà vu*. There may also be facial grimacing, rotation of the head and eyes, and often sucking and chewing movements.

The affected person may perform tasks with no memory of them after the attack. An attack may last for minutes or hours before full consciousness returns.

In some cases a temporal lobe seizure progresses after several seconds or minutes to a generalized grand mal seizure.

DIAGNOSIS AND TREATMENT

The principles of investigation and drug treatment for temporal lobe epilepsy are the same as for other types of epilepsy. Surgery has been used with success in some cases of temporal lobe epilepsy. The operation is designed to remove the part of the lobe containing the irritating focus for the attacks. Operations are performed only in severe cases that have not responded to drug treatment because of the possible effects on other important functions of the brain.

Temporomandibular joint syndrome

Pain and other symptoms affecting the head, jaw, and face that are believed to result when the temporomandibular joints (jaw joints) and the muscles and ligaments that control and support them do not work together correctly.

CAUSES

The most common cause of the temporomandibular joint syndrome is spasm of the chewing muscles. Frequently, this is due to habits such as clenching or grinding the teeth, usually as a result of emotional ten-

LOCATION OF THE TEMPOROMANDIBULAR JOINT
The head of the mandible (jawbone) fits into a hollow on the underside of the temporal bone of the skull at the joint.

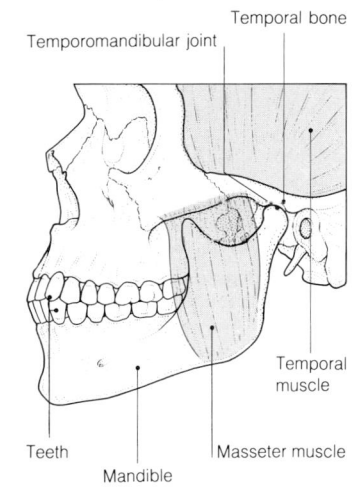

Temporomandibular joint

Temporal bone

Temporal muscle

Teeth

Masseter muscle

Mandible

sion. An incorrect bite, which places additional stress on the muscles, may be a contributing factor.

Temporomandibular joint problems may also be caused by displacement of the joint as a result of jaw, head, or neck injuries. In rare cases, *osteoarthritis* is a cause.

SYMPTOMS

Headaches, tenderness of the jaw muscles, and dull, aching facial pain with severe exacerbation in or around the ear are common symptoms of temporomandibular joint syndrome. Other symptoms may include clicking or popping noises when the mouth is opened or closed, difficulty opening the mouth, jaws that "lock" or get stuck, or pain brought on by yawning, chewing, or opening the mouth wide.

TREATMENT

In most cases, treatment is aimed at eliminating muscle spasm and relieving pain. This may be done by applying moist heat to the face, taking muscle-relaxant drugs, massaging the muscles, eating soft, nonchewy foods, or using a bite splint (a device that fits over the teeth at night to prevent clenching or grinding). Counseling, *biofeedback training*, and *relaxation exercises* may also help.

The bite may need to be corrected by selective grinding of teeth or by the use of braces or other *orthodontic appliances*. In severe cases, surgery on the jaw joint is required.

T

Tenderness

Pain or abnormal sensitivity in a part of the body when it is pressed or touched during medical palpation (examination by touch) or contact with objects in daily living. Tenderness is usually a sign of *inflammation*. For example, *appendicitis* (inflammation of the appendix) causes tenderness of the abdomen; *arthritis* (joint inflammation) causes tenderness around the affected joint. Tenderness is usually associated with swelling, redness, and warmth of the affected part.

Tendinitis

Inflammation of a tendon, usually caused by injury. Symptoms include pain, tenderness, and, occasionally, restricted movement of the muscle attached to the affected tendon. A common example is *painful arc syndrome*, which causes pain in the shoulder when the arm is raised above a certain angle.

Treatment of tendinitis may include *nonsteroidal anti-inflammatory drugs* (NSAIDs), *ultrasound treatment*, or an injection of *corticosteroid drugs* around the tendon.

Tendolysis

An operation performed to free a tendon from *adhesions* (fibrous bands) that surround it and limit its free movement. The adhesions are usually caused by *tenosynovitis* (inflammation of the inner lining of a tendon sheath).

The procedure consists of making a skin incision over the tendon and then splitting open its fibrous sheath. The adhesions are cut away from the tendon surface and the incisions in the sheath and the skin are stitched. Despite surgery, symptoms of tenosynovitis sometimes recur because adhesions form again.

Tendon

A fibrous cord that joins muscle to bone or muscle to muscle. Tendons are extremely strong, flexible, and inelastic. Most are cylindrical, but some, such as those attached to the flat muscles of the abdominal wall, consist of wide sheets of fibers known as aponeuroses.

Tendons are made up principally of bundles of collagen (a white, fibrous protein) and contain some blood vessels. The larger tendons (but not the aponeuroses) also have a nerve supply. Squeezing the tendon hard causes pain; stretching it triggers a *reflex* contraction of the adjoining muscle (e.g., the quadriceps jerk).

FINGER TENDONS

Finger bending and extension are controlled by tendons on either side of the finger; the tendons originate from forearm muscles.

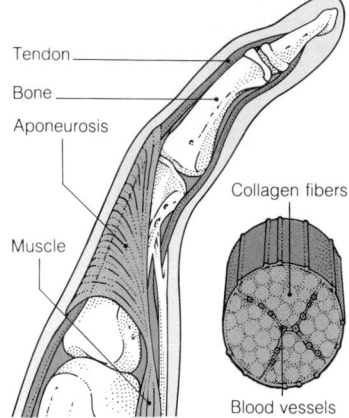

Tendon
Bone
Aponeurosis
Collagen fibers
Muscle
Blood vessels

Internal structure
A cross section of a tendon (inset) shows that it consists of numerous parallel bundles of collagen fibers along with some blood vessels.

The tendons in the hands, wrists, and feet are enclosed in synovial sheaths (fibrous capsules) and bathed in a lubricating fluid secreted by the lining of the sheath. These tendons require this additional protection because they do not move in a straight line and, without the fluid, might be subjected to excessive friction.

DISORDERS
Rupture of the *Achilles tendon* can occur during sprinting and jumping as a result of sudden contraction of the calf muscles stretching the tendon. Rupture of a tendon on the back of a finger, resulting in deformity of the fingertip, may be caused by a direct blow to the end of the finger (see *Baseball finger*). In many cases, however, because tendons are so strong, severe stress pulls off a piece of bone where the tendon is attached to it rather than tearing the tendon itself.

The long tendon of the biceps muscle in the upper arm may become weakened as a result of repeated rubbing against the humerus (upper arm bone) and may rupture under even moderate stress. Rupture of tendons in the hands can occur as a complication of *rheumatoid arthritis*.

Tendons in the hand are commonly severed by a deep cut with a knife or piece of glass; *tendon repair*, using a graft taken from a tendon elsewhere in the body, may be required.

Tendinitis, inflammation of a tendon, may follow an injury. *Tenosynovitis*, inflammation of the inner lining of a tendon sheath, usually results from overuse; it affects tendons in the hands and wrists. If the outer wall of a tendon sheath is inflamed, the gliding movement of the tendon through the sheath may be restricted (as in *trigger finger*).

Tendon release

See *Tendolysis*.

Tendon repair

An operation to join the cut or torn ends of a *tendon* or to replace a damaged tendon.

If the cut or torn ends can easily be brought together, they are stitched together with sutures. If the ends are widely separated or contained within a sheath, it may be necessary to insert a tendon graft. Tendons for grafting are taken from elsewhere in the body, usually the foot.

Tendon transfer

An operation to reposition a *tendon* so that it causes a muscle to perform a different function. Tendon transfer may be used to restore function impaired by a deformity, such as *talipes* (clubfoot), or by permanent muscle injury or paralysis.

To perform the transfer, the tendon is cut away from its original point of attachment and reattached elsewhere. Tendon transfer causes the muscle to which the tendon is attached to lie in a different position and thus to produce a different body movement when the muscle contracts.

Tenesmus

A feeling of incomplete emptying of the bowel in which the urge to pass feces is accompanied by ineffective straining. Tenesmus may be a symptom of disease of the rectum, such as polyps or cancer, or of severe inflammation caused by *ulcerative colitis* or *dysentery*.

Tennis elbow

A condition caused by inflammation around the epicondyle (bony prominence) on the outer side of the elbow, to which certain forearm muscles are attached by *tendons*. It causes pain and tenderness at the outer side of the elbow and in the back of the forearm. The pain is made worse by lifting a heavy object.

Site of tennis elbow
Pulling of the forearm muscles where they attach to the humerus causes tenderness on the outer side of the elbow.

Humerus
Attachment
Point of tenderness
Tendon
Forearm muscle

Tennis elbow is caused by overuse of the muscles that straighten the wrist and fingers. Inflammation occurs as a result of constant tugging of the tendons at their point of attachment. Activities that can cause the condition include home decorating, gardening, or playing tennis (or other racket sports) with a faulty grip.

TREATMENT
Treatment consists of resting the arm, applying *ice packs*, and taking *analgesic drugs* (painkillers) and/or *nonsteroidal anti-inflammatory drugs* (NSAIDs). *Ultrasound treatment* may help reduce the inflammation. If the pain is severe or persistent, injection of a *corticosteroid drug* may be required.

If the pain has occurred after playing a racket sport, it is wise to take a break from the sport for a week or two to prevent recurrence. It is also useful to consult a professional about your playing technique and the size of the grip on your racket.

Tenosynovitis
Inflammation of the thin inner lining of the sheath that surrounds a *tendon*. Tenosynovitis is usually caused by excessive friction due to overuse; it is often brought on by using a badly designed tool or working in an awkward position to do a job that involves repetitive movements. A rare cause of tenosynovitis is a bacterial infection, such as tuberculosis. The tendons in the hand and wrist are the most commonly affected.

Symptoms include pain, tenderness, and swelling over the tendon. There is also occasionally *crepitus* (a grating noise or sensation) when the tendon is moved. Persistent or recurrent tenosynovitis may lead to restricted movement as a result of *adhesions* (fibrous bands) forming between the tendon and its sheath.

TREATMENT
If infection is the cause, *antibiotic drugs* are prescribed. Otherwise, treatment usually consists of *nonsteroidal anti-inflammatory drugs* (NSAIDs) or an injection of *corticosteroid drugs* around the tendon. The hand and wrist may need to be immobilized in a splint for a few weeks. If the condition does not improve, surgery may be required to release adhesions (see *Tendolysis*).

Tenovaginitis
Inflammation or thickening of the fibrous wall of the sheath that surrounds a *tendon*. The cause is unknown. Tenovaginitis that affects the sheath of one of the tendons that bends a finger results in *trigger finger*.

TENS
The abbreviation for *transcutaneous electrical nerve stimulation*.

Tension
A feeling of mental and physical strain associated with anxiety. Sufferers feel unpleasantly keyed up, cannot relax, and may have feelings of bottled-up anger. Muscle tension accompanies the mental symptoms and may result in headaches and muscular stiffness and pain, particularly in the back and shoulders. Persistent tension is related to *generalized anxiety disorder*. (See also *Stress*.)

Teratogen
An agent that causes physical abnormalities in a developing embryo or fetus. Examples of teratogens include the *rubella* virus and the drug *thalidomide*. For a drug to be categorized as teratogenic, there must be evidence that taking the drug during pregnancy causes an increased incidence of congenital abnormalities that cannot be explained by other factors. Many chemicals that are known to be teratogenic in some species (such as rats) have not been proved to be teratogenic in humans. Drug-regulating agencies usually refuse to license drugs for use during pregnancy if they have been found to be teratogenic for any species.

Teratoma
A primary tumor consisting of cells that bear no resemblance to those normally found in that part of the body. For example, teratomas that develop in the ovary—one of the most common sites for this type of tumor—often form cysts (called *dermoid cysts*) that may contain skin, hair, teeth, or

bone. Other common sites include the testes, the pineal gland in the brain, and the mediastinum (the space between the lungs).

Terbutaline
A *bronchodilator drug* used in the treatment of *asthma*, chronic *bronchitis*, and *emphysema*. Terbutaline also relaxes the muscles of the uterus, making it useful for the prevention of premature labor (see *Prematurity*). Terbutaline is under investigation as a treatment for *heart failure*.

Adverse effects include tremor, nervousness, restlessness, nausea, and, in rare cases, palpitations.

Terfenadine
An *antihistamine drug* used to treat allergic *rhinitis* (hay fever) and allergic skin conditions, such as *urticaria* (hives). Terfenadine has little sedative effect and is therefore useful for people who need to avoid drowsiness. Possible adverse effects include nausea, loss of appetite, and rash.

Terminal care
See *Dying, care of the*.

Termination of pregnancy
See *Abortion, elective*.

Testicle
See *Testis*.

Testicular feminization syndrome
A rare inherited condition in which, despite having the external appearance of a female, the affected individual is genetically a male with internal testes. Testicular feminization syndrome is a form of *intersex* and is the most common form of male *pseudohermaphroditism*.

CAUSE
Testicular feminization syndrome is caused by a defective response of the body's tissues to *testosterone* (male sex hormone), even though a normal male level of the hormone is produced. The genes for testicular feminization syndrome are transmitted on the X chromosome (see *Genetic disorders*); thus, females can carry the genes and transmit them to their sons.

SYMPTOMS AND SIGNS
Affected individuals appear to be girls throughout childhood; female secondary *sexual characteristics* develop in most at puberty. People with testicular feminization syndrome tend to be taller than average and are of normal intelligence. However, menstruation

does not occur because there is no uterus and the vagina is short and blind-ending.

DIAGNOSIS, TREATMENT, AND OUTLOOK

The condition may be diagnosed before puberty if a girl is found to have an inguinal *hernia* or a swelling in the labia that turns out to be a testis. Otherwise, the diagnosis is usually made at puberty during investigations for *amenorrhea* (failure to menstruate).

The diagnosis is made by *chromosome analysis*, which shows the normal male chromosomal status, and by blood tests, which indicate male levels of testosterone.

Treatment involves the surgical removal of the testes (because of an increased risk of testicular cancer) and hormonal therapy with *estrogen drugs*. An affected individual can never be fertile, but can lead an otherwise normal life as a woman.

Testis

One of two male sex organs, also called testicles, that produce *sperm* and the male sex hormone *testosterone*.

The testes are formed within the abdomen near the kidneys early in the growth of the male fetus. In response to hormones produced by the mother and to hormones produced in the testes themselves, the testes gradually descend through the inguinal canal (a tunnel in the groin). At birth, they have usually reached the surface of the body, where they hang suspended in a pouch of skin called the *scrotum*.

STRUCTURE

Within each of the testes are the seminiferous tubules, delicate coiled tubes that produce sperm. The seminiferous tubules lead via the vas efferens (small ducts) to the *epididymis*, a structure lying behind the testis in which the newly formed sperm mature. Interstitial cells between the seminiferous tubules produce the male sex hormone testosterone, which passes into small blood vessels in the testis and then into the circulation.

Each testis is protected by a tough, fibrous capsule, the tunica albuginea, and is attached by the spermatic cord, composed of the *vas deferens* (the tube that transports sperm from the epididymis to the urethra) and a number of blood vessels and nerves.

DISORDERS

A direct blow sometimes tears the wall of the testis, resulting in severe pain and bleeding into the scrotal tissue. An operation may be required to drain the blood and repair the testis.

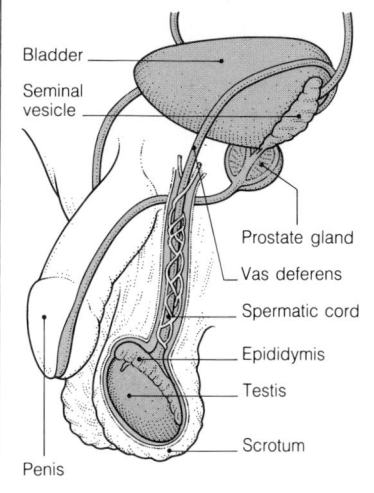

LOCATION OF THE TESTIS
Each testis is suspended in the scrotum by a spermatic cord, which contains the vas deferens, and the arteries, veins, and nerves that supply the testis.

Bladder
Seminal vesicle
Prostate gland
Vas deferens
Spermatic cord
Epididymis
Testis
Scrotum
Penis

Occasionally, a testis fails to develop completely, does not descend fully into the scrotum (see *Testis, undescended*), or descends into an abnormal position (see *Testis, ectopic*). This may lead to reduced or absent sperm production or, if both testes are affected, *infertility*.

Inflammation of the testis, known as *orchitis*, usually results from infection with the mumps virus. Inflammation of the testis and the epididymis occurs in *epididymo-orchitis*, which is usually caused by a bacterial infection.

Painless swelling of the tissues surrounding the testis usually results from *hydrocele* (collection of fluid in the scrotum). Other causes of testicular swelling include *varicocele* (swollen veins within the scrotum), *epididymal cyst* (fluid-filled swelling of the epididymis), and *spermatocele* (a sperm-filled swelling of the epididymis).

Torsion of the testis occurs when the spermatic cord becomes twisted, cutting off the blood supply to the testis; it is most common around puberty (see *Testis, torsion of*).

In rare cases, the testis is affected by cancer (see *Testis, cancer of*).

Testis, cancer of

Malignant growth of the *testis*. Cancer of the testis is rare. It occurs most commonly in young to middle-aged men,

and is very rare before puberty or in old age. The risk is higher in men with a history of undescended testis (see *Testis, undescended*).

TYPES

The most common types of testicular cancer are seminomas and teratomas. Seminomas are made up of a single type of cell (probably developing from the cells that produce sperm). Teratomas consist of several different types of cell. Other cancers affecting the testis are extremely rare and develop from testicular tissue or from lymphatic tissue (see *Lymphoma*) within the testis.

SYMPTOMS AND SIGNS

Testicular cancer most commonly appears as a firm, painless swelling of one testis. In some cases there may be pain and inflammation.

DIAGNOSIS

The physician first examines the testis and may perform tests to exclude other causes of testicular swelling (see *Testis, swollen*).

The diagnosis of testicular cancer can be confirmed only by *orchiectomy* (surgical removal of the testis) and microscopic examination of the testicular tissue. This confirms the presence of cancer and also shows the

SELF-EXAMINATION OF THE TESTIS
A lump that can be felt in the testis must be considered potentially malignant until surgical exploration proves otherwise. Cancers are usually firm to the touch and not tender or painful when pressed.

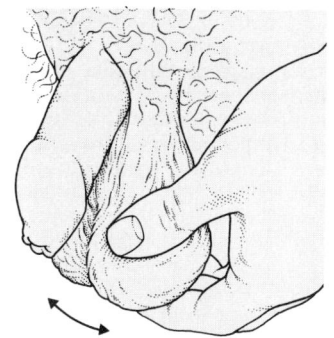

Procedure
Only regular self-examination can detect a tumor early enough to provide assurance of cure. The entire surface of both testes should be felt. The skin over the testes moves freely, making palpation easy.

T

type of cancer that is present. In addition, other tests (including *CT scanning, ultrasound scanning,* and *blood tests*) are performed to look for any signs that the cancer has spread to other parts of the body.

TREATMENT

Orchiectomy may be sufficient to cure testicular cancer in its early stages. However, *radiation therapy* on the remaining testis and on the lymph glands is also usually carried out, even if there are no signs that the disease has spread to these areas. Cancer that has spread beyond the testis is usually treated with *anticancer drugs* in addition to orchiectomy; occasionally, surgery may be needed to remove cancerous tissue from the abdomen.

OUTLOOK

The outlook, which varies according to the type of cancer and how advanced it was when first discovered, is generally good. The cure rate for early testicular cancer is 95 to 97 percent; the cure rate for advanced disease is 80 to 85 percent. Treatment with radiation therapy or anticancer drugs may not cause infertility in the remaining testis.

Testis, ectopic

A *testis* that is absent from the scrotum because it has descended into an abnormal position, usually in the groin or at the base of the penis. An ectopic testis is most often discovered soon after birth during a routine physical examination. Treatment involves an *orchiopexy*, which places the testis in the scrotum.

Testis, pain in the

Even mild injury to the testis may result in pain. Usually, no damage is caused, but a direct blow such as a kick may tear the wall of the testis. In this case, the pain is particularly severe, and an operation may be required to drain any accumulated blood and repair the testis.

Severe pain and swelling are a feature of *orchitis* (inflammation of the testis), *epididymo-orchitis* (inflammation of the testis and epididymis), and torsion of the testis (see *Testis, torsion of*). Cancer of the testis (see *Testis, cancer of*) does not usually cause pain.

Occasionally, pain that seems to come from the testis is actually caused by a small kidney stone lodged in the ureter (see *Calculus, urinary tract*). Sometimes a physician can find no cause for testicular pain; in most of these cases the problem disappears without treatment.

Testis, retractile

A testis that is drawn up high into the groin by a pronounced muscle reflex in response to cold or touch. Retractile testis is normal in young children but usually disappears by puberty. Failure to feel the testis in the scrotum sometimes causes the condition to be confused with undescended testis (see *Testis, undescended*).

Testis, swollen

Swelling of the testis or its surrounding tissues in the scrotum may or may not be accompanied by pain. Most scrotal swellings are harmless and the testis itself is usually not affected. However, swelling of a testis should always be reported to a physician to rule out the possibility of a serious underlying disorder.

PAINLESS SWELLINGS

There are several types of harmless, painless swelling, the most common of which is *hydrocele* (a collection of fluid in the scrotum). Other usually painless swellings include *epididymal cyst* (fluid-filled swelling of the epididymis), *spermatocele* (sperm-filled swelling of the epididymis), *varicocele* (varicose veins in the scrotum), and hematocele (swelling that contains blood and results from injury).

Cancer of the testis (see *Testis, cancer of*) may also cause a painless swelling and requires prompt treatment.

PAINFUL SWELLING

Painful swelling of the scrotum may be caused by a sudden event, such as twisting of the spermatic cord (see *Testis, torsion of*) or a direct blow. When associated with fever, the swelling is usually due to infection of the testis (see *Orchitis*) or of the testis and epididymis (see *Epididymo-orchitis*). In rare cases, a painful swelling is due to cancer of the testis.

Testis, torsion of

Twisting of the spermatic cord, causing acute, severe pain and swelling of the *testis*. Unless treated within a few hours, the testis is damaged permanently and sperm production ceases.

Torsion of the testis is most common around puberty, but may also occur in infants or in young adults. The condition is more likely to occur if the testis is unusually mobile within its covering in the scrotum.

SYMPTOMS AND SIGNS

Pain develops rapidly and is occasionally accompanied by abdominal pain and nausea. The testis becomes swollen and very tender, and the scrotal skin becomes discolored.

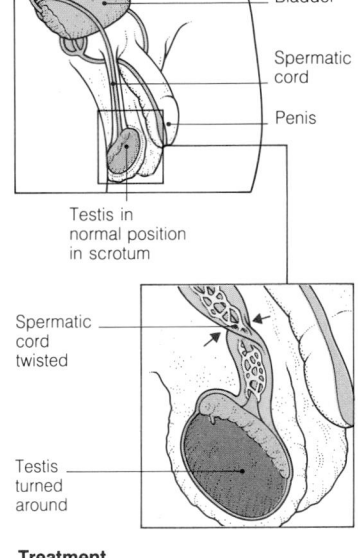

TORSION OF THE TESTIS
If a testis rotates, veins in the spermatic cord become obstructed and there is severe swelling and pain. Torsion of the testis most commonly occurs around puberty.

Bladder

Spermatic cord

Penis

Testis in normal position in scrotum

Spermatic cord twisted

Testis turned around

Treatment
Spontaneous untwisting sometimes occurs but unrelieved torsion is dangerous. Torsion must be treated urgently by manipulation or surgery.

DIAGNOSIS AND TREATMENT

A provisional diagnosis is made from a physical examination; *ultrasound scanning* may also be performed.

Treatment is by surgery. An incision is made in the skin of the scrotum and, if the diagnosis is confirmed, the testis can be immediately untwisted. If blood flow resumes, the testis is anchored in the scrotum with small stitches to prevent torsion from recurring. If irreversible damage exists, *orchiectomy* is performed.

In all cases, the other testis is also anchored to the scrotum to prevent torsion on that side.

OUTLOOK

Recovery from the operation is rapid. If treatment was prompt, the testis recovers completely. Even if one testis was removed, the other is usually capable of maintaining fertility.

Testis, undescended

A *testis* that has failed to complete its normal passage from within the abdomen to the scrotum. Not all testes that

T

are absent from the scrotum are undescended (see *Testis, ectopic*; *Testis, rectractile*). Undescended testis is found in 2 percent of full-term and in up to 10 percent of premature male babies. Usually, only one testis fails to descend. In many cases, the testis descends of its own accord within several months of birth.

CAUSES AND SYMPTOMS

The final descent of the testis through the inguinal canal to the scrotum is controlled by hormones from the mother and from the testis itself. If these stimuli do not have an effect, the spermatic cord (which carries the vas deferens and the blood vessels to the testis) fails to lengthen sufficiently to allow full descent. Alternatively, a normal testis may be prevented from reaching the scrotum by the presence of fibers that interrupt its route and cause it to remain in the groin.

An undescended testis does not develop normally and is not capable of normal sperm production. If both testes are undescended, *infertility* results. A testis that fails to descend normally is at increased risk of testicular cancer (see *Testis, cancer of*).

DIAGNOSIS AND TREATMENT

The diagnosis is made during examination of the newborn or later in infancy. It is rare for the condition to remain unnoticed into adult life.

Treatment is by *orchiopexy*, an operation in which the undescended testis is lowered into the scrotum. Surgery within the first few years of life gives the testis the best chance of developing normally. If the testis is very poorly developed (and the other testis is normal) the undescended testis is removed.

Test meal

A portion of food or a small meal given to determine the functioning of some part of the digestive tract. The meal may contain standardized amounts of various types of food, portions of which are removed at intervals from the stomach. Isotope-labeled food may be given and scanned.

Another type of meal contains a substance that allows the digestive tract to be revealed on an X ray (see *Barium X-ray examinations*).

Testosterone

The most important of the *androgen hormones* (male sex hormones). Testosterone stimulates bone and muscle growth and sexual development. It is produced by the testes and in very small amounts by the ovaries.

DRUG THERAPY

Synthetic or animal testosterone is used to stimulate *puberty* or treat *infertility* in males suffering from deficiency caused by disorders of the testes or *pituitary gland*. Testosterone was once used to treat *breast cancer*, but is rarely used today for this purpose.

Testosterone given to stimulate puberty may interfere with normal growth or cause overrapid sexual development. In males, testosterone may cause *priapism* (painful, persistent erection). In females, high doses of testosterone may cause deepening of the voice, excessive hair growth, or hair loss. Treatment with some oral forms of testosterone may cause liver damage.

Tests, medical

About 10 billion medical tests are carried out each year in the US—about 45 for each man, woman, and child.

TYPES OF MEDICAL TESTS

Body system		

Brain and nervous system	EEG
	Evoked responses
	Hearing tests
	Vision tests
	Lumbar puncture
	Intelligence tests
		Myelography
		Brain imaging
		  CT scanning
		  MRI
		  PET scanning

Skin, bones, and muscles	EMG Biopsy	Bone imaging X rays
Endocrine system and metabolism	Thyroid function tests Thyroid scanning	Blood tests Urinalysis
Blood and immune system	Lymphangiography Blood tests	Skin tests Bone marrow biopsy

Heart and circulation	Heart imaging
	  Chest X ray
	  Angiography
	  Echocardiography
	  Venography
		ECG
		Catheterization, cardiac
		Cardiac stress test

Lungs	Pulmonary function tests
	  Blood gases
	  Peak flow meter
	  Spirometry
		Chest X ray
		Bronchoscopy

Biliary system	Liver function tests Liver imaging Ultrasound scanning Cholangiography	Cholecystography ERCP Liver biopsy
Gastrointestinal tract	Endoscopy Colonoscopy Gastroscopy	Barium X-ray examinations Jejunal biopsy Occult blood, fecal
Urinary tract	Kidney imaging Pyelography Ultrasound scanning	Kidney function tests Cystoscopy Urinalysis
Reproductive system	Hysterosalpingography Mammography Ultrasound scanning Laparoscopy Pregnancy tests	Amniocentesis Cervical smear test Chorionic villus sampling Chromosome analysis Semen analysis

The table above lists some commonly performed medical tests, classified according to the body system they are used to study. Each test listed in the table has its own encyclopedia entry. Only some of the most important imaging techniques for each body organ have been included; a complete list appears in the appropriate imaging article.

Medical tests are usually used to investigate the cause of a person's symptoms to establish a *diagnosis*. In addition, tests are performed on apparently healthy people to find disease at an early stage; this is known as *screening*. The yield from screening is considered small by some, and many unnecessary follow-up procedures may be performed to investigate a falsely positive test result.

To be of value, a medical test must be reasonably accurate in identifying or excluding the presence of a particular disease. The degree of accuracy is based on three factors—sensitivity, specificity, and predictive value.

Sensitivity is the ability of a test to show a positive (abnormal) value when the disease being tested for is actually present. A test that always detects a specific disease is said to have 100 percent sensitivity. One that shows positive results in only 80 people out of a hundred who have the disease is said to have 80 percent sensitivity; the 20 percent of the cases missed on the test reflect the false-negative test results.

The specificity is the extent to which a test shows false-positive results in healthy people. For example, a test that shows false results in 20 percent of the people tested has 80 percent specificity.

Sensitivity and specificity may vary with the controls (known standards) used in different laboratories and with the criteria for normal values.

The third measure of a test's accuracy is its predictive value. It is determined by a mathematical formula that includes the number of times the test is accurate (the true-negative test results plus the true-positive test results) and the total number of tests performed. The predictive value thus determines the probability that a patient with a positive test result actually has the disease or, conversely, that a patient who has a negative test result does not have the disease. The predictive value is dependent on the prevalence of the disease in the group being tested; when a disease is rare, a positive result is much more likely to be significant.

There is tremendous variation in accuracy among tests. For example, the fecal occult blood test (see *Occult blood, fecal*) used to detect cancer of the stomach or intestine is very sensitive; a person whose test results are negative (normal) is unlikely to have the disease. However, the test is not highly specific and many people whose test results are positive (abnormal) do not have the disease. More tests are required to confirm the diagnosis before treatment is performed.

An *ECG* to diagnose acute myocardial infarction (heart attack) is reasonably specific. A person whose test results are positive is almost definitely affected and is admitted to an intensive-care unit for treatment. However, the test is not sensitive; about half the people with severe chest pain who have negative test results may also need treatment.

The best tests have both high specificity and high sensitivity, and therefore high predictive value. Today's tests for syphilis have almost 100 percent predictive value. They almost always show a positive result in someone who has the disease and a negative result in someone who does not have the disease.

Tetanus

A serious, sometimes fatal, disease of the central nervous system caused by infection of a wound with spores of the bacterium CLOSTRIDIUM TETANI.

CAUSES AND INCIDENCE

The spores live mainly in soil and manure, but are also found in the human intestine and elsewhere. If, through a wound, spores enter tissues that are poorly supplied with oxygenated blood, they multiply and produce a toxin that acts on the nerves controlling muscle activity.

About half a million cases of tetanus occur worldwide each year; in the US only about 100 cases are reported annually. All occur in nonimmunized people, mostly in those over age 50. In developing countries, tetanus often causes death in newborn infants as a result of spores contaminating the umbilical stump.

PREVENTION

DPT vaccination—combined immunization against diphtheria, pertussis (whooping cough), and tetanus—is given routinely in the US during childhood, after which tetanus immunization booster shots are needed every 10 years. Any wound, particularly a deep or dirty one, should be cleaned and treated with an antiseptic.

SYMPTOMS AND SIGNS

The most common symptom is *trismus* (stiffness of the jaw, commonly known as lockjaw), which makes it difficult to open the mouth. Other symptoms include stiffness of abdominal and back muscles, and contraction of facial muscles, producing a fixed, mirthless smile. There may also be a fast pulse, slight fever, and profuse sweating. Eventually, painful muscle spasms develop. If they affect the larynx or chest wall, asphyxia may result. The spasms usually subside after 10 to 14 days.

DIAGNOSIS AND TREATMENT

The diagnosis is made from the patient's symptoms and signs, and a course of tetanus antitoxin injections is started. Severe cases may require a *tracheostomy* (insertion of a breathing tube into the windpipe) and maintenance of the person's breathing with a *ventilator*. Given prompt treatment, most people recover completely.

Tetany

Spasms and twitching of the muscles, most commonly those in the hands and feet, although the face, larynx (voice box), or spinal muscles may also be affected. Initially, the spasms are painless; if the condition persists, they tend to become increasingly painful. In some cases, muscle damage eventually results if the underlying cause is not treated. (Tetany, which is a symptom of a biochemical disturbance in the body, should not be confused with *tetanus*, which is an infection.)

The most common cause of tetany is hypocalcemia (a low level of *calcium* in the blood), sometimes due to a diet lacking in vitamin D. Other causes include hypokalemia (a low blood level of *potassium*), which is commonly a result of prolonged diarrhea or vomiting; *hyperventilation* (abnormally deep or rapid breathing), which is most often a result of anxiety; or, more rarely, *hypoparathyroidism* (underactivity of the parathyroid glands). The latter two are also associated with hypocalcemia.

Tetracaine

A local anesthetic (see *Anesthesia, local*). Tetracaine is used to anesthetize the eye before minor surgical procedures; it is also used to facilitate dental treatment, throat examinations, and procedures in which a tube is passed down the throat. Tetracaine is occasionally used for *spinal anesthesia* or *epidural anesthesia* during *childbirth*, and to relieve pain, itching, and inflammation in anal disorders.

POSSIBLE ADVERSE EFFECTS

Tetracaine may cause a localized allergic reaction, which includes burning discomfort, redness, itching, and swelling. Eye preparations may cause dryness or watering of the eyes. High doses may cause anxiety, dizziness, and drowsiness.

T

Tetracycline drugs

COMMON DRUGS

Minocycline Oxytetracycline Tetracycline

A group of *antibiotic drugs* commonly used to treat conditions including *acne, bronchitis, syphilis, gonorrhea, nonspecific urethritis*, and certain types of *pneumonia*. Tetracyclines are also prescribed for some less common infections, such as *cholera, Rocky Mountain spotted fever*, and *brucellosis*.

Possible adverse effects include nausea, vomiting, diarrhea, and, less commonly, rash and itching. Tetracyclines may discolor developing teeth and are therefore not usually prescribed for children under the age of 12 or for pregnant women. Tetracyclines may worsen the condition of the kidneys in people with poor kidney function.

Tetrahydroaminoacridine

A drug under investigation for use in the treatment of *Alzheimer's disease*. In a small clinical trial with the drug, memory loss improved in people with Alzheimer's disease. A large clinical trial intended to establish the effectiveness of tetrahydroaminoacridine was underway until the frequency of adverse drug effects (impaired liver function) became too high.

In Alzheimer's disease, the level of the brain chemical *acetylcholine* is abnormally low. It is thought that tetrahydroaminoacridine increases the production of this chemical. However, the drug does not halt degeneration of brain tissue and thus cannot cure Alzheimer's disease.

Tetrahydroaminoacridine can impair liver function during treatment; the risk of permanent damage from long-term treatment is unknown.

Tetrahydrozoline

A *decongestant drug* used to relieve *sinusitis*, allergic *rhinitis* (hay fever), and the common *cold*. Tetrahydrozoline is also given to relieve redness of the eyes that is caused by minor irritation.

Long-term use may worsen congestion. Other possible adverse effects include headache, restlessness, and palpitations. Eye drops may occasionally cause blurred vision and oversensitivity to light.

Tetralogy of Fallot

A form of congenital *heart disease*, consisting of four coexisting heart anomalies, present from birth (see dia-

NORMAL HEART

Aorta
Pulmonary artery
Right atrium
Left atrium
Left ventricle
Right ventricle
Ventricular septum

TETRALOGY OF FALLOT

Displaced aorta
Narrowed pulmonary valve
Hole in ventricular septum
Thickened wall of right ventricle

Defects in tetralogy of Fallot
The four defects are shown above. Insufficient blood passes to the pulmonary artery and lungs to be oxygenated, and the large volume of blood pumped to the body via the aorta is therefore lacking in oxygen.

gram). The result of the defects is that blood pumped to the body from the heart is insufficiently oxygenated, which leads to *cyanosis* (blue-purple coloration) and breathlessness. Tetralogy of Fallot occurs in about 50 out of 100,000 babies born.

SYMPTOMS AND SIGNS

Affected infants appear normal at birth, although turbulence in the heart can be detected as murmurs by a physician using a stethoscope. There is usually a gradual increase in the degree of cyanosis and breathlessness. Other symptoms include difficulty feeding, failure to gain weight, and poor development.

In older children who remain untreated, *clubbing* of the fingers and toes is usually evident. Another feature in older children is the adoption, after exertion, of a squatting position, with the knees on the chest, to help them recover from breathlessness.

DIAGNOSIS, TREATMENT, AND OUTLOOK

The condition is suspected on the basis of the child's symptoms and a

physical examination. A chest *X ray* shows a characteristic shape of the heart. An *ECG*, echocardiogram (see *Echocardiography*), and in some cases cardiac *catheterization* are performed to determine the extent of the abnormality.

Surgery is necessary for permanent correction of the disorder. The optimal time for surgical repair is before the child starts school. A temporary procedure is usually performed first. A duct is created between the aorta and pulmonary artery so that some of the blood pumped into the aorta is diverted to the lungs. Subsequently, a corrective operation is performed in the course of *open heart surgery*. The narrowed pulmonary artery is widened and the hole in the heart is closed. If successful, no other operation should be necessary.

Thalamus

A structure consisting of two egg-shaped masses of nerve tissue, each about the size of a walnut, deep within the brain. The thalamus sits at the top of the brain stem and is connected by many tracts to all parts of the brain.

FUNCTION

The thalamus is an important relay center for sensory information flowing into the brain. Different clusters of nerve cells within the thalamus receive information from different sense organs (e.g., from the eyes, ears, and, via the spinal cord, from

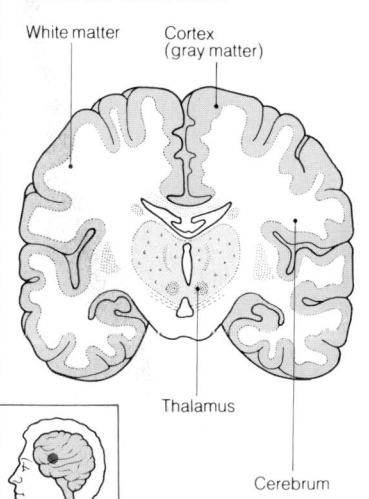

LOCATION OF THE THALAMUS
The thalamus lies deep within the brain, its two lobes located just above the brain stem.

White matter
Cortex (gray matter)
Thalamus
Cerebrum

T

touch and pressure receptors in the skin). Some basic sensations, such as pain, may actually reach consciousness within the thalamus. Other types of sensory information are processed and relayed to parts of the cerebral cortex (outer layer of the brain), where the sensations are perceived.

The thalamus seems to act as a filter, selecting only information of particular importance from the mass of sensory signals entering the brain. This is important for the ability to concentrate on a particular task. Certain centers within the thalamus may also play a part in long-term memory.

DISORDERS

Damage to the thalamus due to *stroke* or *brain tumor* usually causes loss of sensation, but sometimes causes heightened sensitivity to pain, temperature, and other sensory stimuli.

Thalassemia

A group of inherited disorders in which there is a fault in the production of *hemoglobin*, the oxygen-carrying substance that is synthesized in the bone marrow for incorporation into red blood cells. Many of the red cells produced are fragile and rapidly hemolyzed (broken up), leading to hemolytic *anemia*.

Thalassemia is prevalent in the Mediterranean region, the Middle East, and Southeast Asia, and in families originating from these areas.

CAUSES, TYPES, AND INCIDENCE

The hemoglobin of healthy people contains two pairs of globins (protein chains), known as alpha chains and beta chains. In thalassemia, synthesis of either the alpha or the beta chains is reduced, causing an imbalance between alpha and beta chains in much of the hemoglobin produced.

Abnormal hemoglobin production in thalassemia is caused by inheritance of a defective *gene*. Most commonly, it is the production of beta chains that is disturbed, leading to beta-thalassemia. This condition is inherited in an autosomal recessive pattern (see *Genetic disorders*). If a person inherits one defective gene for the disease, he or she is said to have beta-thalassemia minor, or thalassemia trait (which is never severe). If two defective genes are inherited—one from each parent—the result is a much more severe condition called beta-thalassemia major, or Cooley's anemia. If two people with the minor trait have offspring, each child has a one in four chance of suffering from beta-thalassemia major.

Alpha-thalassemia is much less common than the beta type. If there is a severely reduced production of alpha chains, the lack of normal hemoglobin is incompatible with life and an affected infant dies within a few hours of birth. Lesser degrees of alpha-thalassemia also occur.

SYMPTOMS

Beta-thalassemia major produces the symptoms of hemolytic anemia, including fatigue and shortness of breath with jaundice and spleen enlargement due to the rapid break up of red blood cells. These symptoms first appear three to six months after birth. In untreated cases, the bone marrow expands greatly (to compensate for the reduced life span of red cells), which can cause bones to grow abnormally. This leads to an enlargement of the skull in untreated patients. Normal body growth is arrested and, without treatment, death occurs during early childhood.

In the forms of alpha-thalassemia compatible with life, there are also symptoms of anemia but they are generally less severe.

DIAGNOSIS AND TREATMENT

The diagnosis of beta-thalassemia major is made from microscopic examination of the blood, which shows many small, pale red blood cells, and from other blood tests that show reduced levels of adult hemoglobin in the blood.

Treatment is with blood transfusions, which can allow an affected child to grow normally. In addition, the spleen may be removed when the child is older (see *Splenectomy*). However, as each blood transfusion is administered, some iron is absorbed and eventually the internal organs become overloaded with iron. This can lead to liver *cirrhosis*, to gland disorders such as *diabetes mellitus*, and to *heart failure*, which is a frequent cause of death in young adults with the disease.

Research is helping to reduce the iron overload with compounds called *chelating agents*. Efforts have been made to cure the disease with a bone marrow transplant.

OUTLOOK

Parents or other relatives of a child with thalassemia, and any person known to have beta-thalassemia minor (thalassemia trait), may benefit from *genetic counseling*. Beta-thalassemia major can now be diagnosed by *prenatal screening* techniques; parents may choose to have the pregnancy terminated.

Thalidomide

A *sleeping drug* never approved by the FDA for sale in the US. It caused limb deformities in many of the babies born to women who were given this drug during pregnancy.

Thalidomide is currently under investigation for use in treating certain types of *leprosy*.

Thalidomide child
Phocomelia (seal-limb) was a common result of the action of thalidomide on the fetus at an early stage of development.

Thallium

A rare metallic element that does not occur naturally in its pure form but is present (in minute amounts) as various compounds in certain ores of zinc and lead. Thallium 201 (an artificial radioactive isotope of the element) is sometimes used in *radionuclide scanning* of the heart. In this role, it reveals areas of heart muscle that have a poor blood supply or that have been damaged by a *myocardial infarction* (heart attack).

THC

The abbreviation for tetrahydrocannabinol (dronabinol), the active ingredient in *marijuana*. This drug is used to treat the nausea and vomiting of cancer patients undergoing radiation therapy and/or chemotherapy.

Theophylline

A *bronchodilator drug* used primarily in the treatment of *asthma* and to prevent attacks of *apnea* (cessation of breathing) in premature infants. The drug may be used to treat *heart failure* because it stimulates heart rate and increases urine excretion.

Possible adverse effects include dizziness, nausea, vomiting, diarrhea, palpitations, and seizures.

Therapeutic

A term meaning "related to treatment." The therapeutic dose of a drug is the amount required to have a beneficial effect.

T

Therapeutic community

A method of treating antisocial behavior in which patients live together as a group in a nonhospital environment under the supervision of medical staff. Therapeutic communities are used for treating *drug dependence, alcohol dependence,* and certain *personality disorders.*

Staff and patients share all decisions at regular group meetings, and unacceptable behavior and its effects are confronted and discussed openly. All aspects of day-to-day activity thus provide a focus for learning appropriate social and interpersonal skills.

Therapy

The treatment of any disease or abnormal physical or mental condition. Examples of therapy include *radiation therapy* for cancer and *psychotherapy* for psychiatric disorders.

Thermography

A technique in which temperature patterns on the surface of the skin are recorded in the form of an image.

Thermographic image of knees
Areas that have different surface temperatures show up as different shades in the thermographic image.

WHY IT IS DONE

Thermography provides clues to the presence of diseases and abnormalities that alter the temperature of the skin, such as circulation problems, inflammation, and tumors. However, because so many conditions affect skin temperature, further examination and tests are necessary to confirm the underlying cause.

HOW IT IS DONE

Two techniques are used in thermography to detect skin temperature. In one, a special camera or scanner picks up infrared radiation naturally emitted from the skin. In the other, sheets of special temperature-sensitive liquid crystals are applied to the skin; they change color in response to changes in temperature.

RESULTS

Thermography is a safe technique. Results are not sufficiently reliable for thermography to fulfill hopes that it might prove useful as an early screening test for breast cancer.

Thermometer

An instrument used to measure *temperature.* A traditional clinical thermometer consists of a glass capillary (very fine bore) tube sealed at one end and with a mercury-filled bulb at the other. When the bulb is placed in the mouth, the mercury expands up the capillary tube. The thermometer is removed from the mouth and the body temperature—indicated by the level of the mercury—is then read against a scale on the glass. There is a small kink in the capillary tube just above the bulb to prevent the mercury from moving down the tube when the thermometer is removed from the mouth. Before the thermometer can be used again, the mercury must be shaken back down into the bulb.

The capillary tube has a very narrow bore to make the thermometer sensitive to small temperature changes. In addition, the wall of the tube is thickened on one side to form a cylindrical lens that makes the mercury easier to see. Clinical thermometers may be calibrated in *Celsius* (centigrade) or *Fahrenheit* (or sometimes both); different styles may be used in the mouth, armpit, and rectum. A modern version of the traditional clinical thermometer uses an electronic probe connected to a digital readout display.

Recently, there has been a trend toward using disposable skin thermometers that employ heat-sensitive chemicals that change color at specific temperatures. These thermometers are generally less accurate than the mercury or digital types because they are more likely to be affected by external factors, such as the temperature of the environment.

Thiabendazole

An *antihelmintic drug* used to treat *worm infestations,* including *strongyloidiasis, trichinosis,* and *toxocariasis.*

Thiabendazole may cause dizziness, loss of appetite, nausea, vomiting, headache, drowsiness, and diarrhea. In rare cases, an allergic reaction may occur.

Thiamine

See *Vitamin B complex.*

Thiopental

A *barbiturate drug* widely used as a general anesthetic (see *Anesthesia, general*). Thiopental, which is given by intravenous injection, quickly produces unconsciousness. However, because it has a relatively short-lived effect, a different anesthetic agent is used to maintain anesthesia.

Thioridazine

An *antipsychotic drug* used to treat *schizophrenia, mania,* and *dementia.* Although thioridazine does not cure the underlying disorder, its tranquilizing effect suppresses abnormal behavior, reduces aggression, and helps relieve *anxiety* and *depression,* rendering the person more amenable to psychotherapy.

Thioridazine may cause dyskinesia (abnormal movements) but is less likely to do so than some other antipsychotic drugs. Drowsiness, dry mouth, muscle stiffness, and dizziness may occur. High doses of the drug taken over long periods may damage the retina.

Thiothixene

An antipsychotic drug similar to *trifluoperazine.*

Thirst

The desire to drink. Thirst is one means by which the amount of water in the body is controlled (the other is the volume of urine that is produced by the kidneys).

THERMOMETERS
Digital thermometer
Mercury-filled bulb
Fahrenheit scale
Notch
Clinical thermometer
On/off button
Digital display
Temperature-sensitive probe

T

Thirst is stimulated by an increase in the concentration of salt, sugar, or certain other substances in the blood. Particle concentration of the serum (the liquid portion of blood) rises if fluid intake falls or if dietary intake of certain substances (most commonly salt) increases. As the concentrated blood passes through the hypothalamus in the brain, special nerve receptors are stimulated, inducing the sensation of thirst.

Thirst is also stimulated if the volume of blood decreases as a result of sweating, vomiting, diarrhea, severe bleeding, or extensive burns.

In addition, although thirst causes a dry mouth, dryness may also cause thirst, even when a person is adequately hydrated; in such cases, thirst can usually be relieved merely by moistening the mouth.

Damage to the hypothalamus (e.g., as a result of a head injury) may cause loss of the desire to drink and consequent *dehydration*.

Thirst, excessive

A strong and persistent need to drink, most commonly due to *dehydration*. Excessive thirst is a symptom of untreated *diabetes mellitus* and *diabetes insipidus*. Other causes of excessive thirst include *renal failure*, treatment with certain drugs (such as phenothiazine derivatives), and severe blood loss. Abnormal thirst may also be psychological in origin, a condition known as psychogenic polydipsia.

Thoracic outlet syndrome

A condition in which pressure on the *brachial plexus* (the nerve roots that pass into either arm from the neck) causes pain in the arms and shoulders, a pins and needles sensation in the fingers, and weakness of grip and other hand movements.

Pressure on the brachial plexus may result from drooping shoulders; it is made worse by lifting and carrying heavy loads or by an increase in body weight. Severe symptoms are usually caused by a *cervical rib* (an extra rib above the first rib), which is linked to the first rib by a fibrous band of tissue that presses on the brachial plexus.

Treatment usually involves exercises to improve posture. Sometimes *nonsteroidal anti-inflammatory drugs* and *muscle-relaxant drugs* are helpful. Severe cases may be treated by surgical removal of the first rib. Women with large breasts should wear a bra that provides good support.

Thoracic surgeon

A surgeon who specializes in operations on organs within the chest cavity, excluding the heart. These organs include the lungs, esophagus, and trachea (windpipe). Patients generally see a thoracic surgeon only on referral by another physician.

Thoracotomy

An operation in which the thorax (chest) is opened.

WHY IT IS DONE

A thoracotomy is usually performed to allow a surgeon to operate on a diseased heart, lung, or other organ in the chest cavity. It may also be carried out as an emergency procedure following a severe chest injury.

HOW IT IS DONE

There are two types of thoracotomy—lateral and anterior. Both are performed using general anesthesia.

A lateral thoracotomy provides access to the lungs, major blood vessels, and esophagus. A curved incision is made from between the shoulder blades, around the side of the trunk beneath the armpit, to just below the nipple. The underlying muscles are divided to expose the ribs, which are gently spread apart; occasionally, part of a rib is removed. The necessary operation is then performed. Afterward, a drainage tube is inserted into the pleural cavity (the space between the membrane covering the lung and the membrane lining the chest wall) to allow fluid to drain and to prevent the lung from collapsing. The muscles and overlying skin are then closed with stitches.

An anterior thoracotomy provides access to the heart and coronary arteries. A vertical incision is made from between the clavicles (collarbones) at the base of the neck to the lower end of the sternum (breastbone). The sternum is divided with a saw and gently pried apart. The heart is then exposed and the necessary surgery performed. Following insertion of a drainage tube into the pleural cavity, the sternum is closed with strong stitches (sometimes wire) and the overlying skin sewn up.

RECOVERY PERIOD

Despite drainage, secretions in the air passages often cause breathing problems after surgery. To clear the passages, the patient is encouraged to breathe deeply and cough and is given *respiratory therapy*. Within 48 hours after surgery, the drainage tube is usually removed and the patient can begin to move.

Thorax

The medical name for the chest. The thorax extends from the base of the neck to the *diaphragm muscle* and is supported and protected by the *ribs*, *sternum* (breastbone), and vertebrae (see *Spine*). The main structures in the thorax are the *heart, lungs, esophagus*, and large blood vessels such as the *aorta* and pulmonary arteries. (See illustrated box, overleaf.)

Thought

A mental activity that enables humans to reason, form judgments, and solve problems. The essential features of thought are the substitution of symbols (in the form of words, numbers, or images) for objects, the formation of these symbols into ideas, and the arrangement of ideas into a certain order in the mind. A person's thoughts are represented to others by speech, writing, and behavior.

Aspects of thought that can be examined or tested include speed and efficiency, content of ideas, and the logical relationship among ideas. (See also *Thought disorders*.)

Thought disorders

Abnormalities in the structure or content of *thought* as reflected in a person's speech, writing, or behavior.

In the thought disorder characteristic of *schizophrenia*, sometimes referred to as formal thought disorder, associations lose their logical connection. The individual may jump from one subject to another that is apparently unrelated, or may make indirect associations or clang associations (relating words that sound the same rather than connect logically).

Other thought disorders that occur in schizophrenia include inventing new words (*neologisms*), thought blocking (sudden interruption in the train of thought), experiencing thoughts as being inserted into or withdrawn from the mind by some outside force, and auditory *hallucinations*, in which a voice dictates or repeats the subject's thoughts.

An inability to think clearly and coherently occurs in all types of *confusion*, including *dementia* and delirium. Rapidly jumping from one idea to another ("flight of ideas") as a result of loosening of associations is characteristic of *hypomania* and *mania*. In *depression*, the opposite occurs; thinking becomes slow, there is a lack of ideas and associations, and a tendency to dwell in great detail on trivial subjects. Recurrent ideas that seem to

T

ANATOMY OF THE THORAX

The heart, lungs, and large blood vessels, such as the aorta, occupy almost the whole of the thoracic cavity. The extra protection that is afforded to these organs by the rib cage, which also allows breathing movements, reflects their vital importance.

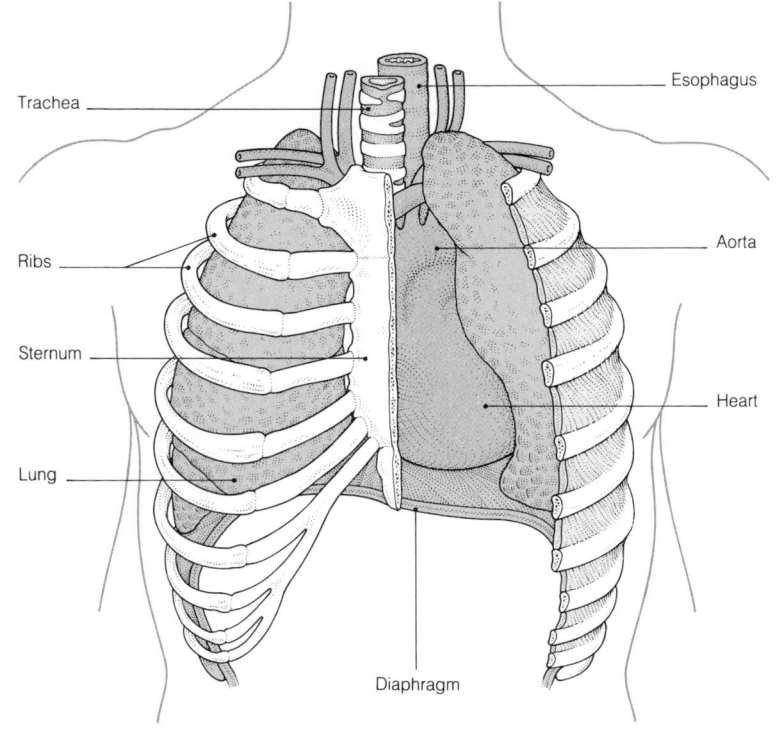

Trachea

Esophagus

Ribs

Aorta

Sternum

Heart

Lung

Diaphragm

come into a person's mind involuntarily are characteristic of *obsessive-compulsive behavior.*

Delusions (false beliefs that do not respond to reasoned argument), which occur in schizophrenia and other psychotic illnesses, may be an expression of distorted thinking.

Threadworm infestation
See *Pinworm infestation.*

Thrill
A vibrating sensation felt when the flat of the hand is held against the front of the chest. It is caused by abnormal blood flow in the heart as a result of a diseased heart valve or due to some form of congenital *heart disease.* An audible heart murmur always coexists.

Throat
A popular term for the *pharynx,* the passage running down from the back of the mouth and nose to the upper part of the *esophagus* and the opening into the *larynx* (voice box). The term is also used popularly to refer to the front of the neck. (See also *Sore throat.*)

Throat cancer
See *Pharynx, cancer of.*

Throat, lump in the
See *Globus hystericus.*

Thrombectomy
The removal of a thrombus (blood clot) that is partially or completely blocking a blood vessel.

Thrombectomy may be performed as an emergency procedure if a thrombus is blocking a major artery (such as one supplying blood to the brain, lungs, or intestines). It may also be performed as a precautionary measure if there is a risk of a fragment (an embolus) breaking off from a thrombus and being carried into the bloodstream to block an artery.

Before surgery, the site of the thrombus is established by *angiography* and the patient is given *anti-coagulant drugs* (drugs that prevent the blood from clotting). Incisions are made (with the use of a general anesthetic) to uncover the affected blood vessel, which is opened, and the thrombus is aspirated (sucked out). The incision is then closed with delicate stitches.

Thromboangiitis obliterans
Another name for *Buerger's disease.*

Thrombocytopenia
A reduction in the number of *platelet* cells in the blood. Because platelets play a vital role in the arrest of bleeding (by plugging any small breaks that develop in the walls of blood vessels), thrombocytopenia causes a tendency to bleed, especially from the smaller blood vessels. The result may be abnormal bleeding into the skin and from other parts of the body (thrombocytopenic purpura).

CAUSES AND SYMPTOMS
Thrombocytopenia may be caused by a reduced rate of production of platelets by the bone marrow or by a fast rate of destruction of the platelets.

In some cases, the underlying cause of the thrombocytopenia is not apparent (idiopathic thrombocytopenia). However, the condition frequently follows a viral infection and may be an *autoimmune disorder* in which the infection triggers destruction of the platelets by the immune system. Idiopathic thrombocytopenia occurs mainly in children and young adults; it usually runs a brief course of a few days to a few weeks before clearing up, although sometimes, particularly in adults, the bleeding tendency recurs from time to time.

The symptoms may include purple bruises or bleeding points in the skin, nosebleeds, *hematuria* (blood in the urine), bleeding in the mouth, and *menorrhagia* (heavy periods). There is a small risk of a *brain hemorrhage,* the warning signs for which are headache and dizziness.

Thrombocytopenia and associated bleeding can also occur as a feature of *leukemia, lymphoma,* some types of *anemia,* systemic *lupus erythematosus,* or *hypersplenism* (overactivity of the spleen). It may also occur after exposure to X rays or radiation, in severe fevers, and as a reaction to certain drugs, such as quinine.

DIAGNOSIS AND TREATMENT
Thrombocytopenia is diagnosed from the patient's symptoms and the presence of low numbers of platelets when a *blood count* is performed. A diagnosis

T

of idiopathic thrombocytopenia is made by excluding possible causes.

If thrombocytopenia is due to some other disease, treatment is of the underlying disease. If a drug is responsible, it is withdrawn. Children with idiopathic thrombocytopenia may not require treatment, but adults are generally given *corticosteroid drugs*. If the condition persists for many weeks or becomes recurrent, *splenectomy* (removal of the spleen) is often performed, giving a lasting cure in about three quarters of the cases.

Thromboembolism

The blockage of a blood vessel by a fragment that has broken off and been carried from a thrombus (blood clot) elsewhere in the circulation. (See also *Thrombosis; Embolism.*)

Thrombolytic drugs

A group of drugs, also known as fibrinolytic drugs, used to dissolve blood clots in *thrombosis, embolism,* and *myocardial infarction* (heart attack). Thrombolytic drugs work by increasing the blood level of plasmin (an enzyme that dissolves fibrin, the main constituent of blood clots).

Treatment is carefully monitored because of the risk of bleeding. An allergic reaction, causing rash and breathing difficulty, may also occur.

Thrombophlebitis

Inflammation of part of a vein, usually near the surface of the body, along with clot formation in the affected segment. Thrombophlebitis can occur after minor injury to a vein (such as after an injection or intravenous infusion) and is particularly common in intravenous drug abusers. It can develop as a complication of *varicose veins* and also in blood vessel disorders such as *Buerger's disease*.

There is obvious swelling and redness along the affected segment of vein, which is extremely tender to the touch. Fever and malaise often occur. Serious complications are uncommon, although sometimes more serious clot formation develops in deeper veins (see *Thrombosis, deep vein*).

Treatment is by gentle support using a crepe bandage and by the use of a *nonsteroidal anti-inflammatory drug* and sometimes *antibiotic drugs* if infection of the vein is suspected.

Thrombosis

The formation of a blood clot (thrombus) within an intact blood vessel. Clotting is a normal response that prevents bleeding when a blood vessel wall is injured. Thrombus formation is abnormal if it occurs when a vessel wall has not been cut or punctured.

A thrombus within an artery may eventually grow to block the artery, preventing blood and oxygen from reaching the organ or tissue supplied by the artery. Thrombi of this type are an important cause of death and disability in the US and other developed countries. A thrombus that forms within one of the arteries supplying the heart muscle (coronary thrombosis) is the usual cause of a *myocardial infarction* (heart attack). A thrombus within one of the arteries supplying the brain (cerebral thrombosis) is a common cause of *stroke*.

Thrombi may similarly block the blood supply to the legs, kidneys, retinas, intestines, and other organs, sometimes causing severe damage and symptoms such as pain and loss of function. Another danger is that a fragment of thrombus—an embolus—may break off and be carried in the bloodstream to block an important blood vessel some distance from its site of origin.

Thrombi may also form in veins—either in inflamed veins near the surface (a condition called *thrombophlebitis*) or in deeper veins (see *Thrombosis, deep vein*). In deep vein thrombosis, the risk of large emboli breaking off and being carried to the heart and lungs is particularly serious.

CAUSES

In the blood there is a fine balance between the mechanisms that encourage and discourage clotting, so there is neither a tendency to bleed nor to form clots (see *Blood clotting*). Thrombosis can occur if there is an upset in favor of clotting.

In arteries, the clotting process may be encouraged by a buildup of atheroma (fatty deposits) on blood vessel walls. Any of the factors that encourage *atherosclerosis*—such as smoking, obesity, *diabetes mellitus,* or *hypertension* (high blood pressure)—is similarly associated with an increased tendency to form clots. Damage to blood vessel walls from inflammation (which occurs in *arteritis* and phlebitis) may also encourage clot formation, as may spread of infection to blood vessels locally or in *septicemia* (spread and multiplication of bacteria through the blood).

A clotting tendency can result from an increase in the level of coagulation factors in the blood; this tendency can occur in pregnancy or when using oral contraceptives. It can result from liver disease that leads to deficient production of antithrombin, an anticlotting factor. It can also result from any cause that slows down blood flow to a certain area (e.g., inactivity during long airplane flights, or general anesthesia induced for a surgical operation).

SYMPTOMS AND DIAGNOSIS

An arterial thrombus may cause no symptoms until it impairs the blood flow through a blood vessel. At this point it may cause reduced function of the organ or tissue supplied by the blood vessel and, in some cases, severe pain. Venous thrombosis may also cause pain and swelling.

When thrombosis is a suspected cause of symptoms, it is investigated by *angiography* or by *venography* (X rays of blood vessels after injection of a radiopaque substance).

TREATMENT

Treatment may include the use of *anticoagulant drugs*, which discourage clotting, or *thrombolytic drugs*, which help break down clots that have already formed. *Nonsteroidal anti-inflammatory drugs* are often given to relieve the inflammation of thrombophlebitis. Other treatment, such as *antibiotic drugs* if infection is the cause of thrombosis, may be necessary. In cases where a clot is life-threatening, surgical removal may be required (see *Thrombectomy*).

Thrombosis, deep vein

Clotting of blood within deep-lying veins, usually in the legs. *Thrombophlebitis* is a condition affecting superficial veins (nearer the surface) when they become inflamed.

CAUSES AND INCIDENCE

Deep vein thrombosis is generally caused by a combination of sluggish blood flow through one part of the body and some factor that increases the tendency of the blood to clot.

Sluggish blood flow occurs when a person lies or sits still for long periods. An increase in the level of coagulation factors in the blood, which occurs after an operation or injury, during pregnancy, and in women taking the birth-control pill, causes an increased tendency for the blood to clot.

An increased tendency to form clots can also occur as a result of *polycythemia* (increased numbers of red cells in the blood), severe infection, liver disease, and certain types of cancer. Deep vein thrombosis is common in people with *heart failure* and in those who have had a *stroke* or who are immobilized for long periods. Other

T

causes include injury to the veins or an extension of thrombophlebitis to deeper veins. Age and obesity both predispose to thrombosis.

SYMPTOMS AND COMPLICATIONS

If the thrombosis is not in a leg, there are often no symptoms. Clots in the leg veins may cause symptoms such as pain, tenderness, swelling, discoloration, and ulceration of the skin, depending on the site of the clots and how extensive they are.

Deep vein thrombosis is not always of serious significance; occasionally, if the clots are extensive, part of a clot may break free and be carried up to the heart and from there to the lungs, where it may block an artery. This is called a *pulmonary embolism* and is always a serious condition.

DIAGNOSIS

The presence and extent of deep vein thrombosis is diagnosed by *venography* (introduction of a radiopaque substance into the veins followed by X rays) and by a type of *radionuclide scanning* called the radioactive fibrinogen test. Doppler *ultrasound scanning* is also sometimes used to help detect certain thrombi.

TREATMENT

Treatment depends on the site and extent of the blood clots. If they are small, confined to the calf, and the patient is mobile, treatment may be unnecessary, as the clots often break up spontaneously. In some cases, *anticoagulant drugs* may be given to prevent extension of the clots. In other cases, *thrombolytic drugs*, which actively dissolve the clots, may be given. If there is a high risk of a clot breaking off and causing a pulmonary embolism, *thrombectomy* may be performed to remove the clot surgically from the vein.

PREVENTION

The incidence of deep vein thrombosis has been reduced by encouraging people to get up as soon as possible after an operation or childbirth. If a person is immobilized for a long period, he or she should wiggle the toes and flex the ankles and knees to keep the blood moving. Blood flow in the legs of an immobilized person may also be stimulated by putting the legs in plastic bags, which are pumped up with air and then deflated.

When an operation is performed on someone thought to be particularly susceptible to deep vein thrombosis, anticoagulant drugs may be given.

Thrombus

A blood clot that has formed inside an intact blood vessel—as distinct from one that has formed to seal the wall of a blood vessel after injury.

DEEP VEIN THROMBOSIS

Thrombi, or clots, tend to form when blood flow is sluggish and in circumstances such as pregnancy where there is a rise in the level of coagulation factors in the blood. Once a clot has formed, it may provide a site for further clotting, so that a long, snaky clot may grow along the length of a vein. Thrombi form most commonly in the leg veins and may interfere with the drainage of blood from a leg (below right), causing signs and symptoms of varying severity.

Normal and obstructed vein
Thrombi tend to form at points where a vein lining is damaged and may then grow to obstruct blood flow. The big danger is that a piece of clot will detach and be carried to the heart and lungs to cause a potentially fatal obstruction.

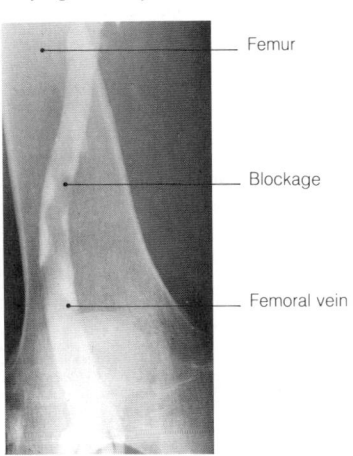

Example of deep vein thrombosis
This venogram shows a thrombus blocking the femoral vein just above the knee.

Calf vein thrombosis
When clots are localized to the calf and popliteal veins, there is usually some pain in the calf but there may be little swelling.

Femoral vein thrombosis
If clots are present in the femoral vein as well as calf veins, there is usually pain and swelling up to the region above the knee.

Iliofemoral vein thrombosis
Clots in the iliac vein may affect drainage of blood from the whole leg, causing severe pain and swelling.

T

A thrombus is life-threatening if it grows to obstruct the blood supply to an organ such as the heart or brain. Even a thrombus in a less vital blood vessel can be dangerous because it may produce gangrene in part of the organ or extremity served, or a fragment of it (an embolus) may break off and be carried to obstruct the blood circulation elsewhere. (See also *Blood clotting; Thrombosis; Embolism*.)

Thrush

A common name for the fungal infection *candidiasis*.

Thumb-sucking

A common habit in young children. For the young child, thumb-sucking provides comfort (especially before falling asleep), oral gratification, amusement if the child is bored, and reassurance, especially during periods of stress, such as the birth of a new baby in the family.

Thumb-sucking tends to decrease after the age of about 3. Only a few children do not grow out of the habit by 6 or 7. In general, it is best for parents to ignore the habit; constant reprimands increase anxiety and may make thumb-sucking worse.

COMPLICATIONS

In most cases, there is no evidence that thumb-sucking is harmful. However, *malocclusion* (incorrect bite) of the second teeth may develop if the habit continues after about age 6. The effect on the teeth is usually only temporary; their position improves considerably or even completely after thumb-sucking stops. In severe cases of malocclusion, repositioning of the displaced teeth with an *orthodontic appliance* may be recommended.

Thymoma

A tumor of the *thymus* gland. Thymomas are rare and are classified according to the type of thymus tissue from which they arise. An epithelial thymoma, arising from *epithelium*, is a slow-growing tumor that rarely spreads to other parts of the body. A lymphoid thymoma arises from lymphoid tissue, eventually resulting in generalized non-Hodgkin's *lymphoma*. A granulomatous thymoma consists of a mixture of epithelial and lymphoid tissue, and closely resembles *Hodgkin's disease*. The other main type of thymoma is a thymic *teratoma* (a tumor consisting of tissue that is not normally found in the thymus), which is usually benign in women but malignant in men.

Thymomas may affect function of the *immune system*, causing increased susceptibility to infection. They are commonly associated with *myasthenia gravis* (an autoimmune disease), which sometimes can be cured by removal of the thymoma.

Thymus

A gland that forms part of the *immune system*. The thymus is situated in the upper part of the chest, behind the breastbone, and consists of two lobes that join in front of the trachea. Each lobe is made up of lymphoid tissue consisting of tightly packed *lymphocytes, epithelium*, and fat.

The thymus plays a part in the body's immune response from about the 12th week of gestation until puberty. The gland gradually enlarges until puberty, when it begins to shrink. Lymphoid and epithelial tissues are gradually replaced by fat, although some glandular tissue remains until after middle age.

The function of the thymus is to cause lymphocytes to become T cells. These T cells play an important part in the body's defense against viruses and other infections.

DISORDERS

Abnormal enlargement of the thymus sometimes occurs in several conditions, including *myasthenia gravis, acromegaly, thyrotoxicosis*, and *Addison's disease*. Myasthenia gravis is also sometimes associated with *thymomas*

LOCATION OF THE THYMUS
At full size, the thymus lies partly in the neck and partly in the chest. It shrinks later in life.

Thymus

Trachea

Lungs

(tumors of the thymus). In children, *immunodeficiency disorders* may arise as a result of abnormal development of the thymus.

Thyroglossal disorders

Congenital defects arising from failure of the thyroglossal duct to disappear during embryonic development. In the embryo, this duct runs from the base of the tongue to the thyroid gland in the neck. Abnormal development may cause the duct to persist in its entirety or partially as a cyst.

Tongue
Thyroglossal duct
Thyroglossal cyst
Thyroid gland

Thyroglossal duct and cyst
The thyroglossal duct, lying between the tongue and the thyroid, sometimes persists after fetal life, and a cyst may form.

A thyroglossal cyst almost always becomes infected and swollen, a condition that may be mistaken for an abscess. Infection may lead to formation of a thyroglossal fistula (abnormal passage between the cyst and the surface of the neck).

Because of the danger of repeated infection, a thyroglossal cyst or fistula should be completely removed surgically, along with any remaining parts of the thyroglossal duct.

Thyroid cancer

Cancer of the *thyroid gland* is relatively rare, accounting for only about 1 percent of all cases of cancer. In most cases, the cause of the condition is unknown, although it is one of the cancers associated with exposure to radioactive fallout. Thyroid cancer has one of the highest cure rates of all cancers.

SYMPTOMS

A thyroid cancer is usually first noticed as a single, firm nodule in the neck, which, on initial physical examination, cannot be distinguished from a benign (noncancerous) mass. For this reason, all single thyroid

T

nodules are imaged (see *Imaging techniques*), sometimes examined with needle *biopsy*, and, when necessary, removed surgically for microscopic examination. If there are several nodules, they are likely to be benign rather than cancerous. The three cell types are papillary (the most common), follicular, and medullary (which secretes *calcitonin*).

Cancerous tumors may grow slowly or rapidly, depending on their type and the age of the patient (growth tends to be slower in younger people). However, in most cases, the cancer spreads to the lymph nodes at an early stage. Advanced cancers are usually hard and irregularly shaped and are often firmly attached to adjacent structures in the neck.

In many cases, thyroid cancers are painless; symptoms arise when they press on other structures in the neck. Such symptoms may include severe hoarseness or loss of voice from pressure on the nerves to the larynx or difficulty swallowing due to pressure on the pharynx (throat).

TREATMENT
Treatment is usually by surgical removal of the entire gland (total thyroidectomy); occasionally, it is necessary to remove surrounding tissues. The loss of thyroid tissue results in a lack of natural *thyroid hormones*, and patients usually need to take hormone supplements for the rest of their lives. Such supplements may also help to control *metastases* (secondary growths).

In virtually all cases, treatment with radioactive iodine is used after surgery. Because it is selectively taken up and concentrated in the thyroid, radioactive iodine has the advantage of destroying any residual cancers while leaving normal body tissue undamaged, minimizing any side effects. This treatment may need to be repeated at one- to five-year intervals if any residual tissue is detected.

If thyroid cancer is diagnosed and treated at an early stage (even if local spread has occurred), the outlook is generally excellent. Papillary cancer is highly treatable; follicular cancer is only slightly less so. Medullary cancer has a less favorable outlook.

Thyroidectomy
Surgical removal of all or part of the thyroid gland.

WHY IT IS DONE
Thyroidectomy is performed to treat *thyroid cancer*, cases of *thyrotoxicosis* (an abnormally high blood level of thyroid

SUBTOTAL THYROIDECTOMY
This operation entails removal of only part of the thyroid. The parathyroids (at the rear of the gland) are left intact.

Thyroid gland

Line of incision

1 After administration of a general anesthetic, an incision is made in the neck. Layers of skin and muscle are then drawn aside to expose the thyroid gland underneath.

Part of thyroid to be removed

Cross section through the neck

2 Once the front of the gland has been detached from its blood supply, much of it is cut away (with care taken not to damage nearby nerves), and bleeding vessels are sealed.

3 Tubes are sometimes placed in the site of the removed gland to drain blood that accumulates. The muscle and skin layers are replaced and the incision closed with sutures or clips.

hormone) that cannot be controlled by drugs, *goiter* that is causing breathing or swallowing difficulties or unsightly swelling, or a benign tumor.

HOW IT IS DONE
The operation to remove part of the thyroid (subtotal thyroidectomy) is shown in the illustration at left.

RECOVERY PERIOD
The wound usually heals quickly. The stitches and drainage tube can usually be removed within a few days of the operation, after which the patient leaves the hospital.

Removal of all—or a large part—of the thyroid gland necessitates lifelong thyroid hormone replacement therapy with thyroxine.

COMPLICATIONS
There is a very small risk of damage to structures close to the thyroid gland. Injury to the nerve supplying the vocal cords can lead to hoarseness; damage to the *parathyroid glands* can result in a low calcium level in the blood and tetany (painful muscle spasms in the hands, feet, and face). After the operation, careful monitoring is required to ensure that hormone levels are in the normal range.

Thyroid function tests
A group of procedures used to evaluate the function of the *thyroid gland* and to detect or confirm any disorder of the gland.

Thyroid function can be measured by carrying out *blood tests* to determine the level of thyroxine (T_4) and triiodothyronine (T_3) in the blood. A sample of blood is taken from the patient's vein and the serum (liquid part of the blood) is tested.

The main function of the thyroid gland is to convert tyrosine (an amino acid) and iodine into T_4 and T_3. One way of measuring thyroid function is therefore to measure the rate at which iodine is accumulated by the gland. This can be done by introducing into the body a radioactive isotope of iodine (or technetium, which behaves in a similar way to iodine) and measuring the level of radioactivity in the gland (see *Thyroid scanning*).

The thyroid secretes T_4 and T_3 into the bloodstream under the direct control of thyroid-stimulating hormone (TSH) from the pituitary gland. Thus measurement of the amount of TSH produced by the pituitary provides a sensitive means of diagnosing thyroid malfunction. Various indices created by ratios of T_3 and T_4 enable the specialist to more accurately diagnose the condition.

Thyroid gland

An important organ of the *endocrine system*. The thyroid gland is situated in the front of the neck, just below the larynx (voice box). It consists of two lobes, one on each side of the trachea (windpipe), joined by a narrower portion of tissue called the isthmus.

STRUCTURE

Thyroid tissue is composed of two types of secretory cells—follicular cells and parafollicular cells (or C cells). Follicular cells make up most of the gland. They are arranged in the form of hollow, spherical follicles, and secrete the iodine-containing hormones thyroxine (T_4) and triiodothyronine (T_3). The space inside the follicles is filled with a semifluid, colloid material that is essential for the production of T_4 and T_3.

Parafollicular cells occur singly or in small groups in the spaces between the follicles. They secrete the hormone *calcitonin*. Also between the follicles are numerous blood capillaries, small lymphatic vessels, and connective tissue. The entire thyroid gland is encased in a thin outer layer of connective tissue.

FUNCTION

T_4 and T_3 play an important role in controlling body *metabolism*. Calcitonin acts in conjunction with parathyroid hormone to regulate calcium balance in the body. (See also *Thyroid gland* disorders box; *Thyroid hormones*.)

Thyroid hormones

The hormones thyroxine (T_4), triiodothyronine (T_3), and *calcitonin*, produced by the *thyroid gland*.

FUNCTION

T_4 (the hormone produced in greatest amounts by the thyroid gland) and T_3 regulate *metabolism* (the chemical activity in cells that releases energy from nutrients or uses energy to create other substances, such as proteins). In children, these hormones are also essential for normal physical growth and mental development.

Calcitonin acts in conjunction with parathyroid hormone (secreted by the *parathyroid glands*) to regulate the level of calcium in the body.

REGULATION

T_4 AND T_3 The secretion of T_4 and T_3 by the thyroid is controlled by a hormonal feedback system involving the *pituitary gland* and *hypothalamus*.

CALCITONIN The secretion of calcitonin by the thyroid is regulated directly by the level of calcium in the blood. Raised blood calcium stimulates calcitonin secretion, stimulating deposition of calcium in bone and thereby reducing the calcium level; decreased blood calcium inhibits calcitonin output to help increase the calcium level. This regulation occurs independently of the pituitary gland or hypothalamus.

DEFICIENCY AND EXCESS

Insufficient thyroid hormone production is known as *hypothyroidism*. Symptoms include tiredness, dry skin, hair loss, weight gain, constipation, and sensitivity to cold. In childhood, deficiency may cause severe growth retardation.

Overproduction of thyroid hormones (*hyperthyroidism*) causes symptoms including fatigue, anxiety,

---

CONTROL OF THYROID HORMONE PRODUCTION

(Raised blood levels of thyroid hormones)

Bloodstream
If blood levels of the thyroid hormones T_3 and T_4 rise, they decrease the sensitivity of the pituitary to thyrotropin-releasing hormone (TRH), secreted by the hypothalamus.

Hypothalamus
Secretes TRH.

Pituitary gland
The pituitary becomes less sensitive to TRH, so it secretes less thyroid-stimulating hormone (TSH).

Thyroid gland
In response to lowered TSH stimulation, the thyroid reduces its production of the hormones T_3 and T_4.

Bloodstream
The blood levels of T_3 and T_4 thus gradually fall back to normal.

(Reduced blood levels of thyroid hormones)

Bloodstream
If blood levels of the thyroid hormones T_3 and T_4 fall, the hypothalamus is stimulated to produce more TRH.

Hypothalamus
Increases secretion of TRH.

Pituitary gland
In response to stimulation by TRH, the pituitary increases production of TSH.

Thyroid gland
In response to increased TSH stimulation, the thyroid increases its production of T_3 and T_4.

Bloodstream
The blood levels of T_3 and T_4 thus gradually rise back to normal.

Why control is necessary
The blood levels of the hormones T_3 (triiodothyronine) and T_4 (thyroxine) produced by the thyroid must be kept within narrow limits, otherwise hyperthyroidism or hypothyroidism may result. The control systems above exist to achieve this balance but certain disorders may interfere with the system.

LOCATION OF THYROID GLAND
This major gland lies at the base of the neck just in front of the trachea (windpipe).

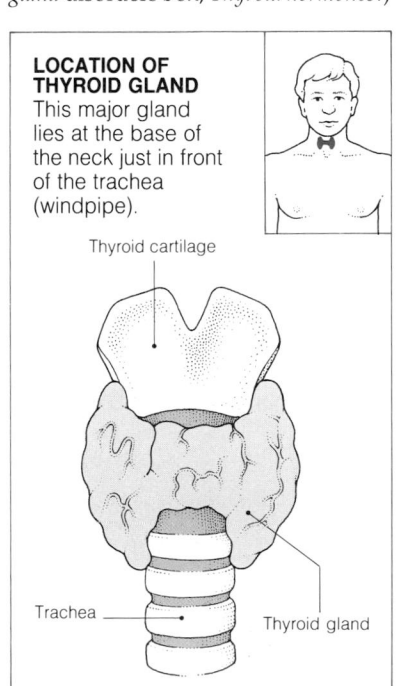

Thyroid cartilage

Trachea

Thyroid gland

T

DISORDERS OF THE THYROID GLAND

The function of the thyroid gland is controlled by both the pituitary gland and the hypothalamus, so thyroid disorders may be due not only to defects in the gland itself, but also to disruption of the hypothalamic-pituitary hormonal control system. Thyroid disorders may cause symptoms due to overproduction of thyroid hormones (*hyperthyroidism*), underproduction of these hormones (*hypothyroidism*), or enlargement or distortion of the gland. Idiopathic (of unknown cause) *goiter* (enlargement of the gland), *Graves' disease*, and *Hashimoto's thyroiditis* are the common disorders of thyroid function. Goiter sometimes occurs without any accompanying abnormality of thyroid function.

CONGENITAL DEFECTS

In rare cases, the thyroid gland is missing completely at birth, producing severe *cretinism*. However, congenital thyroid deficiency more often takes the form of underdevelopment or maldevelopment, in which there is sufficient hormone-producing thyroid tissue to avoid cretinism but insufficient tissue to produce normal amounts of hormones. If untreated, this may lead to juvenile *myxedema*.

Sometimes the thyroid develops in an abnormal position in the neck; in rare cases, this causes difficulty swallowing or breathing.

GENETIC DISORDERS

A genetic disorder may impair the thyroid's ability to secrete hormones. The low blood level of thyroid hormones results in greatly increased secretion by the pituitary gland of thyroid-stimulating hormone (TSH), which, in turn, causes the thyroid to enlarge in an effort to produce more hormone. This is one way in which a goiter may develop.

INFECTION

Thyroid infection is uncommon, but sometimes occurs as a complication of infection elsewhere in the body. The resulting *thyroiditis* may require treatment with antibiotics. If an abscess forms, a minor operation may be necessary to open and drain it. Viral infection of the thyroid can cause temporary hyperthyroidism as well as an extremely painful gland.

Tumors
Lumps in the thyroid are usually benign and some cancers are not highly malignant. Stone-hard, rapidly growing lumps suggest thyroid cancer.

Autoimmune disease
This is the most common cause of thyroid disorders. In Hashimoto's disease, much of the glandular tissue is replaced by masses of lymphocytes.

Goiter
Gland swelling (goiter) is common at puberty due to hormonal disturbance or may be due to autoimmune disease or, rarely, to iodine deficiency.

TUMORS

Thyroid tumors may be benign or malignant. Thyroid *adenomas* are benign tumors that may secrete thyroid hormone, sometimes in sufficient amounts to cause hyperthyroidism. *Thyroid cancers* vary greatly in their malignancy and rate of growth. They are relatively rare but may be suspected if only a single firm or hard lump can be felt in the gland. One particular type of thyroid tumor secretes the hormone calcitonin.

AUTOIMMUNE DISORDERS

Graves' disease is a form of thyroid overactivity whose chief feature is hyperthyroidism. The disease is thought to be due to the body producing an "autoantibody" that stimulates the thyroid to secrete excessive amounts of hormones. Autoantibodies are also believed to be associated with certain other thyroid disorders, notably Hashimoto's thyroiditis, in which the antibodies damage glandular cells.

MYXEDEMA

Deficiency of thyroid hormone (hypothyroidism) may be associated with Hashimoto's thyroiditis or atrophy of the thyroid or be a consequence of treatment for hyperthyroidism. A possible result is myxedema, wherein the skin becomes dry and thickened and facial features become coarse. Constipation, cold intolerance, and fatigue are other common symptoms. In many cases, the cause of myxedema is not known.

HORMONAL DISORDERS

Hormonal changes during puberty or pregnancy are a relatively common cause of a minor degree of goiter, which usually subsides when hormone levels return to normal.

Hyperthyroidism due to excessive production of TSH by the pituitary gland is rare but can occur as a result of a pituitary tumor.

NUTRITIONAL DISORDERS

Because iodine is necessary for the production of thyroid hormone, deficiency of this mineral may lead to enlargement of the thyroid gland (goiter). Severe iodine deficiency in children may cause myxedema. These problems can be avoided by using table salt that contains iodine.

RADIATION

Irradiation of the head or neck (e.g., for acne or enlarged tonsils or thymus gland) increases the likelihood of malignant thyroid tumors, although it may be 25 years or more until such tumors develop.

INVESTIGATION

Suspected disturbances of thyroid function are investigated initially by the taking of a medical history and the performance of a physical examination. Blood samples may also be taken for *thyroid function tests*, in which the levels of thyroid or pituitary hormones are measured, and the gland itself may be imaged by various *thyroid scanning* techniques. In some cases, such as a suspected thyroid tumor, a fine-needle *biopsy* may be carried out to obtain a sample of thyroid tissue for examination under the microscope.

T

palpitations, sweating, weight loss, diarrhea, and intolerance of heat.

DRUG THERAPY

The most commonly used thyroid hormone drugs are the synthetic thyroid hormone preparations levothyroxine and liothyronine. These drugs are used to treat hypothyroidism, to prevent hypothyroidism and reduce thyroid enlargement in certain types of *goiter*, and to treat *thyroid cancer*.

Because a sudden increase in the body's thyroid hormone level may strain the heart, levothyroxine and liothyronine are usually prescribed in low doses that are gradually increased. Since too high a dose may cause symptoms of hyperthyroidism, regular visits to the physician are essential; when necessary, blood tests are carried out to monitor the thyroid hormone level.

Calcitonin is used to treat *Paget's disease*, *osteoporosis*, and *hypercalcemia* (see *Calcitonin*).

Thyroiditis

The medical term for inflammation of the thyroid gland. The condition can be caused by a variety of factors, and occurs in several different forms. The most common form is *Hashimoto's thyroiditis*, an autoimmune disorder causing *hypothyroidism* (underactivity of the thyroid gland).

Subacute thyroiditis is a less common form in which the thyroid becomes tender and painful. Pain, which may be referred (see *Referred pain*) to the jaw, ears, or back of the head, may be accompanied by fever, weight loss, and a general feeling of illness. The condition may persist for several months, but in most cases eventually subsides on its own. In severe cases, treatment with *corticosteroid drugs* may be utilized to reduce the inflammation.

Thyroiditis due to infection is rare; when it does occur, it is usually as a result of an infection that has spread from elsewhere in the body. In some such cases, an abscess forms in the gland, which may require surgical drainage. Rarer still is a condition known as Riedel's thyroiditis (Riedel's struma), in which deposits of dense, fibrous tissue form in the gland and surrounding tissues, resulting in a hardening of the entire area.

Thyroid scanning

Techniques used to provide information about the location, anatomy, and function of the *thyroid gland*. *Radionuclide scanning* is the method

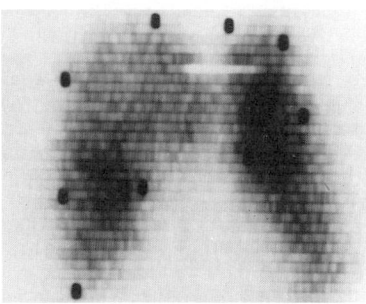

Radionuclide thyroid scanning
In this case, one area of the thyroid has taken up so much of the radioisotope that a diagnosis of a thyroid *adenoma* is likely.

available for investigating thyroid disorders, but *ultrasound scanning* can be useful in some cases.

HOW IT IS DONE

For radionuclide scanning, an injection or an oral dose of a radioisotope substance is given, followed after an interval by the recording of images on a gamma camera. The radioisotope substance usually contains a tiny dose of specially prepared technetium or radioiodine, both of which are taken up avidly by thyroid tissue, but hardly at all by other body tissues.

For the ultrasound scanning, a transducer producing high-frequency sound waves that penetrate tissue is moved back and forth across the skin over the thyroid gland. Echoes of the sound waves are picked up by the transducer and transformed electronically into an image.

WHY IT IS DONE

Radionuclide scanning reveals the position of any functioning thyroid tissue and is therefore useful in showing whether the gland is abnormally located or absent. The scan also shows the amount of the radioisotope substance that is taken up by the gland, thus allowing *hyperthyroidism* (overactivity) or *hypothyroidism* (underactivity) to be detected.

A radionuclide scan may suggest whether a thyroid nodule or tumor is benign or malignant and can show whether it is active or inactive. It can also detect malignant thyroid tissue that has spread to other parts of the body, therefore playing an important part in planning and evaluating the treatment of *thyroid cancer*.

Ultrasound scanning is of more limited use because it can show only the structure of thyroid tissue. It can be useful in showing whether a *goiter* is solid, cystic (fluid-filled), or a mixture of the two.

Thyrotoxicosis

A term for any toxic condition that results from *hyperthyroidism* (overactivity of the thyroid gland). The term thyrotoxicosis is often used as a synonym for *Graves' disease*.

Thyroxine

The most important *thyroid hormone* produced by the *thyroid gland*. Its symbol is T_4.

Tibia

The inner and thicker of the two long bones in the lower leg, also called the shin. The tibia is the supporting bone of the lower leg. It runs parallel to the other, narrower bone, the *fibula*, to which it is attached by ligaments.

The front surface of the tibia lies just beneath the skin and is easily felt. The upper end articulates with the femur (thigh bone) to form the *knee* joint and the lower end forms part of the *ankle joint*. On the inside of the ankle, the tibia is widened and protrudes to form a large bony prominence called the medial malleolus.

FRACTURE

The tibia is one of the most commonly fractured bones. It may break across the shaft as a result of a direct blow to the front of the leg, or at the upper end from a blow to the outside of the leg below the knee. Fracture of the lower end of the tibia may accompany dislocation of the ankle and fracture of

LOCATION OF THE TIBIA
Also called the shin, the tibia is easily felt beneath the skin of the lower leg.

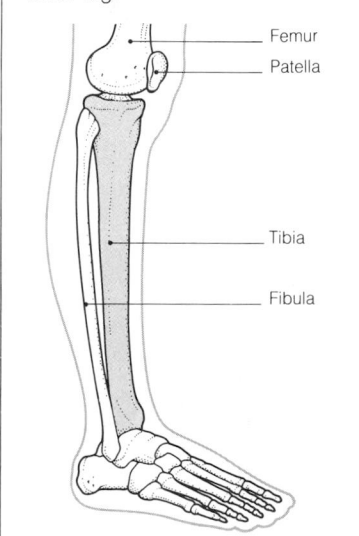

Femur
Patella
Tibia
Fibula

T

the fibula in a *Pott's fracture*, caused by violent twisting of the ankle. Prolonged running or walking on hard ground may cause a *stress fracture* of the tibia.

Some fractures of the shaft heal satisfactorily if the leg is immobilized in a plaster cast, usually for about six to eight weeks. If the bone ends are displaced or unstable, an operation may be needed to fasten them together with a nail or screw.

Tic

A repeated, uncontrolled, purposeless contraction of a muscle or group of muscles, most commonly in the face, shoulders, or arms. Typical tics include pointless blinking, mouth twitching, and shoulder shrugging.

Tics are often a sign of a usually minor psychological disturbance. Most develop in childhood, occurring in as many as a quarter of children and affecting three times more boys than girls. Tics are made worse by stress or by drawing attention to them, but often disappear when the child is deeply absorbed or asleep.

Tics usually stop within a year of onset but in some cases persist into adult life. Most can be controlled for short periods of time by will. However, such control is of questionable value because tics appear to release emotional tension.

In rare cases, tics become so severe that they require treatment with *benzodiazepine drugs* or *antipsychotic drugs*. Examples include involuntary contractions of the diaphragm (the muscle that separates the chest from the abdomen), resulting in grunting noises, and *Gilles de la Tourette's syndrome*, a disorder that is characterized by widespread tics and involuntary noises.

Tic douloureux

Another name for *trigeminal neuralgia*.

Ticks and disease

 Ticks are small, eight-legged animals that can attach themselves to human or animal skin to feed on blood. They are about one eighth of an inch long; when bloated with blood, they may grow much larger. There are two broad categories called soft and hard ticks (hard ticks have a hard shield on their backs). Soft ticks are nocturnal and visit their hosts for relatively short periods to feed; hard ticks may attach themselves for days or weeks.

Ticks may be picked up when a person walks through or reclines in various rural habitats, such as long grass, scrub, woodland, or caves. Ticks can also be brought into the home by dogs. An attached tick may not be noticed for hours; others cause irritation, pain (which is sometimes severe), or bruising.

For walking through tick-infested areas, wear boots and long pants and examine your body afterward. Attached ticks should be encouraged to drop off by applying to them the tip of a lighted cigarette or a pad soaked in chloroform or ether (if a tick is pulled off forcibly, its mouthparts may be left behind and can cause infection). The bite wound should then be washed with soap and water.

Ticks in various parts of the world can spread infectious organisms from animals to humans via their bites. Soft ticks spread *relapsing fever* in parts of North America, South America, and Africa. Hard ticks spread *Rocky Mountain spotted fever*, *Q fever*, *Lyme disease*, *tularemia*, and certain types of viral *encephalitis*, all of which can be contracted in the US.

The prolonged bite of certain female ticks can cause a condition called tick paralysis, in which a toxin in the tick saliva affects the nerves that control movement. In extreme cases, this can lead to paralysis of the respiratory muscles and can be fatal to a young child or elderly person.

Tietze's syndrome

Chest pain localized to an area on the front of the chest wall, usually made worse by movement of the arms or trunk or pressure from the fingers. Tietze's syndrome is caused by inflammation of one or several rib cartilages on their inside edges where they join the sternum (breastbone) or on their outside edges where they join the bony part of the rib. Symptoms may persist for several months.

Treatment is with *analgesic drugs* (painkillers) and *nonsteroidal anti-inflammatory drugs*.

Timolol

A *beta-blocker drug* used in tablet form to treat *hypertension* (high blood pressure) and *angina pectoris* (chest pain due to inadequate blood supply to the heart muscle). Timolol is also among the beta blockers given after a *myocardial infarction* (heart attack) to prevent further damage to the heart muscle. It is also used in eye-drop form to treat *glaucoma*.

Possible adverse effects are typical of other beta-blocker drugs. Eye drops may cause irritation, blurred vision, and headache.

Tinea

Any of a group of common *fungal infections* of the skin, hair, or nails. Most infections are caused by a group of fungi called the dermatophytes and are often called ringworm. Tineal infections may be acquired from another person, from an animal, from soil, or from an inanimate object such as a chair, shower stall, or carpeting.

Physicians commonly use the word tinea followed by the Latin term for the part of the body affected; tinea pedis affects the feet and tinea cruris affects the groin.

TYPES AND SYMPTOMS
The appearance and symptoms of tinea vary according to the site. The most common type is tinea pedis, also called *athlete's foot*. It causes cracking and itching between the toes.

Tinea corporis (ringworm of the body) is characterized by itchy patches on the body that are usually circular with a prominent edge. Tinea cruris (also commonly called jock itch) produces a reddened, itchy area spreading from the genitals outward over the inside of the thigh. It is more common in males.

Tinea capitis (ringworm of the scalp) causes one or several round, itchy, patches of hair loss on the scalp; it occurs mainly in children and is more common in large cities and overcrowded conditions. Ringworm of the nails, also called tinea unguium or onychomycosis, is often accompanied by scaling of the soles or palms. The nails become thick and white or yellow.

DIAGNOSIS AND TREATMENT
Most types of tinea are diagnosed by a physician from their appearances. However, sometimes the diagnosis must be confirmed, and the type of fungus identified, by culture of the organisms in a laboratory. Some scalp infections exhibit fluorescence under a filtered ultraviolet light (Wood's light), but most do not.

For most types of tinea, treatment is with *antifungal drugs* in the form of skin creams, lotions, or ointments. However, for widespread infections or those affecting the hair or nails, an antifungal drug in tablet form (usually griseofulvin) may be taken.

Treatment may be continued for some time after symptoms have subsided to eradicate the fungi and prevent recurrence. For mild infections on the skin surface, there may be four to six weeks of treatment; for toenail infections, treatment may continue for up to one or two years.

Tinea versicolor

A common skin condition that produces patches of white, brown, or salmon-colored finely flaking skin over the trunk and neck. Also known as pityriasis versicolor, it is caused by colonization of the dead outer layer of skin by a fungus that exists unnoticed on most people's skin as a yeast. The condition primarily affects young and middle-aged adults and is more common in men. It is not contagious.

Appearance of tinea versicolor
This fungal infection causes patches of color change in the skin and is particularly common in tropical and subtropical areas.

The condition is usually noticed because of the contrast in color between the affected and surrounding skin. Exposure to sunlight can make it more or less noticeable.

Treatment consists of applying an antifungal cream or lotion at night and washing underclothes and nightclothes thoroughly. It is important to treat the entire trunk, neck, arms, and upper legs (ears to knees) each time the antifungal preparation is applied. Otherwise, a spot may be missed and the fungus will recur. This treatment usually clears the condition, but the spots may take many months to return to normal skin color.

Tingling

See *Pins and needles sensation.*

Tinnitus

A ringing, buzzing, whistling, hissing, or other noise heard in the ear in the absence of environmental noise.
CAUSES
In tinnitus, the acoustic nerve transmits impulses to the brain not as the result of vibrations produced by

external sound waves but, for reasons not fully understood, as the result of stimuli that originate inside the head or within the ear itself. The condition is almost always associated with hearing loss, particularly *presbycusis.*

Tinnitus can occur as a symptom of many ear disorders, including *labyrinthitis, Meniere's disease, otitis media, otosclerosis, ototoxicity,* and blockage of the outer-ear canal with *earwax.* In rare cases, it is a symptom of an *aneurysm* or a tumor pressing on a blood vessel in the head.
SYMPTOMS
The noise in the ear may sometimes change in nature or intensity. In most cases it is present continuously but the sufferer's awareness of it is usually intermittent. Tolerance of tinnitus varies considerably from one person to another and is largely determined by the sufferer's personality. Many people learn to accept the condition without distress, but some find it almost intolerable.
TREATMENT
Any underlying disorder is treated if possible. Many sufferers make use of a radio, television, tape player, or headphones to block out the noise in their ears. Some find a tinnitus masker—headphones that play white noise (sounds produced by frequencies throughout the auditory field)—particularly effective.

Tipped uterus

See *Uterus, tipped.*

Tiredness

A common complaint that is usually the result of overwork or lack of sleep. In some people, persistent tiredness is caused by depression or anxiety. Tiredness may be due to a more serious condition, such as anemia or cancer, but usually there are accompanying symptoms.

Tissue

A collection of *cells* specialized to perform a particular function. Examples of tissues include muscle tissue, which consists of cells that are specialized to contract; epithelial tissue, which forms the *skin* and *mucous membranes* that line the respiratory and other internal tracts; nerve tissue, comprising cells specialized to conduct electrochemical nerve impulses; and connective tissue, which includes blood, adipose tissue (fat), and the various fibrous and elastic tissues (such as tendons and cartilage) that hold the body together.

Tissue fluid

The watery liquid present in the tiny spaces between body cells, also known as interstitial fluid. Tissue fluid is one component of extracellular fluid, which is any body fluid outside the cells, including blood and lymph.

To reach cells, oxygen and nutrients must pass from the blood vessels and into the tissue fluid. Similarly, there is a reverse movement of carbon dioxide and other waste products from the cells into the tissue fluid, and then into the bloodstream.

In addition to nutrients and wastes, tissue fluid also contains *ions.* This fluid contains a much higher level of sodium ions, and a much lower level of potassium ions, than intracellular fluid. It is this difference in ion levels that helps control the movement of water into and out of cells by *osmosis;* ion levels also play a role in the transmission of electrical impulses through nerves and muscles.

Tissue fluid is formed by the filtration of liquid out through the walls of the first part of blood capillaries (that is, the part nearest an arteriole), where it is forced out by the high blood pressure. In the last part of capillaries (nearest to a venule), blood pressure is much lower, and tissue fluid passes back into the capillaries; some tissue fluid is also drained away into the lymphatic vessels. Thus, there is a continual flow that keeps the amount of tissue fluid constant. Various disorders—such as congestive *heart failure*—may disrupt the balance between formation and drainage of tissue fluid, leading to *edema* (excess fluid in tissues).

Tissue-plasminogen activator

A substance produced by body tissues that prevents abnormal blood clotting. Also called TPA, it is produced in small amounts by the inner lining of blood vessels and by the muscular wall of the uterus.
DRUG THERAPY
TPA can be prepared artificially by *genetic engineering* techniques for use as a *thrombolytic drug* (a drug that dissolves blood clots). It is used in the treatment of *myocardial infarction* (heart attack), of severe progressive *angina pectoris* (chest pain caused by inadequate blood supply to the heart muscle), and of arterial *embolism* (blockage of an artery), including *pulmonary embolism.*

Given by *intravenous infusion,* TPA dissolves blood clots by converting plasminogen (a chemical in the blood)

T

to the enzyme plasmin. Plasmin in turn breaks down fibrin, the main constituent of a blood clot.

POSSIBLE ADVERSE EFFECTS

Bleeding or the formation of a *hematoma* (collection of blood) may occur at the site of injection. TPA may also cause bleeding elsewhere in the body but such bleeding can usually be controlled because TPA has a short-lived action. Allergic reaction may occur, although this effect is less likely than with other thrombolytic drugs. (See also *Fibrinolysis*.)

Tissue-typing

The investigation of certain characteristics of the tissues of prospective organ donors and recipients.

WHY IT IS DONE

Tissue-typing is necessary to help match recipient and donor tissues for *transplant surgery*, thus minimizing the risk of rejection of a donor organ by the recipient's *immune system*.

The main features by which a person's immune system distinguishes his or her own tissues from those of other people are called *histocompatibility antigens*. The most important members of this group are called HLAs (human leukocyte antigens), which are present on the surface of the person's cells. A person's set of HLAs is inherited and unique to that person (except for identical twins, who have the same set). Hence, perfect tissue matching is achieved only between identical twins. Nevertheless, close relatives often have closely matching HLA types.

HOW IT IS DONE

A person's tissue type, or HLA "fingerprint," is established by tests in the laboratory on cells from a sample of the person's blood. There are many different possible HLAs and the presence or absence of each must be tested individually.

In one of the simpler methods of tissue-typing, an *antiserum* containing *antibodies* (substances that react with a particular antigen—in this case, a particular HLA) is added to the test specimen. If the antigen is present, it is detected by an observable color or other change.

For organ transplantation, once a recipient has been tissue-typed, a selection is made of a donor whose HLA grouping best matches that of the recipient. This helps reduce the chances of organ rejection after transplantation. It is easiest to find such donors among close relatives, such as brothers or sisters.

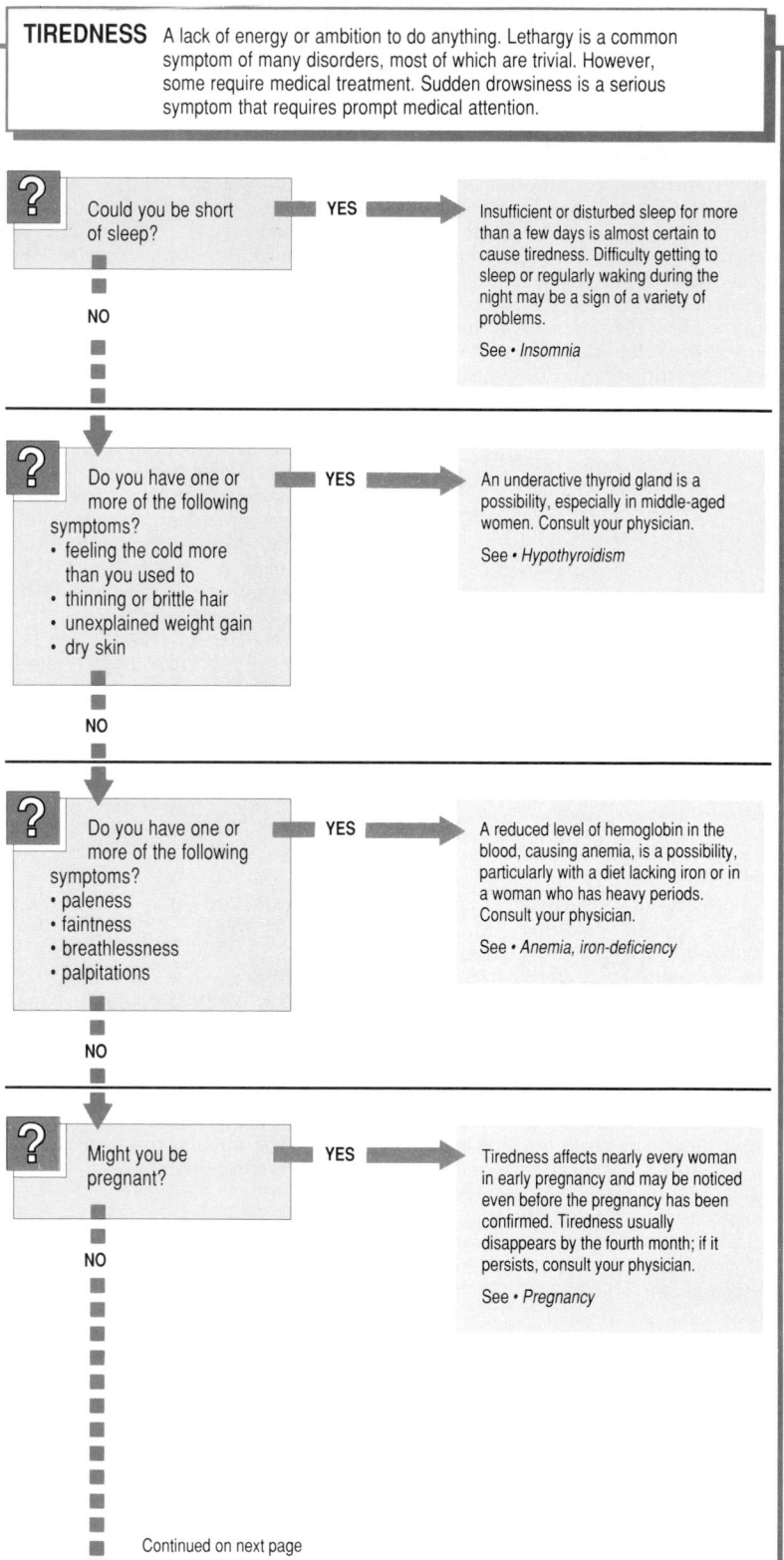

TIREDNESS A lack of energy or ambition to do anything. Lethargy is a common symptom of many disorders, most of which are trivial. However, some require medical treatment. Sudden drowsiness is a serious symptom that requires prompt medical attention.

Could you be short of sleep? — YES → Insufficient or disturbed sleep for more than a few days is almost certain to cause tiredness. Difficulty getting to sleep or regularly waking during the night may be a sign of a variety of problems.

See • *Insomnia*

NO

Do you have one or more of the following symptoms?
• feeling the cold more than you used to
• thinning or brittle hair
• unexplained weight gain
• dry skin

— YES → An underactive thyroid gland is a possibility, especially in middle-aged women. Consult your physician.

See • *Hypothyroidism*

NO

Do you have one or more of the following symptoms?
• paleness
• faintness
• breathlessness
• palpitations

— YES → A reduced level of hemoglobin in the blood, causing anemia, is a possibility, particularly with a diet lacking iron or in a woman who has heavy periods. Consult your physician.

See • *Anemia, iron-deficiency*

NO

Might you be pregnant? — YES → Tiredness affects nearly every woman in early pregnancy and may be noticed even before the pregnancy has been confirmed. Tiredness usually disappears by the fourth month; if it persists, consult your physician.

See • *Pregnancy*

NO

Continued on next page

T

Do you regularly drink more alcohol than the recommended maximum daily intake?

YES → Even in moderate quantities, regular consumption of alcohol can have a depressant effect, making you feel tired. If you find it difficult to reduce your intake or cut out alcohol altogether, consult your physician.

See • *Alcohol dependence*

NO

Do you have one or more of the following symptoms?
• inability to concentrate or make decisions
• lack of interest in sex
• recurrent headaches
• feeling in low spirits

YES → Depression can make you feel tired and run down.

See • *Depression*

NO

Have you been working hard without a break for several weeks, either at your job or in the home?

YES → Overworking for an extended period often causes tiredness, especially if accompanied by stress.

NO

Have you recently recovered from an infectious disease, such as the flu?

YES → It can take several weeks for the body to recover fully from some viral infections. Depression and tiredness are likely during this period.

NO

If you are unable to make a diagnosis from this chart, consult your physician.

Titanium dental implants

Posts surgically embedded in the jaw to form a framework for the attachment of false teeth. Titanium or other synthetic materials that form a bond with the jaw may be used.

Implants are useful for people who have lost all their teeth and who either are unable to tolerate a *denture* or have lost so much tooth-bearing tissue through injury or disease that a denture would not be stable.

FITTING
The procedure for fitting dental implants and attaching a prosthesis is shown in the box on the next page. Some prostheses can be removed only by the dentist; others can be removed by the patient.

TMJ syndrome
See *Temporomandibular joint syndrome*.

Toadstool poisoning
See *Mushroom poisoning*.

Tobacco chewing
See *Snuff*.

Tobacco smoking

Despite its practice in Western countries for more than 400 years—and for much longer in other parts of the world—tobacco smoking has only relatively recently been recognized as a major health hazard. Much of what is known today about the harmful effects of tobacco on the lungs concerns cigarette smoking because cigarette smokers have been studied in much greater depth than pipe or cigar smokers.

HARMFUL EFFECTS
Lung cancer is probably the best known harmful effect of smoking. More than 30 studies in 10 countries have demonstrated a direct link between smoking and lung cancer, a condition that is difficult to treat successfully and which causes about 8 percent of all deaths in men and 4 percent of all deaths in women in the US. Because pipe and cigar smokers tend not to inhale tobacco smoke, they have a slightly lower risk of lung cancer, although the risk is still significantly greater than for nonsmokers. The risk of developing lung cancer begins to diminish as soon as a person stops smoking.

Pipe and cigar smokers have a higher risk of cancer of the oral cavity and upper respiratory tract; tobacco chewers and those who use snuff risk cancer of the oral cavity (see *Nasopharynx, cancer of*).

T

FITTING DENTAL IMPLANTS

Replacement of missing teeth is sometimes carried out by surgically implanting posts into the jaw and then attaching a dental prosthesis to the posts. When all the teeth in the jaw are missing, six posts are usually implanted (below). The procedure is carried out in several stages, with pain prevented by means of a local anesthetic.

Flap of gum tissue

Cover screw

Post

Gum flap stitched

1 Flaps of gum tissue are cut and raised. Holes are drilled in the jaw, posts are inserted, and cover screws fitted.

2 The gum is stitched back over the posts and left for several months to allow time for healing to take place.

3 After the healing period, incisions are made to expose the posts. The cover screws are then removed.

Attachment

Gum

Screw

Dental prosthesis

Attachment

4 Attachments that protrude above the gum are screwed into the posts. The cut edges of the gum are stitched.

5 Several weeks later, when the gums have healed, measurements are taken for the prosthesis. The appliance, which is similar to a *bridge*, is manufactured in the laboratory and then screwed onto the protruding attachments over the posts.

The other important respiratory diseases associated with smoking are chronic *bronchitis* and *emphysema* and combinations of the two. These diseases, features of which include increasing breathlessness and coughing up sputum, account for tens of thousands of deaths annually in the US from respiratory failure. In addition, smoking also increases the risk of *mouth cancer*, *lip cancer*, and throat cancer (see *Pharynx, cancer of*).

The most significant harmful effect of smoking is *coronary heart disease*, which is the most common cause of death in middle-aged men in Western countries. The risk of coronary heart disease in a young man who smokes 20 cigarettes a day is about three times that of a nonsmoker, and the risk increases proportionally with the number of cigarettes smoked.

In addition to its effects on the coronary arteries, smoking damages arteries that supply other parts of the body and also raises blood pressure. Smoking seriously affects the arteries of the legs, leading to *peripheral vascular disease*; in severe cases of peripheral vascular disease, painful *neuropathy*, or *gangrene*, amputation may be necessary. Also affected by smoking are the arteries of the brain, which may result in a *stroke*.

Smoking is extremely harmful during pregnancy. The babies of women who smoke are smaller and less likely to survive than those of nonsmoking mothers. Even after birth, there are hazards for the children of parents who smoke. These children are more likely to suffer from *asthma* or other respiratory diseases and are more likely to become smokers themselves.

There is also evidence that anybody in the vicinity of a smoker is at increased risk of tobacco-related disorders. These "passive smokers" also suffer considerable immediate discomfort in the form of coughing, wheezing, and watering eyes.

HOW SMOKING CAUSES HARM

Tobacco contains a variety of different noxious substances, but the dangers of three of them are particularly important.

Nicotine is the substance that causes addiction to tobacco. It acts as a tranquilizer, but also stimulates the release of *epinephrine* into the smoker's bloodstream, which may explain why some smokers have raised blood pressure.

Tar in tobacco produces chronic irritation of the respiratory system and is a major cause of lung cancer.

Carbon monoxide passes from the lungs into the bloodstream, where, in competition with oxygen, it easily combines with hemoglobin and thus interferes with oxygenation of tissues. In the long term, persistently high levels of carbon monoxide in the blood—which occur in smokers—lead to hardening of the arteries, which increases the risk of *coronary thrombosis*.

STOPPING SMOKING

The most important prerequisite for successfully stopping smoking is an absolute commitment to giving up the habit. The slightest doubt over genuinely wanting to stop is likely to sabotage your efforts. For this reason, simply cutting down the number of cigarettes smoked rarely works; you must decide whether you will continue to smoke or will become a complete nonsmoker.

If you decide to stop smoking, there are many tools that may be helpful. Groups that emphasize behavior modification are effective and may utilize adjuncts such as nicotine-containing chewing gum, *acupuncture*, and *hypnosis*. Those who miss the oral sensation of smoking may find that sucking sweets or chewing gum or toothpicks helps.

Many people worry that they will gain weight as a result of stopping smoking. There is a risk that this will occur, because smoking tends to increase the metabolic rate (the rate at which the body "burns" food) and because many people eat more after they stop smoking. However, most physicians agree that being moderately overweight is far less hazardous to health than smoking.

T

TOBACCO SMOKING

Smoking is a sure way to damage your health; it contributes to about one death in seven in the US. The main harmful effects come from nicotine, carbon monoxide, and tar. The first two contribute to heart disease, while tar causes lung disease and cancer.

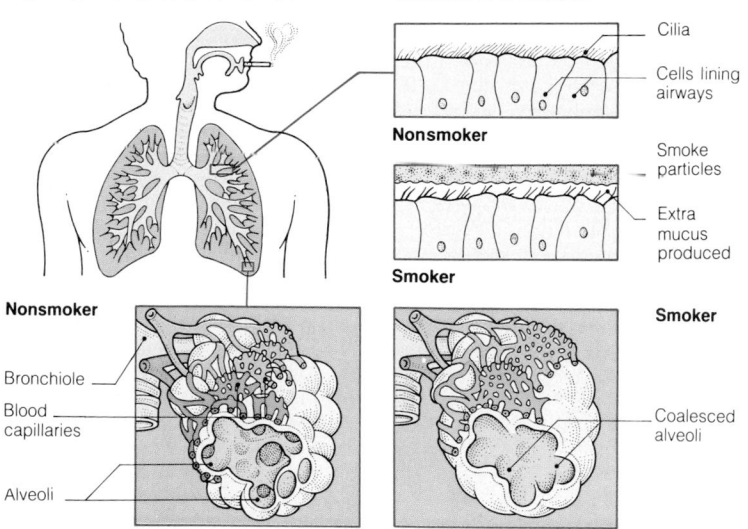

Nonsmoker

Smoker

Bronchiole
Blood capillaries
Alveoli

Smoker

Cilia
Cells lining airways
Smoke particles
Extra mucus produced
Coalesced alveoli

How smoking damages the lungs
Smoke particles irritate the lung airways, causing excess mucus production (top right). They also indirectly destroy the walls of the lungs' alveoli, which coalesce (above left and right). Both factors reduce lung efficiency. In addition, tar in tobacco smoke has a direct cancer-causing action.

SMOKERS AS A PROPORTION OF US ADULT POPULATION

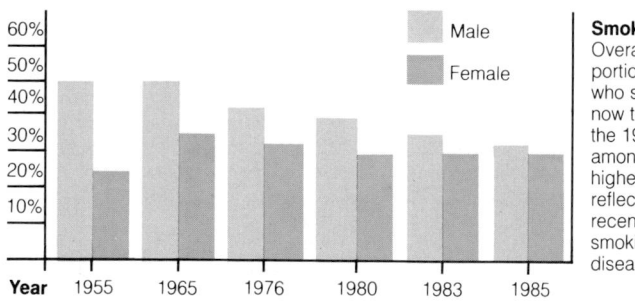

Smoking trends
Overall, the proportion of people who smoke is less now than it was in the 1950s, but among women it is higher. This is reflected in a recent rise in smoking-related disease in women.

SMOKING-RELATED DEATHS BY SEX AND DISEASE IN US IN 1982

	Total	Male	Female
Cancer	139,000	103,000	36,000
Cardiovascular disease	123,000	84,000	39,000
COAD	52,000	35,000	17,000
Total deaths from smoking	314,000	222,000	92,000

Major killers
Most of the deaths result from coronary heart disease (a cardiovascular disease), lung cancer, and chronic obstructive airways disease, or COAD (i.e., chronic bronchitis and emphysema). Male smoking-related deaths far outnumber female deaths because, until recently, many more men than women smoked.

Tobramycin

An *antibiotic drug* used to treat *peritonitis, meningitis,* and severe infections of the lungs, skin, bones, and joints. It is given by injection, usually in combination with a *penicillin drug.* Tobramycin eye drops or ointments are sometimes used to treat *conjunctivitis* and *blepharitis* (inflammation of the eyelids).

High doses given by injection may cause kidney damage, deafness due to inner-ear damage, nausea, vomiting, and headache. Any preparation that contains tobramycin may cause rash and itching.

Tocainide

An *antiarrhythmic drug* that is used to prevent and treat certain ventricular arrhythmias (heart beat irregularities; see *Arrhythmia, cardiac*).

There is a high risk of adverse effects, including nausea, dizziness, tremor, loss of appetite, diarrhea, confusion, and hallucinations. Prolonged treatment may cause blood disorders, such as *thrombocytopenia*.

Tocography

An obstetric procedure for recording the muscular contractions of the uterus during *childbirth*. Tocography is performed in conjunction with *fetal heart monitoring* to assess the quality of labor by measuring the frequency of contractions.

Tocopherol

See *Vitamin E*.

Toe

One of the digits of the foot. Each toe has three phalanges (bones), except for the hallux (big toe), which has two. The phalanges join at hinge joints, which are moved by muscle tendons that flex (bend) or extend (straighten) the toe. A small artery, vein, and nerve run down each side of the toe. The entire structure is enclosed in skin with a nail at the top.

The main function of the toes is to maintain balance during walking. People without hands often learn to use their toes to perform tasks usually performed with the fingers.

DISORDERS
Congenital disorders include *polydactyly* (extra toes), missing toes, *syndactyly* (fused toes), or *webbing* (skin flaps between the toes).

Injuries to a toe are fairly common, particularly a bruise under the skin or a fracture. Inflammation of one or several toe joints, causing stiffness,

T

ANATOMY OF THE TOES

Each hallux, or big toe, has two bones called phalanges, which are connected by hinge joints. All the other toes have three phalanges.

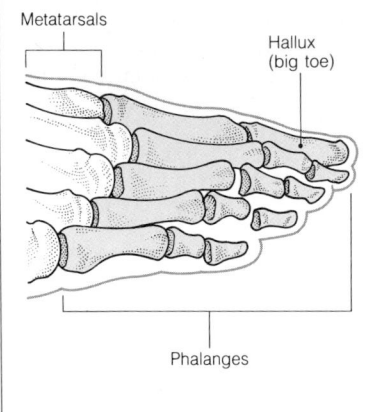

Metatarsals

Hallux (big toe)

Phalanges

pain, swelling, and deformity, may be caused by *osteoarthritis* or *rheumatoid arthritis* as well as other forms of arthritis (e.g., gout).

Infections occur under the nail as a complication of an *ingrown toenail*.

Impaired blood supply, usually due to *peripheral vascular disease* (narrowing of arteries in the legs), causes pain and blueness of the toes and can eventually lead to *gangrene*. Numbness and a pins and needles sensation in the toes may be caused by damage to peripheral nerves, which is common in *diabetes mellitus*.

A common deformity of the big toe is *hallux valgus*, in which the joint at the base projects outward and the top of the toe turns inward. The condition often results in a *bunion* (a firm, fluid-filled swelling over the joint). Abnormality of a tendon in one of the toes may cause the main joint to bend upward (see *Hammer toe*).

Toenail, ingrown

See *Ingrown toenail*.

Toilet-training

The process of teaching a young child to acquire complete bowel and bladder control and make appropriate use of toilet facilities.

WHEN TO START

There is no reason to start toilet-training until the child's nervous system is sufficiently mature. Up to the age of about 18 months, emptying of the bladder and bowel is a totally automatic reaction. The child is not yet able to connect the actions of defecation and urination with their results, and does not have the ability to control these actions at will.

At around 18 months, a child is able to indicate that he or she has passed urine or a bowel movement, but is not yet aware that he or she is about to do so. At this stage, the child is not quite ready to use the potty, but he or she should become familiar with it, be told what it is for, and practice sitting on it. Around the second birthday, the child becomes aware that he or she is about to pass urine or a bowel movement, and says so. At this stage, the child is ready to start using the potty.

USING THE POTTY AND TOILET

Toilet-training should be approached in a relaxed, unhurried manner. The child may rebel if the potty is introduced too early or if he or she is forced to sit on it. Boys initially urinate sitting on the potty but soon learn to urinate standing up.

When the child has gained proficiency using the potty, he or she should be introduced to the toilet. A useful intermediate step is to place the potty near the toilet. The child continues to use the potty for a while, but is taught to wipe with toilet paper and to flush the toilet. When reasonable control has been achieved, the child can be taken out of diapers during the day. However, diapers should continue to be worn at night until the child awakens dry most mornings.

Children vary in the age at which they become toilet-trained and more so in the age at which they are dry both by day and night. A child is unlikely to be completely toilet-trained or be able to empty the bladder on demand before the third birthday. Accidents are common up to age 5, particularly wetting, because a young child can hold on for only several minutes after the urge to urinate starts. Also, children who are toilet-trained may revert to soiling or wetting when anxious or under stress. (See also *Encopresis; Enuresis; Soiling*.)

Tolazamide

An oral hypoglycemic drug (see *Hypoglycemics, oral*) used to treat non-insulin-dependent *diabetes mellitus*. Tolazamide has a mild diuretic action and is therefore useful in treating people with diabetes who have a tendency to retain water.

Tolbutamide

An oral hypoglycemic drug (see *Hypoglycemics, oral*).

Tolerance

The need to take increasingly higher doses of a *drug* to continue producing the same physical or mental effect. Tolerance develops as the result of taking a drug over a period of time and is usually caused either by the liver becoming more efficient at breaking down the drug or by the body tissues becoming less sensitive to it. The most familiar example of tolerance occurs in heavy drinkers who become so tolerant of *alcohol* that they are capable of drinking amounts that would render occasional drinkers unconscious. (See also *Alcohol dependence; Drug dependence*.)

Tolmetin

A *nonsteroidal anti-inflammatory drug* (NSAID) used to relieve pain, stiffness, and inflammation in *osteoarthritis, rheumatoid arthritis,* and *ankylosing spondylitis*. Tolmetin is also given to treat pain caused by minor injuries, such as a ligament *sprain*.

Tolnaftate

An *antifungal drug* used to treat and sometimes prevent the recurrence of types of *tinea*, including *athlete's foot*. Tolnaftate, which is available over-the-counter as a cream, powder, or aerosol, may in rare cases cause skin irritation or rash.

Tomography

An *X-ray* technique that produces a cross-sectional image ("slice") of an organ or part of the body. In tomography, the X-ray camera and film are positioned so that tissue is in focus at one depth only. All background and foreground structures appear blurred.

By taking a series of tomograms it is possible to build an outline image of a part of the body that, on an ordinary X-ray film, would be hidden by other structures. For example, tomography is often used during intravenous *pyelography* to obtain a clear outline of the kidneys (when they would otherwise be obscured by gas or fecal matter in the intestines).

Most tomography today is performed using computerized techniques (see *CT scanning*), which produce extremely accurate, highly detailed pictures.

-tomy

A suffix denoting the operation of cutting or making an incision, as in thoracotomy, a surgical operation in which the thorax (chest) is opened.

T

Tone, muscle

The natural tension in the fibers of a muscle. At rest, all muscle fibers are maintained in a state of partial contraction by nerve impulses from the spinal cord. This resting muscle tone helps control posture, keeps the eyes open, and allows muscles to contract more efficiently.

Abnormally high muscle tone causes *spasticity*, rigidity, and an increased resistance to movement. Abnormally low muscle tone causes floppiness of the body part.

Tongue

A muscular, flexible organ that occupies the floor of the mouth.

STRUCTURE AND FUNCTION

The tongue is composed of a mass of muscles covered by mucous membrane. These muscles are attached to the mandible (lower jaw) and to the hyoid bone above the larynx. Minute nodules called papillae project from the upper surface of the tongue, giving it a rough texture. Situated between the papillae at the sides and base of the tongue are minute sensory organs called taste buds, which are responsible for the sense of *taste*.

Apart from being an organ of taste, the tongue is essential for breaking down food (see *Mastication*), *swallowing*, and *speech*.

ANATOMY OF THE TONGUE

The tongue consists mainly of muscle; on its surface, it has various types of papillae that contain the taste buds.

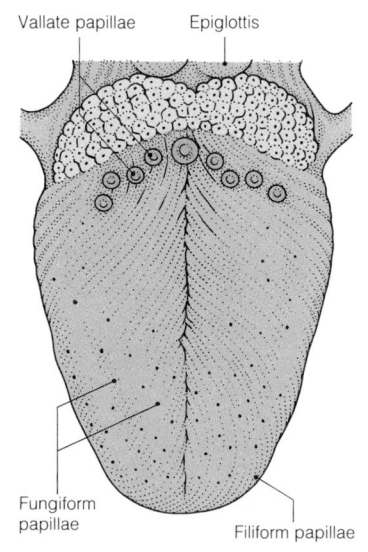

Vallate papillae   Epiglottis

Fungiform papillae

Filiform papillae

DISORDERS

A large tongue is a feature of *Down's syndrome, cretinism*, and *acromegaly*. Temporary swelling occurs in *glossitis*.

Fissures on the tongue are common and usually cause no trouble, but in some cases they are so deep that food particles collect in them, causing discomfort. Unnatural smoothness of the tongue, accompanied by redness and soreness, is a feature of pernicious anemia (See *Anemia, megaloblastic*), iron-deficiency anemia (see *Anemia, iron-deficiency*), *syphilis*, and *glossitis*.

In rare cases, the papillae on the tongue become elongated and turn black or brown, a condition known as black tongue. The disorder, of which the cause is unknown, is harmless but persistent. The unsightly discoloration can be removed by cleaning the tongue twice a day with a toothbrush dipped in an antiseptic mouthwash.

The tongue can be a site for *mouth ulcers* and *leukoplakia* (thickened white or gray patches), a condition that occasionally becomes cancerous (see *Tongue cancer*). Any ulcer or lump on the tongue that does not disappear within about three weeks should be reported to a physician because of the risk of cancer.

Tongue cancer

The most serious type of *mouth cancer* because of its rapid spread. Tongue cancer is one of the two most common types of mouth cancer (the other being *lip cancer*). It primarily affects people over 40. It is usually associated with tobacco smoking and heavy consumption of alcohol; poor oral hygiene is a contributing factor.

SYMPTOMS AND SIGNS

The edge of the tongue is most commonly affected. The first sign may be a small ulcer with a raised margin, a white patch of thickened tissue known as *leukoplakia*, a deep fissure with hard edges, or a raised, hardened mass. Pain is rare until the cancer is advanced, when there is also excessive salivation, stiffness of the tongue, difficulty swallowing, and sometimes offensive breath.

The tumor may become very large, obstructing the throat and occasionally causing asphyxia. It spreads rapidly, to any or all of the following: the gums, the lower jaw, and the lymph nodes in the floor of the mouth and the neck.

DIAGNOSIS AND TREATMENT

Any physical change in the tongue that does not clear up within two or three weeks should be reported to a

Appearance of tongue cancer
The cancer often starts at the edge of the tongue. It may appear (as here) as a raised mass or as a fissure or an ulcer.

physician. Cancer is diagnosed by means of a tongue *biopsy* (removal of a small sample of tissue for microscopic examination).

Small tumors, especially those at the tip of the tongue, are usually removed surgically. Larger tumors or tumors that have spread often require *radiation therapy*. If a tumor is very large and has spread to lymph nodes, the whole tongue, the lymph nodes, and sometimes the lower jaw must be removed. The disease may also be treated with *anticancer drugs*.

OUTLOOK

Unless the cancer is detected very early, its spread makes the outlook poor. In about half of all sufferers, the lymph nodes are involved by the time of diagnosis. About half of affected women but only a quarter of men survive for five years or more.

Tongue depressor

A flat wooden or metal instrument for holding down the tongue against the floor of the mouth to allow examination of the back of the throat.

Tongue-tie

A minor defect of the mouth, also called ankyloglossia, in which the frenulum (band of tissue attaching the underside of the tongue to the floor of the mouth) is too short and extends forward to the tip of the tongue. There are usually no symptoms other than limited movement of the tongue. In rare cases, the condition causes a speech defect, in which case a minor operation is required to divide the frenulum.

Tonic

One of a diverse group of remedies intended to relieve symptoms such as malaise, lethargy, and loss of appetite. Most tonics contain herbal extracts,

T

vitamins, and minerals. Medical evidence suggests that tonics mainly have a *placebo* effect.

Tonometry

The procedure for measuring the pressure of the fluid within the eye. A rise in intraocular pressure is one of the signs of *glaucoma*. Tonometry is usually performed by an *ophthalmologist* during an eye examination.

HOW IT IS DONE

One method of measuring the pressure in the eye is called applanation tonometry. The ophthalmologist applies a drop of quick-acting anesthetic and a trace of *fluorescein* to each cornea; he or she then measures the pressure within the eye by means of a tonometer (measuring device) mounted on a *slit lamp* (light source with a magnifying viewer). The head of the tonometer is illuminated and touched gently against the anesthetized cornea. A visible circle of fluorescein-stained tear film is formed, which the ophthalmologist views through the slit-lamp microscope. The force with which the tonometer head is pressed against the cornea is gradually increased until the area of the circle reaches a fixed standard. The force needed to achieve this degree of corneal flattening, which is read off from a calibrated knob on the tonometer, is a measure of the pressure within the eye. (See also *Eye, examination of.*)

Tonsil

A pair of oval masses at the back of the throat. The tonsils are made up of lymphoid tissue and form part of the *lymphatic system*, which is an important part of the body's defense against infection. Along with the adenoids at the base of the tongue, the tonsils protect against upper respiratory tract infections. The tonsils gradually enlarge from birth, reach their maximum size at about age 7, and then shrink substantially.

Tonsillitis (inflammation of the tonsils) is a common childhood infection. Rarely, *quinsy* (an abscess on the tonsil) may develop as a complication.

Tonsillectomy

Surgical removal of the tonsils.

WHY IT IS DONE

Tonsillectomy was once a common childhood operation; it is now performed only if a child suffers frequent recurrent attacks of severe *tonsillitis*. Less common problems that may necessitate the operation are *quinsy*

LOCATION OF THE TONSILS
The tonsils can be easily seen on either side of the back of the throat. They reach maximum size around the age of 7 years and then shrink.

Nasal cavity — Adenoid

Tongue — Trachea
Tonsil

(an abscess on the tonsil) or a single tonsil considered malignant because it is growing larger or is deeply ulcerated. In rare cases, removal of the tonsils may be advised for adolescents or young adults suffering from recurrent bouts of tonsillitis.

HOW IT IS DONE

The operative technique is shown in the illustration at right.

RECOVERY PERIOD

In the first 24 hours after the operation there may be bleeding from the throat; the patient must lie on his or her side to avoid choking. Postoperative pain in the throat and sometimes the ears is common and may require an analgesic (painkiller). Fluids and soft, easily digestible foods such as ice cream are usually given for a day or two until the patient can eat normally.

Sore throat, particularly at mealtimes, may persist for up to two weeks after the operation. Full recovery usually takes place within three weeks. In some people, late bleeding occurs, requiring examination.

Tonsillitis

Inflammation of the tonsils due to infection. Tonsillitis mainly occurs in childhood, with most children suffering at least one attack.

CAUSES AND INCIDENCE

The function of the tonsils is to help protect the upper respiratory tract against infection. However, some-

times the tonsils themselves become repeatedly infected by the microorganisms they fight. Tonsillitis is most common in children under 9; it infrequently occurs in adolescents and young adults.

SYMPTOMS AND SIGNS

The main symptoms are a sore throat and difficulty swallowing (very young children may refuse to eat). The throat is visibly inflamed. Other common symptoms are fever, headache, earache, enlarged and tender glands in the neck, and unpleasant-smelling breath. Occasionally, the illness causes temporary deafness or *quinsy* (an abscess on the tonsil). If symptoms persist for more than 24 hours or if pus can be seen on the tonsils, a physician should be consulted.

TREATMENT

The illness is treated with bed rest, plenty of fluids, and an *analgesic drug* (painkiller), such as acetaminophen. In some cases, *antibiotic drugs* may also be prescribed.

Tooth abscess

See *Abscess, dental.*

Toothache

Pain coming from one tooth, or from the teeth and gums generally. The pain may be felt either as a dull throb or a sharp twinge.

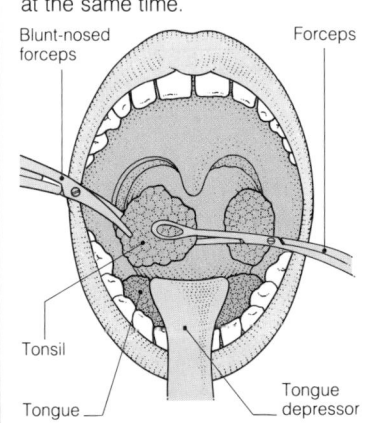

PROCEDURE FOR TONSILLECTOMY
Tonsillectomy is most commonly carried out around the age of 6 or 7. The adenoids may be removed at the same time.

Blunt-nosed forceps — Forceps

Tonsil

Tongue — Tongue depressor

Standard technique
With the patient under a general anesthetic, the tongue is depressed and the tonsils pried from the back of the throat and then cut away.

CAUSES

Early dental *caries* (decay) may cause mild toothache when eating sweet or very hot or cold food. More advanced decay or, less commonly, a fracture in a tooth (see *Fracture, dental*) or a deep, unlined filling (see *Filling, dental*) may result in inflammation of the pulp. This usually causes sharp, stabbing pain, which is often worse when lying down. It is often difficult for the sufferer to locate the painful tooth.

If the inflammation spreads, periapical *periodontitis* (inflammation of supporting tissues around the root tip) may develop, causing localized pain that is brought on mainly by biting and chewing. A dental abscess (see *Abscess, dental*) may also occur. In this case, pain is severe and often continuous, the gum surrounding the affected tooth is tender and swollen, and there may be swelling of the face and neck accompanied by fever.

Chronic periodontitis (inflammation of all the supporting tissues), which causes the gums to recede, results in aching around exposed tooth roots when hot, cold, or sweet food is eaten. Gums around the affected teeth are tender and swollen.

A filling that is not quite level or a blow to a tooth may also result in inflammation of supporting tissues, causing pain when biting.

Sometimes toothache is not caused by a disorder of the teeth or gums. For example, in *sinusitis* (inflammation of the mucous membrane lining the facial air cavities) pain may be referred to the upper molar and premolar teeth (see *Referred pain*).

TREATMENT

Analgesic drugs (painkillers) may provide temporary relief until a visit to the dentist can be arranged. An emergency appointment should be made if the symptoms suggest there is an abscess. The treatment carried out by the dentist depends on the underlying cause.

Toothbrushing

Cleaning of the teeth with a special type of brush to remove plaque and food particles from tooth surfaces. Toothbrushing should be carried out at least once a day using a fluoride *dentifrice* (usually toothpaste); children should brush their teeth after every meal and at bedtime. For complete *oral hygiene*, flossing (see *Floss, dental*) should be performed daily.

A safe and effective toothbrush for general use has an easily gripped handle and soft, round-ended or

---

BASIC TOOTHBRUSHING

Efficient toothbrushing is essential for the preservation of the teeth and the health of the gums. The enemy is plaque, a mixture of food debris, dried saliva, and bacteria, which develops at the gum margins and leads to caries (tooth decay) and gum disease.

1 With the bristle tips set at 45 degrees to the plane of the teeth, scrub gently along the gum line using ¼-inch strokes. The bristle tips should do the work.

2 Keep the bristles angled against the line of the gums and work over the outer and inner surfaces of the upper and lower teeth. Keep the strokes short.

3 Don't forget to scrub over the chewing surfaces of all four sets of premolar and molar teeth. Move slowly over the surfaces, cleaning each tooth in turn.

4 Remember to brush the inside surfaces of the front teeth. Hold the brush almost vertical and scrub with an up-and-down movement.

---

polished bristles. The size and shape must allow every tooth to be reached; children need a smaller toothbrush than adults. Toothbrushes should be rinsed after each use and replaced when the bristles become frayed or bent. Interspace brushes, which have small, round heads, may be useful for cleaning around *bridges* and fixed *orthodontic appliances*. Electric toothbrushes are also available and may make brushing easier for people with some physical disabilities.

Tooth decay

See *Caries, dental*.

Tooth extraction

See *Extraction, dental*.

Toothpaste

See *Dentifrice*.

Tophus

A collection of *uric acid* crystals deposited in the tissues, especially around joints (such as the elbow) but occasionally in other places (such as the ear). A tophus is a sign of *hyperuricemia*, which accompanies *gout*. Tophi may occasionally ulcerate and discharge chalky white material.

Topical

A term describing a *drug* that is applied to the surface of the body, as opposed to being swallowed or injected. Topical refers not only to drugs applied to the skin, but also to those administered into the ear canal, onto the surface of the eye, or as suppositories into the vagina or rectum.

Torsion

A term that means twisting. Almost any structure that is relatively free to move in the body may become twisted, such as the intestine (see *Volvulus*), the spermatic cord from the testis (see *Testis, torsion of*), or a cyst on a stalk. One of the principal dangers of torsion is obstruction of the blood supply to the affected part; if this occurs, pain is usually the first symptom. If the torsion is not corrected, tissue death may develop.

T

Torticollis

Twisting of the neck, causing the head to be rotated and tilted into an abnormal position. Also known as wry neck, torticollis is often accompanied by pain and stiffness in the neck.

Child with torticollis
The muscles on one side of the neck have gone into spasm, pulling the head over to that side and causing pain.

CAUSES
The condition usually results from a minor neck injury that causes irritation of cervical nerves and consequent spasm of neck muscles. Torticollis may also result from muscle spasm caused by sleeping in an awkward position or by anxiety. Injury to a neck muscle at birth can also cause torticollis, as can a burn or other injury that has resulted in heavy scarring and shrinkage of the skin.

TREATMENT
Treatment for torticollis due to muscle spasm may include wearing an orthopedic *collar, heat treatment, ultrasound treatment,* or *physical therapy.* When the cause is birth injury, the muscle is gently stretched several times each day; occasionally, an operation is required to cut the lower end of the muscle. Skin contracture may be treated by *Z-plasty,* which relieves tension in the scar tissue.

Touch

The sense by which certain characteristics of objects, such as their size, shape, temperature, and surface texture, can be ascertained through physical contact.

Many types of touch receptors are present in the skin. In hairy skin areas, some of the receptors consist of webs of sensory nerve cell endings wrapped around the hair bulbs. They are triggered if the hairs are moved. Other receptors are more common in nonhairy areas, such as lips and fingertips, and consist of nerve cell endings that may be free (i.e., naked) or surrounded by bulblike structures.

Signals from touch receptors pass, via sensory nerves, to the spinal cord, from there to the thalamus in the brain, and on to the *sensory cortex,* where touch sensations are perceived.

According to the number and distribution of receptors, different parts of the body vary in their sensitivity to painful stimuli and in touch discrimination (the ability to distinguish between a single pinprick and two pinpricks placed slightly apart). For example, the cornea is several hundred times more sensitive to painful stimuli than are the soles of the feet. The fingertips are good at touch discrimination but relatively insensitive to painful stimuli.

Touch sense becomes much more developed in people deprived of other senses, particularly blind people; it is this capacity for touch development that is used by systems such as braille. (See also *Sensation.*)

Tourette's syndrome

See *Gilles de la Tourette's syndrome.*

Tourniquet

A device placed around a limb to compress blood vessels. A tourniquet may be used to help locate a vein for an intravenous injection or withdrawal of blood. By preventing blood from flowing back to the heart, a tourniquet causes veins in the limb below it to swell and become more prominent.

An inflatable tourniquet, called *Esmarch's bandage,* is used to control blood flow in some limb operations. An inflatable tourniquet also forms part of a *sphygmomanometer,* an instrument for measuring *blood pressure.*

Tourniquets have caused more problems than they have solved. In the past, they were used as a first-aid measure to stop severe bleeding. This use is now discouraged because leaving a tourniquet in place for too long can cause *gangrene* (tissue death). First-aid courses now teach the control of bleeding by pressure over the bleeding site (see *Pressure points*). It is usually effective and safer.

Toxemia

The presence in the bloodstream of toxins (poisons) produced by bacteria. Toxemia may be a feature of *septicemia* (the spread and multiplication of bacteria within the bloodstream from a localized site of infection), but it can also occur without any evidence of bacteria in the blood. Toxemia with or without septicemia is sometimes called blood poisoning.

Toxemia may cause symptoms such as a fever and headache and other symptoms specific to the particular toxin (e.g., muscle spasms caused by the toxin released by *tetanus* bacteria). Toxemia can lead to the highly dangerous condition of *septic shock,* in which there is widespread tissue damage and a drop in blood pressure.

Treatment of toxemia is as for septicemia and septic shock—*antibiotic drugs,* removal of a localized site of infection if one can be found, and measures to treat shock, including *intravenous infusions.* For some types of toxemia, an *antitoxin* may be given.

Toxemia of pregnancy, or *preeclampsia,* has some features common to other forms of toxemia, but no toxin has ever been identified. (See also *Toxic shock syndrome.*)

Toxemia of pregnancy

A disorder of pregnant women characterized by raised blood pressure, tissue swelling, and leakage of protein from the kidneys into the urine (see *Preeclampsia*). If severe, toxemia of pregnancy may progress to seizures and coma (see *Eclampsia*).

Toxicity

The property of being poisonous. The term is also used to refer to the severity of adverse effects or illness produced by a *toxin* (a poisonous protein produced by certain bacteria, animals, or plants), by a *poison,* or by a drug overdose (see *Drug poisoning*).

Toxicology

The study of *poisons,* including their chemical composition, preparation, identification, effects on the body, and antidotes. (See also *Poisoning.*)

Toxic shock syndrome

An uncommon condition linked with the use of certain brands of highly absorbent tampons. Toxic shock syndrome was first recognized in the late 1970s and many cases were diagnosed in young women in the early 1980s. About 70 percent of cases occur in women who are using tampons at the time of onset.

CAUSE
Toxic shock syndrome is caused by a *toxin* produced by the bacterium STAPHYLOCOCCUS AUREUS. Overgrowth of this bacterium in the vagina and increased production of the toxin have been associated with prolonged use of certain brands of highly absorbent tampons (now taken off the market).

THE SENSE OF TOUCH

The skin contains many thousands of specialized cells that respond to external stimuli, such as touch, heat, cold, and pressure. These cells (receptors) are divided into two types. One type of receptor consists only of a thin nerve fiber, which may wrap around an individual hair and respond to its movement. The other type has a specialized structure, known as an end organ, surrounding the nerve ending. Some skin receptors consist of several layers of cells attached to one nerve fiber. Others contain several nerve fibers arranged in a loop or coil. Probably several varieties of receptors play a part in each touch modality.

Merkel's disk

Meissner's corpuscle

Dermis

Free nerve endings

Epidermis

Organ of Ruffini

Pacinian corpuscle

Skin receptors

These receptors vary from free nerve endings to corpuscular or bulblike structures. Individual receptors do not seem to be associated exclusively with any one sensation (e.g., cold or pain).

Delicate touch
The ability to detect light contact between an object and the skin. Areas with more receptors are more sensitive.

Pain
Pain warns the brain about possible injury from an external stimulus and can trigger a reflex withdrawal.

Heat
Some free nerve endings respond specifically to heat. The skin of the wrist is good for testing temperature.

Cold
Cold on the skin is detected by specialized end organs. Extreme cold also stimulates pain receptors.

Pressure
A change in pressure on the skin is detected by specialized end organs called pacinian corpuscles.

TOUCH PERCEPTION

General sensations from various parts of the body are perceived at specific points within the brain's cerebral cortex. Highly sensitive body parts, such as the lips and hands, are represented by correspondingly large regions within the cortex.

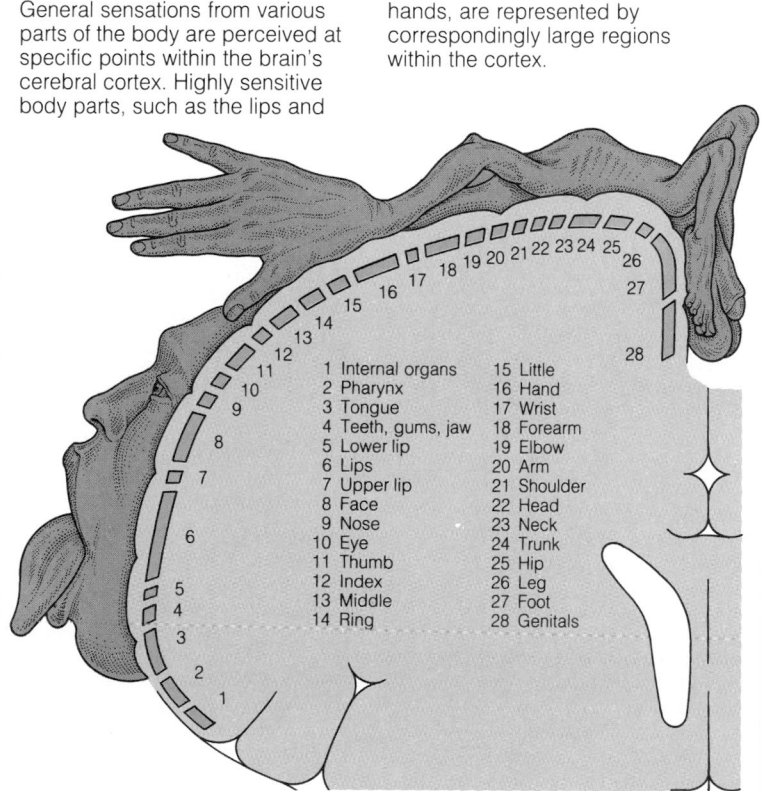

1 Internal organs	15 Little
2 Pharynx	16 Hand
3 Tongue	17 Wrist
4 Teeth, gums, jaw	18 Forearm
5 Lower lip	19 Elbow
6 Lips	20 Arm
7 Upper lip	21 Shoulder
8 Face	22 Head
9 Nose	23 Neck
10 Eye	24 Trunk
11 Thumb	25 Hip
12 Index	26 Leg
13 Middle	27 Foot
14 Ring	28 Genitals

T

Pacinian corpuscle
These receptors are 1 mm to 4 mm long and occur in nonhairy areas of skin, especially the fingers.

Of the cases that do not occur in association with menstruation, some have been linked to use of a contraceptive cap, diaphragm, or sponge. Other cases arise from skin wounds or infections caused by *S. AUREUS* elsewhere in the body.

SYMPTOMS

The onset of toxic shock syndrome is sudden, with high fever, vomiting, diarrhea, headache, muscular aches and pains, dizziness, and disorientation. A skin rash resembling sunburn develops on the palms and soles, and peels within one or two weeks. The blood pressure may fall dangerously low, and *shock* may develop. Other serious complications include *renal failure* and *liver failure*. The mortality is about 3 percent, usually due to a prolonged fall in blood pressure or to lung complications.

TREATMENT

Treatment is with *antibiotic drugs*. *Intravenous infusion* may be necessary to treat shock, and more treatment may be needed for complications.

Recurrence is common; women who have had toxic shock syndrome are advised not to use tampons, caps, diaphragms, or sponges.

Toxin

A poisonous protein produced by pathogenic (disease-causing) bacteria, such as *CLOSTRIDIUM TETANI*, which causes *tetanus*; various animals, notably venomous snakes (see *Snakebites*); or certain plants, such as the death cap mushroom *AMANITA PHALLOIDES* (see *Mushroom poisoning*).

Bacterial toxins are sometimes subdivided into *endotoxins*, which are released only from the inside of dead bacteria; *exotoxins*, which are released from the surface of live bacteria; and *enterotoxins*, which inflame the intestine. (See also *Poison; Poisoning*.)

Toxocariasis

An infestation of humans, usually children, with the larvae of *TOXOCARA CANIS*, a small, threadlike worm that lives in the intestines of dogs. The disease is also known as visceral larva migrans.

CAUSES AND INCIDENCE

The causes and course of an infestation are shown in the illustrated box above right.

PREVENTION

Dogs that live with children should be dewormed—monthly if they are less than 6 months old, when infestation is more likely.

ORIGINS OF TOXOCARIASIS

1 A dog (often a puppy) harboring the small roundworm *TOXOCARA CANIS* in its digestive tract passes large numbers of worm eggs in its feces, which may contaminate soil.

2 Children who play with an infested dog, or with soil contaminated with dog feces, and who then put their fingers in their mouths, may swallow some of the worm eggs.

3 The swallowed eggs hatch in the intestines to liberate larvae, which migrate through the tissues to organs such as the liver, lungs, brain, and eyes. They provoke allergic phenomena such as asthma and may have serious effects, such as loss of vision.

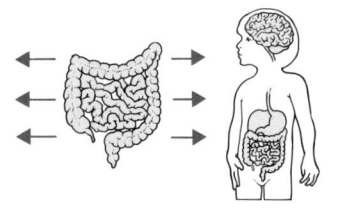

SYMPTOMS AND SIGNS

Usually, infestation causes only mild fever and malaise, which soon clears up. However, following some cases of heavy infestation, *pneumonia* and *seizures* may develop. Another possible complication is loss of vision caused by a larva entering the eye and dying there.

DIAGNOSIS AND TREATMENT

Toxocariasis is diagnosed from sputum (phlegm) analysis, and by a *liver biopsy* (removal of a small sample of the organ for analysis).

Severe cases of toxocariasis require treatment in the hospital, where the patient may be given the *antihelmintic drug* thiabendazole (to control the infestation) and an *anticonvulsant drug* (to control seizures).

Toxoid

An inactivated bacterial *toxin* (poisonous protein). Inactivation, usually by heat or chemicals, removes the toxicity of the toxin but preserves its property of stimulating antibody production by the *immune system*. Certain toxoids are used to immunize against specific diseases, such as *diphtheria* or *tetanus*.

Toxoplasmosis

An infection of mammals, birds, and reptiles that is also common in humans. Toxoplasmosis usually produces no ill effects except when transmitted by a woman to her unborn child or in people with an immunodeficiency disorder.

CAUSES AND INCIDENCE

The infection is caused by the protozoan (single-celled microorganism) *TOXOPLASMA GONDII*. Humans are most commonly infected by eating undercooked meat from infected animals. An estimated 25 percent of pork and 10 percent of lamb eaten by humans contains toxoplasma organisms. In addition, the protozoa multiply in the intestines of cats, and about 1 percent of cats excrete cysts containing toxoplasma eggs in the feces. Infection in humans can occur through failure to wash the hands after handling the cat or its feces.

Toxoplasmosis contracted by a woman during pregnancy is transmitted to the child in about one third of cases, often with severe effects.

Infection is extremely common worldwide. In some areas of the US, *blood tests* show that about half the population have been infected.

SYMPTOMS AND SIGNS

In most cases, the body's *immune system* provides adequate protection against the protozoa, so that the infection produces no symptoms. In some people with a normal immune system, however, the infection causes a feverish illness resembling infectious *mononucleosis*. It may also cause retinitis (inflammation of the retina) and *choroiditis* (inflammation of the blood vessels behind the retina).

Infection of an unborn child during early pregnancy may result in miscarriage or stillbirth. Infants may have enlargement of the liver and spleen, *hydrocephalus*, blindness, mental retardation, and may die during infancy. Infection in late pregnancy usually has no ill effects.

Toxoplasmosis may also take a severe course in people with an immune system deficiency (such as *AIDS*), causing lung and heart damage and severe *encephalitis* (brain inflammation).

DIAGNOSIS AND TREATMENT
The diagnosis is made from blood tests. Treatment is necessary only in pregnant women, in children born with severe symptoms, in people with an immune system deficiency, and in cases of retinitis or choroiditis. Treatment is usually with the antimalarial drug *pyrimethamine* combined with a *sulfonamide drug*.

TPA
The abbreviation for *tissue-plasminogen activator*.

Trabeculectomy
A surgical procedure performed to reduce pressure in the eye. Trabeculectomy is used to control *glaucoma* when medication cannot keep the intraocular pressure within safe limits or when, despite medical treatment, visual field loss and optic nerve damage are progressing.

The procedure provides an alternative outlet route from the eye for aqueous humor (eye fluid) so that a better balance is achieved between the rate of secretion of aqueous humor and its rate of outflow. In this way, the pressure can be kept within normal limits and further damage to the optic nerve fibers prevented.

HOW IT IS DONE
The *conjunctiva* (mucous membrane covering the front of the eyeball) above the upper edge of the *cornea* is opened and a half-thickness flap of *sclera* (white part of the eye) is cut and folded forward. A small block is removed from the inner half near the scleral-corneal junction so that a connection is made into the front chamber of the eye. The outer flap is replaced and secured with a few delicate stitches and the conjunctiva is closed over it.

Trace elements
A group of minerals that is required only in minute amounts in the diet to maintain health. The principal trace elements include *chromium, copper, selenium, sulfur,* and *zinc.* Although tiny amounts of these substances are needed, they are vital to numerous chemical processes in the body. (See also *Nutrition*.)

Tracer
A radioactive substance introduced into the body so that its distribution, processing, and elimination from the body can be followed (by using a radiation detector). Radioactive iodine may be used as a tracer to study the functioning of the thyroid gland.

Trachea
The anatomical name for the windpipe. The trachea begins immediately below the larynx (voice box) and runs down the center of the front of the neck to end behind the upper part of the sternum (breastbone), where it divides to form the two main bronchi.

The trachea consists of fibrous and elastic tissue and smooth muscle. It also contains about 20 rings of cartilage, which help keep the trachea open even during extremes of neck movement. The lining of the trachea includes cells that secrete mucus (called goblet cells) and other cells that bear minute, hairlike cilia. The mucus helps trap tiny particles in inhaled air; the beating of the cilia moves the mucus upward and out of the respiratory tract, thereby helping to keep the lungs and airways free.

DISORDERS
One of the most common disorders is *tracheitis* (inflammation of the lining of the trachea), which is usually caused by an infection (often by a virus) and is frequently associated with *bronchitis* or *laryngitis*. The principal symptoms are difficult, painful breathing and a harsh cough.

Obstruction of the trachea by an inhaled foreign object is rare because the narrowest part of the upper respiratory tract is the larynx, and any objects that pass through it usually continue through the trachea into a bronchus. However, the trachea may become obstructed by a tumor or narrowed as a result of scarring caused by the prolonged presence of a *tracheostomy* tube inserted to create an artificial airway through the front of the neck. Tracheal obstruction produces breathlessness and a loud, harsh, vibrating sound during breathing.

Rarely, a congenital malformation occurs in which a channel forms between the trachea and the esophagus, situated immediately behind it (a condition called a *tracheoesophageal fistula*).

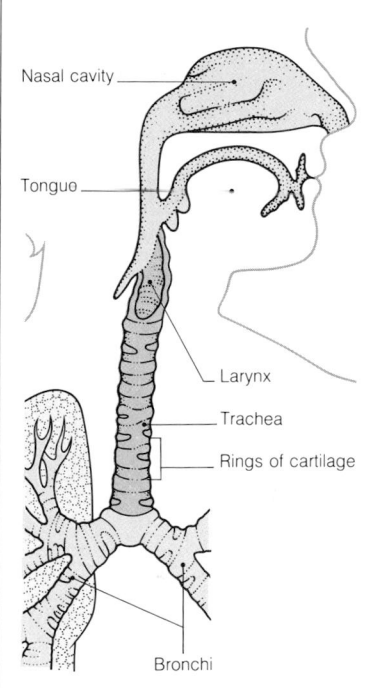

LOCATION OF THE TRACHEA
The trachea extends down from the larynx for 4.5 inches to the point where it divides into the two bronchi.

Nasal cavity

Tongue

Larynx

Trachea

Rings of cartilage

Bronchi

The trachea is sometimes injured by a direct blow or by strangulation. The seriousness of such an injury depends on the extent to which the airway is obstructed. In extreme cases, the trachea may collapse completely, which may be rapidly fatal unless an emergency tracheostomy is performed to reestablish an airway.

Tracheitis
Inflammation of the *trachea* (the windpipe). Tracheitis is usually caused by viral infection and aggravated by inhaled fumes, especially tobacco smoke. It often occurs with *laryngitis* and *bronchitis*, a condition known as laryngotracheobronchitis, which is the most common cause of *croup* in young children.

Typical symptoms of tracheitis include dry cough and hoarseness. In most cases, the condition is short-lived and requires no treatment.

Tracheoesophageal fistula
A rare *birth defect* in which there is an abnormal passage that connects the trachea (windpipe) and the

T

esophagus. About three babies per 10,000 are born with a tracheoesophageal fistula. In the most common form, the lower end of the esophagus connects with the trachea; the upper end is underdeveloped, forming a blind-ending pouch.

SYMPTOMS AND SIGNS

The affected baby cannot swallow saliva, and thus drools constantly. During feeding, food is regurgitated and enters the lungs, causing the baby to choke, cough, and sometimes turn blue because of lack of oxygen. The abdomen becomes distended because inhaled air passes into the stomach through the fistula. The acidic fluid in the stomach passes up into the lungs through the fistula, causing *pneumonia* and *atelectasis* (lung collapse).

DIAGNOSIS AND TREATMENT

In most cases the condition is discovered soon after birth. Milder forms of tracheoesophageal fistula may not be detected until childhood or even adult life, usually after recurrent attacks of pneumonia. The diagnosis is confirmed by *chest X ray*.

Treatment consists of an operation to close the fistula and connect the trachea and esophagus correctly. Before the 1940s, the condition was untreatable; today the survival rate is about 90 percent.

Tracheostomy

An operation in which an opening is made in the trachea (windpipe) and a tube is inserted to maintain an effective airway.

WHY IT IS DONE

Tracheostomy may be performed to treat an emergency or as a planned procedure. Today, acute airway problems are usually handled by an *endotracheal tube* passed via the mouth or nose. However, when the problem (such as a tumor or foreign body) involves the larynx, a tracheostomy is preferable in an emergency.

A planned tracheostomy is most frequently carried out on a person who has lost the ability to breathe naturally and is undergoing long-term *ventilation* (the pumping of air into the lungs by a machine) or who has lost the ability to keep oral and pharyngeal secretions out of the windpipe because of coma or a specific swallowing problem. For this purpose, tracheostomy is performed after passing an endotracheal tube through the nose or mouth and into the trachea. Permanent tracheostomy is necessary after *laryngectomy* (removal of the larynx).

Tracheostomy tube
The tube readily becomes blocked by bronchial secretions; it has a metal inner lining removable for cleaning.

HOW IT IS DONE

The operation is carried out using a local or a general anesthetic.

An incision is made in the skin overlying the trachea, between the Adam's apple and the clavicles (collarbones), the neck muscles are pulled apart, and the thyroid gland, which surrounds the trachea, is usually severed. A small vertical incision (called a "window") is made in the trachea and, in the case of laryngectomy, the cut edges of the trachea are brought forward and stitched to the edges of the skin wound. A metal or plastic tube is then inserted. If the patient cannot breathe unaided, the tube is connected to a ventilator.

RECOVERY PERIOD

For patients able to breathe unaided, the air in the room is humidified to reduce drying of mucus in the airway. Air from a ventilator is humidified before it passes into the tube. Any excessive mucus that accumulates in the airway is sucked away through a catheter inserted into the tube.

While the tube is in place, the patient is usually unable to speak; he or she is provided with a bell or buzzer and pen and paper for communication. After laryngectomy, the tube is removed after several days; a permanent opening remains. In other cases, the tube is removed when the patient has recovered from the condition that necessitated the operation, and the opening soon closes and heals.

Tracheotomy

Cutting of an airway into the trachea. (See also *Tracheostomy*.)

Trachoma

A persistent infectious disease of the *conjunctiva* and *cornea*. Trachoma is caused by an organism, CHLAMYDIA TRACHOMATIS, that is spread by direct contact and possibly by flies (see *Chlamydial infections*). Untreated trachoma leads to complications that may cause blindness.

SYMPTOMS AND SIGNS

Infection by C. TRACHOMATIS causes acute *conjunctivitis*, with pain, *photophobia*, and watering of the eyes. The eyes become red and inflamed and the conjunctiva that lines the lids becomes thickened and roughened with scar tissue and is studded with small lumps called follicles. Damage to the mucus-secreting cells of the conjunctiva and to the lacrimal (tear-producing) glands may lead to *keratoconjunctivitis sicca* (dry eye).

An abnormal growth of blood vessels can extend down from the conjunctiva into the upper part of the cornea, leading to opacity (loss of transparency) and loss of vision. More severe damage to the cornea occurs later when fibrous scarring of the inside of the upper lid causes it to be rolled inward so that the lashes rub against the cornea, causing ulceration and encouraging secondary bacterial infection. The secondary bacterial infection may lead to extensive ulceration, scarring, and even perforation, with spread of infection into the eye and permanent loss of vision.

TREATMENT

Trachoma is treated in the early stages to attempt to eradicate the causative organism, which is sensitive to various *antibiotic drugs* applied to the eye. Antibiotic drugs taken by mouth are also used. Established trachoma with scarring is much more difficult to manage; treatment may involve surgical correction of lid deformities and corneal grafting to restore transparency and vision.

Tract

A group of organs that forms a common pathway to perform a particular function. For example, the urinary tract comprises the kidneys, ureters, bladder, and urethra, which together form a series of connected structures for the removal of waste products from the body.

The term tract also refers specifically to a bundle of nerve fibers that have a common function, as in the pyramidal tract, which carries nerve impulses from the brain to the muscles.

Traction

A procedure in which part of the body is placed under tension to correct the alignment of two adjoining structures or to hold them in position.

T

TRACTION FOR FEMORAL FRACTURE

Because of the power of the thigh muscles and their tendency to go into spasm, fractures of the femur (thigh bone) tend to override.

Without traction to prevent this, the bone would heal with overlapping ends and the leg would be permanently shortened.

Procedure

Traction is usually performed by means of a narrow steel rod through the upper end of the tibia (shin), to which a steel stirrup is attached so that a cord and weight can

be used to apply the force. The other end of the femur must usually be immobilized, or countertraction applied, to keep the fractured bone ends aligned.

WHY IT IS DONE

The most common use of traction is in the treatment of a *fracture* in which muscles around the bone ends are pulling the bones out of alignment. Fractures of the shaft of the *femur* (thigh bone) are most likely to be treated in this way. Traction is also used to align and immobilize unstable fractures of the cervical spine (the neck) when any movement of the vertebrae might injure the spinal cord (see *Spinal injury*).

HOW IT IS DONE

To apply traction to a lower limb fracture, the person lies on a bed with the injured limb supported by attachments from an overhead frame. The upper end of the fractured bone is held immobilized while the lower end is pulled in a straight line away from it by a system of weights and pulleys. The traction grip is obtained by a pin inserted through the tibia (shin) or through a plaster cast applied to the limb. For spinal fractures, the patient lies flat on a firm surface and weights are attached to tongs inserted into holes drilled on either side of the skull. Both limb and spinal fractures are maintained in continuous traction until healing has occurred.

Training

A program of *exercises* to prepare for a particular sport and improve technique. Training may be concentrated on improving skills (e.g., a golfer may practice putting) or on improving physical *fitness*.

Fitness training should include both *aerobic* and anaerobic exercises, which together build strength, flexibility, and endurance (the capacity to exercise for long periods).

Interval training is a type of fitness program in which a particular exercise, such as running a set distance at a timed pace, is repeated several times with a rest period between. Circuit training consists of performing a set number of different exercises, such as push-ups, sit-ups, and step-ups, one after the other.

The selection of an appropriate training program requires specialized assessment and advice. Self-imposed training schedules may be damaging to health; for example, bone and muscle disorders may develop in runners if their training is unsupervised.

Trait

Any characteristic or condition determined by a *gene* or genes (i.e., inherited). Blue or brown eye color, dark or light skin, body proportions, and nose shape are all traits, reflecting the genetic variation among people.

The majority of common traits (such as eye color) have no obvious effect on health; others may have marginally advantageous effects in particular environments (such as dark skin in a sunny climate) or mildly disabling effects (such as color-vision deficiency). Severely handicapping traits, such as *cystic fibrosis* or *osteogenesis imperfecta,* are individually rare, but the fact that there are many different types means that they are collectively quite common (see *Genetic disorders*).

The term trait is also sometimes used in a more restricted sense to describe a mild form of a recessive genetic disorder. For example, a person who inherits the sickle cell gene in a single dose is said to have sickle cell trait. A double dose of the same gene causes the much more serious *sickle cell anemia.*

Trance

A sleeplike state in which consciousness is reduced, voluntary actions are lessened or absent, and bodily functions are diminished. A trance usually results from separation of a group of mental processes from the rest of the mind rather than from any physical brain disturbance.

Trances are claimed to be induced by *hypnosis* and have been reported as part of a group experience, particularly in a religious context. Trances are sometimes a feature of *catalepsy, automatism,* and some forms of petitmal *epilepsy*.

Tranquilizer drugs

Drugs with a sedative effect, subdivided into major tranquilizers (see *Antipsychotic drugs*) and minor tranquilizers (see *Antianxiety drugs*).

Transcutaneous electrical nerve stimulation

A method of pain relief achieved by the application of minute electrical impulses to nerve endings that lie beneath the skin. Transcutaneous electrical nerve stimulation (TENS) seems to work by blocking pain messages to the brain by providing an alternative stimulus. TENS is carried out to relieve severe and persistent pain when it is not satisfactorily controlled by *analgesic drugs*.

HOW IT IS DONE

A TENS unit provides electrical impulses to electrodes that are placed on the skin or sometimes surgically implanted. Adjustments of the unit can be made by the patient to achieve maximal relief.

RISKS

TENS must not be used by anyone with a cardiac pacemaker; the electrical impulses from the transmitter may interfere with the pacemaker's action.

T

TENS is beneficial in about 60 percent of the patients who use it. Pain relief in some people lasts only during stimulation; in others, pain relief persists after treatment.

Transference

The unconscious displacement of emotions from important childhood figures, such as parents or siblings, to people in adult life. Transference is particularly important in *psychoanalysis*, in which the feelings the patient has toward the analyst are explored to show how such projected feelings affect other relationships.

Transfusion

See *Blood transfusion*.

Transfusion, autologous

The use of a person's own blood, donated on an earlier occasion, for *blood transfusion* during surgery. Autologous transfusion is used to avoid the risk that blood from another donor may transmit infection.

Autologous transfusions were first performed on a large scale in the early 1960s for certain major operations, and services continued to develop to some extent during the 1970s. Fear of *AIDS* during the 1980s created a demand for much greater availability and use of this technique.

WHY IT IS DONE
Autologous transfusion eliminates the slight but serious risk of infecting a recipient with HIV (the AIDS virus) or *hepatitis* virus from contaminated blood. It also eliminates the risk of transmitting *cytomegalovirus*, *malaria*, and *syphilis*.

Another advantage of autologous transfusion is the reduced risk of a transfusion reaction occurring as a result of incompatibility between donor and recipient blood.

Autologous transfusion has been used illegally by people associated with professional sports. Carried out just before a sporting event, "blood doping" increases the oxygen-carrying capacity of the circulation and thus improves stamina.

HOW IT IS DONE
Blood can be withdrawn (in the same way as for *blood donation*) in several sessions at least four days apart and up to three days before surgery is planned. A total of up to 8 pints of blood can be removed and stored until required. Iron tablets are prescribed to ensure that the bone marrow produces replacement blood cells.

EFFECT OF CHROMOSOMAL TRANSLOCATION

A translocation is a rearrangement of the chromosomes in body cells. A person carrying a translocation may show no abnormality but there is a risk of his or her child having a *chromosomal disorder*.

Normal cell
A body cell normally contains 22 paired chromosomes (called autosomes) plus two sex chromosomes (XX in women and XY in men). Just two pairs of autosomes—numbers 21 and 14—are shown here.

Example of translocation
In a typical translocation, a large part of one chromosome is joined to a large part of another. Here, most of a chromosome number 21 and a chromosome number 14 have joined.

Balanced translocation (parent)
The remaining bits of chromosomes 21 and 14 disappear. If, as here, the translocation is balanced—that is, the total chromosome complement is normal or near normal—no outward abnormality is seen.

Eggs or sperm produced
A parent with the example translocation makes four types of egg or sperm. They are (from left)—normal, missing a chromosome 21, carrying joined chromosomes 14 and 21, and the same with an extra chromosome 21.

Normal egg or sperm
An egg or sperm from the parent with the translocation combines with one from the other parent, which has one number 21 and one number 14 chromosome. Any of the four outcomes below may result.

Child
The child may have (1) normal chromosomes, (2) a missing chromosome 21 (incompatible with life), (3) a balanced translocation (like the parent), and (4) effectively, an extra chromosome 21, leading to Down's syndrome. In the latter case, the parents may benefit from genetic counseling.

Transient ischemic attack

A brief interruption of the blood supply to part of the brain that results in temporary impairment of vision, speech, sensation, or movement. Typically, the episode lasts for several minutes or, at the most, for a few hours. Any attack that lasts for more than 24 hours is called a *stroke*. Transient ischemic attacks (TIAs) may be the prelude to a full-scale stroke.

CAUSES
Some TIAs occur when an artery supplying the brain becomes temporarily blocked by a flake of clotted blood carried from elsewhere in the bloodstream (see *Embolism*). Other attacks are caused by narrowing of an artery due to *atherosclerosis*.

SYMPTOMS AND SIGNS
Symptoms occur suddenly, and vary widely, according to the site and duration of the interruption to blood flow. They include weakness or numbness in an arm or leg, *aphasia* (disturbance of language functions), dizziness, or partial blindness. An attack is always followed by full recovery.

DIAGNOSIS AND TREATMENT
Diagnostic testing usually includes *CT scanning* to rule out the possibility of a brain tumor or subdural *hematoma* (a swelling containing blood), which sometimes produces TIA-like symptoms. Blood tests to look for blood-clotting abnormalities are also used. Other tests, including *ultrasound scanning*, digital subtraction *angiography*, or conventional angiography, may be used to look at the vessels for evidence of atherosclerosis. In some instances, heart studies are performed to check the heart as a possible source of blood clots.

Treatment is aimed at preventing a major stroke, which occurs within five years in from one fourth to one third of the patients with TIA. Therapeutic options include *endarterectomy, anticoagulant drugs*, or aspirin (an antiplatelet drug). Thus far, only aspirin has been proven effective.

Transillumination

A procedure carried out during physical examination of a lump or swelling. Light from a small flashlight is shined against one side of the lump; if light can be seen on the other side, the physician knows the lump contains clear fluid because fat or other tissue would block the light. For example, a *hydrocele* (fluid-containing swelling in the scrotum) allows light to pass, whereas a *varicocele* (mass of enlarged veins) in the scrotum does not.

Translocation

A rearrangement of the *chromosomes* inside a person's cells. Translocation is a type of *mutation* (change in the genetic material). Sections of chromosomes may be exchanged, or the main parts of two chromosomes may be joined. A translocation may be inherited or acquired as the result of a new mutation.

Often, because there has been no net loss or gain of chromosomal material within the person's cells, a translocation has no outward effect, and causes no abnormality. However, the translocation can mean that some of the person's egg or sperm cells carry too much or too little chromosomal material, which leads to a risk of a *chromosomal abnormality* (such as *Down's syndrome*) in the person's children (see diagram on opposite page).

When a chromosomal abnormality occurs, the child's and the parents' chromosomes are checked to see whether a translocation is the cause (see *Chromosome analysis*). *Genetic counseling* can help determine the risk of another child being affected.

Transmissible

A term meaning capable of being passed from one person to another or from one organism to another of the same or a different species (as in the transmission of disease from an insect to a human). The term is applied to *infectious diseases* and to *genetic disorders*.

Transplant surgery

The replacement of a diseased organ or tissue with a healthy, living substitute. The organ is usually taken from a person who has just died. However, in the US, about one third of transplanted kidneys are taken from living relatives of the patient (see *Organ donation*).

Around the world about 100,000 major organs have been transplanted, mostly in the past 10 to 15 years. About 80 percent of patients are alive and well one year after the transplantation of a major organ (such as the heart or liver) and most survive at least five years.

The earliest successful transplant operation was *corneal grafting*, carried out early this century. The cornea is not affected by the rejection process (the automatic attempt by the body's *immune system* to destroy foreign cells) because it has no blood supply, and therefore no white blood cells and antibodies to bring about rejection after a transplant.

Kidney transplantation was shown to be technically possible in the 1950s, but early transplant operations ended in failure because of rejection. In the 1960s, however, *corticosteroid drugs* and cytotoxic agents (see *Anticancer drugs*) were found to suppress the rejection response, making transplantation practicable. The discovery in the 1970s and introduction in the early 1980s of *cyclosporine*, a more effective *immunosuppressant drug*, substantially improved the success rates for transplant surgery.

Every patient who undergoes an organ transplant operation must take immunosuppressant drugs indefinitely; this damping down of the body's natural defenses exposes him or her to a greater risk of infection, especially with fungi (see *Fungal infections*) and protozoal *parasites*. Patients

TRANSPLANTS PERFORMED IN US IN 1986

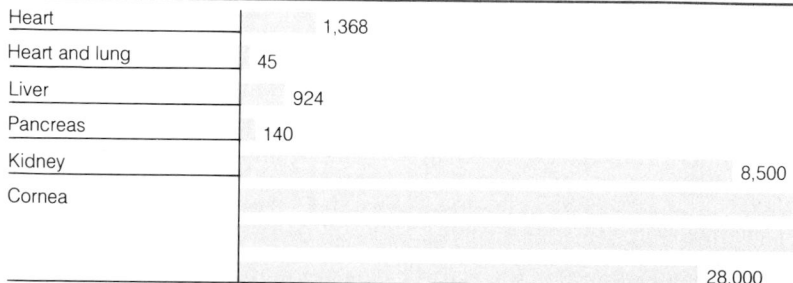

Organ	Number
Heart	1,368
Heart and lung	45
Liver	924
Pancreas	140
Kidney	8,500
Cornea	28,000

Factors affecting transplantation
The number of specific transplant operations performed depends partly on demand (how many people would benefit) and partly on availability. For corneal transplants, there is a high demand and ready availability. But for some other types of transplantation, strict selection is necessary, due to shortages of suitable donor organs or because only a small number of specialist centers can offer the procedure.

T

undergoing long-term immunosuppressant treatment are also at increased risk of certain types of cancer, especially *lymphomas*.

A second important factor in improving the results of transplant surgery has been the steady improvement in techniques for matching the donors and recipients. Organ transplantation proceeds most smoothly when the donor and recipient share most of the same tissue types (see *Histocompatibility antigens*; *Tissue-typing*).

A third factor that has contributed to higher success rates is the development of techniques for organ preservation. After removal from the donor, the organ is washed with an oxygenated fluid and cooled; this reduces the risk of damage due to lack of blood. Nevertheless, it is still important to keep to a minimum the time the organ is deprived of a normal blood supply. In most cases of heart or liver transplantation, the organs are removed from the donor while the heart is still functioning, but after *brain death* has been certified. (See also *Heart transplant*; *Heart-lung transplant*; *Liver transplant*; *Kidney transplant*.)

Transposition of the great vessels

A form of congenital *heart disease* in which the two major vessels that carry blood away from the heart—the aorta and the pulmonary artery—are in each other's normal position. This means that, unless the baby also has a septal defect (hole in the heart) through which blood can flow, insufficient oxygenated blood is supplied to the body's tissues. Transposition of the great vessels occurs in about 40 babies per 100,000 born.

SYMPTOMS, DIAGNOSIS, AND TREATMENT
Cyanosis (blueness of the skin) usually develops and the baby becomes increasingly short of breath, and feeds poorly. Symptoms vary in severity according to the amount of oxygenated blood passing through the septal opening.

A firm diagnosis can be made only after a *chest X ray*, an *ECG* (electrocardiogram), an echocardiogram (see *Echocardiography*), and cardiac *catheterization*, in which a catheter is introduced into the heart.

Once the diagnosis is made, emergency surgical treatment is carried out to create or enlarge a hole in the septum. This allows enough oxygenated blood through to keep the child alive. Later, reconstructive *open*

heart surgery is performed to create normal circulation. The surgery usually allows the child to live a full and normal life.

Transsexualism

A rare psychiatric disorder in which a person feels persistently uncomfortable about his or her anatomical sex.

Usually developing in early adulthood, transsexualism is much more common in men. The condition is often associated with a disturbed child-parent relationship and may follow a period of cross-dressing.

Unlike effeminate homosexual men or masculine lesbians who have no desire to change their anatomical gender, transsexuals wish to live as members of the opposite sex. Frequently, they obsessively seek surgical or hormonal treatment to bring about a physical *sex change*. A careful psychiatric evaluation is used by the physician to rule out a psychotic delusional system, which would make hormonal or surgical treatment extremely risky. Associated features include *personality disorder*, alcohol or drug excess, anxiety, depression, and work problems. Sexual drive is often quite low, although some transsexuals are actively homosexual.

Transsexualism should be distinguished from the delusion (false belief not responding to reasoned argument) of belonging to the other sex, which sometimes occurs in *schizophrenia*. Rare cases of physical intersex (see *Hermaphroditism*), in which there are congenital abnormalities of the sexual structures, are ruled out by the physician during a general and genital examination and by endocrine tests if necessary.

Transvestism

A persistent desire by a man to dress in women's clothing; it is also called cross-dressing. Transvestism most often starts in childhood, usually with the boy dressing in the underwear of a female relative. It is done in private while masturbating. Transvestism should be differentiated from charades or female impersonation, which do not involve the component of sexual arousal.

Transvestism varies from the occasional wearing of female underclothes to constant, public dressing in women's clothes and extensive involvement in transvestite subculture. For some people, cross-dressing serves to relieve anxiety; for others it provides sexual excitement. No

biological factors have been established. Occasionally, transvestism develops into *transsexualism*.

Most transvestites are heterosexual and have a sexual relationship with a female partner who knows and can accept the cross-dressing as a special need. Transvestites rarely seek medical or psychiatric treatment.

An emergency may be created in a couple or family upon accidental revelation of the behavior. Crisis intervention consists of educating the partner and kin that the behavior does not break the law or indicate that the person is dangerous. The situation of the patient (child, teen, or adult) is evaluated carefully to determine why private sexual behavior has become public and therefore a problem.

Tranylcypromine

A monoamine-oxidase inhibitor *antidepressant drug*.

Trapezius muscle

A large, diamond-shaped muscle that extends from the back of the skull to the lower part of the thoracic spine (the part of the spine in the chest) and, at its broadest point, across the width of the shoulders. At the shoulders, the

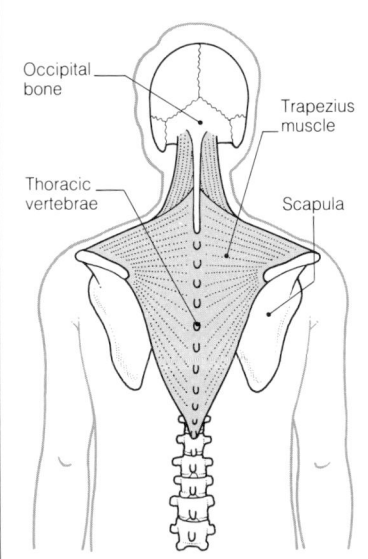

LOCATION OF THE TRAPEZIUS MUSCLE
This extensive, diamond-shaped muscle in the back provides power for activities such as swimming and lifting.

Occipital bone

Thoracic vertebrae

Trapezius muscle

Scapula

T

trapezius is attached to the top and back of the scapula (shoulder blade) and to the outermost part of the clavicle (collarbone). Along its midline, the trapezius is also attached by ligaments to the vertebrae.

The trapezius muscle helps support the neck and spine. It is also involved in movements of the arm. When an arm is raised, the trapezius on that side contracts, thereby causing the scapula to rotate.

Trapped nerve
See *Nerve, trapped.*

Trauma
A physical injury or a severe emotional shock. The psychological condition that can result from physical or emotional trauma is known as *post-traumatic stress disorder.*

Trauma surgery
See *Traumatology.*

Traumatology
Emergency treatment of patients suffering from acute trauma (physical injury), commonly as the result of traffic accidents, industrial accidents, domestic accidents, shootings, or stabbings. In the US, trauma is the most common cause of death in people up to age 30 and the fourth most common cause of death in the population as a whole, accounting for more than 100,000 deaths annually. In addition, more than 1 million more cases of trauma require hospitalization every year.

In cases of life-threatening trauma, the priorities of the trauma surgeon are to maintain a clear airway in the patient and so prevent asphyxia, to arrest bleeding, to treat shock, and to deal with major chest wounds affecting the heart or lungs. If there are abdominal injuries, an exploratory operation called a *laparotomy* or, in the case of head injuries, a *craniotomy,* may be required. Multiple injuries require coordinated treatment by members of many specialities.

Once the patient's condition is stable, other injuries, such as fractures and superficial cuts, are treated.

Travelers' diarrhea
An affliction of people visiting foreign countries. Episodes of diarrhea range in severity from inconvenient to debilitating. Known by a variety of colorful names, such as Montezuma's revenge and the Tokyo trots, all are forms of *gastroenteritis.*

Travel immunization
Any person planning to travel outside of the US, Canada, Europe, Australia, and New Zealand may need immunizations before departure. Few immunizations are now compulsory for international travel. Nevertheless, some immunizations are advisable for the traveler's own protection.

A prospective traveler should consult his or her physician about individual requirements. If necessary, the physician can check with state or local departments of health for the latest immunization recommendations for particular destinations.

The physician needs information on the countries to be visited, the duration and nature of the visit, and the individual's previous immunization history. Most US citizens have received childhood immunization against certain diseases, such as diphtheria, pertussis, tetanus, and polio, so may not need further protection (see *Immunization*). However, in

GUIDELINES FOR TRAVEL IMMUNIZATION

Immunization	Reason for immunization	Effectiveness
Yellow fever	Compulsory for entry to some countries and advisable for visits to others within yellow fever zones in Africa and South America. May also be needed when traveling from yellow fever zones to neighboring states or to some Asian countries.	Near 100 percent protection for at least 10 years. Certificate provided.
Cholera	Occasionally compulsory for entry to some countries in Asia and Africa. Also advisable when traveling to many other Asian and African countries.	Gives moderate protection for six months. Other precautions against cholera needed in epidemic areas.
Typhoid	Recommended when traveling anywhere outside of the US, Canada, Europe, Australia, and New Zealand for anyone who has not received immunization or a booster within the past five years.	Gives moderate protection for about five years, after which a booster is needed.
Tetanus	Advisable for anyone who has not received childhood immunization or a booster within the past 10 years.	Highly effective, with booster needed every 10 years.
Polio	Advisable for anyone who has not received childhood immunization or a booster within the past 10 years.	Highly effective with booster needed every 10 years.
Immune serum globulin	Recommended when traveling to any country where hygiene and sanitary standards are low to protect against viral hepatitis, type A.	Moderate protection for up to three months.
Measles	Advisable for anyone who did not receive childhood immunization and who has not had measles.	Highly effective, lifelong protection.
Diphtheria	Advisable for anyone who did not receive childhood immunization and is shown by a test to be nonimmune.	Highly effective.
Hepatitis B Rabies Meningitis	Recommended only for individuals or groups at special risk through occupation, nature of visit abroad, and so on.	All highly effective.
Smallpox	No longer necessary, as the disease has been eradicated.	

T

some cases, booster doses against tetanus and polio are advisable.

With knowledge of the individual's medical history, the physician can decide if there are grounds for not administering a particular vaccine. Infants younger than 1 year are not usually given certain travel vaccines, notably yellow fever, cholera, and typhoid injections. In general, infants should receive their scheduled immunizations before travel abroad.

After discussion, the physician establishes an appropriate schedule of injections. Some vaccines must be given in two or three doses several weeks apart, so it is wise to consult your physician at least two to three months before departure.

Antimalarial drugs (see *Malaria*) may also be needed for people planning to visit certain destinations.

Trazodone

An *antidepressant drug*. Trazodone has a strong sedative effect and is particularly useful in the treatment of *depression* accompanied by *anxiety* or *insomnia*. Possible adverse effects include drowsiness, constipation, dry mouth, dizziness, and, rarely, *priapism* (painful, persistent erection).

Treatment

Any measure taken to prevent or cure a disease or disorder or to relieve symptoms. Examples include *drug treatment*, *radiation therapy*, *surgery*, and bed rest.

Trematode

The scientific names for any *fluke* or *schistosome* (flattened worms that may parasitize humans).

Trembling

See *Tremor*.

Tremor

An involuntary, rhythmic, oscillating movement in the muscles of part of the body, most commonly the hands, feet, jaw, tongue, or head. Tremor is caused by rapidly alternating contraction and relaxation of the muscles.

Occasional temporary tremors are experienced by almost everyone, usually at times of fear, excitement, or other heightened emotion; they are due to increased production of the hormone *epinephrine*.

A slight persistent tremor unrelated to any disease is common in elderly people. Another type of persistent tremor not associated with disease is essential tremor, a fine-to-moderate tremor (six to 10 movements per second) that runs in families and may be temporarily relieved by a small amount of alcohol or by taking *beta-blocker drugs*. Both these tremors increase with movement of the affected part of the body.

Some types of persistent tremor indicate an underlying disorder. Coarse tremor (four to five muscle movements a second) present at rest but reduced during movement is often a sign of *Parkinson's disease*. Intention tremor (tremor that is worse on movement of the affected part) is a sign of disease of the *cerebellum*. Other disorders marked by tremor include *multiple sclerosis*, *Wilson's disease*, *mercury poisoning*, *thyrotoxicosis*, and hepatic *encephalopathy*.

Tremor may also be caused by drugs, among them *amphetamine drugs*, *antidepressant drugs*, *caffeine*, and *lithium*. It may also be a symptom of drug withdrawal. A tremor can occur in people taking *antipsychotic drugs* for certain psychiatric disorders.

Tremor is also a feature of alcohol withdrawal and, as such, may indicate *alcohol dependence*. The so-called morning shakes occur as blood alcohol levels fall and are relieved by the first drink of the day.

Trench fever

An infectious illness that was common among troops in the trenches during World War I and World War II, but is now rare or unknown in most parts of the world. Like epidemic *typhus*, which it resembles, the disease is caused by rickettsiae (microorganisms similar to bacteria) spread by body lice. The symptoms include headache and muscle pains as well as fever, which may occur in bouts. It is treated with *antibiotic drugs*.

Trench foot

See *Immersion foot*.

Trench mouth

See *Vincent's disease*.

Trephine

A hollow, cylindrical instrument with a saw-toothed edge used for cutting a circular hole, usually in bone. Trephines are most often used to bore holes in the skull to form a removable flap before performing operations on the brain.

Perforating the skull to relieve excess pressure is a recent innovation and is part of conventional surgery. Ancient peoples used trephines on the skull (as evidenced by the skulls found by paleontologists) but the reason they did so is unknown; most likely it was done by witch doctors to encourage the release of evil spirits.

Tretinoin

A drug chemically related to *vitamin A*, used topically to treat *acne* and certain skin disorders characterized by scaling and thickening, such as *ichthyosis*. Tretinoin may aggravate acne in the first few weeks of treatment but usually improves the condition within three to four months.

Tretinoin may cause skin irritation and peeling. Excessive exposure to sunlight may aggravate any irritation and lead to *sunburn*. In rare cases, it may bleach or darken the skin.

Trial, clinical

A test on human volunteers of the effectiveness and safety of a drug, or a systematic comparison of alternative forms of medical or surgical treatment for a particular disorder. Clinical trials are also used to test the usefulness of new medical or surgical appliances, dressings, or equipment.

In the development of new drugs, clinical trials follow animal tests that mainly evaluate toxic effects (see *Animal experimentation*); clinical trials are usually undertaken at a late stage before the manufacturer proceeds to commercial production. The purpose of clinical trials is to demonstrate that the new drug is effective, safe, and superior to, or at least as good as, existing drugs. Such trials are also useful in revealing effects that may not have been suspected from results of the animal tests.

Careful precautions are necessary to ensure that the results of clinical trials are not misleading. Trials that fail to eliminate the effects of personal bias or the *placebo* effect may be of little value. For these reasons, most clinical trials are carried out in the form of randomized, *controlled trials*.

Triamcinolone

CORTICOSTEROID				
Tablet Liquid Injection Cream Ointment Inhaler Dental paste				
📋 Prescription needed				
🔖 Available as generic				

A *corticosteroid drug* used to treat inflammation of the mouth, gums, skin, and joints. Triamcinolone is also

T

used to treat *asthma* and certain blood disorders, such as *thrombocytopenia* and *leukemia*.

Triamterene
A potassium-sparing *diuretic drug*. Triamterene is used with thiazide or loop diuretics to treat *hypertension* (high blood pressure) and *edema* (fluid retention). Possible adverse effects include nausea, vomiting, lethargy, muscle weakness, and rash.

Triazolam
A *benzodiazepine drug* used in the short-term treatment of *insomnia*.

Triceps muscle
The name (meaning "three heads") of the muscle at the back of the upper arm. At the upper end of the muscle, one of its three heads is attached to the outer edge of the scapula (shoulder blade); the other two heads are attached to either side of the upper part of the humerus (the upper arm bone).

The lower part of the triceps is attached by a large tendon to the olecranon process of the ulna (the bony prominence at the back of the elbow). Contraction of the triceps muscle straightens the arm. (See also *Biceps muscle*.)

LOCATION OF THE TRICEPS MUSCLE
This muscle at the back of the arm functions to straighten the elbow joint, thus opposing the action of the biceps at the front of the arm.

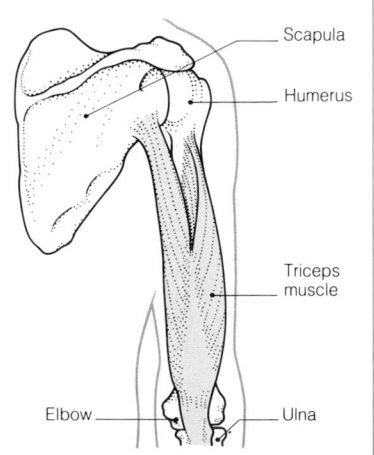

Scapula

Humerus

Triceps muscle

Elbow

Ulna

Trichiasis
An alteration in the direction of growth of the eyelashes in which the lashes grow inward toward the eyeball. The abnormally directed lashes can rub against the eye, causing severe discomfort and sometimes damage to the *cornea*. Trichiasis can result from inflammation and scarring that occurs in *trachoma*. Severe scarring may lead to *entropion* (turning in of the lid margin).

Temporary treatment involves the manual removal of the offending lashes, but the lashes regrow and may again cause pain and damage. Permanent treatment involves destruction of the growth follicles of the offending eyelashes using *electrolysis*.

Trichinosis
 An infestation with the larvae of a tiny worm, *TRICHINELLA SPIRALIS*, usually acquired by eating undercooked pork or pork products, such as ham or sausages.

CAUSES AND INCIDENCE
Worm larvae are present as cysts in the muscles of infested animals, such as rats, dogs, bears, and pigs. If a person eats the raw or undercooked meat of an infested animal, the larvae are released from the cysts and develop into adults in the person's intestines. The adult worms discharge fresh larvae, which travel in the bloodstream to various tissues and organs, including the heart and brain, and to the muscles, where they form cysts.

Infestation of humans is practically confined to pork-eating populations, mainly in North America and Europe. Up to 5 percent of people in the US have had a trichiniferous infestation, but usually without symptoms. The principal preventive measure is thorough cooking of pork and pork products. Freezing to a temperature below 0°F (-18°C) for 24 hours also kills the larvae.

SYMPTOMS AND COMPLICATIONS
Infestation with only a few worms usually causes no symptoms. A heavy infestation may cause diarrhea and vomiting within a day or two of eating infested meat, followed, a week or so later, by more symptoms as new larvae circulate through the body. The symptoms may include fever, swelling around the eyelids, and severe muscle pains, which may last for several weeks. Very rarely, the person becomes seriously ill and may die. In other people, the symptoms subside and gradually disappear.

Biopsy specimen showing trichinosis
This photomicrograph of a section of a patient's muscle shows a cyst formed by a *TRICHINELLA SPIRALIS* larva.

DIAGNOSIS AND TREATMENT
Trichinosis may be suspected by a physician from the symptoms; it is confirmed by *blood tests*, which detect antibodies to the larvae, or by a muscle *biopsy* (sample of tissue), which shows the larvae themselves.

The disease is treated with an *antihelmintic drug* (usually thiabendazole) that kills adult worms in the intestines and attacks larvae in the tissues. *Corticosteroid drugs* are given to reduce inflammation. This treatment generally leads to recovery within a few days to weeks.

Trichomoniasis
 An infection of the vagina, often sexually transmitted, caused by the protozoan (single-celled microorganism) *TRICHOMONAS VAGINALIS*. In addition to being transmitted during sexual intercourse, trichomoniasis is occasionally contracted from an infected washcloth or towel or transmitted by a woman to her baby during childbirth. The infection may also occur in men, affecting the urethra, but usually does not cause any symptoms.

Trichomoniasis is not in itself a serious condition. It is estimated that 3 million people are infected every year in the US.

SYMPTOMS AND SIGNS
The causative organism may inhabit the vagina for years without causing symptoms. If symptoms do occur, they include painful inflammation and itching of the vagina and vulva, and a profuse, yellow, frothy, offensive discharge. Sexual intercourse is usually painful. Men usually have no symptoms but some suffer from urethral discomfort, inflammation of the glans (head) of the penis, and signs of *nonspecific urethritis*.

T

DIAGNOSIS AND TREATMENT

The diagnosis is made from a laboratory examination of a sample of the vaginal discharge or of swabs taken from the urethra. Diagnosis is usually difficult in men.

Treatment is with *metronidazole*, which usually clears up the condition. An infected person's sexual partner or partners should be treated at the same time to prevent reinfection and further spread of infection.

Trichotillomania

The habit of constantly pulling out one's own hair. Trichotillomania is often associated with severe mental subnormality or with a psychotic illness, such as schizophrenia. It may also occur in psychologically disturbed children as an expression of anxiety and frustration.

The sufferer typically pulls, twists, and breaks off chunks of hair from the scalp, leaving bald patches; occasionally, pubic hair is pulled out. Children sometimes eat the removed hair, which may cause a trichobezoar, or hairball (see *Bezoar*).

Treatment may consist of *psychotherapy* and/or *antipsychotic drugs*.

Tricuspid insufficiency

Failure of the tricuspid valve of the heart to close properly, allowing blood to leak back into the right atrium (upper chamber) during contractions of the right ventricle (lower chamber). This lowers the pumping efficiency of the heart.

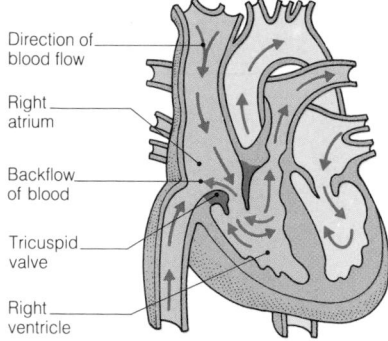

Direction of blood flow

Right atrium

Backflow of blood

Tricuspid valve

Right ventricle

Defect in tricuspid insufficiency
The tricuspid valve lies between the atrium and ventricle in the right side of the heart. Insufficiency means that when the right ventricle contracts, some blood escapes back into the right atrium.

CAUSES AND INCIDENCE

The disorder is usually due to an increased work load on the right side of the heart as a result of *pulmonary* *hypertension* (high pressure in the blood supply to the lungs). This causes the right ventricle to distend and leads to widening of the opening in which the tricuspid valve is situated. In rare cases, tricuspid insufficiency occurs as a result of *rheumatic fever* or, in intravenous drug abusers, as a result of a bacterial infection of the heart; it is then usually accompanied by other heart valve disorders.

SYMPTOMS, DIAGNOSIS, AND TREATMENT

The tricuspid insufficiency causes symptoms of right-sided *heart failure*, notably *edema* (fluid collection and swelling) affecting the ankles and abdomen. The liver is congested with blood and is swollen and tender. Veins in the neck are distended.

The condition is diagnosed from the patient's symptoms, from a characteristic *murmur* heard through a stethoscope, and by tests that may include an *ECG*, *chest X rays*, *echocardiography*, and cardiac *catheterization*.

Treatment for heart failure, with *diuretic drugs* and *ACE inhibitor drugs*, often clears up the symptoms. If symptoms persist, *heart valve surgery* may be performed to repair or replace the malfunctioning valve.

Tricuspid stenosis

Narrowing of the opening of the tricuspid valve in the heart between the right atrium (upper chamber) and right ventricle (lower chamber). Tricuspid stenosis is an uncommon heart valve disorder that occurs mainly in people who have had *rheumatic fever*. It may also occur in intravenous drug abusers as a result of bacterial infection of the heart. It is usually accompanied by other heart valve disorders, such as *mitral stenosis*.

The right atrium must work harder to pump blood through the narrowed valve, causing it to enlarge. The symptoms are very similar to those of *tricuspid insufficiency*; the condition is diagnosed by the same procedures.

Drug treatment is given with *diuretic drugs* to reduce edema and sometimes a *digitalis drug* to increase the force of the heart's contractions. If symptoms persist, *heart valve surgery* may be carried out to repair or replace the valve.

Trifluoperazine

An *antipsychotic drug* used principally in the treatment of *schizophrenia*.

Trifluridine

An *antiviral drug* used to treat and sometimes prevent eye infections caused by the same virus that causes *herpes simplex*. Adverse effects include dryness, stinging, itching, or redness of the eyes, and swollen eyelids.

Trigeminal nerve

The fifth *cranial nerve*. The trigeminal nerve arises from the pons (part of the *brain stem*) and divides into three main branches, which then subdivide into a complex network of nerves. These nerves supply sensation to the face, scalp, nose, teeth, lining of the mouth, upper eyelid, sinuses, and front two thirds of the tongue; control the production of saliva by the salivary glands and of tears by the lacrimal glands; and stimulate contraction of the jaw muscles responsible for chewing.

Damage to, or disease in, one area supplied by a branch of the trigeminal nerve may cause *referred pain* in another area supplied by a different branch of the nerve. For example, sinusitis (infection of the sinuses) may cause toothache.

Trigeminal neuralgia

A disorder of the trigeminal nerve (fifth cranial nerve) in which episodes of severe, stabbing pain affect the cheek, lips, gums, or chin on one side of the face. The pain is very brief (lasting only a few seconds to minutes) but is often so intense that the sufferer is unable to do anything for the duration of the attack. The pain often causes wincing and for this reason is commonly called tic douloureux (literally, "painful twitch").

Trigeminal neuralgia is unusual under the age of 50. When it does occur in younger people, it may be associated with *multiple sclerosis*. Attacks occur in bouts that may last for weeks at a time. Pain-free intervals between attacks tend to become shorter with time.

The cause of trigeminal neuralgia is uncertain. The pain nearly always starts from one trigger point on the face and can be brought on by touching the face, washing, shaving, eating, drinking, or even talking.

Treatment is difficult. *Carbamazepine* suppresses the pain in most sufferers, but resistance to the drug develops in some people or they are unable to tolerate a high enough dosage to relieve the pain. If drug treatment fails, surgical options are available.

Trigger finger

Locking of one or several fingers in a bent position. Forcible straightening of an affected finger usually causes an audible click.

LOCATION OF THE TRIGEMINAL NERVE

The trigeminal nerve splits into three main parts. The ophthalmic nerve supplies most of the scalp, the upper eyelid, tear gland, and cornea; the maxillary nerve supplies the upper jaw; and the mandibular nerve supplies the tongue, lower jaw, and jaw muscles.

Trigger finger is caused by inflammation of the fibrous sheath that encloses the tendon of the affected finger and is accompanied by localized swelling of the tendon. When the finger is bent, the enlarged tendon is forced out of the narrowed mouth of the sheath and is then unable to reenter it. There is usually tenderness at the base of the affected finger. In addition, a small swelling may be felt over the tendon.

Appearance of trigger finger
The disorder is caused by inflammation of one of the tendons involved in controlling the finger's movements.

Treatment of trigger finger involves either the injection of a *corticosteroid drug* into the sheath to reduce inflammation or a surgical procedure to widen the opening.

Trihexyphenidyl

An *anticholinergic drug* often used in conjunction with other drugs that relieve rigidity and tremor in *Parkinson's disease*. Trihexyphenidyl is also occasionally used to relieve the symptoms of *parkinsonism* caused by *antipsychotic drugs*.

Trimeprazine

An *antihistamine drug* used mainly to relieve itching in allergic conditions, such as *urticaria* (hives) and atopic *eczema*. Since trimeprazine has a sedative effect, it is useful in the relief of itching that usually prevents sleep. Trimeprazine is also used as a *premedication* to sedate children before surgery or other medical procedures are performed.

The adverse effects of trimeprazine are typical of other antihistamines, although trimeprazine is more likely to cause drowsiness than some other drugs in this group.

Trimethobenzamide

An *antiemetic drug* promoted for the treatment of nausea and vomiting caused by anesthetics, *radiation therapy*, or *anticancer drugs*. Trimethobenzamide may cause adverse effects such as drowsiness and, rarely, blurred vision, muscle cramps, diarrhea, tremor, rash, and jaundice.

Trimethoprim

An *antibacterial drug* prescribed for a wide variety of infections. Trimethoprim is used to treat *urinary tract infection*, *prostatitis*, and some types of *gastroenteritis*. Combined with another antibacterial drug, *sulfamethoxazole*, trimethoprim is used to treat infections of the urinary tract, ear, and respiratory tract (including *pneumocystis pneumonia*) and *gonorrhea*.

Possible adverse effects include rash, itching, nausea, vomiting, diarrhea, and sore tongue.

Trimipramine

A tricyclic *antidepressant drug*. Trimipramine has a strong sedative effect and is used to treat *depression* accompanied by *anxiety* or *insomnia*.

Possible adverse effects include dry mouth, blurred vision, dizziness, constipation, and nausea.

Triprolidine

An *antihistamine drug* used to treat allergies, such as allergic *rhinitis* (hay fever) and *urticaria* (hives). Triprolidine is also a common ingredient of *cough remedies* and *cold remedies*. It is occasionally given to treat or prevent allergic reactions to *blood transfusions* or certain foods.

Possible adverse effects include dry mouth, dizziness, difficulty passing urine and, in children, *hyperactivity*.

Trismus

Involuntary contraction of the jaw muscles, resulting in the mouth becoming tightly closed, a condition commonly known as lockjaw.

Trismus may occur as a symptom of *tetanus*, *tonsillitis*, *quinsy*, *mumps*, *Vincent's disease*, an abscess around a back tooth, nasopharyngeal cancer (see *Nasopharynx, cancer of*), or *Parkinson's disease*. Occasionally trismus is hysterical in origin (it sometimes occurs in *anorexia nervosa*). Treatment of trismus is directed toward the underlying cause.

Trisomy

The presence, within the cells of a person, of an extra chromosome so that there are three *chromosomes* of a particular number, instead of the usual two. The result can range from the death and spontaneous abortion of an affected embryo to a range of abnormalities in a live-born child.

CAUSES AND INCIDENCE

A trisomy may result from a fault during the formation of an egg or sperm cell by which an extra chromosome gets into the cell. If an affected egg or sperm takes part in fertilization, the resulting embryo also has an extra chromosome, causing trisomy. Trisomy can also result from a *translocation* (a rearrangement of the chromosomes) inherited from one of the parents. Most types of trisomy are more common in older mothers.

Certain trisomies (such as three number 11 chromosomes) have never been observed in live-born babies; if they do occur, such trisomies probably lead to early abortion or stillbirth. By far the most common trisomy in live-born infants is trisomy 21, also called *Down's syndrome*, in which there are three number 21 chromosomes. Much less common are trisomy 18 (Edwards' syndrome) and trisomy 13 (Patau's syndrome). Some others—such as trisomy 8 and trisomy 22—are extremely rare. Partial trisomies, in which only part of a chromosome is in triplicate, have also been found.

Patau's syndrome   Down's syndrome   Edwards' syndrome

Types of trisomy
In all trisomies a child has three, instead of the usual two, chromosomes of a particular number. Down's syndrome is by far the most common trisomy.

SYMPTOMS, DIAGNOSIS, AND TREATMENT
All full trisomies cause multiple abnormalities, such as skeletal and heart defects, facial anomalies, and mental deficiency. The effect of a partial trisomy is variable, depending on how much extra chromosomal material is present. The conditions are diagnosed by *chromosome analysis.*

There is no specific treatment for these conditions. Many children with Down's syndrome survive into adulthood, but babies with other full trisomies usually die early in infancy.

Parents of an affected baby should obtain *genetic counseling* to assess the risk of a future child being affected.

Trisomy 21 syndrome
A set of abnormalities caused when a child has three, instead of the usual two, number 21 chromosomes in each of his or her cells. It is better known as *Down's syndrome*.

Trochlear nerve
The fourth *cranial nerve*. It arises from the midbrain (part of the *brain stem*) and passes through the skull to enter the eye socket through a gap in the skull bones. The trochlear nerve supplies only one muscle of each eye (the superior oblique muscle), the contraction of which rotates the eye outward.

Damage to the trochlear nerve (as a result of a skull fracture, for example) may lead to double vision when trying to look outward.

Trophoblastic tumor
A growth arising from the tissues that develop into the placenta. The most common type of trophoblastic tumor is a benign growth called a *hydatidiform mole*. A malignant trophoblastic tumor that has spread outside the uterus is called a *choriocarcinoma.*

Tropical diseases
Most diseases of temperate areas are also prevalent in the tropics. Many other diseases are virtually confined to tropical areas. In most cases, this is not due primarily to tropical geographic factors (such as temperature, humidity, or disease-carrying insects), but to the fact that large populations in many tropical countries live in poverty.

DISEASES OF POVERTY
Malnutrition is one of the major causes of illness in the tropics. Apart from causing nutritional deficiency disorders, a poor diet weakens the body's ability to fight infectious diseases such as *measles* and *diphtheria*. Overcrowded living conditions are a cause of such diseases as *tuberculosis.*

Low standards of public health administration, food inspection and handling, and a lack of sanitary facilities, which encourage water and soil contamination with human excrement, are the cause of a vast number of diseases including *typhoid fever, shigellosis, cholera, amebiasis,* and *tapeworm infestation*. Most of these diseases were common in temperate zones before improvements in public

LOCATION OF THE TROCHLEAR NERVE
This nerve emerges from the brain and supplies a muscle that rotates the eye down and outward.

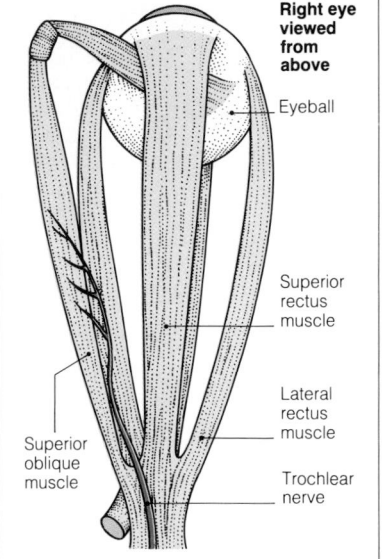

Right eye viewed from above

Eyeball

Superior rectus muscle

Lateral rectus muscle

Superior oblique muscle

Trochlear nerve

health and sanitation. Only some diseases, such as *hookworm infestation* and *schistosomiasis*, appear to be related to temperature or soil conditions found only in the tropics in addition to the lack of community sanitation and walking barefoot.

DISEASES SPREAD BY INSECTS
Some tropical diseases depend on the coincidence of a parasite and a specific insect *vector* (agent responsible for spread) such as a mosquito. These diseases include *malaria, yellow fever, sleeping sickness,* and *leishmaniasis*. It is worth noting, however, that at least some of the relevant insect vectors can survive in temperate zones; malaria was once common in parts of the US.

LIGHT AND HEAT
Certain conditions arise as a result of exposure to tropical sunlight. The most common is skin damage from ultraviolet light, leading to wrinkling, loss of elasticity, and an increased tendency to *skin cancer*, especially in white people with fair coloring. Ultraviolet light also damages the outer tissues of the eye (the conjunctiva and the cornea) and may lead to the development of *pinguecula* and *pterygium*. Overexertion in the tropics, with inadequate water intake

T

and salt replacement, may lead to *heat exhaustion*; prolonged exposure to high temperatures may lead to *heat stroke* in people who are not acclimated to the heat.

Tropical ulcer

An area of persistent skin and tissue loss caused by infection and occurring predominantly in tropical regions. The ulcers are most common in people who are malnourished.

The classic form of tropical ulcer results from contamination of a cut or abrasion (usually on a foot or leg) by a mixture of various types of bacteria. Infections spread beneath the skin, and the affected tissue dies and is shed, leaving the ulcer in place.

Treatment consists of thorough cleaning of the ulcer, which is then dressed; the patient also needs antibiotic drugs and a nourishing, protein-rich diet. With this treatment, the ulcer usually heals, although it may leave some scarring and deformity.

Similar types of ulcer can occur as a result of more specific infections, such as *diphtheria* of the skin, cutaneous *leishmaniasis*, and *yaws*. Treatment is as described above, except that drug therapy may vary.

To avoid tropical ulcers, it is particularly important to wash any cuts, sores, or abrasions thoroughly and cover them with a sterile dressing.

Tropicamide

A drug used to dilate the pupil before an eye examination and, occasionally, before eye surgery. Rare adverse effects include blurred vision, increased sensitivity to light, stinging, dry mouth, flushing, and *glaucoma.*

Trunk

The central part of the body, comprising the chest and abdomen, to which the head and limbs are attached. The term trunk also refers to a large blood vessel or nerve from which smaller vessels or nerves branch off.

Truss

An elastic, canvas, or padded metal appliance used to hold an abdominal *hernia* (protrusion of intestine through a weakened area in the abdominal wall) in place. A truss may be used to treat a hernia that is causing discomfort or is unsightly in people who are waiting for an operation or who are unfit for surgery. The hernia is pushed back through the abdominal wall before the truss is put on, usually while the person lies down.

Trypanosomiasis

A tropical disease caused by protozoan (single-celled) parasites known as trypanosomes. In Africa, trypanosomes spread by tsetse flies are the cause of *sleeping sickness*. In South America, other trypanosomes, spread by beetlelike insects, are the cause of *Chagas' disease.*

Tsetse fly bites

Tsetse flies are found in Africa, where they spread the parasitic disease *sleeping sickness*. They are brown, about the size of houseflies, and each has a proboscis (biting and feeding apparatus) projecting forward at the front. Their bites can be painful. Measures to minimize the risk of bites include use of insecticide sprays and protective clothing impregnated with insect repellent.

T-tube cholangiography

An X-ray procedure, also called operative or postoperative choledochography, performed to exclude the presence of residual gallstones in the common bile duct after removing the gallbladder and exploring the common bile duct (see *Cholecystectomy*).

The procedure is performed in the operating room following removal of the gallbladder eight to ten days after surgery. Contrast medium is injected into the T-tube (a T-shaped rubber tube placed, during surgery, in the common bile duct and brought out through a small abdominal skin incision) and X rays are taken. If there are no residual gallstones on the eighth day, the T-tube is removed. Otherwise, the tube is left until a decision is made concerning treatment to remove the stones.

Tubal ligation

See *Sterilization, female.*

Tubal pregnancy

See *Ectopic pregnancy.*

Tubercle

Any of several small, nodular masses apparent in tissues that have been infected by the *tuberculosis* bacterium. The masses are gray in color and semitransparent.

The term tubercle (or tuberculum or tuberosity) also refers to any small, rounded protrusion on the surface of a bone. For example, the tibial tubercle is a bump at the top of the tibia (main bone of the lower leg), immediately below the knee.

Tuberculin tests

Skin tests used to determine whether or not a person has been previously infected with *tuberculosis*. Tuberculin tests are performed in the diagnosis of suspected *tuberculosis* and are also carried out before *BCG vaccination.*

HOW THEY ARE DONE

The skin of the forearm is first cleansed with alcohol. A small dose of tuberculin (a purified protein extract of tuberculosis bacilli) is then introduced into the skin by one of various techniques. In the Mantoux test, tuberculin is injected into the skin with a needle. In the Sterneedle test, a drop of tuberculin is put on the forearm and a spring-loaded device with a circle of sharp prongs is used to force the tuberculin through punctures in the skin.

RESULTS

The forearm is examined after a few days and the skin reaction at the test site noted. If there is no change in the skin, the reaction is said to be negative. This indicates that the person has never been exposed to and has no immunity against tuberculosis. If a dime-sized area of the skin becomes red, hard, and raised, the reaction is positive. A positive reaction indicates previous exposure to tuberculosis, either through BCG vaccination or through actual infection.

Tuberculosis

An infectious disease, commonly called TB, caused in humans by the bacterium MYCOBACTERIUM TUBERCULOSIS. Tuberculosis was once common worldwide and was a major killer in childhood and early adult life. In Europe, it was responsible for about one quarter of the deaths in the middle 19th century. Its incidence has fallen and continues to fall in developed

Chest X ray showing tuberculosis
The right lung appears normal, but the left shows dense opacities (white areas) adjoining the heart shadow.

T

countries, but tuberculosis remains a major problem in poorer countries.

CAUSES

Infection is passed from person to person in airborne droplets (produced by coughing or sneezing). The bacteria breathed into the lungs then multiply to form an infected "focus." In a high proportion of cases, the body's *immune system* then checks the infection and healing occurs, leaving a scar.

In about 5 percent of cases, however, the primary infection does not resolve. Spread occurs via the vessels of the lymphatic system to the lymph nodes. Sometimes at this stage bacteria enter the bloodstream and spread to other parts of the body; this is called miliary tuberculosis and may occasionally be fatal. In some people, the bacteria go into a dormant state in the lungs and other organs, only to become reactivated many years later. Progressive damage may then occur (e.g., cavities in the lungs).

In some cases, tuberculosis does not primarily affect the lung but may involve the lymph nodes (particularly of the neck), or the intestines, bones, or other organs. Such infections were especially common in bovine tuberculosis, acquired from contaminated cows' milk; this method of transmission has virtually disappeared from developed countries.

INCIDENCE

The incidence of tuberculosis in the US is about eight to 10 new cases per 100,000 population annually and is falling. However, this still represents more than 20,000 new cases in the US per year. The incidence is much higher in certain racial or social groups, such as Hispanics, Haitians, and immigrants from Southeast Asia. The disease is also more common in deprived city areas, in the elderly, in patients with *immunodeficiency disorders*, in diabetics, alcoholics, and in people who are in close contact with a person with tuberculosis.

Worldwide, there are 30 million people with active tuberculosis; about 3 million die of the disease annually. Tuberculosis is most prevalent where resistance has been lowered by malnutrition and other diseases.

PREVENTION

In the US, two types of preventive measures are used against tuberculosis. First is the use of *BCG vaccination* in high-risk groups. Second is *contact tracing*. Relatives and close friends of a tuberculosis victim are examined, X-rayed, and given a skin test so that tuberculosis is detected at

an early stage and the risk of spread to other people is reduced. Any person—especially a child—who has contact in a household with someone who has active tuberculosis is given an antituberculosis antibiotic drug as a preventive measure.

SYMPTOMS AND COMPLICATIONS

Because tuberculosis usually affects the lungs, the main symptoms include coughing (sometimes bringing up blood), chest pain, shortness of breath, fever and sweating (especially at night), poor appetite, and weight loss. The main complications of tuberculosis of the lungs are *pleural effusion* (collection of fluid between the lung and chest wall), *pneumothorax* (air between the lungs and chest wall), and, in some cases, progression of the disease to death.

DIAGNOSIS

The diagnosis is made from the patient's symptoms and signs, and from a *chest X ray* and tests on the sputum and skin. The chest X ray is almost always abnormal. The upper parts of the lung are most commonly affected and may show cavities. Old healed areas of tuberculosis often remain as persistent shadows.

The sputum is examined for tuberculosis organisms. Attempts are also made to grow the bacteria from the sputum or other body fluids, although this procedure can take as long as six weeks. A skin test, called a *tuberculin test*, may be carried out. A positive test result indicates that the person has either been immunized against tuberculosis or has been infected. A strongly positive test result may indicate an active infection. Occasionally, *bronchoscopy* or the removal and examination of a piece of tissue (e.g., from a lymph node) may be necessary to make a firm diagnosis.

TREATMENT AND OUTLOOK

Modern drugs are very effective against tuberculosis, although at least two different antibiotic drugs must be taken to avoid bacterial *resistance* to the drugs. In the US, a common treatment is daily therapy for nine to 12 months with isoniazid and rifampin; other drugs, and sometimes a shorter course of treatment, may also be given. An adverse drug reaction (usually a rash or fever) develops in about 5 percent of patients, who then require a modified course of treatment. Blood tests are performed regularly during treatment to ensure that the drugs are not causing toxic effects on the liver.

Provided the full course of treatment is taken, the majority of patients are fully restored to health and suffer no recurrences.

Tuberosity

A prominent area on a bone to which tendons are attached. The gluteal tuberosity is a ridge on the upper back part of the shaft of the femur (thigh bone) to which tendons of part of the gluteus maximus muscle are attached. Other bones with tuberosities include the ischium (one of the three fused bones that form the pelvis), humerus (upper arm bone), and radius and ulna (lower arm bones).

Tuberous sclerosis

An inherited disorder affecting the skin and nervous system. The most typical skin feature of tuberous sclerosis is adenoma sebaceum (an acnelike condition on the face) but a variety of other skin conditions may also occur. Affected people characteristically suffer from epilepsy and mental retardation, although intelligence may be normal in mild cases. Other associated problems include the development of noncancerous tumors, especially of the brain, kidney, retina, and heart.

There is no cure for tuberous sclerosis. Treatment is aimed at relieving troublesome symptoms, including treatment of epilepsy and removal of tumors. Seriously affected people may not live beyond age 30. *Genetic counseling* is recommended for affected families who are considering children. The gene for tuberous sclerosis can now be detected at an early stage in pregnancy.

Tuboplasty

An operation in which a damaged fallopian tube is repaired to treat infertility. Tuboplasty is performed if a tube has become scarred and blocked, usually following *salpingitis* (tubal infection) or *pelvic inflammatory disease*.

In performing tuboplasty, the gynecologist usually uses *microsurgery* techniques to unblock the delicate tubes. Recently, the use of balloon tuboplasty has been introduced.

The fertility rate following tuboplasty varies from 5 to 50 percent, depending on how badly the tube was damaged to start with and whether other causes of infertility exist. *Ectopic pregnancy* is more common in women who have had diseased tubes or tuboplasty than in those with healthy fallopian tubes.

T

PROCEDURE FOR BALLOON TUBOPLASTY

A blocked fallopian tube may be treated by inserting a balloon catheter into the damaged tube and inflating the balloon. The balloon is then deflated and the catheter withdrawn.

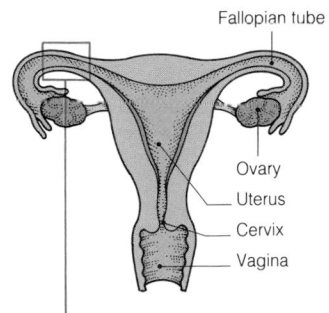

Fallopian tube
Ovary
Uterus
Cervix
Vagina

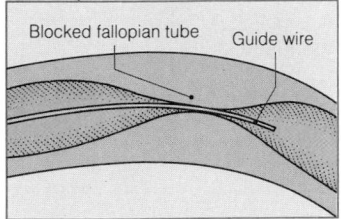

Blocked fallopian tube
Guide wire

1 A thin guide wire is maneuvered along the fallopian tube to the blockage and the tip of the wire is forced through the constricted area.

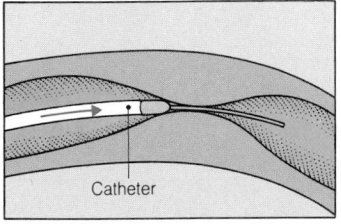

Catheter

2 A balloon-tipped catheter is threaded over the guide wire until the balloon strikes the blockage; the balloon is then inflated.

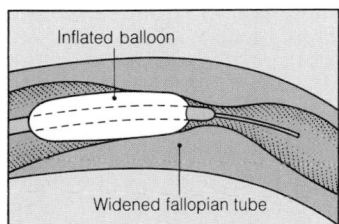

Inflated balloon
Widened fallopian tube

3 The inflated balloon is pushed against the obstructed part. Gradually the blockage widens until the balloon can be pushed through.

Tularemia

An infectious disease of wild animals, such as rabbits, squirrels, and muskrats. Tularemia is occasionally transmitted to humans.

CAUSES AND INCIDENCE

Humans may be infected through direct contact with an infected animal or its carcass, in which case the causative bacteria enter the body via a cut or abrasion in the skin. Tularemia can also be acquired through a bite from an infected tick, flea, fly, or louse or, in rare cases, by eating infected meat.

Tularemia occurs only in North America and some parts of Europe and Asia. A few hundred cases are reported annually in the US. A vaccine is available for people at highest risk, such as hunters, trappers, game wardens, and laboratory workers.

SYMPTOMS, DIAGNOSIS, AND TREATMENT

In most cases, a red spot develops on the skin at the site of infection, grows larger, and forms an ulcer. The lymph nodes in the armpits or groin enlarge and become tender, and there is a fever and often a headache, muscle pains, and malaise. The illness may continue for several weeks. In other cases, the eyes, throat, digestive tract, or lungs are affected.

Tularemia is diagnosed by a blood test that detects antibodies formed against the bacteria. Treatment is with *antibiotic drugs*, such as streptomycin. Without treatment, tularemia is fatal in about 5 percent of cases; with treatment, the fatality rate is less than 1 percent. One attack protects against future disease.

Tumbu fly bites

A cause of *myiasis* (skin infestation with fly larvae) in Africa.

Tumor

By strict definition, any swelling. Also known as a neoplasm, a tumor is an abnormal mass of tissue that forms when cells in a specific area reproduce at an increased rate.

Tumors may be *malignant* or *benign*. Malignant tumors invade surrounding tissues and may also spread via the bloodstream or lymphatic system to form a secondary growth (called a *metastasis*) elsewhere in the body. *Cancer* is the general term used to refer to all types of malignant tumors. A malignant tumor that arises from epithelial tissues (such as skin) is termed a *carcinoma*; one that arises from deep body tissues (such as muscle, bone, or fibrous tissue) is called a *sarcoma*.

Benign tumors usually grow slowly and do not metastasize, although they may sometimes be multiple. They tend to remain confined within a fibrous capsule, making surgical removal relatively straightforward. However, benign tumors may grow large enough to cause damage by pressing on nearby structures, which can be particularly dangerous in confined spaces, such as inside the skull.

At the microscopic level, one essential difference between benign and malignant tumors is that the former retain many of the features of the tissue from which they arose. In contrast, malignant tumors tend to comprise small, rapidly growing cells that form masses of tissue with less recognizable features of the tissue from which they originated.

Tumor-specific antigen

A substance secreted by a specific type of tumor (or class of tumors) that is detectable in the blood. Tumor-specific antigens cannot be used accurately to screen for malignant tumors because most can also be produced in nonmalignant conditions.

Two tumor-specific antigens are carcinoembryonic antigen and *alpha-fetoprotein*. Carcinoembryonic antigen is produced in abnormal amounts by about half of the tumors of the colon, stomach, breast, lungs, and pancreas. Alpha-fetoprotein levels in blood serum are raised in 70 percent of the people who have hepatoma (a primary *liver cancer*) and in most people with teratoma, a type of testicular cancer (see *Testis, cancer of*).

Tunnel vision

Constriction of the *visual field*; only objects straight ahead can be seen.

CAUSES

The most common cause of tunnel vision is chronic *glaucoma*, in which raised pressure within the eye results in destruction of *optic nerve* fibers. Peripheral vision is gradually lost until the visual field is reduced to only a few degrees across.

Tunnel vision may also be caused by a tumor or other brain disorder that interferes with the fibers that connect the *optic nerve* to the brain. Pituitary tumors, for instance, can press on the point where the optic nerves come together, causing loss of the right half of the right eye's field of vision and the left half of the left eye's vision. *Retinitis pigmentosa* (retinal degeneration) may cause the loss of peripheral vision and result in tunnel vision.

T

Turner's syndrome

A disorder caused by a *chromosomal abnormality* that affects only females.

INCIDENCE AND CAUSES

Approximately one in 3,000 live-born girls is born with Turner's syndrome. The chromosomal abnormality may arise in one of three ways. Most affected females have only 45 chromosomes compared with the normal complement of 46, the missing chromosome being one of the X chromosomes. Sometimes, both X chromosomes are present but one is defective. Occasionally, the condition arises as a type of *mosaicism*, in which some cells are missing one X chromosome, some have extra chromosomes, and others have their normal number of chromosomes.

SIGNS

The main features of the syndrome are shortness of stature, webbing of the skin of the neck, absence or very retarded development of secondary sexual characteristics (see *Sexual characteristics, secondary*), absence of menstruation, coarctation (narrowing) of the aorta, abnormalities of the eyes and bones, and a degree of mental retardation. The average adult height is 4 feet 6 inches (135 cm).

TREATMENT

Coarctation of the aorta is treated by surgery at an early age. Menstruation may be induced by *estrogen drugs* but sufferers continue to be infertile.

Twins

Two infants resulting from one pregnancy. Twins may develop from a single ovum (egg) or from two ova.

Monozygotic or monovular (identical) twins develop when a single, fertilized ovum divides completely and equally at an early stage of development; if this division is incomplete it results in *Siamese twins*. Monozygotic twins share the same placenta. Although one is often much bigger than the other at birth, they are always of the same sex and look remarkably alike, hence their common name of identical twins.

Twins from two ova are called dizygotic or binovular twins. The ova from which they develop may be released by the same or different ovaries; fertilization of the two ova occurs simultaneously. Each dizygotic twin has its own placenta. The twins may be of the same or different sexes, and may look quite different.

Twins occur in about one in 90 pregnancies. Dizygotic twins are more likely to occur in older women, in

TWO TYPES OF TWINS

During each menstrual cycle, either one ovum or a small number of ova may be released. If one ovum is fertilized and the two cells formed from its first division develop independently, the result is identical twins. If two ova are fertilized and mature normally, nonidentical twins result.

IDENTICAL TWINS

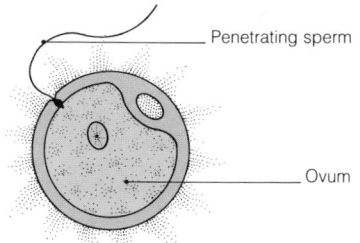

Penetrating sperm

Ovum

Identical twins come from a single fertilized ovum. When the ovum splits, the two cells formed develop independently.

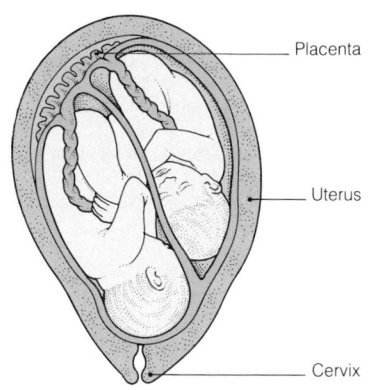

Placenta

Uterus

Cervix

The result is a pair of genetically identical twins sharing the same placenta. They are called monovular or monozygotic.

NONIDENTICAL TWINS

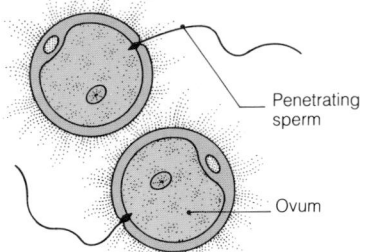

Penetrating sperm

Ovum

Nonidentical twins come from two separate ova that have been fertilized by two separate spermatozoa.

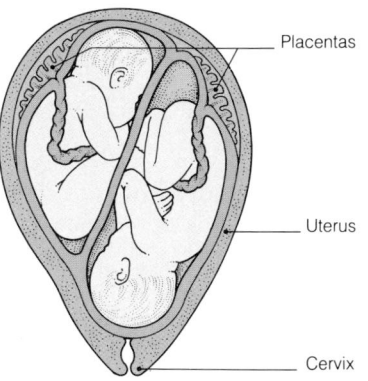

Placentas

Uterus

Cervix

The resulting individuals are genetically distinct and have separate placentas. They are dizygotic, or binovular, twins.

women who have had many previous pregnancies, and in women who have a history of twins in the family; they are also more common in Africa and Asia. These factors do not have any bearing on the incidence of monozygotic twins.

Twins face greater difficulties from the start. Deaths are more frequent before, during, or just after birth. When rearing twins, especially monozygotic twins, it is important to reinforce their importance as separate people. (See also *Pregnancy, multiple*.)

Twins, conjoined

Another name for *Siamese twins*.

Twitch

See *Fasciculation; Tic*.

Tympanometry

A type of *hearing test*, also called impedance audiometry.

Tympanoplasty

An operation to repair a hole in the eardrum and/or ossicles (the tiny bones in the middle ear) to treat hearing loss.

WHY IT IS DONE

In a healthy ear, sound waves are conducted from the eardrum to the oval window of the inner ear by a chain of three bones called ossicles (see *Ear*). Chronic *otitis media* (middle-ear infection) can fuse these bones in position or erode them, in either case interfering with sound conduction and thus causing some degree of conductive hearing loss. In such cases tympanoplasty offers the only chance of restoring some of the lost hearing.

HOW IT IS DONE

An incision is made adjacent to the eardrum (using general anesthesia) to provide access to the middle ear. Viewing the ear through an operating microscope, the surgeon then repositions or repairs the chain of ossicles. This may involve reshaping and transposing one of the bones, replacing an ossicle with a plastic substitute, grafting an ossicle taken from a donor, or fashioning an ossicle from cartilage. The bones are reset in their natural order and the eardrum is repaired.

RESULTS

The operation often improves hearing considerably, but there is no guarantee of success, especially in cases where poor eustachian tube function causes the eardrum to adhere to the ossicles. (See also *Myringoplasty; Stapedectomy*.)

Tympanum

Part of the *ear*, comprising the middle-ear cavity (tympanic cavity) and eardrum (tympanic membrane).

Typhoid fever

An infectious disease contracted by eating food or drinking water that has been contaminated with the bacterium *SALMONELLA TYPHOSA*. An almost identical disease, known as *paratyphoid fever*, is caused by a related bacterium.

CAUSES AND INCIDENCE

The source of infection is the feces of a person who has the disease or is a symptomless carrier of the causative bacteria. In areas of poor sanitation, typhoid is commonly spread by contamination of drinking water with sewage, or by flies carrying the bacteria from infected feces to food. Elsewhere, infection is usually due to handling of food by typhoid carriers. Shellfish that have been contaminated by sewage are an occasional source of typhoid outbreaks.

During the development of the disease, the bacteria pass from the intestines into the blood, and then to the spleen and liver, where they multiply. The organisms are excreted from the liver, accumulate in the gallbladder, and are released in enormous numbers into the intestine. Carriers, after recovering from typhoid fever, may continue to harbor typhoid bacilli in the gallbladder and shed them in the feces for many years.

Typhoid is uncommon in developed countries but epidemics occur regularly in developing countries. There are fewer than 600 cases per year in the US.

PREVENTION

Typhoid is a reportable disease and known cases should be isolated. Immunization against typhoid is recommended for travel anywhere outside of the US and Canada, northern Europe, Australia, and New Zealand. The vaccine is given in two doses, often causing some swelling and pain at the site of injection for one to two days. A booster dose is needed after two to three years. The vaccine does not provide complete protection; travelers at risk should drink only boiled water or bottled drinks and eat well-cooked food.

SYMPTOMS AND SIGNS

Typhoid has an incubation period of seven to 14 days. The course of the infection varies from a mild upset to a major life-threatening illness. The first symptom is usually severe headache, followed by fever, loss of appetite, malaise, abdominal tenderness, constipation, and often delirium. Constipation soon gives way to diarrhea. During the second week of the illness, small, raised pink spots appear on the chest and abdomen for several days; there is also enlargement of the liver and spleen at this time.

The illness usually clears up within four weeks. However, if treatment is delayed, severe, sometimes fatal, complications may develop, including intestinal bleeding, *urinary tract infection, renal failure*, or perforation of the intestine leading to *peritonitis*.

DIAGNOSIS AND TREATMENT

The diagnosis is confirmed by obtaining a *culture* of typhoid bacteria from a sample of blood, feces, or urine, or by a *blood test* that reveals the presence of antibodies against typhoid bacteria.

The *antibiotic drugs* chloramphenicol or ampicillin usually bring the disease under control within a few days; severely ill patients may require brief supplementary treatment with *corticosteroid drugs*.

The complication of intestinal perforation is the principal risk, but can be avoided by adequate control with antibiotics. An operation may be needed if widespread peritonitis or severe bleeding develops.

Given early diagnosis and proper treatment, the outlook is usually excellent. Permanent immunity most often follows an attack of typhoid, although relapses are common if the disease is not fully eradicated by thorough antibiotic treatment.

Typhus

Any of a group of infectious diseases, with similar symptoms, caused by rickettsiae (microorganisms similar to bacteria) and spread by insects or similar animals.

TYPES, CAUSES, AND INCIDENCE

Historically, the most important type was epidemic typhus, spread by body lice. It once occurred in epidemics that killed hundreds of thousands during war, famine, or other natural disasters. Today it is rare except in some highland areas of tropical Africa and South America. Lice ingest the causative organism, *RICKETTSIA PROWAZEKI*, from the blood of infected people and deposit feces containing the microorganisms onto the skin of other hosts, where they enter the blood as the result of scratching.

Endemic, or murine, typhus is a disease of rats that may be spread to humans by fleas. About 50 cases occur in the US each year. Scrub typhus is spread by mites and occurs in India and Southeast Asia. *Rocky Mountain spotted fever* is a disease similar to typhus.

PREVENTION

In crowded conditions following natural disasters, epidemic typhus is prevented through control of human louse infestation with insecticides. A vaccine also exists against the disease.

Other types of typhus are avoided through measures to discourage bites by fleas, mites, or ticks (e.g., the use of protective clothing).

SYMPTOMS AND SIGNS

In epidemic typhus, severe headache, back and limb pain, coughing, and constipation develop suddenly and are followed by high fever, confusion, a rash similar to that of measles, prostration, a weak heart beat, and, often, delirium. Without treatment, death may occur from *septicemia, heart failure, renal failure*, or *pneumonia*.

Other types of typhus have similar symptoms and complications, although endemic typhus is milder.

DIAGNOSIS AND TREATMENT

Particular types of typhus fever are diagnosed by tests that can detect blood products formed in reaction to the rickettsial organisms. Typhus fevers are treated with *antibiotic drugs*. Other measures may be required to relieve severe symptoms and treat complications. Convalescence is often slow, particularly in the elderly.

Typing

See *Tissue-typing*.

T

Ulcer

An open sore on the skin or on a mucous membrane that results from the destruction of surface tissue. An ulcer may be shallow or deep and crater-shaped and is usually inflamed and painful.

Skin ulcers most commonly occur on the leg (see *Leg ulcer*), usually as the result of inadequate blood supply to or drainage from the limb. Among the rarer forms of skin ulcers are those that develop in *basal cell carcinomas*, which are a form of skin cancer.

Ulcers on mucous membranes most commonly develop within the digestive tract, occurring in the mouth (see *Mouth ulcer*), in the stomach or the duodenum (see *Peptic ulcer*), or in the small or large intestine (see *Ulcerative colitis*).

Ulcer on forehead
An ulcer in this skin area is often due to a basal cell carcinoma—a type of skin cancer that is easily treated.

Ulcers in mouth
Aphthous ulcers (canker sores) are common, painful, and are usually precipitated by stress. Most heal well without scarring.

The skin or mucous membranes of the genitalia may also be affected by ulcers (see *Genital ulceration*). Most are caused by sexually transmitted disease. Examples of this type of ulcer are hard and soft chancres (see *Chancre, hard*; *Chancroid*).

Ulcers may also develop on the cornea, the transparent covering at the front of the eyeball (see *Corneal ulcer*).

Ulceration

The formation of one or more *ulcers*.

Ulcerative colitis

Chronic inflammation and ulceration of the lining of the colon and rectum. The disease sometimes begins by affecting the rectum only.

CAUSES AND INCIDENCE
The cause of ulcerative colitis is unknown. In the US, the disease affects between 40 and 50 people per 100,000. It is most common in young and middle-aged adults.

SYMPTOMS AND SIGNS
The main symptom is bloody diarrhea; the feces may also contain pus and mucus. In severe cases, diarrhea and bleeding are extensive and there may be abdominal pain and tenderness, fever, and general malaise. The incidence of attacks varies considerably from person to person. Most commonly, attacks occur at intervals of a few months; however, in some cases, symptoms are either continuous or occur infrequently.

One of the principal dangers of severe ulcerative colitis is *anemia*, caused by loss of blood. Other complications include a toxic form of *megacolon* (a grossly distended colon), which may be life-threatening; rashes; mouth ulcers; *arthritis*; and inflammation of the eye in the form of *conjunctivitis* or *uveitis*. In addition, people whose entire colon has been inflamed for more than 10 years are at increased risk of cancer of the colon (see *Intestine, cancer of*).

DIAGNOSIS
The diagnosis is based on examination of the rectum and lower colon with a viewing instrument (see *Sigmoidoscopy*) or of the entire colon by *colonoscopy* or by a barium enema (see *Barium X-ray examinations*). During sigmoidoscopy or colonoscopy, a *biopsy* (removal of a small sample of tissue for analysis) may be performed. Samples of feces may also be taken for analysis to exclude the possibility of infection (by bacteria or parasites) as a cause of the symptoms. *Blood tests* may be required.

People who have had ulcerative colitis for many years require periodic colonoscopy and biopsy to check for the development of cancer.

TREATMENT
In most cases, medical treatment effectively controls the disease. Treatment usually consists of *corticosteroid drugs* (to control symptoms by reducing inflammation) and the *sulfonamide drug* sulfasalazine (to maintain long-term freedom from symptoms). Newer drug treatments using salicylate derivatives of sulfasalazine have recently become available.

Colectomy (surgical removal of the colon) may be required if inflammation is extensive, severe, and uncontrollable; colectomy is required by most patients who have toxic megacolon. This operation usually produces a dramatic improvement in the patient's health.

Ulcer-healing drugs

COMMON DRUGS
Histamine-2 receptor antagonists *Cimetidine Famotidine Ranitidine*
Others *Sucralfate* *Antacids*

A group of drugs used to treat and prevent *peptic ulcer*.

HOW THEY WORK
Ulcer-healing drugs work in one of two ways.

Histamine-2 receptor antagonists work by blocking the effects of histamine, an action that reduces the secretion of acid in the stomach and thus promotes the healing of ulcers.

Other ulcer-healing drugs, such as sucralfate, are believed to form a protective barrier over the ulcer, thereby allowing the underlying tissues time to heal. *Antacid drugs* taken regularly are also effective.

Ulcer-healing drugs usually relieve symptoms within one to two weeks; in most cases, the ulcer heals within eight weeks. Once healed, a maintenance dose may be prescribed. Without continuing treatment, the chance of an ulcer recurring is between 60 and 70 percent.

POSSIBLE ADVERSE EFFECTS
Adverse effects may include confusion, headaches, and dizziness. Ulcer-healing drugs may mask the symptoms of *stomach cancer*. These drugs are therefore not usually prescribed for periods longer than two months unless the possibility of cancer has been ruled out.

Ulna

The longer of the two bones of the forearm; the other is the *radius*. With the palm facing forward, the ulna is the inner bone (i.e., the bone nearer the trunk) running down the forearm parallel to the radius.

LOCATION OF THE ULNA
The ulna hinges at the elbow on the inner side of the lower end of the humerus (upper arm bone). It is less mobile than the radius.

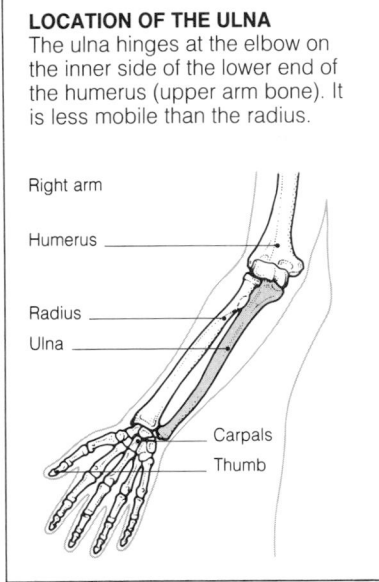

Right arm

Humerus

Radius

Ulna

Carpals

Thumb

The upper end of the ulna articulates with the radius and extends into a rounded projection (called the olecranon process) that fits around the lower end of the humerus (upper arm bone) to form part of the *elbow* joint. The lower end of the ulna is rounded and articulates with the carpals (*wrist* bones) and lower part of the radius.

Ulna, fracture of

Fractures of the *ulna* typically occur across the shaft or at the olecranon process (tip of the elbow).

A shaft fracture is usually caused by a blow to the forearm or a fall onto the hand. In some cases, the radius is fractured at the same time (see *Radius, fracture of*). An operation is usually needed to reposition the broken bone ends and fix them together, using either a plate and screws or a long nail down the center of the bone. The arm is then immobilized in a plaster cast, with the elbow at a right angle, until the fracture heals.

A fracture of the olecranon process is usually caused by a fall onto the elbow. If the bone ends are not displaced, the arm is immobilized in a plaster cast with the elbow at a right-angle. Otherwise, an operation is

needed before immobilization. If the bone ends are displaced, they are fitted together and fixed with a metal screw; if the bone is broken into several pieces, the bone fragments are removed and the triceps muscle reattached to the broken end of the ulna.

Ulnar nerve

One of the principal nerves of the arm, running down its full length into the hand. A branch of the *brachial plexus*, the ulnar nerve controls muscles that move the thumb and fingers. It also conveys sensation from the fifth and part of the fourth fingers, and from the palm at the base of these digits.

DISORDERS

A blow to the *olecranon* process (the bony prominence at the tip of the elbow), over which the ulnar nerve passes, causes a pins and needles sensation and pain in the forearm and fourth and fifth fingers.

Persistent numbness and muscle weakness in the areas controlled by the nerve may be caused by pressure from an abnormal bony outgrowth from the humerus (upper arm bone). Such a growth may be due to *osteoarthritis* or to a fracture of the humerus. If an operation is not performed to relieve the pressure on the nerve, the hand muscles controlled by the nerve may become permanently damaged, resulting in a *clawhand*.

Ultrasound

Sound with a frequency greater than the human ear's upper limit of perception—that is, with a frequency higher than 20,000 hertz (cycles per second). Ultrasound used in medicine for diagnosis or treatment is typically in the frequency range of 1 million to 15 million hertz (see *Ultrasound scanning; Ultrasound treatment*).

Ultrasound scanning

A diagnostic technique in which very high frequency sound waves (inaudible to the human ear) are passed into the body; the reflected echoes are detected and analyzed to build a picture of the internal organs or of a fetus in the uterus. The procedure is considered painless and safe.

Also called sonography, ultrasound scanning was originally a spin-off from naval sonar (used to detect submarines in World War II) and was first used medically in the 1950s. The original ultrasound scanners produced still images; most modern scanners produce moving pictures, which are easier to interpret.

HOW IT WORKS

The illustrated box (next page) explains how ultrasound scanners work and are operated.

WHY IT IS DONE

Ultrasound waves pass readily through soft tissues and fluids, making this procedure particularly useful for examining fluid-filled organs (such as the uterus in pregnancy and the gallbladder) and soft organs (such as the liver). Ultrasound waves cannot, however, pass through bone or gas. They are thus of limited use for examining regions that are surrounded by bone (such as the brain) or that contain gas (such as the lungs or intestines). Nevertheless, ultrasound has been used to examine most parts of the anatomy.

OBSTETRIC USES One of the most common uses of ultrasound is to view the uterus and fetus in pregnancy.

Ultrasound scanning is often performed about 16 to 18 weeks into the pregnancy. If the date of conception is known, the scan shows whether the fetus is of the expected size; fetal size can also help establish the accurate date of conception. The scan also reveals whether there is a multiple pregnancy (see *Pregnancy, multiple*). It is also possible to identify certain gross abnormalities, such as *anencephaly* or *spina bifida*. Congenital *heart disease* can sometimes be detected, enabling the baby to be delivered in a hospital that specializes in correcting such defects. The scan also shows the position of the placenta. If the placenta is in a position that could obstruct normal childbirth (*placenta previa*), delivery by *cesarean section* may be necessary.

Scans earlier in pregnancy may be performed to establish viability (whether the fetus is alive) if the physician suspects an *ectopic pregnancy* (presence of an embryo outside the uterus), *hydatidiform mole* (abnormal tumor in the uterus), impending *miscarriage*, or early fetal death.

Ultrasound is also vital for the procedure of *amniocentesis* (removal of amniotic fluid via a needle for analysis) and is used during *chorionic villus sampling* (removal of tissue from the placenta for analysis). A scan shows the position of the fetus and placenta before the procedure and also helps the physician guide the needle into the uterus.

Later in pregnancy, a scan may be carried out if the growth rate of the fetus seems slow, if fetal movements cease or are excessive, or if the mother experiences vaginal bleeding. For

U

HOW ULTRASOUND SCANNING WORKS

Ultrasound waves are emitted by a device called a transducer, which is placed on the skin over the part of the body to be viewed. The transducer contains a crystal that converts an electrical current into sound waves. The waves used have frequencies in the range of 2.5 to 10 million hertz. At these high frequencies, the waves can be focused into a fine parallel beam, which passes through a "slice" of the body if the transducer crystal is made to oscillate back and forth. Some of the waves are reflected at tissue boundaries, so a series of echoes is returned. The transducer also acts as a receiver, converting these echoes into electrical signals, which are processed and displayed on a screen to give a two-dimensional image of the scanned body slice. By moving the transducer, different slices through the body can be seen.

Operator · Monitor · Arm · Head · Heart · Trunk · Leg · Transducer

Ultrasound has wide applications in medicine and is especially useful in obstetrics. It offers no known risk to the baby. By moving the transducer across the outer wall of the abdomen, views of the growing fetus are obtained from various angles, so it is possible to screen for abnormalities.

Transducer · Monitor · Electronic hardware · Ultrasound wave beams · Image

Parts of an ultrasound scanner
The transducer emits a beam of high frequency waves, which are passed through a slice of the body; the echoes are picked up by the transducer and converted by the electronic hardware into an image displayed on the cathode-ray tube viewing monitor.

Echocardiography is a type of ultrasound technique used to look at the heart; it is particularly useful for investigating congenital heart disease and disorders of the heart valves.

The liver can be clearly viewed by ultrasound, which can be used to diagnose *cirrhosis* and liver cysts, abscesses, or tumors. *Gallstones* in the gallbladder or bile ducts are visible; in a patient with *jaundice*, a scan can help establish whether the jaundice is due to obstruction of the bile ducts or liver disease. The pancreas can be scanned for cysts, tumors, or pancreatitis, and the kidneys for congenital defects, cysts, tumors, and *hydronephrosis* (swelling due to obstruction to the outflow of urine). Other organs that may be scanned by ultrasound for diagnostic purposes (primarily to look for cysts, solid tumors, or foreign bodies) include the thyroid gland, breasts, bladder, testes, ovaries, spleen, and eyes.

Doppler ultrasound is a modified version of ordinary ultrasound that is used for looking at moving objects, such as blood coursing through the blood vessels and the fetal heart beat in pregnancy (see *Doppler effect*).

Ultrasound scanning is also being used more frequently in conjunction with fine needle *biopsy* (inserting a very thin hollow needle into an organ to remove cells, tissue, or fluid for examination) to help guide the needle accurately to a specific spot.

HOW IT IS DONE

For a scan in early pregnancy, the woman is usually asked not to pass urine for a few hours beforehand; a full bladder helps improve the view of the uterus by displacing nearby loops of intestine. For a liver or gallbladder scan, the patient is usually asked to fast for several hours beforehand.

Clothing over the area to be scanned is removed and oil or jelly is smeared over the skin to achieve good contact as the transducer is passed back and forth over the skin. During the scan, which takes about 15 minutes, the patient can usually lie back and watch the images appearing on the screen.

The ultrasonic waves produce no detectable sensation. When a scan is performed in conjunction with a technique involving insertion of a needle, a local anesthetic is used and there is usually little or no discomfort.

Ultrasound treatment

The use of high-frequency sound waves to treat injuries to soft tissues, such as ligaments, muscles, and ten-

high-risk or overdue pregnancies, a predelivery scan may be carried out to check on fetal size, development, and position in the uterus, the amount of amniotic fluid, and to recheck the position of the placenta.

NONOBSTETRIC USES In the newborn child, ultrasound can be used to scan the brain, via a gap (the anterior fontanelle) in the skull, to investigate *hydrocephalus*, or to diagnose a *brain tumor* or brain hemorrhage.

dons. The treatment reduces inflammation and speeds up healing. It is thought to work by improving blood flow through tissues under the skin.

During treatment, there may be a feeling of warmth and a slight tingling sensation. Occasionally, severe pain occurs if the sound waves are pointed at a bone surface just under the skin.

Ultraviolet light

Invisible light from the part of the electromagnetic spectrum immediately beyond the violet end of the visible light spectrum (that is, between visible light and X rays). Long wavelength ultraviolet light (that nearest visible light) is often termed UVA; intermediate wavelength ultraviolet light is designated UVB; and short wavelength ultraviolet light (that nearest X rays) is called UVC.

ELECTROMAGNETIC SPECTRUM

Ultraviolet light in the spectrum
Different types of electromagnetic radiation are defined according to their wavelengths. The diagram shows the different types within the electromagnetic spectrum, together with their wavelength limits (in nanometers, or billionths of a meter). Ultraviolet light falls in the band between visible light and extreme short wavelength radiation, such as X rays.

Ultraviolet light occurs naturally in sunlight, but most of it—including all UVC and much UVB (both of which are potentially harmful)—is absorbed by the *ozone* layer of the atmosphere. The ultraviolet light that reaches the earth's surface, mainly UVA, is responsible for the tanning and burning effects of sunlight and for the production of vitamin D in the skin. However, it is the ultraviolet component of sunlight, particularly the relatively small proportion of UVB, that can cause cataracts and, especially in fair-skinned people, skin cancer (see *Sunlight, adverse effects of*).

Suntanning lamps, which produce ultraviolet light artificially, are designed to emit only UVA rays, although, in practice, they also give off a small amount of UVB light.

A mercury-vapor lamp (Wood's light) can also be used to produce ultraviolet light artificially. This light is used to diagnose certain skin conditions, such as *tinea*, because it causes the infected area to fluoresce.

Ultraviolet light may also be used in *phototherapy* to treat certain skin conditions, including *psoriasis, vitiligo,* and *jaundice* of the newborn.

Umbilical cord

The ropelike structure connecting the fetus to the *placenta* that supplies oxygen and nutrients from the mother's circulation. The umbilical cord is usually 16 to 24 inches (40 to 60 cm) long and consists of a jellylike substance in which two arteries and a vein are embedded.

Several minutes after delivery, the umbilical cord is clamped and then cut about an inch from the baby's abdominal wall. The stump falls off within a couple of weeks, leaving a scar called the *umbilicus* (navel).

DISORDERS

In rare cases, the umbilical cord prolapses (protrudes down) through the mother's cervix during labor. This is a dangerous condition because the baby's oxygen supply can be cut off. Prompt delivery of the infant, either by *cesarean section* or a *forceps delivery*, is necessary. Sometimes the cord pulls tightly around the baby's neck during delivery; it can usually be freed easily by slipping it over the baby's head.

Rarely, there is only one artery in the umbilical cord. This condition may be associated with birth defects.

The newborn baby's umbilical stump sometimes becomes infected and may ooze pus. This condition, called omphalitis, generally begins

Umbilical cord after birth
The cord ceases to function after birth and is clamped and cut; the baby now obtains oxygen through his or her own lungs.

during the first week of life. Treatment involves gently wiping the umbilicus with sterile cotton and water. Treatment with antibiotics may be necessary to prevent serious infection.

Quite commonly, a fleshy protuberance called a *granuloma* grows on the umbilical stump, sometimes as a result of chronic infection. Umbilical granulomas may be removed by local application of *silver nitrate*. Umbilical polyps, also known as umbilical adenomas, are shiny, bright red, raspberrylike growths that also appear in the newborn period. They may require surgical removal.

Umbilicus

The scar on the abdomen that marks the site of attachment of the *umbilical cord* to the fetus. The umbilicus is commonly called the navel.

DISORDERS

An umbilical *hernia* is a soft swelling at the umbilicus caused by protrusion of the abdominal contents through a weak area of the abdominal wall.

Umbilical hernias are quite common in newborns, occurring twice as often in boys. When the baby cries, the

Umbilical hernia
This condition, present from birth, is due to a local weakness in the abdominal wall. Recovery without treatment is usual.

U

swelling increases in size and may cause discomfort. Umbilical hernias usually disappear without treatment by about age 2. They are unlikely to disappear without treatment after about age 4.

Occasionally, umbilical hernias develop in adults, especially in women following childbirth. Surgery may be necessary for large, persistent, or disfiguring hernias.

In rare cases, there may be a discharge from the umbilicus. It can be caused by an infection or by an abnormal connection between the umbilicus and the urinary, biliary, or intestinal tract. The abnormal connection may be due to a birth defect, to cancer, or to tuberculosis. Surgery is used to correct this condition.

Occasionally, benign or malignant tumors develop at the umbilicus. These tumors may be secondary to cancers in the breast, colon, ovary, or stomach. In women, *endometriosis* may in rare cases develop in the umbilicus, which bleeds at periodic intervals. The treatment is surgical excision.

Unconscious

A specific part of the mind in which ideas, memories, perceptions, or feelings that a person is not currently aware of are stored and actively processed. The contents of the unconscious mind are not easily retrievable, in contrast to those of the *subconscious*. *Freudian theory* stresses the importance of the unconscious in determining behavior and causing neurotic symptoms. *Jungian theory* describes a collective unconscious, inherited by every person and derived from experiences in our distant past.

Unconsciousness

Abnormal loss of awareness of self and of the surroundings resulting from a reduced level of activity of the reticular formation in the *brain stem*. Sleep is a normal state of altered consciousness from which a person can be roused easily; an unconscious person can be roused only with difficulty or not at all. Unconsciousness may be brief and light, as in *fainting*, or deeper and more prolonged (see *Coma*). The term *concussion* refers to a brief transient state of unconsciousness following a head injury.

Underbite

A term that describes a type of *malocclusion* in which the lower jaw is set abnormally forward, which causes the lower incisors to overlap the upper incisors.

Unsaturated fats

See *Fats and oils*.

Uranium

A radioactive metallic element that does not occur naturally in its pure form but is widely distributed as various compounds in ores such as pitchblende, carnotite, and uraninite.

Natural radioactive decay of uranium yields a series of radioactive products, including *radium* and *radon*, and progresses ultimately to lead. During the various decay stages, *radiation* is emitted as alpha and beta particles and gamma rays. In addition to its *radiation hazards*, uranium is chemically poisonous in the body, where it damages the urinary system.

Urea

A waste product of the breakdown of proteins and the main nitrogenous (nitrogen-containing) constituent of urine. Proteins in food are digested in the intestine to form *amino acids*, which are absorbed into the bloodstream and transported to the liver. In the liver, amino acids in excess of the body's requirements are converted into urea, which is transported by the bloodstream to the kidneys and excreted in the urine.

The kidneys are usually highly efficient at eliminating urea from the body. A high-protein diet increases the amount of urea produced. Healthy kidneys are able to cope with increased urea production, but *renal failure* impairs the kidneys' ability to eliminate urea and leads to uremia (abnormally high blood levels of urea). For this reason, measuring

FIRST AID: UNCONSCIOUSNESS

DO NOT
- leave an unconscious person alone
- give anyone who is, or has been, unconscious anything to eat or drink

1 Make sure the victim is breathing. If breathing sounds difficult, check the airways and quickly clear the mouth.

2 If the victim is not breathing, start *artificial respiration*. Loosen any tight clothing he or she is wearing.

3 Once normal breathing has resumed, place the victim in the *recovery position*. Cover with a blanket. Seek medical help, but do not leave the victim alone.

U

blood levels of urea is one of the routine kidney function tests.

Urea is also formed in the body from the breakdown of cell proteins. If there is a large increase in urea from this source (e.g., due to severe tissue damage from injury or surgery), the kidneys are sometimes unable to cope and uremia results.

Certain conditions (such as liver damage) may lead to a decrease in the blood level of urea. Blood levels of urea also fall during pregnancy, when the blood is more dilute than usual.

MEDICAL USES

Urea is used in various creams and ointments to moisturize and soften the skin in the treatment of disorders such as *psoriasis*, atopic *dermatitis*, *ichthyosis*, and other conditions in which the skin is dry and scaly. Occasionally, urea is used as an osmotic *diuretic drug*, primarily to reduce pressure in the skull due to cerebral *edema* or pressure in the eye caused by *glaucoma*.

Uremia

The presence of excess urea and other chemical waste products in the blood. Uremia develops as a result of kidney failure (see *Renal failure*).

Ureter

Either of the two tubes that carry urine from the kidneys to the bladder. Each is about 10 to 12 inches (25 to 30 cm) long. The walls of each ureter have three layers—a fibrous outer layer, a muscular middle layer, and an inner membrane. Each ureter is supplied by blood vessels and nerves.

Urine flows down the ureters partly by gravity but mainly by peristalsis, a pumping action as waves of contraction pass several times per minute through the muscle layers in the ureteral walls. Each ureter enters the bladder via a tunnel in the bladder wall, which is angled to prevent reflux of urine back into the ureter when the bladder muscle contracts.

DISORDERS

Some people are born with two ureters on one or both sides. A double ureter is usually accompanied by partial duplication of the kidney on that side. The two ureters may join farther down (to form a Y shape) or may be completely distinct. In many cases, a duplicated ureter causes no problems. However, when the ureters enter the bladder separately, there may be a tendency for urine to reflux up one of the tubes; when a ureter enters the urethra or vagina instead of the blad-

---

ANATOMY OF THE URETER

The ureters are tubes that carry urine from the kidneys to the bladder. They enter the back of the bladder at an angle.

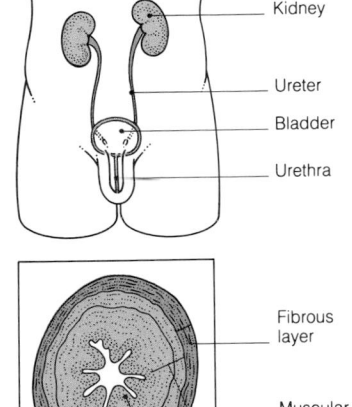

- Kidney
- Ureter
- Bladder
- Urethra

- Fibrous layer
- Muscular layer
- Mucous layer

Cross section
Each ureter has three layers—an outer, fibrous layer, a thick, muscular middle layer, and an inner, mucous membrane.

---

der at its lower end, it can cause *incontinence* or infection. These problems can be corrected surgically.

If a urinary tract *calculus* (stone) passes down or becomes stuck in a ureter, it can lead to spasms of the muscles in the ureteral walls, an extremely painful condition known as *renal colic*.

Ureteritis is an inflammatory condition of a ureter that may be caused by blockage with a stone or by infection spreading up from the bladder.

Ureteral colic

See *Renal colic*.

Ureterolithotomy

The surgical removal of a urinary tract *calculus* (stone) stuck in a ureter (tube that carries urine from a kidney to the bladder). The stone is removed if it is causing recurrent attacks of *renal colic* (severe pain in the loin area) or obstruction to urine flow from a kidney, which can rapidly lead to kidney damage.

Before the operation, intravenous *pyelography* is carried out to locate the stone. An incision is made in the patient's abdomen with the use of a general anesthetic, and the surgeon feels the ureter for the stone. The ure-

---

ter is then opened with a longitudinal cut, the stone is removed with forceps, and a check is made for more stones. The ureter and abdomen are then sewn up, leaving a tube inserted into the abdomen to drain any urine that leaks from the ureter. This tube is removed four or five days later and the patient can then leave the hospital.

Ureterolithotomy is not the only method of dealing with ureteral stones. Stones at the lower end of the ureter can sometimes be removed, after crushing, by means of *cystoscopy* (passage of a viewing tube into the bladder via the urethra). Stones at the top end may be dealt with by shock-wave *lithotripsy* (shattering of stones).

Urethra

The tube by which urine is excreted from the bladder. In females, the urethra is short and opens to the outside just in front of the vagina between the labia minora. In males, the urethra is much longer. It is surrounded by the prostate gland at its upper end and then forms a channel through the length of the penis. The location and relative length of the male and female urethras are shown in the illustrated box (overleaf).

DISORDERS

Although urethral infections, scarring, and congenital abnormalities occur in both sexes, these disorders are much more common and serious in males than in females.

In male infants, a urethral valve is sometimes present. The valve flap arises from the lining of the urethra and impedes the flow of urine. The resulting bottleneck causes back pressure on the kidneys as urine fills the bladder, ureters, and collecting ducts of the kidneys. Permanent and severe damage to the kidneys can occur if the urethral valve is not removed surgically.

Urethritis (inflammation of the urethra) may be due to infection, irritation, or minor injury. Inflammation may be followed by scarring and formation of a *urethral stricture* (a narrowed section of the urethra).

The male urethra is easily damaged in accidents involving pelvic injury and may require surgical repair, again with a risk of a urethral stricture.

Urethral dilatation

Widening of a *urethral stricture* (narrowed urethra) in a male by means of a slim, round-tipped instrument inserted through the opening of the urethra at the tip of the penis.

U

LOCATION OF THE URETHRA

The urethra is the tube through which urine is passed from the bladder. There is no voluntary muscle in the urethra. The flow of urine is controlled by muscles in the bladder wall and outlet.

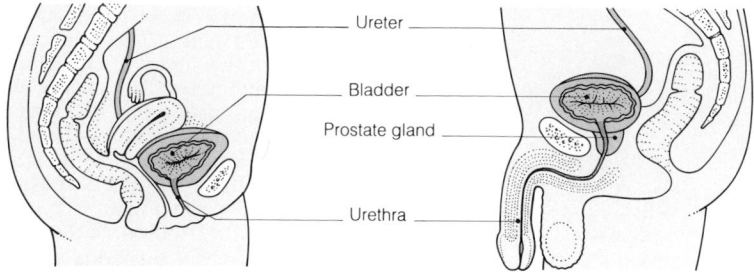

Ureter
Bladder
Prostate gland
Urethra

Urethra in a woman
The female urethra is short—about an inch and a half (4 cm) long—and runs down to open to the exterior just in front of the vagina.

Urethra in a man
The male urethra is about 9 inches (23 cm) long and passes through the prostate gland and along the full length of the penis.

Urethral discharge

A fluid that flows from the urethra in some cases of *urethritis* caused by infection. In gonorrhea, the discharge is yellow and purulent (contains pus); in other types of infection the discharged fluid is clear.

Urethral stricture

An uncommon condition in which the male urethra becomes narrowed and sometimes shortened along part of its length as a result of shrinkage of scar tissue within its walls.

CAUSES AND SYMPTOMS

Scar tissue may form after injury to the urethra or after persistent *urethritis* (inflammation). Urethritis was once most commonly due to *gonorrhea*, but modern antibiotic treatment has made strictures from this cause uncommon.

A stricture can make it difficult or painful to pass urine or to ejaculate and may cause some deformation of the penis when erect. It can also cause damage to the kidneys by back pressure (buildup of fluid) and may encourage the development of a *urinary tract infection*.

TREATMENT

A stricture may be treated by urethral dilatation, in which an attempt is made to stretch and widen the tube by means of an instrument passed into it via the opening at the tip of the penis. This procedure is performed using either local or general anesthesia and may need to be repeated. If dilatation fails, an instrument called a urethrotome may be inserted to cut through the scar tissue. Alternatively, it may be possible to remove the stric-ture altogether and reconstruct the urethra with plastic surgery.

Urethral syndrome, acute

A set of symptoms of uncertain cause experienced by some women and, very rarely, by some men. The symptoms consist of pain and discomfort in the lower abdomen, a frequent urge to pass urine, and, in women, pain around the vulval region. Middle-aged women are the most commonly affected.

Usually, the physician cannot discover any causative infection, and the patient's kidney function and urinary tract anatomy are normal. Emotional and psychological factors may contribute. In women who have gone through the menopause, the symptoms may be due to inflammation of the vulva associated with thinning of tissues (see *Vulvitis*).

There is usually no effective treatment. Cases due to vulvitis may be relieved by use of *estrogen drugs* or *corticosteroid drugs* in cream form. Antiseptic creams and strong soaps should be avoided as they may cause irritation or an allergic reaction that worsens the symptoms. Scrupulous personal hygiene and a high fluid intake are usually recommended.

Urethritis

Inflammation of the urethra, usually due to an infection but sometimes with other causes.

CAUSES

Urethritis may be caused by a variety of infectious organisms, the best known of which is the bacterium that causes *gonorrhea*. *Nonspecific urethritis* may be caused by any of a large number of different types of microorganisms, including bacteria, yeasts, and *chlamydial infection*. Bacteria from the skin or rectum sometimes spread to infect the urethra.

Other causes of urethritis include trauma from an accident or from a surgically introduced catheter or cystoscope (viewing tube for examining the bladder). Irritant chemicals, such as antiseptics and some spermicidal preparations, are other possible causes of urethritis.

SYMPTOMS AND COMPLICATIONS

Urethritis causes a burning sensation and pain when passing urine. The pain can be severe and is sometimes likened to passing small fragments of broken glass. The urine may be blood-stained and, particularly when gonorrhea is the cause, there is often a yellow, pus-filled, discharge.

Urethritis may be followed by scarring and the formation of a *urethral stricture* (narrowing of a section of the urethra), which can make passing urine difficult.

TREATMENT

Gonorrhea is usually cured by penicillin or other *antibiotic drugs*. Treatment of nonspecific urethritis varies according to the causative organism, if it can be identified. Antibiotic treatment may be needed if bacterial infection follows urethritis due to a noninfective cause.

Urethral strictures are treated by the technique of *urethral dilatation*.

Urethrocele

An anatomical abnormality caused by a weakness in the tissues in the front wall of the vagina. This weakness causes the overlying urethra to bulge backward and downward into the vagina. A urethrocele may be congenital (present from birth), may develop after childbirth, or may be associated with obesity.

A urethrocele may cause difficulty emptying the bladder and pain during sexual intercourse (see *Intercourse, painful*). It also increases susceptibility to *urinary tract infection*.

The usual treatment of a urethrocele is a surgical operation to tighten the tissues at the front of the vagina, thus giving the urethra better support (see *Vaginal repair*).

-uria

A suffix relating to urine, as in *proteinuria*, the term for the presence of protein in the urine.

Uric acid

A waste product of the breakdown of *nucleic acids* in body cells. A small amount of uric acid is also produced by the digestion of foods rich in nucleic acids, such as liver, kidneys, sweetbreads, and, to a lesser extent, fish and poultry.

Most uric acid produced in the body passes, via the bloodstream, to the kidneys, which remove the acid from the blood and excrete it in the urine. However, some uric acid passes into the intestine, where it is broken down by bacteria into chemicals that are excreted in the feces.

The kidneys of a healthy person maintain blood levels of uric acid within acceptable limits. When uric acid excretion is disrupted, it may result in *hyperuricemia* (abnormally high levels of uric acid in the blood), which, in turn, may lead to *gout* or kidney stones (see *Calculi, urinary tract*). Causes of hyperuricemia include kidney disease, *leukemia*, hemolytic *anemia*, genetic disorders in which an enzyme involved in uric acid excretion is lacking, and certain drugs, including some diuretic drugs and anticancer drugs.

Urinal

A container for urine, useful for bedridden men (women use a *bedpan*). Also known as a urinal is an appliance for men suffering from urinary *incontinence*; it consists of a thick rubber tube with a hole in the end, connected by a plastic tube to a drainage bag strapped on the leg.

Urinalysis

A battery of tests on a patient's urine, including measurements of the urine's physical characteristics (such as color, concentration, and cloudiness), microscopic examination, and chemical testing. Urinalysis can help check normal kidney function or detect and diagnose urinary tract and other disorders.

Microscopic examination may reveal the presence of red blood cells in the urine, indicating damage to the glomeruli (filtering units) of the kidneys or a disorder of the remaining kidney and upper and lower urinary tract. Microscopic examination of urine may also reveal fragments of protein and kidney cells, called casts, in any of various types of kidney disease; pus or bacteria when there is a *urinary tract infection*; crystals, indicating the possibility of an inborn error of metabolism (see *Metabolism,*

Schistosome egg in urine
The tropical disease schistosomiasis may be diagnosed by the finding of schistosome (fluke) eggs on urinalysis.

inborn errors of) or susceptibility to urinary tract *calculi* (stones); and worm eggs caused by the parasitic disease *schistosomiasis*.

If a single drop of fresh urine is spread thinly on the surface of a nutrient gel and incubated, any bacteria present will multiply and produce colonies. The appearance of these colonies under microscopic examination allows the microbiologist to identify the organism causing a urinary tract infection.

A wide variety of simple stick tests is available to measure substances such as glucose in the urine (a high level usually means that the patient has *diabetes mellitus*). Other substances or properties tested for include blood, protein, bile, the acidity of urine, and its concentration (ratio of dissolved substances to water). These tests rely on a simple color change in a test patch of the stick or strip when it is dipped into the urine.

Detection of human chorionic gonadotropin in the urine is the basis of many *pregnancy tests*. (See also *Kidney function tests*.)

Urinary diversion

Any surgical procedure performed to allow passage of urine when the normal outlet channel, via the bladder and urethra, is obstructed or cannot be used, or when the bladder has been surgically removed.

TEMPORARY DIVERSION

Temporary urinary diversion is commonly required (if an indwelling catheter is not feasible) when passage of urine is blocked by enlargement of the *prostate gland* or by *urethral stricture*. In this case, a small opening is made through the abdominal wall just above the pubic bone and a tube is passed directly into the bladder (see *Catheterization, urinary*). Temporary diversion is also required after some operations on the urinary tract; a small

tube is introduced into the kidney and brought to the abdominal surface, bypassing the ureters and allowing healing to take place.

PERMANENT DIVERSION

Permanent urinary diversion is needed when the bladder has been removed, usually to treat advanced bladder cancer, or when neurological control of the bladder is severely disturbed, such as after severe spinal injury. Permanent diversion may also be required if there is an irreparable *fistula* (opening) between the bladder or urethra and the vagina.

Permanent diversion is usually achieved by creating what is known as an ileal conduit (see illustrated box, overleaf). A section of the ileum is removed to create a substitute bladder. The ureters are implanted into one end of this bladder; the other end is brought out through an incision in the abdominal wall, as in an *ileostomy*. The patient wears a bag attached to the skin to collect urine.

A variant of this method permits the patient to use a catheter to periodically empty the ileal conduit, thereby providing the person with a degree of continence.

Urinary system

See *Urinary tract* and illustrated box on *Urine* formation and excretion.

Urinary tract

The part of the body concerned with the formation and excretion of urine. The urinary tract consists of the *kidneys* (with their blood and nerve supplies), the renal pelves (funnel-shaped ducts that channel urine from the kidneys into the ureters), the *ureters*, *bladder*, and *urethra*.

The kidneys make urine by filtering blood. The urine collects in the renal pelves and then passes down the ureters into the bladder by gravity and by peristalsis (wavelike contractions of the ureteric walls). Urine is then stored in the bladder until a sufficient amount is present to stimulate micturition (passage of urine). When the bladder contracts, the urine is expelled from the body via the urethra.

Urinary tract infection

An infection anywhere in the urinary tract. *Urethritis* (inflammation of the urethra) may be caused by mechanisms other than infection, but *cystitis* (inflammation of the bladder) and *pyelonephritis* (inflammation of the kidneys) are nearly always caused by bacterial infection.

U

URINARY DIVERSION USING ILEAL CONDUIT

This is a standard operation performed when the bladder has been removed or is seriously malfunctioning and beyond hope of repair. A midline incision in the abdomen is used; before making it, the surgeon creates an opening through the abdominal wall in a good position for attaching the future collecting bag.

Midline incision

Opening for collecting bag

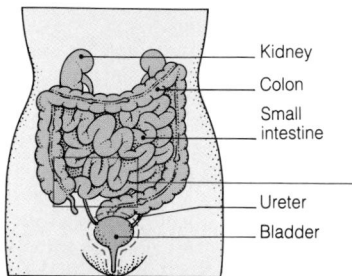

Kidney
Colon
Small intestine
Ureter
Bladder

1 A short length is cut out of the ileum (the lower part of the small intestine), retaining the mesentery (supporting folds of tissue) and the essential blood vessels that supply the freed section.

2 The cut ends of the intestine are stitched together to reestablish continuity. One end of the freed length of intestine is closed and the other end is temporarily clamped.

Umbilicus
Stoma
Ileostomy bag

3 The ureters are now implanted into the isolated length of ileum. The open end of this segment is brought through the abdominal wall and stitched in place.

4 A collecting bag for the reception of the patient's urine is fixed with adhesive around the new stoma (mouth) in the wall of the abdomen.

CAUSES

When urethritis is due to infection, the cause is usually a sexually transmitted disease, such as *gonorrhea* or nonspecific urethritis, often caused by chlamydia organisms. Otherwise, urinary tract infection is usually caused by organisms that have spread from the rectum, via the urethra, to the bladder or kidneys. Infections can also be bloodborne.

Because of the shortness of the urethra in women, infections above the urethra are more common in women than in men. In many women, they occur without any identifiable underlying cause. In most men and some women, however, there is an identifiable cause, usually some factor that impairs the drainage of urine. In men, this may be an enlarged prostate gland (see *Prostate, enlarged*) or a *urethral stricture*.

In either sex, urinary tract infection may be caused by a urinary tract *calculus* (stone), a *bladder tumor*, or a congenital abnormality of the urinary tract, such as a double kidney on one side. Defective bladder emptying as a result of *spina bifida* or spinal cord injury (see *Spinal injury*) leads almost inevitably to urinary tract infection. Urinary tract infection is also more common during pregnancy.

The risks of a urinary tract infection can be reduced by careful personal hygiene, drinking plenty of fluids, and regular emptying of the bladder.

SYMPTOMS AND COMPLICATIONS

Urethritis causes a burning sensation when passing urine. Cystitis causes a frequent urge to pass urine, lower abdominal pain, *hematuria* (blood in the urine), and often general malaise with a mild fever. An infection in the kidneys leads to pain in the loins and high fever.

Urethritis can lead to scarring of the urethra and formation of a urethral stricture. Cystitis, provided there is no upward spread to the kidneys, does not usually produce complications. Without proper treatment, kidney infection can lead to permanent kidney damage, *septicemia* (spread of infective organisms to the blood), and *septic shock*. If a calculus in a kidney is the underlying cause of infection, it may grow rapidly during the course of the infection.

DIAGNOSIS AND TREATMENT

Infection is diagnosed by a *culture* of a few drops of urine. The urine specimen is taken midstream to avoid contamination of the specimen by organisms that normally live in the last part of the urethra.

Further investigation is usually needed for men who have any urinary tract infection or for women suffering from recurrent cystitis or an infection above the level of the bladder. Such investigation is performed by *pyelography* (introduction of a radiopaque dye into the urinary tract, followed by X rays) or by *ultrasound scanning*.

Most urinary tract infections are treated with *antibiotic drugs*; the drug depends on the type of infection.

Urination, excessive

The production of more than about 5 pints (2.5 liters) of urine per day. Excessive urination is known medically as polyuria. It is usually a sign of illness.

CAUSES

Illnesses that cause excessive urination fall into several groups. First, certain psychiatric illnesses can cause a person to drink compulsively. This is called polydipsia and leads inevitably to a high urine output.

Second, a disorder of the pituitary gland that leads to reduced production of *ADH* (antidiuretic hormone) can cause a marked increase in urine volume (ADH acts on the kidneys to concentrate the urine). This is known as central *diabetes insipidus*. Alternatively, normal amounts of ADH may be produced, but the kidneys fail

U

to respond. This is called nephrogenic diabetes insipidus and can result from various diseases or damage to the kidneys.

Third, various diseases may cause abnormal amounts of certain substances to be excreted in the urine; these substances draw water with them, increasing the urine volume. The most important disease in this group is *diabetes mellitus*, in which excess glucose in the blood spills into the urine. Certain kidney diseases, known as salt-losing states, lead to too much salt being lost in the urine, with an accompanying increase in volume.

DIAGNOSIS AND TREATMENT

Any person who passes large quantities of urine should consult a physician, who may use a variety of tests to establish the cause. If the patient's water intake is restricted, urine volume soon drops in the compulsive drinker; however, this does not happen in diabetes insipidus. Central diabetes insipidus improves after administration of synthetic ADH, but nephrogenic diabetes insipidus does not. In patients with diabetes mellitus, the glucose level in the blood and urine is high; in salt-losing patients, excessive sodium is detectable in the urine.

Treatment of excessive urination depends on the underlying cause. (See also *Urination, frequent*.)

Urination, frequent

Passing urine more frequently than usual, also called simply "frequency." Most people pass urine an average of four to six times daily and only occasionally need to urinate at night. A marked increase in this rate constitutes frequency.

In some cases, frequency is the inevitable result of excessive production of urine (see *Urination, excessive*). In other cases, the total volume of urine produced is not high or may even be lower than usual.

Often the cause is *cystitis* (bladder inflammation) due to infection. A common response to this is to drink less. However, the result is a more concentrated (and thus more irritant) urine, which increases urinary frequency. Sufferers from cystitis should drink more than usual, not less.

Anxiety is a common cause of increased frequency. Other causes include *calculi* (stones) in the bladder, an enlarged prostate gland (see *Prostate, enlarged*) in men, and, in rare cases, a *bladder tumor*. Some people with *renal failure* also notice that they

pass urine more frequently, particularly at night. Treatment is always of the underlying cause.

Urination, painful

Pain or discomfort when passing urine, also known medically as dysuria. The pain is often described as having a burning or scalding quality. Sometimes it is preceded by difficulty in starting the flow. Pain after the flow has ceased, with a strong desire to continue, is called strangury.

The most common cause of dysuria is *cystitis* (inflammation of the bladder), especially in women. Dysuria may also be caused by a *bladder tumor* or *calculus* (stone), especially if blood clots or small stones or crystals are passed in the urine. Strangury is usually due to spasm of an inflamed bladder wall; it may also be caused by bladder stones.

Other possible causes of dysuria include *urethritis* (inflammation of the urethra), often due to gonorrhea; in men, *prostatitis* (inflammation of the prostate gland) or *balanitis* (inflammation of the glans of the penis); and in women, vaginal *candidiasis* (thrush) or an allergy to vaginal deodorants.

Mild discomfort when passing urine may be due to highly concentrated urine, which may occur during a fever or after heavy sweating.

Dysuria may be investigated by physical examination, *urinalysis*, and, sometimes, *pyelography*, or *cystoscopy*.

Urine

The pale yellow fluid produced by the kidneys and excreted from the body via the ureters, bladder, and urethra. Urine carries waste products, and excessive water or chemical substances, from the body.

URINE PRODUCTION

Urine is produced by the filtration of blood through the kidneys. The filtering units of the kidneys remove about 230 pints (110 liters) of watery fluid from the blood every day. Nearly all of this fluid is then reabsorbed into the blood; the remainder is passed from the body as urine.

A healthy adult may produce between about 1 and 4 pints (0.5 to 2 liters) of urine per day. The minimum volume of urine needed to remove all waste products is about 1 pint; any volume produced above this level consists of excess water. A high fluid intake increases the amount of urine produced, while a high fluid loss from sweating, vomiting, or diarrhea leads to reduced production.

COMPOSITION OF URINE (g/liter)	
Urea	20.0
Chloride	6.0
Sodium	3.0
Potassium	1.5
Phosphate	1.0
Sulfate	1.0
Creatinine	0.7
Uric acid	0.3
Glucose	0.0
Protein	0.0

Composition of urine
The chart shows normal, average contents of urine, other than water. The main waste products excreted are urea, creatinine, and uric acid. Variable amounts of sodium, chloride, hydrogen, and other ions are excreted to adjust the body's water, salt, and acid-base balance.

COMPOSITION

The average composition of urine excreted by a healthy person is shown in the chart (above).

The volume, acidity, and salt concentration of the urine are carefully regulated by hormones such as *ADH* (antidiuretic hormone), *atrial natriuretic peptide*, and *aldosterone*. These hormones act on the kidneys to ensure that the body's water, salt, and acid-base balance (acidity or alkalinity of the blood and tissue fluids) is kept within narrow limits.

Measurements of the composition of urine are useful in the diagnosis of a wide variety of conditions, from kidney disease and diabetes to pregnancy (see *Urinalysis*).

Urine is normally sterile when passed and has only a faint odor. The unpleasant smell of stale urine is due to the action of bacteria, which causes the release of ammonia. A substance called urochrome, of unknown source, gives urine its yellow color.

Urine, abnormal

Urine may be produced in abnormal amounts or may have an abnormal appearance or composition.

ABNORMAL VOLUME

Production by an adult of more than about 5 pints (2.5 liters) of urine per day is unusual unless he or she is drinking excessively or has a disease (see *Urination, excessive*).

Abnormally low urine production (*oliguria*) of less than about 0.8 pint (0.4 liters) per day may occur in severe

U

THE URINARY SYSTEM

Also known as the urinary tract, the system consists of the kidneys, in which urine is formed to carry away waste materials from the blood; the ureters, which transport the urine from the kidneys; the bladder, where the urine is stored until it can be conveniently disposed of; and the urethra, through which the bladder is emptied to the outside.

The kidneys require a large blood supply and are connected close to the body's main artery, the aorta. More than 2 pints of blood pass through the kidneys every minute.

X ray showing urinary tract

The X ray at left, taken by the technique of intravenous *pyelography*, shows (as lighter areas) the calyces and pelvis of each kidney, the ureters and bladder, as well as the bones of the lower spine and pelvic girdle.

Aorta
Vena cava
Renal vein
Renal artery
Pelvis
Calyces
Medulla
Cortex

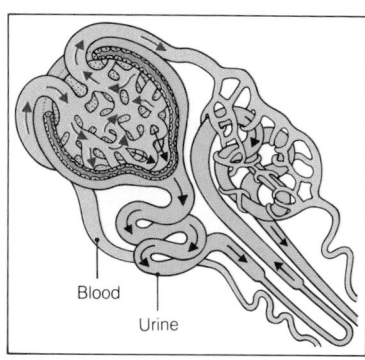

Blood
Urine

The filtering units

Each kidney has about 1 million of these units, which form dilute urine by filtering the blood.

Kidneys

The two kidneys lie within large pads of fat on the inside of the back wall of the abdomen, close to, and on either side of, the spine. Each kidney consists of an outer cortex, an inner medulla, and a urine-collecting system that includes the calyces and the pelvis of the kidney.

COMPOSITION OF URINE

Urine consists mainly of water, with small amounts of urea (the main waste product), other waste products, and salt.

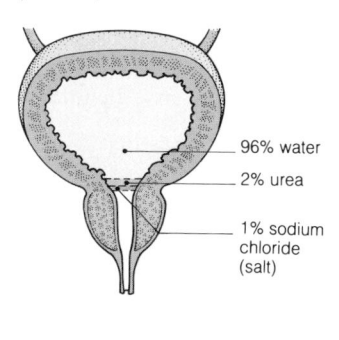

96% water

2% urea

1% sodium chloride (salt)

Collecting system

From the tubules that lead from the filtering units, much of the water and some other substances are reabsorbed into the blood. The remaining, more concentrated, urine runs into collecting ducts and then into the pyramid-shaped calyces of the kidney and the kidney pelvis. From there the urine passes into the ureter.

Ureters

Bladder

The muscular bladder wall can stretch to accommodate about a pint of urine, but at this volume the desire to pass urine is very strong.

Interior of bladder

The two ureteral openings and the urethral orifice form a triangle on the base of the bladder. In males, the urethra runs through the body of the prostate gland situated below the bladder.

Ureteral openings

Urethra

Prostate (male only)

U

dehydration and in cases of acute *renal failure*. It also occurs when the kidneys are not receiving their normal blood supply due, for example, to *heart failure, shock,* or advanced liver disease.

No production of urine by the kidneys (*anuria*) may occur in extreme cases of kidney damage. However, lack of the passage of urine from the bladder is more commonly caused by obstruction in the lower part of the urinary tract as a result of a *bladder tumor, calculus* (stone), or an enlarged prostate gland (see *Prostate, enlarged*).

ABNORMAL APPEARANCE
Cloudy urine may be due to a *urinary tract infection,* in which case it may have an offensive smell. Urinary tract *calculi* (stones) can also produce cloudy urine, which is not necessarily infected. Cloudy urine may be caused by the presence of certain salts, such as phosphates. In rare instances, lymph fluid enters the urine and gives it a milky appearance.

Slight *hematuria* (blood in the urine) produces a smoky appearance. Larger amounts of blood produce easily recognizable red urine, which may contain clots. Red urine is not always due to blood, however. Some dyes used in candy may be excreted in the urine, and a wide variety of drugs can discolor it (rifampin turns urine orange). In some patients with *porphyria,* the urine turns red if it is left to stand; in some patients with *jaundice,* the urine is orange or brown. Frothy urine, particularly if the froth persists after shaking, may contain an excess of protein.

ABNORMAL COMPOSITION
In *diabetes mellitus,* the excess glucose present in the blood spills into the urine, causing *glycosuria.* In *glomerulonephritis* (inflammation of the filtering units of the kidneys) and in the *nephrotic syndrome,* excess protein may be present in the urine (*proteinuria*). In *renal failure,* the total amount of waste products, such as urea, is reduced.

Other kidney disorders, such as *Fanconi's syndrome* and *renal tubular acidosis,* may make the urine too acid or too alkaline, or may cause it to contain excess amino acids, phosphates, salt, or water.

Urine retention
Inability to empty the bladder or difficulty doing so. Urinary retention may be complete, in which case urine cannot voluntarily be passed at all (although some may leak out) or

incomplete, in which case some urine may be passed, but the bladder fails to empty completely.

CAUSES
Retention may be due to an obstruction to the flow of urine. This problem predominantly affects males. Causes include phimosis (tight foreskin), a *urethral stricture, calculus* (stone) in the bladder, *prostatitis* (inflammation of the prostate), or enlargement or a tumor of the prostate (see *Prostate, enlarged; Prostate, cancer of*). In women, urinary retention may result from pressure on the urethra from uterine *fibroids.* In either sex it may be due to a *bladder tumor.*

Alternatively, retention may be due to defective functioning of the nerve pathways concerned with sensing bladder enlargement and triggering bladder emptying. Defective nerve function may be induced by a surgical operation, by a general or spinal anesthetic, by the use of drugs that act on the bladder or the urinary sphincters, or it may be the result of a disease of the spinal cord or damage to the nerve pathways through injury.

SYMPTOMS AND COMPLICATIONS
Except when nerve pathways are defective, complete urinary retention causes discomfort and pain in the lower abdomen, which can be severe. The filled bladder may be felt on examination as a swelling above the pubic bone. Chronic or partial retention, by contrast, may not cause any serious symptoms and the sufferer may be unaware of it.

There is a risk that retention will lead to kidney damage from back pressure up the urinary tract. Incomplete emptying often leads to a *urinary tract infection.*

TREATMENT
Urinary retention is treated by inserting a drainage tube into the bladder, usually via the urethra (see *Catheterization, urinary*). The cause of the retention is then investigated if it is not already known. When obstruction is the cause, it can usually be treated; if nerve damage is the cause, the prospects are less hopeful. Permanent or intermittent catheterization is sometimes necessary.

Urine tests
See *Urinalysis.*

Urography
Imaging of the urinary tract (kidney, ureters, and bladder) by X rays after the introduction of a radiopaque dye. (See *Pyelography.*)

Urokinase
A *thrombolytic drug* prepared from human urine or from a tissue culture of human kidney. Urokinase is given to dissolve blood clots in people who have had a recent *myocardial infarction* (heart attack) or *pulmonary embolism.* Given by injection in the early stages of a myocardial infarction, urokinase may limit the damage caused to the heart muscle.

Treatment with urokinase is strictly supervised due to a risk of excessive bleeding. Urokinase sometimes produces an allergic reaction that causes rash or fever.

Urologist
A specialist in *urology.* A urologist is concerned with the investigation and treatment of such varied disorders or symptoms as *incontinence, cystitis, urine retention, urinary tract infection, calculi* (stones), and *bladder tumors.* In men, the urologist investigates and treats disorders of the prostate gland, testes, and penis.

In addition to a physical examination to establish a diagnosis, the urologist may employ the investigative techniques of *pyelography, cystoscopy, ultrasound scanning, cystometry,* and *urinalysis.* Because many urological problems are treated by surgical operation, most specialists in urology are qualified surgeons.

Urology
A branch of medicine concerned with the structure, functioning, and disorders of the urinary tract in both males and females and of the reproductive tract in males.

Urology is thus concerned with the study of the kidneys, ureters, bladder, and urethra in members of both sexes, and with the testes, epididymis, prostate gland, seminal vesicles, and penis in males.

Ursodeoxycholic acid
A drug under investigation for treating *gallstones* that is prepared from *chenodiol,* a natural acid in bile. Ursodeoxycholic acid seems to be effective in the treatment of small gallstones that do not contain calcium but are largely made up of cholesterol.

Ursodeoxycholic acid works by reducing the amount of cholesterol released by the liver into the bile; it also helps dissolve cholesterol from the surface of gallstones.

Possible adverse effects of ursodeoxycholic acid are diarrhea and temporary impairment of liver function.

U

Urticaria

A skin condition, commonly known as hives, characterized by the development of itchy wheals (raised white lumps surrounded by an area of red inflammation). Wheals vary considerably in size and large ones may merge to form irregular, raised patches. The rash is most common on the limbs and trunk but may appear anywhere on the body. The wheals usually last for no longer than several hours.

Appearance of urticaria
Possible causes are food or drug allergy, contact with certain plants, insect stings or bites, and desensitizing injections.

Dermatographia is a less common form of urticaria in which wheals form after stroking the skin. *Angioedema* is a more severe condition (which sometimes occurs with urticaria) in which the airways become closed.

CAUSES

The cause of urticaria is often unknown. The most common known mechanism is an allergic reaction (see *Allergy*) in which the chemical *histamine* is released from skin cells, causing fluid to leak from capillaries into the skin tissues. Urticaria often results from an allergic reaction to a particular kind of food (such as milk, eggs, shellfish, strawberries, or nuts), food additive (such as some food dyes), or drug (such as penicillin or aspirin).

Less commonly, urticaria occurs in response to sweating brought on by heat or exercise, or to exposure to cold or sunlight.

TREATMENT AND PREVENTION

Itching can be relieved by applying calamine lotion or by taking *antihistamine drugs*. More severe cases may require *corticosteroid drugs*. Identifying and avoiding known trigger factors can help prevent future allergic reactions. Even if the cause cannot be identified, a tendency to urticaria often disappears in time without any treatment.

Uterus

The hollow, muscular organ of the female *reproductive system* in which the fertilized ovum (egg) normally becomes embedded and in which the developing embryo and fetus is nourished and grows.

The uterus is situated in the pelvic cavity behind the bladder and in front of the bowel.

STRUCTURE

The uterus of a nonpregnant woman measures 3 to 4 inches (7.5 to 10 cm) in length and weighs about 2 to 3 ounces (60 to 90 grams). In shape, it resembles an upside down pear. The lower, narrow part of the uterus opens into the vagina at the *cervix* (neck of the uterus); the upper part opens into the *fallopian tubes*.

In most women the uterus is anteverted (tilts forward) at an angle of 90 degrees to the vagina. In about 20 percent of women the uterus is retroverted (tilts backward; see *Uterus, tipped*).

ANATOMY OF THE UTERUS

The nonpregnant uterus lies deep in the pelvis immediately behind and above the urinary bladder and in front of the rectum. It is usually turned forward, at an angle to the vagina, and is curved downward slightly. When the bladder is full, the uterus is pushed up and back.

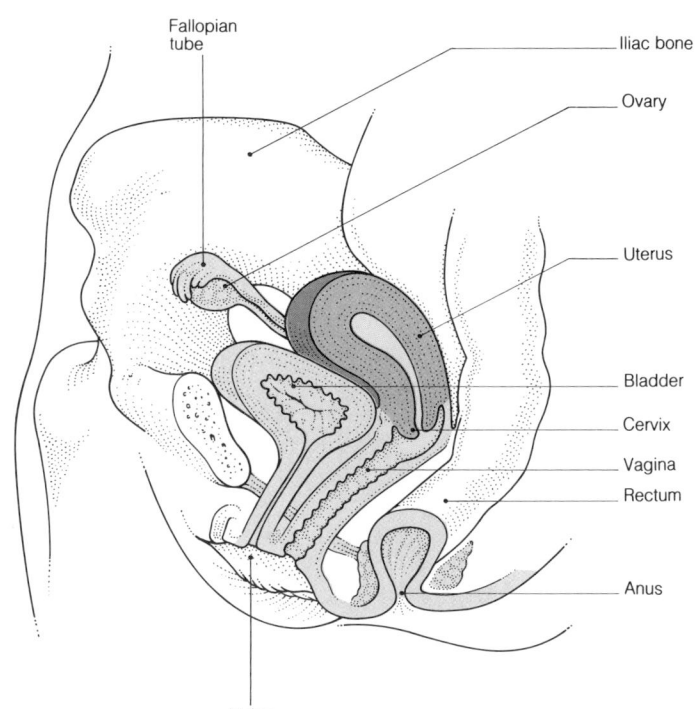

Fallopian tube

Iliac bone

Ovary

Uterus

Bladder

Cervix

Vagina

Rectum

Anus

Vulva

The uterus is a thick-walled organ that consists mainly of muscle. The fallopian tubes enter on both sides of the uterus just below its uppermost point. The small uterine cavity is lined with a mucous membrane called the endometrium, which undergoes changes during the different phases of the menstrual cycle. The cervix is lined with a flatter mucous membrane identical to that of the vagina.

U

DISORDERS OF THE UTERUS

Conditions that affect the uterus include congenital disorders, infection, benign or malignant growths, and hormonal imbalances that may affect menstrual flow.

CONGENITAL DISORDERS

In embryonic life, the uterus develops in two halves, which fuse along the midline. One percent of women have a congenital malformation of the uterus, usually resulting from a fusion error. Malformation is not usually serious, but may predispose a woman to preterm labor, *breech* presentation, or retention of the placenta after childbirth. Less commonly, the uterus may be absent, or there may be separate right and left halves, each with its own cervix and vagina. If a congenital malformation makes it difficult or impossible for a woman to conceive or to carry a pregnancy to term, surgical correction may be necessary.

INFECTION AND INFLAMMATION

Endometritis (infection and inflammation of the lining of the uterus) may originate in the uterus or be caused by infection spreading from elsewhere in the reproductive tract, such as the cervix or fallopian tubes. *Endometritis* may also develop if placental fragments are retained after childbirth or a *miscarriage*.

TUMORS

Benign tumors of the uterus include *polyps* and *fibroids*. Malignant tumors include cancer of the endometrium (see *Uterus, cancer of*).

Endometriosis
The lining of the uterus may grow in abnormal places.

Polyps
Polyps may arise from the cervix or endometrium. If they bleed they require investigation.

Cancer of endometrium
This is the third most common cancer in women and causes abnormal bleeding.

Fibroids
These may cause excessive menstrual bleeding.

Endometritis
This infection of the uterus may be part of a wider infection.

Tumors may also affect placental tissue. Such tumors include *hydatidiform mole*, which is usually benign, and *choriocarcinoma*, which is malignant.

HORMONAL DISORDERS

Excessive production of *prostaglandins* by the uterus may lead to *dysmenorrhea* (painful periods) or *menorrhagia* (heavy periods).

Hormonal disorders affecting the *ovary* or other organs may disrupt the normal buildup of endometrium during the menstrual cycle, causing menstrual disorders (see *Menstruation, disorders of*), especially *amenorrhea* (absence of periods) or irregular, heavy bleeding.

INJURY

Injury to the uterus is rare, except following surgery, particularly an *abortion*. In rare cases, the uterus may be perforated by an *IUD*.

OTHER DISORDERS

The uterus may move from its normal position (see *Uterus, prolapse of*).

Adenomyosis (invasion of the uterine muscle by endometrium) may lead to dysmenorrhea, menorrhagia, and pain during intercourse.

Endometriosis (the presence of endometrium outside the uterus) may be symptomless or may be associated with dysmenorrhea, menorrhagia, painful intercourse, and *infertility*.

INVESTIGATION

A physical examination may be followed by *blood tests*, a *biopsy* (removal of a sample of tissue for microscopic analysis), imaging of the uterus by *hysterosalpingography* or *ultrasound scanning*, or *laparoscopy* (examination of the abdominal cavity through a viewing tube).

The uterus is lined with *endometrium*, which is a specialized tissue that undergoes changes during the menstrual cycle. The endometrium builds up under the influence of hormones from the *ovary*. When hormonal support is withdrawn at the end of each menstrual cycle, the blood supply to the endometrium is cut off and the tissue is shed (see *Menstruation*).

During pregnancy, the uterus expands in size to accommodate the growing baby. Muscle bulk also increases dramatically. At full-term, the uterus weighs about 2 pounds (1 kg), and the powerful uterine muscles expel the baby through the birth canal with great force.

After the *menopause* there is loss of muscle and connective tissue, and the endometrium atrophies (thins). Uterine fibroids almost always shrink after the menopause.

Uterus, cancer of

Malignant growth in the tissues of the uterus. Cancer of the uterus affects two main sites—the cervix (see *Cervix, cancer of*) and the *endometrium* (lining of the uterus). The term uterine cancer usually refers to cancer of the endometrium.

INCIDENCE AND CAUSES

In the US in 1987, there were 35,000 new cases of endometrial cancer (compared to 12,800 new cases of cervical cancer).

Endometrial cancer occurs more commonly in women who have had an excess of estrogen in their systems. Risk factors that raise the estrogen level include obesity, a history of failure to ovulate, or long-term use of estrogen hormones if not balanced by *progesterone hormones*. Excess estrogen is common in women with high blood levels of *estrogen hormones*, particularly if progesterone hormone levels are low.

Unlike cervical cancer, endometrial cancer may occur in women who have not had sexual intercourse; it is more common in women who have had few or no children. Use of the birth-control pill lowers the risk of this cancer.

U

SYMPTOMS AND SIGNS

The first symptom of endometrial cancer in a woman after the menopause is usually a blood-stained vaginal discharge. In a younger woman, the first symptom may be *menorrhagia* (heavy periods), bleeding between periods, or bleeding after sexual intercourse. A variety of other conditions can also cause such bleeding.

DIAGNOSIS

Diagnosis must be made by collecting a sample of uterine lining either by biopsy or dilatation and curettage (*D and C*). A *cervical smear test* (Pap), which screens for cervical cancer, is not an effective screening test for uterine cancer.

TREATMENT

Treatment for very early endometrial cancer is most commonly simple *hysterectomy* and removal of tubes and ovaries. Many surgeons recommend removal of lymph nodes in the pelvis and abdomen to be certain that the cancer has not spread. If the cancer has spread, *radiation therapy* may be recommended. *Chemotherapy* may also be used.

With early treatment, the five-year survival rate is over 80 percent.

Uterus, prolapse of

A condition in which the uterus descends from its normal position down into the vagina. The degree of prolapse varies from only slight displacement to a condition called *procidentia*, in which the uterus can be seen outside the vulva.

Related conditions include *cystocele* and *urethrocele* (in which the bladder and/or urethra bulge along the front wall of the vagina) as well as *rectocele* (in which the rectal wall bulges into the back wall of the vagina). A general term for these conditions is pelvic relaxation. Prolapse of the uterus always occurs with some degree of vaginal relaxation, but vaginal relaxation may occur without any prolapse of the uterus.

CAUSES AND INCIDENCE

Normally, the uterus is kept in position by support ligaments. Stretching of these ligaments (such as during childbirth) is the most common cause of uterine prolapse. In addition, prolapse is more likely if the uterus is retroverted (see *Uterus, tipped*).

Prolapse occurs most commonly in middle-aged women who have had children, although it can occur in childless women. It was far more common earlier this century when women

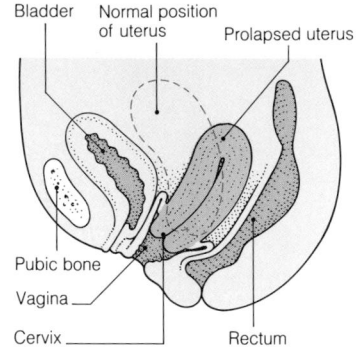

PROLAPSE OF THE UTERUS
This condition is caused by weakening of the various ligaments and muscles that help keep the uterus in position in the lower abdomen.

Bladder — Normal position of uterus — Prolapsed uterus
Pubic bone — Vagina — Cervix — Rectum

First-degree prolapse
In this least severe degree of prolapse, strain causes the cervix (neck) of the uterus to move farther down in the vagina; however, it remains well within the vagina.

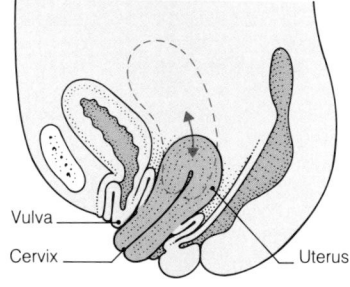

Vulva — Cervix — Uterus

Second-degree prolapse
The cervix projects beyond the vulva during straining, but retracts on relaxation. (In third-degree prolapse, the entire uterus projects permanently.)

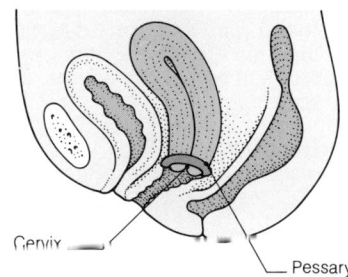

Cervix — Pessary

Treatment of prolapse
The uterus may be held in position by a plastic pessary inserted into the vagina; other patients are treated by hysterectomy or vaginal repair.

had more pregnancies and were in poorer general health. Obesity aggravates prolapse.

SYMPTOMS

There are often no symptoms or the woman may complain of a dragging feeling in the pelvis or a sensation that something is being displaced downward. In severe cases, the uterus is visible from the outside. Other symptoms, such as leakage of urine or difficulty passing urine or feces, may result from an accompanying cystocele, urethrocele, or rectocele.

DIAGNOSIS, PREVENTION, AND TREATMENT

Prolapse of the uterus is diagnosed by physical examination. In some cases, it is discovered during a routine pelvic examination. Evaluation of the urinary system may be necessary if the bladder is also prolapsed.

Pelvic floor exercises strengthen the muscles of the vagina and thus reduce the risk of a prolapse occurring, especially after childbirth.

In severe cases, a vaginal *hysterectomy* (removal of the uterus through the vagina), along with tightening of the support ligaments and, in some cases, *vaginal repair* may be recommended. For women who do not want surgery, or who are not fit enough to undergo general anesthesia, a plastic *pessary* may be inserted into the vagina to hold the uterus in position. The pessary requires periodic changing.

Uterus, retroverted

See *Uterus, tipped*.

Uterus, tipped

A condition in which the uterus inclines backward rather than forward. A tipped, or retroverted, uterus was once believed to be the cause of various gynecological symptoms. It is now generally considered to be a harmless variation of the normal.

CAUSES AND INCIDENCE

About 20 percent of women have a retroverted uterus. Retroversion occurs in some women because the uterus has stayed in the retroverted position usual in infancy rather than becoming anteverted (tilted forward) as it matures. In others, the position of the uterus changes after childbirth—either becoming retroverted when it was previously anteverted, or vice versa. Less commonly, retroversion is caused by a disease, such as a tumor, scarring from *endometriosis*, or *pelvic inflammatory disease*.

SYMPTOMS

Retroversion usually causes no symptoms, but an underlying disease

U

may produce painful periods, painful intercourse, and *infertility*.

DIAGNOSIS AND TREATMENT
A retroverted uterus is diagnosed by physical examination of the pelvis. Treatment is unnecessary if there are no symptoms. In rare cases when there are symptoms, the gynecologist may manipulate the uterus into a forward position and then insert a plastic vaginal pessary to hold the uterus in place. If this relieves the symptoms, surgery may be performed to change the position of the uterus permanently. If underlying gynecological disease is suspected, *laparoscopy* may be suggested.

Uvea
The colored part of the *eye* and the middle, blood vessel-containing layer of the eye. The uvea is a pigmented structure consisting of the *iris* (the diaphragm of the pupil), the ciliary body and its muscle, which focuses the lens, and the *choroid* (the coat of the eye lying just under the retina).

The uvea contains many blood vessels that, in the iris, supply the active muscles that control the opening and closing of the pupil; in the choroid, the blood vessels assist with the nutrition of the retina. The pigment cells of the uvea are concentrated at the back of the iris; in the choroid they are scattered throughout. These pigment cells confer color on the eye and improve its optical efficiency. (See also *Uveitis*.)

Uveitis
Inflammation of the *uvea*, which may seriously affect vision. Uveitis may affect any part of the uvea, including the iris (when it is called iritis), the ciliary body (when it is known as cyclitis), or the choroid (when it is called choroiditis).

The cause of uveitis is most commonly an *autoimmune disorder* rather than an infection.

Treatment involves monitoring the inflammation with a *slit lamp*. *Corticosteroid drugs* in the form of eye drops (or, occasionally, orally or by injection) are given; eye drops containing a substance related to *atropine* are given to block nerve impulses to the muscles of the iris and ciliary body, thus dilating the pupil. Other medications may be given in the rarer cases of uveitis due to an infection.

Uvula
The small, conical, fleshy protuberance that hangs from the middle of the lower edge of the soft *palate* (part of the roof of the mouth). The uvula is composed of muscle and connective tissue, with a covering of mucous membrane.

Some people are born with a bifid (forked) uvula. This is of little significance, but may be associated with *cleft lip and palate*.

U

Vaccination

One of the main types of *immunization* (a procedure to stimulate or bolster the body's *immune system*). Vaccination is another term for active immunization, in which killed or weakened microorganisms are introduced into the body, usually by injection. These microorganisms sensitize the immune system; if disease-causing organisms of the same type later enter the body, they are quickly destroyed through the action of *antibodies* produced by the immune system or by other immune mechanisms.

Vaccination does not encompass the other main type of immunization procedure—passive immunization—in which ready-made antibodies are given by injection to provide short-term immunity.

Vaccine

A preparation given to induce *immunity* against an infectious disease. A vaccine works by sensitizing the body's *immune system* to a particular disease-causing bacterial toxin, virus, or bacterium. If the particular infectious agent invades the body at a later time, the sensitized immune system quickly produces *antibodies* that help destroy either the agent itself or the toxin it produces.

Most vaccines are preparations containing the very organisms (or parts of the organisms) against which protection is sought. So that these organisms themselves do not cause disease, they are killed or weakened. The term "live attenuated organisms" describes strains of organisms that have been rendered harmless either by artificial alteration of their genes or by successively infecting laboratory animals; this leads to changes in the organisms that considerably reduce their ability to cause disease without reducing their ability to induce immunity. Other vaccines contain chemically modified bacterial *toxins*.

Vaccines are now available to protect against a wide variety of infectious diseases. Examples of live attenuated vaccines are those given to protect against *measles, mumps,* and *rubella* (now often combined), *yellow fever,* and Sabin's oral *polio* vaccine. *Diphtheria* and *tetanus* vaccines contain inactivated bacterial toxins. *Cholera, typhoid fever, pertussis, rabies,* viral *hepatitis B, influenza,* and Salk injected polio vaccines contain killed organisms or, in the case of hepatitis B, only a part of the hepatitis B virus.

Vaccines are usually given by injection into the upper arm. Oral polio vaccine is given on a sugar lump or by drops on the tongue. Some vaccines require several doses, spaced some weeks apart; others require only one dose. The effectiveness of vaccines varies from near total protection in most cases, to only partial or weak protection (for typhoid or cholera). The duration of effectiveness also varies from a few months to lifelong. (See also *Immunization.*)

Vacuum extraction

An obstetric procedure to facilitate delivery of a baby. Vacuum extraction was introduced in the 1950s as an alternative to *forceps delivery.* It may be used if the second stage of labor (see *Childbirth*) is prolonged, if the mother becomes exhausted, or if the baby shows signs of *fetal distress.* (Vacuum extraction is also one method used to perform an elective abortion; see *Abortion, elective.*)

HOW IT IS DONE

The procedure is performed using an instrument called a ventouse, or vacuum extractor, consisting of a suction cup connected to a vacuum bottle. The cup is placed on the baby's head in the birth canal and the vacuum machine is turned on; this sucks the

Traction bar

Suction cup

Tube to vacuum bottle

Technique of vacuum extraction
Once the suction cup is attached to the baby's head, the obstetrician pulls on the traction bar during each contraction, and the baby is drawn from the vagina.

baby's scalp firmly into the cup. The obstetrician draws the baby out of the mother's vagina by gently pulling on the cup with each uterine contraction.

Delivery by vacuum extraction is generally slower than with forceps, but there is less risk of damage to the woman's genital tract. The baby is born with a swelling on the scalp, but it is harmless and disappears without treatment within several days. *Cephalhematoma* (localized swelling of the scalp caused by bleeding over a skull bone), which may take two or three weeks to disappear, may develop in some babies.

Vagina

The muscular passage, forming part of the female *reproductive system,* that connects the cervix (neck of the uterus) with the external genitalia.

STRUCTURE

The vagina is 2.5 to 4 inches (7 to 10 cm) in length, the back wall being slightly longer than the front. The vagina is H-shaped in cross section. The muscular walls have a ridged inner surface and are richly supplied with blood vessels. The walls are usually in contact with each other, except during sexual arousal and intercourse when they become engorged with blood.

FUNCTION

The vagina has three functions. It is a receptacle for the penis during *sexual intercourse,* bringing sperm closer to the ova for fertilization; it provides an outlet for blood shed at *menstruation;* and, during *childbirth,* it stretches to allow the baby to pass through.

DISORDERS

Vaginal discharge and *vaginal itching* are very common symptoms; they may indicate a disorder in the vagina, vulva, or cervix.

Congenital abnormalities include vaginal atresia (partial or complete absence of the vagina) and blocking of the external opening of the vagina by an imperforate *hymen.*

Infections (see *Vaginitis*) and prolapse of the vagina (see *Urethrocele; Rectocele*) are the most common disorders. Cancer of the vagina occurs very rarely.

In *vaginismus,* sexual intercourse and pelvic examination are rendered impossible by abnormal spasm of the muscles around the vaginal entrance.

Vaginal bleeding

Bleeding via the vagina that may come from the uterus, the cervix, or from the vagina itself.

STRUCTURE OF THE VAGINA

The vagina has muscular walls, which are highly elastic to allow intercourse and childbirth; it has a ribbed inner lining that secretes a lubricating fluid during sexual excitation and intercourse.

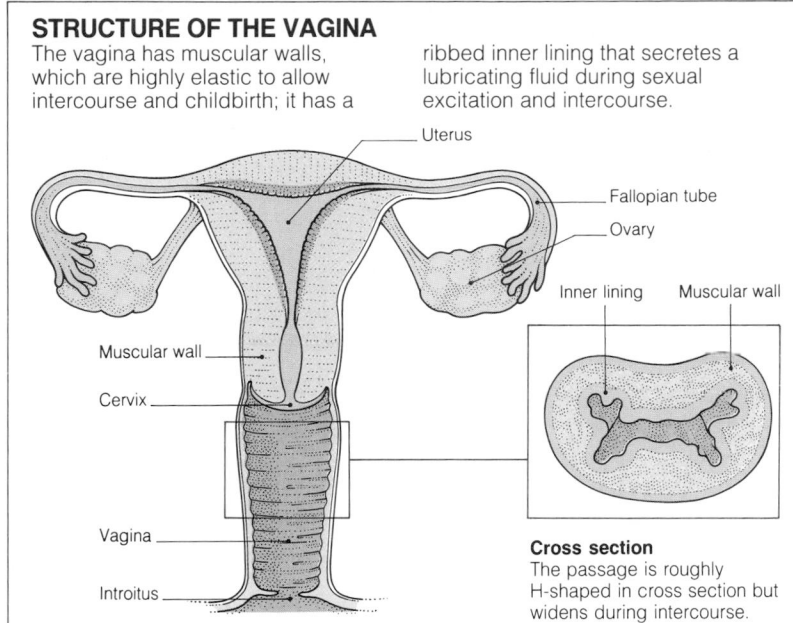

Cross section
The passage is roughly H-shaped in cross section but widens during intercourse.

The most common source of bleeding is the uterus and the most likely reason for it is *menstruation*. From puberty to the menopause, menstrual bleeding usually occurs at regular intervals. However, problems may occur either with the character or timing of the bleeding (see *Menstruation, disorders of*).

Possible causes of nonmenstrual bleeding from the uterus include *endometritis* (infection of the lining of the uterus) and endometrial cancer (see *Uterus, cancer of*). These conditions can also occur after the menopause. In addition, use of hormones (such as use of oral birth-control pills) can result in spotting, usually requiring dosage adjustment. Bleeding from the uterus may occur during pregnancy. In the early months, bleeding may be a sign of threatened *miscarriage*. Later in pregnancy, it may indicate serious fetal or maternal problems.

Bleeding from the cervix may be due to *cervical erosion*, in which case it may occur after sexual intercourse. *Cervicitis* (infection of the cervix) and *polyps* may also cause bleeding. More seriously, bleeding from the cervix may be a sign of cervical cancer (see *Cervix, cancer of*).

Vaginal bleeding, originating from the walls of the vagina, is less common than bleeding from the uterus or the cervix. The most likely cause is injury during intercourse, especially after

the menopause, when the walls of the vagina become thinner and more fragile. In extreme cases, bleeding may occur without any apparent precipitating cause. Occasionally, severe *vaginitis* causes vaginal bleeding. In rare cases, vaginal bleeding is caused by cancer of the vagina.

Any bleeding not caused by menstruation should be investigated to exclude a serious cause. Infections can be treated with *antibiotic drugs*; fragile vaginal walls can be helped by use of a cream containing *estrogen drugs*. Growths, such as polyps, *fibroids*, or cancer of the uterus or cervix, may need surgical treatment.

Vaginal discharge

Some mucous secretion from the walls of the vagina and neck of the cervix is normal in a woman of reproductive years. The amount and nature of the discharge varies considerably among women and at different times in the menstrual cycle. The birth-control pill can increase or decrease the discharge, and secretions are usually greater during pregnancy. Sexual stimulation, with or without intercourse, also produces increased vaginal discharge.

Discharge may be abnormal if it is excessive, offensive smelling, yellow or green, or if it causes itching. Abnormal vaginal discharge often occurs in *vaginitis*. Infection with the fungus CANDIDA ALBICANS causes a thick,

white discharge (see *Candidiasis*); the protozoan parasite TRICHOMONAS VAGINALIS causes a profuse green-yellow discharge (see *Trichomoniasis*). A retained pessary or forgotten tampon may cause a profuse and highly offensive secretion. Very rarely, a vaginal discharge may occur in childhood before the beginning of menstruation; this is usually the result of infection or a foreign body. Abnormal vaginal discharge is often accompanied by itching of the vagina and the vulva.

Treatment depends on the cause. Infections are treated with an *antibiotic drug* or *antifungal drug*. Foreign bodies are removed.

Vaginal itching

Intense irritation and tickling in the vagina and external genital area, also known as pruritus vulvae. Most commonly, vaginal itching is due to an allergic reaction to chemicals that are present in deodorants, spermicides, creams, and douches.

Also very common is itching after the *menopause* due to low estrogen levels. Vaginal infections may also cause itching (see *Vaginitis*). A group of vaginal skin changes, collectively called vulvar dystrophies, can make the skin itch. One form of vulvar dystrophy causes the skin to appear pale and white. Alternatively, the skin may be thickened and scarred.

Treatment for vaginal itching may be in the form of *antibiotic drugs* or hormones, sometimes taken orally and sometimes applied in cream form.

Vaginal repair

An operation, also known as colporrhaphy, to correct prolapse (displacement) of the vaginal wall.

TYPES

There are two different forms of vaginal repair operations—anterior colporrhaphy and posterior colpoperineorrhaphy. Either type may be accompanied by a vaginal *hysterectomy* if the uterus is also prolapsed (see *Uterus, prolapse of*).

ANTERIOR COLPORRHAPHY This operation is performed for prolapse affecting the front wall of the vagina. The repair is performed through the vagina.

A triangle of vaginal skin is removed, with its base lying upward toward the uterus. Supporting stitches are inserted through the skin at one side of the triangle, across the gap, and through the skin at the other side. The tissues are then drawn together, narrowing the vagina.

V

After the operation, a catheter may be inserted into the bladder to drain urine for about 24 hours.

POSTERIOR COLPOPERINEORRHAPHY This procedure is performed for prolapse of the back wall of the vagina (see *Rectocele*). The repair is performed through the vagina using general anesthesia.

Triangles of skin are removed from the vagina and from the perineum (the area between the genitals and the anus), with the bases of the triangles at the vaginal opening. The perineal muscles are stitched tightly together and the skin on each side of the triangles is brought together and stitched, narrowing the vagina.

Vaginismus

Painful, involuntary spasm of the muscles that surround the vaginal entrance, interfering with sexual intercourse. When penetration is attempted, the woman's pelvic floor muscles tighten and virtually close the vaginal entrance, making penetration very painful; her legs may straighten and come together. This spasm usually also occurs when a physician attempts a vaginal examination, which may require anesthesia.

CAUSES
Vaginismus usually occurs in women who fear that penetration will be painful. Often they have been previously unable to insert a tampon or a finger into the vagina. Any traumatic experience with painful penetration, such as rape or a history of sexual molestation as a child, may predispose a woman to vaginismus. Chronic *vaginitis* may result in painful intercourse and lead to vaginismus. Sufferers may also be particularly sensitive to the stretching sensation that occurs during penetration, which may trigger a spasm when intercourse is first attempted. A vicious circle of anxiety and spasm is then established.

In some women, a contributing factor may be underlying guilt or fear associated with the sexual act due to a restrictive upbringing or an inadequate sex education.

DIAGNOSIS AND TREATMENT
The physician first examines the woman to exclude any anatomical abnormalities of the *vagina* that might be causing pain, leading to spasm. Common causes of vaginal pain are infections such as *candidiasis* and atrophy (thinning of the vaginal lining) due to low hormone levels.

Medical problems, such as infection, are corrected; treatment is then by use of a series of graded dilators, which the woman introduces into her vagina. Starting with the smallest size, she practices inserting and removing the instrument, also learning to relax and tighten her vaginal muscles with the dilator in place. Over the course of several treatment sessions, the size of the dilator is gradually increased until the woman is comfortable with the largest size (about the size of the average erect penis). Intercourse can then be attempted.

Results of treatment are usually excellent, with the woman experiencing no discomfort during penetration. (See also *Intercourse, painful.*)

Vaginitis

Inflammation of the vagina. Vaginitis may be caused by infection, allergic reaction, hormone deficiency associated with aging, or a foreign body, such as a forgotten tampon.

Vaginal infection is commonly caused by the fungus CANDIDA ALBICANS (see *Candidiasis*) and the protozoan parasite TRICHOMONAS VAGINALIS (see *Trichomoniasis*), both of which cause irritation and *vaginal discharge*. Vaginitis is also commonly caused by bacteria that are normal inhabitants of the vagina but which, for unknown reasons (possibly stress or a change of sexual partner), multiply and cause an offensive, fishy-smelling discharge; this is called nonspecific vaginitis.

Vaginitis may also be caused by a reaction to spermicidal creams used with barrier contraceptives, to chemicals in vaginal douches, or to soaps, bath oils, or bath salts.

After the menopause, the lining of the vagina becomes thin and dry and prone to inflammation. Such inflammation, known as atrophic vaginitis, is due to a reduction in the production of *estrogen hormones*.

TREATMENT
Infections are treated with *antibiotic drugs* or *antifungal drugs*, as appropriate. In cases of allergy, irritant agents should be avoided. Any foreign body should be removed and any secondary infection treated with drugs. Atrophic vaginitis is treated by giving *estrogen drugs*. (See also *Vulvitis*; *Vulvovaginitis*.)

Vagotomy

An operation in which the *vagus nerve*, which controls production of digestive acid by the stomach lining, is cut to treat a *peptic ulcer*. Excessive production of digestive acid is a major factor in the development of a peptic ulcer. If a peptic ulcer is associated with obstruction of the outlet of the stomach, hemorrhage, or perforation, a vagotomy may be performed to cut the vagus nerve, thus reducing acid production at its source.

HOW IT IS DONE
An incision is made in the upper abdomen, with the use of a general anesthetic, and the two branches of the vagus nerve, which lie in front of and behind the lower esophagus, are exposed. All the nerve fibers are then cut (truncal vagotomy) or, less commonly, some of them are cut (selective vagotomy and highly selective vagotomy).

Since truncal and selective vagotomy cause the stomach to lose its ability to empty itself because muscles of the pylorus (the outlet from the stomach) fail to relax, the operation is usually accompanied by a *pyloroplasty* (surgical widening of the pylorus) or a *gastrojejunostomy* (a surgically created connection between the stomach and jejunum) to allow emptying of the stomach contents.

RECOVERY PERIOD
After the operation the patient is given fluids intravenously (by infusion into a vein) until the gastrointestinal tract can accept swallowed fluids.

TECHNIQUE OF VAGOTOMY
One branch of the vagus nerve acts to increase the secretion of acid and pepsin into the stomach. Vagotomy reduces this secretion and helps to heal peptic ulcers.

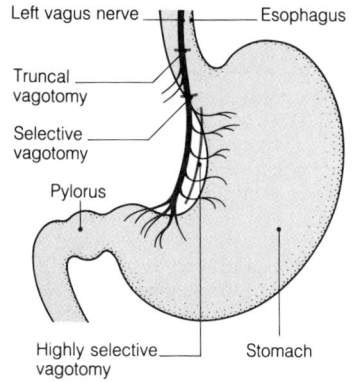

Types
The simplest operation is truncal vagotomy, in which the trunk of the nerve is cut. Selective vagotomy involves cutting only the twigs that supply the stomach.

V

The operation cures peptic ulcers in about 90 percent of cases, but occasionally· there are troublesome side effects, including diarrhea and *dumping syndrome* (premature passing of food from the stomach into the intestine, causing a feeling of weakness and distention after meals).

Vagus nerve

The tenth *cranial nerve* and the principal component of the parasympathetic division of the *autonomic nervous system*. The vagus nerve is the longest of the cranial nerves, and it branches most widely. It emerges from the medulla oblongata (part of the *brain stem*), passes through the neck and chest to the abdomen, and has branches to most of the major organs in the body, including the larynx, pharynx (throat), trachea (windpipe), lungs, heart, and much of the digestive system.

The vagus nerve exerts its effects on target organs by releasing the chemical *acetylcholine*. This causes narrowing of the bronchi and slowing of the heart rate. It also stimulates the production of stomach acid and pancreatic juice; stimulates the activity of the gallbladder; and increases *peristalsis* (the rhythmic, muscular contractions that move food through the digestive tract).

The vagus nerve branches to the larynx and trachea supply the muscles of these structures, thus involving the vagus nerve in swallowing, coughing, sneezing, and speech quality.

DISORDERS
Overactivity of the vagus nerve increases the production of stomach acid, which is a factor in the development of a *peptic ulcer*. Some cases of this type of ulcer may be successfully treated by a *vagotomy* (an operation to cut part of the vagus nerve).

The vagus nerve may be damaged by infection (such as *meningitis*), tumor, or *stroke*. In most such cases, the glossopharyngeal nerve (the ninth cranial nerve) and the spinal accessory nerve (the eleventh cranial nerve) are also affected. Possible effects of such damage include impairment or complete loss of the gag reflex, difficulty swallowing, and hoarseness. In severe cases, death may result.

Valgus

The medical term for outward displacement of a part of the body. For example, in genu valgum (*knock-knee*), the lower leg is displaced outward.

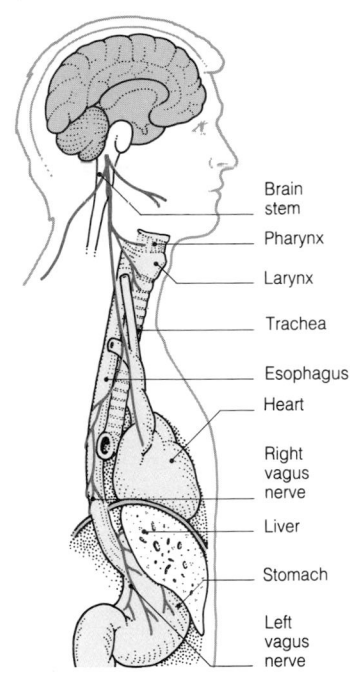

COURSE OF THE VAGUS NERVE
There are two vagus nerves, right and left. The right vagus nerve supplies the rear portion of the stomach; the left vagus nerve supplies the front portion of the stomach.

Brain stem
Pharynx
Larynx
Trachea
Esophagus
Heart
Right vagus nerve
Liver
Stomach
Left vagus nerve

Valproic acid

An *anticonvulsant drug* used to treat *epilepsy*. Although valproic acid has less of a sedative effect than many other anticonvulsant drugs, it occasionally causes drowsiness. Other possible side effects include abdominal discomfort, temporary hair loss, weight gain, and rash. Since prolonged treatment may in rare cases cause liver damage, regular blood tests are usually performed to monitor liver function.

Valsalva's maneuver

A forcible attempt to breathe out when the airway is closed. Valsalva's maneuver may be performed under certain circumstances without conscious effort or it may be carried out as a deliberate action.

Valsalva's maneuver occurs naturally when an attempt is made to breathe out while holding the vocal cords tightly together. This happens when lifting a heavy object, straining on the toilet, and at the beginning of a sneeze.

When performed deliberately by pinching the nose and holding the mouth closed, Valsalva's maneuver is useful in the prevention of pressure damage to the eardrums as it forces air through the ducts leading to the middle-ear cavities (see *Barotrauma*).

Valve

A structure that allows fluid or semifluid material to flow in one direction through a tube or passageway but closes to prevent reflux in the opposite direction. The most important valves in the body are at the exits from the heart chambers and in the veins. By ensuring that blood flows in one direction only, these valves are vital to the circulatory system; without them, the heart would be ineffective as a pump and blood circulation could not occur.

There are also small valves in the vessels of the lymphatic system. The muscular rings at the junction of the stomach and duodenum and between the small and large intestines are also sometimes called valves. In fact, these structures are flow-regulating devices and do not prevent reverse direction flow.

Defects of the *heart valves* include stenosis (narrowing) and/or insufficiency (inability to prevent reflux). Either defect can lead to *heart failure*. Insufficiency of the valves in the veins—most commonly in the legs—causes *varicose veins*.

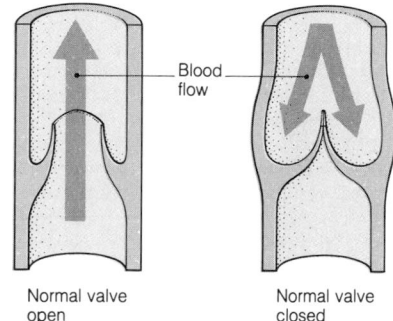

Blood flow

Normal valve open

Normal valve closed

Valves in the circulatory system
The valves are flaps that open to allow blood to flow in one direction but close to prevent counterflow in the other direction.

Valve replacement

A surgical operation to replace a defective or diseased heart valve. (See *Heart valve surgery*.)

Valvotomy

An operation performed to correct a stenosed (narrowed) *heart valve*. Cuts are made, or pressure applied, to separate the flaps of the valve where

V

they have joined and thus reduce the degree of narrowing.

In the past, valvotomy operations were usually performed, with the heart still beating, by means of a dilating instrument or even a finger introduced into the heart via an incision. Today, valvotomy is usually performed with the heart opened up (see *Heart valve surgery*). Balloon *valvuloplasty* is a newer technique for treating a narrowed valve without the need to open the chest.

Valvular heart disease

A defect of one or more of the valves in the heart. (See *Heart valve*.)

Valvuloplasty

A reconstructive or repair operation on a defective heart valve (see *Heart valve surgery*). Valvuloplasty can be performed as an open-heart operation (with the patient connected to a *heart-lung machine* and the heart opened up). However, the newer technique of balloon valvuloplasty makes it possible to treat a stenosed (narrowed) valve without opening the chest. A catheter containing a balloon at its tip is passed through the skin into a blood vessel and from there to the heart. Inflation of the balloon via the catheter may then help separate the flaps of a narrowed valve.

Vancomycin

An *antibiotic drug* used in the treatment of a variety of infections. Vancomycin is usually given to treat infections caused by staphylococci bacteria (see *Staphylococcal infections*) resistant to other antibiotics. It is given by injection to treat *endocarditis, osteomyelitis, pneumonia*, and *meningitis* and by mouth to treat a rare form of infective *colitis*.

Possible adverse effects include tenderness at the injection site, fever, chills, itching, and rash. Taken over a long period in high doses, it may in rare cases cause deafness by damaging the *vestibulocochlear nerve*.

Vaporizer

A device for converting a drug or water into an aerosol so that medication can be taken by inhalation or so that inhaled air can be made more moist. A common example is an *inhaler*, used to administer *bronchodilator drugs* and *corticosteroid drugs* in the treatment of asthma and other respiratory disorders. Vaporizers are also used to moisten air breathed by children with croup.

Varicella

Another name for *chickenpox*.

Varices

Enlarged, tortuous, or twisted sections of vessels, usually veins. Varices is the plural of varix. A vein affected by varices is called a *varicose vein*. Although varicose veins can occur anywhere in the body, they most commonly occur in the legs. *Esophageal varices* are enlarged veins in the lower end of the esophagus.

Varicocele

Varicose veins (abnormally distended veins) that surround the *testis*. Varicocele is a very common condition that affects about 10 to 15 percent of men. It more commonly involves the left testis.

The usual cause of varicocele is failure of the testicular valves. The condition is usually harmless, though there may be an aching discomfort in the scrotum.

Diagnosis is confirmed by examination of the scrotum. The condition may be relieved by wearing an athletic supporter or tight underpants. Further treatment is not usually required. However, an operation to divide and tie off the swollen veins is sometimes performed.

Varicose veins

Twisted, distended superficial veins (just beneath the skin). Varicose veins in the legs are the best known type. Varicosities in other parts of the body include *hemorrhoids* (dilated veins in the anus), *esophageal varices* (in the esophagus), and *varicocele* (collections of varicose veins in the scrotum).

CAUSES

There are two principal systems of veins in the legs—the deep veins, which lie among the muscles and carry about 90 percent of the blood, and the surface veins, which are often visible just under the skin and are less well supported. Once circulating blood has oxygenated the tissues of the legs, it is collected by the veins and, pumped upward by contractions of the leg muscles, it passes, via connecting veins, to veins in the abdomen, which return the blood to the heart.

Valves in the veins prevent blood from draining back down the leg under the force of gravity. However, these valves must support a high column of blood and, in many people, they become defective, causing pooling of blood in the superficial veins,

which become swollen and distorted. Factors that may contribute to the development of varicose veins include obesity, hormonal changes during pregnancy or at the menopause, pressure on pelvic veins when pregnant, and standing for long periods.

Thrombophlebitis (inflammation and clotting of blood in veins) or deep vein *thrombosis* (clotting in the deeper veins) may be associated with varicosities.

INCIDENCE

Varicose veins are extremely common. In the US about 15 percent of adults are affected, women more often than men. The disorder tends to run in families.

SYMPTOMS AND SIGNS

The most common sites for varicose veins are the back of the calf and anywhere on the inside of the leg. The veins are blue, prominent, swollen, and kinked. In some people they cause no symptoms, but others experience a severe ache in the affected area (which is made worse by prolonged standing), swelling of the feet and ankles, and persistent itching of the skin. These symptoms become progressively worse during the day and can be relieved only by sitting with the legs raised. In women, symptoms are often most troublesome just before menstruation.

If backflow of blood is severe enough to cause tissues to become starved of oxygen and nourishment, the skin becomes thin, hard, dry, scaly, and discolored, and *ulcers* may form. They should be treated by cleansing and dressing and facilitating the return of blood to the heart by elevating the legs.

Bumping a large varicose vein may cause severe bleeding. It can be stopped by keeping the affected leg raised and by tying a clean handkerchief around the leg to apply moderate pressure. A physician should then be consulted.

DIAGNOSIS AND TREATMENT

Varicose veins in the legs are diagnosed from a physical examination done while the patient is standing.

In many cases, the only treatment needed is the wearing of elastic support stockings, regular walking, as little standing as possible, and sitting with the feet up.

In more severe cases, *sclerotherapy* may be carried out. An irritant solution is injected into the varicose veins. The consequent scarring and blockage of the vein causes its work to be taken over by other, healthy veins.

VARICOSE VEINS

When valves in the veins work correctly, the weight of the blood column is well distributed. When valves fail, some veins become overfilled with blood and swell.

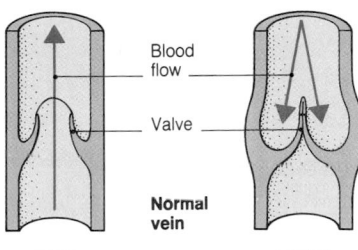

Blood flow

Valve

Normal vein

Blood flow

Valve failure

Varicose vein

How varicosities are caused
In a normal vein, valves stop blood from draining down due to gravity. If valves fail, blood is able to pool downward.

Appearance of varicose vein
This varicosity of the saphenous vein on the inside of the thigh shows the typical tortuous, swollen appearance.

STRIPPING A VEIN

Vein stripping is performed only in severe cases when the valves in the main surface veins are shown to be malfunctioning (and there are symptoms) or the skin is ulcerated. Visible varicosities usually occur in the branches of the vein and these may have to be treated separately.

Site of incision

1 Here the greater saphenous vein and its four main upper branches are exposed through an incision in the groin.

2 The vein is clamped and cut and both free ends tied off. The four branches are also securely tied off and cut. If branches remain, the operation may fail.

3 A small hole is made in the top of the vein and a flexible wire passed down the vein to the calf or ankle and brought out through a small incision.

4 The upper end of the wire has a specially shaped metal head, and the vein is tied firmly to the wire just below it.

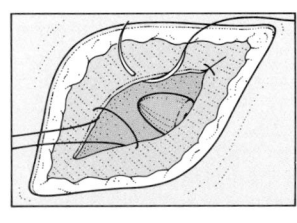

5 The upper incision is closed and the vein is then removed by pulling the wire out through the lower incision. The

vein bunches up on the stripper and its branches tear off as it does so. Bleeding is not usually severe.

If varicose veins are very painful, ulcerated, or prone to bleed, they may require removal by an operation known as stripping (see box). The operation usually takes about half an hour. The patient must keep the leg bandaged for several weeks.

Both sclerotherapy and surgery are usually successful, but varicose veins may later develop elsewhere.

Variola
Another name for *smallpox*. The term variolation was once used to describe smallpox vaccination.

Varus
The medical term for an inward deformity of part of the body. For example, in genu varum (*bowleg*), the lower leg is displaced inward.

Vasculitis
Inflammation of blood vessels. Vasculitis usually leads to damage to the lining of vessels, with narrowing or blockage, so that the blood flow is restricted or stopped. As a result, the tissues supplied by the affected vessels are also damaged, or destroyed, by *ischemia* (lack of blood supply and, therefore, oxygen).

V

Vasculitis is thought to be caused, in most cases, by bodies in the circulating blood known as immune complexes. Immune complexes consist of *antigens* (foreign materials, such as components of microorganisms) bound to *antibodies* that have been formed in response to the antigens. Normally, the immune complexes are destroyed by *phagocytes* (types of white blood cell), but sometimes they settle in the walls of the blood vessels, where they cause severe inflammation. In at least some cases, the causative antigens are known to be viruses.

Vasculitis is the basic disease process in a number of conditions, including *periarteritis nodosa, erythema nodosum, Schönlein-Henoch purpura, serum sickness, temporal arteritis,* and *Buerger's disease.*

Vas deferens

A narrow tube that carries and stores *sperm* released from the *testis* and *epididymis.*

At the base of the bladder, the vas deferens connects to a tube from the seminal vesicles to form the ejaculatory duct. The duct passes into the prostate gland and connects to the urethra. Sperm and seminal fluid are passed through this duct into the urethra during *ejaculation.*

The vas deferens is about 2 feet (60 cm) long. *Vasectomy* involves blocking each vas deferens to prevent the passage of sperm.

LOCATION OF THE VAS DEFERENS

The vas passes from the epididymis at the back of the testis, up and around the bladder, before entering the prostate.

Vas deferens

Seminal vesicle

Bladder

Testis   Epididymis   Prostate gland

HOW VASECTOMY IS PERFORMED

This operation blocks the passage of sperm from the testes but does not prevent the prostate and other glands from secreting the fluids that form most of the semen. Hence it has little effect on the volume of the ejaculate and no effect on orgasm.

Vas deferens

Spermatic cord

Site of incision

Testis

1 Incisions are made on both sides near the root of the penis; the vas deferens is cut free of the spermatic cord. Blood vessels are avoided.

2 A loop of the vas deferens is freed and brought out through the incision. There are now several possibilities; usually, a length of the vas is cut out.

3 To prevent the cut ends from rejoining, they are often bent back and tightly closed with ligatures. They are then pushed back into the cord.

4 The skin incision is now closed with three or four sutures. When the local anesthetic wears off, there is usually a mild, dull, aching pain for a few days.

Vasectomy

The operation of male sterilization. Vasectomy is a minor surgical procedure that consists of cutting the two vas deferens, the ducts that carry sperm from the testes to the seminal vesicles. The man continues to ejaculate as usual, but the semen no longer carries sperm, which are reabsorbed within the testes.

WHY IT IS DONE

Male sterilization provides a method of birth control that is safe and virtually 100 percent effective; the risk of problems or complications is lower than for female sterilization. However, vasectomy is often irreversible, and the decision to have it performed should be carefully considered by the man and his partner.

HOW IT IS DONE

The operation is performed on an outpatient basis using a local anesthetic. The basic steps are shown in the illustrated box (above). The procedure takes 15 to 20 minutes.

RECOVERY PERIOD

The patient should rest in bed for 24 hours. There may be slight bruising of the scrotum and/or bleeding from the external wound for a few days. To relieve any pain, acetaminophen should be taken rather than aspirin, which can prolong bleeding.

Most men return to work within a few days, and sexual relations can be resumed as soon as the man is able, often within a week. For four to six weeks, tight-fitting underpants or a jockstrap should be worn to support the scrotum.

After a vasectomy, a man remains fertile until the sperm already present in the vas deferens are ejaculated or die. Between two and four months after the operation, the man returns to the hospital at least twice with specimens of semen for analysis. It is only when two consecutive specimens are found to be sperm-free that he is considered sterile. Until that time, either he or his partner needs to use some form of contraception.

OUTLOOK

In rare cases, a vasectomy fails because the severed parts of a vas deferens reunite. If this occurs, the man can safely undergo another vasectomy operation.

Although most men who have a vasectomy experience no sexual problems as a result, the operation occa-

V

sionally causes psychological problems that affect sexual performance. If counseling or psychotherapy fails to clear up these problems (or if a man strongly regrets that he has been sterilized) it may be possible to have the operation reversed. About half of reversal operations are successful in restoring fertility.

Vasoconstriction

Narrowing of blood vessels, causing reduced blood flow to a part of the body. Vasoconstriction under the skin occurs in response to cold and reduces heat loss from the body. It also occurs due to a fall in blood pressure in physiological *shock*. Vasoconstriction is also caused by *decongestant drugs*, which relieve nasal congestion by reducing blood flow to the lining of the nose.

Vasodilatation

Widening of blood vessels, causing increased blood flow to a part of the body. Vasodilatation under the skin occurs in response to hot weather and increases heat loss from the body. It also occurs as a response to *vasodilator drugs* and *alcohol*.

Vasodilator drugs

A group of drugs that widens blood vessels. Vasodilator drugs include *ACE inhibitor drugs, calcium channel blockers, nitrate drugs,* and *sympatholytic drugs*.

WHY THEY ARE USED
Vasodilator drugs are used to treat disorders in which abnormal narrowing of blood vessels reduces blood flow through tissues, impairing the supply of oxygen. Such disorders include *angina pectoris* (chest pain caused by inadequate blood supply to heart muscle) and *peripheral vascular disease.*

Vasodilator drugs are also used to treat *hypertension* (high blood pressure) and *heart failure* (reduced pumping efficiency). Drugs of the vasodilator group are also occasionally prescribed in the treatment of senile *dementia*, although they rarely improve symptoms.

HOW THEY WORK
Vasodilator drugs widen blood vessels by relaxing surrounding muscles within the walls of the vessels; calcium channel blockers and nitrate drugs have a direct action on these muscles; sympatholytic drugs block the nerve signals that stimulate muscular contraction; and ACE inhibitors interfere with enzyme activity in

the blood—an action that reduces the production of angiotensin II (a chemical that narrows blood vessels).

POSSIBLE ADVERSE EFFECTS
All vasodilator drugs may cause flushing, headaches, dizziness, fainting, and swollen ankles.

Vasopressin

An alternative name for *ADH* (antidiuretic hormone).

Vasovagal attack

Temporary loss of consciousness due to sudden slowing of the heart beat. A vasovagal attack, which is a common cause of *fainting* in healthy people, is a result of overstimulation of the *vagus nerve*, which helps to control breathing and blood circulation. A vasovagal attack is usually brought on by severe pain, stress, shock, or fear. The loss of consciousness is commonly preceded by sweating, nausea, dizziness, ringing in the ears, dimmed vision, and weakness. A person experiencing these symptoms can sometimes avoid fainting by putting his or her head between the knees.

This cause of fainting is often attributed to instances where no other cause can be found.

VD

The abbreviation for venereal disease, another name for *sexually transmitted disease*.

Vector

An animal that transmits a particular infectious disease. A vector picks up disease organisms from a source of infection (such as an infected person's or animal's blood or feces), carries them within or on its body, and later deposits them where they infect a new host, directly or indirectly.

Mosquitoes, fleas, lice, ticks, and flies are the most important vectors of disease to humans. When an organism develops or completes part of its life cycle inside a vector, this vector is called a biological vector. For example, mosquitoes are biological vectors for malarial parasites, which develop and multiply inside the insect and are injected into the blood of a new host by the mosquito's bite.

TYPES OF VASODILATOR DRUGS

The different types of vasodilator drugs work in various ways to prevent or reduce the contraction of muscle cells in blood vessel walls, thus helping to widen the blood vessels.

Constricted   Dilated

Action
A blood vessel is shown contracted and dilated (above). Vasodilators widen vessels, improving blood flow (below).

Nerve fiber ending

Synaptic cleft

Drug

Muscle cell

Sympatholytic drugs
Muscles in blood vessel walls are made to contract by the action of neurotransmitters. Sympatholytic drugs block the sites where neurotransmitters act.

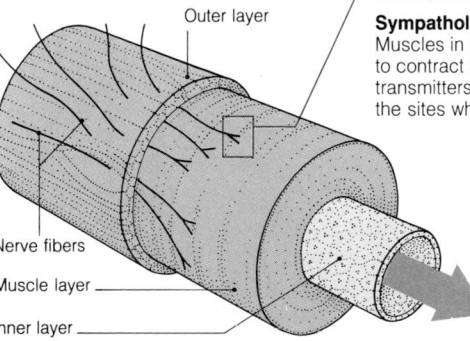

Outer layer

Nerve fibers

Muscle layer

Inner layer

Calcium channel blockers and nitrates
These drugs act directly on the contracted muscle cells in blood vessel walls, causing them to relax.

ACE inhibitors
These drugs work by blocking the activity of a particular enzyme in the blood—an action that reduces the production of angiotensin II, a chemical that acts to narrow blood vessels.

V

When a vector is not essential to the life cycle of a disease organism, it is called a mechanical vector. For example, flies may act as mechanical vectors of *shigellosis* (bacterial dysentery) by carrying the bacteria on their legs from infected feces to food.

Vegetarianism

Eating a diet (see *Nutrition*) that excludes meat and fish, and sometimes all other animal products. A large proportion of the world's total population is vegetarian or primarily vegetarian. Humans do not need to eat meat or animal products to maintain health as long as the various nutrients supplied by plant foods provide a balanced diet.

TYPES
Vegetarian diets can be classified into four types according to the foods that are eaten or are excluded (see chart, below).

EATING A BALANCED DIET
All vegetarians, but especially vegans, must ensure that they eat a sufficient amount of *protein*. It is also necessary to eat different types of protein-containing foods. Whereas animal proteins are complete (containing all the essential *amino acids* needed for good health), individual plant proteins are incomplete (lacking a variety of essential amino acids). Plant proteins must therefore be eaten in combination if they are to provide all the body's amino acid requirements. A balanced vegetarian diet should consist of a wide selection of grains, dried beans and peas, nuts, and seeds. Rice and beans contain different essential amino acids; when eaten together they form a complete protein.

Vitamin B_{12} is plentiful in all animal products. Vegetarians other than vegans are unlikely to suffer deficiency, but vegans should ensure that they are obtaining the vitamin from fortified food sources (such as soy milk or breakfast cereals) or from a vitamin B_{12} supplement, often given by injections since vitamin B_{12} is absorbed poorly when it is taken by mouth in tablet form.

Vegetarians should also receive adequate amounts of vitamin C, which helps the absorption of iron from plant foods.

Milk and milk products are rich in calcium. Lactovegetarians therefore receive a plentiful supply, but vegans must rely on grains, legumes, nuts, seeds, and dark green, leafy vegetables for this mineral. Vitamin D is important for calcium absorption from food in the intestinal tract. It is manufactured by our bodies from the action of sunlight on the skin or may be supplied by a supplement.

ADVANTAGES OF A VEGETARIAN DIET
Vegetarians tend to eat a high-fiber diet. This may help protect them from certain intestinal diseases, such as cancer of the intestines and diverticular disease. Provided they do not eat a lot of high-fat dairy products, vegetarians have a reduced risk of coronary artery disease, high blood pressure, obesity, and non-insulin-dependent diabetes compared to nonvegetarians. Women who are vegetarians have been found to suffer less from *osteoporosis* (brittle bones).

Vegetative state
A term sometimes used to describe a type of indefinite deep *coma*. Although the eyes may be open and occasional random movements of the head and limbs may occur, there are no other signs of consciousness and no responsiveness to stimuli. Only the basic body functions, such as breathing, heart beat, and body temperature, are maintained.

Vein
A vessel that returns blood toward the heart from the various organs and tissues of the body.

The majority of veins carry deoxygenated (blue) blood. This blood collects in small vessels called venules in the tissues. The venules join to form veins, which deliver the blood to the two largest veins in the body, the venae cavae. The venae cavae then carry the deoxygenated blood to the right side of the heart to be pumped to the lungs.

The main exceptions to this design are the pulmonary veins in the chest, which carry oxygenated blood from the lungs to the left side of the heart. Another special vein is the portal vein, which carries nutrient-rich blood from the intestines to the liver.

The walls of veins, like those of arteries, consist of a smooth inner lining, a muscular middle layer, and a fibrous outer covering. However, blood pressure in veins is much lower than it is in arteries. Correspondingly, the walls of veins are thinner, less elastic, less muscular, and weaker. Veins collapse when empty, while arteries remain extended.

V

TYPES OF VEGETARIANISM

Semivegetarian

This diet includes milk, eggs, milk products such as cheese, cream, and yogurt, and allows occasional fish and poultry but no red meat.

Lacto-ovovegetarian

This diet allows milk, eggs, and milk products such as cheese, but excludes all types of fish and poultry as well as red meat.

Lactovegetarian

This is similar to the lacto-ovovegetarian diet except that eggs are excluded in addition to fish and meat. Milk and milk products are allowed.

Vegan

This is the most rigid form of vegetarianism; it excludes all foods of animal origin. Vegans must obtain all the nutrients they need from plant sources.

The inner linings of many veins contain folds, which act as valves, ensuring that blood can flow only toward the heart. The blood is helped on its way through the veins by pressure on the vessel walls from the contraction of surrounding muscles.

Veins, disorders of

The most common vein disorder is a *varicose vein*—swelling, distortion, and twisting of a vein. Varicose veins occur most commonly in the legs, where they are caused by failure of the valves farther up the vein. *Esophageal varices* are varicose veins in the lower part of the esophagus; they commonly result from back pressure through the circulation from *cirrhosis* of the liver. *Hemorrhoids* are varicose veins in the anus.

Inflammation of a vein is called phlebitis. It is almost always associated with a tendency to blood clotting in the affected vein, in which case it is called *thrombophlebitis*. Clot formation in the small veins near the surface is not significant, although clots may cause swelling and tenderness. However, if clots form in deeper, larger

STRUCTURE OF A VEIN AND AN ARTERY

Like arteries, the walls of veins have a smooth, inner layer, a muscular, middle layer, and a fibrous, outer layer. However, the walls are thinner and less muscular than those of arteries.

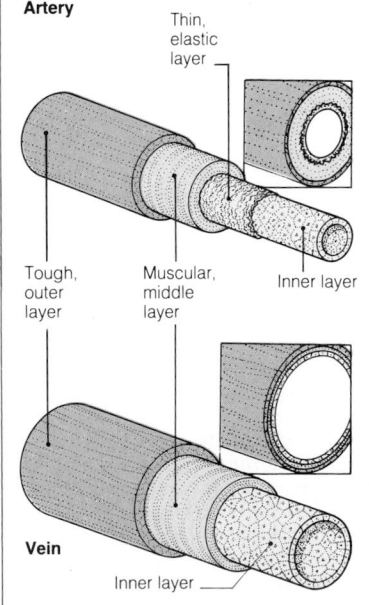

Artery

Thin, elastic layer

Tough, outer layer

Muscular, middle layer

Inner layer

Vein

Inner layer

LOCATION OF THE VENAE CAVAE

All the circulating blood, after being pumped to the body, returns to the heart via the venae cavae. The superior vena cava collects blood from the whole of the upper trunk, head, neck, and limbs. The inferior drains blood from all parts of the body below the chest.

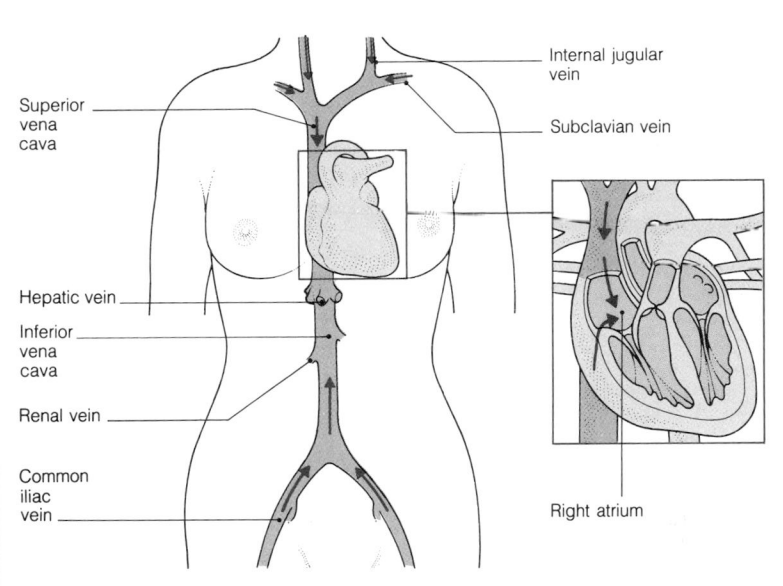

Superior vena cava

Internal jugular vein

Subclavian vein

Hepatic vein

Inferior vena cava

Renal vein

Common iliac vein

Right atrium

veins—a condition called deep vein thrombosis (see *Thrombosis, deep vein*)—they may become widespread and there is a risk that part of the clot will break off and cause blockage of the pulmonary artery.

The blood pressure in veins is much lower than in arteries; an injured vein will thus bleed much more slowly than an artery of the same size. Light pressure on an injured vein is usually sufficient to stop bleeding. Raising an injured part above the level of the heart will also stop bleeding from veins, though not from arteries.

Vena cava

Either of two very large veins into which all the circulating venous (deoxygenated) blood drains. The venae cavae deliver this blood to the right atrium (one of the upper chambers of the heart) for pumping to the lungs. The veins are each nearly an inch in diameter and are situated deep within the chest and abdomen.

The superior vena cava starts at the top of the chest, behind the lower edge of the right first rib and close to the breastbone. It travels some 3 inches (7.5 cm) downward, passing through the pericardium (outer lining of the heart) before connecting to the right atrium. It is formed from the

right and left brachiocephalic veins, which themselves are formed from union of the subclavian veins (draining blood from the arms), the jugular veins (draining blood from the head), and several minor veins. The superior vena cava also receives blood from the azygos vein, which drains much of the chest. The superior vena cava thus collects blood from the whole of a person's upper trunk, head, neck, and limbs.

The inferior vena cava starts in the lower abdomen, in front of the fifth lumbar vertebra, and travels some 10 inches (25 cm) upward in front of the spine, behind the liver, and through the diaphragm before joining to the right atrium. It is formed from the union of the two common iliac veins, which receive blood from the legs and pelvic organs. The inferior vena cava also receives blood from the hepatic vein and from the renal veins, which drain the liver and the kidneys, respectively.

Venereal diseases

See *Sexually transmitted diseases*.

Venereology

The medical discipline concerned with the study and treatment of *sexually transmitted diseases*.

V

Venesection

The process of withdrawing blood from a vein, also called phlebotomy, for *blood donation* or for therapeutic bloodletting. Regular bloodletting is used in the treatment of *polycythemia* (a disorder in which the blood is too thick); in *hemochromatosis* (a disorder of body iron chemistry) to reduce the amount of iron in the body; and very occasionally in some types of *heart failure* to reduce the blood volume and ease the heart's work load.

Venipuncture

A common procedure in which a vein is pierced with a needle to withdraw blood or inject fluid. It is usually performed on a vein in the forearm.

HOW IT IS DONE

A tourniquet is applied to the upper arm, causing the veins to become distended. A suitable vein, usually a large one that can be easily felt through the skin, is selected. The overlying skin is cleansed with a swab soaked in alcohol, and a sterile needle is inserted into the vein. For taking blood or injecting medication, a syringe is attached to the needle. For *intravenous infusion*, a cannula (hollow tube) is inserted into the vein via the needle; the needle is then withdrawn, and tubing for the fluid to flow through is attached to the cannula.

After the required amount of fluid has been injected or withdrawn, the needle or cannula is removed. The area is then covered with a piece of cotton and firm pressure applied for a minute or two until bleeding stops.

The procedure is not usually painful but it may cause some discomfort. Slight bruising may appear at the site of the venipuncture, although such bruising usually subsides within a few days.

Venography

A diagnostic procedure, also known as phlebography, that enables veins to be seen on an X-ray film after they have been injected with a substance opaque to X rays.

WHY IT IS DONE

Venography is used to detect anatomical abnormalities or diseases of the veins themselves—such as narrowing or blockage from *thrombosis* (abnormal clot) or tumor—as well as disease or injury in organs that are supplied by the veins. It is also used to evaluate the extent of disease so that treatment can be planned.

The veins most frequently studied are those in the leg, usually because of

Venogram showing veins within the skull
This X-ray image of a skull shows both the veins and the venous sinuses (dark areas), which are wide blood drainage channels.

suspected deep vein thrombosis (see *Thrombosis, deep vein*). Other commonly studied veins include the axillary veins in the arm, the superior and inferior venae cavae (the main veins leading to the heart), and the renal veins (leading from the kidney).

HOW IT IS DONE

Contrast medium is injected either through a needle directly into the veins to be examined or, if the veins are not readily accessible, through a catheter that has been guided, under X-ray control, along the venous system to the required vein. A sequence of X-ray pictures is taken so that blood flow along the veins can be studied. Leg venography takes about 20 minutes to perform; other types may take longer.

The newer technique of digital subtraction *angiography* adds to the information obtained through use of computer analysis to process images and remove unwanted shadowing.

Venomous bites and stings

Many animals carry poison, or venom, which they can inject into other animals or humans via their mouthparts (bites) or by some other injecting apparatus (stings). Often, these venoms are carried for purely defensive purposes (to discourage predators). Sometimes they are used to kill or immobilize prey. It is rare for a venomous animal to attack a person unless cornered, provoked, stepped on, or otherwise disturbed.

Specific *antivenins* are available to treat many, though not all, animal venoms. In cases of serious poisoning, administration of antivenin can sometimes be lifesaving.

TYPES OF VENOMOUS ANIMAL

For the better known types of venomous bites and stings, see *Snakebites, Spider bites, Insect stings, Scorpion*

stings, and *Jellyfish stings.* Other venomous animals include certain species of lizards, centipedes, millipedes, and fish.

LIZARD BITES Two types of biting lizard are found in the southwestern US and Mexico. A bite causes severe local pain, shock, and other symptoms such as vomiting. Some fatal bites have been reported. Treatment is with powerful *analgesic drugs* (painkillers).

CENTIPEDES AND MILLIPEDES Centipede bites can cause severe pain and local swelling but are not a danger to life. Certain millipedes secrete, and sometimes squirt out, an irritating liquid that may be dangerous if it enters the eyes. First aid is by thorough irrigation with water.

FISH STINGS Venomous fish inflict stings via certain fins or specialized spines on their bodies. These fish include stingrays (found in many parts of the world, including the coast of California), weeverfish (European waters), and scorpion fish, lionfish, and stonefish (throughout the Indian and Pacific oceans). They are a danger to swimmers, waders, snorkelers, and scuba divers.

The effects of a fish sting may include excruciating pain, shock, vomiting, sweating, and cardiac *arrhythmias.* Occasional fatalities occur. Stinging spines should be removed from the wound, which should be thoroughly washed. A useful first-aid procedure is to immerse the stung body part in hot water; the heat inactivates some of the components of the venom and relieves the intense pain. Alternatively, a physician may inject a local anesthetic. In some cases, *cardiopulmonary resuscitation* and life-support procedures are necessary.

Ventilation

The use of a machine called a *ventilator* to take over respiration (and thus maintain life) in a person who has lost or who lacks the ability to breathe naturally.

WHY IT IS DONE

Arrested or severe impairment of breathing may be caused by damage to the respiratory center in the brain stem due to head injury, brain disease, or an overdose of narcotic drugs. Breathing difficulties may also be due to damage to or malfunctioning of the breathing mechanism as a result of chest injury, respiratory disease, a nerve or muscle disorder, or major chest or abdominal surgery. Occasionally, difficulties arise as a result of

V

TECHNIQUE OF ARTIFICIAL VENTILATION

Machine-assisted breathing may be needed when a person has lost the ability to breathe naturally—often following a severe head injury, narcotic overdose, or in various other emergency situations. It may also be needed when a muscle relaxant has been given during an operation as part of a general anesthetic.

Connector to endotracheal tube

In/out pipes

Patient

Valve

Ventilator

Bellows

Speed and stroke volume controls

Procedure
The air is delivered to the patient's lungs via a tube inserted into the windpipe. After each inflation, the air is expelled by the natural elasticity of the lungs. Fluids and drugs must be given to the patient by intravenous infusion.

Air out

Weight

Bellows

Air to patient

Ventilator

Valve

Air in

Air or mixture of gas and air

Pressure gauge

Ventilator components
The pump part of the ventilator consists of a bellows, which is expanded by an electric motor and compressed by a weight. The air (or other gas mixture) is driven through a humidifier and delivered via a hose and valve to the patient. The stroke volume, stroke rate, and oxygen content of the gas mixture can be varied according to the needs of the individual patient.

During ventilation the amount of oxygen and other gases in the patient's blood is checked by analyzing blood samples. X rays are taken to assess the state of the lungs; the pulse, blood pressure, heart rhythm, and temperature are monitored.

The patient is unable to eat or drink when connected to the ventilator. Fluids are therefore given by *intravenous infusion*. Drugs may need to be given in the same way.

The patient's inability to cough may cause secretions to accumulate in the lungs. They are removed by suction apparatus, and intensive *respiratory therapy* is given to prevent the secretions from building up again.

When the patient begins to recover, he or she is disconnected from the ventilator and allowed to breathe naturally for increasingly longer and more frequent periods. After the blood gases have returned to a normal level during spontaneous breathing, the patient is taken off the ventilator permanently.

Ventilator
A device, also known as a life-support machine or respirator, used to take over respiration (and thus maintain life) in a patient who lacks or has lost the ability to breathe naturally.

A ventilator is an electrical pump connected to an air supply that works like bellows. The pump can be adjusted to vary the proportion of oxygen in the pumped air and to regulate the amount of air delivered. The air is first pumped through a humidifier, which adds sterile water vapor to prevent the lungs from drying out; the air is then directed through a tube that has been passed down the patient's trachea (see *Ventilation*). After the lungs have been inflated, the air is expelled by the natural elasticity of the lungs and rib cage. A valve on the ventilator prevents the expelled air from reentering the lungs.

Artificial ventilation is usually carried out in an *intensive-care* unit.

Ventouse
See *Vacuum extraction*.

Ventral
Relating to the front of the body, or describing the lowermost part of a body structure when a person is lying facedown. In human anatomy, the term ventral means the same as anterior. The opposite of ventral is dorsal (or posterior).

V

problems during anesthesia. Severely premature babies with *respiratory distress syndrome* may also need ventilation for a period until their lungs develop sufficiently to cope with breathing unaided.

HOW IT IS DONE
The patient is connected to the ventilator by means of an *endotracheal tube* passed through the nose or mouth into the trachea (windpipe); if prolonged ventilation is likely to be required, a tube is inserted into an opening made in the trachea, an operation called a *tracheostomy*. Conscious patients, and those nearing the end of anesthesia, are usually given muscle-relaxant and sedative drugs to prevent them from resisting the insertion and irritant presence of the tube.

LOCATION OF VENTRICLES

The location of the ventricles in the brain (seen from above) and in the heart are shown below. Of the heart ventricles, the right ventricle pumps blood to the lungs, the left pumps blood to the rest of the body.

VENTRICLES IN THE BRAIN

Together, these irregularly shaped cavities contain about a glassful of cerebrospinal fluid.

Cerebrum

Ventricles

1
2

3
4

VENTRICLES IN THE HEART

The ventricles of the heart are the large, lower chambers, separated by a muscular wall, the septum.

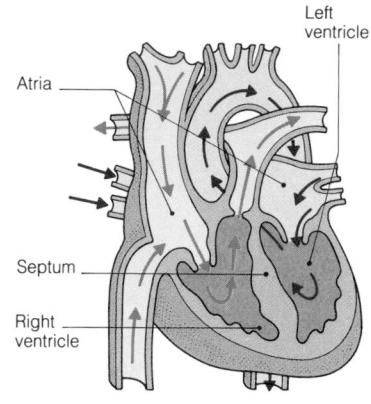

Left ventricle

Atria

Septum

Right ventricle

Ventricle

A cavity or chamber. Both the *heart* and *brain* have anatomical parts known as ventricles.

There are four ventricles in the brain—one in each of the two cerebral hemispheres (which make up the cerebrum, or main mass of the brain), a third at the center of the brain, above the brain stem, and a fourth situated between the brain stem and the cerebellum. These cavities are filled with cerebrospinal fluid and are linked by ducts so that the fluid can circulate through them. The cavities are lined in part with tuftlike clusters of blood vessels called the choroid plexus, which secrete the cerebrospinal fluid.

In the heart, there are two ventricles. They are the lower, pumping chambers, which receive blood from the atria (upper heart chambers) and pump it to the lungs and to the rest of the body.

Ventricular ectopic beat

An abnormal heart beat that has been initiated from electrical impulses in the ventricles (lower heart chambers) rather than the sinoatrial node in the right atrium (upper heart chamber). Many people, especially older people, have occasional ventricular ectopic beats that do not cause symptoms. Ventricular ectopic beats may also be caused by a *myocardial infarction* (heart attack) or *digitalis drugs*.

Occasionally, a ventricular ectopic beat causes the sensation that the heart has stopped for a second and then restarts with a thump.

Ventricular ectopic beats may be detected on an *ECG* (measurement of electrical activity of the heart) as a broad, bizarre-looking wave (see illustrated box, opposite).

If a person has frequent ventricular ectopic beats that cause symptoms or beats that arise from more than one site in the ventricles, treatment with an *antiarrhythmic drug* may be required.

Ventricular fibrillation

Rapid, ineffective, uncoordinated contractions of the heart. Ventricular fibrillation is caused by abnormal heart beats initiated by electrical activity in the ventricles (lower heart chambers). It is a common complication of *myocardial infarction* (heart attack) and may also be caused by electrocution or drowning. The heart ceases to pump blood effectively and the condition is fatal unless the normal heart rhythm is quickly restored. Diagnosis is confirmed by *ECG* (measurement of electrical activity of the heart), which shows broad, irregular waves (see illustrated box, opposite).

Treatment is with *cardioversion* (administration of an electric shock to the heart) and *antiarrhythmic drugs*.

Ventricular tachycardia

A serious cardiac *arrhythmia* (abnormal heart beat) in which each heart beat is initiated from electrical activity in the ventricles (lower heart chambers) rather than the sinoatrial node in the right atrium (upper heart chamber). The result is an abnormally fast heart rate of between 140 and 220 beats per minute.

Ventricular tachycardia is caused by serious heart disease, such as a *myocardial infarction* (heart attack) or *cardiomyopathy*. It may last for a few seconds or several days. Diagnosis is confirmed by *ECG* (recording of the electrical activity of the heart), which shows broad, regular abnormal waves (see box, opposite).

Emergency treatment is with *cardioversion* (administration of an electric shock to the heart) or by injection of an *antiarrhythmic drug*, such as lidocaine. Use of the drug is usually continued by mouth for several months. Untreated ventricular tachycardia may cause heart failure and death.

Ventriculography

An outdated procedure that enables the ventricular cavities within the brain to be seen on X-ray film after the introduction of air or a contrast medium (a substance opaque to X rays). Ventriculography is performed very infrequently; *CT scanning* and *MRI* have largely taken its place.

Verapamil

A *calcium channel blocker drug* used in the treatment of *hypertension* (high blood pressure), *angina pectoris* (chest pain due to inadequate blood supply to heart muscle), and certain types of *arrhythmia* (irregular heart rhythm).

Possible adverse effects include headache, facial flushing, dizziness, ankle swelling, and constipation.

Vernix

The pale, greasy, cheeselike substance that covers the skin of a newborn baby. Vernix consists of fatty secretions and dead cells. It is thought to protect the baby's skin and insulate against heat loss before birth.

Verruca

The medical term for a *wart*.

Version

A change in the direction in which a fetus lies so that a *malpresentation* (abnormal presentation), most often *breech* (bottom down), becomes the normal cephalic (head down) presen-

V

TYPES OF VENTRICULAR ARRHYTHMIA

The ventricles (lower chambers) of the heart usually beat regularly in response to excitatory waves spread from the upper chambers. If rhythm disturbances (which may be associated with heart disease) occur, they are visible on an electrocardiograph (ECG) recording.

Normal heart beat

Normal heart beat
This is the normal ECG appearance of the heart beat. The regular spikes coincide with beats of the ventricles (lower heart chambers). The small rises before each spike coincide with contractions of the atria (upper chambers).

Ventricular ectopic beat

Ventricular ectopic beat
Here there is an abnormal beat, which has a broad, bizarre-looking wave form on the ECG; it occurs just before the expected normal beat. To the patient, the heart may seem to stop at time A and restart with a thump at time B.

Ventricular tachycardia

Ventricular tachycardia
Here there is a rapid succession of abnormal beats, caused by an abnormal focus of electrical activity in a ventricle. It usually indicates serious underlying heart disease. The rate of beating may be very high—up to 220 beats per minute.

Ventricular fibrillation

Ventricular fibrillation
This pattern is seen only when the heart is in a state of virtual arrest, usually after a heart attack, with the ventricles twitching in a rapid and totally irregular manner. Unless a normal rhythm can be restored, the condition is quickly fatal.

tation. Version is also the term for the obstetric procedure used to change the presentation of a fetus.

Many breech babies undergo version spontaneously, especially before the 34th week of pregnancy. If this does not occur, the obstetrician may be able to manipulate the fetus into the cephalic position by a procedure called external version. With one hand on the mother's abdomen over the baby's head and the other over the baby's buttocks, the obstetrician very gently attempts to rotate the baby, bringing its head down into the mother's pelvis. External version is performed between the 34th and 37th week of pregnancy and can be done with or without general anesthesia. Drugs may be used to relax the uterus.

Though effective if properly performed, external version carries small risks of inducing premature labor or rupture of membranes, antepartum hemorrhage, or knotting of the umbilical cord. The risks of external version must be weighed against the risks of vaginal breech delivery and the risks of *cesarean section*.

Internal version is the turning of a fetus by an obstetrician by reaching inside the uterus. Internal version is rarely done except in the case of a second twin who is malposed (not in the normal position) after delivery of the first twin.

Vertebra

Any of the 33 approximately cylindrical bones that form the *spine*, or vertebral column. There are seven vertebrae in the cervical spine in the neck; 12 vertebrae in the thoracic spine in the chest; five vertebrae in the lumbar spine in the lower back; five fused vertebrae in the *sacrum*; and four fused vertebrae in the *coccyx* (see box, overleaf). Between each pair of separate vertebrae is an intervertebral disk (see *Disk, intervertebral*).

Vertebrobasilar insufficiency

Intermittent episodes of dizziness, double vision, weakness, and difficulty speaking caused by reduced blood flow to the brain stem and cerebellum in the brain.

The obstruction to blood flow is usually caused by *atherosclerosis* (narrowing of arteries with deposits of fat) involving the basilar and vertebral arteries and other arteries in the base of the brain.

Vertigo

An illusion that one's surroundings or self are spinning, either horizontally or vertically. Vertigo is a common complaint, but only rarely is it a sign of an underlying disorder. The term is sometimes used erroneously to describe *dizziness* or faintness.

CAUSES
Vertigo results from a disturbance of the semicircular canals in the inner ear or the nerve tracts leading from them. It can occur in healthy people when sailing, on amusement park rides, or

V

LOCATION AND STRUCTURE OF THE VERTEBRAE

The 33 vertebrae are arranged as shown. Apart from the top two, they all have a similar structure. The topmost cervical vertebra (the atlas) has no body. The second (the axis) forms a pivot on which the atlas can rotate, allowing the head to be turned in all directions.

The spine

Cervical vertebrae (7)

Thoracic vertebrae (12)

Lumbar vertebrae (5)

Sacral vertebrae (5)

Coccygeal vertebrae (4)

Cervical vertebrae

Transverse process

Spinous process

Foramen

Body

Thoracic vertebrae

Transverse process

Spinous process

Foramen

Body

Lumbar vertebrae

Transverse process

Spinous process

Foramen

Body

Arrangement
The vertebrae fall into five groups—cervical, thoracic, lumbar, sacral, and coccygeal. The top 24 are separated by disks of cartilage.

Structure
Three typical vertebrae are shown above. The foramen in each is the channel through which the spinal cord runs. The processes serve as muscle attachments.

even when watching a movie. Astronauts in zero gravity experience vertigo when moving their heads.

Severe vertigo, usually accompanied by other symptoms, may indicate a number of diseases. *Labyrinthitis* (inflammation of the semicircular canals) causes sudden vertigo accompanied by vomiting and unsteadiness. It often occurs in conjunction with an infection such as influenza or *otitis media* and usually clears up as the infection subsides. *Meniere's disease* is a more serious condition charac-

terized by attacks of vertigo that are sometimes severe enough to cause the sufferer to fall to the ground. The attacks of vertigo are accompanied by severe vomiting, *tinnitus* (ringing in the ears), *nystagmus* (jerky eye movements), and unsteadiness.

Elderly people with *atherosclerosis* often suffer from vertigo upon sudden movement of the head. Vertigo is less commonly caused by a tumor of the brain stem or by *multiple sclerosis*. Vertigo may also be psychological in origin, in which case it is usually associated with *agoraphobia* (fear of open spaces).

INVESTIGATION AND TREATMENT
If disease is the suspected cause of vertigo, the physician performs an examination of the ears, eyes, and nervous system, sometimes including *CT scanning* of the brain.

TREATMENT
Vertigo that comes on suddenly is usually assumed to be due to labyrinthitis and is treated with bed rest and *antihistamine drugs* or *anticholinergic drugs*. If vertigo persists for more than a few days, the sufferer should walk as much as possible to allow the body to develop compensatory measures. Antihistamine drugs may be prescribed to prevent recurrent attacks.

Vesicle
A small skin blister, usually filled with clear fluid, that forms at the site of skin damage. Vesicle also refers to any small saclike structure in the body; the seminal vesicles are small sacs in which seminal fluid is stored.

Vestibulocochlear nerve
The eighth *cranial nerve* concerned with *balance* and *hearing*. It carries sensory impulses from the inner *ear* to the brain, which it enters between the pons and the medulla oblongata (parts of the *brain stem*).

The vestibulocochlear nerve consists of two parts—the vestibular nerve and the cochlear nerve (also sometimes known as the acoustic, or auditory, nerve). The vestibular nerve carries sensory impulses from the semicircular canals in the inner ear to the cerebellum in the brain, which, in conjunction with information from the eyes and joints, controls balance. The cochlear nerve carries sensory impulses from the cochlea (the snail-shaped part of the inner ear responsible for detecting sound) to the hearing center in the brain, where the impulses are interpreted as sounds.

V

DISORDERS

A tumor of the cells that surround the vestibulocochlear nerve (see *Acoustic neuroma*) may cause loss of balance, *tinnitus* (noises in the ear), and *deafness*. Damage to the vestibulocochlear nerve (e.g., due to an infection such as *meningitis* or *encephalitis*) or an adverse reaction to a drug (such as streptomycin) may also cause deafness.

Viability

The capability of independent survival and development. It is widely accepted that a normal human fetus is viable from 28 weeks' gestation onward. However, today, fetuses born as early as the 23rd to 24th week can often survive after care in a neonatal intensive-care unit.

Vibrator

A mechanical device applied to the body to tone or relax muscles and to massage the skin.

Vibrators may also be used as an aid to sexual stimulation or as an alternative to sexual intercourse for inducing orgasm. They are sometimes used as an aid in *sex therapy*. (See also *Orgasm, lack of*; *Ejaculation, disorders of*.)

LOCATION OF THE VESTIBULOCOCHLEAR NERVE

The nerve conducts sensory impulses concerned with hearing and balance from different parts of the inner ear to the brain.

Cerebrum

Brain stem

Inner ear

Semicircular canals

Vestibulo-cochlear nerve

Cochlea

Villus

One of the countless millions of minute fingerlike projections that occur on the mucous lining of the small intestine. Although villi are present in all three sections of the small intestine, they are largest and most numerous in the duodenum and jejunum (the first and second parts), where most of the absorption of food occurs.

Microvilli in the intestine
This scanning electron micrograph shows numerous villi projecting from a single cell in the lining of the small intestine.

STRUCTURE

Each villus contains a small lymph vessel and a network of capillaries. The outer surface of each villus is covered with hundreds of hairlike structures (microvilli) that increase the surface area of the small intestine to an area approximately equal to that of a tennis court.

FUNCTION

The function of the villi is to provide a large intestinal surface area for the absorption of food molecules into the blood and lymphatic systems. Food particles that are broken down into small molecules by digestive enzymes reach the bloodstream via the capillaries of the villi.

Vincent's disease

Painful bacterial infection and ulceration of the gums, also known as acute necrotizing ulcerative gingivitis, trench mouth, or Vincent's stomatitis.

CAUSES AND INCIDENCE

The condition is caused by abnormal growth of microorganisms that usually exist harmlessly in small amounts in gum crevices. Predisposing factors include poor *oral hygiene*, smoking, throat infections, and emotional stress. In many cases Vincent's disease is preceded by *gingivitis* or by *periodontitis*. The condition is relatively rare, primarily affecting young adults aged 15 to 35.

SYMPTOMS

The symptoms appear over the course of a day or two. The gums become sore and inflamed and bleed at the slightest pressure. Craterlike ulcers, which bleed spontaneously, develop on the gum tips between teeth, and there is a foul taste in the mouth, bad breath, and sometimes swollen lymph nodes. As the disease advances, ulcers spread along the gum margins and into deeper tissues. Occasionally, the infection spreads to the lips and the lining of the cheeks, resulting in destruction of tissues (see *Noma*).

TREATMENT

The dentist usually prescribes a mouthwash containing hydrogen peroxide to relieve pain and inflammation. After a few days, when the gums are less tender, scaling (see *Scaling, dental*) is performed to remove calculus (a hard mineral deposit) and plaque from the teeth. In severe cases, the antibacterial drug *metronidazole* may be prescribed to control infection.

Regular follow-up visits to the dentist may be necessary. Counseling may focus on maintaining oral hygiene, giving up smoking, or learning to cope with stress.

Viremia

The presence of virus particles in the blood. Viremia can occur at certain stages in a variety of viral infections.

Some viruses, such as those responsible for viral hepatitis, yellow fever, and poliomyelitis, may simply be carried in the bloodstream, which is used solely as a means of spreading. Symptoms arise when virus particles enter and start multiplying in target tissues rather than from the viremia.

Other viruses, such as the rubella virus and HIV (the AIDS virus), exist within lymphocytes (types of white blood cell), which they use as a place to multiply as well as for spreading.

If viremia is a feature of a viral infection, there is a risk that the infection may be transmissible in blood or blood products (as is the case with the AIDS virus) or by blood-feeding insects (as is the case with yellow fever).

Virginity

The physical state of not having experienced *sexual intercourse*.

Virilism

Masculine characteristics that affect the physical appearance of a woman. Virilism is caused by excessive levels of androgens. Androgens are male sex hormones that, in women, are normally secreted in small amounts by the adrenal glands and ovaries. Raised levels of these hormones induce

V

various changes in women, including *hirsutism* (excessive hair growth); a male-pattern hairline with balding at the temples; disruption or cessation of menstruation; enlargement of the clitoris; loss of normal fat deposits around the hips; development of the arm and shoulder muscles; and deepening of the voice as a result of enlargement of the larynx. (See also *Virilization*.)

Virility

A term used to describe the quality of maleness, especially sexual characteristics and performance.

Virilization

The process by which *virilism* occurs in women due to overproduction of androgens (male sex hormones) by the adrenal glands and/or ovaries. This process, in turn, may be caused by various underlying conditions, such as certain tumors of the adrenal glands (see *Adrenal glands* disorders box); some types of ovarian cysts (see *Polycystic ovary*); or congenital *adrenal hyperplasia*, a rare genetic disorder.

Virion

A single, complete, virus particle. (See *Viruses*.)

Virology

The study of *viruses* and the *epidemiology* and treatment of diseases caused by viruses. In a more restricted sense, virology also means the isolation and identification of viruses to diagnose specific viral infections. To achieve this, a tissue or fluid sample (such as a specimen of feces, sputum, blister fluid, blood, urine, cerebrospinal fluid, or even brain biopsy specimen, depending on the suspected virus) is needed.

Unlike bacteria, viruses cannot be grown in a suitable culture medium; they can multiply only within living cells. Therefore, viruses must be grown in cultures of cells, which can be any of many types of animal or human cell that are easily made to multiply in test tubes. The culture is exposed to the specimen or fluid containing the virus, and the cells are then observed for distinctive changes that occur when they are infected with certain viruses.

Alternatively, virus particles or components of viruses can sometimes be detected directly in specimens by the use of staining techniques or an electron microscope. Sometimes, the virus particles must first be made to

clump together by adding an *antiserum* (antibodies obtained from the blood of someone who has had the viral infection, and which will bind to the virus particles). *Immunoassay* techniques, in which "labeled" antibodies are added to the specimens and detected if they have bound to virus cell components, are another possibility.

Another method of diagnosing viral infections is to look for antibodies produced by the immune system to combat the viruses. A rapidly rising level of antibodies to a particular virus can provide good evidence of infection. Antibodies can be detected by types of immunoassay and other laboratory techniques (see *Serology*).

Virulence

The ability of a microorganism to cause disease. Virulence can be assessed by measuring what proportion of the population exposed to the microorganism develops symptoms of disease, how rapidly the infection spreads through body tissues, or by the mortality from the infection.

Viruses

The smallest known types of infectious agent. Viruses are about one half to one hundredth the size of the smallest bacteria, from which they differ in having a much simpler structure and method of multiplication. Viral infections range from the trivial and harmless, such as *warts*, the common cold (see *Cold, common*), and other minor respiratory tract infections, to extremely serious diseases, such as *rabies, AIDS*, and probably some types of *cancer*.

NATURE OF VIRUSES

It is debatable whether viruses are truly living organisms or just collections of large molecules capable of self-replication under very specific favorable conditions. Their sole activity is to invade the cells of other organisms, which they take over to make copies of themselves. Outside living cells, viruses are wholly inert. They are incapable of activities typical of life, such as metabolism (internal processing of nutrients).

The number of different kinds of virus probably exceeds the number of types of all other organisms. They parasitize all recognized life-forms—mammals, birds, reptiles, insects, plants, algae, even bacteria. Not all viruses cause disease, but many do.

STRUCTURE AND REPLICATION OF VIRUSES

A single virus particle (virion) consists simply of an inner core of *nucleic acid*

Rotavirus particles
This particular virus is a common cause of stomach upsets and diarrhea in infants. Each white sphere is a virus particle.

surrounded by one or two protective shells (capsids) made of protein. These capsids are built from a number of identical protein subunits arranged in a highly symmetrical form, usually either as a 20-faced solid (an icosahedron) or as a spiral tube. Surrounding the outer capsid may be another layer called the viral envelope. This layer also consists primarily of protein. In many cases, the viral envelope is lost when the virus invades a cell.

The nucleic acid at the core is called the genome; it consists of a string of *genes* that contain coded instructions for making copies of the virus. Depending on the type of virus, the nucleic acid may be either DNA, in which there are two complementary, intertwined strands of nucleic acid (the double helix), or RNA, consisting of a single strand.

The basic process by which a virus replicates is shown in the illustrated box (right). Different viruses employ different strategies, some highly complex, to make copies of themselves once they have invaded a host cell. During replication of the viral nucleic acid, the viral genes may first have to code the manufacture of special enzymes called polymerases or transcriptases to assist in replication, or may borrow these enzymes from the host cell. Sometimes the viral genome must invade the nucleus of the host cell and incorporate itself into the cell's chromosomes before it can replicate.

Sometimes, if the viral genome invades the nucleus of the host cell, it may not at first replicate but may "hide" there, sometimes becoming reactivated months or years later. It may also interact with the cell's chromosomes—a process that may convert the cell into a tumor cell.

V

VIRUSES AND DISEASE

All viruses have the same basic structure (right), but they come in various shapes and sizes. Examples from the main families are shown below (some in cross section). All are tiny (from about one millionth to one hundred thousandths of an inch in diameter) and most cannot be seen even with a powerful light microscope. All types of viruses can multiply only after invading the cells of their human or other host (far right).

Structure of a typical virus particle
Nucleic acid in the center is surrounded by one or more capsids made of protein subunits.

VIRAL REPLICATION

The sequence below shows how a virus multiplies. The signs and symptoms of viral infection are caused by the virus interfering with or destroying the host's cells.

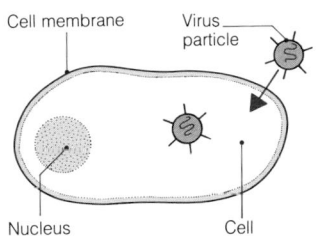

1 The virus particle first attaches itself to and then injects itself into the host cell.

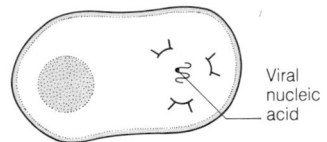

2 The viral capsid breaks down and the viral nucleic acid (DNA or RNA) contained inside is released.

3 The viral nucleic acid replicates itself; the new copies are made from raw materials within the host cell.

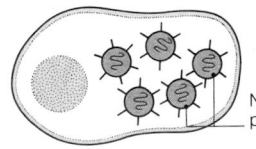

4 Each of the new copies of the viral nucleic acid now directs the manufacture of a capsid for itself.

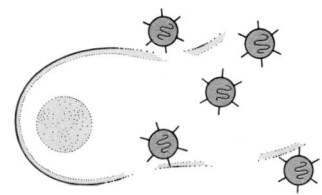

5 The newly formed viral particles are released in large numbers, and the host cell may be destroyed.

TYPES OF VIRUS

Family	Examples of conditions or diseases
Papovaviruses	Warts
Adenoviruses	Respiratory and eye infections
Herpesviruses	Cold sores, genital herpes, chickenpox, herpes zoster (shingles), glandular fever, congenital abnormalities (cytomegalovirus)
Poxviruses	Cowpox, smallpox (eradicated), molluscum contagiosum
Picornaviruses	Poliomyelitis, viral hepatitis types A and B, respiratory infections, myocarditis
Togaviruses	Yellow fever, dengue, encephalitis
Orthomyxoviruses	Influenza
Paramyxoviruses	Mumps, measles, rubella
Coronaviruses	Common cold
Arenaviruses	Lassa fever
Rhabdoviruses	Rabies
Retroviruses	AIDS, degenerative brain diseases, and (possibly) various kinds of cancer

V

TYPES

Viruses that cause human disease are grouped into more than 20 large families; the most important are shown in the table (previous page).

In recent years, special attention has been paid to the family of retroviruses, which include *HIV* (human immunodeficiency virus), the agent responsible for AIDS. HIV is an RNA virus and, after invading a cell, first manufactures an enzyme called reverse transcriptase, which it needs to make copies of itself. Research into this enzyme may reveal a means of attacking HIV.

HOW VIRUSES CAUSE DISEASE

Viruses gain access to the body by all possible entry routes. They are inhaled in droplets; swallowed in food and fluids; and passed through the punctured skin in the saliva of feeding insects or rabid dogs or accidentally on the needles of tattooists, those who pierce ears, or even physicians. Viruses are accepted directly by the mucous membranes of the genital tract during sexual intercourse and by the conjunctiva of the eye after accidental contamination.

Many viruses begin to invade cells and multiply near their site of entry. Some enter the lymphatic vessels and may spread to the lymph nodes, where many are engulfed by white blood cells. Some, such as HIV, invade and then multiply within *lymphocytes* (a type of white cell). Many pass from the lymphatics to the blood and within a few minutes are spread to every part of the body. They may then invade and start multiplying within specific target organs such as the skin, brain, liver, or lungs. Other viruses travel along nerve fibers to their target organs.

Viruses cause disease in a variety of ways. First, they may destroy or severely disrupt the activities of the cells they invade, possibly causing serious disease if vital organs are affected. Second, the response of the body's *immune system* to viral infection may lead to symptoms, such as fever and fatigue, or to a disease process. In particular, antibodies produced by the immune system may attach to viral particles and circulate as immune complexes in the bloodstream. The antibodies may then be deposited in various parts of the body and cause inflammation and severe tissue damage. Third, by interacting with the chromosomes of their host cells, viruses may cause cancer. Fourth, a virus may cause disease by weakening the cell-mediated arm of the immune system (i.e., the activity of T-*lymphocytes*). This is how HIV works, invading and disrupting one type of T-lymphocyte so that the normal defenses to a wide range of infections are lost.

VIRUSES AND CANCER

The chromosomes in all normal body cells contain 50 or more genes (known as oncogenes) that are necessary for the growth or *differentiation* of the cells. Certain retroviruses contain almost identical oncogenes. In the process of replication, these viruses may modify the chromosomes of the host cells. A small mutation in these can "switch on" the oncogenes inappropriately, thus prompting the cell to begin unrestrained division, leading to cancer.

To date, this process has been found to cause many cancers in animals but only one type of cancer in humans. The virus responsible is similar to the AIDS virus and can cause leukemia in the person it infects. However, other viruses are known to be at least potentially cancer-producing in humans; this is a major area of research.

RESISTANCE TO VIRUSES

The immune system deals fairly rapidly with most viruses. Each mechanism of the immune system may be involved in resisting a viral attack—including white cells (macrophages) that engulf the viral particles, and lymphocytes that produce antibodies against the virus or attack virally infected cells. This leads to recovery from most viral infections within a few days to weeks. Furthermore, the immune system is often sufficiently sensitized by the infection to make a second illness from the same virus rare (as is the case with measles).

With some viruses, however, the speed of the attack is such that serious damage or even death may occur before the immune system can adequately respond (as is the case with rabies and some cases of poliomyelitis). In other cases, a virus is able to dodge or hide from the immune system, so the infection becomes chronic or recurrent. This is common with many herpes virus infections (such as genital herpes and shingles) and with viral hepatitis B. Finally, the AIDS virus, by weakening the immune system, leaves the body open to many *opportunistic infections*.

FIGHTING VIRAL DISEASE

Viruses are more difficult than bacteria to combat with drugs because it is difficult to design drugs that will kill viruses without also killing the cells they parasitize. Nevertheless, there has been remarkable progress in the development of antiviral agents, especially against the herpes group of viruses (see *Antiviral drugs*). Such drugs may work by helping to prevent viruses from entering cells or by interfering with their replication in cells.

Interferon refers to a group of natural substances, produced by virus-infected cells, that protects uninfected cells. Some interferons can now be produced artificially and have been tried in the treatment of various viral infections, including the common cold and viral hepatitis B.

Otherwise, treatment of viral infections depends largely on alleviating the patient's symptoms and trusting the body's immune defenses to bring about a cure.

A much more fruitful area in the fight against viruses is *immunization*. One viral disease, smallpox, has already been eradicated worldwide through a coordinated vaccination program. Highly effective vaccines are also now available to prevent many others, including poliomyelitis, measles, mumps, rubella, hepatitis B, yellow fever, and rabies.

Viscera

A collective term used to describe the internal organs.

Viscosity

The resistance to flow of a liquid or gas; the "stickiness" of a fluid. The viscosity of the blood affects its ability to flow through small blood vessels. An increase in the viscosity of the blood—caused by an increase in the proportion of red blood cells—increases the risk of *thrombosis* (abnormal clot formation).

Vision

The faculty of sight. Vision involves two main components—the *eye* and the *brain*.

When light rays reach the eye, most of the focusing is done by the *cornea*. However, the eye also has an automatic fine-focusing facility, called *accommodation*, that operates by altering the curvature of the crystalline *lens*. Together, these two systems provide sufficient optical power to form an image on the *retina*. The light-sensitive rods and cones in the retina convert the elements of this image into nerve impulses that, after preliminary processing in the retina, pass into the brain via the *optic nerves*. The rods,

V

THE SENSE OF VISION

Vision starts in the retina, the membrane at the back of the eye that contains the light-sensitive rod and cone cells. Much of the rest of the eye is concerned with focusing light, in the right quantities, onto the retina. Huge amounts of data are sent from the retina via the optic nerves to the brain for analysis.

Cross section through the eye

Pathways to the brain
Signals pass from the eyes along the optic nerves to the optic chiasma and then to the visual cortices in the brain. There is some crossover of nerve fibers at the optic chiasma, so both sides of the brain receive signals from both eyes.

Stereoscopic vision
The two eyes receive slightly different views of all but the most distant objects; information from the two images is compared and processed in the brain to give a single 3-D interpretation of the object.

IMAGE RECEPTION

The light rays from an object stimulate a group of receptors in the retina within an area that has the same shape as the object but is upside down. The brain automatically interprets the image the right way up.

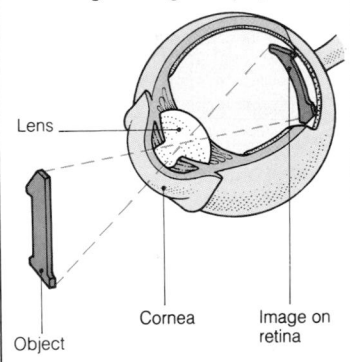

EYEBALL MOVEMENTS

To maintain the image of any moving object on the center of the retina, precise eyeball movements, are achieved by the six muscles shown below, are necessary. The muscles act to swivel the eyeball in the directions indicated (the right eye is shown). The muscles always act in groups.

Inferior oblique
Upward, outward, and anticlockwise rotation

Lateral rectus
Outward

Superior oblique
Downward, outward, and clockwise rotation

Superior rectus
Upward, inward, and clockwise rotation

Medial rectus
Inward

Inferior rectus
Downward, inward, and anticlockwise rotation

V

which are proportionately more concentrated at the periphery of the retina, are highly sensitive to light but not to color. The color-sensitive cones are concentrated more at the center of the retina (see *Color vision*).

Accurate alignment of the two eyes is achieved by coordination of the motor nerve impulses to the six tiny muscles that move each eye. This coordination is achieved in the brain, which correlates information from several sources, taking into account the brain's perception of the images, the position of the head, the position of the eyes relative to the head, and the position of the two eyes relative to each other.

Accurate alignment of the two eyes allows the brain to fuse the images from each eye, but because each eye has a slightly different view of a given object, the brain can interpret solidity or depth. This stereoscopic vision is important in judging distance.

Vision, disorders of

The most common visual disorders are due to simple errors of *refraction*, such as *myopia, hyperopia*, and *astigmatism*. The blurring of vision from refractive errors can almost always be corrected by *glasses*. Defects of vision that cannot be eliminated in this way may have any of a wide variety of causes, including loss of binocular fusion (which can cause *double vision* or *amblyopia*), disorders of the eye or optic nerve, disorders of the nerve pathways that connect the optic nerves to the brain, and disorders of the brain itself.

VISUAL DEFECT FROM EYE AND OPTIC NERVE DISORDERS

Eye or optic nerve disease often affects vision only on the side involved; it can affect one or both sides, often to different degrees. Any interference with the transparency of the eye affects vision. Loss of transparency may result from corneal opacities (opaqueness of the cornea) following infection, ulceration, or injury; from *cataract* (opacification of the crystalline lens); or from *vitreous hemorrhage* (bleeding into the gel of the eye behind the lens).

Defects near the center of the retina cause loss of the corresponding parts of the *visual field* of the affected eye. This is especially serious if the central part of the retina (where sharp *visual acuity* exists) is involved (see *Macular degeneration*). Peripheral retinal damage, which occurs in the early stages of chronic simple *glaucoma* or

retinitis pigmentosa, may not cause noticeable visual disturbance if sharp central vision is unaffected.

Floaters (freely moving shadows perceived in the field of vision) are usually of no significance, but necessitate an eye examination. Floaters may signify a retinal tear or a hemorrhage. Floaters may herald a *retinal detachment*, especially if accompanied by bright flashing lights at the periphery of the field of vision.

A defect in the optic nerve in front of the optic nerve crossing causes visual disturbance in one eye only. It often takes the form of a central *scotoma* (a blind spot in the center of the field of vision). This condition can be due to *optic neuritis*, which is sometimes a sign of *multiple sclerosis*.

VISUAL DEFECT FROM NERVE PATHWAY DISORDER

Disorders of one of the nerve pathways behind the optic nerve crossing always affect both eyes. This is because half of the fibers from each optic nerve—those from the inner half of each retina—cross over before they run back to the back of the brain. Each pathway thus has contributions from both eyes and any interruption thus causes loss of part of the visual field of each eye.

VISUAL DEFECT FROM BRAIN DISORDER

Severe damage to one side of the visual area of the brain, such as from loss of blood supply (stroke), causes loss of the inner half of the field of vision of the eye on the same side and of the outer half of the field of the other eye. This is called *hemianopia*, in which the sufferer has only half of the field of vision.

Visual disturbance may also arise from involvement of the areas of the brain concerned with the psychological and associational aspects of vision. Disorders of these functions may cause visual *agnosia* (failure to recognize objects), visual perseveration (in which a scene continues to be perceived after the direction of gaze has shifted), and visual hallucinations.

Vision, loss of

An inability to see, which may develop slowly or suddenly. Vision loss may affect one or both eyes. It can cause complete blindness, or may affect only peripheral vision or only central vision. Loss of vision may be temporary or permanent, depending on the cause.

SLOW VISION LOSS

A progressive loss of visual clarity is common with advancing age as a

result of loss of transparency of the crystalline lenses of the eyes (see *Cataract*). Other common causes of gradual loss of vision are *macular degeneration, diabetes mellitus*, and *glaucoma*. Gradual visual loss may also be due to progressive opacity of the cornea from *keratopathy* (disease of the cornea) of any kind, or to progressive distortion from *keratoconus* (a conical deformity of the cornea). *Retinitis pigmentosa* causes a variable degree of visual loss in both eyes.

SUDDEN VISION LOSS

Sudden loss of vision may be caused by optical or neurological disorders. *Hyphema* (bleeding into the aqueous humor) usually results from injury; the blood can block the normal passage of the light to the retina. Severe *uveitis* (inflammation of the uvea) may cause serious reduction in vision. *Vitreous hemorrhage* (bleeding into the gel of the eye) and retinal disorders, such as *retinal detachment* and *retinal hemorrhage*, may also reduce vision suddenly.

Optic neuritis (inflammation of the optic nerve) can severely reduce vision in one eye. Any damage to the nerve connections between the eyes and the brain, or to the visual area of the brain itself, can cause loss of peripheral vision. Damage to the visual nerve pathways may sometimes be a result of *ischemia* (inadequate blood supply), tumor, injury, or inflammation.

Vision tests

The part of an *eye examination* that determines if there is any reduction in the ability to see. Most vision tests are tests of *visual acuity* (sharpness of central vision). *Visual field* (side vision) tests may also be performed to assess disorders of the eye and the nervous system. Refraction tests are done to discover whether the patient has a refractive error (that is, an error that can be corrected with glasses), such as *hyperopia, myopia*, or *astigmatism*. Refraction tests also show whether there is a deficiency in the power of *accommodation* (see *Presbyopia*).

VISUAL ACUITY TESTS

Visual acuity is tested, one eye at a time, using *Snellen's chart*. An attempt is made to read letters of standard sizes from a standard distance, classically 20 feet (6 meters).

REFRACTION TESTS

These tests may be done in several ways. In one technique (retinoscopy) a narrow beam of light is projected into the eye, from a distance of about

V

TYPES OF VISION TESTS

These tests are performed to measure a number of variables—the acuity of a patient's distance vision and the power of the lenses he or she may need (visual acuity and refraction tests), the extent of peripheral vision (visual field tests), and the ability to focus on objects close up (accommodation tests).

VISUAL ACUITY TESTS

These tests use the familiar Snellen's chart. Visual acuity is measured according to how far down the chart the patient can read accurately.

ACCOMMODATION TESTS

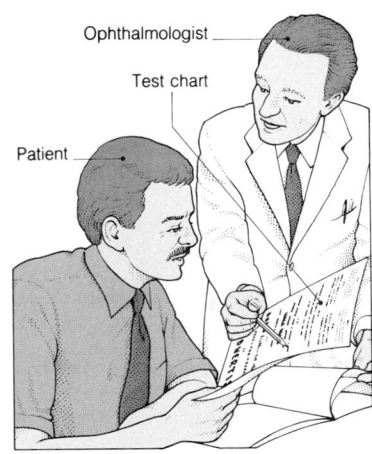

After any distance-focusing ability has been corrected, the ability to read small print close up is measured to test the patient's accommodation.

REFRACTION TESTS

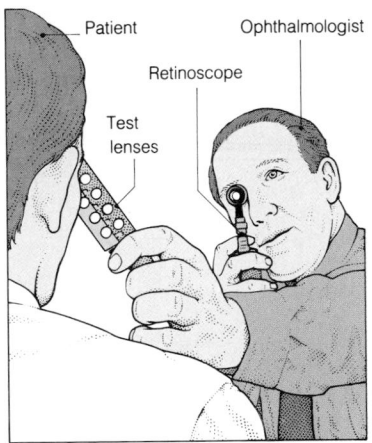

The effect of lenses on movements of light reflected from the eye (as the light source is moved) is observed to help calculate the corrective glasses needed.

VISUAL FIELD TESTS

One eye is fixed straight ahead, the other covered, and lights are shined onto a white bowl or screen in front of the patient to find the field of vision of each eye.

ACCOMMODATION TESTS

The power of accommodation (ability to focus on near objects) may be measured by correcting any refractive error with *glasses*, and then determining the nearest distance at which very small print can be read. Most people at age 45, unless nearsighted, need some assistance (e.g., glasses) with accommodation to read small print up close.

VISUAL FIELD TESTS

Visual field tests can indicate disorders of the peripheral parts of the retinas, of the optic nerves, or of the optical pathways that convey nerve impulses from the eyes to the back of the brain. Most visual field tests involve the use of large black screens or white hollow bowls. The patient's head is secured, one eye is covered, and the other is directed to a point at the center of the inside of the bowl. Small spots of light are projected onto the inner surface of the bowl; the spots appear for brief periods in various places or are moved inward from the periphery. The person being tested responds when he or she sees the spot.

Visual acuity

Sharpness of vision. Visual acuity is not concerned with the extent or clarity of the peripheral vision but with sharpness (discrimination) of central vision (see *Visual field*). A person's visual acuity is measured during a *vision test*.

Refractive errors (errors that can be corrected with glasses) are the most common cause of poor visual acuity. They include *myopia, hyperopia*, and *astigmatism*. Poor visual acuity for near objects occurs in *presbyopia*.

Visual field

The total area in which visual perception is possible while looking straight ahead. The visual fields normally extend outward over an angle of about 90 degrees on either side of the midline of the face, but are more restricted above and below, especially if the eyes are deep-set or the eyebrows are prominent. The visual fields of the two eyes overlap to a large extent so that a defect in the field of one eye may be concealed if both eyes are open (see box, overleaf).

The level of *visual acuity* (sharpness of vision) in the visual field is much lower in areas remote from the point at which one is looking directly. For instance, it is impossible to read fine print as little as 5 degrees to one side of the fixation point. This is especially

26 inches (65 cm), by an instrument that allows the tester to observe the light reflected back through the pupil from the retina. Small movements of the light are made in various directions. The appropriate correction can be determined from the power and type of lenses needed to neutralize the movement of the light. Refinements of the refraction (correction with glasses) can be achieved by determining the person's subjective response to changes made in his or her vision by slight changes in the lenses.

V

THE VISUAL FIELDS

The field of vision of each eye (with the head and eyes immobile) extends through an angle of about 130 degrees and is divided into an area that overlaps with the visual field of the other eye (binocular vision) and an area that can be seen with only the one eye.

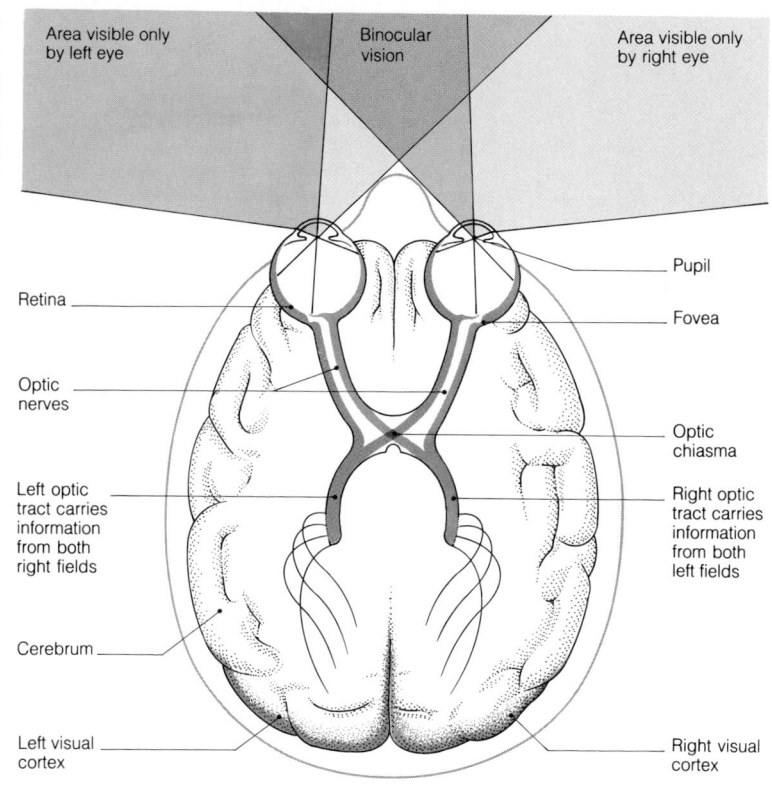

Area visible only by left eye

Binocular vision

Area visible only by right eye

Retina

Optic nerves

Left optic tract carries information from both right fields

Cerebrum

Left visual cortex

Pupil

Fovea

Optic chiasma

Right optic tract carries information from both left fields

Right visual cortex

Route of visual signals
Note that all light from the fields left of center of both eyes (gray) falls on the right sides of the two retinas; and information about these fields goes to the right visual cortex. Information about the right fields of vision (pink) goes to the left cortex. Data about the area of binocular vision go to both cortices.

apparent to people with *macular degeneration*, who have no central vision and must use other parts of the visual field.

Partial loss of visual field is less obvious than loss of central vision; even people with extensive visual field loss, as from *glaucoma* or *stroke*, may be unaware of it if they retain sharp central visual acuity. (See also *Vision, disorders of*; *Vision tests*.)

Vital sign

An indication that a person is still alive. Vital signs include chest movements caused by breathing, the presence of a pulse (which indicates that the heart is beating) at the neck or wrist, and the constriction of the pupil of the eye when it is exposed to a bright light. A physician certifies *death* on the basis of the absence of all these signs. Additional tests, such as measurement of brain activity, may also be required in certain circumstances, notably if the patient is on a life-support system.

Vitamin

Any of a group of complex chemicals that are essential for the normal functioning of the body. With few exceptions (notably vitamin D), the body cannot manufacture these substances itself, making it necessary to obtain them from the diet. There are 13 major vitamins—A, C, D, E, K, B_{12}, and the seven B-complex vitamins. Most are required only in extremely small amounts, and each vitamin is present in many different foods. Vitamin D is also produced in the skin when it is exposed to sunlight.

A balanced diet that includes a variety of different types of foods is likely to contain adequate amounts of all the vitamins, and supplements are not usually necessary. However, a physician may recommend *vitamin supplements* in certain circumstances, such as for a person taking certain *lipid-lowering drugs* (which reduce intestinal absorption of vitamins) or for some women who are pregnant or breast-feeding.

TYPES
Vitamins can be categorized into fat-soluble vitamins and water-soluble vitamins.

FAT-SOLUBLE VITAMINS The fat-soluble vitamins (A, D, E, and K) are absorbed with fats from the intestine into the blood and then stored in fatty tissue (mainly the liver). They are not normally excreted in the urine.

Body reserves of some of these vitamins may last for several years and a daily intake is thus not usually essential; in fact, an excessive intake of a fat-soluble vitamin may cause harmful levels to accumulate in the body. For most people, a balanced diet ensures a sufficient supply.

Deficiency of a fat-soluble vitamin is usually due to a disorder in which intestinal absorption of fats is impaired (see *Malabsorption*) or to a prolonged poor or restricted diet.

WATER-SOLUBLE VITAMINS The water-soluble vitamins are C, B_{12}, and the members of the B complex. Most of these vitamins are stored in the body for only a short period and are rapidly excreted in the urine if taken in greater amounts than the body requires. Vitamin B_{12} is an exception, in that it is stored in the liver. It may take five or six years for deficiency symptoms to appear.

Deficiencies of the water-soluble vitamins are more likely to occur than fat-soluble vitamin deficiencies. Foods that contain water-soluble vitamins should therefore be eaten daily; moreover, prolonged cooking, preserving, and processing tend to destroy these vitamins, so fresh or lightly cooked foods are the best sources. Plain, frozen fruits and vegetables can also be a good source of water-soluble vitamins. Taking very large amounts of water-soluble vitamins does not usually cause toxic effects; adverse reactions to very large doses of vitamin C and vitamin B_6 (pyridoxine) have been reported.

V

FUNCTION

The role of vitamins in the body is not fully understood; most knowledge about them is based on evidence provided by symptoms that occur as a result of deficiency. Most vitamins have been found to have several important actions on one or more body systems or functions; many are involved in the activities of *enzymes* (substances that promote chemical reactions in the body). See also articles on individual vitamins.

Vitamin A

A *vitamin* essential for normal growth and for the formation of strong bones and teeth in children, for normal vision and cell structure, for protecting the linings of the respiratory, digestive, and urinary tracts against infection, and for healthy skin.

Many foods contain vitamin A. Particularly rich sources of this vitamin include liver, fish-liver oils, egg yolk, milk and other dairy products, margarine, and various vegetables and fruits, such as carrots, winter squashes, kale, broccoli, spinach, apricots, and peaches.

DEFICIENCY

Vitamin A deficiency is rare in developed countries. In most cases, it is due to failure of the intestine to absorb enough of the vitamin, which may occur as a result of *cystic fibrosis, bile duct obstruction,* or long-term treatment with certain *lipid-lowering drugs.* Dietary deficiency occurs only in people who have an exceptionally poor diet; it is most common in some developing countries.

The effects of vitamin A deficiency include poor night vision; dry, inflamed eyes; dry, rough skin; loss of appetite; diarrhea; and lowered resistance to infection. Severe deficiency may cause weak bones and teeth, corneal ulcers, and, in extreme cases, *keratomalacia* (an eye disorder in which there is severe corneal damage that can lead to blindness if untreated).

EXCESS

Prolonged, excessive intake of vitamin A can result in a condition called hypervitaminosis A, the symptoms of which include headache, tiredness, nausea, loss of appetite, diarrhea, dry and itchy skin, hair loss, and, in women, irregular menstruation. In extreme cases, there may also be bone pain and enlargement of the liver and spleen. Excessive intake during pregnancy may cause birth defects.

Contrary to popular belief, excessive intake of carotene (e.g., through eating huge amounts of carrots) does not cause hypervitaminosis A, but produces carotenemia (high blood levels of carotene), the most noticeable feature of which is a deep yellow coloration of the skin.

RETINOIDS

Synthetic, vitamin A-like compounds called retinoids have been reported to reverse some of the skin wrinkling, roughness, and mottled pigmentation caused by chronic sun exposure.

Clinical testing of retinoids, which are applied directly to the skin, was begun in 1987.

Vitamin B

See *Vitamin B₁₂*; *Vitamin B complex.*

VITAMINS AND THEIR SOURCES IN THE DIET

Fat-soluble	Good sources
Vitamin A	Liver, fish-liver oils, egg yolk, milk and dairy products, margarine, various fruits and vegetables (such as carrots and apricots)
Vitamin D	Fortified milk, oily fish (such as sardines, herring, salmon, and tuna), liver, dairy products, egg yolk
Vitamin E	Vegetable oils (such as corn, soy bean, olive, and sunflower oils), nuts, meat, green leafy vegetables, cereals, wheat germ, egg yolk
Vitamin K	Green leafy vegetables (especially cabbage, broccoli, and turnip greens), vegetable oils, egg yolk, cheese, pork, liver

Water-soluble	
Thiamine (vitamin B₁)	Wheat germ, bran, whole-grain or enriched cereals and breads, brown rice, pasta, liver, kidney, pork, fish, beans, nuts
Riboflavin (vitamin B₂)	Liver, milk, cheese, eggs, green leafy vegetables, whole grains, enriched breads and cereals, brewer's yeast
Niacin (nicotinic acid)	Liver, lean meat, poultry, fish, whole grains, enriched breads and cereals, peanuts, dried beans
Pantothenic acid	Liver, heart, kidney, fish, egg yolk, skimmed milk, brewer's yeast, wheat germ, most vegetables
Pyridoxine (vitamin B₆)	Liver, chicken, pork, fish, whole grains, wheat germ, bananas, potatoes, dried beans, peanuts
Biotin	Liver, kidney, peanuts, dried beans, egg yolk, mushrooms, cauliflower, bananas, grapefruit, watermelons
Folic acid	Green leafy vegetables (such as spinach and broccoli), mushrooms, liver, nuts, dried beans, peas, egg yolk, whole-wheat bread
Vitamin B₁₂ (cyanocobalamin)	Liver, kidney, chicken, beef, pork, fish, eggs, cheese, butter, yogurt, other dairy products
Vitamin C	Citrus fruits, tomatoes, potatoes, green leafy vegetables, green peppers, strawberries, cantaloupe

Vitamin needs
A varied diet usually provides all vitamin needs. For vegans (who eat no animal products), vitamins B₁₂ and D may be lacking; these vitamins can be obtained from supplements or, in the case of vitamin D, through adequate exposure to sunlight.

V

Vitamin B$_{12}$

Also known as cyanocobalamin, a *vitamin* that plays a vital role in the activities of several *enzymes* (substances that promote chemical reactions in the body). Vitamin B$_{12}$ is important in the production of the genetic material of cells (and thus in growth and development), in the production of red blood cells in bone marrow, in the utilization of folic acid (a constituent of the *vitamin B complex*) and carbohydrates in the diet, and in the functioning of the nervous system.

Foods rich in vitamin B$_{12}$ include liver, kidney, chicken, beef, pork, fish, eggs, and dairy products.

DEFICIENCY AND EXCESS

A balanced diet contains sufficient amounts of vitamin B$_{12}$ for the body's needs. Deficiency of vitamin B$_{12}$ is almost always due to an inability of the intestine to absorb the vitamin, most commonly as a result of pernicious anemia (see *Anemia, megaloblastic*). In rare cases, deficiency of vitamin B$_{12}$ may result from following a vegan diet (one that excludes all kinds of animal products).

The principal effects of vitamin B$_{12}$ deficiency are megaloblastic anemia, a sore mouth and tongue, and symptoms caused by damage to the spinal cord, such as numbness and tingling in the limbs. There may also be depression and loss of memory.

No harmful effects are known to occur as a result of a high intake of vitamin B$_{12}$.

Vitamin B complex

A group of *vitamins* that consists of thiamine (also known as vitamin B$_1$), riboflavin (vitamin B$_2$), niacin (nicotinic acid), pantothenic acid, pyridoxine (vitamin B$_6$), biotin, and folic acid. *Vitamin B$_{12}$* is not usually included in this group.

THIAMINE

This vitamin plays a vital role in the activities of various *enzymes* (substances that promote chemical reactions in the body) involved in the breakdown and utilization of carbohydrates and in the functioning of the nerves, muscles, and heart.

Thiamine is present in most unrefined foods. Particularly good sources of thiamine include wheat germ, bran, whole-grain or enriched cereals and breads, brown rice, pasta, liver, kidney, pork, fish, beans, nuts, and eggs.

A balanced diet usually provides adequate amounts of thiamine. Those susceptible to deficiency include elderly people on a poor diet, people with very high energy requirements (such as manual workers or people involved in high-level endurance activities), or those suffering from *hyperthyroidism* (overactivity of the thyroid gland), those with *malabsorption* disorders, and those with severe *alcohol dependence*. Deficiency may also occur as a result of severe illness, surgery, or serious injury.

Mild thiamine deficiency may cause tiredness, irritability, loss of appetite, and sleep disturbances. Severe deficiency may produce *beriberi*, abdominal pain, constipation, depression, memory impairment, and, in people who are severely dependent on alcohol, *Wernicke-Korsakoff syndrome*.

Excessive intake of thiamine is not known to cause harmful effects.

RIBOFLAVIN

Riboflavin is essential for the activities of various enzymes involved in the breakdown and utilization of carbohydrates, fats, and proteins, the production of energy in cells, the utilization of other B vitamins, and the production of hormones by the adrenal glands.

Riboflavin is found in a wide range of foods. Particularly good sources of riboflavin are liver, milk, cheese, eggs, green leafy vegetables, whole grains, enriched breads and cereals, and brewer's yeast.

A balanced diet usually provides adequate amounts of riboflavin. People susceptible to deficiency include people taking phenothiazine *antipsychotic drugs*, tricyclic *antidepressant drugs*, or estrogen-containing *oral contraceptives*; those with *malabsorption* disorders; or those with severe *alcohol dependence*. Deficiency may also occur as a result of serious illness, surgery, or severe injury.

Prolonged deficiency of riboflavin may cause chapped lips, soreness of the tongue and corners of the mouth, and certain eye disorders, such as nutritional *amblyopia* (poor visual acuity) and *photophobia* (abnormal sensitivity to light).

Excessive dietary intake of riboflavin is not known to produce any harmful effects.

NIACIN

This vitamin plays an essential role in the activities of various enzymes involved in the metabolism of carbohydrates and fats, the functioning of the nervous and digestive systems, the manufacture of sex hormones, and the maintenance of healthy skin.

The principal dietary sources of niacin include liver, lean meat, poultry, fish, whole grains, nuts, and dried beans.

A balanced diet usually provides adequate amounts of niacin. Most cases of deficiency are due to *malabsorption* disorders or to severe *alcohol dependence*. Prolonged niacin deficiency causes *pellagra*, the principal symptoms of which include soreness and cracking of the skin, inflammation of the mouth and tongue, and mental disturbances.

Excessive intake of niacin is not known to cause harmful effects.

PANTOTHENIC ACID

Pantothenic acid is essential for the activities of various enzymes involved in the metabolism of carbohydrates and fats, the manufacture of corticosteroids and sex hormones, the utilization of other vitamins, the functioning of the nervous system and adrenal glands, and normal growth and development.

Pantothenic acid is present in almost all vegetables, cereals, and animal foods. Particularly rich sources of this vitamin include liver, heart, kidney, fish, egg yolks, brewer's yeast, and wheat germ.

A balanced diet generally provides adequate amounts of this vitamin. Deficiency usually occurs as a result of *malabsorption* disorders or severe *alcohol dependence*. Deficiency may also sometimes occur as a result of severe illness, surgery, or serious injury. The principal effects of deficiency include fatigue, headaches, nausea, abdominal pain, numbness and tingling, muscle cramps, and susceptibility to respiratory infections. In severe cases, a *peptic ulcer* may also result.

Excessive intake of pantothenic acid is not known to have harmful effects.

PYRIDOXINE

This vitamin plays a vital role in the activities of various enzymes and hormones involved in the breakdown and utilization of carbohydrates, fats, and proteins, in the manufacture of red blood cells and antibodies, in the functioning of the digestive and nervous systems, and in the maintenance of healthy skin.

Good dietary sources of pyridoxine include liver, chicken, pork, fish, whole grains, wheat germ, bananas, potatoes, and dried beans.

A balanced diet contains adequate amounts of pyridoxine; it is also manufactured in small amounts by intestinal bacteria. Those susceptible to deficiency include some breast-fed

V

infants, elderly people on a poor diet, those with a *malabsorption* disorder, people with severe *alcohol dependence*, people being treated with certain drugs (including *penicillamine* and *hydralazine*), and women taking estrogen-containing *oral contraceptives*.

Deficiency of pyridoxine may cause weakness, irritability, depression, skin disorders, inflammation of the mouth and tongue, cracked lips, anemia, and, in infants, seizures.

Excessive intake—100 times or more above the normal daily intake—has been reported to cause *neuritis*.

BIOTIN

Biotin is essential for the activities of various enzymes involved in the breakdown of fatty acids and carbohydrates and for the excretion of the waste products of protein breakdown.

Biotin is present in many foods. Particularly rich sources of this vitamin include liver, peanuts, dried beans, egg yolks, mushrooms, bananas, grapefruit, and watermelon.

A balanced diet provides enough biotin for the body's needs; biotin is also manufactured by intestinal bacteria. Deficiency may occur during long-term treatment with *antibiotic drugs* or *sulfonamide drugs*. Raw egg whites contain a substance that interferes with the intestinal absorption of biotin, and prolonged, high consumption has resulted in deficiency in several cases. The principal symptoms of biotin deficiency include weakness, tiredness, poor appetite, hair loss, depression, inflammation of the tongue, and eczema.

Excessive intake of biotin is not known to have harmful effects.

FOLIC ACID

This vitamin plays a vital role in the activities of various enzymes involved in the manufacture of nucleic acids (the genetic material of cells) and therefore in growth and reproduction, in the production of red blood cells, and in the healthy functioning of the nervous system.

The principal dietary sources of folic acid include green, leafy vegetables, broccoli, spinach, mushrooms, liver, nuts, dried beans, peas, egg yolk, and whole-wheat bread.

A varied diet that includes fresh vegetables and fruit generally provides enough folic acid for the body's needs. Mild deficiency is relatively common, but can usually be corrected by increasing the daily consumption of foods containing folic acid. More severe deficiency may occur during pregnancy or breast-feeding, in premature or low birth weight infants, in people undergoing *dialysis*, with certain blood disorders, with *psoriasis*, with *malabsorption* disorders, with severe *alcohol dependence*, and in people taking certain drugs, including *anticonvulsant drugs*, antimalarial drugs, estrogen-containing *oral contraceptives*, and some *analgesic drugs* (painkillers), *corticosteroid drugs*, and *sulfonamide drugs*.

The principal effects of folic acid deficiency include anemia, sores around the mouth, a sore tongue, and, in children, poor growth.

Excessive intake of folic acid is not known to have harmful effects.

Vitamin C

Also known by its chemical name, ascorbic acid, a vitamin that plays an essential role in the activities of various *enzymes* (substances that promote chemical reactions in the body). It is important for the growth and maintenance of healthy bones, teeth, gums, ligaments, and blood vessels; in the production of certain *neurotransmitters* (chemicals responsible for the transmission of nerve impulses between nerve cells) and of adrenal gland hormones; in the immune response to infection; in wound healing; and in the absorption of iron from the digestive tract.

The principal dietary sources of vitamin C are fresh fruits and vegetables. Citrus fruits, tomatoes, green leafy vegetables, potatoes, green peppers, strawberries, and cantaloupe are particularly rich sources.

DEFICIENCY

A balanced diet usually provides enough vitamin C for the body's requirements. However, slight deficiency may occur as a result of a serious injury or burn, major surgery, use of *oral contraceptives*, fever, or continual inhalation of carbon monoxide (a constituent of tobacco smoke and traffic fumes). More pronounced deficiency is usually caused by a poor diet.

Mild deficiency may cause weakness, general aches and pains, swollen gums, and *nosebleeds*. Severe deficiency leads to *scurvy* and *anemia*.

EXCESS

Large doses of vitamin C are taken by some people in the belief that they prevent colds, but there is no convincing evidence to support this. Excessive intake of vitamin C is not usually harmful unless the daily dose is more than about 1 gram, when it may cause nausea, stomach cramps, diarrhea, and, occasionally, kidney stones.

Vitamin D

The collective term for a group of related substances—including calciferol (also known as ergocalciferol or vitamin D_2) and cholecalciferol (vitamin D_3)—that play several vital roles in the body. The vitamin helps regulate the balance of calcium and phosphate, aids the absorption of calcium from the intestine, and is essential for strong bones and teeth.

The richest dietary source of vitamin D is fortified milk. Other good sources include oily fish, such as sardines, herring, salmon, and tuna; liver; dairy products; and egg yolks. Vitamin D is also formed by the action of ultraviolet rays in sunlight on chemicals in the skin.

DEFICIENCY

The body requires only small amounts of vitamin D, which are provided by a balanced diet and normal exposure to sunlight. Deficiency may occur in people on a poor diet or on a vegan diet (one that excludes animal products); in premature infants; in those deprived of sunlight, such as night workers; and in dark-skinned people, particularly those living in foggy urban areas, who do not absorb enough ultraviolet rays.

Deficiency also occurs in certain disorders, most commonly those in which intestinal absorption of the vitamin is impaired (see *Malabsorption*). Other causes include liver disorders, kidney disorders, and some genetic defects. Prolonged use of certain drugs, such as the *anticonvulsant drug* phenytoin, may also result in vitamin D deficiency.

Long-term deficiency of vitamin D leads to low blood levels of calcium and phosphate, which results in softening of the bones. This condition is known as *rickets* in children and as *osteomalacia* in adults.

EXCESS

Excessive intake of vitamin D may cause weakness, abnormal thirst, increased urination, gastrointestinal disturbances, and depression. Over a long period, too much vitamin D disrupts the balance of calcium and phosphate in the body, which may lead to abnormal calcium deposits in the soft tissues, kidneys, and blood vessel walls, and sometimes retarded growth in children.

Vitamin E

The collective term for a group of substances—of which alpha-tocopherol is the most important—that play several vital roles in the body.

V

Vitamin E is essential for normal cell structure, for maintaining the activities of certain enzymes, and for the formation of red blood cells. It also protects the lungs and other tissues from damage by pollutants and helps prevent red blood cells from being destroyed by poisons in the blood. In addition, vitamin E is believed to slow aging of cells.

The principal dietary sources of vitamin E are vegetable oils, nuts, meat, green leafy vegetables, cereals, wheat germ, and egg yolks.

DEFICIENCY

A balanced diet provides adequate amounts of the vitamin. Deficiency usually occurs only in disorders that impair intestinal absorption (see *Malabsorption*), in certain liver disorders, and in premature infants.

Vitamin E deficiency leads to the destruction of red blood cells, which eventually results in *anemia*. In infants, deficiency causes irritability and edema (accumulation of fluid in body tissues).

EXCESS

Prolonged, excessive intake of vitamin E may cause abdominal pain, nausea and vomiting, and diarrhea. It may also reduce intestinal absorption of vitamins A, D, and K, which, in severe cases, may produce symptoms of deficiency of these vitamins.

Vitamin K

A *vitamin* that is essential for the formation in the liver of substances that promote blood clotting.

The principal dietary sources of vitamin K are green leafy vegetables (especially cabbage, broccoli, and turnip greens), vegetable oils, egg yolks, cheese, pork, and liver. Vitamin K is also manufactured by bacteria that normally live in the intestine.

DEFICIENCY AND EXCESS

The combination of a balanced diet and the activity of intestinal bacteria usually provides enough vitamin K for the body's needs. Deficiency may develop as a result of prolonged treatment with antibiotics (which destroy intestinal bacteria), disorders in which intestinal absorption is impaired (see *Malabsorption*), certain liver disorders, and chronic diarrhea. Newborn infants lack the intestinal bacteria that produce vitamin K and are therefore given supplements to prevent deficiency.

Deficiency of vitamin K reduces the ability of the blood to clot. This may cause nosebleeds, seeping of blood from wounds, and bleeding from the gums, intestine, and urinary tract. In rare, very severe cases, brain hemorrhage may result.

Excessive intake of vitamin K has no known harmful effects.

Vitamin supplements

A group of preparations containing one or more *vitamins*.

Most people who eat a balanced diet (see *Nutrition*) do not usually need vitamin supplements. Eating a variety of foods provides adequate amounts of all vitamins. Excessive amounts of some vitamins (especially A and D) may actually be harmful, and supplements should be taken only on the advice of a physician. Some multivitamin preparations contain up to five times the recommended daily intake of certain vitamins.

MEDICAL USES

Vitamin supplements are used to treat diagnosed vitamin deficiency, to prevent vitamin deficiency in susceptible people, and to treat certain medical disorders.

In developed countries, deficiency most commonly occurs in people on a poor diet, such as those with severe *alcohol dependence* or *drug dependence*, those on a low income, and elderly people who do not eat properly. A vegan diet (one that excludes not only meat and fish, but also all other animal products, such as eggs and dairy foods) may sometimes result in vitamin deficiency. Deficiency may also result from *malabsorption* (a disorder in which intestinal absorption of nutrients is impaired), *liver disorders*, and *kidney disorders*.

Supplements are used to prevent deficiency during periods of increased requirements, such as pregnancy, breast-feeding, and infancy. They are also given to people who are taking certain drugs (such as *lipid-lowering drugs* and *sucralfate*) that may impair the absorption of vitamins, to those suffering from serious illness or injury, or to people who have had major surgery. People who are being fed intravenously or via a tube (see *Feeding, artificial*) are also likely to need vitamin supplements. In most cases, the vitamin dosage used to prevent deficiency is lower than that needed to treat a deficiency.

Certain vitamins are used to treat some conditions that are not specific deficiency disorders. Vitamin D, for example, is used in the treatment of *osteoporosis* and vitamin A derivatives (retinoids) are now prescribed for severe *acne*.

Although vitamin B_6 is given to treat *premenstrual syndrome* and it has been claimed that high doses of vitamin C help cure the common cold and that vitamin E improves well-being, such claims have not been clearly substantiated by medical evidence.

Vitiligo

A common disorder of skin pigmentation in which patches of skin lose their color. Depigmented white patches are particularly obvious in dark-skinned people, occurring most commonly on the face, hands, armpits, and groin. Affected skin is particularly sensitive to sunlight.

Vitiligo affecting right hand
Loss of pigment is the only skin change that occurs. The usual remedy is to mask the white patches with makeup.

Vitiligo is thought to be an *autoimmune disorder* that causes an absence of melanocytes, the specialized cells responsible for secreting the skin pigment *melanin*. The condition may occur at any age but usually develops in early adulthood. It affects about one in 200 people. Spontaneous repigmentation occurs in about 30 percent of cases.

TREATMENT

Makeup may be used to disguise areas of vitiligo; in mild cases, no further treatment may be necessary. *Phototherapy* using *PUVA* induces significant repigmentation in more than 50 percent of cases, but many treatments are required. Creams containing *corticosteroid drugs* may also help. If areas of vitiligo are extensive, chemicals may be used to remove pigment from remaining areas of normal skin.

Vitreous hemorrhage

Bleeding into the *vitreous humor*, the gellike substance that fills the main cavity of the eye between the crystalline lens and the retina. A common cause of vitreous hemorrhage is diabetic *retinopathy*, in which new, fragile blood capillaries that bleed readily form on the retina.

Any bleeding into the vitreous humor is likely to affect vision; a major hemorrhage into the center of the gel causes very poor vision for as long as the blood remains. Blood released into the periphery of the vitreous humor may be absorbed and the transparency of the gel restored, but a large hemorrhage is likely to persist for weeks or months or may never clear.

Vitreous humor

The transparent, gellike body that fills the large rear compartment of the eye between the crystalline *lens* and the *retina*. The vitreous humor consists almost entirely of water. Under certain conditions, it can exert sufficient pull on the retina to cause *retinal tears* and *retinal detachment*.

The vitreous humor tends to shrink with age; in most people over 65, it has separated from the retina, leaving a water-filled space. This separation is usually harmless but often causes numerous annoying *floaters* to be seen in the field of vision. The floaters usually disperse with time but at their onset should be evaluated by an ophthalmologist.

Vivisection

Strictly, the performance of a surgical operation on a live animal, particularly for research purposes. However,

---

LOCATION OF THE VOCAL CORDS

The vocal cords are located at the top of the larynx (voice box). Their top edges stretch between the thyroid cartilage at the front and the arytenoid cartilages at the back. If brought close together, the cords vibrate and emit sounds as air passes between them.

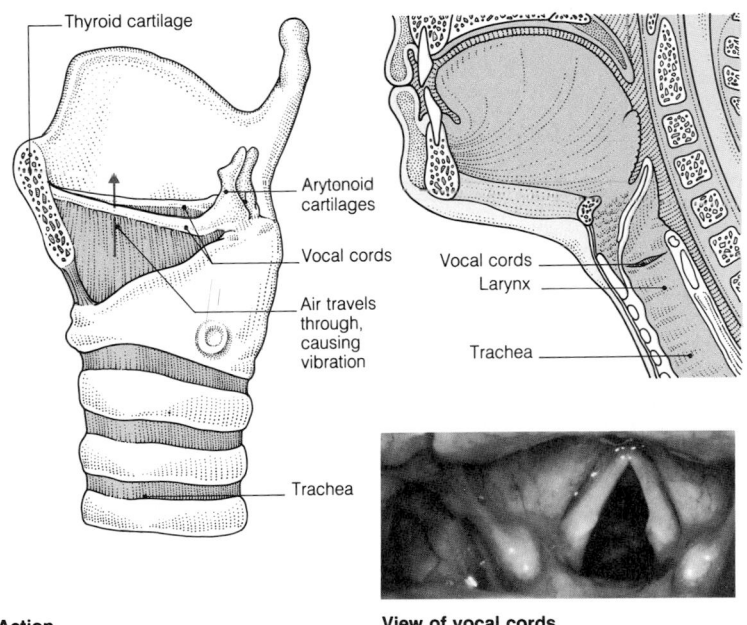

- Thyroid cartilage
- Arytenoid cartilages
- Vocal cords
- Air travels through, causing vibration
- Trachea

- Vocal cords
- Larynx
- Trachea

Action
For voice production, the cords are brought close together by muscles that act on the arytenoid cartilages.

View of vocal cords
This photograph shows the two vocal cords in their position at rest, spaced apart to give a V shape.

LOCATION OF THE VITREOUS HUMOR

The vitreous humor occupies the large rear chamber of the eye, bounded by the back of the crystalline lens and the inner surface of the retina.

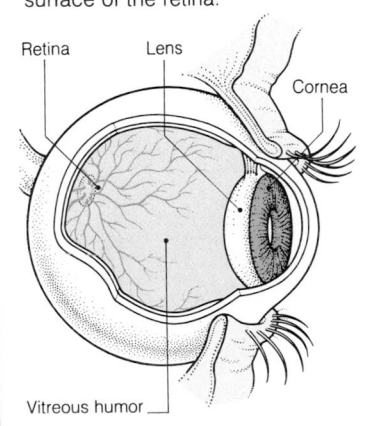

- Retina
- Lens
- Cornea
- Vitreous humor

---

the term vivisection is often popularly used to refer to *animal experimentation* of any kind, even when surgery is not involved.

Vocal cords

Two fibrous sheets of tissue in the *larynx* (voice box) that are responsible for voice production. The cords are attached at the front to the inner surface of the thyroid cartilage (Adam's apple) and at the rear to the arytenoid cartilages.

The so-called true vocal cords are the cords that vibrate and make sound; the false vocal cords are folds in the larynx that have nothing to do with sound production.

Most of the time the vocal cords lie apart, forming a V-shaped opening called the glottis through which air is breathed. Vocal sounds are produced when the cords tighten, close, and vibrate as air expelled from the lungs passes between them. Alterations in the tension of the cords produce sounds of different pitch, which are modified by the tongue, palate, and lips to produce *speech*. (For disorders that affect the vocal cords, see *Larynx, disorders of*.)

Voice box
See *Larynx*.

Voice, loss of

Partial loss of voice, also known as dysphonia, is fairly common and may be caused by any condition that interferes with the normal working of the vocal cords.

Temporary loss of voice frequently results from straining the muscles of the *larynx* (which control the vocal cords) through overuse of the voice. Temporary dysphonia also often results from inflammation of the vocal cords in *laryngitis*.

Persistent or recurrent dysphonia may be due to *polyps* (benign growths) on the vocal cords, thickening of the vocal cords due to *hypothyroidism*, or, less commonly, to interference with the nerve supply to the muscles of the larynx as a result of cancer of the larynx (see *Larynx, cancer of*), thyroid gland (see *Thyroid cancer*), or esophagus (see *Esophagus, cancer of*). In rare cases, nerves or the vocal cords themselves may be accidentally damaged during surgery performed to treat thyroid cancer, resulting in permanent dysphonia.

Total loss of voice, known as *aphonia*, is rare and usually of psychological origin. (See also *Hoarseness; Larynx, disorders of*.)

Volkmann's contracture

A disorder in which the wrist and fingers become permanently fixed in a bent position. It occurs as a result of ischemia (inadequate blood supply) in the forearm muscles that control them.

CAUSES

Ischemia in the forearm muscles may be caused by damage to the brachial artery that results from a displaced fracture of the humerus (upper arm bone) or dislocation of the elbow. Ischemia may also follow any forearm injury that leads to *edema* (retention of fluid within tissues), with consequent swelling of tissues and compression of blood vessels.

SYMPTOMS

Initially, the fingers become cold, numb, and white or blue. Finger movements are weak and painful, and no pulse can be felt at the wrist. Unless treatment is started within a few hours, the characteristic wrist and finger deformity develops.

TREATMENT

Any displaced bones are first manipulated back into position, using a general anesthetic. If blood flow to the hand fails to improve, an operation is performed in which the tissues in the forearm are cut open to relieve pressure on the underlying muscles. Blockage of the artery may be relieved by injecting a *vasodilator drug* or

Appearance of Volkmann's contracture
The wrist is permanently bent due to formation of scar tissue and tautness affecting the forearm muscles.

by cutting open the artery and removing part of the lining. Occasionally, a section of damaged artery is cut out and replaced by a graft taken from a vein.

If there is permanent deformity, *physical therapy* may restore function to an acceptable level. In severe cases, surgery may be required to shorten the bones in the forearm, cut away damaged muscle, and transplant healthy muscle from another part of the forearm. This procedure is sometimes accompanied by *arthrodesis* (fusion) of the wrist joint.

Volvulus

Twisting of a loop of intestine or, in rare cases, of the stomach. Volvulus is a serious condition that causes obstruction of the passage of intestinal contents (see *Intestine, obstruction of*) and a risk of *strangulation*. Symptoms of volvulus are severe *colic* followed by vomiting.

Volvulus may be present from birth or may be a result of *adhesions* (bands

of scar tissue). It is more common in Africa and Asia than in the US or Europe, possibly because of an association with an exceedingly high-fiber diet.

Surgical correction is usually necessary to treat the condition.

Vomiting

Involuntary forcible expulsion of stomach contents through the mouth. Vomiting is usually preceded by nausea, pallor, sweating, excessive salivation, and a reduction in the heart rate.

MECHANISM

Vomiting occurs when the vomiting center in the brain stem is activated. Activation of the vomiting center may occur as the result of information passing directly to it from the frontal lobes of the brain, the digestive tract, or the balancing mechanism in the inner ear when these mechanisms are either damaged or disturbed. The center may also be activated by the chemoreceptor trigger zone, also in

---

THE VOMITING REFLEX

Many situations can provoke vomiting—including the presence of irritants in the stomach, high levels of certain substances in the blood, pressure within the skull, or disturbances of balance.

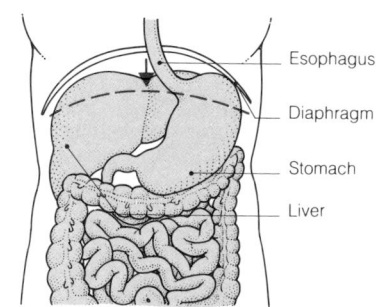

1 In each case, a vomiting center in the brain stem is activated, causing nerve messages to pass toward the abdomen.

2 The messages cause the diaphragm to press down on the stomach and the abdominal wall muscles to contract.

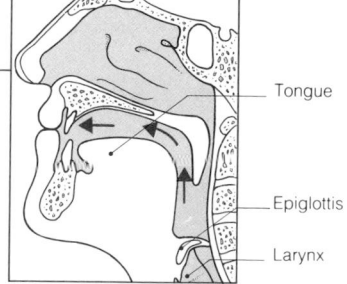

3 The sphincter between the stomach and the esophagus relaxes and the stomach contents are propelled upward

via this sphincter toward the mouth. The epiglottis closes over the larynx to prevent vomit from entering the trachea.

V

VOMITING Forceful expulsion of stomach contents that usually has a simple explanation, such as irritation of the stomach by infection or overindulgence in food or alcohol. However, it may be a sign of a more serious disorder, particularly if there are accompanying symptoms. Vomiting may or may not be preceded by nausea.

Have you had severe abdominal pain that has not been relieved by the vomiting?

YES

☎ **EMERGENCY!**
GET MEDICAL HELP NOW!
A serious abdominal condition, such as appendicitis or a perforated duodenal ulcer, may cause such symptoms.

See • Appendicitis

NO

Have you vomited red blood, or black or dark brown matter that resembles coffee grounds?

YES

Treatment for vomiting
If you have been vomiting, provided you suspect no serious cause, try the following self-help measures:
• Eat no solid food until your nausea and vomiting subside.
• Drink plenty of clear (nonalcoholic) fluids in small sips even if you cannot keep anything down for long.
• Do not smoke.
• Do not take aspirin.

If you vomit repeatedly for more than 24 hours, or if more symptoms develop, consult your physician.

☎ **EMERGENCY!**
GET MEDICAL HELP NOW!
This could be caused by bleeding somewhere in the digestive tract.

NO

Do you have diarrhea OR is your temperature 100°F (38°C) or above?

YES

This may be caused by an infection of the digestive tract. If symptoms persist, consult your physician.

See • Gastroenteritis

NO

In the past few hours, have you done any of the following?
• overeaten
• eaten large amounts of rich, creamy, or spicy food
• consumed a large amount of alcohol

YES

Inflammation of the stomach lining often occurs as the result of overindulgence. Consult your physician if you have recurrent attacks.

See • Gastritis

NO

Have you eaten anything that may have gone bad or to which you may be allergic?

YES

Poisoning by food contaminated by bacteria or by poisonous chemicals or by food to which you are allergic may be responsible for the vomiting.

See • Food poisoning

NO

Continued on next page

V

?

Do you have a headache? — **YES** → Have you had a head injury within the past 24 hours? — **YES** → ☎ **EMERGENCY!**
GET MEDICAL HELP NOW!
You may have a brain injury.

NO (down from head injury)

Do you have one or more of the following symptoms?
- pain when you bend your head forward
- dislike of bright light
- drowsiness or confusion

YES → ☎ **EMERGENCY!**
GET MEDICAL HELP NOW!
These symptoms suggest the possibility of a serious brain disorder.

See • *Meningitis*
 • *Subarachnoid hemorrhage*

NO

Was your headache preceded by visual distortion, weakness of an extremity, and/or nausea AND is the headache one-sided (sometimes with blurred vision and nasal stuffiness)?

YES → The symptoms are probably due to a migraine attack. Consult your physician.

See • *Migraine*

NO

NO (from headache)

?

Do you have severe pain in or around one eye AND is your vision blurred? — **YES** → ☎
Consult your physician without delay!
These symptoms suggest the possibility of acute glaucoma, in which excess fluid causes increased pressure in the eye.

See • *Glaucoma*

NO

?

Before you vomited, did everything around you seem to spin? — **YES** → Disorders of the inner ear cause vomiting and dizzy spells. Consult your physician.

See • *Labyrinthitis*
 • *Meniere's disease*

NO

Vomiting and the Pill
If you are taking the birth-control pill and suffer from an attack of vomiting, your protection against conception may be reduced. Continue to take your pills as usual, but use an extra form of contraception until you start a new packet of pills.

V

Continued on next page

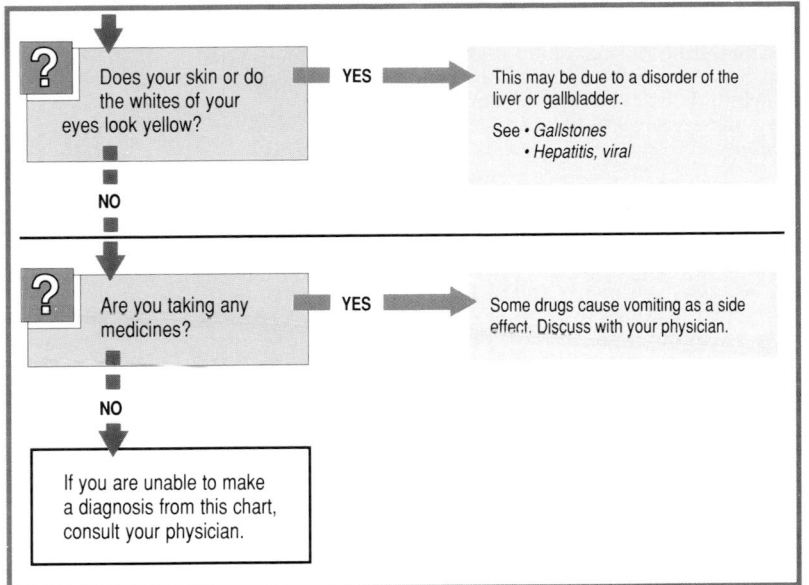

Does your skin or do the whites of your eyes look yellow?

YES → This may be due to a disorder of the liver or gallbladder.

See • Gallstones
• Hepatitis, viral

NO

Are you taking any medicines?

YES → Some drugs cause vomiting as a side effect. Discuss with your physician.

NO

If you are unable to make a diagnosis from this chart, consult your physician.

the brain stem, which is itself stimulated by the presence in the blood of poisons or other substances.

Once activated, the vomiting center sends messages to the diaphragm (the sheet of muscle separating the chest from the abdomen), which presses sharply downward on the stomach, and to the wall of the abdomen, which presses inward. Simultaneously, the pyloric sphincter between the base of the stomach and the intestine closes and the region between the top of the stomach and the esophagus relaxes. As a result, the stomach contents are expelled upward through the esophagus. As this happens, the larynx (voice box) is tightly closed by the epiglottis (the flap of cartilage at its entrance) to prevent vomit from entering the trachea (windpipe) and causing choking.

CAUSES

Vomiting commonly happens after overindulgence in food or alcohol. It is also a common adverse effect of many drugs and often follows general anesthesia (see *Anesthesia, general*).

Vomiting may also result from disorders of the stomach or intestine that result in inflammation, irritation, or distention of either organ. Such disorders include *peptic ulcer*, acute *appendicitis*, *gastroenteritis*, and *food poisoning*. Less commonly, vomiting is a symptom of intestinal obstruction due to *pyloric stenosis*, *intussusception*, or a tumor (see *Intestine, cancer of*).

Vomiting may also be caused by inflammation of organs associated with the digestive tract, such as the liver (see *Hepatitis*), pancreas (see *Pancreatitis*), and gallbladder (see *Cholecystitis*).

Another possible cause of vomiting is raised pressure within the skull, which may be due to *encephalitis*, *hydrocephalus*, a *brain tumor*, or a *head injury*. When the rise is rapid, it causes sudden, extremely forceful vomiting, often without any prior nausea. Vomiting is a common feature of *migraine* as well.

Vomiting is also a common feature of disorders affecting the balancing mechanism within the inner ear, such as *Meniere's disease* and acute *labyrinthitis*, or of disturbance of the mechanism by unusual movement, such as that experienced on a boat (see *Motion sickness*).

Disorders of the *endocrine system*, such as *Addison's disease*, may cause vomiting, as do disturbances of hormone production in early pregnancy (see *Vomiting in pregnancy*).

Vomiting is sometimes a symptom of a metabolic disorder, such as ketoacidosis (excessive production of ketones and acids), which may be due to poorly controlled *diabetes mellitus*.

Internal bleeding from the esophagus, stomach, or duodenum, or swallowing blood from a nosebleed, can also result in vomiting (see *Vomiting blood*).

Vomiting sometimes occurs as a reaction of disgust to a situation or food. It may also be a symptom of a psychological or emotional problem or

be part of the psychiatric disorders *anorexia nervosa* or *bulimia*.

INVESTIGATION AND TREATMENT

Persistent vomiting requires investigation by a physician. Treatment depends on the underlying cause. Do not eat or drink or take any unnecessary medication during the active phase of vomiting. *Antiemetic drugs* may be prescribed.

Vomiting blood

Known medically as hematemesis, vomiting blood is a symptom of bleeding from within the digestive tract. It usually occurs as a result of a serious disorder of the esophagus, stomach, or duodenum.

Vomiting blood may be caused by a tear at the lower end of the esophagus (see *Mallory-Weiss syndrome*), bleeding from *esophageal varices* (widened veins in the esophagus and upper stomach), severe erosive *gastritis* (inflammation of the stomach lining), *peptic ulcer*, or, in rare cases, a malignant stomach tumor (see *Stomach cancer*). Blood can also be vomited if it is swallowed from a nosebleed.

Vomited blood may be dark red, brown, black, or resemble coffee grounds (as a result of the action of stomach acid). Depending on the extent of internal bleeding and the quantity of stomach contents, the blood may either streak the vomit or constitute a major part of it. Vomiting blood is often accompanied by melena (black, tarry feces).

The underlying cause of vomiting blood is investigated by *endoscopy* (passing a viewing tube into the esophagus and stomach) or by *barium X-ray examinations*. If the loss of blood is severe, blood transfusion may be necessary and surgery may be required to stop the bleeding.

Vomiting in pregnancy

Nausea and vomiting in early pregnancy are extremely common. It is experienced by about half of all pregnant women.

The vomiting usually starts before the sixth week of pregnancy and continues until about the 12th week; in some cases it occurs throughout pregnancy. The probable cause is activation of the vomiting center in the brain due to changed hormone levels during pregnancy.

The vomiting occurs most frequently in the morning, often after waking (hence its common name, morning sickness), but can occur at any time. It is sometimes precipitated

V

by emotional stress, traveling, or food. Sufferers may find it helpful to eat small, regular meals.

In rare cases, the vomiting becomes severe and prolonged, a condition known as hyperemesis gravidarum. This can cause dehydration, nutritional deficiency, alteration in blood acidity, liver damage, and weight loss. Immediate hospital admission is required to replace lost fluids and chemicals by *intravenous infusion*, to rule out any serious underlying disorder, and to control the vomiting.

Von Recklinghausen's disease

Another name for *neurofibromatosis*.

Von Willebrand's disease

An inherited lifelong *bleeding disorder* with similarities to *hemophilia*.

CAUSES AND INCIDENCE

Von Willebrand's disease is caused by a defective *gene* and is usually inherited in an autosomal dominant pattern (see *Genetic disorders*). A person needs to inherit only one copy of the defective gene to suffer from the disease. As many as one person in 1,000 is believed to have the gene but its effects are variable. Unlike hemophilia, the disease affects equal numbers of men and women.

The gene defect leads to a reduced concentration in the blood of a substance called von Willebrand factor. This factor plays a dual role in the arrest of bleeding. It helps platelets in the blood to plug injured blood vessel walls, and it forms part of the substance *factor VIII*, which is vital to blood coagulation. In the absence of von Willebrand factor, neither blood coagulation nor platelet plug formation can proceed normally, so there is a bleeding tendency.

SYMPTOMS

The symptoms may include excessive bleeding from the gums and from cuts, nosebleeds, and, in women, *menorrhagia* (excessive menstrual bleeding). In the most severe forms, deep bleeding into joints and muscles may be a problem.

DIAGNOSIS

The disease is diagnosed by *blood-clotting tests*, which show a long bleeding time, and by measurements that reveal reduced levels of von Willebrand factor in the blood.

TREATMENT

There are various treatments available for the disease. One is to administer desmopressin (an *ADH*-like substance), which raises the body's natural production of von Willebrand

factor. Another treatment is to give cryoprecipitate (a preparation obtained from normal blood plasma), which is a rich source of von Willebrand factor. These treatments are generally successful in preventing bleeding episodes.

Voyeurism

The repeated observation of unsuspecting people who are naked, in the act of undressing, or engaging in sexual activity. Commonly called Peeping Toms, voyeurs become sexually aroused through the act of looking and have no wish to engage in sexual activity. Voyeurs achieve orgasm (usually by masturbation) while watching or remembering the witnessed events. In its severe form, voyeurism is the only way in which orgasm is achieved.

Vulva

The external, visible part of the female genitalia. The vulva comprises the *clitoris* and two pairs of skin folds called *labia*.

The most common symptom of a disorder affecting the vulva is itching, known medically as pruritus vulvae. Itching of the vulva often occurs with *vaginal itching*.

Various skin disorders, such as *dermatitis*, commonly affect the vulva and

---

ANATOMY OF THE VULVA
The outer skin folds (labia majora) are usually in contact. If parted, they reveal the clitoris and inner folds (labia minora), which enclose the urethral and vaginal openings.

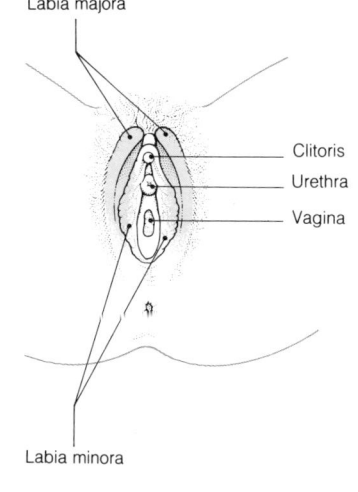

Labia majora

Clitoris

Urethra

Vagina

Labia minora

---

are usually easily relieved. More serious conditions include genital warts (see *Warts, genital*), *vulvitis*, *vulvovaginitis*, and cancer (see *Vulva, cancer of*).

Vulva, cancer of

A rare disorder that most commonly affects postmenopausal women. It may be preceded by vulval itching but often no preliminary symptoms occur before the appearance of a lump or painful ulcer on the vulva.

Diagnosis is made by a biopsy (removal of a small sample of tissue for laboratory analysis).

Treatment of vulval cancer is by surgical removal of the affected area. The outlook depends on how soon the cancer is diagnosed and treated.

Vulvitis

Inflammation of the *vulva* with a variety of different causes.

Infections causing vulvitis include *candidiasis*, genital herpes (see *Herpes, genital*), and warts (see *Warts, genital*). Infestations with *pubic lice* or *scabies* are other possible causes.

Vulvitis may occur as a result of changes in the vulval skin. These changes tend to affect women after the menopause, although there is no apparent cause. They may take the form of red or white patches and/or thickened or thinned areas that may be inflamed. Formerly called a variety of names, such as kraurosis vulvae and lichen sclerosus et atrophicus, the condition is now generally known as vulval dystrophy.

Other possible causes of vulvitis are allergic reactions to soap, cream, or detergent, excessive vaginal discharge, or urinary incontinence (see *Incontinence, urinary*).

TREATMENT

Treatment depends on the cause; a combination of creams applied to the vulva along with good hygiene is the usual remedy. In some cases of vulval dystrophy, a *biopsy* (removal of a small sample of tissue for laboratory analysis) may be carried out to exclude the possibility of cancer. (See also *Vulvovaginitis*; *Vaginitis*.)

Vulvovaginitis

Inflammation of the vulva and vagina. Vulvovaginitis is usually due to the infections *candidiasis* or *trichomoniasis*, which cause a profuse infected vaginal discharge that also affects the vulva.

Treatment of vulvovaginitis is with an *antifungal drug* or an *antibiotic drug*. (See also *Vaginitis*; *Vulvitis*.)

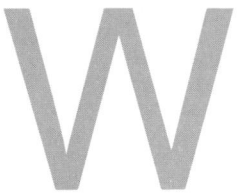

Walking

Movement of the body in one direction by lifting the feet alternately and bringing one foot into contact with the ground before the other starts to leave it. The manner in which a person walks, known as gait, is determined by body shape, size, and posture; it often reflects the individual's personality. A normal pattern of walking is shown in the illustrated box below.

Walking is controlled by nerve signals from the motor cortex (part of the *cerebrum* of the brain) and by signals from the *basal ganglia* and the *cerebellum,* located at the back of the brain. The signals are sent via the spinal cord to nerve cells and from there are carried by nerve fibers to the muscles. In response to changes in position, the cerebellum also receives information from the muscles, joints, eyes, and the balance organ in the inner ear. This information is used to adjust new signals sent to the muscles by the brain centers to ensure balance and coordinated movement.

Some of the nerves that control walking are located in a very primitive part of the brain. This may account for the walking reflex that occurs in newborn babies in which the legs move automatically in a walking motion when the child is held upright (see *Reflex, primitive*). The age at which children walk varies enormously.

DISORDERS
Abnormal gait may be caused by muscle weakness, by abnormalities of the skeleton, or by joint stiffness, causing immobility in the lower limbs or spinal column. Abnormal gait may also be the result of neurological disorders that affect the central control of locomotion and the balance and input of information to the nervous system from muscles and joints.

The different causes affect walking in a variety of ways; the physician can often gain clues to the underlying cause of a disorder by observing the way in which a person walks.

MUSCULAR CAUSES Any condition that causes wasting or loss of any of the muscles connected to the legs or feet may cause abnormal walking. In *muscular dystrophy*, the legs are held wide apart and the person waddles because of weakness of the buttock muscles. In *poliomyelitis* or after severe muscle injury, weakness of individual groups of muscles may cause limping because of unbalanced muscle action.

SKELETAL CAUSES Congenital deformities of the foot, such as *talipes* (club-foot), may prevent normal walking. In talipes equinovarus, for example, the heel cannot be brought to the ground and a characteristic limping gait results. Congenital dislocation of the hip (see *Hip, congenital dislocation of*) that has not been detected in infancy may be noticed only when the child starts to walk—the foot on the affected side is placed flat on the ground while the opposite knee is flexed. *Scoliosis* (deformity of the spine) can also result in abnormal gait.

During a stage in their growth, *knock-knee* or *bowleg* often develops in children. These conditions may produce a strange walk, but both disappear within several years.

Synovitis of the hip is a common cause of limping in children, most often boys aged 2 to 12 years. The limp, which is accompanied by pain of varying severity, starts suddenly and lasts for only a few days or weeks. Another common cause of limping in boys, usually between the ages of 5 and 10, is *Perthes' disease*. The limp may or may not be painful. A painful

---

THE MECHANICS OF WALKING

Many different muscles take part in the walking process. They contract in a complex, rhythmic sequence in response to programs of signals sent from the motor cortex in the brain. Feedback of information from the muscles and joints to the brain helps to ensure that the gait is smooth, steady, and coordinated.

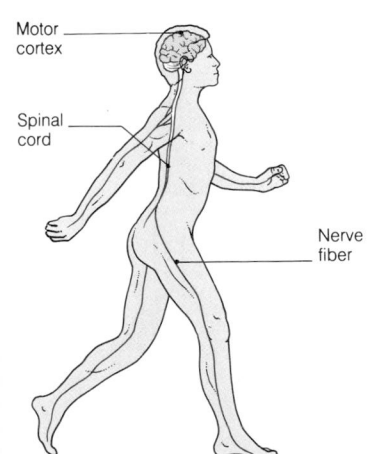

Motor cortex

Spinal cord

Nerve fiber

Route of the signals
The signals for walking originate in the motor cortex and are carried via the spinal cord and nerve fibers to muscles.

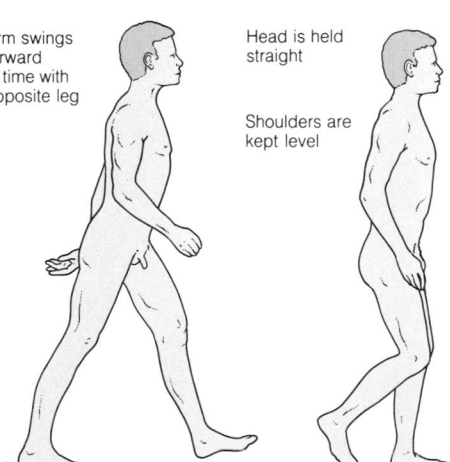

Arm swings forward in time with opposite leg

1 As the left foot contacts the ground, the right arm swings forward and the right foot shifts onto tiptoe.

Head is held straight

Shoulders are kept level

2 Once the left foot is fully planted on the ground and supporting the body, the right foot is raised.

Each step is an equal length

3 A sequence of muscle contractions advances the right leg, and the left arm swings forward.

limp may develop in young adolescents as a result of a slipped epiphysis (see *Femoral epiphysis, slipped*).

Other causes of limp include a painful *bone tumor* and *arthritis*.

Bone shortening may follow fracture or disease of one of the long bones of the leg; this condition always causes an abnormal gait, usually with a dip of the body to the shortened side.

NEUROLOGICAL CAUSES Among the most common of the neurological causes is *stroke*, which frequently results in *hemiplegia* (paralysis or weakness of one side of the body). Because the affected leg is held stiffly extended, it must be swung outward and forward in walking. When both legs are affected by weakness (a condition known as paraparesis), they are held extended and pressed together at the thighs so that only short steps are possible and the toes scrape along the ground. In some people with paraparesis, the legs cross with each step, which produces a characteristic scissors movement.

In *parkinsonism* there is difficulty starting to walk; the body is bent forward at the waist and hips, with bending at the knees and ankles. The steps are short and shuffling with the feet barely clearing the ground. As progress continues, the steps become more and more rapid, and the person may eventually fall unless assisted.

Other disorders, including severe peripheral *neuritis*, *multiple sclerosis*, tertiary *syphilis*, and various forms of *myelitis*, may damage the sensory nerves or the spinal cord. The damage causes loss of information to the brain about the position of the joints, resulting in an easily recognized gait. The body is bent forward and the eyes are fixed on the ground, the legs are held wide apart, and the feet are carried much higher than normal and thrown forward with sudden movements. People affected in this way are critically dependent on vision for walking; the gait becomes even worse if vision is defective.

Disease of the cerebellum or of the balancing mechanisms in the inner ears, such as *Meniere's disease*, may cause severe loss of balance and instability so that the affected person walks cautiously, with the legs apart, sometimes lurching to one side as though intoxicated (see *Ataxia*). In *chorea*, the gait may be bizarre and dancelike, with sudden thrusting movements of the hips and twisting of the trunk and limbs. The steps are irregular and of varying length.

WALKING AIDS

Various types of walking aids are available for different forms and degrees of disability. The choice depends on factors such as whether the person is usually healthy or chronically disabled and whether the disability affects one or both of the person's legs.

Walker

Cane

Elbow crutches

Full-length crutches

Walkers and canes
Walkers are useful for people affected by weakness on both sides, canes for those who have one-sided weakness or pain.

Elbow and full-length crutches
Elbow crutches are often useful for people recovering from strokes, full-length crutches for those with leg injuries.

HOW TO USE CRUTCHES

Crutches are suitable only for people who are able to support their weight on at least one leg.

There are various ways of using crutches, as shown in the illustrations below.

FOUR-POINT WALKING

The feet and crutch tips are well separated, and one point is moved at a time. There are two possible sequences—

right crutch, left foot, left crutch, right foot (above) or right then left crutch, right then left foot.

THREE-POINT WALKING

The crutches are advanced together while the person balances on one or both feet; the weight is then borne by the crutches while the feet are moved.

TWO-POINT WALKING

In two-point walking with crutches, the person moves the left foot and right crutch forward together, followed by the right foot and left crutch.

W

Walking aids

Equipment for increasing the mobility of people who have a disorder that affects *walking*. Support from a walking aid may be required by people with *arthritis* or other diseases affecting mobility, by those recovering from an injury (such as a *fracture* or *sprain*), or by those who are waiting to be fitted with a prosthesis after an amputation.

WALKERS

Walkers provide a very stable form of support and may be useful for people with severe balancing problems or for those who are affected by weakness, pain, or stiffness on both sides. However, walkers tend to get in the way of the feet, allowing only slow progress.

Walkers are usually made of a light, strong alloy and have rubber-tipped legs to prevent sliding. They can be supplied with wheels on the front legs to make maneuvering easier.

CRUTCHES

Crutches provide greater mobility than a walker, but they are suitable only for people who are able to support their own weight. Crutches are often used by people who need to avoid placing weight on an injured leg or foot while healing takes place.

Body weight may be borne by the hands with full-length crutches or by the elbows with elbow crutches. Full-length crutches are usually used by otherwise healthy people who have suffered a fracture or a severe strain or sprain of a bone, joint, or ligament or tendon of a lower extremity.

Elbow crutches are particularly useful for people recovering from *stroke* because they allow gradual progression from a high degree of support to almost natural walking. People with arthritis in their upper limbs should not use elbow crutches because the additional strain on the joints may make the arthritis worse.

Like walkers, crutches are usually made of a light alloy and are rubber-tipped. There are various ways of using crutches (see the illustrated box opposite).

CANES

Canes are most commonly used by people who have weakness, pain, or stiffness on one side. They are usually made of wood and have various types of handles to suit different grips. For extra stability, canes can be supplied with three or four small feet on the end of the shaft.

It is important for a cane to be of the correct length; an upright posture should be achieved with the elbow slightly bent. It is generally best to walk with the cane on the strong side so that the cane is forward when the foot on the weak side comes forward. However, if one side is very weak, the cane may be held on the weak side, close to the leg, and moved with it, acting as a type of splint.

ELECTROMUSCULAR STIMULATION

Computer-controlled electromuscular stimulation of the leg muscles to facilitate walking in quadriplegics and paraplegics was, as of 1988, an investigational procedure.

Walking, delayed

Ninety percent of normal children walk by 14 or 15 months of age. Delayed walking may be suspected if the child is unable to walk alone by 18 months. (See *Developmental delay*.)

Walleye

A form of *strabismus* in which the affected eye turns outward.

Warfarin

WARNING

Always check with your physician before taking any other drug with warfarin since many drugs interfere with its anticlotting effect.

An *anticoagulant drug* used to treat and prevent abnormal blood clotting. Warfarin is used to treat *thrombosis* and to prevent *stroke* or treat *transient ischemic attack*. It is also prescribed to prevent blood clotting after heart valve replacement (see *Heart valve surgery*), in some *heart valve disorders*, or in chronic *atrial fibrillation*. Because warfarin is fully effective only after several days, a faster-acting anticoagulant, such as *heparin*, is usually also prescribed during this period.

POSSIBLE ADVERSE EFFECTS

Warfarin may cause abnormal bleeding in different parts of the body; regular blood-clotting (prothrombin time) tests are therefore carried out to monitor treatment. Warfarin may also cause nausea, loss of appetite, abdominal pain, and rash.

Wart

A contagious, harmless growth on skin or mucous membranes. Warts are caused by the papillomavirus, of which there are 30 types.

Warts infect only the topmost layer of skin. They do not have roots, seeds, or branches. The black dots that are sometimes evident are capillaries that have become clotted due to the rapid skin growth caused by the wart virus.

TYPES

All warts are essentially the same but their appearance may be modified according to their position on the body. They are usually symptomless.

COMMON WARTS These are firm, sharply defined, round or irregular, flesh-colored to brown growths, up to about one quarter inch (6 mm) in diameter. They often have a rough surface. Common warts usually appear on sites subject to injury (e.g., the hands, face, knees, and scalp), particularly in young children.

Common warts on hand
Warts often grow in crops. In time, they disappear spontaneously but can be removed by freezing.

FLAT WARTS Flat-topped, flesh-colored papules that occur mainly on the wrists, the backs of the hands, and the face; they may itch.

DIGITATE WARTS Dark-colored growths with fingerlike projections.

FILIFORM WARTS Long, slender growths that occur on the eyelids, armpits, or neck usually in overweight, middle-aged people.

PLANTAR WARTS These are warts on the sole of the foot (see *Plantar warts*). They are flattened simply because of the pressure placed on them; otherwise, they are just like other warts.

Typical plantar wart
This type of wart may need treatment—a physician may pare it down with a scalpel and apply a corrosive paint.

W

GENITAL WARTS These extensive, pink, cauliflowerlike areas may occur on the genitals of men or women (see *Warts, genital*). Genital warts need prompt treatment. There is some evidence that warts infecting a woman's cervix may predispose her to cervical cancer. It is important that both sexual partners be checked and rechecked since the infection can travel back and forth between them. Condoms can prevent the transfer of warts. Warts present around the genitals of young children may be a sign of sexual abuse.

TREATMENT

About 50 percent of warts disappear in six to 12 months without any treatment. With the exception of disabling plantar warts and genital warts, removal can be delayed. Common, flat, and plantar warts can be cured with several different treatments. Most commonly, liquid nitrogen is used to freeze the wart solid. As it thaws, a blister forms, lifting the wart off. Sometimes a blister-producing liquid (cantharidin) or corroding acid liquids or plasters are used. Several treatments may be needed and sometimes the wart returns. Surgical removal with a scalpel, electric needle, or laser may also be used.

Warts, genital

Soft warts that grow in and around the entrance of the vagina and the anus and on the penis. Genital warts are transmitted by sexual contact and are caused by a papillomavirus. There may be an interval of up to 18 months between infection and the appearance of the warts.

Genital warts around the anus
These growths are painless but need treatment—usually by application of podophyllin or surgical removal.

Genital warts have been linked with cases of cervical cancer (see *Cervix, cancer of*). A woman who has had genital warts—or whose partner has had genital warts—should have frequent *cervical smear tests*.

Genital warts may be removed by surgery or by the application of *podophyllin*. There is a tendency for the warts to recur.

Wasp stings

See *Insect stings*.

Water

Although only a simple chemical (consisting of two atoms of hydrogen bonded to one of oxygen—H_2O), water is essential to all forms of life. Some simple life-forms, such as certain microorganisms, can survive in a state of suspended animation for years or decades without water. However, even they require water to carry out functions such as growth and reproduction.

Water is the most common chemical in the human body (and also one of the most abundant substances on earth). About 99 percent of the molecules in the body are water, although it makes up a smaller proportion of body weight (about 60 percent in an average man). Thus, a man weighing 155 pounds (70 kg) contains about 87.5 pints (42 liters) of water, of which about 58 pints (28 liters) are within the body cells themselves; 29 pints (14 liters) are extracellular. Of the extracellular water, about 6.25 to 8.3 pints (3 to 4 liters) are in the blood plasma, lymph, and cerebrospinal fluid; the remaining 21 to 23 pints (10 to 11 liters) are in *tissue fluid*.

ROLE IN THE BODY

Water is essential to life because it provides the medium in which all metabolic reactions take place. It also provides the medium for the transportation of chemical substances dissolved in it, such as *ions*. The blood plasma carries water to all body tissues; it also carries excess water from tissues for elimination from the body by the liver, kidneys, lungs, and skin. The interchange of water between the blood and tissue cells occurs via the tissue fluid, which bathes all the individual cells. The passage of water in the tissue fluid into and out of cells takes place by a process called *osmosis*.

WATER BALANCE

Water is taken into the body not only by drinking, but also in food; in addition, a small amount is actually formed within the body by the metabolism of food.

Water is lost from the body in *urine*, sweat, *feces*, and as water vapor breathed out. However, the amount lost as sweat depends on physical

WATER BALANCE IN THE BODY

INTAKE (PINTS)

Drinks	3.6 / 7.0
Food	0.85 / 0.85
Metabolism	0.85 / 0.85

LOSS (PINTS)

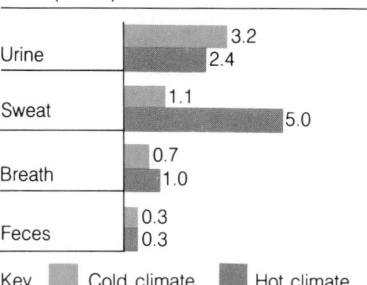

Urine	3.2 / 2.4
Sweat	1.1 / 5.0
Breath	0.7 / 1.0
Feces	0.3 / 0.3

Key   Cold climate   Hot climate

Water intakes and losses
The charts show average intakes of water from various sources and losses in urine, sweat, and so on. In cool climates, people tend to drink more than the amount required to satisfy thirst; the excess water is lost in urine. In hot climates, large amounts of water are lost in sweat, and an increase in fluid intake is essential to avoid dehydration.

activity and the external temperature; the amount passed out of the body in the urine depends largely on the amount of fluid drunk (see chart above).

The amount of water in the body must remain within relatively narrow limits for the proper functioning of metabolic processes; this balance is achieved by the activities of the kidneys, which control the balance between fluid intake and output by regulating the amount of water excreted from the body in the urine. The minimum daily urinary output necessary to remove waste products is about 1 pint (0.5 liters), although most healthy adults usually produce about 3.1 pints (1.5 liters) of urine a day. The amount produced in excess of the minimum is controlled mainly by *ADH* (antidiuretic hormone), which is produced by the posterior portion of the pituitary gland and acts on the kidneys to reduce water excretion.

The body's water balance is also regulated in another way. If there is an excessive amount of any substance (such as sugar or salt) dissolved in the blood that must be excreted by the kidneys, extra water is needed to accomplish this function. This may lead to *dehydration* despite increased production of ADH, but is usually compensated for by increased water intake as a response to *thirst*.

In some disorders, such as *renal failure* or *heart failure*, insufficient water is excreted in the urine, resulting in *edema* (abnormal accumulation of water in body tissues).

Waterborne infection

Water can be a source of infection if it contains infective or parasitic organisms and is drunk, contaminates food, or is played in.

DRINKING WATER

Throughout the world, contamination of water used for drinking is an important means of spread of diseases, including viral *hepatitis A*, many viral and bacterial causes of *diarrhea*, *typhoid fever*, *cholera*, *amebiasis*, and some types of *worm infestation*.

Contamination results from the discharge of human or animal excretory products containing infective organisms into rivers, lakes, reservoirs, or wells used as a source of water supply. The discharge may be direct or in the form of untreated sewage. It can also occur through leakage between sewage and water supply systems. This could happen, for example, in a city affected by a major earthquake.

In developed countries such as the US, the risks of waterborne infection are minimized through measures such as adequate sanitary facilities, sewage treatment and disposal, and the sterilization and testing of water before it is supplied to homes. Tap water is therefore usually safe (unless there is a specific warning not to drink it).

In developing countries, sanitary facilities, sewage disposal, and water treatment may be inadequate. As a consequence, members of the population are more likely to carry the types of disease organisms spread by water. It is therefore best not to drink tap water in poorer countries and always to regard with suspicion any water taken directly from rivers, lakes, and wells.

AVOIDANCE OF INFECTION
The accompanying table summarizes safe and suspect sources of drinking water in developed and developing countries. If safe tap water is unavailable, bottled or canned water or drinks of well-known brand names are usually safe; do not put ice made from suspect water into drinks. Rainwater is usually free of infective organisms provided it is not allowed to stand for a long period before drinking.

SAFETY OF WATER AND OTHER DRINKS FOR CONSUMPTION

	Developed countries	Developing countries
Usually safe	Tap water from public supply; rainwater; canned or bottled drinks; springwater	Canned or bottled drinks of well-known brands; rainwater
Suspect	Water direct from rivers, streams, lakes, ponds, canals, wells	Tap water (cities); springwater
Very suspect	Obviously polluted water, i.e., cloudy in appearance or with an unpleasant smell	Tap water (rural areas); water direct from rivers, streams, lakes, ponds, canals

Safe and suspect water
Any source of water that falls into the suspect or very suspect categories should be sterilized. Techniques include boiling, filtering, and chemical treatment.

Water that may be infected should be sterilized before drinking. The most reliable method is to boil the water for five minutes. Boiling kills any infective organisms present. If boiling is impractical, the alternative is to filter the water and then to sterilize it chemically. Filtering is necessary to remove suspended particles, which can harbor disease organisms and interfere with sterilization. Various types of filters are available; some remove bacteria and other infective organisms as well as inanimate particles. The manufacturer's instructions should be followed carefully. For chemical sterilization, purifying tablets that contain chlorine or iodine are used. Water should be left for 20 to 30 minutes following treatment before it is used.

Vegetables or other food that have been washed in suspect water should not be eaten unless they have been thoroughly cooked.

IMMERSION IN WATER

Swimming in polluted water is liable to cause an ear infection (see *Otitis externa*). The risk can be minimized by shaking the head to the left and the right after swimming to clear water out of the outer-ear canals.

Most swimmers inadvertently swallow some water. If it is contaminated, there is a risk of contracting any of the diseases transmitted in polluted drinking water. It is therefore advisable to avoid swimming in rivers possibly polluted with sewage (e.g., downstream of towns) or in the ocean near large coastal resorts.

Leptospirosis is caused by contact with water contaminated by rat's urine; sewage and canal workers are most at risk.

In tropical countries, swimming or wading in rivers, lakes, and ponds is highly inadvisable due to the risk of *schistosomiasis* (bilharziasis), a serious disease caused by a fluke that can burrow through the swimmer's skin. Swimmers' itch is caused by a similar type of fluke, which burrows into the skin and causes an itchy rash. Outbreaks of swimmers' itch have occurred in the US.

OTHER MECHANISMS OF WATERBORNE INFECTION

Fish (particularly shellfish) that live in polluted water may collect infective organisms in their bodies. They must be expertly cleaned and prepared and then promptly and thoroughly cooked to avoid possible hepatitis, choleralike illnesses, *food poisoning*, or a *tapeworm infestation*.

Legionnaires' disease is caused by a bacterium that can contaminate the water systems of large buildings. It is not apparently contracted from actually drinking contaminated water; the route of infection seems to occur via inhalation from showers or air-conditioning systems. (See also *Food-borne infection*.)

Waterhouse-Friderichsen syndrome

A serious, but very rare, condition caused by infection of the bloodstream by bacteria of the meningococcus group. Thus, meningitis is often associated with this syndrome. The main feature is bleeding into the adrenal glands, which leads to acute *adrenal failure* and *shock*.

The onset of Waterhouse-Friderichsen syndrome is abrupt; the victim collapses within several hours and sinks into a coma. Rapidly enlarging purple spots appear on the skin. The condition is almost invariably fatal unless it is immediately treated in a hospital.

W

Watering eye

An increase in the volume of the tear film, usually producing epiphora (overflow of *tears*). Watering may be caused by excess tear production due to emotion or to conjunctival or corneal irritation. It may also be caused by an obstruction to the channel that drains tears from the eye.

Water intoxication

A condition caused by excessive water retention in the brain. The principal symptoms are headaches, dizziness, nausea, confusion, and, in severe cases, seizures and unconsciousness.

Various disorders can disrupt the body's water balance, leading to accumulation of water in body tissues, including the brain. Such disorders include *renal failure*, liver *cirrhosis*, severe *heart failure*, diseases of the adrenal glands, and certain lung or ovarian tumors that produce a substance with a similar action to antidiuretic hormone (*ADH*).

There is also a risk of water intoxication for about 48 hours after surgery, because the stress of an operation leads to increased ADH production. Water intoxication may also occur during induction of labor with *oxytocin*.

Water-on-the-brain

A nonmedical term for *hydrocephalus*.

Water-on-the-knee

A popular term for accumulation of fluid within or around the knee joint. The most common cause is *bursitis* (inflammation of a bursa, one of the fluid-filled sacs that covers and cushions pressure points in the body). Another cause is fluid within the knee joint (see *Effusion, joint*).

Water tablets

See *Diuretic drugs*.

Wax bath

A type of *heat treatment* in which hot, liquid wax is applied to part of the body to relieve pain and stiffness in inflamed or injured joints. Wax baths are most frequently used to treat sufferers from *rheumatoid arthritis*.

A wax bath is given by dipping the body part, usually a hand or foot, into wax kept at a temperature of 120 to 130°F. The limb is held in the wax for a few seconds and then withdrawn; the wax solidifies, forming a thin layer. The wax may be broken off and the limb redipped or the procedure may be repeated until the wax coating is about half an inch thick. The treated area is then wrapped in a plastic sheet and blanket to retain the heat. After 20 minutes, the wax is peeled off and exercises are performed to encourage movement in the treated joints.

Wax, ear

See *Earwax*.

Weakness

A term used to describe a general lack of vigor or strength, which is a common symptom of a wide range of conditions, including *anemia, emotional problems*, and various disorders affecting the heart, nervous system, bones, joints, and muscles. When associated with emotional disorders (such as depression), weakness may represent a lack of desire or ambition rather than a lack of muscle strength.

More specifically, the term weakness is used to describe loss of power in certain muscle groups, which may or may not be accompanied by muscle wasting and loss of sensation. (See also *Paralysis*.)

Weaning

The gradual substitution of solid foods for milk or formula in an infant's diet (see *Feeding, infant*).

Webbing

A flap of skin between adjacent fingers or toes. Webbing is a common congenital abnormality that may affect two or more digits. Although mild webbing is completely harmless, surgical correction may be performed for cosmetic reasons. In severe cases, adjacent digits may be completely fused (see *Syndactyly*).

Webbing of the fingers
This curious feature is often an inherited trait, appearing in each of several generations of a family.

Wegener's granulomatosis

A rare disorder in which *granulomas* (nodular aggregations of abnormal cells) associated with areas of chronic tissue inflammation due to *vasculitis* (inflammation of blood vessels) develop in the nasal passages, lungs, and kidneys.

CAUSES AND SYMPTOMS
The cause of the condition is unknown, but it is thought to be an *autoimmune disorder* (a disorder in which the body's natural defenses attack its own tissues).

The principal symptoms include a bloody discharge from the nose, coughing (sometimes with the production of bloodstained sputum), breathing difficulty, chest pain, and blood in the urine. There may also be loss of appetite, weight loss, weakness, fatigue, and joint pains.

DIAGNOSIS AND TREATMENT
A diagnosis usually requires the microscopic examination of a *biopsy* sample of abnormal tissue, which may be taken from inside the nose, from a lung, or from a kidney.

Treatment is with a combination of *immunosuppressant drugs*, such as cyclophosphamide or azathioprine, and *corticosteroid drugs* to alleviate the symptoms and in some instances to aid in the induction of a remission in the disease process.

OUTLOOK
With prompt treatment, most people recover completely within about a year, although *renal failure* develops in some sufferers.

Without treatment, various complications may occur, including perforation of the nasal septum, causing deformity of the nose; inflammation of the eyes; a rash, nodules, or ulcers on the skin; and damage to the heart muscle, which may be fatal.

Weight

The heaviness of a person or object, usually measured in pounds or kilograms. Weight is a routine physical measurement of *growth* in children. Accurate scales should be used; ideally, a person should be weighed before breakfast naked or wearing the same amount of clothing each day.

Weight can be compared to charts standardized for an individual's height, age, and sex. If weight is below 80 percent of the standard weight for height, the individual's *nutrition* is probably inadequate as a result of poor diet or disease.

In healthy adults, weight remains more or less stable because calorie intake from the diet matches calorie expenditure used to fuel all body activities (see *Metabolism*). *Weight loss* or weight gain occurs if the net balance is disturbed.

W

WEIGHT TABLE: MEN

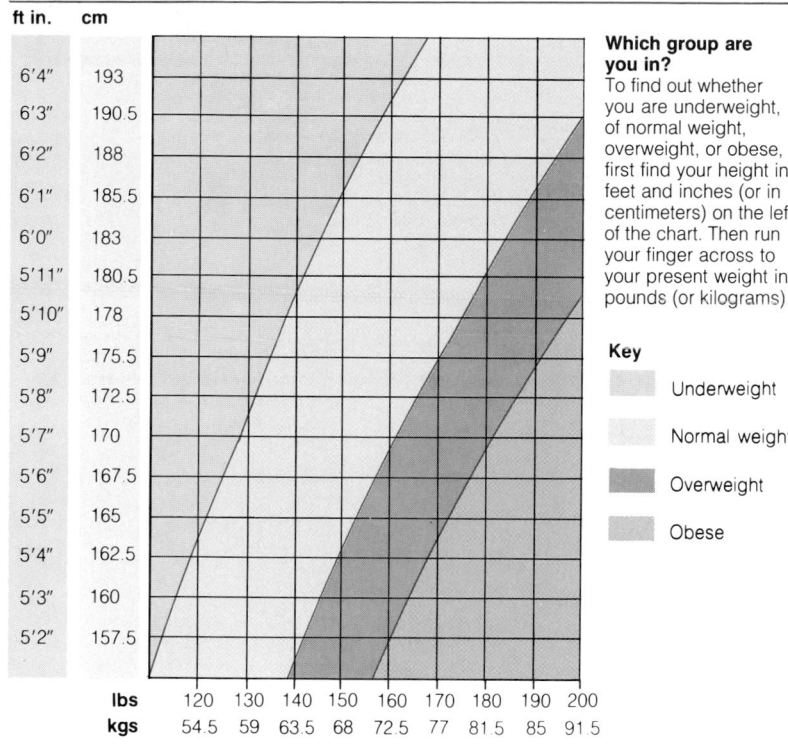

ft in.	cm
6'4"	193
6'3"	190.5
6'2"	188
6'1"	185.5
6'0"	183
5'11"	180.5
5'10"	178
5'9"	175.5
5'8"	172.5
5'7"	170
5'6"	167.5
5'5"	165
5'4"	162.5
5'3"	160
5'2"	157.5

lbs	120	130	140	150	160	170	180	190	200
kgs	54.5	59	63.5	68	72.5	77	81.5	85	91.5

Which group are you in?
To find out whether you are underweight, of normal weight, overweight, or obese, first find your height in feet and inches (or in centimeters) on the left of the chart. Then run your finger across to your present weight in pounds (or kilograms)

Key

☐ Underweight

☐ Normal weight

☐ Overweight

☐ Obese

WEIGHT TABLE: WOMEN

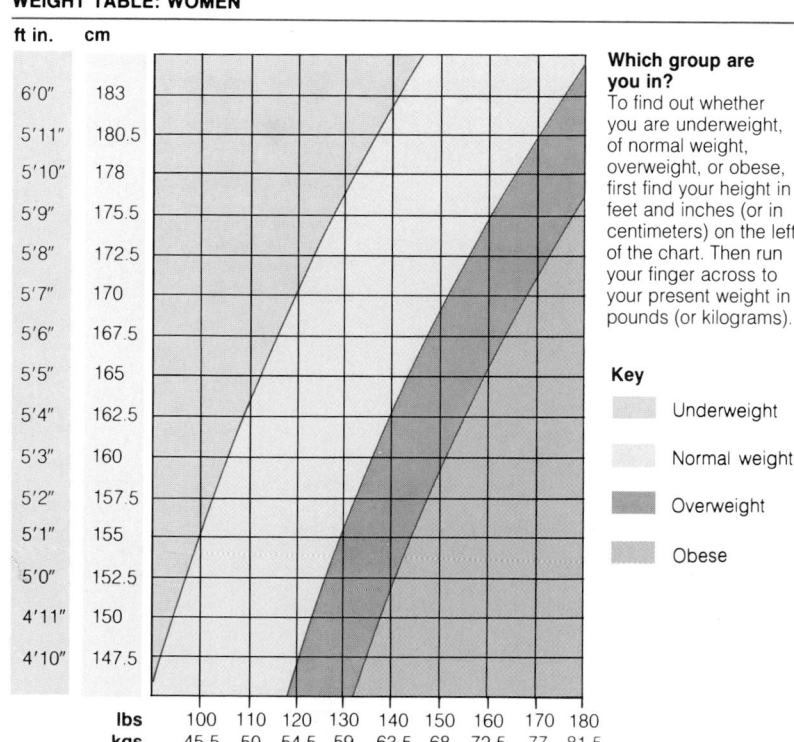

ft in.	cm
6'0"	183
5'11"	180.5
5'10"	178
5'9"	175.5
5'8"	172.5
5'7"	170
5'6"	167.5
5'5"	165
5'4"	162.5
5'3"	160
5'2"	157.5
5'1"	155
5'0"	152.5
4'11"	150
4'10"	147.5

lbs	100	110	120	130	140	150	160	170	180
kgs	45.5	50	54.5	59	63.5	68	72.5	77	81.5

Which group are you in?
To find out whether you are underweight, of normal weight, overweight, or obese, first find your height in feet and inches (or in centimeters) on the left of the chart. Then run your finger across to your present weight in pounds (or kilograms).

Key

☐ Underweight

☐ Normal weight

☐ Overweight

☐ Obese

Obesity can be most easily assessed in terms of weight for height. A person is considered to be obese if his or her weight is 20 percent more than that given in a standard weight-for-height table. An alternative method of assessment is to use the body mass index, which is obtained by dividing weight in kilograms by the square of height in meters; a body mass index above 26 for a woman or 28 for a man constitutes obesity.

Weight loss

Loss of body weight occurs any time there is a decrease in the net balance of caloric intake related to calorie expenditure. This decrease may be due to deliberate *weight reduction*, a change in diet, or change in level of activity; weight loss is also a symptom of a wide range of disorders.

CAUSES

Many diseases disrupt the appetite and may lead to weight loss by reducing the intake of calories. *Depression* reduces the motivation to eat, *peptic ulcer* causes pain and may lead to food avoidance, and *kidney* disorders cause loss of appetite due to the effect of uremia (raised levels of urea in the blood). In *anorexia nervosa* and *bulimia*, complex psychological factors affect the individual's eating pattern.

Calorie intake may also be affected by digestive disorders. Persistent *vomiting* due to *gastroenteritis*, for example, leads to weight loss. Cancer of the esophagus (see *Esophagus, cancer of*) or *stomach cancer* causes loss of weight, as does the *malabsorption* of nutrients that occurs in certain disorders of the intestine or pancreas.

Disorders that increase the rate of metabolic activity in cells cause weight loss by increasing the expenditure of calories. These disorders include any type of *cancer*, chronic infection such as *tuberculosis*, and *hyperthyroidism* (overactivity of the thyroid gland). Untreated *diabetes mellitus* also causes weight loss, initially due to a greater fluid loss from the increase in urine output and as a result of loss of calories from glycosuria (glucose in the urine); eventually, a wasting of tissue mass causes weight loss as fat stores are broken down.

Unexplained weight loss may be a sign of disease and should always be investigated by a physician. A working diagnosis may be established by means of a careful patient history and a physical examination. In some cases, appropriate tests can confirm a specific cause.

W

WEIGHT LOSS Minor fluctuations in weight as a result of temporary changes in the level of exercise taken or the amount of food eaten are normal. More drastic, unintentional weight loss, especially when combined with other symptoms such as loss of appetite, usually requires medical attention.

Is your appetite as good as ever?

YES →

Have you noticed two or more of the following symptoms?
• excessive sweating
• weakness or trembling
• unexplained tiredness
• bulging eyes

YES →

An overactive thyroid gland is a possibility, especially if you are a woman. Consult your physician.

See • *Graves' disease*
    • *Hyperthyroidism*

NO ↓

NO ↓

Have you noticed one or more of the following symptoms?
• unusually frequent or abundant urination
• increased thirst
• unexplained tiredness
• genital itching
• absence of periods

YES →

This may be due to diabetes mellitus, a hormonal disorder in which insufficient insulin is produced by the pancreas.

See • *Diabetes mellitus*

CANCER WATCH
There is a possibility of cancer if weight loss and loss of appetite are combined with abdominal pain OR a change in bowel habits. **Consult your physician without delay!**

NO ▪▪▪▪▪▪ →

If you feel well, there is probably no serious cause for your weight loss. However, if your weight continues to drop, discuss this with your physician to exclude the slight possibility of a serious underlying disorder.

Have you noticed one or more of the following symptoms?
• recurrent bouts of diarrhea
• recurrent constipation
• recurrent abdominal pain
• blood in the feces

YES →

☎
Consult your physician without delay!
A disorder of the digestive tract may be responsible.

See • *Crohn's disease*
    • *Intestine, cancer of*
    • *Irritable bowel syndrome*
    • *Malabsorption*
    • *Peptic ulcer*
    • *Stomach cancer*

NO ↓

Signs of weight loss
If you lose weight without deliberately attempting to slim down, you should always take the matter seriously, especially if other symptoms suggest the possibility of illness. If you do not weigh yourself regularly, the following signs may indicate that you have lost weight:
• people remark on your changed appearance
• your cheeks become sunken
• your pants or skirts become loose around the waist
• your collars fit more loosely
• you need a smaller bra

Continued on next page

W

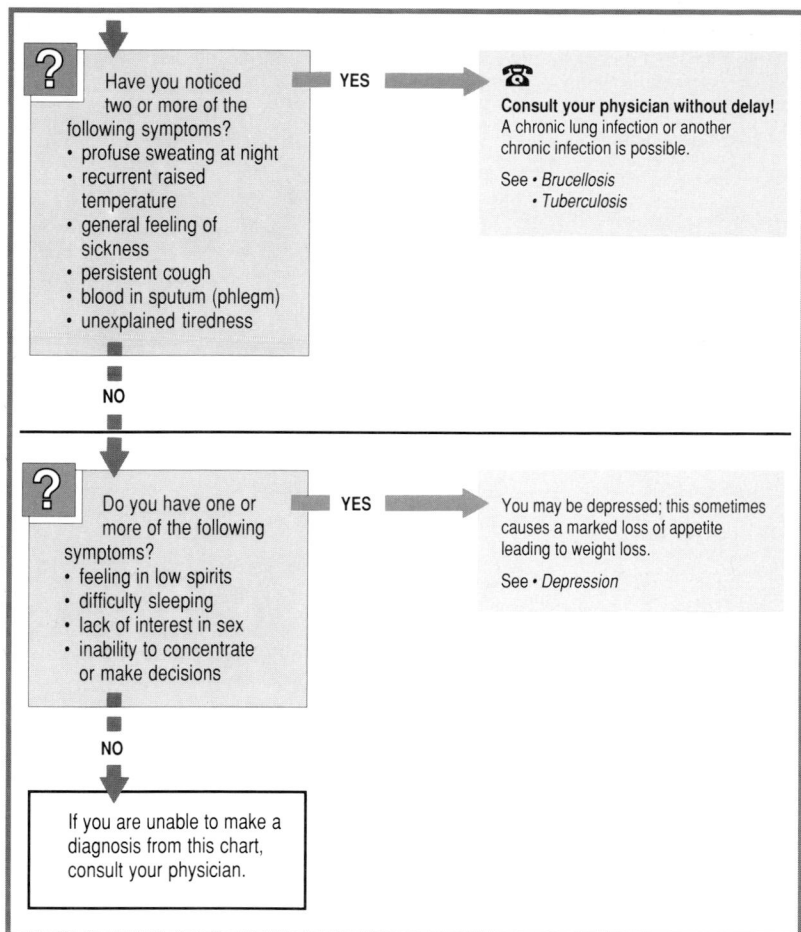

Have you noticed two or more of the following symptoms?
- profuse sweating at night
- recurrent raised temperature
- general feeling of sickness
- persistent cough
- blood in sputum (phlegm)
- unexplained tiredness

YES → ☎ **Consult your physician without delay!** A chronic lung infection or another chronic infection is possible.

See • *Brucellosis*
• *Tuberculosis*

NO

Do you have one or more of the following symptoms?
- feeling in low spirits
- difficulty sleeping
- lack of interest in sex
- inability to concentrate or make decisions

YES → You may be depressed; this sometimes causes a marked loss of appetite leading to weight loss.

See • *Depression*

NO

If you are unable to make a diagnosis from this chart, consult your physician.

RULES FOR WEIGHT REDUCTION

Cut down drastically on all visible fats, such as butter, margarine, cream, and cooking oils, and also on the invisible fats	present in pastries, cookies, and cakes. Choose low-fat milk, cheeses, and yogurts.
Choose lean cuts of meat and avoid processed meat, such as salami. Broil or roast meat without adding fat instead of	frying. Choose fresh fish in preference to the smoked variety.
Eat more boiled legumes (e.g., lentils, peas, and beans); they provide plenty of	protein and are filling but contain very little fat.
Avoid refined carbohydrates such as sugar (dextrose) and cane syrup	(sucrose) as well as refined grain products such as white flour or white rice.
Increase your consumption of unrefined carbohydrates. Eat whole-wheat bread, whole-grain breakfast cereals (without	added sugar), unrefined rice, fresh fruit, and plenty of vegetables.
Reduce intake of alcoholic drinks, which	are high in calories.

Dietary recommendations for weight loss
Careful choice of the right types of food—and, in particular, the avoidance of items with a high calorie content per unit of weight (mainly fats)—makes it easier to achieve a low-calorie diet without necessarily having to reduce the bulk of food you eat.

Weight reduction
The process of losing excess body fat. Weight reduction is usually undertaken by people who are overweight (see *Obesity*) to improve their health or appearance. A person who is severely overweight is more at risk of suffering from various illnesses, such as *diabetes mellitus, hypertension* (high blood pressure), and heart disease.

HOW IT IS DONE
The most efficient way to lose weight is to eat less. To lose weight, people should eat 500 to 1,000 calories a day less than their energy requirements. This should result in a weight loss of approximately 1.5 pounds per week until a desirable weight is achieved. The rate of weight loss may be faster at the beginning of a weight reduction diet, when the body's glycogen and fat stores, which contain water, are being depleted.

Exercise forms an important part of a reducing regime, burning excess calories and improving muscle tone. Some people believe that *aerobics* speed up the metabolism for a short period after exercising and thus make the body more efficient at using energy.

FAD DIETS
Many people who are trying to lose weight want to do so quickly; they may follow fad diets that provide severely restricted calorie intakes. Though there may be a rapid weight loss in the beginning, most of these diets do not work in the long term and the lost weight usually returns.

A number of liquid diets providing about 330 calories per day have been developed. Some physicians are concerned about the effects of these liquid diets. Any diet providing less than 1,000 calories per day should be undertaken only with medical supervision and only briefly or intermittently for short periods.

Weil's disease
Another name for *leptospirosis*.

Welders' eye
Acute *conjunctivitis* and *keratopathy* (corneal damage) that is caused by the intense ultraviolet light radiation emitted by the electric welding arc. Welders' eye is a result of failure to wear adequate eye protection while welding.

Werdnig-Hoffmann disease
A very rare inherited disorder of the nervous system that affects infants. Also known as infantile spinal muscular atrophy, Werdnig-Hoffmann

W

disease is a type of *motor neuron disease*. Werdnig-Hoffmann disease affects the nerve cells in the spinal cord that control muscle movement. Its underlying cause is unknown.

Marked floppiness and paralysis occur during the first few months. Affected babies move less than normal babies and sometimes the mother recalls being aware of reduced fetal movements before the baby was born. Severely affected infants tend to lie still in a froglike position with the knees bent up and turned out. The muscles of the face are unaffected, so the child has an alert expression that is in sharp contrast to his or her physical helplessness. The baby becomes increasingly floppy and deformed over the following few months. The muscles that control breathing and feeding are also affected, which usually causes death before the child is 3 years old.

There is no cure for Werdnig-Hoffmann disease. Treatment aims to keep the affected infant as comfortable as possible.

Wernicke-Korsakoff syndrome

An uncommon brain disorder almost always due to the malnutrition that occurs in chronic *alcohol dependence* or, occasionally, in other conditions, such as cancer with malnutrition.

CAUSES

The factor responsible is deficiency of thiamine (vitamin B_1, see *Vitamin B complex*), which affects the brain and nervous system. The thiamine deficiency is probably caused by the combined effects of poor eating habits and an inherited defect in thiamine metabolism.

SYMPTOMS

The disease consists of two stages— Wernicke's encephalopathy and Korsakoff's psychosis—each characterized by particular symptoms.

Wernicke's encephalopathy usually develops suddenly and produces various abnormal eye movements, *ataxia* (difficulty coordinating body movements, especially walking), slowness, and confusion. Sufferers also usually have signs of *neuropathy*, such as loss of sensation, pins and needles sensation, or impaired reflexes. The level of consciousness progressively falls and may lead to coma and death without treatment.

Korsakoff's psychosis may follow Wernicke's encephalopathy if treatment is not instituted soon enough. Symptoms consist of severe *amnesia* (memory loss), apathy, and disorien-

CAUSE OF WHIPLASH INJURY

This injury to the neck section of the spine may occur when a car is subjected to a sudden violent force and the occupant's body is restrained in the seat but his or her head is not restrained.

Sudden acceleration
Here, there is a sudden force from behind (usually due to another vehicle striking the rear of the car). As the body accelerates forward, the head jerks violently backward relative to the body, stretching and bending the neck; the head then rebounds forward.

Sudden deceleration
Here, there is a sudden violent force from the front toward the back of the vehicle, due, for example, to a collision with a tree. The seat belt restrains the body, but the head continues to move forward, stretching the neck; the head then rebounds backward.

Direction of force

Cervical spine

Ligaments

Direction of force

Cervical spine

Ligaments

tation. Recent memory is affected more than distant memory, sufferers often not being able to remember what they did even a few minutes previously. Confabulation (invention of stories) may occur to make up for gaps in memory.

TREATMENT AND OUTLOOK

Wernicke's encephalopathy is a medical emergency. If the diagnosis is even suspected, high doses of intravenous thiamine are given immediately. This treatment reverses most of the symptoms, often within a few hours.

In the absence of prompt treatment, Korsakoff's psychosis is usually irreversible, leaving the sufferer permanently handicapped by memory loss and in need of continual supervision.

Wernicke's encephalopathy

See *Wernicke-Korsakoff syndrome*.

Wheelchair

A chair mounted on wheels used to provide mobility for a person unable to walk. The simplest type of wheelchair is pushed by an attendant or hand-propelled by the disabled person. Manual wheelchairs have small wheels with casters at the front and large, narrow wheels at the back; these wheelchairs are designed to have metal handles that can be easily gripped.

Powered wheelchairs are battery-operated and controlled electronically by finger pressure or, if necessary, by chin pressure or breath control. The battery provides power for six to eight hours and is recharged overnight by connection to an electrical outlet. Wheels are usually small with wide, low-pressure tires. Several different types of powered chairs are available. Those suitable for outdoor use are capable of negotiating raised obstructions but are usually too wide and long for convenient use indoors; indoor models are lighter and more compact but cannot mount sidewalk curbs.

Wheelchairs may be made of lightweight metal (such as titanium or an alloy) and are often foldable for easy storage in the trunk of a car.

Wheeze

A high-pitched, whistling sound produced in the chest during breathing; it is caused by narrowing of the airways. A wheeze may be loud enough to be heard by those in the room with the sufferer or just audible with a stethoscope. Wheeze is a feature of *asthma* and also occurs in *bronchitis*, *bronchiolitis*, and pulmonary edema (fluid in the lungs). Inhalation of a foreign body, such as a peanut, into the airways may also cause a wheeze. (See also *Breathing difficulty*.)

Whiplash injury

An injury to the soft tissues, *ligaments*, and joints of the cervical spine (neck portion) caused by the neck being bent forcibly and violently forward and then backward or vice versa. Whiplash injury most commonly results from sudden acceleration or deceleration, as in a car collision. However, some degree of whiplash to the neck occurs in all forms of head injury.

Damage to the spine usually involves minor *sprain* of a neck ligament or *subluxation* (partial dislocation) of a cervical joint. Occasionally, a ligament may rupture or there may be a fracture of a cervical vertebra (see *Spinal injury*).

Characteristically, pain and stiffness in the neck are much worse 24 hours after the injury.

Treatment may include immobilization in an orthopedic *collar, analgesic drugs* (painkillers), *muscle-relaxant drugs*, and *physical therapy*. Recovery is usually complete but it can take several weeks before full pain-free neck movement is possible.

Whipple's disease

A rare disorder that may affect many organs. Also called intestinal lipodystrophy, Whipple's disease causes a variety of symptoms and findings. The most common are malabsorption (impaired absorption of nutrients by the small intestine), diarrhea, pain in the abdomen, progressive weight loss, joint pains, swollen lymph nodes, abnormal skin pigmentation, anemia, and fever. The condition most commonly occurs in middle-aged men.

The precise cause of Whipple's disease remains unknown but it is probably due to an unidentified bacterial infection. Diagnosis is by jejunal biopsy (removal of a small sample of tissue from the jejunum for microscopic analysis). Affected tissues are found to contain macrophages (a type of cell) containing rod-shaped bacteria.

Treatment is with *antibiotic drugs* for at least one year. Attempts to correct nutritional deficiencies that have arisen from malabsorption are made with dietary supplements.

Whipple's operation

A type of *pancreatectomy* in which the head of the pancreas and loop of the duodenum are surgically removed. It is named for the US surgeon Allen Whipple (1881-1963).

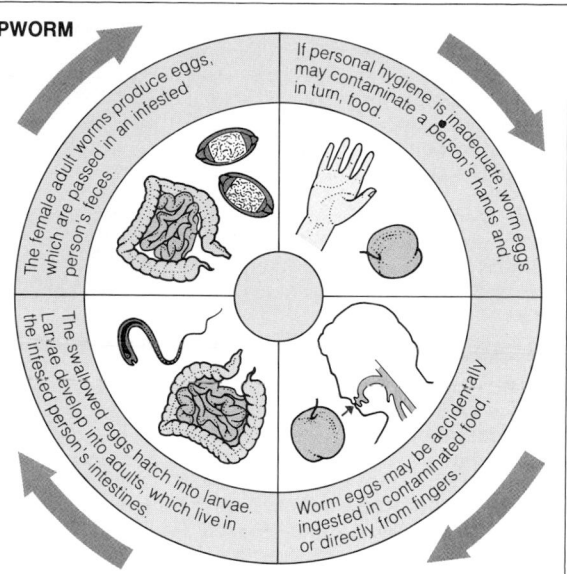

LIFE CYCLE OF WHIPWORM
Whipworm infestation occurs worldwide and is particularly common in the tropics. An estimated 2 million people in the US are affected at any given time—mainly children and residents of mental institutions. Adult worms are 1 to 2 inches in length, with long, whiplike tails; they may live in a person's intestines for up to 20 years. Most infestations do not cause symptoms.

The female adult worms produce eggs, which are passed in an infested person's feces.

If personal hygiene is inadequate worm eggs may contaminate a person's hands and, in turn, food.

Worm eggs may be accidentally ingested in contaminated food, or directly from fingers.

The swallowed eggs hatch into larvae. Larvae develop into adults, which live in the infested person's intestines.

Whipworm infestation

The whipworm is a small, cylindrical worm, 1 or 2 inches (2.5 to 5 cm) long, with a whiplike tail, that can live in human intestines. The life cycle and transmission of infection are shown above.

A light infestation causes no symptoms; a heavy infestation can cause abdominal pain, diarrhea, and sometimes *anemia*, because the worms consume a small amount of the host's blood every day. The condition is diagnosed by finding worm eggs during an examination of feces.

Treatment is with *antihelmintic drugs*, such as mebendazole, which usually bring about a satisfactory cure; heavy infestations may require more than one course of treatment.

Whitehead

A very common type of skin blemish (see *Milia*).

Whitlow

An abscess on the fingertip or, rarely, on the toe. A whitlow causes the finger to swell and become extremely painful and sensitive to pressure and touch. It may be caused by the virus that causes *herpes simplex* or by a bacterium, which usually enters the body through a cut.

A whitlow caused by bacterial infection may be treated with *antibiotic drugs* or, if the infection is severe, by incision and drainage in a minor surgical procedure using local anesthesia.

A whitlow caused by the virus that causes herpes simplex is treated by application of an *antiviral drug*; such whitlows should not be incised and drained because of the high risk of spreading the infection.

A very rare complication of untreated whitlow is *osteomyelitis*, a serious bacterial infection of bone and bone marrow.

Herpetic whitlow
This extremely painful finger infection, caused by the herpes simplex virus, may be helped by applying an antiviral ointment.

Whooping cough

See *Pertussis*.

Wife beating

See *Spouse abuse*.

Will, living

A written declaration, signed by an adult person of sound mind, that instructs his or her physicians to withhold or withdraw life-sustaining treatment if the person suffers from an incurable and terminal condition.

The written declaration must be signed with the same type of formality as a regular will, hence the description of the document as a "living will."

W

In 1987, 38 states and the District of Columbia had enacted laws giving legal effect to living wills. Although the terms and provisions of the laws vary from state to state, in general they require the physician and the hospital to honor the patient's living will or to transfer the care of the patient to another physician who will honor the living will.

The law also provides legal immunity from liability for the physician and the hospital honoring the patient's wishes as expressed in his or her living will.

Wilms' tumor
A type of *kidney cancer*, also called nephroblastoma, that occurs mainly in children.

Wilson's disease
A rare, inherited disorder in which copper accumulates in the liver and is slowly released into other parts of the body. Eventually, Wilson's disease causes severe damage to both the liver and the brain.

SYMPTOMS AND SIGNS
Symptoms vary in severity from person to person; they usually first appear in adolescence but sometimes occur as early as 5 or as late as 50. The toxic effects of copper on the liver can cause various disorders, progressing from *hepatitis* to *cirrhosis*. Accumulation of copper in the brain causes progressive problems ranging from mild intellectual impairment to crippling rigidity, tremor, and dementia.

DIAGNOSIS AND TREATMENT
The diagnosis is based on analysis of blood and urine and a liver *biopsy* (removal of a small amount of tissue for microscopic analysis) to discover the amount of copper in the body.

Wilson's disease requires lifelong treatment with penicillamine, a drug that binds with copper and thus enables it to be excreted. If started soon after the onset of symptoms, penicillamine can sometimes improve liver and brain function. If the disease is discovered before toxic effects produce symptoms, the drug may be able to prevent symptoms from developing.

Windpipe
A common name for the *trachea*.

Wiring of the jaws
Immobilization of the jaws by means of metal wires to allow a fracture of the jaw to heal or as part of a treatment for *obesity*.

Wired jaws
A total of eight pairs of teeth have been wired together to immobilize the jaw while a fracture heals.

In the most commonly used method, thin, hairpin-shaped wires with a central eyelet (closed loop) are wound around pairs of adjacent teeth; about six wires are fixed to teeth in the upper and lower jawbones. Wires are then threaded through opposing pairs of upper and lower eyelets and twisted together to hold the jaws in a rigid position.

When a fracture of the jaw is being treated, the jaws are kept wired in a fixed position for about six weeks. As a means of achieving weight loss, the jaws are wired for as long as a year. In both cases, the person can take only a liquid or semiliquid diet, which for weight loss is calorie controlled. This form of diet treatment, though effective while the jaws are wired, usually fails when the overweight person resumes his or her previous eating habits.

Wisdom tooth
One of the four rearmost *teeth*, also known as third molars. In most people, the wisdom teeth erupt between the ages of 17 and 21. However, in some people, one or more may neither develop nor erupt. In many cases, wisdom teeth are unable to emerge fully from the gum as a result of overcrowding (see *Impaction, dental*).

Crown
Cusps
Neck
Roots
Biting surface of tooth

Structure of wisdom tooth
Like other molars, each wisdom tooth has strong roots and a bulky crown with many cusps and an extensive grinding surface.

Witches' milk
A thin, white discharge from the nipple of a newborn infant. Witches' milk occurs quite commonly and is usually accompanied by enlargement of one or both of the baby's breasts. The discharge is caused by maternal hormones that entered the fetus's circulation through the placenta. Witches' milk is a harmless sign that usually disappears within a few weeks.

Withdrawal
The process of retreating from society and from relationships with others. Withdrawal is usually indicated by aloofness, lack of interest in social activities, preoccupation with one's own concerns, and difficulty communicating with others.

Withdrawal is also a term applied to the psychological and physical symptoms that develop upon discontinuation of a substance to which a person had become addicted (see *Withdrawal syndrome*).

Withdrawal bleeding
Vaginal blood loss that occurs when the body's level of *progesterone* or *estrogen hormones* drops suddenly. *Menstruation* (sloughing of the uterine lining, which takes place each month that fertilization and implantation of an ovum do not occur) is a form of withdrawal bleeding because it is preceded by the withdrawal of both estrogen and progesterone in the menstrual cycle. The withdrawal bleeding that occurs at the end of each cycle of combined *oral contraceptive* pills mimics menstruation, but is usually shorter and lighter. Discontinuation of an estrogen-only preparation also produces bleeding, which may differ from normal menstruation in amount and duration.

Withdrawal method
See *Coitus interruptus*.

Withdrawal syndrome
A set of unpleasant mental and physical symptoms experienced when a person stops using a drug on which he or she is physically dependent (see *Drug dependence*).

In general, any drug that causes euphoria or that relieves pain or anxiety can cause dependence and withdrawal symptoms of varying degrees. Withdrawal syndromes most commonly result from *alcohol dependence*, *narcotic drug* dependence, *tobacco smoking*, or regular use of *tranquilizer drugs*. Other drugs that may

W

FIRST AID: WOUNDS

```
DO NOT
■ attempt to remove the
  object from the wound.
```

FOREIGN BODY

1 Apply direct pressure above and below the object. Lay the victim down and raise and support the limb.

2 Lightly drape a piece of gauze over object and wound and place a ring pad over it. Or use a roll of cotton to build up a pad around the wound. It should be high enough to prevent pressure on the object.

Ring pad

1 Place a narrow bandage across one hand. Wind one end once or twice around your fingers to make a loop.

2 Bring the other end through the loop, wind it repeatedly around the loop, pulling it tight each time.

3 Secure with a roller bandage. Make two straight turns, overlapping the pad, on either side. Then continue with diagonal turns until the pad is held firmly. Take the victim to the hospital.

DEEPER WOUNDS

1 Examine the wound for foreign bodies; if there are none, apply direct pressure to control bleeding by pressing on the wound with the fingers or palm. Lay the victim down and raise the injured part higher than the chest and heart.

2 Put a sterile, unmedicated dressing over the wound so that it extends well beyond its edges. Secure it firmly with a bandage.

3 If the blood seeps through, do not remove the bandage, but put more dressing and another bandage on top. Watch for *shock* and seek medical aid.

CUTS AND SCRAPES

1 Rinse the wound under cold, running water. Then, using a roll of cotton, gauze, or antiseptic wipes, clean around the wound. Work outward, using a clean pad for each stroke.

2 Remove any loose foreign bodies, such as metal, glass, or gravel, with the gauze, cotton, or tweezers.

3 Dry the surrounding area and dress the wound. If it is small, use an adhesive bandage. Otherwise, make a dressing with a piece of gauze and a piece of cotton. Secure with a bandage.

W

lead to withdrawal symptoms include *amphetamine drugs*, *cocaine*, *marijuana*, and *caffeine*.

TYPES

ALCOHOL Withdrawal symptoms start six to eight hours after the last drink and may last four to seven days. Common symptoms include trembling of the hands and tongue, sweating, nausea, anxiety, and sometimes cramps and vomiting. More severe symptoms include seizures (see *Delirium tremens*), confusion, and hallucinations. Withdrawal symptoms may be frightening and frequently result in a resumption of drinking. Many alcohol-dependent people need a drink in the morning to ward off the withdrawal syndrome.

NARCOTIC DRUGS *Heroin* or *morphine* withdrawal syndrome starts eight to 12 hours after the last dose and may last for seven to 10 days. At first, a craving for the drug is the most prominent feature, accompanied by restlessness, sweating, runny eyes and nose, and yawning. As the syndrome progresses, a variety of other symptoms appear, including diarrhea, vomiting, abdominal cramps, dilated pupils, loss of appetite, gooseflesh (the origin of the term "cold turkey"), irritability, tremor, weakness, and depression.

Other narcotic drugs, such as *codeine* and some prescription analgesics, cause withdrawal symptoms similar to those produced by heroin or morphine, but, if the doses have not been too high, these withdrawal symptoms may be less intense and may develop more slowly.

TRANQUILIZERS Withdrawal syndrome from *barbiturate drugs* and *meprobamate* begins from 12 to 24 hours after the last dose and has many similarities to alcohol withdrawal. The first symptoms are usually tremor, anxiety, restlessness, and weakness sometimes followed by delirium, hallucinations, and, in some cases, seizures. A period of prolonged sleep occurs just before the symptoms clear up, which is between three and eight days after onset, depending on the individual drug.

Withdrawal from *benzodiazepine drugs* may begin much more slowly (up to 14 days after the last dose) and can in some cases be life-threatening.

TOBACCO SMOKING Withdrawal symptoms from *nicotine* (the substance in tobacco responsible for dependence) develops gradually over 24 to 48 hours. In addition to a desperate desire to smoke, the most common

DRUGS USED TO TREAT WORM INFESTATIONS

Infestation	Drugs
Pinworm	Mebendazole, pyrantel
Common roundworm (ascariasis)	Mebendazole, pyrantel, piperazine
Whipworm	Mebendazole
Hookworm	Mebendazole
Strongyloidiasis	Thiabendazole
Toxocariasis	Mebendazole, thiabendazole
Tapeworms	Niclosamide, praziquantel
Filariasis	Diethylcarbamazine
Schistosomiasis	Praziquantel

Antihelmintic drugs
Drugs such as those listed above are the main treatment for worm infestations. Usually just one or two doses are required but sometimes longer treatment is needed. Laxatives may also be given to aid expulsion of worms living in the intestines.

symptoms are irritability, difficulty concentrating, frustration, headaches, and restless anxiety.

OTHER DRUGS Discontinuation of an amphetamine or cocaine results in lethargy, extreme tiredness, and dizziness. Cocaine withdrawal may also lead to severe depression, and sometimes other physical symptoms, such as tremor and sweating.

Chronic marijuana users have reported various withdrawal symptoms, including tremor, sweating, nausea, vomiting, diarrhea, irritability, and sleep disturbances.

Symptoms of caffeine withdrawal, consisting of tiredness, headaches, and irritability, may occur in people accustomed to drinking large quantities of tea, coffee, or caffeine-containing soft drinks. The onset of these symptoms usually occurs several hours after the last drink of caffeine-containing liquid.

TREATMENT

Severe withdrawal syndromes require medical treatment. Symptoms may be suppressed by giving the patient small quantities of the drug he or she was using. More commonly, however, a substitute drug is given, such as *methadone* for narcotic drugs or *diazepam* for alcohol. The dose of the drug is then gradually reduced. This substitution process requires careful adjustment and can be safely managed only in a medical setting.

Womb
See *Uterus*.

Word blindness
See *Alexia*; *Dyslexia*.

World Health Organization
The World Health Organization (WHO) was established in 1948 as an agency of the United Nations with responsibilities for international health matters and public health. Its headquarters is in Geneva, Switzerland; there are also regional offices for Europe, Africa, North America, South America, Southeast Asia, the Eastern Mediterranean, and the Western Pacific (including Australia).

The WHO has campaigned effectively against certain infectious diseases, notably smallpox (which was officially declared as eradicated throughout the world in 1980), tuberculosis, and malaria. Its other functions include sponsoring medical research programs, organizing a network of collaborating national laboratories, and providing expert advice to its 160 member states on matters such as health service organizations, family health, the use of medicinal drugs, the abuse of drugs, and mental health. The organization's current strategy is described in its campaign "Health for all by the year 2000." The plan gives specific targets for basic public health measures, such as the provision of piped water supplies and other basic sanitation, the universal provision of immunization of children against infectious diseases, and reductions in the use of tobacco and alcohol.

W

Worm infestation

Several types of worm, or their larvae, can exist as parasites of humans. They range in size from the microscopic to many feet in length and may live in the intestines, blood, lymphatic system, bile ducts, or organs such as the liver. Worms are more common than is realized; in many cases, they cause few or no symptoms, and a person may have an infestation for many years without realizing it. Other worms can cause chronic, sometimes severe and debilitating, illness.

There are two main classes of worm—the *roundworms*, which have long, cylindrical bodies, and the platyhelminths, which have flattened bodies. The platyhelminths are further subdivided into the cestodes (tapeworms) and trematodes (flukes).

Worm diseases found in developed countries, such as the US, include *pinworm infestation, ascariasis, whipworm infestation, toxocariasis*, and *trichinosis* (all caused by different types of roundworm), *liver fluke*, and some types of *tapeworm infestation*. Important types in tropical regions include *hookworm infestation, filariasis*, and *guinea worm disease* (caused by roundworms), and *schistosomiasis* (caused by a type of fluke).

Worms may be acquired by eating undercooked, infected meat, by contact with soil or water containing worm larvae, by accidental ingestion of worm eggs (via fingers or food), from soil contaminated by infected feces, or in day-care centers where hygiene may be compromised.

The diagnosis of a worm infestation may be alarming but most types can be easily eradicated with *antihelmintic drugs* (see box opposite).

Wound

Any damage to the skin and/or underlying tissues caused by an accident, act of violence, or surgery. Wounds in which the skin or mucous membrane are broken are called open; those in which they remain intact are termed closed.

TYPES

Wounds can be divided into the following broad categories—an incised wound (an injury in which the skin is cleanly cut, or a surgical *incision*); an abrasion (a graze in which surface tissue is scraped away); a *laceration* (a wound in which the skin is torn, such as an animal or human *bite*); a penetrating wound (such as a stab or gunshot wound); and a contusion (a wound in which the underlying

Abrasion on arm
Abrasions usually result from sliding falls and may contain dirt. They should be carefully cleaned and dressed.

Knife wound down side of face
This is a deep, incised wound, cleanly cut, and likely to heal with minimal scarring once the edges have been sutured.

tissues are damaged by a blunt instrument). This type of soft tissue injury may include damage to subcutaneous tissue, muscle, bone, blood vessels, and/or nerves. When the wound lies over the thorax or abdomen, internal organs may also be bruised or more severely damaged. Considerable bleeding can occur with little outward evidence.

Many penetrating wounds and some contused wounds are deceptive in appearance, showing little external sign of damage but involving serious internal injury. Low-velocity gunshot injuries cause tissue damage all along the path of the projectile. High-velocity gunshot injuries may also damage distant structures as a result of shock waves traveling through tissues. In stab wounds, vital organs may be perforated or major blood vessels severed. In contusions, the liver, spleen, or kidney may be ruptured and cause internal bleeding.

TREATMENT

Many minor wounds can be treated by first-aid measures (see *Bleeding, treatment of; Dressings*; and first-aid box on previous page). More extensive or deeper wounds require professional treatment.

If the wound contains any foreign material or dead tissue, it is removed; the wound is then cleansed with an antiseptic solution to decrease the risk of *wound infection*.

Clean, incised wounds may be closed by *suturing* if the wounds are fresh; they usually heal with minimal scarring. Lacerations may need to have the jagged skin edges cut away before they are stitched. Contaminated wounds are usually not closed.

Wounds in which there is extensive tissue damage and/or a high risk of infection are usually filled with layers of sterile gauze and covered with a bandage for four or five days. If, after this time, there is no sign of infection and the skin edges can be brought together without tension, the wound may be stitched. Otherwise, the wound may be left open and allowed to heal on its own.

Penetrating wounds or contusions may require an exploratory operation of the abdominal cavity (see *Laparotomy*) or the chest cavity (see *Thoracotomy*). Damage to blood vessels, nerves, or bones often necessitates repair by specialized surgical techniques, such as *microsurgery*. *Skin grafting* may also be required. (See also *Healing*.)

Wound infection

Any type of wound is susceptible to the entry of bacteria; the resultant infection can delay healing, result in disability, or cause death. Complications of wound infection may result in local spread of the infection to adjacent organs or tissue or distant spread via the blood.

SURGICAL WOUNDS

About 5 to 10 percent of surgical wounds become infected. Primary infection—occurring during the operation itself or while dressing the wound afterward—is a common occurrence despite routine *aseptic technique* (the creation of a germ-free environment). *Antibiotic drugs* are therefore administered as a preventive measure for 24 hours after surgery. Infection is more likely to develop in obese patients and in patients with reduced natural defenses against infection, such as the elderly and those suffering from cancer.

For surgery in which there is a higher-than-average risk of infection (such as an intestinal operation) or in which infection would have particularly serious consequences (such as a joint replacement operation), the patient is given antibiotic drugs as a preventive measure.

NONSURGICAL WOUNDS
Nonsurgical wounds most likely to become infected are wounds sustained in an agricultural accident or by soldiers in battle. There is a risk of the soilborne bacterium CLOSTRIDIUM TETANI causing the serious, sometimes fatal, infection tetanus or of related bacteria, such as CLOSTRIDIUM PERFRINGENS, causing gas gangrene.

In dealing with any serious nonsurgical wound, the physician attempts to prevent infection by removing any foreign material or dead tissue from the wound, thoroughly cleaning it with an antiseptic solution, and giving antibiotics. In addition, if there is a risk of the wound being contaminated with soil, an antitetanus injection is given unless the patient has received one within the previous five years.

SIGNS AND TREATMENT
The signs of infection in a wound are redness, swelling, warmth, pain, and sometimes the presence of pus. Pus is usually accompanied by an exquisitely tender dark swelling (an abscess) that either is draining pus or must be incised to permit drainage.

Once infection is discovered, a sample of blood or pus is taken and the patient is given an antibiotic drug. When a culture of the causative bacteria has been grown, treatment may need to be switched to a more appropriate antibiotic. Any abscess should be drained surgically.

Wrinkle
A furrow in the skin. Wrinkling is a natural feature of aging caused by a reduction in collagen production and consequent loss of skin elasticity. Wrinkles are most obvious on the face and other exposed parts of the body but occur all over the skin. Premature deep wrinkling is usually caused by overexposure to sunlight.

Despite the claims made for various "rejuvenating" skin preparations, treatments do not permanently restore skin elasticity. A face-lift smoothes out wrinkles by stretching the skin, but the effects last only about five years. Vitamin A derivatives are currently being evaluated as a means of reducing wrinkling.

STRUCTURE OF THE WRIST
The wrist is a complex joint that allows the hand to be bent forward and backward relative to the arm (through an angle of almost 180 degrees) and also moved side to side (through about 70 degrees).

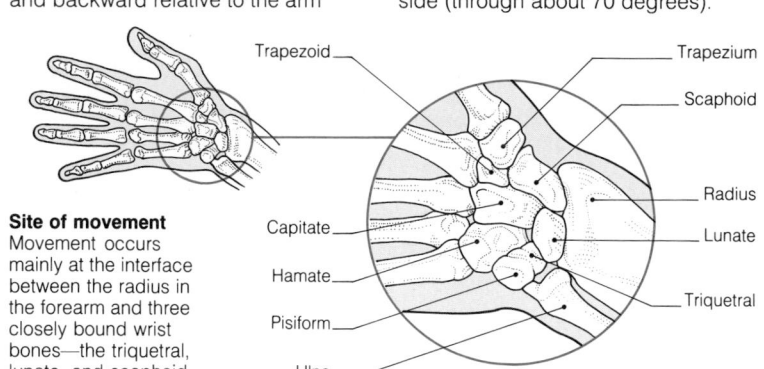

Site of movement
Movement occurs mainly at the interface between the radius in the forearm and three closely bound wrist bones—the triquetral, lunate, and scaphoid.

Trapezoid
Trapezium
Scaphoid
Radius
Lunate
Triquetral
Capitate
Hamate
Pisiform
Ulna

Wrist
The joint between the hand and the arm. The skeleton of the wrist consists of eight bones (known collectively as the carpus) arranged in two rows—the scaphoid, lunate, triquetral, and pisiform bones, which articulate with the radius and ulna (bones of the forearm); and the trapezium, trapezoid, capitate, and hamate, which are connected to the bones of the palm. The bones of the carpus articulate with each other.

Many tendons, which connect the forearm muscles to the fingers and thumb, run across the wrist. The extensor tendons, which straighten the fingers, are on the back of the wrist; the flexor tendons, which bend the fingers, are on the front. These tendons pass under ligaments to prevent them from springing away from the wrist. The gap between the ligaments and tendons at the front of the wrist is known as the carpal tunnel. Also passing across the wrist are the arteries and nerves supplying the muscles, bones, and skin of the hand and fingers.

DISORDERS
Wrist injuries may lead to serious disability by limiting hand movement. This is especially likely with fractures of the scaphoid bone, which often fail to heal, and with cutting injuries involving the tendons or nerves.

A common wrist injury in adults is Colles' fracture, in which the lower end of the radius is fractured and the wrist and hand are displaced backward. In young children, similar displacement results from a fracture through the epiphysis (growing end) of the radius.

Sprain of ligaments at the wrist joint can occur but is usually not severe.

Pressure on the median nerve as it passes through the carpal tunnel causes numbness, tingling, and pain in the thumb, index, and middle fingers (see Carpal tunnel syndrome). Damage to the radial nerve, which may be caused by fracture of the humerus (upper arm bone), results in wristdrop (inability to straighten the wrist).

Other conditions that may affect the wrist include tenosynovitis (inflammation of the inner lining of a tendon sheath) and osteoarthritis.

Wristdrop
Inability to straighten the wrist, so that the back of the hand cannot be brought horizontal with the back of the forearm. This causes weakness of grip because the hand muscles can function efficiently only when the wrist is held straight.

Wristdrop is caused by damage to the radial nerve, usually at a point where it passes beneath the armpit or where it winds around the humerus (upper arm bone). The radial nerve may be damaged by prolonged pressure in the armpit (see Crutch palsy) or by a fracture of the humerus (see Humerus, fracture of).

Treatment involves holding the wrist straight. This may be achieved with a simple splint. However, if damage to the radial nerve is permanent, the usual treatment is arthrodesis (fusion) of the wrist bones.

Wry neck
See Torticollis.

X

Xanthelasma

Yellowish deposits of fatty substance in the eyelids that are associated with a raised level of cholesterol in the blood. (See also *Xanthomatosis*.)

Appearance of xanthelasma
These fatty deposits around the eyes are common in elderly people but are usually of no more than cosmetic importance.

Xanthoma

A yellow deposit of fatty material in the skin, often on the elbow or buttock. Xanthomas may indicate a lipid (fat) disorder. (See *Xanthomatosis*.)

Xanthomatosis

A condition in which deposits of yellowish, fatty material occur in various parts of the body, particularly in the skin, internal organs, corneas, brain, and tendons. The deposits may occur in the eyelids only, a condition known as *xanthelasma*.

The most important feature of xanthomatosis is the tendency for cholesterol to be deposited in the linings of blood vessels, leading to generalized *atherosclerosis*.

Xanthomatosis is often associated with a range of disorders causing *hyperlipidemias* (raised levels of fats and cholesterol in the blood).

Treatment aims to lower the levels of fats and cholesterol in the blood. This is achieved by means of a diet that is low in cholesterol and high in polyunsaturated fat, and by drugs.

Xeroderma pigmentosum

A rare, inherited skin disease. The skin is normal at birth, but extreme sensitivity to sunlight (see *Photosensitivity*) causes it to become dry, wrinkled, freckled, and prematurely aged by about the age of 5. Various types of benign and malignant skin tumors also develop. Xeroderma pigmentosum is often accompanied by conditions that involve the eye such as *photophobia* and *conjunctivitis*.

Treatment consists of preventing exposure to sunlight by wearing protective clothing and using *sunscreens*. Skin cancers are usually treated by surgical removal or with *anticancer drugs*.

Xerophthalmia

An eye disorder in which vitamin A deficiency causes the conjunctiva and cornea to become abnormally dry. Without treatment, xerophthalmia may progress to *keratomalacia*, a condition in which there is severe damage to the cornea.

Xerostomia

Abnormal dryness of the mouth (see *Mouth, dry*).

Xiphisternum

An alternative name for the xiphoid process, the small, leaf-shaped projection that constitutes the lowest of the three parts of the *sternum* (breastbone).

X-linked disorders

Sex-linked *genetic disorders* in which the abnormal gene or genes—the causative factors—are located on the X chromosome, and in which almost all those affected are males. *Color vision deficiency* and *hemophilia* are examples of this type of disorder. (See also *Fragile X syndrome*.)

X rays

A form of invisible electromagnetic energy of short wavelength that is produced when high speed electrons strike a heavy metal. Discovered in 1896 by Wilhelm Conrad Roentgen, X rays are variably able to penetrate all substances. From the time of their discovery, X rays have been used to an increasingly important degree in medicine for both diagnosis and treatment.

WHY THEY ARE USED

X rays can be used to produce images of bones, organs, and internal tissues. Low doses of X rays are passed through the tissues and cast images—essentially shadows—-onto film or a fluorescent screen. The X-ray image, also known as a radiograph or roentgenogram, shows structural changes in the area being examined.

X rays have the potential to damage living cells especially those that are dividing rapidly. Since cancer cells divide rapidly, high doses of radiation are used (along with other forms of radiant energy) for treating cancer (see *Radiation therapy*).

HOW THEY WORK

X rays are produced artificially by bombarding a small tungsten target with electrons in a device known as an X-ray tube (or cooling tube). The X rays that are emitted travel in straight lines and radiate outward from a point on the target in all directions. In an X-ray machine, the X-ray tube is surrounded by lead casing, except for a small aperture through which the X-ray beam emerges.

Each of the body's tissues absorbs X rays in a predictable way. Bones are dense and contain calcium; they absorb X rays well. Soft tissues—skin, fat, blood, and muscle—absorb X rays to a lesser extent. Thus, when an arm, for example, is placed in the path of an X-ray beam, the X rays pass readily through the soft tissues but penetrate the bones much less easily. The arm casts a shadow on film or a fluorescent screen, with the bone appearing white and the soft tissues dark gray.

THE X-RAY EXAMINATION

When a patient arrives for an X ray, the X-ray technician explains the procedure. The patient undresses to expose the area concerned; care is taken to remove any objects that might produce an image on the film, such as jewelry, hair clips, dentures, and wigs.

The position of the patient when the X ray is taken is carefully chosen to provide the clearest view of the part under examination, although this position may require modification if the patient is sick or in severe pain.

The X-ray film is usually contained in a flat cassette; the patient lies, sits, or stands with the region to be examined in contact with the cassette. Movement must be avoided while the X ray is taken since it results in a blurred image. Every effort is made to keep the patient comfortable and relaxed and to use the shortest possible exposure time—usually just a fraction of a second. If necessary, the region of interest can be supported or immobilized.

When the patient is in the correct position, the film is in place, and the X-ray tube is ready, the technician leaves the room for a few moments

X-RAY EXAMINATION

Probably the best known of all imaging techniques, X rays are also one of the most useful, particularly for imaging the skeleton, the chest, and body conduits such as the blood vessels and digestive tract (after they have had a radiopaque material introduced into them).

Modern X-ray equipment is designed to produce high-quality images at the lowest possible radiation dose to the patient.

Procedure
The technician makes sure the patient is correctly positioned, checks that the X-ray tube is ready, and then goes to a control panel behind a protective screen and presses a button to take the X ray. The technician can see and talk to the patient from behind the screen.

X-ray machine

X-ray technician

Area of coverage of X rays. This is easily adjusted.

Patient

Barium enema
This X ray shows the lower part of the large intestine outlined by a radiopaque contrast medium containing a barium compound.

and presses the exposure button on the control panel to take the X ray.

Once the X-ray film has been developed, it is interpreted by a *radiologist*. Some disorders, such as fractures, are immediately recognizable; others, such as some tumors, may take more time to assess.

SPECIAL X-RAY TECHNIQUES
Hollow or fluid-filled parts of the body often do not show up well on X-ray film unless they first have a contrast medium introduced into them. Such contrast-medium techniques are used to look at the gallbladder (see *Cholecystography*), the bile ducts (see *Cholangiography*), the urinary tract (see *Pyelography*), the gastrointestinal tract (see *Barium X-ray examinations*), the blood vessels (see *Angiography; Venography*), the spinal cord (see *Myelography*), and the joint spaces (see *Arthrography*).

X rays can be used to obtain an image of a "slice" through an organ or part of the body by using a technique known as *tomography*. More detailed and accurate images of a body slice are produced by combining tomography with the capabilities of a computer (see *CT scanning*).

X-RAY SAFETY
It is now understood that large doses of radiation can be extremely harmful (see *Radiation hazards*). Modern X-ray film, equipment, and techniques are designed specifically to produce high-quality images at the lowest possible radiation dose (exposure) to the patient. The possible hazard of genetic damage can be minimized by using a lead shield to protect the patient's reproductive organs from the X-ray beam. X-ray examinations are also generally avoided if there is any possibility of pregnancy.

X-ray technicians and radiologists wear a *film badge* to monitor their exposure to radiation. (See also *Imaging techniques*.)

X rays, dental
See *Dental X rays.*

X-ray technician
A person who prepares patients for *X-ray* examinations, takes and develops X-ray pictures, and assists with other imaging techniques.

The X-ray technician gives the patient any special instructions that he or she must follow during the X-ray examination. Once the examination begins, the technician is responsible for positioning the patient to provide the best possible picture of the part being studied.

X-ray technicians also assist *radiologists* in performing specialized X-ray examinations (such as contrast-medium studies) and carrying out other imaging procedures, such as *radionuclide scanning, ultrasound scanning,* and *MRI.* The sources of energy that produce the images for these last procedures are beta particles or gamma rays from radionuclides, high-frequency sound waves, and electromagnetic waves generated by extremely powerful magnets.

Xylometazoline
A *decongestant drug* used to relieve nasal congestion caused by a common cold, sinusitis, or hay fever (see *Rhinitis, allergic*). Available in nose drops or nasal sprays, xylometazoline works by narrowing the small blood vessels in the lining of the nose.

Excessive use of xylometazoline may cause headache, palpitations, or drowsiness. Long-term use may cause congestion to become worse.

X

USING X RAYS TO LOOK AT THE BODY

X rays are perhaps the most widely used method of imaging the body. When passed through body tissues onto photographic film, X rays cast images of internal structures, allowing alterations in silhouette to be seen. Soft tissues do not show up as well as bone on X rays, but, by using a contrast medium, they too can be visualized. New computer techniques produce even clearer, more detailed images.

3-D CT scan
A computer can transform X-ray images of body slices into a three-dimensional image of part of the body. This scan shows a badly damaged shoulder blade.

CT scan
Combined use of a computer and X rays produces cross-sectional images. In this brain scan, the eyes and nose are seen at the top, the central light area represents the brain stem.

Barium X ray
Introducing barium, which is opaque to X rays, into the large intestine allows it to be visualized.

Chest X ray
This heart appears enlarged due to excess fluid around it.

Venography
This technique for examining veins involves injecting them with a contrast medium before they are X rayed. The femoral vein shown here (in the foreground) is partially blocked by blood clots.

X ray of hip joint
This X ray of an osteo-arthritic hip shows almost complete degener-ation of the cartilage.

X rays of knee joint
The X ray at left shows erosion of bone and cartilage. The parts of an artificial knee are seen in the X ray at right.

X ray of foot
All the bones can be clearly seen in this X ray of a 4-year-old's foot.

Y

Yawning

An involuntary act, usually associated with drowsiness or boredom, in which the mouth is opened wide and a slow, deep breath taken through it. Yawning is accompanied by a momentary increase in the heart rate, slight constriction of some blood capillaries, and, in many cases, watering of the eyes (possibly because of pressure on the tear glands as a result of the facial movements).

The purpose of yawning is unknown, but one theory suggests it is triggered by raised levels of carbon dioxide in the blood; thus, its purpose may be to reduce the blood carbon dioxide level and increase the blood oxygen level.

Yaws

A disease found throughout poorer subtropical and tropical areas of the world that is caused by a spirochete (spiral-shaped bacterium) very similar to that which causes syphilis. Yaws is not, however, a sexually transmitted disease. The infection is almost always acquired in childhood.

Yaws ulcer on leg
Yaws is an infection that mainly affects the skin and bones. Ulceration and tissue destruction may occur in advanced cases.

Three or four weeks after infection, a single, highly infectious, itchy, raspberrylike growth appears at the site of infection. Scratching spreads the infection and leads to the develop-

ment of more growths elsewhere on the skin. Without treatment, the growths heal slowly over the course of about six months. Recurrence of the growths is common.

Yaws can be cured by a single large dose of a penicillin. In about 10 percent of untreated cases, widespread tissue loss eventually occurs. This may lead to gross destruction of the skin, bones, and joints of the legs, nose, palate, and upper jaw.

Yeasts

Types of *fungi*. Certain yeasts can cause infections of the skin or mucous membranes. The most important disease-causing yeast is CANDIDA ALBICANS, which causes *candidiasis*.

Yellow fever

 An infectious disease of short duration and variable severity caused by a virus transmitted by mosquitoes. In severe cases, the skin of the sufferer becomes yellow from jaundice—hence the name yellow fever.

CAUSES
Today, yellow fever can be contracted only in Central America, parts of South America, and a large area of Africa. In forest areas, various species of mosquitoes may spread the infection from monkeys to humans. In urban areas, the disease is transmitted between humans by AEDES AEGYPTI mosquitoes.

PREVENTION
Eradication of the causative mosquito from populated areas has greatly reduced the incidence of yellow fever. Vaccination confers long-lasting immunity and should always be obtained before travel to or through affected areas. A vaccination certificate is required for entry to many countries, including parts of Asia as well as other countries where the disease is prevalent.

A single injection of the vaccine gives protection for at least 10 years. Children under 1 year of age should not be vaccinated. Reactions to the vaccine are rare and usually trivial.

SYMPTOMS AND SIGNS
Three to six days after infection, there is sudden onset of fever and headache, often with nausea and nose bleeding. Characteristically, despite the high fever, the heart rate is very slow. In many cases, the patient recovers in three days.

In more serious cases, the fever is higher and there is severe headache and pain in the neck, back, and legs.

Damage may occur rapidly to the liver and kidneys, causing jaundice and *renal failure*. This may be followed by a stage of severe agitation and delirium, leading to coma and death.

DIAGNOSIS AND TREATMENT
During epidemics, diagnosis is easy. Doubt is resolved by isolating the virus from the blood or by the demonstration of *antibodies* to the virus by a type of *immunoassay*.

No drug is effective against the yellow fever virus; treatment is directed at maintaining the blood volume. Transfusion of fluids is often necessary. In mild and moderate cases, the outlook is excellent and complications are few. Relapses do not occur and one attack confers lifelong immunity. Overall, however, about 10 percent of victims die.

Yin and yang

Fundamental concepts in traditional *Chinese medicine* and philosophy. Yang embodies positive, active, "male" qualities and thus complements yin, which embodies negative, passive, "female" qualities. The concepts of yin and yang are also central to the theoretical basis of *macrobiotics*.

Yoga

A system of Hindu philosophy and physical discipline. The main form of yoga practiced in the West is hatha-yoga, in which the follower adopts a series of poses, known as asanas, and uses a special breathing technique. This maintains flexibility of the body, teaches physical and mental control, and is a useful aid to *relaxation*.

If attempted by people in poor health or practiced incorrectly, yoga may pose health hazards, such as back disorders, *hypertension* (high blood pressure), and *glaucoma* (increased pressure in the eye).

Yoga pose
This photograph shows a stage of the full twist asana, which is excellent for promoting flexibility.

Z

Zidovudine

An *antiviral drug* formerly known as azidothymidine (AZT). Zidovudine was approved for use in the treatment of *AIDS* in April 1987.

WHY IT IS USED

Zidovudine is used to reduce the severity of AIDS-related conditions, such as *pneumocystis pneumonia* and infections of the brain and nervous system caused by the AIDS virus. Zidovudine does not cure these conditions but may improve symptoms or prolong remission. For example, it may reduce lymph gland swelling and promote weight gain. Although zidovudine slows the progress of AIDS, relapse commonly occurs after several months of treatment.

HOW IT WORKS

Zidovudine blocks the action of the enzyme that stimulates the AIDS virus to grow and multiply. Clinical trials have shown that the resultant reduction in virus activity leads to an increase in the production and number of T-helper lymphocytes (a type of white blood cell). This in turn improves the efficiency of the immune system, making the occurrence of *opportunistic infections*, such as candidiasis (thrush), less likely. Zidovudine does not appear to stop the growth of other viruses.

POSSIBLE ADVERSE EFFECTS

By reducing the number of red blood cells produced, zidovudine often causes severe *anemia*, requiring blood transfusion. For this reason, regular blood tests are performed and the drug is withdrawn if the blood count is dangerously low. Too high a dose of zidovudine may cause restlessness, insomnia, and fever.

Zidovudine also impairs the absorption and thus the effectiveness of *trimethoprim* and *sulfamethoxazole*, the antibiotic drugs used to treat pneumonia in people who have AIDS.

Zinc

A *trace element* that is essential for normal growth, development of the reproductive organs, normal func-

tioning of the prostate gland, healing of wounds, and the manufacture of proteins and nucleic acids (the genetic material of cells). Zinc also controls the activities of more than 100 enzymes and is involved in the functioning of the hormone insulin.

Small amounts of the element are present in a wide variety of foods; particularly rich sources include lean meat, whole-grain breads and cereals, dried beans, and seafood.

DEFICIENCY

A balanced diet that contains natural, unprocessed foods provides sufficient zinc for the body's needs, so deficiency is rare; it most often occurs in people who are generally malnourished. Zinc deficiency may also be caused by a disorder that impairs intestinal absorption of the mineral (see *Malabsorption; Acrodermatitis enteropathica*) or by increased zinc requirements due to cell damage (e.g., as a result of a burn or in *sickle cell anemia*). Symptoms of deficiency in-

clude impairment of taste and loss of appetite; in severe cases, there may also be hair loss and inflammation of the skin, mouth, tongue, and eyelids. In children, zinc deficiency may impair physical growth and delay sexual development.

EXCESS

Prolonged, excessive intake of zinc (usually through supplements) may interfere with the intestinal absorption of iron and copper, leading to a deficiency of these minerals and resultant symptoms of nausea, vomiting, fever, headache, tiredness, and abdominal pain.

MEDICAL USES

Zinc compounds, such as *zinc oxide*, are included in many preparations for treating skin and scalp disorders.

Zinc oxide

An ingredient of many skin preparations that has a mild *astringent* (drying) action and a soothing effect. Zinc oxide is used to treat painful, itchy, or

A SELECTION OF ZOONOSES (DISEASES CAUGHT FROM ANIMALS)

Animal	Disease	Animal	Disease
Bat	Histoplasmosis Rabies	Parrot	Psittacosis
Cat	Toxoplasmosis Cat-scratch fever Fungal infections	Pig	Trichinosis Pork tapeworm Brucellosis
Cow	Brucellosis Beef tapeworm Q fever Cowpox	Rabbit	Tularemia
Dog	Rabies Toxocariasis Mite infestations Fungal infections	Rat	Leptospirosis Plague Rat-bite fever
Horse	Glanders Equine encephalitis	Sheep	Liver fluke Anthrax
Monkey	Yellow fever	Turtle	Salmonella infection

Relative importance
With the exception of fungal infections and mites caught from pets, all the above are rare in the US. Some are confined to the tropics—such as yellow fever, which is not caught from monkeys directly, but can be transmitted from monkeys to humans by mosquitoes. Apart from the animals listed, bites from various other species (e.g., skunks, foxes, and mongeese) may transmit rabies to humans in different parts of the world.

moist skin conditions (such as eczema, bedsores, and diaper rash) and to ease the pain caused by hemorrhoids and insect bites or stings. It also blocks the ultraviolet rays of the sun.

Zinc oxide is also used to thicken lotions and creams, making them easier to apply.

Zollinger-Ellison syndrome

A rare condition characterized by severe and recurrent *peptic ulcers* in the stomach, duodenum, and upper small intestine.

Zollinger-Ellison syndrome is caused by a tumor, usually found in the pancreas, that secretes the hormone gastrin; the hormone stimulates the stomach and duodenum to produce large quantities of acid, which leads to ulceration. The high levels of acid in the digestive tract also cause diarrhea and steatorrhea (fat in the feces) in almost half the sufferers.

The condition often goes unrecognized until the surgery for the peptic ulcers is rapidly followed by a recurrence of the ulceration. Once suspicion is aroused, the physician performs blood tests; high levels of gastrin are usually sufficient to confirm the diagnosis.

The tumor (or, more frequently, tumors) is most often cancerous, although of a slow-growing type. If possible, the tumor or tumors are removed surgically; otherwise, total *gastrectomy* (surgical removal of the stomach) is necessary.

Zoonosis

Any infectious or parasitic disease of animals that can be transmitted to humans. Many disease organisms can infect only humans or particular animals, but zoonotic organisms are more flexible and can adapt themselves to many different species.

Zoonoses are usually caught from animals closely associated with humans, either as pets (such as dogs, cats, or parrots), food sources (such as pigs or cattle), or scavenging parasites (such as rats). Examples include *toxocariasis* (from dogs), *cat-scratch fever* and some *fungal infections* (from cats), *psittacosis* (from parrots or other birds), *brucellosis* (from cows, goats, or swine), *trichinosis* (from pigs), and *leptospirosis* (from rats). *Rabies* can infect virtually any mammal, but dog bites are a common cause of human infection worldwide.

Other zoonoses are transmitted from animals less obviously associated with humans, usually by insect

TECHNIQUE OF Z-PLASTY

This relatively simple plastic surgery technique is carried out to revise unsightly scars or to relieve skin tension caused by scar contracture.

It can be particularly useful for dealing with facial scars or ones that cross natural skin creases.

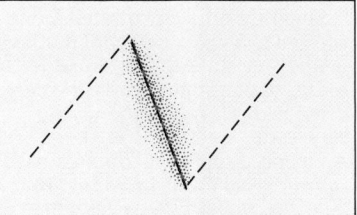

1 Three incisions are made, forming a Z. The central incision is made lengthwise through the scar.

2 Two triangular flaps are developed by cutting skin away from underlying tissue, and the flaps are then transposed.

3 This maneuver creates a new Z, of which the central arm is at right angles to the original direction of the scar.

4 The flaps are sutured in place. With careful planning, the suture lines can be hidden in natural skin creases.

vectors. For example, some cases of *yellow fever* are transmitted from forest monkeys to humans via the bites of mosquitoes. (See also *Dogs, diseases from; Cats, diseases from; Rats, diseases from; Insects and disease*.)

Z-plasty

A technique used in *plastic surgery* to change the direction of a scar so that it can be hidden in natural skin creases or to relieve skin tension caused by scar *contracture*. Z-plasty is especially useful for revising unsightly scars on the face and for releasing scarring across joints, such as on the fingers or in the armpits, that may restrict movement or cause deformity.

A Z-shaped incision is made with the central arm of the Z along the scar. Two V-shaped flaps are created by cutting the skin away from underlying tissue. The flaps are then transposed and stitched. The procedure has the effect of redistributing tension perpendicular to the original defect.

Zygote

The cell produced when a *sperm* fertilizes an *ovum*. A zygote contains all the genetic (hereditary) material for a new person—half coming from sperm and

half from the ovum. Measuring about 4 thousandths of an inch (0.1 mm) in diameter, a zygote is much larger than other body cells. It travels down one of the woman's fallopian tubes toward the uterus, dividing as it does so, but without growing larger. After about a week, the mass of cells (now called a blastocyst) implants into the lining of the uterus, and the next stage of embryological growth begins.

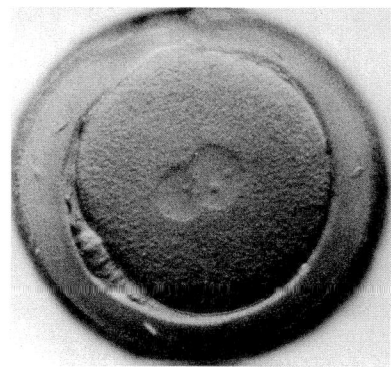

Appearance of zygote
The photograph shows a human egg just after fertilization by a sperm. The two circular areas at center are the nuclei of the sperm and egg merging.

Z

SELF-HELP ORGANIZATIONS, DRUG GLOSSARY, AND INDEX

SELF-HELP ORGANIZATIONS

The following list gives the names and telephone numbers of various organizations and support groups that exist to help people with particular health problems. Even if no specific support group is mentioned for your particular problem, it may be worth contacting one of the more broadly based groups for a referral.

Some numbers offer recorded information, others provide personalized counseling or referrals. In general, diagnoses and recommendations for treatment are not offered.

Portions of this information were derived from the *Healthfinder* booklet published by the US Department of Health and Human Services.

ABORTION AND BIRTH CONTROL

Planned Parenthood Hotline
(800) 223-3303
Provides referrals to local clinics that offer abortion, birth control, pregnancy testing, and obstetrical/gynecological services, and screening for sexually transmitted diseases.

ACQUIRED IMMUNODEFICIENCY SYNDROME (AIDS)

AIDS Information Hotline Public Health Service
(800) 342-AIDS
Provides information to the public on the prevention and spread of AIDS.

National Gay Task Force Crisisline
(800) 221-7044
(212) 529-1604 in NY, AK, and HI
Offers basic information on AIDS, including symptoms, possible causes, and preventive measures. Provides referrals.

ALCOHOLISM

Al-Anon Family Group Headquarters
(800) 356-9996
(212) 245-3151 in NY and Canada
Provides printed materials on alcoholism specifically aimed at helping families.

Alcoholism and Drug Addiction Treatment Center
(000) 302-4357
Refers adolescents and adults to local facilities for help.

National Council on Alcoholism
(800) NCA-CALL
Refers to local affiliates and provides written information on alcoholism.

ALZHEIMER'S DISEASE

Alzheimer's Disease and Related Disorders Association
(800) 621-0379
(800) 572-6037 in IL
Offers information on publications available from the association. Refers callers to local chapters and support groups.

CANCER

AMC Cancer Information
(800) 525-3777
Provides information on causes of cancer, prevention, methods of detection and diagnosis, treatment and treatment facilities, rehabilitation, and counseling services. A service of AMC Cancer Research Center, Denver.

Cancer Information Service (CIS)
(800) 4-CANCER
(808) 524-1234 in Oahu (neighbor islands call collect)
(800) 638-6070 in AK
Answers cancer-related questions from the public, cancer patients and families, and health professionals. No diagnosis made or treatment recommended. Spanish-speaking staff available to callers from the following areas: CA, FL, GA, IL, northern NJ, New York City, and TX. A service of the National Cancer Institute.

CHILD ABUSE

National Child Abuse Hotline
(800) 422-4453
Provides information and professional counseling on child abuse. Gives referrals to local social service groups offering counseling on child abuse.

Parents Anonymous Hotline
(800) 421-0353
(800) 352-0386 in CA
Provides information on self-help groups for parents involved in child abuse.

CHILDREN

National Child Safety Council Childwatch
(800) 222-1464
Answers questions from callers and distributes literature on safety, including drug abuse, household dangers, and electricity. Provides safety information to local police departments.

National Hotline for Missing Children
(800) 843-5678
(202) 644-9836 in DC
Operates a hotline for reporting missing children and sightings of missing children. Offers assistance to law enforcement agents. A service of the National Center for Missing and Exploited Children.

National Runaway Switchboard
(800) 621-4000
Provides counseling and traveler's assistance to runaways. Gives referrals to shelters nationwide. Also relays messages to, or sets up conference calls with, parents at the request of the child.

COOLEY'S ANEMIA

Cooley's Anemia Foundation
(800) 221-3571
(212) 598-0911 in New York City
Provides information on patient care, research, fund-raising, patient-support groups, and research grants. Makes referrals to local chapters.

CYSTIC FIBROSIS

Cystic Fibrosis Foundation
(800) 344-4823
(301) 951-4422 in MD

Responds to patient and family questions and offers literature. Provides referrals to local clinics.

DIABETES

American Diabetes Association
(800) 232-3472
(703) 549-1500 in VA and DC metro area

Provides free literature, newsletter, and information on health education and support group assistance.

Juvenile Diabetes Foundation International Hotline
(800) 223-1138
(212) 889-7575 in NY

Answers questions and provides brochures on juvenile diabetes. Gives referrals to physicians and clinics.

DOWN'S SYNDROME

National Down Syndrome Congress
(800) 232-6372
(309) 452-3264 in IL

Answers questions from parents for assistance with health concerns. Refers to local organizations.

National Down Syndrome Society Hotline
(800) 221-4602
(212) 460-9330 in NY

Offers information on Down's syndrome and gives referrals to local programs for the newborn. Provides free information packet upon request.

DRUG ABUSE

"Just Say No" Kids Club
(800) 258-2766

Responds to questions on how to start a club for 7 to 14 year olds.

National Cocaine Hotline
(800) COCAINE

Answers questions on the health risks of cocaine and provides counseling to cocaine users and their friends and families. Provides referrals. A service of Fair Oaks Hospital, Summit, NJ.

National Federation of Parents for Drug-Free Youth
(800) 554-KIDS
(301) 585-5437 in MD

Provides referrals to parent-support groups for parents of children with drug and alcohol problems. Sends educational materials.

National Parents' Resource Institute for Drug Education (PRIDE)
(800) 241-7946
(404) 658-2548 in GA

Provides a broad range of materials on drug-related issues, including alcohol and legal questions. Refers callers to related organizations for further information.

NIDA Helpline
(800) 662-HELP

Provides general information on drug abuse and on AIDS as it relates to intravenous drug users. Referrals offered. A service of the National Institute on Drug Abuse.

Office of Substance Abuse Prevention
(800) 638-2045
(301) 443-6500 in MD

Offers information and technical assistance to schools, parent groups, business and industry, and national organizations in developing drug abuse prevention activities. Does not provide crisis counseling, intervention treatment referral, or information on the pharmacology or criminal aspects of drugs.

EATING DISORDERS

Anorexia Bulimia Treatment and Education Center
(800) 33-ABTEC
(301) 332-9800 in MD

Answers questions and provides literature on the disorders. A service of Mercy Hospital, Baltimore.

Bulimia Anorexia Self-Help
(800) 227-4785
(800) 762-3334 for 24-hour crisis information

Provides information on bulimia, anorexia, depression, anxiety, and phobias. Refers to local resources.

FITNESS

Aerobics and Fitness Foundation
(800) BE FIT 86

Answers questions from the public regarding safe and effective exercise programs and practices.

GENERAL HEALTH

American Medical Radio News
(800) 621-8094

Offers prerecorded messages that highlight daily health news and feature stories. A service of the American Medical Association.

ODPHP National Health Information Center
(800) 336-4797
(202) 429-9091 in DC

Provides a central source of information for health educators, health professionals, and the general public. No diagnosis made or treatment recommended. Spanish-speaking staff available. A service of the Office of Disease Prevention and Health Promotion, US Department of Health and Human Services.

HANDICAPS
(See also HEARING AND SPEECH and VISION)

HEATH Resource Center
(800) 544-3284
(202) 939-9320 in DC

Provides information on secondary education for the handicapped and on learning disabilities.

Job Accommodation Network
(800) 526-7234
(800) 526-4698 in WV

Offers ideas for accommodating handicapped persons in the workplace and information on obtaining aids and procedures.

Library of Congress National Library Services for the Blind and Physically Handicapped
(800) 424-8567
(202) 287-5100 in DC

Provides both audio and Braille formats for the blind and physically handicapped, or anyone who is unable to read print for any reason, through a network of state libraries.

National Information System for Health Related Services (NIS)

(800) 922-9234
(800) 922-1107 in SC

Makes referrals to specialized services that emphasize diagnosis, treatment, and support for developmentally disabled and chronically ill children.

National Rehabilitation Center

(800) 34-NARIC
(202) 635-5822 in DC

Provides rehabilitation information on assistive devices and disseminates other rehabilitation-related information.

HEADACHE

National Headache Foundation

(800) 843-2256
(800) 523-8858 in IL

Offers membership information and sends literature on headaches and their treatment.

HEARING AND SPEECH

American Cleft Palate Association

(800) 24-CLEFT
(800) 23-CLEFT in PA

Offers basic information to parents and health professionals on cleft palate syndrome. Makes referrals to local support groups and sends information, including lists of plastic surgeons, dentists, and speech pathologists for patients' review. The association does not refer individuals to specific physicians.

Dial a Hearing Test

(800) 222-EARS
(800) 345-EARS in PA

Answers questions on hearing problems and makes referrals to local numbers for a two-minute hearing test, as well as referrals to ear, nose, and throat specialists. Also makes referrals to organizations that have information on ear-related problems, including questions on broken hearing aids.

Grapevine

(800) 352-8888
(800) 346-8888 in CA

Offers information on deafness, including answers for raising and educating a deaf child. Refers callers to parents, professionals, and other resources in their own communities nationwide.

Hearing Helpline

(800) 424-8576
(703) 642-0580 in VA

Provides information on better hearing and preventing deafness. Materials are mailed to callers on request. A service of the Better Hearing Institute.

National Association for Hearing and Speech Action Line

(800) 638-8255
(301) 897-0039 in HI, AK, and MD call collect

Offers information and distributes materials on pathologists and audiologists certified by the American Speech-Language-Hearing Association for hearing and speech problems and hearing aids.

National Hearing Aid Helpline

(800) 521-5247
(313) 478-2610 in MI

Provides information and distributes a directory of hearing aid specialists certified by the National Hearing Aid Society.

HEART DISEASE

Heartlife

(800) 241-6993
(404) 523-0826 in GA

Answers questions on heart diseases and pacemakers and distributes a quarterly periodical entitled *Pulse*.

HOSPITAL CARE

Hill-Burton Hospital Free Care

(800) 638-0742
(800) 492-0359 in MD

Provides a recording on hospitals and other health facilities participating in the Hill-Burton Hospital Free Care Program. A service of the Bureau of Resources Development, US Department of Health and Human Services.

Shriners Hospital Referral Line

(800) 237-5055
(800) 282-9161 in FL

Gives information on free hospital care available to children under 18 who need orthopedic care or burn treatment. Sends application forms to those who meet eligibility requirements for treatment provided by 22 Shriners Hospitals in the US, Mexico, and Canada.

HOSPICE CARE

Hospice Education Institute Hospicelink

(800) 331-1620
(203) 767-1620 in CT

Offers general information about hospice care and makes referrals to local programs. Does not offer medical advice or counseling.

HUNTINGTON'S CHOREA

Huntington's Disease Society of America

(800) 345-4372
(212) 242-1968 in NY

Gives information on the disease and provides referrals to physicians and support groups. Answers questions on presymptomatic testing.

IMPOTENCE

Recovery of Male Potency

(800) 835-7667
(313) 966-3219 in MI

Provides referrals to self-help support groups and other agencies. Distributes an information packet. A service of Grace Hospital, Detroit, and affiliated with 23 hospitals nationwide.

KIDNEY DISEASES

American Kidney Fund

(800) 638-8299
(800) 492-8361 in MD

Grants financial assistance to kidney patients who are unable to pay treatment-related costs. Also provides information on the donation of organs and on kidney-related diseases.

LEARNING DISORDERS
(See also HANDICAPS)

The Orton Dyslexia Society

(800) ABCD-123

Answers questions about dyslexia and about how to become a

member of this society and makes referrals to other members of the society. Written materials are also available.

LEPROSY (HANSEN'S DISEASE)

American Leprosy Missions
(800) 543-3131
(201) 794-8650 in NJ

Answers questions and distributes materials on the disease.

LIVER DISEASES

American Liver Foundation
(800) 223-0179
(201) 857-2626 in NJ

Provides callers with information, including fact sheets. The foundation also makes physician referrals.

LUNG DISEASE

Lung Line
National Asthma Center
(800) 222-5864
(303) 355-LUNG in Denver

Answers questions about asthma, emphysema, chronic bronchitis, allergies, juvenile rheumatoid arthritis, smoking, and other respiratory and immune system disorders. Callers' questions are answered by registered nurses or other health professionals. A service of the National Jewish Center for Immunology and Respiratory Medicine.

LUPUS

Lupus Foundation of America
(800) 558-0121
(202) 328-4550 in DC

Answers basic questions about the disease and provides health professionals and patients and their families with information and literature. Refers callers to local affiliates.

MENTAL HEALTH

American Mental Health Fund
(800) 433-5959
(800) 826-2336 in IL

Makes available via recorded message the AMHF pamphlet that includes general information about the organization, mental health, and warning signs of mental illness.

National Alliance for the Mentally Ill
(703) 524-7600

Self-help advocacy organization for families of people with mental illness. Refers callers to its more than 600 state and local affiliates.

NEUROFIBROMATOSIS

National Neurofibromatosis Foundation
(800) 323-7938
(212) 460-8980 in NY

Responds to inquiries from health professionals and from patients and their families. Makes referrals to physicians on the clinical advisory board.

ORGANS
(See also KIDNEY DISEASES and RETINITIS PIGMENTOSA)

The Living Bank
(800) 528-2971
(713) 528-2971 in TX

Operates a registry and referral service for people wanting to commit their tissues, bones, or vital organs to transplantation or research. Offers information to the public about organ donation and transplantation.

Organ Donor Hotline
(800) 24-DONOR
(800) 552-2138 in VA

Offers information and referrals for organ donation and transplantation. Answers callers' requests for organ donor cards.

PARALYSIS AND SPINAL CORD INJURY
(See also HANDICAPS)

American Paralysis Association
(800) 225-0292
(201) 379-2690 in NJ

Answers questions about research on head and spinal injuries. Raises money to fund research to find a cure for paralysis caused by spinal and head injuries or stroke.

National Spinal Cord Injury Association
(800) 962-9629
(617) 964-0521 in MA

Provides peer counseling to those suffering from spinal cord injuries and makes referrals to local chapters and other organizations. Produces the *National Resource Directory*, which deals with topics that are helpful to people who have handicaps.

Spinal Cord Injury Hotline
(800) 526-3456
(800) 638-1733 in MD

Offers literature on spinal cord injuries, including a quarterly newsletter, and makes referrals to a variety of organizations and support groups. This hotline is a service of the Maryland Institute for Emergency Medical Services Systems.

PARKINSON'S DISEASE

National Parkinson Foundation
(800) 327-4545
(800) 433-7022 in FL
(305) 547-6666 in Miami

Questions about the disease answered by nurses. Also makes physician referrals and provides written materials.

Parkinson's Education Program
(800) 344-7872
(714) 640-0218 in CA

Provides materials such as newsletters, glossary of definitions, and publications catalog, and offers patient-support group information and physician referrals.

PESTICIDES

National Pesticide Telecommunications Network
(800) 858-7378
(806) 743-3091 in TX

Responds to nonemergency questions concerning the effects of pesticides, toxicology and symptoms, environmental effects, waste disposal and cleanup, and safe use of pesticides. The National Pesticide Telecommunications Network is a service of the Environmental Protection Agency and Texas Tech University.

PLASTIC SURGERY

American Society of Plastic and Reconstructive Surgeons
(800) 635-0635

Provides referrals to board-certified plastic surgeons nationwide and from Canada. Offers pamphlets describing plastic and reconstructive procedures and realistic results of some operations.

PREGNANCY

ASPO/Lamaze (American Society for Psychoprophylaxis in Obstetrics)
(800) 368-4404
(703) 524-7802 in VA

Provides list of local certified childbirth educators for people who are interested in this type of birth method. The Virginia number gives information on local Lamaze classes and on becoming a certified Lamaze educator.

Bethany Lifeline
(800) 238-4269

Provides callers with referrals to professional counseling services, adoption services, shepherding home care, and limited group home placement.

The Edna Gladney Home
(800) 433-2922
(800) 772-2740 in TX
(817) 926-3304 (call collect for 24-hour service)

Provides a residential program for unwed, pregnant women in addition to counseling, schooling, and adoption services.

National Pregnancy Hotline
(800) 852-5683
(800) 831-5881 in CA
(213) 380-8750 in Los Angeles

Provides pregnant women with a full range of information, counseling services, and referrals.

Pregnancy Crisis Center
(800) 368-3336
(804) 847-6828 in VA only

Provides a residential program for unwed mothers as well as shepherding homes for those over 18. The center is run by Family Life Services and is also an adoption agency.

RARE DISEASES

National Information Center for Orphan Drugs and Rare Diseases
(800) 336-4797
(202) 429-9091 in DC

Gathers and disseminates information to patients, health professionals, and the public.

RETINITIS PIGMENTOSA

National Retinitis Pigmentosa Foundation
(800) 638-2300
(301) 225-9400 in MD

Covers genetics, current research, and retina donor programs. Responds to questions and makes available an information packet on the disease.

REYE'S SYNDROME

National Reye's Syndrome Foundation
(800) 233-7393
(800) 231-7393 in OH

Provides callers with general information and referrals to families for peer counseling.

SAFETY

Consumer Product Safety Commission
(800) 638-CPSC
(800) 638-8270
(800) 492-8104 in MD

Answers questions and provides material on consumer product safety, including product hazards and product defects and injuries sustained in using products. Covers only products used in and around the home, excluding automobiles, foods, drugs, cosmetics, boats, and firearms.

National Child Safety Council (See CHILDREN)

National Highway Traffic Safety Administration
(800) 424-9393
(202) 366-0123 in DC

Provides information and referral on the effectiveness of occupant protection, such as safety belt use

and child safety seats, and auto recalls. Staffed by experts who investigate consumer complaints and provide assistance to resolve problems. Gives referrals to other government agencies for consumer questions on warranties, service, and auto safety regulations.

National Safety Council
(800) 621-7619 for placing orders
(312) 527-4800 in IL

Provides posters, brochures, and booklets on safety and the prevention of accidents.

SICKLE CELL DISEASE

National Association for Sickle Cell Disease
(800) 421-8453
(213) 936-7205 in CA

Offers genetic counseling and an information packet.

SPINA BIFIDA

Spina Bifida Information and Referral
(800) 621-3141
(301) 770-7222 in MD

Provides information to consumers and health professionals and makes referrals to its local chapters. A service of the Spina Bifida Association of America.

SUDDEN INFANT DEATH SYNDROME

National SIDS Foundation
(800) 221-SIDS
(301) 459-3388 or 3389 in MD

Provides literature on medical information and referrals, as well as information on support groups.

SURGERY

National Second Surgical Opinion Program Hotline
(800) 638-6833
(800) 492-6603 in MD

Helps consumers locate a specialist near them for a second opinion in nonemergency surgery. A service of the Health Care Financing Administration, US Department of Health and Human Services.

TOXIC SUBSTANCES
(See also PESTICIDES)

Asbestos Hotline
(800) 334-8571

Answers questions and maintains a list of laboratories that test consumers' homes for asbestos. Also handles and maintains the US Environmental Protection Agency's bulk sampling analysis program.

TRAUMA

American Trauma Society (ATS)
(800) 556-7890
(301) 328-6304 in MD

Offers information to health professionals and the public on ATS activities. Answers questions about trauma and medical emergencies.

TUBEROUS SCLEROSIS

National Tuberous Sclerosis Association
(800) 225-6872
(312) 668-0787 in IL

Answers questions about the disease and makes parent-to-parent contact referrals. Literature is provided.

URINARY INCONTINENCE

Simon Foundation
(800) 23-SIMON

Provides a recorded message on incontinence and gives ordering information for a quarterly newsletter and other publications.

VENEREAL DISEASES

VD Hotline
(Operation Venus)
(800) 227-8922

Provides information on sexually transmitted diseases and confidential referrals for diagnosis and treatment. The hotline is a service of the American Social Health Association and the United Way.

VISION
(See also HANDICAPS)

American Council of the Blind
(800) 424-8666
(202) 393-3666 in DC

Offers information on blindness. Provides referrals to clinics, rehabilitation organizations, research centers, and local chapters. Also publishes resource lists.

American Foundation for the Blind (AFB)
(800) 232-5463
(212) 620-2147

Gives callers information on visual impairments and blindness and on AFB services, products, and publications.

National Eye Care Project Helpline
(800) 222-EYES

Offers information on free eye examinations. To qualify for this program, people must be financially disadvantaged, at least 65 years old, US citizens, and must not have seen an ophthalmologist in three years.

WOMEN

HERS Foundation
(215) 667-7757

Offers information to women who are considering having, or who have already had, a hysterectomy.

PMS Access
(800) 222-4767
(608) 833-4767 in WI

Provides information, literature, and counseling on premenstrual syndrome (PMS). Gives referrals to physicians and clinics in the caller's locale. A service of Madison Pharmacy Associates, Inc.

Women's Sports Foundation
(800) 227-3988
(212) 972-9170 in AK, HI, and New York City metro area

Provides information on women's sports, physical fitness, and sports medicine.

DRUG GLOSSARY

The drug glossary includes all the most important generic drugs, a broad range of brand-name drugs, and the various vitamins, minerals, and other substances that may be used as drugs. The generic names are the official names for drugs, as approved by the USAN (US Adopted Name) Council. The brand names for drugs are chosen by individual drug manufacturers.

If a generic drug has a separate entry within the encyclopedia, the page number of this entry is given directly after the drug's name. If a drug belongs to a group of drugs that has its own encyclopedia entry, this information is given in the glossary together with the relevant page number. If a generic drug belongs to a drug group that does not have an encyclopedia entry, the glossary tells you the dis-

order or disorders for which the drug you are looking up is most commonly used and gives appropriate page references.

In the case of brand-name drugs, glossary entries give the equivalent generic drug names and appropriate page references to entries within the main part of the encyclopedia. If a brand-name drug contains several generic drugs or if its ingredients do not have separate encyclopedia entries, the glossary will direct you to appropriate drug group or disorder entries.

This selection of drugs is designed to reflect the wide diversity of products available for the treatment or prevention of disease. Inclusion of any drug does not imply AMA endorsement, nor does exclusion indicate AMA disapproval.

A

Accubron a brand name for theophylline 977

Accutane a brand name for isotretinoin 608

Acebutolol 61, a generic beta-blocker drug 165

Acecainide a generic antiarrhythmic drug 114

Aceclidine a generic drug used to treat glaucoma 488

Acetaminophen 61, a generic analgesic drug 97

Acetazolamide 62, a generic diuretic drug 366, used to treat glaucoma 488

Acetic acid 62, an ingredient of antiseptics 119

Acetohexamide 62, a generic hypoglycemic drug 560

Acetophenazine a generic antipsychotic drug 119

Acetylcysteine 62, a generic mucolytic drug 700

Achromycin a brand-name tetracycline drug 976

Acrisorcin a generic antifungal drug 117

Acrivastine a generic antihistamine drug 118

ACTH 65, the abbreviation for adrenocorticotropic hormone

Acthar a brand name for corticotropin 313

Acticort a brand name for hydrocortisone 550

Actidil a brand-name antihistamine drug 118

Actifed a brand-name decongestant drug 336

Activase a brand name for tissue-plasminogen activator 989

Acyclovir 67, a generic antiviral drug 120

Adalat a brand name for nifedipine 727

Adapettes a brand-name artificial tear preparation 966

Adapin a brand name for doxepin 372

Adeflor a brand-name multivitamin 702 containing fluoride 460

Adipex-P a brand name for phentermine 790

Adriamycin a brand name for doxorubicin 372

Adrucil a brand name for fluorouracil 460

Adsorbocarpine a brand name for pilocarpine 795

Advil a brand name for ibuprofen 566

AeroBid a brand-name corticosteroid drug 312

Aerolate a brand name for theophylline 977

Aerolone a brand name for isoproterenol 608

Aeroseb-Dex a brand name for dexamethasone 348

Aerosporin a brand-name antibiotic drug 114

Afrin a brand name for oxymetazoline 761

Afrinol a brand name for pseudoephedrine 829

Agoral a brand-name laxative drug 630

Akarpine a brand name for pilocarpine 795

AK-Cide a brand-name drug containing prednisolone 813 and sulfacetamide 954

AK-Dilate a brand name for phenylephrine 791

Akne-Mycin a brand name for erythromycin 418

AK-Neo-Cort a brand-name drug containing hydrocortisone 550 and neomycin 717

AK-Pred a brand name for prednisolone 813

AK-Sulf a brand name for sulfacetamide 954

AK-Tate a brand name for prednisolone 813

AK-Tracin a brand name for bacitracin 150

AK-Trol a brand name for dexamethasone 348

AK-Zol a brand name for acetazolamide 62

Alatone a brand name for spironolactone 932

Albalon-A a brand-name decongestant drug 336

Albalon Liquifilm a brand name for naphazoline 714

Albuterol 81, a generic bronchodilator drug 215

Alcohol, rubbing 85, a type of antiseptic 119

Alconefrin a brand name for phenylephrine 791

Aldactazide a brand-name drug containing hydrochlorothiazide 550 and spironolactone 932

Aldactone a brand name for spironolactone 932

Aldoclor a brand-name drug containing chlorothiazide 271 and methyldopa 684

Aldomet a brand name for methyldopa 684

Aldoril a brand-name drug containing hydrochlorothiazide 550 and methyldopa 684

Alfacalcidol another name for vitamin D 1059

Algicon a brand-name antacid drug 113

Alka-Seltzer a brand-name analgesic drug 97 containing aspirin 137 and sodium bicarbonate 922

Alkeran a brand name for melphalan 674

Allbee C-800 a brand-name multivitamin 702

Allbee with C a brand-name multivitamin 702

Aller-Chlor a brand name for chlorpheniramine 271

Allerest a brand-name decongestant drug 336

Allerfrin a brand name for triprolidine 1011

Allergen Ear Drops a brand-name analgesic drug 97

Allersone a brand-name preparation containing hydrocortisone 550

Allopurinol 88, a generic drug used to treat gout 495

Alphaderm a brand name for hydrocortisone 550

AlphaRedisol a brand name for hydroxocobalamin 551

Alpha-tocopherol 89, a constituent of vitamin E 1059

Alphatrex a brand name for betamethasone 166

Alphosyl a brand name for coal tar 285

Alprazolam 89, a generic antianxiety drug 114

Alprostadil 89, a generic prostaglandin drug 824 used to treat congenital heart disease 518

Alseroxylon a generic antihypertensive drug 118

ALternaGEL a brand-name antacid drug 113

Alu-Cap a brand-name antacid drug 113

Aluminum acetate a generic astringent 139

Aluminum carbonate a generic antacid drug 113

Aluminum chloride a generic antiperspirant 118

Aluminum hydroxide a generic antacid drug 113

Alupent a brand name for metaproterenol 683

Alurate a brand-name barbiturate drug 157

Alu-Tab a brand-name antacid drug 113

Amantadine 92, a generic antiviral drug 120 now used to treat Parkinson's disease 772

Ambenonium a generic drug used to treat myasthenia gravis 708

Ambenyl a brand-name cough remedy 316

Amcill a brand name for ampicillin 96

Amcinonide a generic corticosteroid drug 312

Amdinocillin a generic penicillin drug 779, a type of antibiotic drug 114

Amen a brand name for medroxyprogesterone 671

Americaine a brand-name local anesthetic 106

Amikacin a generic antibiotic drug 114

Amikin a brand-name antibiotic drug 114

Amiloride 94, a generic potassium-sparing diuretic drug 366

Aminoglutethimide 94, a generic anticancer drug 115

Aminophylline 94, a generic bronchodilator drug 215

Aminosalicylate another name for aminosalicylic acid 94

Aminosalicylic acid 94, a generic drug used to treat tuberculosis 1013

Amiodarone a generic antiarrhythmic drug 114

Amitril a brand name for amitriptyline 94

Amitriptyline 94, a generic antidepressant drug 116

Amobarbital a generic barbiturate drug 157

Amoxapine 95, a generic antidepressant drug 116

Amoxicillin 95, a generic penicillin drug 779, a type of antibiotic drug 114

Amoxil a brand name for amoxicillin 95

Amphojel a brand-name antacid drug 113

Amphotericin B 96, a generic antifungal drug 117

Ampicillin 96, a generic penicillin drug 779, a type of antibiotic drug 114

Amrinone a generic drug used to treat heart failure 519

Amyl nitrite 96, a generic vasodilator drug 1041, formerly used in the treatment of angina pectoris 108, now considered a drug of abuse

Amytal a brand-name barbiturate drug 157

Anacin a brand-name analgesic drug 97 containing aspirin 137 and caffeine 222

Anacin-3 a brand name for acetaminophen 61

Anadrol a brand-name anabolic steroid drug 940

Anamine a brand-name decongestant drug 336

Anaprox a brand name for naproxen 714

Anaspaz a brand-name antispasmodic drug 120

Anatuss a brand-name cough remedy 316

Anavar a brand name for oxandrolone 761

Anbesol a brand-name local anesthetic 106

Ancef a brand-name cephalosporin 248, a type of antibiotic drug 114

Android a brand name for testosterone 974

Anectine a brand-name muscle-relaxant drug 706 used in general anesthesia 104

Anergan a brand name for promethazine 823

Anestacon a brand name for lidocaine 639

Anexsia-D a brand-name analgesic drug 97

Anhydron a brand-name diuretic drug 366

Anisindione a generic anticoagulant drug 116

Anisotropine a generic antispasmodic drug 120 used to treat irritable bowel syndrome 607

Anorex a brand-name appetite suppressant drug 128

Anspor a brand-name cephalosporin 248, a type of antibiotic drug 114

Antabuse a brand name for disulfiram 366

Anthra-Derm a brand name for anthralin 113

Anthralin 113, a generic antimitotic drug used to treat psoriasis 830

Antiminth a brand name for pyrantel 841

Antipyrine a generic analgesic drug 97 used in ear drops

Antispas a brand name for dicyclomine 357

Antivert a brand name for meclizine 669

Anturane a brand name for sulfinpyrazone 954

Anuject a brand-name local anesthetic 106

Anusol-HC a brand-name preparation used to relieve anal itching 608

Apap a brand name for acetaminophen 61

A.P.L. a brand-name gonadotropin drug 494

Apresazide a brand-name drug containing hydralazine 549 and hydrochlorothiazide 550

Apresoline a brand name for hydralazine 549

Apresoline with Esidrix a brand-name drug containing hydralazine 549 and hydrochlorothiazide 550

Aprobarbital a generic barbiturate drug 157

Aquamethyton a brand name for phytonadione 794

Aquasol A a brand name for vitamin A 1057

Aquatag a brand-name thiazide diuretic drug 366

Aquatar a brand-name for coal tar 285

Aquatensen a brand name for methyclothiazide 684

Arachis oil a generic preparation used to treat scaly skin 910

Aralen a brand name for chloroquine 270

Aristocort a brand name for triamcinolone 1008

Aristospan a brand name for triamcinolone 1008

Armour Thyroid a brand name for a thyroid hormone preparation 985

Arnica a generic herbal preparation used to treat bruising 217

Artane a brand name for trihexyphenidyl 1011

Arthropan a brand-name analgesic drug 97

A.S.A. a brand name for aspirin 137

Asbron G a brand-name bronchodilator drug 215

Ascorbic acid 136, another name for vitamin C 1059

Ascriptin a brand-name analgesic drug 97

Asendin a brand name for amoxapine 95

Asparaginase a generic anticancer drug 115

Aspergum a brand-name drug containing aspirin 137

Aspirin 137, a generic analgesic drug 97

Astemizole a generic antihistamine drug 118

Atabrine a brand name for quinacrine 842

Atarax a brand name for hydroxyzine 551

Atenolol 140, a generic beta-blocker drug 165

Ativan a brand name for lorazepam 649

Atracurium a generic muscle-relaxant drug 706 used in general anesthesia 104

Atromid-S a brand name for clofibrate 284

Atropine 143, a generic anticholinergic drug 115

A/T/S a brand name for erythromycin 418

Attenuvax a brand-name measles vaccine 668

Augmentin a brand-name antibiotic drug 114

Auralgan a brand-name analgesic drug 97 in ear-drop form

Auranofin 144, a generic antirheumatic drug 119

Aureomycin a brand-name antibiotic drug 114

Aurothioglucose a generic drug containing gold 494

Aventyl a brand name for nortriptyline 731

Axotal a brand-name analgesic drug 97

Aygestin a brand name for norethindrone 731

Azacitidine a brand-name anticancer drug 115

Azatadine 149, a generic antihistamine drug 118

Azidothymidine another name for zidovudine 1087

Azlocillin a generic penicillin drug 779, a type of antibiotic drug 114

Azmacort a brand name for triamcinolone 1008

Azo Gantanol a brand-name drug containing an analgesic drug 97 and an antibiotic drug 114, used to treat cystitis 328

Azo Gantrisin a brand-name drug containing an analgesic drug 97 and an antibiotic drug 114, used to treat cystitis 328

Azolid a brand name for phenylbutazone 790

Azo-Sulfisoxazole a brand-name drug containing an analgesic drug 97 and an antibiotic drug 114, used to treat cystitis 328

AZT 149, an abbreviation of the former name for zidovudine 1087

Azulfidine a brand name for sulfasalazine 954

Azulfidine EN-tabs a brand name for sulfasalazine 954

B

Bacampicillin 150, a generic penicillin drug 779, a type of antibiotic drug 114

Bacarate a brand-name appetite suppressant drug 128

Baciguent a brand name for bacitracin 150

Bacitracin 150, a generic antibacterial drug 114

Baclofen 153, a generic muscle-relaxant drug 706

Bactine a brand-name skin antiseptic 119 containing lidocaine 639

Bactocill a brand name for oxacillin 761

Bactrim DS a brand-name drug containing sulfamethoxazole 954 and trimethoprim 1011

Balmex ointment a brand-name preparation containing bismuth 174 and zinc oxide 1087

Balneol a cleansing lotion that relieves anal itching 608

Balnetar a brand name for coal tar 285

Bancap HC a brand-name analgesic drug 97

Banflex a brand name for orphenadrine 750

Banthine a brand-name antispasmodic drug 120

Baratol a brand-name antihypertensive drug 118

Barbidonna a brand-name antispasmodic drug 120

Barbita a brand name for phenobarbital 790

Basaljel a brand-name antacid drug 113

Beclomethasone 161, a generic corticosteroid drug 312

Beclovent a brand name for beclomethasone 161

Beconase a brand name for beclomethasone 161

Beepen-VK a brand-name penicillin drug 779, a type of antibiotic drug 114

Belap a brand-name antispasmodic drug 120

Belganyl a brand-name drug used to treat worm 1081 and protozoa infestations 827

Belladenal a brand-name antispasmodic drug 120

Belladonna 164, a generic anticholinergic drug 115

Bellafoline another name for belladonna 164

Bellergal-S a brand-name drug used to treat migraine 688

Beminal-500 a brand-name multivitamin 702

Benacen a brand name for probenecid 822

Benactyzine a generic antianxiety drug 114

Benadryl a brand name for diphenhydramine 361

Bendroflumethiazide 164, a generic diuretic drug 366

Bendylate a brand name for diphenhydramine 361

Benemid a brand name for probenecid 822

Ben Gay a brand-name analgesic drug 97

Benisone a brand name for betamethasone 166

Benoquin a brand-name drug used to treat vitiligo 1060

Benoxinate a generic local anesthetic 106

Benoxyl a brand name for benzoyl peroxide 164

Bentyl a brand name for dicyclomine 357

Benylin a brand-name cough remedy 316

Benzac W a brand name for benzoyl peroxide 164

Benzagel a brand name for benzoyl peroxide 164

Benzalkonium chloride a generic skin antiseptic 119

Benzamycin a brand-name drug containing benzoyl peroxide 164 and erythromycin 418

Benzathine penicillin G a generic penicillin drug 779, a type of antibiotic drug 114

Benzedrex a brand-name decongestant drug 336

Benznidazole a generic drug used to treat trypanosomiasis 1013

Benzocaine a generic local anesthetic 106

Benzoic acid a generic antifungal drug 117

Benzoin an aromatic resin added to inhalations 589

Benzonatate a generic cough remedy 316

Benzoyl peroxide 164, a generic skin antiseptic 119 used to treat acne 63

Benzphetamine a generic appetite suppressant drug 128

Benzquinamide a generic antiemetic drug 117

Benzthiazide a generic thiazide diuretic drug 366

Benztropine a generic drug used to treat Parkinson's disease 772

Benzyl alcohol a generic local anesthetic 106

Benzyl benzoate a generic drug used to treat scabies 881

Benzylpenicillin a generic penicillin drug 779, a type of antibiotic drug 114

Bephenium a generic antihelmintic drug 118

Berocca a brand-name multivitamin 702

Berubigen a brand name for vitamin B$_{12}$ 1058

Beta carotene another name for vitamin A 1057

Betadine a brand-name skin antiseptic 119

Betagan a brand-name beta-blocker drug 165 used to treat glaucoma 488

Betahistine a generic drug used to treat Meniere's disease 674

Betalin 12 a brand name for vitamin B$_{12}$ 1058

Betalin S a brand name for thiamine (vitamin B complex) 1058

Betamethasone 166, a generic corticosteroid drug 312

Betapen-VK a brand-name penicillin drug 779, a type of antibiotic drug 114

Betatrex a brand name for betamethasone 166

Beta-Val a brand name for betamethasone 166

Betaxolol a generic beta-blocker drug 165 used to treat glaucoma 488

Bethanechol a generic drug used to treat urine retention 1029

Betoptic a brand-name beta-blocker drug 165 used to treat glaucoma 488

Bevantolol a generic beta-blocker drug 165

Bezafibrate a generic lipid-lowering drug 642

Bichloracetic acid a generic drug used to treat warts 1069

Bicillin a brand-name penicillin drug 779, a type of antibiotic drug 114

Bicitra a brand-name antacid drug 113

BiCNU a brand-name anticancer drug 115

Biltricide a brand name for praziquantel 812

Biopar Forte a brand-name vitamin B$_{12}$ preparation 1058

Biotin part of the vitamin B complex 1058

Biozyme C a brand-name ointment used to treat skin ulcers 1018

Biperiden a generic drug used to treat Parkinson's disease 772

Biphetamine a brand-name amphetamine drug 95

Bisacodyl a generic stimulant laxative drug 630

Bithin a brand-name antihelmintic drug 118

Bithionol a generic antihelmintic drug 118

Bitolterol a generic bronchodilator drug 215

Blenoxane a brand-name anticancer drug 115

Bleomycin a generic anticancer drug 115

Bleph-10 a brand-name drug used for eye infections 431

Blephamide a brand-name drug used to treat eye infections 431

Blocadren a brand name for timolol 988

Bluboro a brand-name astringent 139

Bonine a brand name for meclizine 669

Bontril a brand-name appetite suppressant drug 128

Borofax a brand-name ointment used to relieve skin irritation 608

Brasivol a brand-name drug used in the treatment of acne 63

Breonesin a brand-name cough remedy 316

Brethaire a brand name for terbutaline 971

Brethine a brand name for terbutaline 971

Bretylium a brand-name antiarrhythmic drug 114

Bretylol a brand-name antiarrhythmic drug 114

Brevicon a brand-name oral contraceptive 747

Brevital a brand-name barbiturate drug 157 used to induce general anesthesia 104

Brexin a brand-name cough remedy 316

Bricanyl a brand name for terbutaline 971

Bromfed a brand-name cold remedy 287

Bromocriptine 213, a generic drug used to treat Parkinson's disease 772

Bromodiphenhydramine a generic antihistamine drug 118

Bromovinyldeoxyuridine a generic antiviral drug 120

Bromphen a brand-name antihistamine drug 118

Brompheniramine a generic antihistamine drug 118

Brondecon a brand-name cough remedy 316 containing a bronchodilator drug 215

Bronkaid Mist a brand name for epinephrine 414

Bronkodyl S-R a brand name for theophylline 977

Bronkolixir a brand-name cough remedy 316 containing a bronchodilator drug 215

Bronkometer a brand-name bronchodilator drug 215

Bronkosol a brand-name bronchodilator drug 215

Bronkotabs a brand-name cough remedy 316 containing a bronchodilator drug 215

Bucladin-S a brand-name antiemetic drug 117

Buclizine a brand-name antiemetic drug 117

Budesonide a generic investigational corticosteroid drug 312

Buff-A Comp a brand-name analgesic drug 97 containing aspirin 137

Bufferin a brand name for aspirin 137

Buf-Oxal 10 a brand name for benzoyl peroxide 164

Bumetanide a generic loop diuretic drug 366

Bumex a brand-name loop diuretic drug 366

Bupivacaine a generic local anesthetic 106

Buprenex a brand-name narcotic drug 715, a type of analgesic drug 97

Buprenorphine a generic narcotic drug 715, a type of analgesic drug 97

Busulfan a generic anticancer drug 115

Butabarbital a generic barbiturate drug 157, a type of sleeping drug 916

Butalbital a generic barbiturate drug 157, a type of sleeping drug 916

Butamben a generic drug used to relieve skin irritation 608

Butazolidin a brand name for phenylbutazone 790

Butesin Picrate a brand-name drug used to relieve skin irritation 608

Butibel a brand-name drug containing belladonna 164

Butisol a brand-name barbiturate drug 157, a type of sleeping drug 916

Butoconazole a generic antifungal drug 117

Butorphanol a generic narcotic drug 715, a type of analgesic drug 97

C

Cafergot a brand-name drug used to treat migraine 688

Caladryl a brand-name drug containing diphenhydramine 361 and calamine 223

Calan a brand-name calcium channel blocker drug 224

Calcet a brand-name drug containing calcium 223 and vitamin D 1059

Calcidrine a brand-name cough remedy 316

Calcifediol another name for vitamin D 1059

Calcimar a brand name for calcitonin 223

Calciparine a brand name for heparin 531, an anticoagulant drug 116

Calcitonin 223, a generic drug used to treat bone disorders 194

Calcitrel a brand-name antacid drug 113

Calcitriol another name for vitamin D 1059

Calcium carbonate a generic antacid drug 113

Calderol a brand name for vitamin D 1059

Caldesene a brand-name preparation used to treat diaper rash 354

Calel-D a brand-name preparation containing calcium 223 and vitamin D 1059

Calmol 4 brand-name rectal suppositories 955 used to relieve anal irritation 608

Caltrate 600 a brand-name antacid drug 113

Cama a brand name for aspirin 137

Camalox a brand-name antacid drug 113

Cambendazole a generic antihelmintic drug 118

Camphor a generic drug used to relieve skin irritation 608

Cannabis 230, a generic central nervous system depressant

Cantharidin a generic drug used to treat warts 1069

Cantharone a brand-name drug used to treat warts 1069

Cantil a brand-name antispasmodic drug 120 used to treat irritable bowel syndrome 607

Capreomycin a generic antibacterial drug 114 used to treat tuberculosis 1013

Captopril 231, a generic ACE inhibitor drug 61

Carafate a brand-name ulcer-healing drug 1018

Caramiphen a generic cough remedy 316

Carbachol 231, a generic drug used to treat glaucoma 488

Carbamazepine 231, a generic anticonvulsant drug 116

Carbamide peroxide a generic preparation used to soften earwax 387

Carbaryl a generic drug used to treat lice 638

Carbenicillin a generic penicillin drug 779, a type of antibiotic drug 114

Carbenoxolone a generic ulcer-healing drug 1018

Carbetapentane a generic cough remedy 316

Carbimide a generic drug used to treat alcohol dependence 81

Carbinoxamine a generic antihistamine drug 118

Carbocaine a brand-name local anesthetic 106

Carbocysteine a generic decongestant drug 336

Carboprost a generic prostaglandin drug 824

Carboxymethylcellulose a generic laxative drug 630

Cardec DM a brand-name cough remedy 316

Cardilate a brand-name drug used to treat angina pectoris 108

Cardioquin a brand name for quinidine 842, an antiarrhythmic drug 114

Cardizem a brand name for diltiazem 361, a calcium channel blocker drug 224

Cardovar a brand-name antihypertensive drug 118

Carisoprodol 238, a generic muscle-relaxant drug 706

Carmol a brand-name drug used to treat dry skin 910

Carmustine a generic anticancer drug 115

Carphenazine a generic antipsychotic drug 119

Casanthranol a generic stimulant laxative drug 630

Cascara a generic stimulant laxative drug 630

Castellani's Paint a brand-name antifungal drug 117

Castor oil 239, a generic stimulant laxative drug 630

Catapres a brand-name antihypertensive drug 118

Ceclor a brand-name cephalosporin 248, a type of antibiotic drug 114

Cefaclor 245, a generic cephalosporin 248, a type of antibiotic drug 114

Cefadroxil a generic cephalosporin 248, a type of antibiotic drug 114

Cefadyl a brand-name cephalosporin 248, a type of antibiotic drug 114

Cefamandole a generic cephalosporin 248, a type of antibiotic drug 114

Cefazolin a generic cephalosporin 248, a type of antibiotic drug 114

Cefizox a brand-name cephalosporin 248, a type of antibiotic drug 114

Cefobid a brand-name cephalosporin 248, a type of antibiotic drug 114

Cefol a brand-name multivitamin 702

Cefonicid a generic cephalosporin 248, a type of antibiotic drug 114

Cefoperazone a generic cephalosporin 248, a type of antibiotic drug 114

Ceforanide a generic cephalosporin 248, a type of antibiotic drug 114

Cefotaxime a generic cephalosporin 248, a type of antibiotic drug 114

Cefotetan a generic cephalosporin 248, a type of antibiotic drug 114

Cefoxitin a generic cephalosporin 248, a type of antibiotic drug 114

Ceftazidime a generic cephalosporin 248, a type of antibiotic drug 114

Ceftizoxime a generic cephalosporin 248, a type of antibiotic drug 114

Ceftriaxone a generic cephalosporin 248, a type of antibiotic drug 114

Cefuroxime a generic cephalosporin 248, a type of antibiotic drug 114

Celestone a brand name for betamethasone 166, a corticosteroid drug 312

Celontin a brand-name anticonvulsant drug 116

Cenocort a brand-name corticosteroid drug 312

Centrax a brand-name antianxiety drug 114

Centrum a brand-name multivitamin 702

Cephalothin a generic cephalosporin 248, a type of antibiotic drug 114

Cephapirin a generic cephalosporin 248, a type of antibiotic drug 114

Cephradine a generic cephalosporin 248, a type of antibiotic drug 114

Cephulac a brand-name laxative drug 630

Cerespan a brand-name vasodilator drug 1041

Cerose-DM Expectorant a brand-name cough remedy 316

Cesamet a brand-name antiemetic drug 117

Cetacaine a brand-name local anesthetic 106

Cetacort a brand-name corticosteroid drug 312

Cetamide a brand name for sulfacetamide 954, an antibacterial drug 114

Cetapred a brand-name drug containing prednisolone 813 and sulfacetamide 954

Cetrimide a type of antiseptic 119

Cevalin a brand name for vitamin C 1059

Chardonna-2 a brand-name drug containing belladonna 164

Chealamide a brand-name chelating agent 258

Chenix a brand name for chenodiol 258

Chenodiol 258, a generic drug used to treat gallstones 474

Cheracol a brand-name cough remedy 316

Chloral hydrate 270, a generic sleeping drug 916

Chlorambucil 270, a generic anticancer drug 115

Chloramphenicol 270, a generic antibiotic drug 114

Chloraseptic a brand-name drug used to treat sore mouth 697 or throat 789

Chlordiazepoxide 270, a generic antianxiety drug 114

Chlorhexidine a type of antiseptic 119

Chlormezanone a generic antianxiety drug 114

Chlorofon-F a brand-name muscle-relaxant drug 706

Chloroform 270, a generic general anesthetic 104

Chloroguanide a generic drug used to treat malaria 659

Chloromycetin a brand-name antibiotic drug 114

Chlorophenothane another name for DDT 333

Chloroprocaine a generic local anesthetic 106

Chloroptic a brand-name antibiotic drug 114

Chloroquine 270, a generic drug used to treat malaria 659

Chlorothiazide 271, a generic thiazide diuretic drug 366

Chlorotrianisene a generic anticancer drug 115

Chloroxylenol a type of antiseptic 119

Chlorphenesin a generic muscle-relaxant drug 706

Chlorpheniramine 271, a generic antihistamine drug 118

Chlorphentermine a generic appetite suppressant drug 128

Chlorpromazine 271, a generic antipsychotic drug 119

Chlorpropamide 271, a generic drug used to treat diabetes mellitus 349

Chlorprothixene a generic antipsychotic drug 119

Chlortetracycline a generic tetracycline drug 976, a type of antibiotic drug 114

Chlorthalidone 271, a generic thiazide diuretic drug 366

Chlor-Trimeton a brand name for chlorpheniramine 271

Chlorzoxazone 271, a generic muscle-relaxant drug 706

Cholecalciferol 272, another name for vitamin D 1059

Choledyl a brand-name bronchodilator drug 215

Cholestyramine 275, a generic lipid-lowering drug 642

Choline magnesium trisalicylate a generic drug used to treat arthritis 132

Choline salicylate a generic drug used to treat arthritis 132

Choloxin a brand-name lipid-lowering drug 642

Chromagen capsules a brand-name vitamin 1060 and mineral supplement 689

Chronulac a brand-name laxative drug 630

Chymopapain an enzyme for chemonucleolysis 258

Chymoral an enzyme used to reduce edema 390

Chymotrypsin an enzyme used in the treatment of cataracts 240

Ciclopirox a generic antifungal drug 117

Cimetidine 280, a generic ulcer-healing drug 1018

Cinnamates a generic sunscreen 955

Cinnarizine a generic antihistamine drug 118

Cinoxacin a generic antibacterial drug 114

Ciprofibrate a generic lipid-lowering drug 642

Cisplatin 283, a generic anticancer drug 115

Citracal a brand name for calcium 223

Citra Forte a brand-name cough remedy 316

Citrocarbonate a brand-name antacid drug 113

Claforan a brand-name cephalosporin 248, a type of antibiotic drug 114

Clemastine a generic antihistamine drug 118

Cleocin a brand name for clindamycin 284

Clerz a brand-name artificial tear preparation 966

Clidinium bromide a generic antispasmodic drug 120 used to treat irritable bowel syndrome 607

Clindamycin 284, a generic antibiotic drug 114

Clinoril a brand-name nonsteroidal anti-inflammatory drug 730

Clioquinol a generic antibacterial 114 and antifungal drug 117

Clobetasol a generic corticosteroid drug 312

Clocortolone a generic corticosteroid drug 312

Cloderm a brand-name corticosteroid drug 312

Clofazimine a generic drug used to treat leprosy 634

Clofibrate 284, a generic lipid-lowering drug 642

Clomid a brand-name drug used to treat infertility 586

Clomiphene 284, a generic drug used to treat infertility 586

Clomipramine a generic antidepressant drug 116

Clonidine 284, a generic antihypertensive drug 118

Clonopin a brand-name anticonvulsant drug 116

Clorazepate 284, a generic antianxiety drug 114

Clotrimazole 284, a generic antifungal drug 117

Cloxacillin 285, a generic penicillin drug 779, a type of antibiotic drug 114

Cloxapen a brand-name penicillin drug 779, a type of antibiotic drug 114

Clozapine a generic antipsychotic drug 119

Clusivol a brand-name multivitamin 702

Clysodrast a brand-name laxative drug 630

Coactin a brand-name penicillin drug 779, a type of antibiotic drug 114

Coal tar 285, a generic ingredient in preparations for skin disorders 910

Cobalt edetate a generic drug used to treat cyanide poisoning 326

Cocaine 285, a generic central nervous system stimulant 942

Codeine 286, a generic narcotic drug 715, a type of analgesic drug 97

Codiclear a brand-name cough remedy 316

Codimal a brand-name cough remedy 316

Cod liver oil 286, a dietary supplement containing vitamin A 1057 and vitamin D 1059

Cogentin a brand-name drug used to treat Parkinson's disease 772

Co-Gesic a brand-name analgesic drug 97

Colace a brand-name laxative drug 630

ColBENEMID a brand-name drug containing probenecid 822 and colchicine 287

Colchicine 287, a generic drug used to treat gout 495

Colestid a brand-name lipid-lowering drug 642

Colestipol a generic lipid-lowering drug 642

Colistin 289, a generic polymyxin 808, a type of antibiotic drug 114

Collyrium a brand-name preparation used to relieve eye irritation 431

Cologel a brand name for methylcellulose 684

Colrex a brand-name cold remedy 287 containing acetaminophen 61

Coly-Mycin a brand name for colistin 289

Colyte a brand-name laxative drug 630

Combid a brand-name drug containing prochlorperazine 822 and an antispasmodic drug 120

Combipres a brand-name antihypertensive drug 118

Comhist LA a brand-name cold remedy 287

Compal a brand-name analgesic drug 97

Compazine a brand name for prochlorperazine 822

Compete a brand-name multivitamin 702 containing iron 606 and zinc 1087

Compound W a brand-name preparation used to treat warts 1069

Comtrex a brand-name cold remedy 287 containing acetaminophen 61

Conar A a brand-name cough remedy 316

Conex DA a brand-name cold remedy 287

Congespirin a brand-name cough remedy 316

Congess a brand-name cough remedy 316

Constant-T a brand-name bronchodilator drug 215

Contac a brand-name cold remedy 287

Cophene PL a brand-name cold remedy 287

Cordran a brand-name corticosteroid drug 312

Corgard a brand-name beta-blocker drug 165

Coricidin a brand-name drug containing aspirin 137 and chlorpheniramine 271

Corilin a brand-name drug containing chlorpheniramine 271 and an analgesic drug 97 similar to aspirin 137

Cortaid a brand name for hydrocortisone 550

Cort-Dome a brand name for hydrocortisone 550

Cortef a brand name for hydrocortisone 550

Cortenema a brand name for hydrocortisone 550

Corticaine a brand-name preparation containing hydrocortisone 550 and a local anesthetic 106 used to treat anal discomfort

Corticotropin 313, another name for ACTH 65

Cortifoam a brand name for hydrocortisone 550

Cortinal a brand name for hydrocortisone 550

Cortisol 313, another name for hydrocortisone 550

Cortisone 313, a generic corticosteroid drug 312

Cortisporin Cream a brand-name preparation containing a corticosteroid drug 312 and an antibacterial drug 114

Cortone a brand name for cortisone 313

Cortrophin Zinc a brand name for corticotropin 313

Coryban-D a brand-name cough remedy 316

Coryztime a brand-name cold remedy 287

Cosyntropin a synthetic form of corticotropin 313

Cotazym a brand name for pancrelipase 767

Cotrim a brand-name drug containing sulfamethoxazole 954 and trimethoprim 1011

CoTylenol a brand-name cold remedy 287 containing acetaminophen 61

Coumadin a brand name for warfarin 1069

Cromolyn sodium 321, a generic drug used for the prevention of asthma 137

Crotamiton a generic drug used to treat scabies 881

Crysticillin a brand-name penicillin drug 779, a type of antibiotic drug 114

Crystodigin a brand name for digitoxin 361

Cuprimine a brand name for penicillamine 779

Curare 325, a generic muscle-relaxant drug 706

Curretab a brand name for medroxyprogesterone 671

Cyanocobalamin 326, another name for vitamin B_{12} 1058

Cyanoject a brand name for vitamin B_{12} 1058

Cyclacillin 326, a generic penicillin drug 779, a type of antibiotic drug 114

Cyclandelate a generic vasodilator drug 1041

Cyclapen-W a brand name for cyclacillin 326

Cyclizine a generic antiemetic drug 117

Cyclobenzaprine 326, a generic muscle-relaxant drug 706

Cyclocort a brand-name corticosteroid drug 312

Cyclomethycaine a generic local anesthetic 106

Cyclopar a brand-name tetracycline drug 976, a type of antibiotic drug 114

Cyclopentamine a brand-name decongestant drug 336

Cyclophosphamide 326, a generic anticancer drug 115

Cycloserine a generic antibiotic drug 114

Cyclospasmol a brand-name vasodilator drug 1041

Cyclosporine 326, a generic immunosuppressant drug 576

Cyclothiazide a generic thiazide diuretic drug 366

Cylert a brand name for pemoline 778

Cyproheptadine a generic appetite stimulant drug 128

Cyronine a brand-name synthetic thyroid hormone 985

Cystospaz a brand name for hyoscyamine 552

Cytadren a brand name for aminoglutethimide 94

Cytarabine a generic anticancer drug 115

Cytomel a brand-name synthetic thyroid hormone 985

Cytosar-U a brand-name anticancer drug 115

Cytosine Arabinoside a brand-name anticancer drug 115

Cytoxan a brand name for cyclophosphamide 326

D

Dacarbazine a generic anticancer drug 115

Dactinomycin a generic anticancer drug 115

Dalalone a brand name for dexamethasone 348

Dalicote a brand name for dexamethasone 348

Dalidyne a brand name for dexamethasone 348

Dallergy a brand-name drug used to treat nasal congestion 715

Dalmane a brand name for flurazepam 460

Damason-P a brand-name cough remedy 316

Danazol 332, a generic drug used to treat endometriosis 404

Danocrine a brand name for danazol 332

Danthron a generic stimulant laxative drug 630

Dantrium a brand name for dantrolene 333

Dantrolene 333, a generic muscle-relaxant drug 706

Daranide a brand-name drug used to treat glaucoma 488

Daraprim a brand name for pyrimethamine 841

Darbid a brand-name antispasmodic drug 120 used to treat irritable bowel syndrome 607

Daricon a brand-name antispasmodic drug 120 used for irritable bowel syndrome 607

Darvocet-N a brand-name drug containing acetaminophen 61 and propoxyphene 824

Darvon a brand name for propoxyphene 824

Darvon Compound 65 a brand-name analgesic drug 97 containing aspirin 137

Daunorubicin a generic anticancer drug 115

Dazamide a brand name for acetazolamide 62

DDAVP a brand-name drug used to treat diabetes insipidus 349

Debrox a brand-name preparation for softening earwax 387

Decaderm a brand name for dexamethasone 348

Decadron a brand name for dexamethasone 348

Deca-Durabolin a brand name for nandrolone 714

Decaject a brand name for dexamethasone 348

Decapryn a brand-name antihistamine 118 sleeping drug 916

Decaspray a brand name for dexamethasone 348

Decholin a brand-name laxative drug 630

Declomycin a brand-name antibiotic drug 114

Deconade a brand-name cold remedy 287

Deconamine SR a brand-name cold remedy 287

Deconsal a brand name for phenylephrine 791

Deferoxamine a generic drug used to treat iron poisoning 606

Dehydrocholic acid a generic laxative drug 630

Dehydroemetine a generic drug used for amebiasis 92

Deladumone a brand-name drug containing estradiol 421 and testosterone 974

Delfen a brand-name spermicide 927

Delsym a brand-name cough remedy 316

Delta-Cortef a brand name for prednisolone 813

Deltasone a brand name for prednisone 813

Demazin a brand-name cold remedy 287

Demecarium a generic drug used to treat glaucoma 488

Demeclocycline a generic tetracycline drug 976

Demerol a brand name for meperidine 680

Demi-Regroton a brand-name drug containing chlorthalidone 271 and reserpine 863

Demulen a brand-name oral contraceptive 747

Depakene a brand name for valproic acid 1037

Depakote a brand name for valproic acid 1037

Depen a brand name for penicillamine 779

Depo-Estradiol a brand name for estradiol 421

Depo-Medrol a brand name for methylprednisolone 684

Depo-Provera a brand name for medroxyprogesterone 671

Depo-Testadiol a brand-name drug containing estradiol 421 and testosterone 974

Deprenyl a generic drug used to treat Parkinson's disease 772

Deprol a brand-name antidepressant drug 116

Dermacort a brand name for hydrocortisone 550

Dermolate a brand name for hydrocortisone 550

Dermoplast a brand-name local anesthetic 106

Desipramine 347, a generic tricyclic antidepressant drug 116

Desonide a generic corticosteroid drug 312

Desoximetasone a generic corticosteroid drug 312

Desoxycorticosterone a generic corticosteroid drug 312

Desoxyn a brand name for a derivative of amphetamine 95

Desquam-X a brand name for benzoyl peroxide 164

Desyrel a brand name for trazodone 1008

Dexamethasone 348, a generic corticosteroid drug 312

Dexatrim a brand name for phenylpropanolamine 791

Dexbrompheniramine a generic antihistamine drug 118

Dexchlorpheniramine a generic antihistamine drug 118

Dexone a brand name for dexamethasone 348

Dextroamphetamine 348, a generic central nervous system stimulant 942

Dextromethorphan a generic cough remedy 316

Dextrothyroxine a generic lipid-lowering drug 642

Dey-Dose Atropine Sulfate a brand name for atropine 143

DHE-45 a brand-name drug used to treat migraine 688

DHS Zinc a brand-name antifungal agent 117 used to treat dandruff 332

DHT a brand name for vitamin D 1059

DiaBeta a brand name for glyburide 493

Diabinese a brand name for chlorpropamide 271

Diacetylmorphine 351, another name for heroin 535

Dia-Gesic a brand-name narcotic cough remedy 316

Dialose a brand-name laxative drug 630

Dialume a brand-name antacid drug 113

Diamidine a generic drug used to treat leishmaniasis 633

Diamox a brand name for acetazolamide 62

Diapid a brand name for lypressin 657

Diazepam 357, a generic benzodiazepine antianxiety drug 114

Diazoxide a generic antihypertensive drug 118

Dibenzyline a brand-name vasodilator 1041 antihypertensive drug 118

Dibucaine a generic local anesthetic 106

Dical-D a brand-name preparation containing calcium 223 and vitamin D 1059

Dichlorphenamide a generic drug used to treat glaucoma 488

Dicloxacillin a generic penicillin drug 779, a type of antibiotic drug 114

Dicumarol 357, a generic anticoagulant drug 116

Dicyclomine 357, a generic antispasmodic drug 120 used to treat irritable bowel syndrome 607

Dideoxycytidine 357, a generic anticancer drug 115 that is being investigated as a treatment for AIDS 76

Didronel a brand-name drug used to treat Paget's disease 762

Dienestrol 357, a generic estrogen drug 421

Diethylcarbamazine a generic antihelmintic drug 118

Diethylpropion a generic appetite suppressant drug 128

Diethylstilbestrol 359, an estrogen drug 421

Diflorasone a generic corticosteroid drug 312

Diflunisal 359, a nonsteroidal anti-inflammatory drug 730

Di-Gel a brand name for simethicone 906

Digitoxin 361, a generic digitalis drug 361

Digoxin 361, a generic digitalis drug 361

Dihydrocodeine a generic narcotic drug 715, a type of analgesic drug 97

Dihydroergotamine a generic drug used to treat migraine 688

Dihydrotachysterol another name for vitamin D 1059

Dihydroxyaluminum a generic antacid drug 113

Diiodohydroxyquin a generic drug used to treat amebiasis 92

Dilantin a brand name for phenytoin 791

Dilatrate-SR a brand name for isosorbide dinitrate 608

Dilaudid a brand-name narcotic drug 715, a type of analgesic drug 97

Dilor a brand-name xanthine bronchodilator drug 215

Diloxanide a generic drug used to treat amebiasis 92

Diltiazem 361, a generic calcium channel blocker drug 224

Dimacol a brand-name cough remedy 316

Dimenhydrinate 361, a generic antihistamine drug 118

Dimercaprol a generic drug used to treat lead poisoning 631

Dimercaptosuccinic acid a generic drug used to treat lead poisoning 631

Dimetane a brand-name antihistamine drug 118

Dimetapp a brand-name cold remedy 287

Dimethindene a generic antihistamine drug 118

Dimethisoquin a generic local anesthetic 106

Dimethyl sulfoxide a generic drug used to treat cystitis 328

Dimethyl tubocurarine a generic muscle-relaxant drug 706 used in general anesthesia 104

Dinoprost a generic prostaglandin drug 824 used to stimulate uterine contractions in childbirth 263

Dinoprostone a generic prostaglandin drug 824 used to stimulate uterine contractions in childbirth 263

Diphenatol a brand-name drug containing diphenoxylate 361 and atropine 143

Diphenhydramine 361, a generic antihistamine drug 118

Diphenidol a generic antiemetic drug 117

Diphenoxylate 361, a generic antidiarrheal drug 117

Diphenylpyraline a generic antihistamine drug 118

Dipivalyl epinephrine another name for dipivefrin, a generic drug used to treat glaucoma 488

Dipivefrin a generic drug used to treat glaucoma 488

Diprolene a brand name for betamethasone 166

Diprosone a brand name for betamethasone 166

Dipyridamole 362, a generic drug used to treat abnormal blood clotting 184

Disalcid a brand-name nonsteroidal anti-inflammatory drug 730

Disipal a brand name for orphenadrine 750

Disodium azodisalicyclic acid a generic investigational drug used to treat inflammatory bowel disease 588

Disophrol a brand-name cold remedy 287

Disopyramide 365, a generic antiarrhythmic drug 114

Disulfiram 366, a generic drug used to treat alcohol dependence 81

Ditropan a brand-name anticholinergic drug 115 used to treat urinary incontinence 579

Diucardin a brand-name thiazide diuretic drug 366

Diulo a brand name for metolazone 684

Diupres a brand-name drug containing chlorothiazide 271 and reserpine 863

Diuril a brand name for chlorothiazide 271, a thiazide diuretic drug 366

Diutensen-R a brand-name drug containing methyclothiazide 684 and reserpine 863

Dobutamine a generic drug used to treat heart failure 519

Docusate a generic laxative drug 630

Dolene a brand-name narcotic drug 715, a type of analgesic drug 97

Dolobid a brand name for diflunisal 359

Dolophine a brand name for methadone 683

Domperidone a generic antiemetic drug 117

Donatussin a brand-name cough remedy 316

Donnagel a brand-name antidiarrheal drug 117

Donnatal a brand-name drug used to treat irritable bowel syndrome 607

Donnazyme a brand-name drug used to treat indigestion 580

Dopamine a natural neurotransmitter 725 used to treat heart failure 519

Dopar a brand name for levodopa 638

Dopram a brand-name drug used to stimulate respiration

Dorcol a brand-name cough remedy 316

Doriden a brand-name sleeping drug 916

Dormalin a brand-name benzodiazepine 164 sleeping drug 916

Doryx a brand name for doxycycline 372

Doss a brand-name laxative drug 630

Dow-Isoniazid a brand name for isoniazid 608

Doxaphene a brand name for propoxyphene 824

Doxapram a generic drug used to stimulate respiration

Doxidan a brand-name stimulant laxative drug 630

Doxorubicin 372, a generic anticancer drug 115

Doxy-II a brand name for doxycycline 372

DOXY-CAPS a brand name for doxycycline 372

Doxycycline 372, a generic tetracycline drug 976, a type of antibiotic drug 114

Doxylamine a generic antihistamine drug 118 sleeping drug 916

Doxy-Lemmon a brand name for doxycycline 372

DOXY-TABS a brand name for doxycycline 372

Dramamine a brand name for dimenhydrinate 361

Drisdol a brand name for ergocalciferol 415

Dristan a brand name for oxymetazoline 761

Drithocreme a brand name for anthralin 113

Dritho-Scalp a brand-name cream containing anthralin 113 and salicylic acid 879

Drixoral a brand-name antihistamine drug 118

Dromostanolone a generic androgen drug 100

Dronabinol a generic antiemetic drug 117 derived from marijuana 664

Droperidol a generic antiemetic drug 117

Drysol a brand-name antiperspirant 118

Dulcolax a brand-name stimulant laxative drug 630

Duofilm a brand name for salicylic acid 879

Duolube a brand-name drug used to relieve dry eyes 615

Duo-Medihaler a brand-name aerosol containing isoproterenol 608 and phenylephrine 791

Duotrate a brand-name nitrate drug 728 used in the treatment of angina pectoris 108

Duphrene a brand-name cold remedy 287

Durabolin a brand name for nandrolone 714

Duracillin a brand-name penicillin drug 779, a type of antibiotic drug 114

Duramorph a brand name for morphine 694

Duraphyl a brand name for theophylline 977

Duraquin a brand name for quinidine 842

Duricef a brand-name cephalosporin 248, a type of antibiotic drug 114

Durrax a brand-name antihistamine drug 118

Duvoid a brand-name drug used to treat urine retention 1029

DV a brand-name estrogen drug 421

Dyazide a brand-name drug containing hydrochloro-thiazide 550 and triam-terene 1009

Dycill a brand-name penicillin drug 779, a type of antibiotic drug 114

Dyclonine a generic local anesthetic 106

Dymelor a brand name for acetohexamide 62

Dynapen a brand-name penicillin drug 779, a type of antibiotic drug 114

Dyphylline a generic xanthine bronchodilator drug 215

Dyrenium a brand name for triamterene 1009

E

Easprin a brand name for aspirin 137

Echothiophate a generic drug used to treat glaucoma 488

Econazole 388, a generic antifungal drug 117

Econochlor a brand name for chloramphenicol 270

Econopred a brand name for prednisolone 813

Ecotrin a brand name for aspirin 137

Edecrin a brand-name loop diuretic drug 366

Edetate calcium disodium a generic chelating agent 258 used to treat metal poisoning 805

Edetate disodium a generic chelating agent 258 used in the treatment of hypercalcemia 552

EDTA a generic chelating agent 258 used to treat hypercalcemia 552

E.E.S. a brand name for erythromycin 418

Effersyllium a brand name for psyllium 834

Eflornithine a generic investigational anticancer drug 115

Efodine a brand-name antiseptic 119

Efudex a brand name for fluorouracil 460

E-Ionate PA a brand name for estradiol 421

Elavil a brand name for amitriptyline 94

Eldopaque a brand-name preparation used to lighten the skin in disorders of pigmentation 794

Eldoquin a brand-name preparation used to lighten the skin in disorders of pigmentation 794

Elixicon a brand name for theophylline 977

Elixophyllin a brand name for theophylline 977

Embolex a brand name for heparin 531

Emcyt a brand-name anticancer drug 115

Emete-con a brand-name antiemetic drug 117

Emetine a generic drug used to treat amebiasis 92

Emko a brand-name spermicide 927

Empirin a brand-name drug containing aspirin 137 and codeine 286

E-Mycin a brand name for erythromycin 418

Enalapril 400, a generic ACE inhibitor drug 61

Enarax a brand-name drug containing hydroxyzine 551 used to treat irritable bowel syndrome 607

Encainide a generic antiarrhythmic drug 114

Encaprin a brand name for aspirin 137

Encare a brand-name spermicide 927

Endep a brand name for amitriptyline 94

Enduron a brand name for methyclothiazide 684

Enduronyl a brand-name antihypertensive drug 118

Enflurane a generic general anesthetic 104

Enovid a brand-name oral contraceptive 747

Entex a brand-name cough remedy 316

Entozyme a brand-name drug used to treat indigestion 580

Entuss a brand-name cough remedy 316

Enuclene a brand-name artificial tear preparation 966

Ephedrine 410, a generic bronchodilator 215 decongestant drug 336

Epifrin a brand name for epinephrine 414

E-Pilo a brand-name drug containing epinephrine 414 and pilocarpine 795

Epinal a brand-name epinephrinelike drug 414

EpiPen a brand name for epinephrine 414

Epitrate a brand name for epinephrine 414

Eppy/N a brand-name epinephrinelike drug 414

Equagesic a brand-name analgesic drug 97 containing aspirin 137

Equanil a brand name for meprobamate 680

Ergocalciferol 415, another name for vitamin D 1059

Ergomar a brand name for ergotamine 416

Ergonovine 416, a generic drug used to stop bleeding after childbirth 263

Ergostat a brand name for ergotamine 416

Ergotamine 416, a drug used to treat migraine 688

Ergotrate maleate a brand name for ergonovine 416

ERYC a brand name for erythromycin 418

ERYC 125 a brand name for erythromycin 418

Erycette a brand name for erythromycin 418

EryDerm a brand name for erythromycin 418

Erymax a brand name for erythromycin 418

Ery-Tab a brand name for erythromycin 418

Erythrityl tetranitrate a generic nitrate drug 728 used to treat angina pectoris 108

Erythrocin a brand name for erythromycin 418

Erythromycin 418, a generic antibiotic drug 114

Esgic a brand-name analgesic drug 97 containing acetaminophen 61

Esidrix a brand name for hydrochlorothiazide 550

Esimil a brand name for hydrochlorothiazide 550

Eskalith CR a brand name for lithium 643

Estar a brand name for coal tar 285

Estinyl a brand name for ethinyl estradiol 422

Estrace a brand name for estradiol 421

Estradiol 421, a generic estrogen drug 421 used to treat symptoms of the menopause 676

Estradurin a brand-name estrogen drug 421 used to treat prostate cancer 824

Estramustine a generic anticancer drug 115

Estratab a brand-name estrogen drug 421

Estratest a brand-name drug containing an estrogen drug 421 and an androgen drug 100

Estrone 422, a generic estrogen drug 421 used to treat symptoms of the menopause 676

Estropipate a generic estrogen drug 421

Estrovis a brand name for quinestrol 842

Ethacrynate sodium a generic loop diuretic drug 366

Ethacrynic acid a generic loop diuretic drug 366

Ethambutol 422, a generic drug used to treat tuberculosis 1013

Ethchlorvynol a generic sleeping drug 916

Ethinamate a generic sleeping drug 916

Ethinyl estradiol 422, a generic estrogen drug 421 used in oral contraceptives 747

Ethionamide a generic drug used to treat tuberculosis 1013 and leprosy 634

Ethopropazine a generic phenothiazine drug 790 used to treat Parkinson's disease 772

Ethosuximide 423, a generic anticonvulsant drug 116

Ethotoin a generic anticonvulsant drug 116

Ethrane a brand-name general anesthetic 104

Ethylestrenol a generic anabolic steroid drug 940

Ethynodiol a generic progesterone drug 823

Etidocaine a generic local anesthestic 106

Etidronate a generic drug used for Paget's disease 762

Etomidate a generic general anesthetic 104

Etoposide a generic anticancer drug 115

Etrafon a brand-name drug containing amitriptyline 94 and perphenazine 786

Etretinate a generic drug used to treat psoriasis 830

Eurax a brand-name drug used to treat scabies 881

Euthroid a brand-name synthetic thyroid hormone 985

Evac-Q-Kit a brand-name stimulant laxative drug 630

Excedrin a brand-name analgesic drug 97

Ex-Lax a brand-name stimulant laxative drug 630

Exsel a brand-name preparation used to treat dandruff 332 and tinea versicolor 989

Extend 12 a brand-name cough remedy 316

Extendryl a brand-name cold remedy 287

F

Famotidine 440, a generic ulcer-healing drug 1018

Fansidar a brand-name drug used to treat malaria 659

Fastin a brand name for phentermine 790

Fedahist a brand-name cold remedy 287

Fedrazil a brand-name decongestant drug 336

Feen-a-Mint a brand-name stimulant laxative drug 630

Feldene a brand name for piroxicam 796

Feminone a brand name for ethinyl estradiol 422

Femiron a brand-name preparation containing iron 606

Femstat a brand-name vaginal cream containing an antifungal agent 117

Fenfluramine a generic appetite suppressant drug 128

Fenofibrate a generic lipid-lowering drug 642

Fenoprofen 445, a nonsteroidal anti-inflammatory drug 730

Fentanyl a generic analgesic drug 97 used in general anesthesia 104

Feosol a brand name for ferrous sulfate 445

Feostat a brand-name preparation containing iron 606

F-E-P Creme a brand-name preparation containing a corticosteroid drug 312 and a local anesthetic 106

Ferancee a brand-name preparation containing vitamin C 1059 and iron 606

Fergon a brand-name preparation containing iron 606

Fer-In-Sol a brand name for ferrous sulfate 445

Fermalox a brand-name drug containing iron 606 and an antacid drug 113

Fero-Folic-500 a brand-name preparation containing iron 606

Fero-Grad-500 a brand-name preparation containing iron 606

Fero-Gradumet a brand name for ferrous sulfate 445

Ferralet Plus a brand-name preparation containing iron 606

Ferro-Sequels a brand-name preparation containing iron 606

Ferrous fumarate an iron salt 606

Ferrous gluconate an iron salt 606

Ferrous sulfate 445, an iron salt 606

Festal II a brand name for pancrelipase 767

Fiberall a brand name for psyllium 834

Fibrinolysin a generic drug used to treat skin ulcers 1018

Fiogesic a brand-name cold remedy 287 containing aspirin 137

Fiorinal a brand-name analgesic drug 97 containing aspirin 137

Flagyl a brand name for metronidazole 684

Flavoxate 458, a generic antispasmodic drug 120 used to treat symptoms of urinary tract infections 1025

Flecainide a generic antiarrhythmic drug 114

Fleet Bisacodyl a brand-name stimulant laxative drug 630

Fleet Relief a brand-name local anesthetic 106

Fletcher's Castoria for Children a brand name for senna 891

Flexeril a brand name for cyclobenzaprine 326

Flexoject a brand name for orphenadrine 750

Flintstones a brand-name multivitamin 702

Florinef a brand-name corticosteroid drug 312

Florone a brand-name corticosteroid drug 312

Floropryl a brand-name drug used to treat glaucoma 488

Florvite a brand-name vitamin supplement 1060

Floxuridine a generic anticancer drug 115

Flucytosine a generic antifungal drug 117

Fludarabine a generic anticancer drug 115

Fludrocortisone a generic corticosteroid drug 312

Fluidil a brand-name diuretic drug 366

Flunisolide a generic corticosteroid drug 312

Fluocinolone 459, a generic corticosteroid drug 312

Fluocinonide a generic corticosteroid drug 312

Fluonid a brand name for fluocinolone 459

Fluoritab a brand name for fluoride 460

Fluorometholone a generic corticosteroid drug 312

Fluoroplex a brand name for fluorouracil 460

Fluorouracil 460, a generic anticancer drug 115

Fluothane a brand name for halothane 505

Fluoxymesterone a generic anticancer drug 115

Fluphenazine 460, a generic antipsychotic drug 119

Flura a brand name for fluoride 460

Flurandrenolide a generic corticosteroid drug 312

Flurazepam 460, a generic benzodiazepine 164 sleeping drug 916

Flurbiprofen a generic nonsteroidal anti-inflammatory drug 730

Flurosyn a brand name for fluocinolone 459

FML a brand-name corticosteroid drug 312

Foille a brand-name topical antibacterial drug 114

Foldan a brand name for thiabendazole 978

Folex a brand name for methotrexate 683

Folic acid 460, a vitamin 1056

Folvite a brand name for folic acid 460

Formula 44 a brand-name cough remedy 316

Fortaz a brand-name cephalosporin 248, a type of antibiotic drug 114

Fostex a brand-name drug used to treat acne 63

Fototar a brand name for coal tar 285

FUDR a brand-name anticancer drug 115

Fulvicin U/F a brand name for griseofulvin 498

Fungizone a brand name for amphotericin 96

Furacin a brand-name antibacterial drug 114

Furadantin a brand name for nitrofurantoin 728

Furazolidone a generic drug used to treat giardiasis 486 and shigellosis 901

Furosemide 471, a generic loop diuretic drug 366

G

Gallamine a generic muscle-relaxant drug 706

Gamimune a brand name for immune serum globulin 570

Gamma benzene hexachloride another name for lindane 641

Gammacorten a brand name for dexamethasone 348

Gantanol a brand name for sulfamethoxazole 954

Gantrisin a brand name for sulfisoxazole 954

Garamycin a brand name for gentamicin 485

Gaviscon a brand-name antacid drug 113

Gelusil a brand name for simethicone 906

Gemfibrozil 478, a generic lipid-lowering drug 642

Gemnisyn a brand-name drug containing acetaminophen 61 and aspirin 137

Genoptic a brand name for gentamicin 485

Gentamicin 485, a generic aminoglycoside, a type of antibiotic drug 114

Geocillin a brand-name antibacterial drug 114

Geopen a brand-name penicillin drug 779, a type of antibiotic drug 114

Geravite a brand-name multivitamin 702

Gerimed a brand-name multivitamin 702 and mineral supplement 689

Geriplex a brand-name multivitamin 702 containing iron 606

Geritol a brand-name multivitamin 702 containing iron 606

Glaucon a brand name for epinephrine 414

Gliclazide a generic hypoglycemic drug 560

Glucamide a brand name for chlorpropamide 271

Glucotrol a brand name for glipizide 490

Glutaral a type of antiseptic 119

Glutethimide a generic sleeping drug 916

Glyburide 493, a generic hypoglycemic drug 560

Glycopyrrolate a generic drug used to treat irritable bowel syndrome 607

Glycotuss a brand-name cough remedy 316

Gold 494, a generic drug used to treat rheumatoid arthritis 870

Gold sodium thiomalate a generic antirheumatic drug 119 containing gold 494

Gramicidin 497, a generic antibiotic drug 114

Grisactin a brand name for griseofulvin 498

Griseofulvin 498, a generic antifungal drug 117

Gris-PEG a brand name for griseofulvin 498

Guaiacolsulfonate a generic cough remedy 316

Guaifed a brand-name cough remedy 316

Guaifenesin a generic cough remedy 316

Guanabenz a generic antihypertensive drug 118

Guanethidine 501, a generic antihypertensive drug 118

Gynecort a brand name for hydrocortisone 550

Gyne-Lotrimin a brand name for clotrimazole 284

Gynogen LA a brand name for estradiol 421

Gynol II a brand-name spermicide 927

H

Halazepam a generic benzodiazepine 164 antianxiety drug 114

Halcinonide a generic corticosteroid drug 312

Halcion a brand name for triazolam 1009

Haldol a brand name for haloperidol 505

Haley's MO a brand-name laxative drug 630

Halofenate a generic lipid-lowering drug 642

Halog a brand-name corticosteroid drug 312

Haloperidol 505, a generic antipsychotic drug 119

Haloprogin a generic antifungal drug 117

Halotestin a brand-name anticancer drug 115

Halotex a brand-name antifungal drug 117

Halothane 505, a generic general anesthetic 104

Haponal a brand-name drug used to treat irritable bowel syndrome 607

Harmonyl a brand-name antihypertensive drug 118

HCG an abbreviation for human chorionic gonadotropin 494

Helmex a brand name for pyrantel 841

Helmizin a brand name for piperazine 796

Hemocyte a brand-name preparation containing iron 606

Hetacillin a generic penicillin drug 779, a type of antibiotic drug 114

Hexachlorophene a type of antiseptic 119

Hexadrol a brand name for dexamethasone 348

Hexocyclium a generic antispasmodic drug 120 used to treat irritable bowel syndrome 607

Hexylcaine a generic local anesthetic 106

Hexylresorcinol a type of antiseptic 119

H-H-R a brand-name antihypertensive drug 118

Hibiclens a brand-name antiseptic 119

Hibistat a brand-name antiseptic 119

Hiprex a brand-name drug used to treat urinary tract infections 1025

Hispril a brand-name antihistamine drug 118

Histabid a brand-name cold remedy 287

Histadyl a brand-name cough remedy 316

Histagesic a brand-name cold remedy 287

Histalet a brand-name cold remedy 287

Histamic a brand-name cold remedy 287

Histaspan a brand name for chlorpheniramine 271

Histex a brand name for chlorpheniramine 271

Historal a brand-name cold remedy 287

Histor-D a brand-name cold remedy 287

Histosal a brand-name cold remedy 287

HMS Liquifilm a brand-name corticosteroid drug 312

Homatropine 544, a generic anticholinergic drug 115

Homicebrin a brand-name multivitamin 702

Humorsol a brand-name drug used to treat glaucoma 488

Humulin a brand name for insulin 594

Hurricaine a brand-name local anesthetic 106

Hyaluronidase an enzyme used topically to reduce bruising 217

Hycanthone a generic antihelmintic drug 118

Hycodan a brand-name cough remedy 316

Hycodaphen a brand-name cough remedy 316

Hycomine a brand-name cough remedy 316

Hycotuss a brand-name cough remedy 316

Hydeltrasol a brand name for prednisolone 813

Hydeltra-T.B.A. a brand name for prednisolone 813

Hydoril a brand name for hydrochlorothiazide 550

Hydralazine 549, a generic antihypertensive drug 118

Hydrea a brand-name anticancer drug 115

Hydrocet a brand-name analgesic drug 97

Hydrochlorothiazide 550, a generic thiazide diuretic drug 366

Hydrocil a brand name for psyllium 834

Hydrocodone a generic narcotic drug 715 used mainly in cough remedies 316

Hydrocort a brand name for hydrocortisone 550

Hydrocortisone 550, a generic corticosteroid drug 312

Hydrocortone a brand name for hydrocortisone 550

HydroDIURIL a brand name for hydrochlorothiazide 550

Hydroflumethiazide a generic thiazide diuretic drug 366

Hydrogen peroxide 550, a type of antiseptic 119

Hydromal a brand name for hydrochlorothiazide 550

Hydromorphone a generic narcotic drug 715, a type of analgesic drug 97

Hydromox a brand-name thiazide diuretic drug 366

Hydropres a brand-name drug containing hydrochlorothiazide 550 and reserpine 863

Hydroprin a brand-name drug containing hydrochlorothiazide 550 and reserpine 863

Hydroquinone a generic drug used to lighten the skin in disorders of pigmentation 794

Hydroserpine a brand-name drug containing hydrochlorothiazide 550 and reserpine 863

Hydrotensin-50 a brand-name drug containing hydrochlorothiazide 550 and reserpine 863

Hydroxocobalamin 551, a synthetic form of vitamin B 1057

Hydroxychloroquine a generic derivative of chloroquine 270

Hydroxyprogesterone 551, a generic progesterone drug 823

Hydroxyurea a generic anticancer drug 115

Hydroxyzine 551, a generic antihistamine drug 118

Hygroton a brand name for chlorthalidone 271

Hyoscyamine 552, a generic anticholinergic drug 115

Hyperetic a brand name for hydrochlorothiazide 550

Hyperstat a brand-name antihypertensive drug 118

Hytakerol a brand name for vitamin D 1059

Hytinic a brand name for iron 606

Hytone a brand name for hydrocortisone 550

I

Iberet a brand-name multivitamin 702 containing iron 606

Iberol a brand-name multivitamin 702 containing iron 606

Ibuprofen 566, a generic nonsteroidal anti-inflammatory drug 730

Idoxuridine 566, a generic antiviral drug 120

Iletin a brand name for insulin 594

Ilosone a brand name for erythromycin 418

Ilotycin a brand name for erythromycin 418

Ilozyme a brand name for pancrelipase 767

Imferon a brand name for iron 606

Imipenem/cilastatin a generic antibiotic drug 114

Imipramine 570, a generic antidepressant drug 116

Imodium a brand name for loperamide 649

Imuran a brand name for azathioprine 149

Inapsine a brand-name antiemetic drug 117

Incremin with Iron a brand-name multivitamin 702 containing iron 606

Indapamide a brand-name diuretic drug 366

Inderal a brand name for propranolol 824

Inderal LA a brand name for propranolol 824

Inderide a brand-name drug containing hydrochlorothiazide 550 and propranolol 824

Indocin a brand name for indomethacin 581

Indomethacin 581, a generic nonsteroidal anti-inflammatory drug 730

Indoramin a generic antihypertensive drug 118

Inflamase a brand name for prednisolone 813

INH a brand name for isoniazid 608

Innovar a brand-name drug containing an analgesic drug 97 and a tranquilizer drug 1003 used in general anesthesia 104

Inocor a brand-name drug used for heart failure 519

Inosiplex a generic investigational antiviral drug 120

Intal a brand name for cromolyn sodium 321

Interferon 598, a generic antiviral 120 and anticancer drug 115

Intron A a brand name for interferon 598

Intropin a natural neurotransmitter 725 used to treat heart failure 519 and shock 901

Iodine 605, an element

Iodo a brand-name antifungal 117 and antibacterial drug 114

Iodochlorhydroxyquin a brand-name antifungal 117 and antibacterial drug 114

Iodoquinol a generic drug used to treat amebiasis 92

Ionamin a brand name for phentermine 790

Ionax a type of antiseptic 119

Ionil a brand name for salicylic acid 879

Iopanoic acid a generic drug used to treat hyperthyroidism 557

Ipecac 606, a generic drug used to induce vomiting in the treatment of drug overdose and poisoning 379

Ipodate a generic drug used to treat hyperthyroidism 557

Ipratropium 606, a generic investigational anticholinergic drug 115 used as a bronchodilator drug 215

Ipsatol a brand-name cough remedy 316

Iromin-G a brand-name multivitamin 702 containing iron 606

Iron 606, an essential mineral

Ismelin a brand name for guanethidine 501

Iso-Bid a brand name for isosorbide dinitrate 608

Isocarboxazid 607, a generic antidepressant drug 116

Isoclor a brand-name drug containing chlorpheniramine 271 and pseudoephedrine 829

Isoetharine a generic bronchodilator drug 215

Isofluorophate a generic drug used to treat glaucoma 488

Isoflurane a generic general anesthetic 104

Isoniazid 608, a generic drug used to treat tuberculosis 1013

Isopropamide a generic antispasmodic drug 120 used to treat irritable bowel syndrome 607

Isoproterenol 608, a generic bronchodilator drug 215

Isoptin a brand name for verapamil 1046

Isopto Carbachol a brand name for carbachol 231

Isopto Carpine a brand name for pilocarpine 795

Isopto Cetamide a brand name for sulfacetamide 954

Isopto P-ES a brand-name drug used to treat glaucoma 488

Isordil a brand name for isosorbide dinitrate 608

Isordil Sublingual a brand name for isosorbide dinitrate 608

Isordil Tembids a brand name for isosorbide dinitrate 608

Isosorbide dinitrate 608, a generic vasodilator drug 1041

Isotretinoin 608, a generic drug derived from vitamin A 1057 used in the treatment of acne 63

Isoxsuprine 608, a generic vasodilator drug 1041

Isuprel a brand name for isoproterenol 608

J

Janimine a brand name for imipramine 570

Jenamicin a brand name for gentamicin 485

K

Kabikinase a brand name for streptokinase 945

Kahlenberg solution a brand-name preparation used to treat warts 1069

Kanamycin a generic antibiotic drug 114

Kantrex a generic antibiotic drug 114

Kaochlor a brand-name potassium supplement 812

Kaolin 614, a generic ingredient of some antidiarrheal drugs 117

Kaon a brand-name potassium supplement 812

Kaopectate a brand-name antidiarrheal drug 117

Karaya gum a generic bulk-forming laxative drug 630

Kasof a brand-name laxative drug 630

Kato a brand-name potassium supplement 812

Kay Ciel a brand-name potassium supplement 812

Keflex a brand name for cephalexin 247

Keflin a brand-name cephalosporin 248, a type of antibiotic drug 114

Kefzol a brand-name cephalosporin 248, a type of antibiotic drug 114

Kemadrin a brand name for procyclidine 822

Kenacort a brand-name corticosteroid drug 312

Kenalog a brand-name corticosteroid drug 312

Keralyt a brand name for salicylic acid 879

Ketamine a generic sedative drug 890 used as a general anesthetic 104

Ketoconazole 616, a generic antifungal drug 117

Ketoprofen 616, a generic nonsteroidal anti-inflammatory drug 730

Ketrax a brand-name antihelmintic drug 118

Kie Syrup a brand-name decongestant 336 cough remedy 316

Kinesed a brand-name antispasmodic drug 120 used in the treatment of irritable bowel syndrome 607

Klebcil a brand-name antibiotic drug 114

Kleer compound a brand-name cold remedy 287

Klonopin a brand-name anticonvulsant drug 116

K-Lor a brand-name potassium supplement 812

Klor-con a brand-name potassium supplement 812

Klorvess a brand-name potassium supplement 812

Klotrix a brand-name potassium supplement 812

K-Lyte a brand-name potassium supplement 812

Kolantyl a brand-name antacid drug 113

Kolyum a brand-name potassium supplement 812

Komed a brand-name preparation used to treat acne 63

Konakion a brand name for phytonadione 794

Kondremul Plain a brand name for mineral oil 689

Konsyl a brand name for psyllium 834

Koromex a brand-name spermicide 927

K-Phos a brand-name mineral supplement 689

Kronofed a brand-name drug containing chlorpheniramine 271 and pseudoephedrine 829

Kronohist a brand-name cold remedy 287

K-Tab a brand-name potassium supplement 812

Kudrox a brand-name antacid drug 113

KU Zyme a brand name for pancrelipase 767

Kwell a brand name for lindane 641

Kwildane a brand name for lindane 641

KY Jelly a brand-name vaginal lubricant 598

L

Labetalol 624, a generic beta-blocker drug 165

LaBID a brand name for theophylline 977

Lac-Hydrin a brand-name preparation used to treat dry scaly skin 910

Lacril a brand-name artificial tear preparation 966

Lacrisert a brand-name artificial tear preparation 966

Lactocal-F a brand-name multivitamin 702

Lactulose 625 a generic laxative drug 630

Lanacort a brand name for hydrocortisone 550

Laniazid a brand name for isoniazid 608

Lanolin 626, a generic preparation used in the treatment of dry skin

Lanorinal a brand-name analgesic drug 97 containing aspirin 137

Lanoxicaps a brand name for digoxin 361

Lanoxin a brand name for digoxin 361

Larobec a brand-name multivitamin 702

Larodopa a brand name for levodopa 638

Larotid a brand name for amoxicillin 95

Larylgan a brand-name analgesic throat spray 97

Lasan a brand name for anthralin 113

Lasix a brand name for furosemide 471

Laudanum 630, a solution of opium 745

Ledercillin VK a brand-name penicillin drug 779, a type of antibiotic drug 114

Lente a brand name for insulin 594

Leucovorin a generic form of folic acid 460

Leukeran a brand name for chlorambucil 270

Leuprolide a generic anticancer drug 115

Levamisole a generic antihelmintic drug 118

Levlen a brand-name oral contraceptive 747

Levobunolol a generic beta-blocker drug 165 used to treat glaucoma 488

Levodopa 638, a generic drug used to treat Parkinson's disease 772

Levo-Dromoran a brand-name narcotic drug 715, a type of analgesic drug 97

Levonorgestrel 638, a generic progesterone drug 823 used in oral contraceptives 747

Levophed a brand name for norepinephrine 730

Levorphanol a generic narcotic drug 715, a type of analgesic drug 97

Levothroid a brand name for levothyroxine 638

Levothyroxine 638, a generic thyroid hormone 985

Levsin a brand name for hyoscyamine 552

Levsinex a brand name for hyoscyamine 552

Librax a brand-name antispasmodic drug 120 used for irritable bowel syndrome 607

Libritabs a brand name for chlordiazepoxide 270

Librium a brand name for chlordiazepoxide 270

Lidex a brand-name corticosteroid drug 312

Lidocaine 639, a generic local anesthetic 106

Lidoflazine a generic drug for angina pectoris 108

Limbitrol a brand-name drug containing amitriptyline 94 and chlordiazepoxide 270

Lincocin a brand name for lincomycin 641

Lincomycin 641, a generic antibiotic drug 114

Lindane 641, a generic drug used to treat scabies 881 and lice 638

Lioresal a brand name for baclofen 153

Liothyronine a generic synthetic thyroid hormone 985

Liotrix a generic synthetic thyroid hormone 985

Lipo-Hepin a brand name for heparin 531

Lipotriad a brand-name multivitamin 702

Liquaemin a brand name for heparin 531

Liqui-Doss a brand-name laxative drug 630

Liquid Pred a brand name for prednisone 813

Liquifilm a brand-name artificial tear preparation 966

Liquiprin a brand name for acetaminophen 61

Lithane a brand name for lithium 643

Lithium 643, a generic drug used to treat manic-depressive illness 663

Lithobid a brand name for lithium 643

Lithonate a brand name for lithium 643

Lithotabs a brand name for lithium 643

Lomotil a brand-name drug containing diphenoxylate 361 and atropine 143

Lomustine a generic anticancer drug 115

Loniten a brand name for minoxidil 689

Lo/Ovral a brand-name oral contraceptive 747

Loperamide 649, a generic antidiarrheal drug 117

Lopid a brand name for gemfibrozil 478

Lopressor a brand name for metoprolol 684

Lopressor HCT a brand name for hydrochlorothiazide 550 and metoprolol 684

Loprox a brand-name antifungal drug 117

Lopurin a brand name for allopurinol 88

Lorazepam 649, a generic benzodiazepine 164 sleeping drug 916

Lorcainide a generic antiarrhythmic drug 114

Lorcet a brand-name analgesic drug 97

Lorelco a brand name for probucol 822

Loroxide-HC a brand name for benzoyl peroxide 164

Lotrimin a brand name for clotrimazole 284

Lotrisone a brand-name drug containing clotrimazole 284 and betamethasone 166

Lotusate a brand-name barbiturate 157 sleeping drug 916

Lovastatin 650, a generic lipid-lowering drug 642

Loxapine a generic antidepressant drug 116

Loxitane a brand-name antidepressant drug 116

Lozol a brand-name diuretic drug 366

Lubrin a brand-name vaginal lubricant 596

Ludiomil a brand name for maprotiline 664

Lufyllin a brand-name bronchodilator drug 215

Lugol's solution a brand-name preparation used to treat hyperthyroidism 557

Lupron a brand-name anticancer drug 115

Luride a brand-name fluoride supplement 460

Lypressin 657, a generic preparation of ADH 68

Lysergic acid another name for LSD 650

Lyteers a brand-name artificial tear preparation 966

M

Maalox a brand-name antacid drug 113

Macrodantin a brand name for nitrofurantoin 728

Mafenide a generic antibacterial drug 114

Magan a brand-name antirheumatic drug 119

Magnesium 658, a mineral 689

Magnesium citrate a generic laxative drug 630

Magnesium gluconate a generic magnesium supplement 658

Magnesium hydroxide a generic antacid drug 113

Magnesium oxide a generic laxative drug 630

Magnesium salicylate a generic antirheumatic drug 119

Magnesium sulfate a generic magnesium supplement 658

Magnesium trisilicate a generic antacid drug 113

Magsal a brand-name magnesium supplement 658 and antihistamine drug 118

Malathion a generic drug used to treat lice 638

Mandelamine a brand-name drug used to treat urinary tract infections 1025

Mandol a brand-name cephalosporin 248, a type of antibiotic drug 114

Mannitol 663, a generic osmotic diuretic drug 366

Mantadil a brand-name drug used to treat skin irritation 608

Maolate a brand-name muscle-relaxant drug 706

Maprotiline 664, a generic antidepressant drug 116

Marax a brand-name drug used to treat asthma 137

Marbaxin-750 a brand name for methocarbamol 683

Marcaine a brand-name epidural anesthetic 412

Marezine a brand-name antiemetic drug 117

Marflex a brand name for orphenadrine 750

Marijuana 664, a generic central nervous system depressant

Marplan a brand name for isocarboxazid 607

Materna a brand-name multivitamin 702

Maxibolin a brand-name anabolic steroid drug 940

Maxidex a brand name for dexamethasone 348

Maxiflor a brand-name corticosteroid drug 312

Maxitrol a brand name for dexamethasone 348

Maxzide a brand-name drug containing hydrochlorothiazide 550 and triamterene 1009

Mazanor a brand-name appetite suppressant drug 128

Mazindol a generic appetite suppressant drug 128

Measurin a brand name for aspirin 137

Mebaral a brand-name anticonvulsant drug 116

Mebendazole 669, a generic antihelmintic drug 118

Mecamylamine a rarely used generic antihypertensive drug 118

Mechlorethamine a generic anticancer drug 115

Meclan a brand-name drug used to treat acne 63

Meclizine 669, a generic antihistamine 118 and antiemetic drug 117

Meclocycline a generic drug used to treat acne 63

Meclofenamate 669, a nonsteroidal anti-inflammatory drug 730

Meclomen a brand name for meclofenamate 669

Medicone a brand-name drug used to treat skin irritation 608

Medigesic a brand-name analgesic drug 97

Medihaler-Epi a brand name for epinephrine 414

Medihaler-Ergotamine a brand name for ergotamine 416

Medihaler-Iso a brand name for isoproterenol 608

Mediplast a brand name for salicylic acid 879

Mediquell a brand-name cough remedy 316

Medrol a brand name for methylprednisolone 684

Medrol Enpak a brand name for methylprednisolone 684

Medrol Oral a brand name for methylprednisolone 684

Medroxyprogesterone 671, a generic progesterone drug 823

Medrysone a generic corticosteroid drug 312 used to treat eye inflammation

Mefenamic acid 671, a generic nonsteroidal anti-inflammatory drug 730

Mefoxin a brand-name antibiotic drug 114

Megace a brand name for megestrol 672

Megestrol 672, a generic progesterone drug 823

Melanex a brand-name preparation used to treat pigmentation disorders 794

Melarsoprol a generic drug used to treat worm infestation 1081 and protozoa infestation 827

Melfiat a brand-name appetite suppressant drug 128

Mellaril a brand name for thioridazine 978

Melphalan 674, a generic anticancer drug 115

Menadiol another name for vitamin K 1060

Menadione another name for vitamin K 1060

Menest a brand-name estrogen drug 421

Menogaril a generic anticancer drug 115

Menotropins 677, a generic drug used to treat infertility 586

Menthol an extract from mint used in inhalations 589 and for skin irritation 608

Mepenzolate a generic antispasmodic drug 120 used to treat irritable bowel syndrome 607

Mepergan a brand-name drug containing meperidine 680 and promethazine 823

Meperidine 680, a generic narcotic drug 715, a type of analgesic drug 97

Mephenytoin a generic anticonvulsant drug 116

Mephobarbital a generic anticonvulsant drug 116

Mephyton a brand name for phytonadione 794

Mepivacaine a generic local anesthetic 106

Meprobamate 680, a generic antianxiety drug 114

Meptazinol a generic analgesic drug 97

Mequitazine a generic investigational antihistamine drug 118

Mercaptopurine 681, a generic anticancer drug 115

Merthiolate a brand-name antibacterial skin preparation 114

Mesantoin a brand-name anticonvulsant drug 116

Mescaline 681, a generic hallucinogenic drug 504

Mesoridazine a generic antipsychotic drug 119

Mestinon a brand name for pyridostigmine 841

Mestranol 681, a generic estrogen drug 421

Metamucil a brand name for psyllium 834

Metandren a brand-name androgen drug 100

Metaprel a brand name for metaproterenol 683

Metaproterenol 683, a generic bronchodilator drug 215

Metaraminol a generic drug used to treat shock 901

Metatensin a brand-name drug containing reserpine 863 and a diuretic drug 366

Metaxalone a generic muscle-relaxant drug 706

Meted 2 a brand-name preparation containing salicylic acid 879 and sulfur 954

Methacycline a generic antibiotic drug 114

Methadone 683, a generic narcotic drug 715, a type of analgesic drug 97

Methamphetamine a generic amphetamine drug 95

Methanol 683, a type of alcohol

Methantheline a generic antispasmodic drug 120 used to treat irritable bowel syndrome 607

Metharbital a generic anticonvulsant drug 116

Methazolamide a generic drug used to treat glaucoma 488

Methdilazine a generic antihistamine drug 118

Methenamine a generic drug used to treat urinary tract infection 1025

Methergine a brand-name drug used to induce labor 263

Methicillin a generic penicillin drug 779, a type of antibiotic drug 114

Methimazole 683, a generic drug used to treat hyperthyroidism 557

Methocarbamol 683, a generic muscle-relaxant drug 706

Methohexital a generic sedative drug 890 used to induce general anesthesia 104

Methotrexate 683, a generic anticancer drug 115

Methoxsalen 683, a generic psoralen drug 829

Methoxyflurane a generic drug used to induce general anesthesia 104

Methscopolamine a generic antispasmodic drug 120

Methsuximide a generic anticonvulsant drug 116

Methyclothiazide 684, a generic diuretic drug 366

Methylbenzethonium a generic antiseptic preparation 119

Methyl-CCNU a generic anticancer drug 115

Methylcellulose 684, a generic bulk-forming laxative drug 630

Methyldopa 684, a generic antihypertensive drug 118

Methylergonovine a generic drug used to induce labor 263

Methyl-glyoxalbisguanyl-hydrazone a generic anticancer drug 115

Methylphenidate a generic central nervous system stimulant 942

Methylprednisolone 684, a generic corticosteroid drug 312

Methyl salicylate a generic analgesic drug 97 in cream form used for muscle and joint pain 132

Methyltestosterone a generic androgen drug 100

Methyprylon a generic sleeping drug 916

Methysergide 684, a generic drug used to prevent migraine 688

Meticorten a brand name for prednisone 813

Metimyd a brand-name drug containing prednisolone 813 and sulfacetamide 954

Metoclopramide 684, a generic antiemetic drug 117

Metocurine a generic muscle-relaxant drug 706 used during general anesthesia 104

Metolazone 684, a generic diuretic drug 366

Metoprolol 684, a generic beta-blocker drug 165

Metreton a brand name for prednisolone 813

Metronid a brand name for metronidazole 684

Metronidazole 684, a generic antibiotic drug 114

Metryl a brand name for metronidazole 684

Metyrapone a generic investigational drug for Cushing's syndrome 325

Metyrosine a generic antihypertensive drug 118

Mevacor a brand name for lovastatin 650

Mexate a brand name for methotrexate 683

Mexiletine 684, a generic antiarrhythmic drug 114

Mezlocillin a generic penicillin drug 779, a type of antibiotic drug 114

Micatin a brand name for miconazole 684

Miconazole 684, a generic antifungal drug 117

Micrainin a brand-name analgesic drug 97 containing aspirin 137

Micro-K a brand-name potassium supplement 812

Micronase a brand name for glyburide 493

Micronefrin a brand name for epinephrine 414

Micronor a brand-name oral contraceptive 747

Midamor a brand name for amiloride 94

Midazolam a generic benzodiazepine drug 164 used for premedication 818

Midol 200 a brand name for ibuprofen 566

Midrin a brand-name drug containing an analgesic drug 97 and a sedative drug 890, used for migraine 688

Milkinol a brand-name laxative drug 630

Milk of Magnesia a brand-name antacid drug 113

Milpath a brand-name drug used to treat irritable bowel syndrome 607

Milprem a brand-name drug containing an estrogen 421 and an antianxiety drug 114

Milrinone a generic digitalis drug 361

Miltown a brand name for meprobamate 680

Minipress a brand name for prazosin 812

Minocin a brand name for minocycline 689

Minocycline 689, a generic tetracycline drug 976, a type of antibiotic drug 114

Minoxidil 689, a generic vasodilator drug 1041

Mintezol a brand name for thiabendazole 978

Miochol a brand name for acetylcholine 62

Mitomycin a generic anticancer drug 115

Mitotane a generic anticancer drug 115

Mitrolan a brand-name laxative drug 630

Mity-Quin a brand-name preparation containing hydrocortisone 550, an antifungal drug 117, and an antibacterial drug 114

Mixtard a brand name for insulin 594

Moban a brand-name antipsychotic drug 119

Mobidin a brand-name antirheumatic drug 119

Mobigesic a brand-name analgesic drug 97

Modane a brand-name laxative drug 630

Modicon a brand-name oral contraceptive 747

Modrastane a brand-name corticosteroid drug 312

Moduretic a brand-name drug containing amiloride 94 and hydrochlorothiazide 550

Molindone a generic antipsychotic drug 119

Mol-Iron a brand-name iron supplement 606

Monistat a brand name for miconazole 684

Monobenzone a generic drug for removal of normal skin pigmentation in severe vitiligo 1060

Monocid a brand-name antibiotic drug 114

Mono-Gesic a brand-name nonsteroidal anti-inflammatory drug 730

Monosodium glutamate 694, a food additive 461

Monosulfiram a generic drug used for scabies 881

Motrin a brand name for ibuprofen 566

Moxalactam a generic antibiotic drug 114

MS Contin a brand name for morphine 694

Mucomyst a brand name for acetylcysteine 62

Murine Plus a brand name for tetrahydrozoline 976

Murocel a brand name for methylcellulose 684

Murocoll-2 a brand name for phenylephrine 791

Muromonab CD3 a generic immunosuppressant drug 576

Muro's Opcon-A a brand-name preparation used to treat conjunctivitis 297

Muro Tears a brand-name artificial tear preparation 966

Mutamycin a brand-name anticancer drug 115

Myadec a brand-name multivitamin 702

Myambutol a brand name for ethambutol 422

Mycelex a brand name for clotrimazole 284

Mycifradin a brand name for neomycin 717

Myciguent a brand name for neomycin 717

Mycitracin a brand-name drug containing bacitracin 150 and neomycin 717

Mycolog a brand name for triamcinolone 1008

Mycolog II Cream a brand-name preparation containing nystatin 737 and triamcinolone 1008

Mycostatin a brand name for nystatin 737

Myco-Triacet a brand-name drug containing triamcinolone 1008 and nystatin 737

Mydfrin a brand name for phenylephrine 791

Mydriacyl a brand name for tropicamide 1013

Myidil a brand name for triprolidine 1011

Myidone a brand name for primidone 822

Mykinac a brand name for nystatin 737

Mylanta a brand-name antacid drug 113

Myleran a brand-name anticancer drug 115

Mylicon a brand name for simethicone 906

Myobid a brand name for papaverine 768

Myochrysine a brand-name drug containing gold 494

Myoflex a brand-name cream containing an analgesic drug 97

Mysoline a brand name for primidone 822

Mysteclin-F a brand-name drug containing amphotericin 96 and tetracycline 976

Mysteclin-F Syrup a brand-name syrup containing amphotericin 96 and tetracycline 976

Mytrex a brand name for triamcinolone 1008

N

Nabilone a generic antiemetic drug 117

Nadolol 714, a generic beta-blocker drug 165

Nafcillin a generic penicillin drug 779, a type of antibiotic drug 114

Nalbuphine a generic analgesic drug 97

Naldecon a brand-name cough remedy 316

Nalfon a brand name for fenoprofen 445

Nalidixic acid 714, a generic antibiotic drug 114

Naloxone 714, a generic drug that blocks the action of narcotic drugs 715

Naltrexone 714, a generic drug that blocks the action of narcotic drugs 715

Nandrolin a brand name for nandrolone 714

Nandrolone 714, a generic anabolic steroid drug 940

Naphazoline 714, a generic decongestant drug 336

Naphcon a brand name for naphazoline 714

Naprosyn a brand name for naproxen 714

Naproxen 714, a generic nonsteroidal anti-inflammatory drug 730

Naqua a brand-name thiazide diuretic drug 366

Naquival a brand-name drug containing reserpine 863 and a thiazide diuretic drug 366

Narcan a brand name for naloxone 714

Nardil a brand name for phenelzine 790

Nasahist a brand-name cold remedy 287

Nasalcrom a brand name for cromolyn sodium 321

Nasalide a brand-name corticosteroid nasal spray 312

Natabec a brand-name multivitamin 702

Natafort a brand-name multivitamin 702

Natalins a brand-name multivitamin 702

Natamycin a generic antifungal drug 117

Naturacil a brand name for psyllium 834

Nature's Remedy a brand-name laxative drug 630

Naturetin a brand name for bendroflumethiazide 164

Navane a brand name for thiothixene 978

ND-Stat a brand-name antihistamine drug 118

Nebcin a brand name for tobramycin 993

NegGram a brand name for nalidixic acid 714

Nembutal a brand name for pentobarbital 780

Neo-Calglucon a brand-name calcium supplement 223

Neo-Cortef a brand-name drug containing hydrocortisone 550 and neomycin 717

NeoDecadron a brand name for dexamethasone 348

Neomycin 717, a generic antibiotic drug 114

Neo-Polycin a brand name for neomycin 717

Neoquess a brand name for dicyclomine 357

Neosar a brand name for cyclophosphamide 326

Neosporin a brand-name preparation containing antibacterial drugs 114

Neostigmine 718, a generic drug used to treat myasthenia gravis 708

Neo-Synalar a brand-name drug containing fluocinolone 459 and neomycin 717

Neo-Synephrine 12 Hour a brand name for oxymetazoline 761

Neo-Tears a brand-name artificial tear preparation 966

Neotep a brand-name cold remedy 287

Neothylline a brand-name bronchodilator drug 215

Nephrocaps a brand-name multivitamin 702

Neptazane a brand-name drug used to treat glaucoma 488

Nestabs FA a brand-name multivitamin 702

Netilmicin 720, a generic antibiotic drug 114

Netromycin a brand name for netilmicin 720

Neutrogena a brand-name soap containing coal tar 285

Niacin a member of the vitamin B complex 1058

Niacinamide a form of niacin, a member of the vitamin B complex 1058

Niclocide a brand name for niclosamide 727

Niclosamide 727, a generic antihelmintic drug 118

Nico-400 a brand name for niacin, a member of the vitamin B complex 1058

Nicobid a brand name for niacin, a member of the vitamin B complex 1058

Nicotine 727, a stimulant drug found in tobacco 991

Nico-vert a brand name for dimenhydrinate 361

Nifedipine 727, a generic calcium channel blocker 224

Niferex a brand-name multivitamin 702

Nifurtimox a generic drug for trypanosomiasis 1013

Nilstat a brand name for nystatin 737

Nimodipine a generic calcium channel blocker 224

Nitro-Bid a brand name for nitroglycerin 729

Nitrodisc a brand name for nitroglycerin 729

Nitro-Dur a brand name for nitroglycerin 729

Nitrofurantoin 728, a generic antibacterial drug 114

Nitrofurazone a generic antibacterial drug 114

Nitrogen mustard a generic anticancer drug 115

Nitroglycerin 729, a generic vasodilator drug 1041

Nitrol a brand name for nitroglycerin 729

Nitrolingual spray a brand name for nitroglycerin 729

Nitropress a brand-name vasodilator drug 1041

Nitrospan a brand name for nitroglycerin 729

Nitrostat a brand name for nitroglycerin 729

Nitrous oxide 729, a gas used to induce general anesthesia 104

Nizoral a brand name for ketoconazole 616

Noctec a brand name for chloral hydrate 270

Nolahist a brand-name antihistamine drug 118

Nolamine a brand-name cold remedy 287

Noludar a brand-name sleeping drug 916

Nolvadex a brand name for tamoxifen 963

Nonoxynol 9 a generic spermicide 927

Norcet a brand-name cough remedy 316

Nordette a brand-name oral contraceptive 747

Norepinephrine 730, a type of hormone 547

Norethindrone 731, a generic progesterone drug 823

Norethynodrel a generic progesterone drug 823 used in oral contraceptives 747

Norflex a brand name for orphenadrine 750

Norgesic a brand-name analgesic 97 containing aspirin 137

Norgestrel 731, a generic progesterone drug 823

Norinyl a brand-name oral contraceptive 747

Norlestrin a brand-name oral contraceptive 747

Norlutate a brand name for norethindrone 731

Norlutin a brand name for norethindrone 731

Normodyne a brand name for labetalol 624

Norpace a brand name for disopyramide 365

Norpace CR a brand name for disopyramide 365

Norpramin a brand name for desipramine 347

Nor-Q-D a brand name for norethindrone 731

Nortriptyline 731, a generic antidepressant drug 116

Noscapine a generic cough remedy 316

Nostrilla a brand name for oxymetazoline 761

Notezine a brand-name antihelmintic drug 118

Novafed a brand name for pseudoephedrine 829

Novafed A a brand-name cold remedy 287

Novahistine DMX a brand-name cough remedy 316

Novocain a brand name for procaine 822

Novolin L, N, R brand-name preparations of insulin 594

NPH Insulin a brand-name preparation of insulin 594

Nubain a brand-name narcotic drug 715, a type of analgesic drug 97

Nucofed a brand-name cough remedy 316

Numorphan a brand-name analgesic drug 97

Nupercainal a brand-name local anesthetic 106

Nuprin a brand name for ibuprofen 566

Nutracort a brand name for hydrocortisone 550

Nutraplus a brand name for urea 1022

Nydrazid a brand name for isoniazid 608

Nylidrin a generic vasodilator drug 1041

Nystatin 737, a generic antifungal drug 117

Nystex a brand name for nystatin 737

O

Obermine a brand name for phentermine 790

Obetrol a brand-name appetite suppressant drug 128 containing amphetamine drugs 95

Occlusal a brand name for salicylic acid 879

Octoxynol a brand-name spermicide 927

Ocusert PILO a brand name for pilocarpine 795

Ogen a brand-name estrogen drug 421

Olive oil 742, a type of oil used to treat cradle cap 317

Omeprazole a generic investigational drug for peptic ulcers 780

Omnipen a brand name for ampicillin 96

Omnipen-N a brand name for ampicillin 96

Oncovin a brand-name anticancer drug 115

Ophthaine a brand-name local anesthetic 106 for eye surgery

Ophthetic a brand-name local anesthetic 106 for eye surgery

Ophthochlor a brand name for chloramphenicol 270

Ophthocort a brand-name preparation containing an antibiotic drug 114 and a corticosteroid drug 312 used to treat eye infections 431

Opium 745, a naturally occurring narcotic drug 715, a type of analgesic drug 97

Opti-Clean a brand-name contact lens cleaning solution 300

Opticrom a brand name for cromolyn sodium 321

Optigene 3 a brand name for tetrahydrozoline 976

Optilets-M-500 a brand-name multivitamin 702

Optimine a brand name for azatadine 149

Optimyd a brand-name drug containing prednisolone 813 and sulfacetamide 954

Orabase HCA a brand name for hydrocortisone 550

Orajel a brand-name local anesthetic 106 gel used to treat toothache 996 and mouth and lip irritation 697

Oramide a brand name for tolbutamide 994

Orap a brand name for pimozide 795

Orasone a brand name for prednisone 813

Orazinc a brand-name zinc supplement 1087

Oretic a brand name for hydrochlorothiazide 550

Oreticyl a brand-name drug containing hydrochlorothiazide 550 and reserpine 863

Oreton Methyl a brand-name androgen drug 100

Orgatrax a brand name for hydroxyzine 551

Orinase a brand name for tolbutamide 994

Ornade a brand-name cold remedy 287

Ornex a brand-name cold remedy 287 containing acetaminophen 61

Orphenadrine 750, a generic muscle-relaxant drug 706

Ortho-Novum 1/35 a brand-name oral contraceptive 747

Ortho-Novum 1/50 a brand-name oral contraceptive 747

Ortho-Novum 7/7/7 a brand-name oral contraceptive 747

Ortho-Novum 10/11 a brand-name oral contraceptive 747

Orudis a brand name for ketoprofen 616

Os-Cal a brand-name drug containing calcium 223 and vitamin D 1059

Osmoglyn a brand name for glycerin 493

Otic-HC a brand-name solution used to treat infections of the external ear 385

Otobiotic a brand-name drug containing hydrocortisone 550 and a polymyxin 808 antibiotic drug 114 used to treat infections of the external ear 385

Otocort a brand-name solution used to treat infections of the external ear 385

Otrivin a brand name for xylometazoline 1084

Ouabain a generic digitalis drug 361

Ovcon a brand-name oral contraceptive 747

Ovral a brand-name oral contraceptive 747

Ovrette a brand-name oral contraceptive 747

O-V Statin a brand name for nystatin 737

Ovulen a brand-name oral contraceptive 747

Oxacillin 761, a generic penicillin drug 779, a type of antibiotic drug 114

Oxalid a brand-name nonsteroidal anti-inflammatory drug 730

Oxandrolone 761, a generic anabolic steroid drug 940

Oxazepam 761, a generic benzodiazepine drug 164

Oxprenolol a generic beta-blocker drug 165

Oxsoralen a brand name for methoxsalen 683

Oxtriphylline 761, a generic bronchodilator drug 215

Oxybenzone a generic drug used in sunscreen preparations 955

Oxybutynin a generic anticholinergic drug 115 used to treat urinary incontinence 579

Oxycodone 761, a generic narcotic drug 715, a type of analgesic drug 97

Oxymetazoline 761, a generic decongestant drug 336

Oxymetholone a generic anabolic steroid drug 940

Oxymorphone a generic narcotic drug 715, a type of analgesic drug 97

Oxyphenbutazone a generic nonsteroidal anti-inflammatory drug 730

Oxyphencyclimine a generic antispasmodic drug 120 used to treat irritable bowel syndrome 607

Oxyphenonium a generic antispasmodic drug 120 used to treat irritable bowel syndrome 607

Oxytetracycline 761, a generic tetracycline drug 976, a type of antibiotic drug 114

Oxytocin 761, a type of hormone 547

P

P-200 a brand name for papaverine 768

Pabalate a brand-name analgesic drug 97

Pamabrom a brand-name diuretic drug 366 used to treat premenstrual syndrome 818

Pamelor a brand name for nortriptyline 731

Pamine a brand-name antispasmodic drug 120

Pancrease a brand name for pancrelipase 767

Pancuronium a generic muscle-relaxant drug 706

Panmycin a brand-name tetracycline drug 976, a type of antibiotic drug 114

Panoxyl, Panoxyl AQ brand-name preparations containing benzoyl peroxide 164

Panthenol a form of pantothenic acid, a member of the vitamin B complex 1058

Pantopon a brand-name narcotic drug 715 containing morphine 694, used as an analgesic 97

Panwarfin a brand name for warfarin 1069

Papaverine 768, a generic vasodilator drug 1041

Para-aminobenzoic acid 768, a generic drug used in many sunscreen preparations 955

Paraflex a brand name for chlorzoxazone 271

Parafon Forte a brand-name drug containing acetaminophen 61 and chlorzoxazone 271

Paraldehyde a generic anticonvulsant drug 116

Paramethadione a generic anticonvulsant drug 116

Paramethasone a generic corticosteroid drug 312

Paregoric a generic narcotic 715 antidiarrheal drug 117

Parlodel a brand name for bromocriptine 213

Parmine a brand name for phentermine 790

Parnate a brand name for tranylcypromine 1006

Paromomycin a generic antihelmintic drug 118

Parsidol a brand-name drug used to treat Parkinson's disease 772

Pathibamate a brand name for meprobamate 680

Pathocil a brand-name penicillin drug 779, a type of antibiotic drug 114

Pavabid a brand name for papaverine 768

Pavacen a brand name for papaverine 768

Paveral a brand name for codeine 286

Pavulon a brand-name muscle-relaxant drug 706

Paxipam a brand-name antianxiety drug 114

PBZ a brand-name antihistamine drug 118

PCNU a generic investigational anticancer drug 115

Pediacof a brand-name cough remedy 316

Pediaflor a brand name for sodium fluoride 460

Pediamycin a brand name for erythromycin 418

Pediazole a brand-name drug containing erythromycin 418 and sulfisoxazole 954

Peganone a brand-name anticonvulsant drug 116

Pemoline 778, a generic stimulant drug 942

Penapar VK a brand-name penicillin drug 779, a type of antibiotic drug 114

Penbutolol a generic beta-blocker drug 165

Penecort a brand name for hydrocortisone 550

Penfluridol a generic antipsychotic drug 119

Penicillamine 779, a generic antirheumatic drug 119 and chelating agent 258

Penicillin V a generic penicillin drug 779, a type of antibiotic drug 114

Penntuss a brand-name cough remedy 316

Pentaerythritol a generic nitrate drug 728

Pentamidine a generic drug used to treat trypanosomiasis 1013, leishmaniasis 633, and pneumocystis pneumonia 803

Pentazocine 780, a generic narcotic drug 715, a type of analgesic drug 97

Pentids a brand-name penicillin drug 779, a type of antibiotic drug 114

Pentobarbital 780, a generic barbiturate drug 157

Pentostatin a generic anticancer drug 115

Pentothal a brand name for thiopental 978

Pentoxifylline 780, a generic drug used to treat peripheral vascular disease 784

Pentrax a brand-name shampoo containing coal tar 285

Pen-Vee K a brand-name penicillin drug 779, a type of antibiotic drug 114

Pepcid a brand name for famotidine 440

Peppermint oil 780, used as a flavoring in some drug preparations

Pepto Bismol a brand-name antidiarrheal drug 117

Percocet a brand-name drug containing acetaminophen 61 and oxycodone 761

Percodan a brand-name drug containing aspirin 137 and oxycodone 761

Percogesic a brand-name analgesic drug 97

Percorten a brand-name preparation of synthetic ACTH 65

Perdiem a brand name for psyllium 834

Pergolide a generic investigational drug used to treat Parkinson's disease 772

Pergonal a brand name for menotropins 677

Periactin a brand-name antihistamine drug 118

Peri-Colace a brand-name laxative drug 630

Peritrate a brand-name nitrate drug 728

Permapen a brand-name penicillin drug 779, a type of antibiotic drug 114

Permethrim a generic drug used to treat lice 638

Permitil a brand name for fluphenazine 460

Perphenazine 786, a generic phenothiazine-type drug 790 used as an antipsychotic drug 119 and an antiemetic drug 117

Persa-Gel a brand name for benzoyl peroxide 164

Persantine a brand name for dipyridamole 362

Pertofrane a brand name for desipramine 347

Pertussin a brand-name cough remedy 316

Peruvian balsam an ingredient of some preparations used to treat hemorrhoids 530

Petrogalar a brand-name laxative drug 630

Petrolatum another name for petroleum jelly 788

Petroleum jelly 788, a greasy substance used as an emollient 399

Pfizerpen VK a brand-name penicillin drug 779, a type of antibiotic drug 114

Phazyme a brand name for simethicone 906

Phenacemide a generic anticonvulsant drug 116

Phenaphen a brand name for acetaminophen 61

Phenazine a brand-name appetite suppressant drug 128

Phenazopyridine 790, a generic analgesic drug 97

Phenelzine 790, a generic monoamine oxidase inhibitor antidepressant drug 116

Phenergan a brand name for promethazine 823

Phenergan-D a brand-name drug containing promethazine 823 and pseudoephedrine 829

Phenformin a generic investigational drug used to treat diabetes mellitus 349

Phenindamine a generic antihistamine drug 118

Pheniramine a generic antihistamine drug 118

Phenobarbital 790, a generic barbiturate drug 157

Phenol a type of antiseptic 119

Phenolphthalein a generic laxative drug 630

Phenoxybenzamine a generic antihypertensive drug 118

Phenprocoumon a generic anticoagulant drug 116

Phensuximide a generic anticonvulsant drug 116

Phentermine 790, a generic appetite suppressant drug 128

Phentolamine a generic antihypertensive drug 118

Phenurone a brand-name anticonvulsant drug 116

Phenylbutazone 790, a generic nonsteroidal anti-inflammatory drug 730

Phenylephrine 791, a generic decongestant drug 336

Phenylpropanolamine 791, a generic decongestant drug 336

Phenyltoloxamine a generic antihistamine drug 118

pHisoHex a brand-name antiseptic 119

Phospholine Iodide a brand-name drug used to treat glaucoma 488

Phrenilin a brand-name drug containing an analgesic 97 and a sedative drug 890

Phyllocontin a brand name for aminophylline 94

Physostigmine 794, a generic drug used to treat glaucoma 488

Pilocarpine 795, a generic drug used to treat glaucoma 488

Pilocel a brand name for pilocarpine 795

Pilopine HS Gel a brand name for pilocarpine 795

Pimozide 795, a generic drug used to treat Gilles de la Tourette's syndrome 487

Pindolol 795, a generic beta-blocker drug 165

Piperacillin a generic penicillin drug 779, a type of antibiotic drug 114

Piperazine 796, a generic antihelmintic drug 118

Piperonyl butoxide a generic drug used to treat skin parasites 771

Pipracil a brand-name penicillin drug 779, a type of antibiotic drug 114

Pirenzepine a generic ulcer-healing drug 1018

Pirmenol a generic antiarrhythmic drug 114

Piroxicam 796, a generic nonsteroidal anti-inflammatory drug 730

Pitocin a brand name for oxytocin 761

Pitressin a brand name for ADH 68

Placidyl a brand-name sleeping drug 916

Plaquenil a brand-name drug used to treat malaria 659

Platinol a brand name for cisplatin 283

Plegine a brand-name appetite suppressant drug 128

Plicamycin a generic anticancer drug 115

Podophyllin 805, a generic drug used to treat genital warts 1070

Polaramine a brand-name antihistamine drug 118

Polycarbophil calcium a generic bulk-forming laxative drug 630

Polycillin a brand name for ampicillin 96

Polyestradiol a generic estrogen-containing anti-cancer drug 115

Polyethylene glycol an ingredient of some skin preparations and certain laxative drugs 630

Poly-Histine CS a brand-name cough remedy 316

Poly-Histine D a brand-name decongestant drug 336

Poly-Histine DM a brand-name cough remedy 316

Polymox a brand name for amoxicillin 95

Poly-Pred a brand name for prednisolone 813

Polythiazide a generic thiazide diuretic drug 366

Poly-Vi-Flor a brand-name multivitamin 702 containing fluoride 460 and iron 606

Polyvinyl alcohol an ingredient of artificial tear preparations 966

Poly-Vi-Sol a brand-name multivitamin 702 containing iron 606

Pondimin a brand-name appetite suppressant drug 128

Ponstel a brand name for mefenamic acid 671

Pontocaine a brand name for tetracaine 975

Posture a brand-name drug containing calcium 223 and vitamin D 1059

Potassium 812, a mineral 689

Potassium chloride a generic potassium supplement 812

Potassium citrate a generic antacid drug 113

Potassium clavulanate a generic drug used to enhance the activity of some penicillin drugs 779

Potassium gluconate a generic potassium supplement 812

Potassium iodide a generic antifungal drug 117, also used to treat hyperthyroidism 557

Potassium permanganate 812, a substance used as an antiseptic 119 and astringent 139

Povan a brand-name antihelmintic drug 118

Povidone-iodine a generic antiseptic 119

Pragmatar a brand-name preparation containing coal tar 285

Pralidoxime a generic drug used to treat poisoning with parathion 771 and certain other pesticides 788

Pramet a brand-name multivitamin 702

Pramilet a brand-name multivitamin 702

Pramosone a brand-name corticosteroid drug 312

Pramoxine a generic local anesthetic 106

Prax a brand-name local anesthetic 106

Praziquantel 812, a generic antihelmintic drug 118

Prazosin 812, a generic vasodilator drug 1041

Precef a brand-name cephalosporin 248, a type of antibiotic drug 114

Pred Forte a brand name for prednisolone 813

Pred Mild a brand name for prednisolone 813

Prednisolone 813, a generic corticosteroid drug 312

Prednisone 813, a generic corticosteroid drug 312

Prefrin a brand name for phenylephrine 791

Pregnyl a brand name for human chorionic gonadotropin 494

Prelone a brand name for prednisolone 813

Prelu-2 a brand-name appetite suppressant drug 128

Preludin a brand-name appetite suppressant drug 128

Premarin a brand-name estrogen drug 421

Prenalterol a generic drug used for heart failure 519

Prenate 90 a brand-name multivitamin 702

Presalin a brand-name analgesic drug 97 containing aspirin 137 and acetaminophen 61

Prilocaine a generic local anesthetic 106

Primaquine 821, a generic drug used to treat malaria 659

Primatene Mist a brand name for epinephrine 414

Primaxin a brand-name antibacterial drug 114

Primidone 822, a generic anticonvulsant drug 116

Principen a brand name for ampicillin 96

Pro-Banthine a brand name for propantheline 824

Probenecid 822, a generic drug used to treat gout 495

Probucol 822, a generic lipid-lowering drug 642

Procainamide 822, a generic antiarrhythmic drug 114

Procaine 822, a generic local anesthetic 106

Procan SR a brand name for procainamide 822

Procarbazine 822, a generic anticancer drug 115

Procardia a brand name for nifedipine 727

Prochlor-Iso a brand-name antiemetic drug 117

Prochlorperazine 822, a generic phenothiazine 790 and an antiemetic drug 117

Proctocort a brand name for hydrocortisone 550

Proctofoam HC a brand-name corticosteroid drug 312

Procyclidine 822, a generic anticholinergic drug 115

Progens a brand-name estrogen drug 421

Progestasert a brand-name progesterone drug 823

Progestin 823, another name for a progesterone drug 823 or hormone 823

Proglycem a brand-name antihypertensive drug 118

Progynon a brand name for estradiol 421

Pro-Iso a brand name for prochlorperazine 822

Prolamine a brand name for phenylpropanolamine 791

Prolixin a brand name for fluphenazine 460

Proloprim a brand name for trimethoprim 1011

Promazine 823, a generic phenothiazine 790, a type of antipsychotic drug 119

Promethazine 823, a generic antihistamine drug 118

Promist a brand-name cough remedy 316

Prompt a brand name for psyllium 834

Pronestyl-SR a brand name for procainamide 822

Propacet 100 a brand-name drug containing acetaminophen 61 and propoxyphene 824

Propafenone a generic antiarrhythmic drug 114

Propantheline 824, a generic antispasmodic drug 120

Prophene 65 a brand name for propoxyphene 824

Propine a brand-name drug used to treat glaucoma 488

Propoxyphene 824, a generic narcotic drug 715, a type of analgesic drug 97

Propranolol 824, a generic beta-blocker drug 165

Propylene glycol a substance used as an emollient 399

Propylhexedrine a generic decongestant drug 336

Propylthiouracil 824, a generic drug used to treat hyperthyroidism 557

Prorex a brand name for promethazine 823

ProSobee a brand-name multivitamin 702

Prostaphlin a brand name for oxacillin 761

Prostigmin a brand name for neostigmine 718

Prostin/15M a brand-name prostaglandin drug 824

Prostin VR a brand-name prostaglandin drug 824

Protostat a brand name for metronidazole 684

Protriptyline 828, a generic antidepressant drug 116

Protropin a brand name for growth hormone 501

Proventil a brand name for albuterol 81

Provera a brand name for medroxyprogesterone 671

Pseudo Bid a brand-name cough remedy 316

Pseudoephedrine 829, a generic decongestant drug 336

Pseudohist a brand-name cold remedy 287

Psilocybin 829, a hallucinogenic drug 504

Psorigel a brand-name preparation containing coal tar 285

Psyllium 834, a generic laxative drug 630

Purinethol a brand name for mercaptopurine 681

Purodigin a brand name for digitoxin 361

P.V. Carpine a brand name for pilocarpine 795

P-V-Tussin a brand-name cough remedy 316

Pyocidin-Otic a brand-name drug containing hydrocortisone 550 and a polymyxin 808

Pyrantel 841, a generic antihelmintic drug 118

Pyrazinamide 841, a generic drug used to treat tuberculosis 1013

Pyrethrins a generic drug used to treat skin parasites 771

Pyridiate a brand name for phenazopyridine 790

Pyridium a brand name for phenazopyridine 790

Pyridium Plus a brand-name analgesic drug 97 used for urinary tract infections 1025

Pyridostigmine 841, a generic drug used to treat myasthenia gravis 708

Pyridoxine 841, a member of the vitamin B complex 1058

Pyrilamine 841, a generic antihistamine drug 118

Pyrimethamine 841, a drug used to treat malaria 659 and toxoplasmosis 1000

Pyrroxate a brand-name cold remedy 287

Pyrvinium a generic antihelmintic drug 118

Q

Quadrinal a brand-name drug used in the treatment of asthma 137

Quazepam a generic benzodiazepine 164 sleeping drug 916

Quelidrine a brand-name cough remedy 316

Questran a brand name for cholestyramine 275

Quibron a brand-name drug used to treat asthma 137

Quibron-T/SR a brand name for theophylline 977

Quinacrine 842, a generic drug used to treat giardiasis 486

Quinaglute a brand name for quinidine 842

Quinamm a brand name for quinine 842

Quindan a brand name for quinine 842

Quinestrol 842, a generic synthetic estrogen drug 421

Quinethazone a generic thiazide diuretic drug 366

Quinidine 842, a generic antiarrhythmic drug 114

Quinine 842, a generic drug used to treat malaria 659

Quinora a brand name for quinidine 842

Quiphile a brand name for quinine 842

R

R & C a brand-name shampoo used to treat lice 638

Racet a brand-name drug containing hydrocortisone 550 and a drug that is both antibacterial 114 and antifungal 117

Ranitidine 849, a generic ulcer-healing drug 1018

Raudixin a brand-name antihypertensive drug 118

Rauwiloid a brand-name antihypertensive drug 118

Rauwolfia serpentina a generic antihypertensive drug 118

Rauzide a brand-name antihypertensive drug 118

Redisol a brand name for vitamin B$_{12}$ 1058

Regitine a brand-name antihypertensive drug 118

Reglan a brand name for metoclopramide 684

Regonol a brand name for pyridostigmine 841

Regroton a brand name for chlorthalidone 271

Rela a brand name for carisoprodol 238

Remegel a brand-name antacid drug 113

Remsed a brand name for promethazine 823

Renese a brand-name thiazide diuretic drug 366

Rescinnamine a generic antihypertensive drug 118

Reserpine 863, a generic antihypertensive drug 118

Resorcinol a generic preparation used to treat acne 63, dermatitis 345, and fungal infections 470

Respbid a brand name for theophylline 977

Respinol-G a brand-name cough remedy 316

Restoril a brand name for temazepam 968

Retet a brand-name tetracycline drug 976, a type of antibiotic drug 114

Reticulogen a brand-name drug used in the treatment of iron-deficiency anemia 102

Retin-A a brand name for tretinoin 1008

Retinoic acid a derivative of vitamin A 1057

Retinol 868, the principal form of vitamin A 1057

Retrovir a brand name for zidovudine 1087

Rhindecon a brand name for phenylpropanolamine 791

Rhinolar a brand-name cold remedy 287

Rhinosyn a brand-name cold remedy 287

Ribavirin a generic antiviral drug 120

Riboflavin 874, another name for vitamin B$_2$ 1058

Rid a brand-name preparation used to treat lice 638

Ridaura a brand name for auranofin 144

Rifadin a brand name for rifampin 874

Rifamate a brand-name drug containing isoniazid 608 and rifampin 874

Rifampin 874, a generic antibacterial drug 114

Rimactane a brand name for rifampin 874

Rimactane INH a brand-name drug containing isoniazid 608 and rifampin 874

Ritalin a brand-name central nervous system stimulant 942

Ritodrine 875, a generic drug used to delay premature labor 263

Robaxin a brand name for methocarbamol 683

Robaxisal a brand-name drug containing aspirin 137 and methocarbamol 683

Robicillin VK a brand-name penicillin drug 779, a type of antibiotic drug 114

Robimycin a brand name for erythromycin 418

Robinul a brand-name anticholinergic 115 and antispasmodic drug 120

Robitet a brand-name tetracycline drug 976, a type of antibiotic drug 114

Robitussin a brand-name cough remedy 316

Rocaltrol a brand-name drug used to treat low blood calcium 223

Rocephin a brand-name cephalosporin 248, a type of antibiotic drug 114

Roferon-A a brand name for interferon 598

Rolaids a brand-name antacid drug 113

Ronase a brand name for tolazamide 994

Rondec a brand-name cold remedy 287

Rondomycin a brand-name antibiotic drug 114

Roxanol a brand name for morphine 694

RP-Mycin a brand name for erythromycin 418

Rubramin a brand name for vitamin B$_{12}$ 1058

Rufen a brand name for ibuprofen 566

Ru-Tuss a brand-name cold remedy 287

Ru-Vert-M a brand name for meclizine 669

Rynatan a brand-name cold remedy 287

Rynatuss a brand-name cough remedy 316

S

Safeguard a brand-name antibacterial soap 114

SalAc a brand-name preparation containing salicylic acid 879

Salicylic acid 879, a generic keratolytic drug 615

Salicylsalicylic acid a generic nonsteroidal anti-inflammatory drug 730

Saligel a brand-name preparation containing salicylic acid 879

Salsalate a generic nonsteroidal anti-inflammatory drug 730

Saluron a brand-name thiazide diuretic drug 366

Salutensin a brand-name drug containing a diuretic drug 366 and reserpine 863

Sandimmune a brand name for cyclosporine 326

Sanorex a brand-name appetite suppressant 128

Sansert a brand name for methysergide 684

Sarna Lotion a brand-name preparation used to treat skin irritation 608

SAS 500 a brand name for sulfasalazine 954

SAStid a brand-name preparation containing salicylic acid 879 and sulfur 954

Satric 500 a brand name for metronidazole 684

Savacort-50 a brand name for prednisolone 813

Scabene a brand name for lindane 641

Schamberg's Lotion a brand-name preparation used to treat skin irritation 608

Scopolamine 887, a generic antispasmodic drug 120

Scot-Tussin a brand-name cough remedy 316

Sebulex a brand-name preparation containing salicylic acid 879 and sulfur 954

Sebulon a brand-name shampoo used to treat dandruff 332

Secobarbital 889, a generic barbiturate drug 157

Seconal a brand name for secobarbital 889

Sectral a brand name for acebutolol 61

Sedapap-10 a brand-name analgesic drug 97 containing acetaminophen 61 and a barbiturate drug 157

Seffin a brand-name cephalosporin 248, a type of antibiotic drug 114

Seldane a brand name for terfenadine 971

Selegiline a generic investigational drug used to treat Parkinson's disease 772

Selenium sulfide an agent used to treat dandruff 332 and tinea versicolor 989

Selsun a brand-name preparation used to treat dandruff 332 and tinea versicolor 989

Semets a brand-name local anesthetic 106

Semicid a brand-name spermicide 927

Semustine a generic anticancer drug 115

Senna 891, a generic stimulant laxative drug 630

Senokot a brand-name stimulant laxative drug 630

Septisol a brand-name antiseptic 119

Septra a brand-name drug containing sulfamethoxazole 954 and trimethoprim 1011

Ser-Ap-Es a brand-name antihypertensive drug 118

Serax a brand name for oxazepam 761

Serentil a brand-name antipsychotic drug 119

Serophene a brand name for clomiphene 284

Serpasil a brand name for reserpine 863

Serpasil-Apresoline a brand-name drug containing hydralazine 549 and reserpine 863

Serpate a brand name for reserpine 863

Sevin a shampoo containing a generic drug used to treat lice 638

Silain Gel a brand-name antacid drug 113

Silvadene a brand name for silver sulfadiazine 906

Silver nitrate 906, an astringent 139

Silver sulfadiazine 906, a generic antibacterial drug 114

Simeco a brand name for simethicone 906

Simethicone 906, a generic drug used to relieve flatulence 458

Simron a brand-name iron preparation 606

Sine-Aid a brand-name drug containing acetaminophen 61 and pseudoephedrine 829

Sinemet a brand-name drug used to treat Parkinson's disease 772

Sinequan a brand name for doxepin 372

Singlet a brand-name cold remedy 287

Sinubid a brand-name cold remedy 287 containing acetaminophen 61

Sinufed a brand name for pseudoephedrine 829

Sinulin a brand-name cold remedy 287

Sinutab a brand-name cold remedy 287

Skelaxin a brand-name muscle-relaxant drug 706

Slo-bid a brand name for theophylline 977

Slo-Phyllin a brand name for theophylline 977

Slo-Phyllin GG a brand-name drug for asthma 137

Slow FE a brand name for ferrous sulfate 445

Slow-K a brand name for potassium 812

Sodium bicarbonate 922, a generic antacid drug 113

Sodium citrate a generic antacid drug 113

Sodium fluoride a type of fluoride 460

Sodium iodide a type of iodine 605 used to treat hyperthyroidism 557 and thyroid cancer 983

Sodium nitrite a generic drug used to treat cyanide poisoning 326

Sodium salicylate 922, a generic nonsteroidal anti-inflammatory drug 730

Sodium thiosulfate a generic drug used to treat acne 63, tinea versicolor 989, and cyanide poisoning 326

Solatene a brand name for vitamin A 1057

Solfoton a brand name for phenobarbital 790

Solganal a brand-name drug containing gold 494

Solu-Cortef a brand name for hydrocortisone 550

Solu-Medrol a brand name for methylprednisolone 684

Soma a brand name for carisoprodol 238

Soma Compound a brand-name drug containing aspirin 137 and carisoprodol 238

Somophyllin a brand name for aminophylline 94

Somophyllin-CRT a brand name for theophylline 977

Somophyllin-T a brand name for theophylline 977

Soothe a brand name for eye drops containing tetrahydrozoline 976

Soprodol a brand name for carisoprodol 238

Sorbitrate a brand name for isosorbide dinitrate 608

Sotalol a generic beta-blocker drug 165

Sparine a brand name for promazine 823

Spectazole a brand name for econazole 388

Spectinomycin a generic antibiotic drug 114

Spectrobid a brand name for bacampicillin 150

Spectrocin a brand-name drug containing gramicidin 497 and neomycin 717

Spironolactone 932, a potassium-sparing diuretic drug 366

Spirozide a brand name for spironolactone 932

S-P-T a brand name for thyroid hormone 985

SSKI a generic antifungal drug 117 also used to treat hyperthyroidism 557

Stadol a brand-name narcotic drug 715, a type of analgesic drug 97

Stanozolol 938, a generic anabolic steroid drug 940

Staphcillin a brand-name penicillin drug 779, a type of antibiotic drug 114

Staticin a brand name for erythromycin 418

Statobex a brand-name appetite suppressant 128

Statrol a brand-name antibacterial drug 114 used to treat eye infections 431

Stelazine a brand name for trifluoperazine 1010

Sterane a brand name for prednisolone 813

Stibocaptate a generic antihelmintic drug 118

Stibogluconate a generic drug used to treat leishmaniasis 633

Stilphostrol a brand name for diethylstilbestrol 359

Stoxil a brand name for idoxuridine 566

Streptase a brand name for streptokinase 945

Streptokinase 945, a generic thrombolytic drug 981

Streptomycin 945, a generic antibiotic drug 114

Streptozocin a generic anticancer drug 115

Stuart Natal, Stuart Prenatal brand-name multivitamin 702 and mineral 689 preparations

Succinylcholine a generic muscle-relaxant drug 706

Sucralfate 952, a drug used to treat peptic ulcer 780

Sucrets Cold Decongestant Formula a brand name for phenylpropanolamine 791

Sudafed a brand name for pseudoephedrine 829

Sufentanil a generic narcotic analgesic drug 97

Sulamyd a brand name for sulfacetamide 954

Sulf-10 a brand name for sulfacetamide 954

Sulfabenzamide a generic antibacterial drug 114

Sulfacetamide 954, a generic antibacterial drug 114

Sulfacet-R a brand name for sulfacetamide 954

Sulfacytine a generic antifungal drug 117

Sulfadiazine a generic antifungal drug 117

Sulfadoxine a generic drug used to treat malaria 659

Sulfamethizole a generic sulfonamide 954, a type of antibacterial drug 114

Sulfamethoxazole 954, a generic antibacterial drug 114

Sulfasalazine 954, a generic anti-inflammatory drug 118

Sulfinpyrazone 954, a generic drug used to treat gout 495

Sulfisoxazole 954, a generic antibacterial drug 114

Sulfoxyl a brand-name drug containing benzoyl peroxide 164 and sulfur 954

Sulfur 954, a mineral 689

Sulindac 954, a generic nonsteroidal anti-inflammatory drug 730

Sulphrin a brand name for prednisolone 813

Sulqui a brand name for niclosamide 727

Sultrin a brand-name drug used to treat vaginitis 1036

Sumox a brand name for amoxicillin 95

Sumycin a brand-name tetracycline drug 976, a type of antibiotic drug 114

Supen a brand name for ampicillin 96

Suramin a generic drug used to treat sleeping sickness 916

Surbex a brand-name multivitamin 702

Surmontil a brand name for trimipramine 1011

Sus-Phrine a brand name for epinephrine 414

Sustaire a brand name for theophylline 977

Sutilains an enzyme used to treat infected burns 219 and skin ulcers 1018

Syllact a brand name for psyllium 834

Symmetrel a brand name for amantadine 92

Synacort a brand name for hydrocortisone 550

Synalar a brand name for fluocinolone 459

Synalgos-DC a brand-name analgesic drug 97 containing aspirin 137

Synemol a brand name for fluocinolone 459

Synkayvite a brand name for vitamin K 1060

Synophylate a brand name for theophylline 977

Synthroid a brand name for levothyroxine 638

Syntocinon a brand name for oxytocin 761

T

Tabloid a brand-name anticancer drug 115

Tabron a brand-name multivitamin 702 and mineral 689 preparation

Tacaryl a brand-name antihistamine drug 118

TACE a brand-name anticancer drug 115

Tagamet a brand name for cimetidine 280

Talacen a brand-name analgesic drug 97 containing acetaminophen 61 and pentazocine 780

Talbutal a generic barbiturate 157 sleeping drug 916

Talwin a brand name for pentazocine 780

Talwin Nx a brand-name drug containing naloxone 714 and pentazocine 780

Tambocor a brand-name antiarrhythmic drug 114

Tamoxifen 963, a generic anticancer drug 115

Tandearil a brand-name nonsteroidal anti-inflammatory drug 730

Tapar a brand name for acetaminophen 61

Tapazole a brand name for methimazole 683

Taractan a brand-name antipsychotic drug 119

Tavist a brand-name antihistamine drug 118

Tazicef a brand-name cephalosporin 248, a type of antibiotic drug 114

Tazidime a brand-name cephalosporin 248, a type of antibiotic drug 114

Tear-Efrin a brand name for phenylephrine 791

Tearisol a brand-name artificial tear preparation 966

Tears Naturale a brand-name artificial tear preparation 966

Tedral a brand-name drug containing ephedrine 410 and theophylline 977

Teebacin a brand name for aminosalicylic acid 94

Teebaconin a brand name for isoniazid 608

Tegafur a generic anticancer drug 115

Tegison a brand-name drug used in the treatment of psoriasis 830

Tegopen a brand name for cloxacillin 285

Tegretol a brand name for carbamazepine 231

Tegrin a brand name for coal tar 285

Teldrin a brand name for chlorpheniramine 271

Temaril a brand name for trimeprazine 1011

Temazepam 968, a generic benzodiazepine drug 164

Tempra a brand name for acetaminophen 61

Teniposide a generic anticancer drug 115

Tenoretic a brand-name drug containing atenolol 140 and chlorthalidone 271

Tenormin a brand name for atenolol 140

Tenuate a brand-name appetite suppressant drug 128

Tepanil a brand-name appetite suppressant drug 128

Teramine a brand name for phentermine 790

Terazosin a generic antihypertensive drug 118

Terbutaline 971, a generic bronchodilator drug 215

Terfenadine 971, a generic antihistamine drug 118

Terpin hydrate a generic cough remedy 316

Terra-Cortril a brand-name drug containing hydrocortisone 550 and oxytetracycline 761

Terramycin a brand name for oxytetracycline 761

Tessalon a brand-name cough remedy 316

Testolactone a generic anticancer drug 115

Testosterone 974, an androgen hormone 100

Testred a brand name for testosterone 974

Tetrabenazene an investigational generic drug used to treat movement disorders 699

Tetracaine 975, a generic local anesthetic 106

Tetrachloroethylene a generic drug used to treat hookworm infestation 545

Tetracyn a brand-name tetracycline drug 976, a type of antibiotic drug 114

Tetrahydroaminoacridine 976, a generic investigational drug used to treat Alzheimer's disease 91

Tetrahydrozoline 976, a generic decongestant drug 336

Tetrex a brand-name tetracycline drug 976

Texacort a brand name for hydrocortisone 550

T/Gel a brand name for coal tar 285

Thalidomide 977, a generic sleeping drug 916

Thalitone a brand name for chlorthalidone 271

Theo-24 a brand name for theophylline 977

Theobid a brand name for theophylline 977

Theoclear a brand name for theophylline 977

Theo-Dur a brand name for theophylline 977

Theolair a brand name for theophylline 977

Theo-Organidin a brand name for theophylline 977

Theophyl a brand name for theophylline 977

Theophylline 977, a generic bronchodilator drug 215

Theospan a brand name for theophylline 977

Theostat a brand name for theophylline 977

Theovent a brand name for theophylline 977

Theozine a brand name for hydroxyzine 551

Theragran a brand-name multivitamin 702 containing iron 606

Thiabendazole 978, a generic antihelmintic drug 118

Thiamylal a generic barbiturate drug 157 used in general anesthesia 104

Thiethylperazine a generic antiemetic drug 117

Thimerosal a mercury compound 681 used as an antiseptic 119 and as a disinfectant 364

Thioguanine a generic anticancer drug 115

Thiopental 978, a generic barbiturate drug 157

Thioridazine 978, a generic antipsychotic drug 119

Thiosulfil a brand name for sulfamethizole, a sulfonamide antibacterial drug 954

Thiosulfil-A a brand-name drug containing phenazopyridine 790 and sulfamethizole, a sulfonamide antibacterial drug 954

Thiotepa a generic anticancer drug 115

Thiothixene 978, a generic antipsychotic drug 119

Thiuretic a brand name for hydrochlorothiazide 550

Thorazine a brand name for chlorpromazine 271

Thymoxamine a generic drug used to treat glaucoma 488

Thyrar a brand name for thyroid hormone 985

Thyroid Strong a brand-name thyroid hormone 985

Thyrolar a brand-name thyroid hormone 985

Ticarcillin a generic penicillin drug 779, a type of antibiotic drug 114

Ticlopidine a generic drug used to prevent blood clotting 184

Tigan a brand name for trimethobenzamide 1011

Timentin a brand-name penicillin drug 779, a type of antibiotic drug 114

Timolide a brand-name drug containing hydrochlorothiazide 550 and timolol 988

Timolol 988, a generic beta-blocker drug 165

Timoptic a brand name for timolol 988

Tinactin a brand name for tolnaftate 994

Tindal a brand-name antipsychotic drug 119

Tinidazole a generic drug used to treat amebiasis 92

Tinver a brand-name drug used to treat tinea versicolor 989

Tioconazole an investigational generic antifungal drug 117

T-Ionate P.A. a brand name for testosterone 974

Tiopronin an investigational generic drug used to treat urinary tract calculi 224

Tissue-plasminogen activator 989, a generic thrombolytic drug 981

Tixocortol an investigational generic drug for inflammatory bowel disease 588

Tobramycin 993, a generic antibiotic drug 114

Tobrex a brand name for tobramycin 993

Tocainide 993, a generic antiarrhythmic drug 114

Tocopheryl acetate another name for vitamin E 1059

Tofranil a brand name for imipramine 570

Tolazamide 994, a generic hypoglycemic drug 560

Tolazoline a generic drug used to treat pulmonary hypertension in the newborn 836

Tolbutamide 994, a generic hypoglycemic drug 560

Tolectin a brand name for tolmetin 994

Tolinase a brand name for tolazamide 994

Tolmetin 994, a generic nonsteroidal anti-inflammatory drug 730

Tolnaftate 994, a generic antifungal drug 117

Tonocard a brand name for tocainide 993

Topicort a brand-name corticosteroid drug 312

Topicycline a brand-name tetracycline drug 976

Topsyn a brand-name corticosteroid drug 312

Torecan a brand-name antiemetic drug 117

Tornalate a brand-name bronchodilator drug 215

Totacillin a brand name for ampicillin 96

TPA the abbreviation for tissue-plasminogen activator 989

Trancopal a brand-name antianxiety drug 114

Trandate a brand name for labetalol 624

Transderm-Nitro a brand name for nitroglycerin 729

Transderm-Scop a brand name for scopolamine 887

Tranxene a brand-name benzodiazepine 164 antianxiety drug 114

Tranylcypromine 1006, a generic monoamine-oxidase inhibitor antidepressant drug 116

Trasicor a brand-name beta-blocker drug 165

Travase a brand-name enzyme-containing preparation used to treat infected burns 219 and skin ulcers 1018

Trazodone 1008, a generic antidepressant drug 116

Trecator-SC a brand-name drug used to treat tuberculosis 1013 and leprosy 634

Tremin a brand name for trihexyphenidyl 1011

Trental   a brand name for pentoxifylline 780

Tretinoin   1008, a generic drug used to treat acne 63

Trexan   a brand name for naltrexone 714

Triacetin   a generic antifungal drug 117 used to treat tinea 988

Triad   a brand-name analgesic drug 97

Triafed-C   a brand name for triprolidine 1011

Triamcinolone   1008, a generic corticosteroid drug 312

Triaminic   a brand name for phenylpropanolamine 791

Triamterene   1009, a generic potassium-sparing diuretic drug 366

Triaprin   a brand-name analgesic drug 97

Triavil   a brand-name drug containing amitriptyline 94 and perphenazine 786

Triazolam   1009, a generic benzodiazepine drug 164

Trichlormethiazide   a generic thiazide diuretic drug 366

Trichloracetic acid   a generic treatment for warts 1069

Triclocarban   a type of antiseptic 119

Triclosan   a type of antiseptic 119

Tricodene   a brand-name cold remedy 287

Tridesilon   a brand-name corticosteroid drug 312

Tridihexethyl chloride   a generic antispasmodic drug 120 for irritable bowel syndrome 607

Tridil   a brand name for nitroglycerin 729

Tridione   a brand-name anticonvulsant drug 116

Trientine   a generic chelating agent 258 used to treat Wilson's disease 1078

Triethylenetetramine   a generic chelating agent 258 used to treat Wilson's disease 1078

Trifluoperazine   1010, a generic antipsychotic drug 119

Triflupromazine   a generic antipsychotic 119 and antiemetic drug 117

Trifluridine   1010, a generic antiviral drug 120

Trigesic   a brand-name analgesic drug 97 containing aspirin 137

Trihexane   a brand name for trihexyphenidyl 1011

Trihexyphenidyl   1011, a generic anticholinergic drug 115

Tri-Hydroserpine   a brand-name vasodilator drug 1041

Trilafon   a brand name for perphenazine 786

Tri-Levlen   a brand-name oral contraceptive 747

Trilisate   a brand name for sodium salicylate 922

Trilostane   a generic synthetic corticosteroid drug 312 for Cushing's syndrome 325

Trimazosin   a generic antihypertensive drug 118

Trimeprazine   1011, a generic antihistamine drug 118

Trimethadione   a generic anticonvulsant drug 116

Trimethaphan   a generic antihypertensive drug 118

Trimethobenzamide   1011, a generic antiemetic drug 117

Trimethoprim   1011, a generic antibacterial drug 114

Trimipramine   1011, a generic tricyclic antidepressant drug 116

Trimox   a brand name for amoxicillin 95

Trimpex   a brand name for trimethoprim 1011

Trinalin   a brand-name drug containing azatadine 149 and pseudoephedrine 829

Trind   a brand-name cold remedy 287

Tri-Norinyl   a brand-name oral contraceptive 747

Trinsicon   a brand-name multivitamin 702 and mineral 689 preparation

Trioxsalen   a generic psoralen drug 829 used in PUVA treatment 839

Tripelennamine   a generic antihistamine drug 118

Triphasil   a brand-name oral contraceptive 747

Triphed   a brand name for triprolidine 1011

Tri-Phen-Chlor   a brand-name cold remedy 287

Triple antibiotic   a generic antibiotic drug 114

Triple Sulfas   a brand-name sulfonamide drug 954

Triprolidine   1011, a generic antihistamine drug 118

Trisoralen   a brand-name psoralen drug 829 used in PUVA treatment 839

Tri-Vi-Flor   a brand-name multivitamin 702 containing fluoride 460

Tri-Vi-Sol   a brand-name multivitamin 702

Trobicin   a brand-name antibiotic drug 114

Trofan   a brand-name nonbenzodiazepine, nonbarbiturate sleeping drug 916

Trolamine   a generic drug used as drops to remove earwax 387

Troleandomycin   a generic antibiotic drug 114

Tromethamine   a generic drug used to treat urinary tract calculi 224

Tronolane   a brand-name local anesthetic 106

Tronothane   a brand-name local anesthetic 106

Tropicacyl   a brand name for tropicamide 1013

Tropicamide   1013, a generic drug used to dilate the pupil

Trymex   a brand name for triamcinolone 1008

Trypsin   an intestinal enzyme used to treat indigestion 580

Tryptophan   a generic nonbenzodiazepine, nonbarbiturate sleeping drug 916

Trysul   a brand-name sulfonamide drug 954

T-Stat   a brand name for erythromycin 418

Tubocurarine   a generic muscle-relaxant drug 706 used in general anesthesia 104

Tuinal   a brand-name barbiturate 157 sleeping drug 916

Tums   a brand-name antacid drug 113

Tussagesic   a brand-name cough remedy 316

Tussanil   a brand-name cold remedy 287

Tussar   a brand-name cough remedy 316

Tussend   a brand-name cough remedy 316

Tussionex   a brand-name cough remedy 316

Tussi-Organidin   a brand-name cough remedy 316

Tussi-Organidin DM   a brand-name cough remedy 316

Tussirex   a brand-name cough remedy 316

Tuss-Ornade   a brand-name cold remedy 287

Twin-K   a brand-name cough remedy 316

Tylenol   a brand name for acetaminophen 61

Tylox   a brand-name drug containing acetaminophen 61 and oxycodone 761

Tympagesic Otic Solution   a brand-name analgesic drug 97 used to treat otitis externa 757

Tyzine   a brand name for tetrahydrozoline 976

U

Ultracef   a brand-name cephalosporin 248, a type of antibiotic drug 114

Undecylenic acid   a generic antifungal drug 117 used to treat athlete's foot 141

Unibase   a brand-name emollient 399

Unilax   a brand-name laxative drug 630

Unipen   a brand-name penicillin drug 779, a type of antibiotic drug 114

Uniphyl   a brand name for theophylline 977

Unipres   a brand-name antihypertensive drug 118

Unisom   a brand-name antihistamine 118 sleeping drug 916

Unproco   a brand-name cough remedy 316

Urecholine   a brand-name drug used to treat urine retention 1029

Urex   a brand-name drug used to treat urinary tract infection 1025

Urised   a brand-name drug used to treat urinary tract infection 1025

Urispas   a brand-name antispasmodic drug 120

Uritabs   a brand-name drug used to treat urinary tract infection 1025

Urobiotic-250   a brand-name drug containing oxytetracycline 761 and phenazopyridine 790

Urodine   a brand name for phenazopyridine 790

Urogesic   a brand-name analgesic drug 97 used for urinary tract infection 1025

Urokinase   1029, a generic thrombolytic drug 981

Uro-Phosphate   a brand-name drug used to treat urinary tract infections 1025

Ursodeoxycholic acid   a generic drug used to treat gallstones 474

Uticillin VK   a brand-name penicillin drug 779, a type of antibiotic drug 114

Uticort   a brand name for betamethasone 166

Utimox   a brand name for amoxicillin 95

V

Vacon   a brand name for phenylephrine 791

Vaginex   a brand-name cream containing an antihistamine drug 118 used to relieve genital irritation 608

Vagitrol   a brand-name vaginal cream containing a sulfonamide antibacterial drug 114

Valdrene   a brand name for diphenhydramine 361

Valergen   a brand name for estradiol 421

Valertest   a brand-name drug containing estradiol 421 and testosterone 974

Valisone   a brand name for betamethasone 166

Valium   a brand name for diazepam 357

Valmid   a brand-name sleeping drug 916

Valpin 50   a brand-name antispasmodic drug 120 used to treat irritable bowel syndrome 607

Valrelease   a brand name for diazepam 357

Vancenase   a brand name for beclomethasone 161

Vanceril   a brand name for beclomethasone 161

Vanoxide-HC   a brand-name drug containing benzoyl peroxide 164 and hydrocortisone 550

Vanseb   a brand name for salicylic acid 879

Vaponefrin   a brand name for epinephrine 414

Vaseline Petroleum Jelly 788, a brand name for petroleum jelly 788

Vasocidin   a brand-name drug containing prednisolone 813 and sulfacetamide 954

VasoClear   a brand name for naphazoline 714

Vasocon   a brand name for naphazoline 714

Vasocon-A   a brand-name drug used to treat allergic conjunctivitis 297

Vasodilan   a brand name for isoxsuprine 608

Vasosulf   a brand name for sulfacetamide 954

Vasotec   a brand name for enalapril 400

Vatronol   a brand name for ephedrine 410

V-Cillin K   a brand-name penicillin drug 779, a type of antibiotic drug 114

Vecuronium   a generic muscle-relaxant drug 706

Veetids   a brand-name penicillin drug 779, a type of antibiotic drug 114

Velban   a brand-name anticancer drug 115

Velosef   a brand-name cephalosporin 248, a type of antibiotic drug 114

Velosulin   a brand name for pork insulin 594

Velvachol   a brand-name preparation containing lanolin 626 and petroleum jelly 788

Ventolin   a brand name for albuterol 81

Vepesid   a brand-name anticancer drug 115

Vermox   a brand name for mebendazole 669

Verrex   a brand-name drug containing podophyllin 805 and salicylic acid 879

Verrusol   a brand-name preparation used to treat warts 1069

Vesprin   a brand-name antipsychotic 119 and antiemetic drug 117

Vibramycin   a brand name for doxycycline 372

Vibra-Tabs   a brand name for doxycycline 372

Vicks   a brand-name cold remedy 287

Vicodin   a brand-name analgesic drug 97

Vicon-C   a brand-name multivitamin 702

Vidarabine   a generic antiviral drug 120

Vi-Daylin   a brand-name multivitamin 702

Viloxazine   a generic central nervous system stimulant 942

Vinblastine   a generic anticancer drug 115

Vincristine   a generic anticancer drug 115

Vindesine   a generic anticancer drug 115

Vioform   a cream containing a generic antibacterial drug 114 and an antifungal drug 117

Viokase   a brand name for pancrelipase 767

Vira-A   a brand-name antiviral drug 120

Viranol   a brand name for salicylic acid 879

Virazole   a brand-name antiviral drug 120

Viroptic   a brand name for trifluridine 1010

Visine   a brand name for tetrahydrozoline 976

Visken   a brand name for pindolol 795

Vistaril   a brand name for hydroxyzine 551

Vitron-C   a brand-name preparation containing iron 606 and vitamin C 1059

Vivactil   a brand name for protriptyline 828

Vivalin   a brand-name central nervous system stimulant 942

Vontrol   a brand-name antiemetic drug 117

Vosal   a brand name for acetic acid 62

VoSol HC   a brand-name drug containing hydrocortisone 550 and acetic acid 62

Voxsuprine   a brand name for isoxsuprine 608

Vytone   a brand-name drug containing hydrocortisone 550 and an antibiotic drug 114

W

Wans   a brand-name drug containing pentobarbital 780 and pyrilamine 841

Wart-Off   a brand-name preparation for warts 1069

Wehless   a brand-name appetite suppressant 128

Wellcovorin   a brand name for folic acid 460

Westcort   a brand name for hydrocortisone 550

Whitfield's Ointment   a brand-name preparation used to treat warts 1069

Wigraine   a brand name for ergotamine 416

Wigrettes   a brand name for ergotamine 416

Wilpowr   a brand name for phentermine 790

Winstrol   a brand name for stanozolol 938

Witch hazel   a generic mild astringent 139

Wyamycin S   a brand name for erythromycin 418

Wyanoids   brand-name rectal suppositories used to relieve anal itching 608

Wycillin   a brand-name penicillin drug 779

Wydase   a brand-name enzyme used to reduce bruising 217

Wygesic   a brand-name analgesic drug 97

Wymox   a brand name for amoxicillin 95

Wytensin   a brand-name antihypertensive drug 118

X

Xanax   a brand name for alprazolam 89

Xerac   a brand-name antiperspirant 118

Xerac BP   a brand name for benzoyl peroxide 164

X-Otag   a brand name for orphenadrine 750

X-Prep   a brand name for senna 891

X seb   a brand name for salicylic acid 879

Xylocaine   a brand name for lidocaine 639

Xylometazoline   a generic decongestant drug 336

Y

Y-Itch   a brand name for tetracaine 975

Yocon   a brand-name antihypertensive drug 118

Yodoxin   a brand-name drug used to treat amebiasis 92

Yohimbine   a generic antihypertensive drug 118

Yohimex   a brand-name antihypertensive drug 118

Yomesan   a brand name for niclosamide 727

Yutopar   a brand name for ritodrine 875

Z

Zantac   a brand name for ranitidine 849

Zarontin   a brand name for ethosuximide 423

Zaroxolyn   a brand name for metolazone 684

Z-Bec   a brand-name multivitamin 702

Zeasorb-AF   a brand name for tolnaftate 994

Zemo   a brand-name preparation used to relieve skin irritation 608

Zenate   a brand-name multivitamin 702 and mineral 689 preparation

Zentinic   a brand-name multivitamin 702 containing iron 606

Zentron   a brand-name multivitamin 702 containing iron 606

Zephiran Chloride   a brand-name antiseptic 119

Zephrex   a brand-name cough remedy 316

Zetar   a brand name for coal tar 285

Zide   a brand name for hydrochlorothiazide 550

Zidovudine   1087, a generic antiviral drug 120

Zinacef   a brand-name cephalosporin 248, a type of antibiotic drug 114

Zincfrin   an astringent 139

Zinc gluconate   a generic compound of zinc 1087

Zincon   a brand-name antifungal drug 117 used to treat dandruff 332

Zinc pyrithione   a generic antifungal drug 117 used to treat dandruff 332

Zinc sulfate   an astringent 139

Ziradryl   a brand name for diphenhydramine 361

Zone-A   a brand-name corticosteroid drug 312

Zorprin   a brand name for aspirin 137

Zyloprim   a brand name for allopurinol 88

Zymenol   a brand name for mineral oil 689

INDEX

This index covers the three major sections of the encyclopedia: **Medicine Today**; the **A to Z of Medicine**; and the **Drug Glossary**. **Self-help Organizations** (see pages 1090-1095) are not included in the index.

Index entries begin with either a capital or a lower-case letter. Most index entries with an initial capital correspond to titles of entries in the **Medicine Today** or the **A to Z of Medicine** sections. Other index entries with an initial capital refer you to a **Drug Glossary** entry. With the exception of a few capitalized abbreviations or eponyms, all other index entries have a lower-case first letter.

Index entries that correspond to the titles of encyclopedia entries usually refer you to the page on which the encyclopedia entry starts. (In the case of encyclopedia entries that are simple cross-references to other encyclopedia entries, the index refers you directly to the cross-referenced entries or to major index entries.) Other index entries and all index subentries refer you to the title of an encyclopedia entry or to an illustration title, accompanied by a page number. This number refers to the page where the index topic appears.

Index entries, subentries, or page numbers in *italic* type refer you to illustrations.

1128

J

O

1163

T

ILLUSTRATIONS AND ADDITIONAL DESIGN